clinical chemistry

J. Stanton King, *Executive Editor*
P.O. Box 5218
Winston-Salem, N. C. 27103
(Tel. 919/725-0208)

Journal of the American Association for Clinical Chemistry

Volume 22
1976

Business Office Tel. (202) 833-3590
1725 K St., NW
Washington, D. C. 20006

January: pages 1–140

February: pages 141–298

March: pages 299–412

April: pages 413–576

May: pages 577–710

June: pages 711–956

July: pages 957–1242

August: pages 1243–1422

September: pages 1423–1554

October: pages 1555–1774

November: pages 1775–1954

December: pages 1955–2114

Volume 22 Number 1
January 1976

CLCHAU 22 (1), 1–140 (1976)
ISSN 0009-9147

clinical chemistry

Journal of the American Association for Clinical Chemistry

1 **INFORMATION FOR AUTHORS**

5 **REVIEW: Recently Discovered Hypothalamic–Pituitary Hormones**
William B. Malarkey

16 **GUEST EDITORIAL: Potentialities of an Inexpensive Computer System for Analysis of Clinical Amino Acid Data: Forecast and Speculation**
Donald M. Schoengold, Roberta H. deFiore, David J. Miner, and Paul B. Hamilton

19 **A Computerized System for Storage and Statistical Analysis of Clinical Amino Acid Data**
Donald M. Schoengold, David J. Miner, Roberta H. deFiore, and Paul B. Hamilton

25 **Simultaneous High-Pressure Liquid-Chromatographic Determination of Some Anticonvulsants in Serum**
Reginald F. Adams and Frank L. Vandemark

32 **Simultaneous Determination of Five Sex Hormones in Human Serum by Radioimmunoassay after Chromatography on Lipidex-5000**
D. Apter, O. Jänne, P. Karvonen, and R. Vihko

39 **Effect of Time and Temperature of Blood P_{50} and 2,3-Diphosphoglycerate Measurements**
Stanley Hellerstein and Tasanaporn Bunthraungroj

42 **Quantitative Fractionation of Alkaline Phosphata Isoenzymes According to Their Thermostability**
Claude PetitClerc

49 **Organic Acids in Urine from Human Newborns**
Lars Björkman, Catherine McLean, and Göran Steen

53 **Measuring Picogram Amounts of Aluminum in Biological Tissue by Flameless Atomic Absorption Analysis of a Chelate**
Gary R. LeGendre and Allen C. Alfrey

57 **Electrophoretic Amylase Fractionation as an Aid in Diagnosis of Pancreatic Disease**
Mark E. Legaz and Margaret A. Kenny

63 **Creatine Kinase Isoenzymes in Baboon Tissues and Organs**
Walid G. Yasmineh, Robert B. Pyle, Naomi Q. Hanson, and Bonita K. Hultman

67 **Improved Microscale Assay for Purine Phosphoribosyltransferase Activities**
Rainer Schmidt, Martine Forêt, and Uwe Reichert

70 **Thermodynamic Aspects of Some Radioassays**
Paul M. Keane, William H. C. Walker, Jack Gauldie, and Guy E. Abraham

74 **Evaluation of a Reagent-Strip Method for Glucose in Whole Blood, as Compared with a Hexokinase Method**
Thomas C. Stewart

79 **Spectrophotometric End-Point Method for Assay of Serum Cystyl-aminopeptidase in Pregnancy**
Brian H. Durham

83 **Comparison of Four Kits for Enzymatic Determination of Ethanol in Blood**
Helmut M. Redetzki and William L. Dees

87 **Atypical Increase in Serum Creatine Kinase Activity in Hospital Patients**
Sylvan M. Sax, John J. Moore, Joseph L. Giegel, and Muriel Welsh

92 **Improved Separation of Creatine Kinase Cardiac Isoenzyme in Serum by Batch Fractionation**
Leo G. Morin

SCIENTIFIC NOTES

98 **Enzymatic Determinations of Cholesterol in High-Density-Lipoprotein Fractions Prepared by a Precipitation Technique**
Bernard W. Steele, Donald F. Koehler, Miguel M. Azar, Thomas P. Blaszkowski, Kanta Kuba, and Mary E. Dempsey

101 **Convenient Method for Checking Detector Response of Spectrophotometers at Three Wavelengths**
Christopher S. Frings, Vincent I. Muscat, and Nancy T. Waldrop

103 **Effect of Storage in the Cold on Activity of Gamma-Glutamyltransferase in Serum**
Douglas P. Rhone and Florence M. White

SELECTED METHOD

105 **Procedure for Mechanized (Continuous-flow) Measurement of Serum Ascorbic Acid (Vitamin C)**
H. Sauberlich, W. C. Goad, J. H. Skala, and P. P. Waring

HISTORY

111 **The Chicago Section, AACC**
Albert A. Dietz

LETTERS

116 **Relationship between Alkaline Phosphatase and Creatine Kinase Activity**
Swei H. Tsung

118 **Reuse of Disposable Sephadex Columns for a Triiodothyronine Uptake Test**
C. H. Bastomsky, D. B. Frenkel-Leith, and J. Lamoureux

120 **Creatine Kinase Isoenzyme BB in Serum of Renal-Disease Patients**
Robert S. Galen

120 **Further Use of the Sure-Sep Technique for Serum-Plasma Separation**
Ralph E. Bernstein

122 **Optimal γ-Glutamyltransferase Assay?**
C. P. Price, J. O'Meara, and P. R. Wenham

122 **Dissenting View on Computer Systems**
Samuel Raymond

124 **Effect of Urobilinogen on Urinary Estrogen Determination**
Sophie Heiberg, Donald J. Campbell, and Jiri Frohlich

BOOK REVIEWS

126 William C. Purdy, A. W. Renuart, and Paul B. Hamilton

130 **THE CLINICAL CHEMIST**
J. S. King

clinical chemistry

J. Stanton King, *Executive Editor*
P.O. Box 5218
Winston-Salem, N. C. 27103
(Tel. 919/725-0208)

Journal of the American Association for Clinical Chemistry

Business Office Tel. (202) 833-3590
1725 K St., NW
Washington, D. C. 20006

General Information: Manuscripts, editorial inquiries, and books for review should be addressed to the Executive Editor (address above). All subscription and circulation inquiries should be sent to the Business Office (address above). **Information for Authors** appears in the January issue.

Subscription: CLINICAL CHEMISTRY is issued monthly. Price per year, $25.00 in the U.S.A. and possessions; $26.00 in North America outside the U.S.; $35.00 elsewhere. Members, domestic and foreign, $12.50 (included in dues). All subscriptions before Oct. 1 start with the first issue of the current volume. Single copies of current-volume issues $5.00; ask Special-Issue Sales for back-issue prices. Claims for missing numbers will not be allowed (*a*) if received more than 60 days from date of issue plus time normally required for postal delivery of journal and claim, (*b*) if notice of a recent change of address has not been received, or (*c*) if the reason for claim is "missing from files." All advertising inquiries should be sent to Scherago Associates, Inc., 11 W. 42nd St., New York, N.Y. 10036. Second class postage paid at Washington, D. C. 20006 and additional mailing offices. Published monthly by the American Association for Clinical Chemistry, Inc., P. O. Box 5218, Winston-Salem, N. C. 27103. Printed at 20th and Northampton Sts., Easton, Pa. 18042.

Volume 22 Number 2
February 1976

CLCHAU 22 (2), 141–298 (1976)
ISSN 0009-9147

clinical chemistry

Journal of the American Association for Clinical Chemistry

141 **Determination of the Molar Absorptivity of NADH**
Robert B. McComb, Lawrence W. Bond, Robert W. Burnett, Richard C. Keech, and George N. Bowers, Jr.

151 **Molar Absorptivities of β-NADH and β-NADPH**
Joachim Ziegenhorn, Martin Senn, and Theodor Bücher

161 **Erythrocyte Porphyrin Analysis in the Detection of Lead Poisoning in Children: Evaluation of Four Micromethods**
Thomas L. Hanna, David N. Dietzler, Carl H. Smith, Santosh Gupta, and Harold S. Zarkowsky

169 **Colorimetry of Carbohydrates with *m*-Aminophenol, and Its Proposed Use in Measurement of Serum Amylase Activity**
Jesse F. Goodwin

173 **Creatine Kinase Isoenzyme Patterns in Human Tissue Obtained at Surgery**
Swei H. Tsung

176 **Sample Stability: A Suggested Definition and Method of Determination**
Ralph E. Thiers, Gaw T. Wu, Allen H. Reed, and Lawrence K. Oliver

184 **Analysis for Indole Compounds in Urine by High-Performance Liquid Chromatography with Fluorometric Detection**
Anthony P. Graffeo and Barry L. Karger

188 **An Integrated Approach to Lipid Profiling: Enzymatic Determination of Cholesterol and Triglycerides with a Centrifugal Analyzer**
Peter W. Wentz, Robert E. Cross, and John Savory

193 **Evaluation of Two Digoxin Radioimmunoassay Procedures in which ^{125}I-Labeled Digoxin Is Used**
Z. Jerry Kuczala and Gurjit S. Ahluwalia

198 **Double-antibody Enzyme Immunoassay Applied to Human α_1-Fetoprotein**
Luc Belanger, Diane Hamel, Didier Dufour, and Marcel Pouliot

205 **Evaluation of a Dipstick Test for Glucose in Urine**
Jørn Dyerberg, Lissi Pedersen, and Ole Aagaard

211 **Evaluation of a Discrete-Sample Computer-Directed Clinical Analyzer**
Roger L. Forrester, Willa Collinge, Pattie Hashimoto, and Jackie Worrall

217 **Effect of Halothane Anesthesia on Muscle, Liver, Thyroid, and Adrenal-Function Tests in Man**
Robert E. Johnstone, Eric M. Kennell, Walter Brummund, Jr., Leslie M. Shaw, and Richard C. Ebersole

221 **Rapid Micromethod for Blood Lead Analysis by Anodic Stripping Voltammetry**
George Morrell and Giri Giridhar

224 **Cholesterol in Amniotic Fluid, Determined by Gas Chromatography**
Valerie M. Jones Owen, Frank K. Ho, Angelo Mazzuchin, Terrance A. Doran, Seigren Liedgren, and C. John Porter

227 **High-Performance Colorimeter with an Electronic Bubble Gate for Use in Miniaturized Continuous-Flow Analyzers**
William E. Neeley, Stephen C. Wardlaw, Tad Yates, William G. Hollingsworth, and Maurice E. T. Swinnen

232 **Improved Assay for Urinary 17-Hydroxycorticosteroids**
Yutaka Ariyoshi and Yoshio Osawa

235 **Assessment of a Serum Separator Device for Obtaining Serum Specimens Suitable for Clinical Analyses**
Ronald H. Laessig, James O. Westgard, R. Neill Carey, David J. Hassemer, Thomas H. Schwartz, and Donald H. Feldbruegge

240 **Cation-Exchange Chromatography of Guanidine Derivatives in Plasma of Patients with Chronic Renal Failure**
Guido Perez, Alberto Rey, Michael Micklus, and Israel Stein

243 **Enzymatic Method for Determination of CO_2 in Serum**
Roger L. Forrester, Lester J. Wataji, Donald A. Silverman, and Kenneth J. Pierre

246 **Measurement of Diphenylhydantoin in 0.1-ml Plasma Samples: Gas Chromatography and Radioimmunoassay Compared**
Michael L'Estrange Orme, Olof Borgå, Clarence Edgar Cook, and Folke Sjöqvist

250 **Radioimmunoassay of Plasma Renin Activity**
Frej Fyhrquist, Pertti Soveri, Liisa Puutula, and Ulf-Håkan Stenman

257 **Improved Method for Measurement of Inorganic Phosphate in Serum with a Centrifugal Analyzer**
Peter W. Wentz, John Savory, and Robert E. Cross

SCIENTIFIC NOTES

261 **Parallel Electrophoretic Fractionation of Alkaline Phosphatase and Serum Protein on Cellulose Acetate Strips: Clinical Evaluation**
Angelo Burlina and Lauro Galzigna

263 ***p*-Hydroxybenzoic Acid Hydrazide Procedure for Serum Glucose Adapted to the Technicon "SMA 12/60," and Compared with Other Glucose Methods**
John J. Ferraro, Francis A. Caccavo, and Abraham Saifer

267 **Complement C3 in Serum and Plasma, as Measured by Radial Immunodiffusion with Four Commercial Kits**
Adrian O. Vladutiu and Barbara M. Winiarski

270 **Long-Term Quality-Control Charting: A Simple Method**
Arthur W. Gottmann, Jerome S. Nosanchuk, and Gail S. Anderson

273 **Direct Determination of Serum Chloride with a Semiautomated Discrete Analyzer**
Stanley S. Levinson

275 **Lipoamide Dehydrogenase in Serum: A Preliminary Report**
John W. Pelley, Gwynne H. Little, Tracy C. Linn, and Frank F. Hall

SPECIAL REPORT

278 **Clinical Chemistry in the Peoples Republic of China Today**
Lilla Sun

LETTERS

282 **Adjustment of Serum Calcium for Protein**
R. W. Pain and P. J. Phillips
(Reply)
Harry Husdan, Abraham Rapoport, Sandra Locke, and Dimitrios Oreopoulos

283 **Drug Interference with Creatinine Assay**
Alan Bye

284 **Defect in the Methodology of Aspartate Aminotransferase Determination with SMAC**
N. M. Chang, B. Davis, and R. Cavaliere
(Reply)
Jack Levine

285 **When Is a Reference Method a Reference Method?**
D. W. Neill and J. R. Doggart
(Reply)
S. S. Brown, J. Büttner, F. L. Mitchell, M. Rubin, and G. R. Cooper

286 **Digoxin Immunoassay with Use of [^{3}H]Digoxin vs. [^{125}I]Tyrosine-methyl-ester of Digoxin**
Susan L. Pippin and Frank I. Marcus

BOOK REVIEWS

288 J. S. King, Lena A. Lewis, and Fred P. Abramson, Earl W. Sutherland, III, and Mario Werner

294 **The Chemyst's Tale**

295 **THE CLINICAL CHEMIST**
J. S. King

clinical chemistry

J. Stanton King, *Executive Editor*
P.O. Box 5218
Winston-Salem, N. C. 27103
(Tel. 919/725-0208)

Journal of the American Association for Clinical Chemistry

Business Office Tel. (202) 833-3590
1725 K St., NW
Washington, D. C. 20006

The contents of advertisements or articles in CLINICAL CHEMISTRY are not to be construed as official statements, evaluations, or endorsements by the Board of Editors or the American Association for Clinical Chemistry.

General Information. Manuscripts, editorial inquiries, and books for review should be addressed to the Executive Editor (address above). All subscription and circulation inquiries should be sent to the Business Office (address above). **Information for Authors** appears in the January issue.

Subscription: CLINICAL CHEMISTRY is issued monthly. Price per year, $25.00 in the U.S.A. and possessions; $26.00 in North America outside the U.S.; $35.00 elsewhere. Members, domestic and foreign, $12.50 (included in dues). All subscriptions before Oct. 1 start with the first issue of the current volume. Single copies of current-volume issues $5.00; ask Special-Issue Sales for back-issue prices. Claims for missing numbers will not be allowed (*a*) if received more than 60 days from date of issue plus time normally required for postal delivery of journal and claim, (*b*) if notice of a recent change of address has not been received, or (*c*) if the reason for claim is "missing from files." All advertising inquiries should be sent to Scherago Associates, Inc., 11 W. 42nd St., New York, N. Y. 10036. Second class postage paid at Washington, D. C. 20006 and additional mailing offices. Published monthly by the American Association for Clinical Chemistry, Inc., P. O. Box 5218, Winston-Salem, N. C. 27103. Printed at 20th and Northampton Sts., Easton, Pa. 18042.

Volume 22 Number 3
March 1976

CLCHAU 22 (3), 299–412 (1976)
ISSN 0009-9147

clinical chemistry

Journal of the American Association for Clinical Chemistry

299 **Use of Polyethylene Glycol in Separating Bound from Unbound Ligand in Radioimmunoassay of Thyroxine**
Marian C. Cheung and W. Roy Slaunwhite, Jr.

305 **Changes in Electrophoretic Mobilities of α- and β-Lipoproteins as a Result of Plasma Delipidation**
Bill E. Cham and Brian R. Knowles

310 **Simultaneous Quantitation of 4-Hydroxy-3-Methoxymandelic (Vanilmandelic) and 4-Hydroxy-3-Methoxyphenylacetic (Homovanillic) Acids in Human Urine**
Somasundaram Addanki, Elmer R. Hinnenkamp, and Juan F. Sotos

315 **Determination of Apolipoprotein A and Its Constitutive A-I and A-II Polypeptides by Separate Electroimmunoassays**
Michael D. Curry, Petar Alaupovic, and C. Alan Suenram

323 **Use of Enzyme-loaded Erythrocytes in In-Vitro Correction of Arginase-Deficient Erythrocytes in Familial Hyperargininemia**
Karel Adriaenssens, Denise Karcher, Armand Lowenthal, and Heinz G. Terheggen

327 **Evaluation of Methods of Coenzyme Activation of Erythrocyte Enzymes for Detection of Deficiency of Vitamins B_1, B_2, and B_6**
Riad A. Bayoumi and Sidney B. Rosalki

336 **Polarographic Method for Rapid Microdetermination of Cholesterol with Cholesterol Esterase and Cholesterol Oxidase**
Akio Noma and Keiko Nakayama

341 **Gas-Chromatographic Analysis for Succinimide Anticonvulsants in Serum: Macro- and Micro-Scale Methods**
James Bonitati

346 **Comparison of Results for 13 Clinical Laboratory Determinations with Three Automated Analytical Systems**
Eric J. Sampson, Dennis D. Derck, and Laurence M. Demers

350 **Statistical Characterization of the Random Errors in the Radioimmunoassay Dose–Response Variable**
David Rodbard, Robert H. Lenox, H. Linton Wray, and Douglas Ramseth

359 **Nonchromatographic Radioimmunoassay of Unconjugated Estriol in Plasma, with Polyethylene Glycol as Precipitant**
Harvey S. Schiller and Margaret A. Brammall

364 **Measurement of 25-Hydroxyvitamin D_3 in Serum**
Roger Bouillon, Piet Van Kerkhove, and Pieter De Moor

SCIENTIFIC NOTES

369 **Simple Fluorometric Determination of Aldosterone in Urine without Use of Isotopes or Chromatography**
William R. Whigham

372 **Glucose Oxidase Chemiluminescence Measurement of Glucose in Urine Compared with the Hexokinase Method**
David C. Williams, Glenn F. Huff, and W. Rudolf Seitz

374 **Evaluation of Contemporary Methods for Serum CO_2**
Jack A. Lustgarten, Ronald J. Creno, Charles G. Byrd, and Robert E. Wenk

379 **Modified Colorimetric Method for Procainamide in Plasma**
Daniel S. Sitar, Donald N. Graham, Robert E. Rangno, Louis R. Dusfresne, and Richard I. Ogilvie

381 **Improved Method for Measuring Fibrinogen in Plasma, with Use of a Plasmin Inhibitor**
Loren W. Steffen and Barbara W. Steffen

SPECIAL REPORT

384 **Provisional Recommendation (1974) on IFCC Methods for the Measurement of Catalytic Concentration of Enzymes**
G. N. Bowers, Jr., H. U. Bergmeyer, and D. W. Moss

LETTERS

393 **Drug Screening for Employment Purposes: The Importance of Telling It Like It Is**
Donald R. Wilkinson, Patricia Jensen, and Doris Winsley

393 **Further on Light Scatter vs. Turbidimetry**
T. O. Tiffany

394 **Instrument Control by Computer an Improvement?**
Samuel Raymond
(Reply)
James E. Davis and John W. Lewis

394 **Laboratory Computers: On- or Off-line?**
Samuel Raymond

395 **Determination of Salicylate and Its Metabolites in Urine**
Gerhard Levy and Josephine Procknal

396 **Improved Detection of Morphine on TLC Plates**
Joyce A. McIntyre and Arlene E. Armandi

396 **Triiodothyronine Radioimmunoassay: Incubation Time, Temperature, and Antisera**
J. C. Standefer
(Reply)
Paul H. Lenz, George H. Wien, and Janice M. Toth

398 **Effective Quality Control**
John W. Eastman

399 **Volatiles and Osmometry**
Richard M. Rocco

BOOK REVIEWS

400 George G. Guilbault and Morton K. Schwartz

403 **THE CLINICAL CHEMIST**
J. S. King

clinical chemistry

J. Stanton King, *Executive Editor*
P.O. Box 5218
Winston-Salem, N. C. 27103
(Tel. 919/725-0208)

Journal of the American Association for Clinical Chemistry

Business Office Tel. (202) 833-3590
1725 K St., NW
Washington, D. C. 20006

General Information. Manuscripts, editorial inquiries, and books for review should be addressed to the Executive Editor (address above). All subscription and circulation inquiries should be sent to the Business Office (address above). **Information for Authors** appears in the January issue.

Subscription: CLINICAL CHEMISTRY is issued monthly. Price per year, $25.00 in the U.S.A. and possessions; $26.00 in North America outside the U.S.; $35.00 elsewhere. Members, domestic and foreign, $12.50 (included in dues). All subscriptions before Oct. 1 start with the first issue of the current volume. Single copies of current-volume issues $5.00; ask Special-Issue Sales for back-issue prices. Claims for missing numbers will not be allowed (*a*) if received more than 60 days from date of issue plus time normally required for postal delivery of journal and claim, (*b*) if notice of a recent change of address has not been received, or (*c*) if the reason for claim is "missing from files." All advertising inquiries should be sent to Scherago Associates, Inc., 11 W. 42nd St., New York, N. Y. 10036. Second class postage paid at Washington, D. C. 20006 and additional mailing offices. Published monthly by the American Association for Clinical Chemistry, Inc., P. O. Box 5218, Winston-Salem, N. C. 27103. Printed at 20th and Northampton Sts., Easton, Pa. 18042.

Volume 22 Number 4
April 1976

CLCHAU 22 (4), 413–576 (1976)
ISSN 0009-9147

clinical chemistry

Journal of the American Association for Clinical Chemistry

413 **Fluorometry of Plasma Amino Nitrogen, with Use of Fluorescamine**
Bernard Klein and Fontaine Standaert

417 **γ-Glutamyltransferase: Substrate Inhibition, Kinetic Mechanism, and Assay Conditions**
Johan H. Strømme and Liv Theodorsen

422 **Method for Monitoring Plasma Progesterone Concentrations in Pregnancy**
Per Winkel, Preben Gaede, and Jørgen Lyngbye

429 **Adaptation of Blank-Corrected Methods for Measurement of Total and Conjugated Bilirubin and Uric Acid to the Centrifugal Analyzer**
Robert E. Cross, M. Geraldine Heintges, John Savory, and Peter W. Wentz

434 **Clinical Laboratory Evaluation of the Perkin-Elmer KA-150 Enzyme Analyzer**
Eugene Hardin, Richard B. Passey, Ronald L. Gillum, John B. Fuller, and Debbie Lawrence

439 **Electrophoretic Pattern of Amylase Isoenzymes in Serum and Urine of Normal Persons**
Makoto Otsuki, Susumu Saeki, Hosai Yuu, Mitsuo Maeda, and Shigeaki Baba

445 **Stability of Fatty Acids in Hyperlipoproteinemic Plasma During Long-Term Storage**
Eugene Z. Hirsch, Sandra Slivka, and Austin P. Gibbons

449 **Development of an Aqueous Temperature-Indicating Technique and Its Application to Clinical Laboratory Instrumentation**
Lemuel Bowie, Fred Esters, Jeffrey Bolin, and Nathan Gochman

456 **Preparation of Optically Clear Lyophilized Human Serum for Use in Preparing Control Material**
Gary J. Proksch and Dean P. Bonderman

461 **New Techniques for Ion-Selective Measurements of Ionized Calcium in Serum after pH Adjustment of Aerobically Handled Sera**
H. Donald Schwartz

468 **Automated Separation and Measurement of Lactate Dehydrogenase Isoenzymes**
Michael G. Busby, Paul J. Kudirka, R. Neill Carey, and E. Clifford Toren, Jr.

471 **High-Pressure Liquid-Chromatographic Separation of Lactate Dehydrogenase Isoenzymes**
Paul J. Kudirka, Ronald R. Schroeder, Thomas E. Hewitt, and E. Clifford Toren, Jr.

475 **Expression of Random Analytical Error as a Percentage of the Range of Clinical Interest**
John H. Glick, Jr.

484 **Direct Radioimmunoassay for Serum Estriol during Pregnancy**
Jim Standefer

489 **Performance Studies on the Technicon "SMAC" Analyzer: Precision and Comparison of Values with Methods in Routine Laboratory Service**
James O. Westgard, R. Neill Carey, Donald H. Feldbruegge, and Lola M. Jenkins

497 **Immunofixation. I. General Principles and Application to Agarose Gel Electrophoresis**
Robert F. Ritchie and Rosemary Smith

500 **On the Design of Clinical Chemistry Quality-Control Sera**
George F. Grannis and W. Greg Miller

513 **Comparison of Three Procedures for Isolating Human Ferritin, for Use as a Standard in an Immunoradiometric Assay**
Lorraine M. Gonyea, Colleen M. Lamb, R. Dorothy Sundberg, and Amos S. Deinard

SCIENTIFIC NOTES

519 **Fast, Economical Technique for Separating Serum from Blood Samples**
Gurjit S. Ahluwalia, Z. Jerry Kuczala, and Lanny R. Carlson

520 **Evaluation of a New Enzymatic Kit for Serum Triglycerides**
Timothy Carter, Paul J. Martin, Peter Wilding, and David M. Goldberg

524 **Serum Iron Determination in Patients Receiving Therapy with Iron Dextran ("Imferon")**
Max E. McIntosh, Jerry K. Lynn, Norma Meyerriecks, and Irene Contant

CASE REPORT

528 **Effect of Tobramycin on Urinary γ-Glutamyltransferase Activity: Studies in a Case of Renal Carcinoma**
Peter Richard Beck, M.Sc., M.B., Ch.B., and Ajay K. R. Chaudhuri

SPECIAL REPORTS

532 **Provisional Recommendation on Quality Control in Clinical Chemistry**
J. Büttner, R. Borth, J. H. Boutwell, and P. M. G. Broughton

541 **Report of the Second Conference on Education in Clinical Chemistry (and a list of training programs)**

LETTERS

550 **Plasma P_i Erythrocyte 2,3-Diphosphoglycerate Concentrations of Non-Acidotic Diabetics in Various Degrees of Metabolic Control**
Jφrn Ditzel and Eberhard Standl

551 **Thyroid-function Tests in Diphenylhydantoin-treated Patients**
P. J. Phillips and R. W. Pain
(Reply)
Melvin R. Stjernholm, Robert N. Alsever, and Merritt C. Rudolph

552 **"The Case of the Latex Gloves" in Scintillation Counting**
P. B. Dewhurst and J. C. Travis

552 **Poor Separation of Creatine Kinase Isoenzymes with Column-chromatographic Kits**
Donald Mercer
(Reply)
Richard J. L. Bondar and Gerald A. Moss

556 **Turbidimetry vs. Light Scattering in Immunochemistry**
Gregory J. Buffone

556 **Interbatch Variability in Measurement of Urinary Amylase with a Commercial Kit**
G. M. B. Berger and W. Liesching
(Reply)
Rida M. Ali and Eva Cederberg

558 **Faster Continuous-flow Analysis for Triglycerides and Cholesterol**
Hillard Zyman, Franz Gabl, and Peter M. Bayer

558 **A Lipase Problem in an Enzymatic Procedure for Serum Triglycerides**
Eric J. Sampson, Laurence M. Demers, and Arthur F. Krieg

558 **Effect of Glutamate on γ-Glutamyltransferase Activity**
B. J. Gibson, I. Farrance, and P. M. Dennis

559 **Bichromatic Analyses with the ABA-100—A Critical Assumption**
J. Richard Pearson and Thurston Matsuura

560 **"Albumin-Titratable Bilirubin" as an Index to Bilirubin Binding**
Rodney L. Levine
(Reply)
W. J. O'Sullivan, G. K. Brown, and G. N. B. Storey

561 **Misuse of Calibration Sera in Automated Laboratory Testing Instruments**
Robert G. Hoffmann

565 **THE CLINICAL CHEMIST**
J. S. King

clinical chemistry

J. Stanton King, *Executive Editor*
P.O. Box 5218
Winston-Salem, N. C. 27103
(Tel. 919/725-0208)

Journal of the American Association for Clinical Chemistry

Business Office Tel. (202) 833-3590
1725 K St., NW
Washington, D. C. 20006

General Information. Manuscripts, editorial inquiries, and books for review should be addressed to the Executive Editor (address above). All subscription and circulation inquiries should be sent to the Business Office (address above). **Information for Authors** appears in the January issue.

Subscription: CLINICAL CHEMISTRY is issued monthly. Price per year, $25.00 in the U.S.A. and possessions; $26.00 in North America outside the U.S.; $35.00 elsewhere. Members, domestic and foreign, $12.50 (included in dues). All subscriptions before Oct. 1 start with the first issue of the current volume. Single copies of current-volume issues $5.00; ask Special-Issue Sales for back-issue prices. Claims for missing numbers will not be allowed (*a*) if received more than 60 days from date of issue plus time normally required for postal delivery of journal and claim, (*b*) if notice of a recent change of address has not been received, or (*c*) if the reason for claim is "missing from files." All advertising inquiries should be sent to Scherago Associates, Inc., 11 W. 42nd St., New York, N. Y. 10036. Second class postage paid at Washington, D. C. 20006 and additional mailing offices. Published monthly by the American Association for Clinical Chemistry, Inc., P. O. Box 5218, Winston-Salem, N. C. 27103. Printed at 20th and Northampton Sts., Easton, Pa. 18042.

Volume 22 Number 5
May 1976

CLCHAU 22 (5), 577–710 (1976)
ISSN 0009–9147

clinical chemistry

Journal of the American Association for Clinical Chemistry

577 **GUEST EDITORIAL: Standardization of Human Immunoglobulin Quantitation: A Review of Current Status and Problems**
Charles B. Reimer and Shirley E. Maddison

583 **REVIEW: Theoretical Approaches to Estimation of Plasma Renin Activity: A Review and Some Original Observations**
Suzanne Oparil

594 **REVIEW: Normative Values of Serum Immunoglobulins by Single Radial Immunodiffusion: A Review**
Shirley E. Maddison and Charles B. Reimer

602 **Radioimmunoassay of Bile Acids in Serum**
Laurence M. Demers and Gershon Hepner

607 **Kinetic Determination of Serum Lipase Activity with the Abbott ABA-100**
Ronald D. Feld, David L. Witte, and David A. Barrett II

611 **Rapid Radioimmunoassay of Total Urinary Estriol**
Dennis W. Anderson and Uwe Goebelsmann

616 **Improved Specificity of Serum Albumin Determination and Estimation of "Acute Phase Reactants" by Use of the Bromcresol Green Reaction**
Jan E. C. Gustafsson

623 **Gas–Liquid Chromatographic Profile of Neutral and Acidic Metabolites in Cerebrospinal Fluid from Newborns and Infants**
Richard D. Malcolm and Richard Leonards

627 **Improved Determination of Prostatic Acid Phosphatase (Sodium Thymolphthalein Monophosphate Substrate)**
Lilian M. Ewen and Ralph W. Spitzer

633 **Evaluation of Lipase Activity in Serum by Radial Enzyme Diffusion**
Jack M. Goldberg and Peter Pagast

638 **Diagnostic Use of Pancreatic Lipase Determination by Radial Enzyme Diffusion, and Design of a Routine Pancreatic Profile**
Jack M. Goldberg

643 **The Anion Gap: Its Use in Quality Control**
David L. Witte, John L. Rodgers, and David A. Barrett II

647 **Decreased Radioassay Values for Folate after Serum Extraction When Pteroylglutamic Acid Standards Are Used**
Gary A. Mitchell, Sharon P. Pochron, Philip V. Smutny, and Rogelia Guity

650 **Creatine Kinase in Serum: 1. Determination of Optimum Reaction Conditions**
Gabor Szasz, Wolfgang Gruber, and Erich Bernt

657 **Profile Analysis of Blood Proteins with a Centrifugal Analyzer**
Mogens Blom and Niels Hjorne

663 **Technical Pitfalls in Measurement of Venous Plasma NH_3 Concentration**
Glynda G. Gerron, Joseph D. Ansley, James W. Isaacs, Michael H. Kutner, and Daniel Rudman

667 **Method for Measuring the Concentration of Urinary Proteins According to Their Molecular Size Category**
Amadeo J. Pesce, A. Hsu, C. Kornhauser, K. Sethi, B. S. Ooi, and V. E. Pollak

673 **Interference of Fatty Acids in the Competitive Protein-Binding Assay for Serum Thyroxine**
William Shaw, Ivey Lois Hubert, and Francis W. Spierto

SCIENTIFIC NOTES

679 **Chemistry of the Kober Reaction**
Ronald W. A. Oliver, Soren B. Jensen, and Gordon Crossley

681 **Specificity and Reproducibility of Acetone Precipitation in Identifying Surface-Active Phosphatidylcholine in Amniotic Fluid**
L. L. Penney, Dwain D. Hagerman, and Catherine A. Sei

683 **Four Commercial Urease Reagents and a Laboratory-Prepared Reagent Compared for Analysis of Blood Urea Nitrogen with the Beckman Analyzer**
Norbert S. Norkus, Norman P. Kubasik, and Harrison E. Sine, Jr.

685 **Use of Blood Specimens Collected on Filter Paper in Screening for Abnormal Hemoglobins**
Robert M. Schmidt, Effie M. Brosious, Solomon Holland, Jane M. Wright, and Graham R. Serjeant

LETTERS

689 **Methaqualone Assay by Radioimmunoassay and Gas Chromatography**
R. O. Bost, C. A. Sutheimer, and I. Sunshine

690 **Enzymatic Determination of Total Serum Cholesterol with the Vickers D-300 Analyzer**
Francesco Zoppi and Domenico Fenili

691 **Collection of Blood Uncontaminated with Ca, Cu, Mg, or Zn, for Trace-Metal Analysis**
Robert O. Hughes, Dorothy F. Wease, and Raymond G. Troxler

692 **Nonleakage of Radioiodide through Plastic**
William W. Miller

692 **Plasma Renin Activity and Radioimmunoassay of Angiotensin I (cont.)**
Herman Rutner and Sidney Gutcho

694 **Ethchlorvynol Interference with Oxidimetric Determination of Ethanol in Urine**
James M. White

694 **Computer Program for Serum Protein Electrophoresis Calculations**
Arthur L. Levy

694 **Interference with Serotonin Determination**
Gregory S. Duboff

695 **Effects of Medication on Plasma Vitamin A Concentrations**
Jerry L. Curtis and Wynette Swicord

695 **Enzymatic Determination of Cholesterol in High-Density Lipoprotein Fractions Prepared by Polyanion Precipitation**
Gerhard M. Kostner

BOOK REVIEWS

697 James F. Glenn and Donald S. Young

699 **THE CLINICAL CHEMIST**
J. S. King

clinical chemistry

J. Stanton King, *Executive Editor*
P.O. Box 5218
Winston-Salem, N. C. 27103
(Tel. 919/725-0208)

Journal of the American Association for Clinical Chemistry

Business Office Tel. (202) 833-3590
1725 K St., NW
Washington, D. C. 20006

The contents of advertisements or articles in CLINICAL CHEMISTRY are not to be construed as official statements, evaluations, or endorsements by the Board of Editors or the American Association for Clinical Chemistry.

General Information. Manuscripts, editorial inquiries, and books for review should be addressed to the Executive Editor (address above). All subscription and circulation inquiries should be sent to the Business Office (address above). **Information for Authors** appears in the January issue.

Subscription: CLINICAL CHEMISTRY is issued monthly. Subscriptions are to be paid in advance; payment should accompany the order. Price per year, \$25.00 in the U.S.A. and possessions; \$26.00 in North America outside the U.S.; \$35.00 elsewhere. Members, domestic and foreign, \$12.50 (included in dues). All subscriptions before Oct. 1 start with the first issue of the current volume. Single copies of current-volume issues \$5.00; ask Special-Issue Sales for back-issue prices. Claims for missing numbers will not be allowed (*a*) if received more than 60 days from date of issue plus time normally required for postal delivery of journal and claim, (*b*) if notice of a recent change of address has not been received, or (*c*) if the reason for claim is "missing from files." All advertising inquiries should be sent to Scherago Associates, Inc., 11 W. 42nd St., New York, N. Y. 10036. Second class postage paid at Washington, D. C. 20006 and additional mailing offices. Published monthly by the American Association for Clinical Chemistry, Inc., P. O. Box 5218, Winston-Salem, N. C. 27103. Printed at 20th and Northampton Sts., Easton, Pa. 18042.

Volume 22 Number 6
June 1976

CLCHAU 22(6), 711–956 (1976)
ISSN 0009-9147

clinical chemistry

Journal of the American Association for Clinical Chemistry

Special Issue on Monitoring Drugs in Biological Fluids

711 **EDITORIAL: A New Role for the Clinical Chemist**
J. S. King

712 **REVIEW: Detection of Drugs of Abuse by Radioimmunoassay: A Summary of Published Data and Some New Information**
R. Cleeland, J. Christenson, M. Usategui-Gomez, J. Heveran, R. Davis, and E. Grunberg

726 **REVIEW: Radioimmunoassay of Antibiotics and Chemotherapeutic Agents**
Alan Broughton and James E. Strong

733 **REVIEW: Quantitative Enzyme Immunoassay: Current Status**
Simon L. Scharpé, Walter M. Cooreman, Walter J. Blomme, and Gert M. Laekeman

739 **Analytical Toxicology: Applications of Element-Selective Electrolytic Conductivity Detection for Gas Chromatography**
Brian E. Pape

749 **Radioimmunoassay, Enzyme Immunoassay, Spectrophotometry, and Gas–Liquid Chromatography Compared for Determination of Phenobarbital and Diphenylhydantoin**
Vina Spiehler, Lilla Sun, Don S. Miyada, Steve G. Sarandis, E. Richard Walwick, Marston W. Klein, Dennis B. Jordan, and Barbara Jessen

754 **Efficacy of Activated Charcoal Hemoperfusion in Removing Lethal Doses of Barbiturates and Salicylate from the Blood of Rats and Dogs**
John B. Hill, Frank L. Palaia, J. Lawrence McAdams, Phyllis J. Palmer, and S. Melissa Maret

761 **Rapid Radioisotopic Procedure for Determination of Nortriptyline in Plasma**
K. P. Maguire, G. D. Burrows, J. P. Coghlan, and B. A. Scoggins

765 **Gas-Chromatographic Micro-Scale Procedure for Theophylline, with Use of a Nitrogen-Sensitive Detector**
Charles J. Least, Jr., George F. Johnson, and Harvey M. Solomon

769 **Simultaneous Gas-Chromatographic Analysis for Phenobarbital, Diphenylhydantoin, Carbamazepine, and Primidone in Serum**
Chempithera V. Abraham and Harry D. Joslin

772 **Gas-Chromatographic Determination of 5-Fluorocytosine in Human Serum**
Sally A. Harding, George F. Johnson, and Harvey M. Solomon

777 **Gas-Chromatographic Analysis for Therapeutic Concentrations of Amitryptyline and Nortriptyline in Plasma, with Use of a Nitrogen Detector**
David N. Bailey and Peter I. Jatlow

782 **Liquid Chromatographic Method for Monitoring Therapeutic Concentrations of L-Dopa and Dopamine in Serum**
Ralph M. Riggin, Richard L. Alcorn, and Peter T. Kissinger

785 **Enzymatic Assay for Methotrexate in Serum and Cerebrospinal Fluid**
Larry C. Falk, Dennis R. Clark, Sumner M. Kalman, and Thomas F. Long

789 **Relative Merits of Some Methods for Amphetamine Assay in Biological Fluids**
Robert O. Bost, Craig A. Sutheimer, and Irving Sunshine

802 **Automated Enzymic Determination of Ethanol in Blood, Serum, and Urine with a Miniature Centrifugal Analyzer**
T. P. Hadjiioannou, S. I. Hadjiioannou, J. Avery, and H. V. Malmstadt

806 **Gas-Chromatographic Determination of an Antifibrinolytic Drug, ε-Aminocaproic Acid**
Thomas R. Keucher, Elizabeth B. Solow, John Metaxas, and Robert L. Campbell

810 **Serum Quinidine Concentrations: Comparison of Fluorescence, Gas-Chromatographic, and Gas-Chromatographic/Mass-Spectrometric Methods**
David H. Huffman and Charles E. Hignite

813 **Rapid Radioimmunoassay for Methotrexate in Biological Fluids**
Jørn Hendel, Lydia J. Sarek, and Eigill F. Hvidberg

817 **Determination of Clomipramine and Desmethyl-Clomipramine in Plasma or Urine by the Double-Radioisotope Derivative Technique**
G. Carnis, J. Godbillon, and J. P. Metayer

824 **Simultaneous Measurement of Phenobarbital, Diphenylhydantoin, and Primidone in Blood by High-Pressure Liquid Chromatography**
Pokar M. Kabra, George Gotelli, Robert Stanfill, and Laurence J. Marton

828 **Radioimmunoassay for Clindamycin**
Terry J. Gilbertson and R. P. Stryd

832 **Tabulation of Therapeutic, Toxic, and Lethal Concentrations of Drugs and Chemicals in Blood**
Charles L. Winek

837 **Assessment of Interference by Aspirin with Some Assays Commonly Done in the Clinical Laboratory**
Joseph I. Routh and William D. Paul

843 **Results on a Nine-Laboratory Survey of Forensic Toxicology Proficiency**
Eugene C. Dinovo and Louis A. Gottschalk

847 **Analysis of Results of Toxicological Examinations Performed by Coroners' or Medical Examiners' Laboratories in 2000 Drug-Involved Deaths in Nine Major U. S. Cities**
Eugene C. Dinovo, Louis A. Gottschalk, Frederick L. McGuire, Herman Birch, and Jon F. Heiser

851 **Serum Theophylline Analysis by High-Pressure Liquid Chromatography**
Merle A. Evenson and Brenda L. Warren

856 **Rapid Micromethod for Measuring Anticonvulsant Drugs in Serum by High-Performance Liquid Chromatography**
S. J. Soldin and J. Gilbert Hill

860 **Rapid Gas-Chromatographic Measurement of Anticonvulsant Drugs in Serum**
Floyd Dorrity, Jr. and Markku Linnoila

Continued on page 4A

863 **Method for Alcohol Determination in Biological Liquids by Sensing with a Solid-State Detector**
Kurt M. Dubowski

868 **REVIEW: Pharmacokinetic Interpretation of Data Gathered during Therapeutic Drug Monitoring**
Barry H. Dvorchik and Elliot S. Vesell

879 **Gas-Chromatographic Method for Acetaminophen (*N*-Acetyl-*p*-Aminophenol) Based on Sequential Alkylation**
Walter A. Dechtiaruk, George F. Johnson, and Harvey M. Solomon

884 **Quantitative Gas-Chromatographic Flame-Ionization Method for *p*-Chlorophenoxyisobutyric Acid in Human Serum and Saliva**
John N. Connor, George F. Johnson, and Harvey M. Solomon

889 **Diazepam Abuse: Incidence, Rapid Screening, and Confirming Methods**
Thomas A. Rejent and Kenneth C. Wahl

892 **Measurement of Clomipramine, *N*-Desmethylclomipramine, Imipramine, and Dehydroimipramine in Biological Fluids by Selective Ion Monitoring, and Pharmacokinetics of Clomipramine**
Jean-Pierre Dubois, Werner Küng, Walter Theobald, and Bernard Wirz

SCIENTIFIC NOTES

898 **Gas-chromatographic Quantitation of Theophylline in Small Volumes of Plasma**
Donald Perrier and Evangeline Lear

901 **Primidone Analyses: Correlation of Gas-Chromatographic Assay with Enzyme Immunoassay**
Lilla Sun and E. Richard Walwick

903 **Improved Micro-Radioimmunoassay of Digoxin in Serum, with Use of ^{125}I-Labeled Digoxin**
Benjamin Calesnick and Annette Dinan

905 **Adaptation of "EMIT" Technique for Serum Phenobarbital and Diphenylhydantoin Assays to the Miniature Centrifugal Analyzer**
Sheldon D. Brunk, Themis P. Hadjiioannou, Semi I. Hadjiioannou, and Howard V. Malmstadt

908 **Simplified Fluorometric Assay for Diphenylhydantoin in Plasma**
Wesley A. Dill, Amy Leung, Arlyn W. Kinkel, and Anthony J. Glazko

911 **Assay of Phenytoin: Adaptation of "EMIT" to the Centrifugal Analyzer**
Paul R. Finley, R. Jane Williams, and James M. Byers III

CASE REPORTS

915 **Monitoring Drug Concentrations in a Case of Combined Overdosage with Primidone and Methsuximide**
George F. Johnson, Ph.D., Charles J. Least, Jr., M.S., James W. Serum, Ph.D., Elizabeth B. Solow, M.S., and Harvey M. Solomon, M.D.

922 **Beta-Carotene Content of Certain Organs from Two Patients Receiving High Doses of Beta-Carotene**
Micheline M. Mathews-Roth, M.D., Andreas A. Abraham, M.D., and Thomas G. Gabuzda, M.D.

LETTERS

925 ***N*-Acetylglucosaminidase and γ-Glutamyltransferase in Urine of Patients with Renal Transplants: Not an Early Indicator of Rejection**
J. W. Keyser, G. Ll. Watkins, and J. R. Salaman

926 **Calibration of Glucose Methods with Lyophilized Materials: A Caution**
R. R. Swain, R. M. Carpenter, and S. L. Briggs

926 **Decomposition of 1,3-Dimethylphenobarbital in Trimethylanilinium Hydroxide**
Patrick S. Callery and James Leslie

927 **Procedures Compared for Extracting Benzodiazepines from Blood**
Alan W. Missen

928 **Quench-Correction Techniques in Liquid Scintillation**
Kent Painter
(Reply)
Edith Zak Helman

929 **Use of an Inhibitor in Kinetic Determination of Glucose with a Centrifugal Analyzer by the Glucose Dehydrogenase Reaction**
R. A. Lutz

929 **Evaluation of the Chemical Activation Procedure (Rao's Method) for the Measurement of the MB Isoenzyme of Creatine Kinase**
R. M. Balkcom, Michael Sheehan and Kenneth Leipper, B. K. Hultman and W. G. Yasmineh, and F. Muschenheim
(Reply)
Parinam S. Rao and Hiltrud S. Mueller

933 **Interference in Drug Screening Assays**
L. P. Hackett and L. J. Dusci

933 **More on Adjusting Serum Ca for Protein**
Harry Husdan, Abraham Rapoport, Sandra Locke, and Dimitrios Oreopoulos, and R. B. Payne and A. J. Little

934 **Bilirubin Standard Solutions**
Arthur M. Zebelman, Margaret A. Kenny, and Catherine G. Sunday

935 **Effect of Mannitol (Osmitrol) Intoxication of Serum "Triglyceride" Values**
Herbert K. Naito, Vytenis J. Gatautis, and Kathryn L. Popowniak

936 **Effect of Two New Serum-Separating Devices on Results for Cholesterol and Triglyceride**
Herbert K. Naito and Vytenis J. Gatautis

937 **Data Handling and Reporting**
L. Brown and R. Feld
(Reply)
Roger L. Forrester, Willa Collinge, Pattie Hashimoto, and Jackie Worrall

939 **Increased Purine-Nucleoside Phosphorylase Activity in Erythrocytes of Gouty Patients**
Lucile Gerbaut, Elisabeth Rey, and Georges Olive

BOOK REVIEWS

943 Theodore Peters, Jr., Richard A. Anderson, and Robert B. McComb

954 **THE CLINICAL CHEMIST**
J. S. King

Information for Authors

Clinical Chemistry, issued monthly, is published under the direction of an Editorial Board appointed by the Board of Directors of the American Association for Clinical Chemistry, Inc. The Editors give equal consideration to original manuscripts in English from any country, whether or not the author is a member of the Association.

Excellent scientific work deserves excellent presentation—but frequently suffers a lack of it. The aim of these suggestions is to expedite publication by making it easier for the potential author to present his work in a form that will minimize editorial revision and delay.

Copies are available on request.

Scope

Clinical Chemistry welcomes contributions on the application of chemistry to the understanding of the human organism in health and disease. Articles submitted for publication should contain original information, experimental or theoretical, that advances the science of clinical chemistry. This includes basic materials or principles, analytical techniques, instrumentation, data processing, statistical analyses of data, clinical investigations in which chemistry has played a major role, and experimental (laboratory animal) investigations of chemically oriented problems of human disease.

Other appropriate contributions include reviews, case reports, scientific notes, and letters to the editor. Prospective contributors should consult recent issues of *Clinical Chemistry* to determine the appropriate category for their contribution, as well as for examples of acceptable style.

Submission of Manuscripts

Manuscripts and other editorial correspondence should be addressed to J. Stanton King, Ph.D., Executive Editor, *Clinical Chemistry,* Box 5218, Winston-Salem, N. C. 27103.

Manuscripts are considered for publication with the understanding that no paper presenting the same information—other than an abstract or preliminary report—has been or will be published elsewhere. *Clinical Chemistry* is copyrighted by the Association. Permission to reproduce copyrighted material for scholarly use can be arranged through the Executive Editor.

An original typescript and one copy of the manuscript are to be submitted, double-spaced (preferably triple-spaced) *throughout* (including abstract, references, tables, figure legends, and footnotes), on one side of paper 22 × 28 cm (no larger), with 4-cm margins. Each copy must include all figures and tables. An abstract precedes the body of the manuscript; a separate sheet should be used for the title page, with authors' names and affiliations, and for the abstract. References, tables, figure legends, and footnotes should be grouped on separate sheets, in that order. Every page, beginning with the title page, should be numbered. All sheets should carry the last name of the author(s) in the upper right corner. If the current address of any author differs from that where the work was done, it will be included as a footnote; if reprints are to be requested from someone other than the first author, or from an address other than that where the work was done, a footnote should include this comment.

Review of Manuscripts

Manuscripts will be evaluated by two anonymous persons, who will be either members of the Editorial Board or qualified invited reviewers. Manuscripts are considered privileged information by the reviewers, who are expected to disqualify themselves before reviewing papers in cases where there may be a possible conflict of interest.

When reviewers clearly disagree on the merits of a manuscript, a referee will generally be asked to examine it. A résumé of the reviewers' critiques will be sent to the author when he is notified of the disposition of the manuscript (usually not later than six weeks from receipt) by the Executive Editor. If the manuscript is rejected, the author may appeal in writing, giving his reasons why the manuscript should be reconsidered.

The principal desiderata for an acceptable paper are:

- subject matter that is original and significantly advances the state of knowledge of clinical chemistry
- conclusions that are justified from the design of the experiments and the data presented
- information that is sufficiently detailed to permit repetition of the work by a competent clinical chemist
- clear, concise, and grammatical writing.

Manuscript Preparation

The principal guides for the author should be the "ACS Handbook for Authors" (*1*), and the "Council of Biology Editors Style Manual" (*2*), with the former taking precedence where there is disagreement. Only critical preparation of the manuscript can enable the author to avoid obscure wording, neologisms, "laboratory slang," and unfamiliar (and undefined) terminology (*3*).

There is no rigid prescription for organization of papers acceptable for publication in *Clinical Chemistry,* but manuscripts should be arranged generally into the following sections: title, abstract, introduction, materials and methods, results, discussion, and references.

Title

The title should be specific, informative, and concise, incorporating appropriate keywords, to facilitate indexing. Symbols, formulas, or arbitrary abbreviations should not be included in the title, except chemical symbols to indicate the structure of isotopically labeled compounds.

Abstract

An abstract, intelligible by itself, should be included in all contributions to *Clinical Chemistry* except letters to the editor. The abstract, not to exceed 150 words, summarizes the plan, procedures, results, and conclusions of the investigation. Remember that the abstract will be the most widely read portion of the paper and is the main source of material for the various abstracting services.

The Executive Editor will select "Additional Keyphrases" not found in the title.

Introduction

This should indicate the importance of the work, its relation to previous work, and (if it is a method) reasons why it is preferable to older methods.

Materials and Methods

The material to be presented dictates the way in which this section is written. Whatever the arrangement, the following topics are usually present:

Apparatus. All apparatus should be identified, including manufacturer's name and address (city, zip code), and model number if different versions exist. Further details are necessary only when the equipment is not standard. If standard apparatus has been modified or new apparatus built, lists of components and their sources should be provided along with directions from which the equipment can be duplicated.

Reagents. All reagents used may be listed; only special or unusual ones need be described in detail, and their source mentioned. If purity or stability of reagents is critical, particulars about the source, degree of purity, and preservation should be included. Only novel details of preparation or purification of reagents need be described.

The pH and composition of buffers should be unambiguous; a standard reference can often be cited. The temperature at which critical pH measurements are made should be stated. Make clear whether the concentrations in a reaction mixture represent final concentrations or the original concentration of the solutions added.

Procedures. Use of the imperative mood here is both clearer and more succinct. Standard procedures should be cited but not described, except where a brief résumé of the principle of a method is appropriate. Only modifications of a published procedure need be described. Adequate details of critical steps (e.g., collection and storage of samples), standardization, calibration, and calculation of results are necessary to permit the work to be repeated by a competent clinical chemist. Mention any potential hazards in the procedure.

Results

These should be presented in concise and simple language, with the use of tables or graphs for clarification if necessary.

Discussion

This section should discuss significance of results, and lead to a valid conclusion. Results and conclusions should be compared and contrasted with those of reference methods or previous studies. Interpret the results here but do not recapitulate them. Such matters as special problems, interferences, effect of order of reagent addition, and color stability are appropriate to this section. Sometimes clarity is improved if discussion is intermingled with results in a single section, but if this is done the author should clearly distinguish speculation and fact.

Acknowledgments

Acknowledgments of financial support, gifts, technical help, or other assistance (especially that rendered by a company in evaluation of a product) are made in a brief paragraph preceding the References. A statement regarding possible conflicts of interest appears in this issue (p 4), and is available on request.

References

References to the literature should be listed by number in the order of their appearance in the text. The appropriate positions in the text should be indicated by underlined Arabic numerals in parentheses. Reference examples:

Journals

1. Klein, B., and Lucas, L. B., Application of Fe(II)-5-pyridyl benzodiazepin-2-ones to the manual or automated determination of serum uric acid. *Clin. Chem.* **19,** 67 (1973).

Books and monographs (except serial volumes, which are treated as journals)

2. Henry, R. J., *Clinical Chemistry: Principles and Technics,* Hoeber, New York, N. Y., 1964, p 364.

3. Schmidt, E., Schmidt, F. W., Horn, H. D., and Gerlach, U., The importance of measurement of enzyme activities in medicine. In *Methods of Enzymatic Analysis,* Section C, H.-U. Bergmeyer, Ed. Academic Press, New York, N. Y., 1963, pp 651–655.

It is the author's responsibility to verify the accuracy and adequacy of reference information. This is where most errors appear—and persist, because the editorial office does not routinely check references. Only essential references should be cited; include review articles when appropriate.

Avoid listing references to unpublished work, manuscripts in preparation, verbal reports given at meetings, and personal communications. This type of information should be mentioned parenthetically in the text. References to papers in press may be included among the references; it is advisable to send copies of such papers to the Editor, to assist in the evaluation of the manuscript. Citations of published abstracts must appear as text footnotes, but should be avoided whenever possible.

Abbreviations

This journal discourages the unnecessary use of new abbreviations, such as acronyms. A few such abbreviations may aid readability; a profusion of them does not. If more than two are used, all nonstandard abbreviations must be defined in a single footnote in the text at the point where the first is used. Abbreviations, if previously defined, may be used in figures, tables, and equations. Letter combinations that form words or that are already in current use as conventional abbreviations must be avoided. Abbreviations listed in the recommended references (*1, 2*) may be used, but internationally-agreed-upon biochemical symbols and abbreviations are to be found in most biochemical journals [e.g., *J. Biol. Chem.* **241,** 527 (1966); **245,** 5171 (1970); **247,** 323 and 977 (1972)].

The Association has officially accepted (*4*) the recommendations of the Commission on Clinical Chemistry of the IUPAC and the IFCC on a standard international (SI) system of units. The following examples include abbreviations appearing most commonly in the journal; others can be found elsewhere (*5*). Examples of abbreviations that are no longer acceptable are also given. Consistently use the proper units in text, figures, and tables. Notice that periods do not follow the abbreviations.

Prefixes for decimal factors:

10^3	kilo-	k	10^{-6}	micro-	μ
10^{-1}	deci-	d	10^{-9}	nano-	n
10^{-2}	centi-	c	10^{-12}	pico-	p
10^{-3}	milli-	m	10^{-15}	femto-	f

Length: m, cm, mm, μm, nm (not acceptable: in., ft., yd., Å, mμ).

Area: m^2, cm^2, mm^2, μm^2 (not acceptable: sq. in., in.^{2}, u^2).

Volume: liter, ml, μl, nl, pl (not acceptable: pint, gallon, cc, ccm, λ, μμl). Where the word "liter" is used in the text, it should be written out in full to avoid confusion with the numeral 1; it will usually be desirable to do so in tables and figures as well.

Mass: kg, g, mg, μg, ng, pg (not acceptable: oz., lb., Kg, gr, gm, gms, mgm, mgms, mgs).

Mass concentration: kg/liter, g/liter, mg/liter, μg/liter (not acceptable: %, g/ml, ppm, mg %).

Substance concentration: mol/liter, mmol/liter, μmol/liter, mmol/liter (not acceptable: M, N, mEq/l).

Temperature: °C (not acceptable: °, C, K).

Time: s, min, h, d, and a.

Density: kg/liter.

Relative density: This term replaces "specific gravity."

Absorbance: A

Radioactivity: Ci, mCi, μCi.

International (IUB) units of enzymatic activity: U (amount), U/liter (concentration).

Coefficient of variation: CV.

Illustrations

Use figures only when they have real utility. Mathematical formulas or a statement of numerical values may often substitute for a figure.

All line drawings and halftones (and such material as computer printouts) should be submitted as camera-ready copy (glossy prints). Illustrations should not be mounted or attached in any way to sheets of paper. Photographs or prints must not be larger than 22 × 28 cm or smaller than 5 × 8 cm. If it is necessary to submit original figures, rather than the preferred glossy prints, they should be drawn with India ink on white drawing paper, blue tracing paper, or coordinate paper ruled in blue only. Gridlines that are to show in the final engraving should be inked in black. Letters, numerals, data points, and other marks should be made neatly *and of such size that the smallest will be readable when the figure is reduced to one- or two-column size.* Avoid wasted space in illustrations; several curves may often be shown clearly on the same graph, for example. The word "top," the figure number, and the author's name should be lightly written in pencil on the back of each illustration. Do not paperclip illustrations together.

A reasonable financial allowance is made to each paper for illustrations and tabular composition. If this allowance is exceeded or if illustrations in color are required, special arrangements must be made with the Executive Editor. Current issues of *Clinical Chemistry* illustrate acceptable figures. Each illustration must have a caption that makes it intelligible by itself. Number in Arabic numerals.

Tables

Each table should be on a separate page and numbered consecutively with Arabic numerals in order of mention in the text. Each table should have a descriptive heading that makes it intelligible without reference to the text; footnotes to the table should appear on the same sheet as the table. Each column should have a heading with clearly defined units. Lengthy tabulations are expensive to set; unless essential, they should be avoided and replaced by statistical statements. Figures and tables should not be used to illustrate the same data; use whichever is clearer, or omit entirely if the information can be stated concisely in the text.

Text Footnotes

Footnotes are used sparingly, for auxiliary or explanatory material that cannot be incorporated into the text without seriously disrupting the train of thought. The position of a footnote in the text is indicated by a *superscript* Arabic numeral. Footnotes should be typed on a separate sheet of paper, with the appropriate number and page number for each. On the first page of each published article, the following information will be printed routinely as footnotes; laboratory affiliation(s) of the author(s) and the dates on which the manuscript was received and accepted for publication. Footnotes to tables are independent of other footnotes, and should be indicated by superscript lower-case italic letters in alphabetical order, reading across the table.

Description of Analytical Methods and Results

Acceptable manuscripts dealing with the development and performance of methods and instruments should discuss sensitivity, specificity, day-to-day precision, within-run precision, accuracy, comparison studies, and normal range of the proposed method. The paper should document the advantages of the new or modified method over existing methods. Totally original analytical methods must be thoroughly tested and should be scrutinized during daily use under routine laboratory conditions.

Standardization and linearity: If the working curve obtained for the method is linear, then the least-squares statistical description of the data suffices: slope, x and y intercepts, and reproducibility (±2 SD limits) of the calibration points. If the working curve is nonlinear, a graphic presentation (also illustrating ±2 SD) is recommended.

Precision: Studies must include "within-day" as well as "day-to-day" estimates of precision. Each should be determined at low-normal and above-normal concentrations in a biological fluid matrix. Within-run studies should be performed with other samples interspersed between the precision samples and should include at least 20 measurements at each of the three concentrations. In day-to-day studies, accumulate one value per day for at least 20 days.

Accuracy: Data should be included concerning recovery, interference, comparison with other methods, and normal range. (*a*) *Studies of recovery* involve mixtures of standard solutions with the biological fluids in which the measurement will be performed. Pathological samples should be included as well as samples from healthy individuals. Percentage recovery is defined as (amount found of added/amount added) × 100. (*b*) *Interference* studies should be performed to ascertain the effects if the serum (e.g.) is lipemic, icteric, turbid, hemolyzed, or otherwise abnormal. Exogenous substances, such as commonly used drugs that might interfere with the determination, should be added to the usual sample matrix. (*c*) In *comparison* studies, results by the new method should be compared with the results by a reference method or other generally accepted method of analysis, desirably with use of 100 to 200 different samples. The concentration range should include the entire range of normal and abnormal values likely to be encountered in samples from patients. (*d*) Depending on the conclusions of the accuracy studies, modification of the existing normal range may be indicated. The "normal range" proposed must include details such as method of selection of the subjects, their number, age, and sex distribution, and other factors that would influence the values obtained.

Statistical data: For *precision* studies, the statistical measures of standard deviation, coefficient of variation, mean, mode, and median are applicable. For *comparison* studies, the least-squares results for slope, intercepts, and standard error should be included. Specific information on applications and interpretation of comparison data is given in detail in a recent paper (*6*). Values for t (Student's t-test), F (F-test), and r (correlation coefficient) are often misused (*7*), hence considerable caution is necessary in their interpretation. In stating the normal range, specify the definition and statistical technique. Distributions must be gaussian if a ± 2 SD range is to be considered the normal range. For examples of nongaussian distributions, and the use of nonparametric techniques to obtain the values for the normal range, several statistical methods are available. Statistical methods should be properly applied (*6*) to the data.

Chromatograms. These are not published unless they show novel features that cannot be described in the text. The method for preparing sample and plates or columns, media, or adsorbent binders should be presented, as well as indicators, activation conditions, duration of migration, and drying and spraying conditions. Migration should be expressed in terms of R_F (or retention times for columns). Temperature conditions should be stated. Solvents or carriers and their order of use should be described in detail. Similar information should be included for electrophoresis.

Enzymatic methods. The effects of certain factors are customarily described in methods for measurement of catalytic activity: temperature, pH, substrate concentration, enzyme concentration, order of reaction, inhibitors, activators, buffers, chelators, and the like. Representative calculations deriving the results must usually be shown, because pure enzymes are seldom obtainable for standardization of the method. Enzymes must be identified by their Enzyme Commission number (*8*) when first mentioned.

References

1. *Handbook for Authors.* American Chemical Society Publications, Washington, D. C. 20036, 1967.
2. Council of Biology Editors, *CBE Style Manual,* 3rd ed., American Institute of Biological Sciences, Washington, D. C. 20016, 1972.
3. *American National Standard for the Preparation of Scientific Papers for Written or Oral Presentation (Z39.16 1972).* American National Standards Institute, Inc., 1430 Broadway, New York, N. Y. 10018, 1972.
4. *Clin. Chem.* **15,** 427 (1969).
5. (a) Dybkaer, R., and Jorgensen, K., *Quantities and Units in Clinical Chemistry.* Williams and Wilkins, Baltimore, Md., 1967. (b) Dybkaer, R., Nomenclature for quantities and units. *Stand. Methods Clin. Chem.* **6,** 223 (1970). (c) *The International System of Units (SI).* C. H. Page and P. Vigoureux, Eds. National Bureau of Standards Special Publication 330 (periodically revised; for sale by the Superintendent of Documents, U. S. Gov't. Printing Office, Washington, D. C. 20402; order by SD Catalog No. C 13.10:330).
6. Westgard, J. O., and Hunt, M. R., Use and interpretation of common statistical tests in method-comparison studies. *Clin. Chem.* **19,** 49 (1973).
7. Reed, A. H., Henry, R. J., and Mason, W. B., Influence of statistical method used on the resulting estimate of normal range. *Clin. Chem.* **17,** 275 (1971).
8. *Enzyme Nomenclature, Recommendations 1972 of the International Union of Biochemistry.* Elsevier, New York, N. Y., 1973.

Statement of Interest

It is usual practice for journals to include a statement of financial support for work done under the auspices of a government agency or private foundation. Indeed, many funding agencies stipulate that such acknowledgments should be included when the supported work is published. In *Clinical Chemistry* such acknowledgments are usually included in the acknowledgments section.

Much of the research performed in the field of clinical chemistry involves assessment of new equipment, reagents, or kits, and the costs of such evaluation are often directly or indirectly underwritten by the manufacturer. When an author of a paper concerned with the evaluation of a product is employed by the manufacturer, readers are normally able to assess any interest that the author may have in the product because of the journal's practice of including the address of the author. When authors who receive consulting or other fees from a manufacturer publish a favorable report on one of the manufacturer's products, they may do their work (and themselves) a disservice by failing to disclose an interest that conceivably could alter their objectivity. If a business address is not used by an employee of a commercial organization, readers will have grounds for questioning the work, even though it may have great scientific merit.

We hope that authors will declare their interest in publications that involve evaluations of commercial products. Such interest would include not only personal financial gain, but also the manufacturer's donation or loan of equipment, reagents, and the like. A brief statement concerning the interest should be included in the acknowledgments to be published with the scientific paper.

No paper will be rejected by *Clinical Chemistry* solely because no such statement has been made. Nevertheless, we strongly encourage our contributors to do this to provide reviewers and readers with additional information of use in assessing publication. At present, we are unaware of any instance in which a reader has felt misled because of his lack of knowledge of a background interest by an author in an appraised product. Nonetheless, we believe that a full disclosure will be of value to our readers and prevent any future misunderstandings.

CLIN. CHEM. 22/1, 5-15 (1976)

review

Recently Discovered Hypothalamic–Pituitary Hormones

William B. Malarkey

In recent years a variety of peptide hormones have been isolated from the mammalian hypothalamus and pituitary. Several hypothalamic hormones, including thyroliberin (thyrotropin-releasing factor), luliberin (luteinizing hormone-releasing factor), and somatostatin (somatotropin release-inhibiting factor), have been characterized and synthesized. The subsequent development of radioimmunoassays for these hormones has made possible the study of their physiology. The measurement of prolactin in serum and the release of pituitary hormones after the administration of the hypothalamic hormones has proved to be useful in clinical diagnosis. The use of hypothalamic hormones in treating various clinical disorders and the isolation and characterization of new releasing and inhibiting hormones in the hypothalamus are actively being investigated.

Additional Keyphrases: *assay, physiology, clinical utility • thyroliberin, luliberin, somatostatin, prolactin*

Introduction

Background—The last five years have been amazingly productive in the field of endocrinology as new hormones have been characterized from the thyroid, intestinal tract, pineal body, hypothalamus, and pituitary. This advance has been made possible by important methodologic contributions in the areas of peptide chemistry and radioimmunoassay. This review will deal primarily, however, with the physiology and the clinical utility of the newly recognized hypothalamic/pituitary hormones: thyrotropin-releasing factor (thyroliberin),[1] luteinizing hormone-releasing hormone (luliberin), growth hormone release-inhibiting factor (somatostatin), and prolactin (Table 1). The data presented in this survey represent the research efforts of many investigators throughout the world; because of space limitations, some of their work will not be cited except as found in the referenced review articles.

Hypothalamic/pituitary regulation. In order to place this review in proper perspective, some comments about the regulation of the endocrine system seem pertinent. Since Harris (*1*) first proposed that the hypothalamus and pituitary function as a unit, investigators have been attempting to isolate and characterize hypothalamic hormones. A hierarchy of control has now been firmly established for most of the peptide hormones of the central nervous system; the hypothalamic hormone produces release of the pituitary hormone, which in turn promotes the secretion and (or) synthesis of the target-organ hormone (see Table 2). This latter secretory product can then produce either negative or positive feedback on endocrine secretion by the hypothalamus and (or) pituitary.

The peptide hormones appear to exert their physiologic effects by combining with an endocrine receptor in the plasma membrane of the target tissue. This receptor-hormone binding activates adenyl cyclase cyclic AMP formation, which, via a specific protein kinase, eventuates in a biological response characteristic for that hormone (*2*).

A recent and most intriguing observation is that the endocrine membrane receptor number is not static but can be altered by the concentration of hormone in the perfusing media. For example, the number of insulin receptors on lymphocytes appears to decline in the face of increased insulin concentrations (*3*).

Department of Medicine, Division of Endocrinology and Metabolism, The Ohio State University Hospitals, 410 West 10th Ave., Columbus, Ohio 43210.

[1] See Table 1.

Received Oct. 1, 1975; accepted Oct. 20, 1975.

Table 1. Nomenclature of Peptide Hormones[a]

Trivial name	Other name(s)
Corticoliberin	Corticotropin-releasing factor
Folliberin	Follicle-stimulating-hormone-releasing factor
Luliberin	Luteinizing hormone-releasing factor
Melanoliberin	Melanotropin-releasing factor
Melanostatin	Melanotropin release-inhibiting factor
Prolactoliberin	Prolactin-releasing factor
Prolactostatin	Prolactin release-inhibiting factor
Somatoliberin	Somatotropin-releasing factor; growth hormone-releasing factor
Somatostatin	Somatotropin release-inhibiting factor
Thyroliberin	Thyrotropin-releasing factor
Corticotropin	Adrenocorticotropic hormone
Follitropin	Follicle-stimulating hormone
Lutropin	Luteinizing hormone (interstitial cell-stimulating hormone)
Prolactin	Mammatropic hormone; mammatropin; lactotropic hormone; lactotropin
Somatotropin	Somatropic hormone; growth hormone
Thyrotropin	Thyrotropic hormone

[a] According to the IUPAC-IUB Commission on Biochemical Nomenclature Recommendations (1974), *J. Biol. Chem.* **250**, 3215 (1975). The trivial name will be used in this review, as based on the following principles: (*a*) new names for hormones of the adenohypophysis bear the ending "tropin"; (*b*) hypothalamic releasing factors (hormones) bear the ending "liberin"; and (*c*) hypothalamic release-inhibiting factors (hormones) bear the ending "statin".

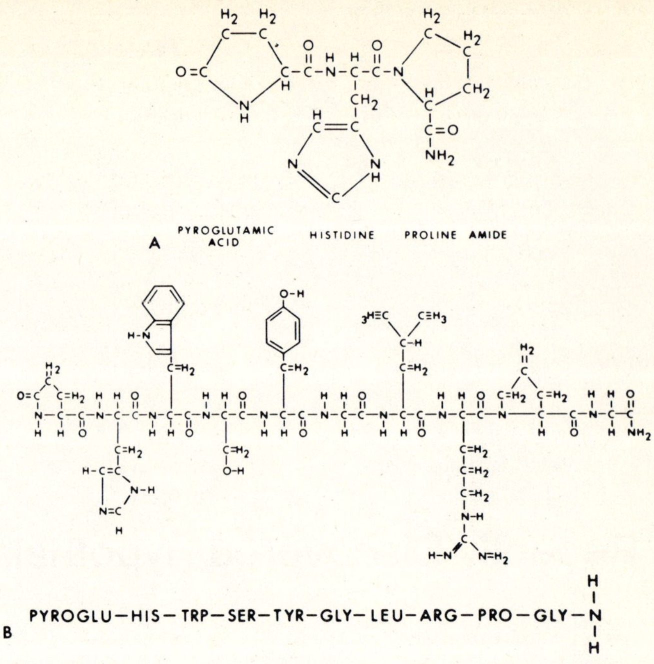

Fig. 1. *A*. Structure of thyroliberin, which promotes pituitary thyrotropin and prolactin secretion. *B*. Structure of luliberin, which releases both pituitary lutropin and follitropin

Therefore it appears that the hormone receptor serves as another modulating factor in endocrine regulation.

With this brief review of endocrine control systems, let us turn to the consideration of the new hypothalamic/pituitary hormones.

Thyroliberin

Background. Guillemin's laboratory (*4*) first reported the isolation of 1 mg of pure thyroliberin from fragments of 300 000 sheep hypothalami. It was found to be composed of three amino acids (pyroglutamyl-histidyl-prolineamide), and it was soon synthesized (see Figure 1). Schally's group (*4*) found a similar structure for porcine thyroliberin that also promotes pituitary thyrotropin release. At this time there is no evidence of major species specificity for synthetic thyroliberin, for it is active in all mammals so far examined. As yet, however, no meaningful data have been acquired in man concerning the regulation of its secretion.

Assay. A radioimmunoassay for thyroliberin has been recently developed (*5*). This assay has proven useful in determining concentrations of the hormone in tissue, but not in serum because thyroliberin is rapidly inactivated by serum (*6*). It has been suggested that this rapid enzymatic destruction may be prevented by sampling in cooled syringes containing benzamidine (*7*).

Another method of assay, proposed by Mitnick and Reichlin (*8*), involves measuring radioactive thyroliberin that has been formed by the action of a thyroliberin synthetase in incubation mixtures of hypothalamic extracts under various experimental conditions.

Physiology. When thyroliberin is infused by vein, thyrotropin is quickly released (*9, 10*), reaching a peak about 20 min after an intravenous bolus (Figure 2). The magnitude of the peak is influenced by age (*10*) and in women by the menstrual cycle (*11*). In 1971, thyroliberin was reported (*12*) to promote prolactin secretion by rat pituitary tumors cultured in vitro. It was soon demonstrated in man (*13–15*) that intravenously administered thyroliberin also promoted prolactin secretion, with a time course of release similar to that of thyrotropin (Figure 2). These observations therefore suggested that, physiologically, thyroliberin was the releasing hormone for secretion of both thyrotropin and prolactin. However, there is information that is not in harmony with this postulate: prolactin release often occurs independently of thyrotropin secretion (*16*), the rat hypothalamus contains prolactin releasing activity that is not thyroliberin related (*17*), and thyroid hormone

Table 2. Hormonal Interrelationships

Hypothalamus	Anterior pituitary	Target organ	Function
Thyroliberin[a]	→ ↑ Thyrotropin ⇌ [b]	T_4+T_3, in thyroid	increase basal metabolic rate
Somatostatin[c] Somatoliberin	→ ↓ Somatotropin → ↑ Somatotropin } →	somatomedin[d], in liver	promote growth
Luliberin Luliberin	→ ↑ Lutropin ⇌ → ↑ Follitropin ⇌	estrogen, progesterone, testosterone } ovary, testes	induce ovulation spermatogenesis secondary sex characteristics
Corticoliberin	→ ↑ Corticotropin ⇌	cortisol, androgens, aldosterone } adrenal	cellular effects weak masculinizing effect sodium balance
Melanoliberin Melanostatin	→ ↑ Melanotropin → ↓ Melanotropin →	melanin formation } skin	darkening of skin
Prolactostatin	→ ↓ Prolactin →	— } breast, ovary	milk production decrease progesterone synthesis

[a] An infusion will also increase prolactin secretion.
[b] ⇌ feedback regulation (T_4 = thyroxine; T_3 = triiodothyronine).
[c] Somatostatin has also been shown to inhibit other endocrine secretion.
[d] Previously called sulfation factor; it is the active factor that produces growth.

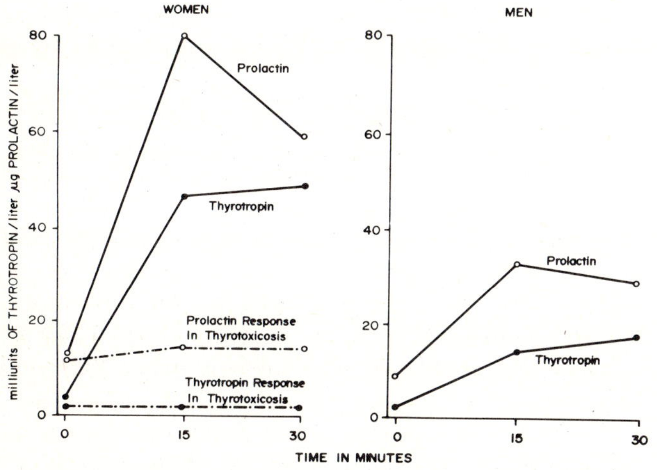

Fig. 2. Prolactin and thyrotropin secretion after an injection of thyroliberin

Note the greater prolactin and thyrotropin release in women and the inhibition of prolactin and thyrotropin release produced by increased thyroid-hormone concentrations. (Reproduced, with modification, from: Reichlin, S., Neuroendocrinology. In *Textbook of Endocrinology,* 5th ed., R. H. Williams, Ed., W. B. Saunders Co., Philadelphia, Pa., 1974, p 789)

administration does not appear to affect serum prolactin concentrations in man (*18*). Thyroliberin can also promote secretion of growth hormone in patients with renal failure (*19*) and acromegaly (*20*), but this is not a normal physiological response in man. Although it is quite clear that thyroliberin promotes pituitary hormone secretion, it has not yet been shown that it directly affects hormone synthesis.

Recent reports detail the presence of thyroliberin in the brain stem, cerebellum, and cerebral cortex of a wide variety of species (*21, 22*). These observations not only suggest an important phylogenetic role for thyroliberin but also raise questions concerning its role in other biochemical events besides hormone release. For example, thyroliberin administration may have an anti-depressant effect in man (*23*)—a finding that has not been supported by other workers using different psychological testing procedures (*24, 25*). Another postulated role for thyroliberin is that of activating pathways in the brain that lead to heat conservation (*26*).

As mentioned earlier, the rapid inactivation of thyroliberin by serum (*6*) has retarded progress in understanding the regulation of its secretion. Mitnick and Reichlin (*8*), however, measured labeled thyroliberin in hypothalamic explants after addition of thyroid hormone. They observed that more thyroliberin was synthesized in the presence of thyroxine, which suggests that the primary site at which thyroxine inhibits thyrotropin secretion is the pituitary. The accordingly increased hypothalamic store of thyroliberin would therefore be ready to promote thyrotropin release when the concentration of thyroxine in serum becomes too low to inhibit pituitary thyrotropin secretion. However, Montoya et al. (*27*) were unable to show any change in hypothalamic thyroliberin content after maneuvers affecting thyrotropin secretion, an observation that casts doubt on the importance of thyroliberin in physiological thyrotropin regulation.

As stated above, a hormone may be able to modulate the number of endocrine receptors in the tissue where it exerts its biological effect. This has been demonstrated for thyroliberin (*28*); increasing concentrations of thyroliberin in tissue culture media decreased the number of its receptors in the pituitary plasma membrane.

Clinical utility. The ability of thyroliberin to promote pituitary thyrotropin and prolactin secretion is the basis of its use in diagnosis of various disorders (*29–32*). An obvious use for thyroliberin was to help differentiate hypothalamic- and pituitary-produced hypothyroidism; failure of a patient to respond to a thyroliberin infusion suggests a pituitary defect, whereas a normal thyrotropin secretory response suggests a hypothalamic abnormality (*29*). Snyder et al. (*32*) have recently demonstrated that a thyroliberin infusion with concomitant measurement of serum thyrotropin and prolactin could be used to detect abnormalities in human hypothalamic/pituitary function that otherwise were not detectable.

Patients with hypo- or hyperthyroidism also have abnormal thyrotropin responses to thyroliberin. Individuals who are hypothyroid have "delayed" but excessive secretion of thyrotropin, whereas thyrotropin release is markedly suppressed in hyperthyroid individuals (*31*).

Administered intravenously, intramuscularly (*33*), or orally (*34*), thyroliberin produces detectable increases in serum thyrotropin concentrations. Other potential clinical uses for thyroliberin have been explored on the basis of the increase in serum prolactin that follows its administration. Tyson et al. (*35*) demonstrated that chronic injections of thyroliberin affect the quantity and quality of the milk in lactating mothers. Because lactation is associated with decreased fertility, thyroliberin has also been investigated for contraceptive properties. Preliminary evaluation in man, however, does not suggest that thyroliberin administration reproducibly inhibits ovulation (*36*).

It is unfortunate that a compound that has been so thoroughly studied around the world and found relatively free of side effects has still not been released for general clinical use in the USA.

Luliberin

Background. Schally et al. (*37*) succeeded in isolating a peptide from 165 000 pig hypothalami that, in nanogram quantities, produced pituitary lutropin and follitropin secretion both in vitro and in vivo. Later, Burgus et al. (*38*) reported that ovine luliberin is a decapeptide and that the synthetic peptide possesses the same biological activity as native luliberin. It also stimulates lutropin and follitropin release from the pituitaries of various species (*39*). Thus luliberin, like thyroliberin, is not species specific.

It is not yet clear whether there is a physiologically separate folliberin or if lutropin and follitropin release is affected by a single hypothalamic hormone. Recent data (*40*) suggest the existence of a distinct folliberin, but this observation is not yet confirmed.

Assay. A bioassay for luliberin in human plasma was reported by Malacara et al. (*41*). They injected human plasma extracts into the jugular vein of anesthetized rats and then determined lutropin by radioimmunoassay of 10-min blood samples obtained from the contralateral jugular vein. More recently, a sensitive and specific radioimmunoassay for luliberin in human plasma has permitted assay of picogram quantities (*42, 43*).

Physiology. Luliberin originates in the hypothalamus, and its synthesis has been demonstrated by hypothalamic tissue in vitro (*44*). Enzymatic inactivation of luliberin has also been demonstrated in the central nervous system (*45*). The curve for disappearance of luliberin from plasma has three components; the half time of disappearance of the three ranges between 2–4 min and 600–1300 min (*46, 47*).

Factors that have been reported, from animal studies, to promote luliberin secretion are dopamine (*48*) and acetylcholine (*49*), whereas serotonin has been considered an inhibitory neurotransmitter for luliberin (*50*). Recent evidence also suggests that there is a hypothalamic luteinizing inhibiting hormone that decreases the lutropin and follitropin secretory response to luliberin (*51*).

Seyler and Reichlin (*52*) investigated luliberin in human plasma by bioassay of successive 10-min blood samples and noted episodic secretion with rapid changes in serum concentrations. They also found that increased serum luliberin concentrations in castrated men were further increased by estrogen administration (*53*). This finding suggested a positive feedback of estrogen in the hypothalamus. The serum lutropin concentrations in these patients, however, were decreased, which suggested a diminished pituitary responsiveness to luliberin (*53*).

By radioimmunoassay, Kelch et al. (*54*) were unable to detect a relationship between serum lutropin and follitropin concentrations and luliberin concentrations. This finding was somewhat influenced by the fact that concentrations in many plasma samples were below the sensitivity of the radioimmunoassay.

In the last few years at least 100 articles have appeared detailing the response of serum follitropin and lutropin after the administration of luliberin intravenously, subcutaneously, intramuscularly, or intranasally (*55, 56*). The response to an intravenous infusion reveals a linear-log dose–response curve (*57*) (see Figure 3), and the serum follitropin and lutropin response to luliberin is influenced by estrogen (*58*), progestins (*58*), sex (*59*), age (*59*), degree of sexual maturation (*54*), phase of the menstrual cycle (*60, 61*), and thyroid status (*62*).

Luliberin has also been found in the pineal body of several species, where its concentration is four- to 10-fold that found in the hypothalamus (*63*). The biological significance of this observation remains to be determined.

The only role now suggested for luliberin besides that of gonadotropin release is the induction of mating behavior in rats (*64*).

Clinical utility. After acute or chronic luliberin

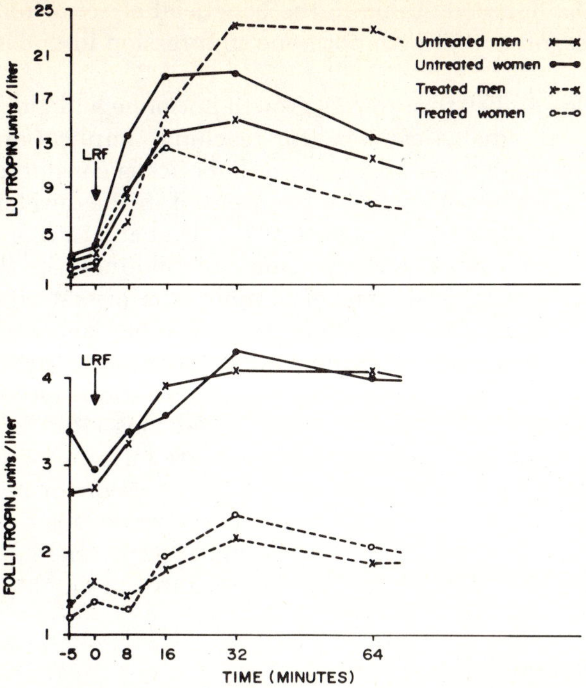

Fig. 3. Mean plasma lutropin and follitropin concentrations after intravenous administration of synthetic luliberin to four groups of subjects

[Reproduced, with modification, from: Kastin, A. J., Schally, A. V., Gual, C., et al., Release of lutropin and follitropin after administration of synthetic luliberin. *J. Clin. Endocrinol. Metab.* **34**, 753 (1972)]

infusion it is possible to differentiate between hypothalamic and pituitary hypogonadotropism (*65–67*). Primary amenorrhea and low basal concentrations of lutropin and follitropin in the serum, which increase after luliberin infusion, support a diagnosis of a hypothalamic defect. Conversely, a lack of response to luliberin suggests a primary pituitary defect.

The secretory responses to luliberin in amenorrheic women are quite variable; however, the magnitude of the lutropin and follitropin response is usually directly related to the fasting hormonal concentrations (*68*).

Twenty-six patients with functional secondary amenorrhea (no demonstrable organic lesion in patients with previous menses) all responded with increased lutropin secretion to a luliberin infusion (*69*). Sixteen of the women also had a normal follitropin response, which suggested hypothalamic rather than pituitary dysfunction in this group with the most common form of secondary amenorrhea.

In patients who have a primary gonadal defect, infusion of luliberin induces augmented release of lutropin and follitropin (*65, 70*), which suggests that in the absence of gonadal hormone feedback, pituitary stores of readily releasable lutropin and follitropin are increased.

In males with hypogonadotropic hypogonadism (decreased testosterone and gonadotropin production), luliberin frequently promotes lutropin and follitropin secretion. Thus a hypothalamic defect may be the most common abnormality in such patients (*71*).

Although luliberin is most often used for diagnostic purposes, there are now several reports of successful pregnancies in infertile women treated with the releasing hormone (*56, 72*). Several groups are also attempting to produce an analog to luliberin that will serve as an antifertility agent by competing with the endogenous pituitary luliberin receptor site and thus prevent the midcycle ovulatory surge of lutropin (*73*).

At this time, however, clinical testing in the USA with luliberin is still confined to investigational use.

Somatostatin

Background. In 1973, Brazeau et al. (*74*) described a tetradecapeptide isolated from ovine hypothalamus, which inhibited growth hormone secretion in vitro and in vivo. This important discovery was stimulated by the observation that certain hypothalamic extracts from previous chromatographic fractions used for the isolation of thyroliberin and luliberin inhibited growth hormone secretion. Since the synthesis of this peptide three years ago, a host of papers have described its physiological effects in man and animals (*75, 76*). This proliferation of data was greatly aided by the rapid dissemination of the synthetic material from the laboratory of Guillemin to various investigators.

Assay. Recently, a radioimmunoassay for somatostatin was reported (*77*), but it contained no data on plasma and tissue concentrations in humans. Hence, most of the information concerning somatostatin has been acquired after its administration in vitro or in vivo.

Physiology. It has now been demonstrated in both man and animals that somatostatin can inhibit growth hormone secretion produced by L-dopa (*78*), arginine (*79*), insulin-induced hypoglycemia (*80*), prostaglandins (*81*), electrical stimulation (*82*), exercise (*83*), sleep (*84*), and morphine (*85*). Somatostatin has now been found in other parts of the central nervous system besides the hypothalamus (*77*) and is also located in gastrointestinal and pancreatic cells (*86*).

Somatostatin not only inhibits growth hormone secretion but secretion of glucagon (*87*), insulin (*88*), gastrin (*89, 90*), thyrotropin (*91*), and possibly prolactin (*92*), and it acts directly on the parietal cell of the stomach to decrease gastric acid secretion (*89*).

The mechanism of the diverse hormonal effects of somatostatin is not clear. However, it decreases anterior pituitary cyclic AMP concentrations (*93*), whereas pituitary cyclic GMP accumulation is increased (*94*); this suggests that part of its action is mediated via alterations in cyclic nucleotide metabolism.

Clinical utility. The observation that a peptide in the central nervous system can inhibit the secretion not only of growth hormone but also of pancreatic in-

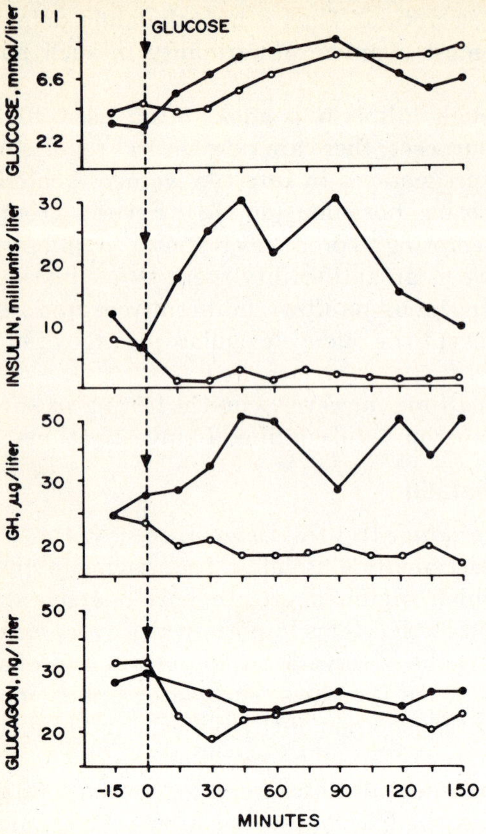

Fig. 4. Changes in plasma glucose, insulin, somatotropin (growth hormone, *GH*), and glucagon in an acromegalic (somatotropin-secreting pituitary tumor) patient during a saline control (●—●) and a 6.7 μg/min somatostatin infusion (O—O), with 50 g glucose given orally

[Reproduced, with modification, from: Mortimer, C. H., Carr, D., Lind, T., et al., Effects of growth-hormone release inhibiting hormone on circulating glucagon, insulin, and growth hormone in normal, diabetic, acromegalic, and hypopituitary patients. *Lancet* **i**, 697 (1974)]

sulin and glucagon is of great clinical interest. A year after the original description of somatostatin, papers appeared (*91, 95, 96*) that detailed the ability of this peptide to decrease growth hormone in acromegalics (Figure 4). The inhibition of growth hormone secretion in these patients, however, ended soon after the infusion was stopped. A method of prolonging the duration of action of the peptide is being sought in order to provide a medical therapy for this difficult-to-manage clinical entity. Recently, somatostatin has been found useful in inhibiting insulin and gastrin hypersecretion in a patient with pancreatic islet cell carcinoma (*97*). Also, its failure to decrease insulin secretion in patients with an insulinoma forms the basis of a diagnostic test for this disorder (*98*).

Glucagon secretion is inhibited by somatostatin, and this is a useful tool for studying glucagon physiology (*99*), as demonstrated by a recent report that glucagon suppression by somatostatin affords protection against the development of ketoacidosis (*100*). It has also been shown in diabetics that glucose tolerance improves during infusion of somatostatin, even though insulin secretion declines (*101*). This effect is probably attributable to the beneficial effect of both glucagon and growth hormone suppression in diabetics.

The ability to suppress growth hormone and glucagon in diabetics has far-reaching implications. Growth hormone secretion in diabetics is considered by many investigators to be essential in the development of diabetic retinopathy (*76*). Diabetic retinopathy is the most common cause of blindness in the USA, and clinical trials of chronic administration of somatostatin are planned. One must be concerned, however, about the chronic administration of such a potent compound. For example, somatostatin reportedly inhibits platelet function in baboons (*102*), and one group has reported that an acute infusion of somatostatin can also affect platelet function in man (*103*), but another study has not confirmed this finding (*104*). Hence, it would appear that there are many exciting chapters of somatostatin research yet to be written.

Prolactin

Background. Until five years ago the lactogenic properties of the pituitary in man were felt by many to reside in the growth hormone fraction of the gland. Many endocrine investigators were not satisfied with this explanation, and in 1970 and 1971 several laboratories presented firm immunological and biochemical evidence demonstrating the existence of prolactin in man (*105–108*). The prolactin radioimmunoassays that were subsequently developed (*105, 109, 110*) permitted detailed investigation of the control of pituitary prolactin secretion in health and disease. Concurrent with these advances were reports from human and animal studies that suggested a function for prolactin in such diverse areas as salt and water regulation (*111*), breast cancer (*112*), and steroidogenesis (*113*). These findings suggested a role for prolactin besides that of promoting lactogenesis.

A new frontier for prolactin investigation has recently been reported by Shiu et al. (*114*), who described its lactogenic receptor in liver plasma membranes. They demonstrated that prolactin—as well as several steroid hormones that effect its secretion—can increase the number of tissue prolactin receptors and thereby modify the tissue response to the hormone.

Assay. Early studies on human prolactin were based on data acquired by bioassay in which prolactin concentration was evaluated by its ability to stimulate the pigeon crop sac (*115*). More recently, several laboratories have reported bioassays by use of mouse breast, based on morphologic changes (*108*), *N*-acetyllactosamine (*106*), or specific milk-protein synthesis (*107*) as end points to evaluate serum prolactin concentrations. Major problems with such bioassays are their variable precision and the time involved in performing the analyses.

Appearing in the literature at about the same time as the bioassays were radioimmunoassays for human prolactin, which confirmed the existence of this hormone and provided a convenient way to study its physiology. The initial homologous radioimmunoassays for prolactin were reported by Hwang et al. (*105*) and Sinha et al. (*110*), and a heterologous radioimmunoassay was described by Jacobs et al. (*109*). This latter radioimmunoassay was based on the similar structure of prolactin obtained from the pituitaries of various species and consisted of a porcine prolactin tracer, a guinea pig anti-ovine antibody, and a human prolactin serum standard. The homologous radioimmunoassay, however, appears to provide a greater sensitivity and precision, and it has been accepted by the Pituitary Program of the National Institutes of Health for general distribution to investigators.

Physiology. There are several excellent recent reviews on the physiology of prolactin in animals (*116*) and man (*117*); therefore I will attempt only to summarize the highlights of data presently available in man. Normal basal prolactin concentrations are slightly higher in women than in men (*117*), and prolactin is secreted periodically throughout the day with a nadir at approximately 10:00 hours and with marked augmentation of secretion occurring between 1 and 2 h after the initiation of sleep (*118, 119*). The most rapid half-times of prolactin disappearance range from 15 to 25 min (*118*). Serum prolactin increases during pregnancy (*120*), and concentrations in the third trimester are about 20-fold what they are in the normal nonpregnant fasting woman. These values decrease after delivery, but quickly increase after suckling (*120*). Breast stimulation in normally menstruating women and in men (*121*) will also produce increases in serum prolactin. Exercise (*122*), various stresses (*123*), and sexual intercourse (*124*) are also associated with an increase in serum prolactin concentrations (Table 3).

Table 3. Causes of Increased Concentrations of Prolactin in Serum

Physiological	Pathological	Pharmacological
Pregnancy	Pituitary tumors	Various drugs (e.g., chlorpromazine)
Stress (e.g., surgery)	Pituitary stalk section	Oral contraceptives
Sleep	Hypothalamic disorders, e.g., sarcoid infiltration	Estrogens
Suckling	Chiari–Frommel syndrome	Thyrotropin-releasing hormone
Exercise	Renal failure	Insulin-induced hypoglycemia
Sexual intercourse	Hypothyroidism	Arginine
	Nelson's syndrome	
	Adrenal insufficiency	
	Ectopic production by tumors	

Numerous other pharmacological and physiological stimuli—including phenothiazines (*125*), insulin induced hypoglycemia (*122*), thyroid-releasing factor (*13–15*), estrogens (*126*), and arginine (*127*)—also promote prolactin secretion. Stimulation of prolactin secretion by phenothiazines, as well as by reserpine and α-methyldopa (*125*), appears to be exerted via competition with the alpha receptors of the adrenergic system leading to a probable decrease in prolactostatin secretion from the hypothalamus.

Prolactin, unlike the other pituitary hormones, appears to be primarily controlled by an inhibiting factor, and an attempt is also being made to isolate a physiological prolactoliberin. We have previously mentioned that thyroliberin infusion can increase serum prolactin; however, its role in promoting physiological prolactin secretion has been challenged by several reports (*16, 18*). Hence the identity of the hypothalamic factor(s) that control prolactin secretion awaits further investigation.

Several pharmacological agents—including L-dopa (*108, 128, 129*), bromergocryptine (*130*), and methanesulfonate (*131*)—reportedly induce a prompt decrease in serum prolactin. Inhibition of prolactin secretion has also been attributed to glucocorticoids (*132*). Suppression of serum prolactin by these agents may occur indirectly via a hypothalamic effect, or by direct pituitary inhibition of secretion, or by both.

Prolactin has not been shown to promote the secretion of another hormone from a distant endocrine gland that then inhibits its secretion by feedback. Therefore it has been suggested that prolactin inhibits its own secretion, and results of animal studies suggest that this inhibition is effected via the hypothalamus (*116*).

The biological role of prolactin in man is just now beginning to be defined. It possesses an amazing number of actions in various vertebrate species: mammotropic, lactogenic, osmoregulatory, diabetogenic, hematologic, and luteotropic (*133*). A role for prolactin in lactogenesis in man is reasonably well established (*134*); there is also evidence that it may have an antidiuretic effect when injected into man (*111*). This latter finding is somewhat difficult to interpret, however, because some animal prolactin preparations are contaminated with vasopressin (posterior pituitary antidiuretic hormone) (*135*).

Prolactin also produces lipolysis in man, with marked increases in serum free fatty acids, glycerol, acetoacetate, and 3-D-β-hydroxybutyrate being observed about 60 min after its intravenous infusion (*136*).

Prolactin may also play a role in regulating ovarian function, as McNatty et al. (*113*) have shown that progesterone production in human ovarian follicles grown in tissue culture can be diminished by prolactin in the media.

Although these reports suggest potentially important roles for prolactin in human physiology, investigative efforts are still in their infancy, and the next few years will probably bring forth other functions for this peptide hormone.

Clinical utility. The development of the prolactin radioimmunoassay (*105, 109, 110*) has made it possible to evaluate prolactin secretion in a wide variety of clinical states. The syndromes of non-pregnancy-induced lactation (nonpuerperal galactorrhea) in women were initially evaluated. It was shown that lactation associated with pituitary tumors (*137–139*), oral contraceptive therapy (*140*), certain drugs (*125*), ectopic tumors (*141*), hypothyroidism (*117*), sarcoidosis (*142*), and adrenal insufficiency (*143*) was associated with abnormally high prolactin concentrations in serum. The latter four disease entities, however, are infrequently associated with increased prolactin in the absence of lactation (*117, 144*) (see Table 3). It has also been reported that abnormal lactation can occur in the presence of normal prolactin secretion (*140*), which challenges our present concepts of the physiology of lactation.

There is now much interest in the role of prolactin secretion in cancer of the breast (*112*). It has been shown in animals that suppressing prolactin secretion inhibits the growth of mammary cancer (*112*); however, another report suggests that prolactin does not promote mammary tumor growth (*145*). Many laboratories are presently working to solve this problem, and it is to be hoped that the role of prolactin in breast cancer will be clarified in the next few years.

Conclusion

Clinical information on these hypothalamic–pituitary hormones is rapidly accumulating. Other hypothalamic hormones are actively being sought, and by the time one reads this review yet another may be characterized and synthesized.

If an analog of luliberin proves effective in fertility control and if somatostatin proves effective in preventing diabetic retinopathy, then the past and future research of the new hypothalamic and pituitary hormones may strongly influence the clinical practice of medicine.

References

1. Harris, G. W., *Neural Control of the Pituitary Gland,* Williams and Wilkins, Baltimore, Md., 1955, p 1.

2. Liddle, G. W., and Hardman J. G., Cyclic adenosine monophosphate as a mediator of hormone action. *New Engl. J. Med.* **285,** 560 (1971).

3. Gavin, J. R., Roth J., Neville, D. M., Jr., et al., Insulin-dependent regulation of insulin receptor concentrations: A direct demonstration in cell culture. *Proc. Nat. Acad. Sci. USA* **71,** 84 (1974).

4. Guillemin, R., The hormones of the hypothalamus. *Am. J. Med.* **57,** 591 (1974).

5. Bassiri, R. M., and Utiger, R. D., The preparation and specificity of antibody to thyrotropin releasing hormone. *Endocrinology* **90,** 722 (1972).

6. Bassiri, R., and Utiger, R. D., Serum inactivation of the immunological and biological activity of thyrotropin-releasing hormone (TRH). *Endocrinology* **91,** 657 (1972).

7. Jeffcoate, S. L., and White, N., Use of benzamidine to prevent the destruction of thyrotropin-releasing hormone (TRH) by blood. *J. Clin. Endocrinol. Metab.* **38,** 155 (1974).

8. Mitnick, M., and Reichlin, S., Enzymatic synthesis of thyrotropin-releasing hormone (TRH) by hypothalamic "TRH synthetase". *Endocrinology* **91,** 1145 (1972).

9. Anderson, M. S., Bowers, C. Y., Kastin, A. J., et al., Synthetic thyrotropin-releasing hormone: A potent stimulator of thyrotropin secretion in man. *New Engl. J. Med.* **285,** 1279 (1971).

10. Snyder, P. J., and Utiger, R. D., Response to thyrotropin releasing hormone (TRH) in normal man. *J. Clin. Endocrinol.* **34,** 380 (1972).

11. Sanchez-Franco, F., Garcia, M. D., Cacicedo, L., et al., Influence of sex phase of the menstrual cycle on thyrotropin (TSH) response to thyrotropin-releasing hormone (TRH). *J. Clin. Endocrinol. Metab.* **37,** 736 (1973).

12. Tashjian, A. H., Jr., Barowsky, N. J., and Jensen, D. K., Thyrotropin releasing hormone: direct evidence of stimulation of prolactin production by pituitary cells in culture. *Biochem. Biophys. Res. Commun.* **43,** 516 (1971).

13. Bowers, C. Y., Friesen. H. G., Hwang, P., et al., Prolactin and thyrotropin release in man by synthetic pyroglutamyl-histidylprolinamide. *Biochem. Biophys. Res. Commun.* **45,** 1033 (1971).

14. Jacobs, L. S., Snyder, P. J., Wilber, J. F., et al., Increased serum prolactin after administration of synthetic thyrotropin releasing hormone (TRH) in man. *J. Clin. Endocrinol.* **33,** 996 (1971).

15. Lister, R. C., Underwood, L. E., Marshall, R. N., et al., Evidence for a direct effect of thyrotropin-releasing hormone (TRH) on prolactin release in humans. *J. Clin. Endocrinol. Metab.* **39,** 1148 (1974).

16. Gautvik, K. M., Tashjian, A. H., Kourides, I. A., et al., Thyrotropin-releasing hormone is not the sole physiologic mediator of prolactin release during suckling. *New Engl. J. Med.* **290,** 1162 (1974).

17. Valverde-R, C., Chieffo, V., and Reichlin, S., Prolactin-releasing factor in porcine and rat hypothalamic tissue. *Endocrinology* **91,** 982 (1972).

18. Malarkey, W. B., and Beck, P., Twenty-four-hour prolactin profiles in normal and disease states: Failure of thyroxine to modify prolactin secretion. *J. Clin. Endocrinol. Metab.* **40,** 708 (1975).

19. Gonzalez-Barcena, D., Kastin, A. J., Schalch, D. S., et al., Responses to thyrotropin-releasing hormone in patients with renal failure and after infusion in normal men. *J. Clin. Endocrinol. Metab.* **36,** 117 (1973).

20. Samaan, N. A., Leavens, M. E., and Jesse, R. H., Jr., Serum growth hormone and prolactin response to thyrotropin-releasing hormone in patients with acromegaly before and after surgery. *J. Clin. Endocrinol. Metab.* **38,** 957 (1974).

21. Jackson, I. M. D., and Reichlin, S., Thyrotropin-releasing hormone (TRH): Distribution in hypothalamic and extrahypothalamic brain tissues of mammalian and submammalian chordates. *Endocrinology* **95,** 854 (1974).

22. Brownstein, M. J., Palkovits, M., Saavedra, J. M., et al., Thyrotropin-releasing hormone in specific nuclei of rat brain. *Science* **185,** 267 (1974).

23. Prange, A. J., Jr., Wilson, I. C., Lara, P. P., et al., Effects of thyrotropin-releasing hormone in depression. *Lancet* **ii,** 999 (1972).

24. Mountjoy, C. Q., Price, J. S., Weller, M., et al., A double-blind crossover sequential trial of oral thyrotrophin-releasing hormone in depression. *Lancet* **i,** 958 (1974).

25. Coppen, A., Montgomery, S., Peet, M., et al., Thyrotrophin-releasing hormone in the treatment of depression. *Lancet* **ii,** 433 (1974).

26. Wei, E., Sigel, S., Loh, H., and Way, E. L., Thyrotrophin-releasing hormone and shaking behaviour in rat. *Nature* **253,** 739 (1975).

27. Montoya, E., Seibel, M. J., and Wilber, J. F., Thyrotropin-releasing hormone secretory physiology: Studies by radioimmunoassay and affinity chromatography. *Endocrinology* **96,** 1413 (1975).

28. Hinkle, P. M., and Tashjian, A. H., Decrease in the number of receptors for thyrotropin releasing hormone (TRH) in GH_3 pituitary cells after prolonged incubation with TRH (abstr. Endocrine Society, June 1975), p 3.

29. Costom, B. H., Grumbach, M. M., and Kaplan, S. L., Effect of thyrotropin-releasing factor on serum thyroid-stimulating hormone. *J. Clin. Invest.* **50**, 2219 (1971).

30. Fleischer, N., Lorente, M., Kirkland, J., et al., Synthetic thyrotropin releasing factor as a test of pituitary thyrotropin reserve. *J. Clin. Endocrinol.* **34**, 617 (1972).

31. Hershman, J. M., Clinical application of thyrotropin-releasing hormone. *New Engl. J. Med.* **290**, 886 (1974).

32. Snyder, P. J., Jacobs, L. S., Rabello, M. M., et al., Diagnostic value of thyrotrophin-releasing hormone in pituitary and hypothalamic diseases. *Ann. Intern Med.* **81**, 751 (1974).

33. Azizi, F., Vagenakis, A. G., Portnay, G. I., et al., Pituitary-thyroid responsiveness to intramuscular thyrotropin-releasing hormone based on analyses of serum thyroxine, tri-iodothyronine and thyrotropin concentrations. *New Engl. J. Med.* **292**, 273 (1975).

34. Haigler, E. D., Jr., Hershman, J. M., and Pittman, J. A., Jr., Response to orally administered synthetic thyrotropin-releasing hormone in rat. *J. Clin. Endocrinol. Metab.* **35**, 631 (1972).

35. Tyson, J. E., Friesen, H. C., and Anderson, M. S., Human lactational and ovarian response to endogenous prolactin release. *Science* **177**, 897 (1972).

36. Jewelewicz, R., Dyrenfurth, I., Warren, M., et al., Effect of thyrotropin-releasing hormone (TRH) upon the menstrual cycle in women. *J. Clin. Endocrinol. Metab.* **39**, 387 (1974).

37. Schally, A. V., Arimura, A., Baba, Y., et al., Isolation and properties of the FSH and LH-releasing hormone. *Biochem. Biophys. Res. Commun.* **43**, 393 (1971).

38. Burgus, R., Butcher, M., Amoss, M., et al., Primary structure of the ovine hypothalamic luteinizing hormone-releasing factor (LRF). *Proc. Nat. Acad. Sci. USA* **69**, 278 (1972).

39. Schally, A. V., Arimura, A., Kastin, A. J., et al., Gonadotropin-releasing hormone: One polypeptide regulates secretion of luteinizing and follicle-stimulating hormones. *Science* **173**, 1036 (1971).

40. Bowers, C. Y., Currie, B. L., Johansson, K. N. G., and Folkers, K., Biological evidence that separate hypothalamic hormones release the follicle stimulating and luteinizing hormones. *Biochem. Biophys. Res. Commun.* **50**, 20 (1973).

41. Malacara, J. M., Seyler, L. E., Jr., and Reichlin, S., Luteinizing hormone releasing factor activity in peripheral blood from women during the midcycle luteinizing hormone ovulatory surge. *J. Clin. Endocrinol.* **34**, 271 (1972).

42. Nett, T. M., Akbar, A. M., Niswender, G. D., et al., A radioimmunoassay for gonadotropin-releasing hormone (Gn-RH) in serum. *J. Clin. Endocrinol. Metab.* **36**, 880 (1973).

43. Arimura, A., Kastin, A. J., Schally, A. V., et al., Immunoreactive LH-releasing hormone in plasma: Midcycle elevation in women. *J. Clin. Endocrinol. Metab.* **38**, 510 (1974).

44. Johansson, N. G., Hooper, F., Sievertsson, H., et al., Biosynthesis *in vitro* of the luteinizing releasing hormone by hypothalamic tissue. *Biochem. Biophys. Res. Commun.* **49**, 656 (1972).

45. Marks, N., and Stern, F., Enzymatic mechanisms for the inactivation of luteinizing hormone-releasing hormone (LH-RH). *Biochem. Biophys. Res. Commun.* **61**, 1458 (1974).

46. Yukitaka, M., Mecklenburg, R. S., Hansen, J. W., and Lipsett, M. B., Metabolism of ^{125}I-luteinizing hormone-releasing hormone. *J. Clin. Endocrinol. Metab.* **37**, 63 (1973).

47. Virkkunen, P., Lybeck, H., Partanen, J., et al., Plasma disappearance of injected synthetic LRH in man as measured by bioassay and radioimmunoassay. *J. Clin. Endocrinol. Metab.* **39**, 630 (1974).

48. McCann, S. M., Neurohormonal correlates of ovulation. *Fed. Proc.* **29**, 1888 (1970).

49. Simonovic, I., Motta, M., and Martini, L., Acetylcholine and the release of the follicle-stimulating hormone-releasing factor. *Endocrinology* **95**, 1373 (1974).

50. Frohman, L. A., Clinical neuropharmacology of hypothalamic releasing factors. *New Engl. J. Med.* **286**, 1391 (1972).

51. Johansson, N. G., Greibrokk, T., Currie, B. L., et al., Factor C-LHIH which inhibits the luteinizing hormone from basal release and from synthetic LHRH and studies on purification of FSHRH. *Biochem. Biophys. Res. Commun.* **63**, 62 (1975).

52. Seyler, L. E., Jr., and Reichlin, S., Episodic secretion of luteinizing hormone-releasing factor (LRF) in the human. *J. Clin. Endocrinol. Metab.* **39**, 471 (1974).

53. Seyler, L. E., Jr., and Reichlin, S., Feedback regulation of circulating LRF concentrations in men. *J. Clin. Endocrinol. Metab.* **39**, 906 (1974).

54. Kelch, R. P., Clemens, L. E., Markovs, M., et al., Metabolism and effects of synthetic gonadotropin-releasing hormone (GnRH) in children and adults. *J. Clin. Endocrinol. Metab.* **40**, 53 (1975).

55. Gonzalez-Barcena, D., Kastin, A. J., Schalch, D. S., et al., Synthetic LH-releasing hormone (LH-RH) administered to normal men by different routes. *J. Clin. Endocrinol. Metab.* **37**, 481 (1973).

56. Taymore, M. L., The use of luteinizing hormone-releasing hormone in gynecologic endocrinology. *Fert. Steril.* **25**, 992 (1974).

57. Kastin, A. J., Schally, A. V., Gual, C., et al. Dose-response relationship of luteinizing hormone to luteinizing hormone-releasing hormone in man. *J. Clin. Invest.* **50**, 1551 (1971).

58. Vandenberg, G., DeVane, G., and Yen, S. S. C., Effects of exogenous estrogen and progestin on pituitary responsiveness to synthetic luteinizing hormone-releasing factor. *J. Clin. Invest.* **53**, 1750 (1974).

59. Hashimoto, T., Miyai, K., Izumi, K., and Kumahara, Y., Gonadotropin response to synthetic LH-RH in normal subjects: Correlation between LH and FSH. *J. Clin. Endocrinol. Metab.* **37**, 910 (1973).

60. Nillius, S. J., and Wide, L., Variation in LH and FSH response to LH-releasing hormone during the menstrual cycle. *J. Obstet. Gynaecol. Br. Commonw.* **79**, 865 (1972).

61. Wang, C. F., and Yen, S. S. C., Direct evidence of estrogen modulation of pituitary sensitivity to luteinizing hormone-releasing factor during the menstrual cycle. *J. Clin. Invest.* **55**, 201 (1975).

62. Distiller, L. A., Sagel, J., and Morley, J. E., Assessment of pituitary gonadotropin reserve using luteinizing hormone-releasing hormone (LRH) in states of altered thyroid function. *J. Clin. Endocrinol. Metab.* **40**, 512 (1975).

63. White, W. F., Hedlund, M. T., Weber, G. F., et al., The pineal gland: A supplemental source of hypothalamic-releasing hormones. *Endocrinology* **94**, 1422 (1974).

64. Moss, R. L., and McCann, S. M., Induction of mating behavior in rats by luteinizing hormone-releasing factor. *Science* **181**, 177 (1973).

65. Roth, J. C., Kelch, R. P., Kaplan, S. L., and Grumbach, M. M., FSH and LH response to luteinizing hormone-releasing factor in prepubertal and pubertal children, adult males and patients with hypogonadotropic and hypergonadotropic hypogonadism. *J. Clin. Endocrinol. Metab.* **35**, 926 (1972).

66. Yen, S. S. C., Rebar, R., Vandenberg, G., and Judd, H., Hypothalamic amenorrhea and hypogonadotropinism: Responses to synthetic LRF. *J. Clin. Endocrinol. Metab.* **36**, 811 (1973).

67. Bell, J., Spitz, I., Slonim, A., et al., Heterogeneity of gonadotropin response to LHRH in hypogonadotropic hypogonadism. *J. Clin. Endocrinol. Metab.* **36**, 791 (1973).

68. Keller, E., Dahlen, H. G., Friedrich, E., et al., Human pituitary gonadotropin index. I. standardized LRH test criteria for evaluation of functional amenorrhea. *J. Clin. Endocrinol. Metab.* **40**, 959 (1975).

69. Nillius, S. J., and Wide, L., The LH-releasing hormone test in 31 women with secondary amenorrhea. *J. Obstet. Gynecol.* **79**, 874 (1972).

70. Siler, T. M., and Yen, S. S. C., Augmented gonadotropin response to synthetic LRF in hypogonadal state. *J. Clin. Endocrinol. Metab.* **37**, 491 (1973).

71. Jorgensen, F. S., Kampmann, J., Micic, S., et al., LH and FSH in serum after intramuscular administration of LH/FSH-releasing hormone in normal and hypogonadal men. *Acta Endocrinol.* (Copenhagen) **78**, 1 (1975).

72. Nakano, R., Katayama, K., Mizuno, T., and Tojo, S., Induction of ovulation with synthetic luteinizing hormone-releasing hormone. *Fert. Steril.* **25**, 471 (1974).

73. Guillemin, R., Physiology and chemistry of the hypothalamic releasing factors for gonadotropins: A new approach to fertility control. In proceedings of the *VIIth World Congress on Fertility and Sterility,* Tokyo, October 17–25, 1971.

74. Brazeau, P., Vale, W., Burgus, R., et al., Hypothalamic polypeptide that inhibits the secretion of immunoreactive pituitary growth hormone. *Science* **179**, 77 (1973).

75. Brazeau, P., and Guillemin, R., Somatostatin: Newcomer from the hypothalamus. *New Engl. J. Med.* **290,** 963 (1974).

76. Cahill, G. F., Jr., and Soeldner, J. S., Diabetes, glucagon and growth hormone. *New Engl. J. Med.* **291,** 577 (1974).

77. Brownstein, M., Arimura, A., Sata, H., et al., The regional distribution of somatostatin in the rat brain. *Endocrinology* **96,** 1456 (1975).

78. Lovinger, R., Boryczka, A. T., Shackelford, R., et al. Effect of synthetic somatotropin release inhibiting factor on the increase in plasma growth hormone elicited by L-dopa in the dog. *Endocrinology* **95,** 943 (1974).

79. Siler, T. M., Vandenberg, G., Yen, S. S. C., et al., Inhibition of growth hormone release in humans by somatostatin, *J. Clin. Endocrinol. Metab.* **37,** 632 (1973).

80. Hall, R., Besser, G. M., Schally, A. V., et al., Action of growth-hormone-release inhibitory hormone in healthy men and in acromegaly. *Lancet* **ii,** 7829 (1973).

81. Hertelendy, F., Todd, H., and Yeh, M., Inhibition by somatostatin of prostaglandin stimulated growth hormone release and cyclic AMP accumulation in rat pituitary glands. *IRCS Libr. Compend.* **2,** 1216 (1974).

82. Martin, J. B., Inhibitory effect of somatostatin (SRIF) on the release of growth hormone (GH) induced in the rat by electrical stimulation. *Endocrinology* **94,** 497 (1974).

83. Hansen, A. P., Orskov, H., Seyer-Hansen, K., and Lundbaek, K., Some actions of growth hormone release inhibiting factor. *Br. Med. J.* **ii,** 523 (1973).

84. Parker, D.C., Rossman, L. G., Siler, T. M., et al., Inhibition of the sleep-related peak in physiologic human growth hormone release by somatostatin. *J. Clin. Endocrinol. Metab.* **38,** 496 (1974).

85. Martin, J. B., Audet, J., and Saunders, A., Effects of somatostatin and hypothalamic ventromedial lesions on GH release induced by morphone. *Endocrinology* **96,** 839 (1975).

86. Polak, J. M., Pearse, A. G. E., Grimelius, L., and Bloom, S. R., Growth-hormone release-inhibiting hormone in gastrointestinal and pancreatic D cells. *Lancet* **i,** 1220 (1975).

87. Gerich, J. E., Lorenzi, M., Schneider, V., et al., Effects of somatostatin on plasma glucose and glucagon levels in human diabetes mellitus. *New Engl. J. Med.* **291,** 544 (1974).

88. Chideckel, E. W., Palmer, J., Koerker, D. J., et al., Somatostatin blockade of acute and chronic stimuli of the endocrine pancreas and the consequences of this blockade on glucose homeostasis. *J. Clin. Invest.* **55,** 754 (1975).

89. Mortimer, C. H., Thorner, M. O., Besser, G. M., et al., Inhibition of gastrin and gastric-inhibiting hormone. *Lancet* **i,** 1106 (1974).

90. Hayes, J. R., Johnson, D. G., Koerker, D., and Williams, R. H., Inhibition of gastrin release by somatostatin *in vitro*. *Endocrinology* **96,** 1374 (1975).

91. Siler, T. M., Yen, S. S. C., Vale, W., and Guillemin, R., Inhibition by somatostatin on the release of TSH induced in man by thyrotropin-releasing factor. *J. Clin. Endocrinol. Metab.* **38,** 742 (1974).

92. Yen, S. S. C., Siler, T. M., and DeVane, G. W., Effect of somatostatin in patients with acromegaly. *New Engl. J. Med.* **290,** 935 (1974).

93. Borgeat, P., Labrie, F., Drouin, J., et al., Inhibition of adenosine 3′, 5′-monophosphate accumulation in anterior pituitary gland in vitro by growth hormone-release inhibiting hormone. *Biochem. Biophys. Res. Commun.* **56,** 1052 (1974).

94. Kaneko, T., Oka, H., Munemura, M., et al., Stimulation of guanosine 3′,5′-cyclic monophosphate accumulation in rat anterior pituitary gland in vitro by synthetic somatostatin. *Biochem. Biophys. Res. Commun.* **61,** 53 (1974).

95. Besser, G. M., Mortimer, C. H., Carr, D., et al., Growth hormone release inhibiting hormone in acromegaly. *Br. Med. J.* **i,** 352 (1974).

96. Hall, R., Besser, G. M., Schally, A. V., et al., Action of growth-hormone-release inhibitory hormone in healthy men and in acromegaly. *Lancet* **ii,** 7829 (1973).

97. Curnow, R. T., Carey, R. M., Taylor, A., et al., Somatostatin inhibition of insulin and gastrin hypersecretion in pancreatic islet-cell carcinoma. *New Engl. J. Med.* **292,** 1385 (1975).

98. Lorenzi, M., Gerich, J. E., Karam, J. H., and Forsham. P. H., Failure of somatostatin to inhibit tolbutamide-induced insulin secretion in patients with insulinomas: A possible diagnostic tool. *J. Clin. Endocrinol. Metab.* **40,** 1121 (1975).

99. Goodner, C. J., Somatostatin leads to glucagon's renaissance. *New Engl. J. Med.* **292,** 1022 (1975).

100. Gerich, J. E., Lorenzi, M., Bier, D. M., et al., Prevention of human diabetic ketoacidosis by somatostatin. *New Engl. J. Med.* **292,** 985 (1975).

101. Gerich, J. E., Lorenzi, M., Schneider, V., et al., Effects of somatostatin on plasma glucose and glucagon levels in human diabetes mellitus. *New Engl. J. Med.* **291,** 544 (1974).

102. Koerker, D. J., Harker, L. A., and Goodner, C. J., Effects of somatostatin on hemostasis in baboons. *New Engl. J. Med.* **293,** 476 (1975).

103. Besser, G. M., Paxton, A. M., Johnson, S. A. N., et al., Impairment of platelet function by growth-hormone release-inhibiting hormone. *Lancet* **i,** 1166 (1975).

104. Mielke, C. H., Jr., Gerich, J. E., Lorenzi, M., et al., The effect of somatostatin on coagulation and platelet function in man. *New Engl. J. Med.* **293,** 480 (1975).

105. Hwang, P., Guyda, H., and Friesen, H., A radioimmunoassay for human prolactin. *Proc. Nat. Acad. Sci. USA* **68,** 1902 (1971).

106. Loewenstein, J. E., Mariz, I. K., Peake, G. T., and Daughaday, W. H., Prolactin bioassay by induction of N-acetyllactosamine synthetase in mouse mammary gland explants. *J. Clin. Endocrinol. Metab.* **33,** 217 (1971).

107. Turkington, R. W., Measurement of prolactin activity in human serum by the induction of specific milk proteins in mammary gland in vitro. *J. Clin. Endocrinol. Metab.* **33,** 210 (1971).

108. Kleinberg, D. L., and Frantz, A. G., Human prolactin: measurement in plasma by in vitro bioassay. *J. Clin. Invest.* **50,** 1557 (1971).

109. Jacobs, L. S., Mariz, I. K., and Daughaday, W. H., A mixed heterologous radioimmunoassay for human prolactin. *J. Clin. Endocrinol.* **34,** 484 (1972).

110. Sinha, Y. N., Selby, F. W., Lewis, U. J., and Vanderlaan, W. P., A homologous radioimmunoassay for human prolactin. *J. Clin. Endocrinol. Metab.* **36,** 509 (1973).

111. Horrobin, D. F., Burstyn, P. G., Lloyd, I. J., et al., Actions of prolactin on human renal function. *Lancet* **ii,** 352 (1971).

112. Smithline, F., Sherman, L., and Kolodny, H., Prolactin and breast carcinoma. *New Engl. J. Med.* **292,** 784 (1975).

113. McNatty, K. P., Sawers, R. S., and McNeilly, A. S., A possible role for prolactin in control of steroid secretion by the human Graafian follicle. *Nature* **250,** 653 (1974).

114. Shiu, R. P. C., Kelly, P. A., and Friesen, H. G., Radioreceptor assay for prolactin and other lactogenic hormones. *Science* **180,** 968 (1973).

115. Apostolakis, M., Prolactin. *Vitam. Horm.* **26,** 197 (1968).

116. Meites, J., Lu, K. H., Wuttke, W., et al., Recent studies on functions and control of prolactin secretion in rats. *Recent Prog. Horm. Res.* **28,** 471 (1972).

117. Frantz, A. G., The regulation of prolactin secretion in humans. In *Frontiers in Neuroendocrinology, 1973.* W. F. Ganong and L. Martini, Eds. Oxford University Press, Oxford, England, 1973, p 337.

118. Sassin, J. F., Frantz, A. G., Weitzman, E. D., and Kapen, S., Human prolactin: 24-hour pattern with increased release during sleep. *Science* **177,** 1205 (1972).

119. Parker, D. C., Rossman, L. G., Vanderlaan, E. F., Sleep-related, nyctohemeral and briefly episodic variation in human plasma prolactin concentrations. *J. Clin. Endocrinol. Metab.* **36,** 1119 (1973).

120. Tyson, J. E., Hwang, P., Guyda, H., and Frieson, H. G., Studies of prolactin secretion in human pregnancy. *Am. J. Obstet. Gynecol.* **113,** 14 (1972).

121. Kolodny, R. C., Jacobs, L. S., and Daughaday, W. H., Mammary stimulation causes prolactin secretion in non-lactating women. *Nature* **238,** 284 (1972).

122. Frantz, A. G., Kleinberg, D. L., and Noel, G. L., Studies on prolactin in man. *Recent Prog. Horm. Res.* **28,** 527 (1972).

123. Noel, G. L., Suh, H. K., Stone, J. G., and Frantz, A. G., Human prolactin and growth hormone release during surgery and other conditions of stress. *J. Clin. Endocrinol. Metab.* **35,** 840 (1972).

124. Stearns, E. L., Winter, J. S. D., and Faiman, C., Effects of coitus on gonadotropin, prolactin and sex steroid levels in man. *J. Clin. Endocrinol. Metab.* **37,** 687 (1973).

125. Turkington, R. W., Prolactin secretion in patients treated with various drugs. *Arch. Intern. Med.* **130,** 349 (1972).

126. Yen, S. S. C., Ehara, Y., and Siler, T. M., Augmentation of prolactin secretion by estrogen in hypogonadal women. *J. Clin. Invest.* **53,** 652 (1974).

127. Rakoff, J. S., Siler, T. M., Sinha, Y. N., and Yen, S. S. C., Prolactin and growth hormone release in response to sequential stimulation by arginine and synthetic TRF. *J. Clin. Endocrinol. Metab.* **37,** 641 (1973).

128. Malarkey, W. B., Jacobs, L. S., and Daughaday, W. H., Levodopa suppression of prolactin in nonpuerperal galactorrhea. *New Engl. J. Med.* **285,** 1160 (1971).

129. Friesen, H., Guyda, H., Hwang, P., et al., Functional evaluation of prolactin secretion: A guide to therapy. *J. Clin. Invest.* **51,** 706 (1972).

130. Del Pozo, E., Varga, L., Wyss, H., et al., Clinical and hormonal response to bromocriptin (CB-154) in the galactorrhea syndromes. *J. Clin. Endocrinol. Metab.* **39,** 18 (1974).

131. Cleary, R. E., Crabtree, R., and Lemberger, L., The effect of Lergotrile on galactorrhea and gonadotropin secretion. *J. Clin. Endocrinol. Metab.* **40,** 830 (1975).

132. Copinschi, G., L'Hermite, M., Leclercq, R., et al., Effects of glucocorticoids on pituitary hormonal responses to hypoglycemia: Inhibition of prolactin release. *J. Clin. Endocrinol. Metab.* **40,** 442 (1975).

133. Bern, H. A., and Nicoll, C. S., The comparative endocrinology of prolactin. *Recent Prog. Horm. Res.* **24,** 681 (1968).

134. Tyson, J. E., Khojandi, M., Huth, J., and Andreassen, B., The influence of prolactin secretion on human lactation. *J. Clin. Endocrinol. Metab.* **40,** 764 (1975).

135. Malarkey, W. B., George, J. M., and Baehler, R. W., Evidence for vasopressin contamination of ovine and bovine prolactin. *IRCS Med. Sci.: Endocrine System; Kidneys and Urinary System; Physiology* **3,** 291 (1975).

136. Berle, P., Finsterwalder, E., and Apostolakis, M., Comparative studies on the effect of human growth hormone, human prolactin and human placental lactogen on lipid metabolism. *Horm. Metab. Res.* **6,** 347 (1974).

137. Tolis, G., Goldstein, M., and Friesen, H. G., Functional evaluation of prolactin secretion in patients with hypothalamic-pituitary disorders. *J. Clin. Invest.* **52,** 783 (1973).

138. Boyar, R. M., Kapen, S., Finkelstein, J. W., et al., Hypothalamic-pituitary function in diverse hyperprolactinemic states. *J. Clin. Invest.* **53,** 1588 (1974).

139. Malarkey, W. B., and Johnson, J. C., Pituitary tumors and hyperprolactinemia. *Arch. Intern. Med.,* in press.

140. Malarkey, W. B., Nonpuerperal lactation and normal prolactin regulation. *J. Clin. Endocrinol. Metab.* **40,** 198 (1975).

141. Turkington, R. W., Ectopic production of prolactin. *New Engl. J. Med.* **285,** 1455 (1971).

142. Turkington, R. W., and Macindoe, J. H., Hyperprolactinemia in sarcoidosis. *Ann. Intern. Med.* **76,** 545 (1972).

143. Refetoff, S., Block, M. B., Ehrlich, E. N., and Friesen, H. G., Chiari-Frommel syndrome in a patient with pituitary adrenocortical insufficiency. *New Engl. J. Med.* **287,** 1326 (1972).

144. Malarkey, W. B., and Kataria, Y. P., Sarcoidosis and hyperprolactinemia. *Ann. Intern. Med.* **81,** 116 (1974).

145. Hill, R., *Prolactin and Carcinogenesis, Proceedings of the Fourth Tenovus Workshop,* Alpha Omega Publishing Co., Cardiff, Wales, U. K., 1972, p 181.

guest editorial

Potentialities of an Inexpensive Computer System for Analysis of Clinical Amino Acid Data: Forecast and Speculation

Donald M. Schoengold, Roberta H. deFiore, David J. Miner,[1] and Paul B. Hamilton

In routine clinical analysis, data are collected that often have applications beyond the immediate use of describing the specific health of the patient(s) involved. Although many applications in the fields of medical and biochemical research are obvious, it is not always realized that mathematical analysis of the data can also be used in computerized feedback studies to extend and enhance the reliability of the clinical analyses as applied to individuals or to groups of individuals. Finally, because the data are frequently from individuals of diverse ethnic, economic, and social backgrounds, the relationships between these factors and the unique biochemistry of an individual can be studied. This last application might have social implications if it could be shown that nutritional requirements were related to an individual's ethnic or racial background.

Unfortunately, clinical chemical data do not seem to be utilized further in this way, probably because of the time consumed in extracting it from the records and subjecting it to the appropriate statistical analyses. It is possible to store, have access to, and to process the data by using commercially available systems for data-base management, but such systems are expensive ($150 000). However, with minicomputers and inexpensive bulk-storage media, a cost-effective computerized filing and analysis system can be set up to make such data accessible and usable.

In this laboratory, we have implemented such a system for handling quantitative data on 27 amino acids and related compounds obtained from the column-chromatographic analysis of plasma amino acids (*1*). The computer equipment needed currently costs between $12 000 and $15 000. The system gives random access to complete patient files from a large data base or to data within files, which can then be followed by extensive analysis of the data. The program handles all transfers of data from the file recovery portion of the program to the analysis portions, so there is no need to keep track of intermediate results. Analytical tests include programs for normalization and ratio calculations, for boundary test studies and for F- and t-test comparisons, for a χ^2-test for normal distribution, and for correlation and regression analyses.

We first wish to consider the potential application of such a data management system in the fields of clinical chemistry, biochemistry, and nutrition. Hardware and software needed to support the system will be discussed later.

Clinical data is typically reported as a result followed by a normal range. If the result lies outside the normal range, the test is reported as positive (regardless of sign). This implicit assumption that the test result can be defined solely on the basis of a fixed boundary limit is reliable only if the result does not lie near the limits. If the result lies close to (either within or without) the upper or lower boundary limits, the result is more ambiguous. The problem involved therefore resides in a definition of normality. This problem has been discussed in a recent review (*2*) in which it was concluded that a large amount of data was necessary to understand all the variables involved. For example, in one study that was considered, results of 12 tests on 3000 individuals were examined. The statistical analysis of such a vast amount of data requires a lot of time and manpower. We feel that our computerized system overcomes this

The Thomas R. Brown Memorial Laboratories, the Alfred I. du Pont Institute, Wilmington, Del. 19899.

[1] Current address: Department of Chemistry, Purdue University, West Lafayette, Ind. 47906.

data processing bottleneck and can increase the reliability of clinical results. Also, the boundary test programs that we use would enable the clinician to make retrospective tests of old data to see if proposed new boundary limits might reduce the number of false positives or negatives in a test.

The ability of a computerized system to do correlation studies on a large volume of clinical laboratory data presents a way of minimizing the number of false results. Combinations of tests, if chosen carefully, can provide more meaningful results than those of a single test. However, it is important to note that if the tests are chosen at random, the probability of false positives or negatives will increase, not decrease. A correlation program would enable the clinician to determine which tests can be combined.

The initial incentive for setting up this system came from the accumulation of a very large file of data from ion-exchange chromatographic analyses for free amino acids in plasma. Gross changes in amino acid values were obvious, but we speculated that there was additional useful information that was not being revealed because of inadequacies of time and manpower. With the computerized system, these limitations were no longer a concern. Some specific applications can be considered.

For example, in children with phenylketonuria (PKU) it is of interest to compare their plasma amino acid composition before a corrective dietary regimen is begun with that of normal children. Thereafter, further comparisons with the pre-dietary results would reveal the progress toward a new metabolic equilibrium. We found (*1*) that several amino acids besides phenylalanine changed significantly after the corrective diet was started. None of them had any obvious relationship to blockage of the phenylalanine to tyrosine conversion. These results suggest hitherto unsuspected metabolic interrelationships that might give new insights into the total derangement, which at present suffers from a rather simplistic and perhaps superficial understanding. Explicitly, why do some children suffer from hyperphenylalaninemia, but do not develop those other characteristics associated with classical PKU?

More sophisticated analyses involving correlation or regression studies can be done as easily as the simple example just outlined. Using our PKU studies again, it might be interesting to attempt to correlate the age at which a child is put on a restricted diet with the extent of mental retardation suffered. Making such a correlation by manual computation would be a monumental undertaking. With our system, all the files that fit the variables of the study can be recovered from the main files and the equation can be determined in a few minutes. A graphic plot that makes the relationship more immediately apparent is readily available.

We recognize that a computerized system such as ours does not provide the investigator with results that could not have been obtained by manual methods. However, it does facilitate the manipulation of large numbers of files, extraction of pertinent data, and the statistical analysis. This advantage, which appears to be just an increase in speed, is not trivial. Because the investigator can now rapidly interact with a large data base without worrying about the mechanics of how the results are obtained, he is likely to try to check interesting ideas that might have been too difficult to attempt.

This easy interaction also means that unplanned experiments may be undertaken from which unanticipated profits may be derived. For example, we have data tapes in our files on the plasma amino acids of newborn children before their first feeding (*3*) and also data tapes on normal fasting adults. One of our programs enables us to correlate each of the amino acids in a group of samples with each and every other amino acid in the same group. The correlation patterns obtained for the newborn infants' group were completely different from the correlation patterns of the adult group. The number of significant correlations for the adults was much greater than for the infants and the amino acids involved in the correlations were different. The significance of this observation escapes us at the moment, but it suggests an area for future work that would not have been discovered manually because there would have been no reason to develop the correlation. We believe that this type of unplanned analysis of data can provide great long-term advantages because it obviously suggests new areas of research.

In addition to the examples just discussed, one can project applications in fields that have important social implications. For example, relationships between nutritional requirements of children and their ethnic, economic, or social background might be studied.

Our major interest in this editorial has been to describe types of investigations suggested by the capabilities of our programs. However, the capabilities of any computer system are in part defined by the hardware and software used, and so some discussion should be devoted to this subject. The entire files of a clinical laboratory could be computerized with a large data-base management system, but the cost of these systems is high ($150 000), by reason of the complex software required and the extensive core and disc memory needed to support the system's versatile, open-ended file structure.

We recommend that a data-management system that employs a fixed-file structure be used instead. Also, instead of attempting to computerize all the tests run by the laboratory with a single program, we feel that only a limited number (in our case, one) should be handled at one time. These simplifications make the fixed-file structure practicable. They also make it easier to write the file-management programs and the analysis programs, thus saving software development costs.

The fixed-file structure of the data-management system does present the problem that after the files are created it is impractical to make any program modifications that involve changing the basic file structure, because this will require that the entire data base be changed. We have avoided this inflexibility by including a keyword coding section as part of each file. Because a keyword list is open-ended and new keywords can be added at any time, this allows for future expansion of the filing system within the fixed-file constraints. Also, the computer algorithm to create and search a keyword file is easy to implement.

By careful programming, it is possible to implement a system such as ours on hardware consisting of an 8k minicomputer, cassette or floppy disc bulk storage, and a teletype for a total hardware investment of about $12 000. We recommend a slightly more expensive package with 16k of memory to provide programming flexibility and a 30-character-per-second terminal instead of the teletype. This system currently costs about $16 000.

A few final thoughts are germane, perhaps not to the mechanics of operations, but to the underlying philosophical speculations that are involved. These may be considered under two broad categories.

The first is the elucidation of disease, particularly the chemical aspects at a molecular level, so that the treatment of disease becomes as rational and as effective as possible. Translated into gross economics, it is likely that the economic existence of our hospitals and health care facilities may not only find these sophisticated aids advantageous, they may find them necessary to exist at all.

In the second broad aspect, a knowledge on a molecular level of the nutritional needs, at any age, for any ethnic group, in any traditional nutritional pattern, but particularly at critical ages when mental capabilities might develop to their maximum potential, offers an avenue to the improved quality of individuals who are going to have to share the burden and legacy of our imperfect knowledge.

References

1. Schoengold, D. M., Miner, D. J., deFiore, R. H., and Hamilton, P. B., A computerized system for storage and statistical analysis of clinical amino acid data. *Clin. Chem.* **22,** 19 (1976).

2. Werner, M., and Marsh, W. L., Normal values: Theoretical and practical aspects. *Crit. Rev. Clin. Lab. Sci.* **6,** 81 (1975).

3. Dickinson, J. C., Rosenblum, H., and Hamilton, P. B., Ion exchange chromatography of the free amino acids in the plasma of the newborn infant. *Pediatrics* **36,** 2 (1965).

A Computerized System for Storage and Statistical Analysis of Clinical Amino Acid Data

Donald M. Schoengold, David J. Miner,[1] Roberta H. deFiore, and Paul B. Hamilton

We have developed a system of computer programs to expedite analyses of amino acid data obtained in a clinical environment. The system contains a program for building and maintaining libraries of chromatogram data, and a program for retrieval of data on the basis of any of its associated biographical characteristics. Several programs have been written that work with data drawn from the libraries. They provide for easy presentation, manipulation, or statistical analysis of the data. Included are comparison of population means and variances and intra-population correlation analyses. A minicomputer that has 12K of core storage is adequate for use with the system.

Any laboratory that runs large numbers of amino acid analyses immediately encounters the problem of how to efficiently handle the large amount of data generated. This problem can be divided into two parts: analog data reduction and file handling. Many systems have been designed to handle the first problem (*1–5*). Very little has been done on the second (*6*), especially from the viewpoint of the clinical chemist.

Normally, the final quantitative report is filed, on paper, by either date, run number, or patient. If filing is done this way, it is unwieldy to use accumulated data for statistical comparisons. The data from each run of interest must be located and copied before the analysis can be done. Also, each time the data is copied, the probability of making an error increases. Another problem with a paper-oriented file system is that it is difficult to retrieve files except on the basis of how they were first filed. If, for example, filing is done by chromatogram number, it is difficult to get data on all patients with a specific disease without searching through all the files or using a cross-indexed record system. This tends to discourage maximum use of the data in the file.

Brown Memorial Laboratories, Alfred I. du Pont Institute, Wilmington, Del. 19899.

[1] Current address: Department of Chemistry, Purdue University, West Lafayette, Ind. 47906.

Received August 25, 1975; accepted September 22, 1975.

If the results were stored on a computerized file system, these problems could be avoided. It is easy to retrieve records from a computer bulk-storage device, and a computerized system can easily be made to be random access. The availability of inexpensive minicomputers and low-cost bulk storage makes a computerized records system practical and affordable, even for a small laboratory.

Using tape cassettes for bulk storage and a minicomputer, we have established a viable records system. It runs on a Hewlett-Packard 2100A computer with 12K of core and a 3-deck Dicom tape cassette unit. The software is written in FORTRAN II with the special tape-handling software that is standard with a Hewlett-Packard 5932A gas chromatograph–mass spectrometer data system.[2]

Program Philosophy

Before any software was written, the goals of the system were carefully evaluated. We report quantitative results on 27 amino acids or related compounds. Although each sample is identified by a sample number, it is also necessary to identify each chromatogram by a separate, unique, chromatogram number, because a sample may be run several times. Thus, each separate chromatogram, or file, on tape was to be identified by a sample number and a unique chromatogram number. It was important to be able to enter additional information about the sample onto the file.

The system was to be completely conversational and self-correcting. It was also to be impossible for an operator error to destroy a file tape. Files were to be accessible in any sequence, not just the order in which they were entered. Although normal access to a file was to be through its unique chromatogram number, it was also to be accessible through any combination of that file's identifying or descriptor parame-

[2] Complete program listings, documentation, and test data may be obtained from the authors or from the Editorial Office of this journal.

```
OPTION CODES:

      TYPE 1 TO ENTER ARTICLES ON TAPE
      TYPE 2 TO OBTAIN A LISTING
      TYPE 3 TO EDIT SINGLE FILES
      TYPE 4 TO EDIT ONE CHARACTERISTIC OF A GROUP OF FILES
      TYPE 5 TO TERMINATE THIS PROGRAM


      ENTER OPTION CODE
2
      DO YOU WANT TO LIST THE COMPLETE DATA FOR EACH FILE(TYPE 1) OR
      THE SAMPLE ID DATA FOR ALL THE FILES ON THE TAPE(TYPE 0).
1
      ENTER THE CHROMATOGRAM # OF THE FIRST AND LAST SAMPLES
      YOU WISH TO HAVE IN THE LIST (SEPARATE THEM WITH A COMMA)
2020,2024

      THE AMINO ACID IDENTIFICATIONS ARE SHOWN BELOW:

  TAU      UREA       HYP       ASP       THR       SER       ASN
    GLN       PRO       GLU       CIT       GLY       ALA       ABU
      VAL       CYT       MET       ILE       LEU       TYR       PHE
        ETH       ORN       LYS       HIS       TRP       ARG

RECORD #1 —SAMPLE  211;  CHROM  2020;  SEX 1;  AGE 73;  DIAGNOSIS  2
          ┌   2.56    777.00     -1.00        .45     26.50     27.60     -1.00
          │    66.10    32.90      8.02      2.74     29.60     45.10      2.91
RECORD #2 ┤      37.20     2.75      6.97      5.41     11.90      5.41     -1.00
          │        -1.00    11.70     27.00      5.99      3.97      3.73
          └TOTAL AMINO ACIDS  1143.51
RECORD #3 —DESCRIPTOR NUMBERS:   1 26 27 28  0  0  0

           SAMPLE  216;  CHROM  2024;  SEX 1;  AGE 73;  DIAGNOSIS  2
              4.20    371.00     -1.00        .75      7.50     16.70     -1.00
               59.70    21.70      9.10      1.20     18.80     30.80      1.65
                 25.80     3.50      2.28     10.00     15.30      8.17    170.00
                   -1.00     7.64     17.30      8.20      5.04      5.62
           TOTAL AMINO ACID$   821.95
           DESCRIPTOR NUMBERS:   1 27 28  0  0  0  0
```

Fig. 1. Program ENTRY. List output

```
                   ENTER SAMPLE
RECORD #1 —211,2020,1,73,2
          ┌2.56, 777, -1, .45, 26.5, 27.6, -1, 66.1, 32.9, 8.02, 2.74
RECORD #2 ┤29.6, 45.1, 2.91, 37.2, 2.75, 6.97, 5.41, 11.9, 5.41, -1, -1
          └11.7, 27, 5.99, 3.97, 3.73
RECORD #3 —1,26,27,28,0,0,0
                   OK?
       YES  1
                   ENTER SAMPLE
          ┌216, 2024, 1, 73, 2
          │4.2, 371, -1, .75, 7.5, 16.7, -1, 59.7, 21.7, 9.1, 2
SAMPLE #2 ┤18.8, 30.8, 1.65, 25.8, 3.5, 2.28, 10, 15.3, 8.17, 170, -1
          │7.64, 17.3, 8.2, 5.04, 5.62
          └1,27,28,0,0,0,0
                   OK?
        NO  0
              216    2024   1  73   2
                   OK?
       YES  1
             4.20 371.0 -1.00   .75  7.50 16.70 -1.00 59.70 21.70  9.10  2.00
                   OK?                                       correction
        NO  0
CORRECTED LINE  4.2, 371, -1, .75, 7.5, 16.7, -1, 59.7, 21.7, 9.10, 1.2
            18.80 30.80  1.65 25.80  3.50  2.28 10.00 15.30  8.17 170.0 -1.00
                   OK?
       YES  1
             7.64 17.30  8.20  5.04  5.62
                   OK?
       YES  1
              1  27  28   0   0   0   0
                   OK?
       YES  1
                   ENTER SAMPLE
TERMINATION FILE  -1
                   ARE YOU SURE THAT WAS THE LAST INPUT?
       YES  1


                   ENTER OPTION CODE
    LIST OPTION  2
                   DO YOU WANT TO LIST THE COMPLETE DATA FOR EACH FILE(TYPE 1) OR
                   THE SAMPLE ID DATA FOR ALL THE FILES ON THE TAPE(TYPE 0).
                0
                ┌211     2020   1  73   2
1ST RECORD LIST ┤216     2024   1  73   2
                └ -1       -1  -1  -1  -1
                   DO YOU WISH TO LIST OTHER PORTIONS OF YOUR FILE?
                0
```

Fig. 2. Program ENTRY. File creation and first record of file list

ters. Files were to be capable of being edited after they were on the tape cassette without affecting any other files on the tape. The system was to be so designed that new statistical tests or analytical procedures could be added easily. Finally, the output was to be readily understandable and attractive.

These goals were achieved by writing a package of several stand-alone programs. It was done this way instead of with subroutines because the system was not large enough to support the entire package if subroutines were used. The programs were broken up into three functionally different groups: file creation and management, file searching, and data analysis. The file creation and management program (ENTRY) is used to generate and edit the master file tape containing all the chromatographic data. The file searching program (SERCH) generates from the master tape a secondary file tape containing only chromatograms of interest. The data analysis programs use the file tape generated by SERCH. They include a normalization and ratio program, a boundary test program, an F- and t-test program, a chi-square test for normal distribution program, and a correlation program.

File Organization

Each file on tape (Figure 1) contains the data from one chromatogram and consists of three records. The first record contains the sample identification data: sample number; chromatogram number; and code numbers representing the sex, age, and diagnosis of the patient. The next record contains results for the 27 amino acids, followed by the figure for total amino acids. It is not necessary for the operator to calculate the total amino acids, because this is done by the program. The last record consists of seven descriptor numbers that can be used to code additional useful data about the sample. We have included such data as treatment, race, symptoms, and time of sampling.

File Creation

Program ENTRY is essentially four subprograms: file creation, file list, and two file edit subprograms. File creation (Figure 2) is straightforward. The operator enters one line of identifying information, three lines of amino acid results, and seven descriptor numbers. Before the file is written on the master file tape, the operator is given the chance to correct entry mistakes. If he answers zero (or no) to the computer query "OK?", the file just typed is listed line-by-line for correction (Figure 2). In the system, unknown concentrations are differentiated from those known to be zero, by representing them as −1. Amino acids with a concentration of −1 are not used by the analysis programs.

The file list subprogram has two options. Normally, selected files identified by their chromatogram number are listed (Figure 1). Alternatively, the file identification record only (Record 1) for every file on the master file tape can be listed (Figure 2). This gives a quick summary of the contents and order of files on the tape.

The two edit subprograms represent two approaches to editing the file tape. If a single file is to be edited, the file is located on the master file tape by its chromatogram number and typed line-by-line on the teletype. The correction dialog is similar to the file entry correction (Figure 2).

This method is unwieldy if the same record in a continuous series of files is to be edited. Instead, the chromatogram number of the first and last files in the group and the record type (file identification, amino acid result, or keyword) is entered (Figure 3). If an amino acid result is to be corrected, the amino acid number is also entered. The proper record for each file in the group is printed on the keyboard for

```
                 ENTER OPTION CODE
          4
                 PLACE A SCRATCH TAPE IN DECK 3
                 ENTER THE CHROMATOGRAM #'S OF THE FIRST AND LAST FILES OF
                 THE GROUP OF FILES TO BE EDITED (SEPARATE THEM BY A COMMA)
          2020,8840
                 IF YOU WISH TO CHANGE I.D. DATA TYPE 1
                 TO CHANGE AN AMINO ACID RESULT TYPE 2,COMMA,ITS NUMBER (1-27)
                 TO CHANGE DESCRIPTOR NUMBERS TYPE 3
CHANGE AMINO  2,7
     ACID #7     AFTER EACH LINE OF DATA 'OK?' WILL BE TYPED.
                 IF THE DATA IS CORRECT TYPE 1. IF IT ISN'T TYPE
                 0 AND THEN THE CORRECTED LINE

                 SAMPLE CHROMATOGRAM # 2020
          ACID NUMBER  7 IS  -1.00
                 OK?
          1
                 SAMPLE CHROMATOGRAM # 2024
          ACID NUMBER  7 IS  -1.00
                 OK?
          0
  CORRECTION  4.23
                 SAMPLE CHROMATOGRAM # 6155
          ACID NUMBER  7 IS  -1.00
                 OK?
          1
                 SAMPLE CHROMATOGRAM # 7493
          ACID NUMBER  7 IS  -1.00
                 OK?
          0
  CORRECTION  5.0
                 SAMPLE CHROMATOGRAM # 8840
          ACID NUMBER  7 IS   5.32
                 OK?
          1
                 DO YOU WISH TO EDIT ANY MORE FILES?
          0
```

Fig. 3. Program ENTRY. Single characteristic edit

correction if necessary. If an amino acid result is to be edited, the value of the single amino acid, not all 27, is printed (Figure 3).

Both edit options were written so that the master file tape always remains the same tape and tapes do not have to be relabeled.

File Search

Statistical analyses are done with data read off a secondary tape generated from the master tape by use of program SERCH. This approach simplifies data access by the analysis programs and increases system flexibility.

Secondary tapes can be generated two ways: consecutive file and random-access search. If the files of interest are in consecutive positions on the master file tape, the initial and final files to be copied from the master file tape are entered and all the files between these file numbers are copied onto the secondary tape.

The random-access search is much more flexible. It does a field by field comparison of the first record (sample identification) and a logical AND comparison of the third record (descriptor number). It only copies on the secondary tape the files that satisfy operator-specified parameters. For example, by typing in the appropriate codes (Figure 4) it is a simple matter to get the data on all samples of one- to six-month-old (age code = 73) Caucasian (descriptor number = 1) males (sex code = 1) who suffer from phenylketonuria (diagnosis code = 2) and show brain damage (descriptor number = 27) and behavioral problems (descriptor number = 28). Only two of the 150 files in the master file tape fitted all these variables.

The computer recognizes that it is at the end of the data files when it reads a termination file with a sample number of −1. In SERCH, the termination file is not written until specifically requested. This allows construction of composite secondary file tapes. If the

```
   OPTION 1 COPIES GROUPS OF CONSECUTIVE FILES ONTO ANOTHER TAPE
   OPTION 2 COPIES FILES THAT MATCH CERTAIN PARAMETERS ONTO ANOTHER TAPE
   OPTION 3 LISTS THE SCRATCH TAPE
   OPTION 4 TERMINATES THIS PROGRAM


   ENTER OPTION NUMBER
 2
   DOES YOUR SCRATCH TAPE HAVE PERTINENT FILES ON IT ALREADY?
 0
   ENTER THE VALUES CALLED FOR BY THE COMPUTER, IF YOU
 ARE NOT INTERESTED IN A CHARACTERISTIC ENTER -1
 ANY FILES ON YOUR MASTER TAPE WHICH MATCH ALL
 OF THE VALUES YOU PROVIDE WILL BE COPIED ONTO DECK 3.

   SEX CODE?
 1
   AGE CODE?
 73
   DIAGNOSIS CODE?
 2
   DESCRIPTOR NUMBERS?  (ENTER 7, SEPARATED BY COMMAS)
 1,27,28,0,0,0,0

     2 FILES COPIED

   ENTER OPTION NUMBER
 3
 THE AMINO ACID IDENTIFICATIONS ARE SHOWN BELOW:
  TAU      UREA      HYP      ASP      THR      SER      ASN
    GLN      PRO      GLU      CIT      GLY      ALA      ABU
      VAL      CYT      MET      ILE      LEU      TYR      PHE
        ETH      ORN      LYS      HIS      TRP      ARG


 SAMPLE  211:  CHROM  2020:  SEX 1:  AGE 73:  DIAGNOSIS  2
       2.56    777.00    -1.00      .45     26.50     27.60    -1.00
        66.10    32.90     8.02     2.74     29.60     45.10     2.91
          37.20     2.75     6.97     5.41     11.90     5.41    -1.00
            -1.00    11.70    27.00     5.99     3.97     3.73
 TOTAL AMINO ACIDS:  1143.51
 DESCRIPTOR NUMBERS:   1  26  27  28   0   0   0

 SAMPLE  216:  CHROM  2024:  SEX 1:  AGE 73:  DIAGNOSIS  2
       4.20    371.00    -1.00      .75      7.50     16.70    -1.00
        59.70    21.70     9.10     1.20     18.80     30.80     1.65
          25.80     3.50     2.28    10.00     15.30     8.17   170.00
            -1.00     7.64    17.30     8.20     5.04     5.62
 TOTAL AMINO ACIDS:   821.95
 DESCRIPTOR NUMBERS:   1  27  28   0   0   0   0
```

Fig. 4. Program SERCH. Random-access search

```
       ENTER OPTION CODE
 2
       DO YOU NEED INSTRUCTIONS?
 0


 ENTER 5 LINES OF RATIO REQUESTS:
 PHE21TYR20
 PHE21TRP26
 ILE18LEU19
 PRO 9HYP 3
 HYP 3PHE21

 SAMPLE   CHROM.   PHE/TYR   PHE/TRP   ILE/LEU   PRO/HYP   HYP/PHE
 NUMBER   NUMBER
   211     2020      .000      .000      .455      .000      .000
   216     2024    20.808    33.730      .654      .000      .000
  1226     6155    22.181    26.462      .531     9.047      .012
 AVERAGE RATIOS    21.495    30.096      .546     9.047      .012
```

Fig. 5a. Program NORML. Ratio option

consecutive file option is used, several groups of noncontiguous consecutive files can be combined on a single secondary file tape. With the random access option, files that satisfy several different groups of identification codes and descriptor number can also be combined. This allows identification codes or descriptor numbers to be highly specific without losing the ability to do searches under general topics. The files on the secondary tape can be listed by using SERCH or they can also be used for further analysis.

Data Analysis

Data analysis is done off the secondary file tapes created by SERCH. There are currently five data-analysis programs running routinely: TTEST, NORML, HISTO, LIMIT, and COREL. The analysis programs can be divided into two groups, those that work with data within a single chromatogram file and those that do statistical analyses of groups of files.

NORML and LIMIT comprise the first group. NORML is used to calculate ratios of amino acids (Figure 5*a*) or to normalize all the amino acids in a

```
                      ENTER OPTION CODE
                  1
                      ENTER THE NUMBER (1-27) OF THE AMINO ACID YOU WANT
                      THE OTHER ACIDS NORMALIZED TO
                  21
                      THE AMINO ACID I.D.'S ARE SHOWN BELOW:
                   TAU     UREA     HYP     ASP     THR     SER     ASN     GLN
                     PRO     GLU     CIT     GLY     ALA     ABU     VAL     CYT
                       MET     ILE     LEU     TYR     PHE     ETH     ORN     LYS
                         HIS     TRP     ARG


AMINO ACID # 21   FILE DISREGARDED - CHROMATOGRAM # 2020
ZERO OR UNKNOWN
                  SAMPLE #  216;  CHROM # 2024;  SEX 1;  AGE 73;  DIAGNOSIS  2
                    .025   2.182  -1.000    .004    .044    .098  -1.000    .351
                      .128    .054    .007    .111    .181    .010    .152    .021
                        .013    .059    .090    .048   1.000  -1.000    .045    .102
                          .048    .030    .033
                  TOTAL ACIDS:  821.95
                  DESCRIPTOR NUMBERS:  1 27 28  0  0  0  0


                  SAMPLE # 1226;  CHROM # 6155;  SEX 1;  AGE  7;  DIAGNOSIS  2
                    .120   2.199    .012    .007    .041    .070  -1.000    .349
                      .106    .033    .018    .150    .244    .009    .129    .031
                        .012    .048    .090    .045   1.000  -1.000    .022    .071
                          .049    .038  -1.000
                  TOTAL ACIDS:  442.73
                  DESCRIPTOR NUMBERS:  1 27 28  0  0  0  0


                  THE AVERAGES OF THE NORMALIZED DATA ARE:
                    .073   2.191    .012    .006    .043    .084    .000    .350
                      .117    .043    .012    .130    .213    .009    .141    .026
                        .013    .053    .090    .047   1.000    .000    .033    .087
                          .049    .034    .033
```

Fig. 5b. Program NORML. Normalization option

sample to a single amino acid (Figure 5*b*). For both options, the average of the results is also calculated. Impossible or meaningless calculations such as normalization or ratioing to an unknown or zero concentration amino acid are checked and avoided.

LIMIT (Figure 6) is used to determine if the amino acids in a sample lie within boundary limits. The upper and lower boundary limits are read from a standards tape that is generated in an option of LIMIT. The program has a clinically oriented option, which scans only a single file, and a more general option, which scans an entire secondary tape. The clinically oriented option (Figure 6) prints the number and amount of any amino acid in the file that lies outside the limits, and the limits used to make the test. The second option (Figure 6) is more general and versatile. It scans all the files on secondary tape, not just a single file. It provides the ability to check against only upper limits, only lower limits, or both. The entire group of 27 amino acids, selected groups, or only single amino acids can be checked. The chromatogram number of each file with unacceptable amino acids and the identifying numbers of all the acids for which the results are unacceptable are printed. In addition, the complete file for each chromatogram with unacceptable amino acids can be dumped on a scratch tape if desired.

The second group of programs is HISTO, TTEST, and COREL.

HISTO is a utility program used to determine if the amino acid data forms a normal population. This is necessary because statistical tests assume that the distribution of the population being tested is normal. It uses a chi-square test to compare the experimental data with a fitted normal curve. It prints out the theoretical and observed distribution, a histogram of the experimental distribution, and the value of chi-square and the number of degrees of freedom. HISTO is normally run only once for each set of data to check for normality.

```
              LIMIT CHECK PROGRAM

      PLACE YOUR FILE TAPE IN DECK 2, AND YOUR STANDARDS TAPE IN DECK 3
      ANSWER QUESTIONS WITH 'Y'ES OR 'N'O

OPTION CODES:  OPTION A DOES A CLINICAL CHECK
               OPTION B SCANS A FILE TAPE
               OPTION C BUILDS,LISTS, OR EDITS STANDARDS TAPES
               OPTION D TERMINATES


ENTER OPTION CODE: A
ENTER CHROM # OF RUN TO BE EVALUATED: 9046

ACID #       VALUE       NORMAL LIMITS

   5         10.70       11.40 - 33.50
  12         20.70       22.40 - 51.40
  13         23.10       23.60 - 41.00
  18          6.67        2.67 -  5.26
  19         11.00        4.65 - 10.90
  21         67.00        4.18 - 11.00
  22          1.74        2.62 -  9.17


ENTER OPTION CODE: B

DO YOU WISH TO CHECK UPPER LIMITS ONLY? N
LOWER LIMITS ONLY? N

DO YOU WISH TO CHECK ALL 27 ACIDS? Y

DO YOU WISH TO DUMP UNACCEPTABLE FILES? N

CHROM #     ACIDS OUTSIDE LIMITS

  1675      21
  1623      10 21
  1695      10
  1699      10
  8339       6  8 10 16 20
  8643       4 10 11 15 16 20
  8689       8 11 12 13 14 16 20
  8672      26 27

ENTER OPTION CODE: D
```

Fig. 6. Program LIMIT

ENTER LEVEL OF SIGNIFICANCE - .05

A.A.	F	VARIANCES DIFF?	T	MEANS DIFFERENT?
TAU	.43	.00	-.07	.00
UREA	.63	.00	-3.81	1.00
HYP	2.23	.00	-.47	.00
ASP	.43	.00	.70	.00
THR	.20	.00	-2.04	1.00
SER	1.34	.00	.02	.00
ASN	.00	.00	.00	.00
GLN	.87	.00	-.60	.00
PRO	.31	.00	-1.32	.00
GLU	.24	.00	-.67	.00
CIT	.69	.00	-1.17	.00
GLY	.90	.00	-.74	.00
ALA	.22	.00	-3.17	1.00
ABU	.65	.00	-2.45	1.00
VAL	.44	.00	-1.76	.00
CYT	.63	.00	.14	.00
MET	.51	.00	-.87	.00
ILE	.49	.00	-.38	.00
LEU	.20	.00	-1.32	.00
TYR	.35	.00	.08	.00
PHE	10.70	1.00	5.68	1.00
ETH	2.63	.00	.01	.00
ORN	.51	.00	.37	.00
LYS	.37	.00	-2.10	1.00
HIS	1.08	.00	-1.08	.00
TRP	.31	.00	-1.80	.00
ARG	.69	.00	-1.26	.00
SUMS	.95	.00	-2.34	1.00

Fig. 7. Program TTEST. Comparison of plasma amino acids in a phenylketonuric, before and after treatment

TTEST has two options. It can be used to calculate the mean, variance, and standard deviation of one group of files. The second option (Figure 7) compares two groups of files. It calculates the mean, variance, and standard deviation of each acid in each group and then calculates the F and t values for the 27 amino acids. The program automatically identifies amino acids that have significantly different means and variances at a significance level specified by the operator.

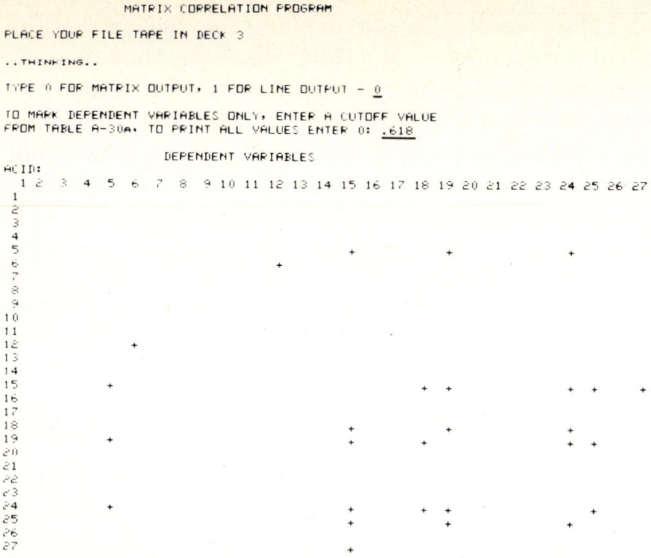

Fig. 8a. Program COREL. Dependent amino acid pairs in normal newborn infants

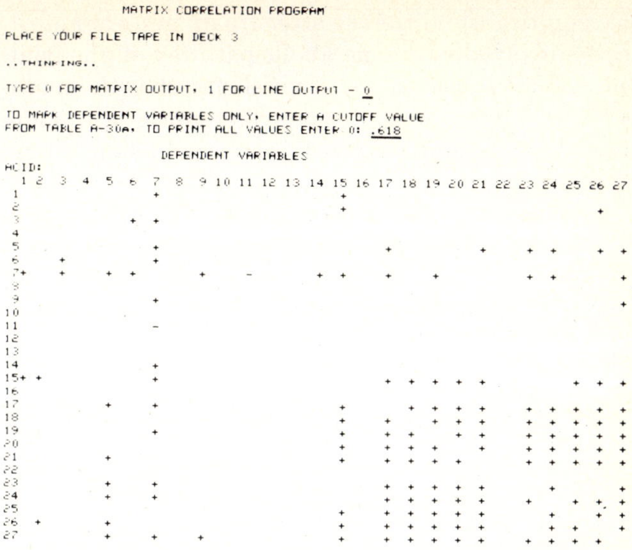

Fig. 8b. Program COREL. Dependent amino acid pairs in normal adults

The last program now in the system is COREL. Given a group of files, it calculates a correlation coefficient r(a,b) for each amino acid with every other amino acid. An r(a,b) of ±1.0 indicates complete dependence; a value of 0.0 complete linear independence. From the value of r(a,b), one can statistically reject the hypothesis that two amino acids are linearly independent. If this hypothesis is rejected, the two amino acids must have some degree of linear dependence on each other. However, r(a,b) is only an indication of the degree of dependence, not a statistically valid measure of it.

COREL has four output options. It is possible to print the values of r(a,b) for all paired amino acids. If a rough idea of the numerical value of each r(a,b) is needed, it can be obtained with a matrix output consisting of one-digit indication of r(a,b) scaled over the range ±10. Amino acid pairs that have an r(a,b) greater than a cutoff value, and thus are linearly dependent upon each other, can be identified in a matrix format (Figures 8*a*, *b*). The amino acid number corresponds to their order of printout in Figure 7. The correlation coefficient of each amino acid with itself (1.0) is not printed. Because a "+" instead of the numerical value of r(a,b) is printed for each dependent pair, it is easy to visually compare different groups of samples. The value of the cutoff chosen depends on the number of variables and the degree of confidence of the test (*7*). It is also possible to print the numerical value of r(a,b) for all pairs for which r is less than the cutoff value. These pairs are probably, but not necessarily, independent.

Results

Any computerized data system can be evaluated from the viewpoint of how well the system operates and from the viewpoint of the validity of the data generated. The system goals we set up were met almost completely. The programs are conversational and self-instructing. If an operator enters an impossible answer to a question, he is either informed of his error and told to re-answer the question or his answer is ignored. Although it is possible to make a mistake that would make output meaningless, it is almost impossible to cause the only irreversible disaster, destruction of the master file tape.

The program options in SERCH and the data-analysis programs cover all the current needs of this laboratory. However, because all the programs are independent, new ones can be written without any interaction with programs now running.

Because all the analysis programs make use of secondary file tapes containing only files of interest, not the master file tape, it is very easy to write programs to do quick one-shot analyses of a group of files. For example, a program to calculate the sum of a group of amino acids would consist of only about 10 lines of FORTRAN programming.

The results of extensive analyses of data with these programs will be published later. However, the following are some examples of useful data that can be generated easily and quickly with these programs.

As part of our studies of amino acid changes in children with phenylketonuria, we have data on amino acid concentrations in the plasma of children before and after treatment. Using TTEST, it was a simple matter to compare the two groups to see which amino acids were significantly different (Figure 7). (To our knowledge, a comparison of this type for these 27 amino acids has not been published.) The number of samples in the pre-treatment group is small (*6*), so conclusions drawn from the results are only preliminary. However, it is interesting to note that the amino acids other than phenylalanine that are significantly different after treatment are not directly involved in the metabolic pathway of phenylalanine. This suggests, not surprisingly, that the metabolic derangements in phenylketonuria are more complex than simply a blockage of conversion of phenylalanine to tyrosine.

In some respects, the determination of whether the variances are different can be as useful as determining whether the means are different. If the two groups of samples were run by the same technique, the amino acids with different variances are probably more sensitive to experimental conditions. The calculation can also be used to compare the scatter of two different analytical techniques by running the same sample by both techniques, generating two secondary tapes, and running TTEST on the tapes.

Results from a correlation analysis must be interpreted with care, because statistical correlation does not necessarily mean a direct causal connection. However, using the combination of matrix printout for dependence and numerical printout of $r(a,b)$ with a high cutoff value, an interesting set of results was generated on a set of samples from 25 newborn infants (*8*). These samples were taken just after birth, before the first feeding. We also have on our master file tape a set of runs on eight normal adults. The output from the matrix test for dependence clearly shows that more amino acid pairs are dependent upon (i.e., correlated with) each other in the adults than in the infants. The numerical printout option was next run. Only two of the pairs for the newborn infants had $r(a,b)$ values greater than 0.80, while 35 pairs in the adult samples have an $r(a,b)$ exceeding 0.80.

These results do not explain the reason for the greater dependence in adults. However, they do indicate results that might warrant further study. We speculate that the reason for the difference between the infants and adults is that the infants have not completed the transition from *in utero* nutrition to dependence upon external food supplies, i.e., many of the pathways that operate in an adult have simply not become operative yet.

We thank Mr. Robert M. Clemick for photographic art work and Miss Susan Keenan for typing the manuscript. We also thank Mr. Mark Vogel for helpful suggestions on the manuscript.

References

1. Buchan, N., Computer analysis of amino acid chromatograms. *J. Chromatogr.* **103,** 33 (1975).

2. Owen, J. M., and Dale, A. D., Analysis of data from amino acid and other automated analyzers. II. Simple Fortran program for identification and quantitation of amino acids. *J. Chromatogr.* **107,** 207 (1975).

3. Young, B. D., A computer technique for the analysis of amino acid chromatograms. *J. Chromatogr.* **92,** 113 (1974).

4. Taylor, R., and Davies, M. G., A Fortran IV computer program for automatic calculation of amino acid composition. *Anal. Biochem.* **51,** 180 (1973).

5. Spitz, H. D., Henyon, G., and Sivertson, J. N., A computer program for amino acid analyses. *J. Chromatogr.* **68,** 111 (1972).

6. Fox, M. A., Programs for use with automatic amino acid analyzer to identify, compute and correlate amino acid concentrations in biological samples. *J. Chromatogr.* **89,** 61 (1974).

7. Dixon, W. J., and Massey, E. J., *Introduction to Statistical Analysis.* McGraw-Hill, New York, N. Y., 1969, p 204.

8. Dickinson, J. C., Rosenblum, H., and Hamilton, P. B., Ion exchange chromatography of the free amino acids in the plasma of the newborn infant. *Pediatrics* **36,** 2 (1965).

9. Grams, R. R., Johnson, E. A., and Benson, E. S., Laboratory data analysis system: Section I—Introduction and overview. *Am. J. Clin. Pathol.* **58,** 177 (1972). (reference added in proof).

Simultaneous High-Pressure Liquid-Chromatographic Determination of Some Anticonvulsants in Serum

Reginald F. Adams and Frank L. Vandemark

We describe procedures for simultaneously determining some anticonvulsants (phenobarbital, diphenylhydantoin, primidone, ethosuximide, methsuximide, carbamazepine) in serum by high-pressure liquid chromatography. The drugs, together with an internal standard, phenacetin, are adsorbed from serum onto charcoal and eluted from it with organic solvent. The eluate is analyzed isocratically on a reverse-phase column with a mobile phase consisting of acetonitrile/water (17/83 by volume). The eluted drugs are detected by their absorption at 195 nm, and quantities estimated from their peak areas as compared with those of extracted standards. Results are reproducible to about 6%. Sensitivities, for 0.5-ml serum samples, of 0.1 mg/liter for all the drugs analyzed except ethosuximide (0.5 mg/liter) are attained routinely. Correlation of results with gas chromatography was 0.912 for phenobarbital, 0.982 for diphenylhydantoin, 0.886 for primidone, and 0.966 for ethosuximide. Amobarbital and secobarbital interfere with the analysis; chlordiazepoxide, methaqualone, salicylate, diazepam, and oxazepam do not. Including extraction, analysis time for a single sample is 20 min.

Additional Keyphrases: *comparison with gas chromatography • metabolite of diphenylhydantoin • drug assay • toxicology*

High-pressure liquid chromatography has particular advantages for analysis of the common anticonvulsant drugs in that compounds may be analyzed without an initial derivatization, ultraviolet detection at 195 nm provides excellent sensitivity, and drugs may be collected unchanged from the column eluate for further analysis.

Here, we used high-pressure liquid chromatography with a reverse-phase column to simultaneously determine concentrations of phenobarbital, diphenylhydantoin, primidone, ethosuximide, methsuximide, and carbamazepine in serum. The reverse-phase column provided, in our hands, greater analytical flexibility than does the adsorption column, giving shorter analysis times and permitting use of a largely aqueous mobile phase consisting of aqueous acetonitrile. To shorten pretreatment time we have developed a micro-scale extraction procedure based on charcoal adsorption (*1*) that obviates evaporating large volumes of extraction solvent. The addition of an internal standard before pretreatment increases the overall accuracy by compensating for extraction and injection variations. The procedure is rapid and accurate, offering a useful alternative method in the routine analysis of anticonvulsant drugs.

The Perkin-Elmer Corp., Main Ave., Norwalk, Conn. 06856.
Received July 21, 1975; accepted Sept. 29, 1975.

Materials and Methods

Apparatus

We used a high-pressure liquid chromatograph (Perkin-Elmer Model LC 601) equipped with a reverse-phase column (ODS-Sil-x I) 0.5 m × 2.6 mm, together with a variable-wavelength spectrophotometer (Perkin-Elmer Model LC 55) to monitor the column effluent. The data were processed with a Perkin-Elmer PEP-II data processor. Special glassware included 10 × 75 mm disposable culture tubes and 16 × 75 mm culture tubes (screw-caps with Teflon liners).

Reagents

Acetonitrile: Acetonitrile (ultraviolet grade), distilled in glass, was from Burdick and Jackson Laboratories, Inc., Muskegon, Mich. 49442.

Mobile phase: This is a solution of 85 ml of acetonitrile in 415 ml of de-ionized water. Both liquids should be degassed by cautious application of reduced pressure (water aspirator) immediately before gentle mixing.

Methanol: "Spectroquality" grade.

Charcoal: Norit A, Neutral, from Amend Drug and Chemical Co., Irvington, N. J. 07111.

Mixed solvent: Dichloromethane/isopropyl alcohol/diethyl ether, 65/10/25 by vol. Spectroquality solvents must be used.

Drug standards: We obtained carbamazepine (as "Tegretol") from Geigy Pharmaceuticals, Ardsley, N. Y. 10502. Methsuximide (as "Celontin") was obtained from Parke, Davis and Co., Detroit, Mich. 48232. Other drugs were obtained from Applied Science Laboratories, State College, Pa. 16801. Individual solutions in methanol of each drug were prepared to a final concentration of 10 g/liter. These solutions were used to determine retention times of the individual drugs and for preparation of standard concentrations in serum. A chromatography standard mixture was prepared as follows: 10 mg each of phenobarbital, diphenylhydantoin, primidone, methsuximide, carbamazepine and 20 mg ethosuximide were dissolved in 5 ml of methanol and the volume was exactly adjusted to 10 ml. The solutions are stable at 4 °C for at least two months.

Internal standard: Dissolve 5 mg of phenacetin (Applied Science Laboratories) in 10 ml of methanol.

Procedure

Transfer 0.5 ml of serum, 2 ml of water, 10 μl of internal standard (equal to 5 μg of phenacetin), and about 8 mg of charcoal to a 16 × 75 mm tube. Mix the contents of the tube for 30 s with a vortex-type mixer. Centrifuge (2000 rpm, 1 min) and aspirate the aqueous phase. Add 300 μl of the mixed solvent to the tube. Using a vortex-type mixer, mix the tube contents vigorously for 30 s. Centrifuge (2000 rpm, 1 min) and decant the solvent into a 10 × 75 mm disposable culture tube. Evaporate the solvent in a gentle current of air (rate not greater than 50 ml/min) at 40 °C. Dissolve the residue in 20 μl of methanol and aspirate 4 μl into a syringe and inject directly onto the column. Table 1 gives the instrumental conditions for chromatography. The order in which the compounds emerge from the column is shown in Figure 1.

Results

Standards. To ascertain the adequacy of the chromatographic conditions, we applied to the column aliquots of the internal standard (phenacetin) plus the standard mixture described above. Also included was the *para*hydroxylated metabolite of diphenylhydantoin. The quantities injected were 1 μg of each compound except ethosuximide, which was 2 μg. The recorder was operated at 10 mV (0.2 absorbance unit full scale). Figure 1 shows a chromatogram of a standard run. Analysis time from time of injection of the sample was about 14 min.

A mixture of drug-free serum plus known quantities of ethosuximide (40 mg/liter), primidone (25 mg/liter), phenobarbital (20 mg/liter), methsuximide (10 mg/liter), diphenylhydantoin (10 mg/liter), and carbamazepine (10 mg/liter) was taken through the procedures. Figure 2 shows the resulting chromatogram. The drugs were identified by retention time. As a control, similar chromatograms were obtained daily.

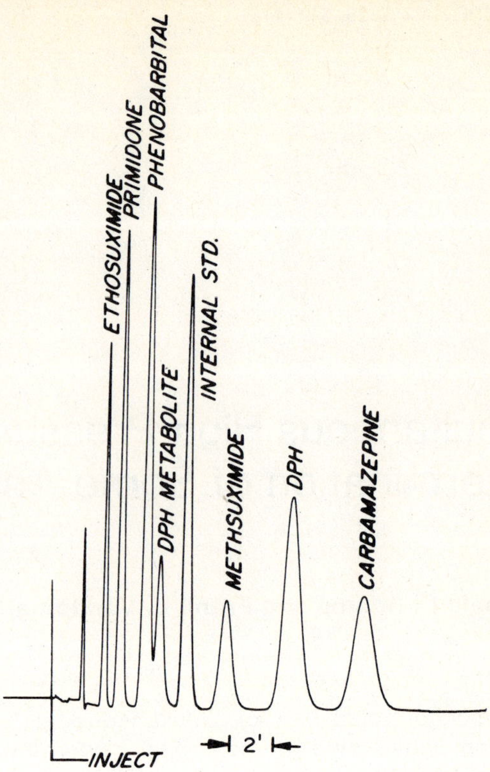

Fig. 1. Chromatogram of a standard mixture of drugs
Quantity chromatographed was 1 μg each except ethosuximide, which was 2 μg. *DPH*, diphenylhydantoin; *DPH metabolite*, 5-(*p*-hydroxyphenyl)-5-phenylhydantoin

Table 1. Chromatographic Conditions

Column	0.5 m × 2.6 mm (o.d.) (Sil-x-1)
Mobile phase	Acetonitrile/water (17/83 by vol)
Flow rate	1.5 ml/min
Pressure	6.21×10^6 Pa (900 psi)
Oven	40 °C
Detector wavelength	195 nm
Recorder	10 mV

Quantitation. Quantitation was done by computer, by use of peak area ratios of drug to internal standard. For the compounds studied, a linear relationship between peak area ratios and concentration was obtained for the range 1–150 mg/liter. Figure 3 shows plots obtained for primidone, phenobarbital, and diphenylhydantoin (to 100 mg/liter).

It was also verified that sufficient accuracy was obtained by peak height ratio calculation. The ratio of the peak height of each drug to that of the internal

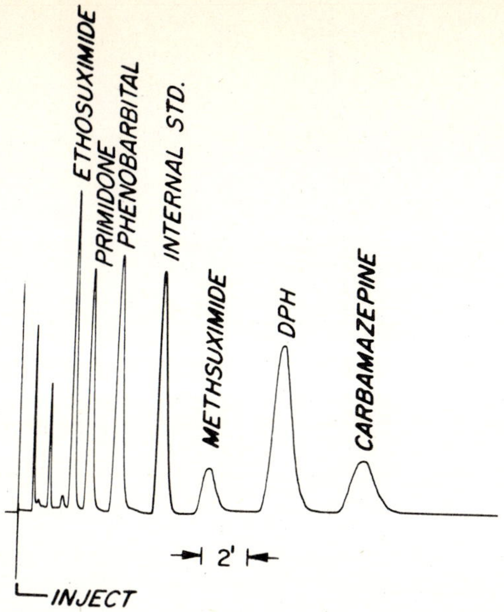

Fig. 2. Chromatogram of an extract of a mixture of serum and drugs

Ethosuximide, 40 mg/liter; primidone, 25 mg/liter; phenobarbital, 20 mg/liter; methsuximide, diphenylhydantoin, carbamazepine, each 10 mg/liter. *DPH*, diphenylhydantoin

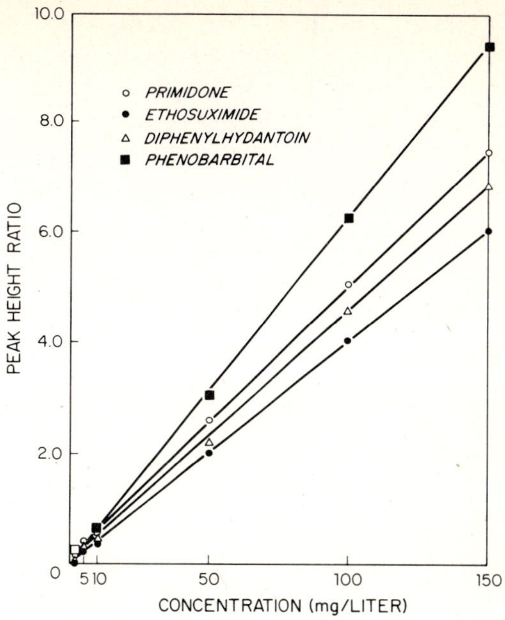

Fig. 4. Peak height ratio vs. concentration: calibration curve for ethosuximide, primidone, phenobarbital, and diphenylhydantoin

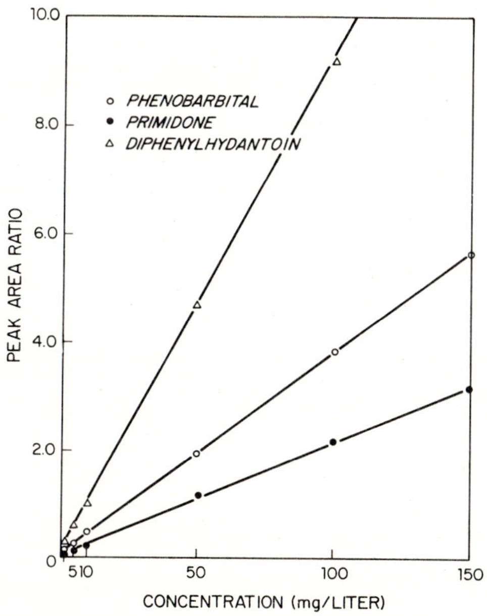

Fig. 3. Peak area ratio vs. concentration: calibration curve for primidone, phenobarbital, and diphenylhydantoin

standard was calculated for several concentrations of the drugs and plotted vs. the concentrations. The relationship was linear in the range 1–150 mg/liter. Figure 4 shows such plots for phenobarbital, primidone, diphenylhydantoin and ethosuximide. The quantity of drug in a sample was determined by calculation of the peak height ratio and determining the corresponding concentration from the plot. Both peak area and peak height ratio measurements should be re-checked routinely with controls and whenever columns or reagents are changed. The lower range of concentration (1–50 mg/liter) should be plotted separately on an expanded scale, to improve the accuracy with which the curve can be read in this region.

Sera. Sera from subjects on anticonvulsant therapy were extracted and chromatographed as described above. Figure 5 shows a typical chromatogram: the primidone concentration was calculated to be 26 mg/liter; phenobarbital, 66 mg/liter; and diphenylhydantoin, 6.8 mg/liter. Figure 6 is from a serum collected from a subject on ethosuximide therapy. The ethosuximide concentration was 42 mg/liter (phenobarbital, 108 mg/liter; diphenylhydantoin, 9.2 mg/liter).

Analytical Variables

Reproducibility. Data on within-run precision were obtained by taking 20 aliquots of pooled sera from patients receiving primidone, phenobarbital, and diphenylhydantoin, and processing aliquots through the complete procedures during one day (Table 2). The mean concentrations (mg/liter) were: primidone, 14.6 (CV, 4.2%); phenobarbital, 31.4 (CV, 4.8%); and diphenylhydantoin, 16.2 (CV, 4.8%). Similar studies were done on pooled sera with added ethosuximide, carbamazepine, and methsuximide. The mean concentrations of these drugs were 12.4 (CV, 6.6%), 10.1 (CV, 5.5%), and 15.2 mg/liter (CV, 6.0%), respectively.

Table 3 summarizes day-to-day precision data for another such serum pool, duplicate aliquots of which, stored frozen until use, were processed during each work-day over a four-week period. The mean concentrations found for the drugs were: ethosuximide, 15.1

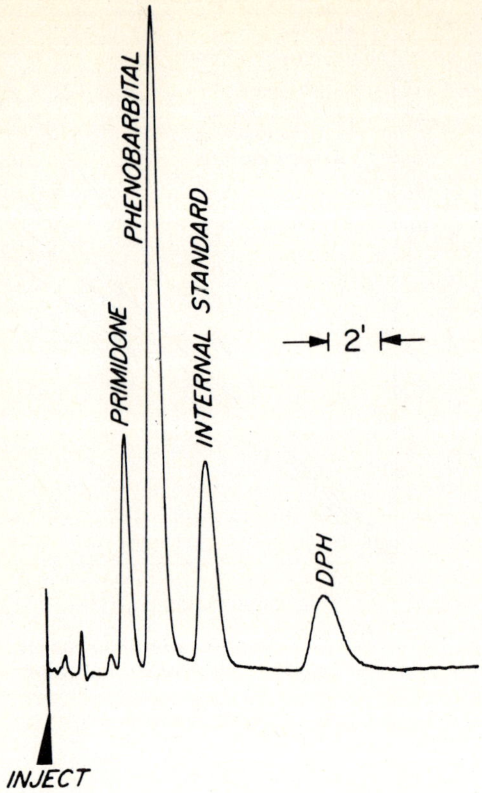

Fig. 5. Chromatogram of a serum extract

Aliquot injected equal to 100 μl serum. *DPH*, diphenylhydantoin. Concentrations were calculated to be: primidone, 26 mg/liter; phenobarbital, 66 mg/liter; DPH, 6.8 mg/liter

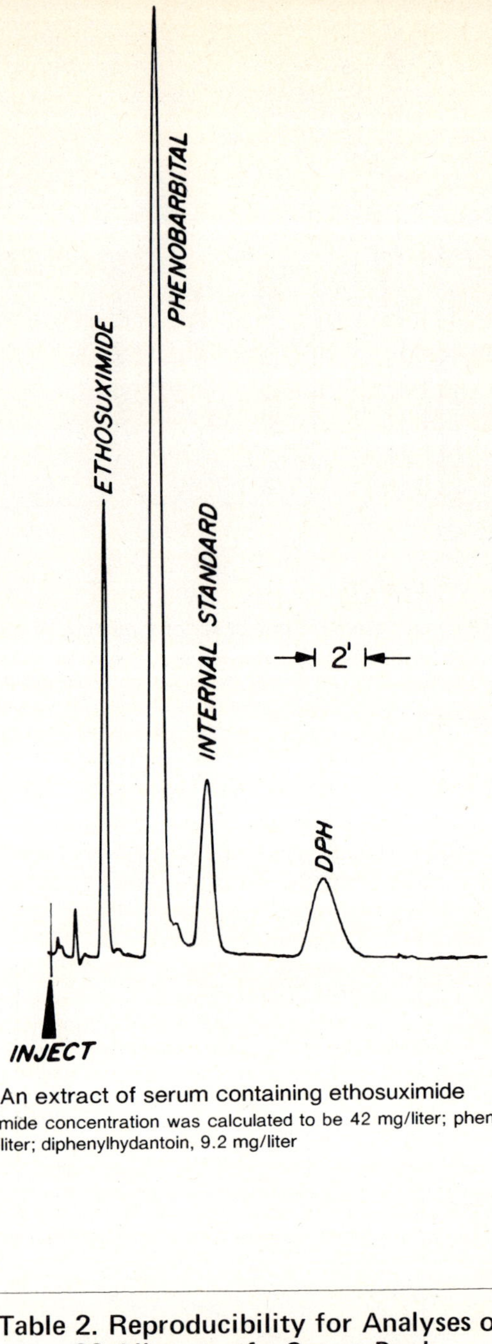

Fig. 6. An extract of serum containing ethosuximide

Ethosuximide concentration was calculated to be 42 mg/liter; phenobarbital, 108 mg/liter; diphenylhydantoin, 9.2 mg/liter

mg/liter (CV, 7.3%); primidone, 11.8 mg/liter (CV, 6.3%); phenobarbital, 35.9 mg/liter (CV, 5.3%); diphenylhydantoin, 14.7 mg/liter (CV, 6.8%); carbamazepine, 9.8 mg/liter (CV, 7.4%); and methsuximide, 16.4 mg/liter (CV, 5.8%).

Background. When processed by our procedure, sera that were known to be drug-free yielded chromatograms with various degrees of background. Instrumental noise sometimes appears as background. Background contamination was also contributed by glassware and solvents; the rest comes from the matrix of the sample itself and is related to the extraction procedure used. To obtain data on the amount of background appearing at elution times corresponding to those of the drugs of interest, we took 20 sera, known to be drug-free, with added internal standard (phenacetin) through the complete procedure. A range of values were calculated for background peaks appearing at the retention time intervals of ethosuximide, primidone, phenobarbital, methsuximide, diphenylhydantoin, and carbamazepine. Aliquots of the same sera were processed without phenacetin but with added phenobarbital to provide an internal standard for the calculation of background appearing at the elution time for phenacetin. Ultraviolet-absorbing background, so expressed, ranged from about 0.00–0.06 mg/liter (Table 4).

Sensitivity. The sensitivity of the procedure is lim-

Table 2. Reproducibility for Analyses of 20 Aliquots of a Serum Pool

Drug	Mean (mg/liter)	SD (mg/liter)	CV, %
Within-run			
Ethosuximide	12.4	0.82	6.6
Primidone	14.6	0.61	4.2
Phenobarbital	31.4	1.50	4.8
Methsuximide	15.2	0.91	6.0
Diphenylhydantoin	16.2	0.78	4.8
Carbamazepine	10.1	0.55	5.5
Day-to-day			
Ethosuximide	15.1	1.10	7.3
Primidone	11.8	0.74	6.3
Phenobarbital	35.9	1.90	5.3
Methsuximide	16.4	0.95	5.8
Diphenylhydantoin	14.7	1.00	6.8
Carbamazepine	9.8	0.72	7.4

Table 3. Day-to-day Precision during Four Weeks for Identical Pooled Serum Containing Six Anticonvulsants

Drug	Mean[a] (mg/liter)	SD (mg/liter)	CV, %
Ethosuximide	15.1	1.10	7.3
Primidone	11.8	0.74	6.3
Phenobarbital	35.9	1.90	5.3
Methsuximide	16.4	0.95	5.8
Diphenylhydantoin	14.7	1.00	6.8
Carbamazepine	9.8	0.72	7.4

[a] n = 20

Table 4. Range of Background Values for 20 Drug-free Sera

Background at retention time for	Range, mg/liter[a]
Ethosuximide	0.01–0.06
Primidone	0.01–0.04
Phenobarbital	0.03–0.02
Phenacetin	0.01–0.04
Diphenylhydantoin	0.01–0.04
Carbamazepine	0.00–0.03
Methsuximide	0.01–0.04

[a] Expressed in terms of the respective drug.

ited largely by serum volume, extraction efficiency, and background. With a 0.5-ml sample volume, the compounds can be detected in concentrations as low as 0.1 mg/liter, except for ethosuximide (0.5 mg/liter).

Recoveries. We studied the analytical recovery of drugs from serum by adding known quantities of ethosuximide, primidone, phenobarbital, methsuximide, diphenylhydantoin, and carbamazepine to pooled serum known to be drug-free. Half-milliliter aliquots of the serum without internal standard were taken through the extraction procedure. After cautious drying, the extracts were reconstituted in 20 μl of methanol containing 5 μg of phenacetin. Aliquots of the solutions were chromatographed, and peak areas were computed to quantitate the chromatogram. Because the phenacetin was not taken through the extraction procedure, it was used to correct for volumetric error in sample injection. Results were expressed as percentages of the peak areas obtained by direct injection of pure standards. Recoveries were calculated for phenacetin but with phenobarbital as the correction standard. Results were calculated for drugs recovered from duplicate serum samples containing drugs added to give concentrations equivalent to 1 or 10 mg/liter. The recovery figures (Table 5) reflect the losses inherent in the micro-scale extraction procedure used. The recovery may be improved by combining a second elution of the charcoal with the first. If serum-based standards are used (serum to which the drugs have been added) and an internal standard is used, adequate correction will be obtained.

Table 5. Recovery Data[a]

Concn, mg/liter	Mean recovery, %
Ethosuximide	
1.0	42
10.0	45
Primidone	
1.0	65
10.0	65
Phenobarbital	
1.0	73
10.0	72
Phenacetin	
1.0	68
10.0	71
Diphenylhydantoin	
1.0	69
10.0	71
Carbamazepine	
1.0	58
10.0	60
Methsuximide	
1.0	44
10.0	41

[a] Obtained for use of the charcoal extraction procedure on aliquots of a mixture of serum and drugs. Duplicate aliquots of each concentration were extracted.

Comparison with Gas Chromatography

Gas chromatography was used as a comparison method. Sera from subjects on anticonvulsant therapy were processed and drug concentrations determined by the gas-chromatographic procedures described by Solow et al. (*2*). Additional aliquots of the same sera were analyzed by the present method. Concentrations of phenobarbital, diphenylhydantoin, primidone, and ethosuximide determined by the two procedures were compared. Figure 7 shows results for phenobarbital in 42 sera. The coefficient of correlation was 0.912; slope, 0.922; y-intercept, +2.07. The estimated standard error (S_r) was 0.065. Results of similar calculations for other drugs were: diphenylhydantoin, (n = 40), coefficient of correlation, 0.982 (slope, 0.938; y-intercept, −0.356; estimated standard error, 0.031); primidone (n = 40), coefficient of correlation, 0.886 (slope, 1.119; y-intercept, −1.65; estimated standard error, 0.075); and ethosuximide, (n = 38), coefficient of correlation, 0.966 (slope, 0.972; y-intercept, +1.48; estimated standard error, 0.043).

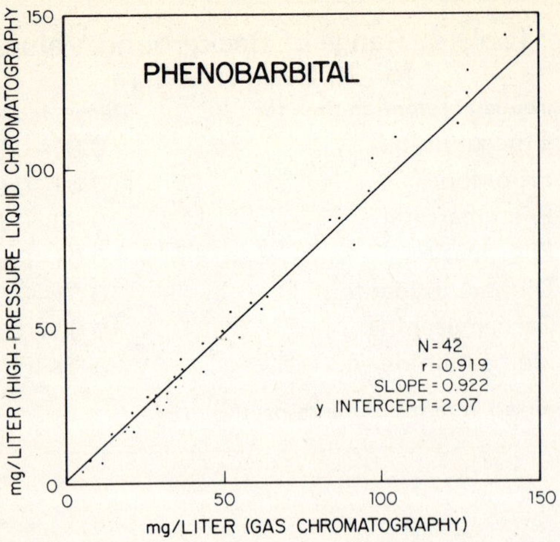

Fig. 7. Comparison of results obtained for 42 sera analyzed for phenobarbital by high-pressure liquid chromatography and by gas chromatography

The number of sera from subjects on therapy including carbamazepine or methsuximide was not sufficient to make similar comparisons on these drugs.

Drugs Other Than Anticonvulsants

To determine the potential usefulness of the procedures and to investigate possible interferences, we studied several other ultraviolet-absorbing drugs by chromatographing pure standards: secobarbital, amobarbital, salicylate, pentobarbital, methaqualone, chlordiazepoxide, glutethimide, propoxyphene, diazepam, and oxazepam. Chlordiazepoxide, diazepam, and oxazepam were not eluted from the column under the conditions used. Methaqualone emerges from the column at 21.4 min, and if it may be present in a sample this must be taken into consideration. Amobarbital emerged from the column with the methsuximide peak; secobarbital, glutethimide, and propoxyphene emerged with diphenylhydantoin. Acetylsalicylic acid and salicylic acid eluted immediately after the solvent peak and before ethosuximide, and thus did not interfere with the analysis. Pentobarbital emerged from the column with methsuximide. It will therefore interfere with methsuximide analysis. Retention times for the compounds tested are given in Table 6. No study of the drugs in physiological samples has been made.

Metabolite of Diphenylhydantoin

We studied the major metabolite of diphenylhydantoin 5-(*p*-hydroxyphenyl)-5-phenylhydantoin. Analytical recovery of the compound added to drug-free sera was 38–44%. The chromatographic conditions used gave a retention time sufficient to allow it to appear immediately after phenobarbital. Concentrations of this metabolite in 90 sera found to contain diphenylhydantoin ranged from undetectable to 0.13 mg/liter.

Table 6. Retention Times (from Time of Injection) for Solutions of Pure Compounds

Compound	Retention time, min
Salicylate	1.68
Ethosuximide	2.20
Primidone	2.93
Phenobarbital	3.98
5-(*p*-hydroxyphenyl)-5-phenylhydantoin	4.51
Phenacetin	5.51
Methsuximide	7.48
Pentobarbital	7.51
Amobarbital	7.50
Secobarbital	10.15
Propoxyphene	10.15
Glutethimide	10.21
Diphenylhydantoin	10.25
Carbamazepine	13.40
Methaqualone	21.40
Oxazepam	did not elute
Diazepam	did not elute
Chlordiazepoxide	did not elute

Discussion

The above results indicate that this high-pressure liquid chromatographic method is adequately sensitive and precise for measuring these anticonvulsants in serum, if most other drugs are absent. Results obtained by gas chromatography and high-pressure liquid chromatography on the same sera correlated well for primidone, phenobarbital, diphenylhydantoin, and ethosuximide. Analysis time and resolution when a reverse-phase column is used are related to the concentration of the organic solvent in the mobile phase. In practice, choice of temperature and varying the acetonitrile concentration provide a considerable opportunity to make the analysis optimal. The temperature (40 °C) and acetonitrile concentration (17% by vol) used in the procedures were chosen because our concern was to adequately separate all the compounds studied within a 15-min analysis time. We found that overall analysis time was affected by temperature of the column oven and by the concentration of acetonitrile in the mobile phase. Retention time for diphenylhydantoin chromatographed at 25 °C was 14 min. At 60 °C, the retention time was 8.5 min. Retention time for diphenylhydantoin eluted at 40 °C with 10% acetonitrile was 13 min. With 20% acetonitrile, the retention time was 8.6 min. An important separation was considered to be that of phenobarbital from the *para*-hydroxylated metabolite of diphenylhydantoin. At 40 °C, the separation factor for these compounds was 1.14; at 60 °C, it was 1.04, a figure unacceptable to us because of potential interference by the diphenylhydantoin metabolite with phenobarbital quantitation. The oven operating temperature, 40 °C, also avoided variations associated with a varying ambient temperature.

The analytical recoveries for the compounds studied are somewhat low because the charcoal adsorption is imperfect. However, this is offset to a large extent by the convenience afforded by the small volume of solvent required.

High-pressure liquid chromatography largely avoids problems of adsorption on the column packing, problems that often are significant with gas chromatography. A great advantage is that low concentrations of drugs may be analyzed without first making a derivative of the compounds. Carbamazepine may be quantitated in serum extracts without the precautions associated with gas-chromatographic procedures (*3*). The high-pressure liquid-chromatographic detection system is nondestructive, permitting the compounds to be recovered for further examination.

The detection wavelength, 195 nm, although relatively nonselective, is sufficiently sensitive for all the drugs tested. The lack of selectivity is compensated for by the chromatographic separation of the drugs. In theory, ultraviolet-absorbing materials extractable from the sample matrix could cause interference. However, as shown, interferences have been negligible.

The number of samples that may be analyzed before the column packing is replaced depends on several factors: gradual loss of column efficiency because matrix material carried over in the extract has coated the column packing (evident as loss of resolution and shortened retention times) and increasing back-pressure. The back-pressure increase is caused by particles from the sample or septum clogging a porous plug sealing the end of the column. We routinely replaced the plug every 100 analyses. We have used one column for 600 analyses without significant loss of resolution. The chromatography time for each analysis was 14 min, with an additional 6 min required for sample preparation.

We are indebted to J. Meola, Associate Director, Clinical Chemistry Department, Albany Medical Center, Albany, New York, for generously providing sera. We thank W. Slavin for advice with this report and G. Schmidt for competent technical assistance.

References

1. Meola, J. M., and Vanko, M., Use of charcoal to concentrate drugs from urine before analysis. *Clin. Chem.* **20,** 184 (1974).

2. Solow, E. B., Metaxas, J. M., and Summers, T. R., Anti-epileptic drugs: A current assessment of simultaneous determination of multiple drug therapy by gas liquid chromatography—on column methylation. *J. Chromatogr. Sci.* **12,** 256 (1974).

3. Perchalski, R. J., and Wilder, B. J., Rapid gas–liquid determination of carbamazepine in plasma. *Clin. Chem.* **20,** 492 (1974).

CLIN. CHEM. 22/1, 32–38 (1976)

Simultaneous Determination of Five Sex Hormones in Human Serum by Radioimmunoassay after Chromatography on Lipidex-5000

D. Apter, O. Jänne, P. Karvonen, and R. Vihko

We describe a method for determination of pregnenolone, progesterone, 17α-hydroxyprogesterone, testosterone, and 5α-dihydrotestosterone in 1–2 ml of serum from male or female. Using microcolumns of Lipidex-5000 (hydroxyalkoxypropyl Sephadex, 0.5 g) and light petroleum/chloroform (97/3) as the solvent during chromatography, we resolved these five steroids into four fractions, with pregnenolone and 5α-dihydrotestosterone eluting together. By use of selected antibodies, the latter two steroids were also determined specifically. Use of microcolumns allowed minimization of solvent volumes and sample transfers. Consequently, blank values for all the five steroids were negligible. Lowest measureable concentrations (in ng/liter) were: pregnenolone 100, progesterone 25, 17α-hydroxyprogesterone 50, testosterone 25, and 5α-dihydrotestosterone 25. Intra-assay and inter-assay coefficients of variation ranged from 5 to 9% and 10 to 15%, respectively, for the five steroids. Serum concentrations of these steroids are given for women in the follicular and luteal phases of the menstrual cycle and for women on oral contraceptives of the combination type, as well as for normal men.

Additional Keyphrases: *diagnosis of endocrine disorders • Lipidex-5000 • column chromatography • reference values • sex-related differences*

The diagnosis of various endocrine disorders—such as congenital adrenal hyperplasia, hirsutism and virilism, and menstrual disorders, among others—significantly depends on steroid analyses. Recent achievements in the application of radioimmunological techniques to assays of serum steroid hormones are rapidly producing clinical chemical techniques for more accurate diagnosis of these disorders. Thus, it is now possible to develop specific, sensitive, and even rapid assays for the more clinically important steroids that were previously beyond detection owing to their minute concentrations in blood.

Department of Clinical Chemistry, University of Oulu, SF-90220 Oulu 22, Finland, and Steroid Research Laboratory, Department of Medical Chemistry, University of Helsinki, SF-00170 Helsinki 17, Finland.

Address correspondence to: Dr. R. Vihko, Department of Clinical Chemistry, University of Oulu, SF-90220 Oulu 22, Finland.

Received Sept. 26, 1975; accepted Oct. 3, 1975.

In this communication we wish to report a method for determination of serum pregnenolone, progesterone, 17α-hydroxyprogesterone, testosterone, and 5α-dihydrotestosterone. The potentially high separation capacity of a highly lipophilic Sephadex derivative, "Lipidex-5000" (hydroxyalkoxypropyl Sephadex), has been used to fractionate serum steroids before their radioimmunological measurement with antisera of carefully checked specificity. The method has already proved useful in the evaluation of abnormal testicular endocrine function (*1*), differential diagnosis of various forms of congenital adrenal hyperplasia (*2*) and for following hormonal changes during puberty (*3*). The present method is based on our previous method for determination of plasma testosterone, progesterone, and 17α-hydroxyprogesterone (*4*).

Materials and Methods

Materials

Solvents and reagents. Diethyl ether (analytical grade; Merck AG, Darmstadt, the Federal Republic of Germany) was twice distilled. Chloroform (Merck) was distilled, 10 ml of ethanol added per liter, and stored in a dark bottle. Light petroleum (BDH, Ltd., Poole, England) was distilled and the fraction boiling at 64–69 °C was used. Succinic anhydride (Fluka AG, Buchs SG, Switzerland), tributylamine (BDH), isobutylchloroformate (Sigma Chemical Co., St. Louis, Mo.), O-(carboxymethyl)-hydroxylamine (Pfalz and Bauer, Inc., Flushing, N. Y.), 2-ethoxy-6,9-diaminoacridine lactate (Rivanol; University Pharmacy, Helsinki, Finland) were used as supplied.

Glassware used in routine analysis was disposable.

Lipidex-5000 (hydroxylalkoxypropyl Sephadex) was either kindly donated by Mr. V. Tarkkanen, Packard-Becker, B.V., Chemical Operations, Groningen, The Netherlands, or prepared according to Ellingboe et al. (*5*), with Sephadex LH-20 (Pharmacia, Uppsala, Sweden) as the starting material.

Steroids and steroid derivatives. Nonlabeled steroids were obtained from Ikapharm, Ramat-Gan, Israel, or Steraloids, Inc., Pawling, N. Y., and were purified on Lipidex-5000 before use. [7-^{3}H]Pregnenolone (specific activity, 18 kCi/mol), [1,2,6,7-^{3}H]progesterone (82 kCi/mol), [1,2-^{3}H]-17α-hydroxyprogesterone (45 kCi/mol), [1,2,6,7-^{3}H]testosterone (87 kCi/mol), and [1,2-^{3}H]-5α-dihydrotestosterone (46 kCi/mol) were purchased from the Radiochemical Centre, Amersham, U. K. 5α-Dihydrotestosterone-17β-hemisuccinate was purchased from Steraloids Inc. and pregnenolone-20-carboxymethyl oxime prepared as described by Erlanger et al. (*6*). These steroid derivatives were linked to bovine serum albumin by the mixed anhydride method (*6*). The preparation of progesterone, 17α-hydroxyprogesterone, and testosterone antigens has been detailed previously (*4*).

Antisera. All the antisera were raised in rabbits. The immunization procedures were conducted as described previously (*4*). The equilibrium association constants of the antibodies were 6×10^9 and 3×10^9 liter/mol at +4 °C for 5α-dihydrotestosterone and pregnenolone, respectively, as measured from a Scatchard-type plot (*7*). Other steroid antisera were the same used previously (*4*). The antisera against 5α-dihydrotestosterone and pregnenolone were diluted 3000- and 1000-fold, respectively.

Material for analysis. Blood samples were drawn from apparently healthy women and men volunteers. Almost all were people working in our institutions. The samples were drawn, before noon, into glass tubes, allowed to clot, and then centrifuged. The serum was stored at −20 °C until analyzed.

Procedure

Extraction. Serum, 1–2 ml, was pipetted into a disposable glass tube (100 × 12 mm) and 3 ml of diethyl ether added. The tube was closed with a plastic stopper and shaken for 15 min in a three-dimensional mixer (Desaga, Heidelberg, the Federal Republic of Germany) in a horizontal position. After transfer of the organic phase into another test tube, the extraction was repeated. The combined ether phases were evaporated under nitrogen.

Chromatography equipment. The chromatography system (Figure 1) consisted of a 5-liter flask, 15 50-ml pipettes, and a corresponding number of chromatography columns. The 5-liter flask was placed slightly above the 50-ml pipettes and served as reservoir for the solvent (light petroleum/chloroform, 97/3 by vol). Lipidex-5000 columns were eluted with the aid of 100-cm hydrostatic pressure. Chromatography usually required about 3 h.

The connection tube from the 5-liter flask to the 50-ml pipette was joined to a disposable plastic tip. This arrangement (Figure 1) was better than a three-way stopcock, because there was no air leakage from hydrostatic pressure in the present construction. The connection tube was open during the washing period and closed during chromatography of the samples. Fifty-milliliter pipettes acted as solvent reservoirs for the chromatography columns. By use of their scale it was possible to follow the volume of the solvent eluted through the column. Consequently, disposable

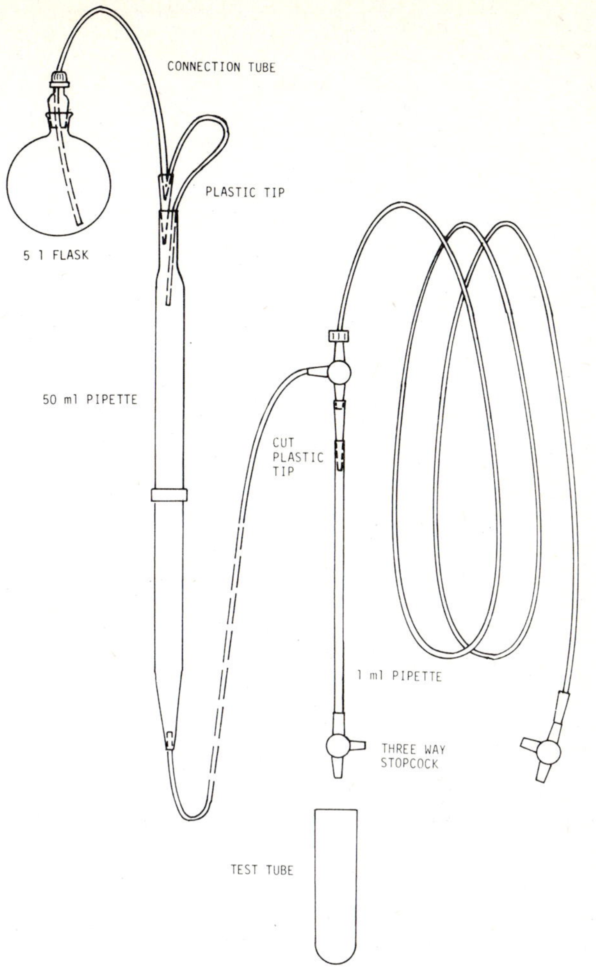

Fig. 1. Chromatography column setup for separation of plasma unconjugated neutral steroids on "Lipidex-5000"

test tubes without a volume scaling could be used for fraction collection. The elution profile was very reliable, because the total volume of solvent passing through the column could be monitored exactly.

The connection tube (VYGON Code 1155-10 Lectrocath, 100 cm; Vygon, BP7-95440, Ecouen, France) from the 50-ml pipette to the chromatography column was fitted tightly to the orifice of the 50-ml pipette.

With use of capillary columns and organic elution solvents, air bubbles forming in the tubes and connections during chromatography—and especially during washing procedures—created problems. These air bubbles easily passed into and air-locked the column. This problem was solved by connecting the top of the column to a blind end loop of Lectrocath (100 cm), which removed air bubbles during washing. The solvent evaporated through the wall of the tube and consequently, the solvent was slowly aspirated constantly into the loop together with any air bubbles. A small stopper was cut away from the three-way stopcocks (Pharmaseal, K-75 three-way stopcock; Pharmacia, Uppsala, Sweden) to allow the solvent to pass into both the column and loop at the same time.

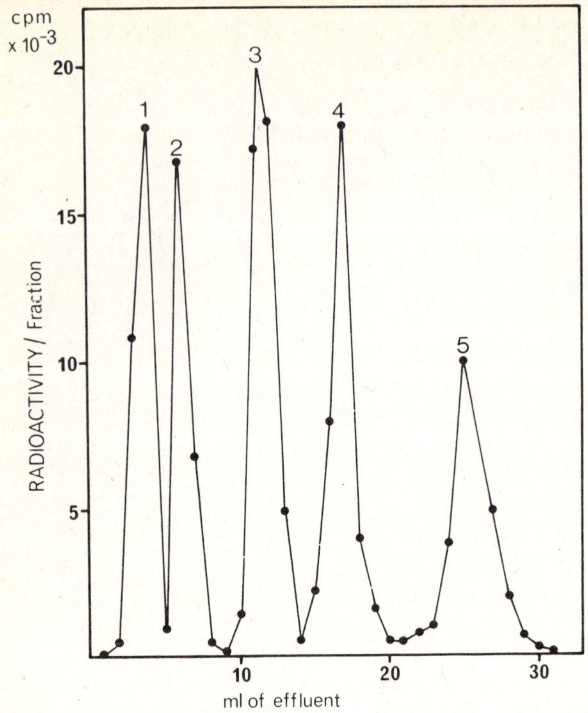

Fig. 2. Elution of progesterone (*1*), cholesterol (*2*), pregnenolone and 5α-dihydrotestosterone (*3*), testosterone (*4*), and 17α-hydroxyprogesterone (*5*) from a 0.5-g column (bed height 320 mm, internal diameter of the column 2.6 mm) of Lipidex-5000 in light petroleum/chloroform, 97/3 by vol

The chromatography columns used were small capillary columns made from conventional 1-ml pipettes and three-way stopcocks, which were fitted to the lower end of the pipette by forcing a gently prewarmed pipette into the stopcock.

The total length of the pipette/stopcock combination was 36 cm and the internal diameter of the pipette 2.6 mm. The column was filled with 0.5 g of Lipidex-5000 to give a bed height of 32 cm.

Lipidex-5000 chromatography. The dry residue after extraction was dissolved in two 0.2-ml portions of light petroleum/chloroform (97/3 by vol) and applied onto a Lipidex column packed in the same solvent. Progesterone was eluted between 2–5 ml; pregnenolone and 5α-dihydrotestosterone, 9–14 ml; testosterone, 14–21 ml; and 17α-hydroxyprogesterone, 21–30 ml of effluent (Figure 2). The fractions were evaporated under a stream of nitrogen and dissolved in 1 ml of ethanol in the same test tubes. The elution profile of each steroid was checked with radioactive tracers once a month.

Saturation analysis was performed as detailed previously (*4*). Bound and unbound radioactivities were separated by treatment with dextran-coated charcoal. The aliquots of the ethanol solution taken for the actual radioimmunological assay are given in Table 1.

Radioactivity was measured with an LKB-Wallac Model 81000 (Wallac, SF-20520 Turku 52, Finland) or Packard Tri-Carb (Packard Instrument Company, Inc., Downers Grove, Ill.) liquid-scintillation spectrometer. "Insta-Gel" (Packard) was used as the scintillation fluid and samples were counted for 10 min, or until a maximum of 10 000 counts had accumulated.

Table 1. Aliquots of Steroid Fractions after Lipidex-5000 Chromatography (Dissolved in 1 ml of Ethanol) Taken for Assay[a]

	Aliquot for assay, %	
Steroid	Females	Males
Pregnenolone	10, 20	10, 20
Progesterone	5[b], 10[b]; 1[c], 2[c]	5, 10
17α-Hydroxyprogesterone	5[b], 10[b]; 2[c], 5[c]	2, 5
Testosterone	5, 10	1, 2
5α-Dihydrotestosterone	10	10

[a] The volume of serum taken for extraction and Lipidex chromatography was 2.0 ml.
[b] Follicular phase.
[c] Luteal phase.

Calculation of the results. The standard curves were linearized by a logit plot method (*8*). In every series of analyses, a new standard curve was constructed by pipetting 0, 5, 20, 30, 50, 100, 200, 500, and 1000 pg samples of the steroid in question in duplicate into disposable polystyrene tubes and processing them identically with unknown samples. Figures 3 and 4 show the standard curves for the radioimmunoassay of pregnenolone and 5α-dihydrotestosterone, respectively.

Statistical procedures. Results from different groups were compared by means of Student's *t*-test or the Mann–Whitney U-test.

Results and Discussion

Our aim was to devise a radioimmunological method for the specific determination of clinically important steroid hormones by combining the high resolving power of hydroxyalkoxypropyl Sephadex (Lipidex-5000) with the use of selected antisera with carefully checked specificities. The current column chromatographic set-up has several advantages in comparison with our previous separation system (*4*). The use of longer capillary columns afforded better separation of the steroids (Figure 2, Table 2), and owing to the smaller bed volume of the column, individual steroids were recovered in less than a third of the volume of our previous method. This enabled us to take the sample through the entire fractionation procedure in a single disposable glass tube. The small solvent volumes also diminished possibly deleterious effects of solvent impurities in the final radioimmunoassay. The present construction lends itself easily to a simultaneous assay of a great number of serum samples (usually 15).

The properties of the antisera used in the determination of progesterone, 17α-hydroxyprogesterone,

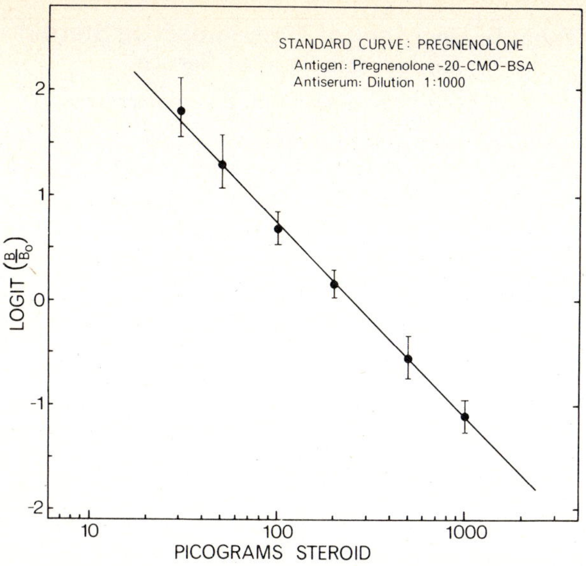

Fig. 3. Standard curve for radioimmunoassay of pregnenolone
Each point is the mean of five duplicate analyses, done during five months. The bars indicate ±2 SD

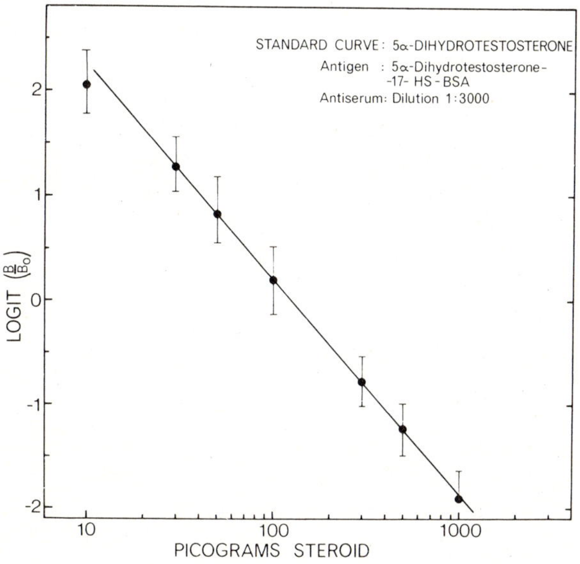

Fig. 4. Standard curve for radioimmunoassay of 5α-dihydrotestosterone
Each point is the mean of six duplicate analyses, done during five months. The bars indicate ±2 SD

and testosterone have been characterized and reported previously, along with the specificity obtained by our original methodology (*4*). With regard to the assay of these three steroids, the current method revealed identical properties with those of the previous system. The antiserum against pregnenolone-20-carboxymethyl oxime/bovine serum albumin displayed a slight cross reactivity with some 3β-hydroxy-5-ene steroids (Table 3). All compounds with this structure we tested—5-androstene-3β,17β-diol, dehydroepiandrosterone, and cholesterol—were excluded from the "pregnenolone" fraction on Lipidex chromatography (Table 2, Figure 2). Only 5α-dihydrotestosterone (1% cross-reactivity with pregnenolone antiserum) was eluted in the same fraction. Thus the available information indicates that the present method is highly specific for determination of serum pregnenolone.

One of the advantages of Lipidex-5000 chromatography is the complete separation of testosterone and 5α-dihydrotestosterone. The antiserum against 5α-dihydrotestosterone-17β-hemisuccinate/bovine

Table 2. Relative (to Progesterone) Elution Volumes of Some Steroids on Lipidex[a]

Compound	Elution volume
5β-Pregnane-3,20-dione	0.71
5α-Pregnane-3,20-dione	0.86
Progesterone	1.00
4-Androstene-3,17-dione	1.14
Cholesterol	1.50
Deoxycorticosterone	2.34
20β-Hydroxy-4-pregnen-3-one	2.43
20α-Hydroxy-4-pregnen-3-one	2.64
Pregnenolone	2.94
5α-Dihydrotestosterone	2.94
5β-Dihydrotestosterone	3.30
Dehydroepiandrosterone	3.69
Testosterone	4.25
Epitestosterone	4.29
17α-Hydroxyprogesterone	6.25
17α-Hydroxypregnenolone	20.00
5α-Androstane-3α,17β-diol	>12
5α-Androstane-3β,17β-diol	>12
5-Androstene-3β,17β-diol	>12
Aldosterone	>20
Cortisol	>20

[a] Column length, 36 cm; internal diameter, 2.6 mm; bed height, 32 cm; dry Lipidex weight, 0.5 g. Solvent: light petroleum (bp 64–69 °C)—chloroform, 97/3 by vol.

Table 3. Relative Affinity of the Antiserum to Pregnenolone-20-carboxymethyl oxime/ Bovine Serum Albumin for Some Steroid Ligands

Steroid	Relative affinity
Pregnenolone	1.00
Dehydroepiandrosterone	0.034
5-Androstene-3β,17β-diol	0.14
5α-Dihydrotestosterone	0.011[a]
Testosterone	0.000070
20α-Hydroxy-4-pregnen-3-one	0.00068
20β-Hydroxy-4-pregnen-3-one	0.0031
Progesterone	0.0060
17α-Hydroxyprogesterone	<0.0034
Cortisol	≪0.00034
Cholesterol	0.0024

[a] Eluted in the "Pregnenolone fraction" on Lipidex.

Table 4. Relative Affinity of the Antiserum to 5α-Dihydrotestosterone-17β-hemisuccinate-BSA for Some Steroid Ligands

Steroid	Relative affinity
5α-Dihydrotestosterone	1.00
Testosterone	0.125
Epitestosterone	0.14
4-Androstene-3,17-dione	0.125
5α-Androstane-3α,17β-diol	0.0033
5α-Androstane-3β,17β-diol	0.022
5-Androstene-3β,17β-diol	0.0042
Pregnenolone	0.0019[a]
Progesterone	0.033
17α-Hydroxyprogesterone	0.0024
Deoxycorticosterone	0.030
Cortisol	0.00013
Cholesterol	0.0005

[a] Eluted in the "5α-Dihydrotestosterone fraction" on Lipidex.

Table 5. Recovery of Nonradioactive Steroids Added to a Pool of Serum[a]

Steroid	Concn, µg/liter		No. analyses	Recovery		CV, %
	Original	Added		ng	%	
Pregnenolone	1.81	—	10	—	—	6.1
		1.5	10	1.29	86	5.2
		3.0	10	2.55	85	7.8
Progesterone	0.74	—	10	—	—	5.9
		0.5	10	0.41	83	6.3
		1.0	10	0.89	89	6.2
17α-Hydroxyprogesterone	0.66	—	10	—	—	6.3
		0.5	10	0.51	102	7.6
		1.0	10	0.86	86	7.8
Testosterone	2.36	—	10	—	—	5.2
		1.0	10	0.94	94	5.5
		2.0	10	1.76	88	6.2
5α-Dihydrotestosterone	0.56	—	10	—	—	7.3
		0.5	10	0.41	83	8.5
		1.0	10	0.76	76	7.1

[a] A mixed pool of serum from men and women. The five steroids were added into samples of this pool, 2-ml aliquots from each sample were analyzed in the same series.

serum albumin gave a 12–14% cross-reaction with testosterone, epitestosterone, and 4-androstene-3,17-dione (Table 4). All these compounds were excluded from the "5α-dihydrotestosterone" fraction during the chromatography. 5α-Dihydrotestosterone and pregnenolone were eluted together; however, the latter cross-reacted only slightly (0.19%, Table 4) with the antiserum against 5α-dihydrotestosterone-17β-hemisuccinate/bovine serum albumin. Therefore, the 5α-dihydrotestosterone determination also seems to be highly specific.

The precision of the method was investigated by repeated analyses of the five steroids from pools of human serum. The intra-assay coefficient of variation was 5–9% (Table 5). The inter-assay coefficient of variation, computed from results accumulated over four months, ranged from 10 to 15% for all five steroids.

The accuracy of the method was evaluated by recovery experiments. Known amounts of nonradioactive steroids were added to a pool of serum and the recovery of the compounds added was measured. Depending on the steroid in question, the recovery varied from 76 to 102% (Table 5). The amounts added covered a wide concentration range (Tables 5 and 6). The inter-assay coefficient of variation in the recovery experiments was 5–9%.

The sensitivity and blank values in the determination of progesterone, 17α-hydroxyprogesterone, and testosterone have been reported previously for our original method (*4*). Similar or increased sensitivity was obtained with the present method without increased blank problems. This can be accounted for by the smaller solvent volumes needed and fewer transfers of the eluates. On taking 2-ml aliquots of quartz-distilled water through the entire procedure and using the largest aliquots shown in Table 1, we found the blank values for all the five steroids to be negligible. When 2-ml samples of serum were taken for the extraction, the lowest measurable values (in ng/liter) were as follows: pregnenolone, 100; progesterone, 25; 17α-hydroxyprogesterone, 50; testosterone, 25; and 5α-dihydrotestosterone, 25.

Concentrations of the five steroids in serum were determined in groups of young women and men (Table 6). The concentrations of progesterone, 17α-hydroxyprogesterone, and testosterone have been discussed exhaustively recently in connection with the description of our previous assay method (*4*). In spite of the fact that different groups of people were studied here, the present method gave similar values for these three steroids, which are therefore not discussed further here (Table 6). With regard to 5α-dihydrotestosterone, a number of reports have appeared in recent years on its concentration in the serum of normal women and men (*9–13*). In these studies, either competitive protein binding or radioimmunoassay has been used as the final assay technique. There is a considerable variation in the values reported in different studies, at least partly because of the small number of subjects investigated in each study referred to, and because the interindividual variation in serum 5α-dihydrotestosterone concentration is large (Table 6), as is the case with many other steroid hormones in blood. Our values for males are very similar to those published by Ito and Horton (*9*), Barberia and Thorneycroft (*11*), and Purvis et al. (*13*), but are considerably lower than those published by Coyotupa et al. (*10*) and higher than those by Bauminger et al. (*12*). The values for

Table 6. Mean Serum Steroid Concentrations in Groups of Normal Women and Men

Steroid	Women: Follicular	Women: Luteal	Women: Oral contraceptives	Men
	μg/liter			
Pregnenolone				
Mean ± SD	1.18 ± 0.60	1.89 ± 0.79	1.00 ± 0.77	1.56 ± 0.81
Range	0.27 – 1.97	0.56 – 2.94	0.32 – 2.57	0.43 – 3.58
n[a] (age)[b]	11 (20–32)	9 (20–31)	8 (20–28)	22 (19–35)
Progesterone				
Mean ± SD	0.20 ± 0.080	3.77 ± 4.05	0.19 ± 0.10	0.24 ± 0.17
Range	0.074 – 0.33	0.38 – 11.17	0.075 – 0.33	0.101 – 0.57
n (age)	11 (20–32)	9 (20–31)	8 (20–28)	14 (19–35)
17α-Hydroxyprogesterone				
Mean ± SD	0.43 ± 0.24	1.04 ± 0.67	0.13 ± 0.034	0.97 ± 0.64
Range	0.15 – 0.94	0.36 – 2.28	0.079 – 0.16	0.40 – 3.26
n (age)	8 (20–25)	8 (20–31)	8 (20–28)	26 (19–35)
Testosterone				
Mean ± SD	0.26 ± 0.15	0.40 ± 0.19	0.17 ± 0.15	4.62 ± 1.99
Range	0.090 – 0.51	0.18 – 0.74	0.027 – 0.51	1.67 – 10.89
n (age)	11 (20–32)	10 (20–31)	8 (20–28)	22 (19–35)
5α-Dihydrotestosterone				
Mean ± SD	0.19 ± 0.082	0.29 ± 0.092	0.23 ± 0.15	0.65 ± 0.24
Range	0.074 – 0.35	0.11 – 0.44	0.037 – 0.45	0.30 – 1.30
n (age)	11 (20–32)	10 (20–31)	8 (20–28)	22 (19–35)

[a] n = no. subjects in the group.
[b] Age (y).

females are very similar in the different reports, including our own. The difference in serum 5α-dihydrotestosterone concentration between males and females (Table 6) is highly significant ($P < 0.001$). The ratio of testosterone to 5α-dihydrotestosterone is much lower in serum from females than from males, being 1.4 and 5.2, respectively. Moreover, the concentration of 5α-dihydrotestosterone in serum is significantly ($P < 0.05$) higher in the luteal than in the follicular phase of the menstrual cycle. This is analogous to serum testosterone concentrations in the female (*4*), and might reflect a secretion of 5α-dihydrotestosterone by the corpus luteum or an increased formation of its precursor, testosterone, during the latter half of the menstrual cycle.

Unconjugated pregnenolone has also been included in recent years among the serum steroids that can be measured (*13–17*). Concentration values published by various authors are in reasonable agreement. Along with a quite recent report by Purvis et al. (*13*), our values for serum pregnenolone in men belong to the highest published, whereas the values for women are very similar to those of other reports. In this series, the luteal serum pregnenolone concentration was significantly ($P < 0.05$) higher than the follicular one, as also reported by Bermudez et al. (*14*) and Abraham et al. (*17*).

There was no significant sex-related difference in the concentration of serum pregnenolone (Table 6). In both sexes, at least part of the pregnenolone originates from the adrenal cortex (*14, 18*). Part of the pregnenolone in the blood of males is of testicular origin (*19*). The presence of comparable amounts of pregnenolone in women's serum before ovulation suggests that the secretion of this steroid also takes place from follicular ovaries. This accords with a previous finding indicating that a very early response, occurring before ovulation, to human menopausal gonadotrophin administration in hypophysectomized women is an increase in plasma pregnenolone and 5-pregnene-3β,20α-diol sulfates (*20*). An enhanced ovarian secretion of this progesterone precursor takes place from the corpus luteum, as indicated by the increased concentration of pregnenolone in the serum during the luteal phase (Table 6). This is further supported by the fact that in women on oral contraceptives of the combination type, the serum pregnenolone concentration is significantly lower than during the luteal phase of the cycle (Table 6).

One technician can analyze all the five steroids from two series of 15 unknown samples along with appropriate controls (low-medium-high control sera and zero samples) in a five-day working period. Thus the current method enables measurement of pregnenolone, progesterone, 17α-hydroxyprogesterone, testosterone, and 5α-dihydrotestosterone in a small (1–2 ml) serum sample with only one chromatographic step. Moreover, Lipidex-5000 columns can be used repeatedly over a period of at least several months if they are washed for 8 h between subsequent runs. The use of antisera with a carefully checked specificity has further increased the reliability of the assays, which have already proved useful in the evaluation of clinical (*1, 2*) and physiological problems (*3*).

The skillful technical assistance of Mrs. Salme Ollikainen and Mrs. Marjatta Tevilin is gratefully acknowledged. This investigation was supported by a grant from the Ford Foundation.

References

1. Jänne, O., Perheentupa, J., Viinikka, L., and Vihko, R., Testicular endocrine function in a pubertal boy with 3β-hydroxysteroid dehydrogenase deficiency. *J. Clin. Endocrinol.* **39,** 206 (1974).

2. Jänne, O., Perheentupa, J., Viinikka, L., and Vihko, R., Plasma pregnenolone, progesterone, 17-hydroxyprogesterone, testosterone and 5α-dihydrotestosterone in different types of congenital adrenal hyperplasia. *Clin. Endocrinol.* **4,** 39 (1975).

3. Apter, D., and Vihko, R., Hormonal changes in puberty: Serum pregnenolone, progesterone, 17-hydroxyprogesterone, testosterone, and 5α-dihydrotestosterone in maturing girls. *Acta Endocrinol.* (Copenhagen) *Suppl. 199,* 122 (1975).

4. Jänne, O., Apter, D., and Vihko, R., Assay of testosterone, progesterone and 17α-hydroxyprogesterone in human plasma by radioimmunoassay after separation on hydroxyalkoxypropyl Sephadex. *J. Steroid Biochem.* **5,** 155 (1974).

5. Ellingboe, J., Nyström, E., and Sjövall, J., Liquid-gel chromatography on lipophilic-hydrophobic Sephadex derivatives. *J. Lipid Res.* **11,** 266 (1970).

6. Erlanger, B. F., Borek, F., Beiser, S. M., and Lieberman, S., Steroid protein conjugates I. Preparation and characterization of conjugates of bovine serum albumin with testosterone and with cortisone. *J. Biol. Chem.* **228,** 713 (1957).

7. Scatchard, G., The attractions of proteins for small molecules and ions. *Ann. N.Y. Acad. Sci.* **51,** 660 (1949).

8. Rodbard, D., and Lewald, J. E., Computer analysis of radioligand assay and radioimmunoassay data. In *Steroid Assay by Protein Binding,* E. Diczfalusy, Ed. Karolinska Institutet, Stockholm, 1970, pp 79–103.

9. Ito, T., and Horton, R., Dihydrotestosterone in human peripheral plasma. *J. Clin. Endocrinol.* **31,** 362 (1970).

10. Coyotupa, J., Parlow, A. F., and Abraham, G. E., Simultaneous radioimmunoassay of plasma testosterone and dihydrotestosterone. *Anal. Lett.* **5,** 329 (1972).

11. Barberia, J. M., and Thorneycroft, I. H., Simultaneous radioimmunoassay of testosterone and dihydrotestosterone. *Steroids* **23,** 757 (1974).

12. Bauminger, S., Kohen, F., Lindner, H. R., and Weinstein, A., Antiserum to 5α-dihydrotestosterone: Production, characterization and use in radioimmunoassay. *Steroids* **24,** 477 (1974).

13. Purvis, K., Brenner, P. F., Landgren, B.-M., Cekan, Z., and Diczfalusy, E., Indices of gonadal function in the human male I. Plasma levels of unconjugated steroids and gonadotrophins under normal and pathological conditions. *Clin. Endocrinol.* **4,** 237 (1975).

14. Bermudez, J. A., Doerr, P., and Lipsett, M. B., Measurement of pregnenolone in blood. *Steroids* **16,** 505 (1970).

15. DiPietro, D. L., Brown, P. D., and Strott, C. A., A pregnenolone radioimmunoassay utilizing a new fractionation technique for sheep antiserum. *J. Clin. Endocrinol.* **35,** 729 (1972).

16. Abraham, G. E., Buster, J. E., Kyle, F. W., et al., Radioimmunoassay of plasma pregnenolone. *J. Clin. Endocrinol.* **37,** 40 (1973).

17. Abraham, G. E., Buster, J. E., Kyle, F. W., et al., Radioimmunoassay of plasma pregnenolone, 17-hydroxypregnenolone, and dehydroepiandrosterone under various physiological conditions. *J. Clin. Endocrinol.* **37,** 140 (1973).

18. Jänne, O., Luukkainen, T., and Vihko, R., Solvolyzable steroid conjugates in human plasma after metyrapone administration. *Eur. J. Steroids* **2,** 457 (1967).

19. Vihko, R., and Ruokonen, A., Regulation of steroidogenesis in testis. *J. Steroid Biochem.* **5,** 843 (1974).

20. Luukkainen, T., Adlercreutz, H., Vihko, R., and Bettendorf, G., Plasma and urinary steroids in hypophysectomized women during treatment with gonadotrophins. In *Clinical Application of Human Gonadotrophins,* G. Bettendorf and V. Insler, Eds. Georg Thieme, Stuttgart, 1970, pp 134–149.

CLIN. CHEM. 22/1, 39-41 (1976)

Effect of Time and Temperature on Blood P_{50} and 2,3-Diphosphoglycerate Measurements

Stanley Hellerstein and Tasanaporn Bunthrarungroj

The oxygen affinity of hemoglobin is affected by various factors, including blood pH and erythrocyte 2,3-diphosphoglycerate. The latter and blood P_{50} values are unchanged when aliquots of blood from normal individuals are permitted to stand at room temperature for as long as 7 h. Our data also show that equilibration in a 37 °C tonometer for times ranging from 0.5 to 1.5 h causes no detectable alterations in P_{50} values.

Additional Keyphrases: *oxygen-dissociation curve* • p_{O_2} • *blood gases*

Measurements of the affinity of hemoglobin for oxygen and of erythrocyte 2,3-diphosphoglycerate concentrations are being done with increased frequency. Because the oxygen affinity of hemoglobin is affected by a variety of factors such as temperature, hydrogen-ion activity, ambient p_{CO_2}, and carbon monoxide and salt concentration, certain technical precautions are recommended to prevent factitious alterations in the oxygen-dissociation curve for hemoglobin. Erythrocyte 2,3-diphosphoglycerate concentrations are altered by changes in blood pH and erythrocyte metabolism, so analytical methods usually stipulate that the blood should be diluted for assay within 5 min or stored in an ice bath for no longer than 2 h (*1-3*).

The points for plotting the oxygen-dissociation curve are commonly located by measuring the p_{O_2} of whole blood and the oxygen saturation of hemoglobin after equilibrating the blood sample with various gas mixtures, at a constant temperature (37 °C) and a fixed ambient p_{CO_2} of about 4.30 kPa (40 mmHg). Changes in hemoglobin and salt concentrations caused by evaporation or condensation are prevented by keeping the humidifier at the same temperature as the tonometer (*4*). The pH of whole blood at 37 °C is measured so that the effective p_{O_2} at a pH of 7.40 can be derived for plotting the oxygen-dissociation curve for hemoglobin.

The Children's Mercy Hospital, 24th at Gillham Rd., Kansas City, Mo. 64108; and the University of Missouri-Kansas City, School of Medicine. Kansas City, Mo. 64108.

Received Aug. 4, 1975; accepted Oct. 6, 1975.

While setting up our procedures for measurement of whole blood P_{50}[1] and erythrocyte 2,3-diphosphoglycerate concentration, we became concerned that alterations in blood samples might arise because of variations in the time required for tonometry. Even after our technicians had become proficient with the equipment, the equilibration time required for determination of a satisfactory P_{50} value varied from 30 to 60 min. (A satisfactory run was defined as three points, more or less equally distributed over the oxyhemoglobin range of 35% to 65%, which defined a line parallel to the normal oxygen-dissociation curve for hemoglobin.) It seemed likely that ongoing metabolic processes in the blood samples might cause the observed P_{50} values to vary while the blood was equilibrating in a 37 °C tonometer. In addition to this technical time variable, we have found it difficult to collect and begin processing blood samples from patients in the clinics or on wards within a fixed time interval, such as within 30 min of drawing the blood.

For these reasons we decided to see how our results would be affected if blood samples were allowed to stand for various times before starting tonometry. In addition, we planned to record the time involved in equilibrating blood for each P_{50} determination in order to evaluate the effect of this variable on the observed P_{50} values.

Materials and Methods

Two sets of experiments were done on blood from eight adult volunteers. About 50 ml of blood were collected in heparinized Vacutainer tubes of 7-ml capacity. In the first four experiments, one sample was run as soon as the blood was drawn, three samples were kept at room temperature, and three samples were kept in the refrigerator. The blood samples at room temperature and those refrigerated were used alternately for measurement of 2,3-diphosphoglycerate and P_{50} values. Aliquots of blood were taken for 2,3-

[1] The P_{50} value serves as a reference point for the location of the oxygen-dissociation curve for hemoglobin. It refers to the partial pressure of oxygen at which hemoglobin is 50% saturated.

Table 1. P_{50} and 2,3-Diphosphoglycerate Measurements

	S.H., ♂, 48-y				J.N., ♀, 51-y				M.K., ♀, 27-y				V.B., ♀, 43-y			
	Time: Since blood was drawn	Time: For doing the P_{50}			Time: Since blood was drawn	Time: For doing the P_{50}			Time: Since blood was drawn	Time: For doing the P_{50}			Time: Since blood was drawn	Time: For doing the P_{50}		
Temp	h	m	P_{50}[a]	2,3, DPG[b]	h	m	P_{50}[a]	2,3-DPG[b]	h	m	P_{50}[a]	2,3-DPG[b]	h	m	P_{50}[a]	2,3-DPG[b]
Room	0	60	27.6	13.5	0	80	25.9	10.2	0	70	28.6	12.4	0	43	27.2	13.1
Room	2	60	27.8	15.0	1½	65	25.5	10.3	1¼	60	28.4	12.4	¾	48	27.4	14.8
Refrig	3	45	29.2	13.1	2½	45	26.3	11.0	2¼	45	28.5	13.4	¾	50	27.6	13.3
Room	5	35	27.3	14.1	3½	35	25.1	10.3	3¼	45	28.4	12.3	2½	47	27.5	13.9
Refrig	5½	35	28.2	14.1	5	30	25.4	8.9	5	35	28.3	14.9	3¼	43	27.8	14.1
Room	6	45	27.8	12.9	5½	65	25.4	9.9	5¾	35	28.8	12.6	5	35	27.3	14.5
Refrig	7	40	27.9	14.3	6½	45	24.9	9.7	6¼	40	28.5	13.6	5¾	55	25.8	14.0
Mean			27.9	13.9			25.5	10.1			28.5	13.1			27.2	14.0
SD			0.6	0.7			0.4	0.6			0.2	0.9			0.6	0.6

	E.K., ♀, 32-y				P.H., ♀, 32-y				B.A., ♀, 46-y				A.Z., ♂, 29-y			
Temp	h	m	P_{50}[a]	2,3-DPG[b]	h	m	P_{50}[a]	2,3-DPG[b]	h	m	P_{50}[a]	2,3-DPG[b]	h	m	P_{50}[a]	2,3-DPG[b]
Room	0	63	26.8	14.9	0	100	27.4	14.7	0	48	27.0	15.5	0	84	27.3	13.6
Room	1	64	26.8	15.8	1	38	27.6	16.1	1	38	27.0	15.2	1½	46	27.6	12.8
Room	2¼	45	27.0	15.2	2¾	39	26.8	15.5	1¾	39	26.8	14.8	2¼	41	27.6	12.5
Room	3	49	27.1	14.2	3½	45	27.7	15.6	2½	39	27.1	15.1	3	46	27.4	12.0
Room	5	43	27.0	14.0	5	42	27.2	15.5	3¼	38	26.8	15.2	4¾	49	26.8	13.1
Room	5¾	37	27.0	14.9	5¾	45	27.8	15.8	5	37	27.3	15.5	5¾	43	27.8	13.2
Room	6½	42	27.4	14.6	6½	38	27.5	15.9	6	37	26.8	15.0	6¾	42	27.3	12.3
Mean			27.0	14.8			27.4	15.6			27.0	15.2			27.4	12.8
SD			0.2	0.6			0.3	0.4			0.2	0.2			0.3	0.5

[a] P_{50}: mmHg at 37 °C, pH = 7.40; 1 mmHg ≈ 133 Pa.
[b] 2,3-DPG: µmol/g of hemoglobin.

diphosphoglycerate determinations at the beginning of each P_{50} determination, and the time that a study was begun and completed was recorded. Data from the first four experiments showed that refrigeration of the sample did not alter the results, so in the last four studies all seven samples were permitted to remain at room temperature.

Erythrocyte 2,3-diphosphoglycerate was measured by the method of Keitt (5), with kit No. 35-UV (Sigma Chemical Co., St. Louis, Mo. 63178) used according to instructions given in their bulletin (6). The change in absorbance when NADH was oxidized to NAD^+ was measured in a Beckman DU Spectrophotometer. The P_{50} values were determined by means of a Blood Gas Analyzer, Gas Mixing System, Tonometer and Co-oximeter (IL 217 Blood Gas System; Instrumentation Laboratory, Inc., Lexington, Mass. 02173). An Instrumentation Laboratory p_{O_2}/pH Nomogram (25151) was used to correct the observed p_{O_2} values to the p_{O_2} at pH 7.40. The P_{50} values were derived from a line through three points parallel to the normal hemoglobin-oxygen-dissociation curve. More than three points were often measured because our criteria for a satisfactory run included the constraint that the three points should be more or less equally distributed over the oxyhemoglobin range of 35% to 65%.

Results

Table 1 gives the data we obtained. The normal range for P_{50} in our laboratory for adult men and women is 3.62 ± 0.93 kPa (27.2 ± 0.7 mmHg) (n = 21, pH = 7.40, T = 37 °C). In the same group, the range for 2,3-diphosphoglycerate is 14.0 ± 1.5 µmol/g of hemoglobin. Except for J.N., a 51-year-old woman who takes 250 mg of methyldopa (Aldomet, Merck Sharp & Dohme) and 0.2 mg of sodium levothyroxine (Synthroid, Flint) per day, the observed mean values for P_{50} and 2,3-diphosphoglycerate among the experimental subjects were within two standard deviations of our normal values.

As the data in Table 1 show, permitting blood to stand for as long as 7 h before starting the analyses resulted in no consistent or significant alteration in either the P_{50} or the 2,3-diphosphoglycerate values. No ice baths were used and refrigeration appeared to make no difference. With two exceptions, the observed values for P_{50} on each subject were within two standard deviations of the mean of the seven determinations done on each subject. The standard deviations of the mean values for the repeated P_{50} determinations were all less than 0.93 kPa (0.7 mmHg), the standard deviation of the mean value in our normal group. Both of the deviant P_{50} values are included in Table 1: the 3-h refrigerated specimen from S.H., and the 5.7-h refrigerated specimen from V.B. Only one of the 2,3-diphosphoglycerate determinations deviated more than two standard deviations from the mean value observed on a single subject. This was the initial value on the blood from subject P.H. (Table 1). The zero-time value was 14.7 μmol/g of hemoglobin and the mean value for the seven determinations was 15.6 ± 0.4 μmol/g. As noted for the P_{50} values, the standard deviations of the mean values for the repeated determinations of 2,3-diphosphoglycerate on each subject were all less than the 1.5 μmol/g standard deviation for the control group.

Duration of tonometry for a P_{50} determination ranged from 30 to 100 min. In a single subject the greatest range was 38 min to 100 min (subject P.H., Table 1). There is no evidence that these variations in equilibration time caused alterations in the observed values for P_{50}.

Discussion

We conclude that there are no significant alterations in P_{50} or erythrocyte 2,3-diphosphoglycerate when blood is permitted to stand, before analysis, at room temperature for periods ranging from 1 to 7 h. The apparent stability of the 2,3-diphosphoglycerate surprised us, because the literature on methodology suggests that analysis should be started promptly or that the blood samples should be chilled in an ice bath until the determination is begun (*2, 3, 6*). The anticipated changes in the oxyhemoglobin dissociation curve were not observed, presumably because erythrocyte organic phosphates were essentially stable during the period of observation (*1*). Of greatest interest and importance are the data showing that the metabolic activities in erythrocytes during equilibration periods varying from 0.5 to 1.5 h do not detectably alter P_{50} values.

We wish to recognize the fine technical assistance of Mrs. Sylvia DiMaggio and Mrs. L. Jean Nicolaisen, and the excellent secretarial help of Mrs. Vivian Brown.

References

1. Duhm, J., Effects of 2,3-diphosphoglycerate and other organic phosphate compounds on oxygen affinity and intracellular pH of human erythrocytes. *Pflügers Arch.* **326,** 341 (1971).

2. Teunissen, A. J., de Leeuw, R. J. M., Boink, A. B. T. J., et al., Comparison of five methods for determination of 2,3-diphosphoglycerate in blood. *Clin. Chem.* **20,** 649 (1974).

3. Atkinson, K. F., Modified automated determination of 2,3-diphosphoglycerate in whole blood. *Clin. Chem.* **18,** 1001 (1972).

4. Torrance, J. D., and Lenfant, C., Methods for determination of O_2 dissociation curves, including Bohr effect. *Respir. Physiol.* **8,** 127 (1969/70).

5. Keitt, A. S., Reduced nicotinamide adenine dinucleotide-linked analysis of 2,3-diphosphoglyceric acid: Spectrophotometric and fluorometric procedures. *J. Lab. Clin. Med.* **77,** 470 (1971).

6. The ultraviolet determination of 2,3-diphosphoglyceric acid in blood at 340 mμ. *Tentative Tech. Bull. No. 35-UV.* Sigma Chemical Co., St. Louis, Mo., 1971.

Quantitative Fractionation of Alkaline Phosphatase Isoenzymes According to Their Thermostability

Claude PetitClerc

Continuous monitoring of heat denaturation of a mixture of alkaline phosphatase isoenzymes at 60 °C and pH 7.5 permits the simultaneous direct identification and quantitation of three isoenzymes: the placental isoenzyme, the L-phenylalanine-sensitive intestinal isoenzyme, and the liver isoenzyme (hepatocytic). The isoenzyme that is principally of bone origin cannot be identified as such without the help of other diagnostic aids and the patient's medical history. All human tissues contain alkaline phosphatase, many organs more than one of the isoenzymes. Liver alkaline phosphatase, which constitutes 40–50% of normal serum alkaline phosphatase activity, was measured in the serum of persons with various liver diseases. Its activity exceeded normal in all types of liver disease; in 80% of cases this increase was accompanied by increased γ-glutamyltransferase activity, but the quantitative correlationship (r = 0.54) was not as good as expected if both enzymes come from the same source and are indices of liver diseases. Liver alkaline phosphatase activity increases in the blood early in liver disease, before most liver tests show abnormalities. The other major isoenzyme of normal serum probably represents a mixture of isoenzymes from bone and reticulo-endothelial and vascular tissues, which all contain the same "very heat-labile" alkaline phosphatase. Cord blood and children's sera contain mostly this very heat-labile isoenzyme.

Additional Keyphrases: *continuous-flow analysis • liver disease • values for cord blood, pregnancy, children, adults • anatomical sources of enzymes • diagnostic aid • γ-glutamyltransferase*

Since the published work of Posen et al. (*1*) on differentiation of alkaline phosphatase (ALP; EC 3.1.3.1) isoenzymes according to their thermostability, many attempts to improve this approach have been proposed (*2–6*). In almost all instances, temperature and incubation time were critical to accuracy and reproducibility. Moreover, such thermofractionation is used to qualitatively assess increased ALP activity in the serum of patients suffering from liver or bone disease.

Department of Biochemistry, Medical School, University of Sherbrooke, Sherbrooke, Canada J1H 5N4.

Current address: Division of Clinical Chemistry, Centre Hospitalier Universitaire, Université de Sherbrooke, Sherbrooke, Canada J1H 5N4.

Presented in part at the scientific sessions of the 26th national meeting of the AACC, Las Vegas, Nev., Aug. 19–23, 1974.

Received July 21, 1975; accepted Oct. 6, 1975.

We describe in this paper a quantitative thermofractionation method that can be used to determine the activities of some ALP isoenzymes in both normal and pathological sera.

Materials and Methods

Analytical Principles

Under a given set of conditions, isoenzymes of different thermostability are denatured at different rates and independently of each other in a mixture. Continuous monitoring of heat denaturation of a mixture of ALP isoenzymes produces a curve that describes the variation of residual activity as a function of time. This curve is in fact a sum of exponentials

$$y = C_1 e^{-k_1 t} + C_2 e^{-k_2 t} + C_n e^{-k_n t} \qquad (1)$$

If three groups of isoenzymes with quite different heat stability are present—very unstable, unstable, and stable—one can easily calculate graphically C_1, C_2, and C_3, and k_1, k_2, and k_3. First or pseudo-first-order processes give straight lines on semilog graphs. The slopes of such graphs give the rate constants and the intercepts at t = 0 give the relative amount of each component in a mixture. The isoenzymes are characterized by the rate constant of denaturation and quantitated by the intercepts on the y axis at t = 0.

The stable component in a mixture of three will have k = 0, reducing equation 1 to

$$y = C_1 e^{-k_1 t} + C_2 e^{-k_2 t} + C_3 \qquad (2)$$

where C_3 = relative concentration of the stable component.

At any time, the residual activity is expressed as a percentage of the original activity by the following:

y = % residual activity = $[(A_t - A\ \ )/(A_0 - A\ \ )] \times 100$
A_t = activity at time t
A_0 = activity at time 0
A = activity at infinite (baseline or stable ALP isoenzyme)

The percentages of residual activity are plotted on a two-cycle semilogarithmic graph as a function of time. Because the more stable enzyme is denatured last, the plot will yield a straight line according to

$$\ln y = -k_2 t + \ln C_2 \qquad (3)$$

where k_2 = slope and C_2 = intercepts on the y axis, in percentage.

$$k_2 = \frac{\ln \%t_1 - \ln \%t_2}{t_2 - t_1}$$

C_2 is found directly from the graph.

As expected, the first part of the graph does not yield a straight line as a function of time. The first exponential can be simply obtained by subtracting, on the graph, the extrapolated straight line (equation 3) from the nonlinear portion of the curve. One will obtain the first exponential, described by

$$\ln y = -k_1 t + \ln C_1 \qquad (4)$$

C_1 is obtained directly from the graph as for C_2.

Because the serum sample cannot reach the desired temperature within seconds, one will find a short time lag before the rate of denaturation is maximal. This will cause the intercepts values of C_1 and C_2 to be higher than they should be. Since C_1 and C_2 should add up to 100%, the true value of C_1 and C_2 are obtained from the apparent C_1 and C_2, according to the ratio: C_1 or C_2 divided by $(C_1 + C_2)_{app.}$.

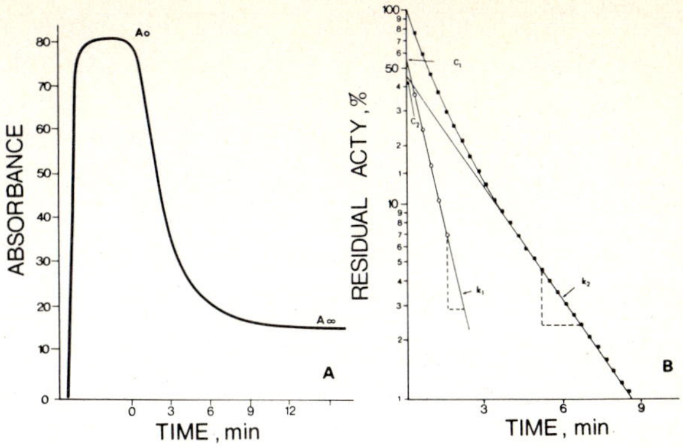

Fig. 2. *A*, Heat-denaturation curve, $[(A_t - A_\infty)/(A_0 - A_\infty)] \times 100 = y = C_1 e^{-k_1 t} + C_2 e^{-k_2 t}$, as it appears on recorder chart

A_0 and A_∞ represent ALP activity before and after denaturation. The difference between the plateaus is a measure of the amount of denaturable ALP activity. Experiments were run at 60 °C in phosphate buffer (20 mmol/liter, pH 7.5) containing NaCl (0.15 mol/liter) and $MgCl_2$ (5 mmol/liter)

B, Semilog graphical representation of percent residual activity, showing the two components of normal serum seen as two curves of different slope

The nonlinear portion is due to simultaneous denaturation of both components at the beginning. The curves are given in $\ln y = -k_1 t + \ln C_1$ and $\ln y = -k_2 t + \ln C_2$ where the slopes k_1 and k_2 are first-order rate constants. C_1 and C_2 are the relative concentrations of each in the mixture (see *Analytical Principles*) obtained directly from the graph, in % of the mixture

Apparatus

The continuous-flow system (Figure 1) for the AutoAnalyzer II (Technicon Instruments Corp., Tarrytown, N. Y. 10591) consists of the following modules: (*a*) circulating water bath with variable temperature control; (*b*) a proportioning pump; (*c*) one modified AutoAnalyzer II alkaline phosphatase cartridge with a 61-cm dialyzer instead of the usual 15.3-cm; (*d*) two AutoAnalyzer II heating blocks (37 °C); (*e*) an AutoAnalyzer II colorimeter; (*f*) a one-pen recorder; and (*g*) a digital printer.

Because the enzyme volume is very small (0.05 ml/min), both incubation time at 37 °C and the dialysis had to be prolonged, to increase sensitivity.

Reagents

Buffer. 2-Amino-2-methyl-1-propanol buffer (625 mmol/liter, pH 10.25 ± 0.05 at 25 °C).

Substrate. Prepare disodium *p*-nitrophenylphosphate hexahydrate (mol wt, 371.2; J. T. Baker Chemical Co., Phillipsburg, N. J. 08865), 5.4 mmol/liter, freshly each day. Add no magnesium to the substrate.

Dialyzing solution. Prepare sodium dihydrogen phosphate monohydrate (mol wt, 137.99; Fisher Scientific Co., Fair Lawn, N. J. 07410), 10 mmol/liter, in 150 mmol/liter sodium chloride and 5 mmol/liter magnesium chloride. Adjust the pH to 7.5 at 25 °C.

Sephadex G-25 (Fine), from Pharmacia, Montreal, Canada.

γ-Glutamyltransferase (EC 2.3.2.2). Statzyme γ-glutamyltransferase from Worthington Biochemical Corp., Freehold, N. J. 07728.

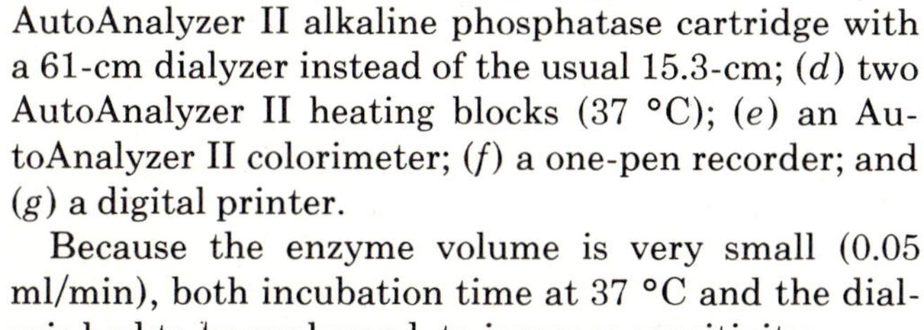

Fig. 1. Continuous-flow diagram

Procedure

Preparation of the serum sample. With the phosphate buffer, 1 ml of serum is washed through a column (1 × 15 cm) containing G-25 Sephadex, and the protein peak, usually diluted two- to threefold by this process, is collected. Alternatively, the serum can be dialyzed overnight in small dialyzing bags, which has the advantage that many samples can be processed simultaneously without diluting the serum.

Heat denaturation. Dialyzed serum, 2 ml, is placed in a Pasteur pipet that has had one end sealed in a flame and that is mounted in a rubber stopper for easy manipulation in the water bath. The digital printer is set to print a reading every 30 s, and the serum is aspirated through the 0.05 ml/min line (Figure 1) for 2 min at room temperature; the pipet is then transferred to the water bath and the time noted as $t = 0$ of denaturation. Aspiration of the specimen is continued until it is gone. The AutoAnalyzer monitors the decrease in residual phosphatase activity at pH 10.25 and the heat denaturation curve appears on the recorder (Figure 2). The difference between the plateaus at A_0 and A_∞ represents the decrease in activity at a given temperature.

Calculation. Values from the digital printer are used for the calculation. The first four or five values represent the plateau of total activity. The succeeding values are those of residual activity at 30-s intervals.

The next operation is to determine the position of the lower plateau. In most cases, this is identical to that of the original baseline, but if the placental or the Regan isoenzyme is present, the lower plateau will be above the baseline. The difference from the baseline is proportional to the activity of these isoenzymes, which can be calculated directly.

Finally, the percentage of residual activity is calculated and plotted as described under *Analytical Principles*. Since by calculation the lower plateau is subtracted, the semilog graph will only yield the thermolabile fractions.

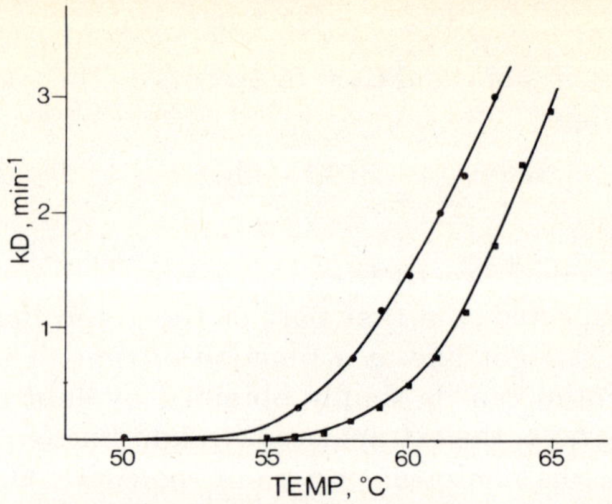

Fig. 4. Effect of temperature on the two ALP fractions that are present in normal serum

Effects measured with sample in phosphate buffer (10 mmol/liter, pH 7.5), in presence of NaCl (0.15 mol/liter) and $MgCl_2$ (5 mmol/liter). *kD* is the denaturation constant calculated for each component from the slopes of semilog graph (see Figure 2 and *Analytical Principles*)

Results

Analytical Variables

When serum or extracts of tissue are dialyzed against tris(hydroxymethyl)aminomethane HCl buffer at pH 7.5, or chromatographed on a Sephadex G-25 column equilibrated with the same buffer, all alkaline phosphatase isoenzymes become more resistant to heat denaturation (Figure 3 and ref. *5*). To identify the cause of such a stabilizing effect of dialysis, we examined various dialyzable components of serum and extracts of tissue.

Sodium chloride increased the heat sensitivity, probably through its contribution to ionic strength (*7*). However, at physiological concentration (0.15 mol/liter), it had no appreciable effect. Nevertheless, sodium chloride was added to the buffer to avoid changes in ionic strength during dialysis and thermodenaturation.

Removal of magnesium by dialysis did not result in an increased thermolability, nor did its addition improve thermostability. Although we consistently observed that removal of magnesium caused the relative activities of the isoenzymes to change, the very heat-labile one becoming more active. To avoid artefacts we routinely added magnesium to the dialyzing buffer.

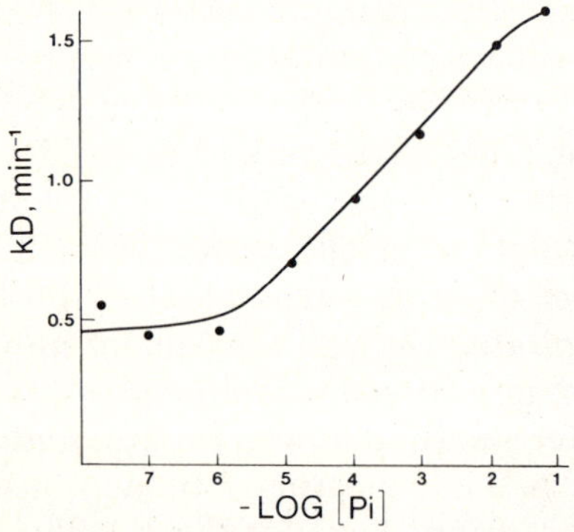

Fig. 3. Effect on dialyzed human serum of increasing inorganic phosphate (P_i) concentration

Only the very heat-labile isoenzyme is shown. The heat-labile isoenzyme is affected similarly. Effect was measured with sample in tris(hydroxymethyl)-aminomethane buffer (0.1 mol/liter, pH 7.5), at 60 °C. *kD* is the denaturation constant calculated from the slope of curves on the semilog graph (see Figure 2 and *Analytical Principles*)

Removal of inorganic phosphate by dialysis strikingly improved the heat stability of all ALP isoenzymes tested. Figure 3 shows the effect of increasing inorganic phosphate concentration on the rate of heat denaturation of the dialyzed heat-labile isoenzyme from normal human serum. A more detailed report on this subject will be published elsewhere.

Of all the dialyzable substances in the serum that affect the heat stability of ALP isoenzymes, inorganic phosphate alone is responsible for more than 90% of this effect. The concentration of inorganic phosphate in normal serum is 1 mmol/liter; thus, even slight variations in serum phosphate concentration will affect thermodenaturation (Figure 3).

To avoid undesirable effects, we used inorganic phosphate (10 mmol/liter) as the dialyzing buffer, at a concentration far exceeding physiological concentration.

For no special reason other than to keep it within the physiological range, the pH was adjusted to 7.5. Phosphate has a good buffering capacity at this pH and is not affected by temperature. In any event, the thermolability of all ALP isoenzymes tested was unchanged between pH 7.0 and 8.5.

Figure 4 shows the temperature dependency of the denaturation constant for the two major components of ALP activity of human serum. At 56 °C, the usual temperature at which thermodenaturation is done, these components are fairly stable. The more unstable fraction is more affected by temperature variation between 55 and 60 °C.

The higher heating-bath temperature, 60 °C, was selected rather than the usual 56 °C because the time required for a complete denaturation at 56 °C was much too long, which resulted in too great a consumption of serum. At 60 °C, the two components are

Table 1. Accuracy of Quantitative Estimation of ALP Isoenzymes

(A) Time at 60 °C (s)	ALP (U/liter), residual activity	Isoenzymes (% total) Expected: Very heat labile[a]	Expected: Heat labile[b]	Found: Very heat labile[a]	Found: Heat labile[b]
0	180			52	48
30	153	31	69	35	65
60	125	19	81	26	74
75	97	15	85	14	86
90	83	11	89	10	90

(B)	Isoenzymes (% total) Expected: Heat labile	Expected: Less heat labile	Found: Heat labile	Found: Less heat labile
$xC + yD$ = total activity	83	17	80	20
C: Heat labile	61	39	62	38
(k: 0.31 min^{-1})	45	55	48	52
D: Less heat labile	19	81	20	80
(k: 0.05 min^{-1})				

(A) [a] Very heat labile: $k = 1.03\ min^{-1}$
[b] Heat labile: $k = 0.34\ min^{-1}$
At $t = 0$, the serum is denatured and isoenzymes calculated. Samples of the same serum are then denatured 30, 60, 75, and 90 s. The residual activity is measured and a complete denaturation is run for each sample. Knowing the rate constant of each component the relative amount of each is predicted as a function of time.
(B) Complete denaturation was run and isoenzymes calculated.

denatured within 10 min and the constants of denaturation are easily calculated. Nonetheless, temperature variations become more likely, which could change the values for denaturation constants, especially that of the more labile component. However, these variations do not affect the calculated activity of each component.

Table 1 summarizes a recovery study done to prove the accuracy and sensitivity of the method. Mixtures of various quantities of two sera with ALP activities of different heat stability gave results in good agreement with expected values for both isoenzymes (Table 1*B*). It is also shown that when a mixture of two isoenzymes of different heat stability is denatured at 60 °C, the more stable enzyme is relatively enriched as a function of time. This table also demonstrates that the two enzymes denature independently and that the amount of any component can be calculated accurately at a given time (Table 1*A*).

The same performance could be achieved with serum or extracts of tissues of low or high ALP activity. However, an ALP isoenzyme has to comprise at least 10% of the activity if it is to be quantitatively estimated. It is much easier to accurately measure low activities of more stable isoenzymes; we have been able to measure as little as 5% of the intestinal isoenzyme in a mixture of this enzyme with the liver isoenzyme.

That the method is quite precise is shown by the quality-control data. For more than 200 determinations on pooled normal serum, heat denaturation constant values for both ALP isoenzymes were found to be: for the very heat-labile one, $k_1 = 1.20 \pm 0.15\ min^{-1}$, and for the heat-labile one $k_2 = 0.36 \pm 0.1\ min^{-1}$; the relative activity of both isoenzymes was found to be, respectively, 51 and 49% ± 7%.

Alkaline Phosphatase Isoenzymes of Human Serum

Table 2 compares data for serum from normal adults, cord blood, normal children, normal pregnant women, and from patients with various liver diseases.

Three isoenzymes (or more precisely, analytical groups of isoenzymes) could be identified in human serum, and these are defined as very heat labile, heat labile, and heat stable, according to their rates of denaturation.

Normal adult serum contains two ALP isoenzymes in an activity ratio of 1:1; we never saw a heat-stable component in these sera.

The ALP activity of cord blood consisted almost exclusively of the very heat-labile isoenzyme.

On the other hand, the serum of normal children contains the two isoenzymes of adults, but in a ratio of 5:1 in favor of the very heat-labile fraction.

With pregnancy serum, the situation is not quite as clear. About half the ALP activity is due to the placental isoenzyme and the rest consists either of the two isoenzymes of the adult serum (50% of cases) or of only one of the two isoenzymes found in serum from nonpregnant adults.

Finally, in proven cases of various liver diseases, the serum with high or normal ALP activity shows a significantly increased heat-labile fraction. Very often, this is the only ALP isoenzyme found.

Source of Serum Alkaline Phosphatase Isoenzymes

Table 3 summarizes data obtained with extracts of human tissues. The tissues have been grouped according to their respective embryologic germ layers (e.g., entoderm or mesoderm).

In the mesodermal series, there seems to be only one class of ALP isoenzymes, which could not be distinguished from each other by the criterion of heat stability. Although, many organs contain ALP, it is often restricted to the capillaries or the adventitia of blood vessels.

Obviously, all entodermal tissues are mixed with mesodermal ones (capillaries, blood vessels, and connective tissue), and this is reflected in the heat-stability pattern of ALP isoenzymes from various organs. Notice that the very heat-labile fraction is similar to the one found in the mesodermal series, and is probably identical, because ALP is also found in capillaries and blood vessels.

The true (hepatocytic) liver isoenzyme was always

Table 2. ALP Isoenzymes of Human Serum

Condition	No. determinations	Mean acty. (U/liter)	Isoenzymes at 60 °C (% total): Very heat labile[a]	Heat labile[b]	Heat stable[c]
Normal adults	200	30–90	45 ± 7[d]	55 ± 7[d]	—
Cord blood	36	130	⩾95	⩽5	—
Pediatric blood	22	226	79 ± 10	21 ± 7	—
Pregnancy blood	7	164	0	61 ± 10	39 ± 10
Pregnancy blood	6	167	50 ± 14	0	50 ± 14
Pregnancy blood	16	151	35 ± 12	27 ± 10	38 ± 15
Liver disease (all types)	135	90–500	15 ± 10	85 ± 10	—

[a] Very heat labile: $k_d = 1.2 \pm 0.2\ \text{min}^{-1}$
[b] Heat labile: $k_d = 0.36 \pm 0.15\ \text{min}^{-1}$
[c] Heat stable: $k_d = 0\ \text{min}^{-1}$
[d] SD is 1 standard deviation.
See Table 3 for tissue source of these isoenzymes.

found to have a stability intermediate to that of the intestinal ALP (stable component) and that of tissues of the mesodermal series. Of all human tissues studied, it is the only one with an ALP isoenzyme of such a heat stability. This isoenzyme accounts for 50% of the heat-labile ALP of normal human serum. It is also the only isoenzyme with increased activity in serum from patients with liver diseases (Table 2). Thus we think it very likely that the heat-labile fraction in the blood originates from the liver.

Intestinal isoenzyme. With electrophoretic techniques, the intestinal isoenzyme is often found to be an important fraction of ALP of normal serum. This isoenzyme can also be identified by virtue of its inhibition by L-phenylalanine.

We have shown that human duodenum contains two isoenzymes of very different thermostability (Table 3). Figure 5 shows that, by the assay described here, the relatively heat-stable isoenzyme is also the only one that is significantly inhibited by L-phenylalanine. On the other hand, the heat-labile isoenzyme is similar to the one found in many other tissues, in that it is little inhibited by L-phenylalanine.

If one defines the intestinal isoenzyme as a relatively heat-resistant and L-phenylalanine-sensitive enzyme, we found no measurable activity of such an isoenzyme in normal sera, but if the heat-labile intestinal isoenzyme were to enter the circulation, it would be absolutely indistinguishable from the bone isoenzyme and certain other isoenzymes (Table 3).

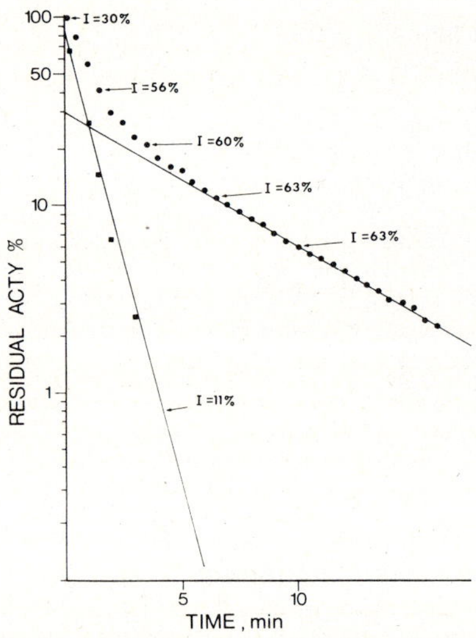

Fig. 5. Heat-denaturation curves for a human duodenum extract prepared from scrapings from the mucosa

At time intervals shown by *arrows* as denaturation proceeds, residual ALP was assayed with and without L-phenylalanine present. Assay conditions were: pH 10.25, 25 °C, 625 mmol/liter 2-amino-2-methyl-1-propanol, 10 mmol/liter L-phenylalanine. D-Phenylalanine was added in control experiments. Notice the two curves with different slope, indicating the presence of two isoenzymes with different thermolability. *I*: percentage inhibition by L-phenylalanine. *I* = 30% at the beginning; as denaturation proceeds, *I* values increase until it reaches a plateau, *I* = 63%, the maximal inhibition for the less heat-labile isoenzyme. *I* = 11%, is the inhibition of the very heat-labile isoenzyme

Alkaline Phosphatase Isoenzymes and Diseases

Fractionation according to thermostability allows isoenzymes to be classified into four groups: placental origin (k = 0), the L-phenylalanine-sensitive isoenzyme of intestinal origin (k = 0.1), liver origin (k = 0.4), and those found elsewhere (bone, marrow, vacular, etc ... (k = 1.2–1.5). It is not now possible to identify the source of the more heat-labile ALP without the aid of the patient's medical history and other diagnostic procedures. In our experience with 600 cases for whom ALP fractionation was requested, 20% of them showed an increased total ALP activity in the serum and a definite increase of the very heat-labile ALP. Such an increase was never found in serum with normal ALP activity. Moreover, γ-glutamyltransferase activity was normal in all cases. In most cases, a diagnosis of primary or secondary bone disease was compatible with the medical history and other diagnostic aids.

Table 3. Tissue Distribution of Heat-Labile Isoenzymes of Human Alkaline Phosphatase

Tissue	Heat-denaturation rate k: min^{-1}	% of total Iso-enzymes	Localization
Placenta	0	100	Trophoblast.
Entoderm derivatives:			
Intestine	1.0	50	Enterocytes: brush
	0.11	50	borders, lateral membranes, Golgi. Capillaries.
Liver	1.2	60	Hepatocytes: Biliary
	0.32	40	canalicules, sinusoids. Blood vessels.
Mesoderm derivatives:			
Bone	1.5	>98	
Bone marrow	1.23	>95	
Leukocytes	1.5	100	
Lymph nodes	1.3	100	Lymphocytes, connective tissue.
Spleen	1.1	100	Capillaries and venous sinuses. Macrophages.
Lung[a]	1.0	>95	Capillaries. Adventitia of arteries. Connective tissue of bronchi.
Heart	1.0	>95	Capillaries.

All tissues were pre-washed in physiological saline, and homogenized in 10 mmol/liter tris(hydroxymethyl)aminomethane HCl containing 0.15 mol/liter NaCl, 10 μmol/liter $ZnCl_2$, and 1 mmol/liter $MgCl_2$. The plasma membranes and mitochondria were collected by centrifugation and ALP was solubilized with *n*-butanol. The aqueous phase was chromatographed on Sephadex G-25 vs. 10 mmol/liter phosphate buffer containing 0.15 mol/liter NaCl and 5 mmol/liter $MgCl_2$.

[a] Lung is primarily an entodermal derivative, but it is mixed with mesodermal one to a great extent. Classification of tissues in this table is according to B. Patten, *Human Embryology,* McGraw-Hill, N.Y., 1968.

During the same study, we found that 65% of the submitted sera were from patients highly suspected of having liver disease or already diagnosed as having liver disease. Even though the increase in total ALP activity was quite variable (1.5- to 10-fold), the liver isoenzyme (k = 0.4) always accounted for 85–100% of total activity. In all instances, γ-glutamyltransferase activity was increased but the correlationship between the increase in the activities of liver ALP and γ-glutamyltransferase in the serum was not as good as expected.

We selected sera with 100% liver ALP from cases of liver diseases and determined γ-glutamyltransferase (Figure 6). In 20% of the cases, both total ALP activity and γ-glutamyltransferase activity were within the normal range; on the other hand, many cases were found with low ALP and high γ-glutamyltransferase (Figure 6).

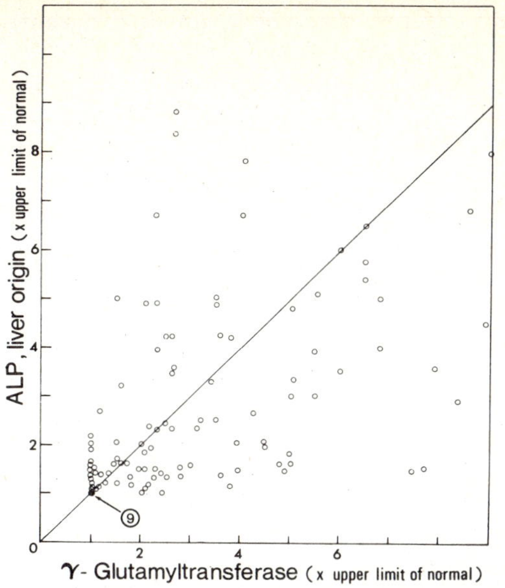

Fig. 6. Relation between liver ALP and γ-glutamyltransferase activities of serum from persons with liver diseases (n = 82)
Perfect correlation is shown by the line, drawn as a reference. Upper limit of normal for adults was set at 80 U/liter for ALP at 37 °C; for γ-glutamyltransferase, it was set at 31 and 38 U/liter for males and females, respectively, at 30 °C. Results given as number on axis times upper limit of normal. The correlation coefficient, r, = 0.54

Discussion

The kinetic approach to the study of thermodenaturation of ALP isoenzymes offers several advantages over existing techniques of isoenzyme analysis:

- Easy to perform with an AutoAnalyzer, the continuous monitoring of the thermodenaturation assures complete control of the reaction path from the very beginning.
- Graphical analysis of kinetic data permits a simultaneous direct identification and quantitation of three isoenzymes in a mixture—e.g. placenta, liver, and bone.
- The method is very sensitive and could be applied to sera and extracts of tissues with low ALP activity.
- Temperature variations will proportionally affect every isoenzyme in a mixture without changing the relative amount of each isoenzyme.
- It is possible to quantitate accurately an isoenzyme that represents as little as 10% of the total activity.

There is a need for standardization of the procedure. Because inorganic phosphate content of the sample is critical, a good phosphate buffer is necessary, especially if one wishes to intercompare tissue extracts, or to compare them with sera or with purified ALP. However, variation in phosphate content of the sample will equally affect the denaturation rates of most isoenzymes but will not change the relative amount of each in the mixture.

A histochemical study of ALP distribution, run in parallel, has shown that most tissues contain ALP and that organs such as liver and intestine have more than one isoenzyme, which can be differentiated by physical means and specific inhibition.

In our hands, specific inhibition of ALP isoenzyme by amino acids has not given additional clues as to how to improve the identification of the tissue from which serum ALP originates in an individual.

In view of our results, we agree that identification of ALP isoenzymes is a complex problem, but we do not feel that another approach will yield better results.

The true liver isoenzyme (i.e., that originating from hepatocytes) evidently has an intermediate thermostability that renders it easy to identify and measure. In normal adults, this isoenzyme accounts for half the total ALP activity of serum. The other major contributors to normal serum ALP are far more difficult to identify, because almost all tissues contain a thermolabile fraction. The latter is certainly easier to identify in a disease state with the help of medical history and other diagnostic aids.

Extensive studies with sera from cases of various liver diseases led us to conclude that the liver isoenzyme is always present in abnormally high activity, whatever the total ALP activity. Although liver ALP activity in the blood varies greatly, it is found in all types of liver diseases (*8*). Increased liver ALP activity is often accompanied by increased γ-glutamyltransferase activity, but the quantitative correlation is not as good as expected, on the basis that both enzymes come from the same tissue and are indicators of liver diseases. In 20% of cases, liver ALP was the only abnormal test. The frequently encountered differences between increases in liver ALP and γ-glutamyltransferase could reflect liver diseases at different time of evolution or different histopathological disorders. This aspect is now under study in our laboratory.

One thing is sure: increased liver ALP activity can be found in the blood at a very early and subclinical stage of liver disease, at a time when most liver tests are normal. It is therefore suggested that both liver ALP and γ-glutamyltransferase should always be measured concurrently whenever liver disease is suspected.

I thank Dr. N. Brière for histological studies done in his laboratory, Messrs. Y. Racine, D. Cloutier, and J. C. Dubois for technical assistance, and Mr. Jack Levine (Technicon) for instrumental assistance. This research was supported in part by the Medical Research Council of Canada (MA-4663).

References

1. Posen, S., Neale, F. D., and Clubb, J. S., Heat inactivation in the study of human alkaline phosphatases. *Ann. Intern. Med.* **62,** 1234 (1965).

2. Ratliff, C. R., Hall, F. F., Culp, T. W., et al., The differentiation of hepatic and skeletal alkaline phosphatase by thermofractionation. *Am. J. Gastroenterol.* **58,** 22 (1972).

3. Diot, M. N., Ronesse, J., and Bohuon, C., Dénaturation thermique des isoenzymes de la phosphatase alcaline sérique: Son intérêt dans l'étude des cancers métastasiques. *Ann. Biol. Clin.* **29,** 309 (1971).

4. Cadeau, B. D., and Malkin, A., A relative heat stability test for the identification of serum alkaline phosphatase isoenzymes. *Clin. Chim. Acta* **45,** 235 (1973).

5. Mestery, D., Leroux, M. L., and Perry, W. F., Effect of dialysis on tissue and serum alkaline phosphatase heat stability. *Clin. Biochem.* **8,** 18 (1975).

6. Moss, D. W., and Whitby, L. G., A simplified heat inactivation method for investigating alkaline phosphatase isoenzymes in serum. *Clin. Chim. Acta* **61,** 63 (1975).

7. PetitClerc, C., A kinetic study of heat stability of alkaline phosphatases. Application to sera with 'normal' alkaline phosphatase activities. Abstracts of 26th national meeting of the AACC, August 1974, Las Vegas, Nevada. *Clin. Chem.* **20,** 888 (1974).

8. PetitClerc, C., and Brière, N., Les isoenzymes de la phosphatase alcaline dans les maladies du foie. *Union Med. Can.* **103,** 2132 (1974).

CLIN. CHEM. 22/1, 49–52 (1976)

Organic Acids in Urine from Human Newborns

Lars Björkman, Catherine McLean, and Göran Steen

The pattern of organic acids in urine from 15 normal newborn infants was investigated by gas chromatography/mass spectrometry of trimethylsilylated derivatives. The urine contains large amounts of succinic, fumaric, 2-ketoglutaric, and 3-hydroxy-3-methylglutaric acids, which are all fairly small components of urine from adults. On the other hand, hippuric acid is a small component in the urine from newborn infants, but a large component later in life. An additional number of differences can be seen. Some previously unrecognized aliphatic dicarboxylic acids were also observed, which are present to some extent in urine from adults.

Additional Keyphrases: *pediatric chemistry • gas chromatography • mass spectrometry • new acids identified in urine*

For the diagnosis of organic acidurias, gas chromatography/mass spectrometry seems to be the method of choice, and several procedures for urine extraction and derivatization have been published in the last few years (*1–5*).

Severe metabolic disease often occurs shortly after birth. In spite of this there is a lack of information concerning the normal pattern of organic acids in urine from newborns, as seen by gas chromatographic/mass spectrometric methods. According to our experience, the newborn pattern is largely different from that of the adult.

We used the method of Sternowsky et al. (*5*), which depends on ethyl acetate extraction of the urine, followed by preparation of oximes and trimethylsilylation. The method is simple to perform, avoids multiple peaks from keto acids, and gives derivatization of hydroxyl groups as well as carboxyl groups.

Materials

Succinic, 3-hydroxy-3-methylglutaric, 2-ketoglutaric, aconitic, citric, isocitric, 4-hydroxy-3-methoxyphenylacetic, 4-hydroxy-3-methoxy mandelic, 5-hydroxy indoleacetic acids, and hydroxylamine hydrochloride were from Sigma Chemical Co., St Louis, Mo. 63178. Oxalic, fumaric, malic, and stearic acids were from Merck, Darmstadt, Germany. 2-Hydroxy-3-methyl benzoic acid was from Merck-Schuckardt, München, Germany.

Pyridine and *N,O*-bis(trimethylsilyl)-trifluoracetamide (BSTFA) were from Pierce Chemical Co., Rockford, Ill. 61105, and ethyl acetate (Analar) was from BDH Chemicals, Poole, England. 3% OV-17 coated on 100–120 mesh Gas Chrom Q was from Applied Science Lab., State College, Pa. 16801.

Methods

Urine samples were collected from healthy newborn infants within the first 24 h after birth. Some of the infants had been fed with breast milk before urine collection. The urines were rapidly frozen to −20 °C until analyzed. An aliquot was taken for creatinine determination by an automated Jaffé method.

Extraction and derivatization was performed essentially according to Sternowsky et al. (*5*) with the following modifications. As internal standard, we used 100 μg of 2-hydroxy-3-methyl benzoic acid, added to 2 ml of urine before extraction. This compound was selected because it was not likely to occur as a metabolite and because it did not co-chromatograph with any major normal compound. Trimethylsilylation was performed with 50 μl of BSTFA at room temperature for 30 min, and 2–4 μl of the reacted mixture was injected into the gas chromatograph.

We used a Model 5750 gas chromatograph (Hewlett-Packard Instruments, Avondale, Pa. 19311) with a flame ionization detector. The column was a 2 m × 4 mm (i.d.) glass column, packed with 3 % OV-17. Helium (30 ml/min) was used as carrier gas, and the temperature was programmed from 100 to 270 °C at 4 °C/min. For gas chromatography/mass spectrometry, an LKB 9000 instrument (LKB-Produkter, Solna, Sweden) was used, equipped with a glass column of the same length and with the same packing as above. Ion source temperature was 270 °C, electron energy 70 eV, and acceleration voltage 3.5 kV.

Peak areas were determined by triangulation. Urinary concentrations and excretions in relation to creatinine were calculated from peak area ratios vs. internal standard. No correction factors were applied for extraction efficiency or detector response. After

Department of Clinical Chemistry, University of Gothenburg, Sahlgren's Hospital, S-413 45 Gothenburg, Sweden.
Received Aug. 22, 1975; accepted Oct. 7, 1975.

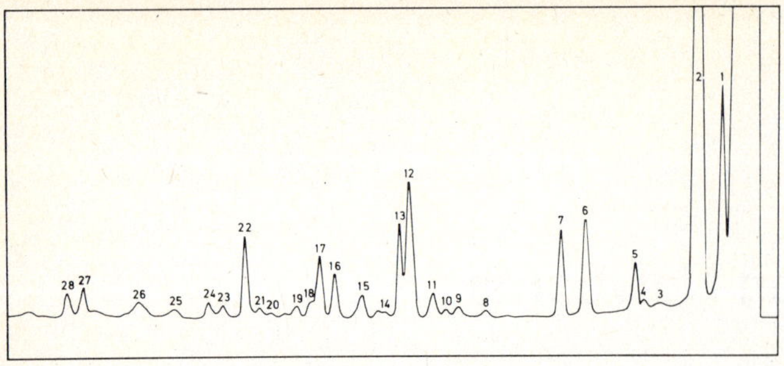

Fig. 1. Gas chromatogram of the extract containing organic acids from the urine of a normal newborn

gas chromatography/mass spectrometry of all samples, all mass spectra from a certain peak were compared visually, and the ions were grouped according to their co-variation and compared to reference spectra.

Results

A gas chromatogram of a urine sample is shown in Figure 1. The peaks have been given numbers, referred to in Table 1. This table includes those ions of the mass spectra that have the highest distinguishing value. The mass spectra of some peaks were found to be highly variable, because they contain several compounds in variable proportions. Therefore, quantitative determinations are of limited value for many peaks, but nevertheless facilitate evaluation of chromatograms from patients. Owing to the complexity of many peaks, it is also inconvenient to express values in moles. All values have been related to creatinine excretion.

Most of the acids mentioned in Table 1 have been identified by comparison with mass spectra from reference compounds. Some acids were identified by means of published information, especially a recent paper by Thompson and Markey (*6*). From their report, phosphoric acid (in peak 6) and glucuronic acid (in peak 22) were recognized and subsequently identified by reference analysis. Also, based on their report, erythronic or threonic acid should be present in peak 8. Hexonolactone may be part of peak 18, but it is too small to give a good spectrum. The hydroxyphenylhydroxypropionic acid of peak 19 is probably identical with *m*-hydroxyphenylhydracrylic acid, described by Armstrong and Shaw (*7*).

A number of previously unidentified components were observed, especially aliphatic dicarboxylic acids. The identity of these acids has been established by studies on methyl esters, which are better suited for preparative work. The structure of 3-methylglutaconic acid (in peak 8) was determined by catalytic hydrogenation and osmium tetroxide oxidation (to be published). The mass spectrum of this substance as trimethylsilyl derivative is dominated by ions at *m/e* 273 (M—CH_3), 198 (M—TMS-OH), 183 (M—CH_3—TMS-OH) and 170 (M—CO-O-TMS—H).

The octenedioic acid of peak 15 is actually part of more than five isomers, where the two major ones are *cis*-3 and *cis*-4 straight chain components (to be published). The present mass spectrum contains ions at *m/e* 301 (M—CH_3), 185 (M—CH_2-CO-O-TMS), 169 (M—[TMS-O-TMS—CH_3]) and 136 (M—2TMS-OH).

Peak 22 contains 5-decynedioic acid, likely to be a metabolite from acetylenic fatty acids. Details on this structure have been published elsewhere (*8*). The major ions of the trimethylsilyl derivative have *m/e*-values 342 (M), 327, (M—CH_3), 252 (M—TMS-OH), 237 (M—CH_3—TMS-OH), 224 (M—CO-O-TMS—H), 211 (M—CH_2-CO-O-TMS), 195 (M—[TMS-O-TMS—CH_3]) and 163 (M—TMS-O—TMS-OH).

The recently discovered 3,4-methylene hexanedioic acid (*9*) is present in very small amounts in peak 12. This acid is a metabolite from cyclopropane fatty acids (Greter, J., Lindstedt, S. and Steen, G., to be published).

Part of peak 14 is likely to be a dihydroxyheptanoic acid, containing a primary hydroxyl group. The mass spectrum contains ions at *m/e* 378 (M), 363 (M—CH_3), 275 (M—CH_2-O-TMS), 273 (M—CH_3—TMS-OH) and 247 (M—CH_2-CO-O-TMS).

The hydroxydecanedioic acid of peak 24 is only tentatively identified based on ions at *m/e* 419 (M—CH_3), 377 (M—C_3H_5O), 329 (M—CH_3—TMS-OH), 317 (M—CO-O-TMS), 303 (M—CH_2-CO-O-TMS), 287 (M—[TMS-O-TMS—CH_3]) and 274 (M—2 TMS—CH_2). The proposed hydroxydodecanedioic and hydroxydodecenedioic acids of peak 26 are analogous with respect to mass-spectral peaks.

A few blank peaks dominate in the first part of the chromatogram (peaks 1–5). The normally occurring small amounts of lactic and 3-hydroxybutyric acids hide within these peaks, but when present in large amounts, they have been easy to find.

As can be seen from a comparison between Tables 1 and 2, the organic acid composition of urine from newborns is largely different from that of adults. When the excretion is related to creatinine, the newborn appears to excrete at least 10-fold more succinic, fumaric, 3-hydroxy-3-methylglutaric and 2-ketoglutaric acids. We do not find such striking differences for citric acid. The values for newborns are a few times higher for aconitic, isocitric, octanedioic, octenedioic, and hexanedioic acids. 4-Hydroxyphenylacetic acid and the mixture of hydroxyphenylhydroxypropionic + 4-hydroxy-3-methoxyphenylacetic-acids did not differ much. Hippuric acid, finally, is usually the dominating peak in a gas chromatogram of an adult urine, while almost absent in the newborn urine.

Discussion

Most of the organic acids found in the urine of normal newborns have been detected before in gas-chromatographic/mass-spectrometric studies of adult human urine (*1–6, 10, 11*) although in other propor-

Table 1. Organic Acids in Urine of Human Newborns (n = 15)

Peak no.	Most distinguishing ions (*m/e* values)	Identity	Excretion, mg/g creatinine: Mean	Range
1	208, 193, 143, 122	Blank		
2	249, 234, 148, 147, 133, 119	Blank (major part)		
	219, 191, 190, 147, 117	Lactic		
3	280, 265, 215, 173	Blank (major part)		
	233, 191	3-Hydroxybutyric		
4	219, 190, 147	Oxalic		
	208, 193, 143, 122	Blank (major part)		
5	293, 278, 147	Blank		
6	204, 189, 171, 147, 100	Urea (major part)		
	314, 299	Phosphoric		
7	247, 147	Succinic } (varying proportions)	86	14–350
	245, 147, 143	Fumaric		
8	273, 198, 183, 170	3-Methylglutaconic } (varying proportions)	11	2–46
	409, 292, 220	Erythronic or threonic		
	335, 245, 233, 191, 190, 189	Malic		
9	275, 185, 172, 159, 141, 111	Hexanedioic	11	1–34
10	289, 199, 186, 173, 155, 125	3-Methyl-hexanedioic	9	3–29
11	363, 273, 247, 231, 199, 115	3-Hydroxy-3-methylglutaric	38	9–105
12	281, 223, 207, 149	2-Hydroxy-3-methylbenzoic (int. standard)		
13	377, 362, 260, 244, 170, 156	2-Ketoglutaric	53	5–312
14	296, 281, 252, 179, 164	4-Hydroxyphenylacetic (major part)	12	2–21
	378, 363, 275, 273, 247	Dihydroxyheptanedioic		
15	303, 187, 171, 139	Octanedioic	22	8–42
	301, 185, 169, 137, 136	Octenedioic (major part)		
	175	Unidentified		
16	375, 346, 285, 229, 211	Aconitic } (varying proportions)	31	13–62
	392, 306, 305, 217, 204	Unidentified		
17	465, 375, 363, 347, 273	Citric	71	12–287
18	465, 375, 363, 347, 319, 305, 273, 245	Isocitric (major part)	32	9–58
	287, 233, 217, 204	Unidentified		
19	398, 383, 280, 267	Hydroxyphenylhydroxypropionic } (varying proportions)	28	5–71
	326, 311, 209, 179	4-Hydroxy-3-methoxyphenylacetic		
20	398, 383, 355, 308, 293, 292, 281, 179	4-Hydroxyphenyllactic } (varying proportions)	8	3–12
	331, 215	Decanedioic		
21	414, 399, 371, 297	4-Hydroxy-3-methoxymandelic (major part)	18	3–37
	333, 217, 204	Unidentified		
22	464, 449, 333, 305, 292, 217, 204	Glucuronic (half-acetal) } (varying proportions)	27	6–59
	342, 327, 252, 237, 224, 211	5-Decynedioic		
	195, 163, 162			
23	236, 206, 105	Hippuric (major part)	17	5–48
	328, 313	Palmitic		
24	419, 377, 329, 317, 303, 287, 274	Hydroxydecanedioic? } (varying proportions)	19	4–44
	233, 217, 204	Unidentified		
25	223, 205, 149	Plasticizer		
26	447, 405, 357, 331, 315	Hydroxydodecanedioic?	18	2–31
	445, 403, 355, 329, 313	Hydroxydodecenedioic?		
	233, 217, 204	Unidentified		
27	407, 392, 290	5-Hydroxyindoleacetic (3 TMS)	24	7–59
28	335, 320, 218	5-Hydroxyindoleacetic (2 TMS)		

Table 2. Some Organic Acids in Urine of Adult Humans (n = 10)

Peak no.	Identity	Excretion (mg/g creatinine) Mean	Range
7	Succinic + fumaric	5	2–9
9	Hexanedioic	5	2–9
10	3-Methylhexanedioic	5	2–14
11	3-Hydroxy-3-methylglutaric	2	1–4
13	2-Ketoglutaric + hydroxyphenylacetic	4	1–7
14	4-Hydroxyphenylacetic	15	7–30
15	Octanedioic + octenedioic	6	2–10
16	Aconitic	15	9–22
17	Citric	46	20–123
18	Isocitric	13	8–20
19	Hydroxyphenylhydroxypropionic + 4-hydroxy-3-methoxyphenylacetic	33	8–106
23	Hippuric	398	209–626

tions. This is true for, e.g., succinic, fumaric, 2-ketoglutaric, aconitic, citric, isocitric, 4-hydroxyphenylacetic, 4-hydroxy-3-methoxyphenylacetic, 4-hydroxy-3-methoxy-mandelic, and 5-hydroxy-indoleacetic acids.

On the other hand, 3-hydroxy-3-methylglutaric acid has not been discovered among the peaks, probably owing to its relative paucity in adult urines. Furthermore, we have found 3-methylglutaconic, octenedioic, and 5-decynedioic acids, previously unidentified in human urine. These are present in adult urines, too, although in somewhat smaller amounts. The tentatively identified hydroxylated aliphatic dicarboxylic acids have not been detected in adult urines.

A recent study on organic urinary acids was published by Aksu et al. (*12*), who used silicic acid column chromatography. These workers did not report such large differences between newborns and adults as those we have found. Most of the differences were of the same kind, however—e.g., higher excretions of fumaric, succinic, 2-ketoglutaric, and aconitic among the newborns, and no difference in citric acid. In contrast to our results, they did not find any difference in hippuric acid excretion. These workers compared groups of age 0–29 days, 1–23 months, and 2–14 years, respectively, which may explain why the differences found in our study are more pronounced.

After a gas chromatographic/mass spectrometric analysis of the urine from a patient, we use Table 1 for a rapid evaluation of the mass spectra obtained. Whenever doubt arises concerning identity, full scale reference mass spectra may be referred to. In addition, it is useful to have a list of inborn errors that are accompanied by organic aciduria, such as that recently published by Watts et al. (*13*).

References

1. Horning, E. C., and Horning, M. G., Human metabolic profiles obtained by GC and GC/MS. *J. Chromatogr. Sci.* **9**, 129 (1971).

2. Jellum, E., Stokke, O., and Eldjarn, L., Screening for metabolic disorders using gas–liquid chromatography, mass spectrometry and computer technique. *Scand. J. Clin. Lab. Invest.* **27**, 273 (1971).

3. Mamer, O. A., Crawhall, J. C., and Tjoa, S. S., The identification of urinary acids by coupled gas chromatography mass spectrometry. *Clin. Chim. Acta* **32**, 171 (1971).

4. Chalmers, R. A., and Watts, R. W. E., The quantitative extraction and gas liquid chromatographic determination of organic acids in urine. *Analyst* (London) **97**, 958 (1972).

5. Sternowsky, H. J., Roboz, J., Hutterer, F., and Gaull, G., Determination of α-keto acids as silylated oximes in urine and serum by combined gas chromatography–mass spectrometry. *Clin. Chim. Acta* **47**, 371 (1973).

6. Thompson, J. A., and Markey, S. P., Quantitative metabolic profiling of urinary organic acids by gas chromatography–mass spectrometry: Comparison of isolation methods. *Anal. Chem.* **47**, 1313 (1975).

7. Armstrong, M. D., and Shaw, K. N. F., The occurrence of (-)-β-*m*-hydroxyphenylhydracrylic acid in human urine. *J. Biol. Chem.* **225**, 269 (1957).

8. Lindstedt, S., and Steen, G., 5-Decynedioic acid, an acetylenic compound in human urine. *Clin. Chem.* **21**, 1964 (1975).

9. Lindstedt, S., Steen, G., and Wahl, E., 3,4-Methylene hexanedioic acid—a previously unknown compound in human urine. *Clin. Chim. Acta* **53**, 143 (1974).

10. Mamer, O. A., and Tjoa, S. S., 2-Ethylhydracrylic acid: A newly described urinary organic acid. *Clin. Chim. Acta* **55**, 199 (1974).

11. Witten, T. A., Levine, S. P., King, J. O., and Markey, S. P., Gas-chromatographic–mass-spectrometric determination of urinary acid profiles of normal young adults on a controlled diet. *Clin. Chem.* **19**, 586 (1973).

12. Aksu, A., Morrow, G., and Barness, L. A., Urinary excretion of non-nitrogenous organic acids by healthy infants and children. *Clin. Chem.* **20**, 603 (1974).

13. Watts, R. W. E., Chalmers, R. A., and Lawson, A. M., Abnormal organic acidurias in mentally retarded patients. *Lancet* **i**, 368 (1975).

CLIN. CHEM. 22/1, 53–56 (1976)

Measuring Picogram Amounts of Aluminum in Biological Tissue by Flameless Atomic Absorption Analysis of a Chelate

Gary R. LeGendre[1] and Allen C. Alfrey[2]

We describe a flameless atomic absorption method for aluminum determination in ethylenediaminetetraacetate extracts of biological tissues. Picogram quantities can be detected, and the technique appears to be more sensitive than other methods of aluminum determination used for biological samples. The extraction simplifies the method and virtually eliminates contamination with extraneous aluminum during the analysis. The extraction method might be useful for separating various other trace elements from biological tissues before analysis.

Additional Keyphrases: *toxicology • trace elements • neurotoxicity • uremia • absorption of Al*

Aluminum-containing antacids have been widely used in therapy for peptic ulcer, and oral phosphate-binding aluminum gels are now routinely prescribed for nondialyzed and dialyzed uremic patients as a method of controlling serum phosphorus concentrations (*1*). Although it has been assumed that the oral aluminum salts form insoluble aluminum phosphates in the gut and are not absorbed, studies by Clarkson et al. (*2*) show that some aluminum is absorbed by uremic patients receiving these compounds. Because analytical methods for aluminum determination are not widely available, there are few studies (*2–4*) on the relation between administration of oral aluminum salts and tissue aluminum content. Because aluminum has neurotoxic effects (*5–7*) this element, if absorbed from the orally administered salts, could represent a potential health hazard.

Renal Section, Denver Veterans Administration Hospital, and the Division of Renal Medicine, University of Colorado Medical Center, Denver, Colo. 80220.

[1] Current address: Western States Chiropractic College, Portland, Oregon.

[2] Address reprint requests to this author at the Renal Section, V.A. Hospital, 1055 Clermont St., Denver, Colo. 80220.

Received July 21, 1975; accepted Oct. 13, 1975.

Here, we describe a flameless atomic absorption method for determination of aluminum in tissues. Its excellent sensitivity makes it an improvement over most other methods currently available for aluminum analysis. Little tissue is required; biopsy specimens are usually adequate. By using the described extraction method in association with the graphite furnace, tissue handling is minimized and most potential sources of external aluminum contamination during the analysis are avoided.

Methods

Tissue Preparation and Aluminum Extraction

Muscle and bone samples were obtained from patients by biopsies or at time of autopsy, and brain samples were obtained at autopsy. The samples were frozen until analyzed.

Muscle and brain were dried for 16 h at 130 °C. The dried muscle was ground to a fine powder and extracted four times with 2 ml of equal volumes of ether and petroleum ether (solvents were Al-free). The residues were redried at 130 °C for an hour and reweighed.

For brain aluminum analysis a 25-mg aliquot of whole brain, as well as gray and white matter separately, was ashed at 400 °C for 16 h in 10-ml Pyrex beakers.

Bone was sampled from the iliac crest and adhering tissue and periosteum removed by scraping with a scalpel. The bone marrow was removed by washing in a jet of de-ionized water. After air drying at room temperature, the bones were ground in a Wiley mill, passed through a 20-mesh sieve, and partially defatted by rinsing four times with petroleum ether (bp 30–60 °C). The bone was reground and passed through a 60-mesh sieve.

Samples of 10 to 25 mg of the dry defatted bone and muscle and the ashed brain were placed into 5 ml of a saturated solution of disodium ethylenediaminetetracetate (EDTA) and mixed for 2 to 4 h. With an Eppendorf pipet, we injected 25 μl of the supernate directly into the graphite furnace for analysis. All glass and plastic containers and plastic pipet tips were pre-rinsed with Na_2EDTA to eliminate surface aluminum contamination.

The saturated EDTA solution used for extraction, preparation of the aluminum standards, and equipment rinsing was made from Na_2EDTA (Fisher Scientific Co., Fair Lawn, N. J. 07410) and de-ionized water. The EDTA was present in great excess of the available metals, including aluminum.

All analyses were performed on a Model 305B atomic absorption spectrophotometer, equipped with a deuterium background corrector and a HGA-2100 flameless system (all from Perkin-Elmer, Norwalk, Conn. 06856). The HGA-2100 control module was electronically modified with a device for gradually increasing the temperature for the char cycle (Sienco, Inc., Morrison, Colo. 80465). With this modification, the time for the rod to achieve the preset char temperature can be varied from 0 to 240 s. All absorption measurements were monitored on a strip-chart recorder. Settings for the 305B and the HGA-2100 are:

305B	HGA-2100
Al hollow-cathode lamp, 309.3 nm @ 25 mA	Dry cycle, 15 s @ 100 °C
	Char cycle, 20 s to 1550 °C
	Atomize cycle 4 s @ 2650 °C
Slit width, 1 mm (0.7-nm bandpass)	Argon gas purge, 60 ml/min
	Sample vol, 25 μl
Absorption mode	Gas flow, interrupt

Results

Validation of the Extraction

To verify the completeness of the extraction with EDTA, we performed two studies on the tissue samples.

First, three different weights of each type of tissue were added to 5 ml of EDTA solution, and the assay was completed. The linearity of the results (Figure 1) shows that a constant amount of aluminum was extracted from each sample and that the working range was appropriate.

Secondly, the extraction efficiency was examined by analyzing EDTA extracts of replicate samples of tissues prepared by alternative methods. In the case of bones the replicate samples were extracted immediately after air drying or after ashing at 400 °C for 16 h in a 10-ml Pyrex beaker. Aluminum in muscle was analyzed in dry defatted tissue and in tissue ashed at 600 °C in platinum crucibles after EDTA extraction. Replicate brain samples were extracted with EDTA after ashing at 400 °C in Pyrex beakers or at 600 °C in platinum crucibles. Results are shown in Table 1. There was good agreement in all cases between the values found for the replicate samples. These studies suggest that the aluminum present in the dry muscle and bone tissue is readily available to EDTA chelation.

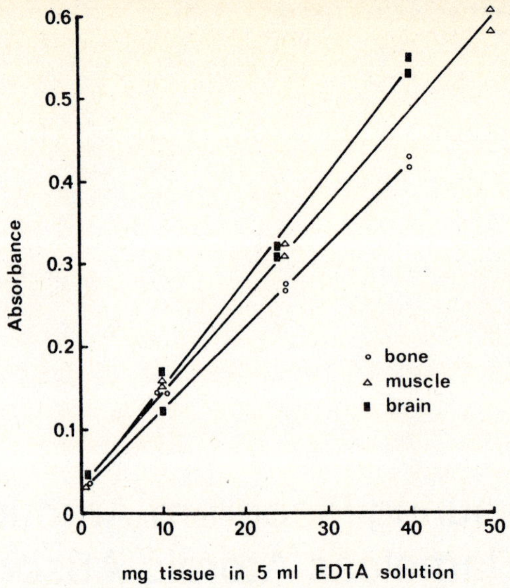

Fig. 1. Absorbance vs. working range of concentrations for three types of tissue

The linearity suggests a constant extraction throughout the range

Analytical Methods

All of the aluminum standards (0, 10, 20, 50, and 100 μg/liter) were made from a 1 mg/liter aluminum stock and prepared in the saturated Na_2EDTA matrix. New standards were prepared for each day's analyses. The sample volume injected was 25 μl. The standard curve was linear from 3 to 100 μg/liter. The standard error of estimate (σ) for the curve, as determined by a least-squares regression, is 3.2 μg/liter. The instrumentation produces no detectable electronic noise, so that both accuracy and precision are evidently limited mainly by reproducibility of sample injection. The sensitivity as defined by 44 milliabsorbance units, is 1.1 μg of aluminum per liter (27 pg/25 μl). However, 3.2 μg/liter (σ) is probably a more reasonable value for this variable. The detection limit, defined as twice the noise level, which is also limited by the σ of the standard curve, is about 6 μg/liter or, for the 25-μl samples, about 150 pg. Similarly, the detection limit as calculated by the equation of Slavin et al. (*8*) was 5 μg of aluminum per liter. The chart recorder records 1 absorbance unit (1.0 *A*) full scale, and a 10 mV input. No scale expansion was used. To ensure that the concentration was within the linear range, all samples were diluted to about 50 μg/liter (0.23 *A*) or less.

To evaluate the effects on absorbance of the respective matrices of the various tissues examined, we added known amounts of aluminum to each type of sample—gray and white matter, cortical and trabecular bone, and muscle—as follows. All samples were prepared in the usual way and 25 mg of each were di-

Table 1. Results of Replicate Aluminum Analyses

	Al, mg/kg of dried tissue		
Drying conditions:	Dry in plastic	400 °C, in Pyrex	600 °C, in Pt
Muscle, 5 samples	3.6	—	3.7
	7.4	—	6.2
	3.9	—	8.8
	21.9	—	20.2
	0.9	—	0.9
Bone, 5 samples	3.5	2.9	—
	1.4	1.1	—
	31.3	29.4	—
	17.7	14.2	—
	184.	212.	—
Brain, 10 samples	—	1.7	2.0
	—	5.1	5.2
	—	2.5	2.5
	—	14.8	14.0
	—	1.0	2.4
	—	2.2	3.8
	—	2.5	1.4
	—	7.4	5.0
	—	7.0	9.0
	—	1.7	1.4

Table 2. Analytical Recovery of Added Al from Various Tissues

	Al present	Al added	
	μg/liter of sample extract		Recovery, %
Trabecular bone	12	50	106
Cortical bone	2	50	100
Trabecular bone	51	50	98
Muscle	5	50	97
Brain, gray matter	37	50	97
Brain, white matter	45	50	95

Table 3. Values Reported for Tissue Aluminum

	Muscle	Brain	Bone
	Al, mg/kg dry weight		
Present study			
Mean	1.22	1.30	3.88
SD	0.72	0.68	1.73
Tipton & Cook (*8*)			
Mean	1.55	1.40	—
SD	3.60	3.00	—
Crapper et al. (*9*)			
Mean	—	1.10	—
Range		(0.23–2.7)	

luted in 5 ml of EDTA solution. After an initial analysis, 25 μl (0.25 μg) of aluminum was added, corresponding to the addition of 50 μg/liter to the sample solutions. The samples were re-analyzed and the results appear in Table 2. If two such aliquots were added (corresponding to 100 and 150 μg/liter), the absorbances deviated slightly from linearity. As mentioned, these concentrations are well above our working range, but the data suggest that the matrix of the samples does exert an 8 to 10% suppressive effect at concentrations greater than 100 μg/liter in the sample.

The effect of various ions on aluminum absorption spectroscopy was also evaluated by adding, per liter, 1 g of Ca^{2+}, Sr^{2+}, Mg^{2+}, k^{+}, La^{3+}, Na^{+}, Cl^{-}, SO_4^{2-}, and PO_4^{3-} to a 100 μg/liter aluminum solution. None of these ions had any significant effect.

The values we found for muscle and brain aluminum concentrations in control subjects were similar to values previously reported by Tipton and Cook (*9*), who used emission spectroscopy, and by Crapper et al. (*10*), who used flame atomic absorption (Table 3). There are too few values reported for bone for us to make a comparison.

Discussion

With this method we have been able to show that uremic patients who are receiving aluminum salts orally have a significantly increased aluminum in brain, muscle, and bone (*11*).

This method of aluminum analysis has a number of advantages over previously described techniques. The sensitivity of aluminum analysis with this flameless atomic absorption method is 175 pg as compared to 4 ng with neutron activation analysis (Gulf General Atomic, San Diego, Calif.) and a reported sensitivity of 50–500 ng for emission spectroscopy (*12, 13*). In our hands, the detection limit for aluminum with flame atomic absorption with use of nitrous oxide and acetylene has been 0.1 mg/liter. Similarly a colorimetric method for aluminum analysis in which Ferron (8-hydroxy-7-iodo-5-quinolinesulfonic acid) is used was found to be too insensitive, susceptible to interferences from other ions, and contamination-prone as a result of the large amounts of reagents used.

Although the flameless atomic absorption system offers a method with the desired sensitivity, matrix effects are a problem. Various chemical reactions occur in the injected sample when the graphite tube is heated and the resulting absorption is affected by the composition and structure of the salt in which the element of interest is precipitated. As a result of the above or additional effects we found that tissue prepared in a nitric acid digest gave erratic results for aluminum with the graphite furnace. Because of the fact that the ethylenediaminetetraacetate anion forms nondissociated water-soluble complexes with a number of metals and has a high formation constant with aluminum ($10^{-16.13}$), as compared to Ca ($10^{-10.70}$) and Mg ($10^{-8.69}$), EDTA extraction (*14*) of the tissues was used as a substitute for the nitric acid digestion, to decrease the chances for sample contamination. Although there is no biological Standard Reference Material (such as SRM 1577, bovine liver) with reported aluminum values for use in verifying the accuracy of this method, there is considerable evidence presented here that suggests that the aluminum present in the tissue samples is completely extracted. First, when different weights of tissue were extracted with EDTA the concentration values found for all samples were similar. Secondly, alternative methods of preparation of tissue samples, drying and ashing, yielded similar results. It seems unlikely that the extraction efficiency could be so similar if extraction were less than 100% complete. Finally, our values for muscle and brain from control subjects are similar to those reported by other authors who used other extraction techniques and other analytical methods (*9, 10*).

Because EDTA also chelates other trace elements, including lead, mercury, cadmium, zinc, copper, and nickel (*14*), this method may be useful in extracting various elements for analysis by flameless atomic absorption techniques. Extraction with EDTA solution offers a number of advantages over other methods of solubilizing biological samples, such as wet and dry ashing: tissues can be lyophilized or dried at low temperature for preparation and extraction, obviating the volatilization of certain elements that could occur with high-temperature ashing; acids that can interfere with the determination of various elements by flameless atomic absorption are not used in this procedure; the method is simple; and external trace-element contamination is largely eliminated. Whether EDTA extraction will prove to be useful for all tissues is unknown, but we are currently studying additional trace elements and tissues with this method.

This study was supported by NIH contract No. 1-AM-4-2217, General V.A. Research support, and a grant from the Rocky Mountain Kidney Foundation. We thank Dottie Goodman and Daisy Rodarte for their secretarial assistance.

References

1. Rubini, M. E., Coburn, J. W., Massry, S. G., et al., Renal osteodystrophy: Some therapeutic considerations relative to long-term dialysis and transplantation. *Arch. Intern. Med.* **124,** 663 (1969).

2. Clarkson, E. M., Luck, V. A., Hynson, W. V., et al., The effect of aluminum balances, the serum parathyroid hormone concentration and the aluminum content of bone in patients with chronic renal failure. *Clin. Sci.* **43,** 519 (1972).

3. Berlyne, G. M., Ben-Ari, J., Pest, D., et al., Hyperaluminaemia from aluminum resins in renal failure. *Lancet* **ii,** 494 (1970).

4. Parsons, V., Daview, C., Goode, C., et al., Aluminum in bone from patients with renal failure. *Br. Med. J.* **4,** 273 (1971).

5. Kopeloff, L., Barrera, S., Kopeloff, N., Recurrent convulsive seizures in animals produced by immunologic and chemical means. *Am. J. Psychiatry* **98,** 881 (1942).

6. Klatzo, I., Wisniewski, H., and Streicher, E., Experimental production of neurofibrillary degeneration. *J. Neuropathol. Exp. Neurol.* **24,** 187 (1965).

7. Miller, C. A., and Levine, F. M., Effects of aluminum salts on cultured neuroblastoma cells. *J. Neurochem.* **22,** 751 (1974).

8. Slavin, S., Barnett, W. B., and Kahn, H. L., The determination of atomic absorption detection limits by direct measurement. *At. Absorpt. Newsl.* **11,** 37 (1972).

9. Tipton, I. H., and Cook, M. J., Trace elements in human tissue. Part II. Adult subjects from the United States. *Health Phys.* **9,** 103 (1963).

10. Crapper, D. R., Krishnan, S. S., and Dalton, A. J., Brain aluminum distribution in Alzheimer's disease and experimental neurofibrillary degeneration. *Trans. Am. Neurol. Assoc.* **98,** 17 (1973).

11. Alfrey, A. C., LeGendre, G. R., and Kaehny, W. D., The dialysis encephalopathy syndrome—possible aluminum intoxication. Accepted for publication, *New Engl. J. Med.*

12. Indraprasit, S., Alexander, G. V., and Gonic, H. C., Tissue composition of major and trace elements in uremia and hypertension. *J. Chronic Dis.* **27,** 135 (1974).

13. Tipton, I. H., Cook, M. J., Steiner, R. L., et al., Trace elements in human tissue. Part I. Methods. *Health Phys.* **9,** 89 (1963).

14. Diehl, H., *Calcein, Calmagite, and 1,1-Dihydroxyazobenzene: Titrimetric, Colorimetric and Fluorometric Reagents for Calcium and Magnesium.* G. Frederick Smith Chemical Co., Columbus, Ohio, 1964, pp 1–4.

CLIN. CHEM. 22/1, 57-62 (1976)

Electrophoretic Amylase Fractionation as an Aid in Diagnosis of Pancreatic Disease

Mark E. Legaz and Margaret A. Kenny[1]

Six α-amylase (EC 3.2.1.1) isoenzymes have been resolved electrophoretically on cellulose acetate membranes in a discontinuous buffer system. The fastest migrating isoenzymes are of salivary origin (S1, S2, S3), the slower ones of pancreatic origin (P1, P2, P3). We determined the amylase isoenzyme distribution in the sera of 240 subjects. A specific pancreatic isoenzyme (P3) was observed in all clinically diagnosed cases of acute or chronic pancreatitis as well as in 15 of 40 renal-transplant patients. Moreover, P3 isoenzyme activity declined during apparent recovery from pancreatitis. The P2 isoenzyme appeared in 95% of all specimens, P1 in only 2%. The pancreatic isoenzymes were preferentially excreted in the urine of both renal-transplant patients and normal individuals. The major salivary isoenzyme, S1, was observed in 95% of all serum and urine samples; however, the S2 and S3 appeared less consistently. Our method is simple and rapid, and quite applicable for use in clinical evaluation of patients with pancreatitis or with certain nonpancreatic dysfunctions.

Additional Keyphrases: *anatomical origin of isoenzymes • various patterns of isoenzymes in serum from various disorders • renal transplant • extraction of amylase from pancreas • normal values*

Evaluation of α-amylase (EC 3.2.1.1; 1,4-α-D-glucan glucanohydrolase) activity in serum and urine is frequently useful in the diagnosis of acute pancreatic disease. The usefulness is enhanced by identifying the source of the activity, because amylase can enter the circulation from several extrapancreatic sites (*1, 2*). Many disorders—such as intestinal obstruction or inflammation, common-duct stones, hepatitis, and facial or abdominal trauma—can produce an abnormally high amylase activity in the serum (*3*). Separating amylase isoenzymes from one another is the first step in identifying the tissue source, and can be done with column chromatography (*4*) or by electrophoresis on polyacrylamide gel (*5*) or cellulose acetate (*6, 7*).

The electrophoretic methods have been most popular with researchers (*5, 6, 8*). We used electrophoretic separation on cellulose acetate membranes in this study because of its adaptability as a routine clinical chemistry procedure. Because little is known as yet about the potential diagnostic utility of amylase isoenzyme evaluation, we applied the method to the problem of distinguishing pancreatic from extrapancreatic diseases.

The amylase in human serum and urine can be separated into six distinct isoenzymes by electrophoresis on cellulose acetate membranes. These isoamylases migrate anodally in the γ- to β_1-globulin regions and have activities consistent with those of pancreatic amylases (P1, P2, P3) and salivary amylases (S1, S2, S3). Most specimens of serum or urine contain fewer than four of the possible six isoenzymes. Furthermore, the predominance of either pancreatic or salivary components in a given sample may reflect either the extent of cellular damage or an inherited trait in a healthy individual.

In this investigation we measured the relative activities of the amylase isoenzymes present in serum or urine (or both) of normal persons and of individuals whose amylase activity was abnormally high. We especially tried to correlate acute pancreatic disease with the presence of increased activity of a particular isoenzyme. Finally, we report our findings on the applicability of measuring amylase isoenzymes in cases of nonpancreatic disorders.

Department of Laboratory Medicine, SB-10, University of Washington School of Medicine, Seattle, Wash. 98195.
[1] Address correspondence to this author.
Received Aug. 4, 1975; accepted Oct. 13, 1975.

Materials and Methods

Procedure for Isoenzyme Separation

The amylase isoenzymes were separated by a modified version of the method described by Benjamin and Kenny (7). All buffers were prepared with chemicals of reagent-grade (or better) purity and dissolved in de-ionized, doubly-distilled water. The various amylase isoenzymes were fractionated on cellulose acetate membranes (Sartorius, 34 Gottingen, West Germany) in a standard "Microzone" electrophoresis cell (Beckman Instruments, Fullerton, Calif. 92634). The isoenzymes were best resolved at 4 °C by using a discontinuous buffer system with tris(hydroxymethyl) aminomethane (0.15 mol/liter, titrated to pH 9.15 with boric acid) in the anodal chamber, and sodium barbital (30 mmol/liter, pH 8.6) in the cathodal chamber.

We fully wetted the cellulose acetate strip with a mixture of equal volumes of anodal and cathodal buffer containing 10 g/liter of bovine serum albumin (Miles Laboratories, Kankakee, Ill. 60901) and carefully blotted it between paper towels before placing it in the electrophoresis apparatus. It was necessary to minimize overheating during the electrophoresis by surrounding the cell with ice. We applied the samples with a 0.25-μl applicator (Beckman), the number of applications depending on the total amylase activity of the sample. Three 0.25-μl applications sufficed for serum of normal amylase activity (0.8–3.2 U/liter), fewer for samples with above-normal amylase activity. We tried to keep the amount of total activity applied for each sample within 3 U/liter, to allow for an equal total color development with the chromogenic substrate at the end of the electrophoresis. We placed a control serum in any of the eight troughs, to check the accuracy and precision of the run. A constant current of 3.0 mA was applied for 1.25 h.

Some Analytical Variables

The duration of the electrophoresis, a constant current, and a large potential gradient are critical to reproducible and reliable amylase isoenzyme fractionation. Too prolonged electrophoresis results in smeared isoenzyme bands, and overheating results if the current is too high, which can denature the enzyme.

The electrophoresis buffer can be used for three runs. The anodal buffer is stable for six months at 4 °C, but the cathodal buffer is stable for only six weeks at 4 °C. Benjamin and Kenny (7) described conditions for assessing the location and relative concentration of the amylase isoenzymes by using Phadebas tablets (Pharmacia, Piscataway, N. J. 08854), dissolved in an agarose (10 g/liter) matrix, as the chromogenic substrate. It is critical that the chromogenic substrate be embedded carefully in the agarose. When it has cooled to 45 °C, this mixture should be poured into a 6 × 10 cm tray; if poured while it is at a higher temperature, the substrate will settle to the bottom of the tray and will not be available for contact with the enzyme.

Measurement of Activity

After their electrophoretic separation and staining, we measured the amylase isoenzymes with a Beckman Model R110 Densitometer equipped with a 594-nm interference filter. This instrument integrates the area under each peak and prints out the proportion of each isoenzyme as a percentage of the total.

The total amylase activity of each specimen was quantitated by the amyloclastic starch/iodide procedure described by Rice (*9*). In this procedure, one measures the amount of starch remaining after a 15-min enzymatic hydrolysis at 37 °C. All sera found to have abnormal amylase activity were electrophoretically fractionated. Each patient's medical record was examined to determine the primary medical diagnosis. In 15 of the 40 patients studied who had pancreatitis, the diagnostic evidence was complemented by histological examination of tissue specimens obtained surgically or at autopsy.

Each specimen was stored at −20 °C in glass test tubes before isoenzyme fractionation. Serum amylase isoenzymes were stable for as long as six months at −20 °C; in contrast, amylase in urine was unstable and had to be quantitated within a day of its collection. The control serum we used as a source of amylase isoenzymes was Hyland unassayed serum (Travenol Laboratory, Costa Mesa, Calif. 92626) supplemented with serum from a pancreatitis patient and with diluted normal human saliva obtained by parotid gland cannulation. The activity of the control serum was 6.2 U/liter. The control serum was stable for six months when stored at −20 °C (in 250-μl conical polyethylene centrifuge tubes).

The pancreatic tissue extract we used as a comparison material was prepared from 15 g of human pancreas obtained at autopsy. The tissue, cut into small pieces, was homogenized in a Virtis "45" homogenization apparatus (Virtis Co., Gardiner, N. Y. 12525) at full speed for 5 min in the presence of 25 ml of sodium phosphate buffer (50 mmol/liter, pH 7.5) containing 0.15 mmol of NaCl per liter, at 4 °C. The resulting homogenate was then centrifuged (7000 × *g*, 10 min, 4 °C) to remove particulate matter. The supernate had an activity of about 3000 U/liter and was stable indefinitely at −20 °C.

Results

Five of the six electrophoretically resolvable amylase isoenzymes are shown on the stained cellulose acetate membrane in Figure 1. The corresponding densitometer tracing of the isoenzymes shown there appears in Figure 2. The direction of migration of the isoenzymes is from right to left, with the P2 and S3 components being the most cathodal and most anodal migrating species, respectively. The origin is not shown in Figure 2, but is approximately at 18 cm on

Fig. 1. Amylase isoenzyme pattern of an amylase-supplemented control serum, electrophoresed on a cellulose acetate membrane
The anode is at the bottom

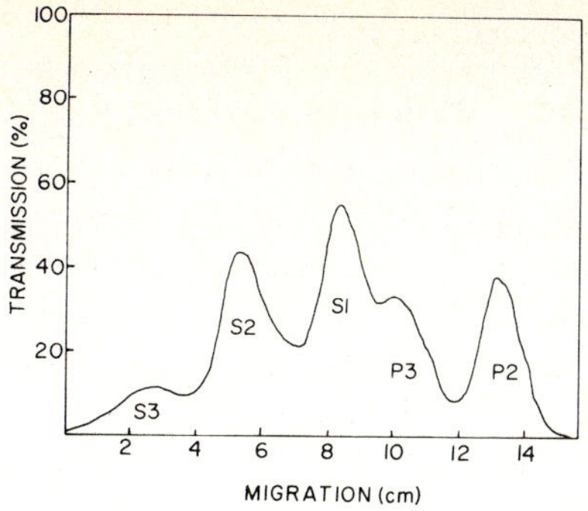

Fig. 2. Densitometer tracing of the amylase isoenzymes shown in Figure 1
The anode is at the left

the abscissa, directly preceding the position where P1 is ordinarily found. The P1 isoenzyme appeared in fewer than 2% of all patients studied, and because of its rarity, was not included in the precision studies. The isoenzymes most commonly observed in serum were the P2, S1, and S2 components. Only the P2 isoenzyme was observed in the supernate from two normal pancreatic homogenates at various dilutions from 1.0 to 20 U/liter. The pancreatic fluid obtained during surgical drainage of a pancreatic cyst contained the fastest moving P3 isoenzyme, along with P2. All three of the salivary isoenzymes shown in Figure 2 were present in saliva obtained by cannulation of a patient's parotid gland. The presence of 50 mmol/liter disodium ethylenediaminetetraacetate in the Phadebas agarose matrix totally inhibited color production. This experiment was performed to eliminate the possibility that one or more of the bands shown in Figure 1 might be an α-glucosidase, which is not inhibited by ethylenediaminetetraacetate.

Between-day precision for the electrophoretic separation of amylase isoenzymes was evaluated by electrophoresing eight 0.25-μl samples of the control serum on a single membrane; this was repeated on 15 consecutive days. Within-day precision for the fractionation procedure was evaluated from five runs done on the same day. Table 1 summarizes results of these precision studies. The mean activity for the individual isoenzymes shown was obtained by multiplying the relative area under each peak (%) by the total activity of the sample (i.e., 6.2 U/liter). The areas under each peak were measured by integrating between the minima of each peak.

To determine the diagnostic usefulness of this procedure, we fractionated the amylase isoenzymes in 240 sera. Each serum was specifically screened for the presence of the fastest migrating (P3) isoenzyme; the results are summarized in Table 2. The P2 and S1 isoenzymes were those most commonly present in the normal blood-donors' sera, with a mean frequency of 55 ± 12% and 47 ± 9%, respectively. The group of 85 patients with abnormally high amylase activity and with no demonstrable P3 had various clinical diagnoses, including cholecystitis, bowel obstruction and inflammation, ruptured ectopic pregnancy, abdominal trauma, peptic ulcer, hepatitis, or short bowel syndrome with hyperalimentation.

The P3 isoenzyme was detected in all patients with a clinical diagnosis of either chronic or acute pancreatitis, as well as in 15 of the 40 renal-transplant patients.

The renal-transplant patients had, as a population, relatively lower total serum amylase than those with pancreatic disease. The renal-transplant patients also had greater salivary isoenzyme activity (Table 3).

Table 1. Between-day and Within-day Precision of the Amylase Isoenzyme Fractionation Method

	Between-day (n = 15 runs)			Within-day (n = 5 runs)		
	Mean activity	SD		Mean activity	SD	
Isoenzyme	U/liter		CV %	U/liter		CV %
P2	1.2	0.05	4.2	1.3	0.04	3.5
P3	1.0	0.06	6.0	1.0	0.04	5.2
S1	1.8	0.04	2.2	1.8	0.03	2.5
S2	1.6	0.04	2.5	1.5	0.04	2.0
S3	0.6	0.12	20.0	0.6	0.10	7.7

Table 2. Presence of the P3 Isoenzyme in the Sera of Various Subject Groups

Group	No. specimens	Mean activity, U/liter	No. sera containing P3 isoenzyme
Normal donors	25	1.6 ± 0.7	0
Inpatients	50	2.0 ± 0.8	0
Renal failure and kidney transplant recipients	40	2.7 ± 1.3	15
Inpatients with facial trauma, bowel obstruction, etc.	85	6.2 ± 2.8	0
Pancreatic disease[a]	40	19.2 ± 7.6	40

[a] The diagnosis of 15 of the 40 was confirmed at surgery or autopsy.

Table 3. Comparison of Serum Amylase Activity and Isoenzyme Distribution in Patients with Pancreatic and Renal Disease

	Serum amylase, U/liter	% of total amylase activity		
		P2	P3	Salivary
Renal disease	2.7 ± 1.3	51 ± 16	14 ± 4	34 ± 16
Pancreatic disease	19.0 ± 7.6	73 ± 10	22 ± 9	6 ± 7

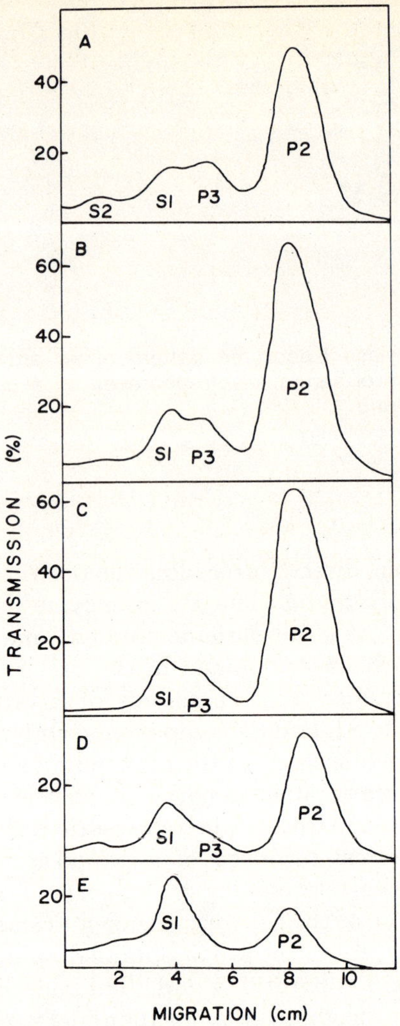

Fig. 3. Densitometer tracings of amylase isoenzymes in serum samples taken from the patient with chronic pancreatitis outlined in Table 4

A, Day 1; *B*, Day 2; *C*, Day 4; *D*, Day 11; *E*, Day 17

Four patients with parotitis and 10 who had sustained facial trauma of various severities were also studied. The combined salivary isoenzyme activity in the sera of these patients represented greater than 85% of the total amylase activity. A single patient with clinically diagnosed macro-amylasemia had a normal isoenzyme distribution in her serum.

Serum from a two-month-old infant who according to endocrinologic and histologic criteria was born without a functional pancreas had an amylase activity half the value for the lower normal limit. No pancreatic isoenzymes were detected; the salivary isoenzyme contribution was 93.6% S1 and 6.4% S2. This low total activity is consistent with other reports that amylase activity is low at birth and increases during the first two years. The absence of any pancreatic isoenzyme activity in this infant may be remarkable, but we are not aware of serum isoenzyme studies in newborns.

Three patients with pancreatitis were studied during the course of their acute attacks, and the increase and decrease in their P3 activity correlated well with their clinical condition. Figure 3 illustrates the appearance and disappearance of the P3 isoenzyme as observed in one of these patients; Table 4 summarizes the activity and relative percentages of his various isoenzyme components. In this patient, a chronic alcoholic with a long history of chronic pancreatitis, the serum amylase isoenzyme distribution served as ancillary documentation of pancreatitis, along with radiographic and roentgenogram evidence.

We examined the amylase isoenzyme distribution in both serum and urine from 15 renal-transplant patients and 10 normal patients. There was a distinguishable increase in the urinary P2 isoenzyme activity, compared with the activity in serum in both the renal-transplant and normal subjects, as seen in Figure 4. The mean P2 isoenzyme activity was 20.7% greater in the urine of the renal-transplant patients than in their serum, whereas the same mean for normal subjects was 19.7% greater for urine than for serum.

In six of the 15 renal-transplant patients in whom both urine and serum were studied, the P3 isoenzyme was detected in the serum but not in the urine; in three, P3 was detected in both serum and urine, with a 15% higher proportion in the urine. In both the renal-transplant and normal patients, the total amy-

Table 4. Distribution of Serum Amylase Isoenzymes for a Patient during an Episode of Chronic Pancreatitis

	Isoenzyme, %					
Day	P2	P3	S1	S2	S3	Total amylase, U/liter
1	74.0	12.4	9.8	2.6	1.2	17.9
2	72.7	11.2	13.6	2.5	0	20.8
4	73.8	9.6	13.4	3.4	0	14.9
11	64.7	4.5	29.6	1.2	0	9.9
17	42.7	0	54.1	3.2	0	1.8

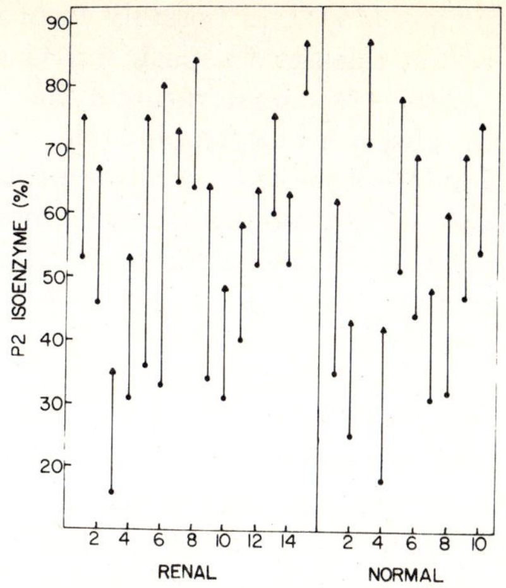

Fig. 4. Comparison of the P2 isoenzyme in serum and urine of renal-transplant patients and normal persons

Dots represent values for activity of isoenzyme P2 in serum. *Triangles* represent urinary isoenzyme P2 activity values

lase activity was within the normal range, and the activity in the serum was always slightly higher (0.3–0.8 U/liter) than in the urine.

Discussion

Many investigators have assessed the amylase isoenzymes in human serum and urine with the intention of finding a potential clinical significance (*8, 10, 11*). Our method, a modified version of the cellulose acetate electrophoresis system outlined by Benjamin and Kenny (*7*), more completely resolves the three pancreatic and three salivary amylase isoenzymes. The overall procedure is simple, rapid, and quite suitable for use in a routine clinical chemistry laboratory.

Because this procedure was designated as a qualitative test that would provide complementary information along with the total amylase activity, the linearity of the method was not fully determined. Peak area and activity were linearly related, however, from 0.8 to 4.8 U/liter when the area under the P2 isoenzyme was used as a reference. The precision, a measurement of the reproducibility of the method, was quite good, both within-day and between-days.

The variability of isoenzyme distribution among normal individuals precluded defining a "normal distribution" for each isoenzyme. Gross elevation of the total salivary isoenzyme components or the presence of the P3 isoenzyme seemed to have the greatest diagnostic usefulness. Moreover, the P3 isoenzyme was present in the sera of all patients studied who had been clinically diagnosed as suffering from pancreatitis. The presence of P3 in 15 of 40 renal-transplant patients is unexplained at this time. Penn et al. (*12*), however, have reported observing an induced pancreatitis and hyperamylasemia in renal-homograft recipients at various times after transplantation. Although none of the renal patients in our study had been positively diagnosed as suffering from pancreatitis, the possibility of a subclinical pancreatitis in the 15 renal-transplant patients who demonstrated the P3 isoenzyme cannot be disregarded. Alternatively, medication used in supportive management of the transplant recipients might induce abnormal secretion of pancreatic isoenzymes.

The isoenzyme pattern shown in Figure 3, which demonstrates the appearance and disappearance of the P3 isoenzyme during the clinical course of a patient's pancreatitis, was also observed in two other cases of acute pancreatitis. The presence of the P3 isoenzyme seemed to coincide well with the overall condition of each, and the average half-life of the observed appearance of P3 activity was about 10 days. In general, the patients with pancreatitis had grossly elevated serum amylase activity, attributable almost exclusively to amylase of pancreatic origin, as shown in Table 3. Furthermore, during the course of pancreatic disease, the activity of the salivary isoenzymes was constant.

Recently, attention has been directed toward the specificity of increased renal clearance of amylase in the diagnosis of acute pancreatitis, in response to a paper published by Warshaw and Fuller (*13*), who reported an apparent increase in the ratio between amylase clearance and creatinine clearance in patients with pancreatitis. Furthermore, they did not detect a similar increase in this clearance ratio in patients with hyperamylasemia attributable to diseases of nonpancreatic etiology. Because of the inflammatory nature of pancreatitis, they suggested that a possible minor proteolysis of pancreatic amylase might account for a smaller, more rapidly cleared amylase. Although our data are consistent with an enhanced clearance of pancreatic amylase isoenzymes relative to salivary-type isoenzymes, they do not indicate an altered clearance mechanism in pancreatitis patients. The electrophoretic mobilities of amylase isoenzymes were the same in the serum and urine of a given patient. Levine et al. (*14*) observed an increased amylase/creatinine clearance ratio in disorders other than pancreatitis.

Some recent indications support the hypothesis that the increased amylase activity observed in diabetic ketoacidosis (*15*), and possibly in other disorders, could reflect release of hepatic amylase after its interaction with lysosomal proteolytic enzymes. Whether the observed electrophoretic variants of pancreatic amylase arise from enzyme proteolysis in the microsomes or represent a true polymorphism is still unclear. However, the presence of both P2 and P3 in the pancreatic fluid of a patient with pancreatitis, along with the observed total absence of these same isoenzymes in a newborn devoid of a functional pancreas, strongly supports the theory that they actually originate in the pancreas. Because amylase requires ionic calcium as a cofactor, and α-glucosidases do not, the assumption that the colored electrophoretic bands actually represent amylase isoenzymes is supported by the finding that 50 mmol of ethylenediaminetetraacetate per liter totally inhibited color development.

The somewhat conflicting reports of Levine et al. (*14*) and of Warshaw and Fuller (*13*) exemplify the shortcomings of evaluating an activity without discriminating the source of enzyme release. Moreover, an evaluation of the various amylase isoenzymes would appear to be a more reliable approach to the study of selective permeability of pancreatic amylase in the kidney. Amylase isoenzyme fractionation studies should appreciably clarify the present controversy regarding the selective glomerular permeability of pancreatic amylase during acute pancreatic disease.

This work was supported in part by NIGMS Training Grant in Clinical Chemistry 5T01-GM00776-12 and by USPHS Research Grant 1-F32-CA05170-01 from the National Cancer Institute.

References

1. Berk, J. E., Searcy, R. L., Hayashi, S., and Ujihira, I., Distribution of serum amylase in man and animals. *J. Am. Med. Assoc.* **192,** 389 (1965).

2. Meites, S., and Rogols, S., Serum amylases, isoenzymes, and pancreatitis. *Clin. Chem.* **14,** 1176 (1968).

3. Meites, S., and Rogols, S., Amylase isoenzymes. *Crit. Rev. Clin. Lab. Sci.* **2,** 103 (1971).

4. Fridhandler, L., Berk, J. E., and Ueda, M., Isolation and measurement of pancreatic amylase in human serum and urine. *Clin. Chem.* **18,** 1493 (1972).

5. Tackeuchi, R., Matsushima, T., Sugimura, T., and Kosu, T., A rapid, new method for quantitative analysis of human amylase isoenzymes. *Clin. Chim. Acta* **54,** 137 (1974).

6. Spiekerman, A. M., Perry, P., Hightower, N.C. and Hall, F. F., Chromogenic-substrate method for demonstrating multiple forms of alpha-amylase after electrophoresis. *Clin. Chem.* **20,** 324 (1974).

7. Benjamin, D. R., and Kenny, M. A., Clinical value of amylase isoenzyme determinations. *Am. J. Clin. Pathol.* **62,** 752 (1974).

8. Taussig, L. M., Wolf, R. O., Woods, R. E., and Deckelbaum, R. J., Use of serum isoenzymes in evaluation of pancreatic function. *Pediatrics* **54,** 229 (1974).

9. Rice, E. W., Improved spectrophotometric determination of amylase with a new stable starch substrate solution. *Clin. Chem.* **5,** 592 (1959).

10. Aw, S. E., and Hobbs, J. R., Human isoamylases. *Biochem. J.* **99,** 16P (1966).

11. Kauffman, D. L., Zager, N. l., Cohen, E., and Keller, P. J., The isoenzymes of human parotid saliva. *Arch. Biochem. Biophys.* **137,** 325 (1970).

12. Penn, I., Durst, A. L., Marchado, M., and Groth, C. G., Acute pancreatitis and hyperamylasemia in renal homograft recipients. *Arch. Surg.* (Chicago) **105,** 167 (1972).

13. Warshaw, A. L., and Fuller, A. F., Specificity of increased renal clearance of amylase in diagnosis of acute pancreatitis. *New Engl. J. Med.* **292,** 325 (1975).

14. Levine, R. I., Glauser, F. L., and Berk, J. E., Enhancement of the amylase-creatinine clearance ratio in disorders other than acute pancreatitis. *New Engl. J. Med.* **292,** 329 (1975).

15. Belfiore, F., and Napoli, E., Interpretation of hyperamylasemia in diabetic coma. *Clin. Chem.* **19,** 387 (1973).

CLIN. CHEM. 22/1, 63-66 (1976)

Creatine Kinase Isoenzymes in Baboon Tissues and Organs

Walid G. Yasmineh, Robert B. Pyle, Naomi Q. Hanson, and Bonita K. Hultman

We determined the activity of the isoenzymes of creatine kinase in homogenates of fresh tissues from six baboons. Twenty-six tissues were removed from each baboon and the isoenzymes in them were separated by chromatography on diethylaminoethyl-Sephadex A-50. Total activity was greatest in skeletal muscle (2600 U/g wet weight) followed by myocardium (800 U/g), brain (180 U/g), and the bladder and tissues of the gastrointestinal tract (about 100 U/g). Ten tissues had total activities of less than 20 U/g: trachea, lung, kidney, thyroid, gall bladder, liver, spleen, pancreas, common bile duct, and adrenal. Skeletal muscle contained only the MM isoenzyme; myocardium contained 81% MM isoenzyme, 18% MB isoenzyme, and 1% BB isoenzyme. Except for thyroid and pancreas, all other tissues contained mainly the BB isoenzyme. Tissues of the gastrointestinal tract contained significant (7 to 17%) MB isoenzyme activity.

Although recent investigations indicate that information on the activity of the MB isoenzyme of creatine kinase (EC 2.7.3.2, CK) in serum is extremely useful in diagnosis of myocardial infarction and estimation of infarct size (*1-8*), there is little information concerning its specificity in human tissues. A major reason for this is the fact that reliable techniques for separating and measuring the activities of the isoenzymes have only recently become available (*3, 9-12*). A second major reason is the obvious problem of obtaining normal fresh human tissues for study.

In the present investigation, we used a sensitive technique recently developed in our laboratory (*11*) to determine the CK isoenzyme activity of various tissues of the baboon (*Papio cynocephalus*), a species closely related to man.

Our results indicate that the myocardium is the major source of the MB isoenzyme, although significant MB isoenzyme activity is found in tissues of the gastrointestinal tract. Despite the bulk of the latter tissues, however, there should be no confusion as to the source of the MB isoenzyme in serum after myocardial damage, because the principal CK isoenzyme in gastrointestinal tissues is the BB isoenzyme, in contrast to myocardium, in which MM is the predominant isoenzyme.

Departments of Laboratory Medicine, Pathology, and Surgery, University of Minnesota Medical School, Box 198, Mayo Memorial Building, Minneapolis, Minn. 55455.

Received Aug. 29, 1975; accepted Oct. 16, 1975.

Material and Methods

Animals and Tissues

In this study, we used six baboons ranging in weight from 10 to 20 kg. The animals were anesthetized with ketamine hydrochloride and phencyclidine hydrochloride. In each case, the heart was the first tissue to be excised because the baboons were part of another study involving measurement of infarct size after experimental induction of myocardial infarction.[1] The remaining tissues were removed during the next 35 to 45 min. After excision, each tissue was immediately washed in ice-cold water, thoroughly dried with gauze, weighed, immersed in powdered solid CO_2, and stored at −70 °C until processed.

Homogenization of Tissues and Assay of CK Isoenzyme Content

Tissues were thawed in homogenizing medium at 4 °C and then homogenized, and the cellular debris was removed by centrifugation as previously described (*11*). CK isoenzymes in the supernatant fluids were separated by discontinuous gradient elution from micro-columns of DEAE-Sephadex A-50. CK activity was measured by the method of Rosalki, with a centrifugal analyzer (*11*).

In tissues for which the CK activity was primarily the BB isoenzyme (such as those of the gastrointestinal tract), the MB isoenzyme fraction was recycled by discontinuous gradient elution from another micro-column of the anion exchanger, to ensure that it was not contaminated with BB isoenzyme. In these tissues, the presence and amount of the MB fraction was further ascertained by its behavior on continuous gradient elution from the anion exchanger and electrophoresis on cellulose acetate (*11*).

Results

Table 1 summarizes, in descending order, the total CK activity in 26 tissues from each of the six baboons. Except for a few tissues that will be discussed below, the range of values for each tissue from the six baboons was reasonably close, so that the average values are meaningful, and fall into two rather distinct groups: those with activities greater than 20 U/g

[1] Pyle, R. B., Nicoloff, D. M., and Yasmineh, W. G., Determination of myocardial infarct size in the baboon. In preparation.

Table 1

Total CK Activity in Baboon Tissues

(Units per Gram Wet Weight)

Baboon No.	1	2	3	4	5	6	Mean	% CV
GROUP I								
Skeletal muscle	2682.2	1543.0	3136.8	1481.4	2871.0	3715.9	2571.7	34.7
Heart	598.8	749.4	723.0	1041.3	794.6	824.6	788.6	18.6
Esophagus	166.0	153.6	200.9	373.4	278.8	300.9	245.6	35.2
Cerebellum	194.9	194.5	134.0	241.5	130.8	196.6	182.1	23.3
Cerebrum	135.6	237.1	160.5	186.4	192.9	155.1	177.9	20.1
Stomach (antrum)	122.3	108.0	115.4	145.2	118.1	161.2	128.4	15.9
Transverse colon	102.2	151.2	106.6	108.1	118.4	118.7	117.5	15.1
Bladder (urinary)	136.6	90.4	100.7	109.7	143.2	116.9	116.2	17.6
Duodenum	58.7	124.4	78.7	99.0	174.2	130.5	110.9	37.1
Spinal cord	76.1	149.5	118.8	141.2	76.2	96.5	109.7	29.1
Ileum	90.7	133.9	103.8	113.8	94.4	111.9	108.1	14.5
Prostate	-	60.2	130.7	240.0	21.7	62.4	103.0	83.6
Jejunum	70.2	88.6	70.1	87.7	97.1	146.4	93.4	30.1
Rectum	80.3	80.2	95.5	98.2	69.6	-	84.8	14.0
Stomach (body)	137.1	-	53.4	38.8	42.0	68.9	68.0	59.3
Cecum	57.8	71.3	57.8	64.3	82.0	73.2	67.7	14.1
GROUP II								
Gall bladder	16.6	15.7	13.5	17.5	25.9	19.0	18.0	23.7
Spleen	8.7	16.1	9.7	18.2	11.3	17.1	13.5	30.3
Common bile duct	9.3	6.1	20.5	7.2	7.2	12.1	10.4	51.8
Kidney	4.9	5.1	6.0	12.6	8.7	14.0	8.6	46.2
Trachea	-	-	-	6.0	6.8	9.6	7.5	25.3
Adrenal gland	5.8	-	6.7	11.3	5.2	7.2	7.2	33.1
Lung	4.8	3.7	-	5.4	5.2	7.1	5.2	23.5
Thyroid	-	3.1	8.0	4.5	3.1	5.0	4.7	42.8
Liver	3.0	3.8	5.2	7.2	2.9	4.9	4.5	36.2
Pancreas	1.5	1.0	1.2	3.8	2.6	0.7	1.8	65.4

Table 2

CK Isoenzyme Activity in Baboon Tissues

	Mean Total CK[a] (U/g)	Mean % MM	Mean % MB	Mean % BB
GROUP I				
Skeletal muscle	2571.7	100.0[b]	<0.1	0.0
Heart	788.6	81.3	17.8	0.8
Esophagus	245.6	22.3	2.7	75.0
Cerebellum	182.1	1.8	1.3	96.8
Cerebrum	177.9	1.7	0.9	97.4
Stomach (antrum)	128.4	2.4	7.3	90.3
Transverse colon	117.5	2.5	9.7	87.8
Bladder (urinary)	116.2	1.1	0.7	98.2
Duodenum	110.9	4.0	17.1	78.9
Spinal cord	109.7	2.3	2.3	95.5
Ileum	108.1	2.8	13.3	84.0
Prostate	103.0	52.6	1.0	46.4
Jejunum	93.4	3.4	14.7	81.9
Rectum	84.8	2.8	6.6	90.6
Stomach (body)	68.0	3.1	2.3	94.6
Cecum	67.7	2.2	7.4	90.4
GROUP II				
Gall bladder	18.0	10.9	2.4	86.7
Spleen	13.5	10.8	0.4	88.8
Common bile duct	10.4	15.0	4.7	80.3
Kidney	8.6	26.2	1.1	72.7
Trachea	7.5	19.6	2.1	78.2
Adrenal gland	7.2	13.4	5.3	81.3
Lung	5.2	19.2	5.3	75.6
Thyroid	4.7	55.3	9.1	35.6
Liver	4.5	23.1	3.3	73.5
Pancreas	1.8	40.2	7.7	52.1

a) These values were carried over from Table I for comparison.

b) Approximately 20 U of CK activity was applied to the column. Following elution of the MM isoenzyme with 0.1 mol/liter NaCl-Tris buffer, the column was washed with two 15-ml aliquots of the same buffer to avoid subsequent contamination of the MB fraction with MM isoenzyme.

wet weight (Group I), and those with less (Group II). Within the first group, the greatest mean activity was found in skeletal muscle (2572 U/g), followed by heart tissue (789 U/g), brain (180 U/g), bladder (116 U/g), and prostate (103 U/g). Tissues of the gastrointestinal tract are also included in this group and contain collectively, except for the esophagus, about the same mean activity (68 to 128 U/g).

High-activity Tissues

Although most of the ranges of CK activity of the tissues in Group I were reasonably close (<30% CV), skeletal muscle, esophagus, body of the stomach, duodenum, jejunum, and prostate showed CV values greater than 30%. In the case of skeletal muscle, the high value is due mainly to two of the six specimens, for which total CK values were low compared to the rest, probably owing to autolysis. Autolysis is also undoubtedly responsible for the high CV values in the body of the stomach, the duodenum, and the jejunum, where proteolytic enzymes abound. In fact, the specimens from the body of the stomach showed an interesting correlation between total CK activity and time of sampling after death, samples with high activity were removed early while those with low activity were removed toward the end of the sampling period. In the case of the esophagus, the high CV value was principally attributable to elevated MM isoenzyme activities in three of the baboons (baboons No. 4, 5, and 6). These baboons were very small (about 10 kg), and therefore portions of the esophagus distal to the stomach (the pars cervicalis and pars thoracica), which are known to contain striated muscle, may have been included in the specimens (*13*). As Table 2 shows, this is reflected in the high percentage of MM isoenzyme activity in esophagus (22%), when compared with the other tissues of the gastrointestinal tract (2 to 4%). The relatively high CK activity (240 U/g) of one prostate specimen was due primarily to its relatively high MM isoenzyme activity. Because not all portions of the prostate could be removed in most cases, this specimen may have included a substantial proportion of cross-striated muscle fibers that exist in the pubic region of the prostate (*13*). The low CK value of one prostate specimen (22 U/g) may have been caused by autolysis.

Within Group II, mean CK values ranged from 2 to 18 U/g.

Table 2 shows the relative proportions of the three CK isoenzyme activities in baboon tissues. Because of the large number of specimens that were processed, we have listed in this table only the mean percentage values obtained for the six individual determinations on each tissue. As previously reported (*3, 4, 11, 14*), CK activity in skeletal muscle and brain was almost exclusively attributable to MM and BB isoenzyme, respectively. In the case of skeletal muscle, no (<0.1%) MB isoenzyme could be detected, even when relatively large amounts (35 g) of muscle were processed. The proportion of MB activity in

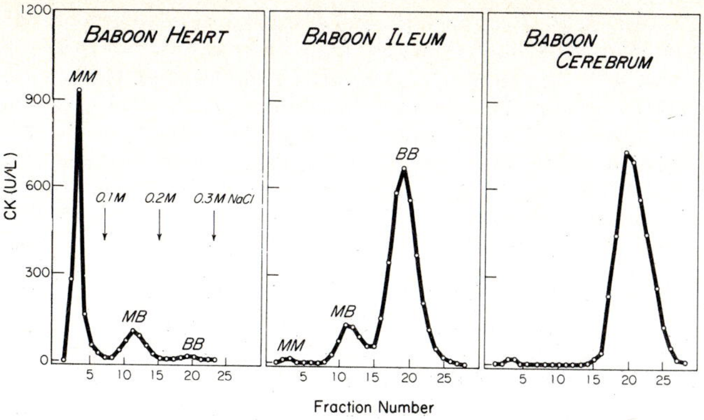

Fig. 1. Separation of CK isoenzymes from baboon heart, ileum, and cerebrum by continuous gradient elution from a column containing DEAE-Sephadex A-50

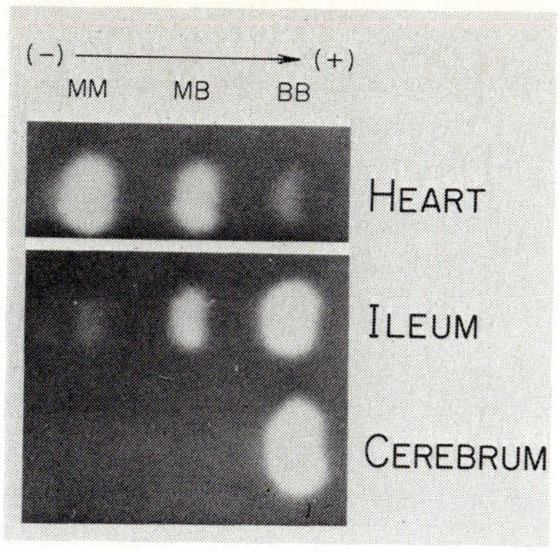

Fig. 2. Separation of CK isoenzymes from baboon heart, ileum, and cerebrum by electrophoresis on cellulose acetate

heart tissue is comparable to that previously reported for humans (*15–17*). In the tissues of the gastrointestinal tract the BB isoenzyme predominates, but they also contain significant amounts of MB isoenzyme activity, smallest in esophagus (2.7%) and stomach (2.3%), more in the antrum of the stomach (7.3%) and small intestine (13.3 to 17.1%), and less in the colon (9.7%) and rectum (6.6%). The presence of MB isoenzyme in gastrointestinal tissues was corroborated by continuous gradient elution on DEAE-Sephadex A-50 and electrophoresis on cellulose acetate (*11*). Typical results by these techniques are illustrated with extracts of baboon ileum (13% MB fraction), heart (18% MB fraction), and cerebrum (1% MB fraction), in Figures 1 and 2, respectively. The proportion of MB activity in the ileum extract as determined from the area under the curve was identical to that obtained after discontinuous elution chromatography and recycling of the MB fraction (11%).

The last two tissues in Group I, bladder and prostate, contain primarily the BB isoenzyme, although, as indicated earlier, the prostate contains an appreciable amount of MM isoenzyme because of the presence of striated muscle.

Low-activity Tissues

Tissues in Group II (Table 2) primarily contain (>70%) the BB isoenzyme, except for thyroid and pancreas, in which MM and BB activities are about equal. The MB activity of the tissues in Group II ranged from 0.4% for pancreas to 9.1% for thyroid. Because the total CK activity of these tissues is small, these percentages correspond to negligible activities of this isoenzyme.

As indicated above, each of the values in Table 2 represents the mean of six separate determinations. There was less variation in this group, especially in the case of the major isoenzyme components in any one tissue. For example, the CV values for the MM and MB isoenzymes of baboon myocardium were 8.8 and 15.2%, respectively, that of the BB isoenzyme of cerebrum 1.4%, and of the MM isoenzyme of skeletal muscle <0.1%.

Discussion

We have determined the CK isoenzyme activity of 26 tissues of the baboon, mainly to establish whether the MB isoenzyme predominates in the myocardium. We worked with the baboon because of its phylogenetic closeness to man, the necessity of using fresh tissues, and the virtual absence (<2 U/liter) of the MB isoenzyme from normal baboon serum.

Our results for the baboon compare well with those of Gowda et al. (*17*), who, to the best of our knowledge, have conducted the only study of CK isoenzymes in fresh human tissues. They reported values for CK isoenzymes in six tissues: brain, heart, skeletal muscle, intestine, lung, and kidney. Values for total CK (in U/g wet weight) from their and our laboratory are: respectively, 180 vs. 200, 800 vs. 900, 2600 vs. 3200, 110 vs. 180, 5 vs. 15, and 9 vs. 9. The isoenzyme patterns of these tissues were also similar, with one exception: they found no MB isoenzyme activity in human intestine, whereas we found it to comprise about 15% and 10% of the total activity in the small and large intestines, respectively, of the baboon. This difference may reflect a species difference, but in view of the close agreement between the results for the other tissues, it is probably due to a more sensitive assay procedure (*11*).

We cannot overemphasize the need for fresh tissues if results are to be valid. In this study, this has been best illustrated by the appreciable degradation of total CK activity in the body of the stomach in some specimens within 35 to 45 min after death. Sobel et al. (*18*) have also reported appreciable loss of CK activity from samples of human myocardium obtained 4 h after death. Comparison of our results with those of another study (*16*), in which the specimens were obtained 12 to 23 h after death, suggests that about 70% of CK activity was lost. For example, in this study (*16*), the mean total CK values reported for skeletal muscle, heart, and brain were 1085, 190, and 71 U/g, respectively.

The virtual absence of MB isoenzyme from skeletal muscle that we found needs comment, because several investigators have reported the presence of MB isoenzyme in serum from normal individuals and in patients with muscular disorders (*11, 19, 20*). Using chromatography on DEAE-Sephadex A-50, Mercer and Varat (*21*) recently reported that as much as 1% of the total activity in human skeletal muscle was attributable to MB isoenzyme, detectable when relatively large amounts of tissue were processed. In the present study, we found that less than 0.1% of the activity was due to MB isoenzyme in 8- to 35-g samples of baboon skeletal muscle. It should be noted, however, that we have found it necessary to use two 15-ml washes to elute residual MM isoenzyme from our columns, to avoid contamination of the MB fraction with MM isoenzyme (see Table 2). We bring up this issue at this point because we think it is important in identifying the source of MB isoenzyme in normal individuals and in patients with muscular disorders. In both groups of individuals, the proportion of MB isoenzyme in serum is frequently greater than 1%, and therefore the possibility that the heart is somehow involved cannot be excluded.

In conclusion, in the baboon the MB isoenzyme of CK is present predominantly in the heart, and to a lesser extent in tissues of the gastrointestinal tract. Because the latter tissues contain mainly BB isoenzyme, however, the presence of MB isoenzyme should not impair the sensitivity or specificity that has been presumed for MB isoenzyme determinations in serum in diagnosis of myocardial damage.

References

1. Wagner, G. S., Roe, C. R., Limbird, L. E., et al., The importance of the identification of the myocardial-specific isoenzyme of creatine phosphokinase (MB form) in the diagnosis of acute myocardial infarction. *Circulation* **47**, 263 (1973).

2. Oldham, H. N., Roe, C. R., Young, W. G., and Dixon, S. H., Intraoperative detection of myocardial damage during coronary artery surgery by plasma creatine phosphokinase isoenzyme analysis. *Surgery* **74**, 917 (1973).

3. Klein, M. S., Shell, W. E., and Sobel, B. E., Serum creatine phosphokinase (CPK) isoenzymes after intramuscular injections, surgery, and myocardial infarction. *Cardiovasc. Res.* **7**, 412 (1973).

4. Mercer, D. W., Separation of tissue and serum creatine kinase isoenzymes by ion-exchange column chromatography. *Clin. Chem.* **20**, 36 (1974).

5. Galen, R. S., Reiffel, J. S., and Gambino, S. R., Diagnosis of acute myocardial infarction. *J. Am. Med. Assoc.* **232**, 145 (1975).

6. Clejan, S., Rabinowitz, B., Doman, J., and Neufeld, H. N., Creatine phosphokinase isoenzymes in myocardial infarction with atypical enzyme profile. *Clin. Chem.* **21**, 974 (1975). Abstract.

7. Mercer, D. W., and Varat, M. A., Cardiac specific creatine phosphokinase isoenzyme in the diagnosis of acute myocardial infarction. *Circulation* **51**, 855 (1975) [abstract: *Clin. Chem.* **21**, 974 (1975)].

8. Smith, A. F., Radford, D., and Wong, C. P., Creatine kinase isoenzyme studies in myocardial infarction. *Clin. Chem.* **21**, 975 (1975).

9. Roberts, R., Ambos, H. D., Carlson, E. M., and Sobel, B. E., Improved quantification of myocardial infarction based on analysis of serum CPK isoenzymes. *Am. J. Cardiol.* **35**, 166 (1975).

10. Roberts, R., Henry, P. D., Witteveen, S. A. G. J., and Sobel, B. E., Quantification of serum creatine phosphokinase activity. *Am. J. Cardiol.* **33**, 650 (1974).

11. Yasmineh, W. G., and Hanson, N. Q., Electrophoresis on cellulose acetate and chromatography on DEAE-Sephadex A-50 compared in the estimation of creatine kinase isoenzymes. *Clin. Chem.* **21**, 381 (1975).

12. Nealon, D. A., and Henderson, A. R., Separation of creatine kinase isoenzymes in serum by ion-exchange column chromatography (Mercer's method, modified to increase sensitivity). *Clin. Chem.* **21**, 392 (1975).

13. Bloom, W., and Fawcett, D. W., *A Textbook of Histology*, Saunders, Philadelphia, Pa., 1962.

14. Eppenberger, H. M., Dawson, D. M., and Kaplan, N. O., The comparative enzymology of creatine kinase. *J. Biol. Chem.* **242**, 204 (1967).

15. Smith, A. F., Separation of tissue and serum creatine kinase isoenzymes on polyacrylamide gel slabs. *Clin. Chim. Acta* **39**, 351 (1972).

16. Jockers-Wretou, E., and Pfleiderer, G., Quantitation of creatine kinase isoenzymes in human tissues and sera by an immunological method. *Clin. Chim. Acta* **58**, 223 (1975).

17. Gowda, K. S., Roberts, R., and Sobel, B. E., Detection of myocardial infarction with serum CPK isoenzymes in surgical patients. *Circulation* **46**, 640 (1972).

18. Sobel, B. E., Breshahan, G. F., Shell, W. E., and Yoder, R. D., Estimation of infarct size in man and its relation to prognosis. *Circulation* **46**, 640 (1972).

19. Silverman, L. M., Mendell, J. R., and Gruemer, H. D., Creatine kinase isoenzymes in muscular dystrophy. *Clin. Chem.* **20**, 865 (1974).

20. Browhlow, K., and Eleviteh, F. R., Serum creatine phosphokinase isoenzyme (CPK_2) in myositis. *J. Am. Med. Assoc.* **230**, 1141 (1974).

21. Mercer, D. W., and Varat, M. A., Detection of cardiac specific creatine kinase isoenzyme in sera with normal and slightly elevated total creatine kinase. *Clin. Chem.* **21**, 1088 (1975).

CLIN. CHEM. 22/1, 67–69 (1976)

Improved Microscale Assay for Purine Phosphoribosyltransferase Activities

Rainer Schmidt, Martine Forêt, and Uwe Reichert

We describe an improved and rapid filter-type assay for purine phosphoribosyltransferase activities. ^{14}C-labeled purine bases are used as substrates, and the equipment includes a sampling manifold and glass-fiber filters coated with polyethyleneimine-cellulose. The method is especially suited for assay of a large number of samples, and may be useful for other enzyme activity measurements.

The purine phosphoribosyltransferases play an important role in the reutilization of purines by liver and other tissues (*1*). They catalyze the following reactions:[1]

$$\text{Hypoxanthine (or guanine)} + \text{PRPP} \xrightarrow{\text{H-PRT}} \text{IMP (or GMP)} + \text{PP}_i$$

$$\text{Adenine} + \text{PRPP} \xrightarrow{\text{A-PRT}} \text{AMP} + \text{PP}_i$$

One of these enzymes, H-PRT, is deficient in erythrocytes and fibroblasts of patients suffering from the Lesch–Nyhan syndrome (*2, 3*), and this deficiency is accompanied by an increased activity of A-PRT (*4*).

The need to measure H-PRT and A-PRT activities has prompted development of a wide variety of procedures for doing so. Besides paper electrophoresis, thin-layer chromatography, and spectrophotometric methods (*5–8*), a filter technique with use of diethylaminoethyl-cellulose paper discs was described (*6, 9*). The procedure proposed in this paper is an improvement of this filter technique.

It has the relative advantage that, without loss of sensitivity, many samples can be quickly assayed. The method is suitable for routine laboratory use.

Materials and Methods

Reagents. [^{14}C]Adenine (54 Ci/mol), [^{14}C]guanine (54 Ci/mol), [^{14}C]adenosine-5′-monophosphate (60 Ci/mol), and [^{14}C]guanosine-5′-monophosphate (58 Ci/mol) were obtained from the Radiochemical Centre Amersham (Amersham Buchler, D-3301 Wenden, G.F.R.). PRPP was purchased from Boehringer Mannheim, D-6800 Mannheim 61, G.F.R.; polyethyleneimine-cellulose for thin-layer chromatography (no. 2336) from Merck, D-6100 Darmstadt, G.F.R.; glass-fiber filters, type GF 92, from Schleicher and Schüll, D-3354 Dassel, G.F.R.; and "Omnifluor" from NEN Chemicals, D-6072 Dreieichenhain, G.F.R. The sampling manifold type 3025 is a product of the Millipore Filter Corp., Bedford, Mass. 01730.

Preparation of glass-fiber filters. Place the filters on the sampling manifold, and coat them evenly with polyethyleneimine-cellulose by passing through each filter 5 ml of a suspension containing polyethyleneimine-cellulose (8 g/liter) in ammonium acetate (1 mmol/liter, pH 5). Wash the filters with a wash solution containing about 5 ml of ammonium acetate (1 mmol/liter, pH 5) and guanine or adenine (100 μmol/liter).

Assay. Prepare the reagent solution containing tris(hydroxymethyl)aminomethane hydrochloride (0.2 mol/liter, pH 7.5), $MgCl_2$ (10 mmol/liter), PRPP (1 mmol/liter), and [^{14}C]adenine or [^{14}C]guanine (40 μmol/liter, 54 Ci/mol). For the measurement of specific enzyme activities at higher concentrations of purine bases, unlabeled compound may be added.

Pipette 60 μl of the reagent solution into small reaction tubes and add 10 μl of a preparation of the respective purine phosphoribosyltransferase. Incubate the samples for different times at constant temperatures, e.g., 25 °C. Thereafter add about 5 ml of the above-described wash solution to the reaction mixture and pass it immediately through the prepared filters. Wash the tubes once with the same solution. Dry the filters completely (about 15 min at 100 °C) and assay for radioactivity, using, for example, a liquid-scintillation counter and a scintillation mixture consisting of 4 g of Omnifluor per liter of toluene.

Remarks on the keeping properties of the reagents. The polyethyleneimine-cellulose powder used for the experiments was about three years old. In suspension, polyethyleneimine-cellulose did not lose binding activity when stored for two months at 4 °C.

Stock solutions of adenine and guanine may be kept in air-tight vials at −35 °C for at least one year.

Although an aqueous solution of PRPP did not decompose significantly when stored frozen for one week, we preferred to prepare it freshly each day and keep it on ice.

Zentralinstitut für Biochemie und Biophysik, Freie Universität Berlin, Ehrenbergstrasse 26-28, D-1000 Berlin 33, Germany.

[1] Nonstandard abbreviations used: PRPP, 5-phosphoribosyl-1-pyrophosphate; H-PRT, hypoxanthine phosphoribosyltransferase (EC 2.4.2.8); A-PRT, adenine phosphoribosyltransferase (EC 2.4.2.7); and PP_i, inorganic pyrophosphate.

Received Sept. 8, 1975; accepted Oct. 14, 1975.

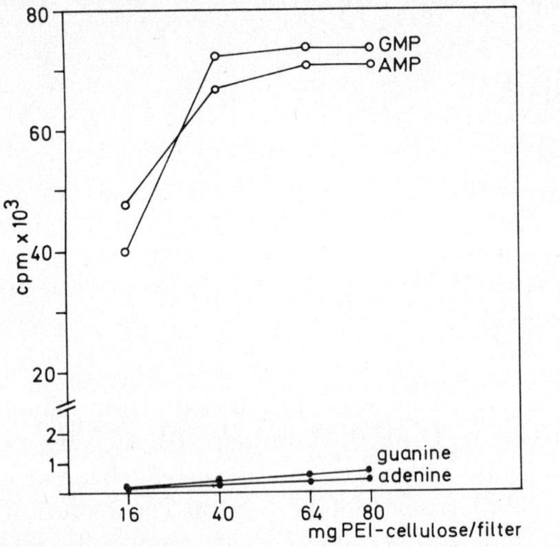

Fig. 1. Adsorption of [^{14}C]purine bases and [^{14}C]nucleoside-5′-monophosphates to different amounts of polyethyleneimine-cellulose per filter

About 100 000 cpm of each compound were passed through the filters as described for the enzyme assay

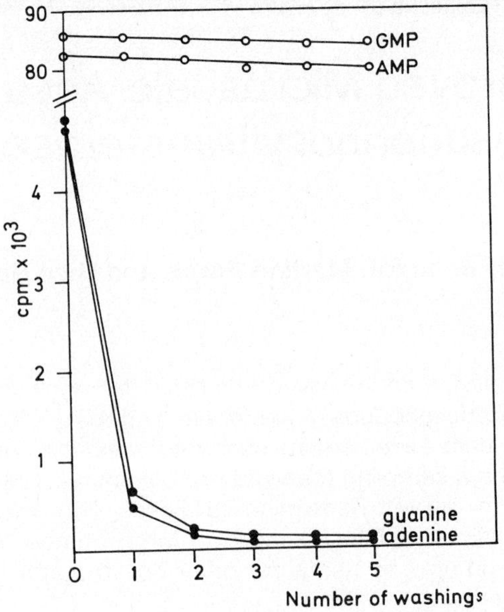

Fig. 2. Retention of [^{14}C]purine bases and [^{14}C]nucleoside-5′-monophosphates relative to the number of washings

About 100 000 cpm of each compound were passed through the filters that had been coated with 40 mg of polyethyleneimine-cellulose

Results

Optimization of the Assay

The rate of conversion of purine bases into the corresponding nucleoside-5′-monophosphates is a measure of the enzyme activity. Because our assay is based on the measurement of radioactivity, the radiolabeled substrate and the radiolabeled product must be well separated. To determine the amount of polyethyleneimine-cellulose necessary for maximum binding of the reaction product without significant adsorption of the labeled substrate, we coated the filters with different amounts of polyethyleneimine-cellulose. Solutions of [^{14}C]adenine, [^{14}C]guanine, [^{14}C]AMP, or [^{14}C]GMP (about 100 000 cpm) were passed through the filters. The filters were washed once with the wash solution and assayed for radioactivity. As shown in Figure 1, 40 mg of polyethyleneimine-cellulose per filter retained the nucleotides almost completely, without significant binding of the bases. Washing the filters more than once did not result in better separation (Figure 2). The linearity of the assay was proved by passing solutions, containing [^{14}C]guanine and [^{14}C]GMP, in various ratios, through the filters (Figure 3).

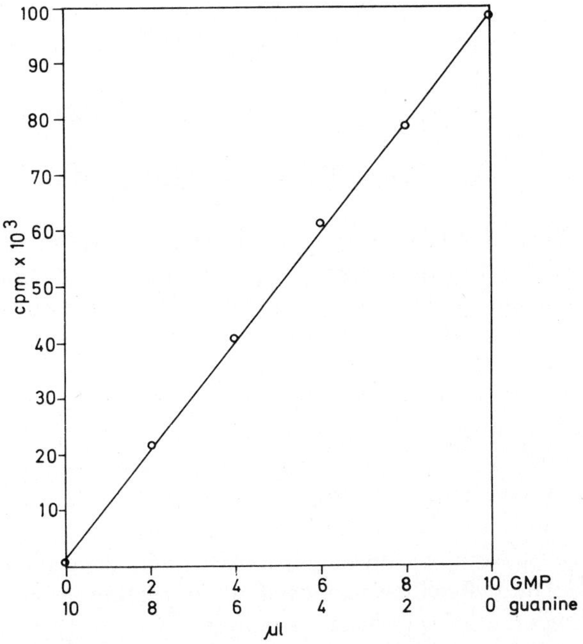

Fig. 3. Calibration curve

Ten µl of solutions (100 µmol/liter) containing [^{14}C]guanine (54 Ci/mol) and [^{14}C]GMP (58 Ci/mol) in different ratios were passed through the filters as described for the enzyme assay

Application of the Assay

Two examples will illustrate the wide range of application for this assay. In the first experiment (Figure 4) we measured the time course for the formation of AMP and GMP from their bases by a cell-free extract of human erythrocytes prepared according to the method of Fujimoto and Seegmiller (*5*).

In the second experiment, a crude extract from the yeast *Saccharomyces cerevisiae,* prepared according to the method of Schmidt et al. (*10*), was fractionated by isoelectric focusing in a polyacrylamide gel according to the method of Söderholm et al. (*11*) with minor modifications. After focusing had been completed, the gel was cut into 80 slices, which at intervals of 15 s were placed into small tubes containing the reaction mixture with [^{14}C]guanine as substrate. The tubes were allowed to stand at 25 °C for 45 min and then their contents were poured onto the filters, as described in *Materials and Methods.* Figure 5 shows the activity profile of H-PRT obtained with this assay and the pH gradient as measured with a surface electrode (type LoT 403-30, Ingold, D-6000 Frankfurt 1, G.F.R.), from which the isoelectric point of the yeast enzyme may be determined as being about pH 5.2.

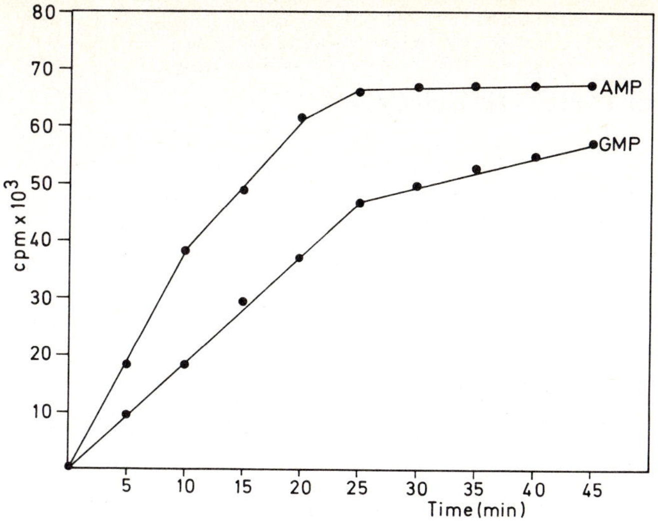

Fig. 4. Time course for conversion of [^{14}C]adenine and [^{14}C]guanine to the corresponding nucleoside-5′-monophosphates at 25 °C by cell-free extracts (1.3 mg of hemoglobin/reaction tube) of human erythrocytes

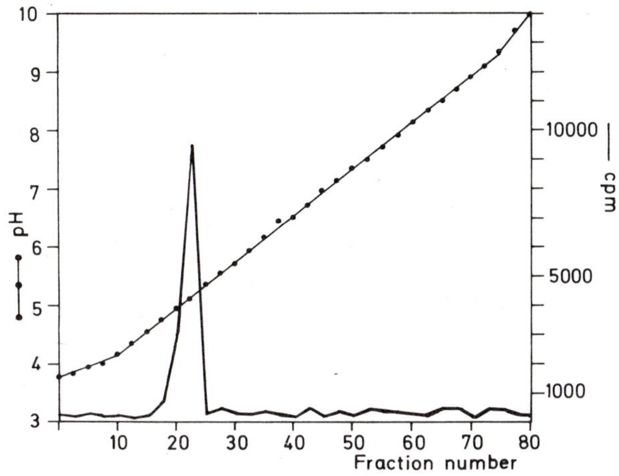

Fig. 5. Assay for HG-PRT activity in a crude extract of yeast that had been subjected to isoelectric focusing in polyacrylamide gel

Discussion

The filter method—introduced by Atkinson and Murray (*9*), simplified by de Bruyn et al. (*6*), and improved in this paper—is the fastest and easiest for determining purine phosphoribosyltransferase activities in micro quantities. Replacing diethylaminoethyl-cellulose paper discs with polyethyleneimine-cellulose-coated glass-fiber filters obviates passing the reaction mixture several times through the same filter (*9*). The main advantage of our improvement is that, without loss of sensitivity, as little as 10 ml of wash solution is sufficient to release adsorbed purine bases almost completely from the filters, whereas the original procedure requires 1600 (*9*) to 600 ml (*6*) per sample. Considering that the passage of 100 ml solution through the filters takes about 1 min (*6*) it is evident that our procedure saves time. Because the labeled substrate is extremely diluted by the addition of the wash solution and because reaction substrates and products are separated within a few seconds it is not necessary to introduce an additional step, such as heating, to stop the reaction.

We suppose that the use of glass-fiber filters coated with ion-exchange cellulose may be also a useful tool for measuring the activity of various other enzymes. Its simplicity and rapidity makes this kind of method especially suitable for clinical or research laboratories where a large number of samples must be assayed.

References

1. Pritchard, R. B., Chavez-Peon, F., and Berlin, R. D., Purines: Supply by liver to tissues. *Am. J. Physiol.* **219,** 1263 (1970).
2. Lesch, M., and Nyhan, W. L., A familial disorder of uric metabolism and central nervous system disfunction. *Am. J. Med.* **36,** 561 (1964).
3. Seegmiller, J. E., Rosenbloom, F. M., and Kelley, W. N., Enzyme defect associated with a sex-linked human neurological disorder and excessive purine synthesis. *Science* **155,** 1682 (1967).
4. Kelley, W. N., Greene, M. L., Rosenbloom, F. M., Henderson, J. F., and Seegmiller, J. E., Hypoxanthine-guanine phosphoribosyl transferase deficiency in gout. *Ann. Intern. Med.* **70,** 155 (1969).
5. Fujimoto, W. Y., and Seegmiller, J. E., Hypoxanthine-guanine phosphoribosyl transferase deficiency: Activity in normal mutant and heterozygote-cultured human skin fibroblasts. *Proc. Nat. Acad. Sci. USA* **65,** 577 (1970).
6. de Bruyn, C. H. M. M., Oei, T. L., and ter Haar, B. G. A., Studies on hair roots for carrier detection in hypoxanthine-guanine phosphoribosyl transferase deficiency. *Clin. Genet.* **5,** 449 (1974).
7. Becker, J. L., Métabolisme des purines dans des cellules de *Drosophila melanogaster* en culture *in vitro:* Interconversion des purines. *Biochimie* **56,** 1249 (1974).
8. Kong Chong, M., and Parks, R. E., Jr., Human erythrocytic hypoxanthinguanine phosphoribosyl transferase: Effect of pH on the enzymatic reaction. *Mol. Pharmacol.* **10,** 648 (1974).
9. Atkinson, M. R., and Murray, A. W., Inhibition of purine phosphoribosyl transferases of Ehrlich ascites tumor cells by 6-mercaptopurine. *Biochem. J.* **94,** 64 (1965).
10. Schmidt, R., Seipel, S., Reichert, U., and Forêt, M., Attempts to isolate purine binding proteins from yeast cells. In *Proceedings of the Fourth International Symposium on Yeasts,* Vienna, Part I H9 (1974).
11. Söderholm, J., Allestam, P., and Wadström, T., A rapid method for isoelectric focusing in polyacrylamide gel. *FEBS Lett.* **24,** 89 (1972).

CLIN. CHEM. 22/1, 70-73 (1976)

Thermodynamic Aspects of Some Radioassays

Paul M. Keane,[1] William H. C. Walker,[1] Jack Gauldie,[1] and Guy E. Abraham[2]

In a number of radioimmunoassays and radiotransin assays, effective equilibrium constants have been measured at different temperatures in order to define the relative contributions of changes of entropy and enthalpy to the change in free binding energy. In systems with a large enthalpy component, the lowest possible incubation temperature maximizes sensitivity, and control of temperature throughout the assay is important. Conversely, when enthalpy change is small, a high temperature allows rapid attainment of equilibrium without loss of sensitivity. At a theoretical level, the thermodynamic characteristics of binding may allow some insight into the nature of the binding process.

Additional Keyphrase: *entropy, enthalpy, and free binding energy*

The temperature dependence of effective equilibrium constants for specific binding proteins (transins) and antibodies in reaction with their target ligands can be used to derive entropy and enthalpy contributions to the free energy change at equilibrium. Data for many antigen/antibody reactions has been reviewed by Karush (*1*), with discussion of the insights provided by such data into the nature of the binding process. In the area of immunoassay, similar data have been reported for estradiol antibodies (*2, 3*), estradiol/uterine cytosol (*4*) and for transcortin (*5*). We have extended these observations to other binding proteins and indicate their practical importance in assay design.

Materials and Methods

Derivation of binding constants: Standard curves for each assay were set up at 4, 25, and 37 °C to yield values of apparent bound/total counts = y'. In addition, extra tubes were set up to define the upper limit (α) and lower limit (β) for y' which differ respectively from unity and zero because of misclassification errors in the separation of bound and free. A zero tube with a 50-fold increase in antibody concentration defines α; a standard tube with 20-fold the upper limit of the working range of unlabeled hormone defines β. Zero and first-order misclassification errors of both bound and free fractions are eliminated by calculating $y = (y' - \beta)/(\alpha - \beta)$ (see Appendix). The mass of labeled ligand (L^*) in the assay tubes was obtained by setting up zero standard tubes with twice, fourfold and sixfold the regular mass of labeled ligand to give values y'_1, y'_3, and y'_5, corresponding to one, three, and five extra aliquots of labeled ligand, which were evaluated in terms of unlabeled ligand by reading off the standard curve.

With y and L^* defined, the standard curves were plotted as Scatchard plots (*6*) with bound/free = $y/(1 - y)$ as ordinate, and bound = $y(L^* + L_a)$ as abscissa, where L_a is the concentration of added ligand in the standard tubes. All binding proteins reported here exhibited functional homogeneity over the temperature range used, as shown by linearity of the Scatchard plots. A representative example is shown in Figure 1.

Minus the slope of the plot yields equilibrium constant in reciprocal units of the abscissa. This is converted to units of litres/mole (K) and then to the dimensionless moles water/mole solute by multiplying by 55.5 to give the unitary free energy change (*7*): $\Delta G_u = -RT \ln 55.5K$. Since $\Delta G_u = \Delta H° - T\Delta S_u$; $R = 1.93$ cal/mol/degree Kelvin. $1.93 \ln 55.5K = -\Delta H° T^{-1} + \Delta S_u$, and a plot of $1.93 \ln 55.5K$ as ordinate and T^{-1} as abscissa will yield a linear relationship with slope $-\Delta H°$ and intercept ΔS_u. Values for enthalpy change, $\Delta H°$, and unitary entropy change, ΔS_u relate to the specific assay conditions used for determining K: ionic strength, pH, buffer ions, etc. Since the values of $\Delta H°$ and ΔS_u may be temperature dependent because of the effects of binding on the partial molal heat capacity of the protein molecule, these values apply only to the range of temperatures tested.

Assay procedures: We defined the temperature de-

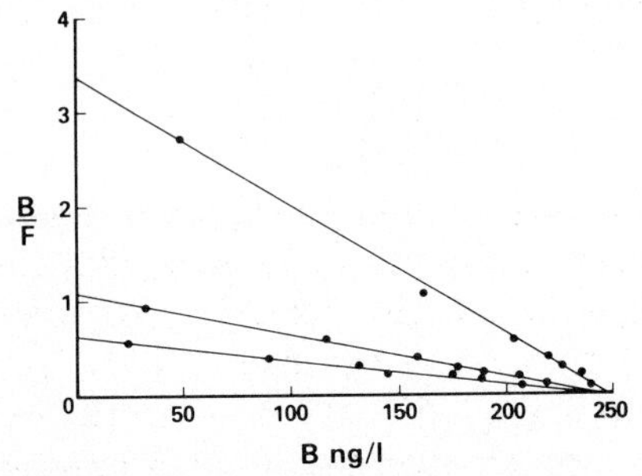

Fig. 1. Scatchard plots for angiotensin I antibody interaction
The upper, middle, and lower lines represent 4, 25, and 37 °C, respectively

[1] Department of Pathology, McMaster University Medical Centre, 1200 Main Street West, Hamilton, Ontario, L8S 4J9, Canada.

[2] Department of Obstetrics and Gynecology, Division of Reproductive Biology, Harbor General Hospital, 1000 West Carson St., Torrance, Calif. 90509.

Received Sept. 1, 1975; accepted Oct. 20, 1975.

Table 1. Apparent Equilibrium Constants for Some Ligand-Binding Proteins

Ligand	Binding protein	T, °C	$K \times 10^{-9}$, l/m	ΔH°, kcal/mol	ΔS_u, cal/mol/K
Group A					
Aldosterone	antibody	5	5.0	−3	42
		25	3.6	(0.1)	(0.4)
		37	2.9		
Digoxin	antibody	5	0.88	+1.6	55
		25	1.1	(0.1)	(0.5)
		37	1.2		
		56	1.2		
Estradiol	antibody	6	34	−4.6	40
(ref. *2*)		25	20		
Estriol	antibody	4	2.1	0	51
		25	2.0	(0.1)	(0.9)
		37	2.1		
Testosterone	antibody	4	8.9	−1	50
		25	8.0	(0.1)	(0.3)
		37	7.3		
Thyroxine	antibody	4	0.69	0	48
		25	0.72	(0.2)	(1.6)
		36	0.65		
Group B					
Angiotensin I	antibody	5	14	−9	22
		25	4.5	(0.2)	(1.2)
		37	2.5		
Angiotensin II	antibody	5	90	−9	27
		25	40	(0.9)	(5.7)
		37	16		
Gastrin	antibody	5	590	−8	32
		25	230	(0.2)	(1.5)
		37	120		
Insulin	antibody	5	120	−7	34
		25	68	(0.9)	(6)
		37	31		
Thyroxine	binding	18	2.7	−9	22
(ref. *19*)	globulin	21	2.4	(1.8)	(13)
		24	2.1		
		27	1.9		
		37	1.0		
Group C					
Cortisol	transcortin	4	0.52	−16	−10
(ref. *5*)		37	0.024		
Estradiol	uterine	5	22	−16	0
(ref. *4*)	cytosol	20	5.8	(2)	(12)
		37	1.0		
Progesterone	binding	5	0.12	−10	9
	globulin	25	0.06	(1.9)	(11)
		37	0.016		

pendence of K by using the quoted procedures for the following radioimmunoassays: aldosterone (*8*), angiotensin I (*9*), angiotensin II (*10*), digoxin (*11*), estriol (*12*), gastrin (*13*), insulin (*14*), testosterone (*15*), and thyroxin (*16*); we also used the quoted procedure for radiotransin assay for progesterone (*17*). In addition, data were obtained from the literature for the following ligand-binding reagents: cortisol-transcortin (by ultrafiltration and dialysis) (*5*), estradiol/estradiol antibody (*2*), estradiol/uterine cytosol (*4*), and thyroxine/thyroxine-binding globulin (*18*).

Results

The apparent equilibrium constants at specified temperatures for each ligand-binding protein are listed in Table 1 with their derived enthalpy ($\Delta H°$) and entropy (ΔS_u) changes (standard error for each parameter in parentheses).

Discussion

Definition of the temperature dependence of an equilibrium constant has practical and theoretical implications. At the practical level, a temperature-dependent binding protein requires control of temperature throughout all stages of an assay, including the separation of bound from free ligand. When maximum sensitivity (the least amount of ligand distinguishable from zero) is required, a low incubation temperature must be used with prolongation of incubation to allow for the slower attainment of equilibrium at low temperature. Delayed addition of the labeled ligand may also be appropriate (*19*). With a temperature-independent binding protein, a high incubation temperature should be used for rapid and complete equilibration, and temperature control in the separation stage may be unimportant.

At the thermodynamic level, do the relative magnitudes of enthalpy and entropy change have validity and can they yield insights into the nature of the ligand/protein interaction? The equilibrium constants have been calculated from Scatchard plots by a least-squares procedure without weighting of the data points. The data of the standard curve have been shown to be heteroscedastic, although this is much less marked when a Scatchard plot is used than with a logit-log plot where statistical weighting must be used (*20*). With triplicate assay values for each data point, precision was sufficient to yield correlation coefficients of 0.990 or greater for all assays studied.

The separation of bound and free imposes a disequilibrium on the ligand-binding protein system and will tend to lead to dissociation of the bound fraction. Because reaction rates increase with temperature, dissociation will be more marked at higher temperatures, with consequent lowering of the apparent equilibrium constant. The observed temperature dependence of the equilibrium constant with some binding proteins could therefore be an artefact of the separation system, being apparent only in those systems that were readily reversible. There are two reasons why this explanation is unlikely. First, the cortisol/transcortin temperature dependence is well documented (*21*) by use of ultrafiltration techniques that leave the equilibrium position undisturbed. Secondly, some temperature-sensitive assay systems are effectively irreversible—for example, angiotensin (*9*) and insulin (*22*)—as demonstrated by the failure of a large excess of unlabeled ligand to displace labeled ligand that is already protein bound.

A more serious problem is posed by the heterogeneity of the matrix in which the binding reaction occurs. The binding protein is present in a complex protein mixture; it may itself have several species of binding sites, with the choice of separation system determining which of these are revealed (*23, 24*). Marked changes in binding avidity may result from changes in pH, ionic strength, and the nature of the buffer anions. The derived equilibrium constant is therefore relevant only to the specific environment of the assay.

Despite these provisos, it is likely that the effect of temperature on protein/ligand interaction indicates at least qualitatively the relative influence of entropy and enthalpy changes in driving the reaction to equilibrium.

It is possible to divide the reactions studied into three classes whose free energies of binding are derived from (*a*) predominantly positive entropy changes, (*b*) combined entropy and enthalpy changes, or (*c*) predominantly negative enthalpy changes. These physical characteristics correspond to structural features of the reactants, the first group comprising antibodies and small relatively apolar ligands; the second, antibodies and peptides; and the third, biological binding proteins and small ligands.

In group *a*, the small enthalpy changes with large entropy changes indicate that bond formation is probably of the hydrophobic type (*1, 25*). The free energies of these reactions derive from a large increase in entropy, which may be the result of release of organized water molecules both from the apolar ligand and from the binding site.

Antibodies to peptides show a greater enthalpy change when they react with their target ligands (Group *b*). The more complex structure of the ligand probably allows a better fit at the binding site, with more extensive bond formation. The entropy and enthalpy contributions are approximately equal and both hydrophobic and Van der Waals interactions may be involved.

When biological binding proteins (Group *c*) react with their target ligands the reactions are enthalpy driven with small entropy changes. This contrasts strikingly with the entropy driven binding of the same ligands to antibodies. The biological binding proteins appear to react with their target ligands with such a goodness of fit that multiple bonds, probably of the Van der Waals type, are formed. It may be that this goodness of fit is facilitated by conformational change in the binding proteins when their binding sites are occupied. Some support for this hypothesis comes from the increased resistance of transcortin to heat inactivation in the presence of excess cortisol (*26*). Direct evidence for conformational change with binding has been obtained by Stroupe and Westphal (*27*) with progesterone-binding globulin. Evidence has recently been presented suggestive of conformational change following the binding of cytosine monophosphate to ribonuclease A associated with large negative enthalpy change (*25*).

We conclude that the magnitude of temperature dependence of the equilibrium constant has important implications for assay design and should be defined with each new antibody. As a general rule, naturally occurring binding proteins are highly temperature dependent, antibodies reacting with peptides are less temperature dependent, and antibodies reacting with steroids show little or no temperature dependence.

Confirmation of enthalpy change estimates by direct calorimetric measurement are needed. The thermodynamic data for antigen/antibody interactions conforms to the findings of previous workers. The data for biological specific binding proteins suggests that conformational changes in the protein molecule result from occupation of their binding sites.

Appendix

If b_0 and b_1 are fixed and proportional (zero and first order) misclassifications of bound/total counts (y); and f_0 and f_1 are fixed and proportional misclassifications of free/total counts $(1 - y)$ (b_1 also allows for first-order reversal of equilibrium state); then

apparent bound/total counts =

$$y' = y + f_0 + f_1(1 - y) - b_0 - b_1 y$$

and

$$y = (y' - f_0 - f_1 + b_0)/(1 - f_1 - b_1)$$

when added ligand $H_a = \infty$; $y = 0$; let $y' = \beta$

$$y' = \beta = f_0 + f_1 - b_0$$

when antibody concentration Ab = ∞; $H_a \ll$ Ab; $y = 1$; let $y' = \alpha$

$$y' = \alpha = 1 + f_0 - b_0 - b_1$$

Hence

$$y = (y' - \beta)/(\alpha - \beta)$$

References

1. Karush, F., Immunologic specificity and molecular structure. *Adv. Immunol.* **2,** 1 (1962).

2. Abraham, G. E., and Odell, W. D., In *Immunologic Methods in Steroid Determination,* F. G. Peron and B. V. Caldwell, Eds. Appleton-Century-Crofts, New York, N.Y., 1970, p 87.

3. Malvano, R., Rolleri, E., and Rosa, U., Standardisation and control of steroid radioimmunoassay. In *Radioimmunoassay and Related Procedures in Medicine* **2,** International Atomic Energy Agency, Vienna, 1974, p 119.

4. Sanborn, B. M., Rao, B. M., and Korenman, S. G., Interaction of 17β-estradiol and its specific uterine receptor. *Biochemistry* **10,** 4955 (1971).

5. Westphal, U., *Steroid-Protein Interactions,* Springer-Verlag, New York, 1971, p 348.

6. Scatchard, G., The attractions of proteins for small molecules and ions. *Ann. N.Y. Acad. Sci.* **51,** 660 (1949).

7. Tanford, C., Protein denaturation. *Adv. Protein Chem.* **24,** 21 (1970).

8. Drewes, P. A., Demetriou, J. A., and Pileggi, V. J., Measurement of urinary aldosterone by a simplified radioimmunoassay procedure. *Clin. Biochem.* **6,** 88 (1973).

9. Viol, G. W., Keane, P. M., Speed, J. F., and Smith, E. K. M., Assay of plasma renin activity using commercially available reagents. *Clin. Biochem.* **5,** 251 (1972).

10. Nussberger, J., Beckerhoff, R., Vetter, W., et al. Simplified immunoassay for plasma angiotensin II. In *Radioimmunoassay and Related Procedures in Medicine* **1,** International Atomic Energy Agency, Vienna, 1974, p 429.

11. Smith, T. W., Radioimmunoassay for serum digitoxin concentration: Methodology and clinical experience. *J. Pharmacol. Exp. Ther.* **175,** 352 (1970).

12. YoungLai, E. V., Two-hour plasma estrogen assay. *Am. J. Obstet. Gynecol.* **117,** 584 (1973).

13. Yalow, R. S., and Berson, S. A., Radioimmunoassay of gastrin. *Gastroenterology* **88,** 1 (1970).

14. Morgan, C. R., and Lazarow, A., Immunoassay of insulin using a two-antibody system. *Proc. Soc. Exp. Biol.* **110,** 29 (1962).

15. Coyotupa, J., Parlow, A. F., and Abraham, G. E., Simultaneous radioimmunoassay of plasma testosterone and dihydrotestosterone. *Anal. Lett.* **5,** 329 (1972).

16. Dunn, R. T., and Lowell, B. F., Radioimmunoassay of thyroxine in unextracted serum by a single-antibody technique. *Clin. Chem.* **19,** 1063 (1973).

17. Pichou, M.-F., and Milgrom, E., Competitive protein binding assay of progesterone without chromatography. *Steroids* **21,** 335 (1973).

18. Elewaut, A., Determination of the binding of thyroxine to plasma proteins by competitive protein binding analysis. *Clin. Chim. Acta* **45,** 37 (1973).

19. Rodbard, D., Ruder, H. J., Vaitukaitis, J., and Jacobs, H. S., Mathematical analysis of kinetics of radioligand assays: Improved sensitivity obtained by delayed addition of labelled ligand. *J. Clin. Endocrinol. Metab.* **33,** 343 (1971).

20. Rodbard, D., and Hutt, D. M., Statistical analysis of radioimmunoassays and immunoradiometric (labelled antibody) assays. In *Radioimmunoassay and Related Procedures in Medicine,* **1,** International Atomic Energy Agency, Vienna, 1974, p 165.

21. Goldie, D. J., Hasham, N., Keane, P. M., and Walker, W. H. C., Temperature dependence of cortisol binding to plasma proteins. *Nature* **217,** 852 (1968).

22. Keane, P. M., Pearson, J., and Walker, W. H. C., Dextran coated charcoal immunoassay of insulin. *Diabetologia* **4,** 339 (1968).

23. Abraham, G. E., Characterisation of anti-steroid antisera. In *Steroid Immunoassay,* E. H. D. Cameron, S. G. Hillier, and K. Griffiths, Eds. Alpha Omega Publishing, Cardiff, U.K., 1975, p 74.

24. Rolleri, E., Malvano, R., Gandolfi, C., and Rosa, U., Effects of irreversible adsorbents on the dissociation of the antigen-antibody complexes. *Horm. Metab. Res.* **6,** 57 (1974).

25. Flogel, M., and Biltonen, R. L., The pH dependence of the thermodynamics of the interaction of 3′-cytidine monophosphate with ribonuclease-A. *Biochemistry* **14,** 2610 (1975).

26. Doe, R. P., Fernandez, R. N., and Seal, V. S., Measurement of corticosteroid binding globulin in man. *J. Clin. Endocrinol.* **24,** 1029 (1964).

27. Stroupe, S. D., and Westphal, U., Conformational changes in the progesterone binding globulin–progesterone complex. *Biochemistry* **14,** 3296 (1975).

CLIN. CHEM. 22/1, 74–78 (1976)

Evaluation of a Reagent-Strip Method for Glucose in Whole Blood, as Compared with a Hexokinase Method

Thomas C. Stewart

The hexokinase method (I) for glucose in biological fluids, proposed by the FDA as a potential national standard method, is compared with the Eyetone/Dextrostix/Control method (II) for measurement of glucose in whole blood. I used a new, two-step calibration procedure based on a 1.30 g/liter standard for the **II** system. The correlation coefficient for results by the two methods was 0.99 for 142 assays in duplicate. Recovery values were near 100% (**I**, range 100.0 to 106.2%; **II**, range 100.8 to 105.1%), and the coefficients of variation were respectively ±4.1% and ±4.5%. Considering the close correlation between the two methods, together with the simplicity, speed, and convenience of **II**, I conclude that it has great clinical utility, particularly in emergency situations. The precision and accuracy of **II** depends greatly on proper calibration and control procedures and on adequate training of the operator.

Additional Keyphrases: *pediatric chemistry* • *emergency procedure*

The need for a simple, rapid test for glucose to meet special applications such as those found in the emergency room or pediatric wards, as well as to relieve the demands on overtaxed laboratory personnel, has been frequently suggested. However, the clinical utility of simple tests has frequently been restricted by inherent limitations in their precision and accuracy (*1–4*). Recent changes in the "Dextrostix" (Ames Co.) system prompted our renewed interest in evaluating the technical capabilities of this 60-s test for glucose in whole blood.

Major changes in the strip and its associated instrument system include an improved reflectance meter ("Eyetone") and new two-step calibration that incorporates a 1.30 g/liter standard to correct systematic variables. The standard is a preparation containing gravimetrically determined quantities of pure D-glucose in a matrix that essentially duplicates the reactive characteristics of whole blood when used with Dextrostix. Taken together, the changes offered considerable potential for improved precision and accuracy in the overall system.

At about the time that the Eyetone/Dextrostix/Control (EDC) system was to be evaluated, the Food and Drug Administration coincidentally proposed several techniques, including a hexokinase (EC 2.7.1.1) procedure, as potential national standard methods for measurement of glucose in biological fluids (*5*). Because hexokinase procedures are specific for glucose and generally quite precise and accurate, and because the FDA procedure in particular is rigorously defined to achieve "state-of-the-art" accuracy in glucose determinations, this method was chosen as the comparison method against which to judge precision and accuracy of the improved strip system.

Materials and Methods

Eyetone/Dextrostix/Control method (EDC), Ames Co., Division Miles Laboratories, Elkhart, Ind. 46514. The Dextrostix contains the glucose-specific enzyme, glucose oxidase (EC 1.1.3.4), to promote the reaction between glucose and oxygen producing gluconic acid and hydrogen peroxide. Peroxidase (EC 1.11.1.7) then catalyzes the reaction between the hydrogen peroxide and a chromogen system, giving a characteristic color that can be read in the Eyetone Reflectance Colorimeter. Because the color development is a continuing reaction, the test strip must be washed and blotted at exactly 60 s and read as soon as possible thereafter to assure proper results.

The Eyetone is an improved version of the older (*6*) Reflectance Meter. The new meter includes a single scale (as opposed to three) for simpler, less error-

Earl K. Long Memorial Hospital, Baton Rouge, La. 70805.
Received April 28, 1975; accepted Oct. 27, 1975.

prone reading, a two-point calibration to control the slope of the response curve, and more stable electronics. The most significant improvement of the system, however, is a synthetic standard, simulating whole blood, used for calibration, This solution closely resembles whole blood and can be used in exactly the same manner; it contains 1.30 g (±0.7%) of D-glucose (National Bureau of Standards) per liter. To duplicate the reactive characteristics of whole blood, the solution also contains polyvinylpyrrolidone, to give proper viscosity; sodium chloride, to match the osmotic pressure of blood; benzoic acid, as a preservative; and red coloring, to give a visual index to proper washing of the reagent strip.

After the instrument was basically calibrated by use of the color chips provided for setting the extremes of the range (equivalent to 500 to 4000 mg/liter), a reagent strip was reacted with the standard solution; at exactly 60 s, the standard was washed from the strip and the strip was blotted and immediately inserted in the roughly calibrated instrument. With a thumbwheel adjustment, the instrument was then set to read exactly 1.30 g/liter. Because the same procedure is used with this calibration strip as with strips reacted with a sample of a patient's whole blood, the systematic errors of the procedure are controlled. All tests with the EDC system in this evaluation were conducted by using this "Two-Step" calibration of the instrument, a procedure that can be used with the older Reflectance Meter as well.

Hexokinase method. In the hexokinase procedure, as detailed in the *Federal Register* (*5*), D-glucose is phosphorylated with ATP in the presence of yeast hexokinase and magnesium ion to yield ADP plus D-glucose-6-phosphate, which reacts with NAD^+ in the presence of glucose-6-phosphate dehydrogenase (EC 1.1.1.49) to yield 6-phosphoglucono-Δ-lactone and NADH, and the latter is measured via its absorbance at 340 nm. The reaction goes essentially to completion and the results for unknown samples are calculated by comparison with standards run at the same time, so timing is not critical and sources of systematic error are essentially eliminated.

Sample Handling

I used whole blood in this evaluation because the EDC system is designed for such samples. Evacuated blood-collection tubes containing ethylenediaminetetraacetic acid were routinely used to collect blood specimens from in-patients and out-patients. After thorough mixing by inversion, the samples were refrigerated at 2 °C until used. Hyperglycemic samples were simulated by adding 0.25 to 0.75 ml of a 10.0 g/liter aqueous solution of glucose; hypoglycemic specimens were simulated by allowing glycolysis of blood samples. After warming to room temperature, samples were tested with the EDC system by using a procedural modification (*7*) in which the strip is dipped into the whole-blood sample. One effect of using whole blood in the procedure would be to change the expected glucose values (*4, 8–10*), because of the diluting effect of the erythrocytes. Immediately after this test, a Somogyi filtrate was prepared (*5*) for the hexokinase procedure, which requires a cell- and protein-free sample. Although in the procedure as described in the *Federal Register* it apparently is assumed that the Somogyi filtrate is prepared from a plasma or serum sample, the procedure is equally effective for whole blood.

Results and Discussion

Dextrostix Reagent Strips have been used since 1964 for visually interpreted, semiquantitative glucose determinations, and the ordinary accuracy of the procedure has been well documented (*11–15*); the Reflectance Meter gave an improvement in precision, but results were still variable (*1–3, 16*), and the lack of an independent standard had been noted (*2*). Our first objective, then, was to evaluate the precision of the method incorporating the new instrument calibrated against the standard solution.

Because the EDC system is designed for use with whole blood, and a significant amount of glycolysis could be expected during a measurement of 20 samples, I decided to first test the system by use of a pool of synthetic standard in addition to that already described, similar control solutions are available with glucose concentrations of 450, 900, and 2500 mg/liter; the first two solutions were mixed to give a solution with a glucose concentration of about 750 mg/liter.

The reproducibility of the hexokinase procedure was tested by using five serum pools. The results (Table 1) illustrate that the two methods are similarly precise.

The essentiality of the two-step calibration procedure and the standard solution is demonstrated. These data involved five separate runs and five bottles of Dextrostix, representing three manufacturing lots, of which one was nearly two years old. The instrument was calibrated before each run. The reading of the instrument before resetting with the 1.30 g/liter standard is recorded in Table 1. The instrument showed readings of 1.35, 1.14, 130, 132, and 140 g/liter. Whatever the causes, these values suggest that without the calibration procedure based on the standard, an additional bias of +50, −160, 0, +20, and +100 mg/liter, respectively, would have been present in the results.

Within-run precision was next studied, to determine whether similarly precise results could be obtained for a sample of whole blood. A specimen was acquired from the blood bank and 20 consecutive determinations were made with the EDC. Immediately after each EDC assay, a 0.5-ml aliquot was taken and a Somogyi filtrate prepared for the hexokinase procedure. The entire procedure required 27 min. (The 20 filtrates were subsequently assayed in a single batch.) As the data show (Table 2), glycolysis was significant during the run, the value for the last sample being about 10% lower than for the first, as determined by

Table 1. Results of Reproducibility Studies[a]

Batch	Assay values, mg/liter HK	EDC	Dextrostix lot no., date of mfg.	Two-step calibration reset value[b]
1	780	800		
	760	760	1212074	1350
	760	800	July '74	
	770	800		
2	810	820		
	810	810	1093034	
	790	790	March '74	1140
	780	810		
3	850	830		
	840	820	1049012	
	840	780	Jan '72	1300
	840	820		
4	790	810		
	760	790	1212074	
	790	820	July '74	1320
	790	780		
5	760	720		
	760	780	1093034	
	750	690	March '74	1400
	740	740		
Mean	788.5	788.5		
SD	32.4	35.5		

[a] Results of the hexokinase (HK) results are for a serum pool, while EDC results are for a simulated whole blood.

[b] Eyetone instrument reading for the 1300 mg/liter glucose standard before resetting the instrument.

Table 2. Within-Run Precision for a Sample of Whole Blood, Assayed by the EDC Method and the Hexokinase (HK) Method

	EDC (mg/liter)	HK (mg/liter)
	1220	1300
	1220	1290
	1200	1280
	1200	1260
	1200	1240
	1180	1240
	1180	1220
	1180	1230
	1180	1220
	1180	1240
	1160	1230
	1160	1220
	1160	1220
	1160	1210
	1150	1210
	1150	1220
	1140	1210
	1140	1200
	1140	1200
	1140	1180
Mean	1172	1231
Bias	−59	

Effect of glycolysis over duration of test is apparent in both assays.

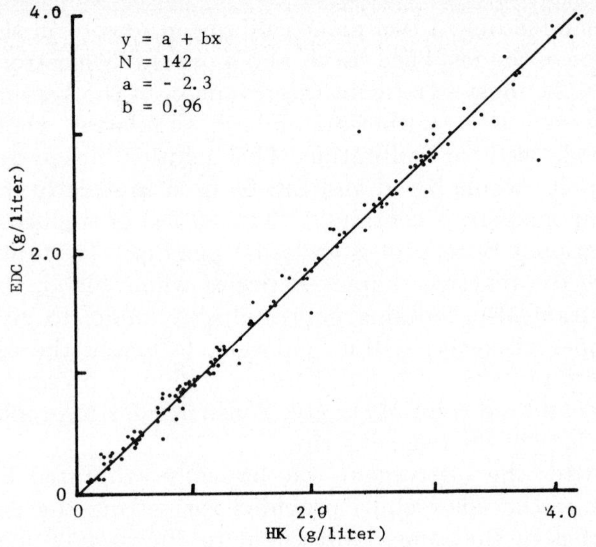

Fig. 1. Relation between blood-glucose values as determined by the hexokinase and EDC assays (142 specimens, assayed in duplicate)

the hexokinase method. Again, the precision of the two methods was nearly the same. Although the data are limited, it appears that the simulated blood does perform with the EDC system much like real blood.

The bias of EDC with respect to the hexokinase method in this run was about −60 mg/liter; this raises a question whether a systematic bias exists in the method or if some interference was present in this particular sample. The results of a comparison of 142 "clinical" specimens (Figure 1) indicates that the bias is probably systematic. Hypoglycemic and hyperglycemic specimens were contrived through glycolysis and the addition of glucose, respectively, to obtain an even distribution of test values over the range between 100 and 4000 mg/liter. The bias across this range, EDC vs. the hexokinase method, proved to be −93 mg/liter.

A better understanding of the correlation between the methods is shown when the data are further divided into three fields as shown in Table 3, which summarizes the major values of a regression analysis applied to each field. It should be noted that the number of samples with values exceeding 3000 mg/liter was too small for precise analysis, but are presented as an indication of the correlation that might be expected in the higher range. In the lower range, the 63 mg/liter bias confirms the systematically lower results given by EDC in the precision study; both of the higher ranges also show a consistently negative bias.

A number of potential interfering substances in whole blood are effectively removed by the Somogyi filtration process (*5, 17*). Although the results of the clinical comparison suggested that interference arising from whole blood constituents was probably not a major problem, the severity of potential interference

Table 3. Correlation of Results by the Hexokinase (HK) and EDC Methods in Each of Three Parts of the Total Range

	100–1500 mg/liter (n = 75)		1500–3000 mg/liter (n = 49)		>3000 mg/liter (n = 18)	
	EDC	HK	EDC	HK	EDC	HK
			mg/liter			
Mean	747	810	2289	2380	3399	3621
Bias	−63		−91		−222	
Regression analysis						
Correlation coefficient, *r*	0.98		0.94		0.98	
a[a]	−2.33		−8.3		−11.2	
b[a]	0.95		1.0		0.97	

[a] These are the values of the regression equation y = a + bx, where y = value of EDC assay, a = y-axis intercept of regression line, b = slope of regression line, x = value of HK assay.

remained a concern. Because the mechanism of interference is much the same in all cases—that is, competition with the chromogen as H^+ donors (*17*)—it was considered sufficient to investigate a few typical interfering substances. Clinical samples containing abnormally high concentrations of bilirubin, creatinine, and uric acid were obtained and the concentration of these constituents determined by the methods of Van den Bergh (Hycel), Jaffé (AutoAnalyzer), and the Caraway modification of the Folin–Denis method (Hycel), respectively. Duplicate assays of each sample were then made by EDC and the hexokinase method; means of the pairs are presented in Table 4 together with the levels of the potentially interfering constituents and the bias between the two glucose methods.

The evaluation of the two methods had already demonstrated a rather consistent negative bias of 6–9% (EDC < the hexokinase method); greater bias would indicate interference. Creatinine apparently does not interfere, and the interference from bilirubin appears to be slight. Uric acid, however, appears to interfere significantly.

In general, the excellent correlation between the improved EDC system and the hexokinase method, combined with the simplicity and speed of the strip test, suggests that it should be very useful in many clinical settings. However, there are some important considerations in the use of the EDC system. Operator variables are critical with Dextrostix, notably timing, washing, and sample application (*2, 4, 18*). Variables in the strips themselves have also been noted, particularly in aged material; the new calibration procedure should control such variables and, in our hands, the precision of the results obtained in this study suggests that it does so effectively.

The simulated whole blood standards—4.5, 1.30, and 2.50 g/liter—are useful because the novice opera-

Table 4. Effects of Same Typical Interfering Substances on EDC Glucose Assay[a]

	Sample 1	Sample 2	Sample 3	Sample 4	Mean
			mg/liter		
Bilirubin, mg/liter	42	96	65	100	72.5
EDC	900	1050	880	1200	1007.5
HK	980	1160	990	1380	1127.5
Bias	−80	−110	−110	−180	−120
Creatinine, mg/liter	84	104	100	105	98
EDC	1150	1800	3100	1000	1762.5
HK	1240	1930	3300	1100	1892.5
Bias	−90	−130	−200	−100	−130
Uric acid, mg/liter	71	133	141	143	123
EDC	1100	860	1300	1100	1090
HK	1220	1100	1490	1310	1280
Bias	−120	−240	−190	−210	−190

[a] All values are means of duplicate assays.

tor can practice with these until the important variables of technique, particularly timing and washing, have been controlled. I have found that nurses and medical technologists who routinely use the method obtain more nearly accurate and reproducible results than do physicians or clinical chemists who only occasionally use it. I therefore recommend that clinical assays be done by a regular operator, for greatest accuracy.

Materials used in this investigation were provided by Ames Co., Division of Miles Laboratories, Elkhart, Ind. 46514.

References

1. Costrini, N. V., Ganeshappa, K. P., Whalen, G. E., and Soergel, K. H., A simple method for regulating and monitoring circulating glucose levels. *J. Lab. Clin. Med.* **82,** 179 (1973).

2. Drury, M. I., Sweeney, E. C., and UaConaill, D., Blood glucose determination by Dextrostix Reflectance Meter System. *Br. J. Med. Sci.* **141,** 181 (1972).

3. Joffe, B. I., and Settel, H. C., Comparison of Dextrostix/Reflectance Meter and AutoAnalyzer methods of blood glucose determination. *S. Afr. Med. J.* **45,** 1200 (1971).

4. Haworth, J. C., Dilling, L. A., and Van Woert, M., Blood glucose determination in infants and children. *Am. J. Dis. Child.* **123,** 69 (1972).

5. Department of Health, Education and Welfare, In vitro diagnostic products for human use: Proposed establishment of product class standard for detection or measurement of glucose. *Fed. Regist.* **39** (126), 24136–24147 (1974).

6. DeLawter, DeW. E., and Moss, J. M., Evaluation of glucose oxidase strip method of blood glucose testing. *Md. State Med. J.* **23,** 43 (1974).

7. Ames Company, Division Miles Laboratories, Alternate Dextrostix procedure, *Technical Services Bulletin 74,* 1 (1974).

8. McDonald, G. W., Fisher, G. F., and Burnham, C. E., Differences in glucose determinations obtained from plasma or whole blood. *Pub. Health Rep.* **79,** 515 (1964).

9. Geeting, D. G., Suther, C. A., and Sylbert, P., Determination of glucose in serum and whole blood: Statistical relationships between values obtained by different methods. *Clin. Chem.* **18,** 976 (1972).

10. Hardy, R., Glucose determinations using Reflectance Meter-Dextrostix and *o*-toluidine methods. *Am. J. Med. Technol.* **37,** 5 (1971).

11. Cohen, S. L., and Legg, S., A bedside method of blood-glucose estimation. *Lancet* **ii,** 883 (1974).

12. Marks, V., and Dawson, A., Rapid stick method for determining blood-glucose concentration. *Br. Med. J.* **i,** 293 (1965).

13. Moss, J. M., The clinical use of the Dextrostix method for blood sugar. *South. Med. J.* **61,** 1089 (1968).

14. Rennie, I. D. B., Keen, H., and Southon, A., A rapid enzyme-strip method for estimating blood-sugar. *Lancet* **ii,** 884 (1964).

15. Schersten, B., Clinical evaluation of a rapid enzyme strip method (Dextrostix) for blood glucose estimation. *Acta Med. Scand.* **178,** 583 (1965).

16. Vickers, M. F., Blood glucose measurement with the Dextrostix Reflectance Meter: An evaluation. *Med. Lab. Technol.* **30,** 235 (1973).

17. Henry, R. J., Cannon, D. C., and Winkelman, J. W., Eds. *Clinical Chemistry, Principles and Technics.* 2nd ed., Harper & Row, New York, N. Y., 1974, p 1271.

18. Spellacy, W. N., Buhl, W. C., Cohn, J. E., and Birk, S. A., Usefulness of rapid blood glucose measurements in obstetrics: Dextrostix/Reflectance Meter System. *Obstet. Gynecol.* **41,** 299 (1973).

CLIN. CHEM. 22/1, 79-82 (1976)

Spectrophotometric End-Point Method for Assay of Serum Cystyl-aminopeptidase in Pregnancy

Brian H. Durham

An optimized end-point method that requires little sophisticated equipment is described for estimating serum cystyl-aminopeptidase during pregnancy. *S*-Benzyl-L-cysteine-4-nitroanilide is used as the substrate.

Additional Keyphrases: *assessing placental integrity • normal values*

Cystyl-aminopeptidase (CAS, α-aminoacyl-peptide hydrolase, EC 3.4.11.3) is an enzyme produced by the placenta that degrades cystine peptides such as oxytocin and vasopressin. During normal pregnancy, serum CAS activity progressively increases, and such measurements can be used to assess placental integrity (*1–3*).

L-Cystine-di-2-napthylamide, the substrate originally used for estimating CAS activity (*4*), is no longer acceptable because of the carcinogenic dangers of napthylamine. Tuppy et al. (*5*) suggested the use of L-cystine-di-4-nitroanilide, but this substrate is very difficult to synthesize and purify and is poorly water-soluble. More recently, *S*-benzyl-L-cysteine-4-nitroanilide has been used, but mostly for kinetic methods (*6–8*); the only end-point method so far described has involved diazotization and coupling of the released 4-nitroaniline (*9*).

This paper describes an end-point method that requires no further color formation after the incubation period has been completed.

Materials and Methods

Reagents[1]

Phosphate buffer, 0.1 mol/liter, pH 7.4 at 37 °C. Dissolve 2.716 g of potassium dihydrogen orthophosphate and 11.413 g of disodium hydrogen orthophosphate in about 0.95 liters of distilled water, adjust to pH 7.4, and dilute to 1 liter with distilled water. Store at either room temperature or 4 °C.

Substrate solution S-benzyl-L-cysteine-4-nitroanilide, 6 mmol/liter in acetone/methanol (10/90 by vol). Dissolve 200 mg of *S*-benzyl-L-cysteine-4-nitroanilide in 10 ml of acetone and dilute to 100 ml with methanol. Store at 4 °C in a dark-glass bottle.

Protein precipitant: Dissolve 100 g of trichloroacetic acid in 1 liter of distilled water.

Stock standard, 4-nitroaniline, 10 mmol/liter. Dissolve 138 mg of 4-nitroaniline in 10 ml of acetone, dilute to 100 ml with methanol. Store at 4 °C in a dark bottle.

Working standard, 4-nitroaniline, 1 mmol/liter. Dilute 1 ml of the stock standard to 10 ml with the phosphate buffer.

Assay Procedure

Allow a mixture of 50 μl of serum and 1.75 ml of buffer to reach a temperature of 37 °C. Equilibrate 1.8 ml of buffer similarly to serve as a blank. Add 0.2 ml of substrate solution to each tube, mix well, and incubate at 37 °C for 20 min. Stop the reaction and precipitate the proteins by adding 1 ml of the trichloroacetic acid solution to each tube. Mix and centrifuge the reaction tubes (3000 rpm, 5 min). Measure the absorbance at 400 nm vs. the method blank. Convert the absorbance into U/liter from the calibration curve.

Calibration curve. Dilute the 4-nitroaniline working standard with buffer and trichloroacetic acid in the proportions shown in Table 1, and read the absorbance of the standards at 400 nm vs. the blank.

Analytical Variables

Protein precipitant. The protein precipitant must be able to stop the reaction and yield, after centrifugation, a clear supernatant fluid that can be decanted without disturbing the packed precipitate, and it must be without effect on the wavelength of maximum absorption of 4-nitroaniline.

Of various commonly used aqueous protein precipitants tested (alkaline zinc salts, tungstic acid, and trichloroacetic acid), the latter was the only one that

Pathology Department, Women's Hospital, Liverpool L8 7NJ, England.

[1] All chemicals were obtained from BDH Chemicals Ltd., Poole, England.

Received Dec. 30, 1974; accepted Oct. 31, 1975.

Table 1. Protocol for Preparation of Calibration Curve

Reagent	Blank	100	200	400	600
	CAS activity, U/liter				
Working standard, ml	0	0.25	0.5	1.0	1.5
Phosphate buffer, ml	5	4.75	4.5	4.0	3.5
Trichloroacetic acid, ml	2.5	2.5	2.5	2.5	2.5

Mix and read absorbance at 400 nm.

Table 2. Effect of 1 ml of Various Trichloroacetic Acid Solutions on the Absorbance of 2 ml of a 4-Nitroaniline Solution (100 mol/liter)

Trichloroacetic acid concn, g/liter	Absorbance, 400 nm	Final pH
20	0.721	2.7
50	0.518	2.0
100	0.335	1.8
150	0.251	1.8
200	0.176	1.8
Buffered 4-nitroaniline	0.777	2.0

fulfilled these criteria. Table 2 shows the absorbances obtained when 2-ml aliquots of a 4-nitroaniline solution (100 μmol/liter) treated with 1 ml of various concentrations of trichloroacetic acid were compared with the absorbance of an aliquot of the 4-nitroaniline solution buffered to the same pH as that of the trichloroacetic acid-treated supernates. Decrease in the molar absorptivity of 4-nitroaniline is a function of the trichloroacetic acid concentration and not of the final pH of the supernate. I used a 100 g/liter solution of trichloroacetic acid because it gave a more compact precipitate button than did lower concentrations.

pH and molarity of the buffer. The phosphate buffer used in the method was studied over the pH range 5.6–8.0 and molarity range 20 to 200 mmol/liter. The source of the CAS was a pool of 30 sera from women who were 36 to 38 weeks pregnant.

The pH optimum was 7.4 and the changes in activity around this pH are more clearly defined than those described for the kinetic method *(6)*. The activity curve flattened near pH 6.0 for every specimen examined. Ryden *(10)* stated that the enzyme activity of other tissues except placental tissue has an optimum at pH 6.0.

The activity is optimum with the 0.10 mol/liter phosphate buffer, but remains reasonably constant for buffer concentrations between 0.10 and 0.16 mol/liter.

Substrate solvent. *S*-Benzyl-L-cysteine-4-nitroanilide has the disadvantage that it dissolves only sparingly in water. A solvent was sought that would readily dissolve it, keep it in solution when diluted 10-fold with a buffer/serum mixture (35/1 by vol), and not inhibit the enzyme activity.

Table 3. Effect of Various Substrate Solvents on Absorbance (CAS Activity)

Acetone/Methanol (ml/dl)	Absorbance, 400 nm
1	0.500
2	0.525
5	0.540
10	0.600
15	0.555
20	0.490
Acetone	0.090
2-Methoxyethanol	0.460

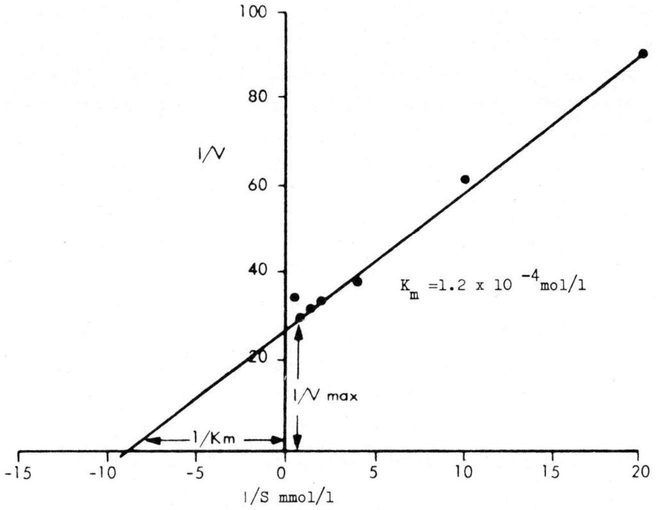

Fig. 1. Lineweaver–Burk plot showing the influence of substrate concentration on reaction velocity with acetone/methanol (10/90 by vol) as the substrate solvent

Tovey et al. *(6)* used 2-methoxyethanol as the solvent for *S*-benzyl-L-cysteine-4-nitroanilide in the manual kinetic method. This solvent, acetone, and various mixtures of acetone/methanol were investigated. CAS activity is inhibited by excess of acetone; to overcome this problem but retain the advantage of the easier solubility, I first dissolved *S*-benzyl-L-cysteine-4-nitroanilide in acetone and then diluted with methanol to the desired concentration and acetone/methanol mixture.

Table 3 shows absorbances obtained when the various solvents were used in the assay procedure, together with the previously mentioned serum pool. CAS activity was highest when an acetone/methanol (10/90 by vol) solvent was used. If the activity obtained by using this solvent is designated 100%, then the activity obtained with 2-methoxyethanol is only 77% as great. For this reason and also the easier preparation of the substrate solution, the acetone/metha-

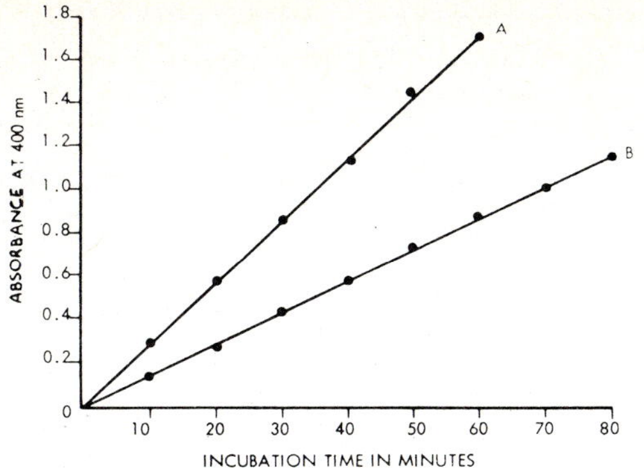

Fig. 2. Progress curves of absorbance (CAS activity) when a 0.6 mmol/liter substrate concentration is used
(*A*) High-activity serum. (*B*) Low-activity serum

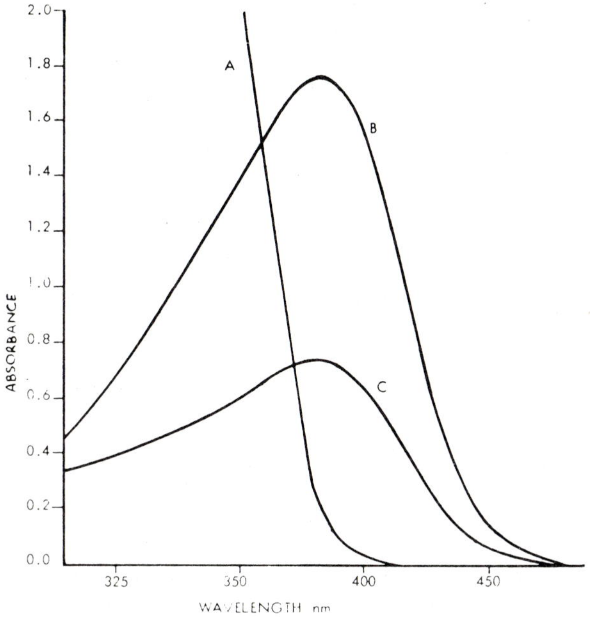

Fig. 3. Ultraviolet absorption spectra
(*A*) 0.6 mmol/liter *S*-benzyl-L-cysteine-4-nitroanilide in trichloroacetic acid-treated phosphate buffer. (*B*) 0.2 mmol/liter 4-nitroaniline in phosphate buffer. (*C*) 0.2 mmol/liter 4-nitroaniline in trichloroacetic acid-treated phosphate buffer

nol mixture was the solvent of choice for this manual method.

Substrate concentration. I investigated the optimum substrate concentration required in the reaction by using final substrate concentrations in the reaction mixture of 0.05 − 2.0 mmol/liter (Figure 1). At the optimum concentration the *S*-benzyl-L-cysteine-4-nitroanilide does not remain completely in solution; 0.65 mmol/liter is its maximum solubility. At 0.60 mmol/liter the velocity of the reaction was 90% of the maximum. When this concentration was used with an extended incubation period the increase in the release of 4-nitroaniline was linear with time over at least a threefold increase in the normal incubation period (Figure 2).

Table 4. Precision of Method at Three Levels of CAS Activity

	Mean (U/liter)	SD (U/liter)	CV, %	n
	Within-batch			
(a)	94	3	3.2	20
(b)	280	6	2.2	20
(c)	398	8	2.0	20
	Between-batch			
(a)	97	4	4.1	10
(b)	278	8	2.9	10
(c)	403	11	2.7	10

Table 5. Serum CAS Activity in the Third Trimester of Normal Pregnancy

Gestational age, weeks	Mean (U/liter)	SD (U/liter)	n
24	86	34	60
28	163	45	60
32	240	63	60
36	305	78	60
40	360	95	60

Choice of wavelength. The wavelength of maximum absorption of 4-nitroaniline is 380 nm, but at this wavelength the reagent blank containing *S*-benzyl-L-cysteine-4-nitroanilide, when measured against the buffer, has an absorbance of approximately 0.500. If the wavelength is changed to 400 nm the absorbance of the blank is decreased to about 0.050 and the absorbance of 4-nitroaniline at this wavelength is 80% of that measured at 380 nm. Because of this decrease in the blank absorbance with only a small decrease in the absorbance of 4-nitroaniline, 400 nm is the wavelength of choice (Figure 3).

Reagent blank vs. serum blank. 100 sera (including hemolyzed, lipemic, and jaundiced samples) were analyzed and read vs. both their own serum blanks and the reagent blank. The mean and standard deviation of the CAS activity, read against the serum blanks, was 318 ± 51 U/liter; when read against the reagent blank it was 320 ± 50 U/liter. From this I concluded that there was no advantage in including individual serum blanks.

Precision of assay. Within-batch precision of the assay was tested by assaying replicates of three pregnancy sera, each with a different activity. Aliquots of the sera, which had been stored at −20 °C, were tested on 10 separate days to obtain data on between-batch precision (Table 4).

Results

Normal Values

Serum CAS activity found in the third trimester of normal uncomplicated pregnancy was established for the described method. Sixty women with uncomplicated and normotensive pregnancies were selected. Blood samples were collected from them every four weeks from 24 to 40 weeks of gestation. Table 5 shows the mean serum CAS activity established for these gestational periods.

Sera from healthy nonpregnant women and from healthy men had values of less than 5 U/liter.

Comparison with the Kinetic Method

Results by the proposed method and the kinetic method (*6*) were compared. Sera from 25 pregnant women, with activities covering the range that could be found in the third trimester, were used. The regression lines were $y = 1.32x + 34.79$ and $x = 0.707y - 11.1$, where y and x are the results from the proposed method and from the kinetic method, respectively. The correlation coefficient was 0.967. The higher values obtained with the proposed method are to be expected because of the increase in CAS activity in the presence of the acetone/methanol solvent over that in 2-methoxyethanol and the optimizing of the molarity of the phosphate buffer.

The proposed method correlates well with the kinetic method and has the advantage that it can be performed without using reaction rate analyzers or other sophisticated equipment.

I thank Drs. R. Rewell and W. Marlow for their useful criticism during the preparation of this method; also Dr. B. Sturgeon of BDH Chemicals Ltd. (Poole, England) for the sample of *S*-benzyl-L-cysteine-4-nitroanilide and for supplying results from the kinetic method.

References

1. Chapman, L., Silk, E., Skupney, A., et al., Spectrofluorimetric assay of serum cystine aminopeptidase in normal and diabetic pregnancy compared with total oestrogen excretion. *J. Obstet. Gynaecol. Br. Commonw.* **78,** 435 (1971).

2. Hurry, D. J., Tovey, J. E., Robinson, D. A., et al., Cystine aminopeptidase in normal and complicated pregnancies. *J. Obstet. Gynaecol. Br. Commonw.* **79,** 788 (1972).

3. Petrucco, O. M., Cellier, K., and Fishtall, A., Diagnosis of intrauterine fetal growth retardation by serial serum oxytocinase, urinary oestrogen and serum heat-stable alkaline phosphate (HSAP) in uncomplicated and hypertensive pregnancies. *J. Obstet. Gynaecol. Br. Commonw.* **80,** 499 (1973).

4. Tuppy, H., and Nesvdba, H., Über die Aminopeptidaseaktivitat des Schwangerenserums und ihre Beziehung zu dessen Vermogen, Oxytocin zu inaktivieren. *Monatsh. Chem.* **88,** 977 (1957).

5. Tuppy, H., Weisbauer, U., and Wintersberger, E., Aminosaure-*p*-nitroanilide als Substrate fur Aminopeptidasen und andere proteolytischer Fermente. *Z. Physiol. Chem.* **329,** 278 (1962).

6. Tovey, J. E., Dawson, P. J. G., and Fellowes, K. P., Evaluation of *S*-benzyl-L-cysteine-4-nitroanilide as a substrate for serum cystine aminopeptidase. *Clin. Chem.* **19,** 756 (1973).

7. Watson, D., and Gibbard, S., Automated determination of serum aminopeptidase. *Clin. Biochem.* **6,** 60 (1973).

8. Chapman, L., Burrows-Peakin, R., Rege, V. P., and Silk, E., Comparison of L-cystine-di-β-napthylamide and *S*-benzyl-L-cysteine-4-*p*-nitroanilide as substrate for the assay of cystine aminopeptidase in pregnancy. *Clin. Chim. Acta* **51,** 335 (1974).

9. Van Buul, T., and Van Oudheusden, A. P. M., Comparative study of recent assays for the determination of cystine aminopeptidase (oxytocinase). *Clin. Chim. Acta* **54,** 263 (1974).

10. Ryden, G., Cystine aminopeptidase and oxytocinase activity in pregnancy. A comparative study in human and rat tissues. *Acta Obstet. Gynecol. Scand.* **45,** *Suppl. 3* (1966).

CLIN. CHEM. 22/1, 83-86 (1976)

Comparison of Four Kits for Enzymatic Determination of Ethanol in Blood

Helmut M. Redetzki and William L. Dees

We compared results obtained with four commercially available kits for the enzymatic (alcohol dehydrogenase) determination of ethanol in blood, in a practical test in which standardized blood samples were used. Each of the kits yielded reliable results with acceptable reproducibility. A tendency to record slightly lower values in the intermediate and high alcohol range is most likely related to incomplete (inhomogeneous) deproteinization. Blood samples containing ethanol plus various concentrations of methanol and isopropanol were analyzed to evaluate the specificity of assays. Highly toxic blood concentrations of methanol (1.5 g/liter) increased apparent ethanol values only insignificantly, but even small concentrations of isopropanol (0.5 g/liter) interfered in all kits to different but substantial extents. The specific technical characteristics of the kits, their advantages and disadvantages are discussed. Costs are compared for analysis of small numbers of samples.

Enzymatic methods for ethanol determination in blood were introduced simultaneously in 1951 by Bücher and Redetzki (*1, 2*) and Bonnichsen and Theorell (*3, 4*). Although not fully specific for ethanol, these methods greatly improved the reliability of assays for ethanol, which at that time were generally done by unspecific reduction methods (*5, 6*). Increasingly, forensic and toxicologic laboratories are using gas chromatography to assay blood alcohol, but many, especially clinical laboratories, continue to use the enzymatic method. Those that have only few such requests often depend on commercial kits, four of which are now available from different companies in the U.S. They differ greatly with respect to use of single enzymes or enzyme combinations, methods of sample deproteinization, incubation time, buffers, and general technical arrangements.

Department of Pharmacology and Therapeutics, Louisiana State University School of Medicine in Shreveport; and Veterans Administration Hospital, Shreveport, La.

Address communications to: P. O. Box 3932, Shreveport, La. 71130.

Received Sept. 8, 1975; accepted Oct. 31, 1975.

Because there are no studies in which these kits have been inter-compared, we have tested the accuracy and specificity of each set, as well as the complexity of the procedures. In addition, data on analysis costs are presented.

Materials and Methods

Blood alcohol reference samples: Three samples with alcohol concentrations of 0.45 g/liter (low), 1.44 g/liter (intermediate), and 3.14 g/liter (high) were prepared by adding measured amounts of ethanol/water (1/4 by vol) to separate aliquots of a uniform pool of human plasma. Concentrations were verified by use of freezing point osmometry according to procedures described by Redetzki et al. (*7, 8*). The samples were stored frozen and again checked osmometrically after thawing before analysis to detect any possible alteration of alcohol content. Osmometry was also used to determine the accuracy of alcohol standards provided with two of the kits.

Specificity was studied by use of a blood sample containing 0.45 g of ethanol per liter, to which 0.50 g and 1.50 g of methanol or isopropanol were added per liter. The kits or reagent sets tested were as follows:

Boehringer Mannheim Corp., New York, N.Y. 10017. Alcohol Test Combination, catalog No. 15425, approximately 50 tests.

Worthington Biochemical Corp., Freehold, N.J. 94080. Ethyl Alcohol Reagent Set, catalog No. 7919, approximately 75 tests.

Sigma Chemical Co., St. Louis, Mo. 63178. Alcohol, Ethyl, Analytical Kit, kit No. 331, approximately 21 tests.

Calbiochem, La Jolla, Calif. 92037. Ethyl Alcohol Stat Pack, catalog No. 869219, approximately 50 tests.

Determinations and calculations were conducted exactly as described in the package inserts. To help assure uniformity of assays, one person did all the procedural steps such as sample deproteinization, pi-

Table 1. Comparison of Blood Alcohol Values Obtained with Four Enzymatic Kits

Supplier	Blood ethanol, g/liter plasma: Sample A, 0.45[a]	Deviation[b] in %	Sample B, 1.44	Deviation in %	Sample C, 3.14	Deviation in %
Boehringer	0.43(±0.02)[c]	−4.5	1.47(±0.02)	+2.1	3.13(±0.06)	−0.3
Worthington	0.44(±0.01)	−2.23	1.39(±0.04)	−3.5	3.00(±0.07)	−4.5
Sigma	0.47(±0.02)	+4.4	1.44(±0.07)	0.0	3.04(±0.06)	−3.2
Calbiochem	0.42(±0.03)	−6.7	1.40(±0.02)	−2.8	2.99(±0.03)	−4.8

[a] Ethanol concentration of samples confirmed by freezing point osmometry.
[b] Deviation from the true alcohol content of the samples.
[c] Each value is the mean of four individual determinations (±SD).

petting, etc. We used an Acta C III spectrophotometer (Beckman Instruments Inc., Fullerton, Calif. 92634.)

Results

Evaluation of the kits was based on analysis of three plasma samples with alcohol concentrations representative of mild, moderate, and severe levels of intoxication. Data on accuracy and precision of assays are presented in Table 1. Standard deviations of the mean were rather uniform for each kit, ranging from 0.01 to 0.07 g/liter. Analytical recovery rates, in terms of deviations from values for reference samples, ranged from 104.4% to 93.3%. Standard curves of the Worthington, Calbiochem, and Boehringer kits remained linear or near linear up to the highest alcohol concentration recommended by the suppliers. The curve for the Sigma kit had a progressively decreasing slope with increasing alcohol concentration. We found it to fit best a power curve function characterized by $y = ax^b$. In all instances, reactions had reached completion at the end of the recommended incubation times.

The two alcohols selected for specificity studies, methanol and isopropanol, are those most often encountered in cases of accidental ingestion or as contaminants of illicitly obtained alcoholic beverages. Table 2 shows our results. The increases in apparent ethanol effected by methanol are insignificant, but isopropanol interferes to various degrees with all four assays, the Worthington kit being less affected than the others.

Table 3 summarizes differences in kit composition and analytical procedures.

Discussion

We have described a practical comparison of four commercially available kits for the enzymatic determination of ethanol. Three of the kits are modifications of the Bücher–Redetzki procedure (*1, 2, 9*) in which yeast alcohol dehydrogenase (EC 1.1.1.1) is the enzyme used, and reduction of NAD^+ (ultraviolet range) is measured in the presence of an aldehyde trapping agent; one kit (Worthington) makes use of a coupled yeast alcohol dehydrogenase/diaphorase (EC 1.6.4.3) system in which a chromogen [2-(*p*-iodophenyl)-3-(*p*-nitrophenyl)-5-phenyl-tetrazolium chloride] is used to reoxidize NADH (*10*). The reduction of this dye to a red formazan allows the reaction to be measured in the visible light range (500 nm) (*11*).

Because two of the kits contain their own ethanol standards, it was necessary to analyze these for accuracy. This is easily accomplished by osmometry (*7, 8*). Although their concentrations were found to be accurate, we recommend this procedure highly, because we have observed deviations in previous measurements of commercially prepared standards of up to 20% from declared values (unpublished data). Osmometry also helped us to confirm the accuracy of

Table 2. Specificity Studies[a]

Supplier	Sample A + methanol, 0.50 g/liter	Deviation[b] in %	Sample B + methanol, 1.50 g/liter	Deviation in %	Sample C + isopropanol, 0.50 g/liter	Deviation in %	Sample D + isopropanol, 1.50 g/liter	Deviation in %
Boehringer	0.48[c](±0.03)	+6.7	0.51(±0.06)	+13.3	0.66(±0.01)	+46.7	0.97(±0.08)	+115.6
Worthington	0.47(±0.02)	+4.4	0.48(±0.01)	+6.7	0.50(±0.05)	+11.1	0.65(±0.04)	+44.4
Sigma	0.48(±0.05)	+6.7	0.47(±0.01)	+4.4	0.69(±0.04)	+53.3	0.81(±0.03)	+80.0
Calbiochem	0.49(±0.03)	+8.9	0.52(±0.04)	+15.6	0.70(±0.04)	+55.6	0.96(±0.06)	+113.3

[a] Ethanol concentration of each sample was 0.45 g/liter, confirmed by freezing point osmometry.
[b] Deviation from the true ethanol content of the samples.
[c] Each value is the mean of four individual determinations (±SD).

Table 3. Composition and Technical Characteristics of the Enzymatic Kits[a]

	Boehringer	Worthington	Sigma	Calbiochem
Deproteinization with	perchloric acid (not included)	barium hydroxide—zinc sulfate (not included)	trichloroacetic acid (included)	perchloric acid (not included)
Buffer	pyrophosphate pH 8.7	pyrophosphate pH 8.9	pyrophosphate pH 9.2	Tris succinate pH 8.8
Trapping agent	semicarbazide (acetaldehyde)	iodonitro tetrazolium violet (NADH)	semicarbazide (acetaldehyde)	aminooxyacetic acid (acetaldehyde)
Diaphorase chromogen system	no	yes	no	no
Wavelength, nm	340 or 366	500	340	340
Incubation time, min	50–70	15	20	8–10
Incubation temp., °C	25–37 (room temp.)	room temp. (>24)	37 (or 30 min at room temp.)	30
Pipetting steps	6	8	4	4
Cost per determination 1 sample (5 samples)[b]	$3.50 ($1.26)	$4.16 ($1.66)	$5.67 ($1.78)	$4.20 ($1.68)
Alcohol standard	not included	not included	included	included

[a] Alcohol dehydrogenase used in all kits.
[b] Sample, blank, and required standards, all in single analysis, no duplicates.

our own standards and plasma alcohol samples directly before each enzymatic assay. With the difficulties encountered in preparation of accurate standards, use of an independent physical method of assay increases the reliability of all data.

The data show that each of the kits offers reasonably good reproducibility. There was a tendency for the results to be low, especially in the high and intermediate alcohol range. Deviations in the low range do not carry as much practical significance. We did not attempt to identify the sources of error, but our previous work with the alcohol dehydrogenase method suggests incomplete deproteinization as the most obvious factor responsible for decreased recovery (*2*).

Our specificity data confirm that isopropanol is oxidized by the enzyme and that methanol does not interfere to any significant degree with the determination (*2*). However, we were surprised that the magnitude of the isopropanol "error" varied greatly among the kits. Each of the package inserts contains brief comments concerning possible interferences by other alcohols. [For a review of the specificity of the alcohol dehydrogenase method, see Bernheim et al. (*12*) and Barron and Levine (*13*).]

The following pertains to technical procedures. All kits contain directions for deproteinization of blood, plasma, or serum samples. The barium hydroxide/zinc sulfate method requires a little more time because it involves two pipetting steps, as compared with the perchloric acid or trichloroacetic acid one-step procedure. With each method it is essential to obtain uniform deproteinization because alcohol may be trapped in coarse protein precipitates.

The general availability of spectrophotometers extending into the ultraviolet range makes it questionable whether the coupled diaphorase/chromogen reaction offers any advantages. Although only the Boehringer kit gives instructions for measurements at 340 nm as well as 366 nm, with the Sigma and Calbiochem kits results can equally well be read at 366 nm. We actually prefer the use of a photometer with mercury lamp (monochromatic line spectrum) over one with a continuous-spectrum light source. The moderate reduction of absorption at 366 nm (absorption maximum, 340 nm) is well compensated by keeping readings in the more accurate, readable range of absorbance scales.

Incubation times required for completion of the reaction vary from 8 to 50 min. The Calbiochem set offers definite advantages if an analysis is requested on an emergency basis. However, if a larger number of samples are to be analyzed, the longer incubation time of the Boehringer set allows continuous and uninterrupted processing of samples. Incubation temperature is not critical with the Boehringer and Worthington sets. Room temperature above 24 °C is sufficient. Instructions for the Sigma kit recommend incubation at 37 °C in a water bath (the procedure followed in this study) but states also that samples may be kept at room temperature if incubation time is prolonged to 30 min. Calbiochem recommends incubation at 30 °C, and indicates that uniformity of temperature is more important than temperature setting. The Calbiochem and Sigma kits require the smallest number of pipetting steps, Worthington's the greatest.

The cost (Table 3) of a single blood alcohol determination varies from \$3.50 to \$5.67. We included three alcohol standards (0.50 g/liter, 1.50 g/liter and 3.00 g/liter) for the Boehringer kit. The others gave specific instructions about the number of standards to be used. The cost per blood sample declines substantially when five samples are analyzed simultaneously (range, \$1.26 to \$1.78). Only two kits provide their own alcohol standards and only one provides the deproteinizing agent, but these add relatively little to the total cost of the assays.

In two of the sets (Calbiochem and Worthington) the reagents are in multi-sample vials which, when activated by addition of fluid, must be used within 4 h. This can result in wastage of unused material and increased cost. The Sigma kit offers the convenience of providing individual test vials that contain aliquots of NAD^+ and enzyme to be activated by addition of buffer. However, one has to rely exclusively on quality-control exerted by the manufacturer, because it is impossible to assure oneself of the proper functioning of an individual vial without conducting duplicate determinations. Vials from different production batches should not be mixed, because enzyme activity often varies with prolonged storage or improper handling. The fact that the slope of the standard curves varies from day to day (differences in room temperature, progressive loss of enzyme activity on storage) does not generally impair the accuracy of the results; however, it makes it mandatory that alcohol standards are run each time assays are conducted. The kits produce reliable results when used according to instructions.

References

1. Bücher, T., and Redetzki, H., Eine spezifische photometrische Bestimmung von Äthylalkohol auf fermentativem Wege. *Klin. Wochenschr.* **29,** 615 (1951).

2. Dotzauer, G., Redetzki, H., Johannsmeier, K., and Bücher, T., Erprobung einer spezifischen Fermentmethode zur Mikrobestimmung von Äthylalkohol. *Dtsch. Z. Gesamte Gerichtl. Med.* **41,** 15 (1952).

3. Bonnichsen, R., and Theorell, H., An enzymatic method for the microdetermination of ethanol. *Scand. J. Clin. Lab. Invest.* **3,** 58 (1951).

4. Brink, N., Bonnichsen, R., and Theorell, H., A modified method for the enzymatic microdetermination of ethanol. *Acta Pharmacol. Toxicol.* **10,** 223 (1954).

5. Redetzki, H., Johannsmeier, K., and Dotzauer, G., Fäulnis und Äthylalkohol. *Dtsch. Z. Gesamte Gerichtl. Med.* **41,** 424 (1952).

6. Harger, R., Ethyl alcohol. In *Toxicology, Mechanism and Analytical Methods.* **II,** C. Stewart and A. Stolman, Eds. Academic Press, New York, N.Y., 1961, pp 86–151.

7. Redetzki, H. M., Koerner, T. A., Hughes, J. R., and Smith, A. G., Osmometry in the evaluation of alcohol intoxication. *Clin. Toxicol.* **5,** 343 (1972).

8. Redetzki, H. M., Use of the osmometer for preparation, analysis and control of alcohol standard solutions. *Q. J. Stud. Alcohol.* **34,** 206 (1973).

9. Redetzki, H., and Johannsmeier, K., Grundlagen und Ergebnisse der enzymatischen Äthylalkoholbestimmung. *Arch. Toxicol.* **16,** 73 (1956).

10. Brower, M., and Woodbridge, J., A rapid colorimetric determination of ethanol in blood. Paper presented at the 22nd national meeting, AACC, 1970. Abstract: *Clin. Chem.* **16,** 539 (1970).

11. Nachlas, M., Margulies, S., Goldberg, J., and Seligman, A., The determination of lactic dehydrogenase with tetrazolium salt. *Anal. Biochem.* **1,** 317 (1960).

12. Bernheim, J., Sachs, V., and Steigleder, E., Systematische Untersuchungen mit dem ADH-Verfahren. Ein Beitrag zur Spezifität der Methode. *Dtsch. Z. Gesamte Gerichtl. Med.* **53,** 28 (1962).

13. Barron, E., and Levine, S., Oxidation of alcohols by yeast alcohol dehydrogenase and by the living cell. The thiol groups of the enzyme. *Arch. Biochem.* **41,** 175 (1952).

CLIN. CHEM. 22/1, 87–91 (1976)

Atypical Increase in Serum Creatine Kinase Activity in Hospital Patients

Sylvan M. Sax,[1] John J. Moore,[1] Joseph L. Giegel,[2] and Muriel Welsh[2]

We use an ion-exchange column-chromatographic technique for separating creatine kinase isoenzymes in serum, and occasionally observe what appears to be sustained increase in the MB fraction. Most patients whose sera show such behavior have myocardial disease, but not necessarily a recent myocardial infarction. Electrophoretic analysis of a small sampling of such sera revealed that the apparent MB migrates atypically, appearing distinctly between isoenzymes MB and MM. In another electrophoretic system, the peak might easily be mistaken for MM. This unusual isoenzyme does not appear to be "macro" creatine kinase. In laboratories that use the ion-exchange technique, the possibility of a falsely positive MB value should be considered in subjects who show persistent increases together with normal or nearly normal values for total creatine kinase activity. A suitable electrophoretic method that clearly demonstrates this unusual isoenzyme should be used in such cases, for confirmation.

Additional Keyphrases: *ion-exchange chromatography • electrophoresis on cellulose acetate • atypical isoenzyme • heart disease*

Many laboratories have confirmed the existence of three isoenzymes of CK,[3] frequently designated as MM, MB, and BB. There are reports of electrophoretically separable bands that do not correspond to any of these three dimers. Although some of the earlier reports have been questioned (*1–4*) because of the separation techniques used or failure to include creatine phosphate-free blanks, later well-controlled studies also report similar CK-active bands. With electrophoresis on polyacrylamide, Smith (*5*) observed splitting of MM and MB, attributed to small conformational changes. Two unusual bands in human serum and tissue extracts, separable on agarose, have been observed (*6, 7*); they may reflect conformational transformation of MB and BB in myocardium and brain, respectively, arising as a result of prolonged ischemia. Sobel et al. (*8*) reported that CK isolated from rabbit heart mitochondria migrates cathodal to MM on cellulose acetate. In serum from a child with Reye's syndrome, a band, considered possibly to be mitochondrial CK, was also seen cathodal to MM on agarose (*9*).

After myocardial infarction the activity of isoenzyme MB in serum typically increases soon after onset and returns to normal in about 48 h. Prolonged elevations have been observed in other subjects when either electrophoresis (*5, 10–14*) or chromatography on DEAE-Sephadex (*15*) was used to effect the separation. Such increases have been noted in various myosites, in muscular dystrophy, and in conditions associated with myoglobinemia (*10, 11*); in subjects with probable myocardial damage, but without documented myocardial infarction (*12, 13, 15*); in an apparently normal person (*5*); in persons with severe myocardial infarction with complications such as cardiogenic shock (*16*); and in patients without acute myocardial infarction, but with chronic atrial fibrillation (*20*). Finally, increased serum MB activity has been reported after CO poisoning (*13*), in malignant hyperthermia (*13*), and in Reye's syndrome (*9*).

We have observed that occasional hospital patients will show persistently elevated MB with normal or minimally increased total CK, when the isoenzymes are separated by chromatography on DEAE-Sephadex (*17*). Application of a newly developed electrophoretic separation kit technique to the same specimens reveals that the apparent MB migrates atypically. In this paper, we describe results for several such specimens analyzed by the two separation techniques.

Materials and Methods

Total CK activity was measured at 30 °C by the Rosalki procedure (*18*) with an ABA-100 analyzer (Abbott Laboratories, Diagnostic Division, Pasadena, Calif. 91030), with use of Abbott's "A-Gent" reagent. Maximum normal value (males) is 100 $U_{30\,°C}$/liter.

We used a column-chromatographic procedure to separate CK isoenzymes (*17*). Activities in the eluates were assessed with the ABA-100 by a procedure differing only in the following details from that described by Mercer and Varat (*15*): we used a 1:11 syringe plate, an incubation temperature of 30 °C, and Abbott's A-Gent reagent. The sensitivity achieved easily permits measurement of MB in sera with normal total CK activity. Normal values for MB are 0–2.4 $U_{30\,°C}$/liter. Isoenzyme resolution was tested

[1] Department of Pathology, The Western Pennsylvania Hospital, 4800 Friendship Ave., Pittsburgh, Pa. 15224.

[2] Dade Division, American Hospital Supply Corp., Box 520672, Miami, Fla. 33152.

[3] Nonstandard abbreviations used: CK, creatine kinase (EC 2.7.3.2); DEAE, diethylaminoethyl; and Tris, tris(hydroxymethyl)aminomethane.

Received Sept. 18, 1975; accepted Oct. 31, 1975.

with a control containing MM, MB, and BB of simian origin ("CPK Isoenzyme Marker"; Dade Division, American Hospital Supply Corp., Miami, Fla. 33152). The eluates of low-, medium-, and high-salt-concentration containing peak activities were examined by the electrophoretic procedure described below; only the single anticipated band was visible in each (see Figure 2). The resolution and sensitivity we found with the column method agree with Mercer (*17*) and Mercer and Varat (*15*) rather than Nealon and Henderson (*19*). A rigorous test for carryover of MM was provided by electrophoresing serum from the victim of a severe electrical burn (45 700 $U_{30\,^\circ C}$ of total CK per liter) through the column, both undiluted and in 100-fold dilution; identical proportions of MM and MB were observed in each case, the MM comprising 99.6% of the total. Sera from 22 patients with above-normal total CK but without evidence of heart disease were examined by column chromatography. The observed 95% range for %MB was 2.4% of total CK; in no case was BB noted. Thus our criteria for suspecting a myocardial source of above-normal MB activity are (*a*) an MB activity >2.4 $U_{30\,^\circ C}$/liter with a normal total value for CK, or (*b*) an MB activity exceeding 2.4% of total CK, when the latter value is above normal.

CK isoenzymes were also separated by an electrophoretic procedure developed by Dade Division (*21*). We separated 1 µl of serum for 15 min at a constant 250 V on cellulose acetate (Beckman Electrophoresis Membranes; Beckman Instruments, Inc., Fullerton, Calif.) in cold (4 °C) Tris barbital buffer, pH 8.8, ionic strength 0.06. For staining we used coupled reactions catalyzed by hexokinase (EC 2.7.1.1) and glucose-6-phosphate dehydrogenase (EC 1.1.1.49); the resulting NADH reacted with nitroblue tetrazolium to yield a blue formazan. The aforementioned "CPK Isoenzyme Marker" (0.25 µl) was run as a control. In some experiments, blank staining reactions, from which creatine phosphate was omitted, were done to differentiate CK from adenylate kinase (EC 2.7.4.3) or from nonspecific staining. In one experiment, electrophoresis was done with use of a kit (CPK Isoenzyme Electrophoresis; Helena Laboratories Corp., Beaumont, Tex. 77704) that depends upon fluorescence of NADH for detection of CK fractions and upon concurrent processing of a CK isoenzyme control provided by Helena for correct location of the bands. We did not attempt to quantify the MB fraction of electrophoretograms.

Approximate molecular weights of serum CK isoenzymes were estimated by use of Sephadex G-100. Serum (0.2 ml), to which was added a combined marker containing Blue Dextran 2000 (Pharmacia Fine Chemicals AB, Uppsala, Sweden) and cytochrome c (Sigma Chemical Co., St. Louis, Mo. 63178), was passed through a 42 × 1 cm column, prepared in Tris HCl (50 mmol/liter, pH 7.2) and eluted with the same buffer. The relative elution volumes were used to estimate molecular weight.

Results and Discussion

Table 1 gives values for total CK and for MB obtained by ion-exchange chromatography of sera from a selected group of hospital patients. All show apparently abnormal MB values for two or more assays over an interval greater than two days, with total CK in the normal or slightly increased range. In most cases, evidence for a concurrent myocardial infarction was not confirmed by electrocardiogram, or by clinical or other laboratory data. In the period between April 9 and July 29, 1975, during which results in Table 1 were obtained, a total of 2215 samples from 519 different patients were tested similarly. Of this population, a third were patients in the coronary care unit at some time during hospitalization. From results for this sample it would seem reasonable to conclude that the occurrence of atypical sustained MB increases, as determined by column chromatography, is not rare. Moreover, a number of the patients not shown gave repeated MB values in the slightly supranormal range, or single, significantly increased MB and normal total CK values, which were not followed serially.

Because supportive evidence for myocardial infarction was lacking in these patients, we attempted to confirm the MB elevations by electrophoresis. Figure 1 shows electrophoretograms for three of the patients shown in Table 1. The patient's serum shown at the top had a single band of activity located midway between MB and MM of the marker. The next patient's pattern (below the diluted marker) also displays a single band, closer to MB, but still unmistakably more cathodal. The final patient shows both MM and intermediate bands. If creatine phosphate was omitted the bands did not appear, confirming that the observed activity does not result from adenylate kinase or nonspecific tetrazolium reduction. Fresh or frozen (for one week) sera from these patients gave identical electrophoretic patterns.

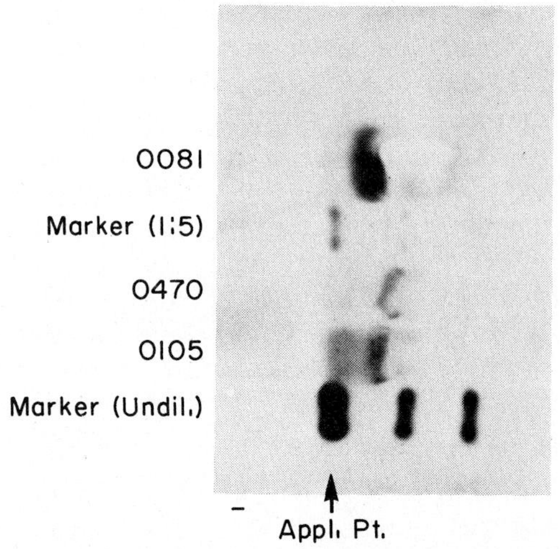

Fig. 1. Electrophoretograms of CK isoenzymes in three selected patients' sera and in Dade "CPK Isoenzyme Marker"
Application point is indicated by arrow in Figures 1–3

Table 1. Data on Selected Patients with Apparently Elevated CK-MB by Ion-exchange Chromatography

Patient no.	Age, yr	Sex	Date (1975)	Total CK, U/liter	MB, U/liter	% MB	Clinical diagnosis and comments
0630	78	F	06/24	29	17	58.6	Fracture of knee; hiatus hernia; asthma-like pulmonary condition; diffuse gastritis. ECG of 06/24 showed ST-T wave changes suggestive of left atrial overload; normal ECG's before and after 06/24.
			06/25	29	15	51.7	
			06/26	26	15	57.7	
0097	70	F	05/24	66	4.7	7.1	Chronic obstructive pulmonary disease with pulmonary emboli; mild congestive heart failure; ASHD with probable old MI; severe left chest pain on admission. ECG did not document a current MI, but indicated atrial fibrillation.
			05/25	65	4.3	6.6	
			05/26	61	3.9	6.4	
			05/27	65	4.7	7.2	
			06/02	31	2.0	6.4	
0530	50	F	05/22	52	3.4	6.5	ASHD; hypertension; cerebral insufficiency. Pacemaker inserted at age 48. ECG's show sinus bradycardia with left ventricular hypertrophy.
			05/25	52	3.9	7.5	
			06/13	68	5.3	7.8	
			06/14	101	4.4	4.4	
0297	53	M	06/16	57	6.5	11.4	ASHD. Internal mammary implant surgery 5 yr. ago. Current admission for intestinal tract disorder. Repeated ECG's and exercise tolerance showed no ischemic changes or angina.
			06/18	38	5.4	14.2	
			06/19	38	5.6	14.7	
0178	64	F	05/21	28	0.9	3.2	Chronic obstructive pulmonary disease; pulmonary emboli; acute bronchitis; ASHD; congestive heart failure. Pt. had dyspnea one week prior to admission.
			05/27	22	2.3	10.4	
			05/28	21	4.1	19.5	
			06/03	28	3.4	12.1	
0418	65	M	06/25	80	5.8	7.2	Gastric ulcer; diabetes; hiatus hernia. Pt. admitted with right pleural effusion with some chest pain.
			06/28	86	5.9	6.9	
0105	53	F	05/17	115	17	14.8	Syncope of questionable etiology; labile hypertension; intermittent ventricular arrhythmia. Repeated ECG's not suggestive of myocardial damage.
			05/18	72	16	22.2	
			05/19	71	15	21.1	
			05/20	62	15	24.2	
			05/21	56	14	25.0	
			05/23	52	13	25.0	
			05/26	55	13	23.6	
0373	59	M	05/23	38	3.7	9.7	Acute URI; ASHD with coronary artery occlusion; osteogenesis imperfecta. Pt. admitted with dyspnea accompanied by mild precordial chest pain and frequent premature ventricular beats.
			05/24	22	2.7	12.3	
			05/25	20	3.1	15.5	
			05/26	17	2.4	14.1	
			05/28	18	3.2	17.8	
			05/29	12	1.9	15.8	
			05/30	20	2.7	13.5	
			07/07	28	3.0	10.7	Pt. readmitted with dyspnea and mild right side chest discomfort. ECG on 07/07 shows sinus tachycardia and on 07/10 shows no changes suggestive of acute MI.
			07/08	26	3.9	15.0	
			07/09	39	9.2	23.6	
			07/10	23	4.3	18.7	
			07/28	23	7.4	32.2	
			07/29	18	6.3	35.0	
0470	63	M	05/12	29	7.9	27.2	Coronary artery disease; old inferior wall MI; chest pains over 1 year prior to this admission. Total occlusion of right coronary artery. Coronary bypass surgery on 06/03.
			05/14	29	7.2	24.8	
			05/16	27	9.7	36.0	
			05/17	31	9.7	31.3	
			05/22	107	8.0	7.5	
			06/03	291	31	10.6	
			06/04	294	8.3	2.8	
			06/05	327	4.9	1.5	
			06/06	247	4.5	1.8	
			06/12	16	3.5	21.9	
			06/13	23	3.9	17.0	
			06/14	21	4.6	21.9	
			06/16	12	4.5	37.5	
0264	48	F	06/08	97	15	15.5	Chest pain of unknown etiology; hypergammaglobulinemia. Pt. admitted with chest pain on 06/08; pain gone next day. Treadmill ECG on 6/20 was painless and showed no evidence of ischemic changes.
			06/09	64	12	18.8	
			06/10	50	12	24.0	
			06/11	46	10	21.7	
			06/12	37	11	29.7	
			06/13	39	10	25.6	

(Continued)

Table 1. *(Continued)*

Patient no.	Age, yr	Sex	Date (1975)	Total CK, U/liter	MB, U/liter	% MB	Clinical diagnosis and comments
0881	46	F	05/10	194	73	37.6	Chest pain; minimal ASHD, type IV hyperlipoproteinemia. Cardiac catheterization on 05/19 showed subocclusion of right coronary artery—believed insufficient to explain chest pain.
			05/11	187	104	55.6	
			05/12	146	91	62.3	
			05/13	154	115	74.7	
			05/14	124	96	77.4	
			05/16	119	82	68.9	
			05/19	123	98	79.7	
			05/20	239	92	38.5	
0288	51	F	04/09	66	39	59.1	ASHD with coronary heart disease; old MI. No evidence of current MI. Cardiac catheterization showed total occlusion of right coronary artery with 75% maximal subocclusion of left anterior descending artery.
			04/10	60	42	70.0	
			04/11	60	39	65.0	
			04/13	55	40	72.7	
			04/14	52	36	69.2	
			05/21	233	28	12.0	New admission. Coronary by-pass surgery on 05/21.
			05/22	303	18	5.9	
			05/23	211	15	7.1	
			05/25	95	9	9.5	
			05/26	77	10	13.0	
			05/27	49	10	20.4	
0421	63	F	06/17	104	34	32.7	Metastatic carcinoma of lung and pleura, confirmed by biopsy. ECG of 06/17 suggestive of recent anteriolateral and high lateral wall injury.
			06/18	80	26	32.5	
0455	44	M	04/27	38	6.1	16.0	Mild type IV hyperlipoproteinemia; chronic chest pain. Cardiac catheterization on 04/30 revealed normal coronary arteries. Resting and treadmill ECG's were normal.
			04/30	42	8.4	20.0	
			05/01	35	7.2	20.6	

Abbreviations: ASHD, arteriosclerotic heart disease: ECG, electrocardiogram; MI, myocardial infarction; Pt., patient; URI, upper respiratory infection.

Figure 2 illustrates electrophoretograms of eluates from DEAE-Sephadex columns. As noted previously, the top three patterns represent the highest activity fractions of the Isoenzyme Marker, eluted in descending order, with low-, medium-, and high-salt buffers. The next three patterns show low-, medium-, and high-salt eluates of serum from patient 0881. Both the low- and medium-salt eluates show single bands located between MM and MB as observed with the unchromatographed serum.

Sera from a patient with a known myocardial infarction, a high total CK, and an elevated MB and from a patient exhibiting an unexplained MB increase with normal total CK gave identical peak activity eluates from Sephadex G-100. The approximate molecular weights were calculated to be 81 000, indicating that the unusual MB fraction is not a macromolecular complex and that it apparently does not differ in molecular weight from the usual MM and MB isoenzymes.

In an attempt to explain the apparent lack of MM in patient 0881 (Figure 2), we mixed two parts of a 100-fold dilution of serum from the previously mentioned patient with a 45 700 U/liter total CK with one part of serum from patient 0881; the mixture was incubated at 37 °C for 30 min, and then electrophoresed by the Dade method. Helena Heart-Muscle Control (Helena Laboratories) and sera from patient 0264 (Table 1) and patient 0560, with a known myocardial infarction and a high total CK, were run simultaneously (Figure 3). Two distinct bands can be seen for the mixture of sera, a band corresponding to the MM of the control, and a band slightly anodal to it. Sample 0264 likewise possesses this unusual band slightly anodal to the MM. Patient 0560 shows a typical MM band. The control has a rather large band cathodal to the MM band, which the manufacturer identifies as myokinase (EC 2.7.4.3). The appearance of a distinct MM band after serum 0881 was incubated with a serum containing a known MM tends to rule out the possibility of a factor in serum 0881 that might bind the usual MM and change its migration.

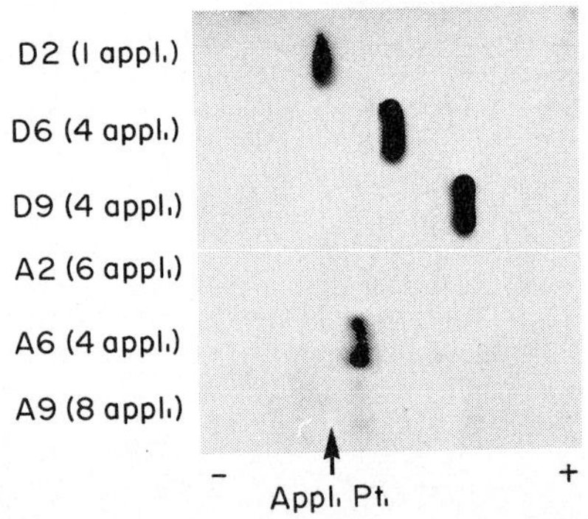

Fig. 2. Electrophoretograms of eluates from DEAE-Sephadex chromatography of Dade "CPK isoenzyme Marker" (*D*) and of serum from patient 0881 (*A*) (*Appl. Pt:* application point)

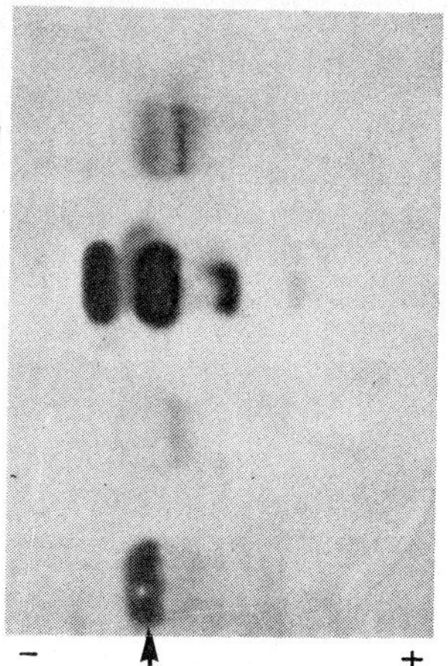

Fig. 3. Electrophoretograms of (*from top*) CK isoenzymes in serum from patient 0881 after incubation with high MM sera; Helena "Heart-Muscle Control," and sera from two selected patients

Electrophoresis of serum No. 0881 and isoenzyme detection with the Helena system resulted in the appearance of a single band slightly cathodal to marker MM. In contrast, with the Dade system the band is anodal to and more discrete from MM.

The possibility that the unusual isoenzyme may be a genetic variant, at least in some of the patients described in Table 1, cannot be ruled out. We have not yet studied family members.

From these experiments, it would appear that the serum of a significant number of patients, most of whom have myocardial disease but not necessarily a recent myocardial infarction, contains a CK isoenzyme of about 80 000 molecular weight that differs from MM, MB, or BB in effective charge or conformation or both. On ion-exchange chromatography this CK is eluted by both low- and medium-salt buffers, but principally by the latter. It could be easily mistaken for MB in the ion-exchange technique. In laboratories that use that technique, a falsely positive MB increase should be considered a possibility in subjects showing persistent apparent above-normal values for MB, with normal or minimally increased values for total CK. We recommend that a suitable electrophoretic method that clearly demonstrates this unusual isoenzyme be used in such cases to confirm or rule out actual increases in MB.

We thank Dr. Fenton Mitchell, Division of Cardiology, The Western Pennsylvania Hospital, for his cooperation and helpful discussions in relation to this study.

References

1. Dawson, D. M., and Fine, I. H., Creatine kinase in human tissues. *Arch. Neurol* (Chicago) **16,** 175 (1967).

2. Somer, H., and Konttinen, A., A method allowing the quantitation of serum creatine kinase isoenzymes. *Clin. Chim. Acta* **36,** 531 (1972).

3. Dawson, D. M., Eppenberger, H. M., and Kaplan, N. O., Creatine kinase: Evidence for a dimeric structure. *Biochem. Biophys. Res. Commun.* **21,** 346 (1965).

4. Somer, H., "Nothing dehydrogenase" reaction as an artefact in serum isoenzyme analyses. *Clin. Chim. Acta* **60,** 223 (1975).

5. Smith, A. R., Separation of tissue and serum creatine kinase isoenzymes on polyacrylamide gel slabs. *Clin. Chim. Acta* **36,** 351 (1972).

6. Madsen, A., Creatine phosphokinase isoenzymes in human tissue with special reference to brain extract. *Clin. Chim. Acta* **36,** 17 (1972).

7. Lim, F., Significance and applications of CPK isoenzyme subbands in the clinical laboratory. *Clin. Chem.* **21,** 975, Abstract No. 181 (1975).

8. Sobel, B. E., Shell, W. E., and Klein, M. S., An isoenzyme of creatine phosphokinase associated with rabbit heart mitochondria. *J. Mol. Cell. Cardiol.* **4,** 367 (1972).

9. Rock, R. C., Dreskin, R., Kickler, T., Wimsatt, T., Creatine kinase isoenzymes in serum of patients with Reye's syndrome. *Clin. Chim. Acta* **62,** 159 (1975).

10. Brownlow, K., and Elevitch, F. R., Serum creatine phosphokinase isoenzyme (CPK_2) in myositis. *J. Am. Med. Assoc.* **230,** 1141 (1974).

11. Roe, C. R., Limbird, L. E., Wagner, G. S., and Nerenberg, S. T., Combined isoenzyme analysis in the diagnosis of myocardial injury: Application of electrophoretic methods for the detection and quantitation of the creatine phosphokinase MB isoenzyme. *J. Lab. Clin. Med.* **80,** 577 (1972).

12. Smith, A. F., Radford, D., and Wong, C. P., Creatine kinase isoenzyme studies in myocardial infarction. *Clin. Chem.* **21,** 975, Abstract No. 178 (1975).

13. Anido, V., Conn, R. B., Mengoli, H. F., and Anido, G., Diagnostic efficacy of myocardial creatine phosphokinase using polyacrylamide disk gel electrophoresis. *Am. J. Clin. Pathol.* **61,** 599 (1974).

14. Wagner, G. S., Roe, C. R., Limbird, L. E., et al., The importance of identification of the myocardial-specific isoenzyme of creatine phosphokinase (MB form) in the diagnosis of acute myocardial infarction. *Circulation* **47,** 263 (1973).

15. Mercer, D. W., and Varat, M. A., Detection of cardiac-specific creatine kinase isoenzyme in sera with normal or slightly increased total creatine kinase activity. *Clin. Chem.* **21,** 1088 (1975).

16. Clejan, S., Rabinowitz, B., Doman, J., and Neufeld, H. N., Creatine phosphokinase isoenzymes in myocardial infarction with atypical enzyme profile. *Clin. Chem.* **21,** 974, Abstract No. 176 (1975).

17. Mercer, D. W., Separation of tissue and serum creatine kinase isoenzymes by ion-exchange column chromatography. *Clin. Chem.* **20,** 36 (1974).

18. Rosalki, S. B., An improved procedure for serum creatine phosphokinase determinations. *J. Lab. Clin. Med.* **69,** 696 (1967).

19. Nealon, D. A., and Henderson, A. R., Separation of creatine kinase isoenzymes in serum by ion-exchange column chromatography (Mercer's method, modified to increase sensitivity). *Clin. Chem.* **21,** 392 (1975).

20. Varat, M. A., and Mercer, D. W., Cardiac specific creatine phosphokinase isoenzyme in the diagnosis of acute myocardial infarction. *Circulation* **51,** 855 (1975).

21. Welsh, M., A simple qualitative method for the visualization of the serum creatine phosphokinase isoenzyme. *Clin. Chem.* **20,** 888 (1974).

CLIN. CHEM. 22/1, 92–97 (1976)

Improved Separation of Creatine Kinase Cardiac Isoenzyme in Serum by Batch Fractionation

Leo G. Morin

I describe a simple, single-tube batch fractionation procedure for separating MM and MB isoenzymes of creatine kinase on a macroporous strong anion exchanger (AG MP-1, Bio-Rad Laboratories). The isoenzymes can be separated in less than 3 min, with a resulting dilution of the serum with no more than an equal volume of buffer. Without sample concentration or spectrofluorometric measurement, the procedure detects 4 U of MB isoenzyme per liter. Sensitivity is limited by the sensitivity and precision of the method of measurement. The CV for the fractionation can be held to less than 4.0% at 65 U of MB per liter. Current fractionation methods are compared to the proposed procedure. With use of a discrete analyzer (Du Pont *aca*) the mean MB activity in a population free of heart disease was 3.2 ± 3.0 U/liter (range, 0 to 8 U/liter). The kinetics and stability of isolated isoenzymes are reported, indicating the advisability of storing or pre-incubating samples with mercaptoethanol.

Additional Keyphrases: *isoenzyme separation on an anion exchanger • heart disease • isoenzyme stability • normal (reference) values • enzyme kinetics*

It has become increasingly apparent that the magnitude of MB[1] isoenzyme activity of CK present in serum is a valid index to the severity of myocardial damage (*1–5*). Consequently, there has been an increasingly urgent need for a simple, rapid, and reliable quantitative procedure that can be used by technicians on a routine basis. Electrophoretic methods (*1–3*) are time consuming and relatively insensitive. Column methods (*5–8*) are intricate, more time consuming, and insensitive unless the sample or eluate has been concentrated, or lyophilized reagent is reconstituted with eluate, or spectrofluorometry is used. The kinetic procedure of Witteveen et al. (*9*) is a complex research method, not suited to routine use. The method of Henry et al. (*10*) is the simplest and most suited to routine use; unfortunately, it involves a 10-fold dilution of the sample, necessitating subsequent reconcentration or use of spectrofluorometry.

I approached the problem from two viewpoints: first, fractionation on the basis of differences in kinetic properties or stability, the results of which will be described briefly, and secondly, fractionation by batch adsorption, analogous to a method developed for hemoglobin A_2 (*11*) and the method of Henry et al. (*10*).

Materials and Methods

Enzyme Activity Measurement

CK activity was measured by four spectrophotometric methods, all based on the Rosalki (*12*) procedure: (*a*) Du Pont's (Wilmington, Del. 19898) procedure for the *aca*, (*b*) Abbott's (South Pasadena, Calif. 91030) procedure for the ABA-100 with Abbott's A-Gent reagent, (*c*) Worthington's (Freehold, N. J. 07728) CPK n-1 two-vial procedure used kinetically with the Beckman Acta III, and (*d*) an in-laboratory-prepared version of Worthington's formulation, except that the components were varied for kinetic studies. All measurements were at 37 °C. The *aca* method gives results about 12–15% higher than those obtained by the other methods.

Laboratory Service, Veterans Administration Hospital; and Department of Pathology and Laboratory Medicine, Emory University School of Medicine, Decatur, Ga. 30033.

[1] Nonstandard abbreviations used: CK, creatine kinase (EC 2.7.3.2; ATP:creatine *N*-phosphotransferase); MM, skeletal muscle CK isoenzyme; MB, cardiac CK isoenzyme (muscle-brain hybrid dimer); BB, brain CK isoenzyme; CP, creatine phosphate; and DEAE, diethylaminoethyl.

Received Oct. 3, 1975; accepted Nov. 3, 1975.

Isoenzyme Purification

Purification and fractionation of isoenzymes from fresh human autopsy tissue (quadriceps femoris, myocardium, cerebrum) was according to Keutel et al. (*13*), except that crude homogenates were prepared in 20 mmol/liter cysteine that had been adjusted to pH 6.9 with $NaHCO_3$ (no additional buffer was used), de-aerated, and stored under nitrogen. Ammonium sulfate precipitation was avoided. Chromatography was fundamentally the same, except for the substitution of DEAE Bio-Gel A (Bio-Rad Laboratories, Richmond, Calif. 94804) for DEAE-cellulose and the omission of mercaptoethanol. Concentration and removal of buffer salts was effected with a Bio-Fiber 80 Beaker (Bio-Rad). Attempts at enzyme crystallization were discontinued because of gross irreversible loss of activity in the presence of sulfates. The purified fractions, with an activity of about 4.0×10^5 U/liter were stored at −70 °C. Percentages of starting activity were about 60% for MM, 52% for BB, and 36% for MB. Small quantities of MB from the frozen concentrate were repurified (to remove MM and BB formed by hybridization in storage) by the discontinuous column method of Nealon and Henderson (*5*), except that DEAE Bio-Gel was used; re-concentration was done with a Minicon B-15 concentrator (Amicon Corp., Lexington, Mass. 02173).

Column Fractionation

Comparisons were made with the column methods of Nealon and Henderson (*5*) and Mercer and Varat (*14*). With the Nealon and Henderson method, I concentrated the eluate rather than the sample. The Mercer and Varat method was used with Worthington reagent and the Beckman Acta III analyzer. The Worthington "Isoenzymes Columns" kit was also compared.

Electrophoresis

Identification of fractions was by electrophoresis on *aci* agarose special-purpose electrophoresis film (Corning *aci*, Palo Alto, Calif. 94306) in cold (about 4 °C) tris(hydroxymethyl)aminomethane hydrochloride buffer (50 mmol/liter, pH 8.6). Electrophoresis was for 10 min at 200 V. The films were developed for 20 min at 37 °C with Worthington reagent, dried, and visually inspected under ultraviolet light (366 nm). For quantitation, appropriate areas of agarose were peeled wet from the film, eluted into 2.5 ml of Worthington reagent, and measured kinetically.

Proposed Method: Batch Fractionation on AG MP-1

Primary buffer. Tris(hydroxymethyl)aminomethane, free base, 90 mmol/liter; HCl, 30 mmol/liter (pH 8.2 ± 0.1 at 25 °C).

Secondary buffer. Tris(hydroxymethyl)aminomethane free base, 600 mmol/liter; HCl 550 mmol/liter (pH 6.9 ± 0.1 at 25 °C).

Preparation of resin. Convert Bio-Rad Laboratories' macroporous strongly basic anion-exchange resin AG MP-1, chloride form, 200–400 mesh, to the free base form in a Büchner funnel by washing with 20 volumes of NaOH (1 mol/liter) and rinsing with at least four volumes of de-ionized water until the effluent water tests slightly acidic with pH paper. Remove the filter cake and suspend it in four volumes of 10-fold concentration of primary buffer and allow to equilibrate for 30 min. Then pour the slurry into a Büchner funnel and wash with four to eight volumes of primary buffer until the pH of the effluent (when passing slowly through the cake) is the same as that of the buffer. Continue draining the cake with reduced pressure until only residual moisture remains and the cake is hard and cracks. Remove the resin to a beaker and to 440 g of resin (recoverable from 1 Bio-Rad package of the resin) add 250–270 ml of primary buffer and mix to fully suspend the resin into a thick latex-like consistency. Pipet 0.5 ml of the well-mixed suspension into each of three 13 × 100 mm tubes; to each of these add 400 μl of an aqueous methylene blue solution (exact concentration is not critical, but should be adjusted to an adsorbance of about 0.8 *A* at 500 nm), mix with the suspension, and obtain the filtrate in Filter Samplers (Unichem, Fairburn, Ga. 30213). Pool the filtrates, centrifuge to remove fines if present, measure the absorbance at 500 nm, and compare to that of the original methylene blue solution. The absorbance of the filtrate should be within ±0.005 *A* of half the absorbance of the original methylene blue solution. If not, the ratio of resin to buffer should be adjusted so that 400 μl of sample is diluted with an equal volume of buffer (i.e., with 500 μl of suspension). Methylene blue is an anionic dye and is not retained on the resin; consequently, it is useful for determining the resin volume that is not available for dilution. Once the proper resin:buffer ratio has been achieved, store the suspension refrigerated until it is used, at which time it should be thoroughly and evenly mixed. It is convenient to prepare enough tubes for several weeks in advance and store them refrigerated, ready for use. Although conventional pipets are satisfactory for dispensing 0.5 ml of suspension into 13 × 100 mm disposable glass tubes, the SMI Micro/Pettor F (Scientific Manufacturing Industries, Emeryville, Calif. 94608) is more convenient and accurate. Place Unichem filters into each tube, stopper the sampler or cover with suitable wrapping film to prevent evaporation, and store refrigerated until ready to use.

Alternatively, and preferably, dilute the adjusted suspension 10-fold with primary buffer, mix, and continue mixing (on a magnetic stirrer), dispense 5 ml to each tube, insert the filter sampler, depress completely, discard buffer, invert on absorbent surface, and apply firm pressure to remove all but residual buffer. Store these refrigerated. The wet weight of the resin in each tube should be 375–400 mg. When using, remove sampler, add 200 μl of primary buffer before adding serum. Still another alternative is to remove the samplers and dry the resin in the tubes in an oven at 70 °C for 2–4 h; replace the dry samplers and store these at ambient temperature. Before using, remove the samplers and add 400 μl of primary buffer to each tube. The dry weight of the resin in each tube should be 75 ± 5 mg.

Procedure. Remove the filter sampler from the resin tube prepared above. Dispense 400 μl of serum (preferably pre-incubated with 10 mmol/liter mercaptoethanol) into the tube, replace the filter sampler and depress it to within 1 cm of the surface, mix well for 1–2 min, depress the sampler into suspension, and pour off the first filtrate, which contains the MM fraction diluted to twice its original volume. Fill the sampler with primary buffer, raise the sampler until the buffer enters the tube below the sampler, allow air bubble to enter, mix well, depress sampler, and discard the wash filtrate. Repeat two or three times (with low CK concentrations, two washes are adequate; with concentrations exceeding 2000 U/liter, three or four washes are advisable). After the final wash, turn the tube downward on an absorbent surface and apply firm pressure, with the tube pushing against the sampler to remove excess buffer. These washes are required to remove, by dilution, MM in the residual fluid. Dispense 600 μl of secondary buffer (300 μl of primary buffer remains trapped under the sampler with the resin) into the filter sampler, raise the sampler, mix the secondary buffer with the resin, depress the sampler again to pick up buffer left behind and avoid dilution, raise the sampler again, and mix thoroughly. Repeat the raising and lowering of sampler with mixing once again. The movement of the sampler should be slow to avoid excessive foaming. Finally, depress the sampler and collect the second filtrate, which contains the MB fraction. The BB fraction is too strongly bound to the resin to be removed by noninhibiting or nondenaturing treatment. The CK activity of the fractions may be determined by any available method and the results multiplied by two. User preference determines which measurements to make. Most probably would prefer to measure total CK and the MB fraction only. Alternatively, the MM and MB fractions may be measured and the total arrived at by addition. In some cases, it may be desirable to measure all three directly. It is not advisable to obtain MB by difference from total CK and MM, because even slight volume or instrument variations could easily lead to misleading results. If proper precautions are taken to control volume and instrument variations, BB may be obtained by difference from total CK and (MM + MB).

Results

Kinetics and Stability of Purified Isoenzymes

The results of substrate affinity for creatine phosphate and adenosine diphosphate (obtained from Lineweaver–Burk plots) and optimum pH are recorded in Table 1. The results indicate that BB is the most active dimer of CK, followed by MB and MM, respectively. The pH optima differ by less than 0.2. The effects of various sulfhydryl activators was studied, and the results recorded in Table 2 indicate that dithioerythritol, dithiothreitol, and mercaptoethanol markedly enhance the activity of BB and MB, as contrasted to glutathione. Acid- and base-lability studies confirmed the results of Keutel et al. (*13*). Heat stability studies demonstrated that MM is relatively stable up to 47 °C, losing about 12% of activity in 30 min. MB and BB, however, become very unstable at 44 °C, losing virtually all activity in 10 min. Although not directly comparable, this appears to be consistent with Mercer (*6*). Unfortunately, MB hybridizes rapidly at this temperature to form the more stable MM and also shows a short-lived increase in activity because of the formation of BB. This was indicated by electrophoresis, after the samples were cooled rapidly in ice at timed intervals. When added to heat-inactivated sera (60 °C for 30 min and cleared by micronfilter filtration), both MB and BB lose activity rapidly, the exact extent varying markedly from serum to serum. The mean loss of activity in 30 sera for MB was 24% in 2 h at ambient temperature (range 6% to 53%), with 84% to 100% loss in 24 h refrigerated. The prompt addition of 10 mmol of dithiothreitol or mercaptoethanol per liter allowed 96% recovery of activity after 24 h refrigeration. A 30-min pre-incubation at ambient temperature with mercaptoethanol allowed about 81% to 89% recovery from sera refrigerated 24 h without preservatives. Measurement without pre-incubation, but with dithiothreitol in the assay formulation, allowed only 38% to 63% recovery. A similar pattern was observed with MM, but usually no more than 15% to 18% of the activity was lost in 24

Table 1. Michaelis Constants and pH Optima for Creatine Kinase Isoenzymes

Isoenzyme, 50 U/liter	K_m (CP)[a]	K_m (ADP)[b]	pH[c]
MM	4.7×10^{-3}	3.0×10^{-5}	6.9
MB	3.5×10^{-3}	2.1×10^{-5}	7.0
BB	2.2×10^{-3}	1.4×10^{-5}	7.1

[a] ADP held at 0.2 mmol/liter.
[b] CP held at 10 mmol/liter.
[c] 2-(*N*-morpholino)ethane sulfonic acid (Na salt) buffer, 100 mmol/liter.

Table 2. Comparison of Sulfhydryl Activation on Isoenzymes[a]

Isoenzymes	Cysteine	DTE	DTT	ME
MM	1.00	1.06	1.05	1.06
MB	1.04	1.40	1.43	1.41
BB	1.03	1.91	1.89	1.92

[a] Expressed as ratio of glutathione activation; all at 10 mmol/liter.
Abbreviation: DTE, dithioerythritol; DTT, dithiothreitol, and ME, mercaptoethanol.

Table 3. Comparison of Mercaptoethanol-Protected and Unprotected Sera

No. sera and description	Mean difference of total CK in protected sera
25 MM (40–322 U/liter)	+0.8%
2 MM (93, 102 U/liter)	+12.2%
5 MM + MB (204–688 U/liter)	+8.4%
8 MM + MB (422–2640 U/liter)	+16.2%
3 MM + MB (96, 112, 132 U/liter)	+89.4%

h, refrigerated and without preservative. Forty patients' sera were divided into unprotected and mercaptoethanol-protected aliquots and measured after 3 h with the Du Pont *aca*. The results (Table 3) are consistent with the results with pure fractions added to sera. Similar results were obtained with other CK reagents, including Worthington's "no lag" reagent.

Isoenzyme Fractionation by Proposed Method

The MM isoenzyme is very loosely bound to AG MP-1 at higher pH (8.6–9.0) and low Cl^- concentration (to 30 mmol/liter). As pH decreases or ionic strength increases, MM is very rapidly released from the resin. MB is retained more strongly, and a lower pH (6.5–7.8) and greater Cl^- concentration (50–800 mmol/liter) is required to elute it. I selected an initial pH (8.2) low enough that all MM would remain unbound with a buffer of relatively low ionic strength, but adequate to give good buffering capacity when diluted with sera. I selected the secondary buffer to be strong enough to overcome the primary buffer, yet at a pH (6.9) low enough to allow complete MB elution without an excessive Cl^- concentration (effective Cl^-, 420 mmol/liter). BB could not be eluted from the resin, except by harsh treatment (citrate buffer, 1 mol/liter, pH 6.0; Cl^-, 3 mol/liter) and with poor recovery, 8% to 20%.

The recovery of active MM added to heat-inactivated sera was 98%, ranging from 96% to 101% for activities from 50 to 4000 U/liter. Likewise, the recovery of added MB was 96%, ranging from 94% to 100% for activities from 5 to 500 U/liter; the presence of MM up to 4000 U/liter did not influence the results. A 1:1 mixture of MM and MB with a total CK of 2.4×10^5 U/liter in serum, yielded 92% recovery, with no cross contamination of fractions detectable by electrophoresis. When BB was obtained by difference [total CK − (MM + MB)], recovery was 104%, ranging from 98% to 110% for activities from 10 to 1000 U/liter of BB and total CK ranging from 140 to 4000 U/liter. Correlation with Nealon and Henderson's (*5*) modification of Mercer's (*6*) chromatographic method was very good (Figure 1). Electrophoretic examination of these fractions also indicated no detectable cross contamination by either method. At lower MB activities the method also compared well (Figure 2) with Mercer and Varat's more recent method (*14*).

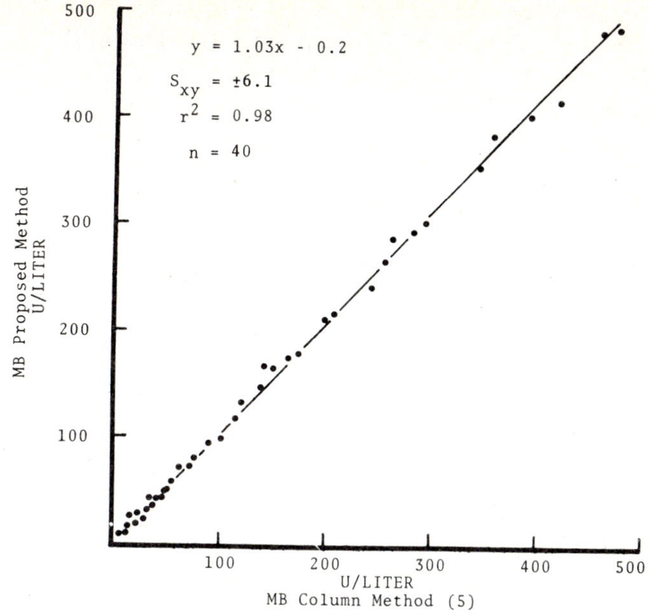

Fig. 1. Comparison of present method with column fractionation

Both methods done with Du Pont *aca;* column eluate measured after concentration with Minicon B-15 concentrator

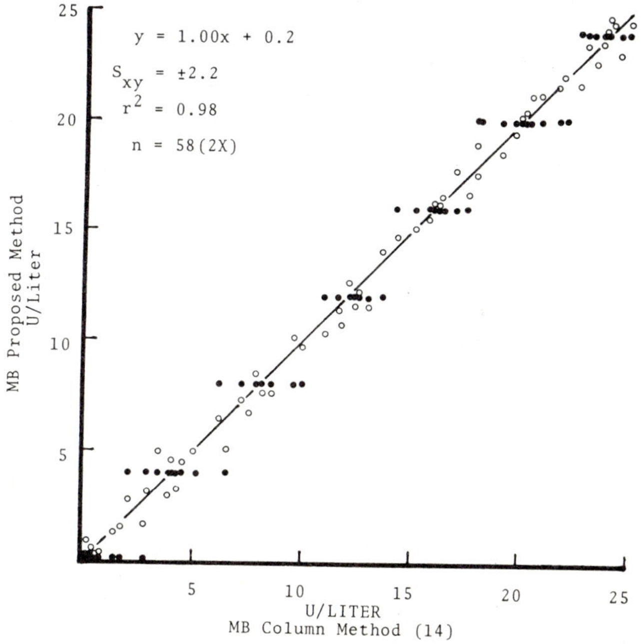

Fig. 2. Comparison of present method with column fractionation, at low activities

● Measured on Du Pont *aca* (counts by 2, and results multiplied by 2, because of dilution; therefore *aca* results are in increments of 4). O Measured manually on Beckman Acta III. Column eluate measured manually on Beckman Acta III with Worthington reagent reconstituted as described by Mercer and Varat (*14*)

Comparisons with a commercial chromatographic method (Worthington's "Isoenzymes Columns") was reasonably good, except that with the kit 4% to 12% of the MB isoenzyme was eluted in the BB fraction. In none of the patient sera examined was BB detected by the proposed method, the method of Nealon and Henderson (*5*), that of Mercer and Varat (*14*), or

Table 4. Precision of Complete Procedure with Measurements on Du Pont *aca*

Mean[a], U/liter			CV, %		
Total CK	MM	MB	CK	MM	MB
92	86	9	3.3	4.7	33
244	204	44	1.6	2.0	6.8
680	628	48	0.6	0.8	6.3
1691	1548	101	<0.1	<0.1	3.9
1948	1445	506	<0.1	<0.1	0.8

[a] Mean of triplicates on 10 different days.

electrophoresis. Only 12 sera (the number of columns available in one kit) were examined by the Worthington kit; consequently, the statistics are inadequate for a valid evaluation.

Precision of the complete method with the Du Pont *aca* was established by triplicate measurements each of total CK, MM, and MB fractions for five sera on 10 different days (Table 4). Precision of the fractionation was determined by 20 repeat determinations, each done at one time, of two sera by manual kinetic measurement, one with a total CK activity of 361 U/liter and the other 2432 U/liter. The mean MM and MB for the first serum were 296 U/liter and 65 U/liter, respectively; standard deviations were ±3.4 U/liter and 2.6 U/liter, respectively (CV = 1.1% and 4.0%). The higher activity serum yielded a CV of 0.16% and 0.42% for MM and MB, respectively, with an MB of 511 U/liter. Thirty-five sera of laboratory personnel and of patients with diagnoses unrelated to heart disease gave a mean MB of 3.2 U/liter (SD = 3.0 U/liter; range, 0–8 U/liter), as measured with the Du Pont *aca*.

Discussion

Although significant differences in kinetics and stability to acid–base and heat were observed between the isoenzymes, none of these characteristics proved amenable to a method for quantitating isoenzymes. Several screening approaches for MB suggested themselves, but all attempts to quantitate proved too complex or impractical. The enhancement of activity by dithioerythritol, dithiothreitol, and mercaptoethanol merits further study, both to determine whether the increased activity merely represents activation of inactive enzyme, a shift in active–inactive enzyme equilibrium, or an enhancement of the activity of already active enzyme, and to further assess its potential as a tool in quantitating isoenzymes.

The results for CK stability in serum, both with purified fractions and patient sera, clearly indicate that sera for CK measurements should have a sulfhydryl protector added as soon as possible, or at the very least that sera be pre-incubated with a sulfhydryl compound; of those examined, dithioerythritol, dithiothreitol, or mercaptoethanol are preferable. The odor of mercaptoethanol is more offensive than the others, but, unlike them, it does not result in clot-like gelling of sera, so that it is preferable for use in storage and pre-incubation. A sulfhydryl agent in the assay medium is clearly inadequate for optimum reactivation of CK, particularly the MB fraction.

The proposed method involves a moderately complex preparation of the resin, but once this is complete, the actual procedure itself is very simple and rapid. Preparation of the resin tubes is markedly less tedious than preparation of columns, and resin tubes are more easily stored in satisfactory condition than columns. This batch method allows a single fractionation to be performed easily in less than 3 min and 36 samples simultaneously, in parallel, in less than 30 min. This compares favorably with column methods (*14*). The only other method that shares its advantage of technical simplicity and rapidity is that of Henry et al. (*10*). That method, however, shares with the chromatographic methods the shortcoming of excessive serum dilution. By contrast, the proposed method involves only a twofold (1:1) dilution, making it possible to measure even normal activities of MB directly by routine spectrophotometric methods. The notorious effects of serum dilution on CK activity is well documented (*5, 15, 16*). The method of Henry et al. (*10*) also does not distinguish MB from BB, and so could give misleading results in those unusual cases where BB does appear in serum (*17*). Although the proposed method does not measure BB directly, it does distinguish it from MB and does allow for its calculation (by difference). Rigorous precautions should be taken to control all volume and instrument variables when obtaining BB by difference. Further, the method of Henry et al. calls for an expensive exchanger, Glycophase-G (Corning Glassworks, Medfield, Mass. 02052), which currently sells for $65.00 for 8 g or 25 ml. The AG MP-1 in the proposed method sells for $51.00 for 453 g (wet) or about 300 g (dry). The resin can be prepared for use in less than 4 h with little reagent expense. Bio-Rad's current service charge for resin conversion is an additional $75.00 for up to 4 kg of resin. The method of Henry et al. requires 300 mg (dry beads)/test, the proposed method only 75 mg (dry resin)/test.

The reason for this resin's superior performance in the presence of relatively high protein concentrations appears from preliminary studies to be the exclusion of most serum proteins from the macropores, making these available for creatine kinase (a relatively small protein) exchange with high efficiency.

The results obtained by this method with non-cardiac-disease subjects are very similar to those obtained by Nealon and Henderson (*5*); the mean results reported by Mercer and Varat (*14*) and Henry et al. (*10*) are about 2 U/liter less. In view of the different methods of fractionation, measurement, and temperature of measurement, such minor discrepancies are negligible. Studies of patients with heart disease will be the subject of a separate publication at a later date.

References

1. Konttinen, A., and Somer, H., Determination of serum creatine kinase isoenzymes in myocardial infarction. *Am. J. Cardiol.* **29,** 817 (1972).

2. Klein, M. S., Shell, W. E., and Sobel, B. E., Serum creatine phosphokinase (CPK) isoenzymes following intramuscular injections, surgery, and myocardial infarction: Experimental and clinical studies. *Cardiovasc. Res.* **7,** 412 (1973).

3. Shell, W. E., Kjekshus, J. K., and Sobel, B. E., Quantitative assessment of the extent of myocardial infarction in the conscious dog by means of analysis of serial changes in serum creatine phosphokinase activity. *J. Clin. Invest.* **50,** 2614 (1971).

4. Wagner, G. S., Roe, C. R., Limbird, L. E., et al., The importance of identification of the myocardial-specific isoenzyme of creatine phosphokinase (MB form) in the diagnosis of acute myocardial infarction. *Circulation* **47,** 263 (1973).

5. Nealon, D. A., and Henderson, A. R., Separation of creatine kinase isoenzymes in serum by ion-exchange column chromatography (Mercer's method, modified to increase sensitivity). *Clin. Chem.* **21,** 392 (1975).

6. Mercer, D. W., Separation of tissue and serum creatine kinase isoenzymes by ion-exchange column chromatography. *Clin. Chem.* **20,** 36 (1974).

7. Yasmineh, W. G., and Hanson, N. Q., Electrophoresis on cellulose acetate and chromatography on DEAE-Sephadex A-50 compared in the estimation of creatine kinase isoenzymes. *Clin. Chem.* **21,** 381 (1975).

8. Leunis, J. C., Séparation chromatographique des isoenzymes de la créatine-phospho-kinase du serum normal et après infarctus du myocarde. *Ann. Biol. Clin.* **31,** 369 (1973).

9. Witteveen, S. A. G. J., Sobel, B. E., and DeLuca, M., Kinetic properties of the isoenzymes of human creatine phosphokinase. *Proc. Nat. Acad. Sci. U.S.A.* **71,** 1384 (1974).

10. Henry, P. D., Roberts, R., and Burton, E. S., Rapid separation of plasma creatine kinase isoenzymes by batch adsorption on glass beads. *Clin. Chem.* **21,** 844 (1975).

11. Morin, L. G., Rapid estimation of hemoglobin A_2 without chromatography or electrophoresis. *Clin. Chem.* **21,** 1490 (1975).

12. Rosalki, S. B., An improved procedure for serum creatine phosphokinase determination. *J. Lab. Clin. Med.* **69,** 696 (1967).

13. Keutel, H. J., Okabe, K., Jacobs, H. K., et al., Studies on adenosine triphosphate transphosphorylases. XI. Isolation of the crystalline adenosine triphosphate-creatine transphosphorylases from the muscle and brain of man, calf, and rabbit; and a preparation of their enzymatically active hybrids. *Arch. Biochem. Biophys.* **150,** 648 (1972).

14. Mercer, D. W., and Varat, M. A., Detection of cardiac-specific creatine kinase isoenzyme in sera with normal or slightly increased total creatine kinase activity. *Clin. Chem.* **21,** 1088 (1975).

15. Graig, F. A., Smith, J. C., and Foldes, F. F., Effect of dilution on the activity of serum creatine phosphokinase. *Clin. Chim. Acta* **15,** 107 (1967).

16. Dobosz, I., The influence of the dilution effect on serum creatine phosphokinase activity in neuromuscular diseases. *Clin. Chim. Acta* **50,** 301 (1974).

17. Nealon, D. A., and Henderson, A. R., Measurement of brain-specific creatine kinase isoenzyme activity in serum. *Clin. Chem.* **21,** 1663 (1975).

scientific notes

CLIN. CHEM. 22/1, 98–101 (1976)

Enzymatic Determinations of Cholesterol in High-Density-Lipoprotein Fractions Prepared by a Precipitation Technique

Bernard W. Steele,[1] Donald F. Koehler,[1] Miguel M. Azar,[1] Thomas P. Blaszkowski,[2] Kanta Kuba,[3] and Mary E. Dempsey[3]

An enzymatic method for cholesterol in serum [*Clin. Chem.* **20,** 470 (1974)] was initially found to be unsatisfactory for measuring cholesterol in high-density-lipoprotein fractions prepared by precipitation with Mn^{2+}. A fine precipitate formed in the cuvette and cholesterol values were falsely increased. We describe a simple, convenient method for circumventing these problems. An ethylenediaminetetraacetate solution is used to reconstitute the enzymatic reagent. Cholesterol values by this procedure correlated with those obtained by the Lipid Research Clinic's procedure for the same lipoprotein fraction preparations (regression slope, .998; *Y*-intercept, 8.9 mg/liter; correlation coefficient, .984; standard error of the estimate, 16.8 mg/liter). Precision of the assay, including the precipitation step, was calculated. The $SD_{\text{within day}}$ was 9.7 mg/liter and SD_{overall} was 23.7 mg/liter. Results for total cholesterol with the modified reagent were linearly related to concentrations exceeding 4 g/liter, thereby permitting determination of high-density-lipoproteins and total cholesterol in a single run.

Determination of plasma lipoprotein fractions provides the clinician with the prognostic, genetic, and therapeutic information necessary for treatment of hyperlipidemic patients (*1, 2*). These fractions are usually measured by continuous-flow colorimetry of isopropanol and zeolite extracts of plasma lipoprotein fractions obtained by ultracentrifugation and precipitation techniques (*3, 4*).

Two recent developments have given promise of simpler and more rapid assay of individual lipoprotein fractions. The first is the determination of the LDL[4] cholesterol by use of the formula of Friedewald et al. (*5*).[5] In this approach, the plasma HDL fraction is prepared by precipitating out the LDL and VLDL fractions with $MnCl_2$ and heparin. The second development is the use of enzymatic reagents for cholesterol determinations (*6, 7*). This method greatly improves specificity and eliminates the need for isopropanol and zeolite extractions.

However, when we tried to combine the two advances, we discovered two problems. First, the manganous chloride formed a visible precipitate with the enzymatic reagent ("A-Gent") and secondly, the presence of manganous chloride in the reaction mixture accounted for a falsely increased cholesterol. We present here a simple and convenient method for circumventing these problems by use of a 4 mmol/liter solution of EDTA to reconstitute the cholesterol reagent.

Materials and Methods

Reagents

Standard. Crystalline cholesterol supplied by the Center for Disease Control, Atlanta, was dissolved in isopropanol (99.9% pure; Baker Chemical Co., Phillipsburg, N.J. 08865) and diluted to make working standards.

Enzymatic cholesterol reagent. The enzymatic cholesterol reagent was "A-Gent," obtained from Abbott Laboratories, South Pasadena, Calif. 91030.

Cholesterol reagent diluent. A 0.2 mol/liter EDTA stock solution (pH 6.7) was prepared by dissolving 4.27 g of disodium EDTA dihydrate (Fisher Scientific Co., Fairlawn, N.J. 07410) and 3.54 g of tetrasodium EDTA dihydrate

[1] Clinical Laboratory Service, Veterans Administration Hospital, Minneapolis, Minnesota, 55417; and Department of Laboratory Medicine and Pathology, University of Minnesota, Minneapolis, Minn. 55455.

[2] National Heart and Lung Institute, National Institutes of Health, Bethesda, Md. 20014.

[3] Department of Biochemistry, University of Minnesota, Minneapolis, Minn. 55455.

Received July 25, 1975; accepted Oct. 13, 1975.

[4] Nonstandard abbreviations used: EDTA, ethylenediaminetetraacetate; HDL, high-density-lipoprotein; LDL, low-density-lipoprotein; and VLDL, very-low-density-lipoprotein.

[5] LDL cholesterol = total cholesterol − (triglyceride/5) − HDL cholesterol.

Table 2. Apparent Cholesterol,[a] mg/liter, with Various Concentrations of EDTA Present

Specimen	EDTA concn, mmol/liter 0	2	4	6	Δ Cholesterol (0–4 mmol/liter EDTA)
HDL reagent-blank[b]	180	30	20	20	160
Plasma HDL fractions (16 subjects)	440	383	376	376	64 (SD = 16.2)
CDC HDL control (alpha Q-2)	600	520	510	510	90
Whole plasmas (12 subjects)	1392	1392	1387	1393	5 (SD = 5.2)
CDC control (target value = 2960 mg/liter)	2870	2890	2850	2850	20

[a] Uncorrected for dilution and HDL reagent-blank.
[b] Diluted 1/51 and assayed by the ABA-100. 183 units of heparin per milliliter and 46 mmol of $MnCl_2$ per liter are contained in the HDL reagent blank.

Table 1. Apparent Cholesterol, mg/liter, in HDL Fraction Reagents with Various Concentrations of EDTA Present

HDL reagent blank[a]	EDTA concn, mmol/liter 0	2	4	6
46 mmol $MnCl_2$ per liter	180	30	20	20
92 mmol $MnCl_2$ per liter	500	40	10	20
No $MnCl_2$	−10	10	0	10

[a] Diluted 1/51 and assayed as a sample with the ABA-100. 183 units of heparin per milliliter is contained in each HDL reagent-blank preparation.

(Matheson, Coleman and Bell, Norwood, Ohio 45212) in 100 ml of de-ionized water.

A 4 mmol/liter EDTA working solution was prepared by diluting the stock solution 50-fold with de-ionized water. The enzymatic cholesterol reagent, when reconstituted with this solution, had a pH of 6.65, which is within the optimum pH range of the reagent (*6*).

Heparin. A heparin solution was prepared by making an eight-fold dilution in saline of aqueous heparin (40 000 units/ml; Riker Laboratories Inc., Northridge, Calif. 91324).

Manganous chloride solution. A 1 mol/liter manganous chloride solution was prepared by dissolving 19.8 g of $MnCl_2 \cdot 4H_2O$, mol. wt. 197.91, (Baker Chemical Co., Phillipsburg, N.J. 08865) in 100 ml of de-ionized water.

Methods

Total plasma cholesterol determinations. These were performed with the Abbott Bichromatic Analyzer (ABA-100; Abbott Laboratories) by the method of Allain et al. (*6*) with the following modifications: First, to increase sensitivity, a 1/51 ratio of specimen to total reaction volume was used instead of the usual 1/101 ratio. Secondly, the cholesterol reagent was reconstituted with the 4 mmol/liter EDTA solution instead of water unless otherwise noted.

Plasma HDL fractions. These were prepared by the method of Burstein and Samaille (*4, 8*). The heparin and $MnCl_2$ were added simultaneously with a Model 25000 Automatic Pipette (Micromedic Systems Inc., Horsham, Pa. 19044).

Plasma HDL cholesterol determinations. The plasma HDL fractions were analyzed for cholesterol by the above modified enzymatic procedure. These cholesterol values obtained were uncorrected for heparin, manganous chloride, and dilution. A sample of saline, prepared with heparin and manganous chloride reagent, was run concurrently as the HDL reagent blank. To correct for dilution, the uncorrected plasma HDL cholesterol minus the HDL reagent blank was multiplied by 1.09.[6]

Results

The enzymatic serum cholesterol method (*6*), used to assay plasma HDL fractions prepared with manganous chloride and heparin (*4*), produced a precipitate in the cuvette and artifactually high values (equivalent to 30 to 90 mg of cholesterol per liter). Eliminating the turbidity of a reaction mixture by rapid filtration did not alter the result as determined on the ABA-100. The pH of the reaction mixture was not significantly altered by the presence of HDL preparation reagents. The addition of 0.01 ml of 46 mmol/liter $MnCl_2$ (the concentration present in plasma HDL fractions) to 0.5 ml of the cholesterol reagent caused a precipitate and a visible color reaction equivalent to 180 mg of cholesterol per liter. Addition of heparin had no effect on the apparent cholesterol value and caused no precipitation.

To eliminate the precipitate, we chelated the Mn^{2+} with EDTA. The added EDTA also decreased the value for apparent cholesterol in the HDL reagent blank to 10 ± 6 (1 SD) mg/liter (Table 1), an error that is constant from 6 mmol to 92 mmol of EDTA per liter. The HDL reagent blank and HDL fractions were run with and without EDTA. The observed differences between the results obtained with and without EDTA were greater for the HDL reagent blank than for the plasmas HDL fractions. The magnitude of the differences varied among clinical specimens (Table 2).

EDTA had no effect on the cholesterol assay of whole plasma (Table 2). Standard concentrations were linearly related to absorbance to 5 g/liter; the cholesterol in the plasma HDL fractions and in whole plasma was linearly related to dilution when assayed with EDTA present (Figure 1).

[6] HDL cholesterol = 1.09 (uncorrected HDL cholesterol − HDL reagent blank).

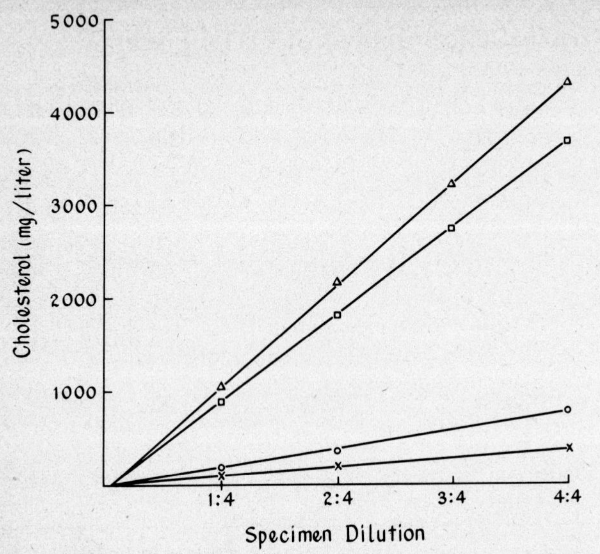

Fig. 1. Dilution and concentration relationship for cholesterol when reagent containing 4 mmol/liter EDTA is used

Plasmas were diluted with saline. Δ and □, plasma cholesterol; O and ×, HDL cholesterol

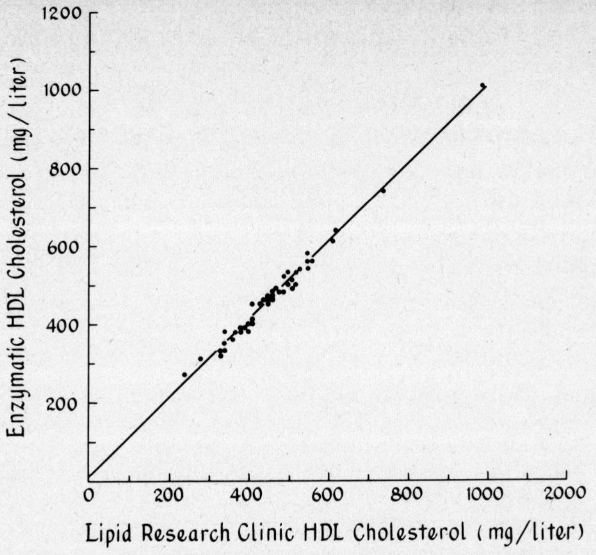

Fig. 2. Cholesterol in 53 HDL fractions, as assayed on the ABA-100 vs. the Minnesota Lipid Research Clinic's method

Slope, .998; *Y*-intercept, 8.9 mg/liter; correlation coefficient, .984; standard error of estimate, 16.8 mg/liter

Table 3. Precision Data[a] for Cholesterol

Specimen	Target value	Mean	Standard Deviation: Overall	Within-day	Between-days
			mg/liter		
CDC HDL[b] control (alpha Q-2)	541[c]	524	23.7 (22.7)[d]	9.7 (16.9)[d]	21.7 (15.1)[d]
HDL reagent blank	—	8.57	7.33	4.9	5.5
CDC normal control	1710	1650	20.5	11.9	16.7
CDC high control	2960	2920	25.3	13.7	21.3
CDC low control	590	567	9.0	6.1	6.6

[a] Based on quadruplicate analysis for 11 weekly runs.
[b] HDL determined after correction for HDL reagent blank and dilution. (CDC, Center for Disease Control)
[c] Value obtained from Minnesota Lipid Research Clinic laboratory (target value not determined by CDC).
[d] Values obtained from Minnesota Lipid Research Clinic laboratory and based on duplicate analyses from 11 weekly runs.

The Minnesota Lipid Research Clinic prepared HDL fractions (*4*) of plasma from 53 subjects. Analyses were begun within 3 h after preparation of the fractions, by the procedures of the Lipid Research Clinic and our (V.A.) procedures. Figure 2 shows the results. The slope was 0.998; the *Y*-intercept, 8.9 mg/liter; the correlation coefficient, 0.984; and the standard error of estimate, 16.8 mg/liter.

This new method for enzymatic HDL cholesterol was used in a clinical situation once weekly for 11 consecutive weeks. Precision data (Table 3) were obtained from the results of weekly quadruplicate determinations; data for both total cholesterol and HDL cholesterol are included. The HDL cholesterol data also includes the variability caused by the precipitation procedure.

Discussion

The source of the interference initially encountered in the enzymatic HDL cholesterol determination was the $MnCl_2$ in the reaction mixture. Presumably Mn^{2+} precipitated with the phosphate buffer of the reagent. The precipitate, however, did not account for the artifactually high values on the ABA-100. (The bichromatic system of the ABA-100 may have corrected for the absorbance caused by the turbidity.) The artifactually high cholesterol values were probably caused by an unknown reaction between $MnCl_2$ and the indicator system.

The accuracy of the enzymatic reagent without EDTA for the determination of total cholesterol in serum has previously been demonstrated (*6, 7*). We have adapted this method to the determination of both HDL cholesterol and total plasma cholesterol in samples having normal and above-normal values. The within-day variability and the overall variability for HDL cholesterols are comparable with such data from the Minnesota Lipid Research Clinic (Table 3). We assumed that a significant portion of the between-day variation for the HDL control from the Center for Disease Control was due to the precipitation procedure: on analysis of the same HDL fractions, there was only a 16.8 mg/liter standard error of estimate between the clinic's procedure and the modified enzymatic procedure.

For improved sensitivity, we decreased the dilution of the specimens. Total cholesterol could be determined in concentrations up to and in excess of 4 g/liter (Figure 1). The EDTA solution described here is for use with a 1:51 syringe plate, and may not be appropriate for use with a 1/101 specimen/reagent dilution ratio.

The procedures outlined offer a means of adapting a highly specific enzymatic cholesterol assay to the determination of individual lipoprotein fractions and phenotyping. When chylomicrons are not present and the plasma triglyceride concentration is less than 4 g/liter, individual lipoprotein fractions can be quantitated by calculation, thereby permitting phenotyping of the vast majority of subjects (*4, 5*).

We thank the Center for Disease Control, especially Dr. Gerald Cooper, for the use of their data. We wish also to thank Dr. Khalil Ahmed and Ms. Diane Hanson of the Minneapolis V.A. Hospital for their technical assistance. This research was supported by V.A. Grant MRIS 0719.

References

1. Fredrickson, D. S., Levy, R. I., and Lees, R. S., Fat transport in lipoproteins—an integrated approach to mechanisms and disorders. *New Engl. J. Med.* **276,** 32, 148, 215, 273 (1967).

2. Stone, N., and Levy, R., Hyperlipoproteinemia and coronary heart disease. *Prog. Cardiovasc. Dis.* **14,** 341 (1972).

3. Rush, R. L., Leon, L., and Turrell, J., Automated simultaneous cholesterol and triglyceride determination on the AutoAnalyzer II instrument. In *Advances in Automated Analysis, Technicon International Congress 1970,* **1,** *Clinical Analysis;* C. E. Barton et al., Eds. Thurman Associates, Miami, Fla. 33132, 1971, p 503.

4. *Manual of Laboratory Operations, Lipid Research Clinics Program, I: Lipid and Lipoprotein Analysis.* National Heart and Lung Institute, National Institutes of Health, Bethesda, Md., 1974; U.S. Government Printing Office, (NIH) 75628.

5. Friedewald, W. T., Levy, R. I., and Fredrickson, D. S., Estimation of the concentration of low-density lipoprotein cholesterol in plasma, without use of the preparative ultracentrifuge. *Clin. Chem.* **18,** 499 (1972).

6. Allain, C. C., Poon, L. S., Chan, C. S. G., et al., Enzymatic determination of total serum cholesterol. *Clin. Chem.* **20,** 470 (1974).

7. Witte, D. L., Barrett, D. A., II, and Wycoff, D. A., Evaluation of an enzymatic procedure for determination of serum cholesterol with the ABA-100. *Clin. Chem.* **20,** 1282 (1974).

8. Burstein, M., and Samaille, J., Sur un dosage rapide du cholesterol lié aux α- et aux β-lypoprotéines du sérum. *Clin. Chim. Acta* **5,** 609 (1960).

CLIN. CHEM. 22/1, 101–102 (1976)

Convenient Method for Checking Detector Response of Spectrophotometers at Three Wavelengths

Christopher S. Frings, Vincent I. Muscat,[1] and Nancy T. Waldrop

We describe the use of a water-soluble dye, available as green food coloring, to check the linearity of detector response of spectrometers and spectrophotometers at three wavelengths. The dye has absorbance maxima at 257 nm, 410 nm, and 630 nm. The advantages of using this solution for this important instrument function check are: one solution with absorption maxima in the opposite ends of the visible spectrum as well as in the ultraviolet region; safe; inexpensive; readily available; easy to use; absorbance not dependent on pH from 2.5 to 10.0 or on temperature from 4 to 56 °C.

An essential part of a quality-assurance program in the clinical chemistry laboratory is certifying that the detector response of spectrometers and spectrophotometers is linear over the range of wavelengths used. The compounds reported for this purpose (*1, 2*) include: oxyhemoglobin at 415 nm, *p*-nitrophenol at 405 nm, cobalt ammonium sulfate at 512 nm, cyanmethemoglobin at 540 nm, and copper sulfate at 650 nm.

Medical Laboratory Associates, A Damon Laboratory, 1025 South 18th St., Birmingham, Ala. 35205.

Presented in part at Ninth International Congress on Clinical Chemistry, Toronto, Canada, July 13–18, 1975.

[1] Postdoctoral trainee in clinical chemistry. Present address: Pathology Laboratory Associates, 241 Cox St., Mobile, Ala. 36604.

Received Aug. 11, 1975; accepted Oct. 30, 1975.

We describe the use of a single water-soluble dye solution, available as green food coloring, to check optical spectrometer or spectrophotometer detector response at three wavelengths (257, 410, and 630 nm).

Materials and Methods

Reagents

French's green food coloring: The commercial product consists of FDC Yellow No. 5 and FDC Blue No. 1, 5 parts yellow to 1 part blue, 25 g/liter in water and propylene glycol (R.T. French Co., Rochester, N. Y. 14609; may be purchased at many local grocery stores).

Stock green dye solution, 0.5 ml/liter: Dilute 0.10 ml of green food coloring to 200 ml with water. This solution is stable for six months in a brown glass bottle at room temperature.

Working green dye solutions: On the day the solutions are to be used prepare serial dilutions of the stock dye solution as follows:

Tube no.	5.0 ml of	5.0 ml of	% of stock concentration
1	stock		100
2	stock	water	50
3	No. 2	water	25
4	No. 3	water	12.5

Table 1. %T Values Selected without Conscious Bias over Twelve Months to Show Adherence to Beer's Law

630 nm				410 nm				257 nm			
Tube 1	Tube 2	Tube 3	Tube 4	Tube 1	Tube 2	Tube 3	Tube 4	Tube 1	Tube 2	Tube 3	Tube 4
27.5	52.0	71.5	84.5	11.0	33.5	58.0	76.5	29.0	53.0	71.0	84.0
28.0	52.5	73.0	86.0	10.5	32.0	57.0	76.0	29.0	53.0	71.5	84.0
27.5	52.0	71.5	84.5	10.0	31.0	53.0	73.0	29.0	52.0	71.5	86.0
27.5	52.0	72.0	85.0	11.5	33.0	56.5	75.5	28.0	52.0	71.0	85.0
26.5	51.0	71.0	83.5	10.5	32.0	56.0	75.5	29.0	52.0	70.5	84.0
28.0	52.5	73.0	86.0	10.5	33.0	55.0	74.5	27.5	52.0	71.0	85.0
28.0	53.0	73.0	85.5	10.5	32.5	56.5	75.5	28.0	51.0	70.0	84.0
26.5	51.5	71.5	85.0	11.0	33.5	58.0	76.5	28.0	51.0	70.5	84.0
28.5	53.0	72.5	85.5	10.0	31.5	54.5	73.5	28.5	52.0	70.0	84.0
29.0	53.5	73.5	86.0	11.0	34.0	56.0	76.5	28.5	51.5	71.0	84.0
28.0	53.0	72.0	85.0	11.0	32.0	56.0	76.0	29.0	53.0	73.0	86.0
29.5	54.5	74.0	86.0	10.5	32.0	55.5	75.5	28.5	52.0	71.0	85.0
27.5	52.5	72.5	85.0	10.0	31.5	56.5	74.5	28.0	52.0	70.5	84.0
29.0	53.5	73.5	86.0	9.5	30.5	55.0	74.5	29.0	53.0	73.0	86.0
28.0	53.0	71.5	85.0	10.0	31.0	56.0	75.0	28.0	52.0	71.0	85.0

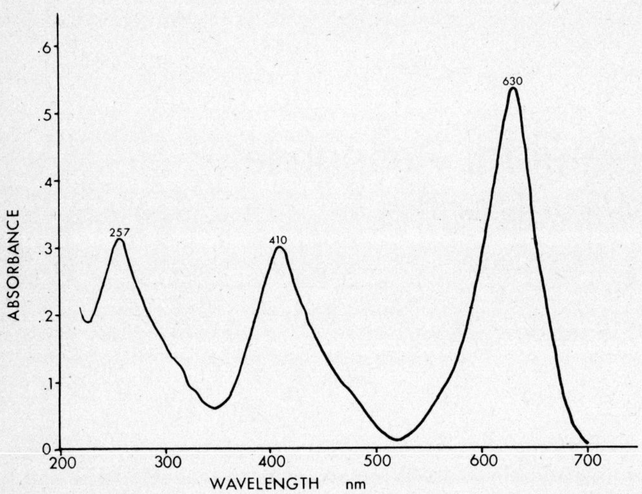

Fig. 1. Absorption spectrum of working green dye solution

Spectrophotometer

All measurements were made with a DBGT Spectrophotometer (Beckman Instruments, Inc. Scientific Instruments Division, Fullerton, Calif. 92634).

Procedure

Measure the transmittance or absorbance of the four working green dye solutions vs. a water blank at 257 nm, 410 nm, and 630 nm. Read all solutions in the same cuvette, starting with the blank and proceeding through the highest concentration. Plot the transmittance (in percent) vs. concentration on semilog graph paper or plot absorbance vs. concentration on coordinate graph paper.

Results and Discussion

French's green food coloring exhibits maximum absorbance at 257, 410, and 630 nm (Figure 1). Two other commercial green food colorings—Durkee (Cleveland, Ohio 44115) and McCormick (Baltimore, Md. 21202)—exhibit identical absorption spectra. No change in absorbance is noted when the pH is varied from 2.5 to 10.0 or when the temperature is varied from 4 to 56 °C. Plots at all three wavelengths follow Beer's law over the entire concentration range (Table 1). Thus, any nonlinear response would indicate either an error in dilution or an instrumental problem.

Table 2. Mean ($\overline{X}$), Standard Deviation (SD), and Coefficient of Variation (CV) of Each Working Green Dye Solution with Corresponding Wavelength (Weekly Determinations, August 1974–October 1975)

	630 nm			410 nm			257 nm		
	$\overline{X}$	SD	CV	$\overline{X}$	SD	CV	$\overline{X}$	SD	CV
Tube 1	27.9	0.8	3.0	10.5	0.5	5.0	28.5	0.5	1.8
Tube 2	52.7	0.9	1.6	32.2	1.0	3.2	52.1	0.7	1.2
Tube 3	72.4	0.9	1.2	56.0	1.3	2.3	71.1	0.9	1.2
Tube 4	85.2	0.7	0.8	75.2	1.0	1.3	84.7	0.8	0.9

The above procedure has been in routine use in our laboratory and in the laboratories of 12 hospitals (ranging in size from 150 to 500 beds) for the past year. Four different lot numbers of French's green food coloring have been used and each gave the same results. Coefficient of variation and the standard deviation of each point indicate excellent precision (Table 2). Weekly linearity checks are performed on the following instruments: Beckman DBGT, Gilford 300 N (Gilford Instrument Laboratories, Inc., Oberlin, Ohio 44074), and B & L Spectronic 70 (Bausch & Lomb, Analytical Systems Division, Rochester, N. Y. 14625).

The advantages of this solution for certifying linear response of detectors are: one solution with absorption maximum in the opposite ends of the visible spectrum as well as in the ultraviolet region; safe; stable; inexpensive; readily available; and easy to use.

References

1. Rand, R. N., Practical spectrophotometric standards. *Clin. Chem.* **15,** 839 (1969).

2. Critique, special topics check sample No. ST-41. Commission on Continuing Education, American Society of Clinical Pathologists, Chicago, Ill., 1969.

CLIN. CHEM. 22/1, 103–104 (1976)

Effects of Storage in the Cold on Activity of Gamma-Glutamyltransferase in Serum

Douglas P. Rhone[1] and Florence M. White

Sera from patients with hepatobiliary disorders were selected to represent a wide range of activity of γ-glutamyltransferase (EC 2.3.2.2). Samples were stored at 4 °C and periodically tested for as long as nine weeks, others at −6 °C for as long as 40 weeks. The frozen-stored samples were thawed and then frozen again after each testing. The activity of the enzyme was essentially unchanged under both conditions of storage. These results are consistent with comments in the literature on the enzyme's stability.

Measurement of the activity of γ-glutamyltransferase [GGT; EC 2.3.2.2; (γ-glutamyl)-peptide:amino-acid γ-glutamyltransferase] in serum has become a useful laboratory tool to aid in the diagnosis of hepatobiliary diseases (*1*). The enzyme is also reported to be abnormally active in sera from patients with myocardial infarction (*2*), intracerebral tumors (*3*), acute pancreatitis, and carcinoma of the pancreas (*1*).

It is often convenient or necessary to store individual specimens of serum until several have been accumulated before analyzing them. Occasionally it is desirable to repeat the determination after the specimen has been refrozen two or three times.

Freezing and thawing of serum samples increases their total alkaline phosphatase activity (*4*, *5*). The effects of freezing and thawing on the activity of GGT have not been reported. Szasz has shown that the activity of GGT is stable in serum that was preincubated in the assay solution for an hour at temperatures ranging from 20 °C to 40 °C; it is also stable when assayed at temperatures from 18 °C to 28 °C (*6*). Several authors have commented on the stability of GGT when serum is stored in the cold (*7–11*). One letter discussed storage for up to 72 h (*12*).

Here, we report the effects of brief and prolonged storage in the cold and of repeated freezing and thawing on the activity of GGT in serum.

Section of Biochemistry, Illinois Masonic Medical Center; and Department of Pathology, Abraham Lincoln School of Medicine, University of Illinois, Chicago, Ill. 60657.

[1] Present address: Department of Pathology, Martin Army Hospital, Fort Benning, Ga. 31905.

The opinions or assertions contained herein are the private views of the authors and are not to be construed as official or as reflecting the views of the Department of the Army or the Department of Defense.

Received May 16, 1975; accepted Oct. 12, 1975.

Materials and Methods

Serum samples. The blood samples were from patients hospitalized with various hepatobiliary disorders. The serum was separated by double centrifugation and the sample was tested immediately. Sera were selected so that a full range of enzyme activity could be studied. The same sera were used for brief and for prolonged storage at two temperatures.

GGT method. GGT was measured by a modification of the Rosalki method (*6*, *7*), in which γ-glutamyl-*p*-nitroanilide is the substrate at a final concentration of 5.6 mmol/liter. The reaction pH was 9.0, incubation time 15 min. Glycylglycine was used as an acceptor and the *p*-nitroaniline produced was quantitated directly in a colorimeter at a wavelength of 405 nm. The coefficient of variation for this method was 3.3%. All measurements were made in duplicate and averaged.

Brief storage. Sera from 10 patients were tested immediately and initial GGT activity was recorded. Each specimen was then equally divided and part was stored in the refrigerator (4 °C) and the other at −6 °C. Enzyme activity was then measured at 6, 24, 48, 72, and 96 h. The frozen sera were thawed and refrozen again after each testing.

Prolonged storage. Sera from 12 patients were tested immediately and the initial GGT activity was recorded. Each specimen was then divided into two equal parts. One part was stored in the refrigerator (4 °C) and aliquots were tested at 1, 2, 5, and 9 weeks. The second part of ten sera was stored in the freezer (−6 °C), and was thawed and tested at 1, 2, 6, 10, and 40 weeks; the specimen was frozen again after each testing.

Statistical analysis. The values obtained for groups of sera stored at various temperatures for given intervals were compared with the initial values for the group. Student's *t*-test was used as a measure of statistical significance.

Results and Discussion

Ten sera were stored for as long as 96 h at 4 °C. They contained initial activity of enzyme ranging from 11 U/liter to 480 U/liter. After six h, two sera showed decreases. Values after 24, 48, 72, and 96 h of storage were similar to those obtained at 6 h. Of the 50 determinations, only 15 showed an increase or decrease that exceeded 10% of the initial enzyme activity.

Table 1. Changes in γ-Glutamyltransferase (GGT) Activity in Sera after Storage at −6 °C and Repeated Thawing

	Activity, U/l, and % of original activity after:												
	I. Brief storage[a]						II. Prolonged storage[b]						
Initial activity	6 h		48 h		96 h		Initial activity	1 wk		6 wk		40 wk	
U/l	U/l	%	U/l	%	U/l	%	U/l	U/l	%	U/l	%	U/l	%
11	11	*100*	13	*118*	11	*100*	12	16	*133*	16	*133*	11	*92*
14	15	*107*	20	*142*	14	*100*	40	49	*123*	41	*103*	42	*105*
16	19	*118*	19	*118*	19	*118*	72	57	*79*	40	*56*	54	*75*
43	36	*83*	36	*83*	36	*83*	84	102	*121*	100	*120*	81	*96*
64	59	*92*	61	*95*	57	*89*	135	121	*90*	121	*90*	108	*80*
94	94	*100*	101	*107*	98	*104*	151	150	*99*	150	*99*	138	*91*
175	184	*105*	178	*101*	181	*103*	167	179	*107*	175	*105*	163	*97*
214	225	*105*	236	*110*	228	*107*	238	252	*106*	265	*111*	210	*88*
352	384	*109*	392	*111*	392	*111*	455	455	*100*	425	*93*	400	*88*
480	536	*111*	544	*113*	508	*106*	730	840	*115*	775	*106*	705	*97*
Mean 146.3	156.3		160		154.4		208.4	222.1		210.8		191.2	

[a] Enzyme activity was also measured after 24 and 72 h.
[b] Enzyme activity was also measured after 2 and 10 weeks.

Twelve sera were stored at 4 °C for nine weeks. Initial activity of enzyme in each serum ranged from 12 U/liter to 810 U/liter. After one week of storage, eight sera showed decreased activity as compared to the initial value and four had increased activities. At five weeks 11 sera showed increased values and at nine weeks increases were seen in nine sera. The mean of initial activity for the group was 243.9 U/liter; after nine weeks of storage the mean activity for the group was 269.4 U/liter.

None of the variations in GGT activity in the sera subjected to either brief or prolonged storage at 4 °C were statistically significant ($P > 0.5$ in all groups).

Table 1 summarizes the effects of brief and prolonged storage at −6 °C and of repeated thawing on GGT activities in serum. Ten sera were stored for as long as 96 h. In 19 of the 50 determinations in this group the variation exceeded 10% of the initial activity. Another 10 sera were stored for as long as 40 weeks. Values similar to those initially recorded were obtained at one, two, and six weeks of storage and after as many as three thawings. At 10 weeks all sera showed increased values. At 40 weeks 10 sera showed decreased values; by this time the samples had been thawed and refrozen five times. In spite of some considerable variations, the changes in GGT activity in sera stored at −6 °C were not statistically significant ($P \geq 0.5$ in all groups).

It has been previously mentioned that activity of GGT in serum is stable at one (*10*) and at six (*8*) weeks when stored at −20 °C. Rosalki et al. (*7*) noted that the enzyme in serum was stable for two months at −18 °C.

Our studies show that GGT activity in serum is stable when the sample is refrigerated (4 °C) or frozen (−6 °C), and that repeated thawing and freezing do not cause statistically significant alterations in the activity of enzyme.

References

1. Lum, G., and Gambino, S. R., Serum gamma-glutamyl transpeptidase activity as an indicator of disease of liver, pancreas, or bone. *Clin. Chem.* **18,** 358 (1972).

2. Ravens, K., Gudbjarnason, S., Cowan, C. M., and Bing, R. J., Gamma-glutamyltranspeptidase in myocardial infarction. *Circulation* **39,** 693 (1969).

3. Ewen, L. M., and Griffiths, J., Gamma-glutamyl transpeptidase: Elevated activities in certain neurologic diseases. *Am. J. Clin. Pathol.* **59,** 2 (1973).

4. Brojer, B., and Moss, D. W., Changes in alkaline phosphatase activity of serum samples after thawing and after reconstitution from the lyophilized state. *Clin. Chim. Acta* **35,** 511 (1971).

5. Massion, C. G., and Frankenfeld, J. K., Alkaline phosphatase: Lability in fresh and frozen human serum and in lyophilized control material. *Clin. Chem.* **18,** 366 (1972).

6. Szasz, G., The effect of temperature on enzyme activity and on the affinity of enzymes to their substrates. *Z. Klin. Chem. Klin. Biochem.* **12,** 166 (1974).

7. Rosalki, S., Rau, D., Lehmann, D., and Prentice, M., Determination of serum gamma-glutamyl transpeptidase activity and its clinical application. *Ann. Clin. Biochem.* **7,** 143 (1970).

8. Orlowski, M., The role of gamma-glutamyl transpeptidase in the internal diseases clinic. *Arch. Immunol. Ther. Exp.* **11,** 1 (1963).

9. Aronsen, K. F., Hanson, A., and Nosslin, B., The value of gamma-glutamyl transpeptidase in differentiating viral hepatitis from obstructive jaundice. *Acta Chir. Scand.* **130,** 92 (1965).

10. Zein, M., and Discombe, G., Serum gamma-glutamyltranspeptidase as a diagnostic aid. *Lancet* **ii,** 748 (1970).

11. Szasz, G., Kinetic photometric method for serum gamma-glutamyl transpeptidase. *Clin. Chem.* **15,** 124 (1969).

12. Juel, R., and Curry, S. N., Stability of gamma glutamyltransferase in serum. *Clin. Chem.* **20,** 914 (1974). Letter to the Editor.

Procedure for Mechanized (Continuous-flow) Measurement of Serum Ascorbic Acid (Vitamin C)[1]

Submitters: H. Sauberlich, W. C. Goad, J. H. Skala, and P. P. Waring, *Department of Nutrition, Letterman Army Institute of Research, Presidio of San Francisco, Calif. 94129*

Evaluators: George E. Nichoalds, *Department of Biochemistry, Vanderbilt University School of Medicine, Nashville, Tenn. 37232*

Jack L. Omdahl, *Department of Biochemistry, School of Medicine, University of New Mexico, Alberquerque, N. Mex. 87106*

Introduction

The two most commonly used procedures for determining ascorbic acid (vitamin C) in serum (plasma) are based on spectrophotometric measurements of either the red product formed from the reaction of 2,4-dinitrophenylhydrazine with dehydroascorbic acid after conversion from ascorbic acid (*11–16*) or the reduction of dichloroindophenol dye by ascorbic acid (*14–16*).

The method presented was designed to provide a means of measuring serum ascorbic acid concentrations in nutrition surveys, field studies, and research studies involving large numbers of samples. The lability of the ascorbic acid warranted a stabilization of the samples and the quantity of samples involved necessitated an automated assay procedure.

The automated method of Garry and Owen (*1*), which follows the manual 2,6-dichloroindophenol dye method described by Henry (*2*), formed the basis for the system, with various modifications and improvements to meet particular needs.

Principle

Ascorbic acid in serum or plasma is stabilized by the addition of metaphosphoric acid immediately after the sample is separated from the cells. This provides a protein-free filtrate that inhibits the catalytic oxidation of ascorbic acid by Fe^{3+} and Cu^{2+}. The filtrate may be stored frozen for several weeks with minimal losses (*17*), or analyzed directly in a continuous-stream automated system without the necessity of dialysis. The elimination of a dialyzer permits a greater concentration of actual sample to be reacted with 2,6-dichloroindophenol (Cl_2Ind) dye (see Note), thus enhancing the sensitivity of the assay while requiring smaller volumes of samples (*18, 19*). When the acid filtrate is buffered to about pH 3.5 with sodium citrate, a color decrease occurs in the presence of ascorbic acid, and it is recorded spectrophotometrically at 505 nm. The reaction is:

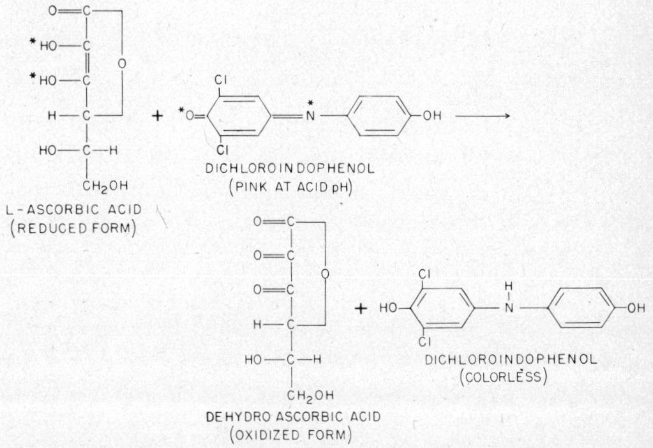

Note: There is inconsistency in the nomenclature of this dye in the literature. 2,6-Dichloroindophenol is the preferred (and CBN-recommended) name, based on Heilbron's (*3*) nucleus for indophenol, Richter's (*4*) condensation preparation, and usage in current chemical catalogs. Other names that have been used: 2,6-dichlorophenolindophenol (*5*), 2,6-dichloro-*N*-(*p*-hydroxyphenyl)-*p*-benzoquinone imine (*6*), 2,6-dichloro-quinonephenolimine (*4*), and 2,6-dichlorobenzenenone-indophenol (*5*).

[1] Mention of sources of equipment, supplies, or chemicals is not to be considered an endorsement of indicated manufacturers, suppliers, or distributors by the United States Army, Letterman Army Institute of Research, or the AACC.

Materials and Methods

Reagents

1. *Stock dye.* 2,6-Dichloroindophenol, 1.00 g/liter of distilled water. Dissolve the dye in hot distilled water. When the solution has cooled to room temperature, adjust the volume to 100 ml and filter, under reduced pressure, through Whatman No. 40 filter paper. The dye is stable for about a month at refrigerator temperature.

Note: Evaluator G.E.N. found that incorporation of a surfactant, Brij-35,[2] into the dye solution helped to ensure the proper color change from blue to pink after the dye was mixed with serum and citrate.
Note: Problems encountered in the automated system (precipitates, baseline noise, and drift) may usually be attributed to either the dye used or the purity and freshness of the metaphosphoric acid.[3]

2. *Working dye.* Dilute 4 ml of stock dye to 200 ml with distilled water just before use each day.
3. *Sodium citrate,* 18 g/liter of distilled water. Dissolve 18 g of sodium citrate ($C_6H_5Na_3O_7{\cdot}2H_2O$) and dilute to 1 liter with distilled water. Then add 1.5 ml of Brij-35 solution and mix. Fresh reagent should be prepared monthly or when cloudiness (mold or bacterial growth) appears.

Note: Brij-35 solution is prepared by dissolving 100 g of Brij-35 in 250 ml of distilled water. Minimal baseline problems and improved peak separation were found with 1.5 ml of Brij-35 per liter of citrate solution.

4. *Metaphosphoric acid wash,* 22.5 g/liter of distilled water. Dissolve 2.25 g of HPO_3 in distilled water and adjust volume to 100 ml.[4] Prepare freshly each day.
5. *Metaphosphoric acid precipitant,* 30 g/liter of distilled water. Dissolve 3 g of HPO_3 in distilled water and adjust the volume to 100 ml. Prepare freshly each day.

Standards

1. *Stock standard.* Ascorbic acid, 1 g/liter. Dissolve 100 mg of ascorbic acid in 20 ml of HPO_3 solution (reagent 5, above) and dilute to 100 ml with distilled water. This stock should be prepared freshly each month.

Note: We find losses of less than 3% for working standards made freshly from six-month-old stock standards, when the latter are stored at 4 °C.

2. *Working standards.* Dilute the following volumes of ascorbic acid stock standard to 100 ml with HPO_3 solution (reagent 4):

Stock standard, ml	Ascorbic acid, mg/dl
0.00	0
0.05	0.05
0.10	0.10
0.20	0.20
0.30	0.30
0.40	0.40
0.50	0.50

At these dilutions, the working standards are fairly stable (about 7–8% loss during one month at 4 °C). However, it is recommended that they be prepared at least weekly.

Apparatus

Figure 1 diagrams the essential components of this automated system, which is readily adaptable for use with basic "AutoAnalyzer I" or "AutoAnalyzer II" (Technicon Instruments Corp., Tarrytown, N. Y. 10591) equipment. The necessary modules include a Sampler, Proportioning Pump, Colorimeter, adjustable range expander, and Recorder.

The components designated on the diagram as AL-177-B004-02 and AL-01-0055-01 (Acculab Div., Precision Technology, Inc., Norwood, N. J. 07648) consist of a Lucite connector block and a 14-turn in-line glass coil, tapped on the 10th turn with a small-bore glass inlet. Minimum lengths of glass tubing are used where they are necessary to connect these components to each other and to the flow cell.

These components facilitate construction and minimize connections, with a resulting improvement in system hydraulics and thus baseline stability. They may be substituted by a type *H3* glass fitting and a 10-turn glass coil joined to a 5-turn coil with a type *A1* glass fitting (Technicon).

The use of Solvaflex pump tubes also improves reagent flow and baseline stability. The acid-wash pump tube and the standard wash reservoirs of

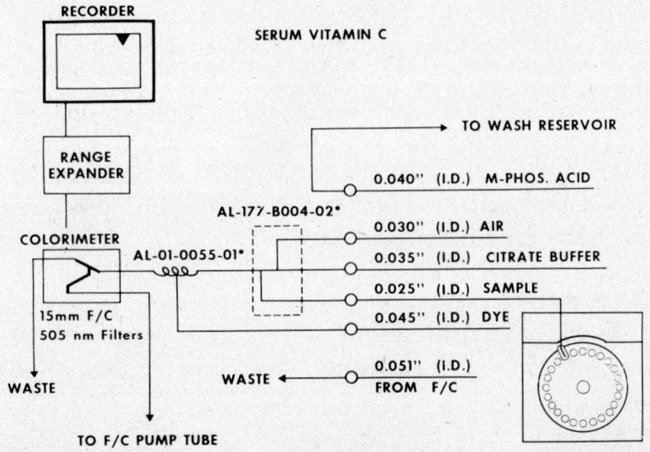

Fig. 1. Flow diagram and essential components adaptable for use with either Technicon basic AutoAnalyzer I or AutoAnalyzer II system

[2] Brij-35 (polyoxyethylene lauryl ether) may be purchased from (e.g.) Nutritional Biochemical Corp., Cleveland, Ohio 44128.
[3] We encountered the fewest difficulties with use of dye purchased from E. H. Sargent & Co., Skokie, Ill.; cat. No. SC 11846 (La Motte Chemical Co., Code 3336).
[4] Mallinckrodt cat. No. 2816, phosphoric acid, meta, AR grade 34–36% HPO_3, 58–62% $NaPO_3$; or Matheson Coleman and Bell, cat. No. PX 1004-CB 521, phosphoric acid, meta, reagent, ACS.

AutoAnalyzer I samplers are more conveniently replaced by Technicon's (or similar) inverted constant volume device (part No. 100-0460-01).

The manifold lines are kept as short as practicable, to minimize the effects of interfering, nonspecific reductants (which react with the dye more slowly than does ascorbic acid), and are of glass where possible, to reduce baseline noise by eliminating the sponge effect of plastic tubing.

Note: Evaluator J.L.O. recommended the use of a dialyzer in the automated system. He found that it leads to a better reproducibility between sequential analyses of standards. Also it requires a twofold dilution rather than a fourfold dilution, thus reducing the dilution error. As noted above, we consider the use of a dialyzer in the described system undesirable and unnecessary. Furthermore, when one is used losses in ascorbic acid occur, because the samples do not receive the benefit of metaphosphoric acid stabilization.

Collection and Handling of Specimens

Blood is drawn for the preparation of either serum or plasma (heparin anticoagulant preferred to ethylenediaminetetraacetate[5]) and kept refrigerated until the cells can be removed by centrifugation, whereupon one volume of serum should immediately be treated with three volumes of HPO_3 precipitant (reagent 5). Ascorbic acid in the frozen serum/HPO_3 mixture is stable for as long as 14 days. Ascorbic acid can be measured in as little as 0.1 ml of serum.

Note: This method was designed for field surveys in which the HPO_3-treated samples are immediately frozen, after mixing, for shipment to a central laboratory for analysis. When analyzed locally, the samples are refrigerated or frozen after mixing, then thawed and analyzed. See also step 3 under *Procedure*.
Note: Evaluator G.E.N. found that protein-free filtrates that have been thawed and re-frozen give an unexplained increase in color production on subsequent analysis, so this should not be done.

Procedure

1. Flush the manifold lines of the AutoAnalyzer system by pumping distilled water for 15–20 min.

2. Pump reagent until the baseline is established, which usually requires 20 to 30 min.

3. Thaw the samples, remove the protein precipitate by centrifugation, and collect supernates for analysis.

Note: For field surveys the samples are prepared in 1.7-ml (½ dram) screw-capped vials (Kimble No. 60910). The samples are thawed, mixed, and about 0.3 ml transferred to polyethylene micro tubes with captive stoppers (Bel Art No. 19928). These are centrifuged for 3 min in a Coleman Model 6-811 micro-scale centrifuge (mean force of 8000 × *g* at 13 000 rpm), or similar micro-scale centrifuge, and the supernates collected for analysis.
Note: Evaluator G.E.N. found that as long as 60 min was required to establish a steady baseline in step 2.

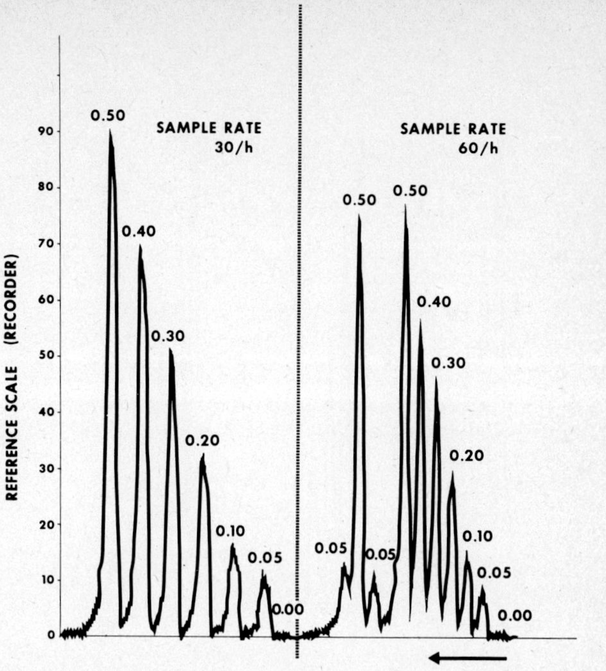

Fig. 2. Recorder chart record for ascorbic acid standards (mg/dl)
Technicon basic AutoAnalyzer I system with scale expansion and a sample/wash ratio of ½; sampling rate, 30 (*left*) and 60 (*right*) per hour

4. Load the sample tray with the standard solutions and the clear sample supernates, with a midrange standard (0.2 or 0.3 mg/dl) every tenth sample to provide a system control and a means of monitoring baseline drift. Several standards should follow the last sample.

5. Samples are analyzed at a rate that may be varied between 30 per hour and 60 per hour, depending on the characteristics of the instruments available (colorimeter stability, range expansion potential, recorder response time, and amplification) and the quality of the dye.

Figure 2 shows a recording for standards assayed with the Technicon AutoAnalyzer I system. The differences in peak heights were produced by a change in the instrument control settings when the sampler cam was changed from a 60/h to a 30/h rate. Figure 3 illustrates reproducibility with this system.

Figure 4 illustrates a recording chart for standards assayed with the Technicon AutoAnalyzer II system.

6. After the last sample appears on the chart, flush the lines with distilled water as in step 1 for 30 min and shut down the system.

Calculations

The ascorbic acid concentrations of the unknown samples are read directly from a standard curve prepared from the working standards, and multiplied by four to take into account the dilution factor of the serum/HPO_3 extract. The flow diagram depicted in Figure 1 was used with both the Technicon AutoAnalyzer I system and the Technicon AutoAnalyzer II

[5] Plasmas prepared with ethylenediaminetetraacetate used as the anticoagulant give slightly smaller peaks as compared with duplicate plasmas prepared with heparin as the anticoagulant or with sera (unpublished data).

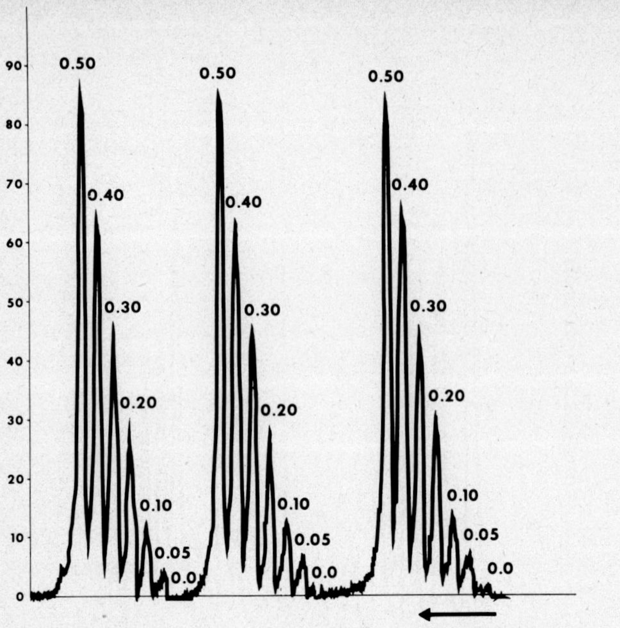

Fig. 3. Reproducibility of ascorbic acid standards (mg/dl)
Technicon AutoAnalyzer I system; sampling rate, 60 per hour; ½ sample/wash cam; recorder set for full-scale response for 5 mg/liter. Recorder pen returned to baseline from maximum deflection; baseline noise equivalent to <0.2 mg/liter

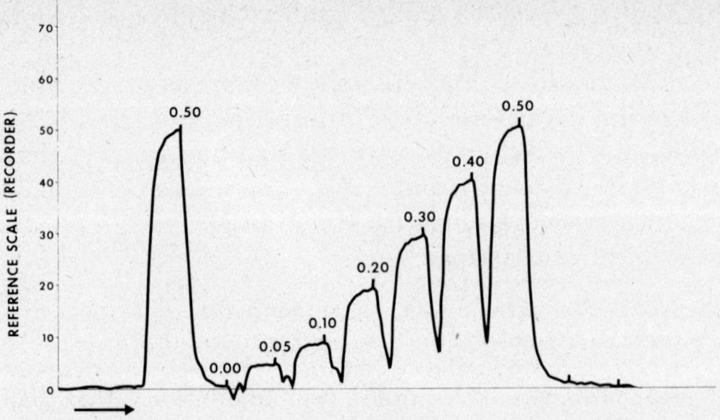

Fig. 4. Recorder chart record for ascorbic acid standards (mg/dl)
Technicon AutoAnalyzer II system. Sampling rate, 60 per hour; wash time, 12 s. Peak heights may be increased or adjusted according to scale expansion selected

system to obtain the standard curves illustrated in Figures 2–4.

Discussion

We studied the stability of ascorbic acid in fresh serum and in frozen serum, with or without HPO_3 treatment. The results are presented in Table 1. [*Ed. note: cf. Clin Chem.* **21,** 1493 (1975)]. Compared with the initial values for the fresh serum, values for untreated frozen serum decreased by 10–15% within 24 h and by 30% at the end of six days, while the frozen HPO_3-treated serum had a mean loss of about 3% during a 13-day storage period. The overall recovery of added ascorbic acid ranged from 92% to 95% (Table 2).

The low standard, 0.05 mg/dl (equivalent to 2.0 mg of ascorbic acid per liter of serum), produces a very readable peak on the recorder chart. Serum ascorbic acid values exceeding this are indicative of acceptable dietary intakes of the vitamin according to the Interdepartmental Committee on Nutrition for National Defense standards. Serum ascorbic acid values of less than 1.0 mg/liter are considered "deficient," while values from 1.0 to 1.9 mg/liter are considered as "low" (7). Occasionally, serum ascorbate values lower than 1.0 mg/liter are difficult to interpret, owing to baseline irregularities caused by the small air bubbles drawn in by the sample probe between sample cup and wash reservoir.

Figure 5 shows reproducibility of standard curves in the analyses of large numbers of human sera. Ascorbic acid standards covering the range from 0.5–5.0 mg/liter were analyzed about every 30 sera; the AutoAnalyzer II system was used at a sampling rate of 60/h. The colorimeter was set to give a 50% recorder scale deflection for the 0.5 mg/dl ascorbic acid

Table 1. Comparison of Ascorbic Acid Stability in Frozen Metaphosphoric Acid Extracts and in Frozen Serum[a]

		Age of extracts (days)								
Sample (no. detns.)		Fresh[b] 0	Frozen[b] 0	1	2	3	4	6	7	13
Frozen HPO_3 extracts (6)	Mean Base	—	—	—	102 ± 3.0	101 ± 2.6	—	—	101 ± 3.6	—
	Range	—	—	—	89–110	89–107	—	—	85–111	—
Frozen HPO_3 extracts (16)	Mean Base	102 ± 1.1	100 ± 0.7		—	—	101 ± 1.5	99 ± 0.8	—	97 ± 1.5
	Range	94–108	94–106		—	—	87–118	95–106	—	90–100
Frozen serum (16)	Mean Base	—	87 ± 1.2		—	—	82 ± 1.7	72 ± 2.2	—	58 ± 2.1
	Range	—	76–92		—	—	71–94	58–87	—	44–74

[a] Values expressed as mean percent (± standard error of mean percent) recovery of the initial (fresh) value as a base with the individual percent recovery range shown below.

[b] Pooled serum sample analyzed immediately (fresh) and aliquots prepared and frozen. Extracts were prepared on a portion of the serum, analyzed immediately, and the remainder divided and frozen.

Table 2. Analytical Recovery of Ascorbic Acid Added to Pooled Plasma

Added (mg/liter)	Found (mg/liter)		Expected	Recovery, % of added		Recovery, % of total	
None	4.3	4.6	—	—		—	
	4.8			—		—	
	4.6			—		—	
5.08	9.2		9.68	90.6	90.6	95.0	95.0
	9.1			88.6		94.0	
	9.3			92.5		96.1	
10.16	13.5		14.76	87.6	90.9	91.5	93.7
	14.1			93.5		95.5	
	13.9			91.5		94.2	
15.24	18.3		19.84	89.9	90.3	92.2	92.5
	18.3			89.9		92.2	
	18.5			91.2		93.2	

[a] 5.08 mg of ascorbic acid was added to 100 ml of pooled plasma. 1-, 2-, and 3-ml aliquots of the ascorbic acid-supplemented plasma were diluted to 10 ml each with the unsupplemented plasma. Time involved for preparation and extraction, about 2 h.

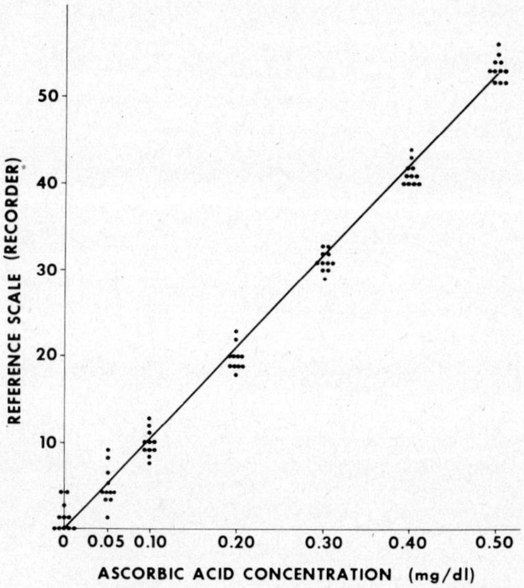

Fig. 5 Correlation between the arbitrary reference scale (recorder chart scale) and the concentration of ascorbic acid standards, as obtained with the Techicon AutoAnalyzer II system

Each point designates a chart reading; the line represents the calculated regression ($y = 1.052x - 0.002$). The correlation coefficient is 0.9956, the standard error of the estimate 0.017

standard. The series of 11 standard curves (77 individual measurements) thus obtained were used to calculate the correlation between the recorder scale values and ascorbic acid concentrations of the standards. Each point on the graph represents an individual value; the line designates the least-squares regression (slope 1.052, intercept 0.002). The coefficient of correlation was 0.9956 and the standard error of the estimate ($S_{y \cdot x}$) was equivalent to 0.17 mg of ascorbic acid per liter.

Table 3. Guidelines for Interpretation of Serum Ascorbic Acid Data

Guideline	Reference	Less than acceptable: Deficient (high-risk)	Less than acceptable: Low (moderate-risk)	Acceptable (low-risk)
		mg/liter		
ICNND (all ages)	*(7)*	<1.0	1.0–1.9	⩾2.0
Ten-State survey (all ages)	*(9, 10)*	<1.0	1.0–1.9	⩾2.0
Canada survey	*(20)*			
0–19 y (♂ & ♀)		<2.0	2.0–6.0	>6.0
20+ y (♂ & ♀)		<2.0	2.0–4	>4.0
Suggested revision (all ages)	*(21)*	<2.0	2.0–2.9	⩾3.0

Interferences from indophenol reducers (sulfhydryl compounds, sulfites and thiosulfates) and phenolic compounds are minimized by keeping the pH of the reaction at about 3.5. Oxyhemoglobin oxidizes ascorbic acid, thus nonhemolyzed sera must be used. Catalytic oxidation of ascorbic acid by Fe^{3+} and Cu^{2+} is inhibited by the metaphosphoric acid (*23*). One problem that may occur with the use of this acid is the preparation of filtrates that show no Tyndall effect, which is sometimes a problem even when fresh reagent, prepared from new bottles of metaphosphoric acid, is used (*8*). The cause and solution of the problem is uncertain.

By the 2,6-dichloroindophenol method, only the reduced form of ascorbic acid is measured. However, dehydroascorbic acid, the oxidized form, is not present in significant concentrations in properly prepared and preserved serum samples (*24*). The 2,4-dinitrophenylhydrazine procedures (*11–16*) measure both ascorbic acid and dehydroascorbic acid. However, for use with serum samples, the procedure is tedious, requires long incubation periods and strong acid, and is less satisfactory for adaptation to an automated system. With properly prepared and preserved serum samples, the two methods provide very nearly the same values.

Normal and Abnormal Values

Guidelines for evaluating serum ascorbic acid data are presented in Table 3. The analytical method outlined has been utilized in a controlled study of human vitamin C deficiency to establish the validity of these guidelines (*22*). The method is employed routinely for vitamin C analysis of serum samples collected during nutrition surveys conducted regularly at this laboratory.

References

1. Garry, P. J., and Owen, G. M., Automated screening technique for vitamin C assay requiring small quantities of blood. In *Automation in Analytical Chemistry, Technicon Symposia 1967,* 1, N. B. Scova et al., Eds., Mediad, White Plains, N. Y., 1968, pp 507–510.

2. Henry, R. J., *Clinical Chemistry: Principles and Techniques,* 1st ed., Hoeber, New York, N. Y., 1964, p 710.

3. Heilbron, I., *Dictionary of Organic Compounds,* **3,** Oxford University Press, New York, N. Y., 1953, p 13.

4. von Richter, R., *The Chemistry of Carbon Compounds,* **3,** Elsevier, New York, N. Y., 1946, p 245.

5. *The Merck Index,* 7th ed., Merck and Co., Inc., Rahway, N. J., 1952, p 331.

6. *The Merck Index,* 8th ed., Merck and Co., Inc., Rahway, N. J., 1968, p 352.

7. *Manual for Nutrition Surveys,* Interdepartmental Committee on Nutrition for National Defense, 2nd ed., U. S. Government Printing Office, Washington, D. C., 1963, p 121.

8. Henry, R. J., *loc. cit.,* p 167.

9. Ten-State Nutrition Survey Reports, **I–V,** Center for Disease Control, Atlanta, Ga. 30330, 1972.

10. O'Neal, R. M., Johnson, O. C., and Schaefer, A. E., Guidelines for classification and interpretation of group blood and urine data collected as part of the National Nutrition Survey. *Pediatr. Res.* **4,** 103–106 (1970).

11. Roe, J. H., and Kuether, C. A., The determination of ascorbic acid in whole blood and urine through the 2,4-dinitrophenylhydrazine derivative of dehydroascorbic acid. *J. Biol. Chem.* **147,** 399–407 (1943).

12. Schaffert, R. R., and Kingsley, G. R., A rapid, simple method for the determination of reduced, dehydro-, and total ascorbic acid in biological material. *J. Biol. Chem.* **212,** 59–69 (1955).

13. Pelletier, O., Determination of vitamin C in serum, urine and other biological materials. *J. Lab. Clin. Med.* **72,** 674–679 (1968).

14. Roe, J. H., Appraisal of methods for the determination of L-ascorbic acid. *Ann. N. Y. Acad. Sci.* **92,** 277–283 (1961).

15. Olliver, M., Ascorbic acid IV. Estimation. In *The Vitamins,* **I,** 2nd ed., W. H. Sebrell, Jr., and R. S. Harris, Eds., Academic Press, New York, N. Y., 1967, pp 338–359.

16. Hove, E. L., Conference on vitamin C methodology: A summary report. *J. Assoc. Off. Agr. Chem.* **48,** 991–996 (1965).

17. Goad, W. C., Skala, J. H., Harding, R. S., and Sauberlich, H. E., A semiautomated technique for the determination of vitamin C (ascorbic acid) in serum or plasma samples. Laboratory Report No. 337, U. S. Army Medical Research & Nutrition Laboratory, September, 1973. Available from: National Technical Information Service, U.S. Dept. Commerce, Springfield, Va. 22161.

18. *Principles of Operation of Basic AutoAnalyzer System.* Technicon Instrument Corp., Tarrytown, N. Y. 10591, 1967.

19. *Programmed Instructions for the Technicon AutoAnalyzer II System.* Publication No. TPI-0170-10, December, 1973, Technicon Instruments Corp., Tarrytown, N. Y. 10591.

20. *Nutrition Canada: National Survey.* Information Canada, 171 Slater St., Ottawa, Canada.

21. Sauberlich, H. E., Dowdy, R. P., and Skala, J. H., *Laboratory Tests for the Assessment of Nutritional Status.* CRC Press, Inc., Cleveland, Ohio 44128, 1974, p 230.

22. Hodges, R. E., Hood, J., Canham, J. E., et al., Clinical manifestations of ascorbic acid deficiency in man. *Am. J. Clin. Nutr.* **24,** 432–443 (1971).

23. Hay, G. W., Lewis, B. A., and Smith, F., Ascorbic acid II. Chemistry. In *The Vitamins,* **I,** 2nd ed., W. H. Sebrell, Jr. and R. S. Harris, Eds., Academic Press, New York, N. Y., 1967, pp 307–320.

24. Woodruff, C. W., Ascorbic acid. In *Nutrition,* **II,** G. H. Beaton and E. W. McHenry, Eds., Academic Press, New York, N. Y., 1964, pp 265–298.

Editor's note: The reader is reminded that Selected Methods do not bear the official imprimatur of the Association. They are methods that seem durable and generally useful, and that have been checked by several evaluators. As detailed elsewhere [Clin. Chem. **19,** 1207 (1973)], *these methods are offered here for criticism by the world community of users, and will be revised appropriately before being collected into a bound volume,* Selected Methods of Clinical Chemistry.

No reprints of these papers will be available, because they are not regarded as necessarily being final versions.

The Chicago Section, AACC[1]

Albert A. Dietz

In December 1948, in New York City, 10 persons gathered for the first formal meeting of the AACC (*1*). Nine of them became charter members of the Association. Less than a year later (September 1949), one of them, Dr. Samuel Natelson, moved to Rockford, Illinois, 85 miles from Chicago. Shortly after arriving in Rockford and after observing the status of clinical chemistry in the area, Dr. Natelson reported (*2*):

"There are very few hospitals in this area which have trained chemists and personnel who are at least college graduates. With the exception of specialists who are engaged in research, the condition, even in the best known hospitals, is unsatisfactory."

He then described the organization of the Chicago Section and noted:

"There is a movement now afoot to raise the standards at which Clinical Chemistry is practiced in the Chicago area and the Middle West."

There being no organization of clinical chemists in the area, Dr. Natelson attended meetings of the Chicago Section of the American Chemical Society (ACS) and soon had it announced that there would be a meeting, following the regular ACS meeting, of those interested in forming a clinical chemist group. This was on January 27, 1950. It is reported that about 50 interested persons remained to hear Dr. Natelson give a sufficiently strong sales talk to inspire the group to meet again on February 17 to form the Chicago Section of the AACC and elect pro tem officers. The group continued to meet with the ACS for the rest of 1950. On September 1, 1950 the Chicago Section AACC received its charter and the pro tem officers became the first officers of the section. The Chicago Section was the fifth local section of the AACC. By the end of 1950, it had 27 members, who can be considered charter members. Of these, seven are still members in 1975.

Officers. The first officers of the Chicago Section were:

Chairman: Dr. Douglas A. MacFayden, who at the time was at Presbyterian Hospital in Chicago. He has now retired from the University of Indiana in Bloomington, where he was Director of Special Education.

Vice-Chairman: Dr. Clarence Cohn, Michael Reese Hospital. Dr. Cohn became the second chairman, and is the only past-chairman of the Chicago Section who is deceased.

Secretary: Dr. Saul Roseman, then at Bob Roberts Memorial Hospital, now Chairman of the Department of Biology and Director of the McCollum–Pratt Institute, The Johns Hopkins University.

Treasurer: Dr. Chi Che Wang, who at the time was with the Research Service, VA Hospital, Hines, Ill. She is now an Emeritus Member of the AACC, having spent a number of years at the VA Hospital in Topeka, Kan.

The officers of the Chicago Section to the present are given in Table 1. At the 25th anniversary meeting of the Chicago Section in May 1975, eight of the 14 chairmen were present, and are shown in Figure 1. One past-chairman is deceased and three are no longer members of the Chicago Section.

Two of the past officers of the Chicago Section, Drs. Melville and Kaplan, were subsequently presidents of the Association, and a third past-officer, Dr. Tietz, is the 1976 president-elect. Another past-president of the Association, Dr. Robert L. Dryer, was a member of the Chicago Section before he moved to Iowa. The section has generated one president of the Association, Dr. Hugh J. McDonald (Figure 1). Dr. McDonald had been most active on the Education Committee of the Association. He was a member of the first Board of Editors for *Clinical Chemistry* and was partly responsible for the arrangements by which Hoeber Publishing Company published the first 15 volumes of this journal. Dr. McDonald was then and still is Chairman of the Department of Biochemistry and Biophysics at the Stritch School of Medicine. He is also the Program Director of an NIH Training Grant in Clinical Chemistry for graduate and postdoctoral students. Dr. Natelson has a similar grant at the postdoctoral level.

Dr. Margaret Kaser was the national treasurer for some six years. Many other persons from the Chicago Section have served faithfully on committees of the Association.

Growth. Figure 2 compares the growth of the Chicago Section to the growth of the Association as a whole. Through much of its history, the membership of the Chicago Section comprised slightly less than 10% of the Association. Its membership lagged in the 1960–1965 period, but was bolstered by the national

Research Service, VA Hospital, Hines, Ill. 60141; and Department of Biochemistry, Stritch School of Medicine, Loyola University of Chicago, Maywood, Ill. 60153.

[1] Presented in part at the 25th anniversary meeting of the Chicago Section, May 25, 1975. Submitted at the request of the Committee on History, AACC.

Received Oct. 14, 1975; accepted Oct. 22, 1975.

Table 1. Officers of the Chicago Section

Year	Chairman	Chairman-Elect[a]	Secretary	Treasurer
1950–52	Douglas A. MacFadyen	Clarence Cohn	Saul Roseman	Chi Che Wang
1952–53	Clarence Cohn	Harry F. Weisberg	Alvin Dubin	Chi Che Wang
1953–55	Harry F. Weisberg	Alvin Dubin	Robert S. Melville	Alex Kaplan
1955–57	Alvin Dubin	G. S. Stewart	Harold Feinberg	Alex Kaplan
1957–59	G. S. Stewart	Harold Feinberg	Alex Kaplan	John F. Polli
1959–61	Harold Feinberg	John F. Polli	Grace Lawrence	Chiadae Chen
1961–63	John F. Polli	Grace Lawrence	Martin Hanke	Norbert W. Tietz
1963–65	Martin E. Hanke	Norbert W. Tietz	Edward W. Bermes	Eleanor Berman
1965–67	Norbert W. Tietz	Edward W. Bermes	Eleanor Berman	Albert A. Dietz
1967–69	Edward W. Bermes	Albert A. Dietz	Donald T. Forman	Stanley Bakshy
1969–71	Albert A. Dietz	Donald T. Forman	Morton B. Epstein	Fred Kimble
1971–73	Donald T. Forman	Morton B. Epstein	Fred Kimble	Herndon G. Shepherd
1973–74	Morton B. Epstein	Fred Kimble	Herndon G. Shepherd	John F. Kachmar
1975	Fred Kimble	Herndon G. Shepherd	Stanley Bakshy	Ramon Stoner

[a] Until 1969 the office was that of vice-chairman.

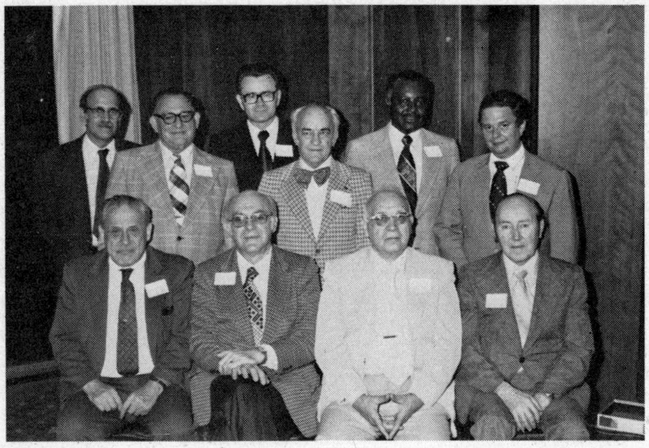

Fig. 1. Persons who helped build the Chicago Section and the AACC

Front row: Samuel Natelson, Charter Member of the AACC and Founder of the Chicago Section; Harry F. Weisberg, Chairman 1953–55; John F. Polli, Chairman 1961–63; Hugh J. McDonald, President of the AACC 1953–55; *Standing:* Morton B. Epstein, Chairman 1973–74; Alvin Dubin, Chairman 1955–57; Norbert W. Tietz, Chairman 1965–67; Albert A. Dietz, Chairman 1969–71; Fred Kimble, Chairman 1975; Edward W. Bermes, Chairman 1967–69 (Photo by P. Kirkpatrick)

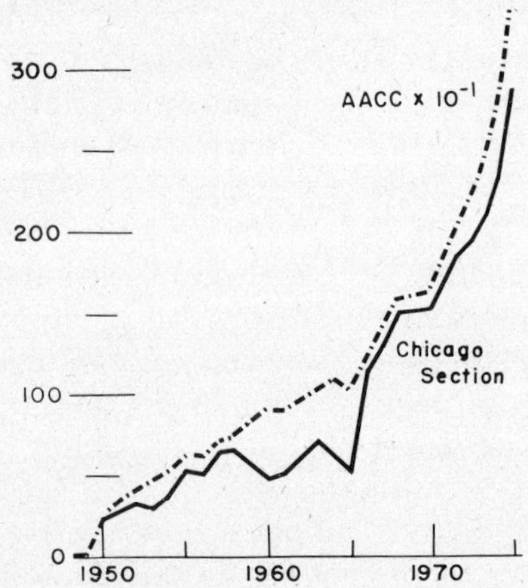

Fig. 2. Growth of the Association and the Chicago Section

The data were taken from many sources. Some are approximations, as accounts were often poor. Most values were obtained from the AACC directories, which were published in any month from January to July, and in many cases the currently unpaid members were included

meeting held in Chicago in 1965, and by an active membership committee. Most remarkable has been the growth of both the section and the Association since 1970, a time when many scientific organizations decreased in membership. In fact, half of the members have belonged to the section for less than 3.5 years (Figure 3).

Meetings. The Chicago Section has been the host for three national meetings. The 4th, in 1952, was held in Milwaukee simultaneously with an ACS meeting. It was the year the first Ernst Bischoff Award (now the AACC Award for Outstanding Contributions to Clinical Chemistry, sponsored by the Ames Co.) was given, going to Dr. Jos Kahn. The meeting was arranged by Dr. Margaret Kaser and the scientific portion was planned by Dr. Saul Roseman. The 5th national meeting, in 1953, was again held in conjunction with an ACS meeting, and was organized by Drs. McDonald and Weisberg. The program was confined to a single day. The Chicago Section also sponsored the 17th national meeting, in 1965. Mr. Alvin Dubin was the chairman of this meeting, which was the first such meeting to have an attendance exceeding 1000 persons. A highlight of the annual dinner was a talk by Lt. Col. Edward C. Knoblock on "Clinical Chemistry in Space," a popular subject at the time. It was the first year of the Warner-Lambert Lectureship, the lecture being given by Dr. Carl-Bertil Laurell, of Sweden. Dr. Natelson received the Ames Award (as it was then called) for his outstanding contributions to clinical chemistry. At this meeting it was learned that Dr. Natelson would be returning to Chicago as director of the clinical chemistry laboratories at Michael Reese Hospital. Dr. Bermes is now organizing the section to plan and administer the 29th national meeting of the Association in 1977.

During the course of its history, the Chicago Section has had joint meetings with some other societies. The section appreciates that many of its early meet-

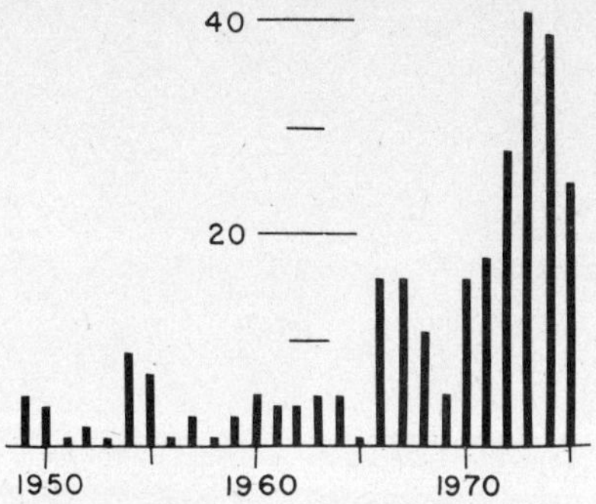

Fig. 3. 1975 membership of the Chicago Section, in terms of the year each member joined
The 1975 figure is only to July 1

ings were in conjunction with meetings of the ACS. In more recent years the section has co-sponsored one meeting each year with the Chicago Section of the ACS. At the 1975 meeting, fully half of those attending represented the AACC, although the local membership of the ACS is 20-fold that of the AACC.

Meetings have also been co-sponsored with the Chicago Pathological Society and the Gas Chromatography Discussion Group. The Chicago Section also organized the AACC activities in AAAS meetings in 1959 and 1970, Alvin Dubin being chiefly responsible for the first and Albert Dietz and Donald Forman for the last.

The section meetings in Chicago have varied considerably and have introduced a number of innovations. Relatively few meetings have featured a single speaker. A forum meeting presenting several points of views is very popular. An example of this was the meeting in January 1974 on "Regulation of in vitro Diagnostic Products," moderated by Dr. Alfred Free, with talks given by Dr. Eloise Eavenson, Mr. Larry Pilot, and Dr. Newton Ressler. [Dr. Eavenson's presentation was published in *Clinical Chemistry* with a summary of the discussion (*3*).] This section was perhaps the first to have a poster session, resulting from an observation made by Dr. Forman when he attended an international meeting in Scandinavia. Dinner meetings are held about twice a year, and have an attendance of 80–110, including guests. Short-paper meetings or workshops are held annually.

Another innovative meeting was the two-day Conference on Amniotic Fluid, held in May 1973. It was a cooperative effort of the Chicago Section of the AACC with the Gynecological, Immunological, and Pediatric Societies of Chicago. The conference, organized by Drs. Natelson, Epstein, and Ressler, was a trial adventure with the AACC Committee on Education. It featured 17 presentations by outstanding persons in the field and was supported by 14 workshops. The workshops, too, were innovative in that each was supported by a different company, but was demonstrated by a clinical chemist. Both the papers and the workshop procedures are now published as the first of a series of books on *Current Topics in Clinical Chemistry* (*4*).

The memberships in Wisconsin and Indiana are now sufficiently large to form new sections, but neither group has yet chosen to do so. Many come to the meetings in Chicago. Wisconsin has formed a clinical chemist club ("WC^3"), which meets regularly, and has a budget allowance from the Chicago Section. In addition, for the past four years, one of the meetings of the Chicago Section has been held in Wisconsin. On several occasions a meeting has been held at Elkhart, Indiana, under the sponsorship of the Ames Company (Dr. Alfred Free is an officer of this company).

Newsletter. In 1953 the Secretary, Dr. Robert Melville, started a newsletter, which continued through his term and that of Dr. Harold Feinberg. A newsletter again emerged in 1968 as the *Chicago Clinical Chemist,* which is now in its 8th volume and is issued in March, September, and December of each year. The first copy resulted from the efforts of Drs. Bermes, Dietz, and Forman; the first two have been the editors since then.

Chicago Awards. Through the efforts of Dr. Norbert W. Tietz, the Chicago Section established two Clinical Chemist Awards in 1967. The Senior Award is given to a member of the Chicago Section for contributions to clinical chemistry and the Association, and has been awarded eight times. A Junior Award (awarded six times) required that a candidate be under 30 (now 35) years of age and that he submit an original research paper that is not part of a thesis.

During its 25 years the Chicago Section has been a leader in the Association. Many of the section members feel that the Association is still faced with problems of professionalism (*5*). Some of its suggestions along these lines are taking fruit in the formation of committees on accreditation, certification, and professionalism that were generated at the 27th meeting of the Association in Toronto. Let us hope the pioneering spirit will continue.

I wish to acknowledge the help received in the form of letters from some of the early members of the Chicago Section (including Alvin Dubin, Alex Kaplan, Margaret M. Kaser, Robert S. Melville, Samuel Natelson, and Chi Che Wang) and information received in conversations with these and many others.

References

1. Reiner, M., The growth of the AACC: 25 years. *Clin. Chem.* **19,** 1409 (1973).

2. Natelson, S., Around the country. Illinois. *The Clinical Chemist* **2** (2), 10 (1950).

3. Eavenson, E., In vitro diagnostic products and FDA regulations. *Clin. Chem.* **20,** 924 (1974).

4. *Amniotic Fluid,* S. Natelson, A. Scommegna, and M. B. Epstein, Eds., John Wiley & Sons, New York, N. Y., 1974.

5. Natelson, S., The clinical chemist as a professional. *Chicago Clin. Chemist* **8,** 16 (1975).

letters

Relationship between Alkaline Phosphatase and Creatine Kinase Activity

To the Editor:

The work of Mueller et al. (*1*) was of great interest to me. In an attempt to confirm their observation, I selected 20 inpatients with abnormally high alkaline phosphatase (AP) values and another 20 with normal values, from the SMA 12/60 list. Creatine kinase (CK) activity was measured in the sera of these patients with a centrifugal analyzer (GEMSAC; Electronucleonics Inc., Fairfield, N. J. 00706) by the kinetic method of Rosalki (*2*), with use of Max-Pack reagents (Calbiochem, La Jolla, Calif. 92037). The results are shown in Figure 1. The normal range of CK in my laboratory is 10–90 U/liter for males, as compared to 5–60 U/liter in Mueller's laboratory. If we can assume that all of my values are 1.5 times greater than his, eight out of 20 (40%) of my patients with abnormally high AP have CK values lower than 30 U/liter, and one of 20 (5%) patients with normal AP has CK lower than 30 U/liter. My results correspond quite well to the six out of 17 (35%) observed in his laboratory (CK lower than 20 U/liter). Mueller et al. indicated that the low CK value in patients with high AP is more pronounced for women. My hospital is one with a patient load that is nearly 100% male, and offers no opportunity to confirm this effect in female patients.

Because patients with high AP values evidently tend to have low CK values, I did further experiments to see whether this effect is caused by AP. The alkaline phosphatase used in the experiments was extracted from placenta by using buffers as formulated by Klein et al. (*3*); the CK was from brain and heart tissue extracted with the same buffer. To study the possible effect of AP on three CK isoenzymes, I obtained these three isoenzymes by discontinuous-gradient elution from DEAE-Sephadex A-50 (Pharmacia Labs. Inc., Piscataway, N. J. 08854) as described by Yasmineh et al. (*4*). An equal amount of eluate containing CK was mixed with an equal volume of heat-inactivated (60 °C for 15 min) placenta extract containing AP and 6 U/liter residual CK and designated "test". CK and AP were assayed in these mixtures. The CK values were compared with those of control, which contained CK eluate and physiological saline instead of placenta extract. As shown in Table 1, addition of 80 to 570 U of AP per liter did not affect the CK isoenzymes. The coefficient of variation for CK determination was 4.2 and 6.1% at activities of 60 and 339 U/liter.

Addition of CK to sera of two patients with liver disease and having AP activities of 1950 and 1600 U/liter showed recovery of 99 and 102%, respectively. This recovery study also indicated that there was no other interfering substance present.

The present work and that of Wearne et al. (*5*) casts considerable doubt that AP can invalidate creatine kinase activity. Mueller et al. also examined the effect of supplementing sera with AP and agreed that AP as such has little effect.

The question still remains as to what does cause the CK activity to be low in the presence of an elevated AP. The possibility of nucleotidase interference can be ruled out, because two patients whose sera was used in the recovery study had an abnormally high serum nucleotidase activity. The enzyme adenosine triphosphatase (EC 3.6.1.3), which catalyzes the dephosphorylation of ATP, reportedly is elevated in patients with liver and bone disease (*6–8*), but we find normal adenosine triphosphatase activity in patients with liver disease.

Bruns et al. (*9*) found a CK lag phase with some sera to be so long that falsely low values would be obtained by most assay techniques. This effect is eliminated by pre-incubation with 2-mercaptoethanol. He stated that glucose phosphate isomerase activity was increased in these sera, but was not responsible for the effect. One might expect some correlation between this enzyme, AP, and glutathione reductase activity in liver disease (*10*). The latter enzyme would interfere if the commercial kit used for CK assay contains glutathione as activator.

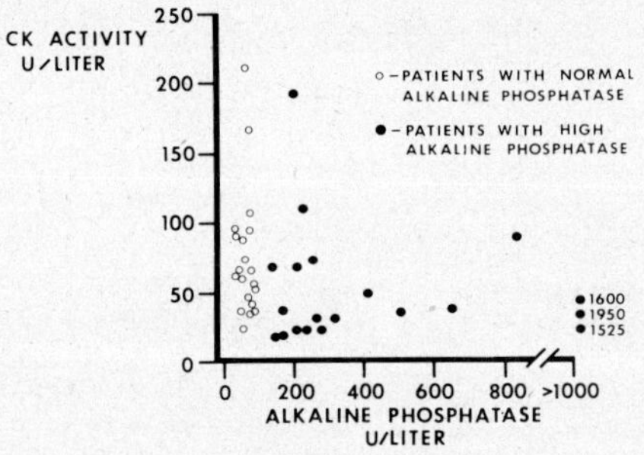

Fig. 1. CPK activity in patients with normal and abnormal AP

References

1. Mueller, R. G., Neville, K., Emerson, D. D., and Lange, G. E., Depressed apparent creatine kinase activity in sera with abnormally high alkaline phosphatase activity. *Clin. Chem.* **21**, 268 (1975). Letter to the Editor.

Table 1. Effect of Alkaline Phosphatase on Activity of CK Isoenzymes

Alkaline phosphatase, 570 U/liter					
MM	MM	MB	MB	BB	BB
T	C	T	C	T	C
66	59	45	38	134	122
Alkaline phosphatase, 360 U/liter					
MM	MM	MB	MB	BB	BB
T	C	T	C	T	C
64	60	45	38	135	124
Alkaline phosphatase, 260 U/liter					
MM	MM	MB	MB	BB	BB
T	C	T	C	T	C
64	61	43	39	136	123
Alkaline phosphatase, 180 U/liter					
MM	MM	MB	MB	BB	BB
T	C	T	C	T	C
65	62	45	40	136	124
Alkaline phosphatase, 80 U/liter					
MM	MM	MB	MB	BB	BB
T	C	T	C	T	C
65	61	43	40	133	125

2. Rosalki, S. B., An improved procedure for serum creatine phosphokinase determination. *J. Lab. Clin. Med.* **69**, 696 (1967).

3. Klein, M. S., Shell, W. E., and Sobel, B. E., Serum creatine phosphokinase (CPK) isoenzymes after intramuscular injections, surgery and myocardial infarction. *Cardiovasc. Res.* **7**, 412 (1973).

4. Yasmineh, W. G., and Hanson, N. Q., Electrophoresis on cellulose acetate and chromatography on DEAE-Sephadex A-50 compared in the estimation of creatine kinase isoenzymes. *Clin. Chem.* **21**, 381 (1975).

5. Wearne, J., Moore, R. W., and Caplan, B., Does alkaline phosphatase affect serum creatine kinase values? *Clin. Chem.* **21**, 1343 (1975). Letter to the Editor.

6. Wachstein, M., and Sigismondi, R., 5'-Nucleotidase activity and adenosine triphosphatase activity in human serums. *Am. J. Clin. Pathol.* **30**, 563 (1958).

7. Meistar, H., Dephosphorylation of adenosine triphosphate by normal and pathological human sera. *J. Clin. Invest.* **27**, 263 (1948).

8. Secchi, G. C., Rezzonico, A., and Gervasini, N., Serum ATP-ase, ADP-ase, and AMP-ase in liver cirrhosis and in hepatic coma. *Enzymologia* **33**, 125 (1967).

9. Bruns, D. E., Ladenson, J. H., and Davis, J. E., Lag phase in creatine phosphokinase (CPK) analysis. *Clin. Chem.* **21**, 987 (1975). Abstract.

10. Bing, R. J., Castellanos, A., and Siegel, A., A diagnostic value of activity of malic dehydrogenase and phosphohexose isomerase. Preliminary report of findings in patients with myocardial infarction and liver disease. *J. Am. Med. Assoc.* **164**, 647 (1957).

Swei H. Tsung

Dept. of Pathology
Medical College of Wisconsin
Milwaukee, Wis. 53233

Reuse of Disposable Sephadex Columns for a Triiodothyronine Uptake Test

To the Editor:

Triiodothyronine (T_3) uptake tests are of great help in elucidating abnormalities in the binding of thyroid hormones to serum proteins. They involve exposure of the test serum to ^{125}I-labeled T_3 and to an insoluble particulate T_3-binding material, such as various resins, coated charcoal, silicate, or Sephadex. Serum proteins and the particulate material compete for binding to the ^{125}I-labeled T_3, and the proportion bound by the particles is determined (*1*).

One such test makes use of Sephadex G-25 (fine) columns, and is available as the "Trilute" kit from Ames Co., Elkhart, Ind. 46514 (*2*, *3*). Because similar Sephadex columns may be regenerated and used repeatedly for the assay of thyroxine (*4* and Bastomsky et al., in preparation) and T_3 (*5*) in serum, we attempted to reuse the columns in the Trilute kit.

The buffer above the kit columns is stated (*2*) to be a phosphate buffer; its pH was 4.8. We therefore prepared 0.2 mol/liter phosphate–0.1 mol/liter citrate buffer, pH 4.8 (*6*). Used Trilute columns were regenerated by washing twice with 6 ml of 0.1 mol/liter NaOH, which removed all but traces of radioactivity. The columns were then washed with 6 ml of water, followed by 6 ml of our buffer. Because it was readily available, we used ^{125}I-labeled T_3 from Abbott Laboratories, North Chicago, Ill. 60064, with specific activity 460 Ci/g (a lower specific activity would probably be satisfactory); 0.03 μCi (68 pg) was added per 0.5 ml of phosphate–citrate buffer.

The same sera were assayed by using fresh columns from the Trilute kit and the ^{125}I-labeled T_3 (unknown specific activity) supplied with the kit and by using regenerated Trilute columns and ^{125}I-labeled T_3 from Abbott Laboratories in phosphate–citrate buffer. We pipetted 0.5 ml of ^{125}I-labeled T_3 onto the column, followed by 0.05 ml of serum. The serum and labeled T_3 were gently mixed by swirl-

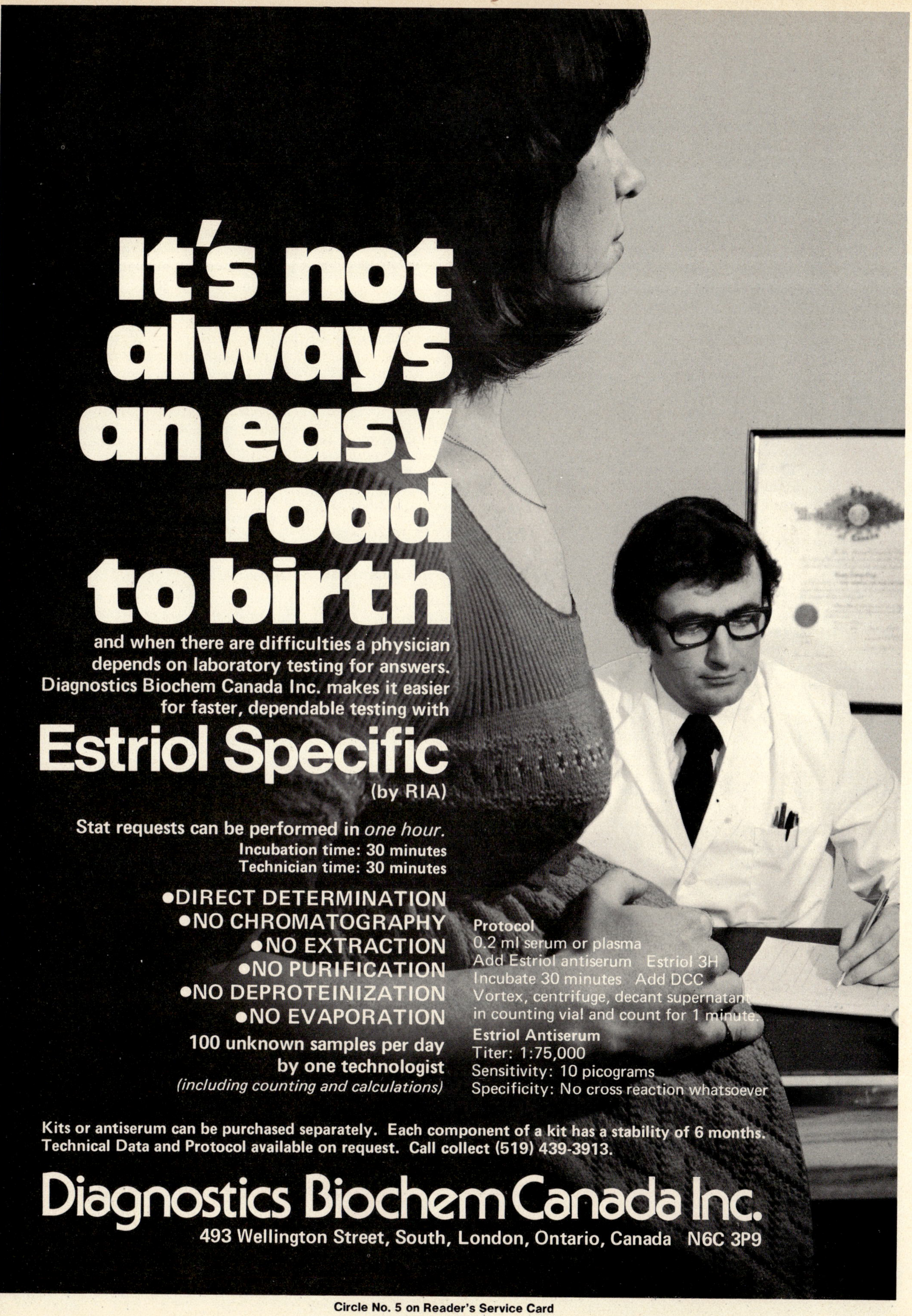

Circle No. 5 on Reader's Service Card

ing, the column was drained, and the effluent was discarded. The column was then washed with 3.0 ml of water. In the kit procedure, we determined the radioactivity retained on the columns and, for total radioactivity applied, on a column to which no serum had been added. When the regenerated columns were used, the radioactivity in the effluent and in 0.5 ml of the ^{125}I-labeled T_3 was measured. In both cases the percentage retention on the Sephadex was calculated. Figure 1 shows that while uptake of ^{125}I-labeled T_3 by Sephadex was greater when regenerated Sephadex columns and Abbott's labeled T_3 were used than when fresh columns and Ames' reagents were used, there was good correlation (r = .905) between the results. The difference may be related to the composition of the buffer, the specific activity of the ^{125}I-labeled T_3, or both. These columns can be regenerated and used repeatedly for more than 2 months (or 40 times) in a competitive protein binding assay for serum thyroxine (Bastomsky et al., in preparation) and could probably be similarly reused for measuring ^{125}I-labeled T_3 uptake. At the end of their useful life the columns can be emptied, refilled with 4.1 ml of a 50% slurry of swollen Sephadex G-25 (fine) in water, and the top porous polyethylene disc replaced. The discs are commercially available (*4*), and prepacked columns of similar dimensions may be obtained from Isolab Inc., Akron, Ohio 44321.

The same sera were also assayed for the uptake of ^{125}I-labeled T_3 by silicate (Tri-tab T_3 uptake kit; Nuclear Medical Laboratories, Dallas, Tex. 75247). Correlation between results with the Tri-tab kit and the Trilute kit was satisfactory (r = .849); correlation between results with the Tri-tab kit and the regenerated column procedure was good (r = .932).

We conclude that it is feasible to reuse Sephadex G-25 (fine) columns to assay T_3 uptake. Normal values would have to be determined for each laboratory, and where room temperature is not constant a temperature correction factor may have to be established (*2*).

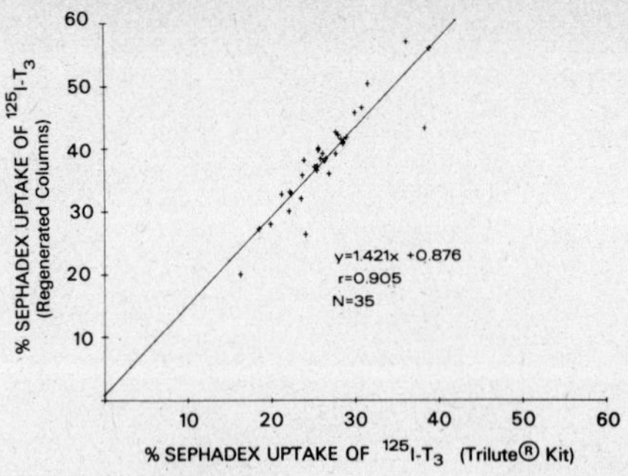

Fig. 1. Comparison of ^{125}I-labeled T_3 Sephadex uptake by Trilute kit and by regenerated columns

References

1. Ingbar, S. H., and Woeber, K. A., The thyroid gland. In *Textbook of Endocrinology*, R. H. Williams, Ed., 5th ed., Saunders, Philadelphia, Pa., 1974, p 137.

2. Instruction Sheet, "Trilute® ^{125}I T-3 Reagent Kit", Ames Co., Division of Miles Laboratories, Elkhart, Ind. 46514.

3. Leonards, J. R., Correlation between results of a new T-3 test and the percentage of free thyroxine in serum. *Clin. Chem.* **16,** 922 (1970).

4. Alexander, N. M., and Jennings, J. F., Analysis for total serum thyroxine by equilibrium competitive protein binding on small, re-usable Sephadex columns. *Clin. Chem.* **20,** 553 (1974).

5. Alexander, N. M., and Jennings, J. F., Radioimmunoassay of serum triiodothyronine on small, reusable Sephadex columns. *Clin. Chem.* **20,** 1353 (1974).

6. McKenzie, H. A., pH and buffers. In *Data for Biochemical Research,* R. M. C. Dawson, D. E. Elliott, W. H. Elliott, and K. M. Jones, Eds., 2nd ed., Oxford University Press, London, 1969, p 484.

C. H. Bastomsky
D. B. Frenkel-Leith[1]
J. Lamoureux

McGill University Clinic
Royal Victoria Hospital and
Division of Nuclear Medicine
Notre Dame Hospital
Montreal, Quebec, Canada

[1] Summer student.

Creatine Kinase Isoenzyme BB in Serum of Renal-Disease Patients

To the Editor:

In their recent study on creatine kinase (CK) isoenzyme separation by batch adsorption on glass beads, Henry et al. (*1*) used a salt concentration that would also desorb the BB isoenzyme. BB activity, if present, would result in a false-positive signal for MB. The authors were not particularly troubled by this, because there have been few reports of BB in human serum.

Ion-exchange procedures, differential inhibition or activation, and immunological approaches to CK isoenzyme separation offer several attractive advantages over electrophoretic procedures. In many of these methods, however, BB and MB are measured as one fraction. It is important, therefore, to collect data documenting the occurrence of BB in serum in various pathological conditions. If its appearance is frequent or widespread, the need to separately identify MB and BB would be critical to avoid the consequences of false-positives.

We wish to report on the presence of CK-BB in serum in patients with renal failure under dialysis. We analyzed serum from 43 such patients for a variety of constituents. CK was assayed by a kinetic ultraviolet-coupled method, and CK isoenzymes were separated on agarose gel, followed by fluorometric scanning. The isoenzyme test was considered positive when the fraction was 3% or more of the total. Of the 43 patients, 20 had total CK values above our laboratory reference range of 125 U/liter. Nineteen of the 20 demonstrated abnormally high BB fractions. Two of those demonstrating BB also had an increased MB fraction; and in each case, BB activity exceeded MB.

The diagnostic value of separating CK isoenzymes is now well established, not only in medical patients (*2*), but in surgical patients and patients undergoing diagnostic procedures as well (*3*). The clinical documentation of this test has been performed by electrophoretic methods, and it behooves all of us working in this area to be aware of the potential pitfalls of alternative methodology.

References

1. Henry, P. D., Roberts, R., and Sobel, B. E., Rapid separation of plasma creatine kinase isoenzymes by batch adsorption on glass beads. *Clin. Chem.* **21,** 844 (1975).

2. Galen, R. S., Reiffel, J. A., and Gambino, S. R., Diagnosis of acute myocardial infarction. *J. Am. Med. Assoc.* **232,** 145 (1975).

3. Galen, R. S., The enzyme diagnosis of myocardial infarction. *Hum. Pathol.* **6,** 141 (1975).

Robert S. Galen

Dept. of Pathology
Columbia Univ. College of
Physicians and Surgeons
New York, N. Y. 10032

Further Use of the Sure-Sep Technique for Serum-Plasma Separation

To the Editor:

Mathies has evaluated the "Sure-Sep" serum-plasma separation (General Diagnostics, Morris Plains, N. J. 07950) for the rapid and efficient separation of cell-free serum or plasma from whole blood (*1*). Since 1958, the separation of serum from blood collected in glass or *inert* plastic containers in this Unit has been by double centrifugation in order to remove all cellular elements, before deep-freeze storage. The final preparation has been examined under oil-immersion phase-contract microscopy (90 × 1.6 × 15) for cellular elements and debris, and by spectrophotometry for serum hemo-

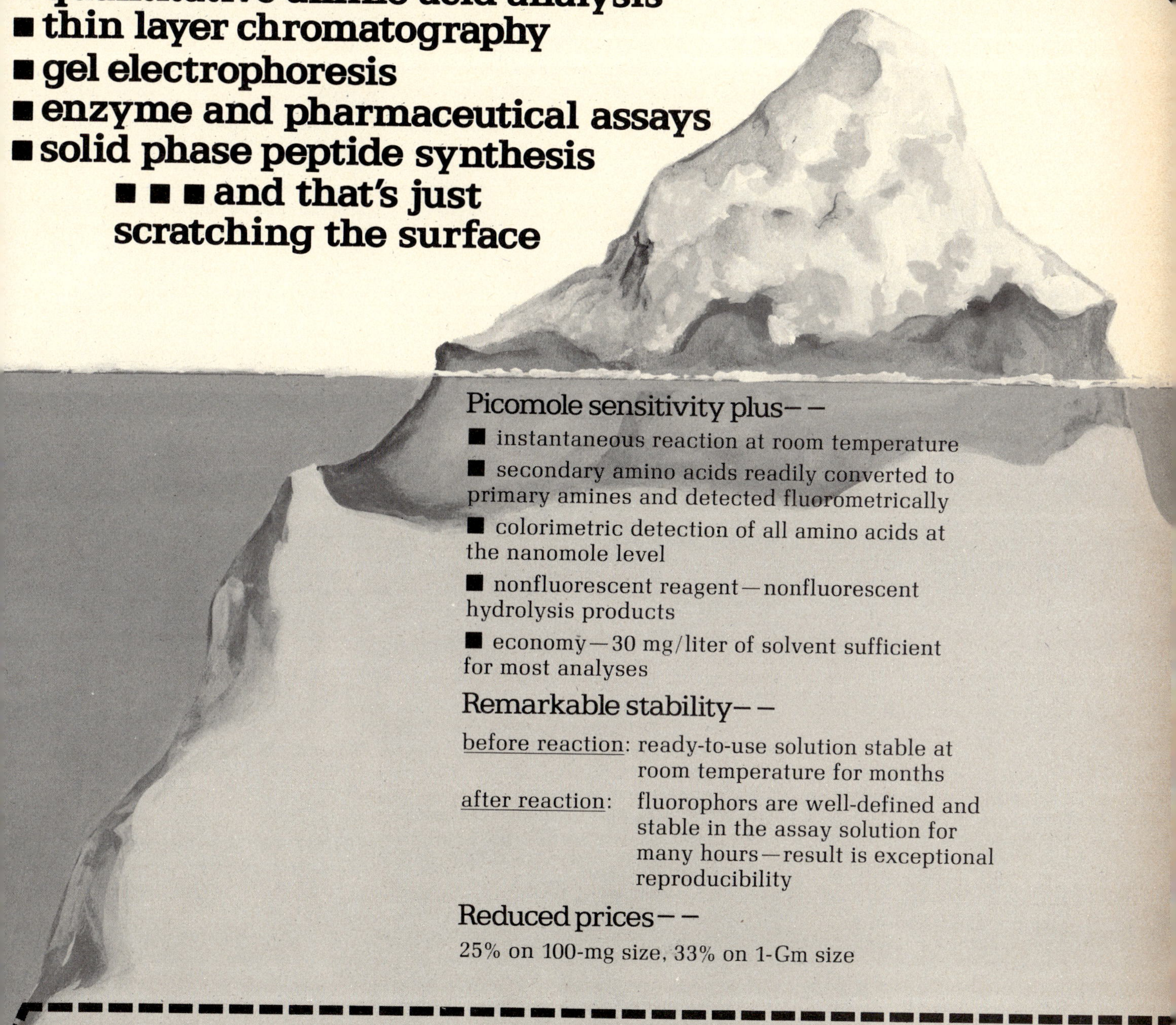

globin. It is essential in any long-term storage of serum to ensure its freedom not only from leukocytes and platelets, but also from erythrocytes, because the latter will undergo hemolysis on freezing during storage and thawing for subsequent analysis. Examination of serum obtained from one-stage "Sure-Sep" separation has revealed complete absence of leukocytes, platelets, erythrocytes, or debris from fragmented cellular elements, as well as very low serum hemoglobin values.

In confirmation of the findings reported (*1*), no statistically significant differences for glucose, total protein, uric acid, and creatine kinase were found after conventional centrifugation, double centrifugation, or the Sure-Sep centrifugal separation. For other enzymes recorded by Mathies—viz., alkaline phosphatase, lactate dehydrogenase, and asparate aminotransferase—values after double centrifugation or Sure-Sep were statistically identical and lower than for the single centrifugation separation. Contributions come from leukocytes and platelets and, to a lesser degree, erythrocytes.

In addition, the following estimations have been performed with and without Sure-Sep, and no statistical significant differences have been found:

(1) cholesterol, enzymatic (*2*); triglyceride, enzymatic (Boehringer Mannheim, W. Germany);

(2) phenylalanine and tyrosine, fluorometric;

(3) enzymes, viz. aldolase; 5-nucleotidase; amylase (Phadebas, Pharmacia, Uppsala, Sweden); β-glucuronidase; oxytocinase; diamine oxidase; and *N*-acetyl-β-glucosaminidase and other hydrolytic lysosomal enzymes, fluorometric, with 4-methylumbelliferone substrates; and

(4) radioimmunoassays, e.g., triiodothyronine uptake; thyroxine; triiodothyronine (*3*); insulin; cortisol, ^{75}Se-labeled (Radiochemical Centre, Amersham); ^{57}Co-Vitamin B_{12}; ^{125}I-folate; and ^{125}I-IgE (Phadebas).

Advantages of the Sure-Sep method were further evidenced by its use in field trips in Southern Africa and for samples collected from members of the South African National Antarctic Expeditions (SANAE Base, 70° 60′ S, 2° 30′ W), where previously the separation of serum entailed a minimum of two centrifugations before storage in an underground storage chamber (−10 to −20 °C). Each annual expedition reaches SANAE in February and leaves the following February, so that samples are stored for as long as 13 months under these conditions; tests have indicated adequate preservation of most constituents under these conditions.

(Supported by the Atomic Energy Board of the Republic of South Africa.)

References

1. Mathies, J. C., Evaluation of a new device for rapidly separating serum or plasma from blood. *Clin. Chem.* **20,** 1573 (1974).

2. Bernstein, R. E., Enzymic assay for serum total cholesterol. *Clin. Chim. Acta,* to be published.

3. Bernstein, R. E., and Clur, P. J. G., Direct radioimmunoassay for serum triiodothyronine. In preparation.

Ralph E. Bernstein

Metabolic Research Unit
South African Institute for Medical Research
Hospital St.
Johannesburg 2001, South Africa

Optimal γ-Glutamyltransferase Assay?

To the Editor:

The assay system for γ-glutamyltransferase (EC 2.3.2.2) optimized at 37 °C presented by Rosalki and Tarlow (*1*) has recently been challenged (*2*). Prior to the observation that the substrate γ-glutamyl-*p*-nitroanilide was readily soluble in dilute hydrochloric acid, we used a kinetic assay procedure with the LKB 8600 reaction rate analyzer, initiating the reaction with the acceptor, glycylglycine. We did not observe any indications of significant "internal transpeptidization" when we compared substrate and acceptor initiation in manual evaluation. The substrate concentration at this time was 4.0 mmol/liter in the reaction mixture.

We have since investigated the substrate optimum, using substrate initiation according to Rosalki and Tarlow, and the results are shown in Figure 1. Other variables were in good agreement with Rosalki and Tarlow. In a comparison of the automated kinetic assay procedure at two substrate concentrations—4.0 mmol/liter (A) and 9.0 mmol/liter (B)—on 30 sera, we obtained a correlation coefficient (*r*) of 0.99 with a regression equation of A = 0.79B − 1.88. In a brief study of 24 sera we compared the techniques of Rosalki and Tarlow (*1*) and Tarbit (*2*) and found a correlation coefficient (*r*) of 0.99, with a regression equation of $y = 0.72\,x + 0.97$ (y = method of Tarbit, x = method of Rosalki and Tarlow).

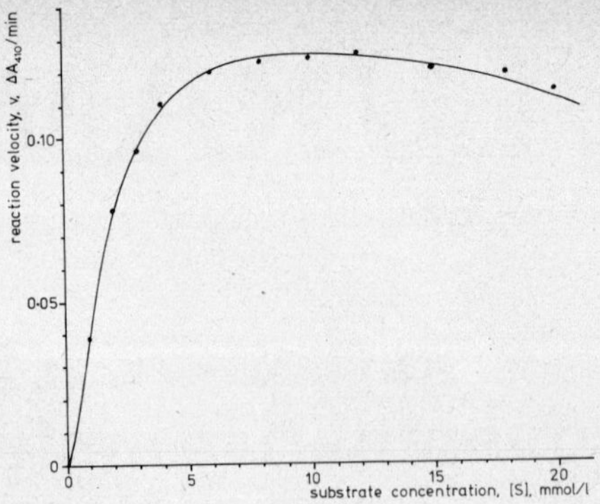

Fig. 1.

Our results agree closely with those of Rosalki and Tarlow, indicating that maximal γ-glutamyltransferase activity is shown as a substrate concentration of 9.0 mmol/liter, although we did not see such a high degree of substrate inhibition at higher concentrations.

References

1. Rosalki, S. B., and Tarlow, D., Optimized determination of γ-glutamyltransferase by reaction-rate analysis. *Clin. Chem.* **20,** 1121 (1974).

2. Tarbit, I. F., More economical γ-glutamyltransferase assay. *Clin. Chem.* **21,** 1548 (1975). Letter to the Editor.

C. P. Price
J. O'Meara
P. R. Wenham

Department of Clinical Chemistry
East Birmingham Hospital
Bordesley Green East
Birmingham B9 5ST, U.K.

Dissenting View on Computer Systems

To the Editor:

The "J. Lloyd Johnson Report" recently reviewed in your pages [*Clin. Chem.* **21,** 1554 (1975)] is sometimes regarded as a complete and authoritative survey of the clinical laboratory computer systems. Because of the importance of the subject, you may perhaps allow your readers to see a dissenting opinion.

The Johnson Report, privately published at $60, is based on an erroneous assumption that vitiates the entire report. This assumption, which is totally unexamined anywhere in the report, is that the principal problem in laboratory computing is *data acquisition.* It

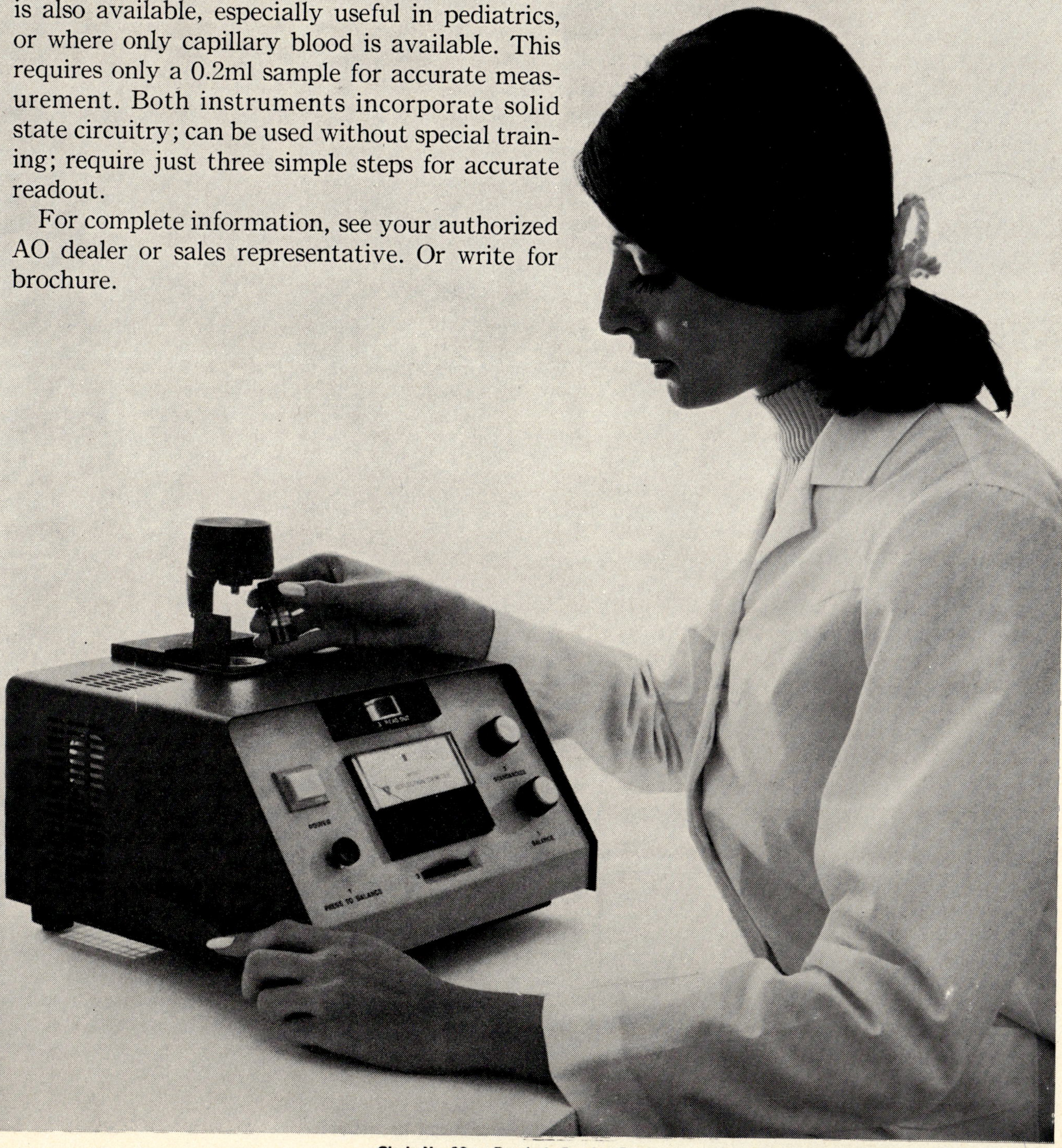

is not: the principal problem is *communication with the physician;* and by ignoring this problem, by directing their attention exclusively to on-line, real-time data-acquisition systems, Johnson Associates have grossly distorted the current picture of laboratory computerization and have done a disservice to clinical laboratories generally.

Not only is on-line real-time data acquisition *not* a legitimate first priority, it is even doubtful whether it should be part of a laboratory system at all. Our experience with the successful operation of a computer system in our laboratory over the last five years has conclusively established that we do not need on-line real-time. Our system is more reliable over all, and costs far less both initially and in total laboratory operating costs, than any of the turn-key systems described in the Johnson Report.

A significant improvement in clinical laboratory service will come when laboratory computer systems are used to provide cost-effective reports to physicians in clinical practice. We need an objective analytical survey of the systems now in use to see how far they meet this objective. The Johnson Report does not satisfy our need.

Samuel Raymond

William Pepper Laboratory
Hospital of the University of Pennsylvania
Philadelphia, Pa. 19104

Effect of Urobilinogen on Urinary Estrogen Determination

To the Editor:

Many substances may interfere with the spectrophotometric determination of urinary estrogens (*1, 2*). In several instances we noticed the presence of a peak at 496 nm when scanning urinary extracts after the development of Kober chromogens. This peak makes it impossible to apply the standard Allen correction to the peak reading at 536 nm and to obtain the correct concentration of estrogens in urine.

Urines exhibiting this phenomenon were found to contain increased amounts of either urobilinogen or urobilin. To test the assumption that the above substances are responsible for the interference, a urine containing 3 Ehrlich units of urobilinogen per 100 ml was used for determination of urinary estrogens by Cohen's method (*3*). A peak at 493 nm was found on scanning.

We then sought ways to correct for this interference. To this end, the urine containing urobilinogen was mixed with different pregnancy urines, the estrogen content of which had been previously determined. Reading of absorbance was made as recommended by Cohen, at 496, 536, and 576 nm (Method A), or at 521, 536, and 551 nm (Method B). Method A gave results that were between 58.9% and 94.1% of the values found originally in equivalent amounts of the urine. It is of interest that the differences were progressively greater with increasing urobilinogen(U):estrogen(E) ratio (EU vs. mg per volume). Thus the 58.9% and 94.1% correspond to U:E ratios of 5.3 and 0.9, respectively. With Method B the values for urinary estrogens in specimens containing urobilinogen were 82 and 100% of equivalent aliquots of the original urine for U:E ratios between 5.3 and 0.9. The losses of estrogens in urobilinogen-containing urines observed by us are far lower than those described by Wood (*4*), who also did not observe any correlation of the low value with the increases in U:E ratio. However, apparently greater amounts of urobilinogen or urobilin (or both) were dealt with.

It is suggested that in urines containing moderate amounts of urobilinogen, the absorbance be read at 521, 536, and 551 nm.

References

1. Adlercreutz, H., paper given at the First European Congress of Clinical Chemistry, Munich, 1974.
2. Adlercreutz, H. In *Proc. Vth International Symposium on Quality Control in Clinical Chemistry,* Geneva, Switzerland, 1973.
3. Cohen, S. L., A method for the rapid colorimetric assay of total estrogens in pregnancy urine. *J. Clin. Endocrinol.* **26,** 994 (1966).
4. Wood, G. P., Urinary estrogen assays and maternal hyperbilirubinemia. *Obstet. Gynecol.* **45,** 133 (1975).

Sophie Heiberg
Donald J. Campbell
Jiri Frohlich

Division of Clinical Chemistry
Vancouver General Hospital
Vancouver, B.C., Canada V5Z 1M9

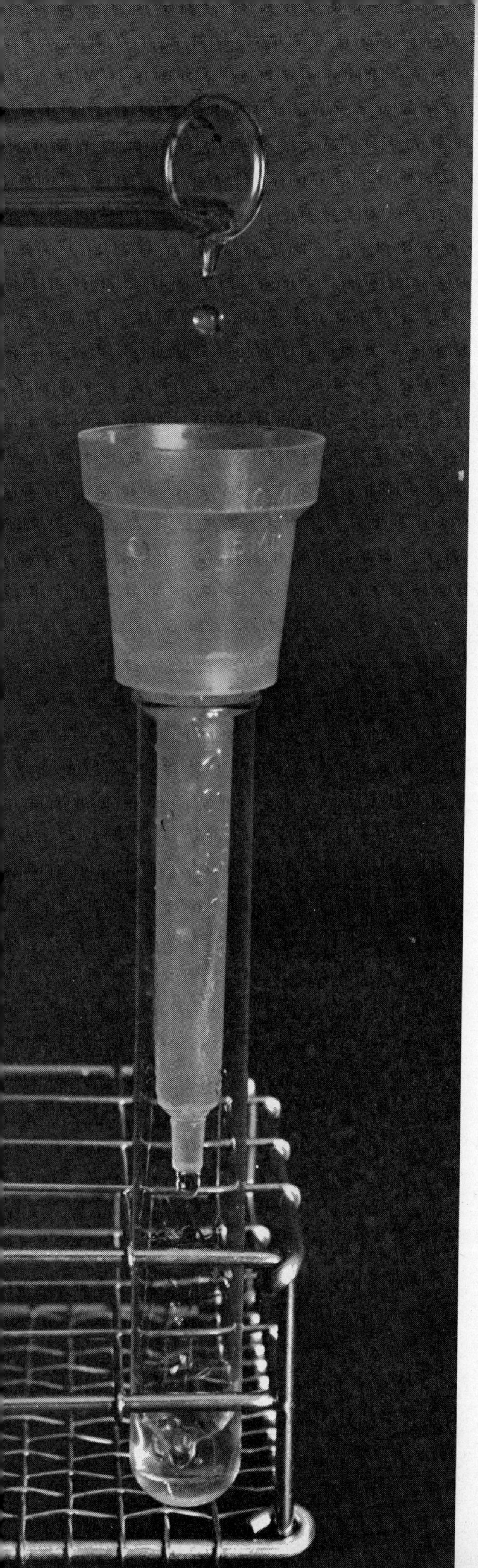

book reviews

Practical Clinical Chemistry. G. Toro and P. G. Ackermann. Little, Brown and Co., Boston, Mass. 02106, 1975, xix + 779 pp.

In the preface to this volume the authors state, "While working in the clinical laboratory, during professional consultations, and in the process of research and teaching medical technology students, we frequently felt the need of a book that would treat the subject of clinical chemistry in greater detail and emphasize at the same time some of the more recent developments in clinical laboratory techniques, such as automation and radioimmunoassay methods. As none of the clinical laboratory texts currently available seemed to fit these needs, the present book was developed."

The authors then devote four chapters to (*a*) laboratory instruments using light measurement, (*b*) physical and other miscellaneous methods, (*c*) chromatography and electrophoresis, and (*d*) normal values, quality control, and units. These chapters are designed to supply the clinical laboratory practitioner with the theoretical background needed for the practice of clinical chemistry. Unfortunately these chapters are a mine of misinformation, sweeping generalizations, and incorrect statements.

In chapter 1 the authors discuss the phenomenon of fluorescence. On page 24 they state, "Since some of the energy is lost in the process of absorption and reemission, the emitted light must always be of longer wavelength (lower energy) than the exciting light." This statement completely neglects *resonance* fluorescence, the type one encounters in the important field of atomic fluorescence.

Chapter 2 is concerned mainly with physical chemistry and methods based on the measurement of physical chemical variables. The first topic the authors introduce is ion-selective electrodes. The opening sentence is, "The use of these electrodes is an electrical method for measuring the concentration of certain ions in solution." Potentiometric electrodes do *not* measure concentration, but activity. The authors mention activity at the bottom of the page (p 27), but fail to define it. Furthermore, the statement "This [activity] will be equal to the concentration in very dilute solutions . . ." will be true only if ionic strength considerations are neglected. In solutions of biological materials where appreciable ionic strengths may be encountered, the activity and the ionic concentration in dilute solutions will be quite different.

The discussion of the oxygen electrode that follows several pages later is completely wrong. The authors suggest that one should make the electrodes and currents small so as not to electrolyze the oxygen too fast. Actually, the current that arises from this amperometric oxygen electrode is proportional to the rate of diffusion of oxygen to the electrode. Two pages later (p 32) the authors describe polarography. It is obvious from their description of the technique that they have never performed a polarographic analysis and have no conception of the underlying theory.

Chapter 2 contains no discussion of reaction kinetics, a topic that the authors touch on in chapter 14, on enzymes. However, the treatment given in chapter 14 makes no mention of reaction order.

Chapter 4 deals with normal values, quality control, and units. The discussion of normal values makes no mention of diurnal variations, although other, less-important factors affecting the results are enumerated. Further, this chapter does not take up the statistical concept of regression analysis even though this is of particular importance in kinetic methods.

Chapter 5, on carbohydrates, makes repeated reference to "blood glucose." However, no mention is made of differences between serum and plasma glucose or about glucose stability in serum samples. On page 114 in this chapter the authors state that glucose may be determined by a coulometric method. This is true, but not by the method they describe. They claim the use of "a coulometric oxygen electrode similar to that used for the measurement of blood P_{O_2}." The Beckman Glucose Analyzer (their ref. 100) makes an amperometric measurement of decreased oxygen tension and determines the glucose concentration from the known kinetics for the oxidation of glucose. Guilbault's method (ref. 97) employs an enzyme electrode consisting of a layer of glucose oxidase-impregnated polyacrylamide over a hydrogen peroxide-sensitive electrode. As hydrogen peroxide is produced a current flows and this current is proportional to the glucose concentration. This is *not* what the authors describe.

Electrolytes is the heading for chapter 9. In the section on "Oxygen Saturation" under a subheading "Coulometric Methods," the reader is greeted by an old friend, the Clark electrode. The determination of oxygen with the Clark electrode involves an amperometric, *not* a coulometric, measurement.

The quotation from the preface that introduced this review emphasized the need for chapters dealing with automation and radioimmunoassay. This latter topic is discussed in chapter 15. The opening sentences read, "The basic principle of both competitive protein binding assay (CPB) and radioimmunoassay (RIA) is the quantitative combination of the substance to be measured with a protein that binds the substance. The three major requirements for all such assays are: availability of a radioactive labeled form of the substance to be measured, a protein that will specifically bind the substance, and a method for separating the protein-bound material from the material that is not bound." CPB does *not* require "a radioactive labeled form of the substance," as is well documented by Savory and others.

Chapter 20 is on hydrogen-ion concentration. This chapter contains a three-page, high school-level discussion of pH and a two-page description of buffer preparation, followed by many helpful tables of buffer mixtures. Even though the authors cite the work of Roger Bates, they cling to the dated (1909) definition of pH which *cannot* be measured. Much has been written about our current understanding of the concept and this information should be given to the practitioners of clinical chemistry. To do otherwise is a disservice.

Countless errors of a less fundamental nature abound in this volume. All of these errors seem to be based on physical chemical principles and the authors' lack of understanding in this area. One example this reviewer could cite is the Nernst equation and the authors' statement that the constant contains the reciprocal of the absolute temperature (the constant is proportional to the first-power of the temperature). Another example is the def-

inition of the freezing point as "the point at which the solid and liquid phases are in equilibrium and hence have the same vapor pressure." This is a common error found in beginning college chemistry texts but not to be found in physical chemistry books.

The chapter on automation (chapter 19) is derived mainly from the manufacturers' descriptions of their own products. Therefore these descriptions tend to point out the advantages of the instrument and omit any disadvantages. It would have been more helpful to the reader if critical user appraisal could have been included for each instrument mentioned.

This book does contain a large number of clinical chemistry procedures, which are well indexed for easy access. A rapid index on the inside front cover is particularly useful. However, the conceptual errors are so numerous that this reviewer cannot recommend purchase of this volume.

William C. Purdy

Department of Chemistry
University of Maryland
College Park, Md. 20742

Laboratory Techniques for the Detection of Hereditary Metabolic Disorders. V. E. Shih. CRC Press, Cleveland, Ohio 44128, 1973, 125 pp. $27.00.

This book is rather exorbitantly priced at $27.00. It offers nothing new on anything that hasn't been published previously. The preface states that the book is "to provide a disease oriented rather than technique oriented approach" and yet this certainly is not evident in the text. The best parts of the book are the tables; the first chapter is an excellent example of this. This book might be useful to the small hospital laboratory that is not familiar with some of these techniques, but otherwise will not find wide acceptance in the medical profession.

A. W. Renuart

Department of Pediatrics
Duke University Medical Center
Durham, N. C. 27706

Chromatography: A Laboratory Handbook of Chromatographic and Electrophoretic Methods, 3rd ed. E. Helfmann, Ed. Van Nostrand Reinhold Co., New York, N. Y. 10001, 1975, xxx + 969 pp. 200 illustrations. $47.50.

The Editor is to be complimented on an exposition of chromatography whose burden is carried by many distinguished authorities in the field. The practicing clinical chemist does not need to know the contents of this book, but if he is complacent in his ignorance of these most important separation techniques he will relegate himself to an unimaginative technician. As the chemical basis of metabolic disease, genetic aberrations, pharmacological action, and nutrition become explainable at a molecular level, the practice and principles of chromatography will become of overwhelming importance. This book is therefore recommended to the clinical chemist for study and inspiration.

Some answer to A.J.P. Martin's interesting foreword to this volume is possible. For example, ion-exchange chromatography is capable today of very high resolution and detection of amino acids, for example, to the 10^{-12} mole quantities or even one or two orders of magnitude less, by means of the earlier ninhydrin reaction or by the more recently introduced fluorescent reactions with fluorescamine or *o*-phthaldehyde. His plea to use various chromatographic techniques in combination is well taken.

There is a valid criticism of this book, in that there are at least two treatments of the theory of chromatography, chapter 3 and chapter 12. The latter chapter makes use of the very sophisticated treatment by E. Gluekauf, whose work was a milestone in the theory of chromatography. However, the random-walk treatment of J. Calvin Giddings, by virtue of its direct flexible and elegant simplicity, should replace all other theories. It also allows highly imaginative approaches to the study of the many variables and parameters that are part of the art of chromatography. Moreover, Giddings' definition of plate height, $H = d(\sigma^2)/d(L)$, keeps one clear of the ambiguities inherent in the older ideas derived from distillation theory.

For the clinical chemist, this text is not easy reading, but it contains a real wealth of information that will grow in relevance to his daily work. The contents are too voluminous to review in detail. There are 14 chapters on fundamentals in liquid-column, paper, thin-layer, gas, gel, and ion-exchange chromatography and on electrophoresis. There are 20 chapters on specific practical applications, e.g., amino acids, lipids, terpenoids, steroids, carbohydrates, drugs, nucleic acids, chlorophylls and phenolic compounds, pesticides, antibiotics, inorganic ions, nonhydrocarbon gases, and hydrocarbons. There is a subject index, but no author index. The price restricts private ownership to the dedicated, but the book should be available for reference.

Paul B. Hamilton

Alfred I. du Pont Institute
Wilmington, Del. 19899

Books Received

Laboratory Manual of Cell Biology. D. O. Hall and S. E. Hawkins, Eds. Crane, Russak and Co., New York, N. Y. 10017. 281 pp. Paperback, $9.75. Pub. 1975.

Chemical Analysis. An Advanced Text and Reference. 2nd ed. H. A. Laitinen and W. E. Harris. McGraw-Hill Company, New York, N. Y. 10020. xv + 611 pp. $19.95. Pub. Jan. 1975.

Biochemistry of Antimicrobial Action, 2nd ed. J. T. Franklin and G. A. Snow. Halsted Press, New York, N. Y. 10016. xii + 224 pp. $16.75. Pub. Aug. 1975.

Collected Tentative Rules and Recommendations of the IUPAC-IUB Commission of Biochemical Nomenclature, 2nd ed. vi + 149 pp. paper bound. $3.00. Pub. June 1975. A compilation of all published tentative rules and recommendations published through May 1975, edited only to eliminate superseded sections, and made available, with the concurrence of the Commission and of the Committee of Editors of Biochemistry, by the American Society of Biological Chemists. Remittance in U. S. dollars must accompany orders to: American Society of Biological Chemists, Inc., 9650 Rockville Pike, Bethesda, Md. 20014.

Concepts of Membranes in Regulation and Excitation. M. Rocha e Silva and G. Suarez-Kurtz, Eds. Raven Press, New York, N. Y. 10036. xi + 226 pp. $16.50. Pub. Aug. 1975.

Advances in Cyclic Nucleotide Research, 6. P. Greengard and G. A. Robison, Eds. Raven Press, New York, N. Y. 10036. 358 pp. $22.50. Pub. Aug. 1975.

The Gangliosidoses. B. W. Volk and L. Schneck, Eds. Plenum Press, New York, N. Y. 10011. xv + 277 pp. $22.50. Pub. 1975.

Advances in Chromatography, 13. J. C. Giddings, E. Grushka, R. A. Keller and J. Cazes, Eds. Marcel Dekker, Inc., New York, N. Y. 10016. xiv + 324 pp. $28.50. Pub. Aug. 1975.

Organophosphorus Stereochemistry, Part I: Origins and P(III and IV) Compounds. W. E. McEwen and K. D. Berlin, Eds. Dowden, Hutchinson & Ross, Inc., Pubs., distributed by Halsted Press, New York, N. Y. 10016. xviii + 387 pp. $30.00. Pub. Aug. 1975.

the clinical chemist

Compiled by J. S. King, Executive Editor

2nd International Symposium on Clinical Enzymology, Chicago, October 27–29, 1975

Three years ago, a Symposium on Clinical Enzymology was held in Chicago at the Mount Sinai Hospital Medical Center. Although on that occasion the participants were mainly from North America, several speakers from overseas ensured that international views were not neglected. Earlier this year the organizer of that Symposium, Dr. Norbert W. Tietz, judged that the time was ripe to reexamine the field of clinical enzymology, again with international participation. The aptness of his timing of this second Symposium (co-sponsored by AACC, ACLPS, ASCP, CAP, CDC, IFCC, and NCCLS) was confirmed by the attendance of more than 300, who were addressed by some 25 invited speakers. Both speakers and audience included representatives of many countries, and discussion was often lively. Three aspects of clinical enzymology were mainly considered: methodology, materials for quality control, and instrumentation.

Methodology. Different analytical approaches to the measurement of alkaline phosphatase, aspartate aminotransferase, and creatine kinase were debated. For all three enzymes, alternative attempts toward "standardization" and current developments in the understanding of the biochemistry of the enzymes were presented.

For alkaline phosphatase it appears that agreement is close as regards the choice of *p*-nitrophenylphosphate as substrate. Use of a phosphorylating buffer gained wide support also. However, arguments as to the relative merits of diethanolamine and AMP showed that the choice of such a buffer is not without its problems.

The main discussion about aspartate aminotransferase was whether or not pyridoxal phosphate should be added to reactivate any apoaminotransferase before measurement. Although well founded on a theoretical basis, several practical problems have to be considered if this additional step is to be included in routine procedures. Also, the clinical interpretation of measurements of the enzyme may be influenced by this change in methodology.

Variables in the three-step coupled reverse reaction for the measurement of creatine kinase now seem to be so well understood that the method can be used with confidence in routine service in most laboratories. Nevertheless, it remains unclear whether addition of *N*-acetyl cysteine or other -SH containing substances will reactivate fully all the creatine kinase after storage in vitro during various periods.

In the section on methodology the proposals for recommended methods put forward by national committees in Europe (Germany, United Kingdom, Scandinavia, and France) and in the USA were presented and compared to each other and to the efforts of the Expert Panel on Enzymes of IFCC. The differences, although still of some importance, are relatively small and are mainly related to the choice of reaction temperatures. Results were presented showing the beneficial effects of method-standardization in some regions (e.g., Scandinavia).

Quality control and materials used for calibration. The approaches used in proficiency surveys in enzymology and their relationship to internal and other kinds of external quality control schemes were presented. The importance of the choice of enzyme preparations and their effects on the results obtained was exemplified for aspar-

Luminaries at the 2nd International Symposium on Clinical Enzymology, Chicago

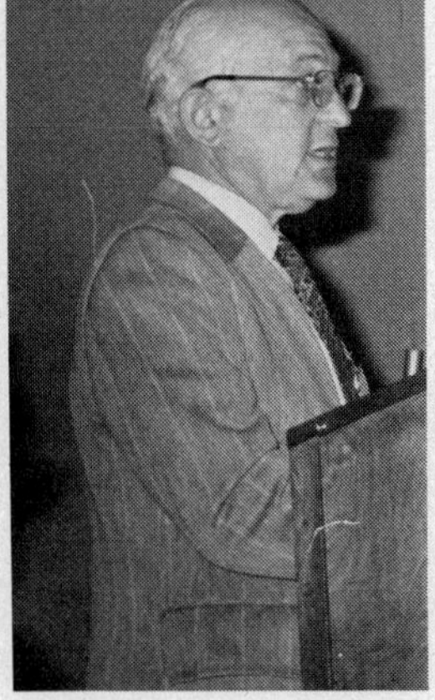

Keynote speaker: David Seligson, M.D., Sc.D., Yale University

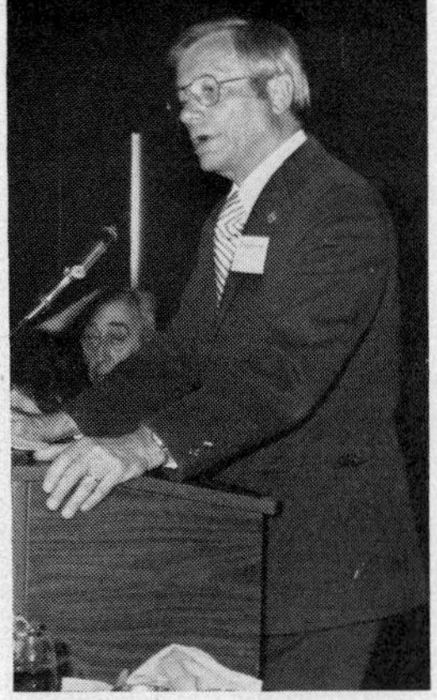

Banquet: Dennis B. Dorsey, M.D., President, College of American Pathologists, addressing seminar participants

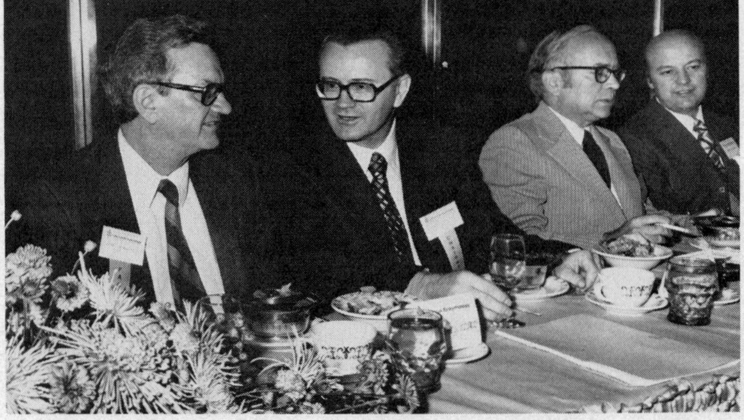

Banquet (*left to right*): Joseph H. Boutwell, Jr., Ph.D., M.D., Acting Assistant Director, Bureau of Labs, CDC; Norbert W. Tietz, Ph.D., Program Director; Royden N. Rand, Ph.D., 1976 President AACC; Donald Moss, Ph.D., Expert Panel on Enzymes, International Federation of Clinical Chemistry

tate aminotransferase and alkaline phosphatase. The requirements for such materials as regards their identity with human enzymes in serum were discussed. It appears that enzymes from animal sources can be used, if their identity with human enzymes in certain kinetic properties is documented. On the other hand, the use of an enzyme from a human source does not of itself guarantee that the material will be appropriate for use in quality control. This was clearly shown for human placental alkaline phosphatase, which in several respects is unlike the alkaline phosphatases that are commonly present in serum.

During this part of the program it was mentioned briefly that the requirements as regards the source of enzyme and the matrix in which it is dissolved vary, depending on the application to which material is to be put; e.g., for internal or external quality control, or for the secondary calibration of methods.

Instrumentation. In the session on instrumentation it was clearly pointed out that the user can only with difficulty test many of the performance parameters of a particular instrument. However, alternative approaches were proposed. Although the principle of the measurement must be that the variables are traceable back to the base units of measurements (i.e., spectrophotometric constants, volumes, and time), this does not necessarily mean that all different steps of the measurement procedure must be available for testing. For example, an overall assessment of the spectrophotometric components (lamp, lenses, amplifier) and the cuvette, by measurement of the absorbance of well-defined, stable reference standards, may be preferable to the separate assessment of each of the above-mentioned components.

For measurements at 340 nm, the production of an accurately known amount of NADH from glucose in the hexokinase-coupled reaction probably is superior to any "calibration" by sequential assessment or to the use of other calibrators such as dichromate.

The need for collaboration between producers and users of instruments became quite clear during the session.

The last session concerned the selection of reaction temperature. Theoretical and practical aspects were presented, especially in favor of 30 and 37 °C. Whereas the provisional choice of the EPE/IFCC of 30 °C seems to be the only temperature usable in *reference* methodology, this does not exclude the use of 37 °C or other temperatures in routine methodology. Data were presented indicating that, if the reaction conditions are identical except for temperature, it is possible to use factors for the transformation of results. It is encouraging, therefore, to see methods published by several semi-official "enzyme committees" for the measurement of more and more enzymes that differ only in the choice of reaction temperature, since this may not be the insuperable barrier to comparison that it once was thought to be. The dispute over reaction temperature has not prevented the development of scientifically founded and experimentally verified methodology, nor has it materially affected the quality of results produced in individual laboratories.

This stimulating Symposium made it quite clear that methodological limitations will not restrict the application of measurements of enzyme activities to clinical medicine. Compared with the first symposium, a much higher standard of information was evident in the debate on all three topics, indicating the steady advance experienced in the field. A further encouraging sign was the willingness of most clinical enzymologists to contemplate the adoption in their laboratories of recommended or standardized methods of various levels of complexity, even though this will entail some loss of freedom of individual scientific choice.

Mogens Hørder

Arhus, Denmark

D. W. Moss

London, England

Ed. note: Plans are underway for publication by AACC of these proceedings in a book. AACC ACCENT credit (20 h) was approved for this program.

Reference Materials

Standard Reference Materials: Glass Filters As a Standard Material for Spectrophotometry—Selection, Preparation, Certification, Use SRM 930 is the title of a 110-p NBS Special Publication 260-51, issued November 1975 (for sale at $1.90 (+ 25% for foreign) by U. S. Govt. Printing Office, Washington, D. C. 20402; cat. No. C13.10:260-51). Authors are R. Mavrodineanu and J. R. Baldwin, of the National Bureau of Standards. Book contains much information on spectrophotometric theory and practice.

Ca Reference Materials. Calcium Serum Reference Materials are available to clinical research laboratories from:

1. the Massachusetts Society of Pathologists Quality Control Program
2. the Illinois Society of Pathologists Quality Control Program

These reference materials, for which the calcium value has been established by the definitive calcium method of the U.S. National Bureau of Standards recently, have been made available to clinical research investigators and others who are interested in the accuracy of serum calcium measurements. The material is available as lyophilized serum. The concentration is known to within 1 SD = 0.17 mg/liter and a CV of 0.18% at the 100 mg/liter concentration.

The definitive isotope dilution/mass spectrometry method for calcium has been established by the Institute of Materials Research of the U.S. National Bureau of Standards. This method, developed originally for atomic-weight research analysis, has now been applied to serum. The two agencies listed below are making available the lyophilized material as technology multipliers of the sophisticated NBS definitive method technique. Analytical data will be supplied with the materials.

For further details, write to:

1. Dr. Jerald M. Rosenbaum, Director
   Massachusetts Society of Pathologists
   Regional Quality Control Program
   Springfield Hospital
   Department of Pathology
   Springfield, Mass. 01107

or

2. Dr. Gerald G. Hoffman, Director
   Illinois Society of Pathologists
   Lake Forest Hospital Laboratory
   660 North Westmoreland Rd.
   Lake Forest, Ill. 60045

Symposium on "Porphyrin Measurements: Laboratory and Clinical Aspects"

This symposium, sponsored by the Capital Section, AACC, and by the NIH, will be held January 22, 1976, at Wilson Hall, NIH, Bethesda, Md. 20014. It is supported by a grant from the American Instrument Co., so there is no registration fee. It features six speakers and a panel discussion. The program has been approved for 5 hours AACC ACCENT credit and for ASMT PACE credit.

For further information: D. E. Uddin, Ph.D., Naval Medical Research Institute, Bethesda, Md. 20014.

"Clinical Laboratory Developments" Reviewed

The increasing recognition of clinical chemistry as a distinct, maturing discipline is most recently exemplified in the November 1975 issue of *Federation Proceedings* (vol. 34, pp 2115–2165), which contains the above Special Topic. Contributors, and their subjects, are: Donald S. Young (introduction, and paper on "Interpretation of clinical laboratory data"), R. Dybkaer ("Nomenclature of laboratory results in medicine"), J. Paul Cali ("Reference materials in clinical chemistry"), Charles D. Scott ("Advanced technology for the clinical laboratory"), Merle A. Evenson ("Developments in therapeutic drug monitoring and alkaloid analysis"), Helen K. Berry ("Screening for genetic disorders"), Robert F. Ritchie ("Specific protein assay"), Martin Fleisher and Morton K. Schwartz ("Hormone analysis: bioassay and immunochemical methodology"), Russell K. Hobbie and Richard L. Reece ("Computer interpretation of laboratory test results"), and David L. Sackett ("Laboratory screening: a critique").

Neither these names nor these subjects are strangers to readers of *Clinical Chemistry*. It is pleasing to see this felicitous overview of clinical chemistry presented to the biological community at large by this panel of experts, who represent the profession well in this distinguished journal.

Plasma Proteins, Second Edition

AACC Editor Theodore Peters, Jr. is the author of a chapter on "Serum Albumin" in the newly issued second edition of the biochemical classic "The Plasma Proteins" (F. W. Putnam, Ed., Academic Press; 2 vol., with a third to come in early 1976).

Awards

Joseph H. Roe Award, Capital Section. Dr. William J. Campbell, AACC Executive Director, received the annual Roe Award from this section on December 10, in ceremonies at the Walter Reed Army Medical Center.

Hycel Young Investigator Award. The Organizing Committee of the 28th national meeting invites significant, original contributions to the science of clinical chemistry to be submitted for the Hycel Young Investigator Award.

The award will consist of an honorarium of $1000 and a scroll, which will be awarded at the 28th national AACC meeting in Houston, Texas. The awardee will be expected to present his/her contribution at that meeting.

Candidates must be a member, associate, or affiliate of the Association and under 35 years of age as of April 1, 1976.

Six copies of the manuscript, prepared by following the guidelines for publication in *Clinical Chemistry* (pp 1–4, this issue) must be submitted to Alan Broughton, M.D., Chairman, Awards Committee, 28th National AACC Meeting, P.O. Box 20661, Astrodome Station, Houston, Tex. 77025, by April 1, 1976. The application form on this page must accompany the entry; additional forms are available from the Chairman of the Awards Committee in Houston.

The successful entrant will be notified by June 30, 1976.

Meetings

AACC national meetings

1976, Houston, Texas, Aug. 1–6
1977, Chicago, Ill., July 17–22
1978, San Francisco, Calif., July 23–28

HYCEL YOUNG INVESTIGATOR AWARD APPLICATION

Name ______________________ Date of birth ____________

Home address ______________________

City ____________ State ____________ Zip ____________

Employer ______________________

Employer's address ______________________

City ____________ State ____________ Zip ____________

Membership Status

____Member

____Associate

____Affiliate

By signing below, the undersigned applicant hereby affirms (1) that the applicant meets the qualifying conditions of this application, (2) that the applicant will submit the research paper to a recognized scientific journal for publication and acknowledges the award in so doing, and (3) that the applicant agrees and understands that Hycel, Inc., the AACC, and any committee or organization which reviews or is associated with this application shall not be held responsible in any manner whatsoever as to selection of the winner or any dispute arising from this application.

____
Signature

1979, New Orleans, La., July 15–20
1980, Boston, Mass., July 20–25
1981, Kansas City, Mo., July 19–24
1982, Southern Calif.
1983, New York City, July 9–15

Therapeutic Drug Monitoring (2nd Pine Mountain Conf. on Clin. Chem.), Calloway Gardens, Pine Mountain, Ga., Mar. 28–Apr. 1, 1976 (Write: Pine Mt. Conf., Box 29134, Atlanta, Ga. 30329 (see details in *Clin. Chem.* **21,** 1696).

Pittsburgh Conference on Analytical Chemistry and Applied Spectroscopy: Cleveland, Ohio, March 1–5, 1976. Includes symposia on history, gas chromatography, future trends in clinical chemistry.

7th International Symposium on Clinical Enzymology, Venice, April 5–7, 1976. (Write A. Burlina, Center for Clinical Enzymology, General Hospital, I-31015 Conegliano, Italy).

Analytika 76, Munich, April 9–13, 1976. (Write: General Secretary Frau Dr. R. Vogel, Klin.-chem. Inst., D-8 München 2, Nassbaumstrasse 20, Germany.

Symposium on Evaluation of Clinical Laboratory Automation in the Americas, March 3–5, 1976, Mexico City. IFCC sponsored. (Write: SECLA Coordination Center, Suite 215, 1025 Connecticut Ave., N.W., Washington, D. C. 20036).

International Symposium on Quantitative Mass Spectrometry in Life Sciences. June 17–18, 1976, Rijksuniversiteit Gent. (Contact: Prof. Dr. A. De Leenheer, Symposium Chairman, Laboratoria voor Medische Biochemie en voor Klinische Analyse, 135 de Pintelaan, B-9000 Gent, Belgium).

Protides of the Biological Fluids, 24th. April 27–May 1, 1976. Brugge, Belgium. (Write: Secretariate, XXIVth Colloquium "Protides of the Biological Fluids," Simon Stevin Instituut, Jerusalemstraat 34, B-8000, Brugge, Belgium.

AAAS, Feb. 18–24, 1976, Boston, Mass.

ASCP/CAP, Mar. 19–25, 1976, Dallas, Tex.

Int. Acad. Pathol. (U. S. and Canadian Div.), March 23–27, Boston, Mass.

ACS, April 4–9, 1976, New York City

FASEB, April 11–16, 1976, Anaheim, Calif.

ASMT, June 20–25, 1976, Chicago

IUB, 10th Int. Congr., July 25–31, 1976, Hamburg

ACS, Aug. 29–Sept. 3, 1976, San Francisco

2nd European Congr. Clin. Chem., Oct. 3–8, 1976, Prague

Xth Int. Congr. Clin. Chem., Feb. 26–Mar. 4, 1978, Mexico City

National Registry in Clinical Chemistry

Dr. Schwartz elected President of NRCC. Dr. Morton K. Schwartz was elected President of the Board of Directors of the National Registry in Clinical Chemistry at the Board's regular fall meeting held in New York City on November 14, 1975. Dr. Schwartz, an NRCC certified Clinical Chemist, has been a member of the Registry Board since 1973, representing the American Society of Biological Chemists. He has also been a member of the Registry's Examination Committee since 1973 and served as its Chairman in 1974. Long active in the field of clinical chemistry, Dr. Schwartz recently completed a one-year term as President of the American Association of Clinical Chemists and currently is Chairman of its Council.

The Registry's new Vice President for 1976 is Dr. A. Wendell Musser, representative of the American Society of Clinical Pathologists. Dr. Musser is Chief of Staff of the VA Hospital in Lexington, Kentucky.

Dr. Marge A. Brewster was elected to a three-year term on the Registry Board as a representative of the American Board of Clinical Chemistry. Dr. Brewster, Assistant Professor of Pathology at the University of Arkansas, was certified by the Registry as a Clinical Chemist in 1971 and became a Diplomate of ABCC in August 1974. She replaces Dr. Robert S. Melville, an original member of the Registry's Board of Directors, who retired after serving three terms.

In other business, the Registry's Board evaluated the results of the October 6, 1975, examination administered to 52 individuals. Those who passed and were certified for 1976 at the Clinical Chemist (CC) and Clinical Chemistry Technologist (CCT) levels are:

Trichey Balsubramanian	CC
Roger R. Calam	CC (Upgraded from CCT)
B. K. Chandrasekhar	CC (Upgraded from CCT)
Ai-Shuan S. Cherng	CC
Linda A. Cranmer	CCT
Walter A. Dechtiaruk	CCT
James K. Fleming	CCT
George V. Foster	CC
Eric Frow	CC
Ann S. Gibson	CCT
Melvin R. Glick	CC
Ronald L. Gombos	CC
Robert J. Heyka	CCT
Pai C. Kao	CC
Navid A. Khan	CCT
Vera Kucera	CC
Sharon K. Laska	CCT
Sharon S. Lin	CCT
Philip B. Menderhausen	CC
M. Gayle Murphy	CC (Upgraded from CCT)
Govindbhai H. Patel	CCT
Raman D. Patel	CCT
Mario J. Peralta	CCT
Bernard A. Selby, Jr.	CCT
Chandrakant K. Shah	CCT
Linda G. Shrader	CCT
Leona E. H. Smythe	CCT
John I. Sup	CCT
Christopher P. Tse	CCT
Teh Y. Wang	CC
Homer R. Yeh	CC
Ernest E. Young	CC (Upgraded from CCT)

One pre-experience candidate from the University of South Florida, James Connolly, took and passed the CCT exam and will be eligible to apply for certification upon completion of one year of acceptable clinical chemistry experience.

In addition, the following students from Dr. Julius Kerkay's clinical chemistry program at Cleveland State University also passed the CCT exam and are eligible for certification upon receipt of their M.S. degree:

David J. Dabbs
Mark W. Johnson
Chin-Chan L. Lee
Ann-Sheng Liu
Henry A. Pawlowski
Sam E. Sato
Nathan T. Scanzillo
Robert C. Wojak
Wuu Shyong Frank Yang

Continuing the policy established during July 1975, candidates requesting their raw scores on the exam will be given the maximum raw score, the range of raw scores, and their raw score for each of the three sections of the exam. The next examination will be given on June 7, 1976.

During its day-long meeting, the Registry Board accepted the proposal of the Examination Committee headed by Miss Sylvia Blatt to begin immediately an item-solicitation drive for questions to be used in future revisions of both Registry examinations. The Committee developed a broad content outline of subject matter to be represented in the pool of questions from which future examinations will be constructed. Areas where questions are particularly needed were highlighted.

Individuals interested in submitting questions for the Registry's examinations, or in obtaining more information on its bilateral certification program, should contact: Mrs. Suzanne B. Roethel, Executive Director, National Registry in Clinical Chemistry, 1155 16th Street, NW, Washington, D. C. 20006, Telephone: (202) 659-9660.

New Societies

AAMI BMET Society. A new society of biomedical equipment technicians has been established in affiliation with the Association for the Advancement of Medical Instrumentation.

The society will provide a means by which the BMET can, nationally, promote the BMET as a professional; institute and implement programs that will further the stature of the BMET; offer guidance and suggestions on the certification of the BMET; promote and sponsor symposia for the advancement and training of the BMET; and further goals of the health-care community.

The Society of Biomedical Equipment Technicians was formed in 1975 by an ad hoc committee of 13 BMETs, located throughout the United States, with support from the Association for the Advancement of Medical Instrumentation.

During the summer of 1975, the ad hoc committee formulated bylaws for the society. These bylaws were circulated to regional groups of BMETs and published in the *BMET News* for comment.

During AAMI's 1976 annual meeting, March 21–25, Atlanta, Ga., the society bylaws, officers, and directors will be ratified.

For further information contact Michael J. Miller, AAMI, 1901 N. Ft. Myer Drive, Suite 602, Arlington, Va. 22209.

Clinical Radioassay Society. Chapter officers of the Clinical Radioassay Society met Tuesday, October 28, 1975, at the Commodore Hotel in New York City. Present were: Dean S. Skelley, John Langan, Robert Grimaldi, Patrick A. Scollin, Jeno P. Bercz, David S. Marsden, Rao Chervu, Grafton D. Chase and Martin Marcus. Their purpose was to merge all chapters into a national organization and plan a joint meeting in the spring of 1976. A pro-tem National Executive Committee was elected with the listed officers:

Martin Marcus Chairman	Fordham Hospital Southern Blvd. & Crotona Ave. Bronx, N.Y. 10458
Grafton Chase Associate Chairman	Philadelphia College of Pharmacy & Science 43rd & Kingsessing Mall Philadelphia, Pa. 19104
Rao Chervu Secretary	Albert Einstein College of Medicine Division of Nuclear Medicine 1300 Morris Park Ave. Bronx, N.Y. 10538
David Marsden Treasurer	Roosevelt Hospital 428 West 59th St. New York, N.Y. 10019

Other members of the Board of Directors are:

John Langan Program Director	Nichols Institute P.O. Box 624 Princeton, N.J. 08540
Peter Bercz Fund Raising	Medical Diagnostic Services Inc. 4531 Reading Road Cincinnati, Ohio 45229
Dean Skelly	Baylor College of Medicine Department of Obstetrics & Gynocology Houston, Tex. 77025
Robert Grimaldi Membership	New England Medical Center 171 Harrison Ave. Boston, Mass. 02111
Patrick Scollin Membership	New England Medical Center 171 Harrison Ave. Boston, Mass. 02111

Chairmen of newly formed chapters will become members of the Board of Directors. The program director will assist new and existing chapters in the selection of speakers for regularly scheduled meetings. This would provide continuing and varied educational programs free from redundancy and leading to audio-visual teaching aids and publication of a proceedings or perspective type journal derived from the lectures.

The society will conduct a two-day symposium on a date in May to be announced. The program will consist of one day dedicated to practical techniques, trouble shooting the assay, quality control procedures, and statistics, and a second day on new procedures, including RIA in cancer diagnosis and therapeutic drug monitoring.

Instrumentation Course

Du Pont Instruments' Scientific & Process Division is offering its customers a formalized instruction program to increase operational efficiencies and to reduce downtime. It is designed to provide a fuller understanding of the practical aspects of instrument technology and maintenance.

The program consists of courses in liquid chromatography, photometric analysis, mass spectrometry, leak detection, and thermal and moisture analysis. Each covers one or more modules on a specific facet of instrumentation and is designed for the knowledgeable operator rather than for the beginner.

The subject matter reviews areas such as circuitry, components, accessories, potential trouble spots, and maintenance. A program can be customized to meet unique customer needs. After an initial counseling, a course outline with appropriate modules is provided.

For additional information, write to Du Pont Co., Instrument Products Division, Wilmington, Del. 19898.

Life Science Separations

Life Science Separations is a new bimonthly publication from Waters Associates. Each issue will explain a different aspect of liquid chromatography as it relates to the analysis or purification of biological/biomedical materials. In addition, a separate page of this publication will contain advance notice of scientific meetings and seminars of interest to the biological/biomedical community and an offering of new literature describing liquid

chromatographic separations of biomedical samples.

For a free introductory copy, write Waters Associates, Inc., Maple Street, Milford, Mass. 01757.

Science Citation Index Now Searchable On-Line

The Institute for Scientific Information (ISI) has announced that it will work with Lockheed Information Systems (LIS) to provide information specialists and researchers with online, interactive, computer searches of the journal literature from the full range of scientific disciplines. Now fully operational, the ISI/LIS service is called SCISEARCH and is designed to give quick, easy, and economical access to one of the world's largest multidisciplinary science literature files. Initiation of the service marks the first time the complete *Science Citation Index (SCI)* data base will be available for on-line searches.

SCISEARCH will cover every significant item (articles, reports of meetings, letters to the editor, editorials, correction notices, etc.) from about 2500 of the world's most important science journals and will offer initially a file of about 800 000 items published from January 1974 to the present. Each month, approximately 40 000 new items will be added. By July 1976, the file will cover the most current 30 months of the literature and will total over one million items.

Searchers will be able to use SCISEARCH 12 to 15 hours each weekday; six hours on the first and third Saturdays of each month. These extensive search periods will be a convenience for searchers in the United States and Canada and will permit Europeans to take advantage of the new service.

For further information, contact Richard Sweet, Product Manager, Data Base Services, Institute for Scientific Information, 325 Chestnut St., Philadelphia, Pa. 19106 (215/923-3300).

NCHLS Elects

The following officers, for calendar year 1976, were elected by the National Council on Health Laboratory Services at its annual meeting in Arlington, Va., on November 8, 1975:

Chairman: Kurt M. Dubowski, Ph.D.; Vice-Chairman: Ralph B. Lingeman, M.D.; Secretary-Treasurer: Dennis W. Weissman.

Immediate past-chairman and a member of the Executive Committee is Mr. David Birenbaum. The newly elected officers represent AACC, American Society of Clinical Pathologists, and American Society for Medical Technology, respectively. Dr. Morton K. Schwartz will retire from his present position as Secretary of NCHLS at the end of this year.

By vote of NCHLS, the membership dues of member organizations were set at $100 for calendar year 1976.

Poster Sessions

A recent Eastman advertisement says it well:

> There is restlessness among the masses who are expected to sit quietly in the gloom fighting off Morpheus while a succession of fellow scientists, terrified or cocky as the case may be, mumble or declaim. The only questions which need to be asked by those familiar with the subject at hand will—likely as not—be turned off by the chair for lack of time, and the speaker will escape to the dark recesses of a concurrent session.
>
> A "poster session" is an adult version of the school science-fair format. The presentation is boiled down to what can be put up in readily legible words and graphics on a board of, say, 8 × 10 feet. It remains up for some hours. The peers drift by and look it over. When discussion ensues, the presenter need feel no embarrassment to learn more from the questioner than vice versa. The occasion is less of a performance and more of an exchange at a mutually agreeable level of discourse among parties fascinated by the topic.
>
> The passerby need not come ready equipped with that fascination. It can be engendered on the spot, right then and there.

Peck Order

Frederick W. Dehme, D.V.M., Ph.D., the editor of *Veterinary Toxicology,* a quarterly publication of the American College of Veterinary Toxicologists, has given us permission to reprint the following instant, but anonymous, classic.

The Order of Things . . .

The Dean

Leaps tall buildings in a single bound
Is more powerful than a locomotive
Is faster than a speeding bullet
walks on water
Gives policy to God.

The Department Head

Leaps short buildings in a single bound
Is more powerful than a switch engine
Is just as fast as a speeding bullet
Talks with God.

Professor

Leaps short buildings with a running start and favorable winds
Is almost as powerful as a switch engine
Is faster than a speeding BB
Walks on water in an indoor swimming pool
Talks with God if special request is approved.

Associate Professor
Barely clears a Quonset hut
Loses tug of war with locomotive
Can fire a speeding bullet
Swims well
Is occasionally addressed by God.

Assistant Professor
Makes high marks on the walls when trying to leap tall buildings
Is run over by locomotives
Can sometimes handle a gun without inflicting self-injury
Treads water
Talks to animals.

Instructor
Climbs the walls continually
Rides the rails
Plays Russian roulette
Walks on thin ice
Prays a lot.

Graduate Student
Runs into buildings
Recognizes locomotives two out of three times
Is not issued ammunition
Can stay afloat with a life jacket
Talks to walls.

Undergraduate Student
Falls over doorstep when trying to enter buildings
Says "look at the choo-choo"
Wets himself with a water pistol
Plays in mud puddles
Mumbles to himself.

Department Secretary
Lifts buildings and walks under them
Kicks locomotives off the tracks
Catches speeding bullets in her teeth and eats them
Freezes water with a single glance
She is God.

Forthcoming Papers

An Integrated Approach to Lipid Profiling: Enzymatic Determination of Cholesterol and Triglycerides with a Centrifugal Analyzer
Peter W. Wentz, Robert E. Cross, and John Savory

Creatine Kinase Isoenzyme Patterns in Human Tissue Obtained at Surgery
Swei H. Tsung

p-Hydroxybenzoic Acid Hydrazide Procedure for Serum Glucose Adapted to thg Technicon "SMA 12/60", and Compared with Other Glucose Methods
John J. Ferraro, Francis A. Caccavo, and Abraham Saifer

Sample Stability: A Suggested Definition and Method of Determination
Ralph E. Thiers, Gaw T. Wu, Allen H. Reed, and Lawrence K. Oliver

Analysis for Indole Compounds in Urine by High-Performance Liquid Chromatography with Fluorometric Detection
Anthony P. Graffeo and Barry L. Karger

Erythrocyte Porphyrin Analysis in the Detection of Lead Poisoning in Children: Evaluation of Four Micromethods
Thomas L. Hanna, David N. Dietzler, Carl H. Smith, Santosh Gupta, and Harold S. Zarkowsky

Rapid Micromethod for Blood Lead Analysis by Anodic Stripping Voltametry
George Morrell and Giri Giridhar

Evaluation of a Discrete-Sample Computer-Directed Clinical Analyzer
Roger L. Forrester, Willa Collinge, Pattie Hashimoto, and Jackie Worrall

Effect of Halothane Anesthesia on Muscle, Liver, Thyroid, and Adrenal-Function Tests in Man
Robert E. Johnstone, Eric M. Kennell, Walter Brummund, Jr., Leslie M. Shaw, and Richard C. Ebersole

Long-Term Quality-Control Charting: A Simple Method
Arthur W. Gottmann, Jerome S. Nosanchuk, and Gail S. Anderson

Direct Determination of Serum Chloride with a Semiautomated Discrete Analyzer
Stanley S. Levinson,

Complement C3 in Serum and Plasma, as Measured by Radial Immunodiffusion with Four Commercial Kits
Adrian O. Vladutiu and Barbara M. Winiarski

Serum Lipoamide Dehydrogenase in Serum: A Preliminary Report
John W. Pelley, Gwynne H. Little, Tracy C. Linn, and Frank F. Hall

High-Performance Colorimeter with an Electronic Bubble Gate for Use in Miniaturized Continuous-Flow Analyzers
William E. Neeley, Stephen C. Wardlaw, Tad Yates, William G. Hollingsworth, and Maurice E. T. Swinnen

Double-Antibody Enzyme Immunoassay Applied to Human α_1-Fetoprotein
Luc Belanger, Diane Hamel, Didier Dufour, and Marcel Pouliot

Determination of the Molar Absorptivity of NADH
Robert B. McComb, Lawrence W. Bond, Robert W. Burnett, Richard C. Keech, and George N. Bowers, Jr.

Parallel Electrophoretic Fractionation of Alkaline Phosphatase and Serum Protein on Cellulose Acetate Strips: Clinical Evaluation
Angelo Burlina and Lauro Galzigna

Improved Assay for Urinary 17-Hydroxycorticosteroids
Yutaka Ariyoshi and Yoshio Osawa

CLIN. CHEM. 22/2, 141–150 (1976)

Determination of the Molar Absorptivity of NADH

Robert B. McComb, Lawrence W. Bond,[1] Robert W. Burnett, Richard C. Keech,[2] and George N. Bowers, Jr.

The molar absorptivity of NADH at 340 nm has been determined by an indirect procedure in which high-purity glucose is phosphorylated by ATP in the presence of hexokinase, coupled to oxidation of the glucose-6-phosphate by NAD^+ in the presence of glucose-6-phosphate dehydrogenase. The average value from 85 independent determinations is 6317 liter mol^{-1} cm^{-1} at 25 °C and pH 7.8. The overall uncertainty is −4.0 to +5.5 ppt (6292 to 6352 liter mol^{-1} cm^{-1}), based on a standard error of the mean of 0.48 ppt and an estimate of systematic error of −2.6 to +4.1 ppt. Effects of pH, buffer, and temperature on the molar absorptivity are also reported.

Oxidation–reduction reactions involving the nicotinamide adenine dinucleotides (NAD^+, $NADP^+$, and their reduced forms) have become a cornerstone in quantitative biochemical analyses. Likewise, in recent years, the prodigious growth of clinical enzymology has to a large extent involved enzymes for which these nucleotides are essential cofactors. Because the nicotinamide adenine dinucleotides are relatively unstable complex compounds with many functional groups, they have not been well characterized. This is particularly true with respect to the molar absorptivity at the analytically sensitive wavelength, 340 nm.

Clinical Chemistry Laboratory, Hartford Hospital, Hartford, Conn. 06115.

Presented in part at the 26th national meeting of the American Association of Clinical Chemists, Las Vegas, August, 1974.

Ed. note: A second paper on this same subject appears in this issue (Zeigenhorn et al.).

[1] Present address: Department of Pathology, St. Vincent Hospital and Medical Center, Toledo, Ohio 43608.

[2] Present address: Department of Pathology, Memorial Hospital Medical Center of Long Beach, Long Beach, Calif. 90801.

Received Sept. 22, 1975; accepted Nov. 6, 1975.

Although estimates of the molar absorptivity had been made prior to 1948 (*1*), it was not until then that Horecker and Kornberg (*2*) performed a series of experiments in which the molar absorptivity of NADH was determined with some degree of certainty. These workers followed changes in absorbance of reaction mixtures in which known amounts of substrate were completely consumed. The average value for six analyses that included three different enzymes and a three-fold range of substrate concentration was 6220 (range, 6110 to 6310). Although several reports of a slightly higher figure have appeared (*3*, *4*), 6220 has remained the authoritative figure for the molar absorptivity for reduced nicotinamide adenine nucleotides during the past three decades.

The availability of high-purity glucose, recently introduced as Standard Reference Material 917 by the National Bureau of Standards, has provided an alternative means of estimating the molar absorptivity of NADH. The method is essentially that proposed by the Subcommittee on Glucose of the AACC Committee on Standards as the Reference Method for glucose, in which the phosphorylation of glucose and subsequent oxidation of the glucose-6-phosphate product is coupled to the reduction of NAD^+ (*5*):

$$\text{D-Glucose} + \text{ATP} \xrightarrow[Mg^{2+}]{\text{hexokinase}} \text{D-glucose-6-phosphate} + \text{ADP} \quad (1)$$

$$\text{D-Glucose-6-phosphate} + NAD^+ \overset{\text{G6PDH}}{\rightleftarrows} \text{D-glucono-}\delta\text{-lactone 6-phosphate} + \text{NADH} + H^+ \quad (2)$$

D-Glucono-δ-lactone 6-phosphate +

$$H_2O \rightleftharpoons \text{6-phosphogluconate} \quad (3)$$

The G6PDH[3] is derived from a bacterial source (*Leuconostoc mesenteroides*) and under optimal conditions catalyzes reaction 2 at a reaction velocity 1.8 times that found when the NAD^+ is replaced with $NADP^+$ (*6*).

Methods

Materials

The following reagents (catalog numbers in parentheses) were obtained from Sigma Chemical Co., St. Louis, Mo. 63178: β-$NADP^+$ (N-0505), β-NAD^+ (D-5755), β-NADH (N-8129), ATP (A-3127), ADP (A2754), Tris (T-1503), glucose-6-phosphate (G-7879), sodium 6-phosphogluconate (P-7977), hexokinase, EC 2.7.1.1 (H-4505, 345 U/mg),[4] and 6-phosphogluconate dehydrogenase, EC 1.1.1.44 (P-0632, 54 U/mg). Placental alkaline phosphatase, EC 3.1.3.1 (catalytic concentration = 7.4 nmol s^{-1} $liter^{-1}$ at pH 10.3 and 30 °C), was kindly supplied by DADE, Miami, Fla. 33152. Glucose-6-phosphate dehydrogenase, EC 1.1.1.49 (from *Leuconostoc mesenteroides* 284 U/mg),[4] was purchased from Worthington Biochemical Corp., Freehold, N. J. 07728. D-Glucose, Standard Reference Material No. 917 (purity 99.9%) and potassium dichromate, Standard Reference Material No. 136b, were obtained from the National Bureau of Standards, Washington, D. C. 20234. [U-^{14}C]-D-Glucose (cat. No. NEC-042X, 234 Ci/mol) was obtained from New England Nuclear, Boston, Mass. 02118.

Apparatus

All spectrophotometric measurements were made with a Cary Model 16 spectrophotometer (Varian Associates, Palo Alto, Calif. 94303), with air in the reference beam. Measurements were made in either a standard 4-ml quartz cuvette (pathlength, 10 mm) or a 2-compartment mixing cuvette (total pathlength, 10 mm; Pyrocell Mfg. Co., Westwood, N. J. 07675).

Radioactivity was measured at 0 °C in a Model 3003 Tri-Carb Scintillation Spectrometer (Packard Instrument Co., Downers Grove, Ill. 60515), with use of 10 ml of "Unogel" scintillation fluid (Schwartz/Mann, Orangeburg, N. Y. 10962).

Fluorometric measurements were made with a MPF2A Spectrofluorometer (Perkin-Elmer Corp., Norwalk, Conn. 06852). The sharp cut-off interference filter was obtained from Chemetrics, San Mateo, Calif. 94401.

Only class-A volumetric glassware was used in these experiments and in all cases this glassware was recalibrated with water to determine the volume delivered or contained at 25 °C. Weighings were done with a Model H20T semimicro balance (Mettler Instrument Corp., Princeton, N. J. 08540).

Procedure

Reaction mixtures for glucose-coupled NADH production were prepared as follows: An appropriate amount of high-purity glucose was weighed and quantitatively transferred to a 2- or 4-liter volumetric flask. The glucose was dissolved and diluted to volume with de-ionized water. This glucose solution was further diluted to working reagent in one of three ways:

A. An aliquot of this stock was transferred with a 10-ml volumetric pipet to either a 50- or a 100-ml volumetric flask. To the same flask was added 2.0, 4.0, or 8.0 ml of a nucleotide stock, which unless otherwise indicated contained ATP, 0.63 mmol/liter; NAD^+, 0.81 mmol/liter; magnesium acetate, 0.125 mmol/liter; and Tris-Tris hydrochloride, 0.125 mol/liter,[5] pH 7.80 ± 0.02 at 25 °C. More 0.125 mol/liter Tris buffer containing 0.125 mmol of Mg^{2+} per liter was added, to adjust to final volume.

B. Aliquots by weight (1 or 2 g) of carefully-prepared stock glucose solutions were transferred to 50- or 100-ml volumetric flasks and diluted with nucleotide stock and Tris/Mg^{2+} buffer as in A.

C. Stock glucose, 100 ml of a 0.4 mmol/liter solution in Tris/Mg^{2+} buffer, was transferred with a volumetric pipet to a 200-ml volumetric flask. Nucleotide stock, 16 ml, was added and the final volume adjusted to 200 ml with Tris-Mg^{2+} buffer as in A. A sequential dilution of 100.0 ml of the new solution was made in exactly the same manner except that an appropriately smaller amount of the nucleotide stock was added to maintain the final NAD^+ and ATP concentrations at 0.65 and 0.5 mmol/liter, respectively.

Exactly 4 ml of each well-mixed reaction mixture prepared by one of the above procedures was transferred at 25 °C to a cuvette, which was placed in a temperature-controlled cell holder of the spectrophotometer. To this mixture was added 1.0 μl of G6PDH (used directly as supplied by the manufacturer; catalytic concentration = 8.8 mmol s^{-1} $liter^{-1}$ at 25 °C and pH 7.8). The absorbance at 340.0 nm of this reaction mixture vs. air was recorded at 1-min intervals for 10 min. To initiate the reaction, 2.0 μl of hexokinase[6] (catalytic concentration = 4.5 mmol s^{-1} $liter^{-1}$ at 25 °C and pH 7.8) was added and thoroughly mixed in. The absorbance at 340 nm was followed until there was a 10-min interval during which no further change was observed.

The completeness of reaction was evaluated as fol-

[3] Nonstandard abbreviations used: G6PDH, glucose-6-phosphate dehydrogenase (EC 1.1.1.49); 6PGDH, 6-phosphogluconate dehydrogenase (EC 1.1.1.43); Tris, tris (hydroxymethyl)aminomethane; ε, molar absorptivity; μ, ionic strength, NBS, National Bureau of Standards; ppt, part per thousand.

[4] See procedure section for experimentally determined activities under the conditions used to determine molar absorptivity.

[5] Here and elsewhere throughout this paper concentration is in terms of moles of ionized and un-ionized tris(hydroxy methyl)aminomethane per liter.

[6] The hexokinase working solution was prepared on the day of the run by dissolving 50 mg of the dry, powdered enzyme in 1.00 ml of water.

lows. Uniformly labeled ^{14}C-glucose was reacted for 30 min under the conditions described above. The reaction mixture was then treated with alkaline phosphatase to convert any residual glucose-6-phosphate to glucose, and an aliquot of this mixture was fractionated by thin-layer chromatography on silica gel. The chromatographed glucose was located and transferred to liquid scintillation vials containing hexokinase, ATP, and G6PDH in order to convert the recovered glucose to 6-phosphogluconate. Finally 6PGDH/NADP$^+$ was added to oxidize the 6-phosphogluconate to CO_2 and ribulose-5-phosphate. Gaseous $^{14}CO_2$ that was released from the acidified reaction mixture was trapped on paper strips that had been presoaked with KOH and suspended over the reaction mixture. The strips were transferred to a scintillation vial and counted.

^{14}C-Glucose at 0.1% of the above radioactivity was taken through the same sequence except that the original hexokinase and G6PDH were omitted. This latter reaction was used to estimate the overall yield of the total system.

Experiments undertaken to verify the linearity of NADH absorption over the range of 1.2 to 0.035 *A* were done as follows. Stock solutions of NADH were prepared directly from commercial material and were precisely diluted in a manner similar to that previously described for glucose (see Method C) except that nucleotide stock and enzyme reagents were omitted. The 340-nm absorbance of these NADH solutions and of the buffer alone was then determined at 25 °C vs. air.

Solutions used to measure pH, buffer, and temperature effects on the molar absorptivity or temperature effects on the wavelength of maximum absorbance were prepared by mixing a NADH solution with appropriate volumes of buffer, to give a solution containing, per liter, 0.1 mmol of NADH, 0.1 mmol of Mg^{2+}, and 0.1 mol of Tris buffer. In several experiments the Tris/Mg^{2+} buffer was replaced by 90 mmol of sodium or potassium phosphate per liter.

The direct effect of NAD$^+$ on the absorptivity of NADH was investigated by measuring the absorbance of the nucleotide at 340 nm in a 10-mm two-compartment mixing cuvette. A 1.000-ml portion of a 0.20 mmol/liter NADH solution was added to one compartment and 1.000 ml of one of several NAD$^+$ solutions, each of different concentration, was added to the other. The absorbance at 340 nm was determined before and after the two solutions were mixed by inversion. Both solutions were prepared in 0.1 mol/liter Tris buffer, pH 7.80, containing magnesium acetate, 0.10 mmol/liter.

It is well known that NADH solutions fluoresce, with maximum emission at about 450 nm. This fluorescence could cause a systematic bias in absorbance measurements at 340 nm if the fluorescent light were of sufficient intensity when it reached the spectrophotometer detector. This effect was evaluated in the following way.

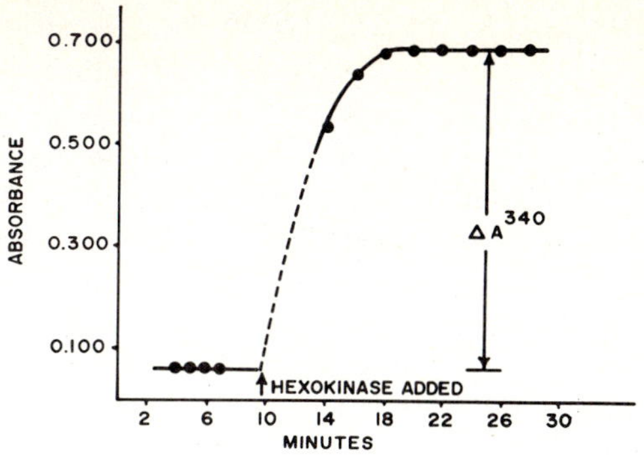

Fig. 1. Time-course of NADH formation by the coupled hexokinase/G6PDH reaction

The fluorescence of a solution of 0.1 mmol/liter NADH in Tris buffer (0.1 mmol/liter, pH 7.8) was compared with that of a solution of 0.1 mmol/liter quinine sulfate in 5 mmol/liter H_2SO_4. Both solutions were excited at 340 nm and the relative fluorescence at their respective emission peaks was measured. Emission was maximal at about 455 nm for NADH and 460 nm for quinine sulfate. Next, measurements were made with the Cary 16 spectrophotometer of the apparent transmittance of a "sharp cut-off" ultraviolet filter, both alone and in series with one of the above solutions in a quartz cell (the one used for the other spectrophotometric determinations). The cell was placed between the filter and the monochromator. This filter had a measured apparent transmittance of less than 0.0002 at 340 nm, 0.75 at 400 nm, and 0.88 at 460 nm. Thus, 340-nm radiation could not reach the detector, but almost all of the fluorescence emitted at 460 nm would be detected.

Results

The time course of a typical hexokinase G6PDH-coupled reaction is shown in Figure 1. We saw no absorbance change in the 10 min before the hexokinase was added, but then NAD$^+$ reduction proceeded rapidly, reaching the equilibrium value in the next 10 to 15 min and changing no further during the next hour.

Further additions of up to 10-fold the usual amounts of hexokinase and G6PDH enzyme reagents to the equilibrium reaction mixture produced no significant side reactions, as indicated by the unchanged absorbance at 340 nm during the next 30 min. Likewise, if 0.1 mmol/liter concentrations of either NADH or 6-phosphogluconate was substituted for glucose in the standard reaction mixture, absorbance at 340 nm was unchanged.

To determine that a slow NAD reduction was not being equally offset by NADH destruction during the critical measurement period, we set up an experiment to evaluate NADH stability under the reaction conditions. The results indicated a ΔA_{340}/h of 0.0005 for 0.1 mmol/liter NADH at 25 °C and pH 7.8 in 0.1 mol/liter Tris/Mg^{2+} buffer. Under the same conditions but at pH 6.8, the ΔA_{340}/h was 0.0013. In 0.09 mol/liter sodium or potassium phosphate buffer (pH 7.8

at 25 °C) the ΔA_{340}/h was 0.0030. Similar rates of destruction at 25 °C in Tris and in phosphate buffers have been given by Lowry and Passonneau (7).

The glucose or glucose-6-phosphate remaining in the reaction mixture when equilibrium was attained was estimated on several occasions by including ^{14}C-labeled glucose in the reaction. Isolation of the residual glucose and measurement of its radioactivity indicated that as much as 0.3% of the glucose or glucose-6-phosphate, or both, might remain after the 30-min reaction. Because of the complexity of the series of reactions needed for this estimation and the possibility of small errors occurring at several different steps, we regard 0.3% as an upper limit for incompleteness of the reaction. However, we do not believe that this number is known with sufficient certainty to warrant correcting the experimentally determined molar absorptivities for this factor, and the values reported are based on the assumption that reactions 1 and 2 go to completion.

The effect of NADH fluorescence on the absorbance reading of NADH was estimated by comparative fluorescence and absorption studies of quinine and NADH. The quinine solution was observed to fluoresce about 45 times more strongly than the NADH solution. In the Cary 16 spectrophotometer, the measured transmittance at 340 nm of the ultraviolet filter plus the cell containing the NADH solution was less than 0.00020, a value that could not be distinguished from the value observed for transmittance of the filter alone. This indicated that the NADH fluorescence was too weak to detect under these conditions. By comparison, when the NADH solution was replaced with the quinine solution the measured transmittance was 0.00053.

Knowing that, under the conditions used, quinine fluoresces about 45 times more strongly than NADH and taking the transmittance of the filter itself into consideration, we calculated the transmittance attributable to NADH fluorescence to be 0.000013. The true transmittance of NADH and the quartz cell was 0.214 at 340 nm, giving a relative transmittance error, $\Delta T/T$, of 0.0607 ppt. This can be converted to the relative absorbance error by using the relationship $\Delta A = -.434\ \Delta T/T$, and $\Delta A/A$ is calculated to be −0.039 ppt. The magnitude of this error increases with increasing absorbance, but is negligible (less than 0.1 ppt) at even the highest NADH concentration we used in the molar absorptivity determinations. Independent experiments indicated that the spectrophotometric cell used in these experiments did not fluoresce. Thus the fluorescence is essentially entirely associated with the NADH solution.

Absorbance changes that may be associated with the change in concentration of species other than NADH were investigated by measuring the absorbance of the individual compounds at 340 nm. These absorbances are shown in Table 1 along with an estimate of ΔA_{340} under reaction conditions. Neither Mg^{2+} nor G6PDH could be shown to affect the absorbance of NADH in solution at the concentrations we used in determining molar absorptivity.

Table 1. Absorbance Change Owing to Compounds Other Than NADH in the Hexokinase/G6PDH Reaction Mixture

Compound	Concn, mmol/liter	A_{340}	Estimated ΔA_{340} in reaction mixture[a]
NAD^+ (*18*)	1.0	0.0026	−0.00026
ATP	5.0	0.0029	−0.00006
ADP	2.0	0.0032	0.00016
Glucose	2.0	0.0006	−0.00003
6-Phosphogluconate	2.0	0.0020	0.00010
		Net ΔA_{340}	−0.00009[b]

[a] After oxidation of 0.1 mmol/liter glucose.

[b] Net $\Delta A/A$ of reaction components = $\frac{-0.00009}{0.63000}$ = −.14 ppt (see ΔA reaction components, Table 3).

Table 2. Molar Absorptivity (ϵ) of NADH at 340 nm

Glucose concn (initial) µmol/liter	ϵ[a]	SD[a]	n	CV, %
25.0	6330	20	10	0.32
50.0	6330	35	20	0.55
100.0	6311	24	39	0.38
200.0	6308	18	16	0.29
All values	6317	28	85	0.44

[a] liter mol^{-1} cm^{-1} at 25°C in Tris buffer (0.1 mol/liter, pH 7.8).

The molar absorptivity (ϵ) of NADH was determined at four different initial glucose concentrations and calculated from the equation below.

$$\epsilon = \frac{(A_F R_F - A_I R_I - \Delta A_{hex})\, MVK}{bW} \qquad (4)$$

A_F and A_I are final and initial absorbances, respectively; R_F and R_I are the appropriate corrections for multiple reflections; ΔA_{hex} is the absorbance change (14×10^{-5} A) caused by the addition of the hexokinase; M is the molecular weight of glucose; W is the weight of glucose used, uncorrected for air buoyancy; V is the effective volume of the glucose solution, corrected for glassware calibration errors and the addition of 3 µl of enzyme solutions to the final reaction mixture in the cell; b is the nominal cell pathlength of 1 cm; and K is a factor to correct for all other systematic errors that we identified and measured. (All errors that were taken into account in the calculation are discussed in the following section.) Table 2 summarizes the mean values obtained at each glucose concentration and Figure 2 shows the

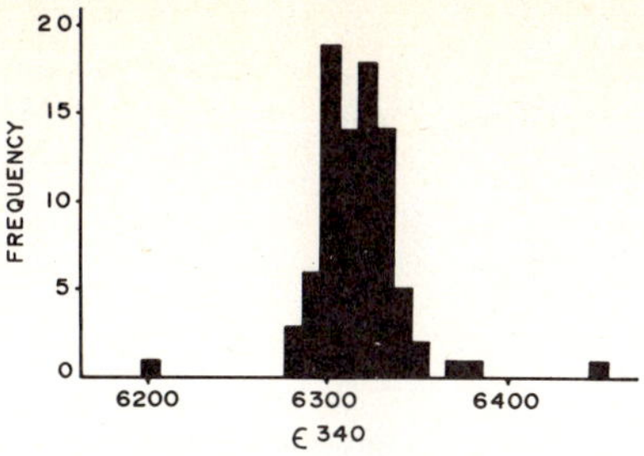

Fig. 2. Frequency distribution of molar absorptivity values for four different concentrations of glucose

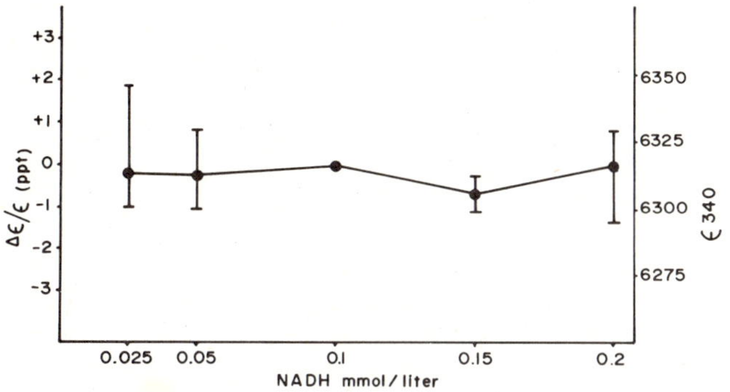

Fig. 3. Effect of NADH concentration on molar absorptivity (sample in 0.1 mol/liter Tris, pH 7.8)

NADH concentrations are not known accurately, but the relative concentrations were established by precise dilutions. Data points indicate mean and range of experimental results

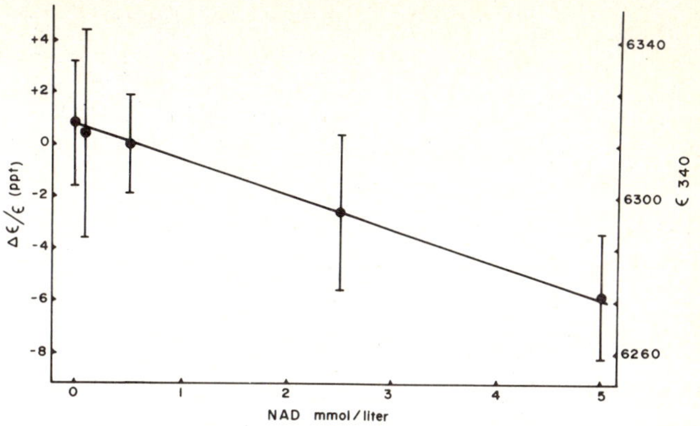

Fig. 4. Effect of NAD^+ concentration on NADH absorption (sample in 0.1 mol/liter Tris, pH 7.8)

Data points indicate mean and range of experimental results. The final NADH concentration was always 0.1 mmol/liter

frequency distribution for all 85 molar absorptivity values. The mean value at 25 °C is 6317 liter mol^{-1} cm^{-1} in Tris-Tris Chloride buffer (0.1 mol/liter, $pH_{25°}$ = 7.8). The standard deviation is 28 liter mol^{-1} cm^{-1}, from which the standard error of the mean was calculated to be 3.04 liter mol^{-1} cm^{-1} (0.48 ppt). The uncertainty in this number is discussed in the following section.

The data of Table 2 suggest a small shift in molar absorptivity as the glucose concentration is decreased. At present we are not certain whether this is a real phenomenon or is merely the result of a systematic error, as yet unascribed, in the measurement procedure. (A systematic absorbance error of less than 0.001 that is independent of the total ΔA could account for the observed differences in mean values of molar absorptivity shown in Table 2.)

Another series of experiments was undertaken to establish that the small differences in molar absorptivity observed at different glucose concentrations were not due to deviations from Beer's law. Direct assessment of the linearity of the NADH concentration/absorbance relationship was made by precise dilutions of a stock NADH solution. Results are shown in Figure 3. All data are normalized to 6317, the average molar absorptivity at 340 nm. No significant deviation from linearity was observed.

In one experiment the initial NAD concentration was increased 10-fold (to 5.6 mmol/liter) to determine whether the glucose-coupled reaction that generates NADH could be driven further toward completion. Unexpectedly the experimental results indicated a decrease of 20 in the value for the molar absorptivity. When NAD^+ was added directly to NADH solutions, to determine whether or not the decrease was nucleotide-related, we observed a significant decrease in the value for molar absorptivity as NAD^+ concentration was increased (Figure 4).

The dependence of molar absorptivity on conditions in the solvent was studied by direct absorbance measurements of a high-purity commercial NADH solution. The effect of pH, ionic strength, and temperature on the molar absorptivity at 340 nm are shown in Figures 5, 6, and 7, respectively. An average decrease in the molar absorptivity of 16 per pH unit was observed in 0.1 mol/liter Tris/Mg^{2+} buffer at 25 °C between pH 6.8 and 8.0. There is a noticeable nonlinearity in this relationship with the $\Delta\epsilon/\Delta t$ greater at pH 6.8 than in the higher pH range. A subsequent experiment, in which the time between dilution of the NADH to pH 6.8 and the absorbance measurement was held to less than 15 min, confirmed the small $\Delta\epsilon/\Delta pH$ previously observed. The results of this latter experiment, corrected for the small decay before measurements as well as for a small ionic strength effect, are represented by the dashed line in Figure 5.

As indicated in Figure 6, for univalent electrolytes increasing ionic strength results in a decrease in molar absorptivity of 66 per mole per liter change in ionic strength. A limited number of experiments with other additives indicated that Na_2SO_4 depressed the molar absorptivity of NADH in a manner similar to that seen for NaCl, while nonelectrolytes such as methanol and sucrose actually elevated the molar absorptivity.

The change in molar absorptivity per degree increase in temperature was −4.2. Part of this change can be accounted for by the increase in solution volume with temperature. Another small increment of

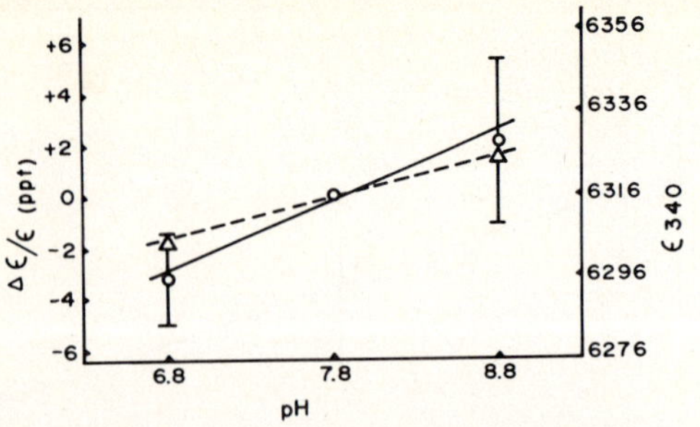

Fig. 5. Effect of pH on molar absorptivity of NADH

The *dashed line* represents one experiment in which corrections were made for effects of ionic strength and time-dependent decay before measurement. Data points indicate mean and range of experimental results

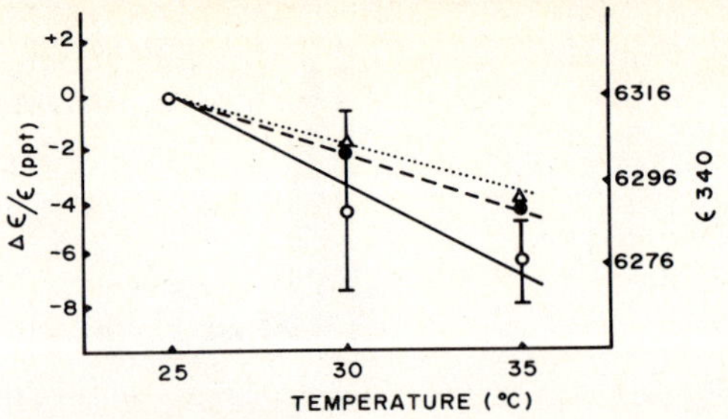

Fig. 7. Effect of temperature on the molar absorptivity of NADH at 0.1 mol/liter and pH 7.8

Broken lines indicate values corrected for volume change related to temperature (- - -), and pH change related to temperature (. . .). *Brackets* indicate range of experimental results for the uncorrected curve

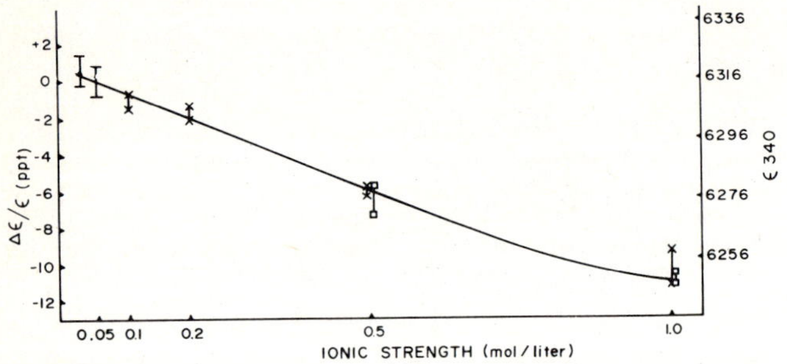

Fig. 6. Effect of ionic strength on the molar absorptivity of NADH

The measurements at 0.05 and 0.025 were in Tris buffer only. At the other values the ionic strengths were established with NaCl (X) or KCl (□) plus the 0.1 mol/liter Tris. Data points indicate range of experimental results

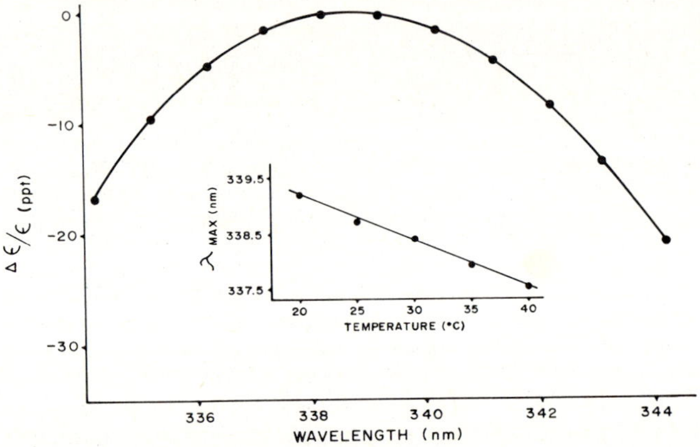

Fig. 8. Effect of wavelength setting on the molar absorptivity of NADH in the 340-nm region

The *insert*, *8A*, shows the effect of temperature on the wavelength maximum of NADH

$\Delta\epsilon/\Delta T$ can be accounted for by the decrease in the molar absorptivity associated with the predicted temperature-induced pH change in the buffer [26×10^{-3} pH units per degree (*8*)]. If molar absorptivity is corrected for these changes, as indicated by the dotted lines in Figure 7, $\Delta\epsilon/\Delta T$ becomes −2.4.

Figure 8 shows the absorption spectrum of NADH in the 340 nm region in Tris/Mg^{2+} buffer, pH 7.8 at 25 °C. Absorbance is maximal under these conditions at 338.8 nm, where it is about 1.0 ppt higher than at 340.0 nm. No difference in λ_{max} was observed between solutions of commercially obtained NADH and solutions of NADH that had been purified chromatographically in our laboratory. As shown in the insert of Figure 8, the change in λ_{max} with temperature was found to be −0.08 nm/°C.

Analysis of Errors

We tried to identify, assess, and correct for all systematic errors that would significantly affect the calculated value for molar absorptivity. We calibrated the various pieces of apparatus before and during the measurements leading to a final molar absorptivity value.

It is shown in the Appendix, by use of propagation of error formulas, that the relative systematic error in molar absorptivity can be obtained by addition or subtraction of the relative errors associated with each of the factors in equation 4. Therefore, all pertinent systematic errors will be expressed in parts per thousand (ppt) with the understanding that these may be added or subtracted to give a resultant relative error in the molar absorptivity. Table 3 lists systematic errors, their magnitudes, the appropriate correction to the molar absorptivity, and the residual uncertainties associated with each of them. The residual uncertainties are our estimates of limiting values for these quantities, except where enough experimental data were available to allow calculation of a standard deviation. For the purposes of the following discussion, a "positive" error is one for which the observed or assumed value is greater than the true value. It can be seen from equation 8 in the Appendix that an error in absorbance or in volume results in an error in the molar absorptivity that has the same sign. The correction term for the molar absorptivity (Table 3, column 2) therefore has the opposite sign. Equation 8 also shows that errors in optical pathlength and in weight have the opposite sign from the resulting errors in molar absorptivity, so the correction term for the molar absorptivity has the same sign as the original error.

Table 3. Systematic Errors and Uncertainties in the Experimentally Determined Molar Absorptivity of NADH

Measurement	Error	Error (parts per thousand)	Correction ϵ (parts per thousand)	Residual uncertainty in ϵ (parts per thousand)
Weight	Air buoyancy	−0.6	−0.6	±<0.1
	Balance calibration	0	0	±1
Volume	Glassware calibration	0	0	±<0.1
Pathlength	Beam convergence	−1.5	−1.5	±.2
	Multiple reflections	*a*	*a*	±<0.1
	Pathlength calibration	−0.2	−0.2	±0.6 (2 SD)
Absorbance	Finite band pass	−0.8	+0.8	0 to −0.2
	Stray light	0	0	0 to +0.1
	NADH fluorescence	0	0	0 to +0.1
	Wavelength calibration	−0.3	+0.3	±0.3
	Absorbance calibration	+0.2	−0.2	±1.8 (2 SD)
Miscellaneous	Glucose purity	+1	+1	±1
	NAD^+ NADH interaction	0	0	0 to +1
	Hexokinase absorbance	*a*	*a*	±0.1
	ΔA of reaction components	−0.1	+0.1	±0.1
	Incomplete reaction	0	0	0 to +3
	Side reactions of NAD^+	0	0	±1
	Decay in NADH (15 min)	−0.2	+0.2	±0.2
	pH not at 7.8	0	0	±0.2
	Temperature not at 25°C	0	0	±0.1
	Ionic strength not at 0.1	0	0	±0.1
	Net correction[b]		+0.1 ppt	
	Net residual uncertainty caused by systematic error			−2.6 to +4.1 ppt

[a] These values may not be expressed as proportional errors but are included in equation 4 and taken into account in each individual calculation.
[b] K of equation 4 = 1.0000 − 0.0001 = 0.9999.

The effect of air buoyancy was considered both for weighings of glucose and for weighings of solutions in certain dilution experiments. The error was calculated in the conventional manner (*9*). The balances were calibrated with class S weights certified by NBS. No systematic error was found in the weight range of interest. The uncertainty in a single weighing was estimated as ±0.1 mg, or ±1 ppt at the lowest weight of glucose used (90 mg).

All volumetric glassware was recalibrated for use at 25 °C. Transfers and absorbance measurements were performed at this temperature. Recalibrated volumes were used directly in calculating V for equation 4.

When the light beam in the cell compartment of the Cary 16 spectrophotometer is focused, there is a small beam-convergence error, because most rays enter the cell obliquely, and the effective pathlength becomes slightly greater than the measured distance between parallel faces of the cell. The most extreme angle of incidence in the vertical plane is about 7.4 degrees.[7] Using the equation given by Burke et al. (*10*) and a solution refractive index of 1.35, we calculated the pathlength error to be −1.5 ppt, the negative sign denoting that the assumed pathlength is less than the actual (effective) pathlength. A small (2°) maximum deviation in the horizontal plane is ignored, because the relatively small proportion of energy carried by these rays results in a negligible bias.

All absorbance readings were corrected for the systematic error owing to multiple reflections of the light beam within the cell. The magnitude of the correction varies with absorbance and ranges from 0.5 ppt at A = 1.3 to 2.6 ppt at A = 0.07. Corrections as tabulated by Burnett (*11*) were applied as R_F and R_I in equation 4.

The pathlength of the single quartz cell used for all absorbance measurements in this study deviated from its nominal 1.000-cm value by approximately 0.2 ppt, determined by comparison of absorbances of both acid dichromate and NADH solutions between the test cell and an NBS SRM No. 932 cell with a pathlength known to within 0.05 ppt (*12*).

The slit width used for all absorbance measurements was 0.5 mm, which provided a spectral bandwidth of 2.44 nm at 340 nm. The natural bandwidth

[7] V. Chupp, Cary Instrument Division, Varian Associates; personal communication.

of NADH is 61 nm and the bandwidth ratio is 0.040, indicating a relative absorbance error of −0.8 ppt (*13*). The actual error is somewhat smaller than this, because the wavelength of maximum absorbance is not exactly 340 nm at 25 °C.

Stray radiation in the double-monochromator spectrophotometer is claimed by the manufacturer to be less than 0.001% at 340 nm. The error in absorbance associated with this amount of stray light is some 10-fold too small for the correction to be significant (*13*).

The accuracy of the wavelength setting for the spectrophotometer was checked several times during the study by measuring the 334.15 nm emission line of mercury (*14*) and the 333.7 and 360.9 nm absorption bands of holmium oxide glass (*15*). Readings averaged 0.2 nm lower than the reference wavelengths values. Absorbances were corrected for this bias based on the assumption of a gaussian-shaped absorbance band centered at 339 nm (Figure 8).

The photometric accuracy of the Cary 16 spectrophotometer was assessed by directly comparing the absorbance of potassium dichromate solutions in perchloric acid solutions at pH 3 between our Cary instrument and the NBS high-performance spectrophotometer (*16*). Measurements were made in the same cell on the same solutions and were corrected for small temperature differences in the two laboratories, beam convergence in the Cary instrument, bandpass difference between the two instruments, and nonlinear response of the NBS instrument. The mean relative absorbance error was 0.2 ppt. The precision of repetitive measurements on the Cary instrument during several days at an absorbance of 0.9 was 0.9 ppt, expressed as one coefficient of variation ($n = 24$).

The accuracy of the molar absorptivity for NADH calculated from these experiments is also directly related to the purity of the glucose to which NAD^+ reduction is coupled. The specifications supplied by NBS for their SRM No. 917 glucose indicate a purity of 99.9 ± 0.1%. A 1 ppt correction was used to correct for impurities in the glucose.

The observed decrease in the molar absorptivity of NADH in one set of experiments in which NAD^+ concentrations were increased up to 10-fold those usually used suggested an NAD^+/NADH interaction might be the cause. The observation that decreases in NADH absorbance were also seen when NAD^+ was added directly to different high-purity NADH solutions lends support to this idea, but direct oxidation of NADH by impurities in the NAD^+ as the cause of the decrease in absorbance cannot be ruled out. For this reason we did not correct for this effect in calculating molar absorptivity.

Because the reaction was started by adding hexokinase, it was necessary to subtract the change in absorbance caused by hexokinase, ΔA_{hex}, from the final absorbance. This term appears in equation 4 and was experimentally determined to be 14×10^{-5}. The change in A_{340} owing to the change in concentration of other reactants was measured and is tabulated in Table 1. The magnitude of this correction is 0.1 ppt.

Although NADH is relatively stable at pH 7.8 and 25 °C, the small decay in absorbance of 0.0005 per hour noted previously should be accounted for in the final molar absorptivity calculation. Accordingly, a value of 0.2 ppt, which corresponds to a 15-min decay period during the absorbance measurement, was included in the systematic error correction in Table 3. The sum of all the above correction factors equals −0.1 ppt, and K in equation 4 is therefore 0.9999.

To express the total uncertainty in the molar absorptivity caused by all of these systematic errors, we chose to compute the square root of the sum of squares of the individual uncertainties, and these values are given in the last column of Table 3. This was done separately for negative and positive contributions, because the sign was known for certain errors. The total uncertainty owing only to systematic errors is considered to be −2.6 to 4.1 ppt.

The overall estimate of uncertainty in the molar absorptivity is now calculated, following the recommendations of Eisenhart (*17*), as the estimated uncertainty owing to systematic errors (−2.6 to +4.1 ppt) plus three times the standard error of the mean. This range is −4.0 to 5.5 ppt.

Discussion

Other investigators (*18, 19*) have recently reported their values for the molar absorptivity of NADH for different conditions of wavelength and temperatures. The values at 340 nm varied from 6280 to 0 °C to 6210 at 38 °C, as determined with the lactate dehydrogenase-catalyzed pyruvate oxidation of NADH. These may be compared with 6317 at 25 °C and in 0.1 mol/liter Tris at pH 7.8, the value we report here.

The rationale for selection of the hexokinase/G6PDH system for generation of NADH rests on the high purity, relatively high stability, and ready availability of SRM D-glucose and the two enzyme reagents. Although several forms of G6PDH are commercially available, the NAD coupled enzyme from *L. mesenteroides* was chosen because of the greater stability of its co-factor, NADH, relative to NADPH (*20*).

pH 7.8 was selected for this reaction because of the favorable equilibrium of NAD^+ reduction at this slightly alkaline pH and the high stability of reaction components under these conditions. Furthermore, pH 7.8 is intermediate to the extremes used in many coupled enzyme assays; e.g., for lactate dehydrogenase, NADH oxidation is optimum at pH 7.35 and NAD^+ reduction is optimum at 8.6 (*21*). All absorbance measurements were made at 340 nm because this has been the reference wavelength for NADH measurements used by most workers, even though the actual absorbance maximum at 25 °C is somewhat lower.

We found no evidence for a nonstoichiometric relation between glucose consumed and NADH produced. The residual glucose and glucose-6-phosphate estimated by radioactive tracer experiments indicated the overall reaction to be at least 99.7% complete. This finding confirms that the final equilibrium is far to the right, as predicted from energy consideration of reactants and products (*22–24*). Absence of NAD^+/NADH coupled side reactions beyond or before the expected product 6-phosphogluconate is indicated by the stable absorbance readings for periods up to 1 h after apparent equilibrium. No detectable changes in absorbance in the presence of up to a 10-fold excess of hexokinase or G6PDH assured a minimal contamination by 6PGDH in either of these enzyme reagents.

As indicated above, the molar absorptivity of NADH is not a constant but depends somewhat on the conditions under which it is measured. pH, ionic strength, and temperature all influence the absorptivity of NADH. The current study confirms the observation by Malcolm (*25*) that absorbance at 340 nm is temperature-dependent, but the $\Delta\epsilon/\Delta T$ we observed is somewhat less than he observed. We have also confirmed the interrelationship between wavelength maxima and temperature as originally reported by Bücher et al. (*19*).

The small effect of pH on the molar absorptivity of NADH observed in this study has, to the best of our knowledge, not previously been reported. A small uncertainty is associated with the absorbance measurements at pH 6.8, because NADH is threefold less stable at pH 6.8 than at pH 7.8; however, repeated confirmation of the decrease in absorbance with pH has convinced us that the effect is real.

Phosphate buffers are often used in enzyme analyses involving NADH-coupled reactions. Our best estimates of the molar absorptivity in phosphate buffer (pH 7.8) indicate a value 2–3 ppt lower in phosphate than in Tris. For two reasons this slightly lower molar absorptivity in phosphate is to be expected. First, the ionic strength of phosphate buffer is much greater than that of Tris under the same conditions, which should result in a slightly lower absorbance. Secondly, NADH is less stable in phosphate than in Tris, resulting in a small decay in 340 nm absorbance before the spectrophotometric measurement. Because of uncertainties associated with these two effects, we do not report a value for the molar absorptivity in phosphate.

We are grateful to Dr. Radu Mavrodineanu of the National Bureau of Standards for making available the NBS high-accuracy spectrophotometer and for helping with the measurements needed to assess the photometric accuracy of our spectrophotometer. We also thank Drs. R. Schaffer, J. Ziegenhorn, W. Gruber, and A. L. Underwood for their critical review of this work.

References

1. Ohlmeyer, P., Darstellung von reiner Dihydroenzymase in Substanz. *Biochem. Z.* **297,** 66 (1938).

2. Horecker, B. L., and Kornberg, A., The extinction coefficients of the reduced band of pyridine nucleotides. *J. Biol. Chem.* **175,** 385 (1948).

3. Beisenherz, G., Bücher, Th., and Garbade, K-H., α-Glycerophosphate dehydrogenase from rabbit muscle. In *Methods in Enzymology* **1,** S. P. Colowick and N. O. Kaplan, Eds., Academic Press, New York, N. Y., 1955, p 391.

4. Hohorst, H. J., Enzymatische Bestimmung von L(+)-Milchsaüre. *Biochem. Z.* **328,** 509 (1957).

5. Duncan, P., Neese, J., Bayse, D., and Stewart, C., A report on the WHO/CDC international glucose-urea standardization program. *Clin. Chem.* **20,** 882 (1974).

6. Olive, C., and Levy, H. R., The preparation and some properties of crystalline glucose-6-phosphate dehydrogenase from *Leuconostoc mesenteroides. Biochem. J.* **6,** 730 (1967).

7. Lowry, O. H., and Passonneau, J. V., *A Flexible System of Enzymatic Analysis,* Academic Press, New York, N. Y., 1972, p 12.

8. Staples, B. R., Certificate of analysis, Standard Reference Materials Tris(hydroxymethyl)aminomethane (922) and Tris(hydroxymethyl)aminomethane hydrochloride (923). National Bureau of Standards, Washington, D. C., June 1971.

9. Lewis, J. E., and Woolf, L. A., Air-buoyancy corrections for single-pan balances. *J. Chem. Educ.* **48,** 639 (1971).

10. Burke, R. W., Deardorff, E. R., and Menis, O., Liquid absorbance standards. *J. Res. Nat. Bur. Stand.* **76A,** 469 (1972).

11. Burnett, R. W., Errors in ultraviolet and visible spectrophotometric measurements caused by multiple reflections in the cell. *Anal. Chem.* **45,** 383 (1973).

12. Mavrodineanu, R., and Lazar, J. W., Standard reference materials: Standard quartz cuvettes for high-accuracy spectrophotometry. *Clin. Chem.* **19,** 1053 (1973).

13. Burnett, R. W., Accurate measurement of molar absorptivities. *J. Res. Nat. Bur. Stand.* **76A,** 483 (1972).

14. *Manual on Recommended Practices in Spectrophotometry,* 3rd ed., American Society for Testing and Materials, Philadelphia, Pa., 1969, p 67.

15. McNierny, J., and Slavin, W., A wavelength standard for ultraviolet-visible-near infrared spectrophotometry. *Appl. Opt.* **1,** 365 (1962).

16. Mavrodineanu, R., An accurate spectrophotometer for measuring the transmittance of solid and liquid materials, *J. Res. Nat. Bur. Stand.* **76A,** 405 (1972).

17. Eisenhart, C., Expression of the uncertainties of final results. *Science* **160,** 1201 (1968).

18. Haid, E., Lehmann, P., and Ziegenhorn, J., Molar absorptivities of β-NADH and β-NAD at 260 nm. *Clin. Chem.* **21,** 884 (1975).

19. Bücher, Th., Krell, H., Lusch, G., et al., Molar extinction coefficients of NADH and NADPH at Hg spectral lines. *Z. Klin. Chem. Klin. Biochem.* **12,** 239 (1974).

20. Lowry, O. H., Passonneau, J. V., and Rock, M. K., The stability of pyridine nucleotides. *J. Biol. Chem.* **236,** 2756 (1961).

21. Gay, R. J., McComb, R. B., and Bowers, G. N., Jr., Optimum reaction conditions for human lactate dehydrogenase isoenzymes as they affect total lactate dehydrogenase activity. *Clin. Chem.* **14,** 740 (1968).

22. Robbins, E. A., and Boyer, P. D., Determination of the equilibrium of the hexokinase reaction and the free energy of hydrolysis of adenosine triphosphate. *J. Biol. Chem.* **224,** 121 (1957).

23. Glaser, L., and Brown, D. H., Purification and properties of D-glucose-6-phosphate dehydrogenase. *J. Biol. Chem.* **216,** 67 (1955).

24. Horecker, B. L., and Smyrniotes, P. Z., Reversibility of glucose-6-phosphate oxidation. *Biochim. Biophys. Acta* **12,** 98 (1953).

25. Malcolm, A. D. B., The temperature dependence of the spectroscopic properties of reduced nicotinamide adenine dinucleotide. *Anal. Biochem.* **55,** 278 (1973).

26. Pugh, E. M., and Winslow, G. H., *The Analysis of Physical Measurements,* Addison-Wesley, Reading, Mass., 1966, p 118.

27. Ku, H. H., Notes on the use of propagation of error formulae. *J. Res. Nat. Bur. Stand.* **70C,** 263 (1966).

Appendix: Derivation of Propagation-of-Error Formula

A function of two variables, $F = f(x, y)$ which has derivatives at all points in an interval containing the point (a, b) may be approximated by a first degree Taylor polynominal

$$F = f(x, y) = f(a, b) + \frac{\partial F}{\partial x}(x - a) + \frac{\partial F}{\partial y}(y - b)$$

where the partial derivatives are evaluated at the point (a, b). This is a useful approximation provided $(x - a)$ and $(y - b)$ are sufficiently small.

Letting $\Delta F = f(x, y) - f(a, b)$, $\Delta x = (x - a)$, and $\Delta y = (y - b)$, the equation may be rewritten as

$$\Delta F = \frac{\partial F}{\partial x} \Delta x + \frac{\partial F}{\partial y} \Delta y \qquad (5)$$

If a value of F is calculated from measured values of x and y, this equation may be used to estimate the error, ΔF, resulting from systematic errors Δx and Δy (*26, 27*).

Equation 4 may be written

$$\epsilon' = \frac{A^*MV}{bW} \qquad (6)$$

where ϵ' is the apparent molar absorptivity, uncorrected for systematic errors, and A^* is the absorbance owing to NADH corrected for multiple reflections and hexokinase absorbance. An expression for $\Delta\epsilon'$ may be derived, following the form of equation 5.

$$\Delta\epsilon' = \left(\frac{MV}{bW}\right) \Delta A^* + \left(\frac{A^*M}{bW}\right) \Delta V - \left(\frac{A^*MV}{b^2W}\right) \Delta b - \left(\frac{A^*MV}{bW^2}\right) \Delta W \qquad (7)$$

Because equation 6 contains only products of variables, a simplification obtains from writing the expression for the relative error, $\Delta\epsilon'/\epsilon'$.

$$\frac{\Delta\epsilon'}{\epsilon'} = \frac{\Delta A^*}{A^*} + \frac{\Delta V}{V} - \frac{\Delta b}{b} - \frac{\Delta W}{W} \qquad (8)$$

Equation 8 expresses the important result that the relative systematic error in molar absorptivity can be calculated by addition or subtraction of the relative errors associated with absorbance, pathlength, and concentration (which has been split into its components, weight of solute and volume of solvent).

If a positive error is defined as one for which the apparent or assumed value is greater than the true value, then the corresponding correction term will have the opposite sign, and the true molar absorptivity, ϵ is given by the expression

$$\epsilon = \epsilon' - \Delta\epsilon' = \epsilon' (1 - \Delta\epsilon'/\epsilon') = \epsilon' K$$

where $K = (1 - \Delta\epsilon'/\epsilon')$ and is the systematic error correction term that appears in equation 4.

CLIN. CHEM. 22/2, 151–160 (1976)

Molar Absorptivities of β-NADH and β-NADPH

Joachim Ziegenhorn, Martin Senn,[1] and Theodor Bücher[2]

Re-investigating the accuracy of the commonly used values for molar absorptivities (ε) of β-NADH and β-NADPH at Hg 334, Hg 365, or 340 nm, we obtained the following results: The maximum of absorbance of NADH is shifted from about 340 nm at 0 °C to about 338.5 nm at 38 °C; the corresponding maxima of NADPH are located at about 0.5-nm longer wavelengths. In addition, the absorption curves of both coenzymes broaden with increasing temperature. For these reasons, the ε-values of NADH and NADPH are generally different from each other, and are temperature-dependent. Only at 334 nm are they almost identical and nearly independent of temperature. Therefore this wavelength is recommended for precise measurements. The ε-values of these coenzymes are influenced by ionic strength and pH. To determine the absolute values of the molar absorptivities, we performed the glutamate dehydrogenase or lactate dehydrogenase assay with carefully purified 2-oxoglutaric acid or pyruvic acid in the presence of excess coenzyme. The purity of the substrates was checked through differential scanning calorimetry, moisture analysis, gas–liquid chromatography, gas chromatography in combination with mass spectrometry, and nuclear magnetic resonance spectroscopy. The ε-values observed under the various conditions are about 1–7% higher than those currently used.

Additional Keyphrases: *effects of temperature, pH • glutamate- and lactate dehydrogenase reactions • reference values • determination of purity of pyruvic acid, 2-oxoglutaric acid • preparation of pure pyruvic acid*

Boehringer Mannheim GmbH, Biochemica Werk Tutzing, Forschungszentrum, 8132 Tutzing, Germany.

[1] Boehringer Mannheim GmbH, Chemische Forschungslaboratorien, 68 Mannheim 31, Germany.

[2] Institut für Physiologische Chemie, Physikalische Biochemie und Zellbiologie der Universität, 8 München 2, Germany.

Based on papers presented at the VIth International Symposium on Quality Control in Clinical Chemistry, Geneva, Switzerland, April 23–25, 1975.

Ed. note: cf. the preceding paper by McComb et al., in this issue.

Received Nov. 20, 1975; accepted Dec. 2, 1975.

At present, for the molar absorptivities of the reduced pyridine nucleotides at 340 nm, Hg 334 nm, or Hg 365 nm, the values 6.22×10^3, 6.0×10^3, or 3.3×10^3 liter·mol^{-1}·cm^{-1} are commonly used. These values are used for both β-NADH and β-NADPH. They are based on experiments of Horecker and Kornberg (*1*), Beisenherz et al. (*2*), and Hohorst (*3*) that date back two to three decades. Already in 1964, one of us presented results that questioned the accuracy of these widely accepted values (*4*). Furthermore, during the past several years, different laboratories reported conflicting results when β-NADPH-dependent reactions were carefully done at Hg 365 nm and results calculated with the ε-value of 3.3×10^3 (*5, 6*). These findings coincided with observations of Boehringer Mannheim control laboratories. Using pyridine nucleotide-dependent assays for the quality control of highly purified products, at Hg 365 nm, concentrations corresponding to more than 100% of the theoretical were obtained with the above ε-value. This, together with other information, prompted us to review the molar absorptivities of the pyridine nucleotides by use of advanced analytical methods. Some of the results have been presented (*7–9*).

Materials and Methods

Apparatus

Gravimetric determinations were done with use of two different precision balances (Model H 20 T, Mettler Instrumente, 8606 Zürich, Switzerland; or Model 404/51, August Sauter, 7470 Ebingen, Germany) that were calibrated with a set of reference weights certified by the Eichamt München (8 München, Germany). The 1-liter measuring flasks and volumetric pipettes (3 ml and 100 μl) used were recalibrated at 20 ± 0.1 °C according to Küster et al. (*10*). Temperature was determined with Tastotherm P4 thermocouples

(Braun Electronic, 6 Frankfurt/Main, Germany), which were calibrated with a reference thermometer (A. H. Thomas, Philadelphia, Pa. 19103). The pH-meters used (Model DIGI 610, WTW, 812 Weilheim, Germany) were calibrated with standard buffers (WTW) of different pH value.

Optical measurements were done with a Cary spectrophotometer (Model 118; Varian Instruments, Monrovia, Calif. 91016) or on four different Eppendorf spectrum line photometers (Model 1101 M and Model 6114; Eppendorf Gerätebau Netheler & Hinz, 2 Hamburg, Germany). The spectrophotometer contained a special quartz-windowed and thermostatted cuvette holder, which could be ventilated with nitrogen to avoid condensation of water at lower temperatures. The spectrum line photometers were likewise equipped with thermostatted cuvette holders. The accuracy of the photometers was checked according to the instructions of the manufacturers. This involved the use of the built-in precision resistances, the use of calibrated glass filters (Carl Zeiss, 7082 Oberkochen, Germany), and the use of a technique at which absolute light intensity was changed at constant absorbance differences. Acid potassium dichromate solutions of different concentrations were used for the intercomparison of the different photometers. The monochromaticity of the light filters of the spectrum line photometers was re-checked by the producer. The wavelength setting of the spectrophotometer was assessed by means of a mercury pencil arc.

The pathlengths of 20 different 1-cm quartz or OS-glass cuvettes used were established at 25 °C with an uncertainty of $\pm 2 \times 10^{-4}$ cm by the originating firm (Hellma, 784 Müllheim, Germany). In some experiments we used special two-compartment mixing cuvettes (total pathlength, 1 cm) or 1-cm cuvettes that contained a built-in water jacket (Hellma).

Differential scanning calorimetry was done with a Model TA 2000 system (Mettler Instruments, 8606 Zürich, Switzerland), which contained the following modules: TA 10 cell, TA 20 power amplifier, TA 30 program controller, TA 31 power supply, and TA 32 temperature controller. The system was interfaced to a HP 9810 computer (Hewlett Packard, Palo Alto, Calif. 94304). For determination of water, we used the moisture analyzer 26-321 (E. I. du Pont de Nemours, Wilmington, Del. 19898).

Gas-liquid chromatography was done with either a Becker 417 chromatograph with thermoconductivity detector or a Becker 409 chromatograph with flame-ionization detector (Packard Instruments, Delft, Holland). The results were evaluated by means of a Model 3352 A data system (Hewlett Packard). Electron-impact mass spectra were obtained by coupling a Model 2740 gas chromatograph (Varian, 28 Bremen, Germany), via a Watson-Biemann separator, to a Varian MAT CH7A mass spectrometer. The spectra were recorded through a Varian MAT SS 100 computer. Chemical-ionization mass spectra were obtained with a Model 9500 gas chromatograph/Model 3300 quadrupole mass spectrometer/Model 6000 computer system (Finnigan Corp., Sunnyvale, Calif. 94086). The system contained a glass jet molecular separator. Nuclear magnetic resonance spectroscopy was done with a Model HFX-8 Fast Fourier Transform spectrometer (Bruker, 7501 Forchheim, Germany).

Reagents

β-NADH, disodium salt, grade I, free of α-NADH; β-NAD, free acid, grade I, free of α-NAD; β-NADPH, tetrasodium salt, grade I; 2-oxoglutaric acid; sodium L-lactate; L-alanine; tris(hydroxymethyl)aminomethane; glutamate dehydrogenase (EC 1.4.1.3) from beef liver; and lactate dehydrogenase (EC 1.1.1.27) from rabbit muscle were products of Boehringer Mannheim, 68 Mannheim, Germany. Pyruvic acid ("purissimum" grade) was bought from Fluka, 9470 Buchs, Switzerland; *N*-trimethylsilyl-imidazole from Macherey & Nagel, 516 Düren, Germany; and deuterated dimethylsulfoxide from Merck Sharp & Dohme, 8 München, Germany. Triethanolamine, NH_4Cl, NaCl, HCl, $(NH_4)_2SO_4$, NaOH, and pyridine (all of "pro analysi" grade) were purchased from E. Merck, 61 Darmstadt, Germany. L-Glutamic acid ("pro analysi" grade), OV 3, and Gaschrom Q were obtained from Serva, 69 Heidelberg, Germany. Porapak PS was bought from Waters Associates, Milford, Mass. 01757. Before use, triethanolamine and pyridine were purified by distillation.

Procedures

Doubly distilled water was used throughout.

Determination of the ratios of molar absorptivities. To compare the ϵ of β-NADH and β-NADPH at 25 °C, we divided a solution of 2-oxoglutarate (80 μmol/liter) and NH_4Cl (150 mmol/liter) in triethanolamine/HCl buffer (0.1 mol/liter, pH 7.6, used throughout) into two parts, to which either β-NADH or β-NADPH (120–160 μmol/liter) was added. The solutions were submitted in parallel to glutamate dehydrogenase assay (see below).

To determine the dependence of ϵ on wavelength and temperature, we used the following procedures: 3.000 ml of a 99 μmol/liter solution of highly purified β-NADH (*11*) in triethanolamine/HCl buffer (0.1 mol/liter, pH 7.6) was pipetted into the cuvette of the Cary spectrophotometer. After sealing the cuvette, we recorded the spectra of the solution at 0 ± 1, 10 ± 1, 25 ± 0.1, or 38 ± 0.1 °C. In the course of scanning, the instrument's wavelength drive was stopped at 334.2, 340, and 365.3, and the digitalized absorbances read. After readjusting the sample to 25 ± 0.1 °C, the β-NADH was oxidized by adding 10 μl of a pyruvic acid solution (40 mmol/liter of the triethanolamine/HCl buffer) and of 10 μl of a lactate dehydrogenase solution (1.1×10^6 U/liter of water). After completion of reaction, the absorbance was recorded. By checking the instrument's wavelength indicator through a mercury pencil arc, the exact wavelengths at the respective scanning stops were determined to be 334.05, 339.85, and 365.1 nm. To get the absorbances at 334.15 nm, we multiplied the readings at 334.05 nm by a factor of 1.0009, which followed from the slope of the absorption curve at this wavelength (0.9% per nm).

In another series of experiments, 150 μmol/liter solutions of highly purified β-NADH (*11*) or β-NADPH[3] preparations in the triethanolamine/HCl buffer were pipetted into a cuvette with built-in water jacket. The cuvette was sealed and the solution brought to 25 ± 0.1 °C within the cuvette holder of a spectrum line photometer. After measuring the absorbances at Hg 334 nm or Hg 365 nm, we heated the water circulating through the jacket, within 5–10 min, to 30 ± 0.1 °C, with shaking of the cuvette, and read the resulting absorbances. The same cuvette was used to determine a blank without coenzyme.

Determination of the effects of pH and ionic strength on ε. 1.000 ml of a solution of highly purified β-NADH or β-NADPH (300 μmol/liter) in the triethanolamine/HCl buffer or tris(hydroxymethyl)-aminomethane/HCl buffer (0.1 mol/liter, pH 7.6) was pipetted into one compartment of a mixing cuvette. To the other compartment, 1.000-ml portions of different solutions free of β-NADH or β-NADPH were added. The composition of these solutions were such as to obtain, after mixing, the conditions noted in the legends of Figures 3 and 4. The cuvette was kept at 25 ± 0.1 °C, and the absorbances were measured at Hg 334 nm before and after mixing. A blank without coenzyme was determined in each case.

Purification of pyruvic acid. Just before each series of experiments, pyruvic acid was purified by three-times-repeated vacuum distillation. The distilling apparatus consisted of a 250-ml round flask, connected to a 50 × 2 cm fractionating column, a water jacket condenser, and an ice-cooled receiver. All operations were done under an atmosphere of dry nitrogen. The heating bath was kept at 40–45 °C. Pyruvic acid fractions were collected at a boiling temperature of 25–27 °C and a pressure of about 1.33 Pa (0.01 Torr). Aliquots of the finally obtained pyruvic acid preparations were accurately weighed and immediately submitted to the determination of their percentage purity and to the assays for ε of β-NADH, respectively.

Determination of the purity of 2-oxoglutaric acid. 2-Oxoglutaric acid, 4–5 mg, was placed into aluminum or gold pans of the differential scanning calorimeter. The starting temperatures were between 99 and 106 °C, the heating rate 1 °C/min. The range was 200 μV. For water analysis, 20 mg of 2-oxoglutaric acid were heated in the moisture analyzer for 20 min at 70 °C.

The silylation of 2-oxoglutaric acid was achieved by adding 50 μl of *N*-trimethylsilyl-imidazole to a solution of 1 mg of the acid in 50 μl of pyridine at 0 °C. Gas–liquid chromatography of the trimethylsilyl derivative was done with a 2 m × 6.4 mm (o.d.) glass column packed with 2% OV 3 on 100–120 mesh Gas-chrom Q. Injection-port temperature was 200 °C, oven temperature 150 °C. The temperature of the flame-ionization detector was 200 °C. Nitrogen at a flow rate of 30 ml/min was used as carrier gas.

For mass spectrometry, 2-oxoglutaric acid was introduced into the ion-source of the Varian MAT CH7A system via a direct solid inlet. The operating conditions were: ionization voltage, 75 eV; ionizing current, 1 mA; accelerating voltage, 3 kV; ion-source temperature, 90 °C; and the temperature of the solid inlet was programmed from 25 to 110 °C.

Nuclear magnetic resonance spectra of a solution of 2-oxoglutaric acid in deuterated dimethylsulfoxide (0.57 mol/liter) were recorded at a field-strength of 21.14 kG and at a frequency of 90 MHz. Spectral width was 1200 Hz, which corresponded to 4096 data points. Pulse width was 3 μs. One hundred pulse interferograms were accumulated.

Determination of the purity of pyruvic acid. Gas–liquid chromatography of pyruvic acid was done under the following conditions: 2 m × 6.4 mm (o.d.) glass column filled with Porapak PS (80–100 mesh); injection port temperature, 180 °C; column temperature, 200 °C; and detector temperature, 240 °C. The column was operated with a helium flow-rate of 60 ml/min when a thermoconductivity detector was used, and with a nitrogen flow-rate of 30 ml/min when a flame-ionization detector was used. For the quantitative evaluation of the gas-chromatographic data, response factors were used.

Likewise, a Porapak PS-filled glass column (2 m × 6.4 mm o.d.) was used for gas chromatography/electron impact mass spectrometry. In this case, the chromatographic separation was performed at a carrier gas (He) flow of 20 ml/min. Injector temperature was 150 °C. The column was held at 140 °C for 6 min, then temperature-programmed to 200 °C at 6 °C/min. The temperature of the molecular separator and interface line was maintained at 100 °C. The mass spectrometer was set up as follows: ionization voltage, 75 eV; ionizing current, 2 mA; accelerating voltage, 3 kV; and ion-source temperature, 80 °C. The spectra were recorded with automatic repetitive scanning (delay after each scan, 2 s) and stored on magnetic tape.

The conditions of the gas-chromatographic separation, done before chemical ionization mass spectrometry, were identical to those for gas chromatography/electron-impact mass spectrometry. The quadrupole mass spectrometer was operated in the following manner: reagent gas, isobutane at 133 Pa (1 Torr); ionization voltage, 70 eV; ionizing current, 200 mA; and ion-source temperature, 130 °C.

Nuclear magnetic resonance spectra of pyruvic acid were obtained under the same experimental conditions as described for 2-oxoglutaric acid.

[3] E. Haid, unpublished.

Determination of the absolute molar absorptivities of β-NADH. An approximate 200-mg portion of 2-oxoglutaric acid was accurately weighed into a 50-ml measuring flask and dissolved in 50 ml of a solution of β-NADH (170 μmol/liter) and NH_4Cl (40 mmol/liter) in the triethanolamine/HCl buffer. After weighing and mixing the solution, 2.5-ml or 5-ml aliquots were pipetted into weighing bottles, weighed, and quantitatively transferred into 1-liter measuring flasks. The flasks were then inserted into a water bath at 20 ± 0.1 °C and filled to volume at this temperature with the above buffer containing β-NADH and NH_4Cl. After careful mixing, 3.000 ml of this solution was pipetted into a 1-cm cuvette and, in the course of 10 min, brought to 25 ± 0.1 °C within the cuvette holder of the photometer. After reading the absorbances $A_1^{Hg\,334}$ and $A_1^{Hg\,365}$, we added 20 μl of a glutamate dehydrogenase solution (1.2 × 10^6 U per liter of the triethanolamine/HCl buffer, 20 ± 0.1 °C), mixed thoroughly, and measured the absorbances $A_2^{Hg\,334}$ and $A_2^{Hg\,365}$ 10 min later, when the reaction was completed. For the purpose of controlling, we observed the absorbances for a further 10-min. In some of the experiments, the cuvette was weighed before and after each pipetting step, to completely eliminate pipetting errors. To determine the self-absorbance of the enzyme, we repeated the above procedure, using the same cuvette, but omitting the addition of 2-oxoglutaric acid. Before and after the enzyme was added the absorbances A_3 and A_4 of the assay solution, respectively, were measured.

If the lactate dehydrogenase assay was used for the determination of ε of β-NADH, then about 120 mg of pyruvic acid was weighed and dissolved in the triethanolamine/HCl buffer containing β-NADH but no NH_4Cl. The reaction was started by adding 20 μl of lactate dehydrogenase solution (1.4 × 10^6 U/liter of the triethanolamine/HCl buffer, 20 ± 0.1 °C). Other experimental conditions were those given for the glutamate dehydrogenase assay.

Determination of the molar absorptivities of 2-oxoglutarate, L-glutamate, pyruvate, L-lactate and β-NAD. These experiments were done as described elsewhere (*11*). However, the triethanolamine/HCl buffer was used as solvent and the optical measurements were made at Hg 334 nm or Hg 365 nm. The concentrations of the 2-oxoglutarate, pyruvate, and L-glutamate solutions used were 13.2–27.1 mmol/liter, 29.2–56.7 mmol/liter, and 25.7–42.0 mmol/liter, respectively. 2-Oxoglutarate and L-glutamate were determined enzymatically (*12, 13*).

Results and Discussion

Ratios of Molar Absorptivities

Figure 1 illustrates that the absorption curve of β-NADH shifts to shorter wavelengths with increasing temperature (*4, 14*). The wavelength of the absorption maximum changes from about 340 nm at 0 °C to about 338.5 nm at 38 °C. The maximum at 25 °C occurs at about 339.0 nm. Although the shapes of the absorption spectra of β-NADH and β-NADPH are almost identical, the corresponding maxima of β-NADPH appear at about 0.5-nm longer wavelengths. Furthermore, the absorption curves of the coenzymes broaden with increasing temperature, as may be seen from Figure 1 in the case of β-NADH. For these reasons, the molar absorptivities of β-NADH and β-NADPH are generally different from each other, and temperature dependent. Only at 334 and about 292 nm are the ε-values for both coenzymes nearly identical. In addition, they are almost independent of temperature at these wavelengths, which could be supposed from the "quasi isobestic points" of the absorption curves of the coenzymes (Figure 1).

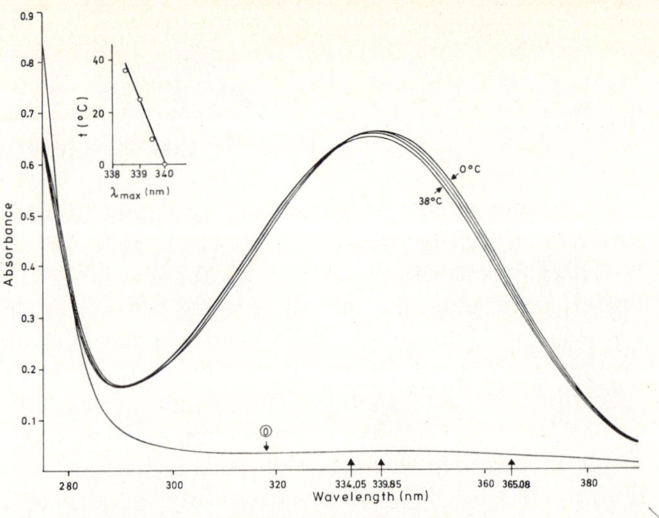

Fig. 1. Sequential recording of absorption spectra of a solution of β-NADH at 0, 10, 25, and 38 °C [from *9*]

Scan speed, 0.2 nm/s; slit width, 0.15 mm; auto gain; period, 1 s. Curve *O* was measured after enzymatic oxidation of β-NADH. At the wavelengths indicated by *arrows*, the scanning procedure was interrupted and the digitalized absorbances noted

To quantify these observations, we used the glutamate dehydrogenase system (equation 1), which allows determination of ε of both pyridine nucleotides with the same test solution because this enzyme exhibits the same activity with β-NADH as with β-NADPH as hydrogen donor. In addition, for the exact determination of the dependence of ε of β-NADH on wavelength and temperature, the lactate dehydrogenase assay (equation 2) was performed. Finally, simple temperature-jump procedures with highly purified β-NADH or β-NADPH preparations were done.

$$\text{L-Glutamate} + \beta\text{-NAD}^+(\beta\text{-NADP}^+) + H_2O \xrightleftharpoons{\text{glutamate dehydrogenase}} \text{2-oxoglutarate} + \beta\text{-NADH}(\beta\text{-NADPH}) + NH_4^+ \quad (1)$$

$$\text{L-Lactate} + \beta\text{-NAD}^+ \xrightleftharpoons{\text{lactate dehydrogenase}} \text{pyruvate} + \beta\text{-NADH} + H^+ \quad (2)$$

When enzymatic methods were used, we computed the ratios of ε-values from the ratios of the corre-

Table 1. Ratios of Molar Absorptivities of β-NADH and β-NADPH[a]

Ratio of ε-values	No. tests	Mean	SEM
β-NADH; Hg 334 nm; 25 °C / β-NADPH; Hg 334 nm; 25 °C	9	1.0007	±0.001
β-NADH; 334.15 nm; 25 °C / β-NADH; 334.15 nm; 0 °C	4	1.0032	±0.0015
β-NADH; Hg 334 nm; 25 °C / β-NADH; Hg 334 nm; 30 °C	10[b]	0.9992	±0.0001
β-NADPH; Hg 334 nm; 25 °C / β-NADPH; Hg 334 nm; 30 °C	10[b]	0.9987	±0.001
β-NADH; Hg 365 nm; 25 °C / β-NADPH; Hg 365 nm; 25 °C	9	0.9751	±0.003
β-NADH; 365.1 nm; 25 °C / β-NADH; 365.1 nm; 0 °C	4	0.9525	±0.003
β-NADH; Hg 365 nm; 25 °C / β-NADH; Hg 365 nm; 30 °C	10[b]	1.0050	±0.0001
β-NADPH; Hg 365 nm; 25 °C / β-NADPH; Hg 365 nm; 30 °C	10[b]	1.0048	±0.001
β-NADH; 340.0 nm; 0 °C / β-NADH; 334.15 nm; 0 °C	5	1.0295	±0.0003
β-NADH; 340.0 nm; 10 °C / β-NADH; 334.15 nm; 10 °C	3	1.0286	±0.003
β-NADH; 340.0 nm; 25 °C / β-NADH; 334.15 nm; 25 °C	4	1.0188	±0.0002
β-NADH; 340.0 nm; 38 °C / β-NADH; 334.15 nm; 38 °C	4	1.0141[c]	±0.003
β-NADH; 365.10 nm; 0 °C / β-NADH; 334.15 nm; 0 °C	5	0.5793	±0.0023
β-NADH; 365.10 nm; 10 °C / β-NADH; 334.15 nm; 10 °C	3	0.5670	±0.0023
β-NADH; 365.10 nm; 25 °C / β-NADH; 334.15 nm; 25 °C	4	0.5517	±0.0005
β-NADH; 365.10 nm; 38 °C / β-NADH; 334.15 nm; 38 °C	4	0.5412[c]	±0.0016

[a] Determined in triethanolamine/HCl buffer (0.1 mol/liter pH 7.6).
[b] Temperature-jump experiments.
[c] Owing to the instability of β-NADH at 38 °C, the ratio is approximate.

sponding absorbance changes to be observed after the conversion of the reactants. The values were corrected for the change of volume in the course of the test procedure, for the self-absorbance of the constituents of the analytical systems (see below), and, if necessary, for the expansion of the cuvette on heating. With temperature-jump procedures, the ratios of molar absorptivities were calculated from the ratios of the absorbances of coenzyme solution before and after heating, and corrected for the extension of solvent and cuvette and for the self-absorbance of buffer plus cuvette. The change of pH of buffer solutions with temperature was not taken into account. The results from this series of experiments (Table 1) substantiated the conclusions we drew above from the absorption spectra.

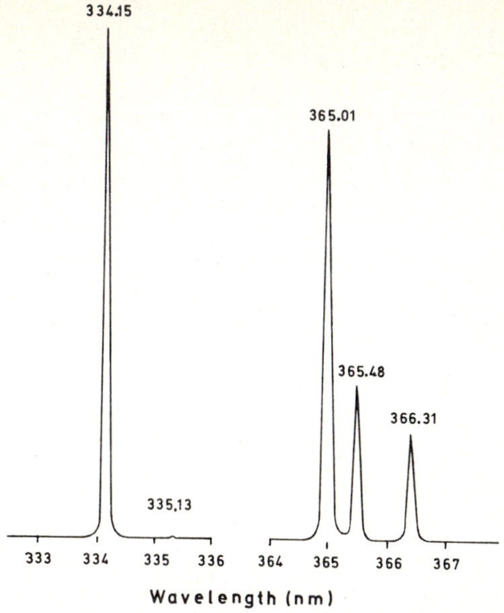

Fig. 2. Relative intensities of mercury emission spectrum lines at 334 nm and 365 nm

The lines at 334 nm were recorded at a 20-fold greater sensitivity of spectrophotometer than were the lines at 365 nm. Light source: mercury lamp No. 15 (Osram, 8 München, Germany). For further details, see *9*

The virtual identity of the molar absorptivities of β-NADH and β-NADPH and their very small dependence on temperature at 334 nm strongly suggest the use of this wavelength if precise analytical results are desired. Fortunately, on modern spectrum line-photometers the sharp and invariant mercury 334-nm line is available in this region of the spectrum.

It is interesting to note that Hg 334 nm actually consists of two spectrum lines, at 334.15 and 335.13 nm (*15*). As Figure 2 shows, however, the relative intensity of the second line is only 0.4% that of the first one. Thus the resulting deviation of the weighted average from 334.15 nm is negligible. The weak line of the mercury emission spectrum at 339.01 nm (relative intensity, 0.8% of that at 334.15 nm; not shown in the figure), which is located next to the line at 334.15 nm, is normally eliminated to about 50% by the light filter of the photometer. Therefore, it likewise can be neglected. In contrast, the triplet structure of Hg 365 (Figure 2) cannot be neglected. In this case, the weighted average depends on the vapor pressure of the mercury lamp and the characteristics of the light filter used. The slope of the absorption curves of the pyridine nucleotides at 365 nm is −5% per nm (Figure 1). Hence, the molar absorptivities of the coenzymes at that wavelength somewhat depend on the type of spectrum line-photometer used. In agreement with the findings of Netheler (*15*), the weighted average of the triplet recorded in Figure 2 is 365.32 nm.

Effects of pH and Ionic Strength on ε

The molar absorptivities of the pyridine nucleotides are influenced by pH and ionic strength of the

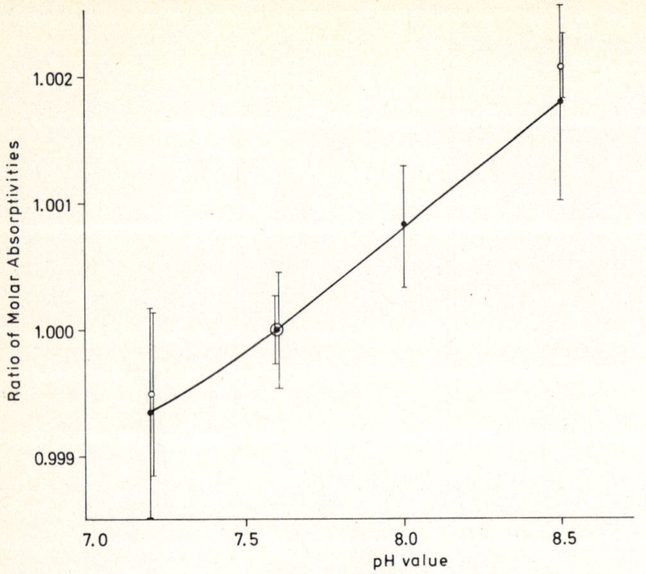

Fig. 3. Effect of pH on ε of β-NADH and β-NADPH at Hg 334 nm and 25 °C

●, β-NADH; O, β-NADPH. The solvent was triethanolamine/HCl buffer. Mean values (±SEM) of 10 replicate determinations of ratios between ε at pH indicated and ε at pH 7.6 are reported

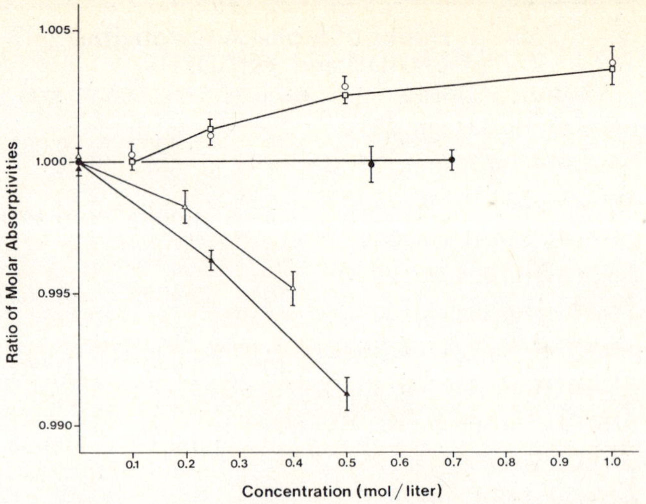

Fig. 4. Effect of ionic strength on ε of β-NADH at Hg 334 nm and 25 °C

O, triethanolamine/HCl buffer, pH 7.6; □, tris(hydroxymethyl)aminomethane-/HCl buffer, pH 7.6; ●, L-alanine; ▲, NaCl; Δ, $(NH_4)_2SO_4$. L-alanine, NaCl, and $(NH_4)_2SO_4$ were dissolved in triethanolamine/HCl buffer (0.1 mol/liter, pH 7.6). Mean values (±SEM) of five replicate determinations of ratios between ε at concentration indicated and ε in triethanolamine/HCl buffer (0.1 mol/liter, pH 7.6) are reported

solution. Figure 3 demonstrates that, in the examined pH range of 7.2–8.5, the ε-values at Hg 334 nm increase with increasing pH. Also, an increase of the molar absorptivities was observed if the concentration of the buffer used was enhanced (Figure 4). The addition of inorganic salts, such as NaCl or $(NH_4)_2SO_4$, to buffered coenzyme solutions, however, caused a decrease in ε (Figure 4). At present, it is still obscure whether in this case the changes measured are really to be explained by the effect of ionic strength. Although only analytical-grade salts were used, we cannot rule out the possibility that they contained traces of oxidizing substances or other material decomposing the coenzyme that we could not detect with the analytical procedure used. Added L-alanine left the ε of β-NADH nearly unchanged (Figure 4).

The effects of temperature, pH, and ionic strength on the molar absorptivities may reflect equilibrium shifts between different conformations of the coenzymes, which presumably differ slightly from one another by their light absorption (*14, 16*).

Absolute Molar Absorptivities

The experiments reported so far provide only information about the relative ε-values of the pyridine coenzymes. To achieve absolute calibration, we determined the molar absorptivities of β-NADH at Hg 334 or Hg 365 nm and 25 °C enzymatically, according to the procedure of Horecker and Kornberg (*1*). As reference materials, we used highly purified 2-oxoglutaric acid or pyruvic acid. With weighed amounts of these substances, the glutamate dehydrogenase or lactate dehydrogenase assay (equations 1, 2) was done in the presence of excess β-NADH. These analytical systems were chosen because of the favorable equilibrium constants of the reactions (*17*), the low absorbance of the enzymes at the wavelengths studied,[4] and the observation that the enzyme–coenzyme complex formed did not alter the absorbance of the coenzyme.[4]

The above approach for the determination of ε is essentially based on precise assessment of the purity of the 2-oxoglutaric acid and pyruvic acid preparations used. For 2-oxoglutaric acid, the absolute purity was determined by means of differential scanning calorimetry aided by moisture analysis, gas–liquid chromatography, mass spectrometry, and nuclear magnetic resonance spectroscopy. The purity of the pyruvic acid was assessed by an indirect procedure, the quantitative estimation of the impurities themselves. The methods used for this purpose included gas–liquid chromatography, gas chromatography in combination with mass spectrometry, and nuclear magnetic resonance spectroscopy.

Purity of 2-oxoglutaric acid. Differential scanning calorimetry could be applied to 2-oxoglutaric acid, because experiments with different sample holders made of aluminum or gold revealed no decomposition of the substance during the melting process (*18, 19*). The molar impurity was found to be 0.74% (n = 9; SEM = ±0.01%),[5] the melting point 114.72 ± 0.04 °C. Moisture analysis (*20*) showed the water content to be 20.0 mg/100 g of substance (n = 3; SEM = ±1.7 mg). These results clearly indicated that 100 ml of the 2-oxoglutaric acid preparation contained 99.26 mol of the acid, 0.16 mol of water, and 0.58 mol of other compounds.

[4] E. Haid and J. Ziegenhorn, unpublished.

[5] Nonstandard abbreviations used: n, number of tests; SEM, standard error of the mean; ppt, part per thousand; ppm, part per million.

Table 2. Gas-Chromatographic Analytical Data for Pyruvic Acid

Substance	No. tests	H_2O	CO_2	Acetic acid	Glyoxylic acid	Methylmaleic anhydride	Pyruvic acid
		g/100 g substance (mean ± range)					
Pyruvic acid 1	3	0.21 ± 0.07	0.13 ± 0.06	0.19 ± 0.04	0.04 ± 0.01	1.00 ± 0.11	98.43 ± 0.30
Pyruvic acid 2	3	0.26 ± 0.04	0.14 ± 0.04	0.48 ± 0.06	0.06 ± 0.01	0.60 ± 0.10	98.46 ± 0.31

Virtually no impurities could be detected in the fast Fourier transform nuclear magnetic resonance spectrum of 2-oxoglutaric acid at lower or higher field than the signals of the compound itself and its satellites.[6] The detection limit for possible impurities was calculated to be of the order of 0.1 mol per 100 mol of substance.

Gas-chromatographic analysis could only be performed after silylation of the substance through *N*-trimethylsilyl-imidazole.[7] The area of the peak obtained for 2-oxoglutaric acid amounted to 99.8% (n = 6; range = ±0.15%) of total peak area. We saw no indication of the presence of higher or lower homologs of 2-oxoglutaric acid. Furthermore, no impurities could be detected by mass spectrometry. Figure 5 shows a typical mass spectrum obtained during a temperature-programmed run.

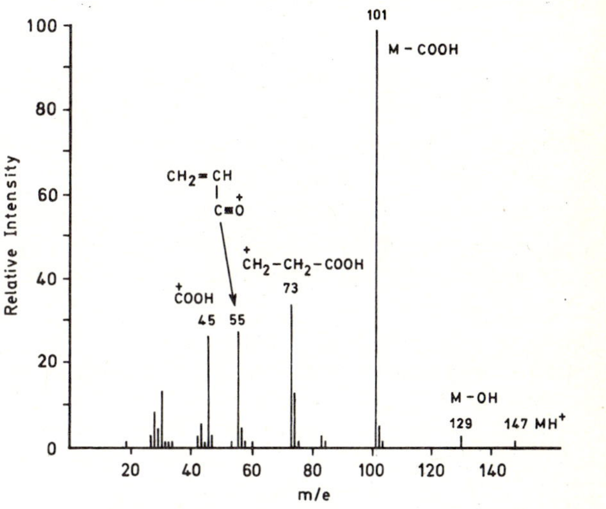

Fig. 5. Typical mass spectrum of 2-oxoglutaric acid obtained during a temperature-programmed run

Taking into consideration all available analytical data and, moreover, assuming a reasonable range of about 50–150 g for the molecular weight of the impurities present in 2-oxoglutaric acid, we calculated the percentage purity of this substance to be 99.6 ± 0.2%.

Purity of pyruvic acid. Differential scanning calorimetry could not be used for pyruvic acid because uniform crystallization of this substance proved to be impossible, presumably because small amounts of the enol form were present. Data on purity could be obtained, however, by gas–liquid chromatography.[7] For this analytical procedure, an all-glass system was used, to avoid decomposition of pyruvic acid caused by contact with metal. Porapak PS was used as the separating phase because it combines a high resolving power with inertness toward organic acids. The analyses were done by means of a flame-ionization detector or a thermoconductivity detector; with use of the latter the water content of the sample could be measured also.

Table 2 presents results of analyses for two different batches of freshly distilled pyruvic acid used in the determination of the molar absorptivities of β-NADH. In both preparations, five impurities could be detected, of which water, carbon dioxide, and acetic acid could be easily identified by comparison with the authentic material. The structure of the remaining two compounds was eludicated through electron impact mass spectrometry and chemical ionization mass spectrometry, respectively.

Identification of glyoxylic acid was based on the presence of a molecular ion at *m/e* 74 in the electron impact mass spectrum and a quasi-molecular ion at *m/e* 75 in the chemical ionization mass spectrum. Moreover, fragments at *m/e* 73 (M-H), 56 ($M-H_2O$), 45 ($COOH^+$), 29 (CHO^+), and 28 (CO^+) could be assigned to glyoxylic acid.

Methylmaleic anhydride was identified by means of a molecular ion at *m/e* 112, a quasi molecular ion after chemical ionization at *m/e* 113, and additional fragments at *m/e* 68

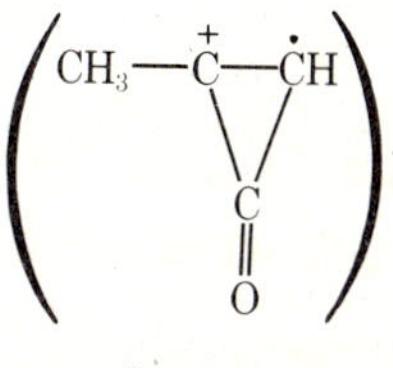

at *m/e* 40 ($CH_3—C^+{=}\dot{C}H$), and at *m/e* 39 ($CH_3—C{\equiv}C^+$).

The absence of acetaldehyde suggests that the carbon dioxide observed did not originate from decarboxylation of pyruvic acid during the analytical procedure. Because heating of the residue after distillation of pyruvic acid liberated considerable amounts of carbon dioxide, it could be assumed that the distilled pyruvic acid also contained traces of dissolved carbon dioxide.

[6] Nuclear magnetic resonance spectra were taken by W. Steingross.

[7] Gas-chromatographic analyses were done by V. Liede.

Additional information about the structure of the impurities present in pyruvic acid was obtained by use of fast Fourier transform nuclear magnetic resonance spectroscopy.[6] The low content of the impurities entailed a limited number of available data points which, in connection with different nuclear relaxation, caused a relative large error for quantitative estimations. The spectrum (Figure 6) exhibits seven signals (3 to 9) in addition to pyruvic acid or solvent proton resonance lines and carbon-13 satellites. By comparison with authentic substances, signal 3 could be assigned to methylmaleic anhydride, signal 4 to acetic acid. Glyoxylic acid could not be detected because its concentration was below the detection limit (about 0.05 mol per 100 mol of substance). The intensity of the signals 5–9 changed if the solvent or the concentration of the sample in deuterated dimethylsulfoxide was varied, an observation that led us to assume that the peaks were produced by associated molecules. Signal 9, at least, could be assigned to a hydrate of pyruvic acid.

Of the impurities present in pyruvic acid, glyoxylic acid reacts at a considerable rate with lactate dehydrogenase (*21*). Therefore, we used the sum of the concentrations of pyruvic acid and glyoxylic acid when calculating ϵ of β-NADH.

Molar absorptivities. Two different quantities of each of the above three substrate preparations were weighed by use of two different balances. With these amounts of substances, in each case, two stock solutions of different substrate content were made that were used in the assays for the determination of ϵ of β-NADH. The measurements were made simultaneously on three different Eppendorf spectrum line photometers.

The test results were evaluated according to equation 3,

$$\epsilon^{\lambda}_{\beta\text{-NADH}} = \frac{\frac{a}{a+b}(A^{\lambda}_1 - A^{\lambda}_3) - A^{\lambda}_2 + A^{\lambda}_4}{\frac{a}{a+b}\cdot c\cdot d} - \epsilon^{\lambda}_{\text{substrate}} + \epsilon^{\lambda}_{\text{product}} + \epsilon^{\lambda}_{\beta\text{-NAD}} \quad (3)$$

where λ = measuring wavelength, a = volume (in ml) of test solution at 25 °C before addition of enzyme, b = volume (in ml) of added enzyme solution at 25 °C, c = molar substrate concentration at 25 °C before addition of enzyme solution, d = pathlength (in cm) of the cuvette at 25 °C, substrate is 2-oxoglutarate or pyruvate, and product is L-glutamate or L-lactate. The measured absorbances were corrected for multiple reflections in the cell (*22*). c was calculated from the weighed quantities of substrates dissolved per liter of test solution at 20 °C, taking into account the percentage purity of the compounds and the expansion of the solution on heating from 20 to 25 °C. In this temperature range, the coefficients of thermal expansion of the solutions used were found to be equal to that of water.[8] In all weighing procedures, we corrected for the buoyancy of the air (*10*). d was corrected for beam convergence: in the spectrum line-photometers used, the angle of aperture of the pencil of rays was 14.8° in the vertical plane and about 0° in the horizontal plane. From this it followed that the actual lightpath was 1.4 ppt longer than the pathlength of the cuvette.[9] We corrected for the self-absorbance of 2-oxoglutarate, pyruvate, L-glutamate, L-lactate, and β-NAD by using the molar absorptivities reported in Table 3 and in a recent communication (*11*). Effects of fluorescence were not taken into consideration.

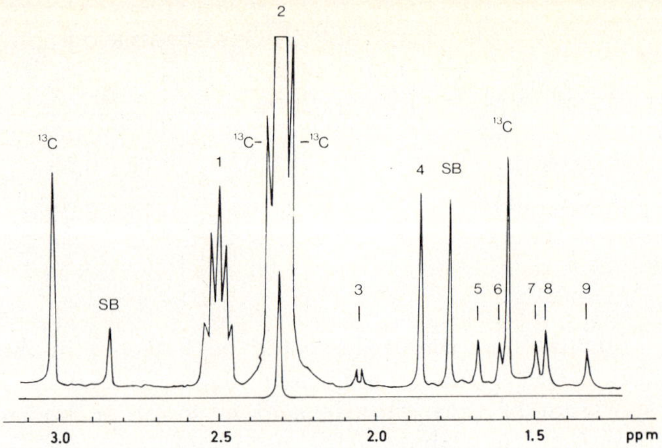

Fig. 6. Nuclear magnetic resonance spectrum of pyruvic acid
Pyruvic acid 2 was used. ^{13}C, carbon-13 satellites; *SB*, side bands; *1*, partly deuterated dimethylsulfoxide; *2*, pyruvic acid; *3*, methylmaleic anhydride; *4*, acetic acid; *5–8*, artefacts; *9*, pyruvic acid hydrate

Following the procedure outlined above, we obtained for β-NADH at Hg 334 nm and Hg 365 nm and at 25 °C the molar absorptivities summarized in Table 4. Examination of this Table reveals slight differences between the outcome of each series of experiments, which we supposed to be chiefly due to errors in the determination of the purity of the substrates. Because in the two analytical systems the same buffer, the same pH value, and an about equal ionic strength was used, the measured values could be combined in each case to yield total mean values. The data shown for the standard error of the mean of the results characterize the precision of the whole enzymatic test procedure, beginning from the weighing of substrates. They were not corrected for the individual errors made at the determination of the respective correction factors, because the exact mathematical relationships between the different errors were unknown. Because the uncertainties associated with all other systematic errors were less than 1 ppt, the uncertainty of the content of the substrates determined the total uncertainty of the final results in the main. Referring to the highest possible or lowest possible content, we estimated the overall range of ϵ at Hg 334

[8] K. Stephani and J. Ziegenhorn, unpublished.
[9] G. Bechtler and D. Bouchain, Eppendorf Gerätebau Netheler & Hinz, personal communication.

Table 3. Molar Absorptivities of Some Compounds at 25 °C[a]

Substance	No. tests	Mean	SEM
		liter·mol^{-1}·cm^{-1}	
Measured at Hg 334 nm			
2-Oxoglutarate	10	19.4	±0.03
Pyruvate	10	19.2	±0.03
L-Glutamate	10	≤0.08	±0.02
L-Lactate	10	≤0.04	±0.001
β-NAD	10	≤2.5	±0.03
Measured at Hg 365 nm			
2-Oxoglutarate	10	3.9	±0.02
Pyruvate	10	4.8	±0.02
L-Glutamate	10	≤0.04	±0.01
L-Lactate	10	≤0.02	±0.001
β-NAD	10	≤1.6	±0.03

[a] Determined in triethanolamine/HCl buffer (0.1 mol/liter, pH 7.6).

Table 4. Absolute Molar Absorptivities of β-NADH at Hg 334 nm or Hg 365 nm and 25 °C[a]

Method	Wavelength, nm	No. tests	Mean	SEM
			liter·mol^{-1}·cm^{-1}	
Glutamate dehydrogenase assay	Hg 334	28	6.179×10^3	±3
	Hg 365	28	3.444×10^3	±2
Lactate dehydrogenase assay, pyruvic acid 1	Hg 334	28	6.162×10^3	±2
	Hg 365	28	3.432×10^3	±2
Lactate dehydrogenase assay, pyruvic acid 2	Hg 334	28	6.187×10^3	±3
	Hg 365	28	3.448×10^3	±2
Total	Hg 334	84	6.176×10^3	±2
	Hg 365	84	3.441×10^3	±2

[a] Determined in triethanolamine/HCl buffer (0.1 mol/liter, pH 7.6).

nm and Hg 365 nm to be ±20 liter·mol^{-1}·cm^{-1} and ±12 liter·mol^{-1}·cm^{-1}, respectively.

By combination of the absolute ϵ-value of β-NADH at Hg 334 nm and 25 °C with the ratios of ϵ (Table 1), the molar absorptivities of β-NADH and β-NADPH at other wavelengths and temperatures can be calculated. Some of the more important data are listed in Table 5.

The Δϵ-values presented in the last column of Table 5 have not been corrected for the self-absorbance of oxidized coenzymes and beam convergence. These values are more suited for practical use. First, with all enzymatic reactions utilizing β-NADH or β-NADPH, β-NAD$^+$ or β-NADP$^+$ are formed and only Δϵ is needed for the calculation of the results. Second, all modern photometers exhibit some beam convergence. At present, it is still unknown whether, in

Table 5. Molar Absorptivities of β-NADH and β-NADPH at Various Wavelengths and Temperatures[a]

Wavelength, nm	Temp., °C	ϵ	Δϵ[b]
		liter·mol^{-1}·cm^{-1}	
β-NADH			
Hg 334	25	6.176×10^3	6.182×10^3
Hg 334	30		6.187×10^3
Hg 365	25	3.441×10^3	3.444×10^3
Hg 365	30		3.427×10^3
339.85 ≈ 340	25	6.292×10^3	6.298×10^3
β-NADPH			
Hg 334	25		6.178×10^3
Hg 334	30		6.186×10^3
Hg 365	25		3.532×10^3
Hg 365	30		3.515×10^3

[a] Determined in triethanolamine/HCl buffer (0.1 mol/liter, pH 7.6).
[b] Values were not corrected for beam convergence and for self-absorbance of oxidized coenzyme.

the near-ultraviolet, β-NADP has the same slight self-absorbance as β-NAD. In calculating the results of Table 1, we assumed the molar absorptivities of the oxidized coenzymes to be identical.

In a previous publication (*11*), we reported relative values for the molar absorptivities of β-NADH and β-NAD$^+$ at 260 nm. The data were computed for the present with the old value of 6.22×10^3 for β-NADH at 340 nm and 25 °C, as the current study was not yet settled. Referring to the new absorption coefficient of β-NADH at 340 nm and 25 °C (Table 5), the ϵ-values of β-NADH or β-NAD at 260 nm and 25 °C were calculated to be 14.25×10^3 liter·mol^{-1}·cm^{-1} or 17.57×10^3 liter·mol^{-1}·cm^{-1}.

The molar absorptivities of the reduced pyridine nucleotides observed at Hg 334 nm, Hg 365 nm, and 340 nm in our laboratories are about 1 to 7% higher than the values commonly used, which essentially confirms earlier findings (*4*). Likewise, a higher ϵ-value has been recently reported for NADH at 340 nm and 25 °C by McComb et al. (*23*).

This study was initiated by Professor Dr. H. U. Bergmeyer. We are grateful to him and to Dr. M. Grassl, W. Gruber, and G. Lettenbauer for helpful discussions. We are greatly obliged to Dr. A. Hagen for his active interest in this work and for critical reading parts of the manuscript. We thank Dr. H. Hindermayr, H. Hoffmann, H. Krell, G. Lusch, and K. Stephani for excellent technical assistance. We are indebted to M. Glocke for mathematical advice and statistical calculations and to Dr. H. Schwab for measuring the mercury emission spectrum. We also thank Dr. W. Seidel (BASF, 67 Ludwigshafen, Germany) for taking the chemical ionization mass spectra and Drs. G. Bechtler and D. Bouchain (Eppendorf Gerätebau Netheler & Hinz, 2 Hamburg, Germany) for providing constructional data on the Eppendorf photometer. This investigation was supported in part by the Deutsche Forschungsgemeinschaft, Sonderforschungsbereich 51, and the Fonds der Chemischen Industrie.

References

1. Horecker, B. L., and Kornberg, A., The extinction coefficients of the reduced band of pyridine nucleotides. *J. Biol. Chem.* **175**, 385 (1948).

2. Beisenherz, G., Bücher, Th., and Garbade, K.-H., α-Glycerophosphate dehydrogenase from rabbit muscle. *Methods Enzymol.* **1**, 391 (1955).

3. Hohorst, H. J., Enzymatische Bestimmung von L(+)-Milchsäure. *Biochem. Z.* **328**, 509 (1957).

4. Bücher, Th., Luh, W., and Pette, D., Einfache und zusammengesetzte optische Tests mit Pyridinnucleotiden. In *Hoppe-Seyler/Thierfelder: Handbuch der Physiologisch- und Pathologisch-chemischen Analyse* **VI/A**, K. Lang and E. Lehnartz, Eds. Springer Verlag, Berlin, Göttingen, Heidelberg, New York, 1964, pp 292–339.

5. Haeckel, R., and Haeckel, H., Die Zuverlässigkeit der automatisierten Aktivitätsbestimmung der Kreatinkinase. In *Fortschritte der Klinischen Chemie: Enzyme und Hormone,* E. Kaiser, Ed. Verlag der Wiener Medizinischen Akadmie, Wien, 1972, pp 115–119.

6. Da Fonseca-Wollheim, F., Enzymatische Glucosebestimmung in hämolysierten Blutproben ohne Störung durch Fructose. *Z. Klin. Chem. Klin. Biochem.* **9**, 497 (1971).

7. Bücher, Th., Krell, H., Lusch, G., et al., Molar extinction coefficients of NADH and NADPH at Hg spectral lines. *Z. Klin. Chem. Klin. Biochem.* **12**, 239 (1974).

8. Haid, E., Lehmann, P., and Ziegenhorn, J., The molar absorption coefficients of β-nicotinamide-adenine dinucleotide. In *Quality Control in Clinical Chemistry,* G. Anido, S. B. Rosalki, E. F. van Kampen and M. Rubin, Eds. Walter de Gruyter, Berlin, New York, 1975, pp 235–240.

9. Bücher, Th., Lusch, G., and Krell, H., Temperature dependence of difference-absorption coefficients of NADH minus NAD^+ and NADPH minus $NADP^+$ in the near ultraviolet. *Ibid.*, pp 301–310.

10. Küster, F. W., Thiel, A., and Fischbeck, K., *Logarithmische Rechentafeln.* Walter de Gruyter, Berlin, New York, 1972, pp 119–120.

11. Haid, E., Lehmann, P., and Ziegenhorn, J., Molar absorptivities of β-NADH and β-NAD at 260 nm. *Clin. Chem.* **21**, 884 (1975).

12. Bergmeyer, H. U., and Bernt, E., 2-Oxoglutarate. In *Methods of Enzymatic Analysis* **3**, H. U. Bergmeyer, Ed. Academic Press, New York, London, 1974, pp 1577–1580.

13. Bernt, E., and Bergmeyer, H. U., L-Glutamate. *Ibid.*, **4**, pp 1704–1708.

14. Malcolm, A. D. B., The temperature dependence of the spectroscopic properties of reduced nicotinamide adenine dinucleotide. *Anal. Biochem.* **55**, 278 (1973).

15. Netheler, H. G., Types of photometer. In *Methods of Enzymatic Analysis* **1**, H. U. Bergmeyer, Ed. Academic Press, New York, London, 1974, pp 184–190.

16. Torreilles, J., and Crastes de Paulet, A., Studies of NAD(H) conformations in solution: A new method using the PMR spectra of cobalt ion-dinucleotide complexes. *Biochim. Biophys. Acta* **362**, 375 (1974).

17. Bergmeyer, H. U., Gawehn, K., and Grassl, M., Enzymes as biochemical reagents. In *Methods of Enzymatic Analysis* **I**, H. U. Bergmeyer, Ed. Academic Press, New York, London, 1974, pp 425–522.

18. Plato, C., and Glasgow, A. R., Differential scanning calorimetry as a general method for determining the purity and heat of fusion of high-purity organic chemicals. *Anal. Chem.* **41**, 330 (1969).

19. DeAngelis, N. J., and Papariello, G. J., Differential scanning calorimetry. *J. Pharm. Sci.* **47**, 1868 (1968).

20. Du Pont (CEC) Bulletin No. 1863/467, Moisture monitor hints. E. I. du Pont de Nemours, Wilmington, Del. 19898.

21. Romano, M., and Cerra, M., The action of crystalline lactate dehydrogenase from rabbit muscle on glyoxylate. *Biochim. Biophys. Acta* **177**, 421 (1969).

22. Burnett, R. W., Errors in ultraviolet and visible spectrophotometric measurements caused by multiple reflections in the cell. *Anal. Chem.* **45**, 383 (1973).

23. McComb, R. B., Bond, L. W., Keech, R., et al., A redetermination of the molar absorptivity of reduced NAD. *Clin. Chem.* **20**, 882 (1974). Abstract. (The paper preceding this one in this issue is the full account.—*Ed.*).

CLIN. CHEM. 22/2, 161–168 (1976)

Erythrocyte Porphyrin Analysis in the Detection of Lead Poisoning in Children: Evaluation of Four Micromethods

Thomas L. Hanna, David N. Dietzler, Carl H. Smith, Santosh Gupta, and Harold S. Zarkowsky

We evaluated four procedures for determination of erythrocyte porphyrin: double extraction with ethyl acetate/acetic acid–HCl, single extraction with ethanol, single extraction with acetone, and direct solubilization with detergent–buffer. The ethyl acetate procedure, when used with two portions of HCl, apparently gives complete recovery of porphyrin and is suitable for reference as a comparison method. The ethanol procedure gives a high and consistent recovery and is technically simpler. The acetone procedure gives low and variable recovery of porphyrin, and the detergent–buffer method is subject to serious hemoglobin interference; neither of these two procedures offers any technical advantage. Stability of samples and methods for standardization were explored. A procedure for expressing results in terms of erythrocyte Zn–protoporphyrin content is given. Because of its stability, coproporphyrin is useful as a daily working standard. The ethyl acetate and ethanol methods are about equally efficient for detecting lead intoxication. Because of its simplicity, the ethanol method seems to be the best for use in screening.

Additional Keyphrases: *screening* • *iron deficiency*

Lead is known to interfere with the synthesis of hemoglobin, and the erythrocytes of children with lead poisoning are known to contain increased porphyrin concentrations (*1*). The interest in erythrocyte porphyrin determination for the detection of lead poisoning in children has resulted in the development of a number of methods of analysis (*2–10*).

Divisions of Clinical Chemistry, and Hematology and Oncology, The Edward Mallinckrodt Department of Pediatrics, Washington University School of Medicine; St. Louis Children's Hospital, St. Louis, Mo. 63110.

Received Aug. 13, 1975; accepted Nov. 5, 1975.

Early procedures were based on the double-extraction method, in which porphyrins were extracted from blood with ethyl acetate/acetic acid and subsequently separated from contaminating substances by re-extraction with HCl. Porphyrins were first measured in the HCl extract spectrophotometrically (*2, 3*) and later were measured fluorometrically, with increased sensitivity and specificity (*4–6*). Subsequently, investigators attempted to simplify the fluorometric determinations by using a one-step extraction with substances such as acetone (*7, 8*) or ethanol (*9*). More recently, a nonextraction fluorometric technique has been reported, in which blood is solubilized in a detergent–buffer solution (*10*). Until then, coproporphyrin I had been used exclusively as a standard and its absorbance or fluorescence was related to that of protoporphyrin IX. With the knowledge that the protoporphyrin IX accumulating in the erythrocyte in lead intoxication is complexed with Zn ion, this Zn–protoporphyrin itself has been recommended for use as a standard (*10, 11*).

Erythrocyte porphyrin concentration, measured fluorometrically in microsamples, has been reported to correlate with blood lead concentration (*1, 4–7*). Because of its simplicity, measurement of porphyrin has been recommended in screening for lead poisoning (*11*). The fluorometric procedures are reportedly sensitive, economical, and practical, yet there are no comparative data to aid in selecting a particular method. We undertook to evaluate the four principal fluorometric methods available: double extraction with ethyl acetate/acetic acid–HCl (*6*), single extraction with acetone (*8*), single extraction with ethanol (*9*), and the direct solubilization of whole blood with detergent (*10*). We have examined analytical characteristics of these methods, explored procedures for their standardization, and assessed their relative usefulness in detection of lead poisoning.

Materials and Methods

Reagents

Coproporphyrin I was obtained in preweighed vials (catalog No. COP 1-5; Sigma Chemical Co., St. Louis, Mo. 63178). Zn–protoporphyrin IX was obtained in preweighed vials from Dr. Bruce Burnham (Porphyrin Products, Logan, Utah 84321). "Ammonyx LO" (dimethyldodecylamine) was obtained from Onyx Chemical Co., Jersey City, N. J. 07302. A stable fluorescent dye (Rhodamine B, cat. No. B1193) was obtained from Matheson, Coleman and Bell, Norwood, Ohio 45212. Aqueous solutions of 40 μg/liter were used daily to check the stability of porphyrin standards. Hemoglobin solutions were prepared by water hemolysis of packed erythrocytes. Erythrocyte membranes were removed by centrifugation at 4 °C and 47 000 × *g* for 30 min. The supernatant fluid was then dialyzed for 24 h at 4 °C vs. a phosphate buffer (0.1 mol/liter, pH 7.4). The concentration of hemoglobin in the supernate was determined with a hemoglobinometer (Coulter Instruments, Inc., Hialeah, Fla. 33010).

Apparatus

Fluorometric measurements were made with a Model A fluorometer (Farrand Optical Co., Inc., Valhalla, N. Y. 10595) equipped with a Honeywell galvanometer, mercury lamp, and RCA No. HP28 photomultiplier tube. Primary filters were Corning No. 5850 and No. 3850; secondary filters were Corning No. 2424 and No. 9788. These combinations of broadbandpass filters yielded maximum transmittance at approximately 408 nm for the primary set and 596 nm for the secondary set. Spectrofluorometric measurements were made with an Aminco Bowman Spectrofluorometer (American Instruments, Silver Spring, Md. 20910). A Beckman Model DU Spectrophotometer (Beckman Instruments, Fullerton, Calif. 92634) was used for all absorbance measurements.

Samples

Blood samples from children suspected of chronic ingestion of lead were obtained from the Lead Evaluation Center, St. Louis Department of Health. Samples from a nonselected population were obtained from the acute-care clinics at St. Louis Children's Hospital, St. Louis. Porphyrin was determined in samples from both groups in the course of the clinical care of these patients.

Procedures

Ethyl acetate/acetic acid porphyrin determinations were performed by the method of Piomelli (*6*) except that 30-μl samples were used and 0.5 mol/liter HCl (*5*) was used in place of the 1.5 mol/liter HCl specified. A coproporphyrin I standard, dissolved in 1.5 mol/liter HCl, was taken through this procedure and used for setting the fluorometer. The concentration of the coproporphyrin standard was calculated by the formula:

$$\text{Coproporphyrin I, mg/liter} = [2A_{401} - (A_{380} + A_{430})] \times 0.817$$

In this formula the correction of Rimington (*12*) is applied, to minimize interference by impurities.

Acetone extractions were performed by the method of Chisholm et al. (*8*).

Determinations with use of detergent buffer were performed by the method of Lamola et al. (*10*).

Ethanol extractions were performed by the method of Murphey (*9*). In this procedure 20 μl of whole blood is pipetted directly into a 12 × 75 mm test tube containing 1.75 ml of ethanol (94% by volume). The contents of the tube are then mixed on a vortex-type mixer for 30 s and centrifuged for 3 min at 1600 × *g*. The supernate is transferred to a 10 × 75 mm test tube and its fluorescence is measured. Coproporphyrin I standards dissolved in 0.1 mol/liter HCl were taken through the ethanol and acetone extraction procedures, and were used for setting the fluorometer. The concentration of these coproporphyrin standards was determined by using the millimolar absorptivity value of 489 at 400 nm, which had previously been determined for coproporphyrin in 0.1 mol/liter HCl (*12*).

The concentration of porphyrin extracted by any of the four methods is:

$$\text{Porphyrin, }\mu\text{g/liter of erythrocytes} = Fu \times Cs/Fs \times 100/\text{Hct} \times 1000$$

Fu = fluorescence of unknown
Fs = fluorescence of standard
Cs = concentration of standard (mg/liter, coproporphyrin I)
Hct = hematocrit

Blood lead determinations were performed by atomic absorption spectroscopy (*13*) in the central laboratory of the St. Louis Department of Health.

Zn–Protoporphyrin Standards

Three procedures for preparation of Zn–protoporphyrin IX standards were investigated.

(*a*) The contents of a preweighed vial of Zn–protoporphyrin IX were dissolved in 100 μl of an organic solvent NH_4OH mixture (Protosol, Porphyrin Products) and diluted to the desired concentration with HCl, 1.5 mol/liter. Because this procedure converts Zn–protoporphyrin IX to protoporphyrin IX, the concentration of this standard was calculated by using the millimolar absorptivity value for protoporphyrin IX of 262 at 408 nm, with 1.5 mol/liter HCl as the solvent (*11*).

(*b*) Zn–protoporphyrin IX was dissolved in a minimum volume of 0.1 mol/liter NaOH and diluted to the desired concentration with de-ionized water according to the instructions of Leonard et al. (*14*). Final concentration was calculated by using a millimolar absorptivity value for Zn–protoporphyrin IX of 87.4 at 412 nm (*14*).

(*c*) The contents of a preweighed vial of Zn–protoporphyrin IX were dissolved in 100 μl of Protosol, and 20-μl aliquots were diluted with 1.5 mol/liter HCl or phosphate buffer (pH 7.4, 0.1 mol/liter). The concentration of this acid solution was determined as described above. Identical amounts of Zn–protoporphyrin in buffer and in 1.5 mol/liter HCl were extracted by the ethyl acetate procedure and their fluorescences compared. The identical fluorescence of the two standards suggested that their concentrations were the same. This third method proved most satisfactory for preparation of standards for the ethanol and ethyl acetate extraction procedures.

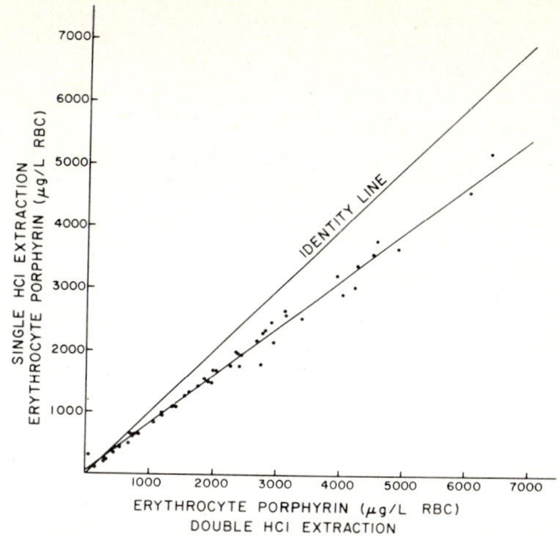

Fig. 1. Recovery of erythrocyte porphyrin with single and double HCl extraction (ethyl acetate method)

Blood samples from 186 patients were assayed by the ethyl acetate method. The regression equation is $y = 0.771x + 4.41$, indicating that recovery with a single extraction approximates 77% of that obtained by double extraction (values based on coproporphyrin)

Results

Completeness of Extraction

Because the ethyl acetate method is based on established extraction procedures, it seemed likely that this method would result in nearly complete extraction of porphyrin from erythrocytes. Completeness of extraction was tested by re-extracting both the erythrocyte residue (with ethyl acetate/acetic acid) and the original ethyl acetate/acetic acid layer (with HCl). The former yielded no additional fluorescence; the latter, however, did yield additional fluorescence. Figure 1 compares the fluorescence yield of a single extraction with HCl with that of two HCl extractions. The double extraction yielded 23% more fluorescence than did a single extraction, but a third and fourth HCl extraction of the same organic phase yielded no additional fluorescence. When 1.5 mol/liter HCl was substituted for 0.5 mol/liter HCl (the concentration we used in this study) the distribution of fluorescence between the first and second extractions was unaltered. In the ethyl acetate extraction method, two HCl extractions apparently completely extract porphyrins from erythrocytes. The values so obtained were regarded as reference values for the purpose of this study.

The erythrocyte porphyrin content of 185 blood specimens was determined by this method, and also by the acetone and ethanol extraction methods. The acetone extraction method yielded between 6 and 17% of the total porphyrin value given by the ethyl acetate method (Figure 2*A*). Because of the threefold variation in extraction efficiency and low rccovery compared to the ethyl acetate procedure, the acetone method was not examined further.

In the ethanol extraction method fluorescence was proportional to zinc protoporphyrin concentration up to 2050 μg/liter of sample (equivalent to 5000 μg/liter of erythrocytes, assuming a hematocrit of 40%). The

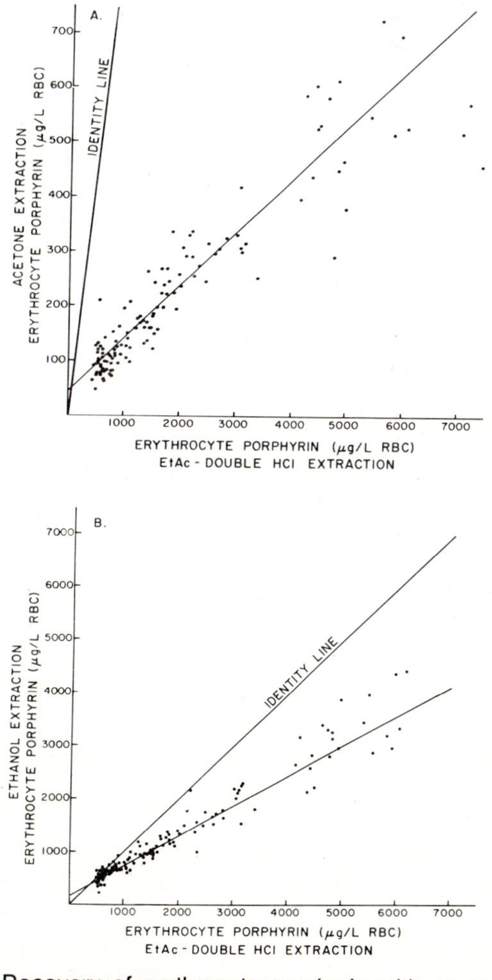

Fig. 2. Recovery of erythrocyte porphyrin with acetone extraction or ethanol extraction compared with ethyl acetate (*EtAc*)–HCl extraction

Blood samples from 186 patients were assayed by the acetone, ethanol, and ethyl acetate-double HCl extraction methods. Calculated values were based on coproporphyrin. *A*, the regression equation is $y = 0.098x + 4.16$; recovery with the acetone method is only 9.8% of the value obtained by double extraction. *B*, the equation of the line is $y = 0.56x + 18.0$; recovery with the ethanol method is 56% of the value obtained by double HCl extraction

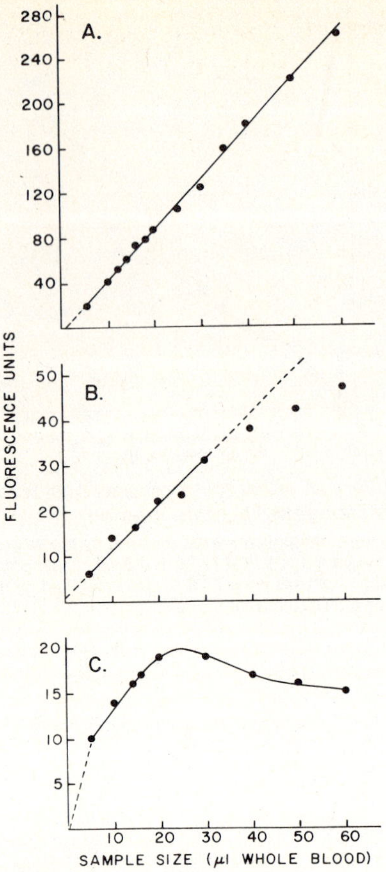

Fig. 3. Relationship of fluorescence to sample volume: three methods of analysis

Samples from individual patients were analyzed by the (*A*) ethyl acetate, (*B*) ethanol, and (*C*) detergent buffer methods. Results are typical in each case of results for samples from three different patients

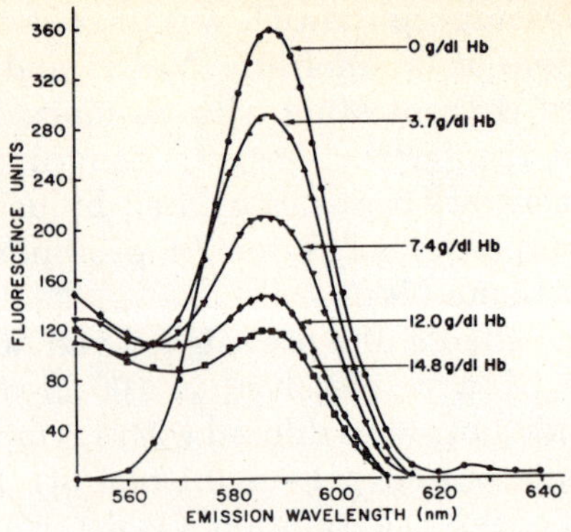

Fig. 4. Hemoglobin (*Hb*) suppression of fluorescence in the detergent/buffer method

A Zn–protoporphyrin solution (1.32 mg/liter, in water) was diluted as in the detergent/buffer method in the presence of various concentrations of added Hb. The lines are labeled with the original Hb concentrations in a blood sample analyzed by the method. Because of the dilution of the sample in the procedure, the final concentration in the assay mixtures is 0.002 the original concentration. Emission spectra of the resulting products are shown. Excitation wavelength was fixed at 416 nm. Hb causes a marked distortion of the fluorescence spectra and suppression of the peak value. Over the usual clinical range of Hb concentration, fluorescence varies markedly (compare 7.4 g of Hb/dl with 14.8 g of Hb/dl)

ethanol method yielded about 56% of the total porphyrin value given by the ethyl acetate method (Figure 2*B*). Re-extraction of the erythrocyte residue with a second volume of ethanol increased the total porphyrin extracted by an additional 17.6 ± 3.2%.[1]

Relationship of Fluorescence Intensity to Sample Volume

With both the ethyl acetate and ethanol extraction methods, fluorescence was proportional to sample size (Figure 3*A*,*B*). The ethyl acetate method demonstrates proportionality with samples as large as 60 µl, and the ethanol method with samples as large as 20 to 30 µl. With the detergent method, fluorescence was not proportional to sample size (Figure 3*C*) over any range of sample volume. Lack of proportionality with this procedure suggested that hemoglobin solubilized by the detergent might be interfering with the porphyrin fluorescence. To evaluate this possibility, we added a constant amount of Zn–protoporphyrin to solutions of detergent–buffer containing various amounts of hemoglobin. As hemoglobin concentration increased, fluorescence markedly decreased (Figure 4). Calculations based on these data show that an initial hemoglobin concentration of 120 g/liter in a sample to be analyzed would decrease porphyrin fluorescence by 59%. Variations in the hemoglobin concentration over the range commonly found in patients' samples would cause marked apparent fluctuations in the porphyrin measured by this procedure.

Identification of Products

Lamola and Yamane (*15*) have identified the substance that accumulates in the erythrocyte in lead intoxication as Zn–protoporphyrin IX. Fluorescence spectra are commonly used in identification of porphyrins extracted from whole blood. We examined the spectra of extracts from the ethyl acetate and ethanol methods, comparing the relative excitation and emission maxima of such extracts with similar extracts of known substances (Table 1). Extraction of whole blood by the ethanol procedure gave values corresponding to those described for Zn–protoporphyrin. Extraction of whole blood or Zn–protoporphyrin solutions by the ethyl acetate method gave values corresponding to those for free protoporphyrin IX.

Stability

Ten samples of whole blood were analyzed immediately by the ethyl acetate and ethanol methods. Aliquots of the same 10 samples were also stored in a Celite/saline suspension (*6*) for re-analysis by the ethyl acetate method, and in 94% ethanol for re-analysis by the ethanol method. After 72 h the former had a mean porphyrin concentration of 97.2 ± 13.8% of their original value whereas the latter had a mean porphyrin concentration of 86.4 ± 6.6% of their original value.

[1] All data presented in this form represent the mean value and standard deviation.

Standardization

Coproporphyrin I has commonly been used as a calibration standard in fluorometry of erythrocyte porphyrin (*4–9*) and Zn–protoporphyrin has recently been identified (*15*) as the major porphyrin accumulating in the erythrocyte in lead intoxication. Therefore, we examined both of these compounds as standards for the ethyl acetate and ethanol procedures.

Solutions of coproporphyrin in 1.5 mol/liter or 0.1 mol/liter HCl demonstrate remarkable stability. When such solutions were stored in the dark their concentrations, determined spectrophotometrically, varied less than 3.0% in 60 days. By comparison with a stable fluorescent dye solution (Rhodamine B, 40 µg/liter), the fluorescence intensity of these solutions was similarly constant over the same interval.

Solutions of coproporphyrin I in either water or 0.1 mol/liter HCl had a fluorescence emission peak at 602 nm when they were diluted with ethanol. When coproporphyrin I was dissolved in concentrations of HCl greater than 0.1 mol/liter and diluted with ethanol, the peak shifted to 592 nm, and the fluorescence intensity increased by more than 1.5-fold. Therefore only solutions of coproporphyrin prepared in 0.1 mol/liter (or more dilute) HCl were used as standards for the ethanol method. In contrast, solutions of coproporphyrin I in HCl in concentrations as great as 1.5 mol/liter behave identically in the ethyl acetate extraction method.

Preparation of Zn–protoporphyrin standards presented a more complex problem. Table 2 outlines the various procedures and difficulties encountered with each of them. We found it necessary to dissolve the Zn–protoporphyrin in Protosol; for use in the ethanol method, this solution must be diluted into buffer, while either buffer or acid may be used in the ethyl acetate method. In both extraction procedures, the spectral characteristics of appropriate Zn–protoporphyrin solutions were identical to those of porphyrin

Table 1. Fluorescence Characteristics of Extraction Products

	Maxima, nm	
	Emission	Excitation
Ethyl acetate method		
Protoporphyrin IX[a]	605	405
Zn–protoporphyrin IX	600	404
Erythrocytes from patients with lead poisoning	600	404
Ethanol method		
Protoporphyrin IX[b]	632	403
Zn–protoporphyrin IX[b]	588	416
Erythrocytes from patients with lead poisoning[b]	588	416
Detergent/buffer method		
Protoporphyrin IX[c]	619	400
Zn–protoporphyrin IX	588	416
Erythrocytes from patients with lead poisoning	588	416

[a] Values from our investigation and literature are in agreement (*1,6*).
[b] Values from our investigation and literature are in agreement (*15*).
[c] Obtained from published data (*15*).

Table 2. Zn–protoporphyrin Standards—Preparation and Properties[a]

Solvent	100 µl Protosol			100 µl NaOH, 0.1 mol/liter		100 µl NH_4OH, 0.1 mol/liter	
Diluent	PO_4^{3-}, 0.1 mol/liter pH 7.4	H_2O	HCl, 1.5 mol/liter	HCl, 1.5 mol/liter	H_2O	PO_4^{3-}, 0.1 mol/liter pH 7.4	HCl, 1.5 mol/liter
Spectrophotometric absorbance peak	416 nm	416 nm	402 nm	no absorbance	416 nm	402 nm	402 nm
Spectrophotometric standardization	unsatisfactory[b]	unsatisfactory[b]	satisfactory[c]	unsatisfactory	satisfactory[d]	unsatisfactory[b]	unsatisfactory[e]
Use in ethyl acetate method	satisfactory[f]	satisfactory[f]	satisfactory	n.a.[g]	unsatisfactory[h]	n.a.	n.a.
Use in ethanol method	satisfactory	unsatisfactory[i]	unsatisfactory[j]	n.a.	unsatisfactory[i]	n.a.	n.a.

[a] Preweighed vials of Zn–protoporphyrin were dissolved in the various solvents. Aliquots of these solutions were diluted to 1 mg/liter with the specified diluents. Spectrophotometric standardization was performed where possible and applications to the two recommended methods are noted.
[b] No published extinction coefficient.
[c] Millimolar absorptivity of 262 at 408 nm, as protoporphyrin IX (*11*).
[d] Millimolar absorptivity of 87.4 at 412 nm, as Zn–protoporphyrin IX (*14*).
[e] Incomplete recovery of the Zn–protoporphyrin; absorbance < 20% of the expected value (*11*).
[f] Concentration based on aliquot diluted in acid (*11*).
[g] Not applicable.
[h] Relationship of fluorescence to calculated concentration not reproducible.
[i] Fluorescence less than a third that of standard diluted with PO_4^{3-} buffer, 0.1 mol/liter.
[j] Zn–protoporphyrin complex dissociated by acid.

extracted from whole blood. Buffered Zn–protoporphyrin was apparently taken through the ethanol extraction as a stable complex; in the ethyl acetate extraction, the Zn–protoporphyrin complex was apparently dissociated and free protoporphyrin IX was produced (Table 1).

Neutral solutions of Zn–protoporphyrin were not stable; their fluorescence decreased by more than 30% in 24 h. In contrast, acid solutions of protoporphyrin IX prepared from Zn–protoporphyrin showed a mean variation in concentration of only 2.8% after 48 h.

Fluorescence-by-weight ratios of coproporphyrin to Zn–protoporphyrin IX were calculated for both the ethanol and ethyl acetate methods. We have determined a ratio of 1/1.21 (Copro/Zn–proto) for the ethanol procedure and a similar ratio, 1/1.26, for the ethyl acetate procedure. The latter factor agrees with earlier values established for protoporphyrin IX (*6*).

Results of Screening

Erythrocyte porphyrin concentration was determined by the ethanol method in an initial study of 672 samples from children who were being evaluated for lead intoxication. None of these children had previously been treated for lead poisoning. All samples were tested within 48 h of collection; porphyrin values were determined without knowledge of blood lead concentrations. Figure 5 shows the median porphyrin concentration and range for each decade of blood lead concentration. All children with a lead concentration greater than 600 μg/liter of blood had an erythrocyte porphyrin concentration exceeding 800 μg/liter of erythrocytes.

Blood samples from a second nonselected population of children were assayed by the ethanol method for screening purposes. Only 15% of those patients had a porphyrin concentration greater than 800 μg/liter of erythrocytes.[2]

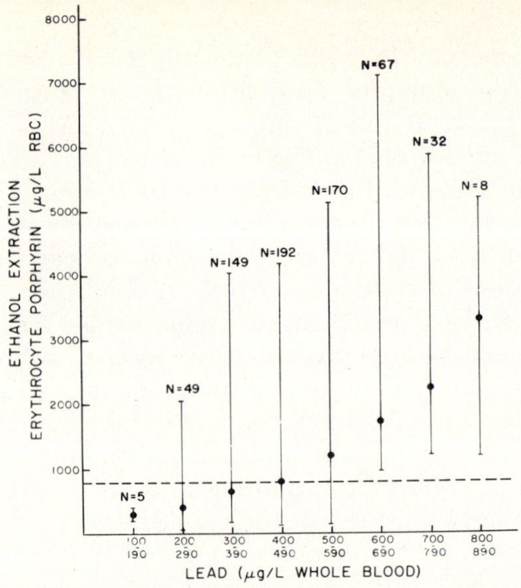

Fig. 5. Correlation of erythrocyte porphyrin (ethanol-extraction method) with blood lead concentration

Samples from 632 patients under evaluation for lead intoxication were assayed by the ethanol method. Median value and range (*bars*) of erythrocyte porphyrin values are shown for each decade of lead concentration. The *dashed line* indicates the porphyrin value adopted as the upper limit for screening purposes (expressed as coproporphyrin I). With this limit, all blood lead concentrations greater than 600 μg/liter were detected

Discussion

Two of the four methods evaluated, the ethyl acetate and ethanol procedures, were satisfactory; the other two presented serious limitations. In the two satisfactory methods porphyrin value is proportional to sample volume, samples can be stored in reagent for 72 h without appreciable loss of porphyrin, and extraction of porphyrin from erythrocytes is relatively complete. Both methods are applicable to capillary-blood samples.

With two extractions with HCl, porphyrin was essentially completely extracted by the ethyl acetate extraction procedure.[3] Such a procedure is recommended if an absolute value rather than technical simplicity is of primary concern. This procedure is suitable as a basic comparison method for reference. With the ethanol procedure, extraction is incomplete but consistent, and the procedure is simpler and more suitable for routine use, particularly when on site determinations are to be performed in the field.

In contrast to these two procedures that we found to be satisfactory, the acetone method extracted only a very low and variable portion of erythrocyte porphyrin (Figure 2*A*). In the detergent method porphyrin value was not proportional to sample volume (Figure 3*C*). Hemoglobin solubilized by the detergent interfered severely with porphyrin fluorometry and introduced serious variability and inaccuracy into the procedure. Dilutions required to overcome this interference limited sensitivity. Thus, both the acetone and detergent procedures demonstrated rather serious drawbacks, and neither was easier to perform than the ethanol method.

Procedures for appropriate standardization were examined. Ideally, a standard should be treated the same as the blood sample throughout the procedure and should be chemically similar to the blood substance assayed. Neither of these criteria has been satisfied in most previous applications. Standards have been diluted directly into acid solutions and their fluorescence recorded, while blood samples have been subjected to more complex extraction procedures before measurement of their fluorescence (*2, 6*). Furthermore, coproporphyrin I has been used as a standard, whereas Zn–protoporphyrin IX is the actual substance present in the erythrocyte.

The first criterion is easily satisfied by taking the standard solution through the same procedure as the

[2] Such patients were referred to the Lead Evaluation Center, St. Louis Department of Health, for further evaluation.

[3] In a recent investigation of ethyl acetate procedures Chisholm and Brown (*16*) also concluded that complete extraction of erythrocyte porphyrin can be achieved.

blood sample, thereby eliminating unnecessary calculations, errors caused by volume changes with extraction, and differential solvent effects on fluorescence. The recent commercial availability of Zn–protoporphyrin has made it possible to satisfy the second criterion, if two appropriate precautions are observed:

(*a*) The Zn–protoporphyrin must be prepared in a form appropriate for the analytical method to be used. An acid standard can be used only in the ethyl acetate method, but a buffered solution is suitable for standardization of both the ethyl acetate and ethanol procedures. Taken through the ethyl acetate extraction, a Zn–protoporphyrin standard in buffer is converted to free protoporphyrin IX, as is the endogenous Zn–protoporphyrin of the erythrocytes. Similarly, ethanol extraction of Zn–protoporphyrin standards in buffer or erythrocytes retains the porphyrin of both sources as a Zn complex.

(*b*) Buffered solutions of Zn–protoporphyrin are markedly labile and must be prepared immediately before use. Routine use of such a solution as a fluorescence standard would therefore be quite expensive and time consuming. Thus this standard is recommended only for primary standardization, while a secondary stable coproporphyrin standard is recommended for routine use as described below.

A suitable procedure for standardization is: (*a*) Prepare the appropriate Zn–protoporphyrin standard as discussed above; determine the ratio of fluorescence of coproporphyrin to Zn–protoporphyrin, and then use the more stable coproporphyrin as a working standard. The fluorescence ratio must be determined in each laboratory because it depends on the particular fluorometer and filters used. (*b*) Check the stability of the coproporphyrin standards during each assay by comparing their fluorescence to that of a highly stable reference compound such as rhodamine B. With these two procedures, the observed porphyrin content of blood samples can be expressed directly as Zn–protoporphyrin, and the stability of standards may be monitored easily.

Both of the recommended procedures can be performed with a general-purpose laboratory fluorometer. Special fluorometers, designed to be used only for porphyrin determinations, have been described (*17, 18, 19*). One of these fluorometers (*18, 19*) utilizes front-surface optics to minimize the interference by hemoglobin found in the detergent/buffer procedure. At present, neither of the special-purpose instruments offers any apparent advantage over the use of the recommended procedures with general-purpose instrumentation. Furthermore, use of a special-purpose instrument necessitates purchase of expensive equipment that will have limited application.

Results of both recommended methods for determining erythrocyte porphyrin correlate similarly with blood lead concentrations. The relative efficiency of screening with each method is shown in Table 3. The larger number of positive results in the range 0–390 μg of lead per liter observed with the ethanol method may be due to two differences in the populations screened by the two studies: (*a*) In the range 0–390 μg of lead per liter the population screened with the ethanol method had a disproportionally large number of patients with lead values exceeding 300 μg of lead per liter [68%, in contrast to 15% in the population screened by the ethyl acetate method (*20*)]. (*b*) The patients screened by the ethanol method came from a population that would be expected to have a high incidence of iron deficiency, a condition that can result in elevated erythrocyte porphyrin in patients with low blood lead concentrations (*21, 22*). In this population approximately a third of the patients with lead values of less than 400 μg/liter and porphyrin values greater than 800 μg/liter also had a hematocrit of 33% or less, suggesting iron-deficiency anemia. Thus, a significant fraction of the "false positives" with lead values of less than 400 μg/liter may have resulted from iron deficiency. As has been pointed out by others (*10*), the ability of the porphyrin screening test to detect iron deficiency as well as lead poisoning is an advantage rather than a disadvantage of the test.

Table 3. Comparison of Screening Efficiency with the Ethyl Acetate and Ethanol Methods

Lead, μg/liter of blood	Ethyl acetate (*20*)	Ethanol
	% positive	
0–390	5.1	25.6
400–490	51.5	50.0
500–590	63.1	73.6
600–690	100	100
700–790	100	100
⩾800	100	100

Most children are not treated on the basis of lead concentration alone unless the value exceeds 600 μg/liter. If a cutoff value of 800 μg of porphyrin per liter of erythrocytes (expressed as coproporphyrin I) is used, all patients whose blood lead concentrations exceed 600 μg/liter are identified by the ethanol extraction procedure. With both methods, 30–50% of the children with intermediate blood lead values (400–600 μg/liter) have porphyrin concentrations that are below the cutoff values. In such children the elevated blood lead value might be an isolated one that does not reflect the burden of soft tissue lead and thus is not associated with metabolic toxicity. By using the porphyrin measurement the emphasis is shifted from identifying children with a single elevated blood lead value to detecting children with evidence of metabolic toxicity, regardless of blood lead concentration. Follow-up studies are needed in order to definitely establish these points.

Results of screening with a nonselected population demonstrated the further advantages of a microscale porphyrin procedure. Only 15% of the patients studied had a porphyrin concentration exceeding 800 μg/

liter of erythrocytes. Therefore, such screening can spare 85% of the population a traumatic venipuncture, and can save the time of trained medical personnel.

The marked simplicity of laboratory procedures for porphyrin determination relative to those for lead analysis makes screening easier and more practical. Of the two recommended methods, the simplicity of the ethanol procedure makes it particularly suitable for use in population screening.

We thank Roberta Kraus for technical assistance in the early phases of this study, and Mrs. Anita Gill and Mrs. Pam Culliton for their help in organizing and correlating data on patients.

References

1. Sassa, S., Granick, S., and Kappas, A., Effect of lead and genetic factors on heme biosynthesis in the human red cell. *Ann. N. Y. Acad. Sci.* **244,** 419 (1975).

2. Schwartz, S., Berg, M. H., Bossenmeier, I., and Dinsmore, H., *Methods of Biochemical Analysis,* D. Glick, Ed., Interscience, New York, N. Y., 1960, p 221.

3. Wranne, L., Free erythrocyte copro- and protoporphyrin. A methodological and clinical study. *Acta Paediatr. Scand., Suppl.* **124,** 49 (1960).

4. Granick, S., Sassa, S., Granick, J. L., et al., Assay for porphyrins, δ-aminolevulinic-acid dehydratase, and porphyrinogen synthetase in microliter samples of whole blood: Applications to metabolic defects involving the heme pathway. *Proc. Nat. Acad. Sci. U. S. A.* **69,** 2381 (1972).

5. Kammholz, L. P., Thatcher, L. G., Blodgett, F. M., and Good, T. A., Rapid protoporphyrin quantitation for detection of lead poisoning. *Pediatrics* **50,** 625 (1972).

6. Piomelli, S., A micromethod for free erythrocyte porphyrins: The FEP test. *J. Lab. Clin. Med.* **81,** 932 (1973).

7. Chisholm, J. J., Mellits, E. D., Keil, J. E., and Barrett, M. B., A simple protoporphyrin assay–microhematocrit procedure as a screening technique for increased lead absorbtion in young children. *J. Pediatr.* **84,** 490 (1974).

8. Chisholm, J. J., Hastings, C. W., and Cheung, D. K. K., Microphotofluorometric assay for protoporphyrin in acidified acetone extracts of whole blood. *Biochem. Med.* **9,** 113 (1974).

9. Personal communication, W. H. Murphey, M.D., Dept. of Pediatrics, University of Oregon, Portland, Ore.

10. Lamola, A. A., Joselow, M., and Yamane, T., ZPP (zinc protoporphyrin): A simple, sensitive screening test for lead poisoning. *Clin. Chem.* **21,** 93 (1975).

11. Equipment and procedures for erythrocyte protoporphyrin (EP) analysis as a screening method for pediatric lead poisoning, Directive from Center for Disease Control, Atlanta, Ga., Feb. 14, 1975.

12. Rimington, C., Spectral absorption coefficients of some porphyrins in the Soret-band region. *Biochem. J.* **75,** 620 (1960).

13. Hessel, D., *Atomic Absorption Newsletter* (Perkin-Elmer Corp.) No. **7,** 55 (1968).

14. Leonard, J. J., Yonetani, T., and Callis, J. B., A fluorescence study of hybrid hemoglobins containing free base and zinc protoporphyrin IX. *Biochemistry* **13,** 1460 (1974).

15. Lamola, A. A., and Yamane, T., Zn-protoporphyrin in the erythrocytes of patients with lead intoxication and iron deficiency anemia. *Science* **186,** 936 (1974).

16. Chisholm, J. J., and Brown, D. H., Micro-scale photofluorometric determination of "free erythrocyte porphyrin" (protoporphyrin IX). *Clin. Chem.* **21,** 1669 (1975).

17. Whittaker Corp. Space Sciences Div., Bulletin TMIA on Space Sciences Micro-porph TM System; Waltham, Mass. 02154.

18. New blood test can screen for lead poisoning. *Chem. Eng. News,* p 18, Feb. 3, 1975.

19. King, J. S., Ed., Lead poisoning tester, (The Clinical Chemist). *Clin. Chem.* **21** (8), 66A (1975).

20. Piomelli, S., Davidow, B., Guinee, V. F., et al., The FEP (free erythrocyte porphyrin) test: A screening micromethod for lead poisoning. *Pediatrics* **51,** 254 (1973).

21. Stockman, J. A., Weiner, L. S., Simon, G. E., et al., The measurement of free erythrocyte porphyrin (FEP) as a simple means of distinguishing iron deficiency from beta-thalassemia trait in subjects with microcytosis. *J. Lab. Clin. Med.* **86,** 113 (1975).

22. McLaren, G. D., Carpenter, J. T., Jr., and Nino, H. V., Erythrocyte protoporphyrin in the detection of iron deficiency. *Clin. Chem.* **21,** 1121 (1975).

CLIN. CHEM. 22/2, 169–172 (1976)

Colorimetry of Carbohydrates with *m*-Aminophenol, and Its Proposed Use in Measurement of Serum Amylase Activity

Jesse F. Goodwin

In the reaction of *m*-aminophenol with carbohydrates in a thiourea/acetic acid reagent, addition of borate suppresses chromogen formation for hexoses and pentoses, and enhances it for disaccharides. All reaction products absorb maximally at 520 nm. The relatively greater intensity of the *m*-aminophenol/maltose reaction product was used in a saccharogenic method for amylase, with low blank readings. This method is compared with two dye/starch procedures.

Aniline and its derivatives react with hexoses and pentoses to form colors with characteristic absorption spectra. A mechanism has been proposed for this type of reaction (*1*), and an investigation of influential factors has been presented (*2*). Hultman (*3*) introduced *o*-toluidine along with 2,5-, and 2,6-dimethylaniline as analytical reagents for aldosaccharides. Earlier, Ek and Hultman (*4*) introduced the use of *m*-aminophenol and *p*-aminobenzoic acid as reagents for measurement of either glucose or fructose. In spite of the relative advantages cited for *m*-aminophenol, I find no additional references regarding its use. Unlike *o*-toluidine, it was reported as being applicable to whole serum and required only a 10-μl sample. In fact, it was one of the earliest "direct" micromethods for serum glucose. Perhaps its introduction at the same time as *p*-aminobenzoic acid as a reagent for hexoses may have overshadowed its distinct advantages.

In this communication, I report observations on the reaction of *m*-aminophenol with hexoses, pentoses, and disaccharides. A study of some factors affecting the reaction of this amine with various carbohydrates is presented, along with preliminary data for its use in amylase measurement.

Division of Laboratories, Detroit Health Department, 1151 Taylor, Detroit, Mich. 48202.

Received Mar. 28, 1975; accepted Nov. 5, 1975.

Materials and Methods

Reagents

Unless otherwise specified, all chemicals are reagent grade and all solutions aqueous. The *m*-aminophenol was twice recrystallized from benzene before use.

Acetic acid/thiourea/borate reagent. Dissolve 1.5 g of thiourea and 10 g of boric acid in glacial acetic acid and dilute to 1 liter.

m-*Aminophenol reagent.* Weigh out 30 g of recrystallized *m*-aminophenol (cat. No. P 1061; Eastman Organic Chemicals, Rochester, N. Y. 14650) and dilute to 1000 ml with the preceding reagent. Store in an amber-colored container. The reagent is stable for one month at room temperature.

Stock maltose standards, 10 g/liter. Dissolve 10.0 g of maltose in a solution of benzoic acid solution and dilute to 1 liter. This solution is stable for a year, stored at room temperature.

Substock maltose standards. Dilute the stock maltose standard with benzoic acid solution to give working standards of 1.0, 2.0, 4.0, and 8.0 g of maltose per liter.

Working maltose standards. Dilute one part of substock with three parts of distilled water. Discard after 24 h.

Buffer/NaCl solution (Tris, 0.1 mol/liter, pH 7.1; NaCl, 0.1 mol/liter). Dissolve 12.11 g of tris(hydroxymethyl)aminomethane and 5.6 g of NaCl in distilled water, adjust the pH to 7.1 with HCl, and dilute to 1 liter.

Starch substrate/buffer solution, 8 g/liter. Dissolve 0.8 g of Merck soluble starch ("after Zulkowsky"; EM Laboratories Inc., Elmsford, N. Y. 10523) in 100 ml of buffer/NaCl solution. Heating is not necessary. This solution should be used for only one day.

Procedures

Amylase estimation. Pipet 0.1 ml of serum into a test tube and incubate it at 40 °C (water bath) for 2–3 min. Add 0.2 ml of the starch substrate/buffer solution, mix, and incubate for 30 min at 40 °C. Stop the reaction by adding 0.1 ml of HCl (0.1 mol/liter) to the tube. A sample blank is prepared just before color development by pipetting 0.2 ml of starch substrate/buffer solution into a test tube, followed by 0.1 ml of HCl (0.1 mol/liter) and 0.1 ml of serum.

Color development. To separate 19 × 105 mm cuvets add 0.2 ml of enzymatic product and 0.2 ml of sample blank. Add 6 ml of *m*-aminophenol reagent to both tubes, mix, and heat the tubes for 15 min at 110 °C in an aluminum heating block. Cool the tubes to room temperature and measure the absorbance of both at 520 nm vs. a reagent blank prepared by heating 0.2 ml of water and 6 ml of reagent in the same manner prescribed for the sample and sample blank.

Standardization. Into separate 19 × 105 mm cuvets, pipet 0.2 ml each of the four maltose working standards. A reagent blank is prepared by pipetting 0.2 ml of water into a 19 × 105 mm cuvet. Develop the color as outlined above, starting with the addition of 6 ml of *m*-aminophenol reagent. Plot concentration vs. absorbance.

Calculations. Net absorbance = A (sample) − A (blank)

Use net absorbance values both in preparing the standard curve and in calculating the maltose concentration of the sample from the plot. For purposes of standardization, maltose (10 mg/liter) is calculated as the equivalent of one Somogyi unit.

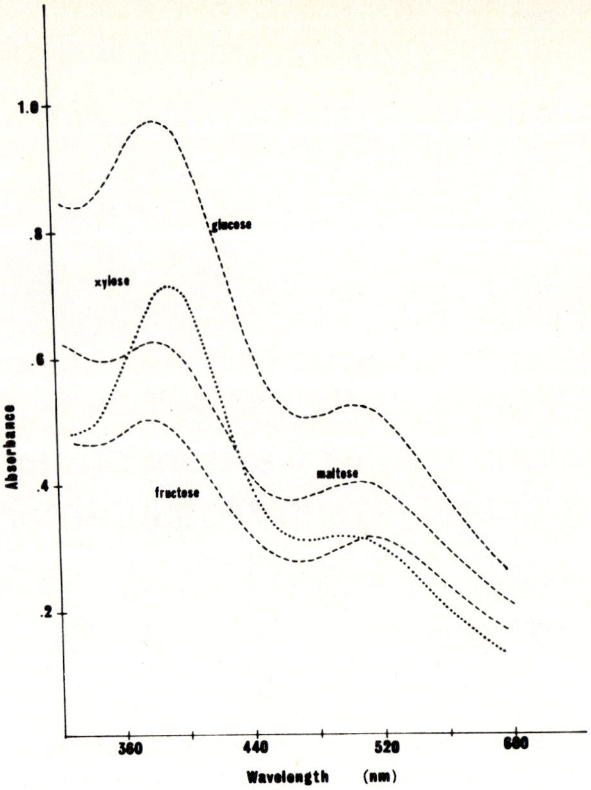

Fig. 1. Absorption spectra of the reaction products of various carbohydrates with *m*-aminophenol

Glucose, 1.0 g/liter; xylose 500 mg/liter; maltose, 2 g/liter; and fructose, 1.0 g/liter

Results and Discussion

Borate intensifies the color produced by the reaction of *o*-toluidine with glucose (*5*). It was suggested that borate enhanced the reactivity of the acyl groups of hexose sugars. Several other aromatic amines gave the same response (*1*). These investigations have been extended to include disaccharides and phenolic amines (*6*). In contrast to *o*-toluidine, I discovered that borate, when added to a solution of 50 g of *m*-aminophenol per liter of acetic acid, significantly decreased the absorbance of the glucose reaction product. In contrast, that of the *m*-aminophenol reaction products of fructose, sucrose, and maltose was enhanced in the presence of borate.

Absorption spectra of the reaction products of glucose, maltose, xylose, and fructose with *m*-aminophenol in thiourea/acetic acid are shown in Figure 1. For all four, there are maxima at 520 nm and at 370 to 400 nm. Glucose and xylose have a larger color yield than do fructose and maltose. The similarity of the absorption spectra of the reaction products of *m*-aminophenol with hexoses and pentoses is significant, because these sugars react with *ortho* substituted aniline derivatives to yield products with quite distinct spectra.

A 10 g/liter concentration of *m*-aminophenol in acetic acid containing thiourea (1.5 g/liter) reacts with maltose and glucose to give maximum color production. For xylose the most intense color is produced when the concentration of *m*-aminophenol is 30 g/liter of reagent. In all cases, color formation reached a maximum and remained constant with this concentration.

Figure 2 shows the effect of various concentrations of boric acid on the *m*-aminophenol reaction with fructose, maltose, glucose, and xylose. Boric acid clearly suppresses color formation with glucose or xylose, while at the same time enhancing color formation with fructose and maltose. These effects are maximum with a boric acid concentration of 10 g/liter in the reagent.

The "glucose color ratios" of several carbohydrates were determined. Glucose color ratio is defined as the absorbance at 520 nm of a carbohydrate reaction product with and without added boric acid (10 g/liter of reagent) divided by the absorbance produced when an equivalent amount of glucose is reacted under identical conditions. All of the hexoses (fructose and galactose) and disaccharides (maltose, sucrose, and lactose) tested produced more color in the presence of boric acid (Table 1). Fucose, a methyl pentose, and xylose, a pentose, formed colors with *m*-aminophenol that were suppressed by boric acid, but relative to glucose the ratios were not significantly altered.

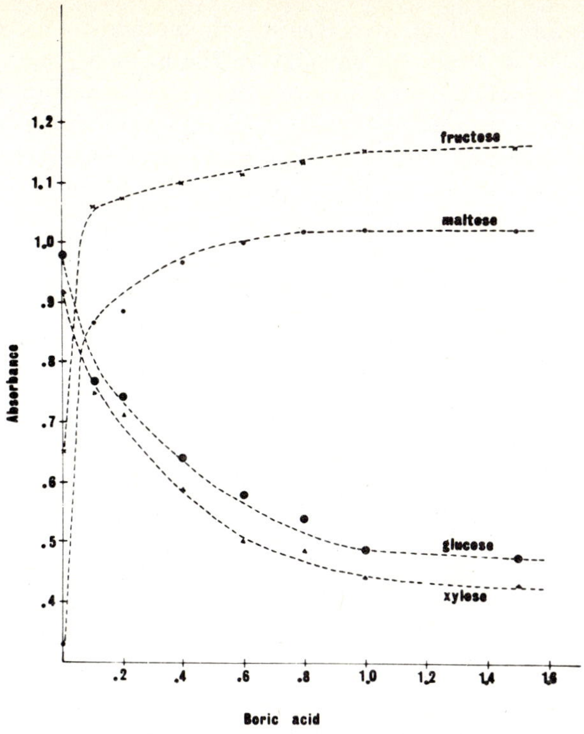

Fig. 2. Effect of boric acid on the reaction of *m*-aminophenol with various carbohydrates

The various carbohydrates indicated (2.0 g/liter) in an aqueous solution were reacted with a 30 g/liter *m*-aminophenol solution in acetic acid/thiourea reagent and various concentrations of boric acid (g/dl)

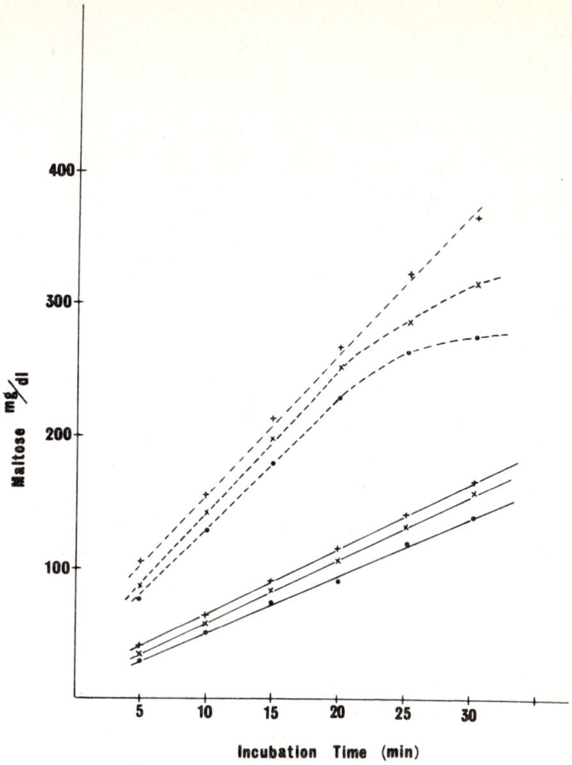

Fig. 3. Effect of soluble-starch substrate concentration on amylase activity, with maltose as an endpoint

Versatol E (- - -), assayed at 300 Somogyi units, and Versatol EN (—), assayed at 140 Somogyi units, were used. Substrate concentrations for each set of curves were (*top to bottom*) 6, 8, or 10 g/liter

Table 1. Relative (to Glucose) Color Yields of Various Carbohydrates with *m*-Aminophenol

Carbohydrate	Glucose ratio: Without boric acid	Glucose ratio: With boric acid
Glucose	1.000	1.000
Fructose	0.648	6.255
Galactose	0.948	3.390
Maltose	0.430	2.040
Sucrose	0.363	4.357
Lactose	0.512	5.124
Xylose	1.178	1.444
Fucose	1.987	1.488
Erythrose	0.780	0.508
Glyceraldehyde	1.390	0.929
2-Deoxyribose	0.245	0.128

Table 2. Amylase Values Obtained by a *m*-Aminophenol Saccharogenic Method, Compared with Two Dye/Starch Methods for Amylase Assay

	m-Aminophenol (y)	Dyamyl (x)[a]	Amylochrome (x)[b]
n		24	26
Mean	142	144.5	—
	141.6	—	112
Range	50–545	37–666	—
	50–545	—	50–295
r		0.97	0.915
$S_{y.x}$		22.1	40.3

[a] $y = 29.1 + 0.80x$.
[b] $y = 53.3 + 1.83x$.
Values are in Somogyi units.

Boric acid also suppressed color formation of the reaction products of shorter-chain carbohydrates.

The color formed by reaction of *m*-aminophenol with hexoses and disaccharides in the presence of boric acid showed greater absorbance as heating time was increased. A 15-min heating time was chosen, because absorbance was linear with time after 10 min.

Maltose is produced by the action of amylase on starch or glycogen. In most saccharogenic methods for amylase estimation, the amount of reducing carbohydrates present after incubation is measured. However, maltose measurement has served as an endpoint for amylase enzyme activity (*7*). The unique property of the *m*-aminophenol/boric acid reagent renders it ideal for maltose measurement. Because of the relatively small amount of chromogen formed by reaction of the amine with glucose, the absorbance of serum blanks is low.

The effect of substrate concentration on the amylase reaction, with maltose as an index to the

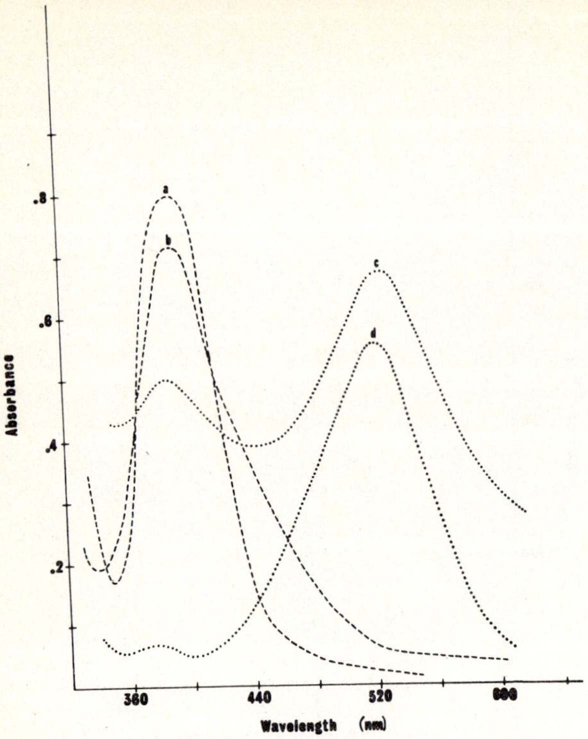

Fig. 4. Absorption spectra of the reaction products of fructose, furfural, acrolein, and formaldehyde with *m*-aminophenol in the presence of borate

Sample concentrations: (*a*) glyoxal (500 mg/liter), (*b*) formaldehyde (1.0 g/liter), (*c*) fructose (1.0 g/liter), and (*d*) furfural (250 mg/liter)

endpoint, is shown in Figure 3 for two enzyme-containing control sera, Versatol EN (1400 Somogyi units/liter) and Versatol E (3000 Somogyi units/liter) (General Diagnostics, Morris Plains, N. J. 07950). The values I obtained using either 6 and 8 g/liter starch solutions agreed well with stated values for both controls. I chose a concentration of 8 g/liter for routine use, because the values obtained more nearly conformed with units established by the Somogyi method (*8*). However, my findings suggest that under optimum substrate conditions (6 g/liter starch concentration), the values obtained with a maltose endpoint will be higher. It also appears that a shorter incubation time ensures better linearity. A 30-min incubation time was used to correlate with the established classical Somogyi method (*8*). Future trials of the method require additional optimization experiments with respect to substrate concentration and incubation time.

Results for amylase assay were compared with those obtained by two dye/starch methods; I used samples of sera selected only on the basis of having been submitted for amylase assay from three local acute-care hospitals (Table 2). The "Dyamyl" method (General Diagnostics) exhibited better correlation than the corresponding "Amylochrome" (Roche Diagnostics, Nutley, N. J. 07110) method. Values for all methods were measured in Somogyi units.

Furfural, a dehydration product of pentoses, reacts extremely rapidly to yield a chromogen with a maximum at 520 nm. This general type of reaction was first described by Stenhouse (*9*). *m*-Aminophenol also reacts with acrolein, formaldehyde, and other alpha-beta unsaturated aldehydes to yield 7-hydroxyquinoline derivatives (*10*). These compounds are highly fluorescent and exhibit spectral maxima in the 360 to 410 nm range. The spectra of the reaction products of fructose, unheated furfural, acrolein, and formaldehyde with *m*-aminophenol in the presence of borate are depicted in Figure 4. Note the similarity of the spectra of the reaction products of furfural, glyoxal, formaldehyde, and fructose.

The role of boric acid and its selective suppression of the color produced by reaction of glucose and shorter-chain carbohydrates with *m*-aminophenol is not fully understood. It may be due to the steric configuration of both *m*-aminophenol and glucose and the accessibility of the reactive sites, or cleavage of the 1,4-glycosidic linkage of maltose may favor a configuration whose reactivity is increased by boric acid.

References

1. Goodwin, J. F., Reaction of aniline and its alkyl derivatives with hexoses and pentoses. *Anal. Biochem.* **48,** 120 (1972).
2. Yee, H. Y., and Goodwin, J. F., Evaluation of some factors influencing the *o*-toluidine reaction with glucose. *Anal. Chem.* **45,** 2162 (1973).
3. Hultman, E., Rapid specific method for determination of aldosaccharides in body fluids. *Nature* **183,** 108 (1959).
4. Ek, J., and Hultman, E., Determination of glucose and levulose in body fluids. *Nature* **181,** 780 (1958).
5. Goodwin, J. F., Method for simultaneous direct estimation of glucose and xylose in serum. *Clin. Chem.* **16,** 85 (1970).
6. Goodwin, J. F., Colorimetric determination of carbohydrates with *m*-aminophenol. *Clin. Chem.* **19,** 660 (1973).
7. Scharpe, S., Determination of a amylase activity in biological fluids. *Clin. Chim. Acta* **37,** 301 (1972).
8. Somogyi, M., Modification of two methods for assay of amylase. *Clin. Chem.* **6,** 23 (1960).
9. Stenhouse, J., Ueber Furfuranilin und Furfurtoludin. *Justus Liebigs Ann. Chem.* **156,** 197 (1870).
10. Alarcon, R. A., Fluorometric determination of acrolein and related compounds with *m*-aminophenol. *Anal. Chem.* **40,** 1704 (1968).

CLIN. CHEM. 22/2, 173–175 (1976)

Creatine Kinase Isoenzyme Patterns in Human Tissue Obtained at Surgery

Swei H. Tsung

Chromatography on DEAE-Sephadex A-50 was applied to study the quantitative distribution of creatine kinase isoenzymes in extracts of human tissue obtained during surgery. The results are compared with those determined by an immunological method [*Clin. Chim. Acta* **58,** 223 (1975)]. Conflicting results for some organs as reported by the two methods are probably attributable to postmortem autolysis.

Additional Keyphrases: *intermethod comparison • column chromatography • reference values • stability in tissues*

Creatine kinase (CK, EC 2.7.3.2) isoenzymes have been intensively investigated, in part because of the recent development of sufficiently sensitive and rapid techniques (*1–4*). However, there is little information regarding the isoenzyme patterns in human tissue. An earlier study by Dawson and Fine (*5*), by a less sensitive technique, reported the presence of CK in a few human organs other than brain, heart, or skeletal muscle. More recently, study by the sensitive immunological method (*6*) showed CK to be ubiquitous in human organs. Unfortunately, the specimens were obtained at autopsy, 12–24 h after death, and the distribution of CK isoenzymes found might not be representative of the situation during life. In this communication, I report the use of a sensitive chromatographic method to study the distribution of CK isoenzymes in tissue obtained during surgery.

Clinical Chemistry Section, Laboratory Service/113, VA Center, Wood (Milwaukee), Wis. 53193; and the Department of Pathology, The Medical College of Wisconsin, Milwaukee, Wis. 53233.

Ed note: cf. the paper by Yasmineh et al., in the January 1976 issue of this journal.

Received Aug. 1, 1975; accepted Nov. 10, 1975.

Material and Methods

Tissue obtained during surgery was homogenized in a Virtis 45 homogenizer (1 g wet weight in 10 ml) within 20 min of its removal. The buffer used was as described by Klein et al. (*7*); per liter it contained 0.25 mol of sucrose, 10 mmol of tris(hydroxymethyl)aminomethane (pH 7.4), 1 mmol of [ethylenebis-(oxyethylenenitrilo)]tetraacetate (pH 7.4), and 1 mmol of mercaptoethanol. Cellular debris was removed by centrifuging twice at 4 °C for 20 min (16 000 × *g*) and the clear supernatant fluid was stored at −20 °C until used.

The supernatant fluid of tissue extracts was chromatographed by discontinuous-gradient elution from DEAE-Sephadex A-50 (Pharmacia Labs. Inc., Piscataway, N. J. 08854) as described by Yasmineh et al. (*2*), with slight modification. One-milliliter aliquots of tissue extracts containing not more than 3 U of CK activity were loaded on 0.6 × 6 cm micro columns of the anion exchanger equilibrated with 0.1 mol/liter NaCl–50 mmol/liter tris(hydroxymethyl)-aminomethane (pH 8.0), CK isoenzymes were consecutively eluted with solutions containing 0.1 mol/liter NaCl–50 mmol/liter tris(hydroxymethyl)aminomethane (pH 8.0), 0.2 mol/liter NaCl (pH 8.0), and 0.4 mol/liter NaCl (pH 7.0). Instead of depending on a fixed elution volume of 15 for isoenzyme MM, 11 for MB, and 8 ml for BB, I determined the elution volume by electrophoresing CK isoenzymes to avoid overdilution of each fraction and to increase the sensitivity. For example, electrophoresis of extracts from stomach showed mainly BB isoenzymes with small peaks of MB and MM; respective elution volumes of

Table 1. Between-run Precision of CK Isoenzymes Assay by Column Chromatography in a Special MB-Fortified Serum Control

	Percentage of			Recovery,
	MM	MB	BB	%
Mean	91.8	7.3	0.9	105.6
SD	1.08	0.78	0.27	2.34
CV, %	1.2	10.6	30.	2.2

n = 25 fortified serum samples with total CK activity ranging from 2295 to 2610 U/liter.

4, 4, and 15 ml were obtained. The electrophoresis was performed at pH 8.8 on argarose film by the CK-isoenzyme procedure of Corning ACI, Palo Alto, Calif. 94303. A 1- to 2-μl sample containing CK was applied and electrophoresed (25 °C, 25 min, 250 V). After electrophoresis, the films were layered with the CK reagent, blotted gently, incubated at 37 °C for 20 min, and dried in an oven at 56 °C. Electrophoretic patterns were scanned with a fluorometer (G.K. Turner Associates, Palo Alto, Calif. 94303). Peak areas were recorded with. a recorder from Beckman Instruments, Inc., Fullerton, Calif. 92634.

CK activity was estimated at 30 °C with a centrifugal analyzer (GEMSAEC; Electronucleonics Inc., Fairfield, N. J. 00706) by the kinetic method of Rosalki (*8*), with reagents from Calbiochem, La Jolla, Calif. 92037.

Results

Column reproducibility was evaluated by repeated analysis of a serum pool fortified with MB isoenzymes from an extract of heart tissue. A sample volume of 1 ml, containing about 2500 U of CK per liter, was applied to each of 25 ion-exchange columns. The results (Table 1) proved satisfactory.

Table 2 summarizes results of the isoenzyme studies on tissue extracts. Skeletal muscle contained the greatest concentration of CK activity, almost exclusively MM isoenzyme, which agreed with previous observations (*2*, *9*). Myocardial tissue contained the second greatest activity, of which 76–78% was MM isoenzyme, 22% MB isoenzyme, and 0–2% BB isoenzyme. CK activity in brain was exclusively attributable to BB isoenzyme. Urinary bladder, lung, prostate, uterus, thyroid, pancreas, stomach, intestine, and kidney contained primarily BB isoenzyme, with activities ranging from 3 to 162 U/g wet weight. In contrast, liver and spleen contained a higher percentage of MM isoenzyme than of BB. Salivary gland and bile contained both MM and BB isoenzymes, with more BB than MM. Placenta was most variable in CK isoenzyme content.

I assessed the stability of CK activity in kidney, stomach, and skeletal muscle. The tissue was stored at room temperature in a Petri dish with sufficient moisture to obviate dehydration. CK activity in kidney and stomach was very stable: only 10% loss 72 h after the specimens were obtained from surgery. At zero time, the isoenzyme distribution was 4% MM, 4% MB, and 92% BB for kidney and 4% MM, 1% MB, and 95% BB for stomach, as compared to 1% MM, 99% BB for both kidney and stomach when analyzed 72 h later. In contrast, skeletal muscle lost half of its CK activity in 10 h.

Table 2. CK Concentration and Isoenzyme Patterns (in Percent of Total Activity CK) in Human Tissue

Tissue	CK activity, U/g wet tissue	MM	MB	BB
			%	
Skeletal muscle (Gastrocnemius)	3281	100	0	0
Skeletal muscle (external intercostal)	1894	99	<1	<1
Heart (right atrium)	402	78	22	0
Heart (right atrium)	356	76	22	2
Brain	157	0	0	100
Urinary bladder	162	2	6	92
Lung	13.4	30	1	69
Lung	9.2	24	1	75
Lung	8.7	16	0	84
Lung	14	35	1	64
Prostate	10	3	4	93
Prostate	8	4	2	94
Uterus	47	2	1	97
Uterus	30	2	3	95
Thyroid	28	26	1	73
Thyroid	36	4	0	96
Pancreas	3	14	1	85
Stomach	86	2	4	94
Stomach	120	3	2	95
Stomach	160	4	1	95
Colon	148	3	1	96
Colon	125	4	0	96
Ileum	161	3	1	96
Kidney	15	12	0	88
Kidney	21	8	0	92
Liver	3.8	90	6	4
Spleen	7	74	0	26
Salivary gland	6	44	0	56
Bile	14.6 (U/liter)	38	2	60
Placenta	1.7	15	22	63
Placenta	2.8	48	6	46

Discussion

The CK isoenzyme distribution I found for some human tissues—such as skeletal muscle, heart, urinary bladder, brain, stomach, and spleen—agreed with that obtained by the immunological method (*6*). However, the values differed somewhat in the case of prostate, uterus, pancreas and intestine, and differed completely for thyroid gland, liver, kidney, and lung. Wretou and Pfleiderer (*6*) found MM isoenzyme predominating in thyroid and kidney; I found BB isoenzyme predominating in these two organs. In contrast to their results, four lung specimens tested contained 60–84% BB isoenzyme with slight variability in CK isoenzyme composition, and one liver specimen contained primarily MM isoenzyme. The conflicting results noted are likely attributable to postmortem autolysis. Sobel et al. (*10*) found low CK activity values in heart autopsy specimens obtained 4–27 h after death and had to extrapolate to the time of death to obtain values comparable to those obtained in fresh surgical specimens. Dawson and Fine (*5*) also encountered the instability of the enzyme activity in autopsy tissue.

My stability study indicates that the BB isoenzyme is more stable than the MM. Our experience with sera from patients with acute myocardial infarct suggests that MB is also less stable than MM. Thus, the number of hours after death at which the autopsy specimens were obtained will affect the isoenzyme pattern in tissue. Moreover, the cause of death may be related to decomposition of organs and a change in isoenzyme pattern—for instance, sepsis.

Reference

1. Mercer, D. W., Separation of tissue and serum creatine kinase isoenzymes by ion-exchange column chromatography. *Clin. Chem.* **20,** 36 (1974).

2. Yasmineh, W. G., and Hanson, N. Q., Electrophoresis on cellulose acetate and chromatography on DEAE-Sephadex A-50 compared in the estimation of creatine kinase isoenzymes. *Clin. Chem.* **21,** 381 (1975).

3. Nealson, D. A., and Henderson, A. R., Separation of creatine kinase isoenzymes in serum by ion-exchange column chromatography (Mercer's method, modified to increase sensitivity). *Clin. Chem.* **21,** 392 (1975).

4. Henry, P. D., Roberts, R., and Sobel, B. E., Rapid separation of plasma creatine kinase isoenzymes by batch adsorption on glass beads. *Clin. Chem.* **21,** 844 (1975).

5. Dawson, D. M., and Fine, I. H., Creatine kinase in human tissue. *Arch. Neurol.* (Chicago) **16,** 175 (1967).

6. Wretou, V. J., and Pfleiderer, G., Quantitation of creatine kinase isoenzymes in human tissue. *Clin. Chim. Acta* **58,** 223 (1975).

7. Klein, M. S., Shell, W. E., and Sobel, B. E., Serum creatine phosphokinase (CPK) isoenzymes after intramuscular injections, surgery and myocardial infarction. *Cardiovasc. Res.* **7,** 412 (1973).

8. Rosalki, S. B., An improved procedure for serum creatine phosphokinase determination. *J. Lab. Clin. Med.* **69,** 696 (1967).

9. Roberts, R., Henry, P. D., Witteeveen, S. A. G. J., and Sobel, B. E., Quantification of serum creatine phosphokinase isoenzyme activity. *Am. J. Cardiol.* **33,** 650 (1974).

10. Sobel, B. E., Bresnahan, G. F., Shell, W. E., and Yoder, R. D., Estimation of infarct size in man and its relation to prognosis. *Circulation* **46,** 640 (1972).

CLIN. CHEM. 22/2, 176–183 (1976)

Sample Stability: A Suggested Definition and Method of Determination

Ralph E. Thiers, Gaw T. Wu, Allen H. Reed, and Lawrence K. Oliver

We propose defining the stability of any chemical constituent of stored samples in terms that are quantitatively related to the precision of the measurement by which it is determined. We suggest that a constituent may be considered stable, for a stated period and under exactly defined conditions, when the average change in its measured value is less than a chosen number, K, of standard deviations of the data obtained by the measuring method over the concentration range in question. Based on this definition a technique utilizing a graphical truncated normal sequential test is presented as the appropriate experimental and statistical design for measuring stability. The statistical basis for the proposal is presented.

Additional Keyphrases: *quality control* • *statistics* • *variation, source of*

In clinical chemistry, stability is a critical consideration, but its assessment seems to have been neglected. We find no literature on an experimental design for doing so. In fact, even an objective definition of stability seems to be lacking.

We propose here a definition of stability that is suitable for clinical chemistry and a method for testing stability as so defined.

We believe that current criteria of stability are frequently relatively superficial, and that conclusions based on them depend on subjective judgment. Measurement errors loom large among the practical problems involved in measuring any change of concentration attributable to instability on storage. Among measurement errors we have observed that inter-day or inter-run biases seem to have been underestimated. These are significant effects that are sometimes disconcertingly obvious, and they tend to be especially serious in measurements of extremely low concentrations for which precision is relatively poor, such as determination of hormones by radioimmunoassay—but where knowledge of stability is nonetheless important.

Bio-Science Laboratories, Dept. of Research, 7600 Tyrone Ave., Van Nuys, Calif. 91405; and (A.H.R.) Management Science Dept., Calif. State Univ. Northridge, Northridge, Calif. 91324.

Received Sept. 12, 1975; accepted Nov. 10, 1975.

In stability studies one routinely seeks differences in measurements made before and after sample storage. In practical terms, and for a given experimental effort, the size of detectable differences is related to the precision of the method of measurement. We, therefore, propose to define stability in terms of analytical precision after Hagebush (*1*) and to utilize experimental designs in which one is used to evaluate the other.

This approach permits a simple definition of stability and a standard method of testing stability that is statistically simple and objective. It is presented here with its supporting derivation. This approach has been tested by application, by comparison with judgments from the literature, and by computer simulation studies, and has been found reliable.

Proposed Definition

A constituent is stable under specified conditions when measurements demonstrate, with prespecified risks of decision-error, that its mean concentration in the tested specimens has changed by less than an amount, δ, where δ is a function of the precision of the method.

Specifically, we suggest setting δ equal to exactly one standard deviation (SD) of the analytical method used, and we suggest setting at 0.05 the probability of deciding that a constituent is unstable (0.025 for positive and 0.025 for negative changes) when it is in fact stable, and setting at 0.05 the probability of deciding that it is stable when it is in fact unstable. Statisticians call these errors of the first and second kind, respectively, and symbolize them α and β.

Re-stated, we are proposing that a constituent be deemed stable under specified storage conditions when its mean concentration is shown to change by less than an amount equal to 1 SD and when we allow 5% risk of error for our decision.

Experimental Design

This definition implies a single duration of storage (if the constituent is unchanged at that time, one may presume that it has been stable until that time).

Also, carefully stated conditions for sample handling and storage must be an integral part of use of this definition. Finally, the definition implies a known, stated, unchanging standard deviation for the analytical method being used, which should be as small as the state of the art permits. Experiments designed to test stability, as defined, should minimize the number of determinations required, minimize the effect of inter-run bias, and be simple to execute.

Sometimes one is fortunate enough to know some set of conditions under which the constituent in question in the given sample matrix is definitely stable. This makes it easy to design experiments that minimize the effects of inter-run bias because one can use the known conditions for comparison. One simply divides each specimen into two aliquots immediately after it is collected and stores one under the conditions of known stability while the other is stored under the test conditions. At the end of the time period being tested the two aliquots are analyzed in the same analytical run. Any number of such aliquot-pairs can be in any given run. Thus both aliquots of each pair are subject to the same inter-run bias and the measured difference in their concentrations should not suffer from this error.

If no set of conditions is known under which the constituent is stable over the time period in question, inter-run bias cannot be avoided, because initial and final determinations on any one sample must be in different runs. Bias can, however, be drastically decreased and minimized by the following experimental design. Each specimen, immediately after it is collected, is divided into two aliquots; one is stored for the designated time and then analyzed, the other is analyzed immediately. All treatment of the aliquots except storage time and starting times for different pairs must be identical. Specimens are collected and analyzed according to a schedule like that exemplified in Table 1, which is a design for determining stability over a two-day period.

Let F represent the measured concentration of the constituent in the control aliquot, whether analyzed at the time of collection or after it has been stored under conditions of stability. Let F_i represent the concentration of the ith such control aliquot. Similarly, let the measured concentration of the ith aliquot "stored" under the test conditions be S_i.

In the case shown in Table 1, aliquot F_1 is assayed on day 0, aliquot F_2 on day 1, and so on. On day 2, the initial assay on specimen 3, F_3, and the final assay on specimen 1, S_1, are run concurrently. On all subsequent days two assays are run, one on a stored and one on a control aliquot. Therefore, in all runs except the first two and the last two, bias that may exist in the runs is compensated by having two aliquots in each run. The effect for one aliquot is on the initial determination (F) and for the other aliquot on the final determination (S). Therefore, the net effect is to substantially cancel the bias in that run. The assumption in Table 1 is that one run is made every day. For a period of other than two days, the schedule would merely have the F and S columns offset by the appropriate number of days corresponding to the length of time desired.

Table 1. Example of Experimental Design—Testing 2-Day Stability

Day no.	Aliquots assayed: Fresh	Stored
0	F_1	
1	F_2	
2	F_3	S_1
3	F_4	S_2
4	F_5	S_3
5	F_6	S_4
6	.	S_5
7	.	S_6
8	.	.
8	.	.
.	.	.
etc.	F_{n+2}	S_n

F_1: analytical result on fresh sample number 1.
S_1: analytical result on stored sample number 1.

Obviously this experimental design demands that an analysis be run every day, or at regular intervals, without regard to weekends or holidays. An effective but slightly less complete cancellation of the effect of inter-run bias can be achieved, where weekends intervene, by spacing the determinations so that either an initial determination on one sample is in the same run with the final of another, or else there is only one sample in any given run. In this case inter-run error is decreased by averaging as well as by some cancellation.

The statistical decision-making process we recommend is the truncated normal sequential test of Schneiderman and Armitage (*2*). We propose that the form in which it is used should be the same for either of the two types of experimental design described above, as follows:

For each successive pair of analytical data F_i and S_i, a test statistic, T.S., is calculated and plotted on a graph (Figure 1) with preset boundaries marked on it.[1] When the statistic crosses a boundary one can decide that the constituent is stable or unstable, depending on which boundary is crossed (as explained below).

The test statistic is:

$$\text{T.S.} = \sum_{i=1}^{N_d} (S_i - F_i)/\text{SD}$$

where

S_i = the measured concentration of the ith sample after storage,

[1] The statistical derivation of this approach and of the decision-boundaries in the various graphs is available to the interested reader from the authors or the Executive Editor of this journal.

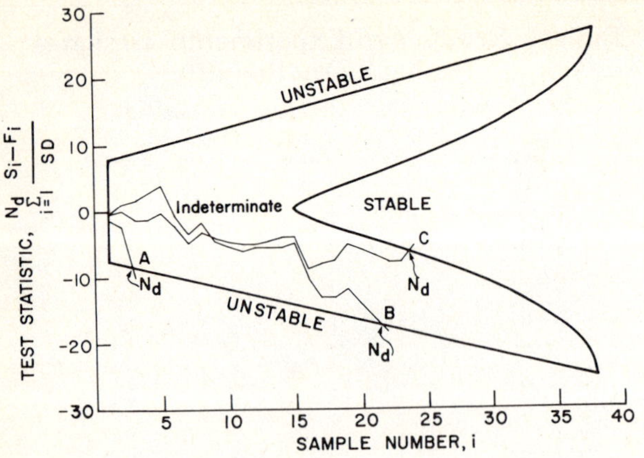

Fig. 1. Graphical presentation of truncated normal sequential test—stability of creatine kinase for 4 days

Line *A*, 30 °C, line *B*, 4 °C, line *C*, −20 °C. Samples were quick-frozen

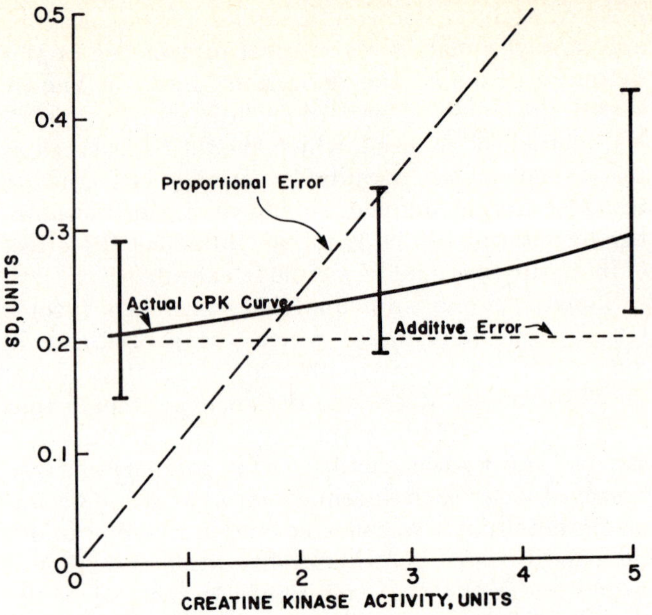

Fig. 2. Relationships of measurement error to concentration (U/liter)

The vertical ranges around the actual curve show the confidence limits for the line at 95% confidence, n = 20

F_i = the measured concentration of the ith sample when fresh, or stored under conditions of known stability (the "control" aliquot).

SD = the overall standard deviation of the analytical method, and

N_d = the number of sample pairs run until a decision is made.

As each pair of analyses is completed, $(S_i - F_i)$/SD is calculated and added to the sum of the previous data. This new sum is plotted on the graph shown in Figure 1. As long as the sum is within the plotted boundaries, no decision can be made regarding stability, and the experiment should be continued. If and when the line crosses either straight-line boundary, the experiment should be ended, because instability in either a rising or falling direction (i.e., an increase or decrease in the constituent) has been demonstrated with $\alpha = 0.025$ (each way) (Figure 1, Line *A*). The straight lines thus represent indices for decisions for instability. On the other hand, if the test statistic crosses the curved boundary line the experiment should be ended because stability has been proved (Figure 1, Line *C*), within the terms of our definition, with $\beta = 0.05$. This is illustrated by the data of Table 2 and Figure 1. Line *A* shows an experiment that demonstrated, after only three pairs of aliquots were assayed, that by our definition creatine kinase (EC 2.7.3.2) was not stable at 30 °C for four days. Line *B* illustrates an experiment that showed, after 22 aliquot-pairs were assayed, that it also is not stable at 4 °C for four days. Line *C* shows, after 24 aliquot-pairs, that with quick freezing and storage at −20 °C it is stable by our definition.

One can argue that we have presented for universal application a test statistic that may be inappropriate because a single value is chosen for SD while a range of concentrations is used, and SD may vary with concentration. As extremes, two conditions actually exist. In one the SD is constant with concentration, error is additive (the additive model), and errors are assumed to be distributed normally. In the other the coefficient of variation (CV) is constant, error is proportional to concentration (the proportion model), and errors are assumed to be distributed lognormally (*3*). These are characterized by the relationships shown in Figure 2.

In the proportional model the test statistic (analogous to that presented above for the additive case) is:

$$\text{T.S.} = \sum_{i=1}^{N_d} \ln (S_i/F_i)/\text{CV}$$

and δ is defined as 1.0 CV rather than 1.0 SD.

These two models were used in the computer simulation studies described below and it was found that the additive model was quite effective for all practical uses.

Experiments, Results, and Discussion

The validity of the proposed approaches was experimentally verified by computer simulation of analytical runs with known conditions of stability or instability and with known amounts and distributions of experimental error. Simulation studies were performed in Fortran IV computer language with a Univac Spectra 70 computer. Values designated f_i and s_i were chosen to represent error-free concentrations of an analyte (control and stored, respectively) under conditions of stability and of different degrees of instability. A gaussian random-number-generating subroutine[2] was used to provide numbers for experimental error, which were combined with the error-free

[2] Random variable generators used were: (1) Random Number Package, Health Science Computing Facility UCLA. (2) IBM System/360 Scientific Subroutine Package. (3) Personal communication from R. B. Koger.

Table 2. Three Examples of Tests of Stability: Creatine Kinase at −20, 4, and 30 °C for Four Days[a]

Sample no. i	Fresh concn. F_i	−20 °C: Stored concn. S_i	−20 °C: Test statistic	4 °C: Stored concn. S_i	4 °C: Test statistic	30 °C: Stored concn. S_i	30 °C: Test statistic
				30 °C experiment			
1	1.5					1.2	−1.5
2	3.3					3.1	−2.5
3	2.1					0.5	−10.5 Unstable, decision after 3 samples
			−20 °C and 4 °C experiment				
1	1.1	1.0	−0.5	1.0	−0.5		
2	4.0	4.1	0.0	4.3	1.0		
3	8.7	8.4	−1.5	8.8	1.5		
4	1.1	1.1	−1.5	1.3	2.5		
5	2.2	2.4	0	2.4	3.5		
6	3.4	2.8	−3.0	2.5	−1.0		
7	5.6	5.1	−5.5	5.1	−3.5		
8	3.4	3.7	−4.0	3.7	−2.0		
9	2.0	1.8	−5.0	1.4	−5.0		
10	2.1	2.0	−5.5	2.0	−5.5		
11	2.8	2.7	−6.0	2.6	−6.5		
12	2.3	2.3	−6.0	2.4	−6.0		
13	1.6	1.7	−5.5	1.6	−6.0		
14	2.3	2.4	−5.0	2.3	−6.0		
15	2.3	2.3	−5.0	2.4	−5.5		
16	5.5	4.5	−10.0	4.5	−10.5		
17	3.7	3.9	−9.0	3.1	−13.5		
18	1.1	1.2	−8.5	1.1	−13.5		
19	3.0	3.5	−6.5	3.2	−12.5		
20	1.5	1.3	−7.5	1.1	−14.5		
21	2.6	2.4	−8.5	2.1	−17.0		
22	0.9	0.7	−9.5	0.6	−18.5		
23	0.9	0.9	−9.5	—	Unstable, decision after 22 samples		
24	1.8	2.3	−5.0	—			
			Stable, decision after 24 samples				

[a] Measured Activity in BSL Units. SD = 0.2 Units.

concentration values to produce simulated analytical data, F_i and S_i. The experiments were divided into simulations of the additive and proportional error situations described above and in each of these two cases various degrees of actual instability were simulated. This was done by assuming that the average difference $E(Z)$ between the expected values of F, designated $E(F)$, and S, designated $E(S)$, was a chosen fraction of SD. The fractions chosen were 0, 0.2, 0.4, 0.6, 0.8, 1.0, 1.2, 1.5, and 2.0. The first of these, of course, represents absolute stability, and the sixth *et seq.* represent instability according to our suggested definition.

In the additive model the computer was programmed to select values of error of F and error of S from a normally distributed population with mean equal to zero and standard deviation equal to 1. In the first case, the difference between $E(F)$ and $E(S)$ was taken as zero ($E(Z) = 0$) and the computer calculated successive values of the test statistic, which in this case is a reflection of only the error terms, and compared the value obtained with values for the inner and outer boundaries. When the test statistic passed any boundary the computer recorded the number, N_d, of aliquot-pairs required to reach a decision in that particular experiment. This number, N_d, and the decision for or against stability were then printed out in a list opposite the serial number of the experiment. Subsequent cases were identical, except that the average differences, $E(Z)$, were taken as 0.2, 0.4, etc., times SD. Table 3 shows an example of one print-out. In each case 1000 experiments were run.

The results of more than 10 000 simulations are shown as Figure 3, Line *A*. When absolute stability existed, the proposed method identified it as stability 97% of the time. When instability to the extent of

Table 3. Computer Simulation, Example of Printout of Results

Experiments with $E(Z) = 0.6 \times$ SD

Exp no.	No. samples run until decision N_d	Decision type: Stability	Decision type: Instability
1	11	X	
2	20		X
3	15		X
4	37		X
5	34	X	
.			
.			
.			
.			
.			
998	21		X
999	27	X	
1000	16		X
No. of runs	1000	504	496

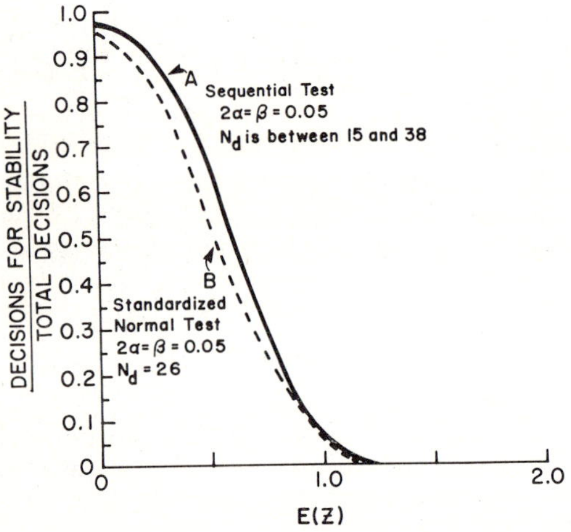

Fig. 3. Fraction of decisions for stability as a function of instability

Instability is expressed as actual change in concentration, $E(Z)$, as a fraction of analytical SD

$E(Z) = 1$ SD existed (by the criterion of $\delta = 1.0$ SD) the proposed method identified it as instability 94% of the time.

In theory, of course, Line *A* of Figure 3 should cross zero abscissa at 95% ($2\alpha = 0.05$) and should cross 1.0 at 5% ($\beta = 0.05$), instead of the 97% and 6% observed. The difference is of no practical significance. However, we repeated thousands of simulation experiments in each of these two cases, with use of random numbers generated by three quite different algorithms, and we continued to get results that differed slightly from the theoretical prediction. This slight discrepancy was also observed, and explained, by Schneiderman and Armitage (*2*).

Figure 3, Line *A* presents the essence of our recommendation because it expresses in quantitative terms the effective meaning of the combination of the suggested definition and the proposed method. The probability of deciding that a constituent is stable is expressed by the percentage of the simulation experiments that give a decision for stability. This probability is shown in Line *A* as a function of actual instability. For example, if the instability under the test conditions exceeds 1.3 SD the probability of deciding for stability is essentially zero. If instability is 0.5 SD the probability of a decision for stability is 0.65, or 65%. Thus the definition and treatment together are quantitative and are more conservative than one might infer from the definition alone—which sounds qualitative—because the definition can be taken to imply that any instability of less than 1.0 SD will be called stability, whereas actually the probabilities of Figure 3 apply.

One can also deduce from Figure 3 the effect of incorrectly estimating the SD of a method. If one overestimates the SD then one greatly improves his chances of deciding for stability, by making the criteria less stringent. Conversely, if one underestimates the SD of the method (this seems to be the more frequent error) then the chances of deciding that a constituent is stable when it actually is not decrease markedly. If the constituent is absolutely stable then errors in estimation of SD should have little effect, on the average, because the expected value of the numerator of the test statistic is zero.

Obviously a statement of the analytical precision of the method must accompany any statements about stability by this definition, an implied requirement of any stability statement.

It is useful to note the frequency distribution of N_d as observed in the simulations (Figure 4), because this enables one to predict the probable duration of any one experiment. As shown in Figure 4*A*, if instability equal to exactly 1 SD exists, the decision is likely to come quickly, with eight being the most likely number of runs required. If the constituent is even more unstable the decision will come even more quickly. If the constituent is absolutely stable ($E(Z)$ = zero) the decision is still likely to come rather quickly, with 16 being the most likely number (Figure 4*B*).

Figure 4 illustrates the greater experimental economy of the sequential statistical approach compared to Student's *t*-test or to U, the standardized normal test (*4, 5*). For example, with the latter, to obtain a β value of 0.05 where $\delta = 1$ SD one would need to run 26 aliquot-pairs. With this number, the relationship shown in line *B* of Figure 3 would hold (*5*).

Incidentally, it is noteworthy in Figure 4 that the incorrect decisions for instability are likely to come late. It is also noteworthy that decisions made at N_d = 37 or 38 tend to be much more prone to error than the average decision. This can be observed in Figure 4, where 13 of the 21 decisions made at $N_d = 38$ are

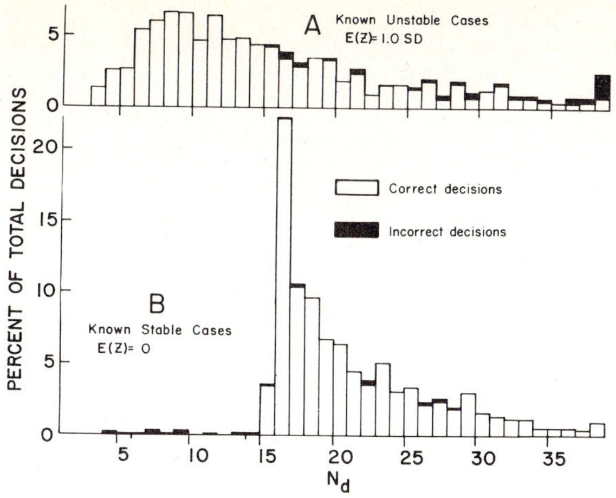

Fig. 4. Frequency distribution of N_d

incorrect, and seven of the 16 at N_d = 37. Such experiments should be repeated.

Simulation tests for the proportional model were run with CV used in place of SD. The logarithmic distribution of errors was obtained by taking exponentials of the random numbers generated by the same basic algorithm as the additive case. The results for the proportional case duplicated exactly those for the additive case (as we realized should be the case after trying it).

The effect of mistakenly using the additive model when in fact the proportional model fits the facts, and vice versa, was tested by simulation. Three sets of 38 simulated glucose concentrations were chosen randomly. All three were from populations with means of 1.20 g/liter. The standard deviations of the population were 180, 300, and 420 mg/liter, respectively. Thus the range of concentrations tested varied more than twofold.

Additive errors were randomly chosen, for each of these concentrations, from a normal population of errors with mean equal to zero and standard deviation equal to 60 mg/liter. For the unstable case a systematic change was chosen such that $E(Z) = 1$. Then the proportional test statistic was applied to the resultant F and S values with CV = 0.05. This CV is, of course, correct only at the mean value, 1.20 g/liter.

Proportional errors were also chosen randomly for each of these concentrations, from a log-normally distributed population mean equal to 1 and CV equal to 0.05. Then the additive test statistic was applied to the resultant F and S values, with SD = 60 mg/liter. This value of SD is, of course, correct only at the mean value.

The results are shown in Table 4. It is clear that choosing the wrong test statistic is not a serious error, especially when the additive statistic is chosen. The values in Table 4 do not depart significantly from 95% until the concentration range gets quite broad indeed.

The effect of various choices of α and β on the truncated sequential test is illustrated by Figure 5 (*2*). In general, the minimum sample size, M, necessary to prove stability is little affected by making these criteria more or less stringent. With $\alpha = 0.005$ and $\beta = 0.01$, $M = 19$. With $\alpha = 0.05$ and $\beta = 0.10$ (10-fold larger), $M = 12$. However, the maximum number that may be run before getting any result in these two cases is 120 and 25, respectively. The effect of α and β on breadth of the patterns is intermediate in its significance. The pattern used in this proposal ($2\alpha = \beta = 0.05$) is the central pattern in Figure 5. In this case the minimum number that must be run to prove stability is 15; the maximum that might be necessary is 38 (Table 5).

The definition, choice of α, β, and δ, and the technique were also tested by use in our laboratory. One example is given in Table 2 and Figure 1. This experiment was designed to test the conditions by which serum samples could be stored long enough to permit coast-to-coast mailing in the U. S. A. A four-day period was chosen since experience in this laboratory indicates that substantially all mailed specimens arrive in four days. The results indicate creatine kinase instability for both room temperature (30 °C was used to simulate summer room-temperature mailing) and 4 °C storage. Quick-frozen samples held at −20 °C proved stable. Samples frozen slowly by placing them casually on solid CO_2 or in a freezer gave extremely variable results. Quick-freezing, by rolling the serum onto the sides of a test tube immersed in solid CO_2/methanol or the equivalent, was necessary.

Our technique for defining and detecting stability

Table 4. Effect of Choosing the Wrong Test Statistic (T.S.) Evaluated by Simulation (1000 Experiments per Case)

Concns. chosen			Proportional error tested with additive T.S.		Additive error tested with proportional T. S.	
			Stable, $E(Z) = 0$	Unstable, $E(Z) = 1$ SD	Stable, $E(Z) = 0$	Unstable, $E(Z) = 1$ CV
Av.	SD	Range	Correct decisions, as % of total			
120	18	93–153	97	95	95	95
120	30	71–175	97	94	91	96
120	42	50–197	95	93	80	97

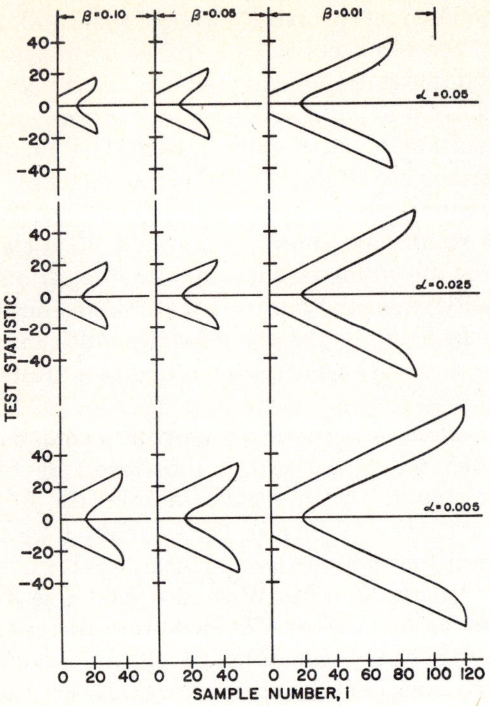

Fig. 5. Relationships of α and β to maximum and minimum sample size for the truncated sequential test

Note that the abscissas and ordinates from Table 4 of ref. *2* have been multiplied by 2 and ±2, respectively, to yield the abscissas and ordinates in this figure

has as a prerequisite a specific method of determination of acceptable known precision for the analyte in question. These conditions should be met in any laboratory that undertakes stability studies, as follows. The method should have been used in the laboratory long enough to have unchanging precision and to be known to be free of "drift" of values with time. The method should be specific for the analyte in question; if it is not, then one may be measuring a cumulative increase in interfering or inhibiting substances. The precision of the method should be good enough to provide knowledge about stability that is useful relative to the acceptable degree of change from (e.g.) a clinical-utility standpoint. It should not be significantly poorer than the state of the art permits. The precision should be known. That is, the relationship between standard deviation and analyte concentration should be known. Such information about methods is surprisingly sparse. It is shown for creatine kinase in Figure 2.

We made four general observations as a result of this study. Although they perhaps are obvious, once stated, they are not implied by the literature or by conventional practice.

(*a*) In general, data on the precision of clinical chemical methods is very incomplete. Typically, precision is measured at one or perhaps two concentrations. No attempt is made to get the complete relationship required by the technique described in this paper.

Table 5. Coordinates of Boundaries of Decision-Making Graph, Assuming $2\alpha = \beta = 0.05$ and $\delta = 1.0$ SD

Straight-line boundaries

$$\text{Upper } \sum_{i=1}^{38} A_i = 7.275 + \tfrac{1}{2} i$$

$$\text{Lower } \sum_{i=1}^{38} A_i = -7.275 - \tfrac{1}{2} i$$

Curved boundaries

Abscissas, i^a	Ordinates, $A_i{}^a$
14.94	±0
15	±0.2
16	±1.6
17	±2.2
18	±3.0
19	±3.6
20	±4.2
21	±5.0
22	±5.6
23	±6.4
24	±7.0
25	±7.8
26	±8.6
27	±9.4
28	±10.2
29	±11.2
30	±12.0
31	±13.0
32	±14.0
33	±15.2
34	±16.4
35	±17.8
36	±19.4
37	±21.6
37.82	±26.2

[a] The abscissas and ordinates from Schneiderman and Armitage's Table 4 (*2*) have been multiplied by 2 and ±2, respectively.

(*b*) Usually CV and SD are given as though they were alternative statements of the same thing instead of ascribing, as they do, quite different properties to the data.

(*c*) Accurate measurements of SD or CV require more work than one usually is willing to apply. Even if one were to run two series of 20 replicate specimens each, the measured values of the respective SD's could differ by almost 50% before the variance ratio test (*4*) would reject them as unlikely at the 0.05 level. Thus statements of SD or CV to more than one significant figure frequently are overinterpreting the data they come from.

(*d*) Reliable demonstrations of stability require more work then one usually is willing to apply. As our theoretical treatment has shown, one cannot prove stability for a single time period to the rather gener-

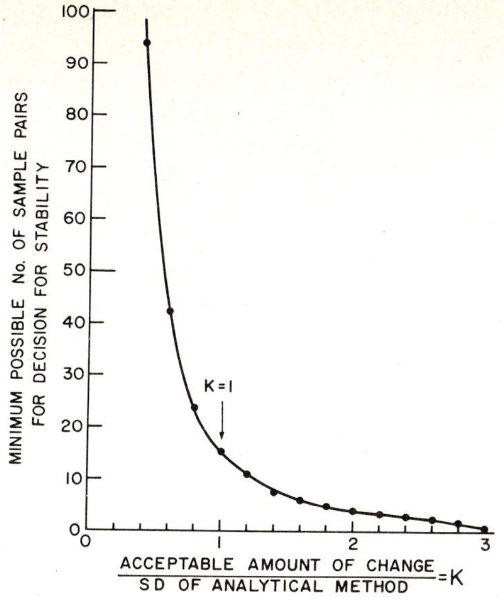

Fig. 6. Relationship between amount of change in concentration acceptable in deciding for stability (expressed as K), and minimum number of sample pairs required to demonstrate stability if it exists

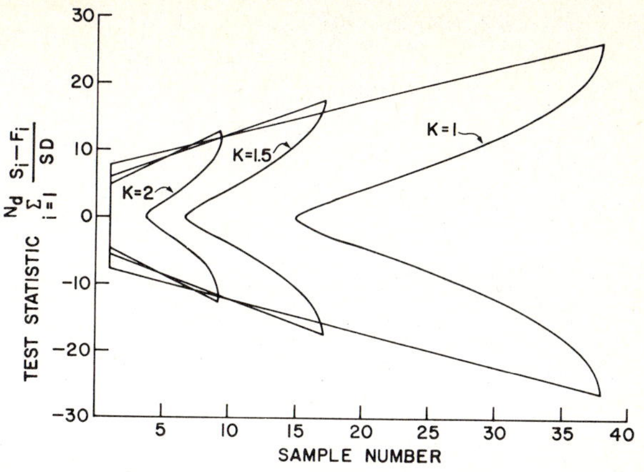

Fig. 7. Graphical presentation of truncated normal sequential test for K = 1, 1.5, 2

ous-sounding limits we propose with fewer than 15 blind-pairs of data by the sequential technique or 26 by conventional tests.

Setting $K = 1$ in the expression $\delta = K \times \text{SD}$ is an arbitrary choice. Whether K should be chosen smaller or larger depends only on the degree of change acceptable in deciding for stability, and fitting $K \times \text{SD}$ to that degree of change.

Figure 6 shows one practical aspect in choosing K, namely the relationship between K and the minimum amount of work required to prove stability, if it exists. This figure illustrates the practicality of choosing $K = 1$.

Values of K other than 1 alter the shape of the graph significantly; increasing values of K increase the probability of reaching a decision for stability. Figure 7 can be used with the test statistic presented here to determine stability to whatever limits desired. For example, one can choose an acceptable degree of change in terms of concentration and relate that to $K \times \text{SD}$ to determine the appropriate K value to use. α and β are also arbitrary numbers and were arbitrarily chosen at $2\alpha = \beta = 0.05$ because they conformed with generally accepted 95% confidence limits, and provided experiments of convenient length. In any given situation, if one wants higher confidence the price to be paid is reflected in the maximum number of samples that may be required to reach a decision (Figure 5).

If the assumption that SD does not vary with concentration is incorrect, this has little effect on the usefulness of the method if the range of values is not too large. The ease of using SD and thus avoiding the logarithms required for the proportional case test statistic led us to recommend the single test statistic presented in this paper. We think that few incorrect decisions will be encountered when this statistic is used, if one chooses reasonable concentration ranges.

When one is using the recommended techniques the accumulation of data may be interrupted at any time and resumed freely, provided only that the experimental conditions regarding handling and analysis of each sample remain unchanged. When specimens are difficult to obtain (abnormal ones, for example), it may be possible to collect data for only one specimen at a time. In case it is not already clear, we strongly recommend using the daily runs in the routine laboratory for stability studies. Although the time elapsing between starting such a study and finishing it can be long, the work load is almost negligible. We have found that the overall time period may not be much longer than the traditional time periods taken to design and do a stability experiment of any duration, because the experimental design is already at hand and quite frequently the experiment ends rather quickly.

We thank Dr. Charles C. Stewart (CDC, Atlanta, Georgia) for several valuable discussions and constructive advice during the development of this work.

References

1. Hagebusch, O. E., Automation in the private practice of laboratory medicine. In *Automation in Analytical Chemistry, Technicon Symposia 1965;* L. T. Skeggs et al., Eds., Mediad, Inc., New York, N. Y. 10017, 1966, p 417.

2. Schneiderman, M. A., and Armitage, P., A family of closed sequential procedures. *Biometrika* **49,** 41 (1962).

3. Aitchison, J., and Brown, J. A. C., *The Lognormal Distribution,* Cambridge Univ. Press. Cambridge, U. K., 1966, chap. 1.

4. Davies, O. L., *The Design and Analysis of Industrial Experiments,* Hafner Pub. Co., New York, N. Y., 1954, chap. 3 and p 596.

5. Dixon, W. J., and Massey, F. J., Jr., *Introduction to Statistical Analysis,* 3rd ed., McGraw-Hill, New York, N. Y., 1969, chap. 14.

6. Lindley, D. V., *Introduction to Probability and Statistics,* Part 2, Cambridge Univ. Press, Cambridge, U. K., 1965, p 137.

7. Mandel, J., *The Statistical Analyses of Experimental Data,* Interscience, New York, N. Y., 1964, pp 72–75.

8. Sobel, M., and Wald, A., A sequential decision procedure for choosing one of three hypotheses concerning the unknown mean of a normal distribution. *Ann. Math. Stat.* **20,** 502 (1949).

CLIN. CHEM. 22/2, 184–187 (1976)

Analysis for Indole Compounds in Urine by High-Performance Liquid Chromatography with Fluorometric Detection

Anthony P. Graffeo[1] and Barry L. Karger[2]

We describe a chromatographic system involving a high-performance chemically-bonded reverse-phase column and fluorescence detection for measurement of indoles in urine. We controlled retention and selectivity by optimizing the methanol content and pH of the mobile phase. Six reference indoles were separated in less than 20 min; three 5-hydroxyindoles were eluted in less than 7 min. About 5–15 ng of aqueous solutions of these compounds can be detected. The combination of selectivity (from use of the chromatographic column) and fluorescence detection permitted analysis for five of the six indoles after a single urine-deproteinization step.

Measurement of indole compounds, especially 5-hydroxyindoles in biological fluids, has been an area of active investigation ever since serotonin was isolated in 1948 (*1*). Many techniques (*2*) have been examined for use in analysis of these substances in physiological fluids. Abnormally high values are associated with (e.g.) malignant carcinoid tumors (*3*) and certain mental deficiencies (*4*).

In most such analyses either individual compounds [e.g., 5-hydroxyindoleacetic acid by its reaction with nitrosonaphthol (*3*)] or a class of compounds [e.g., 5-hydroxyindoles (*5*)] are determined. Chilcote and Mrochek (*6*) analyzed six indole compounds in 50- to 100-ng amounts by using small-particle (12- to 15-μm particle diameter) anion- and cation-exchange resins in columns coupled in series, with fluorescence detection; however, the separation required as long as 3 h. In later work, Chilcote analyzed for several indole acids (*7*) and bases (*8*) by using an appropriate single ion-exchange column, but separation still required 1 h in either case.

Department of Chemistry, Northeastern University, Boston, Mass. 02115.

[1] Present address: Battelle-Columbus Laboratory, Columbus, Ohio 43201.

[2] Author to whom reprint requests should be sent.

Received Sept. 29, 1975; accepted Nov. 10, 1975.

We have examined the separation and analysis of the same six indoles as did Chilcote and Mrochek (*6*). We used a high-performance reverse-phase chromatography column containing a small-particle hydrophobic bonded phase packing. By making optimal the mobile water/methanol phase and the pH, we can discretely separate these compounds in less than 20 min. The use of a filter fluorometer detector results in detection limits of ~5–15 ng per sample (depending on the substance). Moreover, when excited at around 280 nm, indoles fluoresce in the range of 330–380 nm, the precise wavelength depending on their structure. In this region of the spectrum few other compounds in physiological fluids interfere. The combination of separation and detection selectivity permits the simple analysis of the indole compounds in urine with a minimum preliminary treatment of the specimen.

Materials and Methods

Apparatus

The chromatograph we used consisted of a high-pressure pump (Model M/6000; Waters Assoc., Milford, Mass. 01757), a loop injector (Model U6K; Waters Assoc.) and a ultraviolet/fluorescence filter detector (Model 836; Du Pont Instruments, Wilmington, Del. 19898). The fluorescence detector was equipped with a 280-nm interference filter for excitation and a 310-nm cut-off filter for emission. The reverse phase column was a "μ Bondapak C_{18}" column (Waters Assoc.), 30 cm long and packed with particles of 10 μm diameter.

Indoles used as standards were obtained from Sigma Chemical Co., St. Louis, Mo. 63178. The mobile phase was prepared with use of doubly-distilled water and "spectroquality" grade methanol (Burdick and Jackson Laboratories, Inc., Muskegon, Mich. 49422), by preparing a 10 mmol/liter solution of sodi-

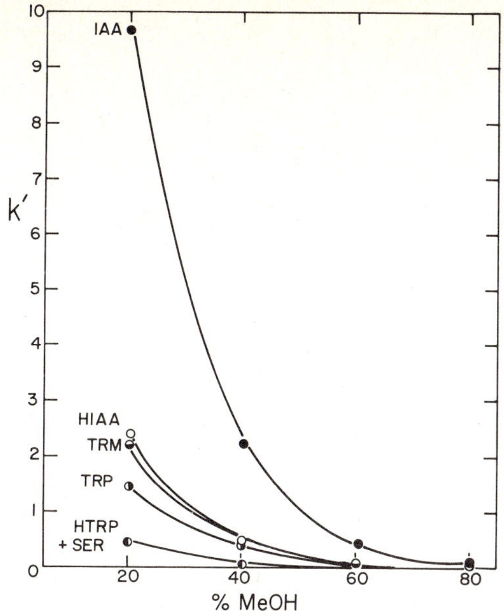

Fig. 1. Effect of percent organic modifier on capacity factor k' values

Mobile phase % methanol in 10 mmol/liter NaAc, pH = 3. Stationary phase, μ Bondpak C_{18}. Abbreviations used in Figures are: *MeOH*, methanol; *HIAA*, 5-hydroxyindoleacetic acid; *IAA*, indoleacetic acid; *SER*, serotonin; *TRM;* tryptamine; *HTRP*, 5-hydroxytryptophan; and *TRP*, tryptophan

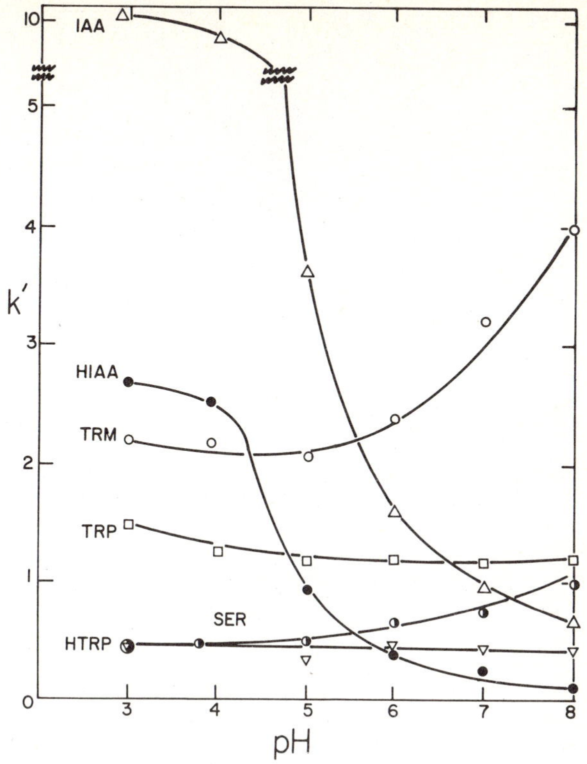

Fig. 2. Effect of mobile phase pH on capacity factor k' values

Mobile phase, 20/80 by vol methanol in 10 mmol/liter NaAc, pH = 3–8. Stationary phase, μ Bondapak C_{18}

um acetate and then adjusting the pH to the desired value with acetic acid; methanol was then added in the desired proportion.

Results and Discussion

Our first goal was to rapidly separate the six indole compounds (5-hydroxyindoleacetic acid, indoleacetic acid, serotonin, tryptamine, 5-hydroxytrytophan, and tryptophan) on a single column. Because they include both weak acids and weak bases, we thought that reverse-phase liquid chromatography offered the best chance for success. Moreover, for rapid analysis we used short (30 cm) columns containing small-particle chemically bonded packings. It is known that the solubility of the substances in the mobile phase plays an important role in retention and selectivity when such hydrophobic chemically bonded phases are used (*9*). We thus tried to make optimum the composition (i.e., water/methanol ratio) and pH of the mobile phase in terms of separation.

We first measured retention (in terms of capacity factor, k') of the six indoles as a function of the amount of methanol in the mobile phase at pH 3 (Figure 1). As expected from solubility considerations, k' decreases in each case as the proportion of methanol increases. Indoleacetic acid has the highest k' value at any methanol composition, as it will be uncharged at pH 3 and does not contain a phenolic group such as is present in 5-hydroxyindoleacetic acid. It is clear from Figure 1 that less than 20 vols. of methanol per 100 vols. should be used, in order that most substances will elute in the optimum k' range of 1.5–5 (*10*).

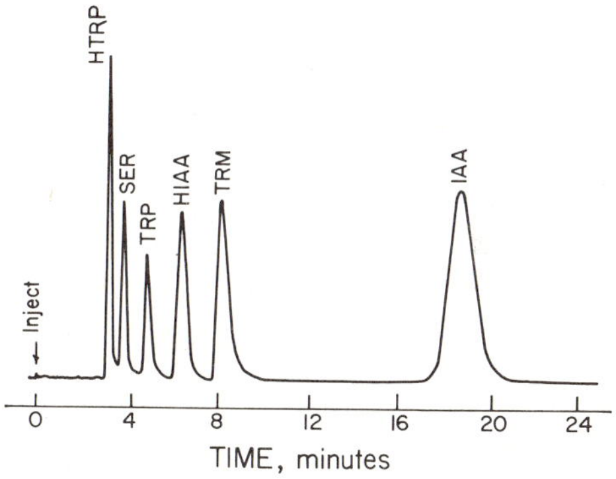

Fig. 3. Separation of standard indoles

Mobile phase, 10/90 by vol. methanol in 10 mmol/liter NaAc, pH = 4.6. Stationary phase, μ Bondapak C_{18}. Flow rate = 2.5 ml/min. Fluorescence detection, atten. = X 64 nA full scale

We next studied the influence of pH on retention and selectivity at a constant methanol/water composition of 20/80 by vol. The pH of the mobile phase was varied from 3 to 8. As expected on the basis of solubility, the extent of ionization of a given indole greatly controls retention (Figure 2). With increasing pH, retention decreases for the acids (5-hydroxyindoleacetic acid and indoleacetic acid) and increases for the bases (serotonin and tryptamine). The amino acids (tryptophan and 5-hydroxytryptophan) are not greatly influenced by changes in pH, as they are amphoteric. Moreover, the inflection point in the sigmoidal curves closely agrees with the pK_a values, e.g.,

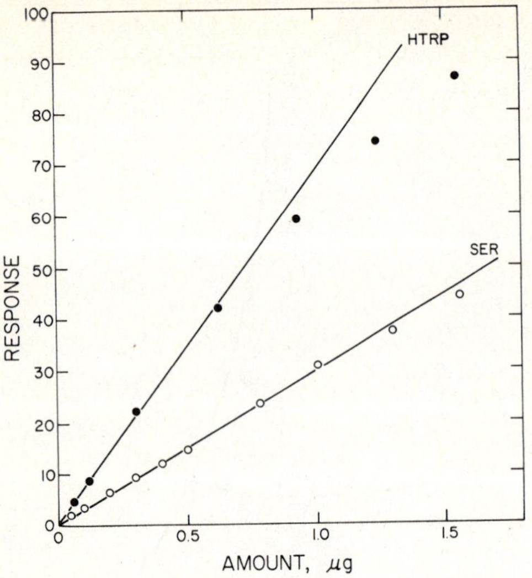

Fig. 4. Fluorescence response vs. amount of indole
Chromatographic conditions as in Figure 3

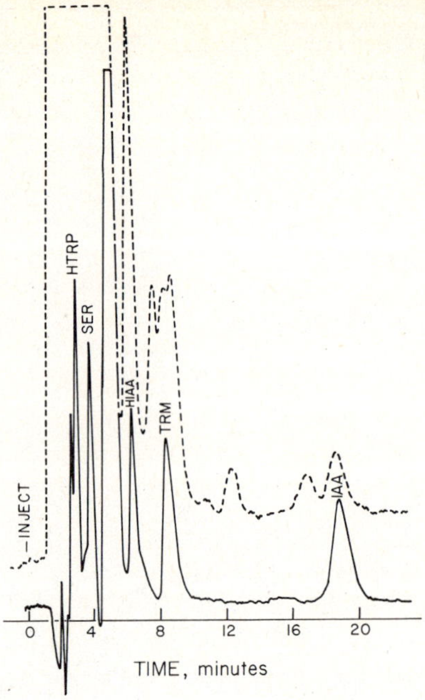

Fig. 6. Chromatograms showing ultraviolet and fluorescence response of deproteinized urine supplemented with 0.4 μmol of standard indoles
Chromatographic conditions as in Fig. 3. 25-μl sample (*dotted line*, ultraviolet; *solid line*, fluorescence). Same attenuation as in Figure 5

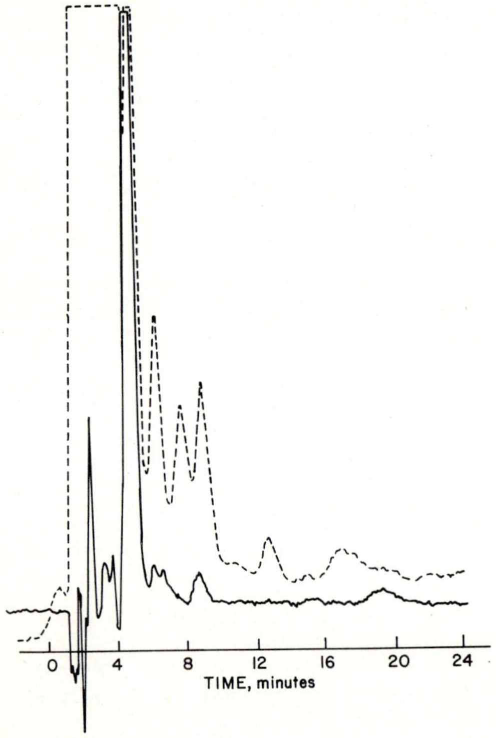

Fig. 5. Chromatograms of ultraviolet and fluorescence backgrounds of deproteinized urine
Chromatographic conditions as in Figure 3. 25-μl sample (*dotted line*, ultraviolet atten. = × .040D; *solid line*, fluorescence atten. = × 16 nA full scale)

the pK_a for indoleacetic acid = 4.75, and the inflection point in Figure 2 is at 4.7. Figure 2 shows that the pH of the mobile phase significantly influences the separation.

At pH values exceeding 7, tailing was observed for serotonin and tryptamine, which are basic compounds. This band asymmetry probably results from adsorption of the amines on unreacted silanol groups on the surface of the silica (*11*). No band asymmetry was observed at acidic pH values, at which the amine groups are protonated. Although small amounts of ammonium carbonate in the mobile phase may decrease tailing of the bases at pH > 7, for simplicity we decided to use a pH of 4.6.

Figure 3 shows the rapid elution of the six indole compounds at pH 4.6. In this case, the absolute retentions of all the indoles were increased by lowering the methanol/water ratio to 10/90 by vol, at which 5-hydroxytryptophan and serotonin were eluted discretely (i.e., because of increase of k' into the optimum range). This separation clearly illustrates the manipulation of methanol concentration to control retention and of pH to control selectivity.

Figure 4 shows typical plots of fluorescence response vs. amount of indole. The relation is linear to ~1 μg of indole per sample (*12*). Because the main use of fluorometry is in trace analysis, the calibration plots are quite adequate for our purposes.

From the noise level of the detector and the response characteristics, we estimated the detection limit to be 5 ng for 5-hydroxytryptophan, 10 ng for 5-hydroxyindoleacetic acid, and 15 ng for serotonin, these being the amounts giving a signal/noise ratio of 2. More practically, twice these sample amounts can be easily analyzed. Detection of such amounts is more than adequate for the clinical investigation of urinary concentrations of indole substances.

The results shown in Figures 3 and 4 were achieved with standard substances and thus represent the best performance of the system. We decided to explore the analysis for the indoles in urine, with use of a simple procedure for sample clean-up.

Table 1. Analytical Recoveries of Added Indoles after Deproteinization of Urine Samples

Compound	Added[a] (ng)	Found (ng)	Recovery, %
Tryptamine	80	80	100
	120	110	92
Serotonin	67	50	74
	100	80	80
5-Hydroxyindoleacetic acid	144	130	90
	217	210	97

[a] per 25 μl of urine, the volume injected into the chromatograph.

A 10-ml sample of normal urine was treated with 1 ml of $ZnSO_4$ (100 g/liter) solution and 0.5 ml of 0.1 mol/liter NaOH, to precipitate the urinary proteins. We used vortex-type mixing, to minimize adsorption on the precipitate. After centrifugation, the supernatant liquid was filtered through a 5-μm (av. pore size) filter (Millipore, Bedford, Mass. 01730). Of the collected solution, 25 μl (an arbitrary volume; larger ones can be used) was injected directly into the column without further pretreatment. Figure 5 presents both the ultraviolet and fluorescence chromatograms of the finally eluted sample. The background for ultraviolet detection is quite high, whereas a much less complex chromatogram is seen for fluorescence.

A 10-ml urine sample was then supplemented with ~0.4 μmol of each indole, to simulate pathological conditions. After the sample clean-up procedure, 25 μl (~150 ng of each indole) was injected into the liquid chromatograph. The resulting chromatograms from ultraviolet and fluorescence detection are shown in Figure 6. Except for tryptophan, which is masked by the large fluorescence peak in the urine background, all the other indoles can be analyzed in amounts of ~1 nmol/25 μl sample without interference, and the three 5-hydroxyindoles (5-hydroxyindoleacetic acid, serotonin, and 5-hydroxytryptophan) can be analyzed in about 6 min. This analysis could not be as readily accomplished with ultraviolet detection because of poorer spectral selectivity.

In a further experiment we determined the analytical recovery of the indole compounds after deproteinization from the supplemented samples of urine. Typical examples of these results are shown in Table 1. The recoveries indicate little sample loss in the deproteinization step. If desired, the method of standard addition can be used to compensate for the less than 100% recovery for each indole substance.

We thank the NIGMS, NIH, USPHS for support of this work under Grant GM-15847.

References

1. Rapport, M. M., Green, A. A., and Page, I. H., Serum vasoconstrictor (serotinin). IV. Isolation and characterization. *J. Biol. Chem.* **176,** 1243 (1948).

2. Lovenberg, S. W., and Engelman, K., Serotonin: The assay of hydroxyindole compounds and their biosynthetic enzymes. In *Methods of Biochemical Analysis,* supplemental vol., D. Glick, Ed., Interscience, New York, N.Y., 1971.

3. Sjoerdsma, A., Weissbach, H., and Udenfriend, S., Simple test for diagnosis of metastatic carcinoid (argentaffinoma). *J. Am. Med. Assoc.* **159,** 397 (1955).

4. Pare, C. M. B. Sandler, M., and Stacey, R. S., 5-Hydroxyindoles in mental deficiency. *J. Neurol. Neurosurg. Psychiat.* **23,** 341 (1960).

5. Nishino, M., Noguchi, T., and Kido, R., Ion-exchange column chromatographic method for the simultaneous separation and determination of 5-hydroxyindoles. *Anal. Biochem.* **45,** 314 (1972).

6. Chilcote, D. D., and Mrochek, J. E., Chromatographic analysis of naturally fluorescing compounds: I. Rapid analysis of nanogram amounts of indoles in physiologic fluids. *Clin. Chem.* **18,** 778 (1972).

7. Chilcote, D. D., Column-chromatographic analysis of naturally fluorescing compounds: II. Rapid analysis of indoleacetic acid and 5-hydroxyindoleacetic acid in biological samples. *Clin. Chem.* **18,** 1376 (1972).

8. Chilcote, D. D., Column-chromatographic analysis of naturally fluorescing compounds: III. Rapid analysis of serotonin and tryptamine. *Clin. Chem.* **20,** 421 (1974).

9. Locke, D. C., Selectivity in reversed-phase liquid chromatography using chemically bonded stationary phases. *J. Chromatogr. Sci.* **12,** 433 (1974).

10. Karger, B. L., Snyder, L. R., and Horvath, C., *An Introduction to Separation Science,* Interscience, New York, N.Y., 1973, chap. 5.

11. Locke, D C., Chemically bonded stationary phases for liquid chromatography. *J. Chromatogr. Sci.* **11,** 120 (1973).

12. Steichen, J. C., A dual-purpose absorbance fluorescence detector for high-pressure liquid chromatography. *J. Chromatogr.* **104,** 39 (1975).

CLIN. CHEM. 22/2, 188–192 (1976)

An Integrated Approach to Lipid Profiling: Enzymatic Determination of Cholesterol and Triglycerides with a Centrifugal Analyzer

Peter W. Wentz, Robert E. Cross, and John Savory

We describe enzymatic methods for determination of cholesterol and triglycerides (triacylglycerols), adapted for use with a centrifugal analyzer. Triglycerides are determined by a two-point kinetic method, which utilizes a single glycerol standard for calibration and provides for a within-run reagent blank correction. The endpoint determination of cholesterol combines the unique blanking capabilities of the centrifugal analyzer to correct for sample and reagent blank interferences. Results correlate well with those obtained by procedures standardized by the Lipid Research Clinics Program for use with a continuous-flow system.

Additional Keyphrases: *continuous-flow method compared* • *high-speed spectrophotometry*

Fully enzymatic methods for determination of serum cholesterol and triglycerides (triacylglycerols) provide the substrate specificity that allows direct analyses to be performed, thus eliminating the tedious pre-analysis extraction and saponification steps that are required in colorimetric and fluorometric procedures to improve accuracy. Several reports have described adapting enzymatic triglyceride methods for use with the centrifugal analyzer (*1–3*). Olson and Brennan (*1*) determined the glycerol produced on saponification of triglycerides by using an enzymatic fixed-time kinetic method. This method was not adequately sensitive in the normal range and involved sufficient sample preparation to render it unsuitable for our purposes. Chong-Kit and McLaughlin (*2*) described a fully enzymatic method for the ENI-GEMSAEC version of the centrifugal analyzer, in which an endpoint program was used; it required 10 min of analyzer running time to follow the reaction to completion. Tiffany et al. (*3*) evaluated both endpoint and nonlinear fixed-time kinetic methods for determination of serum triglycerides. Their fixed-time approach requires less than 3 min for analysis after hydrolysis.

The enzymatic determination of serum cholesterol by use of the enzymes cholesterol esterase (EC 3.1.1.13), cholesterol oxidase (EC 1.1.3.6), and horseradish peroxidase (EC 1.11.1.7) in conjunction with the Trinder reagent has been shown to give results that are in excellent agreement with those obtained by the extraction procedure standardized by the Lipid Research Clinics Program (*4–6*).

We modified Tiffany's method for triglycerides for use with a commercially available centrifugal analyzer system by incorporating a linear fixed-time kinetic program in which a single glycerol solution is used for standardization. In addition, we adapted for use with the same system an enzymatic cholesterol procedure in which sample–reagent blank corrections are combined.

Principles

Triglycerides. Samples are incubated with lipase (glycerol ester hydrolase; EC 3.1.1.3) and α-chymotrypsin (peptidylpeptide hydrolase; EC 3.4.4.5) to convert triglycerides to glycerol. The resulting free glycerol is then determined enzymatically by a series of coupled reactions initiated by the action of glycerol kinase (ATP:glycerol phosphotransferase; EC 2.7.1.30), and culminating in the reduction of pyruvate to lactate. The concomitant decrease in absorbance at 340 nm over a fixed-time interval owing to NADH depletion is measured spectrophotometrically.

Cholesterol. During incubation of serum samples with cholesterol reagent, cholesterol esters are converted to cholesterol by the action of cholesterol esterase. The cholesterol so formed, plus the free cholesterol originally present, is oxidized in the presence of cholesterol oxidase with the simultaneous production of hydrogen peroxide. This reaction is coupled with the peroxidase/phenol/4-aminoantipyrine system, resulting in the formation of a color, which is measured at 520 nm.

Materials and Methods

Apparatus. The centrifugal analyzer we used was the Aminco "Rotochem II" (American Instrument Co., Silver Spring, Md. 20910). The Aminco "Rotofill II" diluter was used for sample and diluent delivery. Reagents were dispensed with Eppendorf microliter pipets (Brinkmann Instruments, Inc., Westbury, N. Y. 11590). Values obtained with the Technicon AutoAnalyzer II for cholesterol and triglycerides were provided by the Lipid Laboratory of Bowman Gray

Departments of Medicine, Biochemistry, Pathology, and Hospital Laboratories, University of North Carolina, Chapel Hill, N. C. 27514.

Received Oct. 27, 1975; accepted Nov. 11, 1975.

School of Medicine and were obtained in accordance with the procedures adopted by the Lipid Research Clinics Program, involving a zeolite/isopropanol extraction and standardization with a serum calibrator supplied by the Center for Disease Control (*4, 7*).

Reagents. Triglyceride reagent, the two-vial "Super Stat-Pack" (Calbiochem, San Diego, Calif. 92112), was prepared by reconstituting vial A, containing the hydrolyzing enzymes, with 12.9 ml of distilled water and vial B, containing the glycerol kinase, with 1.25 ml of distilled water. The single-vial cholesterol reagent (Beckman Microbics, Carlsbad, Calif. 92008), 20-ml size, was reconstituted with 16.0 ml of distilled water.

Standards

Stock triglyceride standard. Accurately weigh about 200 mg of glycerol (Certified Spectranalyzed glycerin; Fisher Scientific Co., Fair Lawn, N. J. 07410) into a tared 100-ml volumetric flask, dissolve, and dilute to the mark with distilled water.

Working triglyceride standard. Prepare a fivefold dilution of the stock triglyceride standard with distilled water to give a working standard with a concentration of about 40 mg of glycerol per deciliter. Calculate the exact concentration, expressed as milligrams of triolein per deciliter, by multiplying the concentration of glycerol (mg/dl) in the working standard by the factor 9.613, which represents the ratio of the molecular weights of triolein to glycerol. Thus, a 200 mg/dl stock standard would give, on fivefold dilution, the equivalent of a 385 mg/dl triolein working standard.

Cholesterol standard. We used, as provided, an aqueous 3.00 g/liter cholesterol standard included as part of a set of six standards (Boehringer Mannheim Corp., New York, N.Y. 10017; Preciset Cholesterol).

Procedures

Triglycerides. Load the sample ring in the following sequence: position 1, a cup containing distilled water; position 2, a cup containing the working triglyceride standard; and in positions 3–14, sample and control cups. Adjust the Rotofill diluter to deliver 10-μl aliquots of the contents of each cup to the corresponding reagent wells of the transfer disc, followed by 60-μl aliquots of saline diluent. After sample loading is completed, manually pipette 500 μl of vial A reagent into each of the reagent wells and allow the enzymatic hydrolysis to proceed for 15 min at room temperature; this sequence of adding reagent to the predispensed sample was shown to provide the most efficient mixing when a manual inverse pipetting technique was used for dispensing reagent. The inverse pipetting technique, characterized by drawing up excess reagent by depressing the pipet push button to the second stop and dispensing reagent by depressing the push button to the first stop, was used exclusively and provided excellent reproducibility. During this hydrolysis period, manually pipette 50 μl of vial B reagent into the sample wells. The reagent well of position zero contains 600 μl of distilled water and serves as the spectrophotometric reference for 100% T. After the 15-min incubation to ensure complete hydrolysis of triglycerides to glycerol, place the transfer disc in the rotor and start the KINETIC RATE III program. Measure absorbance at 340 nm and 30 °C for each cuvet 10 and 130 s after acceleration of the rotor. Computer calculate the results based on comparison of absorbance changes for samples with that of the standard, after correcting for reagent blank (cuvette 1).

Cholesterol. Manually load the reagent well of the zero position with 600 μl of distilled water for both blank and reaction determinations. The loading sequence of the sample ring is identical to that used for the triglyceride measurement, except that position 2 holds a cup containing the cholesterol standard. Adjust the Rotofill diluter to deliver 10-μl aliquots of the contents of each cup to the reagent wells of the transfer disc, followed by 100 μl of saline diluent. After sample loading is completed, manually pipette 400 μl of physiological saline into each of the reagent wells of positions 1 through 14 and use a CUVETTE CALIBRATION program to store sample-blank absorbance data obtained at 520 nm for each of the cuvettes. Then repeat the sample loading process, with use of the same sequence as for the blank determination, and manually pipette 400 μl of cholesterol reagent into each of the reagent wells of positions 1 through 14. After incubation at room temperature for 30 min, start an ENDPOINT II program and automatically correct absorbance measurements obtained at 10 s for sample-blank (CUVETTE CALIBRATION) and reagent-blank (cuvette 1) contributions to the 520-nm absorbance. Base calculations on comparison with the standard (cuvette 2), run in parallel.

Results and Discussion

Linearity

Triglycerides. The range of linearity of the fixed-time kinetic method for triglycerides, which is determined by the range of concentrations over which the overall reaction obeys pseudo-first-order kinetics, was established by using sequential dilutions of a lipemic specimen. A similar calibration curve was obtained with aqueous glycerol standards, with linearity extending to approximately 400 mg/dl in both cases. A single glycerol standard, serving to calibrate each analytical run, may be validly used in the ratiometric calculation of test results for samples with triglyceride concentrations below the upper limit of linearity of the method. A nonlinear fixed-time kinetic program such as that described by Tiffany et al. (*3*) would extend the working range of the method but, by requiring multiple standards for calibration, would limit the number of patient samples that could be analyzed per transfer disc. A working range up to 400 mg/dl is adequate and, to minimize the number of specimens requiring dilutions, those samples that

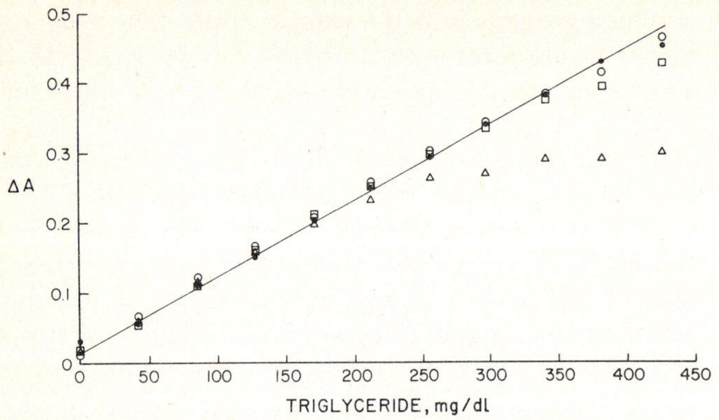

Fig. 1. Effect of glycerol kinase activity on reaction rate (ΔA) and linearity
△, 300 U/liter; □, 600 U/liter; ○, 900 U/liter; ●, 1200 U/liter

are obviously lipemic are diluted with saline before analysis. The ΔA measured between 10 and 130 s corresponds to a change of about 1 milliabsorbance unit per milligram of triglyceride per deciliter and offers reasonable sensitivity in the normal range. We evaluated the effect of varying glycerol kinase activity on the kinetics of the coupled assay for triglycerides, by use of vials of glycerol kinase reconstituted to give different glycerol kinase activities, as calculated from the activity specified in the reagent package insert. Figure 1 illustrates the combined effect on reaction rate (ΔA) and linearity for several glycerol kinase activities. The departure from linearity is quite marked for the reaction catalyzed by glycerol kinase at an activity of approximately 300 U/liter in the final reaction mixture. At an activity of 600 U/liter the linearity is extended to about 350 mg/dl and at higher activities linearity extends to approximately 400 mg/dl. Our choice of 1200 U/liter, an activity obtained by reconstituting vial B with 1.25 ml of distilled water, was based on economy of reagent consumption. Packaged as two-vial sets, reagents in the two vials are used on a nearly 1:1 basis, with each vial providing sufficient reagent for 25 determinations.

Cholesterol. With use of a 10-μl sample, the linearity of the present method extends to 400 mg/dl. This range was determined by using the 400 mg/dl Preciset Cholesterol standard to reconstitute a vial of an elevated cholesterol control serum (General Diagnostics Div., Morris Plains, N.J. 07950; Serachol) to which 50 mg of sodium chloride had been added to enhance solubility.

Standardization

Triglycerides. We chose an aqueous glycerol solution to standardize the enzymatic assay for triglycerides on the basis of its ease of preparation as compared with making an aqueous triolein standard, which requires a surfactant to solubilize the triolein. Chong-Kit and McLaughlin (*2*) have described the preparation of an aqueous triolein standard by using the wetting agent "Triton X-100" (isoctyl phenoxypolyethoxyethanol) to stabilize the solution. The use of an aqueous glycerol standard has the advantage of providing a direct check on the performance of the coupled assay for glycerol. A quality-control sample with an above-normal triglyceride content (Calbiochem, La Jolla, Calif. 92037; Caltrol-340 Abnormal) is included in each analytical run to check the completeness of the pre-analysis hydrolysis of triglycerides by lipase as well as the performance of the coupled assay for glycerol.

Cholesterol. The unique feature of the present method is that the reagent wells of the transfer disc are used as reaction vessels. Initially, we had hoped to increase analysis rate and minimize analyzer running time by doing the incubations in the required number of transfer discs and measuring the final absorbances by taking a 10-s reading after acceleration of the rotor. In this mode, the centrifugal analyzer functions simply as a high-speed spectrophotometer, a capability that deserves greater recognition. In addition to realizing these advantages, however, it readily became apparent that this modification was essential for proper standardization if "Tekit" aqueous cholesterol standard (Searle Diagnostic Inc., Columbus, Ohio 43216) was used, because the cholesterol in the Tekit standard precipitates on dilution with saline or distilled water during dispensing into the transfer disc. If mixing was performed within the analyzer, as is usually the case when sample and reagent occupy the designated sample and reagent wells of the transfer disc, then incomplete transfer would result because cholesterol would be precipitated in the sample well. If the incubation is done in the transfer disc, the direct addition of cholesterol reagent to the reagent well solubilizes the cholesterol and provides a homogeneous reaction mixture. This characteristic feature, however, could be a possible source of operator variability and we preferred to use an aqueous cholesterol standard that was readily miscible with water or saline. The use of Preciset Cholesterol standard obviated this potential source of error. In addi-

Table 1. Cholesterol Values, under Three Sets of Conditions, for Nine Serum Samples[a]

A	*B*	*C*
	Cholesterol, mg/dl	
203	202	196
268	265	261
218	216	213
190	189	187
256	252	247
164	165	158
356	350	350
113	115	110
146	143	139

[a] *A*, 30-min incubation at room temperature, a CUVETTE CALIBRATION program used to correct for sample blanks; *B*, 10-min reaction at 37 °C, with absorbance measurements taken at 6 and 600 s; *C*, 10-min reaction at 37 °C, CUVETTE CALIBRATION program used to correct for sample blanks.

tion, the use of the Preciset standard allows sample and reagent to be mixed within the rotor. It is then possible to follow the reaction course spectrophotometrically as a function of change in absorbance with time. Initial studies suggest that the lag time for the coupled reactions is sufficient that an early absorbance measurement taken 6 s after acceleration of the rotor approximates the absorbance at time zero and provides for a within-run sample-blank correction; this initial absorbance is subtracted from the final absorbance measured when the reaction is completed. Table 1 lists comparative data supporting this. Thus, while the selected adaptation requires a separate sample blank determination, it appears that a within-run correction may be feasible if an early absorbance measurement can be made with the analyzer.

Reaction Time

Triglycerides. The hydrolysis time may be reduced to 10-min if the transfer disc is placed in an incubator at 37 °C.

Cholesterol. Similarly, this endpoint determination would require only 10 min if a 37 °C incubation were utilized. At 10 min the reaction is 95 to 99% complete, as judged from comparison of absorbances measured at 10 min with those obtained after a 30-min incubation at room temperature. Table 1 compares cholesterol values obtained for different temperature-timed incubations. The validity of this approach is based on the observation that the Preciset Cholesterol standard reacts on a time scale similar to serum samples.

Precision. Precision data for the methods (Tables 2 and 3) reflect the excellent reproducibility of direct, discrete sample analyses.

Accuracy

Triglycerides. For 62 patients' sera, the enzymatic Rotochem method was compared with the fluorometric procedure standardized for use with the AutoAnalyzer II (Technicon). The linear regression parameters indicated in Figure 2 suggest an excellent correlation. This precludes the necessity for running sample blanks to correct for endogenous glycerol and pyruvate, and substantiated our initial investigations, which indicated that for a freshly drawn sample of serum the sample blank was usually less than 10 mg/dl. Recoveries, determined by assaying various aliquots of high-value and low-value serum pools, were essentially quantitative as shown in Table 4.

Cholesterol. Comparison of the present method with the Liebermann–Burchard AutoAnalyzer II method, standardized under a protocol established by the Lipid Research Clinics Program, gave statistical agreement as indicated in Figure 3. In Table 4 the

Table 2. Precision of Triglyceride Measurements

	Normal[a]		Abnormal[a]	
	Within-run	Day-to-day	Within-run	Day-to-day
No.	24	30	24	30
Mean, mg/dl	173	179	360	365
SD, mg/dl	4.6	8.0	3.0	7.6
CV, %	2.7	4.4	0.8	2.1

[a] Caltrol control serum.

Table 3. Precision of Cholesterol Measurements

	Within-run	Day-to-day
No.	36	50
Mean, mg/dl	222	140
SD, mg/dl	4.6	5.5
CV, %	2.1	3.9

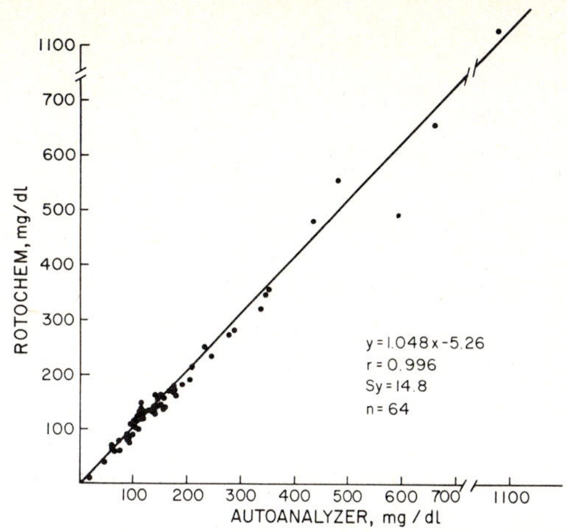

Fig. 2. Comparison of results for triglycerides as obtained by the fluorometric AutoAnalyzer II method and the enzymatic Rotochem procedure

Table 4. Analytical Recovery of Triglycerides and Cholesterol, as Determined by Assaying Mixtures of High- and Low-value Serum Pools

Mixture ratio, high/low	Expected (mg/dl)	Found (mg/dl)	Recovery, %
Triglycerides[a]			
1:1	256	257	100
1:1		254	99
2:1	294	291	99
2:1		292	99
3:1	314	308	98
1:2	217	212	98
1:2		210	97
1:3	190	193	102
Cholesterol[b]			
1:1	238	236	99
1:1		235	99
2:1	263	264	100
2:1		265	101
3:1	276	272	99
1:2	213	218	102
1:2		214	100
1:3	200	197	99

[a] Pool values: high, 372 mg/dl; low, 139 mg/dl.
[b] Pool values: high, 314 mg/dl; low, 162 mg/dl.

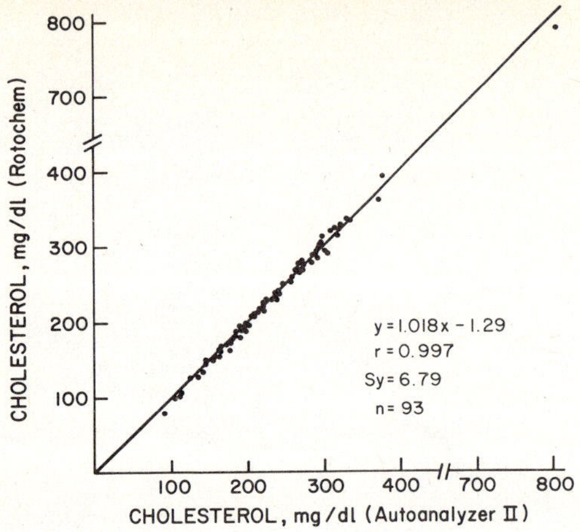

Fig. 3. Comparison of results for cholesterol as obtained by the Liebermann–Burchard AutoAnalyzer II method and the enzymatic Rotochem procedure

analytical recoveries found for samples made by mixing various aliquots of high- and low-value serum pools substantiate the accuracy of the present method.

Interferences

Triglycerides. The instability of the triglyceride reagent, presumably caused by impurities in the enzyme preparations, emphasizes the need for running a reagent blank to correct for nonspecific oxidation of NADH to NAD^+. A reagent blank, run in parallel with each transfer disc, provides an effective within-run correction for the reagent-blank contribution to the absorbance change measured for the glycerol reaction. The comparison study validates the contention that serum blanks need not be routinely run to correct for endogenous glycerol. In fact, as pointed out by Rautela et al. (*8*), the inclusion of serum blank values when reporting the total triglyceride concentration may better reflect the total amount of "neutral fat" in a patient's serum.

Cholesterol. Bilirubin has been shown (*4*) to cause a slight positive interference when cholesterol is determined enzymatically with the Abbott ABA-100 bichromatic analyzer; 1 mg of bilirubin per deciliter is measured as 1–2 mg of cholesterol. Blanking on the Abbott analyzer is provided by its dual-wavelength optical system, which subtracts the absorbance at 600 nm from the absorbance at 500 nm. The higher molar absorptivity of bilirubin at 500 nm than at 600 nm is the source of the slight positive interference. This interference by bilirubin represents a static type of interference that does not undergo chemical change during the analytical reaction, and can be corrected by a simple subtraction process in the case of a centrifugal analyzer. Sample blanks, measured at the same wavelength on the Rotochem as the analytical determination, are true sample blanks and effectively eliminate static interferences.

The methods described represent a conceptual approach to lipid profiling that combines the specificity of an enzymatic assay with the speed and versatility of a centrifugal analyzer. Functioning either in its conceived capacity as a reaction-rate analyzer or as a high-speed spectrophotometer, the centrifugal analyzer offers the flexibility to allow lipid testing to be performed on a daily basis with economical use of reagents, minimal personnel requirements, and excellent precision and accuracy.

This work was supported in part by the National Institutes of Health (Grant GM-92). We are especially grateful to the late Hugh B. Lofland, Ph.D., and to Nina Ann Stokes, M.T. (Department of Pathology, Bowman Gray School of Medicine of Wake Forest University, Winston-Salem, N. C.) for providing the serum samples analyzed by the continuous-flow method that were used in the comparison studies. We are grateful to Ken Pierre, Ph.D., of Beckman Microbics for material support throughout this study. This work was presented in part at the Ninth International Congress on Clinical Chemistry, Toronto, 1975.

References

1. Olson, A. D., and Brennan, R. L., Ratiometric triglyceride analysis by use of a centrifugal analyzer. *Clin. Chem.* **19,** 1060 (1973).

2. Chong-Kit, R., and McLaughlin, P., Fully automated, all-enzymatic tryglyceride method adapted to the GEMSAEC centrifugal analyzer, with use of an aqueous triolein standard. *Clin. Chem.* **20,** 1454 (1974).

3. Tiffany, T. O. Morton, J. M., Hall, E. M., and Garrett, A. S., Jr., Clinical evaluation of kinetic enzymatic fixed-time and integral analysis of serum triglycerides. *Clin. Chem.* **20,** 477 (1974).

4. Witte, D. L., Barrett, D. A., II, and Wycoff, D. A., Evaluation of an enzymatic procedure for determination of serum cholesterol with the Abbott ABA-100. *Clin. Chem.* **20,** 1282 (1974).

5. Allain, C. C., Poon, L. S., Chan, C. S. G., et al., Enzymatic determination of total serum cholesterol. *Clin. Chem.* **20,** 470 (1974).

6. *Manual of Laboratory Operations, Lipid Research Clinics Program, Volume 1, Lipid and Lipoprotein Analysis,* National Heart and Lung Institute, National Institutes of Health, Bethesda, Md. 20014, DHEW Publication No. (NIH) 72-628, May 1974.

7. Rush, R. L., Leon, L., and Turrell, J., Automated simultaneous cholesterol and triglyceride determination on the AutoAnalyzer II instrument. In *Advances in Automated Analysis, Technicon International Congress 1970,* **1,** *Clinical Analysis.* C. E. Barton et al., Eds. Thurman Associates, Miami, Fla. 33132, 1971, p 503.

8. Rautela, G. S., Slater, S., and Arvan, D. A., Assessment of the need for triglyceride blank measurements. *Clin. Chem.* **19,** 1193 (1973).

CLIN. CHEM. 22/2, 193–197 (1976)

Evaluation of Two Digoxin Radioimmunoassay Procedures in Which ^{125}I-Labeled Digoxin is Used

Z. Jerry Kuczala and Gurjit S. Ahluwalia[1]

We present a comparative evaluation of two commercial kits, the "Quantitope" and "GammaCoat," for radioimmunoassay of digoxin in serum. These kits, in which iodine-125 is used as a label, proved to be suitable for digoxin assay as determined by their reproducibility, sensitivity, precision, and a regression analysis. Hemolysis, lipemia, and icterus did not affect results. However, in some cases hypoalbuminemia falsely lowered the assayed digoxin concentration. Recovery of pure digoxin added to native patients' sera having low albumin concentration (24–28 g/liter) ranged from 67–105% with the Quantitope kit and 70–110% with the GammaCoat kit. Low serum albumin concentration did not always decrease the recovery of digoxin; this effect varied from serum to serum, which may indicate that there are factors other than albumin that affect the assay of digoxin.

Additional Keyphrases: *economics of laboratory operation • drug assay*

It has been reported recently that either inadequate digitalization or digoxin toxicity are quite common among patients receiving maintenance doses of digoxin (*1–3*). Consequently, it is important to accurately monitor and regulate the serum digoxin concentrations of these patients (*1, 2, 4*). This has become possible with the recent availability of commercial radioimmunoassay (RIA) kits for serum digoxin determination.

Earlier methods for determining the concentration of cardiac glycosides included bioassay (*4*), chromatography (*5*), polarography (*6*), and ATPase inhibition techniques (*7*)—all either cumbersome or too insensitive. RIA techniques have made it possible to measure cardiac glycosides with sensitivity, specificity, and speed.

Department of Laboratory Medicine, Binghamton General Hospital, Binghamton, N. Y. 13903.
[1] Request reprints from this author.
Received Sept. 24, 1975; accepted Nov. 11, 1975.

Because digoxin is the most widely used cardiac glycoside, various digoxin assay procedures in which tritium or radioactive iodine is used as a label have been reported (*8–10*). It is not practical for most hospital laboratories to produce their own RIA reagents. Consequently, commercially available kits for the radioimmunoassay of digoxin have become popular. Many such kits have been evaluated in the past (*11*).

We report here a detailed evaluation of two iodine-125 digoxin kits: A, the "Quantitope" kit (Kallestad Laboratories, Inc., Chaska, Minn. 55318), and B, the "GammaCoat" kit (Clinical Assays, Inc., Cambridge, Mass. 02142), both currently used in our laboratory. Previously, we have briefly evaluated kits A and B (*12, 13*).

Both kits offer short assay time and eliminate the need for adding an additional reagent after incubation, to separate free and bound fractions. Kit A offers a single-step solid-phase double-antibody precipitation technique in which the first antibody is bound to a second precipitating antibody. This complex binds digoxin and precipitates on centrifugation. In kit B antibody-coated tubes are used to bind digoxin. Bound digoxin is separated simply by decantation, completely eliminating the need for centrifugation.

Materials and Methods

Apparatus

All reagents and patient sera were dispensed with semiautomatic "Lancer" pipettes with disposable plastic tips (Sherwood Medical Industries, St. Louis, Mo. 63103). Polystyrene 12 × 75 mm tubes (Falcon Co., Oxnard, Calif. 93030) served both as the reaction and counting tubes for Kit A. A PR-6000 refrigerated centrifuge (Damon/IEC Division, Needham Hts., Mass. 02194) with a swinging bucket head was used to separate bound and free fractions. Sample counting and data reduction were done with a 1185 automatic gamma counter and pds/3 interfacing computer system (Searle Analytic, Inc., Des Plaines, Ill. 60018).

Reagents

The *digoxin* used for all recovery experiments was obtained from Schwarz/Mann, Orangeburg, N. Y. 10962. All reagents for the measurement of digoxin are supplied in kit form by the manufacturers. They are stored at 2–8 °C and brought to room temperature before use. Both kits contain sufficient digoxin standards for five standard curves in duplicate.

Kit A contains reagents for a total of 100 determinations. The lyophilized reagents include five individual digoxin standards (0.5, 1.0, 2.0, 4.0, and 8.0 ng/ml) in human serum and also digoxin-free human serum. The antibody complex (GR) is goat-antirabbit in a stabilized form. A second antibody complex (G) containing only (goat immunoglobulin to rabbit gamma globulin)–(rabbit gamma globulin) is supplied for the determination of nonspecific binding. The kit also contains 2 μCi of digoxin derivative labeled with iodine-125, in 0.01 mol/liter phosphate buffer. These reagents are reconstituted with distilled water and gently vortex-mixed until the material is in solution. A stock phosphate buffer is also provided which upon 10-fold dilution with distilled water yields 0.01 mol/liter "diluted" phosphate buffer.

Kit B contains reagents sufficient for a total of 50 determinations. Individual standards (0.5, 1.0, 2.0, and 4.0 ng/ml) of digoxin in human serum are provided. An iodine-125 digoxigenin derivative (0.3 μCi) is supplied in tris(hydroxymethyl)aminomethane buffer solution. Stock buffer, 0.36 g in 10 ml, is provided and is diluted 30-fold before use. The polypropylene 12 × 75 mm tubes provided are coated with rabbit anti-digoxin serum.

Control sera. We used commercially available RIA control sera "I" and "II" (Lederle Diagnostics, Pearl River, N. Y. 10965) for assay quality control. These lyophilized control sera were reconstituted with 5 ml of distilled water. Aliquots of 100 μl were stored at −20 °C for three months, and only thawed immediately before use.

Procedure

Blood (2–10 ml) was drawn 6–8 h after the last oral dose of digoxin. This time is necessary to establish an in vivo equilibrium between the concentrations of digoxin in blood and tissues (*14*). Sera not assayed immediately were stored at −20 °C. All specimens were brought to room temperature before assay.

(*A*) *Quantitope Kit*

A 100-μl aliquot of each serum sample was added to the appropriately labeled polystyrene tubes containing 50 μl of ^{125}I-labeled digoxin. To each tube, 500 μl of the well stirred and suspended GR antibody complex was added. After thorough mixing (vortex-type mixer), the samples were allowed to incubate for

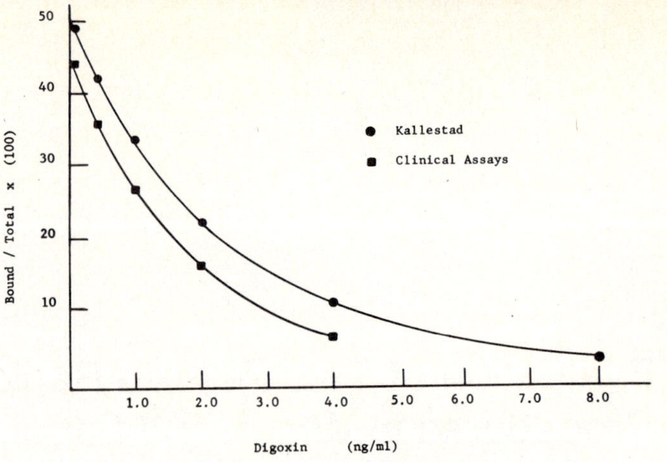

Fig. 1. Digoxin standard curves obtained with kits A and B

Table 1. Analytical Recovery of Digoxin Added to Serum, as Measured with Kits A and B[a]

	Found					
Added	A			B		
	μg/liter					
0.50	0.50		0.50	0.50		0.50
0.25	0.25		0.30	0.25		0.20
0.20	0.20		0.15	0.10		0.15
0.10	0.10		0.10	0.00		0.10
4.0	—	—	—	4.1	4.1	4.2
	—	—	—	3.7	3.9	4.0
8.0	7.9	8.3	8.2	—	—	—
	7.8	7.6	8.0	—	—	—

[a] Pure digoxin was added to a digoxin-free human serum having an albumin concentration of 42 g/liter.

30 min at room temperature (23 ± 3 °C). One milliliter of the "diluted" phosphate buffer was then added and each tube was vortex-mixed for at least 3 s. The tubes were then centrifuged at 4 °C for 20 min at 1000 × *g*. The supernate in each tube was decanted and the tubes were drained for 30 s onto absorbent paper. The radioactivity in the precipitate was then counted. We determined nonspecific binding for the assay by adding 500 μl of the goat antibody suspension (G) to 100 μl of digoxin-free human serum containing 50 μl of ^{125}I-labeled digoxin. Incubation and the following steps were the same as explained above.

(*B*) *GammaCoat Kit*

One milliliter of the buffer was pipetted into each appropriately labeled antibody-coated tube, and 50 μl of the patient's serum was then added. The tubes were gently shaken by hand for 5 s and allowed to stand at room temperature for 15 min. (The contents of the tubes should not be vortex-mixed.) A 100-μl volume of ^{125}I-labeled digoxigenin derivative was then added to all tubes, and they were again gently shaken for 5 s and incubated in a water bath at 37 °C

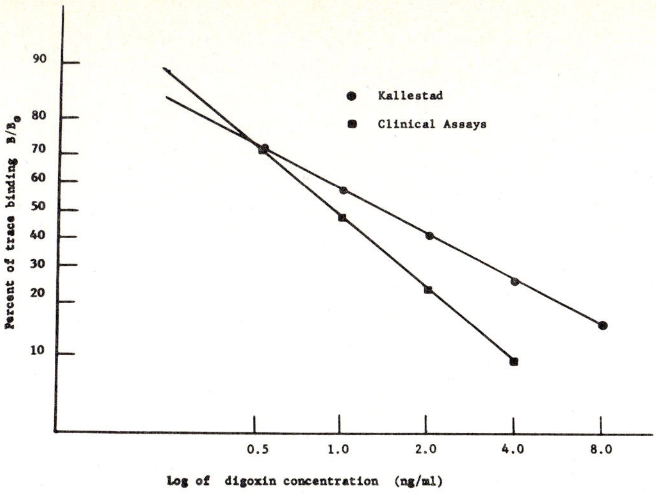

Fig. 2. Logit transformation of digoxin standard curves

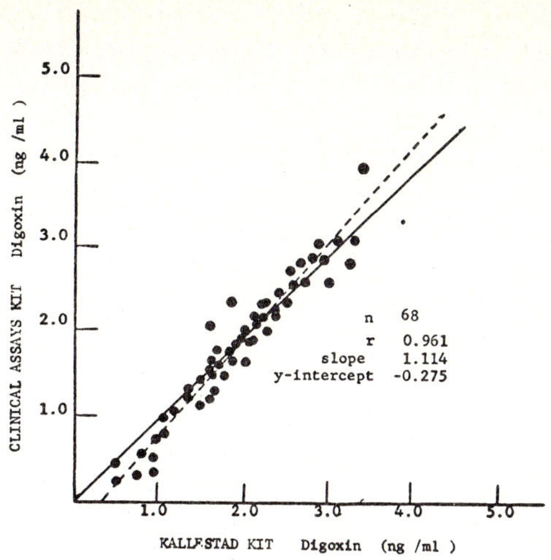

Fig. 3. Regression analysis of kits A and B

Table 2. Analytical Recovery of Digoxin from Patients' Sera with Normal Albumin Concentration

Digoxin added, µg/liter	Sera I	II	III	IV	Cumulative Mean recovery, %
	a Mean recovery, %				
Kit A					
1.0	100	99	100	102	100
2.5	95	95	99	96	96
5.0	81	99	95	90	91
Kit B					
1.0	100	100	101	98	100
2.5	97	94	97	105	98
4.0	93	98	103	93	97

a Each mean recovery is obtained from five different experiments done in duplicate on every serum.

for 45 min. During this period the tubes were shaken for 5 s every 15 min. The contents of all the tubes were then decanted and the tubes were washed twice with 2 ml of the buffer. After the final decantation, the tubes were drained for 1 min onto absorbent paper. The radioactivity in the tubes was then counted.

In both procedures, standards and RIA control sera I and II were treated as were the specimens in each procedure. All assays were done in duplicate.

All samples were counted for the time necessary to obtain 10 000 counts, and the concentration was computed by the interfacing computer system. An RIA computer program provided by the manufacturer automatically corrects all counts for nonspecific binding and interprets the concentration from logit transformation of the experimental data.

$$\text{Logit}(y) = \log_e \frac{y}{1-y}$$

where $y = B/B_0$, B representing the counts per min (cpm) of the sample and B_0 the cpm of the zero standard or the maximum binding obtained in the assay.

Results

Analytical Variables

Figure 1 shows a typical standard curve for each kit, as plotted by the pds/3 system. B_0 for the freshly manufactured kits is about 40–50%, but this progressively decreases with the age of the kits. However, this does not affect the assay during the prescribed life of the kits (approximately 2 months).

From recovery studies with both kits (Table 1) we found assay sensitivity to be 0.25 µg of digoxin per liter, and showed that digoxin concentrations as high as 8.0 and 4.0 µg/liter could be accurately measured with both kits A and B. Additionally, Figure 2 shows the linearity of the relation between sample concentration and binding for each of the kits.

Table 2 shows the analytical recovery of pure digoxin added to four different patients' sera with normal albumin concentration (36–45 g/liter), in five separate experiments. Recovery is comparable for the two kits.

Regression analysis of 68 patients' sera assayed with the two kits is shown in Figure 3.

Interassay variance, intra-assay variance, and the standard deviation (SD) for both kits are shown in Table 3. Two different lots of the RIA control sera I and II were used. With lot *a* a mean of 1.5 µg/liter ± 0.4 (2 SD) (*15*) and 1.6 µg/liter ± 0.4 (*16*) for control serum I and a mean of 3.8 µg/liter ± 0.6 (*15, 16*) for control serum II are listed (package inserts, Lederle Diagnostics) with two other commercial digoxin kits. Means for lot *b* of 1.41 µg/liter ± 0.2 and 3.78 µg/liter ± 0.46 for control sera I and II, respectively, have been reported by Kallestad Laboratories. Our results compare well with these reported values.

Table 3. Intra-assay and Interassay Variance of Kits A and B with Two Different Lots of RIA Control Sera, I and II

	Control serum I		Control serum II		
	$\bar{X}$	2 SD	$\bar{X}$	2 SD	n
	Digoxin, μg/liter				
[a] Lot *a*					
Kit A					
Intra-assay	1.43	0.33	3.35	0.46	20
Interassay	1.33	0.15	3.29	0.32	58
Kit B					
Intra-assay	1.40	0.38	3.52	0.51	25
Interassay	1.41	0.30	3.50	0.46	23
[b] Lot *b*					
Kit A					
Intra-assay	1.42	0.31	3.91	0.76	20
Interassay	1.39	0.35	3.78	0.85	83
Kit B					
Intra-assay	1.40	0.19	3.37	0.51	25
Interassay	1.41	0.37	3.85	0.82	35

[a] Lot *a*: Control serum I, No. 2945-610K1, target value 1.5 ± 0.4
Control serum II, No. 2946-611K1, target value 3.8 ± 0.6
[b] Lot *b*: Control serum I, No. 2945-610R1, target value 1.41 ± 0.20
Control serum II, No. 2946-611R1, target value 3.78 ± 0.46

Table 4. Recovery of Pure Digoxin Added to Patients' Sera with Low Albumin Concentration, with Kits A and B

	Digoxin added, μg/liter					
	1.0		1.5		2.0	
Albumin, g/liter	A	B	A	B	A	B
	Recovery, μg/liter					
24	1.0	0.8	1.5	1.1	2.1	2.1
24	0.7	0.8	1.5	1.1	2.1	1.6
24	0.8	1.0	1.0	1.6	1.7	1.5
24	0.7	0.9	1.1	1.1	1.8	1.5
24	0.8	0.7	1.5	1.3	2.0	2.1
24	0.7	0.7	1.4	1.3	2.0	2.1
24	0.7	0.9	1.5	1.5	2.1	1.9
24	0.9	1.0	1.0	1.3	2.1	2.0
24	0.8	1.1	1.1	1.5	1.8	2.0
24	1.0	1.0	1.1	1.3	1.9	1.5
26	0.9	0.8	1.1	1.3	1.6	1.6
26	0.9	0.7	1.3	1.2	1.4	2.1
26	0.7	1.0	1.4	1.2	1.5	1.7
26	1.0	1.0	1.1	1.3	1.5	1.8
26	0.8	0.7	1.4	1.2	1.5	1.7
27	0.9	0.8	1.0	1.2	1.6	1.4
27	0.8	1.0	1.0	1.2	1.8	1.5
27	0.9	1.1	1.1	1.3	1.6	1.7
27	0.7	0.8	1.1	1.3	1.8	1.8
27	1.0	1.0	1.1	1.5	1.9	2.0
27	0.7	0.9	1.0	1.3	1.6	1.6
28	0.9	0.8	1.0	1.2	1.7	1.9
28	1.0	0.9	1.0	1.6	1.6	1.8
28	1.0	1.0	1.0	1.5	1.6	1.6
28	1.0	0.9	1.5	1.3	2.1	2.0
28	0.8	1.0	1.1	1.1	1.8	1.6
28	1.0	0.9	1.5	1.4	2.0	2.1
28	0.8	0.7	1.0	1.4	1.8	1.4
28	0.7	1.1	1.3	1.3	1.6	1.6
28	1.0	1.0	1.4	1.5	1.7	2.0
$\bar{X}$	0.9	0.9	1.2	1.3	1.8	1.8
Recovery, %	90	90	80	87	90	90

Effect of Hypoalbuminemia

A recent study (*17*) indicates that falsely low values for serum digoxin may be obtained in the case of patients whose serum albumin concentration is subnormal, perhaps because of an increased binding of radioactive label to the antibody. One of the claims made for kit B is that there is no interference with the assay attributable to variation in the protein concentration of the specimen, because of an undescribed additive in the reagents. No such claim has been made for Kit A.

To evaluate the effect of hypoalbuminemia on both kits, we added pure digoxin at concentrations of 1.0, 1.5, and 2.0 μg/liter to each of six different sera (albumin concentration 24–28 g/liter) in five separate experiments; i.e., a total of 30 different sera were tested. All sera were assayed in triplicate. Recovery of digoxin ranged from 67–105% with kit A, 70–110% with kit B (Table 4).

We also investigated the effect of abnormally high concentrations of hemoglobin, bilirubin, and lipids on kits A and B. There was no significant effect on the assay, in both cases, at the concentrations studied (Table 5).

Discussion

We find both kits satisfactory for routine digoxin determination. They are convenient to use, and an assay can be completed within 1.5 h.

Additionally, we found the standard curve obtained with kit A to be reproducible for as long as 3 h after the start of an assay. Late-arriving or emergency specimens can, therefore, be analyzed within this period without repeating a standard curve. This is economical in terms of reagents and technician time. We also observed with kit B that the reproducibility of the standard curve depended on the frequency and method of agitation during the 45-min incubation. A mechanically agitated water bath would provide the necessary uniformity. Kit B eliminates the need for a refrigerated centrifuge and reaction tubes; however, the cost per assay is about double that of kit A.

We demonstrated that, if serum albumin concentration was normal, recovery of the added digoxin ranged from 91–100% with kit A and 97–100% with kit B, slightly decreasing with increasing digoxin concentration. In contrast recovery was more variable and the range significantly lower in the case of hy-

Table 5. Effect of Hemolysis, Icterus, and Lipemia on Results Obtained with Kits A and B

Concn, mg/liter	Digoxin added, μg/liter	Digoxin recovered, μg/liter, Kit A	Digoxin recovered, μg/liter, Kit B	Recovery, %, Kit A	Recovery, %, Kit B
Hemoglobin[a]					
6000	1.50	1.52	1.48	101	99
4000	1.50	1.49	1.49	99	99
2000	1.50	1.47	1.47	98	98
Bilirubin[b]					
210	1.50	1.47	1.52	98	101
170	1.50	1.50	1.48	100	99
150	1.50	1.52	1.46	101	97
Triglycerides[b]					
25 000	1.50	1.46	1.52	97	101
17 500	1.50	1.47	1.50	98	100
10 000	1.50	1.49	1.49	99	99

[a] Pure hemoglobin added to three different sera.
[b] Three different sera.
All these sera had normal albumin concentrations.

poalbuminemic sera. Significantly, low albumin concentration did not always correspond to low recovery; it varied from serum to serum, indicating that there may be factors other than albumin concentration and digoxin concentration in serum that affect the results of digoxin RIA. Similar observations have recently been reported (*17, 18*). Previously, both lower and higher digoxin recoveries were reported for samples with subnormal albumin concentrations (*18, 19*).

With kits A and B, spurious lowering of the results for digoxin on this account may assume importance only in the borderline therapeutic range; a generally accepted therapeutic range is 0.9–1.9 μg/liter. The observed effects of albumin do not negate the general usefulness of these kits, but proper caution must be exercised in interpreting the analytical data if occasionally the assayed abnormal serum digoxin concentration does not parallel the clinical response of the patient with respect to electrocardiogram, serum electrolytes, and other serum analytes (*20, 21*). It may also be advisable for the laboratorian routinely to examine the recent medical records of the patients for their serum albumin concentration. Low serum albumin concentration is not uncommon in patients undergoing digoxin therapy, because many of these patients are elderly and may have impaired renal function (*2*). Thus far in our experience with these two kits we have not been informed by the physicians of any problems in patients arising from the foregoing discrepancies. This would indicate that it may not always be possible to correlate the in vitro adverse effects of low serum albumin concentration on the analytical recovery of digoxin to its in vivo effects.

We conclude that both kits are highly reproducible, analytically sensitive, precise, and show good correlation. Consequently, they are suitable for routine digoxin assay in a hospital laboratory. However, in our opinion, there is still a need for digoxin procedures that are not affected by low serum albumin concentrations. Recently, a digoxin kit marketed by Beckman Instruments, Inc., Fullerton, Calif. 92634 was evaluated by us in this regard. Preliminary studies confirmed the claim of the manufacturer that the results are not affected by low serum albumin concentrations (*22*). A detailed study is in progress.

References

1. Beller, G. A., Smith, T. W., Abelmann, W. H., et al., Digitalis intoxication: A prospective clinical study with serum level correlations. *New Engl. J. Med.* **284,** 989 (1971).
2. Binnion, P. F., Human plasma digoxin levels. *Ir. J. Med. Sci.* **143,** 30 (1974).
3. Smith, T. W., Butler, V. P., Jr., and Haber, E., Determination of therapeutic and toxic serum digoxin concentrations by radioimmunoassay. *New Engl. J. Med.* **281,** 1212 (1969).
4. Moe, G. K., and Farah, A. E., Digitalis and allied cardiac glycosides. *The Pharmacological Basis of Therapeutics,* L. S. Goodman, and A. S. Gilman, Eds., Macmillan, New York, N. Y., 1970, pp 667–708.
5. Jelliffe, R. W., and Blankenhorn, D. A., Gas chromatography of digitoxigenin and digoxigenin. *J. Chromatogr.* **121,** 268 (1962).
6. Hilton, J. G., A polarographic determination of digitoxin. *Science* **110,** 526 (1949).
7. Bentley, J. D., Burnett, G. H., Conklin, R. L., and Wasserburger, R. H., Clinical application of serum digitoxin levels: A simplified plasma determination. *Circulation* **41,** 67 (1970).
8. Berk, L. S., Lewis, J. L., and Nelson, J. C., One hour radioimmunoassay of serum drug concentrations as exemplified by digoxin and gentamicin. *Clin. Chem.* **20,** 1159 (1974).
9. Evered, D. C., Chapman, C., and Hayter, C. J., Measurement of plasma digoxin concentration by radioimmunoassay. *Br. Med. J.* **iii,** 427 (1970).
10. Rombauer, R. B., Frank, C., Doran, M. A., and Piasio, R., Porous glass bead solid phase digoxin radioimmunoassay—a unique approach. *Clin. Chem.* **20,** 870 (1974). Abstract.
11. Gutcho, S., McCarter, H., and Rapun, R., Radioimmunoassay of digoxin: An intercomparison of results with three methods. *Clin. Chem.* **19,** 1058 (1973).
12. Ahluwalia, G. S., and Kuczala, Z. J., Evaluation of an iodine-125 digoxin radioimmunoassay kit. *Clin. Chem.* **21,** 270 (1975). Letter to the Editor.
13. Ahluwalia, G. S., and Kuczala, Z. J., An evaluation of two iodine-125 digoxin radioimmunoassay kits. *Clin. Chem.* **21,** 966 (1975). Abstract.
14. Chamberlain, D. A., White, R. J., Howard, M. R., and Smith, T. W., Plasma digoxin concentrations in patients with atrial fibrillation. *Br. Med. J.* **iii,** 429 (1970).
15. Digoxin (Iodine-125) Radioimmunoassay Kit, Schwarz/Mann Co., Orangeburg, N. Y. 10962.
16. Digoxin Radioimmunoassay Iodine-125 Kit, Curtis Nuclear Corp., Los Angeles, Calif. 90058.
17. Holtzman, J. L., Shafer, R. B., and Erickson, R. R., Methodological causes of discrepancies in radioimmunoassay for digoxin in human serum. *Clin. Chem.* **20,** 1194 (1974).
18. Voshall, D. L., Hunter, L., and Grady, H. J., Effect of albumin on serum digoxin radioimmunoassays. *Clin. Chem.* **21,** 402 (1975).
19. Shaw, W., Radioimmunoassay of digoxin: Effect of albumin. *Clin. Chem.* **21,** 636 (1975). Letter to the Editor.
20. Smith, S. W., Drug therapy, digitalis glycosides. *New Engl. J. Med.* **288,** 719 (1973).
21. Smith, S. W., Drug therapy, digitalis glycosides. *New Engl. J. Med.* **288,** 942 (1973).
22. Ahluwalia, G. S., and Kuczala, Z. J., Effect of albumin on digoxin radioimmunoassay kits. Proceedings of the 16th Annual Meeting of the Southeastern Chapter, The Society of Nuclear Medicine, Atlanta, Ga., Oct. 23–25, 1975. Abstract.

CLIN. CHEM. 22/2, 198–204 (1976)

Double-antibody Enzyme Immunoassay Applied to Human α_1-Fetoprotein

Luc Belanger,[1,2] Diane Hamel,[1] Didier Dufour,[1] and Marcel Pouliot[3]

We report the development of a double-antibody system for enzyme immunoassay of human α_1-fetoprotein. Equilibrium and sequential saturation procedures were evaluated and compared with a similar double-antibody radioimmunoassay. With our method, 3 μg of α_1-fetoprotein per liter can be detected. The dose–response curve covers a 100-fold range of analyte concentrations. Within-run and between-run coefficients of variation are respectively 6.9% and 10.0%. Analytical recovery of added antigen is 99.5 ± 10.6%. Results are routinely obtained in 24 h but can be obtained in less than 8 h. α_1-Fetoprotein was measured in a variety of clinical samples, including sera from 488 pregnant women. The advantages of the present method over radioimmunoassay and other enzyme immunoassay procedures are discussed.

Additional Keyphrases: *radioimmunoassay compared • values for normal persons, and changes in liver disease, pregnancy • equilibrium vs. sequential saturation techniques • cord blood, amniotic fluid, serum*

Recent reports have demonstrated the potential of enzyme labeling of antigens and antibodies for immunoassay purposes (*1–12*). In this paper, we describe the development of a double-antibody method for enzyme immunoassay (E.I.A.) of human α_1-fetoprotein (AFP).[4] Equilibrium and sequential saturation procedures were evaluated and directly compared with a radioimmunoassay procedure performed under identical assay conditions. The sensitivity and reliability of the double-antibody enzyme assay, as well as its practicability and general applicability make this method strongly competitive with radioimmunoassay and with other E.I.A. procedures.

[1] Department of Biochemistry, Faculty of Medicine, Laval University, Quebec G1K 7P4, Canada.

[2] Present address: Department of Pathology, University of California at San Diego, Medical School, La Jolla, Calif. 92037.

[3] Department of Biochemistry, St-Sacrement Hospital, Quebec, Canada.

[4] Nonstandard abbreviations used: E.I.A., enzyme immunoassay; AFP, α_1-fetoprotein; PBS, phosphate-buffered saline; BSA, bovine serum albumin; DEAE, diethylaminoethyl.

Received July 21, 1975; accepted Nov. 12, 1975.

Principles of saturation analyses (*13, 14*) and practical considerations (*15*) are reviewed elsewhere. For a discussion of theoretical and practical aspects of separation techniques in saturation analysis, the reader is referred to Ratcliffe (*16*).

Materials and Methods

Materials

Pure AFP and rabbit anti-AFP serum (first antibody). AFP was purified from pooled cord blood serum by the precipitation method of Nishi (*17*), with use of sheep anti-AFP serum. Preparations were found to be homogeneous on polyacrylamide gel electrophoresis. At 2 mg/ml concentration [as measured by the method of Lowry et al. (*18*)], they yielded no reaction when tested by double diffusion and immunoelectrophoresis with rabbit anti-whole human serum. Enzyme-labeled preparations were not bound by rabbit anti-human albumin and rabbit anti-whole human serum (Figure 1). When used for rabbit immunization, all AFP preparations yielded antisera that revealed only AFP when reacted in immunoelectrophoresis and double diffusion against fetal, cord blood, or tyrosinemic (*19*) or hepatoma sera. Together, these data thus indicate that AFP preparations were free of any significant serum contaminant of human origin. However, it is worth mentioning here that some of the AFP preparations yielded antisera that revealed a weak IgG precipitin line when tested by immunoelectrophoresis with normal sheep serum (this line disappeared after absorption with normal sheep serum, 1 ml to 9 ml of antiserium); furthermore, when used for enzyme labeling, these AFP preparations were significantly bound by rabbit anti-sheep serum (Figure 1). These results show that small amounts of IgG antibodies may contaminate preparations of AFP purified by Nishi's method. As discussed below, such labeled IgG-contaminated AFP preparations can interfere when measuring AFP in rheumatoid factor positive sera.

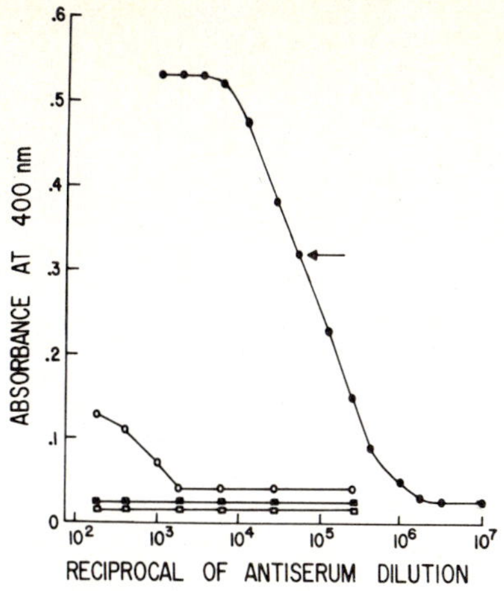

Fig. 1. Titration of rabbit antisera in the presence of optimal concentration of AFP/enzyme conjugate

● anti-human AFP; □ anti-human albumin; ■ anti-human total serum; O anti-sheep total serum. *Arrow* indicates antiserum dilution used for assay. Notice the significant binding with lower dilutions of anti-sheep serum; such a binding is not a constant feature of labeled ligand preparations; when present, it indicates contamination by enzyme-labeled anti-AFP IgG (see text under *Materials*)

Enzyme-labeled AFP. Pure AFP was labeled with Sigma Type VII calf intestinal mucosa alkaline phosphatase (Sigma Chemical Co., St. Louis, Mo. 63178) by use of glutaraldehyde as described by Avrameas (*20*). The specific activity of enzyme stocks we used was 990 U/mg. The labeling procedure can be summarized as follows. Three-tenths milliliter (1.5 mg) of alkaline phosphatase suspension is centrifuged in the cold at 1000 rpm for 10 min. The supernate is discarded and the pellet is dissolved in 0.5 ml of a 1 mg/ml solution of purified AFP. After overnight dialysis against phosphate buffered saline (PBS; 0.15 mol/liter NaCl, 0.05 mol/liter PO_4^{3-}, pH 7.2), the solution is adjusted to 0.75 ml with PBS and 15 μl of glutaraldehyde/PBS (1/5 by vol) is added to the mixture. After 6 h at room temperature, the solution is chromatographed on a Sephadex G-200 column equilibrated in PBS. The excluded peak, which contains the AFP/enzyme conjugate, is stabilized with bovine serum albumin (40 g/liter) and stored at 4 °C, with NaN_3 (200 mg/liter) as preservative. Conjugates can be kept at least 12 months with little loss of activity.

Anti-rabbit IgG (second antibody). Normal rabbit serum IgG was isolated by a combination of ammonium sulfate precipitation and DEAE-cellulose chromatography (*21*). Antisera to rabbit IgG were prepared in sheep.

AFP standards. Standards were prepared in a 10 g/liter solution of bovine serum albumin in PBS (PO_4^{3-}, 0.1 mol/liter; NaCl, 0.15 mol/liter; pH 7.4; NaN_3, 100 mg/liter) either from stocks of pure antigen quantitated by the method of Lowry et al. (*18*) or by serial dilution of a pool of cord blood serum whose AFP content was previously determined (by electroimmunodiffusion) by reference to the World Health Organization standard (kindly supplied by Dr. Ph. Sizaret, International Agency for Research on Cancer, Lyon, France). The concentration of the WHO AFP standard (nominally 50 mg/liter) was found to be 45 mg/liter when referred to our own standard of purified material.

Enzyme substrate and substrate buffer. We used Sigma No 104-105 *p*-nitrophenylphosphate tablets as substrate and sodium carbonate buffer (50 mmol/liter, pH 9.8) containing 1 mmol of $MgCl_2$ per liter as substrate buffer.

"First-antibody solution" and "no-antibody control solution." The first-antibody solution consisted of rabbit anti-AFP serum diluted to a working concentration with barbital buffer (50 mmol/liter, pH 8.6; Fisher Electrophoretic Buffer No 1) containing, per liter, 10 g of BSA, 100 ml of normal goat serum, 8 ml of normal rabbit serum, 0.15 mol of NaCl, and 100 mg of NaN_3. The normal goat and rabbit sera were previously decomplemented by heating at 56 °C for 30 min.

The no-antibody control solution had the same composition but was free of rabbit anti-AFP serum.

There was no advantage to either replacing bovine serum albumin by ovalbumin or by hen serum or to adding a detergent such as "Tween 20" to the solutions.

Assay

The principle of the assay is the same as for the double-antibody radioimmunoassay procedure. Labeled (AFP/enzyme conjugate) and unlabeled (AFP of sample) ligands are incubated with the rabbit anti-AFP serum (first antibody) and the antibody/AFP/enzyme complexes are subsequently precipitated with the sheep anti-rabbit IgG serum (second antibody), with normal rabbit serum as a carrier. The enzyme activity recovered in the precipitate is inversely related to the amount of AFP in sample.

The determination of optimal concentration of labeled ligand and first antibody, the effect of temperature conditions on association and dissociation reactions of labeled AFP with first antibody, the critical steps of the technique, and the performances of different assay procedures will be discussed in the next sections. Routinely, we use a 24-h sequential saturation procedure, performed at room temperature, which can be summarized as follows:

Preparation of samples. Inactivate test and control samples by incubation at 56 °C for 30 min; if required, proceed then to make appropriate dilutions with phosphate-buffered saline (PO_4^{3-}, 0.1 mol/liter; NaCl, 0.15 mol/liter; pH 7.4) containing, per liter, 10 g of bovine serum albumin and 100 mg of NaN_3 (hereafter referred to as BSA–PBS).

First incubation. Distribute 0.8 ml of first antibody solution into a series of 12 × 75 mm glass tubes; add 0.1 ml of BSA–PBS to tubes 1–2 (the zero-dose control) and 0.1 ml of standard, test, and control samples (each in duplicate) to the succeeding tubes. Into two additional tubes, pipet 0.8 ml of no-antibody control solution and 0.1 ml of BSA–PBS. Vortex-mix all tubes and allow to stand for 4 h at room temperature.

Second incubation. Add to all tubes 0.1 ml of labeled antigen diluted to optimal concentration with BSA–PBS. Vortex-mix and allow to stand overnight at room temperature.

Precipitation. Add to all tubes 0.1 ml of second antibody, heat-inactivated and properly diluted in BSA–PBS for optimal precipitation. Vortex-mix and allow to stand for 3 h at room temperature.

Washing. Centrifuge all tubes (22 °C, 10 min, 3000 rpm). Aspirate supernates as completely as possible, being careful not to disturb the pellets. Add 2 ml of the pH 7.4 PBS, vortex-mix, centrifuge as before, and aspirate the supernates. Repeat this operation one time.

Substrate incubation. Transfer the tubes into an ice-water bath. Dissolve *p*-nitrophenylphosphate tablets in substrate buffer (final concentration, 1 mg/ml), add 1 ml of the substrate solution to the tubes and vortex-mix for 2–3 s at high speed. Transfer the rack from the ice-water bath to a 37 °C water bath and incubate for 30 min; shake the rack occasionally during this incubation period. Then transfer the rack back to the ice-water bath and after 5 min stop the reaction by adding 0.2 ml of 1 mol/liter NaOH. Vortex-mix the contents of the tubes and transfer them to room temperature.

Analytical curve, calculation of results. Read the absorbance at 400 nm, using the no-antibody control tubes (the nonspecific background) as blank for zero calibration of the spectrophotometer. From values obtained with standards, construct an analytical curve by plotting either the absorbance (A) or the percentage of maximum binding [$(A/A_0) \times 100$, A_0 being the absorbance recorded in zero-dose control tubes] as a function of the AFP content. The AFP concentration in unknown and control samples is determined from their absorbance or percent maximum binding values by reference to the standard curve.

Speeded procedure. Under the above conditions of assay, results are obtained in 24 h. If AFP measurement is urgent, preliminary results can be obtained in less than 8 h by running the assay at 37 °C: samples are incubated (water bath) with first antibody for 1 h; the label is added and incubated for an additional 3 h; this is followed by an additional 1-h incubation with second antibody; the precipitates are then processed as described above.

Results and Discussion

Optimization of the System

Temperature conditions. The association and dissociation reaction of labeled AFP with first antibody was studied at 4 °C and at 22 °C (room temperature). The results are shown in Figure 2. As expected, association and dissociation reactions are both more rapid at higher temperature. The maximum binding is reached in 16 h at 4 °C and in approximately 8 h at 22 °C, while the dissociation of the AFP/enzyme/

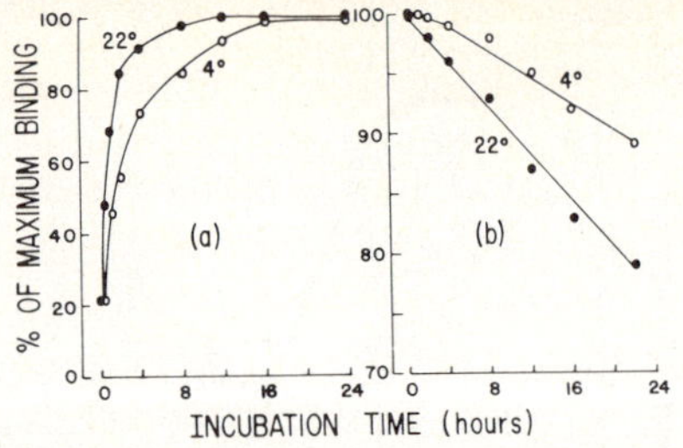

Fig. 2. Association (*a*) and dissociation (*b*) reaction of enzyme-labeled AFP and first antibody at 4 °C and 22 °C (room temperature)

The association rate was determined by measuring the enzyme activity recovered in double-antibody precipitates after incubation periods indicated. Dissociation was evaluated by first allowing the complete formation of the AFP/enzyme/antibody complex at 4 °C; this was followed by the addition of 2000 ng of free AFP and measurement of enzyme activity in the precipitates after incubation periods (at 4 °C or 22 °C) indicated; under these conditions, the chance that enzyme-labeled AFP (10 ng/tube), after having dissociated from its complex with antibody, would again become bound was 1:200 (or less, if we presume that antigenic sites are buried by the coupling with enzyme)

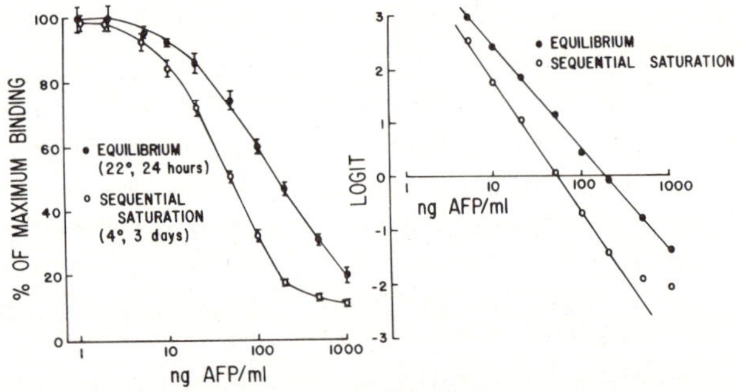

Fig. 3. Dose–response curves obtained by equilibrium and sequential saturation procedures, expressed as percentage of maximum binding or linearized through logit transformation

For equilibrium assay, labeled and unlabeled ligands were mixed first and then incubated with first antibody (overnight at room temperature). For sequential assay, the unlabeled ligand was incubated with first antibody for 24 h; the label was then added and incubated for an additional 24 h; this was followed by an overnight incubation with the second antibody (all incubations at 4 °C). The *bars* represent 2 SD of quadruplicate calibration points

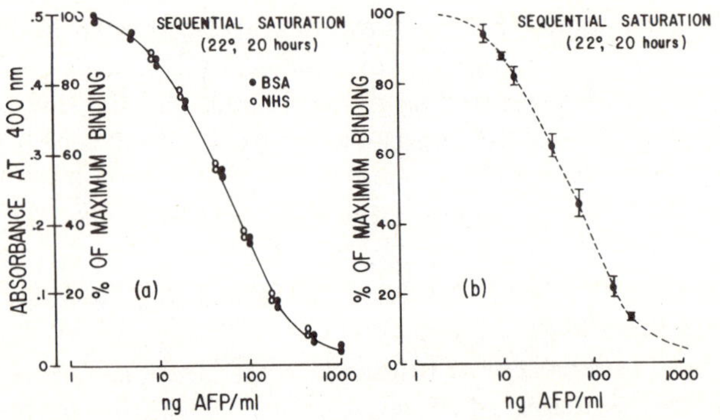

Fig. 4. (*a*) Analytical recovery of AFP after addition of purified antigen to a pool of normal human serum (*NHS*) and to phosphate-buffered saline containing 10 g of BSA per liter (AFP standards)

AFP concentration in native NHS was measured as less than 3 μg/liter. Assay performed as described under *Assay*

(*b*) Reproducibility of five separate AFP determinations on seven different serum samples. Results are $\bar{x} \pm 2$ SD of each value reported on the mean standard curve (*dashed line*) antibody complex after 16 h is about 10% higher at 22 °C than at 4 °C. Because this slightly increased dissociation rate affects neither the sensitivity nor the precision of the system (see Figures 3 and 4), the assay can be conveniently performed at room temperature.

Concentration of labeled ligand and first antibody. On the basis of suitable enzyme measurement, the optimal concentration of labeled AFP has been experimentally determined as being 10 ng of enzyme-tagged antigen per assay tube (assuming that all the initial 500 μg of AFP used for coupling is present in the complexes). Blocking of antigenic sites by enzyme conjugation is probably partly responsible for the high absolute amount of labeled AFP needed in the assay.

The appropriate dilution of rabbit anti-AFP serum is the one that binds 60% of the precipitable label (Figure 1). The antiserum producing the sharpest antibody titration slope provides the most sensitive assay.

Precipitation with second antibody. The amount of carrier is kept small, to minimize nonspecific coprecipitation of labeled antigen (it is probable that the high stability of the tracer further reduces the possibility of separation artefacts). Under our conditions (final concentration of carrier, 0.6%), the no-antibody control background is consistently less than 5% of maximum binding, whether standard, amniotic fluid, or serum is being tested; this eliminates the need for individual blanks.

Decomplementation improves the second-antibody reaction. There is no advantage in prolonging the precipitation step beyond 3 h at room temperature; incubation at 37 °C enhances the reaction but precision is significantly decreased. Compared to standard or amniotic fluid samples, decomplemented serum neither impairs or enhances the precipitation reaction.

Substrate incubation. This is obviously a critical analytical step for all enzyme immunoassay. For optimal performance of the assay, two conditions must be fulfilled. First, incubation time must be selected in such a way that the reaction will proceed with zero-order kinetics in all tubes: under our conditions (37 °C), the absorbance in zero-dose control tubes (maximum binding) increases linearly for 45 min. Secondly, rigorous uniformity (from tube to tube) of temperature conditions and incubation time must be achieved. The successive incubations in water baths at 0 °C (minimal enzyme activity) and 37 °C are admittedly somewhat tedious, but only in this way can maximal precision and accuracy be expected.

Dose–Response Curve: Equilibrium vs. Sequential Saturation Procedures

Figure 3 compares dose–response curves obtained by equilibrium vs. sequential saturation procedures. As could be anticipated from the low dissociation rate of the label and first antibody (Figure 2), the sequential procedure yields an appreciable gain of sensitivity and a shift of the curve toward lower AFP concentrations, whether the assay is performed at 4 °C or at 22 °C (Figure 4). Precision is also generally better in sequential assays, presumably owing to the less-stringent precision required for addition of the label (*cf. 14*).

The logit transformation of equilibrium data yields a linear curve over all concentrations of free AFP while, as also expected (*14*), the sequential saturation data do not fit a straight line at large extremes of unlabeled ligand (Figure 3). When many (eight) standards were used in the assay, we found no significant advantage in using the logit transformation, even in the case of an equilibrium technique.

The sensitivity limit of the 24-h sequential assay, as described under *Assay,* is about 3 μg/liter;[5] the standard dose–response curve adequately covers a two-log range of AFP concentrations. The 8-h, 37 °C sequential assay has a sensitivity threshold of 20 μg/liter; the poor precision of this fast assay precludes its use for routine purposes. However, the use of polyethylene glycol has recently permitted the development of a 5-h sequential procedure that performs favorably as compared to the 24-h assay (R. Daigneault et al., in preparation).

The 3 μg/liter sensitivity limit of the present E.I.A. method compares favorably with that of most radioimmunoassay techniques for measuring human or rat α_1-fetoprotein. Some E.I.A. (*10*) and radioimmunoassay (*22, 23*) procedures achieve a lower detection limit (down to 0.1 μg/liter), but they gain nothing in clinical usefulness and may suffer practical inconveniences such as a limited, low-range analytical curve or prolonged incubation periods.

Reliability

Specificity and accuracy. Specificity and accuracy of the assay were evaluated first by comparing with current published data the results we obtained by E.I.A. in a variety of clinical conditions. We measured AFP in 34 sera from apparently healthy adults. All values were less than 10 μg/liter except two, 11 and 18 μg/liter. None of 75 patients with various extrahepatic malignant or nonmalignant diseases had AFP values exceeding 20 μg/liter. By contrast, higher AFP concentrations were found in eight of eight patients with hereditary tyrosinemia (*19*) and in four of 68 patients with other liver diseases: two of them (100 and 120 μg/liter) had viral hepatitis, one (95 000 μg/liter) had a primary liver cancer and one (1700 μg/liter) was in the acute phase of alcoholic hepatitis complicated by hepatic coma. Data recorded from 488 pregnant women sera showed that the maximal highest mean value for AFP is reached by approximately 32 weeks of gestation; the highest single value measured was 690 μg/liter (see Figure 5). In 62 am-

[5] μg/liter is the SI unit, although ng/ml is the unit now commonly used (as here, in the Figures) in these measurements.—*Ed.*

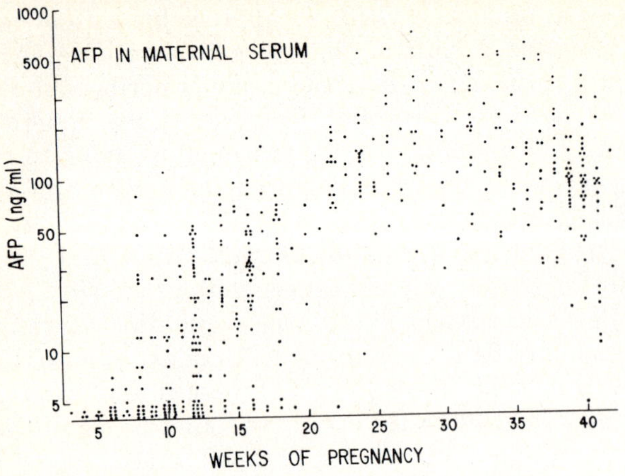

Fig. 5. Distribution of AFP concentrations as determined in sera of 488 pregnant women

"Weeks of pregnancy" are weeks after last menstrual period

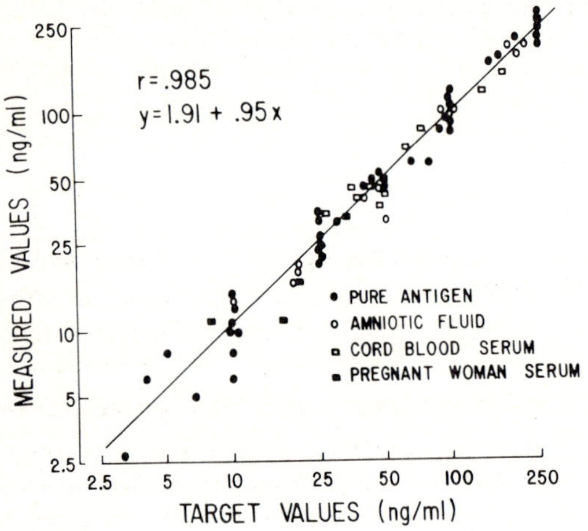

Fig. 6. Analytical recovery of AFP added to 68 different normal serum samples

niotic fluid specimens, AFP values ranged from 280 to 4500 μg/liter between 24 and 30 weeks of pregnancy and from 40 to 1100 μg/liter between 34 and 40 weeks. All these results are in excellent agreement with those obtained by many others (e.g., *25–29*).

Accuracy and specificity of the method were further evaluated by analytical recovery experiments in which either pure antigen, cord blood serum, pregnancy serum, or amniotic fluid was added to various normal and abnormal specimens of serum. As shown in Figure 4*a*, normal serum has no significant effect on the inhibition binding curve. For 68 different normal serum specimens, in the range 5–250 μg/liter (Figure 6), the mean recovery of added AFP (mean % ζ or % ζ) was 99.5% and the coefficient of variation was 10.6% {$\% \zeta = \Sigma\ [(x/\zeta) \times 100] \div n$, where ζ is the true AFP value, x the measured value, and n the number of specimens; the coefficient of variation was calculated as $\sqrt{\Sigma\ (x - \% \zeta)^2 \div (n - 1)}$, by taking x as the individual value in % of true value}. Hemolysis, lipids, bilirubin, and endogenous alkaline phosphatase did not alter the accuracy of the assay, but sera positive for rheumatoid factor had a significantly lowered AFP recovery when sheep IgG-contaminated AFP/enzyme preparations were used as tracer (that is, higher absorbance readings, presumably owing to precipitation of IgG/enzyme complex; see above under *Materials*). Absorption of such sera with normal sheep serum eliminated the interferences, as did the use of more nearly pure AFP/enzyme conjugates (absorption of the label with anti-sheep IgG would probably also eliminate interferences).

Specificity and accuracy of the method were finally assessed by comparing values obtained by enzyme immunoassay and by two types of radioimmunoassay [a double-antibody procedure (Wepsic et al., to be published), and a sodium sulfate procedure (Sell et al.) analogous to the one described in (*30*)]. As shown in Figure 7, E.I.A. and radioimmunoassay results are in excellent agreement, the coefficient of correlation for 42 samples in the range 5–300 μg/liter being 0.99.

Precision. The within-run repeatability was estimated by making two AFP determinations on 25 different amniotic fluid and serum specimens: the duplicate determinations were included in several runs, each pair of duplicates being assayed as nonadjacent samples within a single batch. The coefficient of variation was calculated as $\sqrt{(\Sigma\ d^2)/2n}$, d being the difference in percent between duplicates and n the number of determinations; for the range 10–200 μg/liter, it was 6.9%.

Between-run reproducibility was estimated by running 15 samples on five different days and recording the results each time from a different analytical curve. The coefficient of variation was calculated as $\sqrt{[\Sigma\ (x - \bar{x})2]/(n - 1)}$, by taking $\bar{x}$ (the mean value found for each sample) as 100% and n as number of determinations; it was 10.0% for the range 10–200 μg/liter (see also Figure 4*b*).

Precision and accuracy of the present enzyme assay are thus fully comparable to that achieved by other E.I.A. (*cf. 10*) or radioimmunoassay (*cf. 23, 24*) procedures.

Quality control. The internal control of quality is effected by including in each run a low (10 or 20 μg/liter) and a high (100 or 200 μg/liter) reference sample. The data are used to plot the 2 SD and 3 SD variability limits and to check for drift in between-run precision. When a large assay is set up, within-run drift is monitored by placing standard samples at regular intervals (one out of every 8–10 samples). A control of accuracy is also effected among the few clinical laboratories that are now routinely using the method by submitting to them five to 10 blind known samples each month.

Enzymatic Labeling vs. Isotopic Labeling

To directly compare the performances of the E.I.A. and radioimmunoassay procedures, we labeled pure AFP with ^{125}I by the Chloramine T method (*31*) and developed a double-antibody radioimmunoassay.

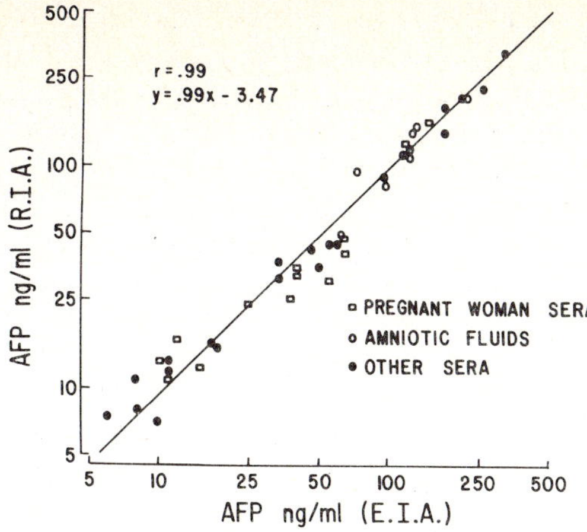

Fig. 7. Comparison between AFP values obtained by E.I.A. and radioimmunoassay

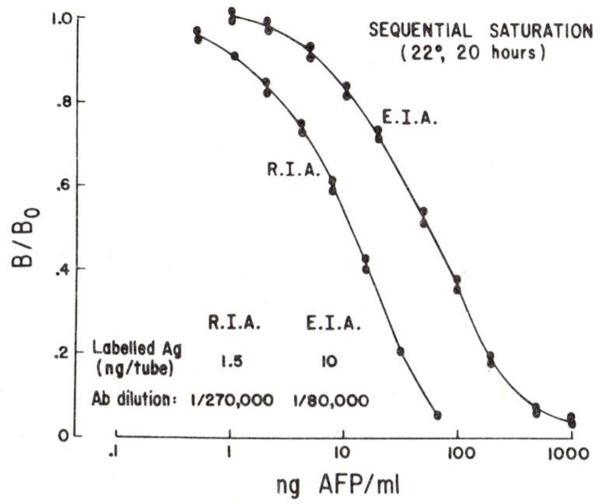

Fig. 8. Comparison of dose–response curves obtained by radioimmunoassay and E.I.A.
Both assays set up under optimal conditions and run as described under *Assay*. B/B_0, percentage bound

(The latter will be published by A. Kirkpatrick et al.) When both procedures were set up under optimal conditions, making use of the same reagents (except for the label) and performed under identical assay conditions, double-antibody radioimmunoassay and E.I.A. differed essentially from each other by the amount of label (1.5 ng per tube for the former vs. 10 ng per tube for E.I.A.) and first antibody (3.5 times less for the radioimmunoassay) used in the assay. These lower concentrations of binder and tracer shifted the radioimmunoassay dose–response curve to the left and resulted in an important (five-fold) gain of sensitivity (Figure 8). These data thus indicate that, under present conditions of assay, the intrinsic capacity of radioimmunoassay is superior to that of E.I.A. However, the use of a label with higher specific enzyme activity will probably improve E.I.A. sensitivity. Furthermore, it is conceivable that the use of fluorometric techniques for detection of enzyme activity would considerably reduce the amount of label needed thus eventually permitting E.I.A. to surpass radioimmunoassay performances.

Table 1. Advantages of Present Double Antibody E.I.A. over Radioimmunoassay (*a*) and Other E.I.A. Procedures (*b*)

a.
1. Eliminates the use of potentially hazardous radioisotopes and the need for expensive counting equipment.
2. Labeling compound inexpensive; required equipment (centrifuge and spectrophotometer) readily available in all clinical chemistry laboratory.
3. Labeled ligand stable for months, possibly for years.
4. Increased potential for multiple simultaneous assays.

b.
1. Simple and practical; provides maximal uniformity and reproducibility of assay conditions.
2. Separation procedure well standardized, easily generalizable.
3. Alkaline phosphatase easily measured; label recovered in the precipitate, thereby eliminating many potential nonspecific interferences.
4. Results obtainable within a few hours.
5. High potential for automation.

Automation

As for any clinical chemical laboratory technique, the enzyme assay procedure has been considerably simplified by use of repeating pipets and sample dilutors (a further improvement would be to use preparation units, such as the Micromedic, to dispense samples and reagents). A further step was to use automated devices for absorbance readings and data listing (we have been currently using the Gilford MicroSample Spectrophotometer 300 N, equipped with data lister). More recently, a computer-based mathematical analysis of the dose–response curve has permitted one to integrate absorbance readings, calculation of the results, and data output (R. Daigneault et al.), thus shortening this manually tedious and time-consuming step to minutes. Development of a fully automated discontinuous system would encounter practical difficulties but, with modifications of the present procedure, is not beyond the realm of technical feasibility.

Conclusion

Optimization of E.I.A. methodology for application in routine clinical laboratory is of great interest. The high stability of the labeled ligand, the elimination of radioisotopes, and the need for only minimal equipment are all unequivocal advantages which should have preference for E.I.A. over radioimmunoassay in selecting a competitive binding assay. In addition, many laboratories now perform hundreds or thousands of assays each day and enzyme assays could greatly add to the efficiency and economy required by modern research and clinical laboratories.

During the past four years, a few types of enzyme immunoassay have been developed. Some of the published methods are based on the solid phase (antibody coated polystyrene tubes) enzyme assay introduced by Engvall and Perlmann (*2*) for the measurement of immunoglobulin G. We have reported a similar immunosorbent assay for rat α_1-fetoprotein (*6*); however, attempts to adapt this solid-phase procedure to human AFP yielded unsatisfactory results. Other enzyme methods, such as those making use of glucose oxidase as labeling agent, may suffer practical problems related to enzyme measurement (*10*). Some solid-phase systems yield other problems: for example, in a "sandwich" immunosorbent E.I.A. recently developed for human and rat AFP by R. Maiolini and R. Masseyeff, rheumatoid factor produces interferences that, if not corrected by previous absorption with aggregated IgG, lead to falsely positive results (personal communication with the authors; to be published).

Table 1 lists the main advantages of present double antibody enzyme assay over radioimmunoassay or other E.I.A. procedures. Because sensitivity and reliability of the method compare satisfactorily to that achieved with other systems, we consider that this type of assay deserves wide acceptance in the routine clinical laboratory.

We gratefully acknowledge the collaboration of Drs. S. Sell and T. Wepsic (Department of Pathology, UCSD Medical School, La Jolla, and Department of Pathology, VA Hospital, La Jolla) and the assistance of D. Stillman and A. Kirkpatrick in comparing the reported method with radioimmunoassay.

Supported by grants from the Medical Research Council of Canada.

Part of this work was conducted in Dr. Stewart Sell's laboratory (Department of Pathology, UCSD Medical School, La Jolla) while L.B. was supported by a postdoctoral fellowship from the Medical Research Council of Canada.

References

1. Van Weemen, B. K., and Schuurs, A. H. W. M., Immunoassay using antigen-enzyme conjugates. *FEBS Lett.* **15**, 232 (1971).

2. Engvall E., and Perlmann, P., Enzyme-linked immunosorbent assay (ELISA). Quantitative assay of immunoglobulin G. *Immunochemistry* **8**, 871 (1971).

3. Avrameas, S., and Guilbert, B., Enzyme-immunoassay for the measurement of antigens using peroxidase conjugates. *Biochimie* **54**, 837 (1972).

4. Rubenstein, K. E., Schneider, R. S., and Ullman, E. F., "Homogeneous" enzyme immunoassay. A new immunochemical technique. *Biochem. Biophys. Res. Commun.* **47**, 846 (1972).

5. Masseyeff, R., Maiolini, R., and Bouron, Y., A method of enzyme immunoassay. *Biomedicine* **19**, 314 (1973).

6. Belanger, L., Sylvestre, C., and Dufour, D., Enzyme-linked immunoassay for alpha-fetoprotein by competitive and sandwich procedures. *Clin. Chim. Acta* **48**, 15 (1973).

7. Van Weemen, B. K., and Schuurs, A. H. W. M., Immunoassay using antibody-enzyme conjugates. *FEBS Lett.* **47**, 215 (1974).

8. Stimson, W. H., and Sinclair, J. M., An immunoassay for a pregnancy-associated α-macroglobulin using antibody-enzyme conjugates. *FEBS Lett.* **47**, 190 (1974).

9. Pesce, A. J., Mendoza, N., Boreisha, I., et al., Use of enzyme-linked antibodies to measure serum anti-DNA antibody in systemic lupus erythematosus. *Clin. Chem.* **20**, 353 (1974).

10. Maiolini, R., Ferrua, B., and Masseyeff, R., Enzymoimmunoassay of human alpha-fetoprotein. *J. Immunol. Methods* **6**, 355 (1975).

11. Alpert, E., Coston, R., and Perroto, J., Immunoenzymatic assay for alpha-fetoprotein. *Lancet* **i**, 626 (1974).

12. Sparacio, R., Hevey, R. C., and Bonacker, L. H., An enzyme-immunoassay for the determination of human alpha-fetoprotein. *Fed. Proc.* **34**, 1024 (1975).

13. Zettner, A., Principles of competitive binding assays (saturation analyses). I. Equilibrium techniques. *Clin. Chem.* **19**, 699 (1973).

14. Zettner, A., and Duly, P. E., Principles of competitive binding assays (saturation analyses). II. Sequential saturation. *Clin. Chem.* **20**, 5 (1974).

15. Skelley, D. S., Brown, L. P., and Besch, P. K., Radioimmunoassay. *Clin. Chem.* **19**, 146 (1973).

16. Ratcliffe, J. G., Separation techniques in saturation analysis. *Br. Med. Bull.* **30**, 32 (1974).

17. Nishi, S., Isolation and characterization of a human fetal α-globulin from the sera of fetuses and a hepatoma patient. *Cancer Res.* **30**, 2507 (1970).

18. Lowry, O. H., Rosebrough, N. J., Farr, A. L., and Randall, R. J., Protein measurement with the Folin phenol reagent. *J. Biol. Chem.* **193**, 265 (1951).

19. Belanger, L., Belanger, M., Prive, L., et al., Alpha-1-fetoprotein in hereditary tyrosinemia. I. Clinical usefulness of alpha-fetoprotein in tyrosinemia. *Pathol.-Biol.* **21**, 449 (1973).

20. Avrameas, S., Coupling of enzymes to proteins with glutaraldehyde. Use of the conjugates for the detection of antigens and antibodies. *Immunochemistry,* **6**, 43 (1969).

21. *Methods in Immunology and Immunochemistry,* **1**, C. A. Williams and M. W. Chase, Eds., Academic Press, New York, N. Y., 1967, p 307.

22. Masseyeff, R., Bonet, C., Drouet, J., et al., Radioimmunoassay of α-fetoprotein. I. Technique and serum levels in the normal adult. *Digestion* **10**, 17 (1974).

23. Chayvialle, J.A.P., and Ganguli, P. C., Radioimmunoassay of alpha-fetoprotein in human plasma. *Lancet* **i**, 1355 (1973).

24. McIntire, K. R., Waldmann, T. A., Moertel, C. G., and Go, V. L. W., Serum α-fetoprotein in patients with neoplasms of the gastrointestinal tract. *Cancer Res.* **35**, 991 (1975).

25. Ruoslahti, E., and Seppala, M., Normal and increases alpha-fetoprotein in neoplastic and non neoplastic liver disease. *Lancet* **ii**, 278 (1972).

26. Delmont, J., Kermarac, J., Lafon, J., et al., Radioimmunoassay of α-fetoprotein. II. Studies in patients suffering from hepatic diseases. *Digestion* **10**, 29 (1974).

27. Garoff, L., and Seppala, M., Alpha-fetoprotein and human placental lactogen levels in maternal serum in multiple pregnancies. *J. Obstet. Gynaecol. Br. Commonw.* **80**, 695 (1973).

28. Purves, L. R., and Purves, M., Serum alpha-fetoprotein. VI. The radioimmunoassay evidence for the presence of AFP in the serum of normal people and during pregnancy. *S. Afr. Med. J.* **46**, 1290 (1972).

29. Hirai, H., Nishi, S., and Watabe, H., Radioimmunoassay of alpha-fetoprotein. *Protides Biol. Fluids* **20**, 579 (1973).

30. Sell, S., and Gord, D., Rat α-fetoprotein. III. Refinement of radioimmunoassay for detection of 1 ng rat α_1F. *Immunochemistry* **10**, 439 (1973).

31. Hunter, W. M., and Greenwood, F. C., Preparation of iodine-131-labeled human growth hormone of high specific activity. *Nature* **194**, 495 (1962).

Evaluation of a Dipstick Test for Glucose in Urine

Jørn Dyerberg,[1] Lissi Pedersen,[2] and Ole Aagaard[2]

As an example of qualitative tests, a dipstick analysis for glucose in urine has been tested for the influence of modifying factors on the test result. Two different types of dipsticks were examined, "Clinistix" and "S-Glukotest." Used according to manufacturer's instructions, the latter is more sensitive and selective. By multivariance analysis the following variables were examined: urine samples, inter- and intra-analyst, exposure to light, and dipstick batch. The first three contributed significantly to the total variation in results, inter-specimen variation being the most important. With knowledge of the frequency of testing urines with a given glucose concentration and the probability of the result at that concentration, an expression of the probability of the glucose content of a urine sample can be obtained. Even with the tests of the type examined having a sensitivity and specificity exceeding 95%, 14 of 100 patients suspected of having diabetes mellitus on the basis of a dipstick examination will be found to have a urinary glucose concentration of <2 mmol/liter. These figures were found when the prevalence of urines with a glucose concentration exceeding 2 mmol/liter was 17.5%.

Additional Keyphrases: *analysis of variance* • *screening*

Tests that give either a positive or a negative result, the so-called qualitative tests, make up a quite considerable part of the diagnostic process. Such tests are used extensively in the clinical chemical field, and as the binary result decides whether the patient will be further examined and possibly treated, it is necessary to know the efficiency and level of discrimination of the basic analyses, as well as what effect modifying factors will have on the test results. Furthermore, these analyses must be controlled, just as quantitative analyses are.

Qualitative tests performed with "dipsticks" are widely used because of their simplicity. However, in our opinion these tests are often performed without sufficient knowledge of the possibilities of misinterpretation and without the necessary measures being taken against modifying factors. We have tried here to illustrate (*a*) which modifying factors may influence results of such tests, and (*b*) what precautions must be taken.

[1] Clinical Chemical Department, Aalborg Hospital North, Box 561, 9100 Aalborg, Denmark.

[2] Clinical Chemical Department, Aalborg Hospital South, Box 365, 9100 Aalborg, Denmark.

Received Sept. 3, 1975; accepted Nov. 12, 1975.

As an example of these tests we have chosen the test for glucose in urine, because this test is one of the most frequently performed. Also, glucose is a well-defined substance that can be quantitated specifically.

Material

We used dipsticks from Ames Co., Miles Lab. Ltd., England ("Clinistix") and from Boehringer Mannheim Corp., Waldhof, Germany ("S-Glukotest"); both were kindly supplied by the manufacturers.

Experimental Design and Results

Factors Affecting Color Change

For both dipsticks, interpretations are based on a change in color to be observed at a fixed time after immersing the dipsticks in urine. Clinistix gives a positive reading when the color changes from red to blue after 10 s. S-Glukotest changes from yellow to green after 30 s. The sensitivity is given as 5–6 mmol/liter for Clinistix and as 2–3 mmol/liter for S-Glukotest. This accounts for the initial color change of the dipstick. Although the manufacturers say it is possible to semiquantify a positive result by the intensity of the color obtained, we used only the results from the initial color change.

The purpose of this part of the study was to establish the effect of modifying factors on the total variation of the color change: variation among samples (*urine factor*), interperson variation (*laboratory technician factor*), intra-person variation (*time factor*), among batches (*batch factor*), and finally, variation of light (*environmental factor*).

The effect of the above factors on color change has been examined by multivariance analysis, in which the interaction terms are presumed to be negligible and where the factors have been picked at random—following a so-called extended Greek Roman square (*1*). Each factor is present in the square at 13 levels. The test plan is illustrated in detail in Figure 1. By such analysis it is possible to decide the relative contribution of a particular factor to the total variation of the system. Any combination of two factors will be encountered only once, and the effect of a particular factor can be compared at different levels because all the other factors make the same contribution at a given level, thus neutralizing each other.

LAB.TECH.

URINE		1	2	3	4	5	6	7	8	9	10	11	12	13
1	T	1	13	12	11	10	9	8	7	6	5	4	3	2
	B	1	13	12	11	10	9	8	7	6	5	4	3	2
	E	1	12	10	8	6	4	2	13	11	9	7	5	3
2	T	2	1	13	12	11	10	9	8	7	6	5	4	3
	B	3	2	1	13	12	11	10	9	8	7	6	5	4
	E	4	2	13	11	9	7	5	3	1	12	10	8	6
3	T	3	2	1	13	12	11	10	9	8	7	6	5	4
	B	5	4	3	2	1	13	12	11	10	9	8	7	6
	E	7	5	3	1	12	10	8	6	4	2	13	11	9
4	T	4	3	2	1	13	12	11	10	9	8	7	6	5
	B	7	6	5	4	3	2	1	13	12	11	10	9	8
	E	10	8	6	4	2	13	11	9	7	5	3	1	12
5	T	5	4	3	2	1	13	12	11	10	9	8	7	6
	B	9	8	7	6	5	4	3	2	1	13	12	11	10
	E	13	11	9	7	5	3	1	12	10	8	6	4	2
6	T	6	5	4	3	2	1	13	12	11	10	9	8	7
	B	11	10	9	8	7	6	5	4	3	2	1	13	12
	E	3	1	12	10	8	6	4	2	13	11	9	7	5
7	T	7	6	5	4	3	2	1	13	12	11	10	9	8
	B	13	12	11	10	9	8	7	6	5	4	3	2	1
	E	6	4	2	13	11	9	7	5	3	1	12	10	8
8	T	8	7	6	5	4	3	2	1	13	12	11	10	9
	B	2	1	13	12	11	10	9	8	7	6	5	4	3
	E	9	7	5	3	1	12	10	8	6	4	2	13	11
9	T	9	8	7	6	5	4	3	2	1	13	12	11	10
	B	4	3	2	1	13	12	11	10	9	8	7	6	5
	E	12	10	8	6	4	2	13	11	9	7	5	3	1
10	T	10	9	8	7	6	5	4	3	2	1	13	12	11
	B	6	5	4	3	2	1	13	12	11	10	9	8	7
	E	2	13	11	9	7	5	3	1	12	10	8	6	4
11	T	11	10	9	8	7	6	5	4	3	2	1	13	12
	B	8	7	6	5	4	3	2	1	13	12	11	10	9
	E	5	3	1	12	10	8	6	4	2	13	11	9	7
12	T	12	11	10	9	8	7	6	5	4	3	2	1	13
	B	10	9	8	7	6	5	4	3	2	1	13	12	11
	E	8	6	4	2	13	11	9	7	5	3	1	12	10
13	T	13	12	11	10	9	8	7	6	5	4	3	2	1
	B	12	11	10	9	8	7	6	5	4	3	2	1	13
	E	11	9	7	5	3	1	12	10	8	6	4	2	13

Fig. 1. Test plan for analysis of the influence of modifying factors on color change

As an example, the diagram should be read as follows: The square in fourth row, column three, means that at time (T) No. 2 laboratory technician No. 3 has to read urine No. 4 with a dipstick from batch (B) No. 5 in environment (E) No. 6

											POINT OF CHANGE MMOL/L	TYPE OF CHANGE
U_A	-	-	-	+	+	+	+	+	+	+	2.5	"NORMAL"
U_B	-	-	+	-	+	+	+	+	+	+	2.5	"DOUBT"
U_C	-	+	-	-	-	+	+	+	+	+	4.5	"FALSE POS."
U_D	-	-	+	+	-	+	+	+	+	+	1.5	"FALSE NEG."
	0	1	2	3	4	5	6	7	8	9 MMOL/L		

Fig. 2. Matrix for interpretation of qualitative results into a point of change, indicating the type of change, i.e. "normal," "doubtful," "false-positive," and "false-negative." U_A, U_B, U_C, **and** U_D **indicate four different urines**

TABLE 1.

THE TEST RESULTS FROM THE TWO SQUARE EXPERIMENTS.
CLINISTIX: A, S-GLUKOTEST: B.

THE FIGURES INDICATE THE POINTS OF CHANGE (MMOL GLUCOSE PER L) READ ACCORDING TO FIG. 2.

LAB.TECH.

URINE		1	2	3	4	5	6	7	8	9	10	11	12	13
1	A	2.8	2.8	2.8	2.8	0.8	2.8	2.8	2.8	0.8	2.8	1.8	2.8	1.8
	B	1.8	0.8	0.8	0.8	0.8	0.8	0.8	0.8	0.8	0.8	0.8	1.8	0.8
2	A	2.0	6.0	3.0	4.0	2.0	4.0	4.0	4.0	3.0	5.0	3.0	5.0	2.0
	B	2.0	2.0	2.0	2.0	1.0	1.0	3.0	2.0	2.0	2.0	3.0	3.0	3.0
3	A	4.0	5.0	2.0	4.0	2.0	4.0	5.0	4.0	2.0	5.0	4.0	5.0	2.0
	B	1.0	2.0	2.0	3.0	2.0	2.0	2.0	2.0	1.0	2.0	3.0	3.0	3.0
4	A	4.9	3.9	2.9	0.9	2.9	2.9	2.9	3.9	2.9	2.9	1.9	3.9	1.9
	B	1.9	1.9	0.9	1.9	1.9	0.9	0.9	1.9	1.9	0.9	1.9	2.9	1.9
5	A	3.5	4.5	4.5	4.5	2.5	3.5	5.5	4.5	2.5	4.5	2.5	6.5	4.5
	B	3.5	3.5	3.4	4.5	3.5	3.5	4.5	3.5	4.5	3.5	4.5	3.5	4.5
6	A	0.7	2.7	1.7	3.7	1.7	1.7	2.7	1.7	3.7	2.7	1.7	2.7	1.7
	B	1.7	1.7	0.7	1.7	0.7	1.7	0.7	1.7	1.7	1.7	1.7	0.7	1.7
7	A	2.5	3.5	4.5	3.5	2.5	4.5	4.5	3.5	1.5	3.5	2.5	3.5	2.5
	B	2.5	2.5	1.5	2.5	2.5	2.5	2.5	1.5	2.5	2.5	2.5	2.5	2.5
8	A	1.7	1.7	1.7	1.7	0.7	1.7	1.7	1.7	0.7	1.7	1.7	1.7	1.7
	B	0.7	0.7	0.7	0.7	0.7	0.7	0.7	0.7	0.7	0.7	0.7	0.7	0.7
9	A	2.8	3.8	3.8	1.8	0.8	2.8	4.8	2.8	3.8	3.8	3.8	1.8	0.8
	B	1.8	1.8	0.8	1.8	0.8	0.8	0.8	0.8	1.8	0.8	1.8	0.8	1.8
10	A	3.1	7.1	3.1	8.1	3.1	5.1	5.1	4.1	4.1	4.1	2.1	4.1	2.1
	B	2.1	2.1	1.1	2.1	1.1	2.1	2.1	2.1	2.1	1.1	2.1	2.1	2.1
11	A	2.9	1.9	1.9	1.9	0.9	3.9	1.9	1.9	0.9	1.9	0.9	2.9	0.9
	B	0.9	0.9	0.9	0.9	0.9	0.9	0.9	0.9	0.9	0.9	0.9	0.9	0.9
12	A	1.5	2.5	1.5	2.5	1.5	2.5	3.5	2.5	2.5	3.5	1.5	0.5	1.5
	B	0.5	0.5	0.5	0.5	0.5	0.5	0.5	0.5	0.5	0.5	0.5	0.5	0.5
13	A	8.8	8.8	5.8	5.8	5.8	5.8	6.8	6.8	6.8	7.8	5.8	2.8	7.8
	B	2.8	2.8	2.8	3.8	1.8	2.8	1.8	2.8	3.8	1.8	3.8	2.8	2.8

The urine factor is represented by 13 night urines selected at random from nondiabetic inpatients. First, the actual glucose content of the urine was determined with an LKB 8600 by use of a hexokinase reagent kit from Boehringer Mannheim (cat. No. 15931). The concentration range was found to be 0–0.6 mmol/liter.

Next, glucose was added to the urine samples, creating 10 different concentrations of the same urine sample, ranging from 0–10 mmol/liter, with intervals of 1 mmol/liter. The samples were then tested in random order.

The laboratory technician factor is represented by 13 laboratory technicians with various degrees of experience in reading Clinistix, but who were not familiar with S-Glukotest.

The time factor indicates the order in which the urine samples were tested by each laboratory technician.

The environmental factor is represented by 13 different locations with various combinations of daylight, neon light, and incandescent lamps.

The batch factor is represented by 13 different batch numbers.

The calculations were based on the average concentrations of the last negative and the following positive reading (Figure 2). In the case of dubious readings, the procedure was as described in Figure 2.

The test was performed twice, first with Clinistix and then with S-Glukotest, under identical conditions. Between the tests the urine samples were kept frozen at −60 °C.

Table 2. Analysis of Variance Table for the Square Experiment with Two Dipsticks

Source of variation	Sum of squares of the deviations	Degrees of freedom	Variance	F	P
		A. Clinistix, read after 10 s			
Urine	4.8251	12	0.40209	18.59	<0.0005
Lab. technician	1.6678	12	0.13899	6.42	<0.0005
Environment	0.6205	12	0.05171	2.39	$0.005 < P < 0.01$
Batch	0.3320	12	0.02767	1.28	$0.1 < P < 0.3$
Time	0.2573	12	0.02144	0.99	$0.3 < P < 0.5$
Remainder	2.3365	108	0.02163		
Total	10.0392	168			
		B. S-Glukotest, read after 30 s			
Urine	9.9036	12	0.82530	71.82	<0.0005
Lab. technician	0.5644	12	0.04703	4.09	<0.0005
Environment	0.2754	12	0.02295	2.00	$0.025 < P < 0.05$
Batch	0.2351	12	0.01959	1.70	$0.05 < P < 0.1$
Time	0.1853	12	0.01544	1.34	$0.1 < P < 0.3$
Remainder	1.2411	108	0.01149		
Total	12.4049	168			

The influence of the factors could now be analyzed, the median point of color change calculated, and the results from the two squares compared by a Wilcoxon test, assuming gaussian-distributed rank sums.

Results

Results of the Variance Analyses

The log-normal distribution was used for the variance analysis of the two test squares. The test results appear in Table 1. Table 2 (*a* and *b*) shows the results of the *F*-test. Evidently, not only the urine factor but also the laboratory technician and environmental factors contribute significantly to the variation in the point of color change. Clinistix read after 10 s and S-Glukotest after 30 s show a median point of color change of 2.8 and 1.8 mmol/liter, respectively. The "95–90" tolerance interval for these points of change was calculated to 0.5–0.8 mmol/liter for Clinistix and 0.5–4.5 mmol/liter for S-Glukotest. Owing to the discrete figure distribution, the tolerance intervals were calculated according to the nonparametric tolerance method (*2*).

Figure 3 shows the distribution of positive/negative answers from 2 × 1690 single results from the test squares, summed up for each of the 10 concentration intervals.

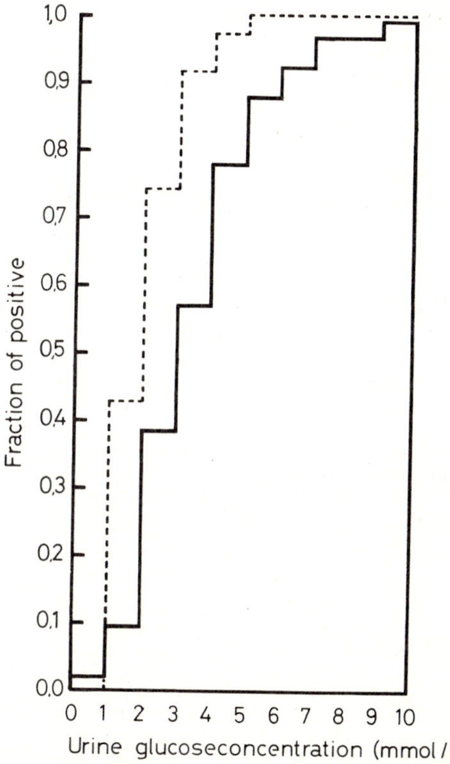

Fig. 3. Distribution of positive results from the 1690 individual results of the two test squares, summed for each of the 10 concentration intervals

Clinistix (—) were read after 10 s, S-Glukotest (- - -) after 30 s

The points of change established by the two test squares, compared by the Wilcoxon test, proved that the sensitivity of Clinistix was significantly poorer than that of S-Glukotest. The rank sum for Clinistix: 36 159 ($P \ll 0.001$). Consequently, we extended the time for reading the Clinistix to 30 s during the succeeding tests, thereby increasing the sensitivity.

As already mentioned, we have arrived at the results presented so far by "translating" the positive/negative answers to a urine glucose concentration. For this we used the matrix shown in Figure 2. Dubious results were obtained only with Clinistix. Among each of the 169 points of change there were 24 "doubtful" cases, four "false-positive" cases, and seven "false-negative" cases. All the results obtained by S-Glukotest were "normal" (Figure 2). This difference in occurrence of dubious answers is statistically significant ($P < 0.01$) according to the binomial distribution.

Level and Ability of Discrimination under Favorable Analytical Conditions

As 13 randomly selected urine samples were not considered representative of all the urine samples tested in a clinical chemical laboratory, and as it was desirable to determine more accurately the discrimination level and ability of the dipsticks, 77 urine samples were enriched with glucose and tested under the most favorable conditions, i.e., by skilled laboratory technicians in the best possible light (neon light and incandescent lamps). For this part of the test, dipsticks of the same batch number were used, and the urine samples were tested before the other analyses that day. The urine samples were collected from nondiabetic inpatients chosen without conscious bias, and the glucose content was determined by the hexokinase kit method. Their glucose concentrations ranged from 0 to 0.9 mmol/liter. The urine samples were enriched with glucose so that six concentrations were prepared from each sample, ranging from 0 to 6 mmol/liter with intervals of 1 mmol/liter, and tested in random order.

As stated above, the point of color change occurred at a considerably higher glucose concentration for Clinistix than for S-Glukotest, but as this difference was lessened by reading the Clinistix after 30 s—and not after 10 s as recommended by Ames—both dipsticks were read after 30 s during this experiment.

Figure 4 shows the distribution of positive/negative results from 77 night urines enriched with glucose at 1 mmol/liter intervals; both Clinistix and S-Glukotest were read after 30 s.

A comparison of Figures 3 and 4 shows the improved sensitivity when Clinistix is not read until after 30 s.

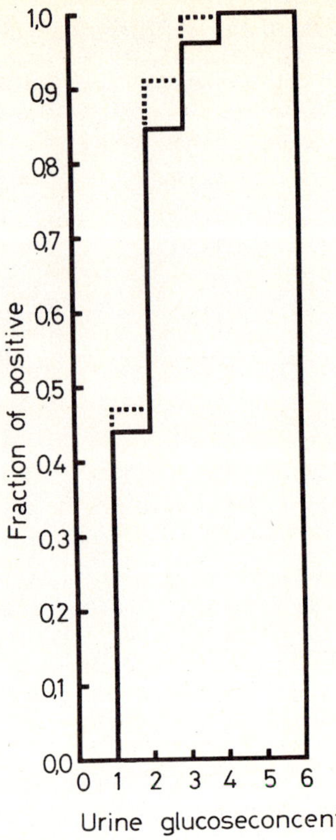

Fig. 4. Distribution of positive results from 77 night urines enriched with glucose (1 mmol/liter intervals), Clinistix (—) and S-Glukotest (- - -), read after 30 s

Interpretation of a Dipstick Result

We used the hexokinase method to measure glucose in urine samples from inpatients, received in the laboratory for glucose screening during one week.

By combining the information about a probable positive/negative dipstick result in the different concentration intervals with the probability of finding urines in the same intervals, we are able to express the value of the information obtained from a dipstick examination, i.e., to predict the probable glucose content of the urine sample. The expression is given by Bayes' formula (*3*):

$$P(C_i \le C < C_{i+1} | \text{neg. statement}) = \frac{P(\text{neg. statement} | C_i \le C < C_{i+1}) \times P(C_i \le C < C_{i+1})}{\Sigma_i P(\text{neg. statement} | C_i \le C < C_{i+1}) \times P(C_i \le C < C_{i+1})}$$

where C_i = 0, 1, 2, 3, ... , n mmol glucose/liter, and C_{i+1} = 1, 2, 3, 4, ... , $(n + 1)$ mmol glucose/liter.

Figure 5 shows the distribution of the glucose concentrations of urines received in the laboratory during one week, as measured by the hexokinase reaction.

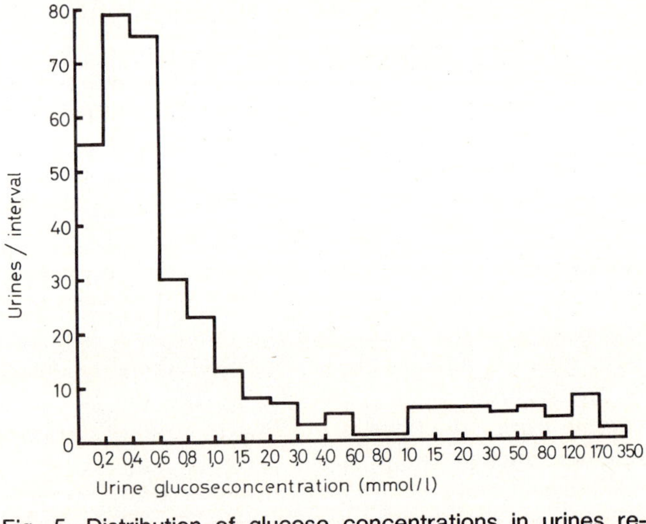

Fig. 5. Distribution of glucose concentrations in urines received in the laboratory from the hospital departments for glucose screening during one week (n = 343)

Table 3 shows the results when Bayes' formula was used to calculate the probability of a urinary glucose value being within certain concentration limits when a negative dipstick reading has been obtained.

The above may picture the capacity of the dipstick method too optimistically because of the relatively large number of normal urines used for the calculation. Thus we have included the same figures in a table of sensitivity and specificity (Table 4).

Table 3. The Probability of Finding the Urine Glucose Content within a Certain Concentration Interval when the Dipstick Reading is Negative[a]

$C_i \leq C < C_i + 1$ (mmol/liter)	$P(C_i \leq C < C_i + 1 \mid$ negative statement$)$ Clinistix[b]	$P(C_i \leq C < C_i + 1 \mid$ negative statement$)$ S-Glukotest[b]
$0 \leq C < 1$	0.953	0.957
$1 \leq C < 2$	0.043	0.041
$2 \leq C < 3$	0.004	0.003
$3 \leq C < 4$	0.0004	0.0001
$4 \leq C$	0	0

[a] For meaning of symbols, see text
[b] Both dipsticks read after 30 s

Table 4. Outline of Specificities at a Selected Discrimination Level of 2 mmol/liter[a]

		< 2 mmol	> 2 mmol	Σ
Negative	Clinistix	79.8	0.4	80.2
	S-Glukotest	79.6	0.2	79.8
Positive	Clinistix	2.7	17.1	19.8
	S-Glukotest	2.9	17.3	20.2
Σ		82.5	17.5	100.0

Sensitivity: Clinistix $\frac{17.1 \times 100}{17.5}$ % = 97.7%; S-Glukotest $\frac{17.3 \times 100}{17.5}$ % = 98.9%

Specificity: Clinistix $\frac{79.8 \times 100}{82.5}$ % = 96.7%; S-Glukotest $\frac{79.6 \times 100}{82.5}$ % = 96.5%

Predictive value: Clinistix $\frac{17.1 \times 100}{19.8}$ % = 86.4%; S-Glukotest $\frac{17.3 \times 100}{20.2}$ % = 85.6%

[a] Figures are percent of total

Discussion

The *F*-test shows that much of the variation in test readings for both types of dipsticks is attributable to inter-sample variation. The lowest positive urine and the highest negative urine had glucose concentrations of 0.3 and 9.3 mmol/liter, respectively.

Like other authors (*4*), we experienced a considerably smaller sensitivity when testing glucose in urine than when experimenting with glucose in water, probably because urine contains a number of compounds that tend to inhibit the analytical reactions applied in the experiment (*4, 5*), particularly certain drugs (*4*). We have not studied the effect of drugs further, as we judge it unwarranted and find it simpler to determine the glucose content of drug-containing urines by quantitative methods.

Unlike the urine factor, the other factors tested can be modified. Among these factors we experienced a significant difference between the laboratory technicians, which illustrates the need for very careful instruction before even as simple a test as the dipstick test is done.

The environment factor has a weak but significant influence on the dipstick readings; it is necessary to do the tests under good and consistent lighting.

However, we found no significant difference between results for various batches of dipsticks or between one particular laboratory technician at different times. We conclude that the two brands of dipsticks are prepared from reasonably consistent compounds and that one laboratory technician can justifiably do analyses in series of up to 130.

However, the similarity between two dipsticks ends here, as illustrated in Figure 3 and by the Wilcoxon test. We conclude that when the two are used according to the manufacturers' instructions, S-Glukotest is more sensitive and gives a more consistent interpretation.

Values in the literature vary greatly on the subject of the physiological limits of glucose in urine. For example, Renschler et al. (*6*) fix the upper limit at 1.67 mmol/liter, and Pileggi and Szustkiewicz (*7*) at 0.55 mmol/liter. The point of change obtained by S-Glukotest is closer to these values than those obtained by Clinistix. By increasing the time before reading the Clinistix to 30 s, we improved its sensitivity to compare with that of S-Glukotest, both now showing an average point of change between 1 and 2 mmol/liter and a range between 1 and 4 mmol/liter (Figure 4).

Another reason for preferring a sensitive method of excluding urines that are normal as far as glucose concentration is concerned is that we have a quantitative method of differentiating all positive tests and thus establishing "false positive" results.

Table 3 states the probable glucose concentration in any particular urine sample when the dipstick test is negative. Note that the calculation has been based on the distribution of urines in Figure 5, which is based on local data and not necessarily universally representative. When a result is negative there is a greater than 95% probability that the glucose concentration is less than 1 mmol/liter and more than 99% probability that it is less than 2 mmol/liter.

The above information seems to justify use of the dipsticks for screening. One must bear in mind, however, that of urine samples with a glucose content of 2 to 3 mmol/liter, Clinistix may give a "negative" answer for 15% and S-Glukotest for 9%. For urines with a glucose content between 3 and 4 mmol/liter, 4% and 2%, respectively, may be so overlooked (Figure 4). This is true even if the sensitivity of Clinistix is improved by reading after 30 s.

On the other hand, the predictive value of the tests is found to be 86%; i.e., 14% of subjects with a "positive" result will have a urinary glucose concentration of less than 2 mmol/liter (Table 4). Suppose that all untreated diabetics have a urinary glucose concentration above and all nondiabetics a concentration below this value—which of course is not quite true—14 of 100 patients suspected to have diabetes mellitus on the basis of a dipstick examination will in fact be healthy.

Generally, we should choose the type of analysis with the highest level of discrimination between well and sick in relation to the consequences of a positive/negative result, and with the greatest ability to discriminate; i.e., with the sharpest change at the appropriate decision value.

Of course, it would be better specifically to measure the glucose in all urine samples, thereby avoiding "false-positive" and "false-negative" results. However, there may be conditions under which only the simple screening test can be done.

One method for increasing the certainty of the decision in the case of a doubtful result is to increase the urine glucose content of the specimen by 2 mmol/liter and observe whether the doubtful reaction, checked at 30 s, now becomes clearly positive. If it is not, the reason may be that inhibitory substances are present, and the glucose must then be checked by other methods.

In any case the consequences of a "false-positive" or "false-negative" result must be considered before choosing the decision value. For example, when a urine sample is tested for glucose, the consequence of a "false-positive" result will usually be only economically detrimental (the cost of a quantitative determination of glucose in urine), plus the fact that the patient may be inconvenienced by an oral glucose-tolerance test. It is quite a different matter with some other qualitative analyses. For instance, to refute a positive result of a dipstick test for protein in urine, one must do several quantitative protein analyses and possibly expose the patient to extensive and trying tests (urography, for example).

When dipsticks are used to screen urines for glucose, there should be quality control of the test system. Because of the great influence of urine composition on dipstick results, we suggest that each day a random series of urines be tested, prepared from a pool of negative urines enriched with glucose to concentration intervals of 1 mmol/liter. When changing to a new batch of dipsticks, results from this batch should be compared with those for old batch by comparing the fraction of positive results obtained when analyzing 20 times at random a control urine with a glucose content corresponding to 0.1 and 0.9 of positive results, respectively.

On the basis of our results we cannot recommend the relatively crude dipstick examination for glucose in urine for quantitative purposes. Differentiating subtle graduations in color intensity at a fixed time will be susceptible to even greater errors than those observed in the "yes or no" situation. As a matter of fact such an attempt was made by the technicians during the study; the results were such that any statistical analysis was impossible. Quick and reliable methods for measuring glucose concentration in urine are at hand. Clinical decisions that imply therapeutic consequences (e.g., alterations in insulin dosage) should be based on information having a validity that justifies these decisions.

References

1. Cox, D. R., *Planning of Experiments.* Wiley, New York, N.Y., 1958.

2. Reed, A. H., Henry, R. J., and Mason, W. B., Influence of statistical method used on the resulting estimate of normal range. *Clin. Chem.* **17**, 276 (1971).

3. Wonnacott, T. H., and Wonnacott, R. J., *Introductory Statistics for Business and Economics.* Wiley, New York, N.Y., 1972, p 363.

4. Jaksch, W., and Tschepper, P., Erfahrungen mit Schnelltests zur Harnuntersuchung beim Hund. *Wien. Tieraerztl. Monatschr.* **61**, 83 (1974).

5. Blaedel, W. J., and Uhl, J. M., Nature of materials in serum that interfere in the glucose oxidase-peroxidase-*o*-dianisidine method for glucose, and their mode of action. *Clin. Chem.* **21**, 119 (1975).

6. Renschler, H. E., Weicker, H., and Baeyer, H. von, Die obere Normgrenze der Glukosekonzentration im Urin Gesunder. *Dtsch. Med. Wochenschr.* **90**, 2349 (1965).

7. Pileggi, V. J., and Szustkiewicz, C. P., Carbohydrates. In *Clinical Chemistry: Principles and Techniques,* 2nd ed., R. J. Henry, D. C. Cannon, and J. W. Winkelman, Eds. Harper and Row, New York, N.Y., 1974, p 1295.

CLIN. CHEM. 22/2, 211–216 (1976)

Evaluation of a Discrete-Sample Computer-Directed Clinical Analyzer

Roger L. Forrester, Willa Collinge, Pattie Hashimoto, and Jackie Worrall

The operational characteristics of the Gilford System 3500 were evaluated for six months as to accuracy, precision, carry-over, reliability, and ease of operation. Accuracy was evaluated by comparison to manual methods of established accuracy. The tests evaluated and their respective correlation coefficients are as follows: glucose (0.99), blood urea nitrogen (0.99), calcium (0.97), total bilirubin (0.99), aspartate aminotransferase (0.97), alkaline phosphatase (0.98), albumin (0.96), and total protein (0.96). Within-run precision (CV) for three commercial calibration sera of differing analyte concentrations (low, intermediate, and high) were respectively: 0.69, 1.02, 1.18; 5.4, 1.2, 1.09; 0.83, 0.77, 0.86; 5.9, 1.0, 0.86; 6.4, 5.2, 2.1; 3.7, 1.5, 1.3; 0.0, 1.4, 0.97; and 1.2, 1.3, 0.75. Day-to-day precision, similarly evaluated during 101–164 days, met accepted criteria for clinically acceptable precision. Carry-over for each of the eight tests was <1%. Instrument reliability has been excellent, and training time is short. In summary, we have found the Gilford System 3500 to be sufficiently precise and fast, easy to operate, highly accurate, and flexible.

We have evaluated the operational characteristics of the Gilford System 3500 Computer-Directed Analyzer during six months for the assay of glucose, blood urea nitrogen, calcium, total bilirubin, aspartate aminotransferase (AST, EC 2.6.1.1), alkaline phosphatase (ALP, EC 3.1.3.1), albumin, and total protein.

The evaluation protocol (*1*) is designed for evaluation of automated instruments in the clinical chemistry laboratory.

Mercy San Juan Hospital, Clinical Chemistry Laboratory, 6501 Coyle Ave., Carmichael, Calif. 95608.

Received Oct. 9, 1975; accepted Nov. 18, 1975.

Materials and Methods

A Gilford System 3500 Computer-Directed Analyzer (serial No. 124; Gilford Instruments, Inc., Oberlin, Ohio 44074) was used to generate all System 3500 data. The manual comparison data were gathered by use of spectrophotometers from Gilford Instruments, Inc. (Gilford 300N); Beckman Instruments, Inc., Fullerton, Calif. 92634 (Model 25); and Varian Instruments, Palo Alto, Calif. 94303 (Model 1200 atomic absorption). Reagents were obtained from various manufacturers. Those for glucose (hexokinase method; cat. No. 7615), alkaline phosphatase (Bowers and McComb, 1966; cat. No. 7085), aspartate aminotransferase (Henry, 1960, and Amador and Wacker, 1962; cat. No. 7052), albumin (bromcresol green; cat. No. 7083), and total protein (biuret; cat. No. 7081) were obtained from Worthington Biochemical Corp., Freehold, N. J. 07728. Those for blood urea nitrogen (BUN; kinetic Urease; cat. No. 89317) were from Smith Kline Instruments, Inc., Palo Alto, Calif. 94306. Those for calcium (methylthymol blue; cat. No. 40895) were obtained from Pierce Chemical Co., Rockford, Ill. 61105. Reagents for total bilirubin (Jendrassik and Grof; cat. No. 9000) were obtained from American Monitor Corp., Indianapolis, Ind. 46268. Lyophilized serum controls—"Versatol Automated Lo," "Lock-in," and "Hi"—were manufactured by General Diagnostics, Morris Plains, N. J. 07950. "Normal" and "Abnormal" unassayed controls were supplied by Hyland Laboratories, Inc., Costa Mesa, Calif. 92626, for the California Society of Pathologists' Quality Assurance Program.

The system 3500 is a complete analytical system,

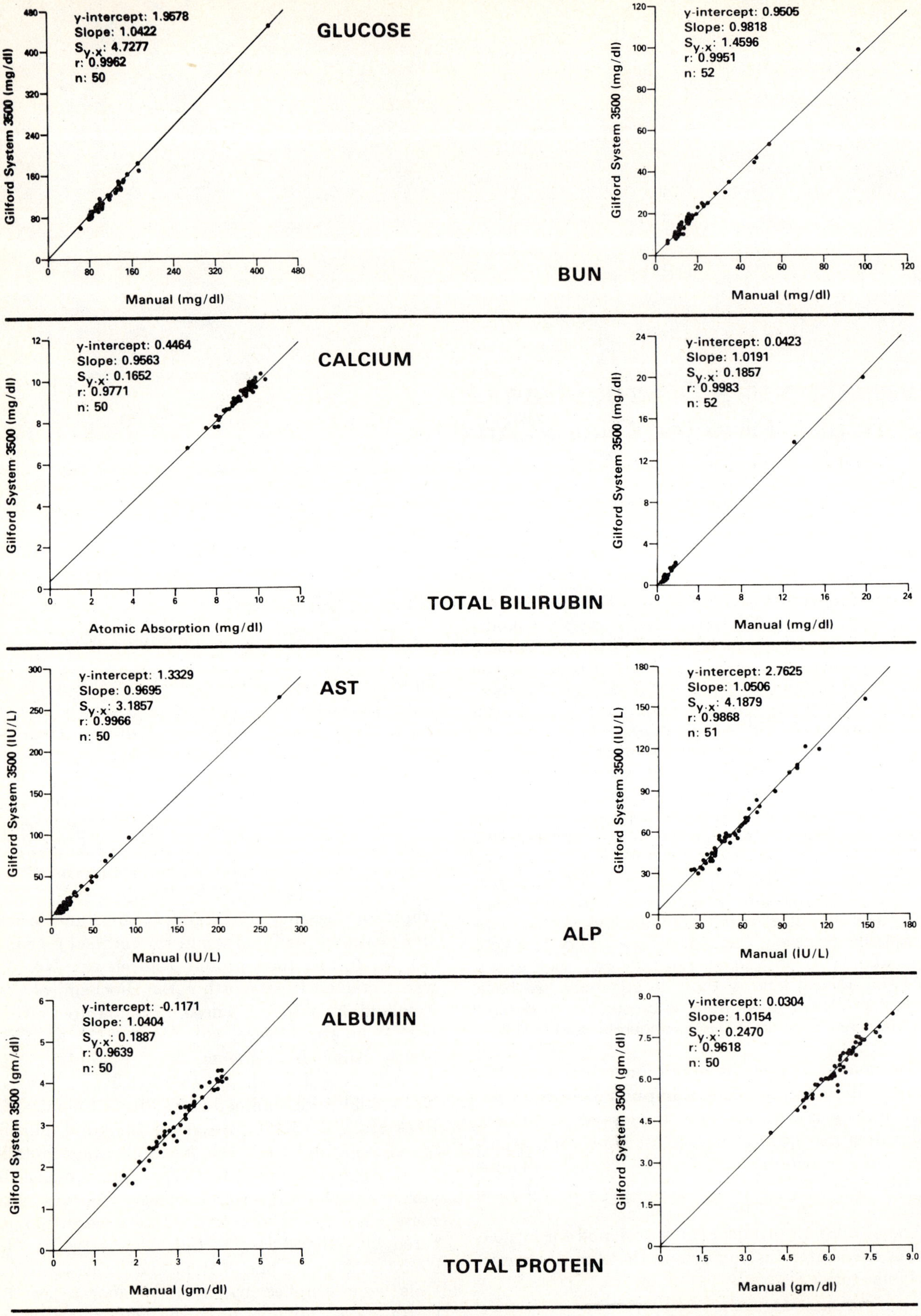

Fig. 1. Comparison of patient values between reference (manual) methods (x) and the Gilford System 3500 (y)

Table 1. Average Percentage Recovery and Upper Limit of Linearity for Each Test

Test	Av % recovery	Upper limit of linearity
Glucose	100.8	5000 mg/liter
Blood urea nitrogen	100.6	1200 mg/liter
Calcium	101.0	150 mg/liter
Total bilirubin	100.7	200 mg/liter
Aspartate aminotransferase	96.3	900.0 U/liter
Alkaline phosphatase	101.2	450.0 U/liter
Albumin	99.8	100 g/liter
Total protein	102.2	100 g/liter

consisting of sample pipetting and reagent dispensing system, a multiple-sample transport system, a precision spectrophotometer, a printer, and a mini-computer programmed by magnetic card to control function of all the other components of the system and calculate results. The sample diluter-dispenser has a sample range of 10 to 100 μl. The outside of the sample probe is cleansed by an aspirated flow of water, and the sample is washed out from the inside by reagent from the first reagent dispenser. The three reagent dispensers are each adjustable in delivered volume from 0.25 to 2.5 ml. The sample syringe and the three reagent syringes are adjusted with fixed-volume stroke stops. The grating spectrophotometer has a continuous wavelength adjustment from 340–700 nm, spectral resolution of 8 nm, low stray-light level, and linear absorbance range of 0 to 2.0000 *A*. The instrument has high sensitivity and low noise, is stable, and is capable of resolving absorbance changes of 0.0002 *A*. The temperature of the micro-cuvette is controlled to ±0.2 °C at 25, 30, 32, or 37 °C by a thermoelectric heating and cooling system. On adjustment, temperature equilibration requires only a few seconds and can be monitored by presentation on the spectrophotometer display. The measured temperature is automatically printed before each set of tests. The alphanumeric printer prints out previously programmed instructions for setup of a test and prints out results, with positive identification of rack and cup number.

Table 3. Day-to-Day Precision at Three Analyte Concentrations for the Gilford System 3500

Test	n	Mean	SD	CV, %
Glucose, mg/liter	162	871	47	5.4
Glucose, mg/liter	164	1,987	70	3.5
Glucose, mg/liter	164	3,451	104	3.0
Blood urea nitrogen, mg/liter	163	126	7	5.6
Blood urea nitrogen, mg/liter	160	601	27	4.5
Blood urea nitrogen, mg/liter	164	813	38	4.7
Calcium, mg/liter	160	77	2.4	3.17
Calcium, mg/liter	164	107	3.2	2.96
Calcium, mg/liter	164	125	3.2	2.59
Total bilirubin, mg/liter	114	6.4	0.6	10.0
Total bilirubin, mg/liter	117	29.6	1.5	5.1
Total bilirubin, mg/liter	118	57.3	2.6	4.6
Aspartate aminotransferase, U/liter	103	24.3	2.1	8.5
Aspartate aminotransferase, U/liter	119	44.7	3.4	7.7
Aspartate aminotransferase, U/liter	101	122.8	7.03	5.7
Alkaline phosphatase, U/liter	158	29.9	2.59	8.66
Alkaline phosphatase, U/liter	148	105.8	4.86	4.59
Alkaline phosphatase, U/liter	140	224.9	9.07	4.04
Albumin, g/liter	162	24.2	1.1	4.52
Albumin, g/liter	164	38.5	1.8	4.69
Albumin, g/liter	164	49.4	2.6	5.28
Total protein, g/liter	159	35.4	1.55	4.38
Total protein, g/liter	160	57.3	2.4	4.13
Total protein, g/liter	163	75.5	2.7	3.61

Table 2. Within-Run Precision for the Gilford System 3500

	Low			Intermediate			High		
Test	Mean	CV, %	n	Mean	CV, %	n	Mean	CV, %	n
Glucose, mg/liter	843	0.69	20	1901	1.02	20	3260	1.18	20
Blood urea nitrogen, mg/liter	122	5.40	20	576	1.20	20	798	1.09	20
Calcium, mg/liter	75	0.83	20	103	0.77	20	125	0.86	20
Total bilirubin, mg/liter	6	5.90	20	30	1.00	20	58	0.86	20
Aspartate aminotransferase, U/liter	19.8	6.40	20	46.0	5.20	20	127.0	2.10	20
Alkaline phosphatase, U/liter	28.6	3.70	20	99.1	1.50	20	217.0	1.30	20
Albumin, g/liter	22	0.00	20	35	1.40	20	45	0.97	20
Total protein, g/liter	35	1.20	20	56	1.30	20	76	0.75	20

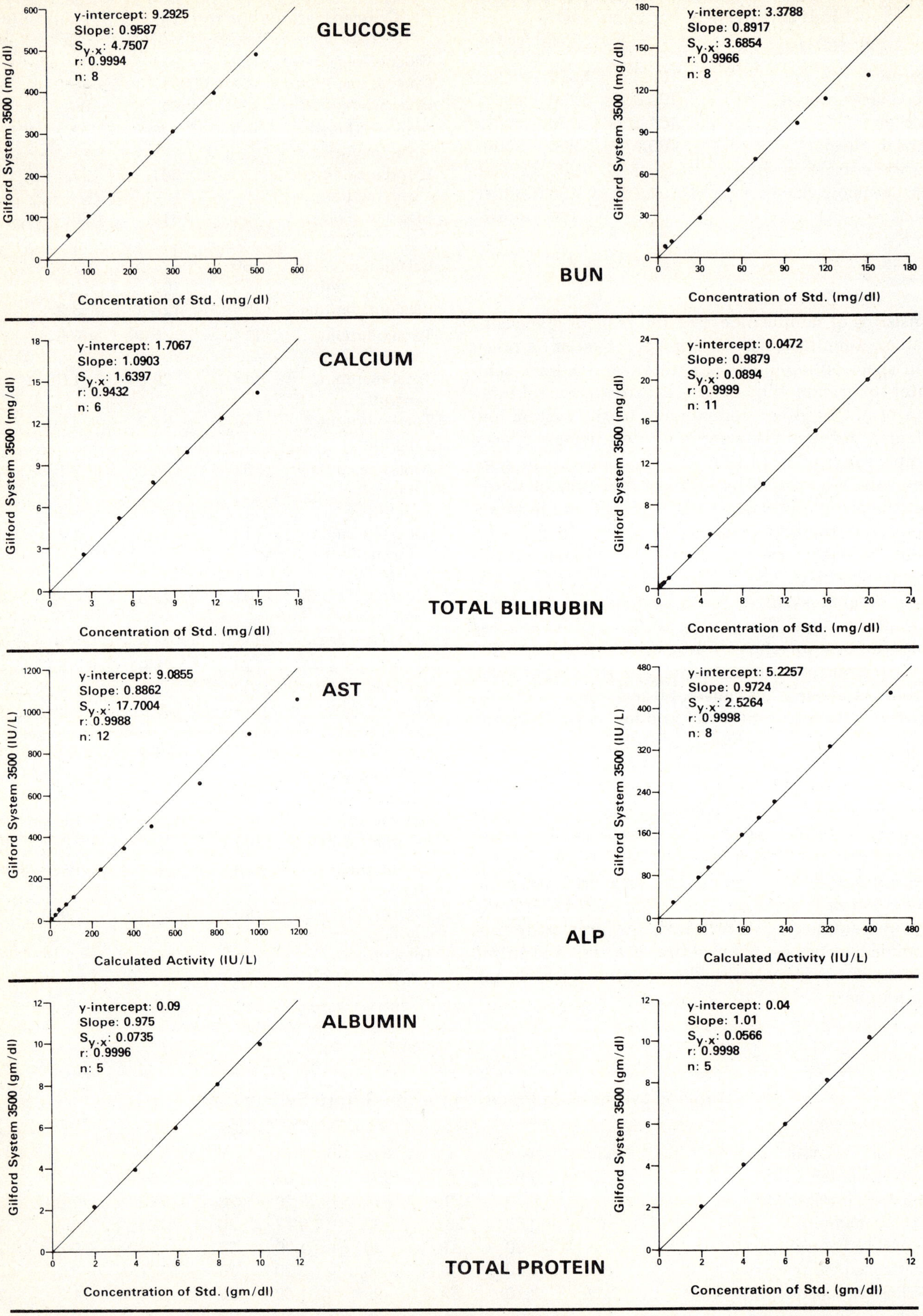

Fig. 2. Linearity of test using aqueous standards and patient sera with high enzyme activity diluted with normal patient sera

Table 4. Comparison of Day-to-Day Precision (for This Laboratory) and Agreement with Other Laboratories Using the Same Control Serum for 30 Days

Test	Gilford System 3500		All Laboratories[a]	
	Mean	CV, %	Mean	CV, %
Glucose, mg/liter	710	3.7	710	2.9
Glucose, mg/liter	1550	2.5	1500	2.4
Blood urea nitrogen, mg/liter	200	5.0	200	4.4
Blood urea nitrogen, mg/liter	460	3.9	450	2.9
Calcium, mg/liter	88	2.9	86	2.6
Calcium, mg/liter	115	2.0	112	2.4
Total bilirubin, mg/liter	13	8.0	14	6.6
Total bilirubin, mg/liter	83	3.9	83	3.4
Aspartate aminotransferase, U/liter	8	25.0	8	21.0
Aspartate aminotransferase, U/liter	52	7.7	47	6.2
Alkaline phosphatase, U/liter	36	7.7	34	7.8
Alkaline phosphatase, U/liter	109	3.9	104	4.6
Albumin, g/liter	31	3.4	32	3.7
Albumin, g/liter	38	3.0	39	3.3
Total protein, g/liter	49	3.8	50	2.0
Total protein, g/liter	62	3.4	63	1.9

[a] Here, the mean, SD, and CV are arithmetic averages of the computer file means, SD's, and CV's.

Results

Accuracy was assessed by comparison to manual methods whose accuracy had already been established by analysis of primary standards, controls, and by recovery studies, except for calcium, which was compared with results of atomic absorption spectroscopy. The results (Figure 1) show excellent agreement between the manual procedure and the 3500 automated procedure. Linearity was measured over the complete concentration range and the data are summarized in Table 1 and Figure 2.

Precision was evaluated at three concentrations of analytes for within-run and day-to-day precision. Within-run precision was evaluated by assaying each of 20 replicate samples three times and averaging the results. Data for within-run precision are summarized in Table 2. Day-to-day precision was evaluated over a period ranging from 101 days to 164 days (Table 3). In addition to the three concentrations used to evaluate within-run and day-to-day precision, one aliquot of each of the California Society of Pathologists' two-concentration unassayed pools was assayed daily as part of our quality-control program. Table 4 compares data for these gathered by our laboratory with data gathered by other laboratories that used the same lot number of these unassayed control sera.

We evaluated overall precision of the pipetting and spectrophotometer system by sampling and diluting two acid potassium dichromate solutions with water and measuring their absorbances at 340 nm. Twenty replicate analyses were made on each solution once per day for three days. Overall precision, expressed as the coefficient of variation, was less than 0.5% in all instances.

Carryover was evaluated by using three aliquots of above-normal patient's serum followed by three aliquots of a normal patient's serum, and three aliquots of above-normal patient's serum followed by three water blanks. "Carryover" is the artifactual excess concentration or enzyme activity measured in the first aliquot of the normal patient's serum or water blank following the above-normal patient's serum. Percentage carryover was calculated according to the following formula:

$$\left(\frac{\begin{array}{c}\text{Normal-value}\\ \text{sample following}\\ \text{abnormal-value sample}\end{array} - \begin{array}{c}\text{normal-value}\\ \text{sample preceding}\\ \text{abnormal-value sample}\end{array}}{\text{Abnormal value sample}}\right) \times 100 = \%\ \text{carryover}$$

Table 5. Carryover Studies: Gilford System 3500

	Value					
	Actual		Obtained	Carryover, %	Value	Carryover, %
	High	Low	Low[a]	To low serum	H_2O[b]	To water
Glucose, mg/liter	3826	855	855	0.0	9	0.27
Blood urea nitrogen, mg/liter	809	121	121	0.0	4	0.49
Calcium, mg/liter	122	74	74	0.0	0.0	0.0
Total bilirubin, mg/liter	70	8	8	0.0	0.0	0.0
Aspartate aminotransferase, U/liter	535	12.1	12.6	0.09	<2	<0.4
Alkaline phosphatase, U/liter	219.6	29.2	28.9	0.0	<2	<0.9
Albumin, g/liter	94	20	20	0.0	0.0	0.0
Total protein, g/liter	97	20	20	0.0	0.0	0.0

[a] For low-concentration sample following high-concentration sample.
[b] For water following a high-concentration sample.

Each experiment was repeated twice with the same samples, and results were averaged. The maximum carryover to serum was 0.09% for aspartate aminotransferase, and to a water blank 0.9% for alkaline phosphatase. Table 5 summarizes data for carryover.

Discussion

Results of correlation studies with the comparison (manual) method were excellent; they indicate that all of the analytes may as validly be measured by the System 3500 as by the comparison method. With the System 3500, the linear range exceeded the published range for the manual method in all cases, and analytical recovery was excellent.

The precision of the instrument was within the manufacturer's specifications. Comparison of our data for a similar system (*2*) is favorable and the criteria for acceptable intralab precision recommended by Tonks (*3*) and Barnett (*4*) are fulfilled. Carryover from samples with high concentration or high concentration or high enzyme activity is negligible.

The reliability of the instrument has been thoroughly tested in our laboratory during the six months of continuous use for 5–6 h per day, six days a week. The only breakdown during this period was a failure of the thermo-cuvette, which was supplied and replaced the next day. Test results have correlated well with clinical findings, and serial test results with successive samples from the same patient have agreed well, as have results for the CSP California Chemistry Pool with those of other laboratories.

We thank Mr. Bob Dulay, of Western Clinical Laboratories, Roseville, California, for performing the calcium analyses by atomic absorption spectroscopy.

References

1. Winstead, M., *Instrument Check Systems,* Lea and Febiger, Philadelphia, Pa., 1971, pp 309–310.

2. Campbell, D. J., The Abbott Biochromatic Analyzer 100—'the instrument of choice for end-point chemistry'. *Lab. Med.* **5,** 24 (1974).

3. Tonks, D. B., A study of the accuracy and precision of clinical chemistry determinations in 170 Canadian laboratories. *Clin. Chem.* **9,** 217 (1963).

4. Barnett, R. N., Medical significance of laboratory results. *Am. J. Clin. Pathol.* **50,** 671 (1968).

CLIN. CHEM. 22/2, 217-220 (1976)

Effect of Halothane Anesthesia on Muscle, Liver, Thyroid, and Adrenal-Function Tests in Man

Robert E. Johnstone, Eric M. Kennell, Walter Brummund, Jr., Leslie M. Shaw, and Richard C. Ebersole

Seven healthy men volunteers received 6.6 ± 1.3 (SD) percent-hours of halothane oxygen anesthesia without surgery. Serum bilirubin, alanine aminotransferase, and aspartate aminotransferase significantly increased after anesthesia, which may indicate subclinical liver-cell damage. Creatine kinase of skeletal muscle origin increased above 90 U/liter in six subjects, indicating subclinical muscle-cell damage. Cortisol, triiodothyronine uptake, thyroxine, and free thyroxine index increased significantly immediately after anesthesia. Serum bromide concentrations had increased by fivefold on the second day after anesthesia, and on the ninth day was still elevated fourfold. Oral temperatures increased 0.7 °C 6 h post-anesthesia, possibly because of increased thyroxine activity. Lactate dehydrogenase, hydroxybutyrate dehydrogenase and γ-glutamyltransferase activities did not change significantly. No drugs administered during the course of this study chemically interfered with any of the test methods used.

In the 20 years since its introduction in 1956, halothane has become the most widely used general anesthetic in the world (*1*). In the United States alone, millions of halothane anesthetics are administered every year. Proven safety and ease of administration are the primary reasons for the wide acceptance of halothane by anesthesiologists (*2, 3*). Despite the unquestioned advantages, halothane and its metabolites do cause toxic side effects, just as other anesthetics do (*4*).

About 1 to 7 of every 10 000 patients receiving halothane anesthesia develop severe hepatotoxicity (*5*). Mild but undiagnosed hepatic damage may occur much more frequently (*6*). A few patients receiving halothane anesthesia have developed hyperpyrexia (*7*). Moreover, we have recently suggested that serum bromide, a metabolite of halothane, may increase to psychoactive concentrations postoperatively, thus contributing to psychosis and psychomotor depression frequently seen after anesthesia (*8*).

Numerous biochemical studies have been made of surgical patients after halothane anesthesia. Biochemical factors known to be changed by halothane anesthesia include bromide, potassium, bilirubin, bromsulphthalein retention, prothrombin time, cortisol, corticotropin, lutropin, testosterone, somatotropin, thyroxine, albumin, and the enzymes AST, ALT, LDH, OCT, and CK[1] (*9–19*). A definitive interpretation of these findings in surgical patients has been obscured by the complex interaction of many variables, including comcomitant use of other anesthetics and drugs, type and extent of surgery performed, and the pathophysiological conditions of the patient (*5*). To more precisely define the effect of halothane on liver, thyroid, and adrenal function tests, we studied the biochemical effects of halothane on normal volunteers.

Materials and Methods

Subjects. We studied seven healthy men volunteers, ages 21 to 25, weights 63 to 92 kg, and heights 170 to 183 cm. All subjects denied taking any medicines. Each subject fasted after midnight preceding the study. On the day of the study, each subject lay on an air cushion. Catheters were inserted into two peripheral veins, a radial artery, and internal jugular vein, and a needle was placed in a jugular bulb. Halothane oxygen anesthesia was induced by mask. An endotracheal tube was passed after administration of curare (0.6 mg/kg body weight), and each subject was mechanically ventilated (125 ml/min). Carbon dioxide was added to the inspired gas to maintain arterial blood p_{CO_2} at 4.32 kPa (40 Torr). After induction, alveolar halothane concentrations varied between 0.5 and 1.5 vol per 100 vol. The mean dose of anesthesia for the seven subjects was 6.6 ± 1.3 (SD) percent-hours, calculated as the product of alveolar concentration and duration of halothane administration. Warming lights kept the rectal temperature of each subject constant. Phenylephrine infusion and blood volume expansion with plasma protein (50 g/liter solution) maintained blood pressure at pre-anesthesia values. Heparin (2000 units), neostigmine (5 mg), atropine (2 mg), indocyanine green (100 mg), and ^{85}Kr were the only other drugs administered. Post-anesthesia recovery was in a quiet room maintained at ap-

The Department of Anesthesia and the William Pepper Laboratory, University of Pennsylvania, 3400 Spruce St., Philadelphia, Pa. 19104.

Reprint requests to: William Pepper Laboratory (Dr. Brummund or Dr. Shaw).

Received Nov. 3, 1975; accepted Nov. 18, 1975.

[1] Nonstandard abbreviations used: ALT, alanine aminotransferase (EC 2.6.1.2); AST, aspartate aminotransferase (EC 2.6.1.1); CK, creatine kinase (EC 2.7.3.2); FTI, free thyroxine index; GGT, γ-glutamyltransferase (EC 2.3.2.2); HBD, hydroxybutyrate dehydrogenase; LDH, lactate dehydrogenase (EC 1.1.1.27); OCT, ornithine carbamoyl transferase (EC 2.1.3.3); T-3, triiodothyronine; T-4, thyroxine.

proximately 22 °C. Oral temperatures were measured hourly for 12 h after anesthesia. Blood was sampled immediately before and after anesthesia, and subsequently in the morning of the 1st, 2nd, 3rd, 6th, and 9th day after anesthesia.

Biochemical analyses. The following biochemical analyses were performed: plasma cortisol (*20*), serum T-3 uptake (*21*), serum T-4 (*22*), FTI (*23*), serum conjugated and total bilirubin (*24*), and the following enzymes: ALT, AST, LDH, HBD, CK, and GGT. Enzyme activities were determined by kinetic photometric methods (*25, 26*) at 30 °C with a CentrifiChem centrifugal analyzer (Union Carbide, Inc.) by use of reagent kits [Boehringer Mannheim Corp; AST (15923), ALT (15925), CK (15721), LDH (15977), HBD (15765), GGT (15794)]. Samples with abnormally high CK values were fractionated by cellulose acetate electrophoresis (*27*). The resulting isoenzyme patterns were compared with those of tissue extracts containing CK isoenzymes of human heart, brain, and skeletal muscle.

The blood sample drawn immediately after anesthesia might have contained drugs administered during anesthesia, which could interfere with the analytical assays. We therefore tested for direct chemical interference with the chemical assays by assaying serum in the presence and absence of drugs used in the study. In this test, the following drugs were incubated with fresh, pooled human serum, at the concentrations indicated: halothane (425 μg/ml), heparin (1 units/ml), neostigmine (0.1 μg/ml), atropine (0.5 μg/ml), and indocyanine green (2.5 μg/ml). These are the maximum drug concentration expected in the serum of individuals receiving these drugs. Bilirubin, enzymes, T-3 uptake, and T-4 assays were performed in duplicate on the pooled serum, with and without the added drugs. The only test affected by this combination of drugs was the total bilirubin test. Subsequent total-bilirubin analyses in the presence of various concentrations of indocyanine green revealed that it causes a 6% increase in apparent total bilirubin when it is present in a concentration of 2.5 μg/ml. However, the half-life of indocyanine green in the blood compartment is 3.8 min (*28*), and the first post-anesthesia blood samples were drawn 30 min after the last 25-mg injection of indocyanine green. If one assumes a 3000-ml plasma volume for each subject, the concentration of indocyanine green remaining in the post-anesthesia serum sample would be less than 50 ng/ml, or one-fiftieth that of the indocyanine green used in the control test. Therefore, we conclude that at the concentrations expected in our study there would be no effect on the total bilirubin test because of indocyanine green.

To test for possible direct chemical effect of halothane on the T-3 uptake, T-4, and FTI values, a control blood sample was divided into three aliquots. One sample received no treatment, oxygen was blown over a second sample, and halothane (2 vol/100 vol) was blown over a third sample. Exposure time was 4 h, during which the temperature of each sample was maintained at 37 °C. T-3 uptake, T-4, and FTI were then determined for each sample. No significant differences occurred among the three samples. In a separate test, we determined that ^{85}Kr did not interfere with the competitive protein binding assays for cortisol, T-3 uptake, or T-4.

All data were analyzed by two-way analysis of variance with critical difference testing at a significance level of $P < 0.05$.

Results

Table 1 summarizes the mean values obtained for each biochemical test.

Serum enzymes were measured in all seven subjects. AST and ALT activities increased significantly, with maximal values on the third post-anesthesia day. Changes in LDH, HBD, and GGT were insignificant. Significant increases in CK values were observed in six of seven subjects on the first or second day after anesthesia, with the highest individual value being 259 U/liter. Electrophoretic analysis of these supranormal CK samples revealed a single band characteristic of skeletal muscle isoenzyme.

Serum bromide concentrations were significantly elevated on each of the post-anesthesia days on which measurements were taken.

Total bilirubin concentrations increased significantly immediately after anesthesia, and remained increased for two days after anesthesia in each of five subjects. Increases in conjugated bilirubin concentrations paralleled the changes in total bilirubin.

Serum cortisol concentrations were measured in four subjects. Values were significantly increased at the end of anesthesia, but returned to normal by the next morning. T-4, T-3 uptake, and FTI were elevated immediately after anesthesia. All three of these values fell below pre-anesthesia levels on the following day. T-4 and FTI remained significantly below pre-anesthesia values on the 2nd, 6th, and 9th days after anesthesia. Oral temperatures increased after anesthesia in four of six subjects, the greatest individual increase being 1.6 °C. Temperatures were maximum 5 to 7 h post-anesthesia. By this time, all subjects could walk to the toilet, and intermittently sat in a chair. No subjects developed either productive coughs or infections at the puncture sites.

Discussion

Our results suggest that halothane or its metabolites, or both, without the added stresses of surgery and disease states, cause direct but subclinical liver-cell damage. This suggestion is based on the increases we saw in ALT, AST, and bilirubin. Maximal ALT and AST values were reached three days after anesthesia, and maximal bilirubin concentrations occurred immediately after anesthesia. Others have reported similar bilirubin and enzyme increases in the serum of surgical patients anesthetized with halothane (*5*).

Table 1. Values for Blood Constituents after Halothane Anesthesia

Mean ± SD for 4 to 7 subjects

Test (units)	Normal range	Pre-anesthesia	Immediately post-anesthesia	Day after anesthesia 1	2	3	6	9
T-4 (μg/dl)	5–13	7.3 ± 0.5	8.3 ± 0.5[a]	5.2 ± 0.4[a]	6.0 ± 1.0[a]	7.0 ± 0.5	6.0 ± 0.6[a]	6.3 ± 0.4[a]
T-3 uptake	0.85–1.15	1.22 ± 0.07	1.44 ± 0.09[a]	1.21 ± 0.07	1.23 ± 0.05	1.28 ± 0.12	1.15 ± 0.09	1.15 ± 0.13
FTI (μg/dl)	4.5–12.0	8.9 ± 0.5	12.0 ± 0.6[a]	6.2 ± 0.2[a]	7.4 ± 1.2[a]	8.9 ± 0.3	7.7 ± 1.4	6.9 ± 0.4[a]
Cortisol- (μg/dl)	5--20	17.7 ± 2.6	28.6 ± 68.8[a]	22.3 ± 3.0	10.0 ± 2.6[a]	10.6 ± 2.6[a]	14.3 ± 3.1	13.3 ± 4.7
Bilirubin (mg/dl)	0.2–1.2	0.50 ± 0.18	1.35 ± 0.28[a]	1.00 ± 0.20[a]	0.97 ± 0.55[a]	0.78 ± 0.38	0.47 ± 0.14	0.50 ± 0.21
LDH (U/l)	140–270	198 ± 55	178 ± 25	196 ± 43	229 ± 40	224 ± 23	203 ± 36	224 ± 61
AST (U/l)	10–25	15 ± 3	15 ± 3	17 ± 3	30 ± 17[a]	34 ± 19[a]	22 ± 3	19 ± 5
ALT (U/l)	9–38	15 ± 7	14 ± 9	13 ± 7	24 ± 11	39 ± 20[a]	14 ± 3	14 ± 7
HBD (U/l)	110–230	139 ± 42	128 ± 22	143 ± 25	156 ± 24	156 ± 21	136 ± 28	152 ± 51
GGT (U/l)	6–40	14 ± 14	14 ± 16	14 ± 14	15 ± 11	15 ± 12	8 ± 2	11 ± 5
CK (U/l)	20–90	65 ± 26	39 ± 17	117 ± 73[a]	96 ± 65	81 ± 37	70 ± 26	80 ± 57
Bromide (mmol/l)		0.65 ± 0.32	0.82 ± 0.28	1.92 ± 0.59[a]	2.98 ± 0.60[a]	2.79 ± 0.58[a]	2.98 ± 0.85[a]	2.41 ± 0.30[a]

[a] Significantly different from pre-anesthesia level, determined by the two-way analysis of variance ($P < 0.05$).

Studies of halothane's effect on experimental animals support the hypothesis that halothane or its metabolites (or both) directly affect the liver. Zimmerman et al. (*29*) monitored serum ALT and AST in rats after intraperitoneal injection of 3.5 mmol of halothane per kilogram of body weight. Three hours after halothane injection, serum ALT activity increased to sixfold the pre-injection values, serum AST to ninefold. Saline-injected control animals showed no elevations in either ALT or AST. In another animal study, Dudley et al. (*30*) observed morphological changes in liver-cell ultrastructure in rats exposed to an atmosphere of 10 and 500 ppm halothane, eight hours per day, five days per week, for four to eight weeks. These concentrations of halothane are comparable to the occupational exposure of anesthetists (500 ppm) and operating room nurses (10 ppm) (*31*). The ultrastructural changes in the liver cells included glycogen depletion, breakup of rough endoplasmic reticulum, mitochondrial changes, indented nuclei, and coagulative necrosis of hepatocytes.

The mean CK value for our subjects increased to about twice the mean pre-anesthesia value on the first day after anesthesia, an increase attributable to CK of skeletal muscle origin. The halothane procedure itself evidently causes some skeletal muscle damage. An increased CK in plasma or serum after surgery is a well-known phenomenon (*16*). In two different studies, CK values were maximum on postoperative day 1 (*16, 32*). These elevations (fourfold the pre-operative value) exceeded those we observed in our subjects. Since CK has a high specific activity in skeletal muscle, muscle trauma incident to surgery has been suggested as the probable source of increased activity of the circulating enzyme (*33*). However, our subjects were not subjected to surgical trauma. Muscle trauma was limited to placing a single needle in a jugular bulb, through the thin platysma muscle of the neck. Consequently, it appears that halothane anesthesia itself may contribute significantly to the increased CK activity observed in patients following surgery.

The mechanism of this effect of halothane anesthesia on muscle is unknown. One possibility is that halothane or its metabolites directly disturb skeletal muscle. Enhanced CK values have been observed after the oral administration of a number of drugs (*34*). Another possible explanation is that muscle damage occurred as a result of the prolonged pressure of each subjects' weight on his muscles. Penn et al. (*35*) proposed that prolonged pressure on dependent muscles or the hypoxia resulting from the compression of major arteries is a probable cause of myoglobinuria in patients who are in coma as a result of drug ingestion (*35*). They observed marked increases in CK activity in the serum of patients with drug induced coma, irrespective of the drug ingested.

It is also possible that the neuromuscular blocking agent used during the anesthesia caused the observed increases in CK. Such increases in anesthetized surgical patients given the neuromuscular blocking agent, succinylcholine, are greater than in patients not given this drug (*16*). In the present study the neuromuscular blocking agent, curare, was administered to each subject. Possibly curare contributed to the CK increases even though it does not cause muscle fasciculations as succinylcholine does.

Elevated corticotropin and cortisol concentrations have been measured previously during and after halothane anesthesia (*11, 12*). The lower cortisol concentrations on the second and third days after anesthesia may be attributed to drawing these blood samples later in the morning. Increases in somatotropin and lutropin released from the pituitary (*11, 13*), together with increases in corticotropin and thyroxine, suggest a general pituitary stimulation.

We thank Ms. J. Ciccarelli, P. Townsend, H. Mason, G. Knee, K. G. Levkovich, and Drs. Bonnie Tompkins and Peter Lief who assisted the study.

Supported in part by USPHS grants 5-T01-00215 and 5-P01-GM-15430 from the NIGMS, NIH.

References

1. Strunin, L., and Simpson, B. R., Halothane in Britain today. *Br. J. Anesth.* **44,** 919 (1972).

2. Reves, J. G., Halothane hepatitis. Current concepts. *Postgrad. Med.* **56,** 65 (1974).

3. National halothane study. Summary of the national halothane study: Possible association between halothane anesthesia and postoperative hepatic necrosis. *J. Am. Med. Assoc.* **197,** 775 (1966).

4. Dawson, B., Adson, M. A., Dockerty, M. B., et al., Hepatic function tests: Postoperative changes with halothane or diethyl ether anesthesia. *Mayo Clin. Proc.* **41,** 599 (1966).

5. Thompson, D. S., and Greifenstein, F. E., Enzyme patterns reflecting hepatic response to anesthesia and operation. *South. Med. J.* **67,** 69 (1974).

6. Klatskin, G., and Kimberg, D. V., Recurrent hepatitis attributable to halothane sensitization in an anesthetist. *New Engl. J. Med.* **280,** 515 (1969).

7. Isaacs, H., and Barlow, M. B., Malignant hyperpyrexia during anesthesia: Possible association with subclinical myopathy. *Br. Med. J.* **i,** 275 (1970).

8. Johnstone, R. E., Kennell, E. M., Behar, M. G., et al., Increased serum bromide concentration after halothane anesthesia in man. *Anesthesiology* **42,** 598 (1975).

9. Rehder, K., Frobes, J., Alter, H. et al., Halothane biotransformation in man: A quantitative study. *Anesthesiology* **28,** 711 (1967).

10. Stevens, W. C., Eger, E. I., Joas, T. A., et al., Comparative toxicity of isoflurane, halothane, fluoroxene, and diethyl ether in human volunteers. *Can. Anaesth. Soc. J.* **20,** 357 (1973).

11. Von Werder, K., Stevens, W. C., Cromwell, T. H., et al., Adrenal function during long-term anesthesia in man. *Proc. Soc. Exp. Biol. Med.* **135,** 854 (1970).

12. Oyama, T., and Takaguchi, M., Plasma levels of ACTH and cortisol in man during halothane anesthesia and surgery. *Anesth. Analg.* (Cleveland) **49,** 363 (1970).

13. Carstensen, H., Amer. I., Wide, L., and Amer, B., Plasma testosterone, LH and FSH during the first 24 hours after surgical operations. *J. Steroid Biochem.* **4,** 605 (1973).

14. Innes, R. K. R., and Stromme, J. H., Rise in serum creatine phosphokinase associated with agents used in anaesthesia. *Br. J. Anaesth.* **45,** 185 (1973).

15. Smith, A. A., Volpitto, P. P., Gramling, Z. W., et al., Chloroform, halothane and regional anesthesia: A comparative study. *Anesth. Analg.* (Cleveland) **52,** 1 (1973).

16. Phornphutkul, K. S., Anuras, S., Koff, R. S., et al., Causes of increased plasma creatine kinase activity after surgery. *Clin. Chem.* **20,** 340 (1974).

17. Oyama, T., Shibata, S., Matsuki, A., and Kudo, T., Serum endogenous thyroxine levels in man during anaesthesia and surgery. *Br. J. Anaesth.* **41,** 103 (1969).

18. Adikman, S. A., Flanagan, T. V., and Landmesser, C. M., A comparative study of serum glutamic pyruvic transaminase changes following anesthesia with halothane, methoxyflurane and other inhalation agents. *Anesth. Analg.* (Cleveland) **45,** 819 (1966).

19. Dawson, B., Adson, M. A., Dockerty, M. B., et al., Hepatic function tests: Post-operative changes with halothane or diethyl ether anesthesia. *Mayo Clin. Proc.* **41,** 599 (1966).

20. Murphy, B. P., Measurement of steroids by competitive protein binding radioassay. *J. Clin. Endocrinol. Metab.* **27,** 973 (1967).

21. Mitchell, M. L., Hardin, A. B., and O'Rourke, M. E., The *in vitro* resin sponge uptake of triiodothyroxine from serum in thyroid disease. *J. Clin. Endocrinol. Metab.* **20,** 1474 (1960).

22. Nakajima, H., Kuramochi, M., Horiguchi, T., and Kubo, S., A new and simple method for the determination of thyroxine in serum. *J. Clin. Endocrinol. Metab.* **26,** 99 (1966).

23. Rosenfeld, L., Free thyroxine index. A reliable substitute for "free" thyroxine concentration. *Am. J. Clin. Pathol.* **61,** 118 (1974).

24. Malloy, H. T., and Evelyn, K. A., The determination of the serum bilirubin with special reference to the prompt reacting and the chloroform soluble type. *J. Lab. Clin. Med.* **30,** 293 (1945).

25. Recommendations of the German Society for Clinical Chemistry. *Z. Klin. Chem. Klin. Biochem.* **10,** 281 (1972).

26. Szasz, G., A kinetic photometric method for serum glutamyl transpeptidase. *Clin. Chem.* **15,** 124 (1969).

27. Sherwin, A. L., Siber, G. R., and Elhilali, M. M., Fluorescence technique to demonstrate creatine phosphokinase isoenzymes. *Clin. Chim. Acta* **17,** 245 (1967).

28. Wiegand, B. D., Ketterer, S. G., and Rapaport, E., The use of indocyanine green for the evaluation of hepatic function and blood flow in man. *Am. J. Dig. Dis.* **5,** 427 (1960).

29. Zimmerman, H. J., Kendler, J., and Koff, R. S., Intraperitoneal halothane administration: Evidence of hepatic and muscle injury. *Proc. Soc. Exp. Biol. Med.* **138,** 678 (1971).

30. *J. Am. Med. Assoc. Med. News* **228,** 1634 (1974).

31. *J. Am. Med. Assoc. Med. News* **226,** 609 (1973).

32. Hobson, R. W., Constant, C., Mahoney, W. D., and Baugh, J. H., Serum creatine phosphokinase. Analysis of postoperative changes. *Am. J. Surg.* **124,** 625 (1972).

33. Sorensen, N. S., Dahl, J. A., and Aastrup, J. E., Creatine phosphokinase and operation. *Ugeskr. Laeg.* **127,** 1431 (1965).

34. King, J. O., and Zapf, P., A review of the value of creatine phosphokinase estimations in clinical medicine. *Med. J. Aust.* **1,** 699 (1972).

35. Penn, A. S., Rowland, L. P., and Fraser, D. W., Drugs, coma, and myoglobinuria. *Arch. Neurol.* (Chicago) **26,** 336 (1972).

CLIN. CHEM. 22/2, 221–223 (1976)

Rapid Micromethod for Blood Lead Analysis by Anodic Stripping Voltammetry

George Morrell and Giri Giridhar[1]

We describe a rapid microscale procedure for blood lead determination by anodic stripping voltammetry. Results correlate well with those obtained by atomic absorption spectroscopy. The procedure involves use of a metal-exchange reagent, which rapidly releases bound lead from its macromolecular binding sites, thus eliminating a long and cumbersome perchloric acid digestion procedure. Reproducibility and analytical recovery of added lead were both excellent. Our results show that anodic stripping voltammetry is a reliable, sensitive micromethod for routine determination of blood lead.

Additional Keyphrases: *trace metals* • *screening* • *comparison with atomic absorption spectroscopy*

Anodic stripping voltammetry with use of a composite mercury/graphite electrode is recognized as a sensitive technique for analyses of lead and other trace metals (*1–4*). Perchloric acid has been used (*3, 4*) to first digest blood samples, to liberate lead bound to erythrocytes. Results correlate well with those obtained by atomic absorption spectroscopy (*5*).

We describe a rapid, simplified procedure of this kind for blood lead, in which the digestion step has been eliminated. A metal-exchange reagent is used instead, which lyses the erythrocytes, releases bound lead from intracellular binding sites, and prevents any rebinding. With this procedure, blood lead can be determined routinely with excellent reproducibility.

Materials and Methods

Instrumentation

Trace Metals Analyzer, Model 3010 (Environmental Science Associates, Burlington, Mass. 01803).

Atomic Absorption Spectrophotometer, Model 5A (Varian Techtron, Palo Alto, Calif. 94303).

Pipets and tips (Scientific Manufacturing Industries, purchased from Scientific Products, Edison, N.J. 08817).

Sonifer, Model W185 (Heat Systems, Ultrasonics, Inc., Plainview, L.I., N.Y.).

Reagents

Lead stock standard, 1 g/liter (Fisher Scientific Co., Fair Lawn, N.J. 07410).

"Triton X-100" surfactant, 50 g/liter (Sigma Chemical Co., St. Louis, Mo. 63178).

Methyl isobutyl ketone (J.T. Baker Chemical Co., Phillipsburg, N.J. 08865).

"Metexchange" reagent (Environmental Science Associates, Burlington, Mass. 01803). This reagent consists of chromium chloride hexahydrate, 10.7 g/kg, calcium acetate monohydrate, 14.30 g/kg, and mercuric ions (Hg^{2+}), 28 mg/kg.

Lead control solution: low (50 μg/liter) and high (1030 μg/liter) controls (Environmental Science Associates).

"TOX-EL" (A. R. Smith Co.), lyophilized blood lead control, 650 μg/liter (purchased from Fisher Scientific Co.).

Procedure

The Analyzer was operated with the following settings: Initial potential, −1090 mV; final potential, −200 mV; sweep rate, 14.00 mV/stp; recorder set point, −700 mv; integration set point, −515 mV.

The instrument was calibrated with the low and high control. Once the instrument is calibrated, 30 to 40 lead samples can be assayed per hour.

We used only heparinized blood samples in this study. All samples were sonicated routinely for about 15 s to break up any small clots that might have been present, and 100 μl was then transferred with an SMI pipet to 2.9 ml of the Metexchange reagent in a cell. The cell contents were mixed and the cell was placed in the cell holder. Lead is plated initially, then stripped. The current generated during this stripping

Center for Laboratory Medicine, 16 Pearl St., Metuchen, N. J. 08840.

[1] Address all communications to G.G.

Received Aug. 29, 1975; accepted Nov. 19, 1975.

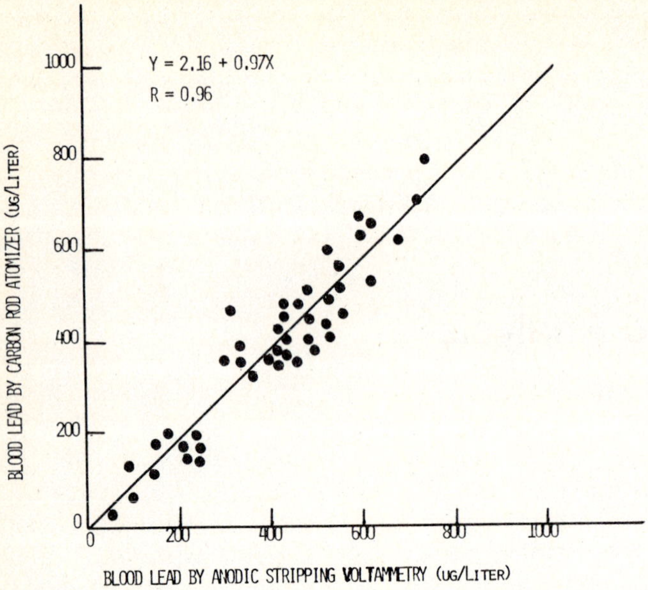

Fig. 1. Comparison of results by the present method and by use of the carbon rod atomizer

Table 1. Comparison of Our Values with Those from Center for Disease Control Lead Survey, 1975

Reference lab mean	Acceptable range	ASV[a]
	μg/liter	
580	493–667	540
164	104–224	170
346	286–406	400
435	370–500	372
300	248–368	288
140	84–204	105
736	626–846	818
453	385–521	470
315	255–375	347.5

[a] anodic stripping voltammetry

Table 2. Analytical Recovery of Lead Added to Pooled Blood as Lead Nitrate

Lead added	Expected	Found		Recovered, %
		Av	(range)	
	μg/liter			
0	—	170	(150–190)	—
100	270	270	(260–280)	100
200	370	380	(380–380)	105.0
300	470	450	(440–460)	93.3
350	520	540	(530–560)	105.7
400	570	580	(580–580)	102.5
500	670	640	(630–660)	94.0
600	770	780	(770–800)	101.6
700	870	850	(850–850)	97.1

Table 3. Values Obtained on Diluting High-Lead Control Sample with Pooled Blood

Sample	Dilutions	n	Expected	Found	
				Av	(range)
			μg/liter		
TOX-EL (control)	—	5	—	640	(630–650)
Pooled blood	—	5	—	250	(250–260)
TOX-EL + pooled blood	1 + 1	5	450	410	(400–420)
TOX-EL + pooled blood	1 + 2	5	380	340	(320–350)
TOX-EL + pooled blood	1 + 3	5	350	330	(320–350)

Table 4. Reproducibility of Blood Lead Values, for Various Concentrations of Lead in 10 Samples of Blood

n	Mean	SD	CV, %
	μg/liter		
	Within-run		
10	340	26	7.8
9	620	24	3.8
13	110	28	25.0
10	690	21	3.1
	Day-to-day (during three weeks)		
14	700	25	3.6
16	350	27	7.6
14	640	24	3.8
14	550	18	3.2
14	1030	18	1.7
14	580	18	3.1

phase is displayed in the read-out display in terms of micrograms per deciliter. For control purposes, every 10th sample analyzed was a TOX-EL control. The results are expressed as the mean of triplicate analyses.

For analysis of blood lead by use of the carbon rod atomizer, we used the following procedure: To a series of polypropylene tubes, 1.0 ml of unknown, control, or standards was added. To each tube was added 0.5 ml of ammonium pyrrolidone dithiocarbamate solution (20 g/liter in the Triton X-100 solution). All tubes were vortex-mixed, and allowed to stand for 10 min. To all tubes, 2 ml of methylisobutyl ketone was added and the capped tubes were rotated on a rotary mixer for 15 min. The tubes were centrifuged for 10 min and 2 μl of the supernate was injected onto the carbon rod. Settings for the atomic absorption spectrophotometer for determination of lead with use of the carbon rod atomizer were: wavelength, 217 nm; spectral bandwidth, 0.6 nm; hollow-cathode lamp, 6 mA; dry, 25 s at 5.0 V; ash, 25 s at 5.0 V; atomize, 2.8

s at 3.0 V. Absorbance peaks were recorded with a strip-chart recorder for both the standards and unknown specimens, and values for the unknown samples were determined from a standard curve prepared by the method of addition.

Results and Discussion

Heparinized blood specimens from 46 patients, selected without conscious bias, from samples we received for blood lead analyses, were assayed both by use of the carbon rod atomizer (*6*) and by anodic stripping voltammetry. The correlation coefficient for the two results was 0.96 (Figure 1).

Table 1 compares results from recent Center for Disease Control blood lead surveys, those obtained by the ASV method vs. the reference laboratory's values—which were obtained by the Delves cup procedure (*7*) or Hessel's procedure (*5*)—and conventional anodic stripping voltammetry (*3, 4*).

Analytical recovery was assessed by adding a known amount of lead nitrate to pooled blood and analyzing for lead. The average recovery of added lead (100 to 700 μg/liter) was 99.9%, with a range of 93.3–105.7% (Table 2). Recoveries of lead nitrate added to individual blood samples (n = 5) were all between 93 and 109%.

As part of the recovery studies, TOX-EL control was diluted one-, two-, and threefold with pooled blood and analyzed. Table 3 shows the results. All values obtained were within ±40 μg/liter of that expected.

Chemical interference was studied by adding various cations and anions to pooled blood. Sodium (200 mmol/liter), potassium (40 mmol/liter), iron (5.0 mg/liter), calcium (5 mmol/liter), magnesium (10 mmol/liter), copper (1.5 mg/liter), chloride (150 mmol/liter), phosphate (50 mg/liter), bicarbonate (30 mmol/liter), and zinc (5.0 mg/liter) were added to pooled blood. We observed no significant interferences by any of these ions in the analyses for blood lead.

Table 4 shows analytical precision for various concentrations of blood lead, within-run and day-to-day. The blood samples were refrigerated for this study, but the samples were homogenized by sonication each day before analyses were performed. Blood lead values in some specimens remained unchanged for as long as six weeks at 4 °C; in others the blood lead values decreased after about a week.

Based on these results as well as the good correlation between anodic stripping voltammetry and other atomic absorption methods (*8–10*), both micro- and macro-scale, shows the anodic stripping voltammetry procedure to be sensitive and specific. Its major advantages are its sensitivity, ease of operation, cost of the instrument, and analysis time. Because there is no sample preparation as in the macro procedure (*5*) or as in the perchloric acid digestion procedure (*3, 4*), loss attributable to sample preparation or contamination is eliminated.

Our procedure requires 100 μl vs. 10 μl for the Delves cup technique, but collection of a 100-μl sample is no more troublesome than collection of a 10-μl sample, and sampling precision is perhaps greater.

The skill required in operating and assaying for blood lead is about the same as that required in the assay of any micro-scale sampling technique. The routine maintenance of the instrument is also fairly simple. Reproducibility was excellent with SMI 100-μl pipets.

We conclude that blood lead can be accurately determined by anodic stripping voltammetry.

References

1. Matson, W. R., Roe, D. K., and Carritt, D. E., Composite mercury graphite electrode for anodic stripping analysis. *Anal. Chem.* **37,** 1594 (1965).

2. Matson, W. R., and Roe, D. K., Trace metal analyses of natural media by anodic stripping voltammetry. *Anal. Instrum.* **4,** 19 (1967).

3. Searle, B., Chan, W., and Davidow, B., Determination of lead in blood and urine by anodic stripping voltammetry. *Clin. Chem.* **19,** 76 (1973).

4. Matson, W. R., Griffin, R. M., and Schreiber, G. B., Rapid subnanogram simultaneous analysis of zinc, cadmium, lead, copper, bismuth and thalium. In *Trace Substances in Environmental Health IV,* Univ. of Missouri, Columbia, Mo., D. Hemphill, Ed., 1971, pp 396–406.

5. Hessel, D. W., A simple and rapid quantitative determination of lead in blood. *At. Absorpt. Newsl.* **1,** 55 (1968).

6. Kubasik, N. P., and Volosin, M. T., Use of carbon rod atomizer for direct analysis of lead in blood. *Clin. Chem.* **20,** 300 (1974).

7. Delves, H. T., A micro sampling method for the rapid determination of lead in blood by atomic absorption spectrophotometry. *Analyst* (London) **95,** 431 (1970).

8. Elser, R. C., Savory, J., and Mushak, P., Measurement of lead in blood by atomic absorption spectrometry. *Clin. Chem.* **15,** 188 (1969).

9. Christian, G. D., and Feldman, F. J., *Atomic Absorption Spectroscopy. Applications in Agriculture, Biology and Medicine.* Wiley-Interscience, New York, N.Y., 1970, pp 407–413.

10. Fernandez, F. J., Micromethod for lead determination in whole blood by atomic absorption with the use of graphite furnace. *Clin. Chem.* **21,** 558 (1975).

CLIN. CHEM. 22/2, 224–226 (1976)

Cholesterol in Amniotic Fluid, Determined by Gas Chromatography

Valerie M. Jones Owen, Frank K. Ho, Angelo Mazzuchin,[1] Terence A. Doran, Seigren Liedgren,[2] and C. John Porter[3]

Cholesterol was extracted from amniotic fluid, saponified, converted to its trimethylsilyl derivative, and gas chromatographed, with cholesteryl acetate as the internal standard. The method is sufficiently accurate and precise for use with the range of concentrations of cholesterol found in amniotic fluid (5 to 46 mg/litre). Total cholesterol was measured in amniotic fluids collected at different stages of gestation. No significant trend or change was observed nor was cholesterol in the amniotic fluid and the mother's serum correlated at any stage of gestation. Thus we conclude that cholesterol is not a useful indicator of fetal age or maturity. Cholesterol concentrations in amniotic fluid from complicated pregnancies were within the range found for normal pregnancies.

Additional Keyphrases: *indexes to fetal maturity • cholesterol in serum • gas chromatography and continuous-flow analysis compared*

The technique of amniocentesis has greatly increased the feasibility of sampling amniotic fluid at different stages of gestation, for use in assessing fetal maturity and status. Of the many chemical constituents investigated, creatinine and lecithin in amniotic fluid have been shown to be useful indicators of fetal maturity (*1, 2*). We decided to measure cholesterol in amniotic fluid and see if this measurement has any clinical significance and application.

Wolf et al. (*3*) and Fennefrohn (*4*) reported that the cholesterol concentration did not change significantly throughout gestation, but it is difficult to see how they measured the cholesterol with precision, because they both used AutoAnalyzer SMA (Technicon) systems but neither reported any modification of the method to allow for the fact that the cholesterol concentration in amniotic fluid is only about one hundredth that in normal serum. Because the usual methods for estimation of serum cholesterol are not appropriate for use with small volumes of amniotic fluid, we developed a gas-chromatographic method for the determination of total cholesterol, and assessed its precision and accuracy.

We then measured cholesterol in amniotic fluid, to see if there is any correlation with other variables such as fetal age or the mother's serum cholesterol concentration.

Amniotic Fluid Study Office 4th Floor, Norman Urquhart Wing, Toronto General Hospital, 101 College St., Toronto, Ontario, M5G 1L7 Canada.

[1] Present address: Laurentian Hospital, Sudbury, Ontario, Canada.

[2] Present address: Ripgatan 20, Linkoping, Sweden.

[3] Present address: Department of Clinical Biochemistry, Toronto General Hospital, Toronto, Ontario, M5G 1L7, Canada.

Received April 1, 1975; accepted Nov. 20, 1975.

Materials and Methods

Samples

Amniotic fluid was obtained by amniocentesis, at cesarian section, by hysterotomy or amniotomy. After centrifugation, those samples that could not be analyzed immediately were frozen. The mother's blood was sampled at the same time as the amniotic fluid, and the serum was analyzed.

Reagents

Cholesterol stock standard. About 25 mg of cholesterol (Fisher Scientific Co., Certified Reagent) was weighed out accurately and diluted to 200 ml with chloroform. Stored refrigerated, this solution can be used for as long as a month.

Cholesteryl acetate standard. This compound was prepared by dissolving cholesterol in anhydrous pyridine and adding anhydrous acetic anhydride.

The solution was refluxed for 30 min, cooled, and water added until white crystals precipitated. The crystals were collected by filtration, recrystallized from ethyl acetate, and dried. Cholesteryl acetate standard was prepared to contain 10 mg of cholesteryl acetate per 100 mg of dry pyridine. The solution can be stored in a fume hood for as long as one month. We also used cholesteryl acetate "Standard for Chromatography" obtained from Sigma Chemical Co., St. Louis, Mo. 63178.

Cholesterol palmitate standard. About 15 mg of cholesterol palmitate (Sigma Chemical Co., "Standard for Chromatography") was weighed out accurately and diluted to 100 ml with chloroform.

Hexamethyldisilane and trimethylchlorosilane were obtained from Sigma Chemical Co.

Pyridine "Spectro grade" was obtained from Eastman Kodak Co., Rochester, N. Y. 14650.

n-*Hexane* was laboratory-reagent grade, from BDH Chemicals, Toronto, Canada.

KOH in ethanol. Ten grams of "Certified Reagent" (Fisher Scientific Co., Montreal, Canada) was dissolved in 20 ml of distilled water and 6 ml of this was diluted to 100 ml with ethanol immediately before use.

Equipment

We used an F and M Scientific 402 High Efficiency Gas Chromatograph with a hydrogen flame-ionization detector (Hewlett-Packard, Avondale, Pa. 19311). The 150-cm column was packed with 3% OV-17 on Gas Chrom Q, 100–120 mesh (Chromatographic Supply, Brockville, Ontario, Canada). The oven temperature was 280 °C, and the carrier gas was helium.

Methods

Cholesterol standards were prepared by pipetting 0.1-, 0.2-, and 0.3-ml aliquots of cholesterol stock standard into test tubes and evaporating under nitrogen. Then 1 ml of a saline solution (NaCl, 8.5 g/litre) was added to each tube.

To 1 ml of either amniotic fluid or the cholesterol standard in saline was added 5 ml of ethanolic KOH and the tube contents were vortex-mixed for 15 s and incubated at 37 °C for 90 min. After the mixture had cooled to room temperature, 10 ml of *n*-hexane was added.

The tubes were vortex-mixed for 1 min and the layers allowed to separate. Seven milliliters of the hexane (upper) layer was removed and evaporated in a stream of air at room temperature. To the residue were added 0.5 ml of cholesteryl acetate in pyridine, 0.2 ml of hexamethyldisilane, and 0.1 ml of trimethylchlorosilane; the tubes were vortex-mixed for 1 min, and the mixture was allowed to stand for 15 min at room temperature. Then we injected 2 μl into the gas chromatograph and measured the heights of the peaks corresponding to the internal standard, cholesteryl acetate, and the trimethylsilyl derivative of cholesterol. A calibration curve was prepared by plotting the cholesterol concentration in the standard vs. the height of the trimethylsilyl-cholesterol peak, divided by the height of the cholesteryl acetate peak. The use of the internal standard corrected for mechanical loss of the sample during preparation and variation in the amount injected into the gas chromatograph.

Maternal serum. The cholesterol concentration in the mother's serum was estimated with the AutoAnalyzer (*5*).

Analytical Variables

Recovery studies. The analytical recovery of cholesterol esters was checked by adding known amounts of cholesterol palmitate to amniotic fluid and estimating the amount of cholesterol in the sample before and after the addition.

Precision. Precision was investigated by analyzing one pool of amniotic fluid 20 times during four days. Also duplicate samples of amniotic fluid were analyzed during several weeks. The duplicates were sometimes run on the same day, sometimes on separate occasions.

Correlation studies. Serum samples were analyzed by using an AutoAnalyzer (*5*). The same serum samples were diluted 100-fold with a saline solution (NaCl, 8.5 g/litre), and analyzed by the gas-chromatographic method. The results obtained by gas chromatography were multipled by 100 and compared with those obtained on the AutoAnalyzer.

Table 1. Analytical Recovery of Cholesterol Added to Amniotic Fluid (as Cholesterol Palmitate)

Cholesterol, Added	Cholesterol, Found	Recovery, %
mg/litre		
0.0	6.8	
8.6	15.4	100.0
17.2	23.2	95.3
25.8	31.1	94.2
34.4	39.9	96.3
		97

Results

The calibration curve was linear up to at least 500 mg of cholesterol per litre.

Table 1 shows that, on average, 97% of the cholesterol added to amniotic fluid in the form of cholesterol palmitate could be analytically accounted for. These results were obtained for cholesterol at the concentrations found in amniotic fluid.

For the pool of amniotic fluid analyzed 20 times, a mean value of 17.3 mg/litre was obtained (SD, 1.2; CV, 7.11%). The SD for the results obtained on the duplicate estimation of 68 samples was 1.6 mg/litre. Comparison of the results of the AutoAnalyzer method (x) with the gas-chromatographic method (y) showed the following results: $y = 1.14x - 191.2$, correlation coefficient = 0.99 (n = 22). The serum samples used were in the range 1000 to 4000 mg/litre.

Table 2 gives the results of the analysis of cholesterol in amniotic fluid collected at different times during gestation. The results for any given time were not normally distributed, being skewed toward the low side. The number of samples collected before 30 weeks of gestation was small and therefore not appropriate for meaningful statistical comparison. The number of samples collected after 30 weeks was greater and the results were compared statistically. The mean value increased after the 31st week of gestation, but not statistically significantly, except for the mean at 31 weeks, which was significantly (P = 0.05) lower than the means obtained later in gestation.

Table 2 shows the distribution of the results for cholesterol in the maternal serum throughout gestation; values are about 100-fold those for amniotic

Table 2. Amniotic Fluid and Maternal Serum Cholesterol Concentrations

Estimated week of gestation	15	19	22	25	28	31	34	37	40	44
Range, weeks	12 to 17.9	18 to 20.9	21 to 23.9	24 to 26.9	27 to 29.9	30 to 32.9	33 to 35.9	36 to 38.9	39 to 41.9	42 and over
Amniotic fluid cholesterol, mg/litre										
n	3	3	—	1	4	8	16	23	33	8
Mean	16.5	12.3	—	34	25.4	9.2	14.4	13.8	16.6	20.5
Standard error of mean	0.85	0.54	—	—	3.54	1.16	2.15	1.43	1.45	2.66
Range	14 to 18	11 to 13	—	—	16 to 36	5 to 11	6 to 34	7 to 28	7 to 46	11 to 38
Maternal serum cholesterol, mg/litre										
n	21	55	8	22	22	18	47	50	80	24
Mean	2032	2164	2576	2573	2577	2571	2430	2467	2513	2428
Standard deviation	302	367	369	398	440	613	525	513	448	382

fluid. We examined the ratio for cholesterol in serum and amniotic fluid for each case in which we had both of these data, but found no correlation at any time of gestation.

We measured cholesterol in amniotic fluid from 28 pregnancies complicated by abnormalities such as hypertension, diabetes, rhesus sensitization, hydramnios, or interuterine growth retardation. Our results were within the range found in normal pregnancies.

In one case, which was excluded from the statistical analysis, the amniotic fluid cholesterol concentration was 139 mg/litre. The corresponding value for serum was 2720 mg/litre, which was within the usual range during pregnancy. No abnormalities were noted in this pregnancy, which was in the 42nd week of gestation when the amniotic fluid was collected. In eight other similar post-mature pregnancies, the mean amniotic fluid cholesterol was 20.5 mg/litre, ranging up to 38 mg/litre.

Discussion

This gas-chromatographic method for estimating cholesterol has been shown to be appropriate for use with amniotic fluid. Our analytical recoveries of a cholesterol ester, cholesterol palmitate, were good at the concentrations of total cholesterol found in amniotic fluid. Serum and serum dilutions were used to show that results of this method are similar to those obtained with a continuous-flow system. Some of the variation in the results obtained on duplicate analysis may be due to the presence of vernix in samples taken late in gestation. The vernix is difficult to separate by centrifugation, and small particles may be inadvertently included in the sample for analysis. Vernix is rich in cholesterol.

We agree with Wolf et al. (*3*) and Fennefrohn (*4*) that the cholesterol concentration in amniotic fluid is not significantly correlated with gestational age. For some stages of gestation the number of cases was small; differences in the means may well have been of greater statistical significance if more cases had been studied, but it is apparent from this limited study that there is a wide overlap in the values for cholesterol in amniotic fluid collected at different stages of gestation. We conclude that cholesterol is not a useful indicator of fetal age or maturity.

The concentration of cholesterol in the maternal serum was 100-fold that in amniotic fluid, an extreme difference that has not been seen in other components of amniotic fluid, such as protein, that we have studied (*6*). The lack of correlation between values for maternal serum cholesterol and amniotic fluid cholesterol suggests that there is no equilibrium or free exchange between the maternal serum and the amniotic fluid cholesterol. Robertson and Sprecher (*7*) report that in guinea pigs the proportion of the fetal serum cholesterol of maternal origin can vary with the mother's diet, but that concentrations of circulating cholesterol in the fetus remain the same whether the mother's diet is cholesterol free or rich in cholesterol. In rats, during early gestation fetal cholesterol is of maternal origin; later, the fetus synthesizes its own cholesterol (*8*).

This work was supported by Ontario Provincial Health Research Grant No. PR 279.

References

1. Doran, T. A., Benzie, R. J., Harkins, J. L., et al., Amniotic fluid tests for fetal maturity. *Am. J. Obstet. Gynecol.* **119,** 829 (1974).

2. Bhagwanani, S. G., Fahmy, D., and Turnbull, A. C., Prediction of neonatal respiratory failure by estimation of amniotic fluid lecithin. *Lancet* **i**, 159 (1972).

3. Wolf, P. L., Block, D., and Tsudaks, T., Biochemical profile of amniotic fluid to assess fetal maturity. *Clin. Chem.* **16,** 843 (1970).

4. Fennefrohn, B. Z., Fruchtwasseruntersuchungen in den letzten Schwangerschaftswochen. *Z. Geburtshilfe Perinatol.* **176,** 233 (1972).

5. Technicon AutoAnalyzer Methodology N24-a, Technicon Instruments Corp., Tarrytown, N. Y. 10591.

6. Benzie, R. J., Doran, T. A., Harkins, J. L., et al., Composition of the amniotic fluid and maternal serum in pregnancy. *Am. J. Obstet. Gynecol.* **119,** 798 (1974).

7. Robertson, A. F., and Sprecher, M., A review of human placental lipid metabolism and transport. *Acta Paediatr. Scand., Suppl.* 183 (1968).

8. Chevallier, F., Transferts et synthese du cholesterol chez le rat au cours de sa croissance. *Biochim. Biophys. Acta* **84,** 316 (1964).

CLIN. CHEM. 22/2, 227-231 (1976)

High-Performance Colorimeter with an Electronic Bubble Gate for Use in Miniaturized Continuous-Flow Analyzers

William E. Neeley,[1] Stephen C. Wardlaw,[4] Tad Yates,[2]
William G. Hollingsworth,[1] and Maurice E. T. Swinnen[3]

We describe a high-performance colorimeter with an electronic bubble gate for use with miniaturized continuous-flow analyzers. The colorimeter has a flow-through cuvette with optically flat quartz windows that allows a bubbled stream to pass freely without any breakup or retention of bubbles. The fluid volume in the light path is only 1.8 μl. The electronic bubble gate selectively removes that portion of the photodetector signal produced by the air bubbles passing through the flow cell and allows that portion of the signal attributable to the fluid segment to pass to the recorder. The colorimeter is easy to use, rugged, inexpensive, and requires minimal adjustments.

Numerous colorimeters and spectrophotometers are commercially available for use with continuous-flow analyzers; most of them are expensive, fragile, bulky, require excessive quantities of fluid, and do not have flow-through cuvettes adequate for the passage of a bubbled stream.

Wishing to construct an efficient, low-cost miniaturized high-speed continuous-flow system (*1*), we found it essential to design and develop a high-performance colorimeter. Our prime considerations in the colorimeter design were:

1. It must be capable of accurate and precise transmittance measurements.

2. The photodetectors and associated circuitry must be highly stable, sensitive, and respond linearly to low light intensities.

3. The flow-through cuvette must employ optically flate quartz windows that allow a bubbled stream to pass without any breakup or retention of the bubbles.

4. An electronic bubble gating system must selectively remove that portion of the photodetector signal caused by the air bubbles passing through the flow cell and allow that portion of the signal from the fluid segment to pass to the recorder.

5. It must be of low cost, easy to use, rugged, require minimal quantities of raw materials, and have minimal adjustments.

Here we describe the design and construction of such a colorimeter.

Colorimeter Construction[5]

General description. Figure 1, a simplified block diagram of the colorimeter, illustrates the main components. The light source is a high-intensity quartz halogen lamp. The light passes from the lamp through an interference filter, a biconvex lens, a flow-through cuvette, and then reaches the photodetector. The photodetector signal is amplified and enters the electronic bubble gate. The electronic bubble gate eliminates that portion of the signal produced by the bubble artifact and allows the signal from the transmittance of the fluid segments to pass to the strip-chart recorder.

The optical feedback (optical servo) system, which continually monitors and controls the lamp intensity, increases stability. The light passes through an aperture and an interference filter to a photodetector. The photodetector signal is amplified and enters the light-regulation circuit that controls the current to

Divisions of Biochemistry,[1] Instrumentation,[2] and Neuropsychiatry,[3] Walter Reed Army Institute of Research, Washington, D. C. 20012; and the Department of Laboratory Medicine, Yale–New Haven Hospital, New Haven, Conn. 06510.[4]

Reference to products by manufacturer does not constitute endorsement by any government agency and is included only for purpose of description.

Received Oct. 1, 1975; accepted Nov. 21, 1975.

[5] Xerographic copies of the colorimeter components, detailed parts listing, and printed circuit board layouts may be obtained on specific request to either the authors or the Editorial Office.

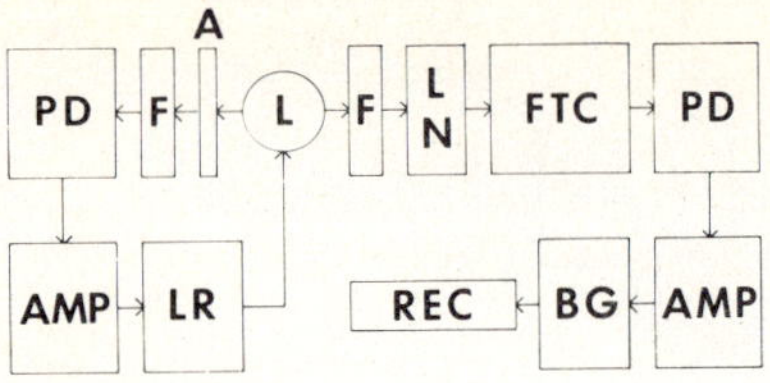

Fig. 1. Block diagram of colorimeter
L = lamp, *F* = interference filter, *LN* = lens, *FTC* = flow-through cuvette, *PD* = photodetector, *AMP* = amplifier, *BG* = electronic bubble gate, *REC* = recorder, *A* = aperture, and *LR* = light regulation circuit

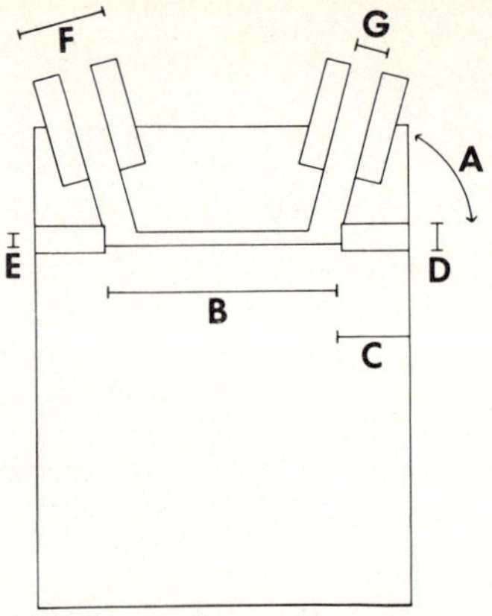

Fig. 2. Cross section of flow-through cuvette
A = 66° 17′ angle from horizontal, *B* = 8 mm (light pathlength), *E* = 0.5 mm (diameter of light path), *C* = 6.35 mm (length of quartz rod), *D* = 1.0 mm (diameter of quartz rod), *G* = 0.79 mm (internal diameter of fluid inlet), *F* = 2.39 mm (external diameter of fluid inlet)

the lamp. A quartz halogen lamp is used because of its high intensity and relatively low power consumption. As noted by Hewitt and Pardue (2), the high-intensity lamp provides a high signal/noise ratio and minimizes the independent and proportional errors in absorbance measurements.

Interference filters. The interference filters (1.3 × 1.3 cm, approximately 0.5 cm thick) are inexpensive (about $4.05 in lots of 20) and have excellent blocking properties in the near-infrared region as required when silicon P.I.N. photodiode detectors are used (Ditric Optics, Inc., Valencia, Calif. 91355).

Lens. In place of an expensive and complicated lens system, excellent results are obtained by the use of a simple biconvex lens ($1.50 each; A. Jaegers, Inc., Lynbrook, N.Y. 11563). The lens holder is a very simple design, yet precise adjustments are easy. The lens is mounted in a holder and a small spring applies upward pressure. Two small adjustment screws are used to position the lens precisely. By adjusting each of the two screws with an adjustment tool, the lens can be easily moved over a small circular area to provide optimal alignment. To align the lens, the flow-through cuvette is filled with water and the adjustment screws are rotated until the voltage output of the photodetector amplifier (Figure 3, *IC2*, pin 6) is maximum. At this point a maximum amount of light is passing through the flow-through cuvette. If at a particular wavelength the light intensity is too great the lens may be slightly defocused to decrease it.

Flow-through cuvette. The flow-through cuvette is constructed from a polyvinyl chloride or Kel-F block. Polyvinyl chloride is satisfactory for most reagents used in the clinical chemistry laboratory and is used in most cases because it is easily machined and inexpensive. A jig was first designed and the flow-through cuvette was constructed in clear acrylic to assure correct internal design. The jig was then used to manufacture the actual flow-through cuvettes in opaque polyvinyl chloride blocks. A cross section of the flow-through cuvette is diagrammatically illustrated in Figure 2. The light path (*B*) is 0.8 cm long and 0.5 mm in diameter (*E*). The volume in the light path is only 1.8 μl. The inlet ports are 0.79 mm in internal diameter (*G*) and approach the horizontal path from an angle of 66° 17′ (*A*). Quartz rods with flat, polished ends (Honde Glass Co., Newark, N.J. 07104) measuring 0.635 cm in length (*C*) and 0.10 cm in diameter (*D*), are press-fitted in the block to provide optically clear windows. Adhesive is not applied to the rods, because it can easily coat the inner face and thus partially block the transmitted light. The great advantage of this flow-through cuvette is that a large amount of light passes through the flow cell because of the quartz windows. Unlike flow cells constructed from bent glass tubing, there is no light reaching the detector through the glass tubing walls. In earlier designs, a major problem arose: small bubble fragments would break off from the larger bubbles and would attach to the interface between the glass ends and the plastic body. In the present design this does not occur. By allowing the quartz rod on each end to protrude slightly into the flow path, a slight turbulence is created as the solution enters the light path over the edge of the quartz rod. This greatly aids in "cleansing" the quartz rod face and prevents bubble entrapment. At the distal end of the light path, the increased fluid velocity and the tendency for bubbles to float upwards aids in preventing bubble entrapment. Alternatively, one can substitute a commercially available flow-cell that is used on the SMAC analyzer (cat. No. 178-B724-02; Technicon Instruments Corp., Tarrytown, N.Y. 10591).

Photodetectors. A silicon P.I.N. photodiode is the photodetector. Used for measurements between 430 and 1000 nm, its advantages are small size, low noise, low cost, long-term stability, linearity over wide ranges of incident light, ruggedness, and low voltage operation (5–15 V d.c.). The particular photodetector we used ($6.25 each) is guaranteed for 10 years by the manufacturer (Monsanto Commercial Products, Cupertino, Calif. 95014). In contrast, photomultipliers are expensive, temperature-sensitive, require high-voltage supplies (1100 V d.c.), extensive and expensive shielding, and complicated electronic circuits, and are easily damaged by excess light.

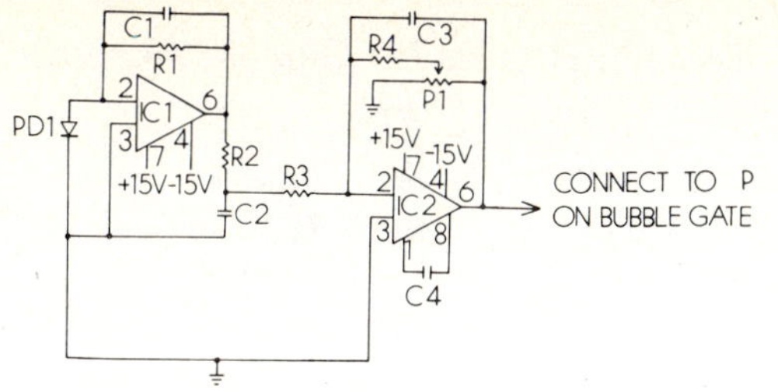

Fig. 3. Photodetector circuit

IC1, FET operational amplifier; *IC2,* operational amplifier; *PD1,* silicon *PIN* photodiode; *C1–4,* disc capacitors; *R1–4,* resistors; *P1,* precision potentiometer, 10-turn

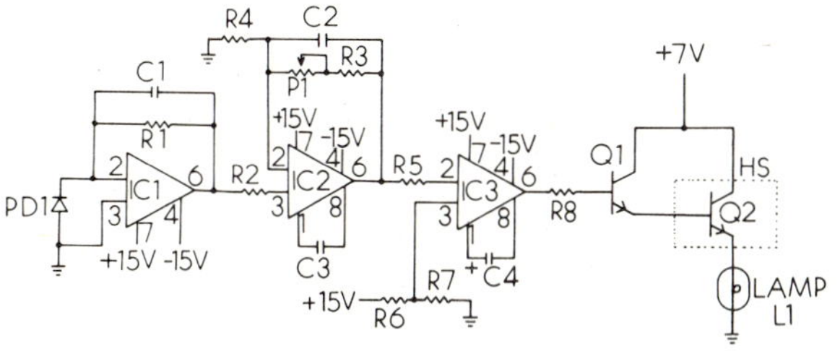

Fig. 4. Light-regulation circuit

IC1, FET operational amplifier; *IC2,3,* operational amplifiers; *Q1,2, NPN* power transistors; *C1–3,* disc capacitors; *C4,* electrolytic capacitor; *R1–8,* resistors; *P1,* trim potentiometer, 10-turn; *HS,* heat sink

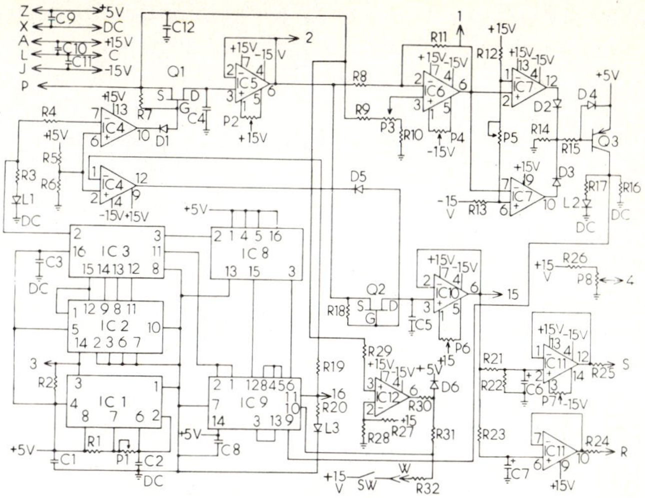

Fig. 5. Electronic bubble gate circuit

Digital commons (d.c.) are specifically indicated; the remaining commons are analog (*C*). Points *A,J,L,P,R,S,W,X,Z,1,2,3,4,15,* and *16* refer to specific contacts on our printed circuit board

IC 1, clock; *IC 2,* decade counter; *IC 3,* BCD-to-decimal decoder; *IC 5,10,* FET operational amplifiers; *IC 6,12,* operational amplifiers; *IC 8,* dual *J-K* flip flop; *IC 9,* quad NAND gate; *Q 1,2,* field effect transistors; *Q 3,* PNP transistor; *L 1–3,* light emitting diodes; *P 1–8,* trim potentiometers, 10-turn; *C 1,2,3,8,9,10,11,* disc capacitors; *C 4,5,* mylar capacitors; *C 6,7,* electrolytic capacitors; *C 12,* tantalum capacitor; *D 1–6,* silicon diodes; *R 1–32,* resistors

The photodiode (*PD1*) is connected to an operational amplifier (*IC1*) with a field-effect transistor input to provide high input impedance (Figure 3). The operational amplifier serves as a current-to-voltage converter. As contrasted with most other photodetectors, the P.I.N. photodiode is operated without bias. This is the correct method of operation in this application, as it ensures zero dark current. Used in this fashion, the diodes are linear over a range of almost twelve decades. The value of the feedback resistor (*R1*) ranges from 200 to 1000 MΩ (Victoreen Instrument Division, Cleveland, Ohio 44104). At low wavelengths (430–540 nm) a 1000-MΩ resistor is used; for higher wavelengths, a 200-MΩ resistor. Capacitor *C1,* used to reduce high-frequency noise, should be carefully selected, because too small a value will result in excessive noise and too large a value will result in a low slew rate, which precludes proper operation of the electronic bubble gate. *PD1, IC1, R1,* and *C1* must be electronically shielded. Power-supply bypass disc capacitors are used (not shown) in close proximity to each operational amplifier. The second operational amplifier (*IC2*) inverts and amplifies the analog signal to provide the necessary 0–8 V input range required by the electronic bubble gate. *P1* is used to adjust the photodetector signal to approximately 8 V for 100% T.

Light-regulation circuit. The light-regulation circuit is based on the earlier work of Pardue et al. (*3, 4*), in which optical feedback was used to stabilize their photometers. The photodetector circuit constantly monitors the lamp output, and if any change in light intensity is detected, the current supply to the lamp is proportionally decreased or increased, resulting in a very nearly constant lamp intensity. Light striking the photodiode *PD1* (Figure 4) produces a small current, which is converted to a voltage by the high-impedance operational amplifier (*IC1*). *IC2* further amplifies the signal and provides an adjustment for the gain. A third operational amplifier (*IC3*) serves as a voltage comparator and controls the base current of transistor *Q1,* which in turn controls the power transistor (*Q2*). A large capacitor (*C4*) prevents oscillation. *Q1* and *Q2* form a Darlington circuit with a large current gain. For example, if the lamp intensity should increase slightly, *PD1* senses this increase. With the elevated voltage signal at the inverting input of the comparator (*IC3*) as compared to the fixed voltage at its noninverting input, the output of the comparator will decrease the base current to transistors *Q1* and *Q2.* This then decreases the current to the lamp. If the lamp intensity should decrease slightly below its set level the circuit will respond to increase the lamp current. With a 7-V lamp power supply, the maximum voltage available to the lamp is about 6.3 V. For the light regulation circuit to operate properly, the lamp voltage is adjusted with *P1* to about 5.8 V.

Electronic bubble gate (Figure 5). The first bubble gate (*5*) allowed a bubbled stream to pass through a colorimeter and, by a specific method not mentioned, would interrupt the photodetector signal to the recorder whenever a bubble would pass through the light path. Later, Habig et al. (*6*) eliminated the need for a debubbler by their design and construction of a device called a "bubble-gated flow cell," which monitored flow cell conductance and deactivated the recorder servo motor whenever bubbles passed through the colorimeter flow cell. They concluded that as a result of the bubble gate system, efficiency was significantly increased but that their particular design, although useful for testing the method, would not withstand daily technician use and abuse. Neeley et al. (*7*) recently described a new, rugged, electronic bubble gate (signal comparator) that would eliminate the bubble artifact from the photodetector signal while allowing the signal produced from the fluid segment to remain intact. This instrument is reliable, easy to use, presently in routine use in a hospital laboratory, and does not require any adjustments by the technician.

Our new electronic bubble gate is based on the principles and logic described in our earlier article (*7*). This electronic bubble gate has been improved by the addition of several newly designed electronic components that provide greater flexibility and a significant reduction in overall cost.

The circuit design, printed circuit board layout, photoetching, and assembly is done entirely within our laboratories. The commercial window comparator has been replaced by a newly designed window comparator constructed from two inexpensive operational amplifier chips, a transistor, and a few passive components. The window width (in millivolts) of the window comparator is fully adjustable upward from a minimum of 1 mV. In addition, the window can be symmetric or adjusted over a wide asymmetric range. The three light-emitting diodes incorporated into the circuit provide a quick visual check to verify proper operation of the circuit at any time. The recorder output can be set to any voltage range from 10 mV to 8 V. An optional bias voltage is provided to allow the use of Bristol (AutoAnalyzer) recorders. A separate analog signal of 0–8 V is provided to facilitate interfacing with any on-line data-processing equipment.

Performance

Linearity. Rather than measure the linearity of individual components, a truer estimate of overall performance is to use the colorimeter in several high-speed continuous-flow systems that are performing actual chemical determinations. Several chemical systems were chosen to represent various portions of the operating spectrum of the instrument. Accurate standards that have been verified against National Bureau of Standards materials were used. A Hewlett-Packard 9810A programmable calculator was used on-line with the continuous-flow system to convert voltage to transmittance and then to absorbance (*8*). Several standards were run and a least-squares linear regression was performed on-line and the correlation coefficient obtained (Table 1).

Stability. Stability of the filter photometer depends highly on the wavelength used, because voltage output of the photodetector amplifier is directly related to the emission of the lamp at the particular wavelength and the particular wavelength response of the photodetector. At the longer wavelengths, the high photodetector output combined with the high emission of the tungsten lamp yields a large output signal, whereas at 430 nm the output signal is relatively low because of the combination of low lamp emission and relatively low photodetector sensitivity. Thus, at longer wavelengths there is maximum stability, owing to the large signal, and at low wavelengths there is minimum stability, owing to the small signal. To describe the stability of the photometer, transmittance measurements were made at 660 nm and at 430 nm by allowing a bubbled stream of fluid to pass through the flow-through cuvette. After a 10-min warmup, drift during 1 h was 0.3% T at 660 nm and 0.7% T at 430 nm. This is a negligible drift when one considers that in this time period, 150 samples could have been analyzed on each channel.

Table 1. Results for Glucose Analyses

Analyte	Method	Wavelength, nm	Concn of standards	Correl. coeff., *r*
Carbon dioxide	Cresol red[a]	430	10, 20, 30, & 40 mmol/liter	0.9999
Glucose	Glucose oxidase[b]	510	500, 1000, 1500, 2000, 2500, 3000 mg/liter	1.0000
Glucose	Glucose oxidase[c]	660	500, 1000, 1500, 2000, 2500, 3000 mg/liter	0.9999

[a] Carbon dioxide procedure for SMA systems, Technicon Instrument Corp., Tarrytown, N.Y. 10591
[b] "GOD/PAP (Trinder)", Boehringer Mannheim Corp., New York, N.Y. 10017
[c] "GOD/PERID", Boehringer Mannheim

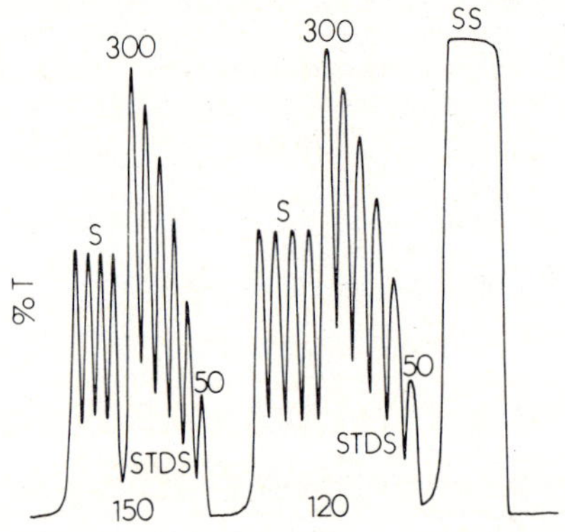

Fig. 6. Glucose analyses at 120 and 150 samples per hour by the Trinder glucose oxidase method

Steady state (*SS*) for 300 mg/100 ml standard. Standards range from 50–300 mg/100 ml, in 50 mg/100 ml increments. Repeated analysis of a single serum sample is shown (*S*)

Evaluation of serum analysis. Figure 6 shows a strip-chart tracing of glucose analyses by the Trinder glucose oxidase method (*9*). At 120 samples per hour the results were: $\bar{x}$ = 1340, SD = ±11 mg/liter, CV = 0.8% (n = 25) and at 150 samples per hour is $\bar{x}$ = 1340, SD = ±1.7 mg/liter, CV = 1.3% (n = 25).

Discussion

We have now expanded the colorimeter from a single channel to four channels by the simple addition of three sets of flow-through cuvettes, interference filters, lens, and photodetectors. These colorimeters are an integral part of our four-channel high-speed continuous-flow systems that are currently performing our routine clinical chemistry determinations. The overall result has been to more than double analysis rates and to decrease reagent consumption by eight- to 10-fold as compared to AutoAnalyzer II or SMA (Technicon) systems. We included on-line programmable calculators to provide automatic calculation and printing of results.[6] The current overall cost is less than $600 for a single-channel colorimeter. In addition to the design and construction of the instruments we are also responsible for their repair. As a result, each colorimeter is totally modular, with great emphasis being placed on ruggedness and simplicity in design. Each four-channel instrument is equipped with its own digital panel meter and a multiposition switch to allow the operator to monitor voltages at strategically located positions throughout the system. Should electronic difficulty develop, it can be accurately diagnosed without extensive test equipment or removal of the surrounding case. Furthermore, all of the circuits are on plug-in printed circuit boards that can be easily and quickly replaced.

[6] Sing, H. C., and Neeley, W. E., Use of programmable desk-top calculator for on-line data acquisition, computing, and printing of results from single and multichannel laboratory instruments. *Clin. Chem.* **20,** 890 (1974). Abstract.

References

1. Neeley, W. E., Wardlaw, S. C., and Sing, H. C., Design and performance of a miniaturized high-speed continuous-flow analyzer. *Clin. Chem.* **20,** 24 (1974).
2. Hewitt, T. W., and Pardue, H. L., Theory of photometric errors applied to the design and evaluation of a high-performance filter photometer. *Clin. Chem.* **21,** 249 (1975).
3. Pardue, H. L., and Rodriguez, P. A., High-stability photometer utilizing optical feedback. *Anal. Chem.* **39,** 901 (1967).
4. Pardue, H. L., and Deming, S. N., High-stability low-noise precision spectrophotometer using optical feedback. *Anal. Chem.* **41,** 986 (1969).
5. Smythe, W. J., and Shamos, M. H., Automated analysis apparatus and method. United States Patent 3,804,593; filed 25 May 1964, granted 16 April 1974; Assignee: Technicon Instruments Corp., Tarrytown, N.Y.
6. Habig, R. L., Schlein, B. W., Walters, L., and Thiers, R. L., A bubble-gating flow cell for continuous flow analysis. *Clin. Chem.* **15,** 1045 (1969).
7. Neeley, W. E., Wardlaw, S. C., and Swinnen, M. E. T., Design and operation of a signal comparator to increase the efficiency of continuous-flow analyzers. *Clin. Chem.* **20,** 78 (1974).
8. Neeley, W. E., and Sing, H. C., Use of a programmable desk top calculator for on-line acquisition, processing, computing, and reporting of data from automated laboratory instruments. *Am. J. Clin. Pathol.* **61,** 804 (1974).
9. Trinder, P., Determination of glucose in blood using glucose oxidase with an alternative oxygen accepter. *Ann. Clin. Biochem.* **6,** 24 (1969).

Improved Assay for Urinary 17-Hydroxycorticosteroids

Yutaka Ariyoshi[1] and Yoshio Osawa[2]

We describe a simple, rapid, reliable method for determining urinary 17-hydroxycorticosteroids. A neutral resin (Amberlite XAD-2), which is a non-ionic cross-linked polystyrene, is used to extract and concentrate the steroids, which are then quantitatively determined with the Porter–Silber reaction. Use of the resin eliminates the need for enzymatic hydrolysis and *n*-butanol extractions, thereby decreasing analysis time considerably; results can be obtained within 3 h of receipt of specimens. Most of the nonsteroidal Porter–Silber chromogens are removed, resulting in a method that is highly specific and sensitive, even at low concentrations (0.6 mg/liter), and so more accurate and reproducible than currently used methods.

Additional Keyphrases: *Porter–Silber reaction • extraction with a resin • pediatric chemistry*

Since Porter and Silber (*1*) reported the specific color reaction of 17,21-dihydroxy-20-ketosteroids with phenylhydrazine and sulfuric acid, many investigators (*2–6*) have adapted it to use with urinary extracts of glucocorticoids purified by their own methods. Osawa and Slaunwhite (*7*) and Chu et al. (*8*) reported the use of Amberlite XAD-2 for the clinical estimation of estrogen conjugates in pregnancy and nonpregnancy urine and Bradlow (*9*) described the extraction of conjugated cortisol metabolites from urine with the resin.

We present here a procedure for clinical determination of 17-hydroxycorticosteroids, in which this resin is used to separate and purify the analyte. It is a simpler, faster, and more reliable method than those currently in use.

Medical Foundation of Buffalo, 73 High St., Buffalo, N. Y. 14203.

[1] Postdoctoral Research Fellow. Present address: Clinical Laboratory, Aichi Cancer Center, Nagoya, Japan.

[2] Address correspondence to this author.

Received Oct. 10, 1975; accepted Nov. 22, 1975.

Material and Methods

Reagents

Neutral resin. Amberlite XAD-2 resin (Rohm and Haas Co., Philadelphia, Pa. 19105), a non-ionic cross-linked polystyrene, is put in a large column and washed successively with three volumes of water, one volume of methanol, and 10 volumes of water. Fine floating particles of resin should be removed by decanting or aspiration. The resin is then stored for use. Alternatively, the washing may be done in the small columns for processing the urine, which may be reused repeatedly after final washing with 15 ml of ethanol and 30 ml of water.

Phenylhydrazine reagent. Dissolve 65 mg of phenylhydrazine hydrochloride (recrystallized twice from ethanol) in 100 ml of sulfuric acid/water (62/38 by vol) (Baker, reagent grade). Prepare this reagent freshly before use.

Kaolin. Activate acid-washed kaolin by heating it at 120 °C for 2 h. Store in a desiccator until use. It will remain active for a period of months.

Other reagents. Sulfuric acid/water (62/38 by vol), aqueous NaOH (400 g/liter), ethanol/water (80/20 by vol), and absolute ethanol were reagent grade or prepared from reagent-grade chemicals.

Methods. Adjust the pH of a 30-ml aliquot of a 24-h urine specimen to pH 2–3 by dropwise addition of the dilute sulfuric acid. Suspend about 0.5 g of dry kaolin in this aliquot and after 3 min of gentle shaking, centrifuge the suspension to remove the kaolin. Adjust a 25-ml aliquot of kaolin-treated urine to pH 7–8 by dropwise addition of the sodium hydroxide solution and pass it through a column (1.5–2 ml/min) containing 3 ml of neutral resin between glass-wool plugs. Wash the column with 10 ml of water and then elute with 12.5 ml of ethanol/water (80/20 by vol, 1.5–2 ml/min), and collect the same volume of eluent

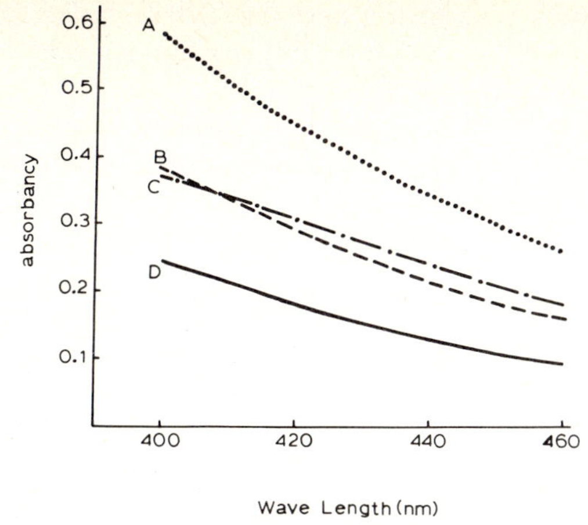

Fig. 1. Influence of pH and kaolin treatment

Each curve represents the absorption spectrum of the ethanolic eluate derived from urine treated: *A*, no kaolin treatment, applied to column at pH 2; *B*, kaolin treatment at pH 2, applied to column at pH 2; *C*, no kaolin treatment, applied to column at pH 7; *D*, kaolin treatment at pH 2, applied to column at pH 7

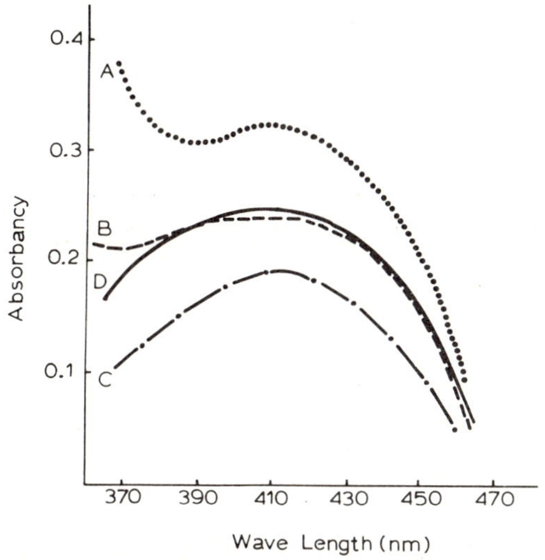

Fig. 2. Absorption spectra of Porter–Silber color obtained from the respective eluates in Figure 1

The corrected absorbances (*A*) were *A*, 0.098; *B*, 0.160; *C*, 0.180; *D*, 0.210

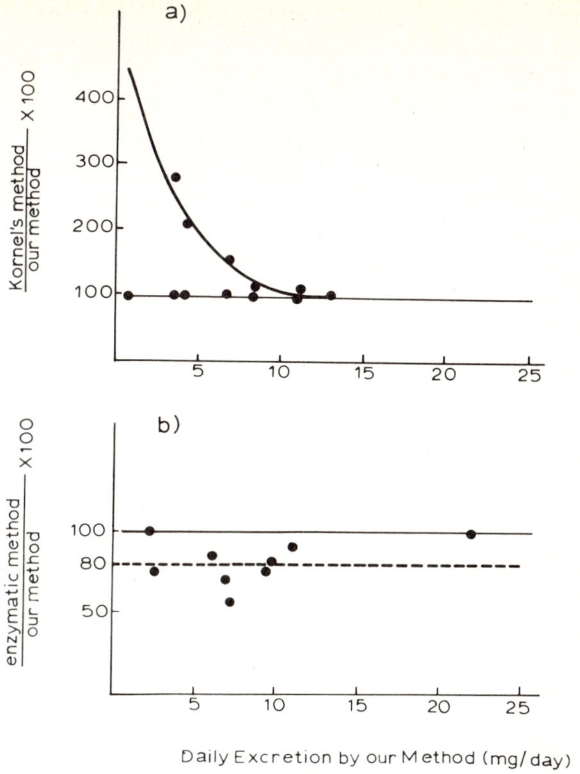

Fig. 3. Comparison of the present method with *a*) that of Kornel and *b*) enzymatic hydrolysis

Values are expressed in percent of those obtained by our method. The dotted line (3*b*) represents the mean of the percentage derived from nine comparisons

in a volumetric cylinder. Place two 2.0-ml aliquots (each equivalent to 4 ml of urine) in test tubes and evaporate under a stream of nitrogen in a water bath set at 60 °C. Then add 1 ml of absolute ethanol and 3 ml of the dilute sulfuric acid to one test tube (reference) and 1 ml of absolute ethanol and 3 ml of phenylhydrazine reagent to the other (sample). Perform this procedure with the tubes in an ice bath, to avoid overheating when the sulfuric acid is added. Mix the contents of the tubes thoroughly and heat them at 60 °C for 15 min, then cool in an ice bath for 5 min to stop the reaction. Read absorbances (*A*) of the sample tubes vs. the reference tube at 452, 412, and 372 nm, and apply the Allen correction (*5*). Estimate urinary corticosteroids in terms of cortisol as: amount per tube, $\mu g = 109 \times A_{(corr.)}$; and 24-h excretion = volume of 24-h urine (ml) × 0.25 × amt. per tube [109 is the factor relating absorbance and weight of analyte; 0.25 is the factor correcting to 1 ml of urine].

Results and Discussion

The reliability of data obtained by the Porter–Silber reaction depends largely on elimination of urinary pigments and nonsteroidal chromogenic compounds. Schopman et al. (*10*) maintained that nonsteroidal contamination of urinary extracts was the major difficulty in obtaining high specificity. In the present study, the ethanol/water eluate containing the 17-hydroxycorticosteroids is relatively free of interfering chromogens. The influence of kaolin treatment and of pH adjustment is indicated in Figure 1. Kaolin removed some nonspecifically absorbing urinary components both at pH 2 and 7. As shown in Figure 2, the resulting absorption spectra after the Porter–Silber reaction are somewhat improved. [^{3}H]Tetrahydrocortisone glucuronide (3α,17α,21-trihydroxy-5β-pregnane-11,20-dione glucosiduronate) and [^{3}H]cortisol were not significantly retained by the kaolin. The ratios of absorbances at 372, 412, and 452 nm for the urinary extract were 0.58/1.00/0.54 as compared to 0.58/1.00/0.51 for pure cortisol.

The reproducibility of the method was demonstrated by repeated (n = 19) assays of the same specimen of urine during three weeks. The mean value for total urinary 17-hydroxycorticosteroids was 8.5 ± 0.3 mg (SD). When the Allen correction was not used the standard deviation was about threefold greater. Aliquots of cortisol were added to a corticosteroid-free urine and assayed. The relationship between weight and absorption conformed closely to Beer's law. The straight line obtained (μg cortisol = 109 × $A_{corr.}$) was used in the estimation of urinary 17-hydroxycorticosteroids. The minimum detectable amount of steroid is 2.4 μg (0.02 $A_{corr.}$), which is equivalent to a concentration in urine of 0.6 mg/liter. It may occasionally be necessary to increase the size of the aliquot of column eluate taken for analysis of a low-titer urine. The aliquot may be increased considerably before interference by the remaining nonspecific chromogens becomes excessive, and is limited only by the amount of such material in the original specimen. Low concentrations in infants' urines are thus reliably measured by this method. Experiments in which [^{3}H]tetrahydrocortisone glucuronide was added to urine from normal individuals showed the mean analytical recovery to be 92% ± 1.8% (n = 8).

Daily excretion of urinary 17-hydroxycorticosteroids was determined by Kornel's method of extraction with *n*-butanol/chloroform (*3*) and by enzymatic hydrolysis. Kornel's method resulted in higher values than ours at low concentrations, but coincided with our values as the concentrations of 17-hydroxycorticosteroids increased (Figure 3*a*). On the other hand, enzymatic hydrolysis yielded values lower than or equal to ours at all concentrations (Figure 3*b*).

Analysis time was drastically reduced. As demonstrated by Osawa and Slaunwhite (*7*), relatively rapid flow rates (0.5 to 5 ml/min) were possible for adsorption, washing, and elution of the urinary steroid conjugates. These operations can be performed sequentially, with no waiting periods. Ten samples can be processed from column preparation to calculation within 3 h.

We think this method will be highly valuable for assay of urinary 17-hydroxycorticosteroids. It is rapid, relatively simple, and requires no special techniques or expensive material and equipment.

This work was supported by the United Health Foundation of Western N. Y. and USPHS Research Grant HD04945. We thank Mrs. M. Cegielski for technical assistance.

References

1. Porter, C. C., and Silber, R. H., A quantitative color reaction for cortisone and related 17,21-dihydroxy-20-ketosteroids. *J. Biol. Chem.* **185,** 201 (1950).

2. Reddy, W. J., Jenkins, D., and Thorn, G. W., Estimation of 17-hydroxycorticoids in urine. *Metabolism* **1,** 511 (1952).

3. Kornel, L., An improved rapid method for free and conjugated 17-hydroxycorticosteroids in urine. *Metabolism* **8,** 432 (1959).

4. Hertoghe, J., Crabbé, J., Duchert-Maichbetsch, A., and Müller, A. P., Improved estimation of the 17,21-dihydroxy-20-ketosteroids by use of the Allen correction in the method of Reddy. *Acta Endocrinol.* (Copenhagen) **20,** 139 (1955).

5. Allen, W. M., A simple method for analyzing complicated absorption curves of use in the colorimetric determination of urinary steroids. *J. Clin. Endocrinol.* **10,** 71 (1950).

6. Glenn, E. M., and Nelson, D. H., Chemical method for the determination of 17-hydroxycorticosteroids and 17-ketosteroids in urine following hydrolysis with β-glucuronidase. *J. Clin. Endocrinol.* **13,** 911 (1953).

7. Osawa, Y., and Slaunwhite, W. R., Studies on phenolic steroids in human subjects. XIII. A rapid assay of urinary estrogen cojugates in pregnancy. *Steroids* **15,** 73 (1970).

8. Chu, T. M., Osawa, Y., and Reynoso, G., Simple assay for urinary estrogens in nonpregnancy. *Clin. Chem.* **17,** 438 (1971).

9. Bradlow, H. L., Extraction of steroid conjugates with a neutral resin. *Steroids* **11,** 265 (1968).

10. Schopman, W., Huisin'tVeld, L. G., van der Vies, J., and Lampe-Hintzen, D. A. V. M., Some experiences with a modification of the method of Reddy, Jenkins and Thorn for the quantitative determination of 17,21-dihydroxy-20-ketosteroids in urine. *Acta Endocrinol.* (Copenhagen) **28,** 153 (1958).

CLIN. CHEM. 22/2, 235-239 (1976)

Assessment of a Serum Separator Device for Obtaining Serum Specimens Suitable for Clinical Analyses

Ronald H. Laessig,[1] James O. Westgard,[2] R. Neill Carey,[2] David J. Hassemer,[1] Thomas H. Schwartz,[3] and Donald H. Feldbruegge[2]

We have evaluated a serum separator device that is designed to effect better separation and isolation of serum from clotted blood. This device consists of an evacuated blood-drawing tube (Vacutainer) containing 1.5 ml of a semi-solid silicon polymer that forms a barrier between serum and clot during centrifugation. We compared test specimens with conventionally processed (Vacutainer) specimens as controls. Eighty-one chemical, toxicological, and immunological reactions, tests, or methods were studied. For several tests we observed changes that are statistically but not clinically significant. The one clinically significant change in serum chemistry values occurred in the case of lactate dehydrogenase, for which values were increased by 5–8% of the upper limit of normal.

Additional Keyphrases: *variation, source of* • *specimen preparation*

Serum for use in clinical chemical determinations is usually prepared by drawing blood into evacuated tubes, allowing the clot to form, centrifuging, then separating and transferring the serum into storage containers. During this process, rapid, clean, and complete separation of the serum from the clot is important (*1–3*). Various studies (*4–6*), including ours,[4] show that values for many serum constituents are changed by extended clot contact as well as by the degree of hemolysis and other processing variables.

Several mechanical devices have been proposed to improve this separation. In some, beads or semi-permeable disks have been used to form a barrier between serum and clot. Another device transfers serum to a plastic container by passage through a tube in a rubber disk. There are also filter devices, which are inserted into the collecting or holding tube to clear serum of fibrin and microclots as well as to effect separation. A recently introduced device consists of a sealed container of semi-solid polymer that is placed in the top of the blood-drawing tube just before centrifugation (*7*). During centrifugation, the polymer decends through the serum and becomes layered on the clot, thereby effecting serum separation. The latest devices include the polymer within the blood-collecting tubes.

The present study evaluates the performance of one of these, the Vacutainer "Serum-Separator Tube" (SST; Becton-Dickinson, Rutherford, N. J. 07070). This integral serum-separator device consists of a semi-solid silicon polymer in the bottom of a conventional 7-, 10-, or 15-ml evacuated blood-drawing tube. When this device is used, blood specimens are drawn in the usual manner. The specimens are allowed to clot for 30–45 min and then centrifuged. During centrifugation, the polymer positions itself between the clot and the serum because its density is midway between the two. The polymer adheres to the wall of the tube, forming a barrier-seal that isolates the serum from further contact with the clot. We assessed the effectiveness of the SST by comparing analytical results with those from conventionally drawn Vacutainer specimens.

Materials and Methods

Test Specimens

Blood specimens from apparently healthy volunteers were used for studying the normal serum constituents. For toxicological analyses, the specimens were control sera (Lederle Toxicology Control 2940-69; Lederle Diagnostics, Pearl River, N. Y. 10965). A pool of normal sera was used to study chromatographic baselines for SST-induced contaminants.

[1] State Laboratory of Hygiene, Department of Preventive Medicine, 465 Henry Mall, University of Wisconsin, Madison, Wis. 53706. Address correspondence to R. H. L.

[2] Department of Medicine, Pathology and Clinical Laboratories, University of Wisconsin Hospitals, Madison, Wis. 53706.

[3] Department of Health and Social Services, State of Wisconsin, Madison, Wis. 53701.

[4] Laessig, R. H., Hassemer, D., Indriksons, A. A., Paskey, T. A., and Schwartz, T. H., Changes in serum chemical values as a result of prolonged contact with the clot. Accepted, *Am. J. Clin. Pathol.*, November 1975.

Received Aug. 1, 1975; accepted Nov. 26, 1975.

Study Protocol

Blood-drawing equipment consisted of regular Vacutainer tubes (15 ml, red-top, cat. No. 4796) and matched 15-ml SST tubes (cat. No. 3810). Control and SST tubes came from the same lot of Vacutainers. Half had been reprocessed to produce the SST device (i.e., polymer added and tubes reevacuated) so that all materials, including stoppers, were uniform throughout the study. We used SST tubes from several such production runs.

Two samples (control and SST) were obtained from each subject from a single venipuncture in the conventional manner, with use of 20-gauge needles. Specimens were collected and analyzed in a pre-arranged format to eliminate sequential effects. Subjects 1, 3, 5 . . . were sampled in the order control–SST, subjects 2, 4, 6 . . . were sampled in the order SST–control. Sera from subjects 1 and 2 were analyzed in the order drawn, sera from subjects 3 and 4 were analyzed in reverse order, and so on. In all processing, the respective pairs were treated as nearly alike as possible, maintaining adjoining positions in the clotting racks, centrifuge, and analysis trays.

During each run (day), eight to 10 subjects were bled within 15 min. The time allowed for clotting was 30–45 min, which simulates times encountered when blood is collected under routine hospital conditions and transported to the laboratory for processing. Stoppers were then removed, and both tubes were centrifuged at 700 × *g* for 15 min without first disengaging the clot from the tube wall. When bicarbonate values were measured, stoppers were in place during centrifugation and were removed immediately before analysis. To check SST function, specimens were visually inspected with reference to four criteria: (*a*) barrier failure (i.e., failure to form an adequate seal), (*b*) visible hemolysis, (*c*) barrier appearance, and (*d*) erythrocytes present in the serum. When quantitating erythrocyte contamination, serum was removed from SST and control tubes with a Pasteur pipette. The processors were instructed to recover the maximum amount of serum consistent with good laboratory practice. These sera were recentrifuged in 15-ml conical centrifuge tubes (700 × *g*, 15 min) and all but 0.5 ml of serum was then carefully aspirated with a Pasteur pipette. The 0.5 ml remaining was diluted to 15 ml with Drabkin's reagent, thoroughly mixed, and its hemoglobin content was determined spectrophotometrically at 540 nm vs. a reagent blank.

Clinical Methods of Analysis

To evaluate SST effects on serum constituents quantitatively, the paired sera were subjected to a variety of chemical analyses. These include "SMAC" (Technicon, Instruments Corp., Tarrytown, N. Y. 10591) analyses for chloride, bicarbonate, glucose, urea nitrogen, calcium, phosphorus, uric acid, cholesterol, lactate dehydrogenase (EC 1.1.1.27; LD), total protein, albumin, total bilirubin, alkaline phosphatase (EC 3.1.3.1), alanine aminotransferase (EC 2.6.1.1; ALT), potassium, and asparate aminotransferase (EC 2.6.1.1; AST); SMA 12/60 (Technicon) analyses for calcium, phosphorus, glucose, urea nitrogen, uric acid, cholesterol, total protein, albumin, total bilirubin, alkaline phosphatase, AST, and LD; SMA 6/60 (Technicon) analyses for cholesterol, glucose, uric acid, total bilirubin, creatinine, and AST; AutoAnalyzer I (Technicon) analyses for glucose, uric acid, urea nitrogen, cholesterol and triglycerides; Du-Pont *aca* (Du Pont, Wilmington, Del. 19898) analyses for glucose, creatine kinase (ED 2.7.3.2; CPK), lactic acid, LD, and pseudocholinesterase; Microzone System (Beckman Instruments, Inc., Fullerton, Calif. 92634) electrophoretic separation and quantitation of (serum proteins) albumin, α_1-globulin, α_2-globulin, β-globulin, and γ-globulin and (serum lipoproteins) beta, pre-beta, alpha, and chylomicrons; flame emission assays for sodium and potassium; coulometric titration of chloride; radioimmunoassay of triiodothyronine (T3) uptake, thyroxine (T-4), cortisol, vitamin B_{12}, digoxin, and folate; radial immunodiffusion assays of immunoglobulins A, G, and M, and α_1-antitrypsin activity; atomic absorption spectrometry of calcium and magnesium; manual assays for iron, unsaturated iron-binding capacity, glucose, γ-glutamyltranspeptidase (EC 2.3.2.2), α-hydroxybutyrate dehydrogenase, and LD; and gas-chromatographic measurements of sera containing ethanol, methyprylon, meprobamate, glutethimide, methaqualone, amobarbital, phenobarbital, diphenylhydantoin, and negative (no drugs present) sera.

The multiple assays of some analytes reflect the various methodological approaches in current use: six different glucose procedures, enzyme assays by end point and kinetic procedures; albumin by three chemical systems; metal ions by dye-binding, electrode, flame absorption and emission; and lipids by direct and extraction techniques. The chemical analyses were selected according to several criteria:

(*a*) tests most often requested (the SST is intended for routine use),

(*b*) tests sensitive to clot mishandling and (or) those adversely affected by clot contact,

(*c*) tests likely to be affected by contact between organic polymer and whole blood, serum, or cells (e.g., reactions dependent on activators or affected by inhibitors that could be depleted by contact with the polymer), those strongly affected by molecular conformation (e.g., enzymatic reactions with high substrate specificity), and those based on immunological reactions,

(*d*) tests susceptible to trace-contaminant interference (particularly gas-chromatographic assays) and those in which low concentrations of endogenous or exogenous constituents might be irreversibly absorbed by the organic polymer.

Statistical Analysis

The data was subjected to paired *t*-test analysis and the bias, standard deviation of the difference, and *t*-value were calculated.

Table 1. Comparison of SST and Control Analyses

Test (SMAC)[a]	SST mean	Control mean	Bias[b]	SD of differences	No. data pairs	*t*-value[c]
1. Chloride	104.6	104.3	0.35	0.98	23	1.70
2. Glucose	84.6	84.7	−0.29	2.23	23	0.19
3. Urea nitrogen	13.2	13.1	0.04	0.21	23	1.00
4. Calcium	9.91	9.93	−0.02	0.11	23	0.96
5. Phosphorus	2.95	2.96	0.004	0.06	23	0.37
6. Uric acid	5.50	5.46	0.01	0.06	23	0.70
7. Cholesterol	199.6	198.9	0.74	5.35	23	0.66
8. Lactate dehydrogenase	154.6	153.6	1.04	17.29	23	0.29
9. Total protein	7.39	7.37	0.02	0.11	23	0.59
10. Albumin	4.56	4.55	0.01	0.09	23	0.44
11. Total bilirubin	0.68	0.69	−0.01	0.08	23	0.52
12. Alkaline phosphatase	62.4	61.7	−0.74	1.51	23	2.34
13. Alanine aminotransferase	18.8	19.5	−0.64	1.29	23	2.31
14. Potassium	3.92	3.96	−0.04	0.17	23	1.21
15. Aspartate aminotransferase (other)	21.6	22.7	−1.07	2.23	14	1.79
16. Lactate dehydrogenase[d]	133.5	117.2	−16.3	8.76	20	8.32
17. Lactate dehydrogenase[e]	55.8	52.1	3.68	2.91	10	4.00
18. Lactate dehydrogenase[f]	124.4	124.9	0.50	21.68	20	0.10
19. α-Hydroxybutyrate dehydrogenase[g]	100.6	94.3	6.26	8.30	20	3.28

[a] All SMAC methods as described in Technicon Publication UA3-0306B10, September, 1974, Units: Cl^-, K^+, mmol/liter; albumin, total protein, g/dl, alkaline phosphatase, ALT, AST, LD, and α-hydroxybutyrate dehydrogenase, U/liter; all others mg/dl.
[b] Bias = SST mean − control mean
[c] Significant *t*-values ($P = 0.05$): n = 10, $t = 2.31$; n = 14, $t = 2.15$; n = 20, $t = 2.10$; n = 23, $t = 2.09$.
[d] Du Pont *aca*.
[e] LDH-UV cat. No. 61631, Boehringer Mannheim Corp. 219 E. 44th St., New York, N.Y. 10017.
[f] SMA 12/60.
[g] Alpha-HBDH Max-Pack, cat. No. 869809; Calbiochem La Jolla, Calif. 92037.

Results

Qualitative

There were no failures in *barrier formation* for the 400 SST tubes we used during the four-month study. Small, pin-head size clumps of erythrocytes could be seen imbedded in the polymer barrier. These cells were occluded in the polymer and were not in direct contact with the serum. *Fibrin strands* were observed in some subjects' sera but appeared to adhere to the SST polymer and were not transferred during separation. SST's that were incompletely filled ("*short-draw specimens*") did not affect performance; the barrier formed on top of the clot independent of volume of blood that was drawn. No *hemolysis* was observed in any SST specimen, though one control specimen that was drawn first showed unexplained hemolysis. *Serum yields* were about equal from both specimen containers.

Quantitative

The volume of *suspended erythrocytes* was about 1 mm^3 in both control and SST sera. The mean values for hemoglobin were about 70 mg/liter for either type of collecting tube, or about 0.02% of the total erythrocytes in a 15-ml specimen of blood. Unhemolyzed suspended erythrocytes corresponding to as much as 0.1% or 1.0% of the total erythrocytes have no appreciable effect on the usual clinical laboratory determinations.[5]

Table 1 summarizes the statistical data for the SMAC analyses and other determinations of critical interest. Similar data for each test or method are on file and available upon request from the Editorial Office of this journal.

Discussion

In designing this study, we chose to draw specimens from a normal, healthy population in order to gain precise control over the many variables involved in sample acquisition and processing. In addition, it was advantageous to sample a homogeneous group in order to control the analytical variations, which tend to be greater at the extreme ends of the ranges of measurement. This approach permitted assessment of small differences between the SST and control specimens.

[5] Laessig, R. H., Hassemer, D., Paskey, T. A., and Schwartz, T. H., The effect of 0.1 and 1.0% of red blood cells and hemolysis on serum chemistry values. Accepted, *Am. J. Clin. Pathol.*, December 1975.

The differences were interpreted by assessing their statistical and clinical significance. Statistical significance ($P = 0.05$, $n = 20$) is indicated when the t-statistic exceeds 2.0, implying that the data are sufficient to be sure that a difference does exist. The size of that difference is estimated by the bias statistic, which represents the average difference between specimen pairs. In addition, the size of individual differences can be estimated from the standard deviation of the differences. These latter two statistics permit assessment of the clinical significance of the observed differences. Therefore, we examine the bias and standard deviation of the differences as well as the t-value. The final interpretation depends on both the statistical and clinical significance of the observed differences.

Changes caused by hemolysis of erythrocytes: For LD, the SST introduced a bias of 4 U/liter for the manual method and 16 U/liter for the *aca* method. This increase corresponds to 5–8% of the value of the upper limit of the normal range. Hemolysis of only 0.1% of the total erythrocytes in a specimen of whole blood increases serum LD values by about 35–40 U/liter,[5] therefore, the observed increase of 16 U/liter (*aca*) represents only 0.03–0.04% hemolysis. α-Hydroxybutyrate dehydrogenase is closely associated with lactate dehydrogenase isoenzymes 1 and 2 and is increased by 6.7% in the SST, confirming that the observed increase in LD is of erythrocyte origin. These findings, if extrapolated to serum isoenzyme studies, indicate that LD isoenzyme 1 and 2 activities would be expected to increase by a total of 6–7% in normal patient patterns (*8*). When serum LD values are abnormally high, the effect on the isoenzyme patterns would be expected to be negligible. Attempts to verify this finding by measuring LD-5 activities were unsuccessful because of precision limitations in the technique. However, the inference of minimal cell damage is supported by the absence of a concurrent increase in potassium values. There is an apparent conflict in the LD data from the different methods; only two of four methods exhibit SST-induced changes. We believe this is a consequence of the low amount of hemolysis responsible for the observed effect. A small variation in blood-processing technique could easily result in insidious hemolysis in one or two control specimens, which would obscure any SST-induced increase.

Changes in protein conformation: Serum enzyme activity measurements (other than LD) and enzyme–substrate reactions did not exhibit any changes attributable to use of the SST. Both types of assays are sensitive to (*a*) induced changes in molecular shape, charge, or conformation of the enzyme, (*b*) similar changes in critical coenzymes and (or) substrates, or (*c*) loss of activators. Protein conformation and other physical properties are also highly critical in the determinations of immunoglobulins G, A, and M and the immunological assay of α_1-antitrypsin activity. No SST-induced changes were observed in the measurement of any of these constituents. In addition, competitive protein binding determinations of thyroxine, cortisol, digoxin, folate, and vitamin B_{12} were not affected.

Changes in (normally) exogenous serum constituents: The potential problem of absorption of small organic molecules was studied by analyzing for drugs by gas-chromatographic/solvent-extraction techniques. Identical aliquots of commercial control sera that contained drugs were placed in SST and conventional tubes for 48 h. Polymer absorption would be reflected by a decrease in the assay value in the SST specimens. Neither ethanol (2.16 g/liter) nor methyprylon, meprobamate, glutethimide, methaqualone, amobarbital, phenobarbital, and diphenylhydantoin (each 20 mg/liter) showed any changes in peak area or alterations in peak shape. Analyses of aliquots of drug-free serum held in conventional tubes and SST tubes for 48 h gave identical negative chromatographic baselines for the acidic and neutral fractions. (These findings should not be generalized to other drugs or other analytical procedures.)

Changes in electrophoretic properties: There were no observed differences in electrophoretic separation and quantitation of serum proteins and lipoproteins on cellulose acetate strips. This suggests there are no alterations in molecular polarity or charge, or any polymer adhesion to the proteins.

Quantitative determinations based on electrode reactions provided an additional means of checking for polymer contaminants in SST-collected sera. Coulometric chloride assays, as well as sodium and potassium measurements with ion-selective electrodes, exhibited no evidence of interference in electrode reactions; such evidence might be expected if polymer contaminants were present.

Changes in serum analyte values: With the exception of LD and α-hydroxybutyrate dehydrogenase, none of the other tests or methods showed SST-induced differences of clinical significance. Alkaline phosphatase, ALT, creatinine, calcium by atomic absorption, and bicarbonate showed biases that were statistically significant by the t-test ($P = 0.05$). Their magnitudes, however, were so small that the differences were not judged to be clinically significant: alkaline phosphatase 0.7 U/liter, or 1.1% of the control mean value; ALT 0.6 U/liter, or 3%; creatinine 0.9 mg/liter, or 9%; calcium 0.5 mg/liter, or 0.6%; and bicarbonate 1.0 mmol/liter, or 4%. None of the 81 determinations listed earlier had a bias greater than 3% of the mean control value.

Routine hospital use: From our data we concluded that the SST was acceptable for routine hospital testing. To evaluate its performance under conditions where abnormal serum chemistry values and atypical whole blood morphologies are encountered, the device was introduced in five hospitals, where paired-specimen comparisons were made. The blood-drawing staff was instructed to obtain a regular specimen (control) and a paired SST specimen when the patient's condition permitted. The specimens were analyzed by each respective laboratory's routine procedures.[6] The data were subjected to paired *t*-test analysis and in addition, a special computation of the data compared only abnormal results. Determinations studied included those listed in Table 1, with the addition of CPK, globulin, and sodium. A total of 100–200 patients' data, of which 40–50 were abnormal, were compiled for each determination. The *t*-test on data from the total and from the exclusively abnormal populations indicated no SST-induced differences that could be attributed to the processing of actual patient specimens. Small differences observed in the study on normal subjects were not confirmed, probably reflecting the loss of tight experimental control. For example, LD data in the field test exhibited a non-statistically significant bias of 1.6 U/liter, with a control mean of 160 U/liter for the total population, and a bias of 3 U/liter and a mean of 285 U/liter for the abnormal group.

[6] Laessig, R. H., Carey, R. N., Westgard, J. O., Hassemer, D. J., and Habig, R., Field evaluation of the Becton-Dickinson SST. Submitted *Health Laboratory Science,* September 1975.

Elsewhere[7] we report on the lack of effect of allowing serum to stand on the barrier for 48 h at 4 °C.

References

1. Henry, R. J., Cannon, D, and Winkelman, J. W., Eds., *Clinical Chemistry Principles and Techniques,* 2nd ed., Harper and Row, New York, N. Y., 1974, pp 374–388.
2. Tietz, N. W., *Fundamentals of Clinical Chemistry,* Saunders, Philadelphia, Pa., 1970, p 44.
3. Davidsohn, I., and Henry, J. B., *Todd-Sanford Clinical Diagnosis of Laboratory Methods,* Saunders, Philadelphia, Pa., 1969, pp 487–493.
4. Caraway, W. T., Chemical and diagnostic specificity of laboratory tests. *Am. J. Clin. Pathol.* **37,** 445 (1962).
5. Martinek, R., Specimens for clinical laboratory analysis-collection and preservation. *Postgrad. Med.* **37,** A46 (1966).
6. Hagebusch, O. E., Automation in the private practice of laboratory medicine. In *Automation in Analytical Chemistry, Technicon Symposia 1965,* L. T. Skeggs, Jr. et al. Eds., Mediad, New York, N. Y., 1966, pp 417–422.
7. Mathies, J. C., Evaluation of a new device for rapidly separating serum or plasma from blood. *Clin. Chem.* **20,** 1573 (1974).
8. Van der Helme, H. J., A simplified method of demonstrating lactic dehydrogenase isoenzymes. *Clin. Chim. Acta* **37,** 124 (1962).

[7] Laessig, R. H., Hassemer, D. J., Westgard, J. O., Carey, R. N., Feldbruegge, D. H., and Schwartz, T. H., Assessment of the Serum Separator Tube as an intermediate storage device within the laboratory. Submitted, *Am. J. Clin. Pathol.,* June 1975.

CLIN. CHEM. 22/2, 240-242 (1976)

Cation-Exchange Chromatography of Guanidine Derivatives in Plasma of Patients with Chronic Renal Failure

Guido Perez, Alberto Rey, Michael Micklus, and Israel Stein

Guanidine derivatives are suspected of contributing to the toxic manifestations of uremia. We describe a method for measurement of guanidine derivatives in 5-ml samples of plasma by liquid chromatography. Concentrations of guanidinosuccinate and guanidinobutyrate in plasma were significantly increased both in undialyzed patients with chronic renal failure (5.54 ± 0.94 and 17.5 ± 4.07 mg/liter) and those undergoing maintenance hemodialysis (2.35 ± 0.41 and 19.4 ± 3.99 mg/liter) when compared to healthy controls (<0.4 and 1.0 ± 0.3 mg/liter, respectively). Creatine and guanidinoacetate concentrations tended to be higher in hemodialysis patients and lower in the undialyzed group of patients with chronic renal failure. This procedure provides a rapid, sensitive, and accurate method for the study of guanidine metabolism in persons with uremia.

Guanidine derivatives are suspected of contributing to the toxic manifestations of uremia. For example, methylguanidine intoxication in experimental animals produces a symptom complex similar to the uremic syndrome (*1*) and guanidinosuccinic acid has been implicated in the qualitative platelet defect responsible for uremic bleeding (*2*). Methodological limitations, however, have hindered attempts to isolate and quantitate guanidines in biological fluids.

This report describes a high-pressure liquid chromatographic system for simultaneous determination of guanidine derivatives. We have measured the plasma concentration of these compounds in healthy volunteers, in patients with far-advanced chronic renal failure, and in patients receiving maintenance hemodialysis.

Materials and Methods

Analytical Methods

The compounds under study were separated by cation-exchange column chromatography. Twenty-five grams of cation-exchange resin (Aminex A-5; particle size, 13 ± 2 μm; BioRad Laboratories, Richmond, Calif. 94804) was washed in 250 ml of sodium citrate buffer (0.2 mol/liter, pH 3.25), stirred for 30 min, filtered through a fritted-glass funnel, and resuspended again in fresh buffer. The resin was then packed into a 0.9 × 23 cm water-jacketed column (Beckman Instruments, Inc., Spinco Division, Palo Alto, Calif. 94304). The column was packed to a height of 19 cm at 58 °C (Lauda circulating water bath, Model K-2, Arthur Thomas Co., Philadelphia, Pa.), at 2020 kN/m^2 (20 atm) (multi-speed transmission pump, Model 600-000; Harvard Apparatus Co., Dover, Mass. 02030). After running 100 ml of the sodium citrate buffer at 40–60 ml/h at the same temperature and pressure, the column was ready for use.

Before chromatography, the proteins in a 5-ml sample of plasma were precipitated with 1.4 ml of a 200 g/liter solution of trichloroacetic acid, and the mixture was centrifuged (2000 rpm, 1 h). The decanted supernate was extracted three times with an equal volume of diethyl ether to remove the trichloroacetic acid, and the pH of the sample was adjusted to 5.5 ± 0.5 with sodium hydroxide 0.2 mol/liter. The sample (5 ml) was then applied to the column. It was eluted in 6 h with 160 ml of a sodium citrate buffer of increasing pH (3.25, 80 ml; 4.25, 40 ml; 5.26, 40 ml), followed by 40 ml of sodium hydroxide (0.2 mol/liter). The effluent was collected in 4-ml fractions with a fraction collector with a drop-counting device, and duplicate samples of the fractions were analyzed colorimetrically by a modification of the Voges–Proskauer reaction (*3*).

Chromatographically pure standards of arginine, guanidinosuccinic acid (Schwarz/Mann, Orangeburg, N. Y. 10962), guanidinoacetic acid, creatine (Sigma Chemical Co., St. Louis, Mo. 63178), and guanidinobutyric acid (Calbiochem, Los Angeles, Calif. 90059) were chromatographed to establish their elution patterns. Their concentrations were determined from calibration curves for these compounds in concentration of 5, 10, 15, 20, and 25 mg/liter. Analytical recoveries were determined after adding 55–125 μg of each compound to 5 ml of plasma. The coefficient of variation for replicate determinations was calculated. The partition coefficients for the various guanidine compounds, between ether and a trichloroacetic acid solution, were also determined.

Experimental Subjects

Eight hospitalized patients on maintenance hemodialysis, and five ambulatory patients with chronic renal failure not requiring hemodialysis were the subjects. Controls were six apparently healthy labo-

Department of Medicine, University of Miami School of Medicine; and Medical and Research Services, Veterans Administration Hospital, 1201 NW 16th St., Miami, Fla. 33125.
Address correspondence to G.P. at the V.A. Hospital.
Received Oct. 28, 1975; accepted Nov. 28, 1975.

Table 1. Concentrations of Guanidine Derivatives in Plasma

	Guanidinosuccinic acid	Creatine	Guanidinoacetic acid	Guanidinobutyric acid	Arginine	Creatinine
	mg/liter					
Controls (C) (n = 6)						
	<0.40	3.82 ± 0.40 (2.12 – 4.85)	0.35 ± 0.06 (0.18 – 0.59)	1.02 ± 0.32 (0.12 – 1.93)	14.4 ± 1.20 (11.9 – 19.2)	10 ± 3 (7 – 16)
Renal failure (RF) (n = 5)						
	5.54 ± 0.94 (2.42 – 8.09)	36.2 ± 21.3 (3.10 – 110.7)[a]	0.75 ± 0.23 (0.20 – 1.44)	17.5 ± 4.07 (4.70 – 25.9)	11.5 ± 1.47 (8.23 – 16.2)	120 ± 10 (80 – 150)
Hemodialysis (H) (n = 8)						
	2.35 ± 0.41 (0.68 – 3.79)	23.1 ± 11.7 (0.66 – 96.5)[a]	1.45 ± 0.48 (0.35 – 3.74)	19.4 ± 3.99 (6.60 – 38.3)	28.2 ± 4.68 (14.7 – 55.8)	150 ± 10 (110 – 170)
Group differences						
H vs. RF	$P < 0.018$[b]	NS	NS	NS	$P < 0.02$	$0.05 < P < 0.1$
H vs. C	$P < 0.001$[b]	NS	$0.05 < P < 0.08$	$P < 0.005$	$P < 0.05$	$P < 0.001$
C vs. RF	$P < 0.004$[b]	NS	NS	$P < 0.005$	NS	$P < 0.001$

Values are mean ± SE and (range); NS, $P > 0.05$.
[a] The patients with serum values of 110.7 and 96.5 mg/liter had clinical evidence of muscle wasting.
[b] Mann–Whitney U test.

ratory workers of similar age, with normal urinalyses, normal serum creatinine concentrations, and no history of renal disease.[1] Hemodialysis was performed with the Dow/Cordis No. 4 Hollow Fiber Artificial Kidney for 5 h per session, three times a week. Those patients being hemodialyzed ingested a diet including 1.25 g of protein per kilogram of body weight; the other patients received a protein-restricted (40–60 g/day) diets. In patients on maintenance hemodialysis, blood specimens were obtained before dialysis and before the first meal of the day.

The data are presented as means ± SE and were statistically evaluated by one-way analysis of variance (Kruskal–Wallis or F test) followed by Student's t-test for parametric indices or by the Mann–Whitney U test for nonparametric indices (*4*).

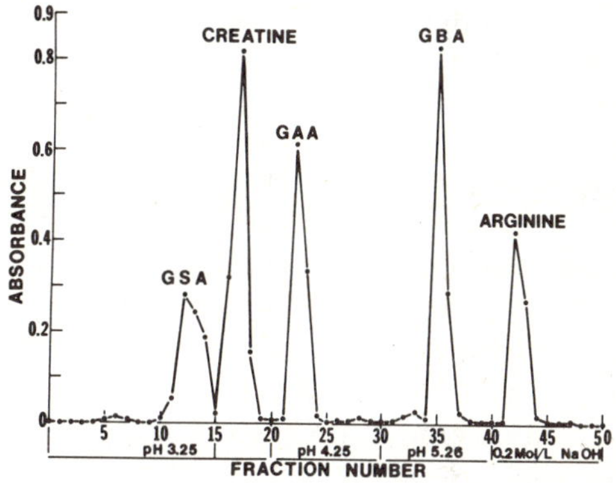

Fig. 1. Fractionation of a synthetic mixture of guanidine derivatives by liquid chromatography

GSA, guanidinosuccinic acid; *GAA*, guanidinoacetic acid; and *GBA*, guanidinobutyric acid

Results

Figure 1 illustrates a typical chromatographic separation of a synthetic mixture of arginine, creatine, guanidinoacetate, guanidinosuccinate, and guanidinobutyrate. In this system, urea was eluted in fractions 4–6 and creatinine in fractions 33–35. Although its elution pattern overlapped somewhat with guanidinobutyrate, creatinine did not interfere with the Voges–Proskauer color reaction in the range of concentrations measured in our patients.

The analytical recovery of added known amounts of guanidines from plasma ranged from 87 to 102%. Experiments designed to measure the partition coefficient of the various guanidine derivatives between diethyl ether and a trichloroacetic solution revealed that less than 1% of each of the compounds under study was extracted into the ether layer. The coefficient of variation for eight replicate determinations of each compound ranged from 3 to 7%. In all cases the individual result ±2 SD overlapped with the corresponding duplicate analysis ±2 SD. The lower limit of sensitivity of the method ranged from 0.1 to 0.4 mg/liter.

The mean plasma concentration of each guanidine compound in control subjects and the two groups of patients is shown in Table 1. Except for arginine in those patients not undergoing hemodialysis, all values were higher in patients than in controls, although not statistically significantly so in the case of creatine and guanidinoacetate. The wide range in plasma creatine concentrations was largely attributable to above-normal values (96.5 and 110.7 mg/liter) found in two patients with marked muscle wasting.

[1] Signed informed consent was obtained from each subject and the protocol was approved by the Committee on Human Experimentation of the Miami Veterans Administration Hospital. The research was done according to the principles outlined in the Declaration of Helsinki.

Guanidinosuccinate concentrations in all the controls were <0.4 mg/liter, the lower limit of sensitivity of the test. When plasma concentrations of guanidinoacetate, guanidinobutyrate, or guanidinosuccinate in all subjects were grouped together and correlated with serum creatinine concentrations, a statistically significant relationship was obtained ($P < 0.05$, $P < 0.001$, and $P < 0.05$, respectively).

The chromatographic elution pattern for uremic plasma was similar to that for normal persons except for the presence of a small unidentified Voges–Proskauer-positive peak corresponding to fractions 31–33. In one patient with combined renal and hepatic insufficiency the concentrations of arginine (8.2 mg/liter) and guanidinosuccinate (2.4 mg/liter) were much lower than was true of the patients with uncomplicated chronic renal failure and comparable serum creatinine concentration.

Discussion

We have described a rapid, sensitive, and accurate method for measuring guanidine derivatives in plasma and confirmed previously reported data on these compounds in the serum of healthy subjects and of patients with chronic renal insufficiency (*1, 5*).

Concentrations of guanidinosuccinate, guanidinoacetate, guanidinobutyrate, and creatine were greater in both groups of patients than in the healthy controls, although not statistically so in the case of guanidinoacetate and creatine. Arginine values tended to be higher in hemodialysis patients and lower in undialyzed renal failure patients.

Arginine values for the patients with chronic renal failure were comparable to those of normal controls (*6, 7*). The above-normal values found pre-dialysis in our hemodialysis patients may be a result of their higher protein intake or perhaps to breakdown of arginine conjugates during sample deproteinization or chromatography at low pH.

In a previous study in patients with chronic renal failure, Cohen (*6*) found values similar to ours for creatine in plasma but much greater concentrations of guanidinoacetate. He postulated that increased values for creatine and guanidinoacetate, caused by renal retention, inhibited L-arginine:glycine amidinotransferase (EC 2.1.4.1) with resulting transfer of the amidino group of arginine to aspartate to form guanidinosuccinate.

The presence of increased amounts of guanidinosuccinate in uremic serum has been reported (*5, 8*); in general, the concentrations we found in our patients are lower. Because guanidinosuccinate in plasma is decreased by hemodialysis (*9*), more efficient and more frequent dialysis in our subjects may explain this difference. Likewise, the use of protein-restricted diets may be responsible for the lower guanidinosuccinate values in our undialyzed patients with chronic renal failure (*8*).

Shainkin et al. (*10*) described a method for simultaneous measurement of guanidine derivatives in biological fluids by use of a modified amino acid analyzer. They found values for guanidinosuccinate similar to ours, but their values for guanidinoacetate and guanidinobutyrate were lower than in our cases. On the other hand, they found increased concentrations of guanidinopropionate in plasma of both dialyzed and undialyzed patients with chronic renal failure. Methylguanidine concentrations, previously reported to be increased in uremia (*11, 12*), were not different from controls. The practical advantage of the present method over that of Shainkin et al. (*10*) lies in its greater simplicity and perhaps lower cost of purchase and operation.

Although the exact role of these compounds in the production of uremic symptoms is difficult to define, it is likely that several guanidine derivatives contribute to the toxicity of uremia (*1, 6*). The application of new analytical techniques for the measurement of these compounds in uremic patients is likely to increase our understanding of guanidine metabolism in chronic renal failure.

We are grateful to Hilda Obaya for her technical assistance and to Charlene Morgan and Linda Haghighy for secretarial help.

This project was supported by a grant from the Veterans Administration (6992-01).

References

1. Giovannetti, S., Biagini, M., Balestri, P. L., et al., Uremic-like syndrome in dogs chronically intoxicated with methylguanidine and creatinine. *Clin. Sci.* **36,** 445 (1969).

2. Horowitz, H. I., Cohen, B. D., Martinez, P., et al., Defective ADP-induced platelet factor 3 activation in uremia. *Blood* **30,** 331 (1967).

3. Micklus, M. J., and Stein, I. M., The colorimetric determination of mono and disubstituted guanidines. *Anal. Biochem.* **54,** 545 (1973).

4. Snedecor, G. W., and Cochran, W. G., *Statistical Methods,* 6th ed., Iowa State University Press, Ames, Iowa, 1968.

5. Stein, I. M., Cohen, B. D., and Kornhauser, R. S., Guanidinosuccinic acid in renal failure, experimental azotemia and inborn errors of the urea cycle. *New Engl. J. Med.* **280,** 926 (1973).

6. Cohen, B. D., Guanidinosuccinic acid in uremia. *Arch. Intern. Med.* **126,** 846 (1970).

7. Young, G. A., and Parsons, F. M., Plasma amino acid inbalance in patients with chronic renal failure on intermittent hemodialysis. *Clin. Chim. Acta* **27,** 491 (1970).

8. Kopple, J. D., Gordon, S., and Wang, M., Effect of chronic uremia, protein intake and hemodialysis (HD) on guanidinosuccinic acid (GSA) levels. *Abstr. Am. Soc. Nephrol.* **5,** 41 (1971).

9. Kamoun, P. P., Pleau, J. M., and Man, N. K., Semiautomated method for measurement of guanidinosuccinic acid in serum. *Clin. Chem.* **18,** 355 (1972).

10. Shainkin, R., Giatt, Y., and Berlyne, G. M., The presence and toxicity of guanidinoproprionic acid in uremia. *Kidney Int.* **7,** S302 (1975).

11. Stein, I. M., Perez, G., Johnson, R., et al., Serum levels and urinary excretion of methylguanidine. *J. Lab. Clin. Med.* **77,** 1020 (1971).

12. Giovannetti, S., Balestri, P. L., and Barsotti, G., Methylguanidine in uremia. *Arch. Intern. Med.* **131,** 709 (1973).

Enzymatic Method for Determination of CO_2 in Serum

Roger L. Forrester,[1] Lester J. Wataji,[1] Donald A. Silverman,[2] and Kenneth J. Pierre[3]

We describe an enzymatic method, requiring only 10 μl of serum, for determining CO_2 as bicarbonate or dissolved gas. Phosphoenolpyruvate carboxylase catalyzes the reaction of HCO_3^- with phosphoenolypyruvate to give oxalacetate. The resulting NADH, in the presence of malate dehydrogenase, is oxidized to NAD^+, and the decrease in absorbance at 340 nm is directly proportional to the amount of CO_2 present in the sample. Reaction is complete in 3 to 6 min under assay conditions, and is linearly related to CO_2 concentrations between 8 and 65 mmol/liter. Analytical recovery is 95–110% (average, 101%). Two laboratories compared values obtained by continuous-flow analysis. The resulting correlation coefficients were 0.966 and 0.987, values for the *t*-test were *t*(paired) = 0.473 and *t*(paired) = 0.334, and average day-to-day precisions (three concentrations) were 3.9% and 4.2%.

Total carbon dioxide content can be measured by the Van Slyke procedure: volumetric, manometric, or by the microchemical modification of Natelson (*1, 2*). The Van Slyke procedure is both cumbersome and time-consuming. Recently a modification of it was developed in which an extraction chamber combined with a modified tuberculin syringe is used (*3*). Although sufficiently accurate and precise for clinical use, it is still rather cumbersome and slow.

Continuous-flow analysis (AutoAnalyzer; Technicon Instruments Corp., Tarrytown, N. Y. 10591), one of the more commonly used methods for determination of carbon dioxide, is precise and reasonably accurate. Several such methods (and modifications of them) have been developed (*4–7*). One of them, the cresol red procedure, has also been adapted to a discrete analyzer (the Beckman Discrete Sample Analyzer; Beckman Instruments, Inc., Fullerton, Calif. 92634) (*8*). Many laboratories either do not have an AutoAnalyzer or do not operate it all day; thus they need a simple, accurate, and precise means of measuring CO_2 content.

The enzymatic method we describe requires little pipetting and only two readings on any spectrophotometer capable of being read at 340 nm and 0–2 *A*, followed by a simple calculation. Our data suggest that the method is more simple, accurate, and precise than older methods and is a valuable back-up method.

[1] Clinical Chemistry Laboratory, Mercy San Juan Hospital, 6501 Coyle Ave., Carmichael, Calif. 95608.

[2] Department of Biochemistry, Hektoen Institute for Medical Research of the Cook County Hospital, 627-637 S. Wood St., Chicago, Ill. 60612.

[3] Beckman Instruments, Inc., 6200 El Camino Real, P. O. Drawer 877, Carlsbad, Calif. 92008.

Received Oct. 9, 1975; accepted Dec. 1, 1975.

Materials and Methods

Instrumentation

We used a Beckman Model 25 Kinetic System, a Model 300-N Spectrophotometer (Gilford Instruments, Inc., Oberlin, Ohio 44074), and a Zeiss PMQ II Spectrophotometer (Carl Zeiss, Oberkochen, West Germany) for all manual assays at 30 °C. A Gilford System 3500 Computer-Directed Analyzer was used for all automated assays at room temperature.

Reagents

Per liter, the reagent contains 1.79 mmol of phosphoenolpyruvate, 0.35 mmol of NADH, 212 U of phosphoenolpyruvate carboxylase (EC 4.1.1.31), and 1250 U of malate dehydrogenase (EC 1.1.1.37). The CO_2 reagent and reconstituting solution, available as single-test vials or five-test vials (CO_2 reagent and reconstituting solution packaged separately), were obtained from Beckman Instruments, Inc., Microbics Operations, Carlsbad, Calif. 92008). The reagent can be used for about 2 h after reconstitution at room temperature if kept sealed, or 4 h at 4 °C.

Procedures

In the *manual assay,* 3.0 ml of reconstituted substrate is pipetted into a 1-cm cuvette and placed in a temperature-controlled spectrophotometer to equilibrate at 30 °C for 5 min. The initial absorbance (A_0) at 340 nm is recorded. Serum, 10 μl, is added to the cuvette, mixed, and allowed to incubate at 30 °C for 5 min. The final absorbance (A_f) is recorded.

Calculation:

$$CO_2\text{, mmol/liter} = \frac{(A_0 - A_f) \times V_t}{6.22 \times V_s}$$

where V_t = total volume, V_s = sample volume, and 6.22 = millimolar absorptivity of NADH at 340 nm.

The automated assay on the Gilford 3500 is done by use of a program designed for the procedure, which requires 1.5 ml of reagent and 5 μl of sample. The result is determined by relating the change in absorbance of unknowns to the change in absorbance of a standard. Analysis rate is 120 determinations per hour.

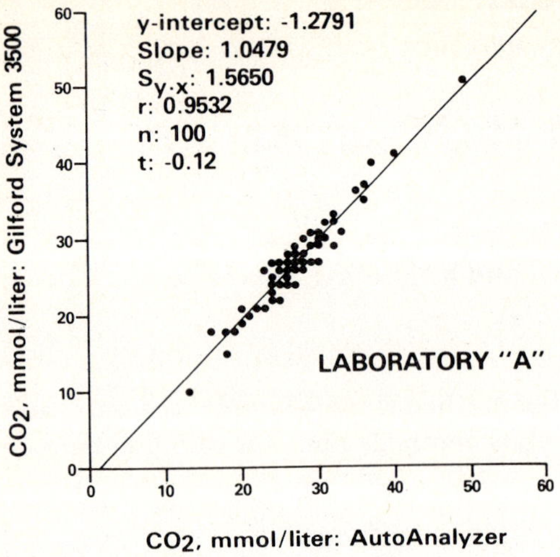

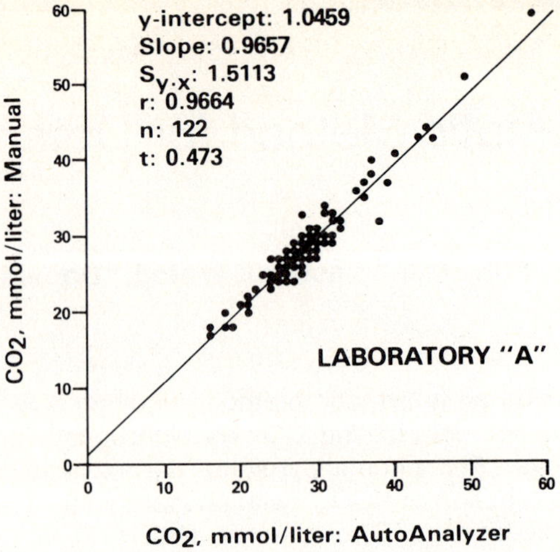

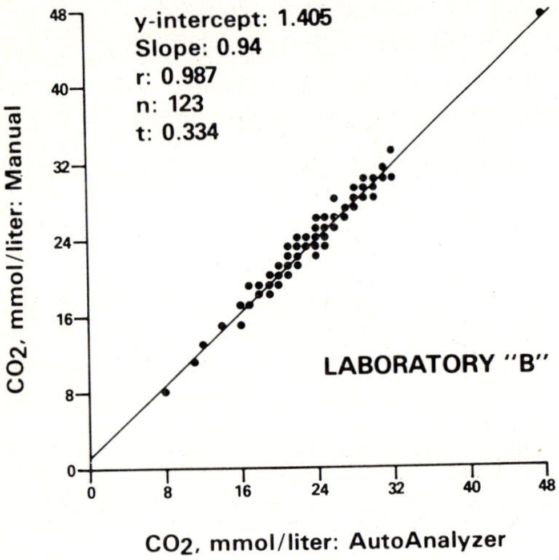

Figure 1.

Comparison of patient values for CO_2 obtained by enzymatic analysis with values obtained on the AutoAnalyzer. Laboratory A: Mercy San Juan Hospital; Laboratory B: Hektoen Institute for Medical Research of the Cook County Hospital.

Table 1. Results of Linearity Study (Serum-Based Comparison Material Used)

Known	Found
CO_2, mmol/liter	
4.0	5.8
8.0	8.7
16.0	15.0
26.0	26.0
36.0	37.0
52.0	51.0
62.0	63.0
72.0	66.0

Results

Regression analysis of three separate sets of data (two manual, one automated) yielded the results shown in Figure 1.

Linearity (Table 1) were determined by adding weighed amounts of sodium bicarbonate to pooled normal serum.

Recovery was determined for three sample concentrations, six replicate determinations at each (Table 2).

Day-to-day precision was determined by the laboratory at Mercy San Juan Hospital by assaying three different concentrations of control materials for 30 days. The laboratory at Hektoen Institute assayed three different concentrations of control material twice a day for 15 days (Table 3).

Discussion

No statistically significant differences were found in any of the correlation studies. In all cases, the t value would have to be greater than 2.0 to indicate a significant difference at the $P = 0.05$ level.

The range of linearity of the test is more than adequate for use in the clinical laboratory.

Analytical recovery was found to be essentially the same for all concentrations of CO_2—whether present as bicarbonate, carbonate, or dissolved gas—reacted with the reagent. Sodium carbonate standards and sodium bicarbonate standards gave the same changes in absorbance. The specificity of the test is satisfactory.

Table 2. Analytical Recovery of Weighed Amounts of Sodium Bicarbonate Added to Control Serum

Low			Normal			High		
Actual	Found	Recovery	Actual	Found	Recovery	Actual	Found	Recovery
mmol/liter		%	mmol/liter		%	mmol/liter		%
Laboratory A								
16	16	100	26	28	107	36	34	94
16	17	106	26	24	92	36	34	94
16	18	113	26	26	100	36	35	97
16	18	113	26	26	100	36	36	100
16	18	113	26	27	104	36	37	103
16	18	113	26	28	107	36	34	94
Laboratory B								
10	9.53	95.3	20	19.17	95.9	30	28.7	95.7
10	10.32	103.2	20	20.53	102.7	30	29.3	97.7
10	10.10	101.1	20	19.87	99.4	30	30.7	102.2
10	9.78	97.8	20	20.53	102.7	30	29.0	96.7
10	9.97	99.7	20	19.62	98.1	30	31.5	104.9
10	105.4	105.4	20	20.22	101.1	30	29.9	99.5

Table 3. Precision Studies for Three Concentrations of Control Material

	Laboratory A				Laboratory B			
Concn	n	Mean	SD	CV, %	n	Mean	SD	CV, %
		mmol/liter				mmol/liter		
Low	30	17.33	0.83	4.79	30	9.62	0.71	7.3
Normal	30	25.87	1.09	4.20	30	20.84	0.63	3.0
High	30	35.47	0.99	2.80	30	42.57	0.94	2.2

Table 4. Comparative Precision of Several Methods for CO_2 in Serum

Method	Mean	SD	Ref.
	mmol/liter		
Van Slyke volumetric	26.9	1.88	Went & Whitehead (*11*)
Van Slyke manometric	19.8	0.41	Went & Whitehead (*11*)
AutoAnalyzer	19.3	0.44	Went & Whitehead (*11*)
AutoAnalyzer	17.0	1.1	Went & Whitehead (*11*)
Enzymatic	17.3	0.83	Lab. A
Enzymatic	25.87	1.09	Lab. A
Enzymatic	20.84	0.63	Lab. B

Went and Whitehead (*11*) reviewed the precision of several methods of carbon dioxide assay (Table 4). The precision of our assay compares well with that of these methods. In our study, the precision in one laboratory was slightly less than in the other, probably because the first used more than one instrument.

The desirable technical features of the enzymatic assay recommend its use as both a routine test and a back-up method for automated methods. By using the enzymatic assay with the Gilford 3500 Computer-Directed Analyzer, many smaller laboratories can afford to automate CO_2 determinations.

References

1. Van Slyke, D. D., and Neill, J. M., The determination of gases in blood and other solutions by vacuum extraction and manometric measurement. *J. Biol. Chem.* **61,** 523 (1924).

2. Van Slyke, D. D., and Plazin, J., *Micromanometric Analysis.* Williams and Wilkins, Baltimore, Md., 1961.

3. Creno, J. J., et al., An evaluation of the Harleco total carbon dioxide apparatus. *Am. J. Med. Technol.* **40,** 50 (1974).

4. Gambino, S. R., and Schreiber, H., The measurement of CO_2 content with the AutoAnalyzer. A comparison of three standard methods and a description of a new method (alkalinization) for preventing loss of CO_2 from open cups. *Am. J. Clin. Pathol.* **54,** 406 (1966).

5. Kenny, M. A., and Cheng, M. H., Rapid automatic simultaneous determination of CO_2 and chloride. *Clin. Chem.* **18,** 352 (1972).

6. Skeggs, L., An automatic method for the determination of carbon dioxide in blood plasma. *Am. J. Clin. Pathol.* **33,** 181 (1960).

7. Van Slyke, D. D., et al., Photometric measurement of plasma pH. *J. Biol. Chem.* **179,** 743 (1949).

8. Sterling, R., and Flores, O., Automated method for micro-scale determination of serum carbon dioxide. *Clin. Chem.* **18,** 544 (1972).

9. Wilson, W., Jesyk, P., Rand, R., and Bevill, R. D., Use of Vickers Discrete Analyzer for enzymatic determination of bicarbonate content of serum. *Clin. Chem.* **19,** 640 (1973). Abstract.

10. Menson, R. C., Narayanswamy, V., Bussian, R. W., and Adams, T. H., A kinetic method for determination of CO_2 in biological fluids. *Clin. Chem.* **20,** 872 (1974). Abstract.

11. Went, J., and Whitehead, T. P., Automated serum carbon dioxide content determinations as a screening test for disorders of the acid-base state. *Clin. Chim. Acta* **26,** 559 (1969).

CLIN. CHEM. 22/2, 246–249 (1976)

Measurement of Diphenylhydantoin in 0.1-ml Plasma Samples: Gas Chromatography and Radioimmunoassay Compared

Michael L'Estrange Orme,[1] Olof Borgå,[2] Clarence Edgar Cook,[3] and Folke Sjöqvist

Concentrations of diphenylhydantoin in 364 plasma samples have been measured both by radioimmunoassay and with a recently developed gas-chromatographic method, which requires only 0.1 ml of plasma per determination. There was an excellent correlation between values obtained by the two methods (r = 0.986), and in only 11 plasma samples did the results differ by more than 20%. Of the investigated samples, 105 were obtained from uremic patients. For these, an equally good agreement was obtained between the two methods. Within-assay variance was 3.1% for the immunoassay and 3.3% for the gas-chromatographic procedure. Without automatic pipetting equipment, the radioimmunoassay procedure took twice as long as the chromatographic assay, and the cost of chemicals was considerably higher. Nevertheless, the better sensitivity of the radioimmunoassay makes it of great value, especially in children, because plasma samples of 10 to 20 μl can be used.

Additional Keyphrases: *Micro-scale gas chromatography • flash methylation • pediatric chemistry • uremia • epilepsy*

There is an increasing need for sensitive, precise, and specific methods for measuring the concentrations of drugs in plasma, both for research purposes and for monitoring therapy (*1, 2*).

A radioimmunoassay for diphenylhydantoin (DPH) was developed by Tigelaar et al. (*3*) but was unspecific in that the main metabolite 5-(4-hydroxyphenyl)-5-phenylhydantoin was detected as sensitively as DPH. This technique also required the antiserum to be used at a final dilution of only eightfold and the lower limit of detectability was relatively high (300 μg/liter of plasma). Although adequate for clinical purposes—the range of therapeutic plasma concentrations is 10–20 mg/liter—this is a relatively low sensitivity for an immunoassay procedure. Cook et al. (*4*) developed an immunoassay that was specific for DPH and showed little cross reactivity with either 5-(4-hydroxyphenyl)-5-phenylhydantoin or with drugs structurally similar to DPH, such as primidone or phenobarbital. The antiserum was used at a dilution of about 14 000-fold, and the limit of sensitivity was of the order of 1 μg/liter of plasma. To evaluate the use of this radioimmunoassay in clinical practice, we decided to compare it with the gas-chromatographic micromethod used for the routine determination of plasma DPH concentrations in this hospital.

Materials and Methods

Plasma Samples

The plasma samples to be analyzed were divided into three groups:

a. Retrospective. All plasma samples coming into the laboratory for routine DPH analysis during one month were analyzed on arrival by the gas-chromatographic method. They were analyzed retrospectively by the immunoassay techniques after a mean storage time at −20 °C of 16 days. DPH in plasma is stable at −20 °C for at least three months (unpublished data from this laboratory).

This group comprised 131 plasma samples, of which 11 samples were also analyzed by both methods on a second occasion.

b. Plasmas from uremic individuals. 105 plasma samples were collected during a year and stored at −20 °C; they were from a group of six patients who were receiving DPH and who also had impaired renal function. The creatinine clearance in these patients varied between 6 and 18 ml/min. Five of these patients had received a single intravenous dose of DPH (2.0 mg/kg body wt), to explore the effect of impaired binding of the drug to plasma proteins on its distribution kinetics (*5*). The other patient was receiving DPH for the treatment of grand mal epilepsy.

Department of Clinical Pharmacology, Huddinge University Hospital, Karolinska Institutet, S-141 86 Huddinge, Sweden.
[1] Wellcome Swedish Fellow.
[2] To whom correspondence should be directed.
[3] Chemistry and Life Sciences Division, Research Triangle Institute, Research Triangle Park, N.C. 27709.
Received Oct. 8, 1975; accepted Dec. 1, 1975.

In patients with impaired renal function, concentrations of both conjugated and unconjugated 5-(4-hydroxyphenyl)-5-phenylhydantoin in plasma are known to increase more than in patients with normal renal function (*6*). If the immunoassay were to measure the metabolites of DPH to any extent, then analysis of such plasma samples provides a good test for the specificity of the immunoassay (by comparison of results with those obtained gas chromatographically).

c. Prospective. In a prospective study, we assessed the practicability of the radioimmunoassay for the routine measurement of plasma DPH in a laboratory not automated for immunoassay work. During four weeks all plasma samples entering the laboratory for DPH analysis were assayed concurrently by gas chromatography and radioimmunoassay. Analyses were started at the same time of day and the time required for the complete analyses was recorded. The plasma samples (n = 128) were analyzed in batches of 20.

Radioimmunoassay of DPH

The radioimmunoassay was done as described by Cook et al. (*4*), with a few modifications. The affinity constant of the antiserum was 3.5×10^9 liter/mol. The plasma samples were diluted 10 000-fold in buffer before analysis and if necessary were re-analyzed on the next occasion at a 1000-fold dilution. The standard DPH samples were prepared from an alcoholic solution (1 g/liter) and diluted serially in buffer so as to give the following quantities per 0.5 ml: 2000, 1000, 500, 200, 100, 50, and 20 pg. Both standard samples and unknown plasma samples were analyzed in triplicate. In addition, two different volumes of the diluted plasmas—0.1 and 0.4 ml—were analyzed. A quality-control solution (20 mg of DPH per liter) was analyzed in each assay as above. (All concentrations of DPH mentioned in this paper refer to the free drug, rather than its sodium salt.)

The range of the standard curve at a plasma dilution of 10 000-fold enables DPH concentrations between 5 and 200 mg/liter to be measured and at a 1000-fold dilution concentrations between 0.5 and 20 mg/liter.

Gas Chromatography of DPH

We used an improved version of the method of Berlin et al. (*7*), a microadaptation of the principles outlined in the method by MacGee (*8*), including on-column methylation of DPH by trimethylanilinium hydroxide and use of the internal standard 5-(4-methylphenyl)-5-phenylhydantoin. The procedure, which omits one of the extraction steps in the original procedure (*7*), was:

To a 100-μl sample of plasma in a 3-ml tapered, glass-stoppered tube, was added 25 μl of NaH_2PO_4 (3 mol/liter) and 2.00 ml of toluene containing 2.40 μg of the internal standard. The tube was gently shaken for 5 min and centrifuged. The toluene (top) layer was transferred to a similar glass tube and 25 μl of a trimethylanilinium hydroxide solution (1 mol/liter) in water/methanol (equal volumes) was added. The tube was shaken vigorously for 1 min (vortex-type mixer) and centrifuged. One microliter of the trimethylanilinium hydroxide (bottom) layer was analyzed on a 1.5 m × 3 mm (i.d.) glass column packed with 3% OV-17 on Gas Chrom Q, 100–120 mesh (Applied Science Labs Inc., State College, Pa. 16801) kept at 220 °C. The injector and detector temperatures were 270 and 265 °C, respectively. The flow rates were: N_2, 25 ml/min; O_2, 200 ml/min; and H_2, 25 ml/min.

Under the above conditions the retention times for DPH and the internal standard were respectively 2.7 and 3.8 min (compared to 8 and 10.9 min in the original publication).

Standard curves were prepared by adding pure DPH to drug-free plasma to produce concentrations of 5, 10, 15, and 20 mg/liter. All standard samples and unknowns were processed in duplicate.

For the plasma samples from uremic patients, which generally contained low concentrations of DPH (*5*), 400-μl samples were analyzed and calculated from standard curves covering concentrations from 0.25 to 4 mg/liter. The lower limit of sensitivity was 0.5 mg/liter for 100-μl samples, 0.2 mg/liter for 400-μl samples.

Results

Reproducibility

The radioimmunoassay gave good repeatability in the analysis of plasma DPH concentrations. A quality control containing 20.0 mg of DPH per liter gave a mean value of 19.00 mg/liter, with a standard devia-

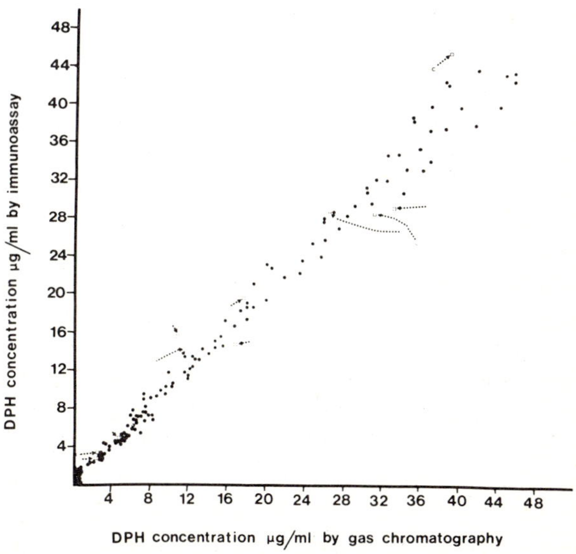

Fig. 1. Comparison between plasma DPH concentrations as measured by gas chromatography and radioimmunoassay in the retrospective study (131 plasmas)

The *dotted lines* join plasma concentrations of DPH in those samples where the analyses were repeated by both methods. The *open circles* indicate the first analysis, and the *open squares* indicate the second analysis tion of 1.02 mg/liter, in 22 determinations. A control plasma containing 2 mg of DPH per liter gave a mean value of 2.00 ± 0.103 mg/liter (SD) (n = 8). Within-assay variance was 3.1% for the immunoassay and 3.3% for the gas-chromatographic procedure.

Correlations

Plasma DPH concentrations as measured by radioimmunoassay and by gas chromatography correlated excellently in all the three parts of the study. In the regression analyses the gas-chromatographic value was arbitrarily chosen as the "independent" variable (x-value).

Retrospective study. In the retrospective study the correlation coefficient (r) was 0.983. The equation for the line was $y = 0.995x + 0.5$. In 11 of the 131 plasma samples there was an apparent disparity between the DPH concentrations found by the two methods. These samples are indicated by arrows in Figure 1. The disparity was largely due to differences in the chromatographic results on the two occasions.

Uremic study. There was a good correlation between the plasma DPH concentrations obtained by the two methods ($r = 0.993$, n = 105). The equation of the line was $y = 0.94x + 0.04$ (Figure 2). The plasma samples all contained less than 5.0 mg of DPH per liter.

Prospective study. There was also a good correlation between the plasma DPH concentrations measured by the two methods in the prospective study ($r = 0.986$, n = 128, $y = 1.02x + 0.04$).

Other Considerations

Assay times and costs. The average time for immunoassay of 20 unknown plasma samples was 8.2 h (not including counting time), while the average time for determination of the same samples by the gas-chromatographic procedure was 4.6 h. Throughout the immunoassay procedure, pipetting was done by hand (using Oxford samplers). The cost of the chemicals (not including the cost of ^{3}H-DPH and antiserum) for the immunoassay as performed was $1.50 per plasma sample (for an assay of 20 plasma samples), and the chief cost was that of liquid-scintillation fluid. The cost and time analysis of the immunoassay were based on triplicate analysis of all samples, and furthermore each unknown plasma sample was analyzed at two dilutions as described in the experimental part. The cost of the gas-chromatographic analysis for DPH was less than $0.25 per plasma sample.

Interference from other drugs. The patients from whom these plasma samples were taken were also being treated with various other anti-epileptic, sedative, and cardiovascular drugs, but in no plasma sample could any disparity between the two methods be ascribed to an interfering drug. In the retrospective and prospective studies combined, 109 plasma samples were from patients taking phenobarbital, 48 from patients receiving carbamazepine, 38 from patients receiving primidone, 25 from patients receiving ethosuximide, and 37 from patients receiving diazepam or nitrazepam. Many patients were receiving more than one drug at the same time (the number of drugs taken averaged 1.96 per patient), including such drugs as digoxin, furosemide, thiazide diuretics, propranolol, orphenadrine, chlorpromazine, thioridazine, and haloperidol.

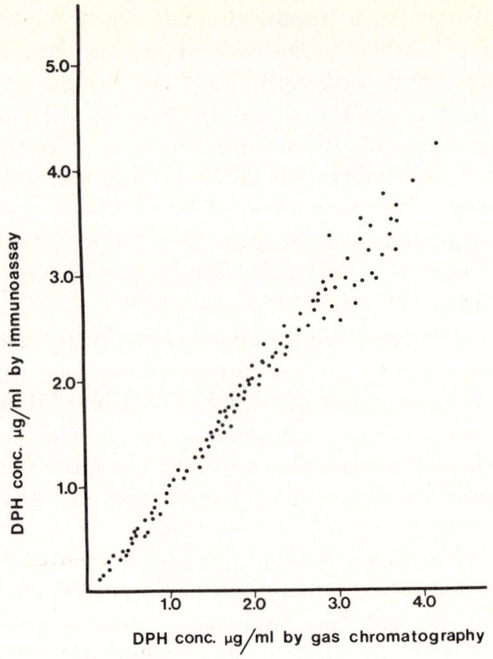

Fig. 2. Comparison between plasma DPH concentrations as measured by gas chromatography and radioimmunoassay in 105 plasma samples taken from six patients with impaired renal function

Discussion

Measurement of diphenylhydantoin is becoming increasingly important, and recent studies have shown that clinical care is improved considerably if DPH concentration is monitored (*9*). Most current analyses are gas chromatographic, but we have shown here that the radioimmunoassay developed by Cook et al. (*4*) gives results identical to those found by gas chromatography in the large majority of analyses. The few discrepancies exceeding 20% seemed to be due to nonsystematic errors rather than specificity problems. No interference has been found in either of the two assay procedures from any of the drugs usually given with DPH, nor have we found any interference from the metabolites of DPH. There was 2% cross-reaction of 5-(4-hydroxyphenyl)-5-phenylhydantoin (added in vitro) with the antiserum used in this study. The cross reactivity to other known metabolites of DPH in man has not been tested in vitro, owing to the lack of reference compounds. There was a cross reaction between 5-(3-hydroxyphenyl)-5-phenylhydantoin and this antiserum of 16%. However, 5-(3-hydroxyphenyl)-5-phenylhydantoin is a DPH metabolite in the dog, but not in man (*10*). It seems unlikely, therefore, that any of the metabolites of DPH in man will interfere with the immunoassay of DPH. This is in contrast to a previous immunoassay for diphenylhydantoin developed by Tigelaar et al. (*3*), in which the antibody used had a 100% cross-reactivity with 5-(4-hydroxyphenyl)-5-phenylhydantoin and thus limited the value of this assay.

As done in this study, the immunoassay procedure took twice as long to perform as the gas-chromatographic assay, but if the immunoassay were in constant use an automatic pipetting station (such as the Micromedic) would result in much time saving. In routine use it should be possible to accept a smaller range for the immunoassay (e.g., 3–36 mg/liter) and thus to analyze only one volume of the diluted plasma. This would essentially halve both labor and costs.

The cost of the immunoassay was also greater than that of the gas-chromatographic procedure. It should be pointed out that the cost quoted is just for the chemicals involved (except ^{3}H-DPH and antiserum) and does not include costs for equipment or labor. Capital costs of the immunoassay are also likely to be greater, because a liquid-scintillation counter is usually much more costly than a gas chromatograph. However, one advantage of the immunoassay is the possibility of using small (capillary-blood) samples, which makes it ideal for pediatric practice. It would also appear to be useful in pharmacokinetic studies in either animals or man where plasma concentrations of DPH of less than 0.5 mg/liter are to be anticipated.

This work was supported by Grant 04X-3902 from the Swedish Medical Research Council. The antiserum and radiolabeled diphenylhydantoin were prepared under Contract No. PH-43-NIGMS-65-1057 between the Pharmacology/Toxicology Program, NIGMS, NIH, USPHS, and Research Triangle Institute.

References

1. Koch-Weser, J., Serum drug concentrations as therapeutic guides. *New Engl. J. Med.* **287,** 227 (1972).

2. Sjöqvist, F., and Bertilsson, L., Plasma concentrations of drugs and pharmacological response in man. In *Biological Effects of Drugs in Relation to Their Plasma Concentration,* D. S. Davies and B. N. C. Prichard, Eds., Macmillan, London, 1973, pp 25–40.

3. Tigelaar, R. E., Rapport, R. L., Inman, J. K., and Kupferberg, H. J., A radioimmunoassay for diphenylhydantoin. *Clin. Chim. Acta* **43,** 231 (1973).

4. Cook, C. E., Kepler, J. A., and Christensen, H. D., Antiserum to diphenylhydantoin: Preparation and characterization. *Res. Commun. Chem. Pathol. Pharmacol.* **5,** 767 (1973).

5. Odar-Cederlöf, I., and Borgå, O., Kinetics of diphenylhydantoin in uremic patients: Consequences of decreased protein binding. *Eur. J. Clin. Pharmacol.* **7,** 31 (1974).

6. Letteri, J. M., Mellk, H., Louis, S., et al., Diphenylhydantoin metabolism in uremia. *New Engl. J. Med.* **285,** 648 (1971).

7. Berlin, A., Agurell, S., Borgå, O., et al., Micromethod for the determination of diphenylhydantoin in plasma and cerebrospinal fluid—a comparison between a gas chromatographic and a spectrophotometric method. *Scand. J. Clin. Lab. Invest.* **29,** 281 (1972).

8. MacGee, J., Rapid determination of diphenylhydantoin in blood plasma by gas-liquid chromatography. *Anal. Chem.* **42,** 421 (1970).

9. Lund, L., Anticonvulsant effect of diphenylhydantoin relative to plasma levels. A prospective three-year study in ambulant patients with generalized epileptic seizures. *Arch. Neurol.* (Chicago) **31,** 289 (1975).

10. Atkinson, A. I., MacGee, J., Strong, J., et al., Identification of 5-*meta*-hydroxyphenyl-5-phenylhydantoin as a metabolite of diphenylhydantoin. *Biochem. Pharmacol.* **19,** 2483 (1970).

CLIN. CHEM. 22/2, 250–256 (1976)

Radioimmunoassay of Plasma Renin Activity

Frej Fyhrquist, Pertti Soveri, Liisa Puutula, and Ulf-Håkan Stenman

We describe a sensitive, simplified radioimmunoassay method for determination of plasma renin activity. Plasma was acidified to the optimal pH (6.0) of angiotensin I generation with the least possible dilution, by using a single addition of hydrochloric acid and the enzyme inhibitor hydroxyquinoline. Recovery of unlabeled angiotensin I added to plasma was 92–97%; that of monoiodinated angiotensin I exceeded 90%, indicating satisfactory protection from proteolytic enzymes. Plasma constituents interfered little with the radioimmunoassay. Blank values for plasma kept at 0 °C were 10.7 ± 2.3 (mean ± SD) percent of the activity values for samples kept at +37 °C (n = 63). In the routine setting, 6.25 pg of angiotensin I or 10^{-6} Goldblatt units of Standard Human Renin was detected. We report results of plasma renin activity measurements and a comparison with seven renin kits, and with bioassay for plasma renin activity.

Additional Keyphrases: *angiotensin I • reference values • "kit" methods • variables affecting the assay • comparison with bioassay • changes in disease • problems of standardization • aldosteronism*

The main problems with current assay methods for plasma renin activity (PRA; EC 3.4.99.19) are insufficient sensitivity (*1, 2*), methodological variations (*3, 4*), and the technical complexity of most methods published so far.

We have developed a method to determine PRA based upon radioimmunoassay of angiotensin I (AI) generated by endogenous renin and renin substrate reacting at +37 °C, pH 6.0, for 1 h. The main advantages of this method are its simplicity of performance (acid and enzyme inhibitor are added in one step), the optimal pH of AI generation (6.0), and the small degree of dilution of plasma during incubation (10%), which minimizes harmful dilution effects.

The Minerva Institute for Medical Research, P.O. Box 819, Helsinki 10, Finland; and the IVth Department of Medicine, University of Helsinki, Finland.

Received Nov. 11, 1975; accepted Nov. 25, 1975.

Materials and Methods

Reagents

Angiotensin I antiserum. Antibodies to AI were generated in rabbits by monthly intramuscular injections of ileu$_5$-AI (Schwarz/Mann, Orangeburg, N. Y. 10962) coupled to human serum albumin (Kabi, Stockholm, Sweden) by carbodiimide condensation (*5*). All of the nine rabbits so injected developed antisera useful in the RIA of AI. The serum chosen showed low cross reaction with ileu$_5$-angiotensin II (<0.2%), 2-8 ileu$_5$-angiotensin II heptapeptide (<0.05%), and 3-8 ileu$_5$-angiotensin II hexapeptide (<0.5%). This antiserum bound 50% of a 100-pg amount of ^{125}I-labeled AI when diluted 400 000 fold.

^{125}I-labeled angiotensin I and isoelectric focusing. Ileu$_5$-AI was iodinated at +4 °C with ^{125}I (IMS 30, Amersham, England) by the Chloramine T method. Reaction time was 10–15 s, pH was 7.5. A 1 × 80 cm column containing diethylaminoethyl-Sephadex A-25 (Pharmacia, Uppsala, Sweden) was used for purification, as described elsewhere (*5*). The first peak of radioactivity, containing the monoiodo-AI, was tested for purity with the isoelectric focusing technique, performed in a 110-ml LKB column at a 100 ml/liter LKB Ampholine (LKB, Bromma 1, Sweden) concentration and a temperature of +4 °C. The column was stabilized with a 500 g/liter sucrose gradient. Focusing time was two days, voltage 450 V. Fractions of 1 ml were collected, and the pH and radioactivity of each fraction recorded.

Purified ^{125}I-labeled AI was diluted and stored in assay buffer at −20 °C, remaining useful in the radioimmunoassay for AI for at least 16 weeks.

Assay buffer. We used a phosphate buffer, 150 mmol/liter, pH 7.5, containing Na$_2$ethylenediaminetetraacetate, 30 mmol/liter; hydroxyquinoline, 3.5 mmol/liter; neomycin sulphate (Upjohn Co., Kalamazoo, Mich. 49001), 200 mg/liter; and human serum albumin, 1.0 g/liter. This buffer remained stable for three weeks at +4 °C, in the dark.

Acid inhibitor mixture. Hydrochloric acid, 760 mmol/liter, and hydroxyquinoline, 70 mmol/liter in ethanol (200 ml/liter), were mixed in equal volumes and stored at +4 °C in the dark, remaining stable for four weeks.

Coated charcoal. Coated charcoal stock was prepared by mixing 0.5 g of Dextran T 70 (Pharmacia, Uppsala, Sweden) and 2.5 g of charcoal (Sigma Chemical Co., St. Louis, Mo. 63178) with 200 ml of phosphate buffer (150 mmol/liter, pH 7.5). This stock was stable for three months at +4 °C.

Special reagents. Ileu$_5$angiotensin I, ileu$_5$2-8 heptapeptide, and ileu$_5$3-8 angiotensin II hexapeptide were from Schwarz/Mann. Standard Human Renin (batch 68/356) was a gift of The National Institute for Medical Research, Hampstead Laboratories, Holy Hill, London NW3 6RB.

Renin-assay kits were from the following sources: Clinical Assays Inc., 237 Binney St., Cambridge, Mass. 02142; Cea-Ire-Sorin, 91190, Gif sur Yvette, France; Mallinkrodt Inc., 675 Brown Rd., Hazelwood, Mo. 63042; New England Nuclear, 15 Harvard St., Worcester, Mass. 01608; Ormonoterapia Richter, Via Chioggia 2, 20125 Milano, Italy; Schwarz/Mann; and Squibb & Sons Inc., New Brunswick, N. J. 08903.

Renin Assay

Collection of blood. Blood samples were collected into ice-chilled tubes containing Na$_2$ethylenediaminetetraacetate, 6 g/liter of blood. Plasma was separated by centrifugation at +4 °C, and stored until assayed at −20 °C.

Generation of angiotensin I. Thawed plasma, 0.9 ml, and acid/inhibitor mixture, 0.1 ml, were added to duplicate tubes in an icebath.

Half of the sealed tubes were transferred to a +37 °C waterbath, and incubated for 60 min. The other half (blanks) were kept on ice. The reaction was stopped by adding 3.0 ml of ice-cold assay buffer, and the mixture transferred to the icebath. Small plasma volumes (e.g., 225 µl) were easily measured by dividing all reagent volumes by four.

Radioimmunoassay of angiotensin I. This was performed by incubating the following mixture at +4 °C for 18–24 h:

1. Samples (37 °C) *or* Blank (0 °C) *or* Standard angiotension I (6.25–1000 pg)	0.2 ml
2. ^{125}I-labeled AI (20000 counts/100 s)	0.2 ml
3. Anti-AI serum (1:200 000)	0.4 ml
Incubation volume	0.8 ml

All reagents were diluted in assay buffer; tubes were run in duplicates. Samples expected to yield high AI values were assayed at additional (10-fold) dilutions. Antibody-bound polypeptide was separated with coated charcoal, 0.4 ml, freshly diluted fourfold from stock with ice-cold phosphate buffer (150 mmol/liter, pH 7.5) on ice. The tubes were shaken with this mixture for 1 min, then centrifuged (2000 rpm, 10 min) at room temperature. Either the charcoal precipitate or 0.7 ml of the supernate was counted in a gamma counter.

Calculation of PRA

After subtraction of background radioactivity, the percent of ^{125}I-labeled AI (B%) was calculated according to the formulas:

1. Supernate counted: B% = (sample or standard counts/corrected total counts) × 100. Corrected total counts = counts in 0.7 ml from tubes containing the total counts in 1.2 ml.

2. Charcoal counted: B% = (total counts − sample or standard counts/total counts) × 100.

Standard curves were constructed on semilog paper, with B% on the ordinate and pg AI on the abscissa. PRA was calculated according to the formula:

3. PRA, µg/liter per hour = AI generated ($\mu g^{+37\,°C} - \mu g^{+0\,°C}$)/(sample volume × incubation time). The values were corrected for known dilution.

Results

Analytical Variables

Incubation pH. Maximal AI was generated at pH 6.0. In 56 clinical plasma samples chosen without conscious bias, the pH after the addition of the acid-inhibitor mixture was 6.03 ± 0.14 (mean ± SD) and remained unchanged during incubation for 1 h at +37 °C. Thus, the pH remained within the optimal pH range throughout the incubation period.

There was a 1.9-fold increase (mean) in PRA when plasma was incubated at pH 6.0 as compared to pH 7.4 (Figure 1). The increase was of the same order in all samples investigated, in both peripheral venous

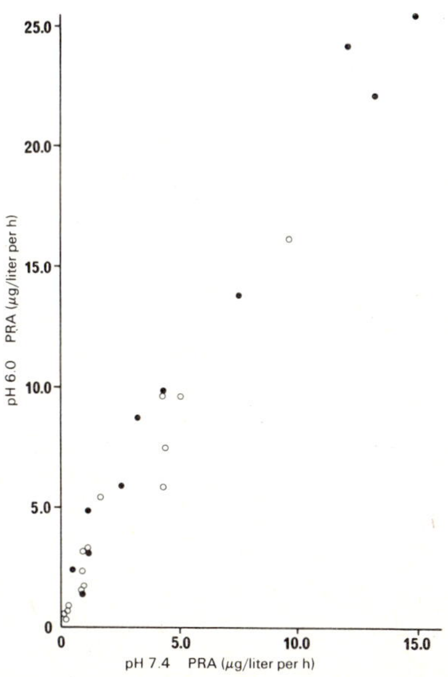

Fig. 1. Correlation between PRA values, plasma incubation at pH 7.4 and 6.0, for the same samples of peripheral venous plasma (*open circles*) and renal venous plasma (*closed circles*)
n = 26, *r* = 0.97

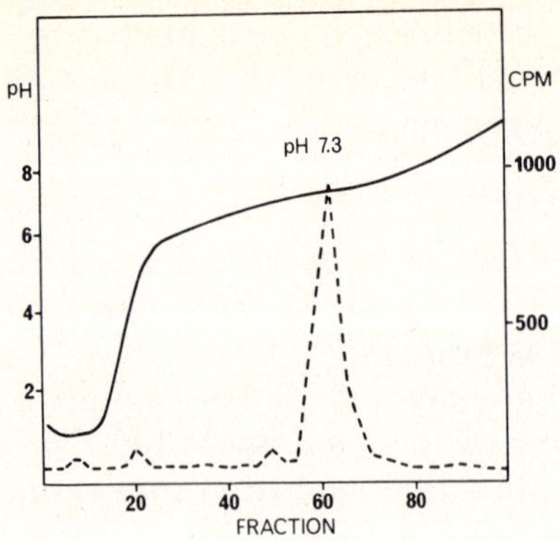

Fig. 2. Result of isoelectric focusing of ^{125}I-labeled angiotensin I after incubation with plasma containing Na_2ethylenediaminetetraacetate and hydroxyquinoline at pH 6.0 for 1 h at +37 °C

Monoiodinated angiotensin I is focused at pH 7.3 (*broken line*). The pH gradient is indicated by the *unbroken line*

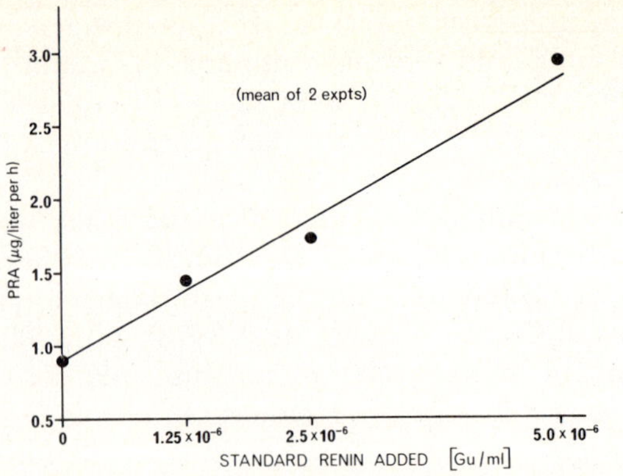

Fig. 3. Recovery of standard human renin added to pooled human plasma

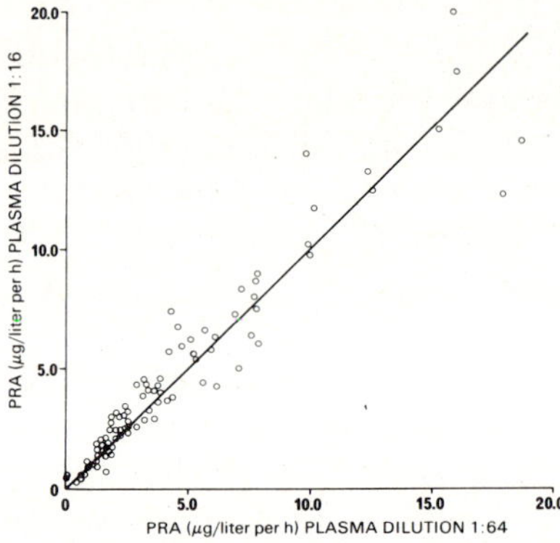

Fig. 4. Correlation between PRA values measured in the same plasma samples diluted 64- (*x*-axis) and 16-fold (*y*-axis)

n = 82, r = 0.91. The line of identity is indicated

and renal venous blood, and at low, normal, and high PRA's as well.

Incubation time and temperature. The amount of AI generated with time increased linearly or almost linearly during the first 120 min of incubation at +37 °C in each of 22 individual samples tested. When the incubation time was further prolonged, the rate of AI generation was gradually decreasing in all samples tested.

Stability of angiotensin I during incubation. When ileu$_5$-AI, 50–2000 pg, was added to plasma before incubation, 94% (range, 92–97%) was recovered by radioimmunoassay after incubation at +37 °C for 1 h as described above (*Materials and Methods*). In six other experiments, 100 pg of monoiodinated ^{125}I-labeled AI was incubated with plasma under the same conditions. The plasma was then boiled for 5 min. Isoelectric focusing of the supernate showed no appreciable breakdown of the ^{125}I-labeled AI (Figure 2).

Analytical recovery of standard human renin. The addition of standard human renin in doubling amounts to pooled low-renin human plasma resulted in linear increases of PRA (Figure 3). Using this preparation of standard human renin and the routine PRA assay setting, we estimated sensitivity to be at least 1.0×10^{-6} Goldblatt units per milliliter of plasma.

Blank. Blank values for plasma kept on ice correspond to 10.7 ± 2.3 (mean ± SD) percent of the PRA values of the same samples kept at +37 °C (n = 63, mean PRA, blank subtracted = 2.38 ± 1.03 μg/liter per hour. The percentage blank values decreased with higher PRA values.

Plasma dilution. Results of AI radioimmunoassay were not significantly affected by plasma dilution exceeding the one we used in the present method. There was an excellent correlation between AI values obtained in the same plasma samples diluted 16- and 64-fold (Figure 4).

Sensitivity, accuracy, and reproducibility. In the routine setting, 6.25 pg of AI consistently produced a deflection greater than 2 SD from zero dose of unlabeled AI in the standard curve. This corresponded to the PRA value 0.16 μg/liter per hour for a 1-h incubation. Thus, all clinically important PRA values, including those of 12 patients with primary aldosteronism (Table 1) were detected.

Within-assay variation (CV) was 6.8% in the low, 5.5% in the intermediate, and 4.0% in the high range of PRA values (n = 20 for each group). Interassay variation was 7.4% in the low, 6.5% in the intermediate, and 4.7% in the high range of PRA (in 18 consecutive assays).

Comparison with bioassay and renin kits. PRA values obtained with the present assay method compared well with those obtained with each of six commercially available kit methods (Table 2), but these kits yielded values for PRA ranging from 27 to 73% of the values obtained for the same plasma samples with the present method.

Isoelectric focusing of the ^{125}I-labeled AI supplied with the kits indicated acceptable purity in most kits. One batch of one kit (Squibb) contained material appearing at three values of isoelectric point (Figure 5). Of these peaks, the one at pH 7.3, corresponding to monoiodinated AI, was of high immunoreactivity.

Table 1. Comparison of PRA Values Obtained with the Present Assay Method with Commercial Renin Kits and with Bioassay

Method	n	Mean percent of the present method	Correlation, *r*	pH during plasma incubation
Present method		100		6.0
New England Nuclear	12	73	0.95	5.5–6.0
New England Nuclear	12	75	0.97	5.5–6.0
Cea-Ire-Sorin	12	57	0.91	5.5–6.0
Cea-Ire-Sorin	12	59	0.68	5.5–6.0
Richter	10	33	0.99	6.4
Richter	10	59	0.88	6.4
Mallinkrodt	10	41	0.87	6.0
Schwarz/Mann	12	34	0.81	7.4
Clinical Assay	16	27	0.98	7.4
Squibb	20	27	0.93	7.4
Bioassay	16	40	0.76	5.5

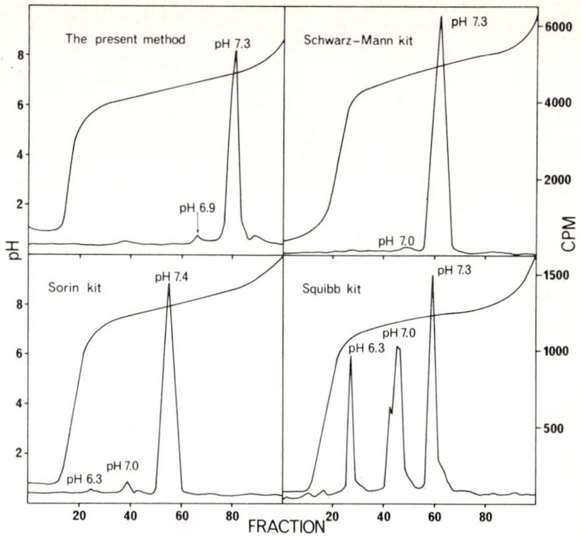

Fig. 5. Results with isoelectric focusing of ^{125}I-labeled angiotensin I supplied with three kit batches, and one batch from the present method

PRA's in Healthy and Diseased Subjects

All clinically important PRA's were detected with the present assay method (Table 2), including those of 12 patients with suppressed PRA's because of primary aldosteronism. PRA values in ambulatory fertile women were greater in the postovulatory than in the preovulatory phase of the menstrual cycle, and were even greater in pregnancy. PRA decreased with age. Forty-two patients with renovascular hypertension all had PRA values exceeding the upper limit of reference values for healthy subjects in the upright posture.

Discussion

There is a lively debate with regard to the optimal conditions for assay of PRA (*1, 2, 4, 6–9*). Several important objections to available PRA assay methods have been stated by Heise (*10*) and discussed at length by (e.g.) Sealey and Laragh (*1, 2*). The present assay method satisfies most of the requirements for an adequate PRA assay method. Thus, in the AI-generation step, we used the optimal pH (6.0) for AI generation, acidification of plasma with minimal dilution, a short incubation (1 h), and maximal simplification of all steps involved. Moreover, by the present method, diluted plasma, stored frozen, may be repeatedly radioimmunoassayed for its AI content with no need for re-incubation of plasma.

Table 2. Values for PRA in Healthy and Diseased Subjects

Condition	n	Daily sodium intake, mmol	Plasma renin activity (mean ± SEM), μg/liter per h: Supine[a]	Upright[b]
Healthy women				
Preovulatory	37	ad lib.	0.74 ± 0.08	
Postovulatory	34	ad lib.	1.18 ± 0.13	
Healthy men				
45–55 years old	470	ad lib.	0.96 ± 0.16	
21–37 years old	14	ad lib.	1.26 ± 0.14	
Control patients[c]	200	100–140	1.34 ± 0.27	3.09 ± 0.41
Essential hypertension	113	100–140	1.21 ± 0.08	1.92 ± 0.17
Primary aldosteronism	12	100–140	0.26 ± 0.04	0.35 ± 0.05
Renovascular hypertension	42	100–140	9.17 ± 1.48	19.5 ± 3.23
Anephric, male	6	80	0.0–0.08 (range)	

[a] After more than 1 h of supine position, at 0800–0900 hours.
[b] After 2 h of upright position, at 1000–1100 hours.
[c] Patients without drugs or diseases assumed to affect the renin–angiotensin system.

Incubation pH. The reaction between renin and renin substrate should preferably take place at optimal pH (5.7–6.2), to ensure maximal generation of AI (*1, 2, 5, 10*). The 1.9-fold increase in PRA observed at pH 6.0 as compared to pH 7.4 agrees well with previous data (*2*). We observed that this increase is of the same magnitude for PRA's in the low, medium, or high range. This also applies to renal venous plasma. The use of optimal incubation pH did not distort proportions between PRA values, an important factor in the evaluation of renal venous PRA (*11*).

It has been suggested that acid proteases generated AI in the plasma from an anephric man, at pH 6.0 (*6*). In agreement with this observation, we observed low (maximally, 0.08 μg/liter per hour) generation of AI in plasma from anephric patients, but none at pH 7.4. For a 1-h incubation period, however, we consider such low renin-like activity negligible. Our results with isoelectric focusing of monoiodinated AI exposed for 1 h at pH 6.0 to plasma containing Na_2ethylenediaminetetraacetate and hydroxyquinoline would indicate excellent protection of the AI generated. This is important, because the pH of plasma incubation may be critical for the efficiency of various enzyme inhibitors (*6*).

We invariably observed increases of PRA when the incubation pH was decreased from 7.4 to 6.0, in agreement with earlier reports (*2, 12, 13*) but opposing the recent report by Oparil et al. (*6*). Differences in enzyme inhibitors, incubation time, or technique of plasma acidification may account for this discrepancy. If plasma is considerably diluted in the course of acidification, the resulting dilution of substrate may decrease PRA more than would be expected from dilution of renin alone, as discussed by Sealey and Laragh (*2*).

In the present assay method, plasma was acidified to pH 6.0 with a single addition of hydrochloric acid, and only a 10% dilution. No change in pH was observed during incubation for 1 h at +37 °C. Thus no buffers in addition to those offered by plasma constituents appeared necessary. A serious problem when incubating nonbuffered plasma at +37 °C, pH 7.4, is the tendency of the pH to increase, resulting in an even lower rate of AI generation (*1, 2*).

Incubation time. Because generation of AI in incubated plasma decreases with time (*12–17*), as confirmed by our data, we consider a short incubation time, 1 h or less, preferable to the long incubation times (e.g., 18 h) recommended for low PRA samples (*1, 2*). Consumption of renin substrate and possible inactivation of renin during prolonged incubation leads one to expect nonlinearity of AI generation with prolonged incubation time. However, linearity of AI generation during 18 h of incubation has been reported (*1, 2*). This problem, although not yet completely solved, appears irrelevant when all clinically important values of PRA can be measured by use of a short (1-h) incubation. The present assay method, like some other methods (*12, 17, 22*), is sensitive enough to allow for a short incubation time, which we do recommend.

Stability of angiotensin I. No known combinations of enzyme inhibitors used in current PRA assay methods provide complete protection of the AI generated (*1, 2, 5, 6, 13, 15*). We have chosen the combination of Na_2ethylenediaminetetraacetate, 30 mmol/liter (or K_2ethylenediaminetetraacetate), and hydroxyquinoline, 3.5 mmol/liter, because at pH 6.0, this resulted in high recovery of unlabeled and monoiodinated AI added to plasma before incubation. The concentration of hydroxyquinoline appeared to be critical. Proteolytic breakdown of added AI increased when hydroxyquinoline concentration was less than 2.5 mmol/liter. Other enzyme inhibitors recommended to be used in renin assays—namely PMSF (*5, 7*), DFP (*1, 2, 6, 7*), and BAL (*5, 6, 7, 15*)—did not improve our method when tested at pH 6.0 in the combinations and at the concentrations recommended (unpublished data). The added neomycin in all buffers protected against bacterial growth during the incubation step of the immunoassay.

Comparison with bioassay and kit methods. Values of PRA obtained with the present assay method correlated well with those obtained with a bioassay according to Boucher et al. (*19*), but our method gave values about 2.5-fold greater, in agreement with previous reports (*3*).

PRA determined with commercially available kits according to the manufacturers' instructions correlated quite well with data obtained with the present assay method. However, they gave lower PRA values than our method (range 27–75%), indicating lower sensitivity. This may be explained by: (*a*) nonoptimal pH of plasma incubation (Clinical Assays, Schwarz/Mann, Squibb), (*b*) dilution of plasma when acidified (Cea Ire Sorin, Mallinkrodt, NEN), (*c*) longer incubation time (Mallinkrodt, Richter, Schwarz/Mann, Squibb), and (*d*) impurities of the labeled AI (Squibb, Figure 5).

Differences in the standard AI supplied with kits were usually small and did not explain the lower values obtained with renin kits. The ^{125}I-labeled AI supplied with kits was usually more than 90% monoiodinated, as tested with isoelectric focusing—monoiodinated, highly immunoreactive material appearing at pH 7.3. Peaks of lower immunoreactivity, focusing at isoelectric pH values 6.9–7.0 and 6.3 (Figure 5)—likely to be products of overiodination—usually did not disturb the radioimmunoassay step.

Immunological and nonspecific interference, blank. The problem of nonspecific interference of plasma proteins (*20*) and other plasma constituents (*21*) that may interfere with the binding of AI to antibody has been circumvented by boiling (*22*) or extracting (*23*) plasma samples after incubation. Like other investigators (*1, 2, 12, 18*), we have used dilution of plasma before radioimmunoassay to minimize interference. Applying dilution with a factor 16 or more, we did not detect serious interference from plasma constituents, and this was further demonstrated by identity of standard curves when plasma diluted 16-fold or plain assay buffer were used as diluents (unpublished results).

The antiserum used in the present assay method showed negligible immunological cross reaction with angiotensin II, des_1-heptapeptide, and $des_{1,2}$-hexapeptide of angiotensin II, known to be present in human blood. With the exception of the des_1-angiotensin I nonapeptide, not demonstrated in human blood, but theoretically a possible product of enzymes acting on renin substrate or AI, immunological cross reaction therefore can be neglected in the present assay method.

Blanks were low, about 10% of the PRA values at +37 °C, if the samples were properly cooled and handled. However, in critical work, particularly when searching for suppressed PRA's, blanks appear advisable. Blanks should correct for both the small amounts of AI present in plasma before incubation, the specific interference, and interference by nonspecific plasma constituents (*20, 21*), which may interact with the angiotensin–antibody binding. The use of blanks requires characterization of the antiserum chosen, because percentage blank values may vary with the antiserum (*2*). We observed increased blank values with decreasing K_a values of five antisera generated against AI, in harmony with the observations of Sealey and Laragh (*2*) (unpublished observation). Thus, high-affinity antisera not only increase the sensitivity of the AI radioimmunoassay, but also appear to decrease nonspecific plasma interference.

Reference standards for renin assays. As long as various procedures for renin assay are used in different laboratories, results are difficult to compare (*2, 3, 9, 10*). This applies particularly to differences in incubation pH (*2, 6*) and time (*1, 2, 12, 15, 17*), and to enzyme inhibitors used (*1, 2, 6, 7, 15*). Until the answers to these questions have been generally agreed upon, comparison and calibration of renin assays may be undertaken by using available sources of Human Standard Renin (The National Institute for Medical Research, Holy Hill, London NW3 6RB). The basic requirement of any renin assay, be it an assay for PRA or plasma renin concentration (*7, 22–25*), is that it provides relevant information on the activity of the renin–angiotensin system. The data therefore ought to reflect blood concentrations of angiotensin II, the main effector of this system at the receptor level. By using a radioimmunoassay for angiotensin II (*26*) and the present PRA assay method, we obtained good correlation between PRA and angiotensin II concentration ($n = 84$, $r = 0.87$) measured in the same plasma samples from randomly chosen hypertensive ward patients (unpublished). This agrees with previous reports (*17*) and shows that the present PRA assay method gives data that reflect the blood concentration of the most active principle of the renin–angiotensin system, angiotensin II.

The use of heterologous renin substrate from sheep (*22, 25*) or swine (*24*) introduces the problem of controlling possible renin inhibitors, activators, and intrinsic renin activity present in such preparations. These circumstances, and the widespread use of PRA in current medical literature, may explain why methods for measuring plasma renin "concentration" have not gained popularity in clinical laboratories, although they offer zero-order kinetics of the renin–renin substrate reaction.

Among the newest problems of renin assay are (*a*) the possible existence of "prorenin" in human plasma (*27*) and (*b*) postulated renin activators (*28*) and inhibitors (*29*). The change of PRA values in plasma stored frozen (*30*) may be associated with these new observations and may have important bearings on PRA assay in general. We believe that these problems should be solved before decisions concerning standardization of renin assays are made.

Note added in proof. The important report of an international collaborative study on renin assay of Bangham et al. (*31*) contains useful information on interlaboratory variations and recommendations made on renin assay procedures as a result of the study.

Plasma renin activity was bioassayed by S. Lahovaara, M.Sc., Department of Pharmacology, Univ. of Helsinki. F.F. was supported by the Finnish National Research Council for Medical Science (1663-3) and the Nordisk Insulinfond, Copenhagen.

References

1. Sealey, J. E., and Laragh, J. H., Searching out low renin patients: Limitation of some commonly used methods. *Am. J. Med.* **55,** 303 (1973).

2. Sealey, J. E., and Laragh, J. H., Radioimmunoassay of plasma renin activity. *Semin. Nucl. Med.* **5,** 189 (1975).

3. Fleming, L. W., Stewart, W. K., and Hutchinson, F., Incubation conditions during the radioimmunoassay of plasma renin activity. *Clin. Chim. Acta* **50,** 215 (1974).

4. Haas, E., and Goldblatt, H., Indirect assay of plasma-renin. *Lancet* **i,** 1330 (1972).

5. Freedlender, A. E., Fyhrquist, F., and Hollemans, H. J. G., Renin and angiotensins. In *Methods of Hormone Radioimmunoassay,* M. B. Jaffe and H. R. Behrman, Eds. Academic Press, New York, N. Y., 1974, pp 455–469.

6. Oparil, S., Koerner, T. J., and Haber, E., Effects of pH on apparent generation of angiotensin I in human plasma. *J. Clin. Endocrinol. Metab.* **39,** 965 (1974).

7. Kodish, M. E., and Katz, F. H., Plasma renin concentration: Comparison of angiotensinase inhibitors and correlation with plasma renin activity and aldosterone. *J. Lab. Clin. Med.* **83,** 705 (1974).

8. Kotchen, T. A., Flamenbaum, W., Cirksena, W., and Gamble, W., Comparison of a biological and an immunological assay for the measurement of plasma renin activity. *J. Clin. Endocrinol. Metab.* **36,** 804 (1973).

9. Latta, J., Improved measurement of plasma renin activity and concentration. *Clin. Chem.* **21,** 1344 (1975). Letter to the Editor.

10. Heise, C. M., Measurement of plasma renin activity. *Clin. Chem.* **21,** 447 (1975). Letter to the Editor.

11. Vaughan, E. D., Bühler, F. R., Laragh, J. H., et al., Renovascular hypertension. Renin measurements to indicate hypersecretion and contralateral suppression, estimate renal plasma flow, and score for surgical curability. *Am. J. Med.* **55,** 402 (1973).

12. Cohen, E. L., Grim, C. E., Conn, J. W., et al., Accurate and rapid measurement of plasma renin activity by radioimmunoassay. *J. Lab. Clin. Med.* **77,** 1025 (1971).

13. Malvano, R., Zuchelli, G. C., Rosa, U., et al., Measurement of plasma renin activity by angiotensin I radioimmunoassay: (I) an assessment of some methodological aspects. *J. Nucl. Biol. Med.* **16,** 24 (1972).

14. Osmond, D. H., McFadzean, P. A., and Scaiff, K. D., Renin activity by radioimmunoassay: The plasma incubation step. *Clin. Biochem.* **7,** 52 (1974).

15. Zucchelli, G. C., Malvano, R., Rosa, U., and Salvetti, A., Control of enzyme systems in plasma renin activity measurements by angiotensin I radioimmunoassay. *J. Nucl. Biol. Med.* **17,** 187 (1973).

16. Gould, A. B., Skeggs, L. T., and Kahn, J. R., Measurement of renin and substrate concentration in human serum. *J. Lab. Invest.* **15,** 1802 (1966).

17. Emanuel, R. L., Cain, J. P., and Williams, G. H., Double antibody radioimmunoassay of renin activity and angiotensin II in human peripheral plasma. *J. Lab. Clin. Med.* **81,** 632 (1973).

18. Haber, E., Koerner, T., Page, L. B., et al., Application of radioimmunoassay for angiotensin I to the physiologic measurement of plasma renin activity in normal human subjects. *J. Clin. Endocrinol. Metab.* **29,** 1349 (1969).

19. Boucher, R., Veyrat, R., DeChamplain, J., and Genest, J., New procedures for measurement of human plasma angiotensin and renin activity levels. *Can. Med. Assoc. J.* **90,** 194 (1964).

20. Page, L. B., Dessaulles, E., Lagg, S., and Haber, E., Interference with immunoassays of angiotensin I and II by proteins in human plasma. *Clin. Chim. Acta* **34,** 55 (1972).

21. Goodfriend, T. L., Fyhrquist, F., Gutmann, F., et al., Clinical and conceptual uses of angiotensin receptors. In *Hypertension '72,* J. Genest and E. Koiw, Eds., Springer-Verlag, New York, N. Y., 1972, pp 549–563.

22. Stockigt, J. R., Collins, R. D., and Biglieri, E. G., Determination of plasma renin concentration measured by angiotensin I immunoassay. *Circ. Res. Suppl. II,* 28 & 29, 175 (1971).

23. Giese, J., Jörgensen, M., Nielsen, M. D., et al., Plasma renin concentration measured by use of radioimmunoassay for angiotensin I. *Scand. J. Clin. Lab. Invest.* **26,** 355, (1970).

24. Waldhäusl, E., and Lewandowski, J. A., Measurement of plasma renin concentration using exogenous substrate and radioimmunoassay. *Eur. J. Clin. Invest.* **3,** 1 (1973).

25. Hummerich, W., and Krause, D. K., Improvement of renin determination in human plasma using a commonly available renin standard in a radioimmunological method. *Klin. Wochenschr.* **53,** 559 (1975).

26. Fyhrquist, F., Kala, R., Standertskiöld-Nordenstam, C-G., and Eisalo, A., Angiotensin II plasma levels in hypertensive patients. *Acta Med. Scand.* **192,** 507 (1972).

27. Day, R. P., Luetscher, J. A., and Gonzales, C. M., Occurrence of big renin in human plasma, amniotic fluid and kidney extracts. *J. Clin. Endocrinol. Metab.* **40,** 1078 (1975).

28. Sambhi, M. P., Eggena, P., Barrett, J. D., et al., A circulating renin activator in essential hypertension. *Circ. Res. Suppl. I,* 36, 28 (1975).

29. Kotchen, T. A., Talwalkar, R. T., Kotchen, J. M., et al., Evidence for the existence of an acetone soluble renin inhibiting factor in normal human plasma. *Circ. Res. Suppl. I,* 36, 17 (1975).

30. Sealey, J. E., and Laragh, J. H., "Prorenin" in human plasma? Methodological and physiological implications. *Circ. Res. Suppl. I,* 36, 10 (1975).

31. Bangham, D. R., Robertson, I., Robertson, J. I. S., et al., An international collaborative study of renin assay: Establishment of the international reference preparation of human renin. *Clin. Sci. Mol. Med.* **48,** 135 (1975).

CLIN. CHEM. 22/2, 257-260 (1976)

Improved Method for Measurement of Inorganic Phosphate in Serum with a Centrifugal Analyzer

Peter W. Wentz, John Savory, and Robert E. Cross

A direct method [*Clin. Chim. Acta* **46,** 113 (1973)] for determination of inorganic phosphate in serum was adapted for use with a centrifugal analyzer. Contamination is minimized and analysis rate maximized by doing the reaction in the reagent wells of the transfer disc and by utilizing the high-speed spectrophotometric and data-reduction capabilities of the centrifugal analyzer. Hemolysis, icterus, and moderate lipemia cause no interference. Grossly lipemic sera and sera from patients with plasma cell dyscrasias can be analyzed by incorporating appropriate blanking and dilution techniques. The method exhibits excellent sensitivity and precision and results correlate well with those from a continuous-flow procedure.

Additional Keyphrases: *Rotochem* • *colorimetry of reduced phosphomolybdate*

Only two methods have been reported for the automated measurement of inorganic phosphate (P_i) in serum and urine with a centrifugal analyzer.

Daly and Ertingshausen have described an endpoint determination for use with the Union Carbide "CentrifiChem" system, involving measurement of an unreduced phosphomolybdate complex at 340 nm (*1*). While a very early absorbance reading is taken to provide a presumed combined sample/reagent blank correction, Pesce and Bodourian (*2*) pointed out that samples, from infants, containing bilirubin in concentrations greater than 30 mg/liter give falsely high results by this method. Furthermore, the procedure requires 12 min of instrument time.

Departments of Medicine, Biochemistry, Pathology and Hospital Laboratories, University of North Carolina, Chapel Hill, N. C. 27514.

Received Oct. 27, 1975; accepted Dec. 2, 1975.

Pesce et al. (*3*) described an endpoint method—also for the "CentrifiChem" system—that involves measurement at 340 nm of the NADPH produced as the result of a series of coupled enzyme reactions. Because glycogen is one of the substrates, however, falsely low values have been reported for certain specimens with abnormally high amylase activity (*4*). In addition, the reaction requires 16 min of instrument time. Although this time may be shortened by increasing the phosphorylase activity in the working reagent, there is a corresponding increase in the cost per test.

We report here a procedure for measurement of inorganic phosphate in serum, developed for use with the Aminco "Rotochem" system. An adaptation of the manual method of Morin and Prox (*5*), the determination involves direct colorimetry of a reduced phosphomolybdate complex at 620 nm. Only 10 μl of serum is required, protein precipitation is not necessary, and sensitivity and precision are excellent. The reagents are inexpensive, and instrument use time is minimal.

Materials and Methods

Instrumentation

A centrifugal analyzer, the Aminco "Rotochem II" (American Instrument Company, Silver Spring, Md. 20910) was used for discrete sample analysis. The Aminco "Rotofill I" dilutor was used for sample and diluent delivery. Reagent was dispensed with a 500-μl Eppendorf pipet (Brinkmann Instruments, Inc., Westbury, N. Y. 11590). Continuous-flow analyses were done with an SMA 12/60 system (Technicon Instruments Corp., Tarrytown, N. Y. 10591).

Reagents

Catalyst reagent. Combine 72 g of polyvinylpyrrolidone (mean molecular weight, 40 000; Arthur H. Thomas Co., Philadelphia, Pa. 19105), 1.2 g of sodium azide, and 11.5 ml of *N,N*-dimethylformamide in a 1-liter glass-stoppered graduated cylinder, and dissolve in about 750 ml of distilled water with vigorous shaking. Dilute to 1 liter with additional water, add 1.2 ml of Triton X-100 surfactant, and mix. The reagent appears to be stable indefinitely at room temperature when stored in an amber-colored bottle.

Acid molybdate reagent. To a 1-liter volumetric flask containing about 500 ml of distilled water, add 268 ml of concentrated sulfuric acid, with cooling. After the solution has cooled to room temperature, add 14.5 g of ammonium molybdate, dissolve, and dilute to 1 liter with water. Stability is the same as for the catalyst reagent.

Reducing reagent. Dissolve 4.5 g of *o*-phenylenediamine dihydrochloride (Eastman Organic Chemicals, Rochester, N. Y. 14650) and 7.5 g of thiourea in 50 ml of *N,N*-dimethylformamide with vigorous shaking (immersing the flask in a sonicator bath greatly shortens the time for solution). The reagent is stable for two weeks at room temperature when stored in an amber-colored bottle.

Working reagent. Add 5.0 ml of acid molybdate reagent and 1.0 ml of reducing reagent to 25.0 ml of catalyst reagent and mix. Freshly prepared working reagent is light green and clear. If freshly prepared working reagent appears cloudy it should be discarded and new reducing reagent prepared for use in the reagent formulation.

Stock phosphate standard, 1.00 g of P per liter. Dissolve 439 mg of reagent-grade potassium dihydrogen phosphate in 100 ml of distilled water.

Working phosphate standard, 5 mg P/dl. Dilute 5.0 ml stock standard to 100 ml with distilled water.

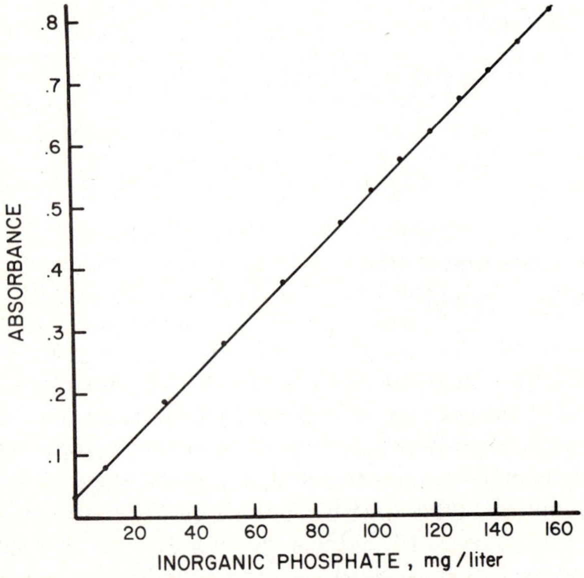

Fig. 1. Standard curve for inorganic phosphate

Table 1. Precision of the Method (with the Rotochem)

	Within-run		Day-to-day	
	Normal	Abnormal	Normal	Abnormal
No.	36	36	30	30
Mean, mg/liter	39.7	90.5	25.9	65.0
SD, mg/liter	0.7	1.2	1.1	1.6
CV, %	1.80	1.35	4.28	2.42

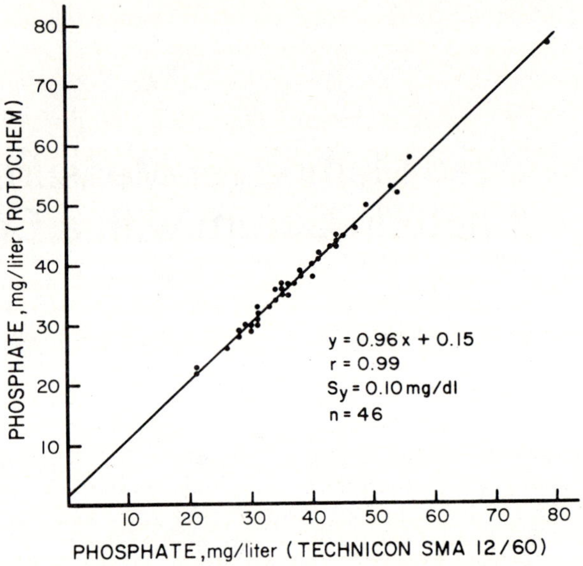

Fig. 2. Comparison between results with the Technicon 12/60 molybdenum blue method and the Rotochem procedure

Procedures

First run a CUVET CALIBRATION program that stores zero-time absorbance corrections based on distilled water for each of the cuvettes. Automatically deliver 10 μl of sample followed by 90 μl of physiological saline diluent to the reagent wells of positions 1–14 of the transfer disc. The sample in position 1 is distilled water, the sample in position 2 is the working standard, and samples in positions 3–14 are patients' specimens and controls. Manually transfer 600 μl of distilled water to the reagent well of the reference position (position 0 of the transfer disc). After completion of sample loading, manually deliver 500 μl of working reagent to the reagent wells of positions 1–14 with an Eppendorf pipet. Allow incubation to proceed for 10 min at room temperature. Then initiate the END POINT II program with a final reading time of 10 s at 620 nm and a temperature of 30 °C. The CUVET CALIBRATION-corrected absorbance of the solution in cuvette 1 serves as a reagent blank correction, and is automatically subtracted from the CUVET CALIBRATION-corrected absorbances for cuvettes 2–14. Calculations are then based on comparison of the reagent blank-corrected sample absorbances with that of the standard.

Results and Discussion

Linearity. The standard curve (Figure 1) is linear to at least 160 mg of P per liter.

Precision and accuracy. Within-run precision was determined by performing 36 replicate analyses (three transfer discs) on serum samples arbitrarily chosen for their values in the normal and abnormal range (Table 1). Day-to-day precision was based on assays of normal and abnormal lyophilized control sera (Hyland, Level I and II) during 30 days (Table 1). Results obtained by the present method for 46 serum specimens correlated well with those obtained by the molybdenum blue method as performed on the SMA 12/60 (Figure 2). Table 2 gives results of analytical recovery studies, performed by mixing appropriate aliquots of the sera of two patients with high and low inorganic phosphate values. Recoveries for serum samples supplemented with known quantities of inorganic phosphate (Table 3) were consistently less than 100%. This observation was reproducible and could not be accounted for by an analytical or arithmetic error. In view of the excellent correlation obtained it does not appear that this obvious discrepancy would create a fundamental liability to the clinical interpretation of the laboratory results. A molecular basis for this finding is not apparent at this time.

Interferences. No spectral interference was observed for hemolyzed, icteric, or moderately lipemic sera, as confirmed by the absence of significant sample blanks for such samples at 620 nm. Grossly lipemic sera may contribute a significant error to test results. Such interference is effectively eliminated, however, by performing a sample-blank correction on a lipemic specimen that has been prediluted threefold with physiological saline. To do this, one measures the absorbance of the diluted sample after substituting an equal volume of blanking solution for the working reagent in an adjacent position of the transfer disc. The blanking solution is prepared by omitting the reducing reagent in the preparation of the working reagent and substituting an equal volume of *N,N*-dimethylformamide. This absorbance is then manually subtracted from the reagent blank-corrected absorbance measured for the color reaction for that sample. Calculation of the result is then based on the absorbance of the standard corrected for the reagent blank.

The sera of two patients with plasma cell dyscrasias (Waldenstrom's macroglobulinemia and IgG multiple myeloma) gave falsely high values for inorganic phosphate (>100 mg of P per liter) when assayed by the present method. It was noted upon visual inspection of the reaction mixtures as they appeared in the transfer disc that the blue molybdenum complex formed was of relatively low intensity, inconsistent with values of 100 mg of P per liter. Sample blanks were determined (by substituting an *o*-phenylenediamine-free working reagent) and indicated that protein was interfering by precipitation. An initial threefold dilution of the sera with physiological saline effectively eliminated the interference and yielded results comparable to those obtained by the manual Fiske–SubbaRow method (*6*), Table 4. The need for this modification of the procedure was somewhat surprising in view of the contention by Morin and Prox (*5*) that as much as 120 g of albumin or 50 g of globulin per liter had no effect on performance.

Table 2. Analytical Recovery for Various Mixtures of High- and Low-phosphate Pooled Sera Assayed for P_i with the Rotochem[a]

Mixture ratio: Low pool		Mixture ratio: High pool	Calculated (mg phosphate/liter)	Found (mg phosphate/liter)	Recovery, %
1	:	1	67.0	68.3	102
1	:	2	75.5	75.6	100
2	:	1	58.4	60.2	103

[a] Assay values: High pool, 92.7 mg P/liter; low pool, 41.3 mg P/liter.

Table 3. Analytical Recovery of P_i Added to Serum

Already present (mg/liter)	Added (mg/liter)	Found (mg/liter)	Expected (mg/liter)	Recovery, %
63.3	38.2	97.2	101.5	89
63.3	73.4	129.4	136.7	90
43.8	31.0	73.0	74.8	94
43.8	58.9	100.7	102.7	97

Table 4. P_i in Sera of Subjects with Plasma Cell Dyscrasias, as Determined by the Present[a] and by the Manual Fiske–SubbaRow Methods

Total protein, g/liter	Present method (mg phosphate/liter)	Manual method (mg phosphate/liter)
101	38	37
93	36	34

[a] Performed on sera diluted threefold with physiological saline.

Table 5. P_i in Sera of Hyperbilirubinemic Subjects, as Determined by the Present and by the Manual Fiske–SubbaRow Methods

Bilirubin, mg/liter	Present method (phosphate, mg/liter)	Manual method (phosphate, mg/liter)
173	37	36
243	34	32
245	63	64

Bilirubin as a source of interference was evaluated by analyzing samples from hyperbilirubinemic subjects by the present method and by the manual Fiske–SubbaRow method. No interference was found (Table 5), attesting to the usefulness of this method for measuring inorganic phosphate in newborns.

The present method for determining inorganic phosphate in serum with a centrifugal analyzer is unique in that the reagent wells of the transfer disc serve as the reaction vessels. Transfer to the curvettes upon rotor acceleration provides a rapid, precise technique for measuring the final absorbance and performing the calculations with a suitable computer program. By minimizing centrifugal analyzer running time, an increased rate of analysis (up to 300 samples per hour) is possible. The approach in the present investigation serves to minimize possible contamination from phosphate buffers, which are used extensively in clinical chemistry tests, by doing the reaction in the transfer disc. It is practical to specify one or more transfer discs in a laboratory for use only with tests in which phosphate buffers are not used. Precision studies indicated that the order of addition to the reagent wells of the transfer disc was important. Adding reagent with a microliter pipette after sample dispensing provided proper mixing. An automated dilutor was not used to deliver the working reagent because of reaction between the caustic working reagent and the stainless-steel piston, the surface of which in time was observed to darken. For the relatively short time (10 s) that the reaction mixture is in contact with the stainless-steel cuvette assembly no corrosion is apparent and even after several months of use no cumulative effect was observed. Indeed, the impetus for utilizing the Teflon transfer disc as the reaction vessel stemmed from its chemical inertness. The advantages of the present adaptation—increased analysis rate and high precision and accuracy—make it the method of choice at the present time for the measurement of inorganic phosphate with a centrifugal analyzer.

This study was supported in part by NIH Grant GM-92. Special thanks go to John A. Bittikofer, Ph.D., of the Clinical Chemistry Department, Duke University School of Medicine, for providing the data from the SMA 12/60. It is a pleasure to acknowledge the help of Lawrence M. Killingsworth, Ph.D., M. Geraldine Heintges, M.T. (A.S.C.P.), Kati Perry, M.T. (A.S.C.P.), and Meena Sonawena, M.T. (A.S.C.P.) during the initial evaluation. This work was presented at the Ninth International Congress on Clinical Chemistry, Toronto, 1975.

References

1. Daly, J. A., and Ertingshausen, G., Direct method for determining phosphate in serum with the "CentrifiChem." *Clin. Chem.* **18,** 263 (1972).

2. Pesce, M. A., and Bodourian, S. H., Bilirubin interference with ultraviolet determination of inorganic phosphate on the "CentrifiChem." *Clin. Chem.* **19,** 436 (1973).

3. Pesce, M. A., Bodourian, S. H., and Nicholson, J. F., Enzymatic method for determination of inorganic phosphate in serum and urine with a centrifugal analyzer. *Clin. Chem.* **20,** 332 (1974).

4. Lustig, V., Enzymatic determination of inorganic phosphate in serum and urine with a centrifugal analyzer. *Clin. Chem.* **20,** 1381 (1974).

5. Morin, L. G., and Prox, J., New and rapid procedure for serum phosphorus using *o*-phenylenediamine as reductant. *Clin. Chim. Acta* **46,** 113 (1973).

6. Fiske, C. H., and SubbaRow, Y., The colorimetric determination of phosphorus. *J. Biol. Chem.* **66,** 375 (1925).

CLIN. CHEM. 22/2, 261–263 (1976)

Parallel Electrophoretic Fractionation of Alkaline Phosphatase and Serum Protein on Cellulose Acetate Strips: Clinical Evaluation

Angelo Burlina and Lauro Galzigna

We describe here a simple, time-saving method for separating alkaline phosphatases on cellulose acetate, with a parallel detection of serum protein pattern. The staining procedure is based on a coupling reaction between the reaction product of α-naphthol with Fast Red Violet LB. The enzymatic reaction is done by bringing the cellulose acetate strip containing the phosphatase band into contact with the surface of a solid agar/substrate mixture. The whole procedure requires 80 min. The method has some features in common with other recently proposed procedures but is more reproducible and rapid because of the choice of the reagents and an improved yield of the coupling step.

Additional Keyphrase: *phosphatase isoenzymes in adults and children, in pregnancy, in hepatic, bone, and neoplastic disease*

The electrophoretic separation of serum alkaline phosphatase (orthophosphoric monoester phosphohydrolase, EC 3.1.3.1) has been described by several authors who used techniques based on different supports and different staining procedures, many of them too cumbersome to be suitable as clinical aids (*1–6*).

Electrophoresis on cellulose acetate has been recommended because it is simple and quick (*4, 5*), although caution has to be used in interpreting the nature of the electrophoretic bands and assigning them to different isoenzymes, because phosphatase molecules tend to aggregate easily.

Materials and Methods

Apparatus

Power supply: (Gelman Instrument Co., Ann Arbor, Mich. 48106) constant current DeLuxe Regulated Power Supply (cat. No 12.38520). *Sample application:* 10-μl Hamilton microsyringe (The Hague, Netherlands). *Electrophoresis cell:* Gelman DeLuxe (cat. No 12.51211). *Cellulose acetate:* 2.5 × 15 cm strips (Cellogel, Labometrics, Milan, Italy; or Sepraphore III, Gelman Instrument Co.). *Disposable trays:* 7.5 × 13 cm plastic trays (Dade, Miami, Fla. 33152). *Densitometer:* Chromoscan, 5-044 green filter (Joyce-Loebl, Gateshead, U.K.).

Reagents

Buffer for migration: Tris(hydroxymethyl)aminomethane/barbital buffer, pH 8.8, 50 mmol/liter (Gelman HR buffer, cat. No 51104). The composition is described in "Gelman Procedures for Special Electrophoresis."

Buffer for enzymatic reaction, 2-amino-2-methyl-1,3-propanediol, pH 10.0, with magnesium sulfate. Dissolve 105.14 g of 2-amino-2-methyl-1,3-propanediol in 1000 ml of de-aerated distilled water. Mix 790 ml of this 1 mol/liter solution with 50 ml of 1 mol/liter HCl and dilute to 1000 ml with distilled water. Add 650 mg of magnesium sulfate heptahydrate (Merck, Darmstadt, Germany). Final pH is 10.0, buffer concentration is 0.79 mol/liter, and magnesium concentration is 2.64×10^{-3} mol/liter.

Agar (Hoechst Italia, Milan, Italy): Dissolve 2 g in 100 ml of buffer at pH 10.0. Distribute 5-ml aliquots in test tubes (16 × 160 mm) and store in a cold room. For use, melt the contents of one tube at 100 °C and add the substrate, after cooling the melted agar to 45 °C.

Substrate: Just before use, dissolve 5 mg of naphthol-AS-phosphate (Sigma Chemical Co., St. Louis, Mo. 63178) in 0.25 ml of pure dimethylsulfoxide (BDH, Poole, England). The final concentration of the substrate is 29 mmol/liter.

Chromogen: Just before use, dissolve 10 mg of Fast Red Violet LB (Sigma) in 25 ml of distilled water. The final concentration is 1.54×10^{-3} mol/liter.

Procedure

Serum samples: We examined the sera of 310 normal men, age 26 to 40 years; 52 children of both sexes, age 2 to 11 years; and 98 women, age 22 to 32 years, in late pregnancy (6th to 8th month).

We also examined sera from 54 patients with cirrhosis, 38 with cholestatic icterus, 27 with chronic hepatitis, and 28 with viral hepatitis, together with 11 sera from osteopathic patients and sera of patients with tumors of the lung (9), stomach (19), uterus (5), and prostate (5). Among the

Center of Clinical Enzymology, General Hospital, 31015 Conegliano, Italy; and Institute of Biological Chemistry, University of Padova, 35100 Padova, Italy.

Received June 30, 1975; accepted Nov. 4, 1975.

clinically normal individuals we found 5 subjects with an abnormally high activity.

Total phosphatase activity was determined in each sample according to the procedure optimized according to recently issued recommendations (*7*). The range of normal values with this procedure was 60 to 170 U/liter for adults, 150 to 470 U/liter for children.

Thermolability was assayed by incubating small volumes of serum in thin-walled test tubes, covered with Parafilm, at 56 ± 0.05 °C for 10 min. Immediately after incubation the tubes were put into iced water (1 to 2 °C), following Moss's procedure (*5*). In some cases the inactivation at 65 °C was studied.

Serum protein fractions: The protein pattern was determined with the same apparatus, the same type of strips, and under the same conditions.

Electrophoresis: Unhemolyzed serum, 5 μl, was applied at the negative electrode end of each of two strips, 2.5 cm from the edges. The two strips were marked with two inked arrows so that a proper alignment could be obtained for comparison after staining. The samples were applied by using the edge of a glass microscope slide as applicator.

The strips were previously soaked with the pH 8.8 buffer. A constant current of 300 V, corresponding to 1 mA/cm, was then applied for 50 min (temperature, 21–25 °C). The contents of one tube containing 5 ml of agar were melted when the electrophoretic separation was nearly over and mixed with 5 ml of buffer and 50 μl of naphthol-AS-phosphate substrate dissolved in dimethylsulfoxide. The mixture was poured into plastic trays and allowed to solidify for 1–2 min at room temperature. The approximate final concentration of components in the mixture, per liter: 10 g of agar, 29 mmol of substrate, 0.39 mol of buffer, and 1.32×10^{-3} mol of magnesium sulfate.

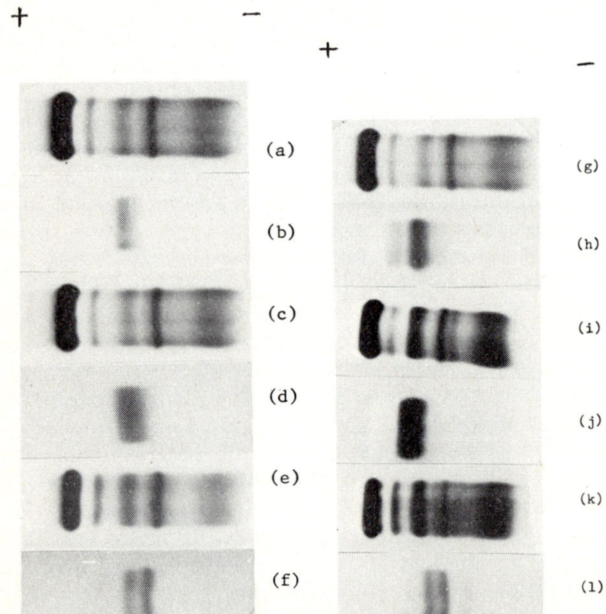

Fig. 1. Electrophoretic pattern for serum protein and serum alkaline phosphatase, respectively, for:
a and *b*, normal man, total alkaline phosphatase 176 U/liter. *c* and *d*, normal child, total alkaline phosphatase 530 U/liter. *e* and *f*, woman in 8th month of normal pregnancy, total alkaline phosphatase 360 U/liter. The band nearer the cathode constitutes 70% of the total. *g* and *h*, man with obstructive icterus, total alkaline phosphatase 680 U/liter. The two bands correspond to 42 and 58% of the total activity. *i* and *j*, man with Paget's disease, total alkaline phosphatase 1100 U/liter. *k* and *l*, man with carcinoma of the lung, total alkaline phosphatase 210 U/liter. 56% of the total activity corresponded to the anodic band. The β-gamma globulin-mobile bands are identified as Regan isoenzyme on the basis of thermolability

At the end of the electrophoretic fractionation one strip was stained for serum protein with Ponceau Red S (BDH, Poole, England), as described in "Gelman Procedure for Special Electrophoresis."

The other strip was removed and placed onto the solid agar/substrate surface, with the side used to deposit serum facing down. After 15 to 30 min at 21–25 °C, the strip was taken from the agar surface and dipped into the freshly prepared chromogen solution. The red-violet bands appear after 1–2 min, and the strip can be stored for two weeks in dilute acetic acid solution (50 ml/liter) without the color fading. The bands were classified on the basis of their comparison with the major serum globulins (α_1, α_2, β, γ).

Results and Discussion

Figure 1 shows a typical electrophoretic pattern of serum protein of a normal adult and of a normal child, and the parallel normally observed alkaline phosphatase band, which is in both cases anodal and migrates at a position corresponding to α_2-globulin. In some adults with high total alkaline phosphatase activity, the intensity of the α_2 globulin band is also increased.

Figure 1 also shows the typical parallel protein-isophosphatase pattern of a normal woman at the 8th month of pregnancy. In this case there are two phosphatase isoenzyme bands; in addition to the normal α_2-globulin-mobile band, a β-globulin-mobile band, stronger than the band at α_2, is present.

Figure 1 shows an example of phosphatase pattern in obstructive icterus, with an α_1-globulin-mobile band and an α_2-band stronger than the normal one. In hepatic cirrhosis in addition to the normal bands at α_2 and α_1, two new bands often appear at the β and γ-globulin position.

Figure 1 also shows a typical large band, appearing between the α_2 and β-globulins in a case of Paget's disease and an example of the pattern found in a lung carcinoma, with an α_2-band and a β-globulin band (Regan isoenzyme).

Incorporation of the chromogen into the agar is to be avoided, because it inhibits the enzymatic reaction (*8, 9*).

The main difference in phosphatase pattern between adults and children is that children show a more pronounced α_2 band.

The second phosphatase band, that observed at the β-globulin position in the case of serum from pregnant women, does not disappear after heating the serum at 65 °C for 30 min.

The results obtained with serum from patients with liver diseases allow one to identify the band at the α_1-globulin position as a hepatic band. It appeared in all cases of obstructive icterus, in some cases of cirrhosis, and in one case of viral hepatitis with icterus. Cirrhosis is characterized by the presence of bands with the mobility of β- and γ-globulin.

In Paget's disease, the α_2-globulin-mobile band is greatly enlarged and this supports the idea that the α_2 band typical of normal serum depends on a enzyme originating from bone, although the size of the band in Paget's disease can result from an overlapping of different bands.

With the present procedure, as in other and more complicated procedures, the main criterion for distinguishing bone and liver phosphatase is thermostability. The mean residual activity after heating at 56 °C was 42 ± 10% for serum of liver-disease patients, 26 ± 8% for serum of normal adults, and 11 ± 7% for serum of patients with bone disease.

The dubious significance of the different normal phosphatase bands observed with different techniques encouraged us to use a method that can give an all-or-none response. In other words, we find that the clinician is much happier with a laboratory result presented in terms of "appearance of abnormal band" than with figures indicating percent increase or decrease of normal bands, particularly in the case of liver disturbances.

This convinced us of the practical value of a quick and simple one-band method in which the phosphatase band is identified by means of a parallel serum protein electropherogram, and the same buffer system and electrophoretic procedure is used for both.

References

1. Korner, N. H., Distribution of alkaline phosphatase in serum protein fractions. *J. Clin. Pathol.* **15,** 195 (1962).
2. Rawstron, J. R., NG, S. H., Rapid electrophoresis of alkaline phosphatase isoenzymes. *Clin. Chim. Acta* **32,** 303 (1971).
3. Johnson, R. B., Jr., Ellingboe, K., and Gibbs, P., A study of various electrophoretic and inhibition techniques for separating serum alkaline phosphatase isoenzymes. *Clin. Chem.* **18,** 110 (1972).
4. Wilkinson, J. H., Clinical applications of isoenzymes. *Clin. Chem.* **16,** 733 (1970).
5. Moss, D. W., Alkaline phosphatase isoenzymes. Technical and clinical aspects. *Enzyme* **20,** 20 (1975).
6. Romel, W. C., Lamancusa, S. J., and Dufrene, J. K., Detection of serum alkaline phosphatase isoenzymes with phenolphtalein monophosphate following cellulose acetate electrophoresis. *Clin. Chem.* **14,** 47 (1968).
7. Recommendations of the German Society for Clinical Chemistry. Standardization of methods for the estimation of enzyme activities in biological fluids. *Z. Klin. Chem. Klin. Biochem.* **10,** 281 (1972).
8. Rhone, D. P., and Mizuno, F. M., Separation of isoenzymes of alkaline phosphatase by substrate-gel imprint after electrophoresis on cellulose acetate. *Clin. Chem.* **18,** 662 (1972).
9. Fritsche, H. A., and Adams-Park, H. R., Cellulose acetate electrophoresis of alkaline phosphatase isoenzymes in human serum and tissue. *Clin. Chem.* **18,** 417 (1972).

CLIN. CHEM. 22/2, 263–266 (1976)

p-Hydroxybenzoic Acid Hydrazide Procedure for Serum Glucose Adapted to the Technicon "SMA 12/60," and Compared with Other Glucose Methods

John J. Ferraro, Francis A. Caccavo, and Abraham Saifer

We adapted the *p*-hydroxybenzoic acid hydrazide procedure for serum glucose for use with the Technicon SMA 12/60 AutoAnalyzer. Like the *o*-toluidine method, this method is based on a general carbohydrate reaction except that it occurs in a mildly alkaline medium and the intense yellow color formed is measured at 400 nm. Advantages of this reagent over *o*-toluidine include lower cost, less toxicity, and higher purity. Aside from those carbohydrates that are present in serum in insignificant quantities, there are no interferences from various physiological compounds or drugs (hypoglycemic agents) found either in normal persons or diabetics. Within-run and day-to-day values had coefficients of variation of 1.39% and 3.44%, respectively; recoveries ranged from 100 to 102% (mean, 101%). Comparative data showed excellent agreement with the hexokinase ($r = 0.998$; $y = 0.950x + 5.91$) and glucose oxidase ($r = 0.996$; $y = 0.986x + 5.34$) enzymatic ("true") glucose methods, and with the *o*-toluidine procedure ($r = 0.998$; $y = 0.979x + 3.14$).

Additional Keyphrases: *continuous-flow analysis • inter-method comparison*

Biochemistry Department, Isaac Albert Research Institute of the Kingsbrook Jewish Medical Center, Brooklyn, N. Y. 11203.

Received Sept. 15, 1975; accepted Nov. 10, 1975.

A new colorimetric reaction for determination of carbohydrates was reported by Lever (*1*) in 1972. Less than 1 μg of glucose (or other reducing sugars) reacts with *p*-hydroxybenzoic acid hydrazide (*p*-HBAH) in mild alkaline solution to give an intense yellow color. Although the reaction is a relatively general one for reducing sugars, the intensity of the color varies with the structure of the carbohydrate. Mechanized methods based on this reaction have been published (*2, 3*) for the routine determination of serum glucose.

Normal blood constituents that interfere with the ferricyanide, glucose oxidase, *o*-toluidine, and copper-neocuproine procedures do not influence glucose values obtained by the *p*-HBAH method (*2, 3*). Although abnormally high protein and bilirubin concentrations in serum give slightly increased color yields in the direct glucose procedure (*1*), the dialysis step in the mechanized methods (*2, 3*) eliminates this interference. Thus, in the mechanized *p*-HBAH procedure, serum glucose concentration and color are linearly related to 3.00 g/liter, the method reportedly is specific for reducing sugars, and results correlate well with those by other methods. Added advantages were stated to be the lack of toxicity of *p*-HBAH and low reagent cost.

We have modified the serum glucose *p*-HBAH method for use with the SMA 12/60 AutoAnalyzer (Technicon Instruments Corp., Tarrytown, N. Y. 10591). Increased linearity—i.e., to more than 3.00 g of glucose per liter—was obtained by suitable manifold changes and by use of protein-containing glucose standards. Our results were compared to those obtained by three different manual procedures that have recently been proposed as reference methods for determination of serum glucose (*4*).

Materials and Methods

Reagents and Solutions

All solvents and chemicals were of reagent grade and were used without further purification. Glucose (Merck & Co., Inc., Rahway, N. J.), ACS grade, had specifications that met the requirements designated for a calibrator (*4*).

Glucose standards. Aqueous glucose working standards were prepared freshly as needed, by appropriate dilution of a glucose stock standard. Commercial control sera—"LederSet," "LederNorm," and "LederTrol"—were obtained from Lederle Diagnostics, American Cyanamide Corp., Pearl River, N. Y. 10965.

Albumin glucose standards. Add bovine albumin (Miles Laboratories, Kankakee, Ill. 60901), 63.0 g, in small portions to about 900 ml of saline [9 g NaCl per liter, containing 100 mg of thimerosal (Merthiolate) per liter] with stirring until dissolved, then dilute to 1 liter with the saline. To 100-ml aliquots of this solution add weighed amounts of glucose to give the desired standards.

Brij-35 solution. Add 1 ml of Brij-35 surfactant (200 g/liter) to a liter of de-ionized, distilled water.

p-*HBAH reagent,* 0.328 mol/liter in 0.5 mol/liter hydrochloric acid. This reagent is stable for several weeks at room temperature.

Sodium hydroxide solution. Prepare a 0.95 mol/liter solution and add 1 ml of the Brij-35 surfactant solution per liter.

Reagents for the manual *o*-toluidine method were as described by Cooper and McDaniel (*5*); for the manual glucose oxidase procedure we used those described by Fales (*6*). These methods and the manual hexokinase method have been proposed as reference methods and are detailed in a U. S. government publication (*4*).

Instrumentation

A Model 2000 spectrophotometer (Gilford Instrument Co., Oberlin, Ohio 44074) was used for the manual determinations. Our flow diagram for the SMA 12/60 (Figure 1) differs from those of Powell and Lever (*2*) and Fingerhut (*3*). Samples from the main sample stream were diluted with water and dialyzed vs. water. After heating at 90 °C, the analytical stream was monitored at 400 nm by the colorimeter with a CE-34-Q phototube. For convenience in phasing, the analytical cartridge was placed in position seven.

Methods

Standardization of the p-*HBAH–SMA 12/60 glucose procedure.* Linearity checks of the *p*-HBAH method were performed with the use of aqueous glucose standards, albumin glucose standards, and pooled sera augmented with known amounts of glucose. With the SMA under normal operating conditions and the mode selector switch on *record,* samples were aspirated and the absorbances, read from the programmer meter as each analytical stream reached the colorimeter, were plotted vs. the known glucose concentrations (Figure 2). Recovery data were obtained from the curve for glucose-augmented pooled serum (Figure 2).

The data in Figure 2 showed concordant results for glucose between the human serum pool and the albumin glucose standard. Therefore, we used a commercial reference

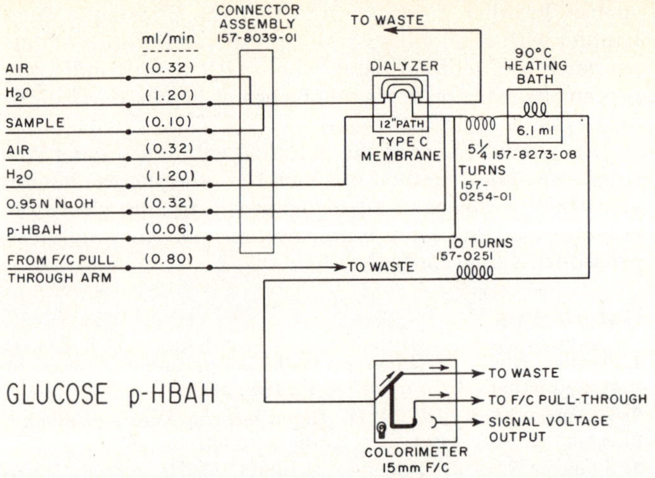

Fig. 1. Flow diagram for the automated measurement of glucose with *p*-hydroxybenzoic acid hydrazide (*p*-HBAH) procedure with the SMA 12/60

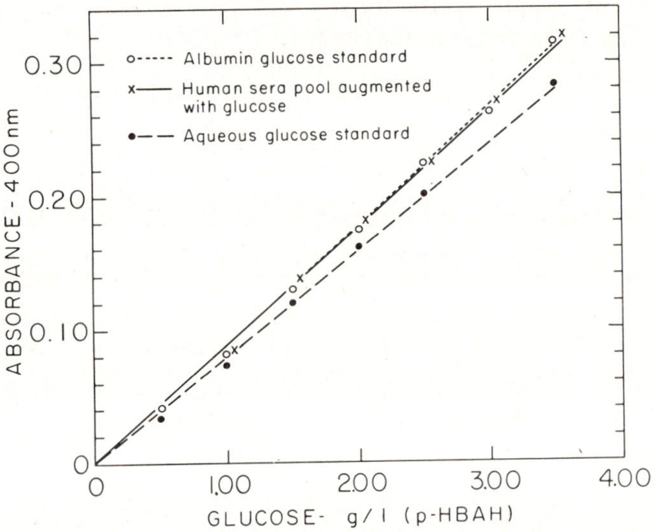

Fig. 2. Linearity of the *p*-HBAH method for aqueous and albumin glucose standards, and glucose-augmented sera with the SMA 12/60

serum, "LederSet," to set the initial SMA glucose value and the readings, in g/liter, were adjusted after every tenth sample.

Sera were then assayed in the usual manner with the SMA 12/60, with use of the glucose cartridge illustrated in Figure 1. From these analyzed sera, about 100 were selected to cover the entire range of normal and abnormal glucose values, and these were then re-assayed with manual glucose procedures based on the *o*-toluidine (*5*), glucose oxidase (EC 1.1.3.4) (*6*), and hexokinase/glucose-6-phosphate dehydrogenase (EC 2.7.1.1/EC 1.1.1.49) reactions as recommended by the Food and Drug Administration (*4*). Each type of assay involved the preparation of protein-free filtrates: trichloroacetic acid filtrates for the *o*-toluidine method and Somogyi filtrates (*7*) for the enzymatic methods. In each, aqueous glucose solutions were used as the primary standards.

The glucose content of the commercial control serum (LederSet) was also determined by each of the three procedures. Each manual procedure gave a slightly different glu-

Table 1. Correlation of the "SMA 12/60" *p*-Hydroxybenzoic Acid Hydrazide Procedure for Serum Glucose with Manual Reference Methods

Methods	Linear regression equation
p-HBAH vs. hexokinase	$r = 0.998$; y(*p*-HBAH) = 0.950 x (hexokinase) +5.91
p-HBAH vs. glucose oxidase	$r = 0.996$; y(*p*-HBAH) = 0.986 x (glucose oxidase) +5.34
p-HBAH vs. *o*-toluidine	$r = 0.998$; y(*p*-HBAH) = 0.979 x (*o*-toluidine) +3.14

cose value for "LederSet" serum, so the patients' serum glucose values obtained with the mechanized *p*-HBAH-SMA 12/60 procedure were adjusted by multiplying their values by a constant factor. Data so obtained for the automated *p*-HBAH method were plotted vs. those obtained for the same sera by the manual hexokinase, glucose oxidase, and *o*-toluidine procedures, and a statistical summary is presented in Table 1.

Within-run and day-to-day precision for the mechanized *p*-HBAH method were established (Table 2) by repeat determinations on more than 40 aliquots from pools of normal and abnormal serum (stored at −20 °C).

Sample-to-sample interaction was negligible during a routine run. The largest detected interaction, less than 1.0%, occurred when a 3.50 g/liter was followed by a 0.50 g/liter glucose sample.

The reactivity of various carbohydrates, reported to be present in trace amounts in normal serum or plasma (*8*), was investigated with the *p*-HBAH reaction by assaying 5.55 mmol of each sugar and measuring its chromogenicity relative to glucose.

Although other investigators (*1–3*) have furnished data on a number of substances normally present in blood, which could conceivably influence glucose values obtained by the *p*-HBAH method, no data were presented on the influence of commonly used oral hypoglycemic agents. We examined the effect of such drugs, in concentrations up to 1000 mg/liter, on serum glucose values obtained by the *p*-HBAH procedure.

Results

The linearity of absorbance readings with glucose concentration was investigated. For this purpose, primary standards were prepared both in distilled water and in 63 g/liter bovine albumin solution shown to be free of carbohydrates (*9*). In addition, secondary standards or calibration materials, i.e., glucose-augmented serum samples, were prepared by the standard addition technique (*10*). Linear results were obtained for glucose values up to 3.50 g/liter for all three kinds of calibration materials. However, results obtained with the albumin/glucose and the glucose-augmented serum samples were the same, whereas the aqueous glucose standards gave appreciably lower absorbance readings. This unexpected finding was confirmed by keeping the glucose concentration constant at 2.50 g/liter while varying the bovine serum albumin concentration between 0 and 100 g/liter. Again, *p*-HBAH color yield decreased with decreasing albumin concentration below 40 g/liter. Other investigators (*11*) have also questioned the reasonableness of using aqueous primary standards in procedures requiring dialysis when the samples to be analyzed contain high amounts of protein, and Koch and Misanik (*9*) proposed the use of primary standards made up of weighed-in constituents dissolved in albumin solution. We conclude that protein/glucose solutions of known composition, rather than aqueous glucose solutions, constitute the only suitable *primary* calibration materials for use in the procedure described here. The validity of their use is verified by glucose addition experiments and by the excellent analytical recoveries (Figure 2).

Many investigators (*8*) consider the enzymatic hexokinase method as the one that most closely approaches a "true" glucose assay; the data given in Table 1 indicate almost perfect correspondence of the *p*-HBAH and the manual hexokinase values over a wide range of glucose values. Similar good correlations were obtained for the manual glucose oxidase vs. *p*-HBAH and for the manual *o*-toluidine vs. *p*-HBAH procedures (Table 1). The within-run and day-to-day precision of glucose values obtained with the mechanized *p*-HBAH method (Table 2) compare favorably with the values reported for the hexokinase (*12*), glucose oxidase (*11*), and *o*-toluidine (*13*) methods.

Westgard et al. (*11, 14*) have defined a "performance standard" as the allowable error at the concentration where critical medical decisions must be made. For glucose, they suggested that the allowable error at 0.50 g/liter and 1.20 g/liter decision levels be ±0.10 g/liter. The allowable error is the sum of systematic and random errors. The systematic error at each decision level is calculated from the slope of the regression line and from the intercept obtained by comparing the proposed method (*p*-HBAH–SMA 12/60) to the reference method, e.g., manual hexokinase. The random error is obtained from the standard deviation of the day-to-day precision studies and is equal to ±2 SD. Thus, assuming that the hexokinase method (*4*) affords "true" glucose values at 0.50 g/liter, the *p*-HBAH method will give a total error of +0.034 g/liter (systematic error) ±0.060 g/liter (random error ±2 SD), or 0.534 ± 0.060 g/liter; at 1.20

Table 2. Within-Run and Day-to-Day Precision of Glucose Values Obtained with the Present Method

	Within-run		Day-to-day	
	Normal pool	Abnormal pool	Normal control	Abnormal control
No. assays	50	45	43	43
Mean (g/liter)	1.48	2.39	0.86	2.94
Standard deviation (±)	0.0207	0.0135	0.0296	0.0596
Standard error (±)	0.0029	0.0020	0.0045	0.0091
Coefficient of variation (%)	1.39	0.56	3.44	2.02

g/liter, −0.001 g/liter (systematic error) ±0.060 g/liter (random error ±2 SD), or 1.20 ± 0.060 g/liter. Results for serum glucose obtained with our method are acceptable in comparison with any of the three proposed manual reference procedures. Glucose reference specimens, furnished by the Center for Disease Control (Atlanta, Ga. 30333), gave values with the *p*-HBAH method within ±3% of the stated mean values of the reference specimens, which had been assayed by the manual hexokinase method (*4*).

On the basis of specificity, the practicing clinical chemist now has a choice of either one of the two mechanized enzymatic glucose procedures (glucose oxidase or hexokinase) or of a relatively specific mechanized chemical glucose method such as *o*-toluidine or the present procedure. Manual versions of the first three methods have been advocated by the Food and Drug Administration (*4*) as reference procedures, or product class standards, for quantitative glucose determinations. After weighing the pros and cons of enzymatic versus nonenzymatic glucose techniques, Pileggi and Szustkiewicz (*8*) state that "It is the opinion of many investigators that when all factors are considered—e.g., susceptibility of enzymatic methods to inhibitors, expense of reagents, stability of reagents, and ease of performance—the *o*-toluidine method, either automated or manual, is the choice for the routine clinical chemistry laboratory."

We believe the advantages of the present method over the *o*-toluidine method include: (*a*) availability of *p*-HBAH as a pure, crystalline compound, which can be used without further purification (*4*); (*b*) nontoxicity of *p*-HBAH as compared to *o*-toluidine (*15*); (*c*) *p*-HBAH reactions occur in a mild alkaline medium as compared to highly acidic conditions needed for *o*-toluidine (*4, 14*); and (*d*) overall cost of the working reagent is even less than that of the *o*-toluidine working reagent (*2*).

Neither the *o*-toluidine nor the *p*-HBAH glucose procedures respond to the "saccharoid" or nonglucose reducing substances present in normal or diabetic blood serum (*1, 2, 8*). Azotemia causes little or no interference with the glucose values obtained by either method (*3, 14*), but causes erroneously high values with reduction methods and low values with some glucose oxidase procedures. Other possible interferences with both the *o*-toluidine and the present methods—e.g., bilirubin, protein, etc.—are removed either by dialysis or by preparing protein-free filtrates (*1, 2*). Galactose and mannose (and to a lesser extent lactose) are the only carbohydrates that are potential sources of error in the *o*-toluidine method (*3, 8*), whereas the *p*-HBAH reagent is somewhat less specific for reducing sugars (*3*). However, sera from some uncontrolled diabetics, and those containing glycosans that are hydrolyzed in hot acid solution, may yield values with the *o*-toluidine method that appreciably exceed their actual glucose content. Various commonly ingested hypoglycemic drugs such as phenformin, tolbutamide, chloropropamide, and acetohexamide, in concentrations up to 1.0 g/liter, had no appreciable effect on results for a pooled serum containing 1.50 g of glucose per liter. The concentrations of carbohydrates other than glucose normally present in serum and plasma (*8*) is about 0 to 40 mg/liter (*16*). The comparative data between the *p*-HBAH method and the hexokinase, glucose oxidase/peroxidase, and *o*-toluidine procedures (Table 1) indicate a slight positive bias for the former method at low glucose concentrations.

Our preliminary studies of the kinetics of the *p*-HBAH reaction indicate that glucose is first isomerized to fructose—i.e., the Lobry de Bruyn transformation (*8*)—before the intermediate is formed that reacts with *p*-HBAH to give the color. Further work on the mechanism of the *p*-HBAH reaction, and on the composition of the colored complex formed, is presently in progress.

References

1. Lever, M., A new reaction for colorimetric determination of carbohydrates. *Anal. Biochem.* **47,** 273 (1972).

2. Powell, J. C., and Lever, M., A new automated procedure for the colorimetric determination of glucose. *Biochem. Med.* **6,** 543 (1972).

3. Fingerhut, B., Automated method for serum glucose with *p*-hydroxybenzoic acid hydrazide. *Clin. Chem.* **19,** 1022 (1973).

4. (*a*) Schmidt, A. M., Proposed establishment of product class standard for detection or measurement of glucose. *Fed. Regist.* **39,** 24136 (1974); (*b*) Bayse, D., Center for Disease Control, Atlanta, Ga. 30333, private communication.

5. Cooper, G. R., and McDaniel, V., The determination of glucose by the *ortho*-toluidine method. *Stand. Methods Clin. Chem.* **6,** 159 (1970).

6. Fales, F. W., Glucose (enzymatic). *Stand. Methods Clin. Chem.* **4,** 101 (1963).

7. Nelson, N., and Somogyi, M., Glucose. *Stand. Methods Clin. Chem.* **1,** 65 (1953).

8. Pileggi, V. J., and Szustkiewicz, C. P., Carbohydrates. In *Clinical Chemistry, Principles and Technics,* 2nd ed., R. J. Henry, D. C. Cannon, and J. W. Winkelman, Eds., Harper & Row, Hagerstown, Md., 1974, pp 1265–1294.

9. Koch, T. R., and Misanik, L. F., Standardization and quality control of the SMA 12/60 and SMA 6/60 using aqueous standards. *Clin. Chem.* **19,** 650 (1973). Abstract.

10. Laessig, R. H., Schwartz, T. H., and Paskey, J. H., Determination of SMA-Mark X set points for bilirubin by standard addition technique. *Clin. Chem.* **18,** 48 (1973).

11. Carey, R. N., Feldbruegge, D., and Westgard, J. O., Evaluation of the adaptation of the glucose oxidase/peroxidase 3-methyl-2-benzothiazolinone hydrazone-*N,N*-dimethylaniline procedure to the Technicon "SMA 12/60", and comparison with other automated methods for glucose. *Clin. Chem.* **20,** 595 (1974).

12. Hasson, W., Penton, J. R., and Widdowson, G. M., Determination of glucose with a research model Aminco Rotochem by the hexokinase reaction. *Clin. Chem.* **20,** 15 (1974).

13. Moorehead, W. R., and Sasse, E. A., An automated micromethod for determination of serum glucose with an improved *o*-toluidine reagent. *Clin. Chem.* **16,** 285 (1970).

14. Westgard, J. O., Carey, R. N., and Wald, S., Criteria for judging precision and accuracy in method development and evaluation. *Clin. Chem.* **20,** 825 (1974).

15. Indriksons, A., Hazards of *o*-toluidine. *Clin. Chem.* **21,** 1345 (1975). Letter to the Editor.

16. Hyvärinen, A., and Nikkilä, E. A., Specific determination of blood glucose with *o*-toluidine. *Clin. Chim. Acta* **7,** 140 (1962).

CLIN. CHEM. 22/2, 267–269 (1976)

Complement C3 in Serum and Plasma, as Measured by Radial Immunodiffusion with Four Commercial Kits

Adrian O. Vladutiu and Barbara M. Winiarski

Quantitation of the C3 component of complement by single radial immunodiffusion is subject to error because the C3 molecule has several antigenic determinants and anti-C3 sera differ in their specificity to these determinants. C3 was measured in plasma (ethylenediaminetetraacetate anticoagulant) and serum, in five normal individuals, by use of four such commercial kits. The effects of ethylenediaminetetraacetate and of incubation at −20, 4, and 37 °C for 1, 2, and 7 days were investigated. We found wide variations in C3 in the same sample, as measured with different kits. Incubation for longer than 48 h at 4 °C changed C3 concentrations as compared to those in fresh samples. Reference sera for C3 assay and standardized procedures for sample processing are both essential to valid results.

Lately, measurement of the C3 component of complement (also known as β1C globulin) in serum has become routine, and such information is useful in monitoring some immune diseases (*1, 2*).

C3 can be measured by a hemolytic assay or by radial immunodiffusion (RID) in which antiserum to C3 is incorporated in agar (*3, 4*). RID is complicated by the fact that the C3 molecule has several antigenic determinants, and with aging of serum there is rapid proteolytic cleavage of the molecule into several fragments. Consequently, some antigenic determinants disappear (*5*), as (*6*) reported for quantitation of C3 by the AutoAnalyzer II nephelometric method—a method still used only in large hospitals.

Several manufacturers now supply kits for C3 assay by RID. Values obtained with different kits could vary considerably, because anti-C3 sera differ with respect to their specificity for the antigenic determinants of the C3 molecule (*7*).

We compared the values for serum C3 obtained with four different kits, three of them in which an antiserum to the whole C3 molecule is used (the so-called anti-β1C/β1A) and one in which the antiserum (anti-β1A) is specific for only one antigenic determinant of C3. We investigated the effect of aging and of the anticoagulant ethylenediaminetetraacetic acid on C3 values obtained with different kits and assessed the comparability of C3 values obtained with them.

Laboratory of Immunopathology, The Buffalo General Hospital, Buffalo, N. Y. 14203.

Received Oct. 13, 1975; accepted Nov. 17, 1975.

Materials and Methods

Blood samples were collected into evacuated glass tubes, plain or with ethylenediaminetetraacetic acid (Vacutainers; Becton-Dickinson, Rutherford, N. J. 07070), from five apparently normal men and women ranging in age from 25 to 35 years. After the samples had stood for 1 h at room temperature the serum or plasma was separated by centrifugation at 4 °C and divided into aliquots. One aliquot of serum or plasma from each subject was assayed immediately; the others were kept at −20, 4, and 37 °C for 24 and 48 h or at −20 and 4 °C for seven days, in polystyrene tubes (Falcon Plastics, Oxnard, Calif. 93030).

RID plates were obtained from four commercial sources (A through D in the tables)[1] in the form of kits for C3 assay, every kit including its own reference sera. Manufacturers A, C, and D recommended an early read-out (*3*); manufacturer B recommended reading the results at antigen–antibody equivalence ("end point") (*4*). Incubation conditions were: kit A, 18 h at room temperature; kit B, 48 h at room temperature; kit C, 18 h at 4 °C; and kit D, 18 h at room temperature; kit C, 18 h at 4 °C; and kit D, 18 h at room temperature. (After this work was completed, manufacturer D changed his kits, providing a choice of both early readout and reading the results at antigen–antibody equivalence). A micropipette with disposable, calibrated glass tips, delivering 5 μl ("Micro Dispenser"; Drummond Scientific, Broomall, Pa. 19008) was used to dispense all samples, regardless of the instructions of manufacturers A, C, and D to simply fill the wells. In the case of the plates from source A, the wells were not completely filled by 5 μl. All of the wells from any one kit were filled in a single operation, to maintain the incubation time constant. The plates were kept in a moist chamber. A pool of normal sera was kept for 14 days at 37 °C, divided into aliquots, and stored at −20 °C. For each test an aliquot of this pool, serving as an "internal" control, was assayed with every kit. Every determination was done in duplicate and the results were averaged. Diameters of the precipitin rings, measured to the nearest 0.1 mm, were compared to the curve obtained with the reference sera supplied with the kits, which was plotted on semi-logarithmic graph paper as antigen concentration

[1] A, Kallestad Laboratories, Inc., Chaska, Minn. 55318; B, Behring Diagnostics, Somerville, N. J. 08876; C, Meloy Laboratories, Springfield, Va. 22151; D, Hyland Laboratories, Costa Mesa, Calif. 92626.

vs. precipitin ring diameter (*3*) for manufacturers A, C, and D; and on linear graph paper as antigen concentration vs. square of the diameter (*4*) for manufacturer B. To assess the C3 concentrations in the standards included in the kits, we reciprocally assayed the three standards from each kit as unknowns in the other kits. (Kit B contained only one standard, from which we prepared three serial dilutions).

Results

We did not obtain multiple precipitin rings or ambiguously hazy circles with any of the kits; however, the rings were more clear in some kits than in others. Although a comparison of the clarity of the precipitin rings among the four kits was not our main purpose, we noted that the plates of kit D gave particularly clear rings. The within-day coefficient of variation in our laboratory for the RID assay of C3 was less than 2% for 10 identical samples of a middle range C3 value; it was less than 3% from day-to-day on 25 consecutive days when the same lot number of the commercial kit D was used.

C3 concentrations for five normal individuals, as measured with the four kits, are given in Tables 1 and 2.

After 24-h storage at 4 or 37 °C, plasma C3 measurements with kit B decreased slightly as compared to fresh plasma. The same was true for seven days at 4 or −20 °C. When kit C was used, apparent C3 concentrations were slightly decreased after plasma was stored for seven days at 4 °C. With kit D only, C3 values were increased for both serum and plasma after 48 h at 37 °C.

Differences between values for C3 in plasma and serum from the same subject, probably attributable to ethylenediaminetetraacetic acid, were seen only in the fresh samples and only when kit B was used. Initially, serum values were lower than plasma values, but after a week at 4 °C the plasma values decreased to match those for the serum.

For any one individual, there were marked differences in the values for C3 in serum, as assayed with the different kits. For example, a fresh plasma sample from subject 1 gave a value of 910 mg/liter when kit A was used and 1590 mg/liter when kit C was used, a difference of 74%. A serum sample from subject 3, after 48 h at −20 °C, gave a value of 640 mg/liter with kit B and 1570 mg/liter with kit C, a difference of 145%.

Each standard had a different value for C3 when tested with different kits. For example, the first standard from kit C gave C3 values of 1250 mg/liter and 2500 mg/liter (expected value, 2900 mg/liter) when tested with kits A and D, respectively. When kit A was used for the assay, C3 values for the standards from kit B approached the stated values, while those from the other two kits had about half the stated values. When kit D was used for the assay, C3 concentrations for the standards of kits A and C were near those expected, but the values for the standards of kit B were much higher. Finally, when kit B was used, C3 values for the standards from kits A, C and D were much lower than expected (Table 3).

In our hands, kits C and D seemed to be better than the other two.

Table 1. C3 Concentrations in Fresh Samples, as Measured with Four Kits (A–D)

Subject	A	B	C	D
	mg/liter			
Plasma				
1	910	1060	1590	1340
2	910	1060	1430	1260
3	1060	1120	1630	1260
4	920	1000	1390	1080
5	1420	1200	1680	1610
Serum				
1	1000	680	1390	1260
2	910	780	1340	1260
3	890	800	1390	1210
4	830	900	1060	1080
5	1490	960	1590	1610

Discussion

There are pitfalls in the assay of C3 by RID, owing both to the method and the properties of C3. One of the most common sources of error is variable filling of the wells. When a calibrated micropipette is used, reproducible results can be obtained. Other causes of error in RID assay are reviewed elsewhere (*8*).

The present study shows that wide variations in C3 values are obtained with different commercial kits. In part these are due to the different specificities of anti-C3 sera for C3 antigenic determinants. C3 (β1C globulin) has at

Table 2. C3 Concentrations in Samples Incubated for Various Intervals at Different Temperatures[a]

	24 h			48 h			7 days	
	−20°	4°	37°	−20°	4°	37°	−20°	4°
Kit	mg/liter							
Plasma								
A	1120	1100	1040	1110	1130	1070	1100	1070
B	890	890	960	720	690	890	760	710
C	1360	1430	1420	1340	1420	1580	1370	1350
D	1350	1480	1520	1310	1470	1620	1340	1500
Serum								
A	1030	1060	1250	1050	980	1290	1080	1000
B	740	800	1000	700	670	1040	700	650
C	1400	1370	1370	1400	1560	1930	1340	1550
D	1380	1300	1670	1390	1340	1820	1410	1470

[a] Each value represents the average of apparent C3 concentrations (which differed widely) of five normal individuals.

Table 3. C3 Concentrations of Reference Sera Tested with Four Kits

Kit used for assay	Source of reference sera: A			B			C			D		
	mg/liter											
A	(3100)[a]	(1500)	(620)	1050	500	250	1250	640	140	1200	600	180
B	2160	1460	760	(1200)	(600)	(300)	1600	1040	120	1460	760	120
C	3460	1670	700	1860	1120	660	(2900)	(1920)	(370)	2420	1050	320
D	3620	1880	680	1740	1180	590	2500	1700	370	(2600)	(1290)	(370)

[a] In parentheses: values claimed by manufacturers.

least 3 antigenic determinants: A, B and D. As serum ages the B determinant disappears and β1C globulin is replaced by β1A globulin (C3c), having a faster electrophoretic mobility and the determinant A, and by α2D globulin (C3d), having the determinant D. There may be another C3 fragment, C3e, not yet characterized. The "conversion" of β1C to β1A and α2D is gradual and depends on temperature and time of storage, inactivating enzymes, and chelating agents (such as ethylenediaminetetraacetic acid). The rate of conversion varies from one serum to another, therefore a correction factor applied to the values obtained on aged sera for the purpose of relating the values to fresh sera is not accurate, unless sera are aged for a very long time. The stability of C3 was increased when the time allowed for clotting was longer and the temperature of incubation during clotting was higher, suggesting that C3-inactivating enzymes were trapped during clotting (L. van Es, WHO Complement Standardization Subcommittee; personal communication). The effect of ethylenediaminetetraacetic acid as a stabilizing agent for C3 is controversial; such an effect was not found for the B determinant (*6*). Incorporation of ethylenediaminetetraacetic acid in the agar of the diffusion plate has been suggested (*10*).

Because the A determinant is present both on the intact C3 molecule and after its breakdown, apparent C3 concentrations might not be influenced by the aging of serum if only this determinant is being measured. However, aged serum consumes more antibody to A antigen than does fresh serum (*9*), suggesting that fresh serum will produce smaller precipitin rings with anti-C3 sera. Surprisingly, when we used kit B, which allegedly measured only the A determinant, we found decreased C3 values in old plasma preserved with ethylenediaminetetraacetic acid as compared to fresh plasma. This shows that aging of samples apparently changes the C3 concentrations even if only one antigenic determinant is measured.

Different C3 values for the same sample, obtained with different kits, are also due to the fact that there are no international standards for C3 assay as there are for immunoglobulins. The standards supplied with the commercial kits had variable amounts of A and B determinants, as we saw by immunoelectrophoresis of standards when anti-whole C3 sera was used. This could explain the discrepancies in the C3 values of the same standard serum when assayed with different kits (Table 3). International standards are now being evaluated to determine the stability of lyophilized C3 (L. van Es, personal communication); such reference sera will permit inter-laboratory comparison of data.

Standardization of the procedures for collecting and storing the samples for C3 assay and establishing a normal range for the local population is of particular importance. Every laboratory should have at least one "internal standard," preferably a pool of human sera aged 14 days at 37 °C, divided into aliquots, and stored frozen. Our data do not show that serum C3 values change much after 48 h incubation at 4 °C, regardless of the kit used to measure them. However, if the C3 assay cannot be done within 48 h after the sample is collected, the serum should be kept frozen at −20 °C and the assay performed on sera stored for the same length of time.

C3 concentrations in the serum of the normal population vary widely; extending this range because of pitfalls in the C3 assay itself could raise doubts about the value of this assay. Crossed antigen–antibody electrophoresis might be a more suitable technique for measuring C3, because it allows C3 breakdown products to be both detected and measured (*11*).

References

1. West, C. D., Northway, J. D., and Davis, N. C., Serum levels of β1C globulin, a complement component in the nephritides, lipoid nephrosis and other conditions. *J. Clin. Invest.* **43,** 1507 (1964).

2. Vallota, E. H., Forristal, J., Davis, N. C., and West, C. D., The C3 nephritic factor and membranoproliferative nephritis: Correlation of serum levels of the nephritic factor with C3 levels, with therapy and with progression of the disease. *J. Pediatr.* **80,** 947 (1972).

3. Fahey, J. L., and McKelvey, E. M., Quantitative determination of serum immunoglobulins in antibody-agar plates. *J. Immunol.* **94,** 84 (1965).

4. Mancini, G., Carbonara, A. O., and Heremans, J. F., Immunochemical quantitation of antigens by single radial immunodiffusion. *Immunochemistry* **2,** 235 (1965).

5. West, C. D., Davis, N. C., Forristal, J., et al., Antigenic determinants of human β1C and β1G globulins. *J. Immunol.* **96,** 650 (1966).

6. Davis, N. C., West, C. D., and Ho, M., Effect of aging of serum on quantitation of complement component C3. *Clin. Chem.* **18,** 1485 (1972).

7. Spath, P., and Gabl, F., Critical factors for the immunochemical quantitation of the third complement component C3. *Protides Biol. Fluids, Proc. Colloq.* **22,** 551 (1975).

8. Berne, B. H., Differing methodology and equations used in quantitating immunoglobulins by radial immunodiffusion—a comparative evaluation of reported and commercial techniques. *Clin. Chem.* **20,** 61 (1974).

9. West, C. D., Winter, S., Forristal, J., and Davis, N. C., Effect of aging of serum on consumption of antibody by β1C-globulin determinants; evidence for circulating breakdown products in glomerulonephritis. *Clin. Exp. Immunol.* **3,** 57 (1968).

10. Stitzel, A. E., and Spitzer, R. E., C3 standards. *Lancet* **ii,** 364 (1975).

11. Kroll, J., and Thambiah, R., Quantitative estimation of electrophoretically heterogeneous proteins by electrophoresis in antibody-containing agarose gel. *Protides Biol. Fluids, Proc. Colloq.* **17,** 533 (1969).

CLIN. CHEM. 22/2, 270–272 (1976)

Long-Term Quality-Control Charting: A Simple Method

Arthur W. Gottmann,[1] Jerome S. Nosanchuk,[2] and Gail S. Anderson[3]

We describe a simple graphing technique for use in long-term quality control of methodologies. It warns of subtle or gross problems, whether they appear gradually or abruptly.

Laboratory accuracy and precision achieved consistently over long periods of time are as important as day-to-day quality control. Unless there is both long-term and daily accuracy and precision, a patient's long-term progress cannot be assessed within the same laboratory, much less between different laboratories. The classic view that the major source of analytical error lies in differences between laboratories (*1, 2*) has recently been refuted by Gilbert (*3*), who found that sources within the laboratory account for two-thirds to three-quarters of all errors. Our own observations on the etiology of errors in a routine hematology laboratory support Gilbert's contention (*4*).

Elegant techniques for analyzing accumulated quality-control data have been presented by Westgard et al. (*5*). However, availability of a simpler technique, requiring no sophisticated tools and demanding only a modicum of additional effort by the laboratory's staff, would be useful. We therefore developed a simple graphic approach to analyze our quality-control programs.

We participate in five extralaboratory check-sample programs and routinely use two concentrations of intralaboratory quality-control pools. The significance of this mass of quality-control data was not always fully appreciated, because there was little or no interprogram-comparison analysis. If one could deduce that some programs are better than others—in general or for a specific purpose—then a quality-control program suited for a specific laboratory could perhaps be selected.

[1] Metropolitan Laboratories and General Rose Memorial Hospital, Denver, Colo.

[2] Department of Pathology, University of Rochester School of Medicine and Dentistry, Rochester, N. Y.

[3] Department of Pathology, General Rose Memorial Hospital, Denver, Colo.

Correspondence should be directed to A. W. G. at Metropolitan Laboratories, 2137 South Birch, Denver, Colo. 80222.

Received Mar. 31, 1975; accepted Nov. 17, 1975.

Method

Results for commonly run tests are graphed and updated each month. The potassium graph (Figure 1) shows the two intralaboratory pooled-sera samples (Control I and II), which are connected by a broken line. In the intralaboratory pools, we use our accumulated monthly values for calculation of the mean, SD, and CV. The bar graph spans ±2 SD about our mean (represented by the "X") and if available, the group mean (identified by the dot). Because we desire to use as many values as possible, the process is reversed for the check samples (we only do a few determinations in our laboratory), and use the group mean (dot) and the group ±2 SD values as the bar graph and identify our values with an "X." In this way, our standard deviations can be visually compared with group standard deviations at various analyte concentrations.

The interprogram comparison is simplified by summarizing the accumulated data in a single consistent, readily readable graphic format. The graphs are appropriately scaled for each test and identified chronologically. The calculated CV is recorded near the bottom of the graph. Comments that might explain significant changes are also written on the graph. Color coding of various samples enhances the graph's utility.

Results and Discussion

Figure 2 shows one of the subtle changes discovered by this technique. Our chloride values in nearly every survey were above the mean, yet usually within ±2 SD. This consistent aberration was undetectable by any single quality-control program result, but was immediately obvious from the graph, which suggested that the value given the standard by the manufacturer was inappropriate or that slight methodological changes had occurred.

The creatinine graph (Figure 3) reflects some interesting findings: First, the CV ranges between 2.2 and 33%. Second, almost half of the check-sample values are between 8 and 15 mg/liter; only three exceed 40 mg/liter. Because most of the smaller CV's are found in either our pool or the CAP check samples, we are alerted to be wary of these two programs for possible bias or data manipulation. Thus, the creatinine graph provoked serious concern about quality

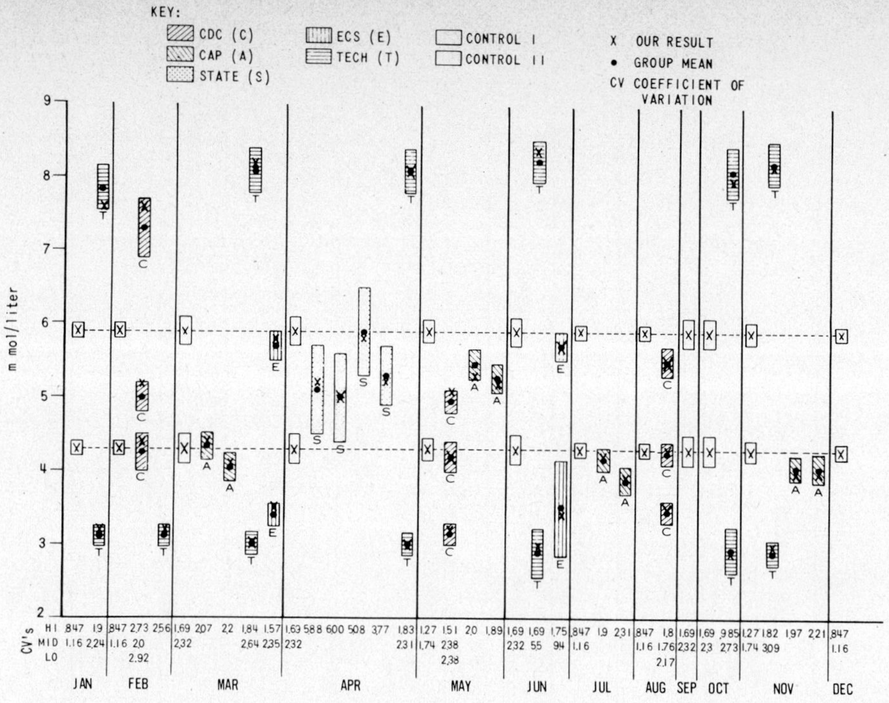

Fig. 1. Graphic display of results for potassium quality-control materials in 1973, including results for intra- and interlaboratory pools (identified in the *key* at the top)

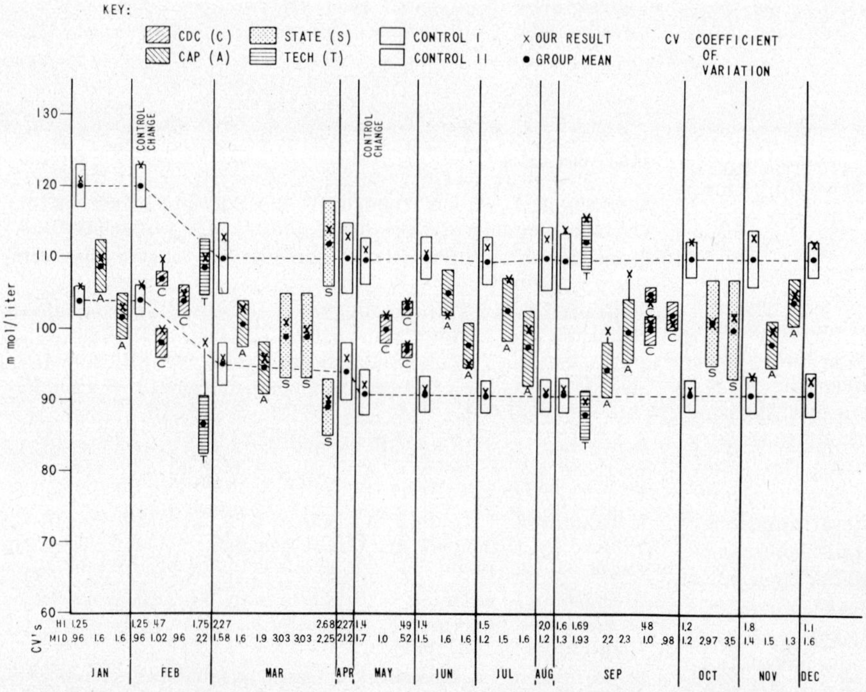

Fig. 2. Graphic display of quality-control data for chloride during 1974

A subtle increase is well illustrated. This aberration is not detected by any single quality-control sample

and linearity of our results, because there were no checks below 8 and only a few above 40 mg/liter. Following the techniques suggested by Grannis et al. (*6*) we re-evaluated our creatinine method (*7*) and discovered that the data were reasonably linear and accurate only in a range between 100 and 10 mg/liter. By assaying serum diluted with distilled water, we discovered that we should probably be reporting low creatinines as "less than 10 mg/liter."

The above example also suggests that we were not correctly calibrating our instruments as well as not running controls at the proper concentrations. Others (*5, 8, 9*) advocate that accuracy and precision should be especially emphasized at the medically significant or decision values, defined by Barnett (*8*) as the most useful values for patient care or the values from which "medical decisions are commonly made concerning the presence or absence of a disease state or the necessity for treatment." Thus, preoccupation with controls in the normal range to the neglect of other values is an inadequate basis for an acceptable quality-control program.

Analysis of our long-term quality-control graphs led to some additional pertinent observations. The Colorado Program and similar types of check-sample programs that test a wide variety of laboratories whose quality-control pro-

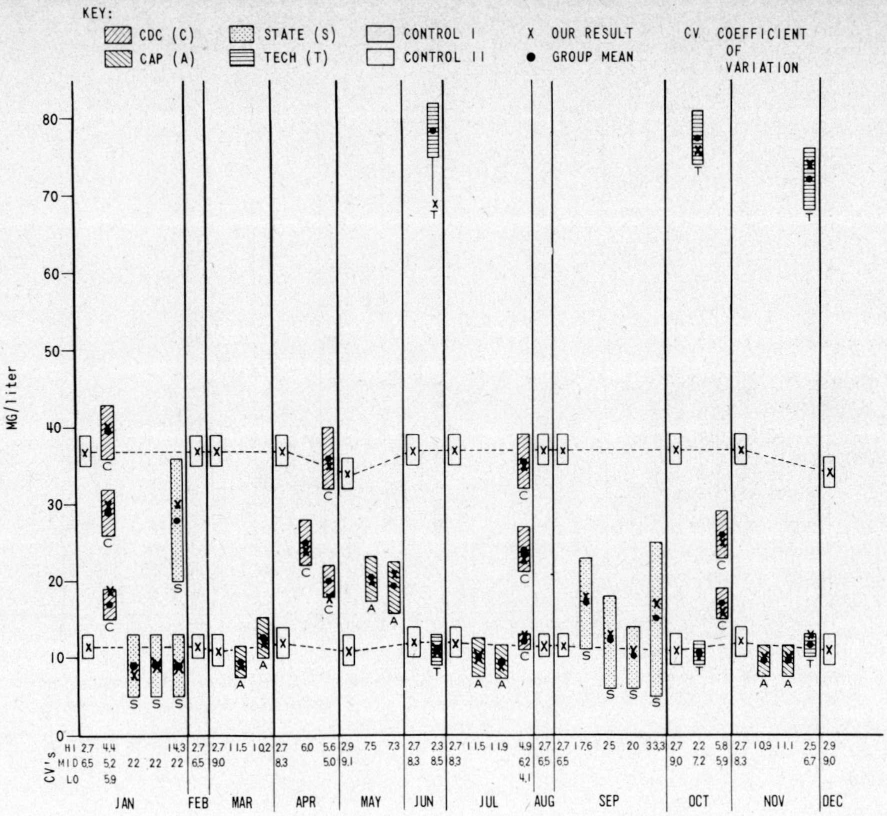

Fig. 3. Graphic display of quality-control data for creatinine

The graph shows the limited range of values tested and the CV achieved in the surveys. The paucity of values provoked us to investigate the quality and linearity of our creatinine method

grams vary from sophisticated to none at all provide information of minimal value; information content could be improved some by providing an analysis of the quality of results. Long-term quality-control analysis reveals that intralaboratory quality may vary significantly; programs that provide check samples only in the normal range and not in the medically significant ranges are of questionable value. Reliance on a single quality-control program is hazardous, as it alone may be inadequate to identify deficiencies.

An important implication is that long-term quality-control programs used in conjunction with methods that produce accurate and precise results during a long time may permit us to narrow our normal ranges and use the patient as his own "normal base," at least for some determinations. Cotlove et al. (*9*) have shown that for certain laboratory tests the individual biological variation is smaller than analytical error. This observation clearly suggests that medically significant shifts in an individual's values may now lie hidden within current "normal" ranges as now calculated. These small but significant shifts might be rendered apparent by the above techniques and might allow (*a*) use of a more narrow normal range, (*b*) establishment of long-term reproducibility, and (*c*) use of the "individual normal base" concept.

References

1. Skendzel, L. P., and Youden, W. J., Systematic versus random errors in laboratory surveys. *Am. J. Clin. Pathol.* **54,** 448 (1970).

2. Youden, W. J., Statistical techniques for collaborative tests. *Assoc. Off. Anal. Chem.,* Washington, D. C., 1967, p 64.

3. Gilbert, R. K., The size and source of analytic error in clinical chemistry. *Am. J. Clin. Pathol.* **61,** 904 (1974).

4. Nosanchuk, J. S., and Gottmann, A. W., CUMS and delta checks: A systematic approach to quality control. *Am. J. Clin. Pathol.* **62,** 707 (1974).

5. Westgard, J. O., Carey, R. N., and Wold, S., Criteria for judging precision and accuracy in method development and evaluation. *Clin. Chem.* **20,** 825 (1974).

6. Grannis, G. F., Lott, J. A., Edison, J. A., and McCabe, W. C., Proficiency evaluation of clinical chemistry laboratories. *Clin. Chem.* **18,** 222 (1972).

7. Chasson, A. I., Grady, H. T., and Stanly, M. A., Determination of creatinine by means of automatic chemical analysis. *Am. J. Clin. Pathol.* **35,** 83 (1961).

8. Barnett, R. N., Medical significance of laboratory results. *Am. J. Clin. Pathol.* **60,** 671 (1968).

9. Cotlove, E., Harris, E. K., and Williams, G. Z., Biological and analytic components of variation in long-term studies of serum constituents in normal subjects III. Physiological and medical implications. *Clin. Chem.* **16,** 1028 (1970).

CLIN. CHEM. 22/2, 273–274 (1976)

Direct Determination of Serum Chloride with a Semiautomated Discrete Analyzer

Stanley S. Levinson

I show how mercuric thiocyanate reagent can be used in assaying serum chloride economically, rapidly, and precisely. I used a semiautomated discrete analyzer with direct concentration read-out capability but the method can easily be applied to many mechanized instruments. Linearity between concentration and color is obtained by adding appropriate amounts of mercuric nitrate to the reagent. As many as 300 samples can be assayed per hour, and the method is excellent for emergency use.

Mercuric thiocyanate/ferric nitrate reagent has long been used for assaying chloride in serum (*1*). Unfortunately, the widely used mechanized version (Technicon AutoAnalyzer) is not as precise as might be desired (*2*), assays only 60 samples per hour, and requires relatively lengthy calculations to obtain the final results, making the instrument impractical for laboratories performing few chloride analyses each day. Accordingly, many laboratories have either adopted expensive coulometric equipment to enable more rapid and precise analysis for chloride or are using (even less precise) manual titration methods for small numbers of analyses and for emergency use.

With the introduction of semiautomated and automated instrumentation with direct concentration read-outs and print-outs, improved precision, and the capabilities of reading absorbances of two or greater, the classical mercuric thiocyanate/ferric nitrate reagent takes on a new perspective for chloride analysis. An abstract describing use of this reagent with semiautomated equipment (*3*) did not give details of the reagent mixture and described its use only with an instrument that requires specifically prepackaged reagents, not applicable for general use.

For use with inexpensive semiautomated equipment without computer interfacing, there must be linearity of absorbance over an appropriate range of concentrations. Such linearity can be achieved by properly adjusting the mercuric nitrate concentration in the reagent (*1*).

Here, I describe appropriate use of a mercuric thiocyanate/ferric nitrate/mercuric nitrate reagent in a way that enables low cost, rapid, and precise analysis of chloride in serum, and which is directly applicable to most analytical instruments capable of a direct concentration read-out. We routinely assay as many as 30 chloride samples each day in less than 5 min. With semiautomated equipment the method is also ideal for emergency work.

Materials and Methods

Apparatus

We used a semiautomated Bichromatic Analyzer, ABA-50 (Abbott Diagnostics Division, South Pasadena, Calif. 91030) and, for pipetting, an Abbott micro-diluter with a 1:101 diluter plate.

Laboratory, Brookline Hospital, Brookline, Mass. 02146.
Received Oct. 10, 1975; accepted Nov. 17, 1975.

Reagents

Stock mercuric thiocyanate (saturated), ferric nitrate (68.5 g/liter) in 0.33 mol/liter nitric acid, and mercuric nitrate (202 g/liter) were purchased from Technicon Instruments Corp., Tarrytown, N. Y. 10591.

Working color reagent is prepared by adding 100 ml of ferric nitrate stock solution to 1000 ml of saturated mercuric thiocyanate stock solution, then accurately adding 0.85 ml of mercuric nitrate stock solution to give a final concentration of 530 μg of mercuric nitrate per liter.

Chloride standards (70, 100, and 125 mmol/liter) are prepared by weighing out 4.092, 5.845, and 7.306 g of sodium chloride (AR, dried at 110 °C), respectively, and dissolving each in 1 liter of de-ionized water.

Method

Instrument-temperature is kept at 37 °C by means of an internal bath. A 500/600 filter is inserted into the instrument. Five microliters of sample and 0.5 ml of substrate are pipetted into labeled cuvettes with the micro-diluter (1:101 dilution). The samples are in the following sequence: into the first cuvette of the series is pipetted 5 μl of water (blank), into the second and third cuvettes 5 μl of 100 mmol/liter standard each, into succeeding cuvettes an appropriate sample or control sera, and into each of the final two cuvettes of the series a 70 mmol and 125 mmol/liter standard, respectively.

A 2-min incubation is allowed while the solutions equilibrate at the 37 °C temperature of the cuvette. The instrument is adjusted with the zero control so that the direct concentration read-out is zero with the water blank in the assay position. The instrument is adjusted with the scalar control so that the 100 mmol/liter standards read 100 on the display. Usually these two standards give readings that are within 2% of one another; if they differ by more than 2%, the other standards are checked to determine which of the 100 standards is the more nearly correct, and the instrument is then adjusted on the better of the two. The samples are read from the display and recorded.

Results

Figure 1 shows the effect of various concentrations of mercuric nitrate on the assay. Our routine concentration, 530 μg/liter, provides linearity between 70 and 140 mmol/liter. Increasing the concentration of mercuric nitrate changes the region of linearity to higher concentrations of chloride, lowering it to 430 μg/liter changes the region of linearity to between 60 and 125 mmol of chloride per liter.

Figure 2 demonstrates the correlation between results for 36 sera assayed by the present method and the same sera assayed, after preparing protein-free filtrates, by a titration method (*4*). The corresponding normal range of the two methods, determined from the regression line, is nearly identical.

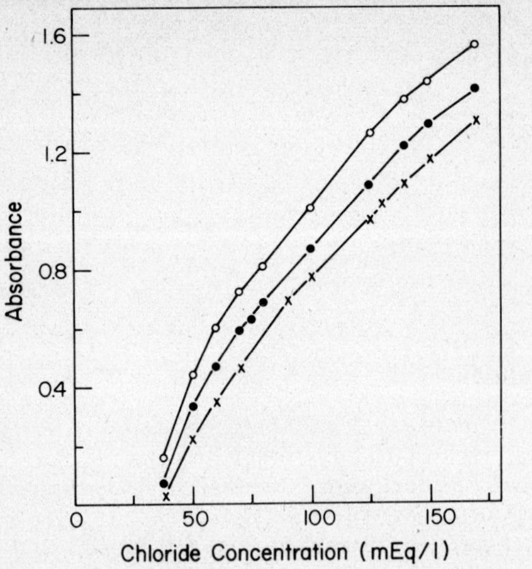

Fig. 1. Relationship between chloride and absorbance with various amounts of mercuric nitrate added to the color reagent

X's represent 620 μg of mercuric nitrate per liter of color reagent, or 1 ml of mercuric nitrate stock solution per 1100 ml of color reagent; *closed circles* represent 530 μg of mercuric nitrate per liter of color reagent, or 0.85 ml per 1100 ml of color reagent; *open circles* represent 440 μg of mercuric nitrate per liter of color reagent, or 0.70 ml per 1100 ml of color reagent

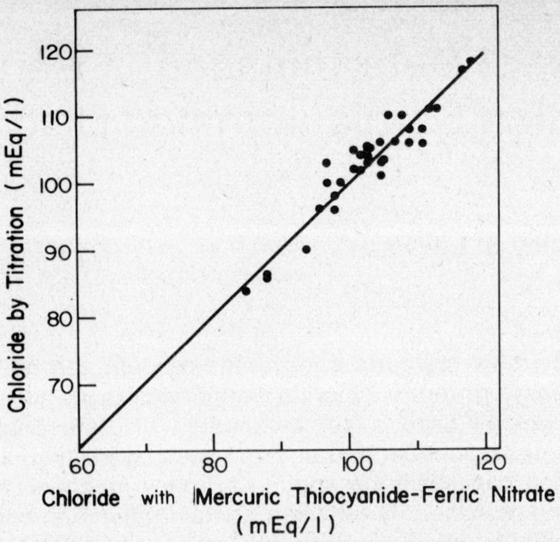

Fig. 2. Relationship between chloride assay by mercuric thiocyanate ferric nitrate reagent with chloride assayed by titration, with use of mercuric nitrate in the presence of diphenylcarbazone (*4*)

Slope, +0.962; *y*-intercept, +3.777; correlation coefficient, 0.951; n, 36

The within-run coefficient of variation, as determined on 10 100-mmol/liter samples, was less than 1% in two different experiments. Day-to-day variation was determined by calculating a coefficient of variation for 10 assays each of normal and abnormal control sera ("Validate-N" and "Validate-A"; General Diagnostics, Division of Warner-Lambert Co., Morris Plains, N. J. 07950) over 10 consecutive days. The coefficient of variation for the normal control was 1.28% and for the abnormal control, 1.24%. The average value for the abnormal control was 85.7 mmol/liter and that for the normal was 104.1 mmol/liter, values nearly the same as those listed (85 and 105 mmol/liter, respectively) by General Diagnostics for the same lots assayed with a Cotlove chloridometer.

Bovine serum albumin (50, 100, or 150 g/liter) and bilirubin (40, 60, or 120 mg/liter) did not significantly alter the readings for 100 mmol/liter chloride samples. Triglycerides in concentrations of 6.0, 4.5, 3.0, or 1.5 g/liter, prepared by adding aliquots from a turbid serum to aliquots from a clear serum, altered the chloride readings less than 1 mmol/liter.

Discussion

With semiautomated instrumentation, use of mercuric thiocyanate/ferric nitrate reagent clearly is a rapid, precise technique for assaying serum chloride. Only a 5-μl sample is needed with the ABA-50, and less reagent is used than is needed in continuous-flow analysis. The working reagents are stable for months.

As indicated in Figure 1, adequate linearity is obtained by adjusting the mercuric nitrate concentration of the reagent. We find the recommended concentration ideal for semiautomated instruments because sera containing less than 70 mmol of chloride per liter can easily be repeated at the end of a series by using a 1/51 dilution of sample to reagent rather than the usual 1/101. This alters the apparent sample concentration back into the linear range. The actual concentration is then obtained by dividing the apparent concentration by 2. Accordingly, concentrations exceeding 140 mmol/liter can be brought into the linear range by a 25-fold dilution. With automated equipment it would be more efficient to use 430 μg of mercuric nitrate per liter of reagent, thereby providing linearity between 60 and 125 mmol of chloride per liter.

The recommended concentration of mercuric thiocyanate and ferric nitrate was purposely selected to give fairly high absorption differences in the linear range (0.6 to 1.2) together with a large dilution of sample, which minimizes the effects of turbidity, bilirubin, etc., and eliminates the need to run serum blanks with each sample. As noted in the *Results* section, bilirubin up to 120 mg/liter does not affect the assay significantly, nor have we noticed any significant effect attributable to serum turbidity.

We perform a battery of 10 tests on the ABA-50 each morning, most of which require a 37 °C incubation. Chloride is measured at 37 °C for convenience only. We have performed the assay with a Perkin-Elmer Coleman 55 spectrophotometer semiautomated system at room temperature without any substantial difference in speed or precision, although the larger cuvette necessitates that the sample and reagent be scaled up to 15 μl and 1.5 ml, respectively.

References

1. Hamilton, R. H., A direct photometric method for assaying chloride in biological fluids employing mercuric thiocyanate and perchloric acid. *Clin. Chem.* **12,** 1 (1966).

2. Tietz, N. W., Electrolytes. In *Fundamentals of Clinical Chemistry,* N. W. Tietz, Ed. W. B. Saunders Co., Philadelphia, Pa., 1970, p 624.

3. Kelley, T. F., Lewis, W. W., Eldrige, C., and Kapteyn, R. J., Determination of serum chloride and magnesium with the Clinicard system. *Clin. Chem.* **20,** 908 (1974).

4. Tietz, N. W., *loc. cit.*, p 622.

CLIN. CHEM. 22/2, 275–277 (1976)

Lipoamide Dehydrogenase in Serum: A Preliminary Report

John W. Pelley, Gwynne H. Little, Tracy C. Linn, and Frank F. Hall

Lipoamide dehydrogenase was identified in serum and the optimal conditions for its assay at 30 °C were defined. The pH optimum in tris(hydroxymethyl)aminomethane buffer is 7.8, and activity is inhibited if buffer concentration exceeds 100 mmol/liter. Saturating concentrations of the substrates NAD^+ and lipoamide are 3 mmol/liter and 5 mmol/liter, respectively. Activity is decreased eightfold when lipoic acid is substituted for lipoamide. Activity is linearly related to enzyme concentration up to a limiting absorbance change of 0.300 at 340 nm, and both within-day and day-to-day precision are satisfactory. Data suggest a normal range (2 SD) of 3–19 kU/liter. The highest value measured in serum was 473 kU/liter. A correlation with direct bilirubin concentrations ($r = 0.435$, $P < 0.01$) was found.

Additional Keyphrases: *reference values • correlation with bilirubin*

We report here for the first time the measurement in serum of activity attributable to lipoamide dehydrogenase (LAD),[1] which catalyzes the following reversible reaction:

$$\text{lipoamide (red.)} + NAD^+ \rightleftharpoons \text{lipoamide (oxid.)} + NADH$$

In this initial report we document the presence of LAD in blood serum, and define the requirements and optimum conditions for its clinical assay. In addition, we have attempted to correlate above-normal LAD activity in serum with some established chemical indices of disease; the only positive correlation found was with values for direct bilirubin in serum.

Materials and Methods

Reagents

LAD I (Tris–NAD^+). Add 432 mg of NAD^+ (N-7004; Sigma Chemical Co., St. Louis, Mo. 63178) to 100 ml of 0.1 mol/liter Tris HCl, pH 7.8, and 40 ml of water. Readjust the pH to 7.8 and dilute to a final volume of 150 ml with water. Divide the solution into 10-ml aliquots and store at −20 °C until used. Thawed solutions are stable for at least three 8-h workdays at 30 °C with overnight storage at −20 °C.

LAD II (Tris–DDT–Lipoamide). Dissolve 40 mg of lipoamide (Sigma) and 60 mg of DTT in 2.0 ml of 95% ethanol. Add 6.0 ml of 50 mmol/liter Tris HCl, pH 8.2, and incubate for 30 min at 30 °C. Divide the solution into aliquots sufficient for one day's use, and store them at −20 °C. This solution is stable for 8 h at 30 °C; leftover amounts can be frozen and reused once without adverse effects.

Procedure

Assays were routinely performed with a Model 24 recording spectrophotometer (Beckman Instruments, Inc., Fullerton, Calif. 92634) with a constant-temperature cell holder equilibrated at 30 °C. Reagents LAD I and LAD II were pre-equilibrated at 30 °C and maintained at this temperature in a constant-temperature apparatus. The assays were done in a 1.4-ml cuvette with a 1.0-cm lightpath, as follows:

1. Add 750 µl of LAD I reagent.
2. Add 50 µl of serum or an appropriate dilution.
3. Preincubate for 10 min at 30 °C. Monitor nonspecific background with the spectrophotometer during this step.
4. Add 200 µl of LAD II reagent.
5. Record the increase in absorbance (A) at 340 nm. Calculate ΔA/10 min, subtracting background activity determined in step 3, as necessary.

The concentration (in mmol/liter) for each component in the 1.0-ml reaction mixture is: Tris HCl (pH 7.8), 0.057; NAD^+, 3; lipoamide, 5; and DTT, 10. LAD values are reported in international (IUB) units per liter (U/liter) when assayed under the conditions described above. The calculation for a 50-µl sample is as follows:

$$\text{U/liter} = (\Delta A_{340}/10 \text{ min}) \times (322 \times 10^3)$$

The factor 322×10^3 takes into account the volume of sample used, the time course of the reaction, and the molar extinction coefficient of NAD^+ (6.22×10^3) at 340 nm.

The sera we used were from both outpatients and inpatients; however, their case histories were not available to us. The normal range for LAD was determined for sera that had no values outside the normal range in the usual SMA 12/60 (Technicon Instruments Corp., Tarrytown, N. Y. 10591) profile.

Results

The LAD assay described has an absolute requirement for DTT, NAD^+, and enzyme (serum). The background reduction of NAD^+ in the absence of lipoamide (lipoamide blank) is generally negligible. The highest LAD activity assayed to date had a net value of 473 kU/liter and the lipoamide blank for this serum was 0.3 kU/liter. Our results lead us to estimate the normal range for LAD in serum to be 3–19 kU/liter, based on results for sera from 100 patients.

Department of Biochemistry, Texas Tech University School of Medicine, Lubbock, Texas 79409 (J. W. P., G. H. L. and F. F. H.); and Department of Biochemistry, University of Texas Southwestern Medical School, Dallas, Texas 75235 (T. C. L.).

[1] Nonstandard abbreviations used, and enzyme identification: LAD, lipoamide dehydrogenase (NADH) [NADH:lipoamide oxidoreductase, EC 1.6.4.3]; DTT, dithiothreitol; and Tris, tris(hydroxymethyl)aminomethane.

Received Sept. 1, 1975; accepted Nov. 17, 1975.

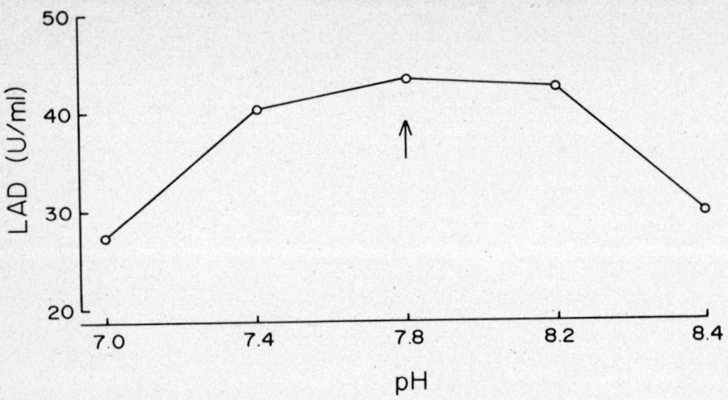

Fig. 1. Serum LAD activity as a function of pH

Assay pH adjusted as indicated. In Figures 1–6, assay conditions were as described in text, except as noted

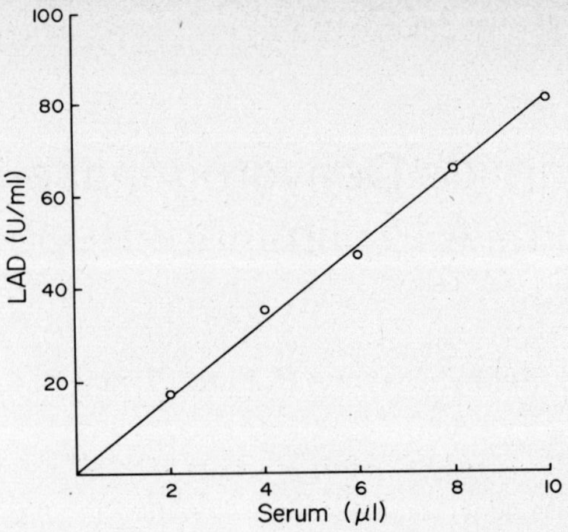

Fig. 3. Serum LAD activity as a function of volume of serum added

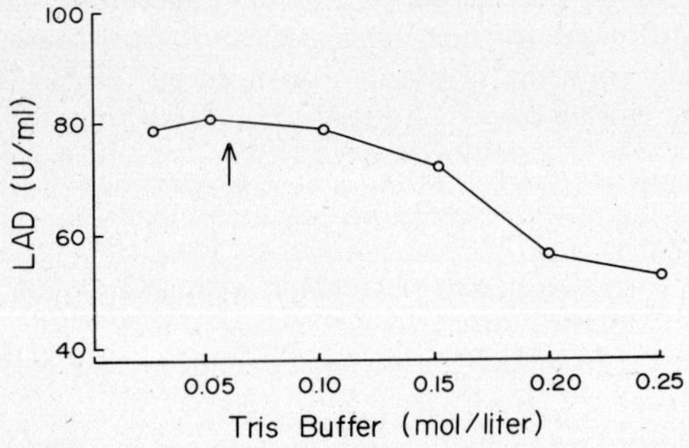

Fig. 2. Serum LAD activity as a function of buffer concentration

Tris buffer added as indicated. *Arrow* indicates buffer concentration used in assay as standardized

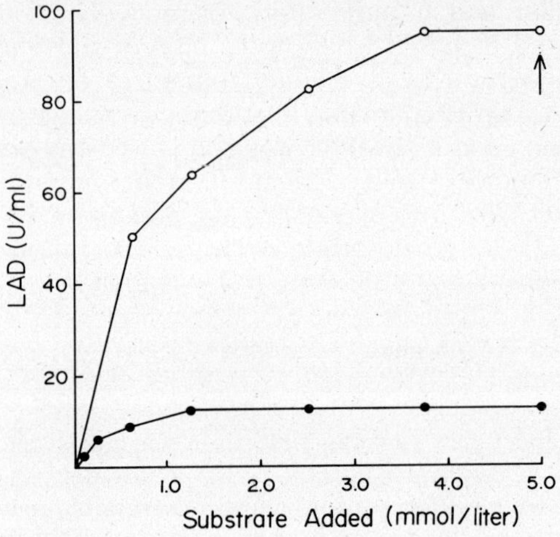

Fig. 4. Serum LAD activity as a function of lipoamide or lipoic acid

Arrow indicates concentration used in assay as standardized

The optimum pH for LAD assay is 7.8 (Figure 1). Background activity is also least at this pH. LAD is inhibited by concentrations of Tris buffer higher than that recommended here (Figure 2). Hemolysis does not interfere.

The assay conditions described here are optimal for measuring LAD at concentrations up to 100 kU/liter (0.300 ΔA_{340}/10 min). Within these limits the reaction rate is directly proportional to the quantity of serum added (LAD activity) (Figure 3). Figures 4 and 5 demonstrate that the reaction is zero order with respect to the substrates, lipoamide, and NAD^+, at the concentrations used. Also illustrated is the lessened (about an eighth) activity of the same sera with lipoic acid substituted for lipoamide. Under optimal conditions, within-day precision and day-to-day precision are satisfactory for both normal and abnormally high values (Table 1).

LAD activity is stable in fresh serum for 8 h at room temperature, for 24 h at 0–3 °C. Thawing and refreezing once does not significantly decrease the activity of LAD in serum. When a serum sample has been thawed it should be kept on ice until assayed.

Serum LAD activity was investigated in sera that had abnormally high values for either creatine phosphokinase [ATP:creatine phosphotransferase, EC 2.7.3.2]; aspartate aminotransferase [L-aspartate:2-oxoglutarate aminotransferase, EC 2.6.1.1]; alanine aminotransferase, [L-alanine:2-oxoglutarate aminotransferase, EC 2.6.1.2]; blood urea nitrogen; alkaline phosphatase [orthophosphoric monoester phosphohydrolase, EC 3.1.3.1]; lactate dehydrogenase [L-lactate:NAD oxidoreductase, EC 1.1.1.27]; or bilirubin (total, direct, and indirect). Figure 6 shows the statistically significant positive correlation between LAD activity and *direct* bilirubin concentration in 39 samples of serum (r = 0.435, P <0.01). Based on results for 15 or more samples each, we found that (possibly excepting alanine aminotransferase) the other serum analyses investigated do *not* correlate with increased serum LAD activity.

Discussion

Lipoamide dehydrogenase is an integral part of the multienzyme α-keto acid dehydrogenase complexes (*2*), where it functions to regenerate oxidized lipoic acid. The natural substrate for LAD is a reduced lipoic acid moiety that is covalently bound to the ϵ-amino group of a lysine residue in one of the other component enzymes of the α-keto acid dehydrogenase complexes. In vitro, an analog, lipoamide, serves as a substitute for the protein-bound lipoyl moiety. The active (dihydro) form of the substrate is generated in slightly alkaline DTT solution (LAD II) before it is added to the assay mixture. By preincubating the serum sample with the NAD^+ reagent (LAD I) the nonspecific background can be monitored before the reaction is started with LAD II. Routinely, background values are so low that this measurement is negligible. However, these data can be easily obtained without performing a separate assay. Previous reports have shown that LAD and diaphorase [NAD(P)H:

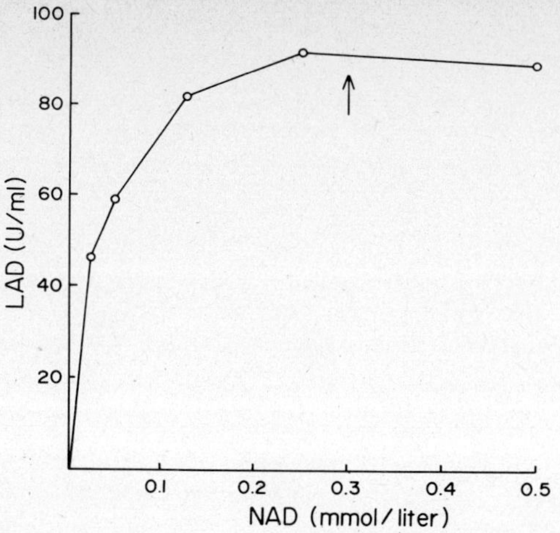

Fig. 5. Serum LAD activity as a function of NAD^+ added
Arrow indicates concentration used in standard assay

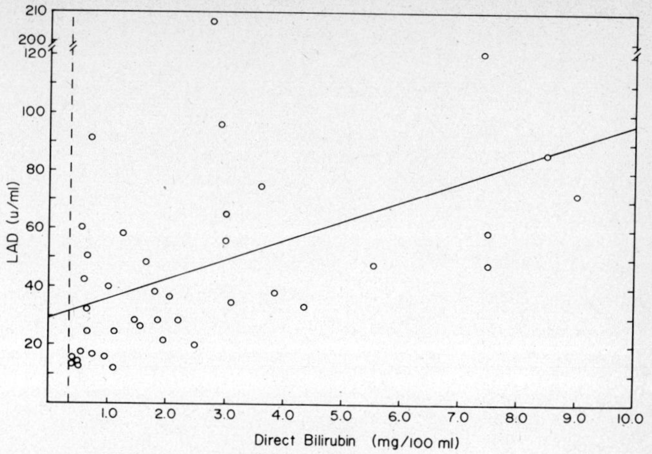

Fig. 6. Serum LAD activity vs. direct bilirubin concentration
The normal limit for direct bilirubin indicated by *vertical dotted line*. Direct bilirubin determined by method of Gambino (*6*)

Table 1. Precision of Serum Lipoamide Dehydrogenase Assay

Within-day precision:[a]

	Serum 1	Serum 2	Serum 3
Mean activity, kU/liter	9.86	48.6	95.3
SD	0.44	1.66	3.06
CV, %	4.5	3.4	3.2

Day-to-day precision:[b]

	Serum 1	Serum 2
Mean activity, kU/liter	11.6	31.5
SD	1.0	2.8
CV, %	8.6	8.9

[a] Versatol reference serum (General Diagnostics, cat. No. 30101; Warner-Chilcott Laboratories, Morris Plains, N.J. 07950) containing given activities of lipoamide dehydrogenase (cat. No. L-2002, Sigma Chemical Co., St. Louis, Mo. 63178) were assayed, 20 replicates of each.

[b] Freshly drawn sera with increased or normal values, divided into aliquots, frozen, and assayed on 15 consecutive workdays.

acceptor oxidoreductase, EC 1.6.99.-], a potential source of background interference, are identical proteins (*3*). It was subsequently shown, however, that diaphorase, an enzyme of no known physiological function, probably is a somewhat denatured form of LAD (*4*).

Most present enzymological methods for serum measure enzymes that originate and are localized either in the cytoplasm (e.g., alanine aminotransferase, lactate dehydrogenase) or in the mitochondria and the cytoplasm (e.g., aspartate aminotransferase). Methods for enzymes localized only in the mitochondrion—for example, glutamate dehydrogenase [L-glutamate:NAD^+ oxidoreductase (deaminating), EC 1.4.1.2]—are fewer, and so studies on their diagnostic, prognostic, and monitoring potential have necessarily also been few (*5*). Enzymes localized exclusively within the mitochondrion should be of unique value for diagnosing acute disease, because tissue damage must be relatively severe before they would be expected to appear in the circulation.

Our method has given satisfactory results in daily use in a private medical-service laboratory without direct supervision from our laboratory. Although LAD activity is normally low or absent in serum, it is increased in certain pathological conditions. A positive correlation with direct bilirubin suggests a potential clinical value of serum LAD determinations, because increased values for direct bilirubin are always associated with liver or biliary tract disease (*7*).

Further studies are needed as to the normal range and clinical significance of serum LAD. We cannot at present pursue this investigation further, but we hope that this report will encourage other laboratories to do so.

We thank Mrs. Laurel Dingrando for expert technical assistance.

References

1. Lusty, C. J., and Singer, T. P., Lipoyl dehydrogenase: Free and complexed form in mammalian mitochondria. *J. Biol. Chem.* **239,** 3733 (1964).
2. Reed, L. J., and Cox, D. J., Macromolecular organization of enzyme systems. *Annu. Rev. Biochem.* **35,** 57 (1966).
3. Massey, V., The identity of diaphorase and lipoyl dehydrogenase. *Biochim. Biophys. Acta* **37,** 314 (1960).
4. Veeger, C., and Massey, V., The reaction mechanism of lipoamide dehydrogenase. *Biochim. Biophys. Acta* **64,** 83 (1962).
5. Batsakis, J. G., Sodeman, T. A., and Deegan, M. J., Enzymatic evaluation of hepatobiliary disease. *Lab. Med.* **5,** 33 (1974).
6. Gambino, S. R., Bilirubin (modified Jendrassik and Grof)—provisional. *Stand. Methods Clin. Chem.* **5,** 55 (1965).
7. Gambino, S. R., Other, A., and Burns, W., Direct serum bilirubin and the sulfobromophthalein test in occult liver disease. *J. Am. Med. Assoc.* **201,** 171 (1967).

special report

Clinical Chemistry in the Peoples Republic of China Today

Ed. note: For some months now, the Editorial Office has been receiving the English version of the Chinese Medical Journal, *published bimonthly by the Chinese Medical Association, the most recent issue (New Series vol. 1, no. 5) having been received in December. This well-illustrated publication gives interesting insights into Chinese medicine. In this report, an AACC member summarizes a recent visit to mainland China. Interested readers may obtain more information on this subject from* China Medicine As We Saw It, *an anthology of articles by scientists who have recently visited mainland China, published by the Fogarty International Center, NIH, Bethesda, Md. 20014, and available on request (limited number). Another intriguing description of medical education and practice in that part of the world appears in a series of two articles on India by Elmer Bendiner, which appeared in the May and September 1975 issues of* Hospital Practice.

In August 1975, I visited the Peoples Republic of China—my first visit "home" in 26 years. While there, I talked with scientists in the biochemical and biophysical institutes and at a cancer-research hospital, observed surgery during acupuncture anesthesia, interviewed doctors working on farm communes, and presented a series of seminars on radioimmunoassay, nuclear counting, and spectrophotometry. I also had an opportunity to exchange ideas with scientists and learn about the new medical-research programs in China.

It was a very informative experience. Most impressive was the self-reliant attitude of the Chinese. Although foreign technologies are welcome in China, they do not intend to depend on them.

In China, political thoughts come first; other considerations, including business, follow. "Serve the people" dominates thought and activity. Chairman Mao's pictures and statues spur China on to greater achievement.

My first tour was to the Shanghai Industrial Exposition in Shanghai, where Shanghai-made clinical instruments were on display, such as single-beam UV spectrophotometers, pH meters, gas and liquid chromatographs, EEG, blood-gas analyzers—more than a dozen of them were in this exhibit on the exposition floor.

I was surprised that complicated clinical instruments could be built in Shanghai. Recalling 26 years ago, I couldn't remember the colleges ever having any such instrument that had not been imported from a foreign country. The instruments I saw in the exposition were not as sophisticated as the ones we have here in the United States. In another area of the exposition, Chinese medicines (herbs) in the form of tablets were displayed. I remembered that when I was a child my parents fed me preparations from plants when I was ill—with always a bitter or unpleasant taste. The old Chinese saying, "Good medicine is always bitter," no longer holds true with this improvement in health remedies.

I visited a large vegetable farm commune in a suburb of Shanghai. The farm has 4300 families, with 28 000 people living in seven units. Besides large apartment complexes and schools up to 12 grades, they also have a 40-bed hospital with a clinical laboratory, pharmacy, and outpatient clinic. Doctors and nurses are on duty 24 hours a day. Usually doctors visit the patient in the patient's home. Doctors are assigned on a rotating basis; they have to work in the communes one to two months a year. Consequently, the Chinese government has achieved an outstanding goal, the aim of which is twofold: (1) it has permitted the doctors to work directly with the farmers and give them medical treatment; (2) it has also made the doctors realize that farmers have an important task in serving their country. The hospital is only for minor diseases or obstetrics. For major cases, patients are moved to the large city hospital. Prenatal care was unheard of on the farms 26 years ago. Now, women from the farm regularly go to the clinic for a checkup. The laboratory is equipped with common instruments for CBC, urinalysis, and microbiology. I

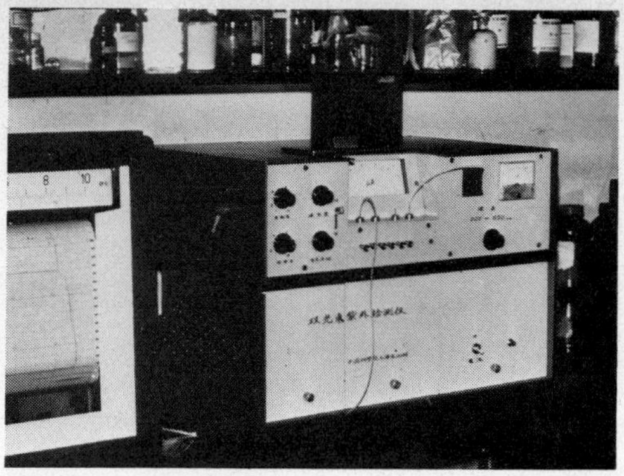

Fig. 1. Shanghai-made double-beam ultraviolet spectrophotometer

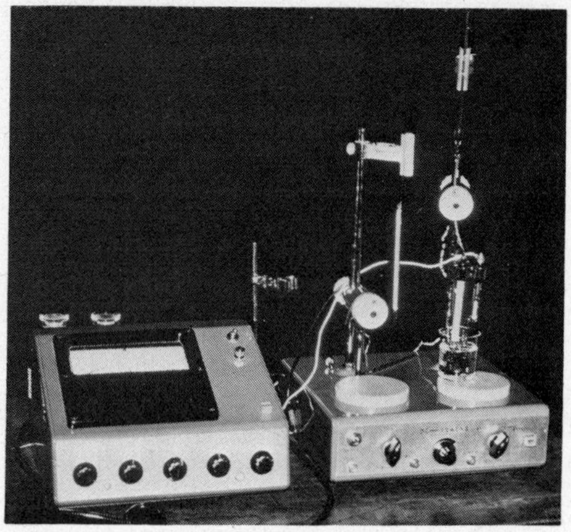

Fig. 2. pH meter made in the instrument shop of Chun Shan Hospital

couldn't believe my eyes—that I had really found a hospital and clinical laboratory in a farm area—because even in the United States, people in some rural areas have to travel miles to find a doctor to get treatment.

While in Shanghai and Peking, I met many scientists from various fields. We had occasion to discuss subjects such as radioimmunoassay, EMIT, clinical enzymology, etc. I found that their research approach is different from that in the United States; for instance, when they are working on radioimmunoassay research, the work force is combined from various institutes, such as nuclear medicine, biology, biochemistry, chemistry (organic and inorganic), vaccine and serum, and biophysics. They all stressed that their research work is done directly for the people. Therefore, research projects are concerned with the most common and frequently found diseases. Cancer is now their number one target. People from farms and factories volunteer for mass screening of cancer disease. In 1974 a national radioimmunoassay conference was held in Shanghai, and most radioimmunoassay applications are concerned with cancer research.

I was invited by Drs. K. Lin and W. Y. Chao from Chun Shan Hospital (about 500 beds) to tour their facilities. I had an opportunity to view two surgical procedures in which acupuncture anesthesia was used. One of them, rather complicated, was ureterolithotomy. During this surgery, the patient was alert and wide awake. When I took a picture of him, he smiled and said "thank you." I toured the hospital clinical laboratories, and the director of the laboratory told me that they are doing most routine clinical chemical procedures as well as some special ones: phenotyping electrophoresis, isoenzymes, urinary hormones, blood gases, etc. Most of the equipment I saw in their laboratory was of the basic sort; some instruments were made by the hospital instrument shop, some were old ones from 1940–50. Radioimmunoassay is done in the Nuclear Medicine Department. A single-well gamma counter with digital readout, built by the hospital, is being used for carcinoembryonic antigen assay and thyroid-function tests. I did not see any fully automated chemistry instrument in any of the laboratories that I visited.

The laboratory in Shanghai Chun San Hospital makes its own reagents. Chemicals are prepared and supplied by other institutes such as inorganic and organic institutes, biochemical institutes, vaccine and serum institutes, etc. I believe that no reagent test kits like those in the United States are marketed in the Peoples Republic of China.

From what I have heard and observed, pathologists are not necessarily the ones in charge of the clinical laboratory in China. The laboratory is usually supervised by a specialist; i.e., a clinical chemical laboratory would be directed and supervised by an experienced clinical chemist, a radioimmunoassay laboratory by a nuclear medicine physician.

In Shanghai, I visited Biochemistry Professor C. W. Shen, of the Institute of the Chinese Academy of Sciences. Prof. Shen, educated in Canada and the United States, is the director of the institute. The institute has three main divisions: Research, Biochemical Reagents and Drugs, and Instrument Shop.

The research division is doing much biochemical research, on subjects such as insulin, amino acids, enzymes, rice germination, and immunology. At the Insulin Research Laboratory I learned that it was in China that insulin was first synthesized by a chemical method six years ago. Now they are working on the relation of insulin to biochemical, physiological, metabolic, and related problems.

The second division produces amino acids and derivatives, nucleic acids and related substances, coenzymes, proteins, enzymes and their inhibitors, carbohydrates, and steroids. These biochemical reagents have immediate practical application. An example is the use of luliberin (luteinizing hormone-releasing factor) to increase the supply of edible fish. They have found that some edible river fish do not lay eggs unless they are in a pond. Therefore, people put the fish from the Yangtse River into a fish pond and feed

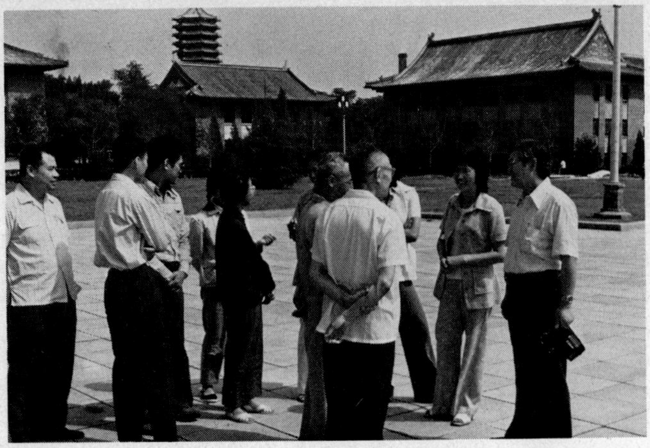

Fig. 3. At Peking University, Ms. Sun (at right) chats with professors and students from the biochemistry and physics departments

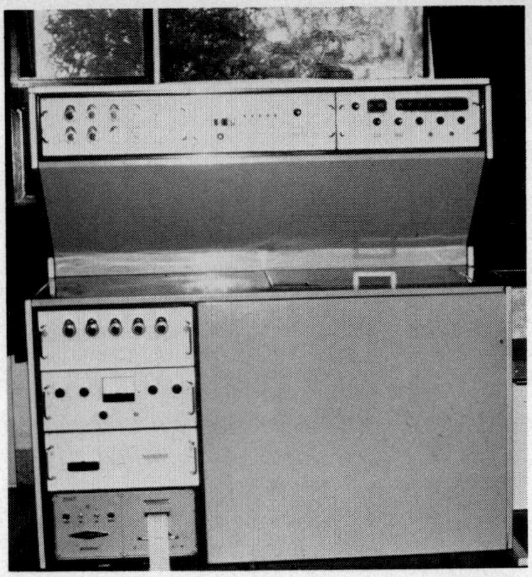

Fig. 4. Liquid-scintillation counter fabricated by the Biophysics Institute, Peking

them with luliberin. Within 10 to 20 hours the fish start to produce young. At this rapid reproduction rate, the large demand for fish can be supplied.

When I traveled to Peking, I met my colleagues from Ohio State University, and also had an opportunity to see a high-school friend. She is now also a clinical chemist and country doctor, working in Northeast China with a special research interest in asthma, mostly in older persons. She is experimenting with a herb treatment for asthma that is very successful.

Peking University is situated on a beautiful campus and is one of the largest and oldest schools in China. I was the guest of professors from the Biochemistry Department and the Physics Department. I learned that they are experimenting with certain programs that cover a variety of fields over a three-year academic period. In order to shorten one school year, they do not repeat and overlap courses. Courses are specialized and concentrated in particular fields. The summer vacation is rather short (4–5 weeks). For science and engineering students, they combine equal parts of theory and practical experiments by letting students actually work in the course-related shops. Students in these shops have built the schools' computers and instruments. If three years are not enough for science and engineering majors, they extend their learning period until the student is ready to finish his major. I understand that there is no degree granted to anyone, but rather an evaluation and assignment. The recently built university library contains a great deal of Chinese history and culture, including reference books on medicine and pharmacology dating back two to three thousand years.

I had a chance to join three doctors in a tour of a Tz Tan cancer hospital. The director of the research lab, a very knowledgeable woman doctor, told us about their research projects, one of which is population mass screening for the liver cancer that occurs among people living in the farm communes.

They have been using the "rocket" electrophoresis method to assess α_1-fetoprotein. Because the electrophoresis system is a very small system, it is easily transported to the commune hospital laboratory. Because there are hundreds of communes in China, the screening data from farms are massive; more than 400 000 cases are now on file. A report on this project was published and reported at a European cancer meeting last year. A project on esophageal carcinoma is also in progress. One doctor demonstrated how esophageal samples are collected from volunteers. He used a very efficient, yet very simple device. This study has also been reported and published.

At the Peking Biophysics Institute I was shown the prototype of a liquid-scintillation counter by a group of scientists from the institute (Figure 4). The instrument is being built by 30 members from the physics, chemistry, and biochemistry departments and the hospitals. I was told that it has taken them 20 months to complete this instrument from the drawing-board stage to the evaluation stage. The instrument has a background of 22 cpm in the ^3H channel and 24 cpm in the ^{14}C channel. Their ^3H counting efficiency is 54.4%, their ^{14}C counting efficiency 92.8%.

I went to the Chinese Medical Association headquarters and met with Dr. Tow, the Vice Secretary, and Dr. Chen, the Director of Foreign Affairs. As a representative of Dr. Martin Rubin, President of IFCC, I delivered a copy of the IFCC annual report and newsletter to Dr. Tow. We discussed the state of the art of clinical chemistry and various related organizations in the United States and abroad. It was there that I learned about the Chinese method of treating patients with burns over 95% of their body by use of traditional Chinese herbs as well as Western drugs, by mouth and as dressings. Equally important are the spiritual persistence, years of experience, and patience of the nurses and doctors. I learned more about acupuncture applications, such as single-needle acupuncture anesthesia in pulmonary resection, and about deaf mutes cured by acupuncture treatment.

In a group discussion, I had an opportunity to meet a few scientists from the Drug and Biological Products Control Institute. They have done many research projects dealing with the relation to clinical chemistry of patients, traditional herbal medicine, and metabolic functions after the patient has taken certain herbs, and with discovering the exact essential and active compound in different herbs. Chinese doctors work closely with farmers and workers. Many of the doctors are well-trained, college science graduates with two years of medical training followed by extensive experience, literally "in the field." They work as laborers in between doctoring, combining first-hand factory or farm job knowledge with their academic training.

All these people that I met seem to have one goal: "to serve the people." Self-reliance is their slogan; they always manifest a hardworking and eager spirit and are proud of their work.

The "barefoot doctors" are actually technicians who have received six months' specialized training after completing one or two years of junior college. They are able to do some basic examinations and perform simple laboratory tests after much observation and practice under supervision.

In the Peoples Republic of China, Chinese herbal medicine and acupuncture are undergoing extensive clinical use and research. Western-trained doctors and herbal doctors are working together and combine their best talents in teaching, research, and patient care. This is contrary to the situation that existed 26 years ago when herbal and Western medicines never mixed together.

The current upsurge of interest in acupuncture in the United States is generated by increasing reports from scientifically-trained Western observers visiting China. As one Chinese doctor told me in Shanghai, "Acupuncture is a very complex subject to study and understand, especially for those without any knowledge of the Chinese old science culture." He also emphasized that even in China, the science of acupuncture is still not completely understood, and more intensive research is required.

China has a great future in clinical chemistry. Perhaps some day, China will find the answer to the number-one enemy, cancer.

I am indebted to Dr. A. O. Beckman and Mr. Harry Graff for their encouragement and arrangements of my visit to the Chinese scientific institutes and hospitals. I also thank Mr. H. Eugene Robbins of *Beckman New Dimensions* for his valuable assistance with the photographic work.

Lilla Sun
Senior Clinical Applications Chemist

Beckman Instruments, Inc.
Scientific Instruments Division
Irvine, Calif. 92713

letters

Adjustment of Serum Calcium for Protein

To the Editor:

The important problem of the interpretation of the serum total calcium concentration when the serum protein concentration is abnormal was discussed recently by Husdan et al. (*1*). These authors advocated the routine adjustment of serum total calcium concentration for the serum total protein concentration according to the formulas of either Parfitt (*2*) or Dent (*3*) and have calculated reference ranges for such adjusted values. While agreeing that some adjustment needs to be made, we wish to submit the following three criticisms of the above authors' approach.

First, both the formulas of Parfitt and Dent use an *average* regression coefficient (binding factor) for serum total calcium concentration on serum total protein concentration. We have previously shown (*4*) that, although the average regression coefficient for serum total calcium concentration on serum albumin concentration is 25 μmol of calcium per gram of albumin, there is more than a sevenfold variation in regression coefficients between individuals, the 95 percentile range being 7 to 53 μmol/g. Thus a patient with serum total calcium and albumin concentrations of 1.65 mmol/liter and 20 g/liter, respectively, would have the following serum calcium concentrations, when adjusted to the mean serum albumin concentration of 48 g/liter: 2.35 mmol/liter with use of an average regression coefficient and 1.85 or 3.13 mmol/liter with use of the lower or upper limits, respectively, of the 95 percentile reference range of regression coefficients. That is, a patient who would be considered normocalcemic when an average factor was used could in fact be either hypo- or hypercalcemic. Hence in situations where knowledge of the "true" or adjusted serum total calcium concentration is important, we advocate establishing the individual's own binding factor by using a 15-min period of venous occlusion, with four blood samples taken at 0, 5, 10, and 15 min (*4*). It is then a simple matter to graph the serum total calcium concentrations vs. the corresponding serum albumin concentrations and to draw the regression line the slope of which is the current regression coefficient for that individual. The suggested period of hemoconcentration allows significant increases in both serum protein and total calcium concentrations (38% and 18%, respectively, compared to 5.8% and 2.4% obtained by Husdan et al.) and the fact that there are four points virtually eliminates any error in drawing the regression line because of analytical variation in the measurements.

Second, the authors calculated "normal adjusted serum total calcium ranges" by using the formulas of Parfitt and Dent, in both of which average regression coefficients are used. For the reasons alluded to above, it would be necessary to determine the *individual* binding coefficients as well as the serum total calcium and albumin concentrations on each of a significant number of normal subjects to establish a valid reference range for adjusted total calcium concentration in serum. This would be quite an undertaking, but one that is essential to the rational "adjustment" of serum total calcium concentration.

Third, we cannot agree that it is preferable to adjust for serum total protein rather than for serum albumin concentration. The authors found (but did not give details) that the estimation of serum total protein concentration by refractometry was more reproducible than that of serum albumin concentration by photometry or by electrophoresis. However in our laboratory, representative within-batch coefficients of variation (CV) for serum total protein and albumin concentrations determined with the Technicon SMA 12-60 are similar, being 1.1% and 1.2%, respectively. While the CV for total protein by refractometry in our laboratory is less (0.7%), the difference is not significant clinically, and in any case refractometry would be unacceptable for routine testing in most laboratories. Moreover Payne et al. (*5*) have shown that in patients with hypergammaglobulinemia the correlation coefficient for the relation between serum total calcium concentrations and serum total protein concentration (r = 0.682) is significantly less than that for the relation between serum total calcium concentration and serum albumin concentration (r = 0.867). Husdan et al. themselves emphasized that the formulas of Parfitt and Dent are not applicable to patients with abnormal concentrations or compositions of globulins, but such patients not uncommonly present diagnostic problems of calcium metabolism. One would have expected this better correlation of calcium with albumin than with total protein on theoretical grounds, because at least 80% (*6*) and perhaps more than 90% (*7*) of bound calcium is bound to albumin. Thus we consider that the serum albumin concentration is more appropriate than the serum total protein concentration as the basis of adjustment of serum total calcium concentration.

In summary, we agree with the authors that some adjustment for serum protein concentration is necessary "to enhance the sensitivity of serum calcium measurements in the diagnosis of disease," but consider that this adjustment should use the *individual's* binding factor to correct for an abnormal serum *albumin* concentration and be compared with an *appropriately determined* reference range.

References

1. Husdan, H., Rapoport, A., Locke, S., and Oreopoulos, D., Effect of venous occlusion of the arm on the concentration of calcium in serum, and methods for its compensation. *Clin. Chem.* **20,** 529 (1974).
2. Parfitt, A. M., Chlorothiazide-induced hypercalcemia in juvenile osteoporosis and hyperparathyroidism. *New Engl. J. Med.* **281,** 55 (1969).
3. Dent, C. E., Some problems of hyperparathyroidism. *Br. Med. J.* **ii,** 1419 (1962).
4. Pain, R. W., Rowland, K. M., Phillips, P. J., and Duncan, B. McL., Current "corrected" calcium concept challenged. *Br. Med. J.* (accepted for publication).
5. Payne, R. B., Little, A. J., Williams, R. B., and Milner, J. R., Interpretation of serum calcium in patients with abnormal serum proteins. *Br. Med. J.* **iv,** 643 (1973).
6. Moore, E. W., Ionized calcium in normal serum, ultrafiltrates, and whole blood determined by ion-exchange electrodes. *J. Clin. Invest.* **49,** 318 (1970).
7. Pedersen, K. O., Protein-bound calcium in human serum. Quantitative examination of binding and its variables by a molecular binding model and clinical chemical implications for measurement of ionized calcium. *Scand. J. Clin. Lab. Invest.* **30,** 321 (1972).

R. W. Pain
P. J. Phillips

Division of Clinical Chemistry
Institute of Medical and Veterinary Science
Frome Road
Adelaide, South Australia 5000

The authors of the paper in question respond:

To the Editor:

We are aware that both the Dent and Parfitt methods of adjusting serum Ca for protein (*1, 2*) have inherent limitations such as result from the use of a mean correlation value rather than the subject's own binding factor. We would therefore agree in principle with the first two criticisms of our paper.

In recent reports dealing with the protein correction of serum Ca values, there has been a tendency to use an albumin factor rather than the total protein factor. A linear relationship is known to exist between total serum Ca and serum albumin and between total serum Ca and serum total protein (*2*). Moore (*3*) claims that 81% of the protein-bound Ca is bound to albumin and the remaining 19% to globulins. In such a case an albumin correction alone would not be expected to completely compensate the Ca changes caused by simultaneous changes in both serum albumin and globulins.

We used a 3-min period of venous occlusion of the arm to show that significant changes occur in the time that would normally be required to take a sample of blood. Had we prolonged this period our changes would, like those mentioned by Pain and Phillips, have been appreciably greater. Their method of obtaining the subject's binding factor, involving a 15-min venous occlusion of the arm and the collection and analysis of four blood samples, seems somewhat impractical, particularly where large numbers of specimens are to be analyzed and automated equipment such as the SMA 12/60 is not available. The methods of compensation described in our paper, however, have simplicity and convenience. Furthermore, prolonged venous occlusion of the arm, especially if the hand is pumped—e. g., for 15 minutes—could lead in some cases to the accumulation of lactic acid and a decrease in pH, with the consequent artificially decreased protein-bound Ca fraction and an increase in ionized Ca.

Our precisions of the values for total serum protein and total serum Ca have previously been reported (*1, 2*). The precisions for albumin and total protein as measured on the AutoAnalyzer appear equally satisfactory, whereas the precision of albumin measurements involving electrophoretic separation and total protein measurement is less than that of the total protein measurement alone. Pain and Phillips have incorrectly quoted our statement (*2*) that "Total proteins are much more reproducibly measured clinically (by the T.S. Refractometer) than is albumin (by photometry *and* electrophoresis) . . ." (italics added).

Both the binding capacity of albumin and globulins as well as the absolute amounts of these protein fractions could vary in disease. A paper to be published by Pain et al. (*4*) in fact points out that the individual's correction factor may also be influenced by pH, drugs, etc. Because patients are frequently receiving drugs and there are large numbers of different drugs, this possibility could be a serious shortcoming in their technique. That is, the binding factor determination might frequently be required when a serum Ca value is requested on patients. In a series of 284 patients for whom 614 simultaneous values for plasma ionic Ca and Parfitt-corrected total serum Ca were obtained on the same specimens, there was agreement in 75% of the specimens. This signifies that normal, low, and high values for ionic Ca were obtained in specimens giving respective normal, low, and high values for corrected total serum Ca. Of the remaining 25%, 12% had normal values for corrected total Ca and high values for ionic Ca; some were hyperparathyroid patients, others were in acidosis. The remaining 13% lacked agreement for various reasons: disease state, drugs, acid-base disturbances, and possibly the use of a correction incorporating a mean factor. The point is that in the 25% lack of agreement, the "fault" frequently lay with the ionic rather than the corrected Ca. When the *uncorrected* total serum Ca values were compared with the plasma ionic Ca values for the above specimens, the agreement between the two decreased from 75 to 65%. This indicates that our method of correcting serum Ca for protein improves our ability to follow the direction of changes in ionic Ca. It remains to be seen whether the method of Pain and Phillips based on their technique and derived normal total Ca range will, in practice, show a significantly better correlation between ionic and corrected total serum Ca values than does ours.

References

1. Husdan, H., Rapoport, A., and Locke, S., Influence of posture on the serum concentration of calcium. *Metabolism* **22,** 787 (1973).
2. Husdan, H., Rapoport, A., Locke, S., and Oreopoulos, D., Effect of venous occlusion of the arm on the concentration of calcium and methods for its compensation. *Clin. Chem.* **20,** 529 (1974).
3. Moore, E. W., Ionized calcium in normal serum, ultrafiltrates and whole blood determined by ion-exchange electrodes. *J. Clin. Invest.* **49,** 318 (1970).
4. Pain, R. W., Rowland, K. M., Phillips, P. J., and Duncan, B. M., Current "corrected" calcium concept challenged. *Br. Med. J.*, accepted for publication.

Harry Husdan
Abraham Rapoport
Sandra Locke
Dimitrios Oreopoulos

Departments of Medicine and Clinical Biochemistry
University of Toronto and Metabolic-Renal Unit and
Laboratory of the Toronto Western Hospital
Toronto, Ontario, Canada M5T 2S8

Drug Interference with Creatinine Assay

To the Editor:

At least two papers (*1, 2*) report that therapy with trimethoprim/sulfamethoxazole (TMP/SMX) causes an increase in serum creatinine. An in-

Table 1. Concentrations of Trimethoprim, Sulfamethoxazole, and Creatinine in the Plasma Samples

Creatinine	Trimethoprim	Sulfamethoxazole
	mg/liter	
9	0	0
9	5	0
9	0	200
9	5	200
45	0	0
45	5	0
45	0	200
45	5	200

crease with time would indicate impairment of renal function during therapy with the drugs "Septrin" and "Bactrim" and would especially limit their benefit in cases of pre-existing damage. We investigated the possibility of erroneous interpretation of results of creatinine assays caused by the presence of TMP or SMX, or both.

We have two assays for creatinine, the usual Jaffé alkaline picrate reaction adapted for a Technicon AutoAnalyzer and a reaction rate method (*3*) adapted for LKB reaction rate analyzers. We used both to estimate creatinine in 20-ml samples of human plasma to which creatinine, TMP, and SMX were added in the proportions shown in Table 1. All samples were assayed in apparatus in routine use so as to estimate the variation to be expected from laboratories not involved in specific work. Plasma came from a single subject with a nominal creatinine concentration of 9 mg/liter. Extra creatinine was added to produce a fivefold increase representing severe renal failure, and TMP and SMX were added to represent the highest values normally encountered in therapy.

The next two tables, with the data in the same order, show the results for the picrate (Table 2) and the reaction rate (Table 3) methods, respectively. Different requirements of sample size account for the different number of replicates offered for the two methods.

For the picrate method the means of the low creatinine concentrations differ significantly ($P < 0.01$) with the addition of TMP and SMX. Plasma creatinine concentrations near 10 mg/liter are overestimated by about 10% by the method in the presence of SMX and (or) TMP. No similar increase is apparent for creatinine concentrations near 45 mg/liter.

For the reaction rate method, the sample means for plasma creatinine concentrations near 10 mg/liter were not affected by addition of either TMP or SMX. At concentrations near 45 mg/liter, there were some differences, inconsistent and possibly therefore owing to a fault that could arise spontaneously in routine laboratory service.

Table 2. Creatinine Values from the AutoAnalyzer (Alkaline Picrate Method)

Creatinine, mg/liter Mean	SD	n	CV, %
8.43	0.178	20	2.1
8.98	0.089	20	1.0
9.85	0.366	20	3.7
9.29	0.055	20	0.6
45.34	0.278	20	0.6
38.31	0.078	17	0.2
45.65	0.69	20	0.2
45.41	0.313	19	0.7

Table 3. Creatinine Values by the Reaction-Rate Method

Creatinine, mg/liter Mean	SD	n	CV, %
8.98	1.109	6	12.3
8.87	0.513	6	5.8
9.57	1.015	6	10.6
10.20	1.539	6	15.1
45.93	5.720	6	12.5
33.35	5.404	6	16.2
42.87	5.461	6	12.7
50.92	2.293	6	4.5

We conclude that the widely used Technicon method for measuring plasma creatinine could result in overestimations of about 10% in the range of normal values as a result of the presence of TMP and SMX. An overestimate of this size is insignificant, however, in the range of abnormally high values seen in renal failure.

References

1. Horn, B., and Cottier, P., Kreatininkonzentration im Serum vor und unter Behandlung mit Trimethoprim-Sulfamethoxazole (Bactrim). *Schweiz. Med. Wochenschr.* **104,** 1809 (1974).

2. Kalowski, S., Nanra, R. S., Matthew, T. H., and Kincaid-Smith, P., Deterioration in renal function in association with co-trimoxazole therapy. *Lancet* **ii,** 394 (1973).

3. Larsen, K., Creatinine assay by a reaction-kinetic principle. *Clin. Chim. Acta* **41,** 209 (1972).

Alan Bye

Wellcome Research Laboratories
Beckenham, Kent, U.K.

Defect in the Methodology of Aspartate Aminotransferase Determination with SMAC

To the Editor:

Proper assay of aspartate aminotransferase (EC 2.6.1.1) requires a preincubation of up to 30 min with NADH (*1*), during which α-keto acids in serum are converted to their reduced forms, catalyzed by endogenous lactate dehydrogenase (EC 1.1.1.27). Many manufacturers add lactate dehydrogenase to their premixed reagents to shorten the necessary preincubation time. However, the methodology for the assay of aspartate aminotransferase used in SMAC (Technicon Corp., Tarrytown, N. Y.) allows for only a 2-min preincubation period before analysis.

We checked whether a significant error was introduced because of the theoretical shortcoming of the methodology used in SMAC for the assay of aspartate aminotransferase. To Technicon's MDH/NADH reagent was added 3 U of lactate dehydrogenase (from pig heart) per milliliter. The values obtained with this modified reagent were then compared with values obtained with unmodified reagent on the same control serum. Table 1 shows that for serum with low activity, there was a significant difference ($P = 0.01$) in assay values. The value obtained for aspartate aminotransferase activity with unmodified reagent is 9 U/ml higher than the manufacturer's stated value. The addition of lactate dehydrogenase to the MDH/NADH reagent brings the SMAC results into good agreement with the manufactur-

Table 1. Effect of Added Lactate Dehydrogenase on Assay of Aspartate Aminotransferase

Control serum	Manufacturer's stated value	Value obtained: with unmodified MDH/NADH reagent[a]	Value obtained: with lactate dehydrogenase added to MDH/NADH reagent
		U/ml	
Versatrol (low)	17	26 ± 2.2	18 ± 1
Versatrol (middle)	91	80 ± 4.3	84 ± 4.3
Versatrol (high)	180	177 ± 2.8	176 ± 6.7

[a] Average of seven determinations ± one standard deviation.

er's stated value. It is to be expected that the extraneous oxidation of NADH will cause a proportionately larger error in serum with low aspartate aminotransferase activity when compared to serum samples with high activity. It is strongly recommended that users of SMAC reexamine the validity of their assay values for aspartate aminotransferase, especially the low ones.

Reference

1. Demetriou, J. A., Drewes, P. A., and Gin, J. B., Enzymes. In *Clinical Chemistry: Principles and Technics*, 2nd ed., R. J. Henry, D. C. Cannon, J. W. Winkelman, Eds., Harper and Row, New York, N. Y., 1974, p 877.

N. M. Chang

Automated Lab. Services of Korea
CPO 494, Seoul, Korea

B. Davis
R. Cavaliere

Automated Laboratory Services
15551 Cabrito Rd.
Van Nuys, Calif.

Technicon Corp. was asked to respond, and did so as follows:

To the Editor:

Several workers brought this problem to our attention and asked us to modify our system accordingly. This work was completed this summer and all SMAC systems shipped since September have included Program 7, which eliminates the problem of endogenous pyruvate. In addition, an active retrofit program is underway, which should bring all SMAC's in the field up to the current state of the art by January.

The use of lactate dehydrogenase into the MDH/NADH reagent utilized in the Technicon SMAC assay for the measurement of aspartate aminotransferase(AST) is one of several improvements that have been incorporated into Program 7. In addition, the analytical cartridge has been modified to incorporate 2.8 min of pre-incubation before the first measurement of absorbance at 340 nm. In SMAC, AST activity at 37 °C is monitored in three successive flow cells over a time interval of 3.4 min.

Examination of selected hospital samples showed a nonlinearity of reaction between the flow cells in the absence of added lactate dehydrogenase. This disappeared when the new formulation was used. Levels of pyruvate as high as 1.5 mmol/liter were added to serum with no apparent change in sample activity.

The problem has been recognized and, more importantly, is now solved.

Jack Levine
Manager, Scientific Relations
Technicon Instruments Corp.
Tarrytown, N. Y. 10591

When Is a Reference Method a Reference Method?

To the Editor:

We have been interested to note that, as part of the effort to improve the quality of work done in hospital laboratories, more clinical chemists are at least paying attention to the need for standardization of methods—a concept that has been accepted for a long time by analysts in other branches of chemistry.

We are, however, worried by two facts. The first is that there appears to be a lack of coordination or direction in the work being done in the field of method standardization; the second is that, as a consequence, methods are published and hailed as "reference" methods before they have been properly validated in a number of countries.

The "reference" method for calcium (*1*) has been shown (*2*) to incorporate a number of features that would tend to prevent its use outside the U. S. A. We would suggest that it should have been published as, e.g., a "Proposed Reference Method" (*cf.* the NCCLS procedure for defining standards) and that its final acceptance as a Reference Method, and that of the two "Reference" Methods presented in July at the Toronto Congress, should follow only after a vetting procedure laid down by the World Health Organization or by a body it designates. We note that it was suggested at the 27th World Health Assembly, in a report on standardization of diagnostic materials, that an important function of WHO could be the co-ordination of different standardization efforts, leading to greater international acceptability of the standardization of diagnostic materials, and that a group should formulate plans for international collaborative studies. At the moment it is uncertain who has the authority to assign the title of "Reference Method"; is it the Editors of "Selected Methods," NBS, NCCLS, IUPAC, IFCC, BCR (in Europe), or a national body of clinical chemists?

When clinical chemists come to the stage of standardizing routine methods we hope that they will ask for and pay attention to the advice of their fellow analysts who have long experience of this approach. Such advice would, we are sure, be readily given by the association of Official Analytical Chemists, the Analytical Division of The Chemical Society, and others.

References

1. Cali, J. P., Bowers, G. N., Jr., and Young, D. S., A reference method for the determination of total calcium in serum. *Clin. Chem.* **19,** 1208 (1073).

2. Pickup, J. F., Jackson, M. L., Price, E. M., and Brown, S. S., Assessment of the referee method for determination of total calcium in serum. *Clin. Chem.* **20,** 1324 (1974).

D. W. Neill
J. R. Doggart

Department of Biochemistry
Royal Victoria Hospital
Belfast, Northern Ireland

The above letter was brought to the attention of some appropriate persons. Their collective response follows:

To the Editor:

During recent years a new concept of reference technology has been evolved, and is now accepted, for the advancement of standardisation of methodology and thereby the improvement of accuracy throughout clinical chemistry. We share the concern expressed by Neill and Doggart over a lack of co-ordination of effort on several aspects of work on this front, and the need for thorough international validation of what are commonly referred to as "reference methods" before they are accepted as such.

Confusion has undoubtedly arisen because of the differing usage of certain terms, and will persist unless firm definitions are accepted and adhered to. The following explanations and definitions have been suggested at various times during the recent congresses in Munich (*1*), Geneva, and Toronto; those marked with an asterisk are based on proposals (*2*) of the IFCC Expert Panel on Nomenclature and Principles of Quality Control. We submit them now for critical appraisal prior to their being adopted by the IFCC (in particular, its Reference Materials and Methods Office) together with editors of journals, etc., for international usage.

*Definitive Method:** One which, after exhaustive investigation, is found to have no known source of inaccuracy or ambiguity.

*Reference Method:** A technique that can be accomplished with generally available equipment and that, after exhaustive investigation, has been shown to have acceptable known inaccuracy in comparison with a definitive method.

Special Reference Method: Because it is not yet possible to establish definitive and reference methods for all substances, it is necessary to have special methods for enzymes and most proteins, etc. This is simply a procedure that is specified in suitable detail so as to produce the best and most useful result.

Selected Method: The application of reference technology will allow the selection of certain routine procedures for satisfactory operation. These may be defined as methods designed for routine use and, in competition with others, selected as being satisfactory on grounds of good accuracy, precision, economy of labor and materials, ease of operation, etc. In the absence of a reference method, selection is by the best criteria available.

Reference Method Value and Ascribed Value. If a reference method is used for an analysis, the results would be termed the *reference method value*. However, until reference technology becomes widely available, it is understood that each nation or group may select its own points of reference, either from existing methods or by developing and validating new ones. If two or three of these methods are equally suitable from a scientific standpoint, each might be accepted until an international consensus can be developed. These methods should be identified as to the country or organisation designating and using them. An *ascribed value* is that derived from a set of results obtained by using such a method.

The thinking behind the hierarchical structure implied by the above definitions is that stated by Cali (*3*) and Rodgerson and Tietz (*4*). An important aspect is a firm understanding that a reference method cannot exist without there being a corresponding definitive method for the analyte concerned.

For the methods defined above to be acceptable, they must have had international exposure to, and testing by, the best minds and facilities available—wherever their location may be. International groups, academic, governmental, institutional, and commercial interests, and individual scientists must all have a clear opportunity to contribute to the final international consensus. It is the intention of the International Federation of Clinical Chemistry (IFCC) to submit reference methods for WHO recommendation after they have been approved by a consensus mechanism to be established.

We would stress that international bodies such as the IFCC can only achieve acceptable solutions in areas such as these if all available evidence is provided. The constituent associations should encourage their members to offer the needed evidence and expose it to the criticism of their international peers. Such exposure might well be through the pages of "Selected Methods" (*5*).

Critiques of the above definitions would be welcomed, and should be sent to S. S. Brown (address below).

References

1. Rinsler, M. G., and Mitchell, F. L., Reference materials and methods in clinical chemistry. *Z. Klin. Chem. Klin. Biochem.* **12,** 558 (1974).

2. Büttner, J., Borth, R., Boutwell, J. H., and Broughton, P. M. G., International Federation of Clinical Chemistry. Provisional Recommendation on Quality Control in Clinical Chemistry. Part 1. General Principles and Terminology. *Clin. Chim. Acta* **62,** F25 (1975).

3. Cali, J. P., Worldwide reference methods. *Clin. Chem.* **21,** 1344 (1975). Letter to the Editor.

4. Rodgerson, D. O., and Tietz, N. W., Selection of "Recommended Methods" for use in a clinical laboratory—some urgent considerations and a suggested approach. *Clin. Chem.* **21,** 1057 (1975). Guest editorial.

5. Cooper, G. R., and Young, D. S., Selected methods. *Clin. Chem.* **19,** 1207 (1973). Editorial.

S. S. Brown
Secretary, IFCC Office of Reference Materials and Methods

Division of Clinical Chemistry
Clinical Research Centre
Harrow, Middlesex HA1 3UJ
England

J. Büttner
President, IFCC Committee on Standards and Past Joint Secretary, Office of Reference Materials and Methods

Medizinische Hochschule Hannover
Institut für Klinische Chemie
3 Hannover-Kleefeld
Karl-Wiechert-Allee 9
West Germany

F. L. Mitchell
Past Joint Secretary, IFCC Office of Reference Materials and Methods

Division of Clinical Chemistry
Clinical Research Centre
Harrow, Middlesex HA1 3UJ
England

M. Rubin
President, IFCC

Georgetown University Hospital
3800 Reservoir Rd., N.W.
Washington, D. C. 20007

G. R. Cooper
Editor-in-Chief, Selected Methods of Clinical Chemistry (*AACC*)

Metabolic Biochemistry Branch
Clinical Chemistry Division
Bureau of Laboratories
Department of HEW
Center for Disease Control
Atlanta, Ga. 30333

Digoxin Immunoassay with Use of [^{3}H]Digoxin vs. [^{125}I]Tyrosine-methyl-ester of Digoxin

To the Editor:

This report compares the accuracy, precision, and sensitivity of a radioimmunoassay for digoxin by use of [^{125}I]tyrosine-methyl-ester of digoxin with that in which the standard [^{3}H]digoxin isotope is used. The ^{125}I method involves immune precipitation of bound radioactivity and does not require addition of dextran-coated charcoal to separate bound from free digoxin.

Table 1. Accuracy, Precision, and Sensitivity of Two Assay Techniques

	Accuracy µg/liter	Precision (SD/mean) × 100	Sensitivity µg/liter
^{3}H method	±0.10	5%	0.16
^{125}I method	±0.12	8%	0.20

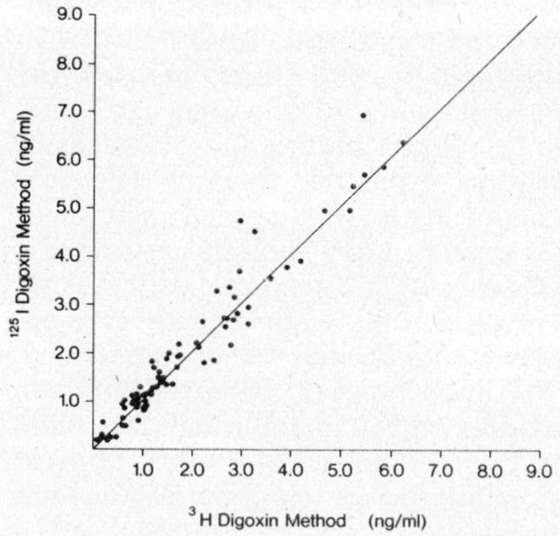

Fig. 1. Plasma digoxin concentrations as determined by the ^{3}H and ^{125}I assay procedures

The diagonal line represents a perfect correlation

The procedure for the tritium-based assay was described previously (*1*). The digoxin antiserum for use in it, purchased from Burroughs Wellcome Co., was stored and reconstituted as recommended. The antiserum (digoxin binding reagent), a double antibody, and the [^{125}I]tyrosine-methylester of digoxin for the ^{125}I assay (Burroughs Wellcome) were stored and reconstituted as suggested. Standards for both assays were prepared from pooled outdated human plasma purchased from the American Red Cross. The standards were stored frozen. The ^{125}I assay was performed as suggested by the supplier.

For the ^{125}I assay, the reciprocals of the cpm of the standards were plotted vs. known concentrations. A linear-regression program was used to provide the best straight line through the data points, and unknowns were then calculated from this plot. For the tritium assay, reciprocal dpm's were plotted instead of reciprocal cpm's.

The results of analysis of plasma from 83 patients who received digoxin showed that comparable values were obtained by the two assay methods (Figure 1). The correlation coefficient was .967, highly significant by the t-test ($P < .001$) (*2*). Thirty-one samples assayed higher by the ^{3}H method, 46 samples assayed lower, and six assayed identically by the two methods.

Table 1 shows the accuracy, precision, and sensitivity of the two methods. The accuracy was determined by assaying seven standards of known concentration in quadruplicate, and was expressed as the mean deviation from the known concentration. Results of the two assays were compared by a paired t analysis. An F test was used to compare the precision of the ^{125}I and ^{3}H assays. The coefficient of variance [(SD/mean) × 100] was calculated for each triplicate analysis of patient's serum. Sensitivity of the ^{3}H and ^{125}I assays was determined from 14 separate assays of pooled digoxin free plasma. An excellent correlation was obtained when patients' samples were assayed for digoxin by the ^{125}I digoxin method and the ^{3}H method. The sensitivity and accuracy were equivalent ($P < 0.8$ and $P < 0.7$, respectively); however, the ^{3}H method was more precise than the ^{125}I method ($P < 0.005$) (*2*).

The ^{125}I digoxin method was the more rapid method because it did not require a second counting after internal standardization. It could be further speeded by incubation at 37 °C for 30 min; results and precision were the same as obtained after 90-min incubation at 25 °C. There were several technical problems with the performance of the ^{125}I assay. Occasionally a patient's sample failed to form a typical pellet; floating material was lost on decanting. Results for such samples were falsely high. In addition, plasma used as the zero standard could not be stored at 4 °C for longer than a few days. The pellet formed did not cling to the tube. Standards prepared from pooled plasma were adequate for both assays for four months when stored frozen.

MacKinney et al. (*3*) analyzed serum digoxin by these two methods, with use of commercial radioimmunoassay kits. They obtained similar assay results with one [^{3}H]digoxin kit but not with another as compared with the ^{125}I method. Therefore, a laboratory that elects to change from a ^{3}H method to the ^{125}I procedure described here should determine for themselves how well the results of the two methods correlate, in order to alert the physicians of a possible change in the assay results.

Supported in part by NIH Grant No. 5-R01-HL-12736-05 and AHA Grant-In-Aid No. 74 1085.

References

1. Marcus, F. I., Ryan, J. N., and Stafford, M. G., The reactivity of derivatives of digoxin and digitoxin as measured by the Na-K-ATPase displacement assay and by radioimmunoassay. *J. Lab. Clin. Med.* **86,** 610 (1975).

2. Bulmer, M. G., *Principles of Statistics.* M.I.T. Press, Cambridge, Mass., 1967.

3. MacKinney, A. A., Burnett, G. H., Conklin, R. L., and Wasson, G. W., Comparison of five radioimmunoassays and enzyme bioassay for measurement of digoxin in blood. *Clin. Chem.* **21,** 857 (1975).

Susan L. Pippin
Frank I. Marcus

Section of Cardiology
Dept. of Internal Medicine
University of Arizona Medical Center
Tucson, Ariz. 85724

book reviews

The Healing Hand. Man and Wound in the Ancient World. Guido Majno, Harvard University Press, Cambridge, Mass., 1975, xxvi + 571 pp, profusely illustrated and annotated; index. $25.

Dr. Majno is a pathologist (Harvard, Université de Genève, and now departmental chairman at the medical school of the University of Massachusetts). As the jacket blurb says, he writes with "a scientist's mind and a detective's eye." Anyone with more than the most trivial interest in the origins of medicine and its allied arts is bound to enjoy this book, which not only is the distillate of the author's painstaking efforts but incorporates those of a large number of other talented people who helped and advised him. The resulting scholarly but vibrant account can be apprehended by any literate person.

As the subtitle suggests, the theme of the book is how the various ancient civilizations dealt with wounds (and inflammation), but the author takes us on intriguing side excursions—intriguing because he is a writer who can make them so. These include (e.g.) weapons, acupuncture, the origins of written language, of pharmacology, and of the scientific approach to treatment.

Beginning with pre-history—the fossil evidence—and then proceeding to scan nine ancient civilizations (not, however, including the MesoAmerican) in as many chapters, the book ends with Galen, after whom "the history of the wound grinds to a halt for at least one thousand years."

With such help, one can begin to appreciate the conceptions and misconceptions under which the art of medicine struggled to become a science, a struggle that still is in progress, but with victory finally in sight (someone has said that only in the last thirty years or so have the chances of a patient actually benefitting from his encounter with the physician been better than fifty-fifty). The author has taken the trouble to test experimentally some of the ancient recommendations.

Misobservations and the weight of mistaken authority often led various aspects of treatment up blind alleys for centuries. It was not unusual for key writings, and even entire libraries, to be lost—the cumulative record of (literally) painful progress—and the recorded experience had to be re-experienced and re-recorded. Superstition and religious beliefs encumbered progress on what seems a Sisyphean journey over the centuries and around the globe to the benefits that we take for granted today as a "right."

The Harvard Press is to be complimented on the esthetics of the book. From binding to typography and layout and proofing, it reflects taste and care and skill.

I urge you to run, not walk, to the nearest bookstore and take a look for yourself. This is a fine scientific account of one aspect of man's ancient history.

J. S. King
Executive Editor, AACC

1829 Meadowbrook Drive
Winston-Salem, N. C. 27104

Intrahepatic Cholestasis. P. Gentilini, U. Teodori, S. Gorini, and H. Popper, Eds. Raven Press, New York, N. Y. 10036, 1975, xi + 187 pp. $15.95.

The book is a summary of an international symposium held in Florence, Italy. Intrahepatic cholestasis, which can be likened to an experiment in nature, has provided excellent material for many approaches of study, which are exemplified in the diversity of material reported. The first four chapters deal with the problem of cholestasis, morphologic aspects, the organelle pathology of cholestasis and the clinical and functional aspects associated with intrahepatic cholestasis. A chapter on neonatal cholestasis points out the difficulty of establishing the etiologic diagnosis in such cases. A useful summary for clinician and clinical chemists is presented that lists appropriate tests to help in the differential diagnoses. The problems that may arise if liver transplantation develops into an effective means of therapy are discussed. An interesting concept that supports the view that primary biliary cirrhosis and active chronic hepatitis can be unified under the term "immune hepatitis" is presented by E. Pisi et al. The chapters by J. Caroli on a new form of cholestatic hepatitis in adults with massive hyperlipidemia, and by D. Seidel and R. Fellin on "behavior of serum lipoproteins in cholestasis" are of interest to the clinical chemist and clinician. Nanetti et al. briefly summarize 50 previously reported cases and describe six additional cases of recurrent intrahepatic cholestasis. The relatively benign nature of the disease and the strong familial clustering are important characteristics that will merit further investigations of this unusual problem. G. Sotgiu and G. Cavalli, in the chapter on morphologic aspects and pathogenetic and therapeutic considerations in intrahepatic cholestasis, broaden the perspective to include some additional morphologic studies and also consideration of possible therapy. The final chapter by H. Remmer, on experimental intrahepatic cholestasis, presents evidence that the cause of increased amounts of bile salts in the liver in experimental models is not understood. The importance of the mixed-function oxidase of the endoplasmic reticulum in the metabolism of drugs that occasionally induce cholestasis was emphasized.

The book presents a general view of the complexity of the problems and the still incomplete understanding of intrahepatic cholestasis. As a source for information of the current status of the problems in intrahepatic cholestasis, clinicians and clinical chemists should find the book useful.

Lena A. Lewis
Cleveland Clinic Foundation
Cleveland, Ohio

Pharmokinetics. M. Gibaldi and D. Perrier. Marcel Dekker, Inc., New York, N. Y. 10016, 1975, xi + 329 pp. $19.50.

Biopharmaceutics and Pharmacokinetics. An Introduction. 2nd ed. R. E. Notari with the assistance of J. L. De Young and R. C. Anderson. Marcel Dekker, Inc., New York, N. Y. 10016, 1975, x + 285 pp. $13.75.

Both books deal with the same general subject and both originate from the same publisher. However, the authors have dealt in rather different ways with their topic.

Gibaldi and Perrier's book is the first volume of a series on Drugs and Pharmaceutical Sciences designed for the pharmacist and others in the health sciences field. Major sections cover the one-compartment model, multicompartment models, multiple dosing, bioavailability, apparent volumes of distribution, kinetics of reversible pharmacologic effects, nonlinear pharmacokinetics, route of administration and drug disposition, and renal impairment. A number of appendices provide details of mathematical methods and a glossary. There are many illustrations. The index is well done.

This book strongly emphasizes formal mathematical analysis and derivation of pharmacokinetic equations. It is unlikely that the clinical chemist benefits from such an approach and the authors' claim that this text is suitable for self-study appears debatable. On the other hand, the chapter on renal impairment is particularly worthwhile.

The major sections of Notari's book cover bioavailability, rate processes in biological systems, principles of pharmacokinetics, biopharmaceutics, and clinical applications of pharmacokinetic parameters, and pharmacokinetic aspects of structural modifications in drug design and therapy. This book evolved from course material presented to pharmacy students. It is a work book, and casual reading will not suffice. The book is meant mainly to provide an introduction into the mathematical underpinnings of pharmacokinetics. Each principle is illustrated by sample problems suitable for self-study, to which the solutions are provided. There are many clarifying figures and tables. This extensively revised edition also contains an expanded and updated bibliography, and the typesetting is a welcome improvement over its predecessor.

Notari's text is highly recommended for pharmacologists. For clinical chemists wishing to have a broader understanding of pharmacokinetics as applied to the monitoring of drug therapy, this book can provide an introduction to a field of science often confusing to the uninitiated. The practical application of pharmacokinetics is the scientific prescription of initial drug regimens and those adjustments that are necessary for the individual patient. While an understanding of pharmacokinetics is not required to develop and apply drug assays in the laboratory, it is a necessity for meaningful consultation at the bedside. The second major area covered in Notari's book, biopharmaceutics, relates to drug trials and is rarely relevant to routine therapy.

Neither text gives the reader a full appreciation of the pharmacokinetics of any individual agent. Gibaldi and Perrier present selected pharmacokinetic data for important drugs such as warfarin, salicylates and propranolol, while Notari emphasizes only certain antibiotics.

Fred P. Abramson
Earl W. Sutherland, III
Mario Werner

The George Washington University Medical Center
Washington, D. C. 20037

Books Received

Drug Interactions, 3rd ed. P. D. Hansten. Lea & Febiger, Philadelphia, Pa. 19106. ix + 405 pp. Paperback. $11.50. Pub. Nov. 1975. The 2nd edition of this book was reviewed in *Clin. Chem.* **19,** 1231 (1973).

Contributions to Nephrology, I, Proteinuria. Series Eds. G. M. Berlyne, & S. Giovannetti; Vol. Eds. G. M. Eisenback, J. Brod, H. Stolte. Karger, Basel, 1975, 166 pp, 80 figures, 18 tables. Plastic-bound. Proceedings of the 2nd Symposium of Nephrology, June 1974, Hannover. $25.00. Papers of interest to clinical chemists include those on glomerular permeability, renal handling of peptides and small proteins, fibrinuria, IgG in urine, clinical value of protein clearance determinations.

What People Eat. An Introduction to Chemistry and Food Sciences. I. Raw, A. Bromley, E. R. Pariser, and J. Vournakis, Eds. William Kaufmann, Inc., Los Altos, Calif. 94022. 328 pp. Paperback. $9.00. Pub. 1975.

Ed. note: Scholars have long wondered if some of *The Canterbury Tales* are not simply undiscovered, rather than unwritten, and indeed such Chaucerian fabliaux come to light now and again. Careful study invariably has revealed them to be mere simulations, but hope springs eternal. The following, in manuscript, came to us recently from the Islets of Langerhans, where it is said to have been found. I present it here for scholarly examination.—**J.S.K.**

The Chemyst's Tale

A Clynycal Chemyst ther was, yclad alle in whyte,
Who diligentte dide worke both daye and nyght.
Contended he with routine and with stat,
And parfait dide he knowe of this and thatte.
Eche subtyle ferment measured he exact
And set the figures downe as solemn fact.
Fluids bubbl'd through the coyles right myrielie,
Boyled in his cauldrons to exact degree.
Balances hadde he that koude weygh precyse,
Counters, and eek other strange devyce.
For him computers wylling did magicks—
With alle wost he of Elektronicks.
Learnèd, he had passed Alchemie's gate—
None better koude makke ethyl formicate.
Alembic and cucurbit he koude wield
(But whan he gotte machines, these he conceeled.)

Lyke in whyte array, swete Maydens dide hym serve,
Possess'd of wondrous traits, y will observe;
Eek buxom was, well rounded in ye hamme,
Ful long of heer, and shapelie in ye gambe,
Cheeks rody, round thè eyes al lyvely hewed;
Eche morn, eche her beautie Avon-newed,
Skins as whit as is the lylye flour.
But naught of daliaunce or paramour;
He *onlie thot of them as beings bryght,*
Adept with leech, and dial, and blynkyng lyght.

One such came up to hym one busie daye,
And seyde semely, Look you, Master, praye;
Ther canne be naught e'er seen the match of this,
So calcick is the serum and the pisse.
Quod Chemyst, By my trouthe, this manne is sick;
Anon speke this to one learn'd in Physick.
But ere we doo so, praye the tests repeate
And enter trewly alle upon the shete.
Take measure of the ferment phosphatase
Yf yts activitie doth go apace,
And assay PTH by RIA,
And telle me anon what these tests doo saye.
(For this the paycioun yette ageyn was bledde;
Ten silver pieces did yt cost; nyne went to Overhedde.)

The Chirurgeon, none was so wyse as he,
Vers'd well in Physick and in Chirurgie;
Attir'd in skullcap, mask, and surplys green,
A bolder figure never man hath seen.
Nature nor art could better or amend
In any wise, as people did contend.
Eke day belyke he digged amongst entrailles
And cast the parts he cutte out into pailles.
He knew also of drugges as well as any can—
For sothe, he learnt it from the Detail Manne.
He cutte for stone with grate dexteritie;
For encore, sometime prostatectomie.

This paycioun he hadde cutte the daye before
And calx stones tuk out from amidst the gore,
Then Historie indited ful exact;
Insurance shetes all filled with grisly fact.
So ful were these of hieroglyph and scrawl,
Alas, was noon koude makke them out at al!
The paycioun from his hed he then dismyst
Until ther came this shete from the Chemyst.
The Chirurgeon, ensconc'd in 'carmin'd coat,
Resolved thereon to cutte this paycioun's throat.
(He doubted not he woud bee payde—
Hail Blue Cross, Medycare, and Medycaide!)

The mediastinum now was ful explor'd
(Excursion round the throat with gun and sword).
Two adenomas bigge as currants fetched to viewe,
Enfolded snug in thyroyd glande tissue.
The paycioun then no longer did repine,
His strength return'd, and he tuk mete and wine.
At last a cler and blyssful slep he got—
More tyme in bedde, and less astride his chambre pot.
Soon woude he able bee to work his fille;
In tyme, enow he'd earn to paye the bill.

When Chemyst met Chirurgeon on the morn
He ne hadde for his labour but a scorn.
He dide, withal with gentil courtesy,
Make him good cheer, enquiring earnestly,
For news of how he fared, to learn by word,
Whatever of the paycioun koude bee heard.
Said Chemyst, May I venture to suppose
Our data changed how one would diagnose?
Quod Chirurgeon, Back to your machines.
What knowes one who has never paycioun seen?
What wenest one of paycicuns must be rude
Who Urine casts and messes with the Blude.
Aye, some the like I felt *betymes was wrong;*
Nay, by my fay, I knew *hyt alle along!*

Thus endes the tale thatte y woude say to thee,
And may God save al this fair companie! Amen.

the clinical chemist

Compiled by J. S. King, Executive Editor

Amazing Grace

Notice to subscribers who have not renewed their subscriptions: In the past, journal delivery has continued ("graced") through March or April, whether or not a renewal was received. This year, both economics and postal regulations preclude such generosity. Thus if you have not renewed your subscription this is the last issue you will receive. Renewals should be addressed to the business (Washington, D. C.) office, *not* the editorial (Winston-Salem) office.

Awards

Ernest S. Cotlove Award, Capital Section, AACC. This award ($50) will be made at the March meeting, and is for the best paper contributed at that 2nd Annual Contributed-papers Meeting. (No restriction to AACC members is mentioned.)

1976 Bernard F. Gerulat Memorial Award, New Jersey Section, AACC. This award goes to Dr. Martin Rubin (Georgetown University, Washington, D. C.) on March 20. Presented annually to that individual who best furthers progress toward the collective charter goals of the Association. For more on Dr. Rubin's achievements, see *Clin. Chem.* **18,** 859 (1972).

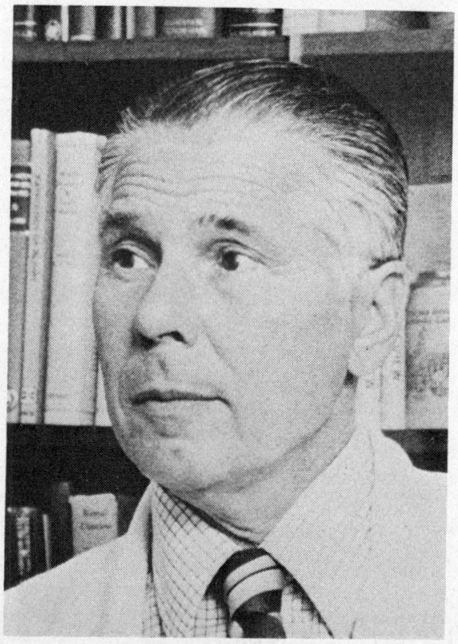

Dr. Martin Rubin

Meetings

Symposium on Evaluation of Clinical Laboratory Automation in the Americas, March 3–5, 1976, Mexico City. IFCC sponsored. (Write: SECLA Coordination Center, Suite 215, 1025 Connecticut Ave., N.W., Washington, D. C. 20036).

Pittsburgh Conference (in Cleveland, Ohio), Mar. 1–5, 1976. Information from: A. J. Kavoulakis, ALKAV Laboratories, Inc., 3000 Grand Blvd., Neville Island, Pittsburgh, Pa. 15225. (412/771-2626).

19th Annual Postgraduate Course in Medical Technology, Kamloops, B. C., Canada, May 17–21, 1976. Write: Glenn M. Martin, M.D., Royal Inland Hospital, Kamloops, B. C.

Seminar on Thyroid Function, Capital Section, AACC, May 8, 1976. Write: Dr. D. E. Uddin, Naval Medical Research Institute, Bethesda, Md. 20014.

Medical Writing

Physician Michael Crichton, better known as author of (e.g.) *Terminal Man,* writes in *The New England Journal of Medicine* (Dec. 11, 1975) on "Medical Obfuscation: Structure and Function," illustrating with examples from three issues of that journal [This same issue contains a review of particular interest to clinical chemists on measurement and interpretation of urinary electrolytes.]

Continuing Education

The AACC national Committee on Education now has available a four-tape audiovisual series on the "Clinical Biochemistry of the Neonate" for loan to local sections or to individual members. These tapes were prepared by Ross Laboratories, who generously allowed the AACC the use of them. The Symposium was sponsored by the Capital Section and was held in Washington, D. C., December 1974. Participants in that conference were taped in several formats, including lecture, panel discussion, and question and answer sessions. The titles and viewing times are listed below.

Loan copies are available from the Executive Director, American Association for Clinical Chemistry, 1725 K Street, N.W., Washington, D. C. 20006. Two formats are available: ½″

Reel	Program time, min	Subject
1–50 min	1–18	History and Folklore of the Placenta and Reproductive Models, P. K. Besch, Ph.D., E. C. Knoblock, Ph.D.
	2–10	Effect of Maternal Nutrition on Fetal Development, P. Rosso, M.D.
	3–13	Enzyme Differentiation in the Neonate, F. Moog, Ph.D.
	4–9	Influence of Maternal Drug Therapy on the Child and Effects of Maternal Addiction on the Neonate, R. M. Hill, M.D., C. Zelson, M.D.
2–55 min	5–14	Protein Metabolism in the Newborn, R. Gutberlet, M.D.
	6–9	Metabolic Problems Associated with the Newborn and High Risk Infant, D. O'Brien, M.D.
	7–19	Failure to Thrive and Problems of Growth in the Neonate, A. Root, M.D.
	8–8	Carbohydrate Metabolism in the Neonate. J. Nicholson, M.D.
	9–5	The Clinical Laboratory and the Newborn Serice, G. Avery, M.D., J. M. Hicks, Ph.D.
3–29 min	10–9	Mucopolysaccharidoses, I. Shafer, M.D.
	11–14	Medical Problems of the Newborn, T. Blumenfeld, M.D.
	12–6	The Pediatric Clinical Laboratory, D. S. Young, M.D., J. M. Hicks, Ph.D.
4–54 min	13–13	Pathogenesis of Neonatal Hyperbilirubinemia, G. Odell, M.D.
	14–9	Hyaline Membrane Disease, M. Renfield, M.D.
	15–32	Immunologic Responses of the Neonate, J. Bellanti, M.D.

reel-to-reel and SONY cassette. To obtain any tape, send a letter to the Executive Director requesting the tape number and specifying the type of equipment available. Also indicate the date you wish to have the tape and an alternate date. The tapes will be sent for a *two-week* period. Prompt return is requested to ensure availability to other interested persons. There is no charge.

Useful Literature

"Physical Properties of Some Organic Solvents" is the title of *Eastman Organic Chemical Bulletin* **47**, no. 1, 1975 (received Dec. 20, 1975). Eight properties of each of 911 solvents are listed.

Unionization

"The American Society for Medical Technology is not a union, has not been a union, and has no plans to become a union," says Executive Director Stephen B. Friedheim in *ASMT News*, in response to inquiries from members. Confusion arose, probably, from ASMT's taking the lead in efforts to form and support the National Economic Council [see *Clin. Chem.* **18**, 733 (1972)], from which it is entirely separate. Their legal counsel explains ASMT's position in a letter that accompanies the report.

Forthcoming Papers

Improved Method for Measuring Fibrinogen in Plasma, with Use of a Plasmin Inhibitor
Loren W. Steffen and Barbara W. Steffen

Comparison of Results for 13 Clinical Laboratory Determinations with Three Automated Analytical Systems
Eric J. Sampson, Dennis D. Derck, and Laurence M. Demers

Statistical Characterization of the Random Errors in the Radioimmunoassay Dose–Response Variable
David Rodbard, Robert H. Lennox, H. Linton Wray, and Douglas Ramseth

Gas-Chromatographic Analysis of Ethosuximide and Other Succinimide Anticonvulsants in Serum: Macro- and Micro-Scale Methods
James Bonitati

Changes in Electrophoretic Mobilities of α and β-Lipoproteins as a Result of Plasma Delipidation
Bill E. Cham and Brian R. Knowles

Determination of Apolipoprotein A and Its Constitutive A-I and A-II Polypeptides by Separate Electroimmunoassay
Michael D. Curry, Petar Alaupovic, and C. Alan Suenram

Use of Polyethylene Glycol in Separating Bound from Unbound Ligand in Radioimmunoassay of Thyroxine
Marian C. Cheung and W. Roy Slaunwhite, Jr.

Simultaneous Quantitation of 4-Hydroxy-3-Methoxymandelic (Vanilmandelic) and 4-Hydroxy-3-Methoxyphenylacetic (Homovanillic) Acids in Human Urine
Somasundaram Addanki, Elmer R. Hinnenkamp, and Juan F. Sotos

Use of Enzyme-loaded Erythrocytes in In Vitro Correction of Arginase-Deficient Erythrocytes in Familial Hyperargininemia
Karel Adriaenssens, Denis Karcher, Armand Lowenthal, and Heinz G. Terheggen

Evaluation of Methods of Coenzyme Activation of Erythrocyte Enzymes for Detection of Deficiency of Vitamins B_1, B_2, and B_6
Riad A. Bayoumi and Sidney B. Rosalki

Use of Polyethylene Glycol in Separating Bound from Unbound Ligand in Radioimmunoassay of Thyroxine

Marian C. Cheung[1] and W. Roy Slaunwhite, Jr.[2]

In most rapid radioimmunoassay methods, absorbents are used that disturb the equilibrium of the ligand–antibody interaction; thus the separation process must be rigidly timed. We show here that polyethylene glycol (mol wt, 6000) abolishes this constraint. We measured γ-globulin precipitation by polyethylene glycol (150 g/liter) in a thyroxine radioimmunoassay system involving use of a sheep anti-thyroxine antiserum, quantitatively and qualitatively, with either normal human serum or bovine γ-globulin as carrier protein. γ-Globulin was completely precipitated at pH 6–9 at 4 and 25 °C, but incompletely if salt concentration was high (1 mol/liter). Specificity of γ-globulin precipitation increased with increasing pH and temperature. All γ-globulin-bound thyroxine was precipitated, and also some not bound to γ-globulin. This was taken into account by including "blank" tubes (no antibody, but with normal sheep serum) in all assays. Because this reaction is predominantly entropic and temperature independent, the entire procedure can be done at 37 °C and room temperature without rigid timing. The assay requires 10 μl of serum, its reproducibility is 4–8% (CV) in the euthyroid and hyperthyroid range, and its accuracy is close to 100%.

Additional Keyphrases: *euthyroid values* • *"kit" methods* • *triiodothyronine*

Various techniques, which have been recently reviewed (*1*), have been used to separate bound and free antigen in radioimmunoassay (RIA).[3] Double-antibody precipitation, adsorption on coated charcoal, and fractional precipitation of bound antigen by organic solvent or salt solution are the more popular ones.

Double-antibody precipitation of bound antigen is time consuming and expensive, requiring days, not hours, to ensure completion of precipitation, a requirement that minimizes the effects of interfering factors in the serum (*2*). Consequently, it is not suitable for use in routine clinical diagnostic RIA systems.

The coated-charcoal adsorption method overcomes these two disadvantages of the double-antibody technique, and it has been used in the RIA of insulin (*3*) and thyroid hormones (*4–7*), and in 66% of steroid hormone assays (*8*). When it is used to separate bound and free antigen, it may disturb the equilibrium and absorb not only the free ligand but also some that had been in the bound state:

$$\begin{array}{c} \text{Antibody} + \text{antigen} \rightleftharpoons \text{antibody-antigen complex} \\ + \\ \text{charcoal} \\ \updownarrow \\ \text{antigen–charcoal complex} \end{array}$$

In minimizing such a likelihood, incubation time and temperature after the charcoal is added to the assay mixture become critical (*9*). The time-dependent nature of this separation technique indirectly influences the number of tubes that can be handled per unit time, and hence the cost of the assay.

For more assay tubes to be handled in a given time, one must resort to a time-independent separation technique: precipitation of the bound fraction with either an organic solvent or a salt solution. Precipitation with ammonium sulfate is used in about 20% of RIA's of steroids (*8*), but it lacks the specificity that is sometimes needed. Polson et al. (*10*) and Iverius and Laurent (*11*) in their investigation of the protein-fractionation properties of polyethylene glycol (PEG) of molecular weight 6000 ("Carbowax 6000") indicated that PEG caused a more nearly quantitative precipitation of γ-globulin than did ammonium sulfate. This precipitation method was used by Desbuquois and Aurbach (*12*) to separate free and bound peptide hormones in RIA's.

Departments of Biochemistry and Pediatrics, Schools of Medicine and Dentistry, SUNY/Buffalo, Buffalo, N. Y. 14214.

[1] Taken from a dissertation submitted by M.C.C. to the State University of New York at Buffalo Graduate School in partial fulfillment of the requirements for the degree of Doctor of Philosophy. Present address: Northwest Lipid Research Clinic, University of Washington, Department of Medicine, 325 9th Ave., Seattle, Wash. 98104.

[2] Address reprint requests to Dr. W. Roy Slaunwhite, Jr., Dept. Biochemistry, SUNY/Buffalo, P.O. Box U, Station B, Buffalo, N. Y. 14207.

[3] Nonstandard abbreviations used: RIA, radioimmunoassay; PEG, polyethylene glycol; T3, triiodothyronine; T4, thyroxine.

Received Oct. 27, 1975; accepted Dec. 7, 1975.

We have reported earlier (*13*) a rapid RIA of triiodothyronine (T3) in which PEG was used in the separation. We wish to report here a further study of the use of PEG in the separation of free and antibody-bound ligand, an RIA for thyroxine (T4) being used as a model.

Materials and Methods

Materials

Sources of materials were as follows: 3,5,3′,5′-tetraiodo-L-thyronine, free acid (thyroxine, T4; Sigma Chemical Co., St. Louis, Mo. 63178); albumin, human fraction V powder (Nutritional Biochemicals Corp., Cleveland, Ohio 44128); γ-globulin, bovine, Cohn fraction II (ICN Biochemicals, Irvine, Calif. 92664); normal human serum (pooled, out-dated serum from hospitals); ^{125}I-labeled thyroxine (research service preparation, Tetramet-125; Abbott Laboratories, North Chicago, Ill. 60064); 1-cyclohexyl-3-(2-morpholinoethyl)-carbodiimide metho-*p*-toluenesulfonate (Morpho CDI; Aldrich Chemical Co., Milwaukee, Wis. 53233); *N,N*,-dimethylformamide, polyethylene glycol (PEG, Carbowax 6000), decolorizing alkaline carbon (Norit A), sodium salicylate (Fisher Scientific Co., Fair Lawn, N. J. 07410); tris(hydroxymethyl)aminomethane (Sigma); Freund's complete adjuvant (Difco Laboratories, Detroit, Mich. 48204); 8-anilino-1-naphthalene sulfonic acid, sodium salt (K & K Laboratories, Plainview, N. J. 11803); 2,4-dinitrophenol, acrylamide, *N,N*-methylenebisacrylamide, *N,N,N′,N′*-tetramethylethylenediamine, bromphenol blue, trichloroacetic acid (Eastman Organic Chemicals, Rochester, N. Y. 14650); ammonium persulfate (J. T. Baker Chemical Co., Phillipsburg, N. J. 08865); Amido Schwarz (Buffalo Black, Naphthol Blue Black) (Allied Chemical Corp., Morristown, N. J. 079601).

Methods

Buffers: Phosphate buffer, 0.05 mol/liter of sodium phosphates, pH 7.5; barbital buffer, 0.05 mol/liter of sodium barbital, pH 8.6.

Production of antibody: Anti-T4 antibody was produced by intradermally injecting conjugate (with human serum albumin; molar ratio 7:1) prepared by the method of Gharib et al. (*14*) into the back of a young ovariectomized Dorset ewe at multiple sites. Antisera were obtained from a jugular vein 5–10 days after a booster injection was given. The dilution that yielded 50% bound in the absence of unlabeled T4 was recorded as the titer of the antibody. The T4 antiserum used in this report had a titer of 3000.

Binding of unlabeled and labeled T4 to the T4-antiserum: In RIA, it is assumed that labeled and unlabeled ligand bind similarly to the antibody. To check this assumption, two sets of assays were performed in parallel. In one assay, 100 μl (about 10 000 cpm) of ^{125}I-labeled T4 of high specific activity (>1000 Ci/g) in phosphate buffer was added to 12 × 75 mm tubes, followed by 100 μl of unlabeled T4 standard solutions in the same buffer. In the other assay, 100 μl (0.32 ng) to 700 μl (2.24 ng) of labeled T4 of relatively low specific activity (about 50 Ci/g) in phosphate buffer was added to each tube. Sheep anti-T4 antiserum, 50 μl, diluted in the same buffer to give about 50% bound in the presence of the smallest amount of the labeled T4 was added to each tube. The total volume of each tube was adjusted to 1 ml with the same buffer. Precounting, incubation, and separation of bound and free T4 were done as described under *Recommended T4-RIA procedure.*

Equilibrium studies: Because in RIA it is also assumed that equilibrium is reached between antigen and antibody binding, the time to reach equilibrium at various temperatures must be established. In these assays, the content of each tube was the same: 350 μl of phosphate buffer, 100 μl of labeled T4 (about 10 000 cpm, 0.1–0.2 ng) in the same buffer, and 50 μl of diluted antiserum. The separation and counting procedures followed the T4-RIA procedure.

Preparation of T4-free serum: Norit decolorizing charcoal, 15 g, was added to 100 ml of pooled human serum. The mixture was stirred for 12 h at 4 °C (*7*). The charcoal was then removed by centrifuging the serum four times at 25 000 × *g* for 1 h each time. Any traces of charcoal still present were removed by filtration.

Preparation of quality control: The T4 samples for quality control were prepared by dissolving 1 mg of T4 (free acid) in ethanolic ammonium hydroxide solution, pH 11.5, and then serially diluting with ethanol to concentrations of 5, 10, and 20 ng/ml. Twenty 100-μl aliquots of each of these T4 solutions were pipetted into 12 × 75 mm disposable glass tubes, and the solvent was evaporated under nitrogen in a water-bath at 37 °C ("N-Evap" analytical evaporator). These tubes were then capped and stored at −20 °C until used.

Preparation of standard solutions: Standard solutions were prepared by dissolving 1 mg of T4 (free acid) in sodium hydroxide (0.1 mol/liter). This was serially diluted with T4-free serum diluted 10-fold with sodium barbital buffer, so that 0.1, 0.2, 0.3, 0.5, 0.8, 1, 2, 3 ng of T4 were contained in 100 μl of each solution.

Recommended T4-RIA procedure: Two hundred and fifty microliters of sodium barbital buffer containing 175 μg of 8-anilino-1-naphthalene sulfonic acid,[4] a binding inhibitor, was pipetted into each tube, including duplicates of "damaged" tubes, "blank" tubes, and quality controls. This was followed by 100 μl of unknown serum (diluted 10-fold) or standard T4 solution prepared in 10-fold diluted T4-free serum, or 10-fold diluted T4-free serum (to the "damaged," "blank," and quality-control tubes). Labeled T4, 100 μl (about 10 000 cpm) in the same

[4] This concentration was shown to be optimal. In our hands, neither 2.8 mg of 2,4-dinitrophenol nor 180 mg of sodium salicylate, saturation concentrations of these two inhibitors, was able to displace T4 completely from thyroxine-binding globulin (*18*).

buffer (without binding inhibitor) was added to each tube. Antiserum, 50 μl (diluted in the same buffer without binding inhibitor to give about 50% bound in the presence of a tracer quantity of labeled T4), was added to all tubes except the "damaged" and "blank" tubes. To these two sets of tubes was added 50 μl of sodium barbital buffer or preimmune sheep serum, respectively. The contents of all tubes were gently vortex-mixed and precounted. After incubation for 30 min at 37 °C, they were cooled to room temperature. To separate the antibody-bound T4 from free T4, 500 μl of aqueous polyethylene glycol (300 g/liter) followed by 50 μl of pooled normal human serum were added to all tubes, which were vortex-mixed vigorously. After centrifugation (1500 × g, 20 min), the supernates were aspirated and the radioactivity in the precipitates was measured in a gamma scintillation spectrometer (Packard Model 578).

Percentage bound was calculated as follows: Let B represent the radioactivity (cpm) that was precipitated, N the radioactivity (cpm) that was nonspecifically precipitated ("blank" tubes), and T the total radioactivity (cpm) in each incubation mixture. Then % bound, $B/T = (B - N)/T \times 100$

Quantitative and qualitative analysis of PEG precipitates: To verify that polyethylene glycol, 150 g/liter, completely separates bound from free T4, we did the following. Precipitates remaining after decantation were redissolved in 0.5 ml of water. One hundred microliters of each supernate and redissolved precipitate solution, as well as samples of normal human serum and ^{125}I-labeled T4, was applied to polyacrylamide gels (75 g/liter) for electrophoresis. Using bromphenol blue as a tracking dye, we allowed the proteins to migrate until the albumin-bound dye was about 1.5 cm from the bottom of the gel. One gel containing normal human serum was stained for proteins. All other gels (each about 7 cm in length) were cut into 5-mm segments, which were assayed for radioactivity.

To study the effect of pH, ionic strength, and temperature on PEG precipitation, we added 50 μl of pooled normal human serum or bovine γ-globulin (60 mg/ml) to 2 ml of PEG in buffer (150 g/liter) at 4 or 25 °C; the contents, after vortex-mixing vigorously, were centrifuged at 1500 × g for 20 min at the temperature of precipitation. The supernate was aspirated and the precipitate was redissolved in a minimal amount of water (0.5–2.0 ml, depending on the buffer condition). Total protein was estimated by a Lowry protein determination. To analyze the precipitates qualitatively, 100 μl of the dissolved precipitate was applied to a polyacrylamide gel (75 g/liter), electrophoresed, and stained for protein with the Amido Schwarz reagent.

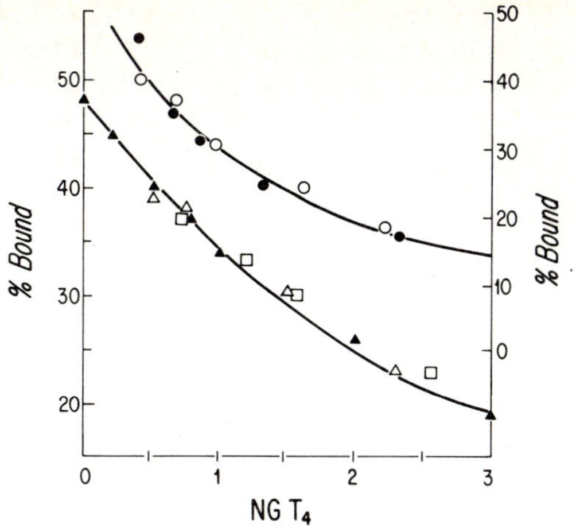

Fig. 1. (*upper curve*): Binding of labeled and unlabeled T4 to sheep T4 antiserum
(●) represents increasing unlabeled T4 in the presence of a constant amount of labeled T4. (O) represents increasing amounts of labeled T4

(*lower curve*): Serial dilution of hyperthyroid serum (△) and T4-free serum with known amounts of T4 added (□), as compared to a standard calibration curve (▲)
The T4 concentration reported by the laboratory which provided the serum was taken as the initial concentration of the hyperthyroid serum

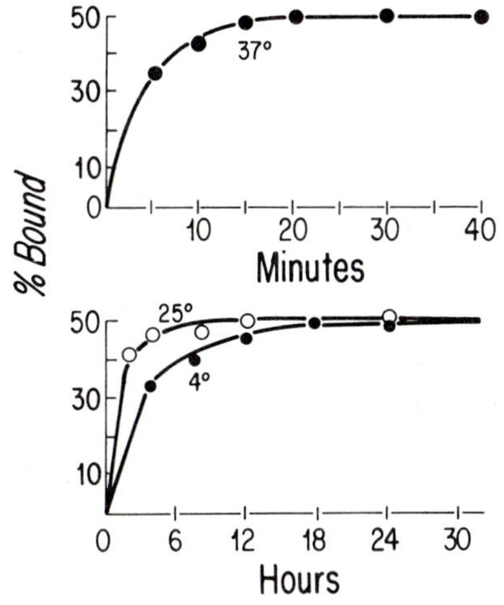

Fig. 2. Equilibrium of binding of T4 to sheep T4 antiserum at various incubation temperatures

Results

The binding curves for two sets of RIA performed in parallel are shown in Figure 1. The assay that used T4 of low specific activity contained labeled and unlabeled T4 in constant proportion but increasing amounts. The assay that used T4 of high specific activity contained a constant amount of labeled T4 with increasing proportions of unlabeled T4. The two curves were practically superimposable, implying that labeled and unlabeled T4 bound similarly to the antibody.

Time required for binding equilibrium to be attained depended on incubation temperature (Figure 2). Equilibration time decreased from 18 h to 12 h to 30 min as the temperature was increased from 4 to 25 to 37 °C. Hence, we chose 37 °C and 30 min as the conditions for our assay.

Table 1. Protein Precipitated from Normal Human Serum and Bovine γ-Globulin by Carbowax 6000

pH of phosphate buffer, 50 mmol/liter	Serum protein pptd., mg		γ-globulin pptd., mg	
	4 °C	25 °C	4 °C	25 °C
4.0	0.38	0.38	—	—
5.5	1.08	—	—	—
6.0	1.63	1.68	2.58	2.65
6.7	1.21	1.09	—	—
7.5	1.26	1.11	2.64	2.67
8.2	1.09	0.73	—	—
9.0	0.98	—	2.65	2.69
9.5	0.39	0.35	—	—
7.5 + 0.15 mol Cl⁻/l	1.18	0.94	—	—
7.5 + 0.5 mol Cl⁻/l	1.01	0.73	—	—
7.5 + 1.0 mol Cl⁻/l	0.91	0.64	2.02	2.02

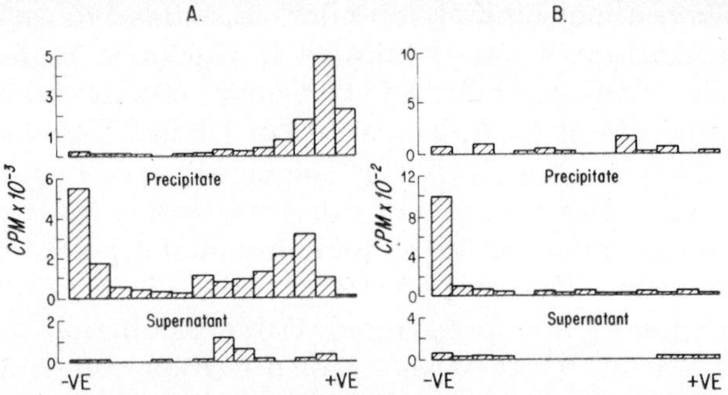

Fig. 3. Polyacrylamide-gel electrophoresis (*−VE*, cathode; *+VE*, anode) of labeled T4 in T4 antiserum after addition of PEG in phosphate buffer with (*A*) normal human serum or (*B*) bovine γ-globulin as carrier protein

Top to bottom: control (*A*, T4 alone; *B*, T4 with BGG), precipitate, supernate

The ability of PEG to precipitate all γ-globulins and thus completely separate bound T4 from unbound T4 was studied at various pH's and salt concentrations at 4 and 25 °C. With pooled normal human serum as a carrier, the amounts of protein precipitated gradually decreased as the pH increased (Table 1). Below pH 6 and above pH 9, the total amounts of protein precipitated were greatly decreased, owing to incomplete precipitation, evidenced by the turbid supernates seen after centrifugation at 1500 × *g*. When the pH was below 4.0 or above 10.0, there was no precipitate. Precipitation was also influenced by the presence of chloride ions; increasing ionic strength decreased the total amount of protein precipitated.

When pH and ionic strength were kept constant, PEG precipitated more protein at 4 than at 25 °C, and this was more noticeable at high chloride ion concentration.

These results prompted the following question: were the different amounts of proteins precipitated attributable to different amount of γ-globulin precipitated and (or) different amounts of non-γ-globulin serum proteins co-precipitated? Polyacrylamide gel electrophoresis of the precipitates, to resolve this question, indicated that in all cases proteins other than γ-globulins were precipitated. When a tracer quantity of labeled T4 was also present, polyacrylamide gel electrophoresis of both supernate and precipitates showed that, on the basis of radioactivity, all the γ-globulin-bound T4 was found in the precipitate formed between pH 6 and 9 at 4 °C. Therefore, the differences in the amounts of protein precipitated between pH 6 and 9 at 4 °C were due to the precipitation of non-γ-globulin proteins.

Further to substantiate this observation, we did experiments on bovine γ-globulin (2.65 mg, as estimated by absorbance at 280 nm) as a carrier. Practically all the γ-globulin was precipitated between pH 6 and 9 at both 4 and 25 °C. Precipitation was incomplete, however, in the presence of a high concentration of salt.

The distribution of radioactivity in the pH 7.5 supernate and precipitate of a RIA in which human serum was used as carrier protein and developed by polyacrylamide gel electrophoresis shows (Figure 3*A*) that substantial amounts of radioactivity were present in fractions of the precipitate other than γ-globulin. Was this radioactivity labeled T4 trapped (or bound) with non-γ-globulin carrier protein or was it γ-globulin T4 that separated during the process of electrophoresis? To answer this question, we again used bovine γ-globulin instead of normal human serum as carrier protein in the precipitation procedure. The distributions of radioactivity in the precipitates and supernates between pH 6 and 9 showed no differences within this pH range (Figure 3*B*). A comparison of these histograms with those in Figure 3*A* showed two differences: (*a*) there was little or no radioactivity in the supernate, and (*b*) although there was some scattering of radioactivity away from the γ-globulin region, it was less than when normal human serum was the carrier protein.

Having obtained this information on the ability of PEG to precipitate the antibody-bound T4 from free T4, we applied it to a T4-RIA. More than 40 serum samples were obtained from four different clinical laboratories that used different methods to measure serum T4 concentration. The T4 concentrations measured by our RIA were compared to those reported by the other laboratories (Figure 4). With respect to a perfect correlation (i.e., a straight line of slope 1 drawn through the origin), it can be seen that most of the T4 readings obtained with the Mallinckrodt kit (euthyroid range, 50–137 μg/liter) and Abbott "Tetrasorb" (euthyroid range, 53–145 μg/liter) were higher. On the other hand, most of the values obtained with the Curtis kit (euthyroid range, 49–99 μg/liter) were slightly lower. The best agreement was obtained with the Nuclear Med Labs "Tetra-Tab" (euthyroid range, 46–115 μg/liter). From our results

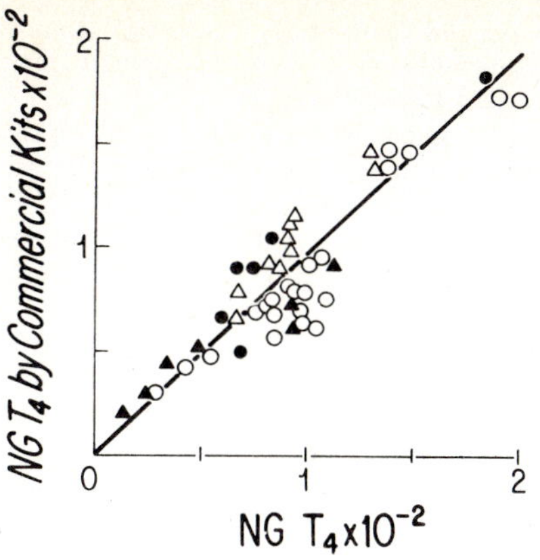

Fig. 4. Correlation of serum T4 measurement between available commercial kits and our T4 RIA

T4 measurements with (▲) Nuclear Med Labs Tetra-Tab, (○) Curtis Nuclear T4 kit, (●) Mallinckrodt T4 kit, and (△) Abbott Tetrasorb

for 39 sera that were reported as euthyroid after using these kits, we derived a tentative euthyroid range of 45–120 μg/liter for our assay.

Accuracy was checked by comparing readings of serially diluted hyperthyroid serum with standard T4 solutions and by assaying serum of known T4 content; the latter was prepared by adding increasing amounts of T4 to "T4-free serum" or to hypothyroid serum. (Using charcoal and the method described in *Methods,* we could remove more than 98% of serum T4 from pooled normal human serum to give "T4-free serum"). Figure 1 shows that the binding curves of all three systems were practically superimposable. Therefore, the accuracy is about 100%.

In agreement with this result is the recovery of T4 when 20, 70, or 140 μg of T4 per liter were added to a hypothyroid serum containing 15 μg of T4 per liter; the percentage recoveries were 100, 104, and 102, respectively. Recovery of radioactivity was also checked. In 50 cases, the radioactivity was measured in both supernates and precipitates; recovery averaged 97%.

By assaying a few samples repeatedly, the intra- and interassay reproducibility, expressed as mean ± standard deviation and coefficient of variation (CV), at different parts of the standard curve were found to be 15 ± 3 μg/liter (20%), 83 ± 7 μg/liter (8%), and 155 ± 10 μg/liter (6%) for intra-assay; and 36 ± μg/liter (17%), 93 ± 4 μg/liter (4%), and 154 ± 8 μg/liter (5%) for interassay comparison.

The extent to which various biological T4 analoges bind to the antiserum was studied by the method described Sekadde et al. (*13*). It can be seen (Table 2) that at their biological concentration, these compounds would not interfere with the T4 assay.

Table 2. Cross-Reactivity of Some Biological Compounds in the T4 Immunoassay

Compound	Cross-reactivity, %
L-Thyroxine (T4) (Sigma)	100
L-Triiodothyronine	18
3,5,3′,5′-Tetraiiodothyroacetic acid ("Tetrac") (Mann)	3.4
3,5,3′-Triiodothyroacetic acid ("Triac") (Warner-Lambert)	3.8

Discussion

Our results show that complete precipitation of γ-globulin with PEG (150 g/liter) was not affected by acidity between pH 6 and 9 or by temperatures between 4 and 25 °C (Table 1). High salt concentration, however, did lead to incomplete precipitation. Comparative studies showed that between pH 6 and 9 and between 4 and 25 °C, specificity of γ-globulin precipitation increased as pH and temperature increased. This is in accordance with the observation of Polson et al. (*10*).

The T4-RIA described here differs significantly from those published (*4, 6, 7, 15*) only in its sensitivity and the separation procedure. Most published T4-RIA's require at least 25 μl of serum sample; this one requires only 10 μl. Owing to the time-independent nature of our precipitation method, we have been able not only to handle over a hundred assay tubes per run, but also to use RIA for doing binding studies. With this separation procedure, a "busy" centrifuge was never a problem to us: once PEG and the carrier protein were added and well mixed, the tubes could be kept at 4 °C until a centrifuge was available. (We prefer keeping the tubes cold as a precaution, because most proteins and labeled materials are more stable at 4 °C).

The thermodynamic constants of the reaction between T4 and *our* T4 antibody indicated that *this* reaction is predominantly entropic and temperature independent (Cheung, Slaunwhite, and Cody, manuscript in preparation), an observation in accord with that of Keane and Walker (*16*). Therefore the entire procedure can be done at 37 °C and room temperature without rigid time constraint.

Desbuquois and Aurbach (*12*) applied PEG precipitation to RIA for separation of bound and free peptides (insulin, parathyroid hormone, growth hormone, and arginine vasopressin) and Barrett and Cohen (*17*) for assay of angiotensin I and digoxin. Our results, together with that of Sekadde et al. (*13*), show that precipitation with PEG is also a good separation procedure for RIA of thyroid hormones. We believe that this separation procedure should also be applicable to steroid RIA's or, for that matter, to RIA's of any small molecules that are not precipitated by PEG at 150 g/liter concentration.

References

1. Ratcliffe, J. G., Separation techniques in saturation analysis. *Br. Med. Bull.* **30,** 32 (1974).

2. Midgley, A. R., Rebar, R. W., and Niswender, G. D., Radioimmunoassays employing double antibody techniques. *Acta Endocrinol.* (Copenhagen) *Suppl. 142,* 247 (1969).

3. Herbert, V., Lau, K. S., Gottlieb, C. W., and Bleicher, S. J., Coated charcoal immunoassay of insulin. *J. Clin. Endocrinol. Metab.* **25,** 1375 (1965).

4. Mitsuma, T., Colucci, J., Shenkman, L., and Hollander, C. S., Rapid simultaneous radioimmunoassay for triiodothyronine and thyroxine in unextracted serum. *Biochem. Biophys. Res. Commun.* **46,** 2107 (1972).

5. Larsen, P. R., Direct immunoassay of triiodothyronine in human serum. *J. Clin. Invest.* **51,** 1939 (1972).

6. Dunn, R. T., and Foster, L. B., Radioimmunoassay of thyroxine in unextracted serum by a single-antibody technique. *Clin. Chem.* **19,** 1063 (1973).

7. Larsen, P. R., Dockalova, J., Sipula, D., and Wu, F. M., Immunoassay of thyroxine in unextracted human serum. *J. Clin. Endocrinol. Metab.* **37,** 177 (1973).

8. Nieschlag, E., and Wickings, E. J., A review of RIA for steroids. *Z. Klin. Chem. Klin. Biochem.* **13,** 261 (1975).

9. Binoux, M. A., and Odell, W. D., Use of dextran-coated charcoal to separate antibody-bound from free hormone: A critique. *J. Clin. Endocrinol. Metab.* **36,** 303 (1973).

10. Polson, A., Potgieter, G. M., Largier, J. F., et al, The fractionation of protein mixtures by linear polymers of high molecular weight. *Biochim. Biophys. Acta* **82,** 463 (1964).

11. Iverius, P. H., and Laurent, T. C., Precipitation of some plasma proteins by the addition of dextran or polyethylene glycol. *Biochim. Biophys. Acta* **133,** 371 (1967).

12. Desbuquois, B., and Aurbach, G. D., Use of polyethylene glycol to separate free and antibody-bound peptide hormones in radioimmunoassays. *J. Clin. Endocrinol. Metab.* **33,** 732 (1971).

13. Sekadde, C. B., Slaunwhite, W. R., Jr., and Aceto, T., Jr., Rapid radioimmunoassay of triiodothyronine. *Clin. Chem.* **19,** 1016 (1973).

14. Gharib, H., Mayberry, W. E., Ryan, R. J., and Hockett, T., Radioimmunoassay for triiodothyronine (T3). I. Affinity and specificity of the antibody for T3. *J. Clin. Endocrinol. Metab.* **33,** 509 (1971).

15. Chopra, I. J., A radioimmunoassay for measurement of thyroxine in unextracted serum. *J. Clin. Endocrinol. Metab.* **34,** 938 (1972).

16. Keane, P. M., and Walker, W. H. C., In *Handbook of Radioimmunoassay,* G. Abraham, Ed., Marcel Decker, New York, N. Y., 1976, in press.

17. Barrett, M. J., and Cohen, P. S., Radioimmunoassay of serum renin activity and digoxin concentrations with use of polyethylene glycol to separate free and antibody-bound ligand. *Clin. Chem.* **18,** 1339 (1972).

18. Cheung, M. C., Characterization of a sheep antibody to thyroxine and its use in radioimmunoassay. Ph.D. thesis, SUNY at Buffalo, 1975.

CLIN. CHEM. 22/3, 305–309 (1976)

Changes in Electrophoretic Mobilities of α- and β-Lipoproteins as a Result of Plasma Delipidation

Bill E. Cham and Brian R. Knowles

A two-phase system containing the ternary mixture butanol/diisopropyl ether/plasma in different proportions yields ordered delipidation of α-lipoproteins, pre-β-lipoproteins, and β-lipoproteins in plasma, as quantitated by densitometry after electrophoresis. As a consequence of delipidation the electrophoretic mobilities of pre-β-lipoprotein and β-lipoprotein increased, that of α-lipoprotein decreased.

Additional Keyphrases: *zonal electrophoresis on agarose • gradual delipidation • immunoelectrophoresis*

In a previous communication (*1*) we reported that the ternary mixture butanol/diisopropyl ether/plasma provides a convenient two-phase system for extraction of unesterified fatty acids, triglycerides, cholesterols, and phospholipids from plasma. When the solvent components are mixed in suitable proportions, plasma or serum are completely delipidated in 30 min. After centrifugation the lipids distribute into the upper, non-polar phase, whereas the proteins and other chemical constituents remain completely soluble in the clear lower phase.

This paper reports that exposure of plasma for 30 min to a two-phase system consisting of these same solvents in different proportions yields ordered delipidation of α-lipoproteins, β-lipoproteins, and pre-β-lipoproteins as quantitated by densitometry after electrophoresis.

These observations may indicate varying affinities of the different apolipoprotein fractions for lipid in plasma. Changes in electrophoretic mobilities after delipidation of these lipoprotein classes are also reported.

Department of Medicine, University of Queensland, Royal Brisbane Hospital, Brisbane, 4029, Australia.

Received Oct. 16, 1975; accepted Dec. 9, 1975.

Materials and Methods

Plasma

We used outdated human acid citrate-dextrose plasma obtained from the district blood bank.

Reagents

Diisopropyl ether was laboratory-reagent grade and was made peroxide free by distilling in the presence of ferrous sulfate; all other reagents were analytical grade.

Procedures

Delipidation. Partially and totally delipidated plasma was prepared by the method of Cham and Knowles (*1*). For the present studies, 10-ml aliquots of plasma were added to 20 ml of organic phase consisting of 0, 2.5, 5, 10, 20, 30, or 40 ml of butanol per deciliter of diisopropyl ether.

The samples were mixed for exactly 30 min at room temperature in a blood-cell-suspension rotator. After removing the aqueous phase from the organic phase, we subjected the samples to quantitative lipid analysis and electrophoresis.

Chemical analysis. The lipids in the plasma, before and after exposure to the organic solvent, were measured by semiautomated continuous-flow methods. Cholesterol and triglyceride (triacylglycerol) were determined in isopropanol extracts. Cholesterol was estimated by method N-24a (*2*), and triglyceride by the method of Lofland (*3*), modified by using Fletcher's (*4*) zeolite mixture instead of the Doucil mixture to absorb phospholipid. Phospholipid was extracted by the method of Folch et al. (*5*) and, after sample digestion, phosphorus was measured by the method of Fiske and SubbaRow (*6*). The factor 25 was used in converting lipid phosphorus values to

Table 1. Delipidation of Human Plasma on 30-min Extraction

Extraction solvent, butanol/diisopropyl ether	Triglycerides	Cholesterols	Phospholipids
		% of control[a]	
None	100	100	100
0/100	80	80	96
	(72–90)	(73–88)	(95–100)
2.5/97.5	57	64	82
	(45–70)	(54–75)	(56–95)
5/95	41	55	73
	(22–52)	(42–71)	(49–85)
10/90	10	27	63
	(4–25)	(17–42)	(40–79)
20/80	0	0	39
			(28–57)
30/70	0	0	18
			(13–21)
40/60	0	0	0

[a] Each value, as percent delipidation, is the mean of five experiments. Range is in parentheses. Range of initial concentrations (mg per deciliter of plasma) were: triglyceride, 100–276; cholesterol, 120–190; phospholipid, 131–276.

phospholipid values. Percentage delipidation was calculated by difference.

Zonal electrophoresis. Zonal electrophoresis on agarose (7) was performed in barbital buffer (50 mmol/liter, pH 8.60). We used Fat Red 7B (Analytical Chemists, Palo Alto, Calif. 94303) and Coomassie Blue (ICI, Australia) to stain lipid and protein, respectively.

Densitometry. After destaining, the gels were scanned with a Quick Scan Jr. Densitometer incorporating a built-in integrator unit (Helena Laboratories, Beaumont, Tex. 77704). We integrated the areas stained with Fat Red 7B in the α-, pre-β-, and β-lipoprotein fractions of plasma, before and after exposure to the organic solvent, by the method of McTaggart and Dwyer (8). The percentage of lipid removed by the organic solvent from each fraction was calculated by difference.

Immunoelectrophoresis. For this we used pre-cast agarose (10 g/liter) slides (Corning-Eel, Halstead, Essex, England). The conditions for electrophoresis and immunodiffusion were described by Keyser (9). Rabbit antisera to human α-lipoproteins and β-lipoproteins were obtained from Behringwerke AG (Farbwerke Hoechst AG, Frankfurt/Main, Germany).

Results

Increasing proportions of butanol in the butanol/diisopropyl ether extraction mixture produce increasing degrees of delipidation of human plasma in 30 min (Table 1). Both triglyceride and cholesterol are completely extracted by butanol diisopropyl ether (20/80 by vol). A 40/60 mixture is required to extract all phospholipids from their plasma lipoproteins into the organic phase.

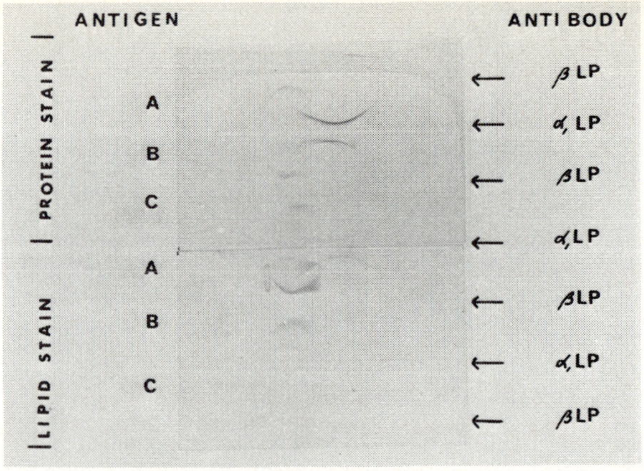

Fig. 1. Immunoelectrophoresis on agarose in control, partially delipidated, and totally delipidated plasma

Antibody troughs contain antisera to human α-lipoprotein or β-lipoprotein. Antigen wells contain control plasma, *A*; plasma, partially delipidated with butanol/diisopropyl ether (10/90 by vol) for 30 min, *B*; plasma, totally delipidated with butanol/diisopropyl ether (40/60 by vol) for 30 min, *C*. Proteins and lipids are stained with Coomassie Blue and Fat Red 7B, respectively. *C* contains no detectable lipid

On immunoelectrophoresis, control plasma showed single precipitin arcs against antisera to α_1- and β-lipoprotein (Figure 1, *A*) and defined the electrophoretic mobility of these fractions under the experimental conditions. The partially and totally delipidated samples undergoing immunoelectrophoresis simultaneously with the control plasma produced precipitin arcs of differing mobility and intensity to the control plasma (Figure 1, *B* and *C*). Specifically, fractions reacting with α_1-lipoprotein antibody moved more slowly in both the protein-stained partially and totally delipidated samples. Additionally, two precipitin arcs were apparent in the partially delipidated plasma. Fractions reacting with β-lipoprotein antibody migrated more rapidly in the partially and totally delipidated plasma than did the corresponding fraction in the control plasma. Lipid-stainable material was demonstrated at sites corresponding to the precipitin arcs in the control and partially delipidated specimens, but no lipid-stainable material was demonstrable at these sites in the totally delipidated plasma.

Figure 2 shows the electrophoretic patterns of partially and totally delipidated samples, obtained after 30-min extraction of plasma aliquots with increasing concentrations of butanol in diisopropyl ether, as well as an unextracted control. When the electrophoretograms were simultaneously stained for protein, it was seen that increasing quantities of lipid removed from the plasma correspond to a broadening in the α-globulin band and a narrowing of the β-globulin band. A second series of electrophoretograms, prepared concurrently from the same samples stained for protein, were simultaneously stained with Fat

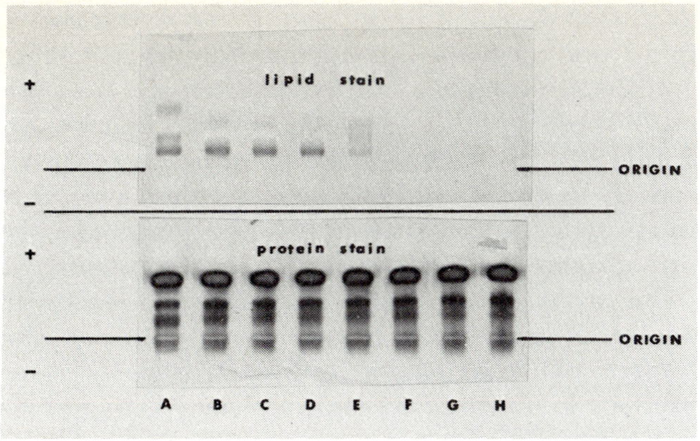

Fig. 2. Agarose electropherograms comparing control unextracted human plasma with human plasma extracted for 30 min with increasing concentrations of butanol in diisopropyl ether

Lipid and protein were stained with Fat Red 7B and Coomassie Blue, respectively. *A*, unextracted control; *B–H*, respective extraction mixtures (butanol/diisopropyl ether) were 0/100, 2.5/97.5, 5/95, 10/90, 20/80, 30/70, and 40/60 by vol. *F* and *G* contained some phospholipid, undetectable with the lipid stain. No lipid was present in sample *H* on quantitative estimation

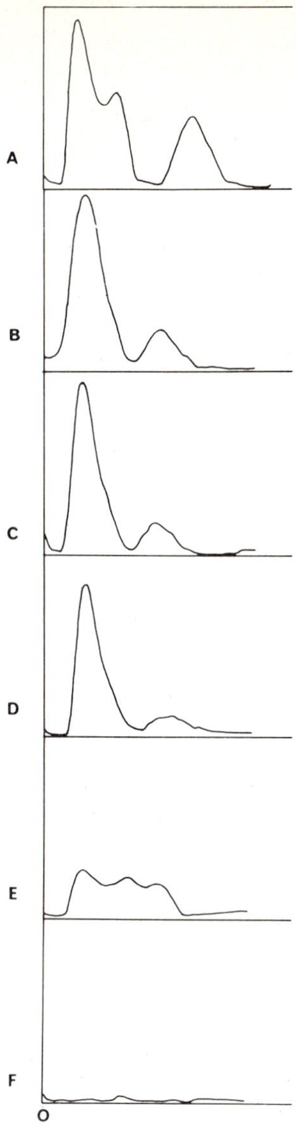

Fig. 3. Densitometric scans of agarose electropherograms, stained for lipid, illustrating the effect on electrophoretic mobility and the degree of delipidation of human plasma on extraction for 30 min with increasing concentrations of butanol in diisopropyl ether

A, unextracted control; *B–F*, respective proportions of solvents in extraction system are 0/100, 2.5/97.5, 5/95, 10/90, and 20/80. *O*, origin. The peaks in *A* are (*left to right*) beta-, pre-beta, and alpha-lipoproteins

Red 7B to demonstrate the lipid bound in the lipoprotein fractions (Figure 2) and scanned with the densitometer, at 520 nm (Figure 3).

As more lipid was removed from plasma, electrophoretic mobilities of the β- and pre-β-lipoprotein fractions increased; that of the α-lipoprotein fraction decreased. Integration of the densitometric scans demonstrates that α-lipoproteins are more readily delipidated by our solvent system than are the β- and pre-β-lipoprotein fractions. In some cases, because of the change in electrophoretic mobilities, it was not possible precisely to distinguish the pre-β-lipoprotein peak, which was masked by incomplete resolution from β-lipoprotein band (Table 2).

Because the lipid components—cholesterols, triglycerides, and phospholipids—add up to give a value almost the same as that for the total lipid present in the α-, β- and pre-β-lipoprotein fractions in plasma, lipid remaining in the various lipoprotein classes after partial delipidation correlated well, whether determined by chemical analysis or by densitometry (Table 3). This correlation did not apply over the whole range of delipidation, because some phospholipid still present in the plasma after 30-min delipidation with butanol/diisopropyl ether (20/80 by vol) was not detectable by Fat Red 7B stain.

Discussion

Application of a biphasic extraction method for plasma lipids, without first precipitating proteins, has permitted a comparative study of the extraction of lipids from the individual lipoprotein fractions in plasma.

Stained protein-bound lipid was directly measured densitometrically after agarose electrophoresis of plasma samples with various degrees of delipidation. An objection to direct densitometry is the nonlinear relationship between concentration of unextracted lipoprotein and density of bound dye (*10*). Nevertheless, Adlersberg et al. (*11*) successfully quantitated lipoproteins by densitometry. Individual pure lipids stain with various intensities, increasing the difficulty of quantitating lipid bound to the lipoprotein fractions. Notwithstanding these inadequacies, densitometry is the method of choice for quantitating serum lipoproteins (*8, 10–13*), in contrast to quantitative estimation of lipid fractions.

Lipids stainable with Fat Red 7B were more readily extracted with butanol/diisopropyl ether from α-lipoprotein than from the pre-β- and β-lipoprotein fractions in plasma. We saw little difference in lipid extractability of β- and pre-β-lipoprotein fractions in

Table 2. Effect on Electrophoretic Mobility of 30-min Extraction of Human Plasma by Various Solvent Mixtures[a]

Extraction solvent, butanol/ diisopropyl ether	Lipo-protein fraction	Distance migrated, mm	Integration units	Lipid extract-ed, %
No extraction	α	61.5	130	0
	pre-β	32	150	0
	β	16	210	0
0/100	α	48	85	35
	pre-β	—)	360)	0
	β	18.7)	)	
2.5/97.5	α	46	50	62
	pre-β	—)	280)	23
	β	19)	)	
5/95	α	46	40	69
	pre-β	—)	230)	36
	β	19)	)	
10/90	α	46	30	77
	pre-β	35	60	60
	β	19	90	58

[a] Electrophoresis in agarose gels, pH 8.6, of α-, β-, and pre-β-lipoprotein fractions. The concentrations of these fractions relative to the corresponding unextracted control plasma lipoprotein fractions are expressed as percent lipid extracted. Percent lipid extracted was derived from densitometric integration units.

plasma. These results compare favorably with those of Scanu and Schiano (*13*), who delipidated serum by a continuous cold-extraction method and obtained precipitated proteins, which were partly soluble in physiological saline. They found that the α-lipoprotein fraction was more easily delipidated than the β-lipoprotein fraction in serum. However, it is possible that all the apolipoprotein fractions obtained in the precipitated form by this continuous cold-extraction method were not soluble in physiological saline, because Tris-HCl buffer at pH 8.2 is required to re-dissolve similarly treated individual lipoprotein fractions that have been separated ultracentrifugally (*14*). Our butanol/diisopropyl ether extraction of lipid from plasma leaves apolipoproteins in solution (*1*). We surmise from our experience with the butanol/diisopropyl ether extraction system that less energy is required to break the bond between the Fat Red 7B stainable lipid and apolipoproteins of the α-lipoprotein fraction than is required for β- and pre-β-lipoprotein fractions, when these are in plasma.

Our extraction of lipid from plasma results in greater electrophoretic mobilities of the pre-β- and β-lipoprotein fractions, as compared with the same fractions in unextracted control plasma. The reverse is true for α-lipoprotein: removal of plasma lipids results in an electrophoretic mobility that is less than that of α-lipoprotein in unextracted plasma. Magnitude of net charge determines the velocity of migration; the sign of the charge dictates the direction of movement; the algebraic sum of the charges on the particle and those surrounding it determines net charge; shape, size, and mass of the molecule influence the absolute rate of migration. At least some of these factors are altered when lipid is extracted from the apolipoprotein moiety.

The demonstration (Figure 1*B*) that partly delipidated α-lipoprotein yields two immunoelectrophoretic boundaries with different mobilities suggests heterogeneity of α-lipoprotein. When delipidation is complete, an apparently uniform electrophoretic mobility occurs, but the precipitin arc is less intense, a difference unlikely to be the result of loss of protein, because protein loss by this delipidation technique is insignificant (*1*). Previous observations on the immunoreactivity of delipidated α-lipoprotein (*1, 15*) are in accord with the current findings.

Electrophoretic mobility of the delipidated forms of the pre-β- and β-lipoproteins in plasma may be increased because of removal of lipid. If the lipids removed are neutral, then one would expect the apolipoproteins to migrate faster than the lipoproteins because they have lost about 80% of their mass. Alternatively, pre-β- and β-lipoprotein in plasma may be

Table 3. Comparison of Chemical Analysis and Densitometry for Lipid Components of Plasma Lipoproteins after Partial Delipidation by 30-min Extraction

Extraction solvent, butanol/ diisopropyl ether	Analysis of plasma lipoprotein-bound lipids: Triglyceride	Cholesterol	Phospholipid	Total lipids determined by chemical analysis[a]	Residual total lipid, %	Total lipids determined by densitometry,[a] integration units	Residual total lipids, %
	mg/dl						
No extraction	164	163	189	516	100	490	100
0/100	130	132	182	444	86	445	90
2.5/97.5	90	105	160	354	69	330	67
5/95	60	90	142	292	57	270	55
10/90	14	42	123	179	35	180	36

[a] Total lipids determined by chemical analysis correspond to the sum of cholesterols, triglycerides, and phospholipids in mg per 100 ml plasma. Total lipids determined by densitometry correspond to the sum of integration units of alpha, beta, and pre-beta-lipoproteins strained by Fat Red 7B after electrophoresis.

dissociated into smaller apolipoprotein units as a result of delipidation with our extraction mixture; β- and pre-β-apolipoproteins evidently contain heterogeneous units (*14, 16*). If the net charge of the parent lipoproteins is not evenly distributed between derived heterogeneous units, then electrostatic forces will also produce differences in migration rate, with the possibility of producing less distinct, or even merging, electrophoretic zones.

Either of these explanations would be compatible with our observations, as also would be a net change in mass, charge, and (or) molecular configuration. A clearer difference in electrophoretic mobility would be anticipated if one were to study separated apolipoproteins containing no other proteins.

Skillful technical assistance by Grant W. Johnson is gratefully acknowledged.

References

1. Cham, B. E., and Knowles, B. R., A solvent system for delipidation of plasma or serum without protein precipitation. *J. Lipid Res.*, in press.

2. Technicon Instrument Corp., Tarrytown, N. Y. 10591; method N-24a.

3. Lofland, H. B., A semiautomated procedure for the determination of triglycerides in serum. *Anal. Biochem.* **9,** 393 (1964).

4. Fletcher, M. J., A colorimetric method for estimating serum triglyceride. *Clin. Chim. Acta* **22,** 393 (1968).

5. Folch, J., Lees, M., and Sloane Stanely, G. H., A simple method for the isolation and purification of total lipids from animal tissues. *J. Biol. Chem.* **226,** 497 (1957).

6. Fiske, C. H., and SubbaRow, Y., The colorimetric determination of phosphorus. *J. Biol. Chem.* **66,** 375 (1925).

7. Noble, R. P., Electrophoretic separation of plasma lipoproteins in agarose gel. *J. Lipid Res.* **9,** 693 (1968).

8. McTaggart, W. G., and Dwyer, J. L., Improved method for densitometry of electrophoretic lipoprotein fractions. *Clin. Chem.* **21,** 183 (1975).

9. Keyser, J., Immunoelectrophoresis—applications and recent developments. *Chem. Br.* **8,** 480 (1972).

10. Jencks, W. P., and Durrum, E. L., Paper electrophoresis as a quantitative method; the staining of serum lipoproteins. *J. Clin. Invest.* **34,** 1437 (1955).

11. Adlersberg, D., Bossak, E. T., Sher, I. H., and Sobotka, H., Electrophoresis and monomolecular layer studies with serum lipoproteins. *Clin. Chem.* **1,** 18 (1955).

12. Straus, R., and Wurm, M., A new staining procedure and a method for quantitation of serum lipoproteins separated by paper electrophoresis. *Am. J. Clin. Pathol.* **29,** 581 (1958).

13. Scanu, A., and Schiano, N., Su di una nuova metodica di estrazione continua a freddo con etere dei lipidi del siero. Applicazione allo studio dei complessi lipoproteici. *Ist. Sierot, Ital.* **29,** 457 (1954).

14. Scanu, A. M., Edelstein, C., and Aggerbech, L., Application of the technique of isoelectric focussing to the study of human-serum lipoproteins and their apoproteins. *Ann. N. Y. Acad. Sci.* **209,** 311 (1973).

15. Levy, R. I., and Fredrickson, D. S., Heterogeneity of plasma high density lipoproteins. *J. Clin. Invest.* **44,** 426 (1965).

16. Shore, V. G., Shore, B., and Hart, R. G., Changes in apolipoproteins and properties of rabbit very low density lipoproteins on induction of cholesterolemia. *Biochemistry* **13,** 1579 (1974).

Simultaneous Quantitation of 4-Hydroxy-3-Methoxymandelic (Vanilmandelic) and 4-Hydroxy-3-Methoxyphenylacetic (Homovanillic) Acids in Human Urine

Somasundaram Addanki, Elmer R. Hinnenkamp, and Juan F. Sotos

We describe a simultaneous analysis for vanilmandelic and homovanillic acids in urine. An aliquot of a final extract, containing phenylpropionic acid as external standard, is dried, an internal standard (resorcinol) is added, and the mixture is silylated and chromatographed. The two compounds are identified from their characteristic retention times and from their elution behavior in relation to four different marker compounds (the external and internal standards and two other naturally occurring compounds, *p*-hydroxyphenylacetic and hippuric acids) and are quantitated from their relative response factors. Within-run precision (CV) varied from 2 to 14% for vanilmandelic acid and 1 to 18% for homovanillic acid. The ratio of the amount of phenylpropionic acid extracted to the amount of added resorcinol found is a useful quality-control index. Values for vanilmandelic acid obtained by this method and by the technique of Pisano et al. [*Clin. Chim. Acta* **7**, 285 (1962)] correlated well (r = 0.844).

Additional Keyphrases: *gas chromatography • diagnosis of pheochromocytoma, dysautonomia, neuroblastoma*

Present methods for measuring 4-hydroxy-3-methoxymandelic acid (vanilmandelic acid, VMA)[1] and 4-hydroxy-3-methoxyphenylacetic acid (homovanillic acid, HVA) in urine are based on spectrophotometry, thin-layer chromatography, paper chromatography, or gas chromatography. Williams and Greer (*1*) reported that the laboratory diagnosis of neuroblastoma can be made more than 95% accurate by simultaneously quantitating VMA and HVA. Their method, however, utilized a toxic and explosive reagent, diazomethane, a fact that impedes the use of their technique in a service laboratory.

By the method reported here, VMA and HVA can be simultaneously measured with better resolution than with the older methods, and many more metabolites in urine can also be detected. Used in our laboratory for more than three years, the method (*2*) assists in the diagnosis of disorders that result in increased excretion of VMA (pheochromocytoma) or HVA (dysautonomia), or both (neuroblastoma).

Materials and Methods

Materials

HVA, VMA, and *p*-hydroxyphenylacetic acid were purchased from Sigma Chemical Co., St. Louis, Mo. 63178; [^{3}H]VMA and [^{3}H]HVA from New England Nuclear Corp., Boston, Mass. 02118; ethyl acetate, methylene chloride, acetone, toluene, and chloroform from Burdick and Jackson, Muskegon, Mich. 49442 (all sold as "distilled in glass"); *N,O*-bis(trimethylsilyl)trifluoro-acetamide containing 10 g of trimethylchlorosilane per liter, pyridine, and dimethyl formamide from Regis Chemical Co., Morton Grove, Ill. 60053; methyl violet 6B from Matheson, Coleman and Bell Co., Norwood, Ohio 45212; phenylpropionic acid from Aldrich Chemical Co., Milwaukee, Wis. 53233; OV-11 silicone fluid from Supelco, Inc., Bellefonte, Pa. 16823; Gas Chrom Q (80–100 mesh), silane-treated glass wool, OV-17 silicone fluid, and Hamilton syringes from Applied Science Laboratories, State College, Pa. 16801; and Dexil 300-impregnated asbestos cord from Analabs, Inc., North Haven, Conn. 06473. Tapered reaction vials (1-, 3-, and 5-ml sizes) and the Teflon "Mininert" valves for them were from Pierce Chemical Co., Rockford, Ill. 61105.

All of the glassware was coated with water-soluble silicone ("Siliclad"; Clay Adams, Parsippany, N.J. 07054).

HCl (6 mol/liter), sodium bicarbonate (100 g/liter), and methyl violet 6B (30 g/liter) were all dissolved in de-ionized distilled water.

Standards for VMA, HVA, and *p*-hydroxyphenyla-

Division of Endocrinology and Metabolism, Departments of Pediatrics and Physiological Chemistry, The Ohio State University College of Medicine; and The Children's Hospital Research Foundation, Columbus, Ohio 43205.

[1] Nonstandard abbreviations used: HVA (homovanillic acid), 4-hydroxy-3-methoxyphenylacetic; VMA (vanilmandelic acid), 4-hydroxy-3-methoxymandelic acid.

Received Aug. 8, 1975; accepted Dec. 16, 1975.

cetic acid were prepared by dissolving 10 mg in 10 ml of ethyl acetate and storing the solution in 5-ml reaction vials with Mininert valves.

The external standard, phenylpropionic acid, was prepared by dissolving 14.6 mg in 10 ml of sodium bicarbonate solution (100 g/liter) and distributing 5-ml aliquots into reaction vials with Mininert valves.

The internal standard, resorcinol, was prepared by dissolving 15 mg in 50 ml of pyridine and distributing 5-ml aliquots into reaction vials with Mininert valves.

Column-packing material: Weigh 2.5 g of OV-11 silicone fluid (stationary phase) into a 250-ml round-bottom flask, add about 100 ml of chloroform, and swirl until the silicone is dissolved. Add 22.5 g of Gas Chrom Q and mix to make a slurry. Connect the flask to a rotary evaporator, keeping the flask half immersed in water at 40 °C. [If toluene is used as a solvent or commercially prepared chromatographic supports (Supelco Inc., Bellefonte, Pa. 16823) are used, the trimethylsilyl derivatives will not be eluted from the column.] Under reduced pressure, evaporate until the odor of the solvent is no longer detectable (yield, 25 g). The 6.1-m column we used takes about 6 g of this support and can be used for 4 to 5 months (400 runs).

Curing of the Column

Pack and install the column into the gas-chromatographic apparatus; use Dexil 300-impregnated asbestos cord and OV-17 to seal the column. Close the oven lid and warm the oven to 100 °C. There will be a rapid baseline rise as the temperature increases, followed by a slower fall as the temperature nears 100 °C. Stepwise, increase the temperature in 50 °C increments; allow time after each increase for the column to clear the rapidly eluted material and resnug the retaining nuts each time, until the curing temperature (310 °C) is reached. The initial baseline will drop slowly to 30 to 40 divisions during three to five days. Snugness of the column retainer nuts should be periodically checked. Indications that the column needs repacking include peak tailing, shortened retention times (less than 11 min for resorcinol), poor peak resolution, and a rise in the baseline.

Analytical Procedures

Extraction of urinary HVA and VMA: Step I: Place a volume of urine equivalent to 1 mg of creatinine or 0.2% of the 24-h volume in a 25-ml screw-cap (Teflon-lined) culture tube (20 × 150 mm), add 25 μl of the phenylpropionic acid solution as external standard, and adjust the volume to 4.0 ml with distilled water. Add two drops of aqueous methyl violet 6B and adjust the pH to 1.0 (brownish green) with HCl. Adjust the total volume to 6 ml with distilled water. Saturate the mixture with about 3 g of sodium chloride. The sample should become bright yellow. Add 12 ml of ethyl acetate and shake for 5 min in a horizontal shaker at low speed (Eberbach Corp., Ann Arbor, Mich. 48106).

Step II: Immediately transfer 10 ml of ethyl acetate layer to another culture tube. Add 3 ml of 100 g/liter sodium bicarbonate, and shake for 5 min (low speed).

Step III: Immediately transfer 2 ml of the sodium bicarbonate layer to another culture tube. Add 1 drop of aqueous methyl violet 6B. Add HCl dropwise until a brownish green color appears (pH 1.0). Add about 1.5 g of sodium chloride, and 4.0 ml of ethyl acetate, and shake the mixture for 5 min (low speed). Immediately transfer 3.0 ml of the ethyl acetate layer to a tapered reaction vial.

The above procedure can be safely interrupted just after any of the three transfers.

Silylation: Evaporate the 3.0 ml of the ethyl acetate layer transferred to the tapered reaction vial by directing a gentle stream of dry nitrogen into the vial for about 20 min. Then add 1.0 ml of methylene chloride and evaporate with a gentle stream of dry nitrogen. This dehydrates the sample. The vial is immediately capped in order to avoid hydration. With a 50-μl Hamilton syringe, add 25 μl of the resorcinol in pyridine into the vial, followed by 25 μl of the *N,O*-bis(trimethylsilyl)trifluoroacetamide/trimethylchlorosilane. Heat the vial in a heating block (we used a Temp-Block; Lab-Line, Melrose Park, Ill. 60160) for 1 h at 60 °C and then cool it to room temperature; aspirate a 3-μl aliquot into a 10-μl Hamilton syringe adapted with a needle 15.2 cm in length and inject the sample onto the column for quantitation. This procedure improves resolution and reduces thermal breakdown of trimethylsilyl derivatives.

Instrumental conditions: The derivatives were quantitated in a Model 1440 gas chromatograph (Varian Associates, Palo Alto, Calif. 93403) with a flame ionization detector. Other accessories included a linear temperature-programmer, a millivolt strip-chart recorder, and a Model 50B automatic attenuator (all from Hewlett-Packard, Palo Alto, Calif. 93404). We filtered nitrogen and hydrogen (each at 25 to 30 ml/min) through gas-drying traps (Guild Corp., Bethel Park, Pa. 15102) before use. Compressed air was used at the rate of 300 ml/min. The injection port, which is kept at ambient temperature, contains a Teflon-backed silicone-rubber septum (Varian). The column was a 6.1-m glass coil (o.d., 3 mm; i.d., 2 mm) packed with OV-11 on Gas Chrom Q, 80–100 mesh (10 g/100 g). Column temperature was programmed from 65–305 °C at 4 °C/min. Several different temperature programs between 2 °C/min and 20 °C/min were tried; 4 °C gave the best compromise between speed and precision. Detector temperature was kept at 340 °C.

Results and Discussion

Response of trimethylsilyl derivatives: The relative response values of derivatives of several pure compounds did not change from 30 min to 72 h after silylation, indicating stability and completeness of derivatization (Table 1). Smaller response values

Table 1. Stability of Trimethylsilyl-Derivatives[a]

Name of compound[b]	Relative response, with respect to phenanthrene, after silylation (h)					
	0.5	1.5	3	72	73	74
VMA	0.67	0.63	0.59	0.69	0.69	0.72
HVA	0.80	0.82	0.80	0.72	0.68	0.76
PHPAA	1.07	1.01	1.05	0.92	0.93	1.10
RS	1.16	1.12	1.19	1.21	1.17	1.28

[a] The silylation mixture was prepared in a valve-stoppered reaction vial and kept at room temperature.
[b] PHPAA, *p*-hydroxyphenylacetic acid; RS, resorcinol.

Table 2. Guidelines for the Identification of Urinary Acids

Name of compound	Relative retention time[a]: Min after the elution of	Min before the elution of	Time span between the two markers, min
PPA[b]	R + 2.86	P − 5.94	8.80
HVA	P + 4.21	H − 4.02	8.23
VMA	P + 5.93	H − 2.40	8.33

[a] R, resorcinol; P, *p*-hydroxyphenylacetic acid; H, hippuric acid.
[b] PPA, phenylpropionic acid.

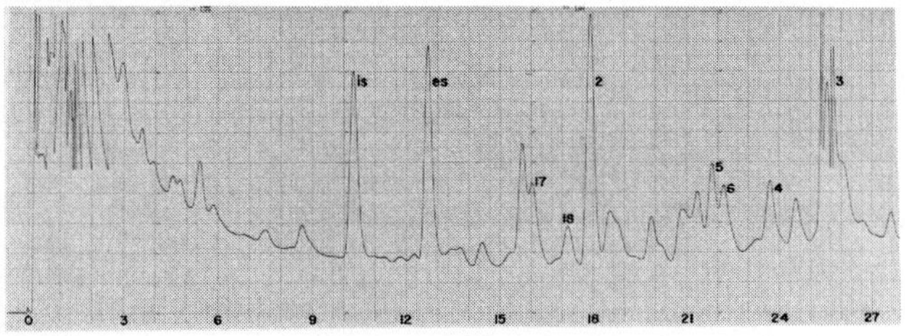

Fig. 1. Gas-chromatographic tracing of a silylated urine extract (82.5 mg of creatinine per deciliter)
Peak identification: *p*-hydroxyphenylacetic acid, 2; hippuric acid, 3; VMA, 4; HVA, 5; homogentisic acid, 6; resorcinol, *is;* phenylpropionic, *es; o*-hydroxyphenylacetic, 17; *m*-hydroxyphenylacetic, 18; (series CXCVII 4 × 10^{-10}, 125 to 295 °C at 4 °C/min, OV-11 on Gas Chrom Q (10 g/100g), 1″/min)

Table 4. Extraction of [^{3}H] VMA from Urine into Various Fractions[a] **(pH = 1.0 and NaCl Saturation)**

Step no.	Percent [^{3}H] VMA extracted (expressed as percent of the original): Ethyl acetate layer (mean ± SD)[b]	Aqueous layer (mean ± SD)
I	85.74 ± 1.39	11.57 ± 0.52
II	0.53 ± 0.03	87.02 ± 2.16
III	75.38 ± 1.01	9.01 ± 0.59

[a] [^{3}H] VMA (194 390 dpm, New England Nuclear Corp., No. NET 339, 1–5 Ci/mmol) was added to a urine aliquot and extracted by the described procedure. [^{3}H] VMA present in the ethyl acetate layer was counted in a toluene-based liquid-scintillation medium, that present in the aqueous layer was counted in a dioxane-based liquid-scintillation medium.
[b] Mean ± 1 SD of six determinations.

were noted as a result of moisture pick-up when the reaction vials were opened several times. The response relative to the trimethylsilyl derivative of resorcinol for the trimethylsilyl derivatives of VMA, HVA, *p*-hydroxyphenylacetic acid, and phenylpropionic acid were 0.50 ± 0.03, 0.57 ± 0.02, 0.71 ± 0.03 and 0.67 ± 0.03, respectively. These values were used to calculate the amounts represented by the area of the peaks in the chromatograms.

Peak identification: Compounds present in the urine extracts were identified from their retention times relative to four marker compounds: the external standard (phenylpropionic acid); the internal standard (resorcinol); hippuric acid, which is the largest peak appearing towards the end of the chromatogram; and *p*-hydroxyphenylacetic acid, which is eluted halfway between the internal standard and hippuric acid and is usually larger than other peaks in the middle of the chromatogram. Retention times (in minutes) were: resorcinol, 30.59 ± 0.40; *p*-hydroxyphenylacetic acid, 39.50 ± 0.39; HVA, 43.78 ± 0.52; VMA, 45.44 ± 0.38; and hippuric acid, 48.16 ± 0.37. Retention times were measured for each com-

Table 3. Effect of pH and Sodium Chloride Saturation on Extraction of [^{3}H] VMA into Ethyl Acetate (Step I)

	Percent [^{3}H] VMA extracted into ethyl acetate[a] (Mean ±SD)[b]				
pH	3.0	2.0	1.5	1.0	0.5
Without NaCl	49.58 ± 2.75	69.90 ± 1.77	64.32 ± 1.91	59.73 ± 2.00	63.32 ± 1.11
With NaCl	81.75 ± 2.69	86.86 ± 3.21	86.48 ± 3.30	80.75 ± 4.95	66.67 ± 1.94

[a] [^{3}H] VMA (265 380 dpm, New England Nuclear Corp., No. NET 339, 1–5 Ci/mmol), was added to a urine aliquot, extracted into the ethyl acetate, and counted in a toluene-based liquid-scintillation medium.
[b] Mean ± 1 SD of four determinations.

Table 5. Ratio of the Area of Peak for the External Standard (Phenylpropionic acid) to That for the Internal Standard (Resorcinol)[a]

No. samples extracted	Phenylpropionic acid/ resorcinol, mean ± SD	CV, %
53	1.016 ± 0.071	6.99
12	1.024 ± 0.091	8.99
8	1.011 ± 0.026	2.57
10	0.972 ± 0.051	5.25
10	1.065 ± 0.051	4.79
9	1.033 ± 0.059	5.71
9	1.151 ± 0.120	10.43
9	1.049 ± 0.069	6.58
6	1.063 ± 0.066	6.21
9	1.041 ± 0.068	6.53
4	1.065 ± 0.049	4.60
8	1.064 ± 0.023	2.16
5	1.070 ± 0.057	5.33
11	1.025 ± 0.026	2.54
7	1.067 ± 0.040	3.75
6	1.027 ± 0.066	6.43
8	1.018 ± 0.035	3.44
9	1.091 ± 0.076	6.97
9	1.033 ± 0.079	7.65

[a] 36.5 μg of phenylpropionic acid was added to each of the urine samples before extraction. 8.34 μg of resorcinol was added to each of the samples during silylation. These observations were made during seven months.

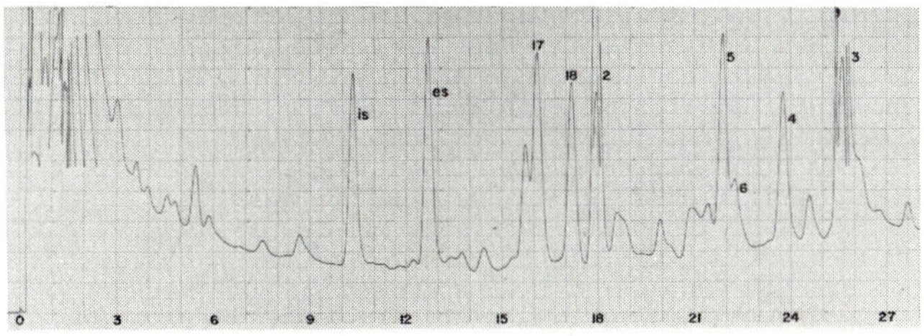

Fig. 2. Gas-chromatographic tracing of a supplemented urine (82.5 mg of creatinine per deciliter)

Supplement: 20 μl of a standard containing 20.0 μg of *o*-hydroxyphenylacetic acid, 20 μg of *m*-hydroxyphenylacetic acid, 20.0 μg of *p*-hydroxyphenylacetic acid, 20.0 μg of HVA, and 20.0 μg of VMA. At the end of extraction, specimen was silylated and a 3-μl sample injected onto the column Peak numbers and conditions correspond to those of Figure 1

pound relative to the other marker compounds (Table 2). The elution pattern could thus be used as a guide for the identification of compounds with other program rates.

Purification of urinary metabolites: Quantitation of urinary metabolites—either by thin-layer chromatography, gas chromatography, or spectrophotometry—requires an initial extraction and purification. Gas-chromatographic tracings of silylated unextracted human urine showed no peaks. Tracings of a one-step extraction showed poor resolution, overlapping of several peaks, and drifts in the baseline. A three-step extraction resulted in good resolution, permitting identification and quantitation of several compounds (Figure 1). Known amounts of standards were added to the same urine, and the resulting tracing is illustrated in Figure 2. The increased height of the peaks corresponding to the added compounds is obvious, as is their sharpness and symmetry.

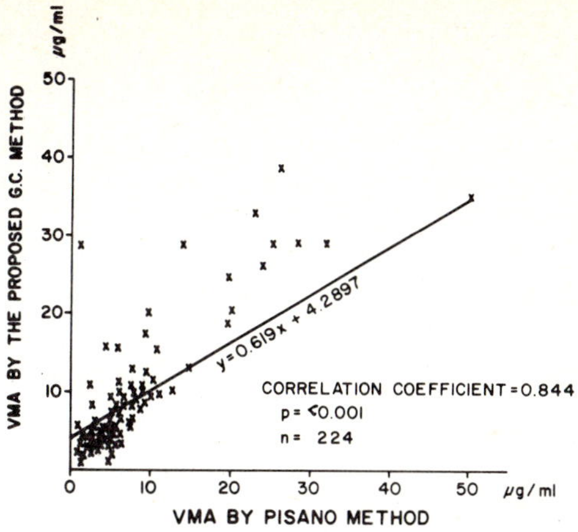

Fig. 3. Relation between VMA values obtained by the technique of Pisano et al. (*3*) and the present method

Analytical recovery of compounds: [^{3}H]VMA was used to evaluate the percentage extraction under the conditions described. The effects of pH (0.5 to 3.0) and sodium chloride saturation on Step I of the extraction are shown in Table 3. Saturation with sodium chloride enhanced the extraction of VMA at each pH value, for example from 49 to 81% at pH 3.0 and from 60 to 81% at pH 1.0. Thus, all of the urine samples were routinely adjusted to pH 1.0 and saturated with sodium chloride before extraction.

The percentage extraction of VMA at each step of the procedure was determined (Table 4). Of the added VMA, 85% was recovered in Step I and 75% at the end of Step III. The percentage extraction of added VMA was linear from 25 μg to 100 μg.

Recovery studies were also performed on different human urine samples to see if it varied from urine to urine. The percentage recoveries (±1 SD) from seven urines were 85 ± 11.00 for VMA and 93.7 ± 19.7 for HVA. The CV for other samples ranged from 2 to 14% for VMA, 1 to 18% for HVA, and 1 to 5% for phenylpropionic acid.

The CVs obtained for a 24-h urine quantitated six times during five weeks were 6.92% for VMA and 9.5% for HVA.

Our VMA values for 224 patients' urines were compared with those obtained by the technique of Pisano et al. (*3*) (Figure 3). The correlation coefficient, *r*, was 0.844. A highly significant ($P < 0.001$) simple linear regression was obtained.

External and internal standards: Some compounds were evaluated as external standards. Resorcinol added to different human urine samples was not extracted by this procedure. Benzoic acid was already present in several urine samples and so was not selected. Phenylpropionic acid was selected and has been used in the assay of more than 500 urine samples because it elutes in the middle of chromatogram, does not interfere with any of the peaks found in tracings of human urines, and is easily extractable (81.7%)—all desirable characteristics for an external standard. The ratio of the area of the phenylpropionic acid peak and that of resorcinol was used as a quality-control index for 26 extractions during seven months (Table 5). All values remained within the 95% confidence limits, indicating that the entire methodology was in control for this period. The CV of this ratio ranged from 2.0 to 10.5%.

Several compounds were tried for their suitability as internal standards. The elution time of estradiol was prolonged and consequently impractical. Phenanthrene dissolved into the reaction vial caps and eluted very near the hippuric peak. Trimesic acid (1,3,5-benzenetricarboxylic acid) eluted with an interfering peak. Similarly, C-19, C-20, and C-21 fatty acids were unsuitable. Resorcinol, the compound we chose as internal standard, should be dissolved in pyridine; if dimethylformamide is used as a solvent it attacks the reaction-vial caps.

Interfering substances: Ingestion of vanillin, coffee, bananas, or chocolate interferes with the determination of VMA by other methods (*4*). Vanillin does not interfere with our quantitation, because only about 10% is extracted by the present method and its retention time is different from VMA and HVA. For similar reasons, drugs such as aspirin and *o*-hydroxybenzoic acid and their metabolites do not interfere. In about 10 cases out of 1500 we observed that large quantities of urinary lactic acid interfered with the resolution of resorcinol from lactic acid dimer. In these instances, results for VMA and HVA were calculated based on the response of phenylpropionic acid. On a few other occasions, increased quantities of *p*-hydroxyphenyllactic acid, and, rarely, homogentisic acid, when present in very large quantity, interfered with VMA and HVA quantitations, respectively.

Different column lengths have been used by different authors: a 1.8-m column by Greer et al. (*5*) and Crawhall et al. (*6*) and a 3.7-m column by Gitlow et al. (*7*). We found a 7.6-m aluminum column to be unsatisfactory because broad, tailed peaks resulted. The 6.1-m glass column we used, longer than those conventionally employed, gives better resolution because of the increased number of theoretical plates.

This investigation was supported by USPHS General Research Support Grant RR 05504, National Science Foundation Grant GB-17634, and J. W. Champion Center, Children's Hospital. We thank Mr. Ronald L. Gombos for technical assistance, Ms. E. F. Freier, Department of Laboratory Medicine and Pathology, University of Minnesota, for determining VMA by Pisano's method, and Dr. Samuel Meites for helpful comments.

References

1. Williams, C. M., and Greer, M., IV, Estimation by gas chromatography of urinary homovanillic acid and vanilmandelic acid in neuroblastoma. In *Methods in Medical Research,* **12,** R. E. Olson, Editor-in-Chief, Year Book Medical Publishers, Chicago, Ill., 1970, pp 106–113.

2. Addanki, S., Hinnenkamp, E. R., Gombos, R. L., and Sotos, J. F., Neuroblastoma-investigation on urinary vanilmandelic (VMA) and homovanillic (HVA) acids by gas liquid chromatography (GLC). *Clin. Chem.* **18,** 691 (1972). Abstract.

3. Pisano, J. J., Crout, J. R., and Abraham, D., Determination of 3-methoxy-4-hydroxymandelic acid in urine. *Clin. Chim. Acta* **7,** 285 (1962).

4. Sunderman, F. W., Jr., Cleveland, P. D., Law, N. C., and Sunderman, F. W., A method for the determination of 3-methoxy-4-hydroxymandelic acid (vanilmandelic acid) for the diagnosis of pheochromocytoma. *Am. J. Clin. Pathol.* **34,** 293 (1960).

5. Greer, M., Anton, A. H., Williams, C. M., and Echevarria, R. A., Tumors of neural crest origin. *Arch. Neurol.* (Chicago) **13,** 139 (1965).

6. Crawhall, J. C., Mamer, O., Tjoa, S., and Claveau, J. D., Urinary phenolic acids in tyrosinemia. Identification by gas chromatography mass spectrometry. *Clin. Chim. Acta* **34,** 47 (1971).

7. Gitlow, S. E., Bertani, L. M., Rausen, A., et al., Diagnosis of neuroblastoma by qualitative and quantitative determination of catecholamine metabolites in urine. *Cancer* **25,** 1377 (1970).

CLIN. CHEM. 22/3, 315–322 (1976)

Determination of Apolipoprotein A and Its Constitutive A-I and A-II Polypeptides by Separate Electroimmunoassays

Michael D. Curry, Petar Alaupovic,[1] and C. Alan Suenram

Electroimmunoassays ("rocket" electrophoresis) are described for human serum apolipoprotein A and its constitutive A-I and A-II polypeptides. Purified lipoprotein A, A-I, and A-II were used to prepare monospecific antisera and to standardize assays. These specific, rapid (5–8 h), precise (the within- and between-assay coefficients of variations are 5 and 7%, respectively), and accurate (by gravimetry) assays are applicable to measurement of these polypeptides in whole serum and in various density classes of lipoproteins. Comparable results are obtained with intact and delipidized lipoproteins. Results correlated well with those obtained by radial immunodiffusion or radioimmunoassay. However, the present procedure is more rapid than the former and simpler than the latter immunoassay. Concentrations of A-I and A-II in the serum of normal men and women were similar (143 ± 24 and 146 ± 78 mg/dl, respectively, for A-I and 78 ± 17 and 83 ± 25 mg/dl for A-II). Subjects with type IIa, IIb, and IV hyperlipoproteinemias had similar concentrations of both polypeptides, while patients with type I disease, lecithin:cholesterol acyltransferase deficiency and LP-A deficiency had lowest concentrations of A-I (0.3–30 mg/dl) and A-II (11–20 mg/dl). The molar ratio of A-I/A-II in the serum and high-density lipoproteins was close to unity.

Additional Keyphrases: *"rocket" electrophoresis • reference values • radial immunodiffusion and radioimmunoassay compared • hyperlipoproteinemia • lecithin:cholesterol acyltransferase deficiency • lipoprotein A deficiency*

Lipoprotein Laboratory, Oklahoma Medical Research Foundation; and Department of Biochemistry and Molecular Biology, University of Oklahoma Health Sciences Center, Oklahoma City, Okla. 73104.

[1]Address correspondence to P. Alaupovic, Ph.D, Head, Lipoprotein Laboratory, Oklahoma Medical Research Foundation, 825 N. E. 13th St., Oklahoma City, Okla. 73104.

Received Nov. 6, 1975; accepted Dec. 18, 1975.

From a chemical viewpoint, the fundamental physical-chemical entities of serum lipoprotein systems are lipoprotein families rather than density or electrophoretic lipoprotein classes. A lipoprotein family is defined as a polydisperse lipoprotein distribution characterized by the presence of a single, distinct apolipoprotein or its constitutive polypeptides (*1–3*). The five currently recognized lipoprotein families are designated as LP-A, LP-B, LP-C, LP-D, and LP-E.[2] They occur as individual separable entities above a density range of 1.019–1.030 g/ml. Below this density range, lipoprotein families exist in the form of association complexes (*1, 4, 5*).

It has already been suggested (*1, 2*) that the proper functioning of the lipid-transport system depends both on the availability and an optimal concentration range of each apolipoprotein or its lipoprotein family. When a favorable concentration balance is disrupted by metabolic or genetic derangements, the defective lipid transport process(es) may be characterized by specific distribution patterns of lipoprotein families. To establish the relative and absolute concentration ranges of lipoprotein families in normal and hyperlipoproteinemic subjects, we used electroimmunoassay (*6*) as the method of measuring apolipoproteins or their constitutive polypeptides.

[2]Nonstandard abbreviations used: LP-A, lipoprotein A, characterized by apolipoprotein A as its protein moiety; LP-B, lipoprotein B, characterized by apolipoprotein B; LP-C, lipoprotein C, characterized by apolipoprotein C; LP-D, lipoprotein D, characterized by apolipoprotein D; LP-E, lipoprotein E, characterized by apolipoprotein E ("arginine-rich" polypeptide); ApoA, apolipoprotein A, consisting of A-I and A-II polypeptides; ApoB, apolipoprotein B; ApoC, apolipoprotein C, consisting of C-I, C-II, and C-III polypeptides; ApoD, apolipoprotein D; ApoE, apolipoprotein E; HDL, high-density lipoproteins.

This paper describes the adaptation of electroimmunoassay to the quantitative determination of apolipoprotein A (ApoA) and its A-I and A-II polypeptides. Studies on the column-chromatographic separation of A-I and A-II have yielded semiquantitative data on their concentrations in HDL fractions (*7–9*). Recently, methods describing quantification of A-I by radioimmunoassay (*10, 11*) and ApoA by electroimmunoassay (*12*) have been reported. Results presented in this paper show that the electroimmunoassays of ApoA and A-I and A-II polypeptides are sensitive, precise, accurate, technically simple, and rapid.

Materials and Methods

Isolation of Lipoproteins and Polypeptides

Lipoprotein density classes were isolated from serum samples of fasting normolipidemic subjects by sequential preparative ultracentrifugation (*13*). LP-A was isolated from HDL according to a previously described procedure (*3*). A-I and A-II polypeptides were isolated and characterized according to procedures described by Kostner and Alaupovic (*14*). HDL was delipidated by the procedure of Scanu (*15*).

Preparation of Antisera

We prepared monospecific antisera to A-I and A-II by immunizing rabbits with two successive intraperitoneal injections of 2 mg of antigen dissolved in 1 ml of 0.1 mol/liter $(NH_4)_2CO_3$ and an equal volume of complete Freund's adjuvant. The rabbits were bled by heart puncture, and the antibodies were detected three weeks after the second injection. The antisera were characterized by immunodiffusion and immunoelectrophoresis against A-I, A-II, ApoB, C-I, C-II, C-III, ApoD, and ApoE ("arginine-rich" polypeptide). Antisera to A-I and A-II only gave positive reactions with their corresponding antigens. The preparation and characterization of an antiserum to LP-A have been described previously (*3*).

Electroimmunoassays of ApoA, A-I and A-II

In the present adaptation of Laurell's electroimmunoassay (*16*), the supporting medium was prepared by melting agarose ("Indubiose" agarose powder; Gallard-Schlesinger, Carle Place, N.Y. 11514) 20 g per liter of diethylbarbiturate buffer (50 mmol/liter, pH 8.4) on a boiling water-bath with continuous stirring. Dextran T10 (Pharmacia Fine Chemicals, Piscataway, N. J. 08854) was added to the agarose solution to give a final concentration of 50 g/liter. Antiserum to either LP-A (0.8 ml), A-I, or A-II (0.3 ml) was thoroughly mixed with 25 ml of the agarose/Dextran solution, which had been allowed to cool to 55 °C. This mixture was then poured into a mold constructed of two glass plates separated by a **U**-frame (205 × 110 × 1.5 mm) and a strip of Cronar Graphic Arts film (clear base, type P-72, 0.007-inch thick; E. I. du Pont de Nemours & Co., Wilmington, Del. 19898) of similar dimensions. The film acted as support for the gel medium throughout the assay and provided a permanent backing after it was dried and stained. After the agarose mixture had congealed, 18 antigen wells of 4 mm diameter were punched out with center-to-center distances of 10 mm. Ten microliters of standard or sample, properly diluted with the buffer, was applied with a Drummond microdispenser. A normal serum usually required a 100- to 200-fold dilution for all three assays. For the electrophoresis we used an electrophoresis apparatus (Farbwerke Hoechst AG, Frankfurt, Federal Republic of Germany) connected to a variable voltage power supply with a maximum of 500 V and 350 mA. A field strength of 10 V cm^{-1} was applied to the electroimmunoassay plate for 4 h for ApoA, 4.5 h for A-I, and 3.5 h for A-II assay; the electrophoresis buffer was that described above. The temperature of water circulating through the electrophoresis platform was maintained at 15 °C with a Lauda K-2/RD refrigerated circulator (Brinkmann Instruments, Inc., Westbury, N. Y. 11590). The assay plate was placed in a bath containing NaCl (9 g/liter) for 1–2 h, blotted with Whatman No. 1 filter paper, and dried with hot air. Immunoprecipitates were stained with a 1.2 g/liter solution of Coomassie Brilliant Blue R (Sigma Chemical Co., St. Louis, Mo. 63178) (Coomassie Brilliant Blue R/water/acetic acid/95% ethanol, 2/2/2/1, by vol) for 10 min, and destained to a clear background in a solution of acetic acid/95% ethanol/water (1/3/5 by vol). The height in millimeters from the center of the antigen well to the apex of the rocket was measured with a microcomparator, millimeter graph paper, or ruler. Results by all three procedures of measurement were comparable, but, for simplicity, measurements were generally made with a ruler to the nearest 0.5 mm.

Radial Immunodiffusion

Radial immunodiffusion was performed by the method of Mancini et al. (*17*). Antiserum to either A-I or A-II (0.3 ml) was added to 25 ml of agarose solution (20 g per liter of the buffer) that had been cooled to 55 °C. This solution was poured into the mold described above and allowed to congeal. Twenty-one antigen wells of 2 mm diameter were punched out, and 5 μl of standard or serum was placed into each well. After this arrangement had been standing for 72–120 h in a humid chamber at 30 °C, the ring-shaped immunoprecipitates were measured.

Protein Analysis

Protein content of the A-I used as standard was determined by the following three methods: (*a*) *Amino acid analysis*—Immunochemically homogeneous polypeptide preparations were dried over P_2O_5 under reduced pressure and weighed on a Cahn electrobalance; the protein content was determined by amino acid analysis of 24- and 72-h hydrolysates

(*18*). (*b*) *Method of Lowry et al.* (*19*)—Protein content was estimated with human serum albumin as standard. (*c*) *Kjeldahl digestion and nitrogen determination with Nessler's reaction* (*20*)—Nitrogen values were converted to protein by using the factor 6.0 (16.76% N) calculated from the amino acid analysis. Although values obtained by all three methods agreed within 5%, those obtained by method *b* were consistently the lowest. For construction of the standard curve, we estimated the protein concentration of A-I from the amino acid analysis.

Protein content of immunochemically homogeneous A-II or LP-A preparations used as standards was also determined from the amino acid composition. Results obtained by method *b* were comparable.

Whole Serum Comparison Material

This was prepared by diluting normal human sera with a solution containing, per liter, 0.25 mole of sucrose, 9 g of NaCl, and 1.0 g of sodium azide in doubly distilled water. Aliquots of diluted serum were frozen (−70 °C alcohol bath), lyophilized, sealed under nitrogen, and stored in 2-ml ampuls at −30 °C. For use in the assays, these lyophilized sera were reconstituted with distilled water. Whole serum prepared and stored in this manner yielded reproducible values for A-I and A-II concentrations for longer than one year. After standard curves were obtained with A-I and A-II polypeptides, subsequent analyses were done with reference serum samples. Use of reference sera prepared at different times provided a check of their stability. Periodic restandardization with purified A-I and A-II polypeptides was undertaken, to evaluate stability of references or to observe any differences among standard curves obtained with different preparations.

Results

Standardization of Assays

Immunochemically homogeneous A-I and A-II polypeptides and LP-A of known protein content were used for constructing the standard curves. The relationship between rocket height (y) and protein concentration (x) was linear for all three assays [A-I, $y = 30x + 3$ ($r = 0.96$); A-II, $y = 17.1x + 4.6$ ($r = 0.98$); ApoA, $y = 6x + 4.5$ ($r = 0.98$)]. There was also a linear relationship between the protein concentration and the areas of immunoprecipitates. The slopes of the linear functions obtained with whole serum, HDL, or LP-A agreed well with the standard curves produced with ApoA polypeptides. For the same concentration of A-I or A-II, the heights and areas of the immunoprecipitates formed with either polypeptides, whole serum, intact HDL, or LP-A were identical. Figure 1 shows the characteristic rocket shapes of A-I and A-II.

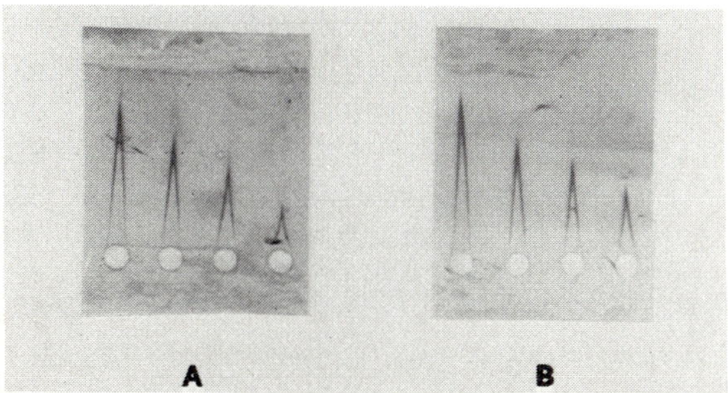

Fig. 1. Immunoprecipitation ("rockets") of A-I (*A*) and A-II (*B*)

Sensitivity of Assays

The assay sensitivity, defined under present experimental conditions as the lowest point of linearity between rocket height and protein concentration, was about 0.2 mg/100 ml of whole serum for both A-I and A-II, and 1.0 mg/100 ml of whole serum for ApoA. These values correspond to 20 ng of A-I or A-II and 100 ng of ApoA applied to the sample well. The sensitivity of assays can be further enhanced by lowering the concentration of antibodies.

Precision of Assays

Within-assay precision—i.e., precision within the same electroimmunoassay plate—was assessed for all three assays. Ten samples, representative of the entire concentration range of standards, were analyzed on separate plates. Each sample was added to several wells at various positions across the plate. The standard deviation (SD) and the coefficient of variation [(SD/mean) × 100] were calculated for each sample. Similarly, between-assay reproducibility—i.e., precision computed from the mean of five separate assays on 10 different samples at one-week intervals—was assessed for ApoA, A-I, and A-II. Within- and between-assay coefficients of variation for A-I, A-II, and ApoA analyses were 5% and 7%, respectively. They were consistent over the entire linear range of the standard curves.

Electroimmunoassay of A-I and A-II in Intact and Delipidized Lipoproteins

Five HDL samples isolated from sera of normal and hyperlipoproteinemic subjects were assayed for A-I and A-II polypeptides in their intact and totally delipidized forms. The results of this experiment (Table 1) indicated that delipidization of HDL neither exposed nor destroyed any antigenic determinants of A-I or A-II polypeptides. These results also demonstrated that any possible changes in the electrophoretic mobility of delipidized HDL had no effect on the concentrations of A-I and A-II polypeptides. The average weight ratio of A-I/A-II for these five preparations was 1.7 (Table 1). A-I accounted for 55% (range, 47–63%) and A-II for 31% (range, 24–36%) of the total protein content of HDL (Table 2). Differences in the relative contents of A-I and A-II in various HDL preparations were due to the number of recentrifugations required to remove albumin and the presence of various concentrations of other lipo-

Table 1. Electroimmunoassay of A-I and A-II Polypeptides in Intact and Delipidized HDL[a]

High-density fraction	A-I	A-II	Weight ratio A-I/A-II
	mg		
Intact HDL (I)	129	80	1.6
Delipidized HDL (D)	128	68	1.9
I	83	53	1.6
D	90	56	1.6
I	116	65	1.8
D	105	53	2.0
I	8	6	1.3
D	8	5	1.5
I	63	36	1.8
D	68	35	1.9
		Mean weight ratio	1.70

[a] Each sample represents a different aliquot of five separate HDL preparations.

Table 2. Relative Content of A-I and A-II Polypeptides in Various HDL Preparations[a]

Total protein (mg/100 ml)	A-I polypeptide	A-II polypeptide	Sum of A-I and A-II (ApoA)
		%	
222	58.0	31.0	89.0
174	52.0	32.0	84.0
225	47.0	24.0	71.0
14.0	57.0	36.0	93.0
108	63.0	32.0	95.0
Range	47–63	24–36	71–95
Mean	55	31	86

[a] Relative content of A-I and A-II polypeptides expressed as percentage of total HDL protein.

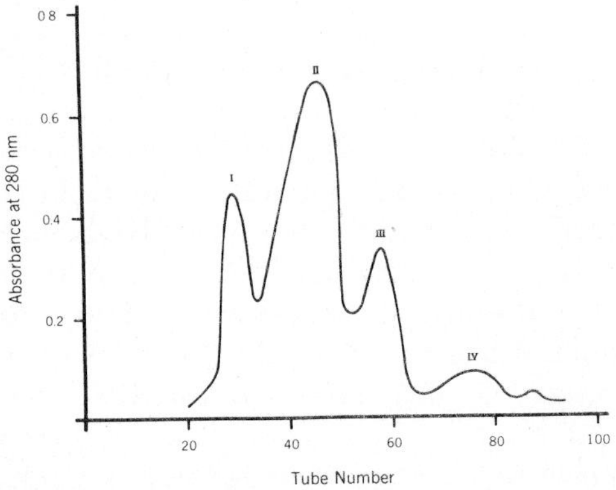

Fig. 2. Fractionation of apoHDL_3 (*d*, 1.13–1.21 g/ml) on a Sephadex G-100 column (2.5 × 100 cm) eluted with acetic acid, 2 mol/liter (5.5 ml/tube)

protein families, including LP-B, LP-C, LP-D, and LP-E.

To provide direct evidence for the accuracy of A-I and A-II estimations, a preparation of totally delipidized HDL_3 was fractionated by column chromatography on Sephadex G-100; the polypeptide content of four fractions (Figure 2) was determined by gravimetry and electroimmunoassays. Results showed (Table 3) that each fraction contained more than one polypeptide. Although fraction II consisted mainly of A-I and fraction III of A-II, both fractions contained measurable amounts of both polypeptides. In addition, fractions III and IV contained ApoD and ApoC polypeptides, which accounted for the remaining protein content of these fractions. Adequate separation of A-I and A-II required more than a single chromatography; additional manipulation of polypeptide fractions resulted in too many sources of experimental error to allow quantitative recoveries. Results were also inconclusive when totally delipidized HDL_3 were fractionated on immunosorbers to A-I and A-II. Either the nonspecific adsorption or protein–protein interactions, or both, prevented a complete separation of A-I and A-II by a single passage over the immunosorbers. Because column-chromatographic procedures proved to be inadequate as a means for assessing the accuracy of electroimmunoassays, the sum of separately determined A-I and A-II concentrations was compared with the gravimetrically measured protein content of HDL_3 (Table 4). Two HDL fractions (*d*, 1.13–1.21 g/ml) were isolated from individual donors and purified by repeated ultracentrifugations until free of albumin. The A-I and A-II concentrations were determined by electroimmunoassay. The total protein content was quantified by gravimetric determination of exhaustively dialyzed and delipidized HDL aliquots. Although these two HDL samples also contained LP-C and LP-D, their contri-

Table 3. Gel-Filtration Chromatography of ApoHDL_3 (*d*, 1.13–1.21 g/ml) on Sephadex G-100 and Distribution of A-I and A-II Polypeptides

Fraction	Protein	A-I	A-II	Total protein as ApoA polypeptides
		mg		%
I	4.4	3.0	1.1	93
II	36.0	29.0	6.8	99
III	14.0	1.5	8.1	68.5
IV	3.2	Not detectable	1.9	59.0
Total	57.6	33.5	17.9	

A-I accounts for 58% protein recovered; A-II accounts for 31% protein recovered; ApoA (A-I + A-II) accounts for 89% protein recovered.

Table 4. Comparison of Electroimmunoassay and Gravimetry for Quantitative Determination of Apolipoprotein A in a HDL Fraction (*d*, 1.13–1.21 g/ml)

Subject	Apolipoprotein A by electroimmunoassay	Protein content by gravimetry
	mg	
1	48	49
2	85	95

Table 5. Comparison of Serum Apolipoprotein A Concentrations Estimated by Single and Separate Electroimmunoassays

Subjects	Apolipoprotein A (electroimmunoassay of ApoA)	A-I + A-II (separate electroimmunoassays)
Male (n = 8)	254 ± 39	246 ± 24
Female (n = 15)	268 ± 75	245 ± 71

Table 6. Concentrations of A-I and A-II Polypeptides in Whole Serum of Normal and Hyperlipoproteinemic Subjects

Subjects			A-I	A-II	A-I/A-II weight ratio
Type	Sex	No.	mg/100 ml ± SD		
Normal	M	19	143 ± 24	78 ± 17	1.83
	F	19	146 ± 78	83 ± 25	1.75
I	M	2	27 ± 7	19 ± 2	1.42
II-a	M	5	140 ± 19	93 ± 14	1.50
	F	7	154 ± 10	96 ± 15	1.60
II-b	M	2	118 ± 2	78 ± 4	1.51
	F	4	138 ± 19	103 ± 27	1.33
IV	M	6	120 ± 6	76 ± 17	1.57
	F	9	152 ± 34	108 ± 31	1.40

bution to the total protein content was small. The sum of A-I and A-II contents as estimated by electroimmunoassay agreed closely with the dry weight of HDL protein (Table 4).

Electroimmunoassay of ApoA

The A-I and A-II polypeptides are integral constituents of apolipoprotein A and its corresponding lipoprotein family LP-A (*1, 3*). To develop an electroimmunoassay for the determination of ApoA, we utilized an antiserum to LP-A (*3*) that contained antibodies to both A-I and A-II polypeptides. Results in Table 5 show that the ApoA concentrations estimated by this assay agree excellently with the sum of A-I and A-II concentrations assayed separately on the same samples.

Quantification of A-I and A-II in Whole Serum and Lipoprotein Density Classes

Results of quantitative determination of A-I and A-II in normal and some hyperlipoproteinemic serum samples from men and women are presented in Table 6. The mean A-I content of normolipidemic serum was 143 mg/100 ml for men and 146 mg/100 ml for women. The corresponding concentrations of A-II were 78 mg/100 ml and 83 mg/100 ml, respectively. Whereas patients with type IIa hyperlipoproteinemia had normal serum concentrations of A-I and A-II, men with type IIb and type IV hyperlipoproteinemias had slightly lower levels of A-I. Owing to a relatively small number of samples, the statistical significance of this trend in A-I values could not be assessed from the results of this study. In contrast to these results, two patients with hyperchylomicronemia (type I disease) were characterized by significantly lower concentrations of both polypeptides in their serum; A-I and A-II accounted for only one-fifth to one-fourth of the normal values. We have already reported (*21*) that patients with lecithin:cholesterol acyltransferase (EC 2.3.1.43) deficiency are also characterized by low concentrations of A-I (40 mg/100

Table 7. Distribution of A-I and A-II Polypeptides among the Lipoprotein Density Classes from Seven Normal Human Sera[a]

Whole serum and density classes, g/ml	A-I polypeptide, mg/100 ml	Percent of total A-I	A-II polypeptide, mg/100 ml	Percent of total A-II	Weight ratio A-I/A-II
Serum	145 ± 5	—	90 ± 11	—	1.6
d < 1.006	0.6 ± .3	0.4	0.3 ± .2	0.3	2.0
1.006–1.019	0.3 ± .2	0.2	.15 ± .1	0.2	2.0
1.019–1.063	0.8 ± .5	0.6	0.4 ± .2	0.4	2.0
1.063–1.13	28 ± 7	19	14 ± 5	16	2.0
1.13–1.21	98 ± 7	68	67 ± 10	74	1.5
d > 1.21	17 ± 9	12	8 ± 6	9.0	2.2

[a] The A-I and A-II concentrations of density classes were adjusted to the serum volume and to 100 percent recovery of the serum apolipoprotein concentrations. Separate experiments indicated that the relative losses of ApoA polypeptides during ultracentrifugation from *d* 1.063–1.13 and *d* 1.13–1.21 were the same.

ml) and A-II (25 mg/100 ml) polypeptides. However, the lowest concentrations of both polypeptides in serum were recorded in a case of LP-A deficiency (*22*) with only trace amounts (0.3 mg/100 ml) of A-I and 11 mg/100 ml of A-II.

The average weight ratio of A-I/A-II in the whole serum of normolipidemic men and women was 1.85 and 1.75, respectively. Corresponding ratios in all forms of primary hyperlipoproteinemia ranged between 1.40 and 1.60 (Table 6).

The distribution of ApoA polypeptides among lipoprotein density classes was determined in unwashed fractions, because preparation of albumin-free lipoproteins by repeated ultracentrifugations resulted in substantial losses (30–40%) of both polypeptides. Although the greatest portion of ApoA polypeptides was present in HDL (87–90%), all major density classes had measurable amounts of A-I and A-II (Table 7). Combined very-low-density and low-density lipoproteins contained about 1% and very-high-density lipoproteins about 10% of the total serum ApoA content. The distribution of A-I and A-II polypeptides among lipoproteins with $d < 1.063$, HDL and VHDL was the same (1%, 88%, and 11%, respectively. There was, however, a small difference in the A-I/A-II ratios between HDL_2 and HDL_3 fractions. The higher A-I/A-II ratio of HDL_2 and very-high-density lipoproteins probably reflected the already established occurrence in these density regions of some LP-A-I (lipoprotein family characterized by the presence of only A-I as its protein moiety) in addition to LP-A (*3, 23*). The molar ratio of A-I and A-II polypeptides in whole serum and HDL_3 was close to unity, indicating a constant polypeptide composition of ApoA regardless of the lipid composition of polydisperse LP-A.

Comparison of Electroimmunoassay and Radial Immunodiffusion

Radial immunodiffusion assays of whole sera and HDL were performed with use of A-I and A-II as standards and the corresponding monospecific antisera. There was a linear relationship between the squared diameter of precipitate rings and amount of protein in the standards. The same samples of whole serum and HDL were assayed by electroimmunoassay. Correlation coefficients, r, for A-I and A-II concentrations by electroimmunoassay vs. radial immunodiffusion were 0.85 and 0.90, respectively. Although both immunological methods yielded comparable results, the coefficients of variation for within- (10%) and between- (15%) assays were greater than those of electroimmunoassay.

Discussion

Results of this study show that ApoA in whole serum or density classes can be quantitatively determined either by an electroimmunoassay of ApoA or by separate assays of A-I and A-II polypeptides. The specificity was substantiated by results of A-I and A-II quantification in patients with hyperchylomicronemia, lecithin:cholesterol acyltransferase deficiency, and in a subject with LP-A deficiency. In hyperchylomicronemia, the low concentrations of A-I and A-II corresponded well with decreased concentrations of HDL cholesterol (*24*). Low concentrations of A-I and A-II polypeptides in lecithin:cholesterol acyltransferase deficiency confirmed previous reports indicating a substantial reduction of ApoA in this familial disease (*21, 25*). The LP-A deficiency (*22*) was characterized by near absence of A-I and severe deficiency of A-II.

Precision of all three electroimmunoassays equalled those of reported radioimmunoassays of A-I (*10, 11*). Our own results showed that the electroimmunoassays were more precise than the radial immunodiffusion assays of ApoA polypeptides.

Results of the accuracy tests showed that the values for ApoA (encompassing A-I and A-II polypeptides) estimated by electroimmunoassay agreed closely not only with the sum of separately determined values for A-I and A-II but also with those estimated gravimetrically. The concentrations of A-I and A-II determined by electroimmunoassay were very similar, if not identical, to those estimated by radial immunodiffusion. Farish et al. (*12*) have recently described an electroimmunoassay of ApoA. Although the assay was based on an HDL_3 preparation and a commercially obtained antiserum to α_1-lipoproteins, the reported values for serum ApoA concentrations agreed well with ours.

The mean value (143 ± 24 mg/100 ml) for the A-I concentration in whole serum compares favorably with a corresponding value for A-I (121 ± 16 mg/100 ml) estimated by one (*11*) of the three recently published radioimmunoassays, but is somewhat higher than the values (102 ± 5 and 100 ± 35 mg/100 ml) reported by Starr et al. (*26*) and Schonfeld and Pfleger (*10*). The relatively low values for A-I reported in the last-cited study may have been caused by the necessity to extract lipoproteins before A-I could be reliably measured. The additional manipulation of samples and incomplete solubilization of delipidized lipoproteins may have accounted for some loss of A-I. In both fully published reports (*10, 11*) on the radioimmunoassay of A-I, the accuracy was only tested by column-chromatographic separation and determination of A-I. In one case (*10*) the values obtained by radioimmunoassay were lower and in the other (*11*) they were higher than those estimated by column chromatography. In general, however, results obtained by electroimmunoassay and radioimmunoassay seem to agree well; some differences among reported values for ApoA polypeptides in serum may be attributable to population differences, or to the relatively small number of analyses performed, or both. Differences among reported HDL concentrations of ApoA may be attributed to isolation effects.

There are no previously reported data for A-II concentrations in the whole serum or density classes that could be compared with results presented in this study. Quantification of A-II by electroimmunoassay and by radial immunodiffusion gave the same results. Although all A-II values were arrived at independently, they agree well with those that can be deduced from results for ApoA and A-I.

Results of quantitative determination of ApoA polypeptides in whole serum of normolipidemic subjects indicated no sex-related difference in values for A-I and A-II. This finding was similar to that of Schonfeld and Pfleger (*10*), but differed from data reported by Farish et al. (*12*) and Starr et al. (*26*). Since age of subjects may have influenced the data in each of these series of experiments, the clarification of contrasting results must await additional studies with larger population samples of well-defined age groups. The concentrations of A-I and A-II in serum were similar in normal subjects and patients with types IIa, IIb, or IV hyperlipoproteinemia. This finding confirms results reported by Schonfeld and Pfleger (*10*), who found no difference in A-I concentrations of normal and hyperlipoproteinemic subjects.

A-I polypeptide accounted on an average for 55% and A-II polypeptide for 31% of the HDL protein. These data confirmed a previous report of ApoA content of HDL (*3*). The weight ratio of A-I and A-II in whole serum and HDL was consistently lower (1.7 ± 0.2) than those (2.5–3.0) based on spectrophotometric estimation of column-chromatographic eluates. More significantly from a structural point of view, these results indicated that the molar ratios of A-I and A-II were close to unity.

Detection of substantial amounts of ApoA polypeptides in the very-high-density lipoprotein fraction has confirmed similar findings by other investigators (*10–12, 23, 27, 28*), who have attributed the presence of A-I in this fraction to the formation of an artifactitious lipoprotein by ultracentrifugation or high salt concentration, or both. It has already been shown that the extent of degradation of ApoA-containing lipoproteins depends on the number of ultracentrifugal runs required for the sequential isolation and purification of HDL (*11, 28*). This degradative effect of ultracentrifugation seems to be the main reason for the discrepancy between serum ApoA values as determined by any of the reported immunoassays and those estimated from the percentage protein content of ultracentrifugally isolated and measured HDL. The protein values calculated from HDL concentrations (*29*) may be 15–40% lower than those of serum ApoA values determined by immunoassays. These results clearly indicate the drawbacks of ultracentrifugal methodology and emphasize the need for an alternative procedure(s) for isolating and measuring ApoA-containing lipoproteins.

Present electroimmunoassays represent the most rapid immunochemical method for quantitative determination of ApoA polypeptides. Even though quantification by radial immunodiffusion is a technically simple procedure, there are at least three aspects of electroimmunoassay that make it the method of choice. Quantification by electroimmunoassay can be accomplished by use of polyvalent antisera. Secondly, the electroimmunoassay can be completed in 5–8 h, whereas radial immunodiffusion requires at least 3 days. Finally, the rocket-shaped immunoprecipitates often provide important clues about the free and associated forms of lipoprotein families. For example, the reaction between LP-A and anti-LP-A was characterized by one and not two rockets, indicating that A-I and A-II are integral components of ApoA or its corresponding lipoprotein family LP-A. On the other hand, a reaction between whole serum or HDL and a mixture of antisera to ApoA and ApoD yielded two separate rockets, indicating that these two apolipoproteins form separate physical-chemical entities or lipoprotein families. These arguments are also applicable to a comparison of electroimmunoassay and radioimmunoassay. More importantly, electroimmunoassay does not require some of the burdensome tasks of radioimmunoassay such as frequent preparations of radioactively labeled antigens with retained immunoactivity, rechromatography of the labeled antigen before each assay, and evaluation of all reagents for nonspecific binding. Unless sensitivities comparable to serum hormone concentrations are required, ApoA polypeptides can be measured with the same precision and accuracy but more rapidly by the electroimmunoassay than by the radioimmunoassay. Electroimmunoassay is especially suited for screening studies of large population samples.

This work was supported in part by USPHS Grant HE-6221 and by Contract NO1-HV-2-2932 from NHLI, NIH. We thank Dr. W. J. McConathy for valuable suggestions in course of these studies. We also thank Mr. J. Fesmire and Mrs. C. Quiroga for valuable technical assistance, Mr. R. Burns for preparing the drawings, and Mrs. M. Farmer for typing the manuscript.

References

1. Alaupovic, P., Conceptual development of the classification systems of plasma lipoproteins. In *Protides of Biological Fluids*, 19th Colloquium. H. Peeters, Ed. Pergamon Press, Oxford & New York, 1971, p 9.

2. Alaupovic, P., Apolipoproteins and lipoproteins. *Atherosclerosis* **13**, 141 (1971).

3. Kostner, G., and Alaupovic, P., Studies of the composition and structure of plasma lipoproteins. Separation and quantification of the lipoprotein families occurring in the high density lipoproteins of human plasma. *Biochemistry* **11**, 3419 (1972).

4. Gustafson, A., Alaupovic, P., and Furman, R. H., Studies of the composition and structure of serum lipoproteins. Separation and characterization of phospholipid-protein residues obtained by partial delipidization of very low density lipoproteins of human serum. *Biochemistry* **5**, 632 (1966).

5. Lee, D. M., and Alaupovic, P., Physicochemical properties of low-density lipoproteins of normal human plasma. Evidence for the occurrence of lipoprotein B in associated and free forms. *Biochem. J.* **137**, 155 (1974).

6. Laurell, C. B., Quantitative estimation of proteins by electrophoresis in agarose gel containing antibodies. *Anal. Biochem.* **15**, 45 (1966).

7. Shore, B., and Shore, V., Heterogeneity in protein subunits of human serum high-density lipoproteins. *Biochemistry* **7**, 2773 (1968).

8. Scanu, A., Toth, J., Edelstein, C., et al., Fractionation of human serum high density lipoprotein in urea solutions. Evidence for polypeptide heterogeneity. *Biochemistry* **8,** 3309 (1969).

9. Rudman, D, Garcia, L. A., and Howard, C. H., A new method for isolating the nonidentical protein subunits of human plasma α-lipoprotein. *J. Clin. Invest.* **49,** 365 (1970).

10. Schonfeld, G., and Pfleger, B., The structure of human high density lipoprotein and the levels of apolipoprotein A-I in plasma as determined by radioimmunoassay. *J. Clin. Invest.* **54,** 236 (1974).

11. Fainaru, M., Glangean, M. C., and Eisenberg, S., Radioimmunoassay of human high density lipoprotein apoprotein A-I. *Biochim. Biophys. Acta* **386,** 452 (1975).

12. Farish, E., Shepherd, J., Lawrie, T. D. V., and Morgan, H. G., Plasma apolipoprotein A levels in healthy human adults. *Clin. Chim. Acta* **62,** 97 (1975).

13. Havel, R. J., Eder, H. A., and Bragdon, J. H., The distribution and chemical composition of ultracentrifugally separated lipoproteins in human serum. *J. Clin. Invest.* **34,** 1345 (1955).

14. Kostner, G., and Alaupovic, P., Studies of the composition and structure of plasma lipoproteins. C- and N-terminal amino acids of the two nonidentical polypeptides of human plasma apolipoprotein A. *FEBS Lett.* **15,** 320 (1971).

15. Scanu, A., Forms of human serum high density lipoprotein protein. *J. Lipid Res.* **7,** 295 (1966).

16. Laurell, C. B., Electroimmunoassay. *Scand. J. Clin. Lab. Invest.* **29,** *Suppl.* **124,** 21 (1972).

17. Mancini, G., Carbonara, A. O., and Heremans, J. F., Immunochemical quantitation of antigens by single radial immunodiffusion. *Immunochemistry* **2,** 235 (1965).

18. Lee, D. M., and Alaupovic, P., Studies of the composition and structure of plasma lipoproteins. Isolation, composition, and immunochemical characterization of low density lipoprotein subfractions of human plasma. *Biochemistry* **9,** 2244 (1970).

19. Lowry, O. H., Rosebrough, N. J., Farr, A. L., and Randall, R. J., Protein measurement with the Folin phenol reagent. *J. Biol. Chem.* **193,** 265 (1951).

20. Williams, C. A., and Chase, M. W., *Methods in Immunology and Immunochemistry* **II,** Academic Press, New York, N. Y., 1968, p 249.

21. Alaupovic, P., McConathy, W. J., Curry, M. D., et al., Apolipoproteins and lipoprotein families in familial lecithin:cholesterol acyltransferase deficiency. *Scand. J. Clin. Lab. Invest.* **33,** *Suppl.* **137,** 83 (1974).

22. Lindeskog, G. R., Gustafson, A., and Enerbäck, L., Serum lipoprotein deficiency in diffuse "normolipemic" plane xanthoma. *Arch. Dermatol.* **106,** 529 (1972).

23. Albers, J. J., and Aladjem, F., Precipitation of ^{125}I-labeled lipoproteins with specific polypeptide antisera. Evidence for two populations with differing polypeptide compositions in human high density lipoproteins. *Biochemistry* **10,** 3436 (1971).

24. Fredrickson, D. S., Levy, R. I., and Lindgren, F. T., A comparison of heritable abnormal lipoprotein patterns as defined by two different techniques. *J. Clin. Invest.* **47,** 2446 (1968).

25. Torsvik, H., Presence of α_1-lipoprotein in patients with familial plasma lecithin:cholesterol acyltransferase deficiency. *Scand. J. Clin. Lab. Invest.* **24,** 187 (1969).

26. Starr, J. I., Juhn, D. J., Mako, M. E., et al., Circulating high density lipoprotein (HDL): Measurement of an apoprotein component by radioimmunoassay. *J. Clin. Invest.* **52,** 81a (1973).

27. Levy, R. I., and Fredrickson, D. S., Heterogeneity of plasma high density lipoproteins. *J. Clin. Invest.* **44,** 426 (1965).

28. Scanu, A., and Granda, J. L., Effects of ultracentrifugation on the human serum high-density ($1.036 < \rho < 1.21$ g/ml) lipoprotein. *Biochemistry* **5,** 446 (1966).

29. Ewing, A. M., Freeman, N. K., and Lindgren, F. T., The analysis of human serum lipoprotein distributions. *Adv. Lipid Res.* **3,** 25 (1965).

Use of Enzyme-loaded Erythrocytes in In-Vitro Correction of Arginase-Deficient Erythrocytes in Familial Hyperargininemia

Karel Adriaenssens,[1] Denise Karcher,[2] Armand Lowenthal,[2] and Heinz G. Terheggen[3]

The capacity of arginase-deficient erythrocytes of patients with familial hyperargininemia to produce urea and to catabolize arginine can be increased in vitro by introducing human liver arginase into their erythrocytes. The results of this study on a specific human model show that it is possible to change the metabolic function of a genetically defective erythrocyte by incorporating exogenous human enzyme. The in vivo application of enzyme-loaded erythrocytes for enzyme replacement therapy of inborn metabolic errors in humans must await in vivo studies on animal models.

Additional Keyphrase: *potential enzymic therapy of certain inherited disorders*

Familial hyperargininemia with arginase deficiency of erythrocytes is an inborn error of the urea cycle described in only two families (*1, 2*). Arginase (EC 3.5.3.1) catalyzes the conversion of arginine to ornithine and urea. Clinically, the disease is characterized by mental retardation, spastic paralysis, seizures, ataxia, tremor, and periodic vomiting. Important biochemical abnormalities are high plasma concentrations of arginine and ammonia and a secondary cystinuria/lysinuria (*3*).

Proteins (*4, 5*) and enzymes (*6*) can be introduced into erythrocytes during hypotonic hemolysis. Using these techniques, we loaded normal human erythrocytes and arginase-deficient erythrocytes from two patients with arginase deficiency and one obligate heterozygote with exogenous arginase and we compared the capacity to produce urea and to catabolize arginine of these arginase-loaded erythrocytes with that of the original erythrocytes. Potential therapeutic implications of some inborn errors of metabolism are proposed in terms of this model.

[1] Provincial Institute for Hygiene and University of Antwerp, Universiteitsplein, 1, 2610 Wilrijk, Belgium.
[2] Born-Bunge Foundation and University of Antwerp, 2610 Wilrijk, Belgium.
[3] Children's Hospital, Cologne, West Germany.
Received October 27, 1975; accepted Dec. 18, 1975.

Materials and Methods

Materials

Blood samples: Citrated blood samples were obtained from normal controls, from two patients, and from one obligate heterozygote with familial hyperargininemia. The plasma was separated by centrifugation and used as described below. Packed erythrocytes were prepared by washing and centrifuging (3000 rpm) the cells three times with five volumes of isotonic sodium chloride solution. Each time, the buffy coat was carefully discarded.

Arginase: Bovine liver arginase prepared by the method of Greenberg with an activity of 5.4 kU/g was purchased from Sigma Chemical Co., St. Louis, Mo. 63178 (lot No. 44 C-8210). Purified human liver arginase was prepared by the method of Schimke (*7*); the activity was 10.4 kU/g.

Procedures

Arginase activity was measured according to the method of Azizi et al. (*8*); one unit equals 1 μmol of urea produced per minute at 37 °C in 0.1 mol/liter arginine at pH 10.14 (glycine buffer) after activation of the enzyme for 20 min in 65 millimolar Mn^{2+} at 55 °C.

Urea was measured by the diacetylmonoxime method of Marsh et al. (*9*).

Arginine was measured by the column-chromatographic method of Efron (*10*).

Arginase loading of the erythrocytes: To prepare the erythrocytes we added one volume of packed cells to 16 volumes of 30 mmol/liter sodium chloride solution (0.2 of isotonic solution) containing various amounts of arginase. After 1 min of this hypotonic hemolysis (*5*), the isotonicity was restored with 3.4 volumes of 750 mmol/liter hypertonic sodium chloride and the membranes were allowed to reseal during 5 to 30 min at 37 °C (*11*). The arginase-loaded cells were then centrifuged (3000 rpm) and washed several times with isotonic sodium chloride. The argi-

Table 1. Values Found for Plasma Arginine and Erythrocyte Arginase

	Human controls	Hyperargininemia patients: Homozygotes (3 patients)	Hyperargininemia patients: Heterozygotes (2 patients)
Plasma arginine, μmol/dl	Mean, 8.17 SD, 1.81	mean, 62.02 (30 samples) range, 45.23–73.32	mean, 18.29 (10 samples) range, 13.2–26.7
Erythrocyte arginase, U/ml	11.6 (12 controls) range, 6–16.8	range, 0–0.5	range, 3.5–3.8

nase activity of packed erythrocytes and hemolyzing solutions is expressed in U/ml (=kU/liter).

Urea production: To measure urea production, we incubated 10 μl of packed erythrocytes for 20 to 60 min at 37 °C and pH 7.4 in 100 μl of their own plasma, adding 1 mmol/liter of arginine to simulate hyperargininemia. Identical volumes of the same, but unincubated, samples served as blanks. The urea production is expressed in μmol/ml of packed cells per hour.

Arginine catabolism: To measure arginine catabolism, we incubated 10 μl of packed erythrocytes for 60 min at 37 °C and pH 7.4 in 200 μl of their own plasma. Various amounts of arginine were added at the start of the incubation and the decrease of arginine was measured. The results are expressed in μmol/dl.

Results

Plasma arginine and erythrocyte arginase activity: Table 1 shows the plasma arginine and the erythrocyte arginase values for the normal controls, the homozygotes, and the heterozygotes with familial hyperargininemia. The inverse correlation of plasma arginine values and erythrocyte arginase activity in the different groups is obvious.

Arginase loading of erythrocytes: Table 2 shows that arginase can be introduced into human erythrocytes and that in patients with arginase deficiency and in the obligate heterozygote the erythrocyte arginase activity can be brought within the normal range.

The amounts of arginase introduced into the erythrocytes correlates with the arginase present in the hemolyzing solutions.

The higher amounts of arginase in the loaded erythrocytes compared to the amounts in the corresponding hemolyzing solutions can be explained by the increase in erythrocyte volume during the hemolysis and by the closure of the transient holes in the erythrocyte membrane before the decrease in the erythrocyte volume when isotonicity was restored.

Urea production: Table 3 shows that the urea production in normal erythrocytes and the very low to nonexistent urea production in arginase-deficient erythrocytes of familial hyperargininemia patients can be increased in vitro by introducing controlled amounts of arginase.

Arginine catabolism: The inability of the arginase-deficient erythrocytes to catabolize arginine can be abolished by loading these erythrocytes with arginase, as shown in Table 4.

Table 2. Arginase Activity Introduced into Erythrocytes

Type of erythrocytes	Original activity (U/ml)	Activity in hemolyzing solution (U/ml)	Activity in loaded erythrocytes (U/ml)
Human controls[a]			
Control 1	16.80	37.20	44.40
Control 2	16.00	27.60	37.40
Control 3	15.80	14.50	18.20
Control 4	8.60	13.80	22.80
Familial hyperargininemia[b]			
Patient 1	0.30	4.40	6.20
		5.00	9.50
		8.10	14.50
Patient 2	0.50	4.40	5.20
		5.00	9.20
		8.10	12.80
Obligate heterozygote	3.50	4.40	6.20

[a] Loaded with bovine liver arginase.
[b] Loaded with human liver arginase.

Stability of arginase-loaded erythrocytes in vitro: The exogenously introduced arginase activity and the increased urea production are maintained in vitro for at least 12 days, when the human erythrocytes are kept at 4 °C in acid citrate–glucose solution. Very little arginase leaks from the cells into the medium. Arginase activity in the cells was 44.4 U/ml initially, 35.9 U/ml 12 days later; corresponding values for the supernate were 0.7 and 2.1 U/ml.

Discussion

The introduction of exogenous enzymes into erythrocytes as a method of treatment of inborn errors, especially Gaucher's disease, has been suggested by Ihler et al. (*12*), who loaded human erythrocytes with rat kidney β-galactosidase and β-glucosidase.

Fiddler et al. (*13*) used the method of Ihler et al. to study in vivo the fate of bovine β-glucuronidase en-

Table 3. Arginase Activity and Urea Production in Erythrocytes: Effect of Arginase Loading

Type of erythrocytes	Arginase activity U/ml packed cells	Urea produced µmol/ml packed cells per h
Original		
Human controls	mean, 11.60 (12 controls) range, 6.00–16.80	mean, 1.80 (9 controls) range, 0.30–3.90
Hyperargininemia		
Patient 1	0.30	0.00 (4 samples)
Patient 2	0.50	0.00 (4 samples)
Arginase loaded		
Human controls (bovine liver arginase)		
Control 1	44.40	7.20
Control 2	32.13	8.40
Control 3	35.59	6.00
Hyperargininemia (human liver arginase)		
Patient 1 sample 1	9.50	16.80
sample 2	14.50	19.80
Patient 2 sample 1	9.20	7.80
sample 2	12.80	15.60

trapped in erythrocytes after injection into β-glucuronidase-deficient mice. They suggested further studies in the mouse system before its use for enzymic therapy in human lysosomal storage diseases.

Our studies show that exogenous human liver arginase can be incorporated into genetically arginase-deficient human erythrocytes.

This is important in view of recent studies that show that highly purified human enzyme must be used if maximal effectiveness and immunological tolerance are to be attained in human enzyme replacement therapy (*14, 15*). Important also is the fact that the urea production and the arginine-degradation studies in vitro indicate that the exogenously introduced arginase was functionally active when in vivo conditions were simulated. In other conditions, higher activities can be obtained; for example, urea production is 10-fold greater in an isotonic bicarbonate buffer at pH 8.5. These conditions are entirely different from the prevailing in vivo situation (our own unpublished results).

The fact that exogenously introduced arginase can be kept for at least 12 days in acid citrate–dextrose solution (a commonly used blood preservative) in a functionally active state in human erythrocytes is promising in the light of further in vivo studies. Indeed, the short half life in vivo of most endogenous or exogenous human enzymes and the difficulty of pro-

Table 4. Plasma Arginine Catabolism in Untreated and Arginase-Loaded Cells

Types of erythrocytes	Arginase activity U/ml packed cells	Plasma arginine, µmol/dl: At start of incubation	Plasma arginine, µmol/dl: Decrease after 1-h incubation	Decrease in percent
Original				
Human control 1	8.60	9.49	−1.16	−12
		91.70	−24.62	−26
		380.86	−28.11	−8
Human control 2	8.00	5.03	−1.29	−25
		109.68	−30.87	−28
		498.52	−153.99	−30
				mean: −21
Hyperargininemia				
Patient 1	0.30	46.41	−0.81	
		356.77	+1.91	No significant decrease
Patient 2	0.50	53.00	+0.77	
		374.88	−5.95	
Arginase loaded[a]				
Hyperargininemia				
Patient 1	14.50	44.90	−21.80	−47
		356.77	−125.25	−35
Patient 2	12.80	50.80	−27.12	−53
		374.88	−128.17	−34
				mean: −42

[a]Human liver arginase.

ducing large amounts of purified human enzyme (*14, 15*) make it clear that the protection of the exogenous enzyme in the erythrocytes will be important in enzyme replacement therapy. The erythrocyte is free from proteolytic enzymes and macromolecules catabolizing lysosomes, and its membrane prevents direct contact between the exogenous enzyme and possible circulating antibodies, which could provoke acute allergic manifestations.

The in vivo fate of enzyme-loaded erythrocytes in men and different animals is not well known. Under certain in vitro conditions, the resealed enzyme-loaded erythrocytes maintain many of the properties of normal cells, such as shape, volume, and transport system. Important factors in vitro are pH; temperature; ionic concentration of sodium, potassium, calcium, and magnesium; and ATP concentration of the hemolyzing solution during the preparation of the loaded erythrocytes (*11, 16–24*).

Suitable animal models for familial hyperargininemia are goats and possibly mutants of monkeys (*25, 26*). For example, the goat has a physiological hyperargininemia with arginase-deficient erythrocytes (*25*).

The very low urea production of goat erythrocytes can be enhanced in vitro by loading the erythrocytes with goat liver arginase in a similar way as described for the loading of erythrocytes from familial hyperargininemia patients with human liver arginase.[4]

Can it be expected that the studies in vivo with the goat as an animal model will resolve some of the remaining problems, so that treatment of inborn errors with enzyme-loaded erythrocytes in humans could be foreseen?

References

1. Terheggen, H. G., Schwenk, A., Lowenthal, A., et al., Argininemia with arginase deficiency. *Lancet* **ii**, 748 (1969).

2. Cederbaum, S. D., Shaw, K. N. F., and Valente, M., Hyperargininemia with red cell arginase deficiency. *Am. J. Hum. Genet.* **25**, 20a (1973).

3. Terheggen, H. G., Lowenthal, A., Lavinha, F., and Colombo, J. P., Familial hyperargininemia. *Arch. Dis. Child.* **50**, 57 (1975).

4. Hoffmann, J. H., Physiological characteristics of human red blood cell ghosts. *J. Gen. Physiol.* **42**, 9 (1958).

[4] Adriaenssens K., and Karcher D., Results presented at the meeting of the European Society for Applied Neurochemistry, Skvode, Sweden, May 14, 1975.

5. Seeman, P. H., Transient holes in the erythrocyte membrane during hypotonic hemolysis and stable holes after lysis by saponin and lysolecithin. *J. Cell Biol.* **32**, 55 (1967).

6. Taverna, R. D., and Langdon, R. G., A new method for measuring glucose translocation through biological membranes and its application to human erythrocyte ghosts. *Biochim. Biophys. Acta* **298**, 412 (1973).

7. Schimke, R. T., The importance of both synthesis and degradation in the control of arginase levels in rat liver. *J. Biol. Chem.* **239**, 11, 3808 (1964).

8. Azizi, E., Dror, Y., and Wallis, K., Arginase activity in erythrocytes of healthy and ill children. *Clin. Chim. Acta* **28**, 391 (1970).

9. Marsh, W. H., Fingerhut, B., and Miller, H., Automated and manual direct methods for the determination of blood urea. *Clin. Chem.* **11**, 614 (1965).

10. Efron, M. L., Quantitative estimation of aminoacids in physiological fluids using a Technicon amino acid analyser. In *Automation in Analytical Chemistry, Technicon, Symposia 1965;* L. T. Skeggs, Jr. et al., Eds. Mediad, New York, N.Y., 1966, p 637.

11. Sen, A. K., and Post, R. L., Stoichiometry and location of adenosine triphosphate dependent sodium and potassium transport in the erythrocyte. *J. Biol. Chem.* **239**, 345 (1964).

12. Ihler, G. M., Glew, R. H., and Schnure, R. W., Enzyme loading of erythrocytes. *Proc. Nat. Acad. Sci. U.S.A.* **70**, 2663 (1973).

13. Fiddler, M. B., Thorpe, S. J., Krivit, W., and Desnick, R. J., Enzyme therapy III: In vivo fate of erythrocyte entrapped bêta-glucuronidase. In *Enzyme Therapy in Lysosomal Diseases.* J. M. Tager, G. J. M. Hooghwinkel, and M. T. H. Daems, Eds. North-Holland Pub. Co., Amsterdam, 1974, p 182.

14. *Enzyme Therapy in Genetic Diseases.* D. Bergsma, Ed., Birth Defects, March of Dimes, IX, March 2, 1973.

15. *Enzyme Therapy in Lysomal Storage Diseases.* J. M. Tager, G. J. M. Hooghwinkel, and W. T. H. Daems, Eds. North-Holland Pub. Co., Amsterdam, 1974.

16. Weed, R. I., La Celle, P. L., and Merrill, E. W., Metabolic dependence of red cell deformability. *J. Clin. Invest.* **48**, 795 (1969).

17. La Celle, P. L., Alternations of the deformability of the erythrocyte membrane in stored blood. *Transfusion* **9**, 238 (1969).

18. Haradin, A. R., Weed, R. I., and Reed, C. F., Changes in physical properties of stored erythrocytes: Relationship to survival in vivo. *Transfusion* **9**, 229 (1969).

19. Palek, J., Curby, W. A., and Lionetti, F. J., Size dependence of ghosts from stored erythrocytes on calcium and adenosine triphosphate. *Blood* **40**, 469 (1972).

20. Palek, J., Stewart, G., and Lionetti, F. J., The dependence of shape of human erythrocyte ghosts on calcium and adenosine triphosphate. *Blood* **44**, 583 (1974).

21. Lefevre, P. G., Persistence in erythrocyte ghosts of mediated sugar transport. *Nature* **191**, 970 (1961).

22. Taverna, R. D., and Langdon, R. G., Glucose transport in white erythrocyte ghosts and membrane derived vesicles. *Biochim. Biophys. Acta* **298**, 422 (1973).

23. Bodeman, H., and Passow, H., Factors controlling the resealing of the membrane of human erythrocyte ghosts after hypotonic hemolysis. *J. Membrane Biol.* **8**, 1 (1972).

24. Lepke, S., and Passow, H., The effect of pH at hemolysis on the reconstitution of low cation permeability in human erythrocyte ghosts. *Biochim. Biophys. Acta* **255**, 696 (1972).

25. Barej, W., and Hill, H., Arginine metabolism in the blood cells of cattle and goats. *Q. J. Exp. Physiol.* **55**, 64 (1970).

26. Shih, V. E., Jones, T. C., Levy, H. L., and Madigan, P. M., Arginase deficiency in macaca fascicularis I. Arginase activity and arginine concentration in erythrocytes and in liver. *Pediatr. Res.* **6**, 548 (1972).

CLIN. CHEM. 22/3, 327–335 (1976)

Evaluation of Methods of Coenzyme Activation of Erythrocyte Enzymes for Detection of Deficiency of Vitamins B_1, B_2, and B_6

Riad A. Bayoumi and Sidney B. Rosalki[1]

We describe optimized, ultraviolet spectrophotometric procedures for determination of erythrocyte transketolase, glutathione reductase, and aspartate aminotransferase activity, and their activation by their respective coenzymes—thiamine pyrophosphate, flavin-adenine dinucleotide, and pyridoxal-5-phosphate—as tests for vitamin B_1, B_2, and B_6 deficiency. With these procedures we have investigated healthy subjects on normal and vitamin-supplemented diets, and a series of (mainly) alcoholic hospital in-patients. The enzyme procedures described have good precision and can be readily carried out in the routine laboratory. Abnormal transketolase activation correlated well with clinical evidence of vitamin B_1 deficiency.

Additional Keyphrases: *ultraviolet spectrophotometry • normal values • enzyme kinetics • transketolase • glutathione reductase • aspartate aminotransferase • thiamine pyrophosphate • FAD • pyridoxal-5-phosphate • alcoholism*

Assessment of vitamin B_1 (thiamine), B_2 (riboflavin), and B_6 (pyridoxine) nutritional status ideally requires direct measurement of the concentrations of these vitamins in tissues. Plasma concentrations reflect current intake rather than tissue stores. Erythrocytes are a conveniently sampled tissue, but direct vitamin measurement in them is not possible in the routine laboratory. However, erythrocytes contain several enzymes for which vitamin B_1, B_2, and B_6 function as coenzymes. Activities of these enzymes are increased by in vitro addition of the coenzymes. The degree of activation of erythrocyte transketolase (TK[2]; EC 2.2.1.1, sedoheptulose-7-phosphate:D-glyceraldehyde-3-phosphate glycolaldehyde transferase), glutathione reductase (GR; EC 1.6.4.2; NAD(P)H: glutathione oxidoreductase), and aspartate transaminase (AST; EC 2.6.1.1; L-aspartate:2-oxoglutarate aminotransferase) by in vitro addition of thiamine pyrophosphate (TPP), flavin-adenine dinucleotide (FAD), and pyridoxal-5-phosphate (PLP), respectively, has been suggested as an indirect measure of their respective vitamin content and to inversely relate to erythrocyte vitamin concentration (*1–3*).

To apply these coenzyme activation procedures to routine clinical chemistry laboratory practice, we examined methods involving ultraviolet reaction-rate (kinetic) analysis with continuous monitoring for each of the enzymes. This permits a uniformity of approach to enzyme and activation measurement and the use of analytical techniques with which most laboratories are familiar.

The procedures chosen for examination were based on the reaction systems originally proposed by Smeets et al. (*4*) for TK, Beutler (*5, 6*) for GR, and Karmen (*7*) for AST. However, published recommendations for measurement of these erythrocyte enzymes and of coenzyme activation effects varied widely, and necessitated a thorough examination of the reaction conditions for each enzyme. We present here the results of these studies, the details of opti-

Department of Diagnostic Chemical Pathology, St. Mary's Hospital, Praed St., London, W.2., England.
[1] Address correspondence to this author.
Received Dec. 1, 1975; accepted Dec. 18, 1975.

[2] Nonstandard abbreviations used: TK, transketolase; GR, glutathione reductase; AST, aspartate aminotransferase; TPP, thiamine pyrophosphate; FAD, flavin-adenine dinucleotide; PLP, pyridoxal-5-phosphate; TIM, triosephosphate isomerase; GDH, glycerol phosphate dehydrogenase; GS–SG, oxidized glutathione; GSH, reduced glutathione; MDH, malate dehydrogenase; Tris, tris(hydroxymethyl)aminomethane; and EDTA, ethylenediaminetetraacetate.

mized conditions that we propose for enzyme and activation measurement, and the results of clinical studies done with the adopted methodology.

Materials and Methods

Preparation of Hemolysate

Fresh heparinized blood is centrifuged (3000 rpm) for 5 min and the plasma and buffy coat are removed. The erythrocytes are washed three times with ice-cold saline (9 g NaCl per liter) and the packed erythrocytes dispensed into 0.5-ml aliquots. Enzyme activities are best assayed immediately, though for some studies packed cells were stored frozen at −18 °C. Erythrocytes in a 0.5-ml aliquot are hemolyzed by adding 2 ml of an aqueous solution (5 ml/liter) of "Sterox SE" (Harleco) for TK assay, or 2 ml of distilled water for GR and AST assays. Cell debris is centrifuged and hemoglobin determined by the cyanmethemoglobin method (*8*). Hemoglobin content is adjusted with distilled water to give a final working hemolysate concentration of 50 g of hemoglobin per liter for TK assay and 10 g of hemoglobin per liter for GR and AST assays.

Apparatus

A Unicam SP800 spectrophotometer with attached recorder was used for enzyme determinations. A wide slit-width, 0.10 mm, was found necessary to reduce noise caused by high absorbance of hemoglobin. Plastic cuvettes of 10 mm lightpath were used and the temperature was controlled with a circulating waterbath.

Erythrocyte Transketolase Assay

Principle: TK activity is measured by minor modification of the nicotinamide-adenine dinucleotide (NADH)-dependent method of Smeets et al. (*4*). Ribose-5-phosphate is used as substrate and the glyceraldehyde-3-phosphate formed (Equation 1) is converted to dihydroxyacetone phosphate by triosephosphate isomerase (TIM, EC 5.3.1.1) (Equation 2). The dihydroxyacetone phosphate formed is reduced to glycerol-1-phosphate by glycerol-3-phosphate dehydrogenase (GDH, EC 1.1.1.8) and NADH (Equation 3), the latter being simultaneously oxidized to NAD^+. The rate of decrease in absorbance at 340 nm consequent upon NADH oxidation provides a measure of TK activity.

$$\text{Ribose-5-PO}_4 + \text{xylulose-5-PO}_4 \xrightleftharpoons{\text{TK}} \text{sedoheptulose-7-PO}_4 + \text{D-glyceraldehyde-3-PO}_4 \quad (1)$$

$$\text{D-Glyceraldehyde-3-PO}_4 \xrightleftharpoons{\text{TIM}} \text{dihydroxyacetone-PO}_4 \quad (2)$$

$$\text{Dihydroxyacetone-PO}_4 + \text{NADH} \xrightleftharpoons{\text{GDH}} sn\text{-glycerol 3-PO}_4 + \text{NAD}^+ \quad (3)$$

Reagents: (1) tris(hydroxymethyl)aminomethane buffer (Tris-HCl) 0.1 mol/liter, pH 7.6 at 37 °C, (2) ribose-5-phosphate, disodium salt (Sigma) 15 mmol/liter in Tris-HCl buffer, (3) thiamine pyrophosphate chloride (Sigma) 10 mmol/liter in Tris-HCl buffer, (4) nicotinamide adenine dinucleotide, reduced form, NADH (Boehringer), 10 mmol/liter in Tris-HCl buffer, (5) glycerol-3-phosphate dehydrogenase/triosephosphate isomerase (GDH/TIM) suspension in ammonium sulfate (Boehringer; activity of GDH, 73 kU/liter; activity of TIM, 1800 kU/liter).

Procedure: To 2.4 ml of buffered ribose-5-phosphate kept at 37 °C, add 50 μl of hemolysate (50 g Hb/liter), 0.01 ml of the GDH/TIM suspension, 50 μl of NADH, and 0.10 ml of TPP, and mix. For the assay of activity without TPP, replace it with 0.1 ml of Tris-HCl buffer. Incubate the mixture at 37 °C for 15 min. Continuously monitor the reaction rate at 340 nm for a further 15 min at 37 °C and note the linear absorbance change (ΔA). Use a mixture of 2.55 ml of Tris-HCl buffer and 50 μl of hemolysate as reference. Activities with and without TPP are always measured simultaneously.

Final concentration of reactants: Ribose-5-phosphate, 14.4 mmol/liter; NADH, 190 μmol/liter; thiamine pyrophosphate, 380 μmol/liter; TIM > 6500 U/liter; and GDH, >250 U/liter.

Calculation of activity: Express TK activity in U/g of hemoglobin and calculate it according to the equation:

$$\frac{\Delta A}{15} \times \frac{2.61 \times 1000}{6.22 \times 0.05} \times \frac{1}{50} = \text{activity, in U/g Hb}$$

where ΔA is the decrease in absorbance at 340 nm during 15 min, 6.22×10^3 is the molar absorbance of NADH at 340 nm, 2.61 is the final volume (ml), and 50 is the final hemoglobin concentration of hemolysate (g Hb/liter).

Erythrocyte Glutathione Reductase Assay

Principle: Erythrocyte GR activity is measured by modification of the method introduced by Beutler (*5*, *6*). GR catalyzes the reduction of oxidized glutathione (GSSG) with simultaneous oxidation of nicotinamide-adenine dinucleotide phosphate (NADPH) (Equation 4). Again, the rate of absorbance decrease at 340 nm provides a measure of enzyme activity.

$$\text{GS-SG} + \text{NADPH} + \text{H}^+ \rightleftharpoons 2\,\text{GSH} + \text{NADP}^+ \quad (4)$$

Reagents: (1) potassium phosphate buffer, 0.1 mol/liter, pH 7.4 at 37 °C; (2) ethylenediaminetetraacetate (EDTA), 80 mmol/liter of distilled water; (3) nicotinamide-adenine dinucleotide phosphate, tetrasodium salt, reduced form, NADPH (Boehringer), 4 mmol/liter of aqueous sodium bicarbonate solution (10 g/liter); (4) disodium flavin-adenine dinucleotide, FAD (Sigma), 250 μmol/liter of distilled water; (5) disodium glutathione, oxidized form (Sigma), 50 mmol/liter of aqueous sodium hydroxide solution (2 g/liter).

Procedure: To 2.0 ml potassium phosphate buffer,

add 50 μl of EDTA, 0.10 ml of hemolysate (10 g Hb/liter), 0.10 ml of oxidized glutathione, and 0.10 ml of FAD, and gently mix. For assay of the activity without FAD, replace it with 0.10 ml of distilled water. Preincubate the mixture at 37 °C for 30 min. Start the reaction by adding 0.10 ml of NADPH solution and monitor the linear absorbance decrease continuously at 340 nm for 5 min at 37 °C. Use a solution of 2.35 ml of phosphate buffer and 0.10 ml of hemolysate as reference. Always measure activities with and without FAD simultaneously.

Final concentration of reactants: Glutathione, 2 mmol/liter; NADPH, 162 μmol/liter; FAD, 10 μmol/liter; and EDTA, 1.6 mmol/liter.

Calculation of activity: GR activity is calculated according to the equation:

$$\frac{\Delta A}{5} \times \frac{2.45 \times 1000}{6.22 \times 0.1} \times \frac{1}{10} = \text{activity, in U/g Hb}$$

where ΔA is the decrease in absorbance at 340 nm for 5 min, 6.22×10^3 is the molar absorbance of NADPH at 340 nm; 2.45 is the final volume (ml), and 10 is the final hemoglobin concentration (in g/liter) of hemolysate.

Erythrocyte Aspartate Aminotransferase Assay

Principle: Erythrocyte AST activity is assayed by a modification of the ultraviolet method of Karmen (*7*) and coenzyme activation by modification of the method of Stanulovic et al. (*9*). We used optimized conditions similar to those recommended for serum AST measurement by the German Society for Clinical Chemistry (*10*) and the International Federation of Clinical Chemistry (*11*). The oxaloacetate produced from L-aspartate and 2-oxoglutarate is reduced by malate dehydrogenase (MDH, EC 1.1.1.37) in the presence of NADH (Equations 5, 6). The rate of NADH absorbance decrease at 340 nm is proportional to AST activity.

$$\text{L-Aspartate} + \text{2-oxoglutarate} \overset{\text{AST}}{\rightleftharpoons} \text{glutamate} + \text{oxaloacetate} \quad (5)$$

$$\text{Oxaloacetate} + \text{NADH} \overset{\text{MDH}}{\rightleftharpoons} \text{malate} + \text{NAD}^+ \quad (6)$$

Reagents: (1) Tris-HCl buffer, 0.1 mol/liter, pH 7.4 at 25 °C. (2) AST substrate mixture, sufficient for 50 tests: (*a*) L-aspartic acid, potassium salt (Sigma), 5.31 g, (*b*) malate dehydrogenase in glycerol/water (equal volumes), with specific activity 720 kU/g (Boehringer), 0.625 mg in 0.125 ml suspension, and (*c*) NADH (Boehringer), 21.3 mg. Adjust the volume to 135 ml with Tris-HCl buffer, gently mix, and dispense in 2.7-ml aliquots. Store frozen; stable for one month. (3) 2-Oxoglutarate, sodium salt (Sigma), 360 mmol/liter of Tris-HCl buffer; stable for one month when frozen. (4) Pyridoxal-5-phosphate (Sigma), 8.2 mmol/liter of Tris-HCl buffer; should be protected from light and freshly prepared before use.

Procedure: Preincubate 10 volumes of hemolysate (10 g Hb/liter) with 1 volume of pyridoxal-5-phosphate (final preincubation concentration, 750 μmol/liter of hemolysate) or with 1 volume of Tris-HCl buffer for 30 min at 25 °C. Add 0.2 ml of this preincubated hemolysate to 2.7 ml of the substrate mixture (aspartate, NADH, and MDH) and incubate for 15 min at 25 °C. Start the reaction by adding 0.10 ml of 2-oxoglutarate and monitor continuously at 340 nm for 5 min. Always measure simultaneously the activities with and without pyridoxal-5-phosphate. Solutions of 2.8 ml of Tris-HCl buffer and 0.2 ml of the corresponding preincubated hemolysate serve as instrument blanks. Set up two reagent blanks from which hemolysate is omitted and run them with each batch of assays: one without pyridoxal-5-phosphate (to detect spontaneous NADH oxidation) and the other with added pyridoxal-5-phosphate (to correct for apotransaminase contamination of MDH) (*12*).

Final concentration of reactants: L-Aspartate, 200 mmol/liter; 2-oxoglutarate, 12 mmol/liter; NADH, 200 μmol/liter; MDH, 3000 U/liter; and pyridoxal-5-phosphate, 50 μmol/liter.

Calculation of activity: AST activity is calculated according to the equation:

$$\frac{\Delta A}{5} \times \frac{3 \times 1000}{6.22 \times 0.2} \times \frac{1}{10} = \text{activity, in U/g Hb}$$

Where ΔA is the decrease in absorbance at 340 nm during 5 min, 6.22×10^3 is the molar absorptivity of NADH at 340 nm, 3 is the final volume (ml), and 10 is the final hemoglobin concentration (g/liter) of the hemolysate.

Calculation of Percentage Activation

Percentage activation resulting from in vitro addition of coenzymes to TK, GR, and AST is calculated according to the following formula:

$$\frac{\text{Activity with coenzyme} - \text{activity without coenzyme}}{\text{activity without coenzyme}} \times 100$$

Statistics

(*a*) Results obtained for enzyme optimization studies (Figures 1 to 6) represent the means of at least four experiments, each on a separate hemolysate examined in duplicate.

(*b*) Coefficients of variation (CV) in Table 2, are calculated from standard deviations (SD) obtained from the difference (*d*) between duplicates by using the formulas:

$$SD = \sqrt{\frac{\sum(d^2)}{n - 1}}$$

Where n is the total number of pairs

$$CV = (SD/\bar{X}) \times 100$$

Where $\bar{X}$ is the mean of all values.

(*c*) Levels of significance of difference (*P* values) in Tables 4 and 5 are obtained by the paired Student's *t*-test. Values of *P* of <0.05 were considered significant.

Results

Transketolase Assay

Substrate: In their transketolase assay, Smeets et al. (*4*) use final substrate (ribose-5-phosphate) concentration of 14 mmol/liter. Examination of the effects of substrate concentration variation, however, revealed progressive increase in TK activity up to the highest concentration tested (150 mmol/liter). The Lineweaver–Burk plot of data obtained was of particular interest (Figure 1). Two slopes were apparent, suggesting hydrolysis of the substrate by two enzymes (*13*) with K_m values of 2.5 mmol/liter (K_{m1}) and 50 mmol/liter (K_{m2}), respectively. For the definitive TK assay, we chose a low final substrate concentration (14.4 mmol/liter), because we found no difference in percentage activation by TPP at low (14.4 mmol/liter) or high (100 mmol/liter) substrate concentration and it was impossible to obtain a substrate concentration appropriate to the higher K_m (K_{m2}) without introducing interference from changes in hemoglobin absorbance at high ribose-5-phosphate concentrations.

In several experiments, the addition of xylulose-5-phosphate to the reaction mixture did not affect TK activity. It is safe, therefore, to assume that xylulose-5-phosphate (Equation 1) is made available to TK through conversion of ribose-5-phosphate by D-ribose-5-phosphate ketol-isomerase (EC 5.3.1.6) and D-ribulose-5-phosphate 3-epimerase (EC 5.1.3.1) present in the erythrocyte hemolysate. Stimulation of this pathway by increasing ribose-5-phosphate concentration possibly accounts for the K_{m2} value obtained above.

Coenzyme: We saw no difference in TK percentage activation by in vitro addition of TPP at final concentrations of 100 to 800 μmol/liter. Smeets et al. (*4*)

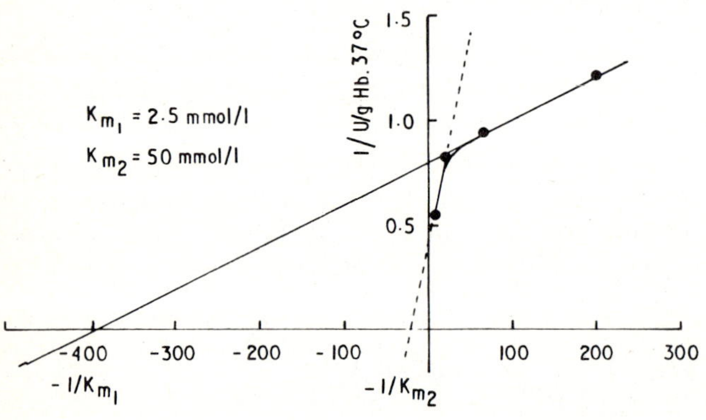

Fig. 1. Lineweaver–Burk plot of effect of variation of ribose-5-phosphate substrate concentration on erythrocyte transketolase activity

Table 1. Final Concentrations of Glutathione, NADPH, and FAD Chosen for Glutathione Reductase Assay by Various Authors

Authors	Glutathione, mmol/liter	NADPH, μmol/liter	FAD, μmol/liter
Present method	2.0	162	10
Beutler (1969)	3.3	100	1
Tillotson and Baker (1972)	0.3	78	11
Hornbeck and Bradley (1974)	2.0	118	4
Nichoalds et al. (1974)	0.3	80	10
Glatzle et al. (1974)	0.2	118	9
Hoorn et al. (1975)	1.0	120	2

used a final concentration of 380 μmol/liter, which we therefore also used.

Blanks: For an instrument blank, 50 μl of hemolysate added to 2.55 ml of Tris-HCl buffer is satisfactory. However, a fairly wide slit-width (0.10 mm) on the Unicam SP 800 spectrophotometer was necessary to reduce noise caused by high absorbance of hemoglobin. Appropriate reagent-blank determinations, omitting ribose-5-phosphate or TIM/GDH, yield negligible absorbance changes, with or without TPP.

Preincubation with TPP: The conditions of preincubation of hemolysate with TPP in the presence of substrate proposed by Smeets et al. (*4*) were found to be satisfactory for maximal activation.

Glutathione Reductase Assay

In view of the widely differing reaction conditions reported by various authors (Table 1), we report here full details of the examination of assay conditions for erythrocyte GR.

Substrate: Figure 2 shows the effect of various oxidized glutathione concentrations on GR activity. The final glutathione concentrations used by Nichoalds et al. (*14*), Tillotson and Baker (*15*), and Glatzle et al. (*16*) (Table 1) were found to be suboptimal. A final concentration of 2 mmol/liter was necessary for optimum assay conditions. This is similar to that used by Hornbeck and Bradley (*17*), but lower than that used by Beutler (*5, 6*).

Coenzyme: With a FAD final concentration of less than 4 μmol/liter, GR was not maximally activated (Figure 3); at 10 μmol/liter, the enzyme was fully activated. Hornbeck and Bradley (*17*) reported enzyme inhibition at this FAD concentration, but we did not observe this. Therefore, this concentration was chosen for the definitive GR assay.

NADPH: A final concentration exceeding 160 μmol/liter was required to obtain a linear reaction rate for a suitable period of time (5 min).

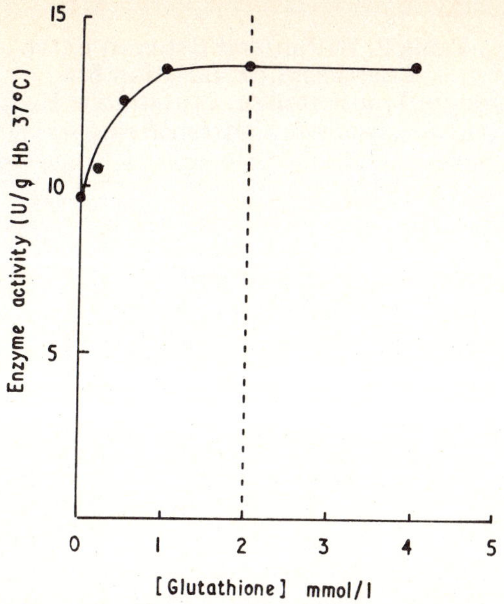

Fig. 2. Effect of variation of concentration of glutathione on erythrocyte glutathione reductase activity

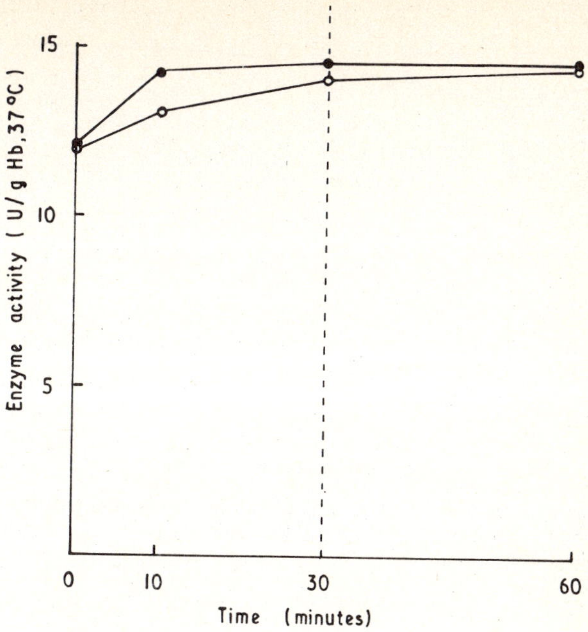

Fig. 4. Effect of variation of preincubation time with coenzyme (FAD) on erythrocyte glutathione reductase activity, when the reaction is started with glutathione (*open circles*) or with NADPH (*closed circles*)

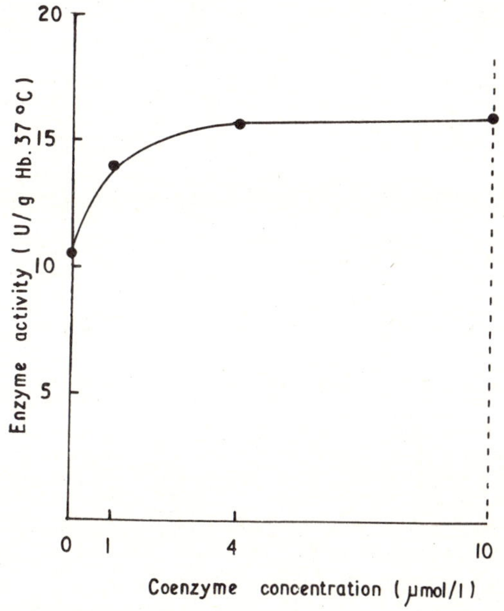

Fig. 3. Effect of variation of FAD coenzyme concentration on erythrocyte glutathione activity

Preincubation of hemolysate with FAD: A 1-h preincubation of hemolysate with FAD was necessary for maximal activation of GR when the reaction was started with glutathione (Figure 4, *open circles*). However, when the reaction was started with NADPH (*closed circles*), the enzyme was activated more quickly, activation being near maximal within 10 min. From then on, activation was almost unchanged for up to 1 h of preincubation. A preincubation time of 30 min was therefore adopted. None of the previous authors, including Nichoalds et al. (*14*), whose procedure has been recommended in the Selected Methods series in *Clinical Chemistry,* have reported the effect of preincubation time of hemolysate with FAD; and only Tillotson and Baker (*15*) and Hoorn et al. (*18*) start the reaction with NADPH.

Aspartate Aminotransferase Assay

Buffer: Because the inhibition of PLP binding to AST apoenzyme by L-aspartate is less in Tris-HCl than in phosphate buffer (*19*), the former was chosen. NADH is also more stable when frozen in Tris-HCl than in phosphate buffer (*20*), permitting bulk preparation and storage of substrate mixture.

Substrates: Rej et al. (*21*) reported similar optimal substrate concentrations for purified erythrocyte AST as for the serum enzyme. For determination of the latter the International Federation of Clinical Chemistry (*11*) has recommended substrate concentrations of 200 mmol/liter for L-aspartate and 12 mmol/liter for 2-oxoglutarate, which are similar to those recommended by the German Society for Clinical Chemistry (*10*) and chosen for this work. Examination of these concentrations verified that they were indeed optimal for the erythrocyte enzyme. The L-aspartate concentration of 38 mmol/liter recently recommended by Hoorn et al. (*18*) for erythrocyte AST measurement was suboptimal.

Preincubation of hemolysate with PLP: Preincubation of hemolysate with PLP rather than including PLP in the determination reagents was preferred for the following reasons: (*a*) In the presence of L-aspartate, binding of PLP to AST apoenzyme is inhibited, and the time for full activation is known to be substantially prolonged. Even when PLP is added directly to the hemolysate, its binding to AST apoenzyme is time-dependent, and maximal activation

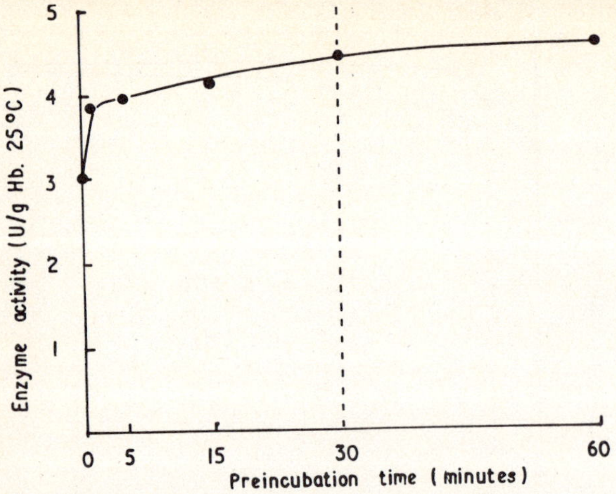

Fig. 5. Effect of variation of preincubation time with coenzyme (pyridoxal-5-phosphate) on erythrocyte aspartate aminotransferase activity

could only be attained with a preincubation of at least 30 min (Figure 5). (*b*) A high concentration of PLP in the hemolysate can be achieved with minimal final absorbance. A PLP concentration of 736 μmol/liter of hemolysate was found to be suitable for maximal activation of erythrocyte AST (Figure 6). Such a concentration of PLP, if present in the reagents, would itself contribute an absorbance value of some 1.4.

Assay Precision Studies

Twenty hemolysates were examined in duplicate during one day. Repeat determinations were also made on 20 hemolysates after storage at −18 °C for 24 h. Within-batch and between-batch precision data (expressed as coefficient of variation) for these specimens are shown in Table 2. Storage instability (see

Table 2. Within/and Between-Batch Coefficient of Variation for Erythrocyte Transketolase, Glutathione Reductase, and Aspartate Aminotransferase Assays

		Activity without coenzyme (n = 20)	Activity with coenzyme (n = 20)
Transketolase	Within-batch	2	2
	Between-batch	7	9
Glutathione reductase	Within-batch	5	4
	Between-batch	8	5
Aspartate aminotransferase	Within-batch	2	3
	Between-batch	9	10

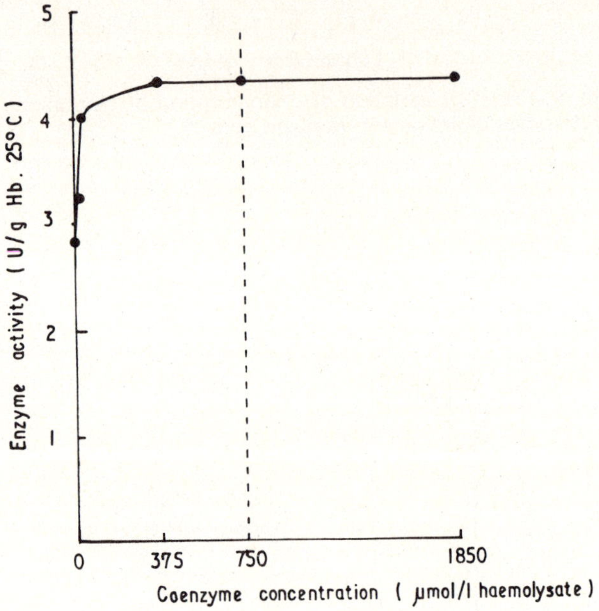

Fig. 6. Effect of preincubation concentration of coenzyme (pyridoxal-5-phosphate) on erythrocyte aspartate aminotransferase activity

Table 3. Erythrocyte Transketolase, Glutathione Reductase, and Aspartate Aminotransferase Activities of Hospital Inpatients, and the Effect of Storage

	Transketolase: Mean activity (U/g Hb) n = 8, Without TPP (Mean ± SD)	With TPP (Mean ± SD)	Mean percentage activation	Glutathione reductase: Mean activity (U/g Hb) n = 8, Without FAD (Mean ± SD)	With FAD (Mean ± SD)	Mean percentage activation	Aspartate aminotransferase: Mean activity (U/g Hb) n = 8, Without PLP (Mean ± SD)	With PLP (Mean ± SD)	Mean percentage activation
Fresh hemolysate	866 (±173)	1000 (±240)	15	11.1 (±2.2)	13.0 (±1.2)	17	1.91 (±0.50)	3.28 (±0.53)	72
Hemolysate stored frozen for 24 h	852 (±125)	964 (±140)	13	10.5 (±2.2)	12.5 (±1.5)	19	1.82 (±0.50)	3.46 (±0.56)	90
Hemolysate stored frozen for 2 w	777 (±226)	838 (±232)	8	9.2 (±2.1)	10.9 (±1.5)	18	1.58 (±0.47)	3.02 (±0.64)	91
Change in acty or activation after 2 w	−89 (−10%)	−162 (−16%)	−7	−1.9 (−17%)	−2.1 (−16%)	+1	−0.33 (−17%)	−0.26 (−8%)	+19

Table 4. Percentage Coenzyme Activation of Three Enzymes, before and after Vitamin Supplementation in Laboratory Workers (n = 15)

	Transketolase		Glutathione reductase		Aspartate aminotransferase	
	Before	After	Before	After	Before	After
Mean	13	6	32	8	83	50
SD	5	3	22	8	24	18
Mean + 2 SD	23	12	76	24	130	86
Signif. of diff.	$P < 0.001$		$P < 0.001$		$P < 0.001$	

later) may partly account for the higher between-batch coefficient of variation of the TK and AST assays, in comparison with the very acceptable within-batch precision.

Hemolysate Storage Stability

Storage of hemolysates at −18 °C for two weeks resulted in a 10% loss of TK activity assayed without TPP and a 16% loss with TPP added. Under the same conditions, GR activity declined by 17% without and 16% with addition of FAD. AST activity declined by 17% when assayed without coenzyme, and 8% with coenzyme (Table 3).

It has been claimed that both TK and GR are stable for three to four weeks at −20 °C (*4, 14, 18*), but this has not been confirmed and is not supported by this study. In respect of AST stability, similar findings to the above have been reported by Rose et al. (*22*).

The percentage activation of GR and AST by in vitro coenzyme addition showed minimal change after two weeks of storage at −18 °C, whereas TK activation decreased by half.

Clinical Studies

Normal subjects: Percentage activation of TK, GR, and AST was studied in healthy laboratory workers (seven women and eight men, between 18 and 45 years old) on an unrestricted diet. Results are shown in Table 4. The upper limits of normal (mean + 2 SD) are: TK, 23%; GR, 76%; and AST, 130%. Higher values were considered to indicate the corresponding vitamin deficiency.

Inpatients. Values for percentage activation of TK, GR, and AST in several hospital inpatients not suffering from nutritional disorders were found to lie within the normal range established above (Table 3).

Normal subjects receiving vitamin supplements: The laboratory workers mentioned above each took oral vitamin supplements of thiamine (45 mg), riboflavin (45 mg), and pyridoxine (30 mg) daily for seven days, and the percentage activation of TK, GR, and AST was estimated on samples of blood obtained at the end of the 7th day. Values obtained before and after vitamin supplementation are shown in Table 4. Activation after vitamin supplementation was significantly ($P < 0.001$) lower for all three enzymes.

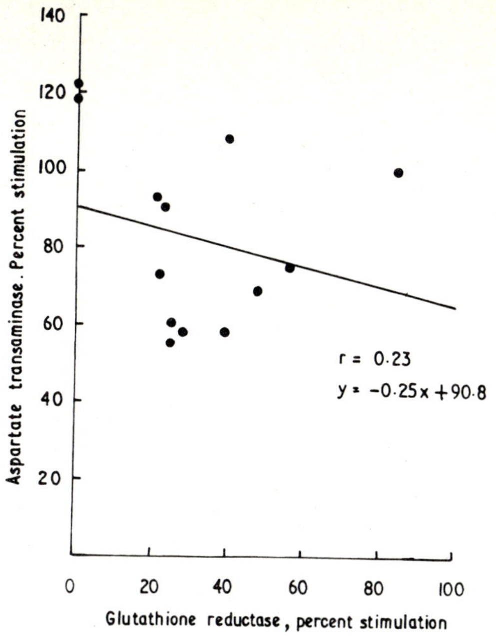

Fig. 7. Relation between stimulation of erythrocyte aspartate aminotransferase by pyridoxal-5-phosphate and glutathione reductase by FAD, in healthy subjects *before* oral administration of vitamins

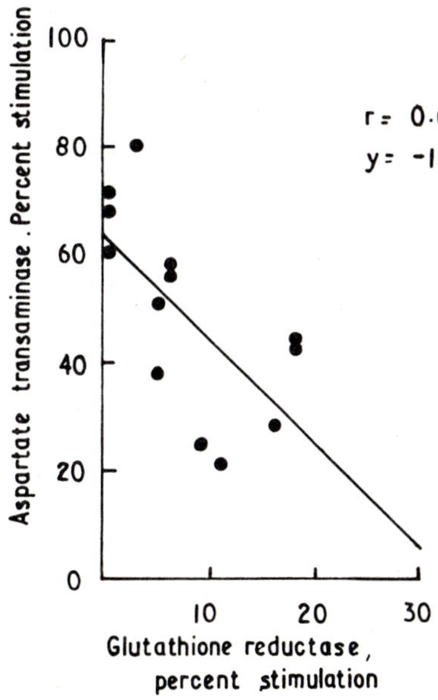

Fig. 8. Same as Figure 7, except *after* oral vitamins

Inhibition of glutathione reductase activity by pyridoxal-5-phosphate: An inverse correlation between activation of AST and of GR was observed in hemolysates obtained from the normal persons after vitamin supplementation (Figures 7 and 8). The lower the AST activation (implying high in vivo pyridoxine concentration), the higher was GR activation. Because of these in vivo effects, we examined the ef-

Table 5. Effect of In Vitro Addition of Pyridoxal-5-phosphate on Glutathione Reductase Activity[a]

	Glutathione reductase activity, U/g Hb		
	Without FAD (Mean ± SD)	With FAD (Mean ± SD)	Percentage activation
Without PLP (n = 8)	9.4 (±1.1)	10.8 (±1.1)	15
With PLP (n = 8)	8.8 (±1.2)	10.7 (±1.0)	22
Signif. of change	$P < 0.01$	$P > 0.1$	

[a] Hemolysates are preincubated with pyridoxal-5-phosphate before glutathione reductase determination, with and without FAD.

Table 6. Analysis of 47 Routine Transketolase Requests

Clinical	No. with abnormal activation
Alcoholics:	
1. Clinical B_1 deficiency: (Neuropathy, psychosis or high output cardiac failure)	8/23
2. No clinical B_1 deficiency	4/10
Geriatric patients:	
No clinical B_1 deficiency	1/7
Others:	
No clinical B_1 deficiency	0/7
Total	13/47

fect of in vitro addition of PLP on GR activity. GR activity was assayed (with and without FAD) in eight additional hemolysates, with and without addition of PLP, at a final concentration of 66 μmol/liter. The results (Table 5) show that this PLP concentration, which is substantially higher than the likely in vivo level, inhibits GR activity by some 6% and increases the percentage activation of GR from 15 to 22%.

Alcoholics: In a preliminary study, the percentage activation of TK, GR and AST was examined in 13 inpatient alcoholics. Four were found to have TK activation greater than 23%, indicating thiamine deficiency. A further two had GR activation greater than 76%, indicating riboflavin deficiency. However, none had AST activation greater than 130%, implying that none was B_6 deficient.

Abnormal TK activation was also observed in 12 of 33 alcoholics with suspected thiamine deficiency. The incidence of abnormality in relation to clinical symptoms is shown in Table 6, which also shows results on nonalcoholics without clinical evidence of B_1 deficiency, but referred for investigation because of their poor diet.

Discussion

We consider it appropriate to comment on methodology in the *Results* section of this paper and to confine our discussion to considering the implication of the results obtained with our chosen methods.

The validity of activation tests for identification of vitamin deficiency states is supported by numerous studies. The inverse relationship between TK activation by TPP and thiamine status was first described by Brin et al. (*1*), and for GR activation by FAD and riboflavin nutrition by Beutler (*5, 6*) and Tillotson and Baker (*15*). An inverse relation between AST activation by PLP and B_6 deficiency was noted by Raica and Sauberlich (*3*) and Hamfelt (*23*), and the latter correlated such activation with erythrocyte vitamin concentration.

In healthy subjects on an unrestricted diet, we obtained reference values (mean + 2 SD) for TK, GR, and AST activation of 23, 76, and 130%, respectively. The reference value for GR (76%) was higher than that reported by Glatzle et al. (*16*), Nichoalds et al. (*14*), or Hoorn et al. (*18*) (50, 30, and 29%, respectively). It was also higher for AST (130%) than that reported by Nobbs (*24*) or by Hoorn et al. (*18*) (25 and 86%, respectively). Our use of optimized procedures presumably accounts for this. For TK, only little modification of the method of Smeets et al. (*4*) was necessary, and the reference values are similar.

Though oral vitamin supplementation to healthy subjects on an unrestricted diet results in reduction in activation for each enzyme (Table 4; also ref. *5, 6,* and *22*), we do not believe that the decreased values should be chosen as normal reference values. To do so would imply that the healthy population is vitamin deficient, which by definition is not true, because an adequate vitamin intake is regarded as the amount sufficient for physiological requirements, i.e., for health. An adequate vitamin intake is not necessarily that required for maintaining erythrocyte enzymes at maximum saturation with cofactors. There is evidence also from this study that vitamin supplementation may produce interaction between activation effects (e.g., between AST and GR). A final point is that the tests are useful in the diagnosis of deficiency states only if the non-vitamin-supplemented range is used for reference. The use of the lower (supplemented) range would yield abnormal values in healthy and deficient alike.

The value of the proposed procedures in relation to clinical deficiency became evident in our initial studies on 13 inpatient alcoholics. Neurological symptoms of B_1 deficiency were present in four of them, and all four showed abnormal TK coenzyme activation. It was also possible to identify, biochemically, two additional patients with riboflavin deficiency.

When results of routine laboratory requests for TK determination in 43 patients referred in a subsequent six months period were analyzed, we could again correlate a high incidence of abnormal TK activation with a high incidence of clinical evidence of vitamin B_1 deficiency (see Table 6).

Clinical vitamin B_2 and B_6 deficiency with classical symptoms and signs is uncommon in the United Kingdom; however, there are many situations where *biochemical* vitamin B_6 deficiency has been postulated. Thus abnormal tryptophan loading tests and lowered blood vitamin B_6 have been reported in gestational diabetes (*25*), and in preliminary studies we have found an increased incidence of abnormal AST activation in this condition. Abnormal AST activation has also been observed in women, B_6 deficient as a consequence of use of oral contraceptives (*22, 26*), and in epileptics on anticonvulsant therapy (*27*). Such studies indicate that the biochemical deficiency of vitamin B_6 that usually precedes the development of the typical clinical deficiency state can be detected by increased erythrocyte AST coenzyme activation, and in animal experiments done in collaboration with Dr. W. R. D. Smith (Middlesex Hospital, London) we have observed significantly increased AST coenzyme activation in rats within a week of commencing pyridoxine-deficient diet and before any clinical abnormality. Presumably the same would apply to the GR coenzyme activation test in vitamin B_2 deficiency.

In contrast to other laboratory procedures for the diagnosis of vitamin B_1, B_2, and B_6 deficiencies, the activation methods we have used can readily and conveniently be used in the routine clinical chemistry laboratory. We believe that this will facilitate a wider application of the tests to the investigation of these deficiency states.

References

1. Brin, M., Shohet, S. S., and Davidson C. S., The effect of thiamine deficiency on glucose oxidative pathway of rat erythrocyte. *J. Biol. Chem.* **230,** 319 (1958).

2. Glatzle, D., Weber, F., and Wiss, O., Enzymatic test for the detection of riboflavin deficiency. NADPH-dependent glutathione reductase of red blood cells and its activation by FAD in vitro. *Experientia* **24,** 1122 (1968).

3. Raica, N., and Sauberlich, H. E., Blood cell transaminase activity in human vitamin B_6 deficiency. *Am. J. Clin. Nutr.* **15,** 67 (1964).

4. Smeets, E. H. J., Muller, H., and De Weal, J., A NADH-dependent transketolase assay in erythrocyte haemolysates. *Clin. Chim. Acta* **33,** 379 (1971).

5. Beutler, E., Effect of flavin compounds on glutathione reductase activity: In vivo and in vitro studies. *J. Clin. Invest.* **48,** 1957 (1969).

6. Beutler, E., Glutathione reductase: Stimulation in normal subjects by riboflavin supplementation. *Science* **165,** 613 (1969).

7. Karmen, A., A note on the spectrophotometric assay of glutamic-oxaloacetate transaminase in human blood serum. *J. Clin. Invest.* **34,** 131 (1955).

8. Dacie, J. V., and Lewis, S. M., *Practical Haematology,* 5th ed., Churchill, London, 1975, p 32.

9. Stanulovic, M, Miletic, D., and Stock, A., The diagnosis of pyridoxine deficiency based on the estimation of the erythrocytic aspartate aminotransferase and its stimulation in vitro with pyridoxal-5-phosphate. *Clin. Chim. Acta* **17,** 353 (1967).

10. Bergmeyer, H. V., Büttner, H., Hillman, G., et al., Recommendations of the German Society for Clinical Chemistry. *Z. Klin. Chem. Klin. Biochem.* **10,** 281 (1972).

11. International Federation of Clinical Chemistry, Expert Panel on Enzymes. IFCC method for aspartate aminotransferase. Draft proposal. *Clin. Chem.* **21,** 797 (1975).

12. Rosalki, S. B., and Wilkinson, J. H., A source of error in serum glutamic-oxaloacetic transaminase determination. *J. Clin. Pathol.* **12,** 138 (1959).

13. Dixon, M., and Webb, E. C., *Enzymes,* 2nd ed., Longmans, London, 1964, p 89.

14. Nichoalds, G. E., Lawrence, J. D., and Sauberlich, H. E., Assessment of status of riboflavin nutriture by assay of erythrocyte glutathione reductase activity. *Clin. Chem.* **20,** 624 (1974).

15. Tillotson, J. A., and Baker, E. M., An enzymatic measurement of the riboflavin status in man. *Am. J. Clin. Nutr.* **25,** 425 (1972).

16. Glatzle, D., Vuillenmier, J. P., Weber, F., and Decker, K., Glutathione reductase test with whole blood, a convenient procedure for the assessment of the riboflavin status in humans. *Experientia* **30,** 665 (1974).

17. Hornbeck, C. L., and Bradley, D. W., Concentrations of FAD and glutathione as they affect values for erythrocyte glutathione reductase. *Clin. Chem.* **20,** 512 (1974).

18. Hoorn, R. K. J., Flikweert, J. P., and Westerink, D., Vitamin B_1, B_2, and B_6 deficiencies in geriatric patients, measured by coenzyme stimulation of enzyme activities. *Clin. Chim. Acta.* **61,** 151 (1975).

19. O'Kane, D. E., and Gunsalus, I. C., The resolution and purification of glutamic aspartic transaminase. *J. Biol. Chem.* **170,** 425 (1947).

20. Ebeling, J., Meijers, C. A. M., and Spijkers, J. B. F., The use of tris buffer for U.V. spectrophotometric assay of GOT and GTP. *Clin. Chim. Acta* **25,** 174 (1969).

21. Rej, R., Vanderlinde, R. E., and Fasce, C. F., Jr., An L-aspartate:2-oxoglutarate aminotransferase reference material from human erythrocytes: Preparation and characterization. *Clin. Chem.* **18,** 374 (1972).

22. Rose, D. P., Strong, R., Folkard, J., and Adams, P., Erythrocyte aminotransferase activities in women using oral contraceptives and the effect of vitamin B_6 supplementation. *Am. J. Clin. Nutr.* **26,** 48 (1973).

23. Hamfelt, A., Pyridoxal phosphate concentration and aminotransferase activity in human blood cells. *Clin. Chim. Acta* **16,** 19 (1967).

24. Nobbs, B. T., Pyridoxal phosphate status in clinical depression. *Lancet* **i,** 405 (1974).

25. Bennink, H. J. T. C., and Schreurs, W. H. P., Improvement of oral glucose tolerance in gestational diabetes by pyridoxine. *Br. Med. J.* **3,** 15 (1975).

26. Adams, P. W., Wynn, V., Rose, D. P., et al., Effect of pyridoxine hydrochloride (vitamin B_6) upon depression associated with oral contraception. *Lancet* **i,** 897 (1973).

27. Reinken, L., Hohenauer, L., and Ziegler, E. E., Activity of red cell glutamic oxalacetic transaminase in epileptic children under epileptic treatment. *Clin. Chim. Acta* **36,** 270 (1972).

CLIN. CHEM. 22/3, 336-340 (1976)

Polarographic Method for Rapid Microdetermination of Cholesterol with Cholesterol Esterase and Cholesterol Oxidase

Akio Noma and Keiko Nakayama

Cholesterol concentrations in serum are enzymatically determined rapidly by use of a polarographic oxygen analyzer with a circuit modified to record simultaneously the amount and rate of oxygen consumption. The final assay system, assessed from the oxygen consumption value that we found to be optimum, consists of 1 ml of sodium phosphate buffer (0.6 mol/liter, pH 7.0) containing NaN_3 (10 mg/liter), Triton X-100 surfactant (10 ml/liter), 0.4 U of cholesterol ester hydrolase, and 0.6 U of cholesterol oxidase. Oxygen consumption and cholesterol concentration are linearly related to 8.0 g/liter, and only 10 μl of serum is required. Replicate analyses of pooled serum by the present method demonstrated the following inter-run precision: mean = 1731 mg/liter, SD = 22.3 mg/liter, CV = 1.3%. Bilirubin and ascorbic acid were without effect on the present method, unlike the enzymatic colorimetric methods.

Additional Keyphrases: *pediatric chemistry • intermethod comparison*

Because of clinical importance and analytical difficulties, determination of serum cholesterol has been the subject of numerous investigations. Colorimetric reactions for cholesterol determination have been plagued with a long list of difficulties: lack of specificity, difficulty in standardization, variable reactivity of esters, unstable and corrosive reagents, and many interfering substances. Recently, the specificity provided by enzyme reagents has been introduced into cholesterol determinations (*1–4*). In the enzymatic cholesterol-measuring systems adopted in the routine assays, hydrogen peroxide resulting from the catalytic action of cholesterol oxidase is measured colorimetrically by the coupled systems involving oxidation of either methanol in the presence of catalase (EC 1.11.1.6) or phenol and 4-aminoantipyrine in the presence of peroxidase (EC 1.11.1.7). These reactions, however, have many disadvantages: lengthy reaction time and interfering substances (most notably bilirubin and ascorbic acid).

This paper presents a new polarographic microdetermination of serum cholesterol with use of two enzymes, based on the method for serum glucose determination (*5–7*).

Division of Clinical Biochemistry, Tokyo Metropolitan Geriatric Hospital, 35-2, Sakae-cho, Itabashi, Tokyo, Japan.
Received Nov. 25, 1975; accepted Dec. 24, 1975.

Materials and Methods

Reagents

All enzyme preparations were from Boehringer Mannheim Yamanouchi K. K., 2-9, Kandatacho, Chiyoda-ku, Tokyo, and were used without further purification. Cholesterol oxidase (EC 1.1.3.6; cholesterol: oxygen oxidoreductase) from *Nocardia erythropolis* had a specific activity of approximately 20 kU/g or 20 kU/liter. Cholesterol esterase (EC 3.1.1.13; sterol-ester hydrolase), with a specific activity of 10 kU/g or 20 kU/liter, was from a microorganism (not specified by the supplier). Glucose oxidase (EC 1.1.3.4; β-D-glucose:oxygen oxidoreductase), 210 kU/g, was of fungal origin, and mutarotase (EC 5.1.3.3; aldose-1-epimerase), with approximately 6000 kU/g or 30 000 kU/liter, was from hog kidney.

Sodium azide, a strong inhibitor for catalase, was dissolved in buffer to give a final concentration in the assay system of 10 mg/liter. Sodium taurocholate and sodium cholate were purchased from Calbiochem, La

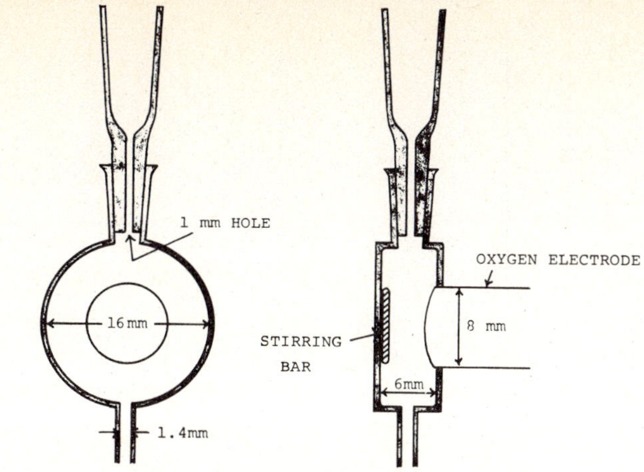

Fig. 1. Reaction cell (1-ml glass cell)

Jolla, Calif. 92037 and used without further purification. Isooctyl phenoxypolyethoxyethanol (Triton X-100) and fatty acid-poor bovine serum albumin were obtained from Sigma Chemical Co., St. Louis, Mo. 63178. Polyoxyethylene sorbitan monooleate (Tween 80), was from Kanto Chemical Co., Inc., Tokyo. Cholesterol standard solution ("Preciset Cholesterol") was a gift from Boehringer Mannheim Yamanouchi K. K., Tokyo. All other chemicals used were of reagent grade.

Apparatus

To measure oxygen consumption, we used a polarographic oxygen analyzer with oxygen electrode (used in all models of the Glucose Analyzer, Beckman Instruments Inc., Fullerton, Calif. 92634) and recorder. A 1.0-ml drumshaped glass cell with small Teflon-coated stir bar (Figure 1) was placed in the thermostatically controlled system. With this apparatus we could monitor and simultaneously record the amount and rate of oxygen consumption. We used microsyringes—10, 25, 50, and 100 μl—to add serum samples and reagents to the reaction mixture.

Procedure

This method is based on the absolutely specific oxidation of free cholesterol, which is formed with cholesterol esterase (CE), with cholesterol oxidase (CO).

$$\text{cholesterol ester} + H_2O \xrightarrow{\text{CE}} \text{cholesterol} + \text{fatty acid} \quad (1)$$

$$\text{cholesterol} + O_2 \xrightarrow{\text{CO}} \text{4-cholesten-3-one} + H_2O_2 \quad (2)$$

If catalase is present in the sample, the hydrogen peroxide formed in equation 2 is decomposed to 0.5 mole of oxygen and 1 mole of water, and the oxygen thus formed may be again used for the oxidation of another molecule of cholesterol by equation 2. To block the action of any catalase present, we added NaN_3, a strong catalase inhibitor, to the reaction mixture.

Determination of true cholesterol concentration of standard solution. In the reaction cell was placed buffer (see below) containing NaN_3 (final concentration, 10 mg/liter), 50 μl of glucose oxidase solution (3150 kU/liter), 40 μl of mutarotase solution (30 000 kU/liter) and 30 μl of cholesterol oxidase solution (20 kU/liter). After setting the meter reading of the oxygen analyzer at a proper position, while continuously stirring with a stirring bar covered with Teflon, we added 10 μl of D-glucose solution (2 mmol/liter) to give an oxygen consumption value (A) corresponding to total D-glucose (α-anomer + β-anomer) in the sample solution. Subsequently, 10 μl of cholesterol standard solution was added to give a further oxygen consumption value (B). Then, the true cholesterol concentration (mmol/liter) of standard solution was calculated as $2 \times (B/A)$.

Measurement of free and esterified cholesterol in serum. In the reaction cell was placed phosphate buffer (0.6 mol/liter, pH 7.0, and containing, per liter, 10 mg of NaN_3 and 10 ml of Triton X-100). After adding 30 μl of cholesterol oxidase and setting the meter reading of the apparatus at a proper position while continuously stirring the mixture, 10 μl of serum sample was added to give an oxygen consumption corresponding to the free cholesterol in the sample. Then 20 μl of cholesterol ester hydrolase (20 kU/liter) was added to give a further oxygen consumption corresponding to the esterified cholesterol in the sample (Figure 2).

Results

Analytical Variables

Optimal pH. The optimal pH for assay system was studied by determining the maximal rate for cholesterol standard solution. A broad pH optimum, between 6.5–8.0, was observed (Figure 3). Subsequent studies were made at pH 7.0.

Buffer concentration. Sodium phosphate, pH 7.0, was used as the buffer at final concentrations ranging

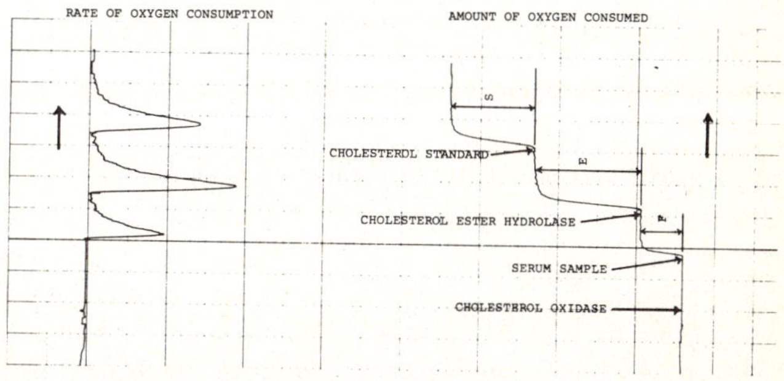

Fig. 2. Determination of free and esterified cholesterol in serum

Values F, E, and S are the amounts of oxygen consumed corresponding to free and esterified cholesterol in the sample, and cholesterol standard solution, respectively. Incubation was at 37 °C

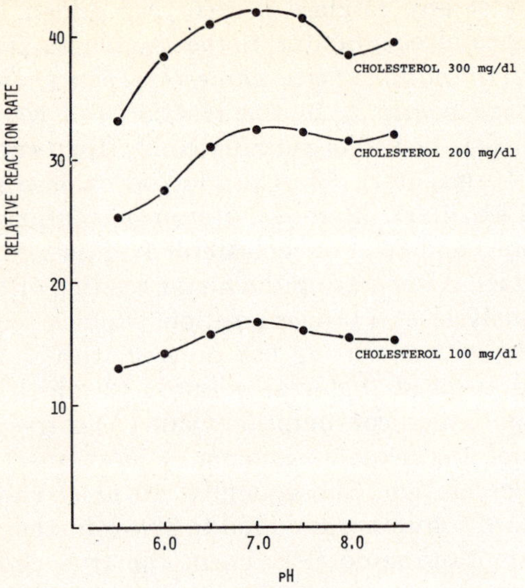

Fig. 3. Effect of pH on the reaction rate of oxygen consumption
0.6 mol/liter sodium phosphate buffer used. Here, and in Figures 4, 5, 7, 8, values on ordinate are oxygen consumption rate

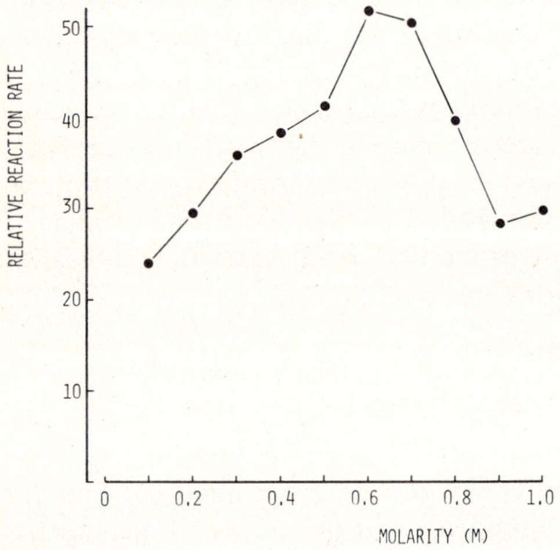

Fig. 4. Effect of phosphate concentration on the rate of oxygen consumption

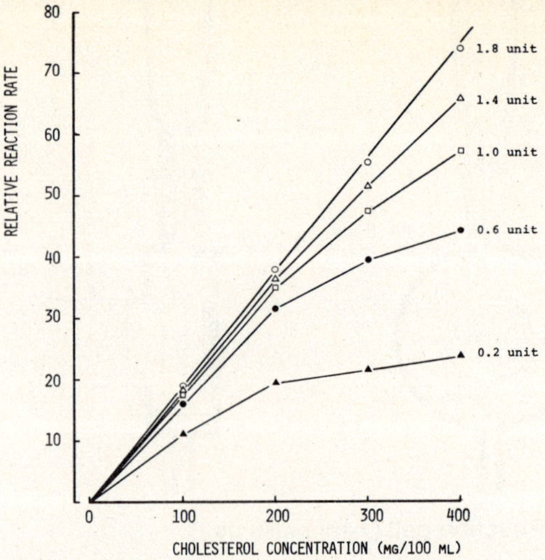

Fig. 5. Effect of amount of cholesterol oxidase on the rate of oxygen consumption

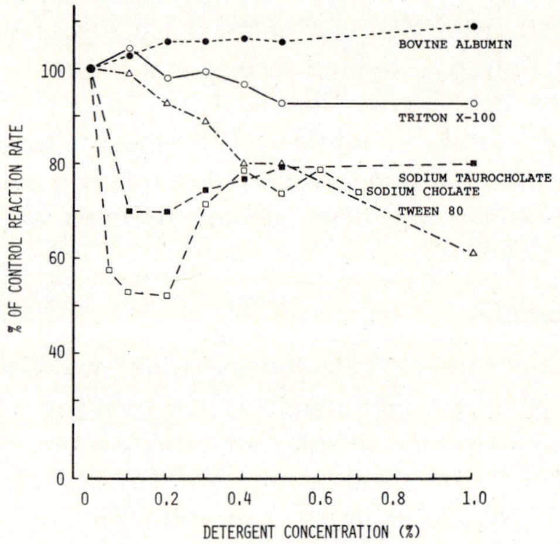

Fig. 6. Effects of various concentrations of detergents on the reaction rate by using cholesterol standard solution

from 0.1 to 1.0 mol/liter, in 0.1 mol/liter increments. A range of 0.6–0.7 mol/liter was found to be optimal (Figure 4).

Cholesterol oxidase concentration. We measured oxygen consumption and reaction rate of the oxidation of free cholesterol with various amounts of cholesterol oxidase at various concentrations of cholesterol standard solution. As shown in Figure 5, reaction rate was linear with respect to enzyme concentration when more than 1.8 U of cholesterol oxidase was present. On the other hand, oxygen consumption was linear with as little as 0.2 U of cholesterol oxidase present. In subsequent measurements of cholesterol concentration, we used oxygen consumption as our measure.

Effects of various detergents. When 10 μl of cholesterol standard solution, containing hydroxypolyethoxydodecane (an unspecified concentration) as detergent, was used, effects of various concentrations of other detergents on the rate of cholesterol oxidase reaction were as shown in Figure 6. Bovine serum albumin slightly activated the reaction, in the concentrations used in this experiment. Triton X-100 slightly inhibited the activity of cholesterol oxidase. Another non-ionic detergent, Tween 80, significantly inhibited the reaction rate. On the contrary, maximal inhibitions were observed when bile salts (1 or 2 g/liter) were present, but the activities increased again as bile salt concentrations were increased above 3 g/liter.

In contrast with serum as the sample, these detergents had different effects. As shown in Figure 7, in the case of buffer without detergent no activity of cholesterol oxidase was recorded. On adding Triton X-100 (final concentration, 1 ml/liter), the activity was sharply increased and reached the maximal rate;

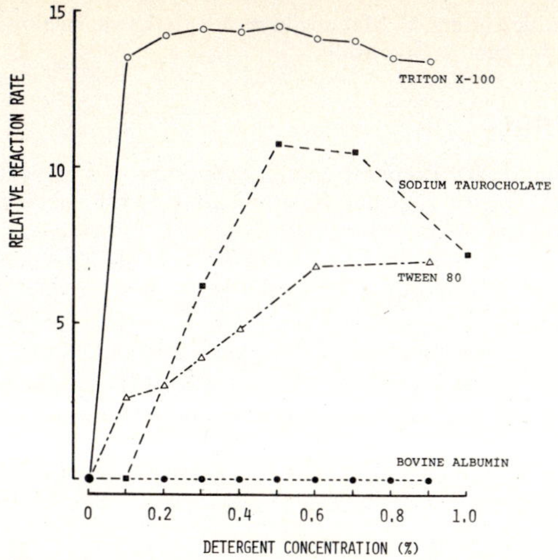

Fig. 7. Effects of various concentrations of detergents on the reaction rate by using serum as a sample

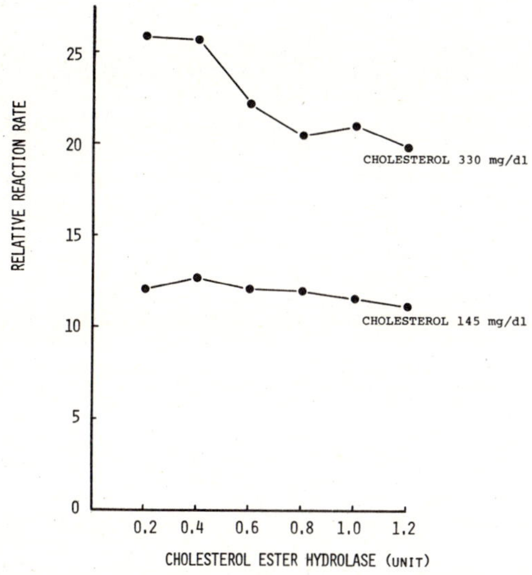

Fig. 8. Effect of amount of cholesterol ester hydrolase on the rate of oxygen consumption with serum samples of low and high cholesterol concentrations

0.6 mol/liter sodium phosphate buffer, pH 7.0, containing 1 ml of Triton X-100 per liter

no further change was observed with up to 10 ml of Triton X-100 per liter. The activity increased gradually with increasing concentrations of bile salt and Tween 80. No activity was observed with bovine serum albumin present in any of the concentrations tested. The rate of the coupled reaction with cholesterol ester hydrolase and cholesterol oxidase also reached the maximal value with 1 ml of Triton X-100 per liter. This concentration of Triton X-100 was used in subsequent studies.

Cholesterol esterase concentration. Under optimal conditions of pH, buffer concentration, detergent concentration, and cholesterol oxidase amount, the effects of various amounts of cholesterol esterase on the reaction rate were studied, with use of serum samples of high and low concentrations of cholesterol. As seen in Figure 8, reaction rates were maximal with 10–20 μl (0.2–0.4 U) of cholesterol esterase. Unexpectedly, greater amounts of the enzyme inhibited the activities. Thus, 20 μl of cholesterol esterase was used in subsequent studies.

Sensitivity. It is apparent from the results of dilution experiments that, with a 10-μl sample, a cholesterol concentration of 125 mg/liter is measurable with the present method.

Linearity. The standard curve prepared with various concentrations of cholesterol standard solution was a straight line up to 8.00 g/liter. Another curve prepared with various volumes of serum sample (total cholesterol, 1540 mg/liter) was linear up to 40 μl of serum, corresponding to a cholesterol concentration of about 6000 mg/liter.

Reproducibility. The precision of the present method was determined by performing 12 replicate assays of pooled serum. The mean was 1731 mg/liter, with a standard deviation of 22.3 mg/liter and coefficient of variation of 1.29%. The day-to-day CV was 1.95%, mean 1696 mg/liter, and standard deviation 33.1 mg/liter.

Correlation with Results by Other Methods

Thirty-two samples were assayed by using the AutoAnalyzer II, with isopropanol extraction, and also by the method of the Boehringer enzymatic color test. Both procedures were those of the manufacturer. The resulting equations are: y (AutoAnalyzer) = $0.793\,x + 17.72$ ($r = 0.94$) and y (enzymatic) = $1.037\,x + 16.15$ ($r = 0.985$). Clearly, there is good agreement between the present method and those compared with it.

Effect of Interfering Substances

A native human serum was mixed with solutions containing either bilirubin or ascorbic acid and analyzed. These substances in concentrations up to 100 mg/liter were without effect on either the amount or the rate of oxygen consumption.

Discussion

Since Kadish and Hall (*8*) reported the determination of D-glucose with an oxygen electrode and β-D-glucose oxidase (EC 1.1.3.4) in 1965, blood glucose has been determined with similar techniques. At present, glucose in serum, plasma, and urine is determined in the routine assay by the glucose oxidase method by use of a polarographic analyzer with a circuit modified to record the rate of oxygen consumption (*9*). However, Okuda et al. (*5–7*) reported a method for determining glucose from the amount of oxygen consumed. As shown in Figure 5, cholesterol determination from the rate of oxygen consumption requires a substantial amount of cholesterol oxidase even if only free cholesterol is being determined. Moreover, the rate of oxygen consumption varies according to the amount of oxygen contained in the reaction cell. Thus, our method for cholesterol determination is based on the amount of oxygen consumed by free cholesterol catalyzed by cholesterol oxidase to 4-cholesten-3-one. Measurement of the amount of oxygen consumed is influenced by the atmospheric oxygen, but in the present method, with the specific cell, diffusion of atmospheric oxygen into the test solution was scarcely observed during the measurement, because the baselines of the chart were absolutely stable.

The present method for determining cholesterol has several advantages: rapidity, sensitivity, and no interference from bilirubin or ascorbic acid. In less than 2 min total cholesterol can be determined in a sample. Free and esterified cholesterol can be successively determined within 4 min. Moreover, the minimum detectable amount of cholesterol by the present method is about 1 μg (10 μl of 125 mg/liter solution). The cholesterol in as little as 1 μl of serum or plasma can be measured.

In conclusion, although the present method is not especially suitable for routine assay of many samples, it has special research and pediatric applications. With the present method we are studying lipoproteins as substrate and the interaction between detergents and lipoproteins or lipid micelles.

We thank Messrs. S. Matsuzaki and Y. Hikawa, Beckman-Toshiba Ltd., for their cooperation.

References

1. Richmond, W., Preparation and properties of a cholesterol oxidase from *Nocardia* sp. and its application to the enzymatic assay of total cholesterol in serum. *Clin. Chem.* **19,** 1350 (1973).

2. Allain, C. C., Poon, L. S., Chan, C. S. G., et al., Enzymatic determination of total serum cholesterol. *Clin. Chem.* **20,** 470 (1974).

3. Tarbutton, P. N., and Gunter, C. R., Enzymatic determination of total cholesterol in serum. *Clin. Chem.* **20,** 724 (1974).

4. Witte, D. L., Barrett, D. A., II, and Wycoff, D. A., Evaluation of an enzymatic procedure for determination of serum cholesterol with the Abbott ABA-100. *Clin. Chem.* **20,** 1282 (1974).

5. Okuda, J., and Okuda, G., A rapid polarographic microdetermination of glucose with glucose oxidase. *Clin. Chim. Acta* **23,** 365 (1969).

6. Okuda, J., and Miwa, I., Polarographic microdetermination of D-glucose anomers with β-D-glucose oxidase. *Anal. Biochem.* **39,** 387 (1971).

7. Okuda, J., and Okuda, G., Rapid and successive microdeterminations of oxygen, D-glucose, and its anomers in blood with β-D-glucose oxidase and oxygen electrode. *Biochem. Med.* **7,** 257 (1973).

8. Kadish, A. H., and Hall, D. A., A new method for the continuous monitoring of blood glucose by measurement of dissolved oxygen. *Clin. Chem.* **11,** 869 (1965).

9. Kadish, A. H., Litle, R. L., and Sternberg, J. C., A new and rapid method for the determination of glucose by measurement of rate of oxygen consumption. *Clin. Chem.* **14,** 116 (1968).

CLIN. CHEM. 22/3, 341–345 (1976)

Gas-Chromatographic Analysis for Succinimide Anticonvulsants in Serum: Macro- and Micro-Scale Methods

James Bonitati

A gas-chromatographic analysis for the succinimide anticonvulsant drugs—ethosuximide, methsuximide, and phensuximide—in 1.0 ml of serum was modified to improve its reliability, speed, and precision. A separate procedure for 10–100 μl of serum was also developed. Neither method requires an initial preparation of derivatives. The working range of each method is about 10–100 mg/liter for the macro-method, 2–100 mg/liter for the micro-method. The methsuximide metabolite, *N*-desmethylmethsuximide, is included in both methods. Concentrations of *N*-desmethylmethsuximide in the blood of two patients with petit mal epilepsy are reported.

Additional Keyphrases: *drug assay • monitoring drug concentrations in serum • therapy for epilepsy*

Several gas-chromatographic methods are available for measuring the circulating concentrations of ethosuximide (2-ethyl-2-methylsuccinimide, "Zarontin"; Parke, Davis & Co., Detroit, Mich. 48232), and the other common succinimide anticonvulsants: methsuximide (*N*,2-dimethyl-2-phenylsuccinimide, "Celontin"; Parke, Davis & Co.), and phensuximide (*N*-methyl-2-phenylsuccinimide, "Milontin"; Parke, Davis & Co.) (*1–9*).

Although these methods appear to be specific and accurate, they tend to be tedious, lengthy, or otherwise not adapted to the rapid manual analysis of multiple samples. For example, several methods (*1–3*) involve extraction with large volumes of solvent, followed by either lengthy evaporation steps or the use of bulky rotary evaporators. In other methods (*4, 5*) the succinimides require a long time to emerge from the chromatographic column. The method of Toseland et al. (*6*) is rapid, simple, and extremely sensitive, but requires a special detector for nitrogen in the gas chromatograph.

Several liquid phases are available for use in gas-chromatographic assay of the succinimides in the free state, so that derivatives of these drugs need not be made, except in schemes that include the concurrent analysis for other anticonvulsant drugs. Furthermore, methsuximide is rapidly *N*-demethylated in the body to *N*-desmethylmethsuximide (*7*), a product that appears to be as strongly anticonvulsive as the parent compound (*7*). Methylation in the gas chromatograph would thus tend to complicate the measurement of methsuximide in the blood.

The method of van der Kleijn et al. (*8, 9*), which includes a single chloroform extraction and does not involve derivative formation, appears to offer a simple and rapid alternative to the foregoing methods. A shortcoming of this procedure, however, is the difficulty and uncertainty of obtaining sufficient serum extract in the final centrifugation step, because sera emulsify to various extents during the extraction step. Also, the syringe may become clogged when drug extract in the bottom phase is retrieved through the emulsified top phase. Finally, precision is decreased at higher concentrations of the drugs.

I have modified the method of van der Kleijn et al. for 1.0 ml of serum, to increase its reliability, speed, and precision. A scaled-down procedure for use with 10–100 μl samples is also presented. *N*-Desmethylmethsuximide, the methsuximide metabolite, is measured in both procedures, and its concentrations in the blood of two patients are reported.

Materials and Methods

Reagents

Chloroform. Analytical reagent grade.

Phosphate buffer. Saturated aqueous solution of KH_2PO_4.

Neurochemistry Division, Harry M. Dent Neurologic Institute, Millard Fillmore Hospital, 3 Gates Circle, Buffalo, N. Y. 14209.
Received Nov. 3, 1975; accepted Dec. 22, 1975.

Standards

Pure samples of ethosuximide, methsuximide, and phensuximide were gifts from Parke, Davis & Co. *N*-Desmethylmethsuximide was a gift from Dr. A. J. Atkinson, Jr., Northwestern Memorial Hospital, Chicago, Ill.

The internal standard was fluorene (*o*-biphenylene-methane), obtained as an analytical-grade reagent from Eastman Kodak Co., Rochester, N. Y. 14650.

Ethosuximide standard solution. An aqueous 500 mg/liter solution.

Mixed drugs standard solution. Ethosuximide, methsuximide, phensuximide, and *N*-desmethylmethsuximide, each 500 mg/liter of water.

Internal standard solutions. Stock solution: fluorene, 625 mg/liter (500 μg/800 μl) in chloroform. *Macromethod standard:* fluorene, 62.5 mg/liter (50 μg/800 μl). Dilute the stock solution 10-fold with chloroform. *Micromethod standards:* Two standard solutions were used: 5 μg/800 μl, and 1 μg/800 μl, for the assay of 50 μl and 10 μl of serum, respectively. These solutions are prepared by diluting the macro-method standard 10-fold and then fivefold with chloroform. All these solutions should be stored refrigerated.

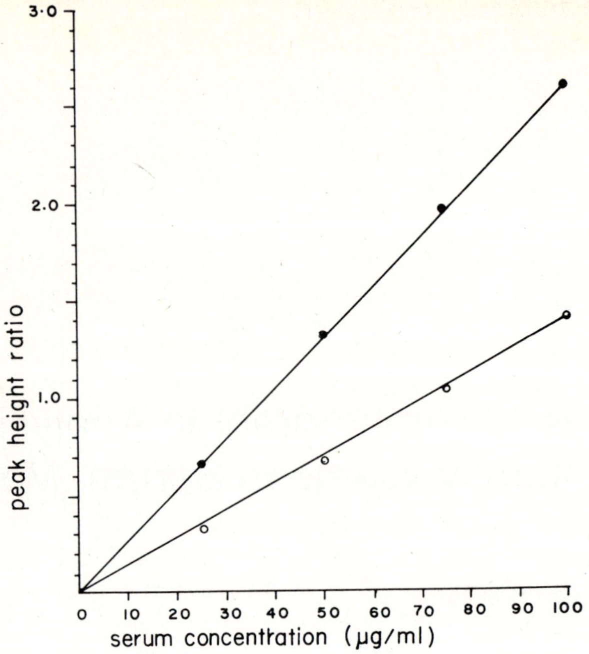

Fig. 2. Calibration curves for ethosuximide in serum by isothermal gas chromatography

Dark circles: micro-method. 10-μl volumes of serum standards were analyzed. *Light circles:* macro-method. 1.0-ml volumes of serum standards were analyzed

Apparatus

A Cliniscreen gas chromatograph equipped with dual flame-ionization detectors (Beckman Instruments, Inc., Irvine, Calif. 92664) was used for chromatography. The column was a 185 cm glass **U**-tube (2 mm i.d.) packed with 5% OV-17 liquid phase on 100–120 mesh Gas Chrom Q (Applied Science Laboratories, Inc., State College, Pa. 16801). Temperature settings were: injector port, 150 °C; detector line, 250 °C; detectors, 275 °C. Two oven temperature modes were used: isothermal heating at 180 °C for samples containing ethosuximide only, and temperature programming for multiple drug analysis: 180 °C for 1.5 min, increased to 230 °C at a rate of 10 °C/min. The carrier gas (helium) flow rate was 50 ml/min. Gas flows (ml/min) to the detectors were: air, 300; hydrogen, 45; and helium, 50. Instrument settings were: range, 1000; recorder attenuation, 1; detector suppression, 3. The response range of the 255-mm (10-inch) chart recorder was 1 mV full scale; chart speed was 12 mm (0.5 inch)/min.

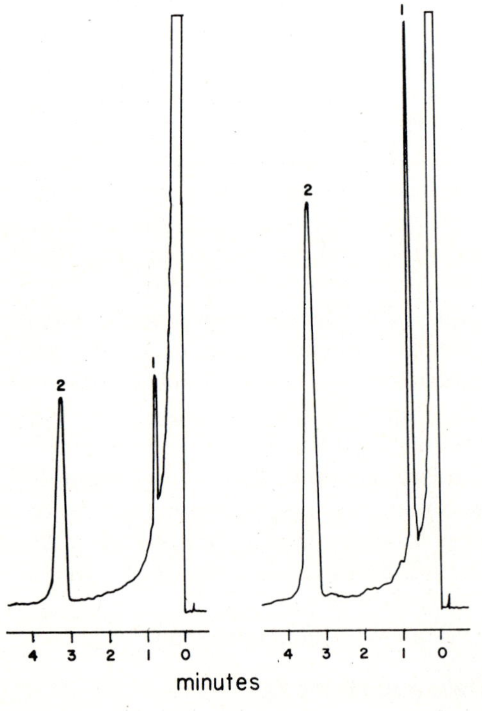

Fig. 1. Isothermal gas chromatography of ethosuximide in serum extracts

(*left*) macro-method. 1.0 ml of serum containing 50 mg of ethosuximide per liter was analyzed. (*right*) micro-method. 10 μl of serum containing 50 mg of ethosuximide per liter was analyzed. *1*, ethosuximide; *2*, internal standard (fluorene)

Procedures

Macro-volume method. To 1.0 ml of serum in a 12-ml conical centrifuge tube add 1.0 ml of phosphate buffer, followed by 800 μl of internal standard solution (delivered with a Pipetman adjustable microliter pipet, 1000-μl model; Rainin Instruments Co., Inc., 1030 Commonwealth Ave., Boston, Mass. 02215). Briskly shake on a vortex-type mixer (two tubes can be mixed at one time), and then centrifuge at 1000 × *g* for 5 min. Aspirate the top layer and inject 2 μl of the clear bottom layer into the gas chromatograph. Ethosuximide samples should be chromatographed isothermally. For mixed-drug samples use the temperature-programmed mode.

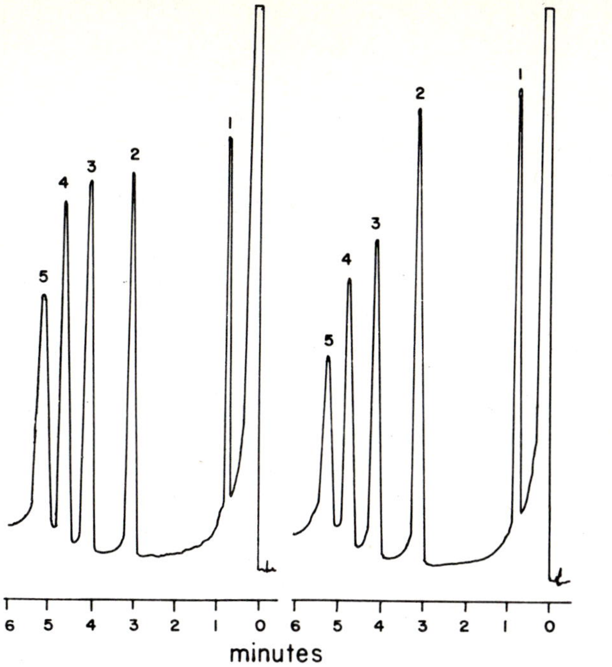

Fig. 3. Temperature-programmed gas chromatography of succinimide anticonvulsants in serum extracts

(*left*) macro-method. Analysis of 1.0 ml of serum containing 100 mg each of mixed drugs per liter. (*right*) micro-method. Analysis of 50 μl of serum containing 100 mg each of mixed drugs per liter. *1*, ethosuximide; *2*, internal standard; *3*, methsuximide; *4*, phensuximide; *5*, *N*-desmethylmethsuximide

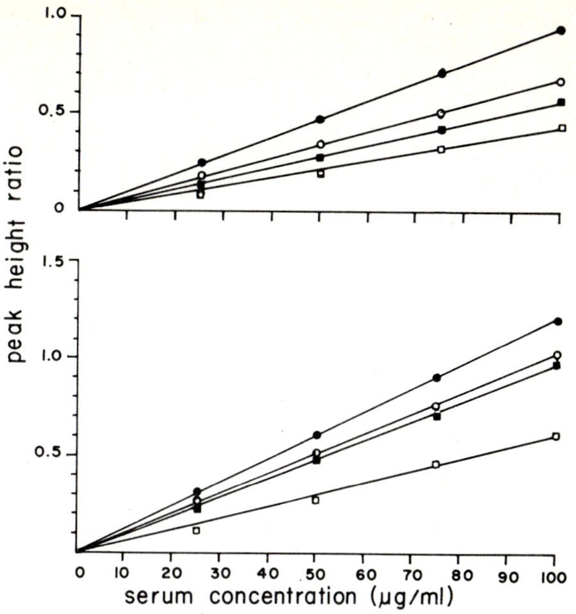

Fig. 4. Calibration curves for succinimide anticonvulsants in serum by temperature-programmed gas chromatography

(*upper*) micro-method. 50-μl volumes of serum standards were analyzed. (*lower*) macro-method. 1.0-ml volumes of serum standards were analyzed. *dark circles*, ethosuximide; *light circles*, methsuximide; *dark squares*, phensuximide; *light squares*, *N*-desmethylmethsuximide

Prepare calibration curves for the drugs in the concentration range 25–100 mg/liter from data on extracts of drug-free pooled serum to which standard solutions are added. Plot peak-height ratios of drug to internal standard vs. drug concentration. Prepare two calibration curves, one for ethosuximide, another for the drug mixture.

Samples containing less than 25 mg of drug per liter can be assayed by concentrating a portion of the extract to a small volume (5–20 μl) at 35 °C in a stream of air.

Micro-volume method. In this method, 10–100 μl of serum can be assayed for ethosuximide alone, and 50–100 μl for mixed drugs. Transfer 0.1 ml of phosphate buffer to a 12-ml conical centrifuge tube. Deliver 10–100 μl of serum for the determination of ethosuximide or 50–100 μl of serum for the determination of mixed drugs. Add 800 μl of internal standard; for 10-μl samples use the 1 μg/800 μl internal standard solution and for 50–100 μl samples use the 5 μg/800 μl solution. Mix and centrifuge as in the macro-method. Remove the top layer and, with Pasteur pipets, transfer the bottom extract to clean centrifuge tubes. Evaporate the samples to 5–20 μl at 35 °C in a stream of air. Inject 1 μl of sample into the gas chromatograph.

Prepare calibration curves for the micro-volume method from data on serum containing drugs in the concentration range 25–100 mg/liter, as in the macro-method.

Results

Analytical Variables

Chromatography and calibration. Figure 1 shows isothermal chromatograms of ethosuximide and fluorene in serum extracts. The fact that ethosuximide elutes almost with the solvent front does not interfere with quantitation. The ethosuximide peak is more sharply defined in the micro-method however, because the solvent peak is smaller than it is in the macro-method. Figure 2 shows calibration curves for extracts of ethosuximide from serum, by both methods.

On isothermal chromatography of methsuximide, phensuximide, and *N*-desmethylmethsuximide, the peaks representing these compounds were broad, with relatively long retention times. Temperature programming produced sharp, well-separated peaks, with shorter retentions (Figure 3). The initial isothermal segment of the temperature program allows ethosuximide to be assayed in combination with the other drugs. Figure 4 shows mixed drug calibration curves for the macro- and micro-methods. Separate calibration curves are required for isothermal and programmed modes, because the elution temperature of the internal standard differs in the two cases.

Precision. Analytical precision within-run was calculated from results of 10 successive assays of the same serum sample. Day-to-day precision was calculated from at least 20 measurements during a 30-day period.

Within-run precision (CV) of macro- and micro-methods for ethosuximide by isothermal chromatography was 4% and 6%, respectively; day-to-day precision was 5% and 8%, respectively.

Within-run precision for temperature-programmed chromatography of mixed drug standards in serum by the macro- and micro-methods was 5% and 7%, respectively, for all drugs; day-to-day precision was 6% and 10%, respectively, for all drugs.

Sensitivity. Analytical sensitivity, expressed as the minimal concentration of drug detectable in serum, was 10 mg/liter for ethosuximide and *N*-desmethylmethsuximide, and 5 mg/liter for methsuximide and phensuximide, in the macro-method. In the micro-method, depending on the serum volume (10–100 μl) assayed, the sensitivity was 2–10 mg/liter for ethosuximide and *N*-desmethylmethsuximide, and 1–5 mg/liter for methsuximide and phensuximide.

The sensitivity of the macro-method can be increased by transferring serum extract to a clean centrifuge tube and evaporating to 5–20 μl before injection into the gas chromatograph. Under these conditions the internal standard peak will be very large compared with the drug peaks and must be selectively attenuated during chromatography. Calibration curves for analysis of 2.5–10 mg of drugs per liter of serum were linear, and they were continuous with the 25–100 mg/liter calibration curves in Figures 2 and 4.

The sensitivities of both the macro- and micro-method can be increased by injecting larger quantities of sample extract into the gas chromatograph, except for ethosuximide, because its peak is obscured by the increased size of the peak representing the solvent under these conditions.

Analytical recovery. Extraction efficiencies for the macro-method, measured by comparing extracted serum standards with standard chloroform solutions of the drugs, were 49.5% for ethosuximide, 67% for *N*-desmethylmethsuximide, and >90% for methsuximide and phensuximide.

In the micro-method recoveries exceeded 90% for all drugs.

Specificity. In concentrations of 1.0 mg/liter none of the following commonly used anticonvulsant drugs interfered with the present methods: diphenylhydantoin (Dilantin), phenobarbital, primidone (Mysoline), and carbamazepine (Tegretol). These drugs are not eluted from the gas-chromatographic column under the present conditions of chromatography.

Internal standards. Two other compounds besides fluorene were examined as internal standards for the assay procedures. The succinimide derivative, 2,2-dimethyl-3-methyl-succinimide, did not separate from ethosuximide in the present chromatographic system. With naphthalene as internal standard, analytical precision was poor. Furthermore, the high chromatographic mobility of this compound required the use of low flow rates of carrier gas, which greatly lengthened the chromatographic runs, and also resulted in broadened drug peaks.

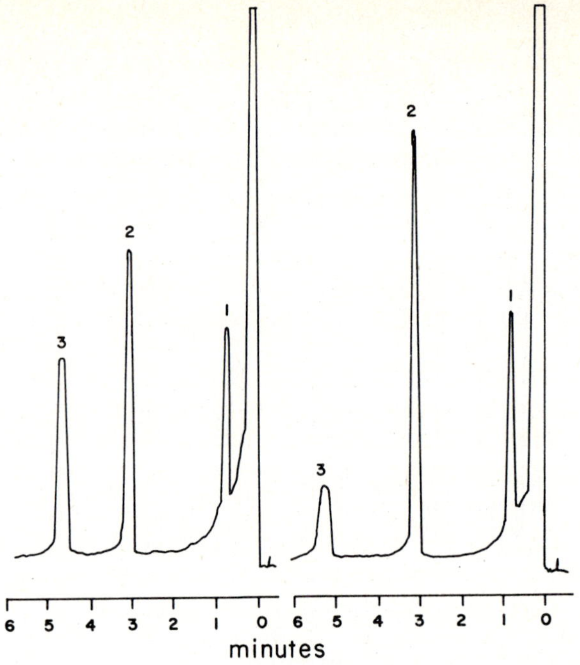

Fig. 5. Gas chromatography of serum extracts from epileptic patients on long-term methsuximide or phensuximide therapy
Left: serum from a woman with petit mal epilepsy controlled on chronic mixed-drug therapy with ethosuximide and phensuximide (250 mg of each drug three times per day). *1,* ethosuximide, 48 mg/liter; *2,* internal standard; *3,* phensuximide, 65 mg/liter. *Right:* serum from a woman with petit mal epilepsy controlled on chronic mixed-drug therapy with ethosuximide and methsuximide (250 mg of each drug three times per day). *1,* ethosuximide, 37 mg/liter; *2,* internal standard; *3, N*-desmethylmethsuximide, 28 mg/liter. A second patient, also a woman, on the same drug regimen had the following concentrations of drugs in her serum: ethosuximide, 42 mg/liter; *N*-desmethylmethsuximide, 15 mg/liter. All three serum samples were assayed by the macro-method

Results for Patients on Methsuximide and Phensuximide

Figure 5 shows tracings for sera from two patients with petit mal epilepsy who were on long-term anticonvulsant therapy with ethosuximide together with either methsuximide or phensuximide. Only ethosuximide and phensuximide were detected in the serum of the patient receiving these drugs. In the patient receiving ethosuximide and methsuximide, however, the methsuximide peak was absent, but a peak for its metabolite, *N*-desmethylmethsuximide, appeared, together with the peak for ethosuximide. This is in agreement with the observations of Strong et al. (*7*), who found, by using a highly sensitive fragmentographic method, that *N*-desmethylmethsuximide concentrations in serum were about 700-fold greater than methsuximide concentrations in methsuximide-treated patients. In line with this, Glazko and Dill (*3*) observed large increases in liver *N*-demethylase activity of rats that had received long-term treatment with methsuximide.

Discussion

Method modifications. The present macro-method, though based on a procedure of van der Kleijn et al. (*9*), differs from it as follows. The extraction solvent volume is increased from 0.1 ml to 0.8 ml, to eliminate emulsification problems and ensure an ample quantity of extract. The larger solvent volume permits removal of the upper emulsified layer after extraction and centrifugation, thus providing a clear extract for sampling without the complication of syringe clogging. With the elimination of serum emulsification and syringe clogging, assays could be performed faster and with greater reliability.

A new internal standard, fluorene, was used.

Use of lower injector port temperature (150 °C vs. 200 °C) increases the precision of the measurements in the present system. For example, repeated injections of the same sample of ethosuximide (100 mg/liter) and internal standard (50 mg/liter) at the two temperatures gave analytical precisions (CV) of 2% and 14%, respectively.

A further difference in assay conditions was the use, in the present methods, of a higher concentration of liquid phase in the chromatographic column—5% instead of 3% OV-17.

In the micro-method introduced here the volume of serum required for analysis is reduced by 10 to 100-fold compared with the macro-method, with only slight loss in precision.

Therapeutic concentrations in serum. The therapeutic concentrations of the succinimide anticonvulsants in serum are not yet firmly established. Tentative values are: 40–80 mg/liter for ethosuximide (*10*), and 20–30 mg/liter for methsuximide, expressed in terms of *N*-desmethylmethsuximide (*7*). These values fall within the scope of the assay methods presented here. Therapeutic values for phensuximide are still under investigation.

Patients' sera were provided by W. R. Kinkel, M.D., and Mrs. R. Ekes.

References

1. Cremers, H. M. H. G., and Verheesen, P. E., A rapid method for the estimation of anti-epileptic drugs in blood serum by gas-liquid chromatography. *Clin. Chim. Acta* **48,** 413 (1973).
2. Meijer, J. W. A., Simultaneous quantitative determination of anti-epileptic drugs, including carbamazepine, in body fluids. *Epilepsia* **12,** 341 (1971).
3. Glazko, A. J., and Dill, W. A., Ethosuximide: Chemistry and methods for determination. In *Antiepileptic Drugs.* D. M. Woodbury, J. K. Penry, and R. P. Schmidt, Eds. Raven Press, New York, N. Y., 1972, pp 413–415.
4. Solow, E. B., Metaxas, J. M., and Summers, T. R., Antiepileptic drugs: A current assessment of simultaneous determination of multiple drug therapy by gas liquid chromatography-on column methylation. *J. Chromatogr. Sci.* **12,** 256 (1974).
5. Solow, E. B., and Green, J. B., The simultaneous determination of multiple anticonvulsant drug levels by gas–liquid chromatography. *Neurology* **22,** 540 (1972).
6. Toseland, P. A., Albani, M., and Gauchel, F. D., Organic nitrogen-selective detector used in gas chromatographic determination of some anticonvulsant and barbiturate drugs in plasma and tissues. *Clin. Chem.* **21,** 98 (1975).
7. Strong, J. M., Abe, T., Gibbs, E. L., and Atkinson, A. J., Jr., Plasma levels of methsuximide and *N*-desmethylsuximide during methsuximide therapy. *Neurology* **24,** [illegible] (1974).
8. van der Kleijn, E., Collste, P., Norlander, B., et al., Gas chromatographic determination of ethosuximide and phensuximide in plasma and urine of man. *J. Pharm. Pharmacol.* **25,** 324 (1973).
9. van der Kleijn, E., Pijnappel, H., van Wijk, C., et al., Pharmacokinetic concepts for chronic treatment with anti-epileptic drugs. In *Methods of Analysis of Anti-epileptic Drugs,* J. W. A. Meijer, H. Meinardi, C. Gardner-Thorpe, and E. van der Kleijn, Eds. American Elsevier, New York, N. Y., 1973, pp 10–11.
10. Penry, J. K., Porter, R. J., and Dreifus, F. E., Ethosuximide: Relation of plasma levels to clinical control. In *Antiepileptic Drugs.* D. M. Woodbury, J. K. Penry, and R. P. Schmidt, Eds. Raven Press, New York, N. Y., 1972, pp 431–441.

CLIN. CHEM. 22/3, 346–349 (1976)

Comparison of Results for 13 Clinical Laboratory Determinations with Three Automated Analytical Systems

Eric J. Sampson, Dennis D. Derck, and Laurence M. Demers[1]

We evaluated the Abbott Bichromatic Analyzer-100 (ABA-100) for use in the routine clinical chemistry laboratory by examining 13 different determinations that can be performed on the instrument. Results with the Du Pont "*aca*" and Technicon continuous-flow systems were compared to the ABA-100 in terms of upper limits of linearity, inter-run coefficient of variation, and results for samples from patients. The upper limits of linearity for the methods on the ABA-100 exceeded all of those for the continuous-flow systems, except for urea nitrogen. Precision of the ABA-100 was as good as or better than that of the *aca* for all determinations, except for glucose in a normal control serum and creatine kinase and creatinine in an above-normal control serum.

Additional Keyphrases: *discrete and continuous-flow analysis • analytical systems • inter-method comparison*

The "Abbott Bichromatic Analyzer" (ABA-100; Abbott Laboratories, South Pasadena, Calif. 91030) is a discrete analyzer possessing several features of interest, including micro-sampling and "bichromatic" measurement that compensates for turbidity and lipemia. Several reports have appeared in the literature on the precision and accuracy of this instrument with both glucose (*1*) and cholesterol (*2*) methodologies. Loeb et al. (*3*) described the effects of a recommended evaporation retardant for the instrument's sample cups, "Sera Seal", on the rates of several enzymatic reactions.

Division of Clinical Pathology, The Milton S. Hershey Medical Center, The Pennsylvania State University, Hershey, Pa. 17033.
[1] Address correspondence to L. M. D.
Received Oct. 3, 1975; accepted Dec. 22, 1975.

We examined 13 different determinations done with the ABA-100, and compared results by these procedures with those obtained with the "*aca*" discrete analyzer (E.I. du Pont de Nemours and Co., Inc., Wilmington, Del. 19898) and continuous-flow systems (Technicon Corp., Tarrytown, N. Y. 10591), with respect to linearity, coefficients of variation, and results for patients' sera. The latter two instrument systems have previously been so compared (*4*).

Material and Methods

ABA-100: The following determinations and methods were examined, Abbott "A-Gent" reagents being used: alkaline phosphatase[2] according to Bessey et al. (*5*), modified with 2-amino-2-methyl-1,3-propanediol as the buffer; urea nitrogen, Talke and Schubert (*6*) (enzymatic), urease modified with phosphate buffer; cholesterol, Allain et al. (*7*) (enzymatic); creatine kinase, Oliver (*8*), activated with L-cysteine and dithioerythritol, modified with bacterial glucose-6-phosphate dehydrogenase and NAD^+; glucose, Richterich and Dauwalder (*9*) (enzymatic), hexokinase modified with NAD^+; aspartate aminotransferase, Henry et al. (*10*); alanine aminotransferase, Henry et al. (*10*); lactate dehydrogenase, Amador et al. (*11*);

[2] Nonstandard abbreviations used and systematic names of enzymes: alkaline phosphatase (orthophosphoric monoester phosphohydrolase, EC 3.1.3.1); creatine kinase (ATP:creatine phosphotransferase, EC 2.7.3.2); aspartate aminotransferase (EC 2.6.1.1); alanine aminotransferase (alanine:2-oxoglutarate aminotransferase, EC 2.6.1.2); lactate dehydrogenase (lactate:NAD oxidoreductase, EC 1.1.1.27); SMA 12/60, *S*equential *M*ultiple *A*nalyzer, Model 12/60 (Technicon Corp.).

and total protein, Gornall et al. (*12*) (biuret). In addition, the following determinations and methods were examined with use of reagents from other manufacturers: calcium, *o*-cresolphthalein complexone/8-hydroxyquinoline (*13*) (Dow Diagnostics, Indianapolis, Ind. 46206); creatinine, Jaffé (*14*) (Harleco, Gibbstown, N. J. 08027); inorganic phosphorus, phosphomolybdate reduced by ferrous ammonium sulfate (*15*) (Hycel, Houston, Tex. 77023); and triglycerides, enzymatic, Bucolo and David (*16*) (Calbiochem, La Jolla, Calif. 92037). All of the above determinations were done according to Abbott procedures at 37 °C, except that creatinine was measured at 30 °C.

aca: With this instrument we used Du Pont reagent packs. The determinations and the methods for them that we examined were essentially the same as those described for the ABA-100, except that creatine kinase was activated with only dithioerythritol and the glucose method makes use of NADP instead of NAD^+. All determinations were done at 37 °C.

Continuous-flow systems: Determinations were performed with Fisher reagents (Fisher Scientific Corp., Fair Lawn, N. J. 07410), except that GOD-Perid reagent from Boehringer Mannheim Corp., New York, N. Y. 10017, was used for glucose. The methods are essentially the same as those described for the ABA-100, with the following exceptions: urea nitrogen, diacetyl monoxime in the presence of thiosemicarbazide and ferric ion (*17*); cholesterol, Levine and Zak (*18*), with extraction (Technicon methodology N-24A); glucose, glucose oxidase/peroxidase (*19*); inorganic phosphorus, phosphomolybdate reduced by stannous chloride and hydrazine (*20*); triglyceride, Kessler and Lederer (*21*), with extraction and fluorometric quantitation (Technicon methodology N-78).

Precision: Day-to-day precision of the ABA-100, *aca,* SMA 12/60, and AutoAnalyzers I and II was evaluated by use of commercially available control products in which the analytes were present in either normal or above-normal concentrations. Coefficients of variation were tabulated from 30 different assayed values, obtained during two months.

Range of linearity: Freshly prepared aqueous standard solutions representing urea nitrogen (urea, NBS), calcium ($CaCl_2$, Fisher), creatinine (NBS), glucose (NBS), phosphorus (Na_2HPO_4, Baker Chemical Co., Phillipsburg, N. J. 08865), protein (albumin, bovine, fraction V; Sigma Chemical Co., St. Louis, Mo. 63178), and triglycerides (glycerol, Baker) were examined, to assess the extent to which concentration and readings are linearly related in the case of the ABA-100. The same solutions were used with the *aca,* except for triglycerides, and with the Technicon systems, except for calcium and phosphorus, which were prepared in bovine serum albumin, 60 g/liter. Cholesterol (NBS) standards were prepared in isopropanol. In the case of the enzymes, we used dilutions of patients' samples with supranormal values.

Comparison of values: Before comparing the results obtained with different instruments for patients' specimens, we calibrated the methods with aqueous standards or, for the enzymatic determinations, by calibrating the different instruments to yield the same values obtained on the ABA-100 for several normal, slightly-above-normal, and much-above-normal samples of patients' sera. Although we recognized the arbitrary nature of this latter calibration procedure, it was necessary if enzyme determinations generated by these laboratory instruments were to be used interchangeably in patient care.

For each comparison, 50 to 100 specimens from patients were examined by dividing the samples and analyzing one aliquot from each instrument. The resulting data were subjected to least-squares analysis, to determine the slope, intercept, and correlation coefficient as compared with such data for the ABA-100.

Results and Discussion

Table 1 summarizes the results obtained with the ABA-100, *aca,* and Technicon systems for upper limit of linearity, day-to-day precision, regression data, and correlation coefficient. Note that enzymatic procedures were used with the ABA-100 for urea nitrogen, cholesterol, and triglyceride, while the corresponding Technicon methods were nonenzymatic. Hexokinase was used in the determination of glucose with the ABA-100 vs. glucose oxidase with the AutoAnalyzer II. In the Technicon instruments, a dialysis step was used in the determination of alkaline phosphatase, urea nitrogen, calcium, creatinine, glucose, aspartate aminotransferase, and inorganic phosphorus. Except for differences in reagent concentration and sample-to-reagent ratio, the methods examined with the ABA-100 and *aca* were similar for each of the determinations investigated. With respect to sample volume, the ABA-100 required a substantially smaller amount. For example, in determining aspartate aminotransferase and alanine aminotransferase activity with the *aca* and cholesterol with the AutoAnalyzer II, the ABA-100 required 0.01 the sample volume.

Compared to the *aca,* the ABA-100 had a greater limit of linearity for creatine kinase, glucose, and inorganic phosphorus; the opposite was true for alkaline phosphatase, urea nitrogen, aspartate aminotransferase, alanine aminotransferase, lactate dehydrogenase, and total protein. The upper limits of linearity on the SMA 12/60 were investigated only to the top of the recording chart. Values were found to be linearly related to concentration throughout this region, except for alkaline phosphatase and lactate dehydrogenase activities, which deviated slightly below the maximum values of 350 and 600 U/liter, respectively. Urea nitrogen was the only determination in which the limit of linearity of the continuous-flow systems exceeded that for the ABA-100.

Table 1 lists inter-run precision data obtained on two commercially available control products. *F*

Table 1. Comparison of Thirteen Determinations on the ABA-100 with Other Automated Analytical Systems

Detn	Instrument	Principle ref. nos.	Sample vol, µl[a]	Upper limit of linearity	Inter-run coefficient of variation, % Normal (mean)	Elevated (mean)	Range[b]	Comparison of methods Slope	Intercept	Corr. Coeff., r
Alkaline phosphatase	ABA	5	5	900 U/l	4.73 (60 U/l)	4.00 (210 U/l)	45-300 U/l			
	SMA	5	300	300 U/l	2.66*	2.68*		1.081	-7.4	0.962
	ACA	5	200	1100 U/l	7.37*	5.89*		0.912	11.1	0.996
Urea nitrogen	ABA	6	2.5	800 mg/l	4.02 (220 mg/l)	2.21 (440 mg/l)	50-320 mg/l			
	SMA	6	40	1000 mg/l	3.24	1.97		1.027	-1.2	0.995
	ACA	17	20	2500 mg/l	5.08	2.69		0.953	0.0	0.995
Calcium	ABA	13	5	200 mg/l	1.81 (90 mg/l)	1.98 (130 mg/l)	80-150 mg/l	9.35[c]	1.07[d]	
	SMA	13	85	150 mg/l	1.51	1.65		9.35	1.26	0.988
	ACA	13	60	200 mg/l	2.48*	2.03		9.16	1.32	0.914
Cholesterol	ABA	7	5	5.0 g/l	7.53 (1.2 g/l)	7.54 (2.5 g/l)	0.9-3.9 g/l			
	AA-II	18	500	4.0 g/l	6.06	7.01		1.160	-35.4	0.962
Creatine kinase	ABA	8	5	2000 U/l	4.23 (120 U/l)	7.29 (580 U/l)	20-250 U/l			
	ACA	8	200	900 U/l	3.39	4.44*		0.961	0.9	0.984
Creatinine	ABA	14	20	350 mg/l	4.59 (10 mg/l)	3.25 (48 mg/l)	6-18 mg/l			
	SMA	14	400	150 mg/l	5.30	1.44*		1.040	0.0	0.994
	ACA	14	200	300 mg/l	6.36*	1.63*		1.000	0.0	0.990
Glucose	ABA	9	10	7.5 g/l	3.21 (0.9 g/l)	1.94 (1.9 g/l)	0.6-2.5 g/l			
	AA-II	19	100	5.0 g/l	2.98	1.81		1.026	-5.0	0.995
	ACA	9	40	6.0 g/l	2.10*	1.86		1.029	-1.3	0.998
Aspartate amino-transferase	ABA	10	5	500 U/l	8.28 (18 U/l)	5.46 (80 U/l)	8-140 U/l			
	SMA	10	200	300 U/l	6.49	3.32*		1.010	-5.2	0.994
	ACA	10	500	800 U/l	14.44*	6.96		1.170	-7.0	0.992
Alanine amino-transferase	ABA	10	5	550 U/l	9.77 (50 U/l)	6.67 (230 U/l)	4-110 U/l			
	ACA	10	500	800 U/l	11.49	6.41		0.932	0.4	0.993
Lactate dehydrogenase	ABA	11	5	550 U/l	2.97 (220 U/l)	5.74 (450 U/l)	90-320 U/l			
	SMA	11	80	500 U/l	5.16*	3.31*		1.084	-12.5	0.978
	ACA	11	200	700 U/l	4.86*	4.84		0.950	3.0	0.997
Inorganic phosphorus	ABA	15	10	90 mg/l	3.94 (30 mg/l)	2.55 (70 mg/l)	15-60 mg/l			
	SMA	20	200	70 mg/l	2.51*	2.63		1.05	0.2	0.947
Total protein	ABA	12	5	100 mg/l	2.77 (48 mg/l)	1.94 (62 mg/l)	50-80 mg/l			
	SMA	12	50	100 mg/l	1.98*	1.69		1.03	-0.2	0.988
	ACA	12	160	120 mg/l	4.35*	2.81*		0.97	0.3	0.943
Triglycerides	ABA	16	10	6.0 g/l	3.51 (0.6 g/l)	3.53 (2.5 g/l)	0.6-4.0 g/l			
	AA-I	21	500	3.0 g/l	10.3*	5.06*		1.05	5.2	0.993

[a] Refers to volumes listed by the various manufacturers. SMA 12/60, AA-I and II values are only approximate volumes, based on average flow rates.
[b] Refers to the range of values obtained on patients' samples.
[c,d] Slope and intercept values calculated from regression analysis were erroneous, because of the patients' values were within a very narrow range, therefore, the values given are the means (b) and standard deviation (c) of 58 samples. t-values indicated no significant difference between the ABA-100 and the SMA or aca, p=0.05.
*Indicates the difference in precision of the method compared to the ABA-100 is statistically significant at p=0.05, 30 df numerator and 30 df denominator.

values were calculated, to compare the precision of the ABA-100 to the other instruments listed. For determination of alkaline phosphatase activity, the precision of the SMA 12/60 appeared to be better than that of the ABA-100 with both controls, which in turn was better than the *aca*. With the normal control, determination of calcium, creatinine, aspartate aminotransferase, and lactate dehydrogenase on the ABA-100 was more precise than for the *aca;* the reverse was true with the above-normal control for creatine kinase and creatinine. The precision for determination of total protein in both controls was better with the ABA-100 than with the *aca*. Similarly, the SMA 12/60 offered better precision than the ABA-100 for the normal control for inorganic phosphorus and total protein and the above-normal control for creatinine and lactate dehydrogenase. The enzymatic triglyceride procedure on the ABA-100 was more precise with both controls than was the method of Kessler and Lederer on the AutoAnalyzer I.

Table 1 summarizes regression data and correlation coefficients calculated from a comparison of methods with the ABA-100 (*y*-axis). For practical purposes only six determinations are discussed. In comparing the diacetyl monoxime method used with the SMA 12/60 and the urease method used with the ABA-100 for determination of urea nitrogen, the small negative intercept, −1.2 mg/dl, may relate to the specificity of the enzymatic vs. the nonenzymatic reactions. Similarly, cholesterol values obtained by the method of Levine and Zak with the AutoAnalyzer II revealed a large negative bias, −35 mg/dl, when compared to the enzymatic method on the ABA-100, which again may reflect the nonspecific nature of the Technicon procedure. Witte et al. (2) noted similar regression data in comparing the enzymatic cholesterol method of Allain to a Technicon SMA 12/60 procedure. In comparing results by the Rosalki method for creatine kinase determination with the ABA-100 and *aca,* it was noteworthy that the creatine kinase reagent used with the *aca* (obtained from the plastic packs) displayed 40% greater activity on patient samples than did the Abbott "A-Gent." In order to use CPK results interchangeably in patient care, the *aca* instrument was initially calibrated against the ABA-100 to obtain the regression data given in

Table 1. For creatinine determination, a kinetic Jaffé method was used with the ABA-100 in which color development was monitored at 500 and 600 nm between 0.5 and 2.0 min after the reaction was initiated. Values were printed at 1.0, 1.5, and 2.0 min and added together to yield the creatinine value. Although the rate of the reaction was changing rapidly during this interval, results obtained by this method appeared to agree well with results obtained with both the SMA 12/60 and *aca*. The hexokinase method for glucose determination from the ABA-100 revealed a negative bias, −5 mg/dl, compared to the glucose oxidase method from the AutoAnalyzer II. Gochman et al. (*1*) recently investigated both methods in terms of possible interfering substances. Finally, the enzymatic method for triglyceride analysis on the ABA-100 was based on the method of Bucolo and David (*16*) requiring two separate reagents, the first being dispensed with the sample in the usual manner and the second being manually dispensed into each cuvette well on the second revolution of the instrument's carousel. Results by this method appeared to agree well with those by the nonenzymatic method of Kessler and Lederer (*21*) on the AutoAnalyzer I.

The ABA-100 has been in routine service in our laboratory for one year. The enzymatic cholesterol and triglyceride methods used with the ABA-100 have replaced the more tedious and time-consuming continuous-flow methods without loss of accuracy or precision. It was not possible to use the results of enzyme determinations on the three instrument systems interchangeably in patient care without initially changing the calibration factors on one system to yield values in agreement with another. In this study we arbitrarily calibrated the *aca* and SMA 12/60 to agree with values obtained on the ABA-100. Our laboratory personnel easily learned to operate the ABA-100 and quickly adapted its use to meet the laboratory's micro-chemistry responsibilities.

This work was supported in part by postdoctoral training grant No. IF 22 AMO2827-01, NIH, USPHS.

References

1. Gochman, N., Ryan, W. T., Sterling, R. E., and Widdowson, G. M., Interlaboratory comparison of enzymatic methods for serum glucose determination. *Clin. Chem.* **21,** 356 (1975).

2. Witte, D. L., Barrett, D. A., and Wycoff, D. A., Evaluation of an enzymatic procedure for determination of serum cholesterol with the Abbott ABA-100. *Clin. Chem.* **20,** 1282 (1974).

3. Loeb, H. G., Tramell, P. R., Szepessy, G., et al., Effect of a sample evaporation retardant on enzyme activity results with the Abbott Bichromatic Analyzer-100. *Clin. Chem.* **18,** 698 (1972).

4. Westgard, J. O., and Lahmeyer, B. L., Comparison of results from the Du Pont "*aca*" and the Technicon "SMA 12/60". *Clin. Chem.* **18,** 340 (1972).

5. Bessey, O. A., Lowry, O. H., and Brock, M. J., A method for the rapid determination of alkaline phosphatase with five cubic millimeters of serum. *J. Biol. Chem.* **164,** 321 (1946).

6. Talke, H., and Schubert, G. E., Enzymatische Harnstoffbestimmung in Blut and Serum im optischen Test nach Warburg. *Klin. Wochenschr.* **43,** 174 (1965).

7. Allain, C. C., Poon, L., Chan, S. G., et al., Enzymatic determination of total serum cholesterol. *Clin. Chem.* **20,** 470 (1974).

8. Oliver, I. T., A spectrophotometric method for the determination of creatine phosphokinase and myokinase. *Biochem. J.* **61,** 116 (1955).

9. Richterich, R., and Dauwalder, H., Vergleichende Bestimmungen der Uringlucosekonzentration mit der Polarimetrie und einer enzymatischen Method (Hexokinase/Glucose-6-phosphat-dehydrogenase). *Schweiz. Med. Wochenschr.* **101,** 860 (1971).

10. Henry, R. J., Chiamori, N., Golub, O. J. and Berkman, S., Revised spectrophotometric methods for the determination of glutamic-oxalacetic transaminase, glutamic-pyruvic transaminase, and lactic acid dehydrogenase. *Am. J. Clin. Pathol.* **34,** 381 (1960).

11. Amador, E. Dorfman, L. E., and Wacker, W. E. C., Serum lactic dehydrogenase activity: An analytical assessment of current assays. *Clin. Chem.* **9,** 391 (1963).

12. Gornall, A. G., Bardawill, C. J., and David, M. M., Determination of serum proteins by means of the biuret reaction. *J. Biol. Chem.* **177,** 751 (1949).

13. Connerty, H. V., and Briggs, A. R., Determination of serum calcium by means of *ortho*cresolphthalein complexone. *Am. J. Clin. Pathol.* **45,** 290 (1966).

14. Jaffé, M., Über den Niederschlag, welchen Pickrinsäure im Normalen Harn erzeugt und uber eine neue Reaktion des Kreatinins. *Z. Physiol. Chem.* **10,** 391 (1886).

15. Horwitt, B. N., Determination of inorganic serum phosphate by means of stannous chloride. *J. Biol. Chem.* **199,** 537 (1952).

16. Bucolo, G., and David, H., Quantitative determination of serum triglycerides by the use of enzymes. *Clin. Chem.* **19,** 476 (1973).

17. Marsh, W. H., Fingerhut, B., and Miller, H., Automatic and manual direct methods for the determination of blood urea. *Clin. Chem.* **11,** 624 (1965).

18. Levine, J., and Zak, B., Automated determination of serum total cholesterol. *Clin. Chim. Acta* **10,** 381 (1964).

19. Werner, W., Rey, H. G., and Weilinger, H., Properties of a new chromogen for the determination of glucose in blood according to the GOD/POD method. *Z. Anal. Chem.* **252,** 224 (1970).

20. Kraml, M., A semi-automated determination of phospholipids. *Clin. Chim. Acta* **13,** 442 (1966).

21. Kessler, G., and Lederer, H., Fluorometric measurement of triglycerides. In *Automation in Analytical Chemistry, Technicon Symposia 1965;* L. T. Skeggs et al., Eds., Mediad, New York, N. Y., 1966, p 341.

CLIN. CHEM. 22/3, 350–358 (1976)

Statistical Characterization of the Random Errors in the Radioimmunoassay Dose–Response Variable

David Rodbard, Robert H. Lenox, H. Linton Wray, and Douglas Ramseth

We have developed practical methods for evaluating the magnitude of the random errors in radioimmunoassay dose–response variables, and the relationship between this error and position on the dose–response curve. This is important: to obtain appropriate weights for each point on the dose–response curve when utilizing least-squares curve-fitting methods; to evaluate whether the standards and the unknowns are subject to error of the same magnitude; for quality-control purposes; and to study the sources of errors in radioimmunoassay. Both standards and unknowns in radioimmunoassays for cAMP and cGMP were analyzed in triplicate. The sample mean ($\bar{Y}$), sample standard deviation, s_Y, and variance (s_Y^2) of the response variable were calculated for each dose level. The relationship between s_Y^2 and $\bar{Y}$ was calculated utilizing several models. Results for standards and unknowns from several assays were pooled, and a curve smoothing procedure was used to minimize random sampling errors. This pooling increased the reliability of the analysis, and confirmed the presence of the theoretically predicted nonuniformity of variance. Thus, the calculation of results from these radioimmunoassays should utilize a *weighted* least-squares curve-fitting program. These analyses have been computerized, and can be used as a "preprocessor" for programs for routine analysis of results of radioimmunoassay.

Additional Keyphrases: *quality control • computer analysis • precision • heteroscedasticity • weighted least-squares regression*

Reproduction Research Branch, National Institute of Child Health and Human Development, National Institutes of Health Bethesda, Md. 20014 (D.R.); and the Depts. of Neuroendocrinology, Endocrinology and Metabolism, and Biometrics, Walter Reed Army Institute of Research, Washington, D. C. 20012.

Received Nov. 12, 1975; accepted Dec. 23, 1975.

Numerous methods have been proposed for the computer analysis of radioimmunoassay (RIA)[1] results. These usually involve use of a least-squares regression, either linear in the case of the logit-log method (*1, 2*), or nonlinear as in the mass action law models (*2*) or the four-parameter logistic model (*3, 4*). In any least-squares method, we need to make assumptions regarding uniformity of variance of the response, or else derive an appropriate weighting function to compensate for nonuniformity of variance. It is clear that the logit transformation introduces severe nonuniformity of variance (*1*). However, controversy has persisted regarding the uniformity or nonuniformity of variance of the radioimmunoassay dose–response variables in the absence of a logit transformation, e.g., when using response variables such as "raw" counts bound, counts free, bound over total (B/T), bound over free (B/F), free over total (F/T), free over bound (F/B), percent bound relative to initial percent bound (B/B_0) or its reciprocal $1/(B/B_0)$. Rodbard et al. have consistently claimed nonuniformity of variance for RIAs for hLH, hFSH, hGH, angiotensin, ferritin, serum hepatitis B virus, and most other assays (*1–4*). This has been confirmed by Midgley et al. (*5*); however, many other workers have implicitly or explicitly made the assumption that there is uniformity of variance (*6–11*) for the RIA response variable. Some workers have

[1] Nomenclature and nonstandard abbreviations: RIA, radioimmunoassay; B/T, bound-to-total ratio for labeled ligand corrected for nonspecific counts; B/F, bound-to-free ratio for labeled ligand corrected for nonspecific counts; B/B_0, normalized fraction bound for labeled ligand, i.e., B/T relative to B/T for zero dose of labeled ligand.

implicitly assumed that there was uniformity of variance for the logarithm of counts bound (*12*). Bliss (*13*) and Duddleson et al. (*14*) have made the assumption that the response variables B/T, B/B_0, or bound counts behave as "Poisson-like" variables, with variance directly proportional to the expectation of the response. Spona (*15*) implicitly assumed uniformity of variance for the logarithm of the logarithm of the counts bound. Others have implicitly assumed that $1/(B/B_0)$ or "B_0/B", or 1/(B/T), or 1/(counts bound) shows uniformity of variance, a clearly untenable assumption (*16*). Chang et al. (*17*) apparently advocate unweighted regression, but with close attention to experimental design in terms of choice of dose levels. However, their own data indicate severe nonuniformity of variance for B/B_0 (their Table I), and their results indicate better performance for a weighted rather than unweighted logit-log regression, in terms of the shape of confidence intervals.

If there were no experimental errors in the pipetting of any of the reagents, nor in the separation of the bound and free fractions, such that the response variable was subject only to the counting error caused by the random radioactive decay process for the isotope, then one should have a true Poisson variance for the observed (raw) counts, governed by the equation $\sigma_Y^2 = E(Y)$, where E(Y) represents the true mean or expectation of Y.[2] Thus, in general, one expects that under ideal assay conditions (where pipetting and misclassification errors are negligible) one would observe nonuniformity of variance. Further, it can be shown theoretically that there is usually severe nonuniformity of variance of the response variable, even in the presence of experimental errors (*1, 18, 19,* and unpublished studies). If we make a series of plausible assumptions (e.g., a random pipetting error for each of the reagents, and random errors in total reaction volume, reaction time, temperature, and rate constants), one can show that $\hat{\sigma}_Y^2$ is nearly linearly related to E(Y) for assay conditions close to an "ideal" (*19,* and unpublished data). These theoretical studies also show that the "misclassification" errors (random errors in the separation of bound and free ligand) may either accentuate, diminish, or eliminate this nonuniformity of variance (*1, 19*). Thus it is not surprising that some assays in some laboratories may show uniformity of variance, while other assays in other laboratories may show severe nonuniformity of variance. We postulate that most claims of uniformity of variance are the result of a failure to use appropriate methods to detect nonuniformity of variance. In many bioassay programs, Bartlett's test is included to test for heterogeneity of variance. However, this test is extremely inefficient in the presence of low degrees of freedom. Further, it is quite insensitive to systematic (as opposed to "random") changes in σ_Y^2 along the dose–response curve.

Previously distributed versions of the logit-log program (*2*) contained subroutines that provided a plot of s_Y^2 vs. $\bar{Y}$ for the standard curve, and provided estimates of the variance at both extreme ends of the curve (% B/B_0 = 0, 100). More recent versions, used in our laboratories for the past two years, display a similar analysis for the unknowns whenever the necessary replicates are present. However, further analyses and decisions were left to the discretion of the user; as a result these data were rarely used appropriately. The present study was undertaken so that appropriate analyses of nonuniformity of variance would be made automatically, and incorporated into a "preprocessor" program before "fitting" the dose–response curve. RIAs for cyclic AMP and cyclic GMP were analyzed in detail, and found to display nonuniformity of variance of the type predicted by theory.

Materials and Methods

Assay Methods

Adenosine 3′:5′-cyclic monophosphate (cAMP) and guanosine 3′:5′-cyclic monophosphate (cGMP) were assayed by a modification of the radioimmunoassay procedure described by Steiner et al. (*20*). These assays are based on competition of the cyclic nucleotide with isotopically labeled cyclic nucleotide derivatives for binding sites on specific antibody. Derivatives of the cyclic nucleotides with high specific activity were prepared by iodinating the tyrosine methyl ester derivative of the succinylated cyclic nucleotide with ^{125}I. Free and antibody bound ^{125}I-labeled cyclic nucleotides were then separated by use of Carbowax (polyethylene glycol). Binding equilibrium is reached in 24 h. All assays were done by the same technician under identical conditions, and both standard and unknown samples were analyzed in triplicate. Similar specific activities, total counts, and antibody concentrations were used in successive assays.

Statistical Methods

Data were analyzed by using the weighted nonlinear four-parameter logistic model as described by Rodbard and Hutt (*3*). A new "preprocessor" program was written, to perform the series of calculations outlined in Table 1. For each set of replicates (triplicates in the present study), the sample mean ($\bar{Y}$), sample standard deviation (s_Y), and the variance (s_Y^2) of the responses were calculated and stored. s^2 was plotted vs. Y, with separate symbols for standards and unknowns. Then, these data were analyzed by least-squares regression, by using the following equations:[2]

---

[2] σ_Y^2 represents "true" or population parameter, in contrast to the experimentally observed s_Y^2. Also, we commonly use Y as generic for the RIA response variable, instead of $\bar{Y}$. Equation 1 is a shorthand method for writing the statistical model,

$$\sigma_Y^2 = \alpha_0 + \alpha_1 \mu_Y$$

or

$$s_Y^2 = \alpha_0 + \alpha_1 \mu_Y + \epsilon_i$$

or

$$\hat{s}_Y^2 = a_0 + a_1 Y$$

$$\sigma_Y^2 = a_0 + a_1 Y \tag{1}$$

$$\sigma_Y^2 = a_0 + a_1 Y + a_2 Y^2 \tag{2}$$

$$\log(\sigma_Y^2) = \log(a_0) + j \log(Y) \tag{3}$$

These three models are designated, for convenience, the "linear", "quadratic", and "log-log" models, respectively. Use of the "log-log" model was suggested for this purpose by Prof. David J. Finney (personal communication). Both weighted and unweighted regression was used to fit the parameters of these equations (see below). For equation 2, the method of orthogonal polynomials was used (*21*). To reduce the sampling error in the calculated sample variances with low degrees of freedom, we "pooled" the individual estimates of s_Y^2 by clustering the data. This was done in either of two ways: (*a*) by dividing the observed range of Y into 10 (or 30) equal segments, or (*b*) by dividing the observed range of Y into unequally spaced regions containing an equal (or nearly equal) number of "points" ($\bar{Y}$, s_Y^2 pairs). The former method resulted in clusters ("bins") with drastically different numbers of points and hence degrees of freedom. This necessitated the use of weighted regression when finding estimates of parameters for equations 1–3. Accordingly, we adopted the second approach to "clustering." The median s_Y^2 was found for each cluster or "bin". We used the median, rather than the mean, in order to minimize the effects of "outliers" in the raw data, and (or) in the calculated s_Y^2. Then the regression analyses for equations 1–3 were repeated on these "smoothed" or "binned" data. In some preliminary studies, we also used the models:

$$\sigma_Y^2 = a_1 Y \tag{4}$$

and

$$\sigma_Y^2 = a_0 Y^j \tag{5}$$

Equation 4 is the "Poisson-like" model, a degenerate case of equations 1–3 or 5. Equation 5 is the explicit form of the "exponential" model proposed by D. J. Finney (personal communication). It is a generalization of equation 4, and it may be viewed as an alternative model to equations 1 or 2. Equation 5 was "fit," with and without weighting, by using the "MLAB" system (*22*) at the NIH Division of Computer Research and Technology. We used weighting, to compensate for the nonuniformity of variance of s_Y^2. The weighting functions included

$$W = df \tag{6}$$

$$W = \frac{df}{s_Y^2} \tag{7}$$

$$W = \frac{df}{(s_Y^2)^2} \tag{8}$$

where df is the degrees of freedom for the local estimate of s_Y^2. The s_Y^2 in the denominator could be the median s_Y^2 in a "bin", or the s_Y^2 predicted from a previous attempt (iteration) at curve fitting. Usually, similar results were obtained for the parameters of models 1–5 irrespective of the weighting used. Nonlinear curve fitting by use of equation 5 with weights given by equations 6–8 often failed to converge and was unsatisfactory for purposes of routine analysis. The use of equation 3 with unweighted regression is nearly equivalent to the use of equation 5 with weights given by equation 8, because the logarithm of the sample variance is asymptotically normally distributed and shows uniformity of variance. Using the log transform does not permit direct comparison of the residual variance for equation 3 with that of the other equations; accordingly, the residual variance for the fit to equation 3 was recalculated in terms of s_Y^2.

Table 1.

(1) Calculate and store s_Y^2, $\bar{Y}$ for each set of replicates.
(2) Plot s_Y^2 vs. $\bar{Y}$ for standards.
(3) Plot s_Y^2 vs. $\bar{Y}$ for unknowns.
(Plots 2 and 3 may be superimposed on the same graph.)
(4) "Pool" the results for standards and unknowns after testing for homogeneity, if sufficient data are available.
(5) "Fit" the relationship between s_Y^2 and $\bar{Y}$ by using three models (linear, quadratic, log-log).
(6) Plot the "fitted" relationships.
(7) Select the "best" model by objective, quantitative criteria (e.g., residual variance, *F* test).
(8) "Bin" the results in local regions of the dose response curve, and repeat steps 2–7.
(9) Pool results over assays, and repeat steps 2–8.

After calculating the several regressions (equations 1–5), we selected the "best" model as the one with the smallest residual variance. In comparing equation 2 (which involves three fitted parameters) with the equations 1 or 3 (which involve two fitted parameters), we used an approximate *F* test:

$$F = \frac{\Delta SS/\Delta df}{MS} \tag{9}$$

where ΔSS is the difference in the sum of squares for the two models, Δdf is the change in number of df, and MS is the Mean Square (residual variance) for the model with the larger number of fitted parameters (equation 2 in this case). Similar considerations apply when comparing model 4 with the others. Also, to be suitable for use as a weighting function in subsequent curve-fitting procedures, the predicted variance (σ_Y^2) must be greater than zero over the allowable or observable range for the assay. If any model resulted in a predicted σ_Y^2 that was zero or negative with Y in the observed range for an assay, then this

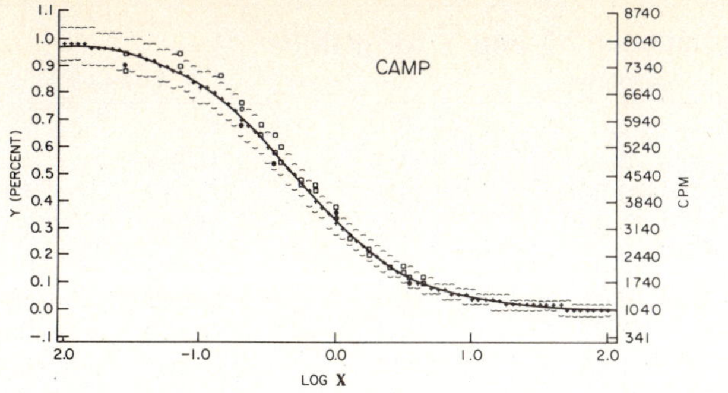

Fig. 1. Representative dose–response curve for cyclic AMP (cAMP)

Abscissa: Dose in picomoles per tube on a logarithmic scale. *Right-hand ordinate:* Counts precipitated. *Left-hand ordinate:* Normalized response variable ranging between zero and unity. The best fitting curve is shown by the heavy line. The *curved brackets* indicate the 95% confidence limits for a single observation around the line, ignoring the uncertainty in the position of the curve itself. *Solid circles* indicate the observed values; *open squares* designate multiple superimposed points. Note the symmetrical smooth **S**-shaped curve satisfactorily described by the logistic function (*3*), and the tapering of the 95% confidence limits corresponding to the nonuniformity of variance

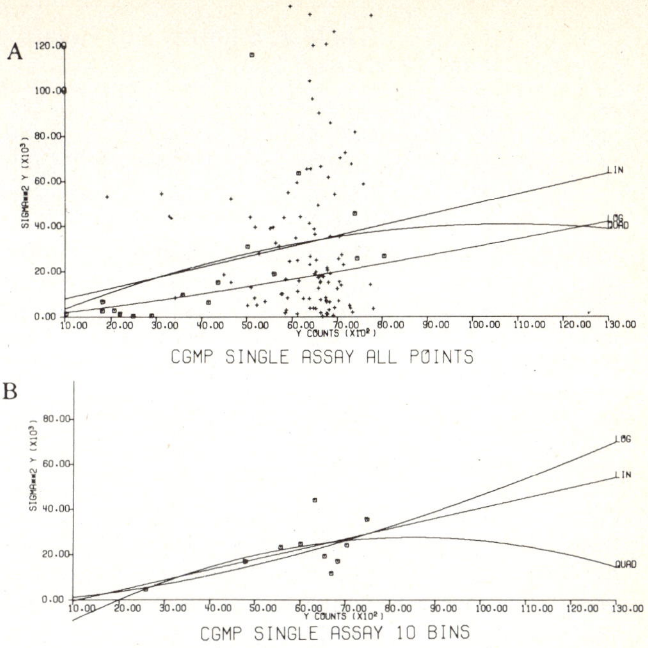

Fig. 2 *A*. Relationship between the variance of the original (nontransformed) response variable, $s_{\bar{Y}}^2$ (designated "SIGMA**2 Y × 10^3," i.e., in units of thousands) on the *ordinate* vs. the mean counts bound (in hundreds of counts) for replicates at any given dose level for a single cGMP assay

The plus signs, +, designate values obtained from replicate unknowns; a plus sign surrounded by a square, ⊠, represents the values obtained from replicate standards. Shown are the regression lines corresponding to a linear (*LIN*), quadratic (*QUAD*), or log-log (*LOG*) relationship

B. The same data as Figure 2*A*, except that individual points have been clustered into 10 "bins" containing approximately 12 observations per bin, and the median value of $s_{\bar{Y}}^2$ within each bin was used. This reduces the sampling error, and the correlation between $s_{\bar{Y}}^2$ and $\bar{Y}$ becomes apparent, irrespective of the regression model used

model was rejected and the next best model was selected.[3] Appropriate calculations for transformed response variables (e.g., B/T, B/F, B/B_0) are given in the Appendix.

Results

Figure 1 shows a representative dose–response curve. Gross inspection suggests the presence of nonuniformity of variance of the response variable (bound counts) in RIAs for both cAMP and cGMP. Figure 2 indicates the relationship between $\sigma_{\bar{Y}}^2$ and Y for the standards and unknowns from a single assay for cGMP. The results for the standards and unknowns appear compatible, so they have been "pooled" for subsequent analyses. This relationship has been fit by a linear model, a quadratic polynomial model, and a log-log model (equations 1–3), designated LIN, QUAD, and LOG, respectively. Each point on this graph represents a sample variance based on only two degrees of freedom (df = N − 1 = 2 for triplicates). Thus, there is enormous sampling error in the sample standard deviation and sample variance and indeed the 95% sampling limits for $s_{\bar{Y}}^2$ are at .025 and 3.69 times the expected results. To simplify the analysis and to make clear the relationship between $\sigma_{\bar{Y}}^2$ and Y, we divided the horizontal axis representing the response variable into 10 segments between the lowest and highest values, such that each segment contains the same number of "points" (and, hence, df in the present case). The median variance in each of these intervals was then calculated. Results from assays for cGMP are shown in Figure 2*B*. Now, each of the points represents an estimate of the variance based on approximately 24 degrees of freedom. The linear, parabolic, and log-log models have been fitted to these data, combining results from standards and unknowns. Note the excellent agreement between the three models utilized over the observed range for the response variable. The results of the three models diverge as one extrapolates from the data. Results from 22 consecutive assays for cGMP are summarized in Table 2. Figure 3 shows what happens when we "pool" results (for $s_{\bar{Y}}^2$ vs. $\bar{Y}$) for 22 cGMP assays. Although Figure 3*A* appears to be completely "random" at first blush, regression analysis shows a definite, significant relationship when equations 1, 2, or 3 are used. By pooling or "binning" and thus obtaining about 400 df for each local estimate of $s_{\bar{Y}}^2$, a very strong underlying relationship is seen (Figure 3*B*). Again, there is an excellent correlation, whether one utilizes a linear, quadratic, or log-log model. Quite clearly, there is nonuniformity of variance with about a fourfold increase in $s_{\bar{Y}}^2$ over the observable range of counts. A similar analysis can be applied separately to the points from the standard curve (Figure 4) or the unknowns (Fig-

[3] A program, written for a CDC 3500 in Fortran IV, is available on request from Douglas Ramseth, Walter Reed Army Institute of Research, Washington, D. C., or from the Editorial Office of this journal.

Table 2. Summary of Relationship between σ_Y^2 and $\bar{Y}$ for cGMP[a]

		Linear		Quadratic			Log-Log	
Assay	N	a_0	a_1	a_0	a_1	a_2 (×10³)	a_0	j
1	122	3376	4.634	−4478	8.41	−0.391	0.461	1.206
2	18	−6904	7.834	−10310	10.20	−0.285	0.017	1.653
3	95	15086	3.184	−25481	26.97	−2.777	0.277	1.296
4	76	19191	4.034	−72820	53.93	−5.936	5.391	0.986
5	42	15505	2.459	−17282	18.67	−1.684	0.548	1.182
6	112	16348	3.543	−29530	27.36	−2.701	57.910	0.686
7	148	12599	2.716	−8938	11.18	−0.747	232.300	0.480
8	133	6244	2.856	−38499	24.73	−2.331	0.194	1.274
9	17	9039	0.929	−17785	18.52	−2.338	113.900	0.501
10	16	24941	3.963	−43608	40.60	−4.020	36.800	0.795
11	22	−5512	7.884	13256	−6.28	1.621	0.137	1.374
12	116	11920	7.207	−2929	21.83	−2.023	1.472	1.174
13	105	8741	5.199	5069	7.38	−0.267	0.859	1.199
14	125	4385	2.488	−365	7.65	−0.906	27.800	0.669
15	95	28116	2.891	−21314	29.70	−2.633	33.380	0.787
16	88	19453	3.555	−13625	17.87	−1.231	60.610	0.688
17	70	23085	3.620	−27863	29.86	−2.566	12.070	0.913
18	148	14961	3.788	−5432	15.15	−1.239	31.630	0.769
19	98	6933	0.587	−1863	7.00	−0.859	49.220	0.579
20	99	14870	2.566	−284	10.42	−0.864	1518.000	0.256
21	90	17954	2.492	23887	0.21	0.187	284.500	0.484
22	88	4166	3.141	−11316	14.64	−1.528	19.510	0.751
Mean		12022	3.708	−14158	18.00	−1.614	113.000	0.896
Pooled		10403	4.056	−4954	13.09	−0.993	3.501	0.999
Pooled and binned		4986	3.027	−1961	7.17	−0.445	8.586	0.917

[a] Results are shown for each of the three regression models for several assays. The means of the coefficients are presented, together with the coefficients obtained by regression analysis for the data pooled over assays ("pooled"), or for data that have been both pooled over assays and "binned" into ten intervals containing the same number of degrees of freedom. It is apparent that the coefficients for the quadratic model are extremely unstable (between assays). Ideally, one should examine these coefficients together with their joint 95% confidence limits.

ure 5). This provides a more refined test for similar behavior of standards and unknowns than simply analyzing the data from one assay (e.g., Figure 2).

The linear regressions for all the cases given above are highly statistically significant, i.e., the slope is significantly different from zero ($P < .01$). In this example it appears that s_Y^2 for the high Y values is approximately four times larger than the variance at the other end of the curve. The intercept (a_0) does not appear to be significantly different from zero. Hence, we are dealing with a Poisson-like variable, and in lieu of the two-parameter linear model, we could utilize a simple linear model forced through the origin, i.e., equation 4. Also, when utilizing the log-log model of Finney, the exponent j does not differ significantly from unity (Table 2). In this particular example, all three of the equations (1–3)—or, for that matter, all five of the models—would have provided a satisfactory model for the nonuniformity of variance. Indeed, in view of the large sampling error, it appears impossible to discriminate between the performance of these five models for the present data. Similar results, summarized in Figure 6*A*, were obtained with the cyclic AMP assay. Figure 6*B* again shows the median variance in each of 10 bins, pooling data from both the standard and the unknowns from 23 assays.

Discussion

Use of the Predicted Variance for Weighted Curve-fitting

The major practical application of these analyses is the use of one of the models to calculate weights for the curve-fitting procedure used to describe the standard curve, and used as a basis for dose interpolation for unknowns. Jacquez and Norusis (*23*) have pointed out that use of empirically determined weights may actually result in a decreased performance of a linear curve-fitting procedure. This is true if the weights are based on a sample variance with a very small number of degrees of freedom (df < 9). Accordingly, in some commercial adaptations of the "logit-log" curve-fitting method, which uses weights based on a sample variance (for logit(B/B_0)) with only one or two df, the use of weights may actually seriously degrade the performance of the curve-fitting procedure. In contrast to Jacquez and Norusis, the approach advocated here and elsewhere (*1–5, 14*) results in an estimate of σ_Y^2 with extremely high degrees

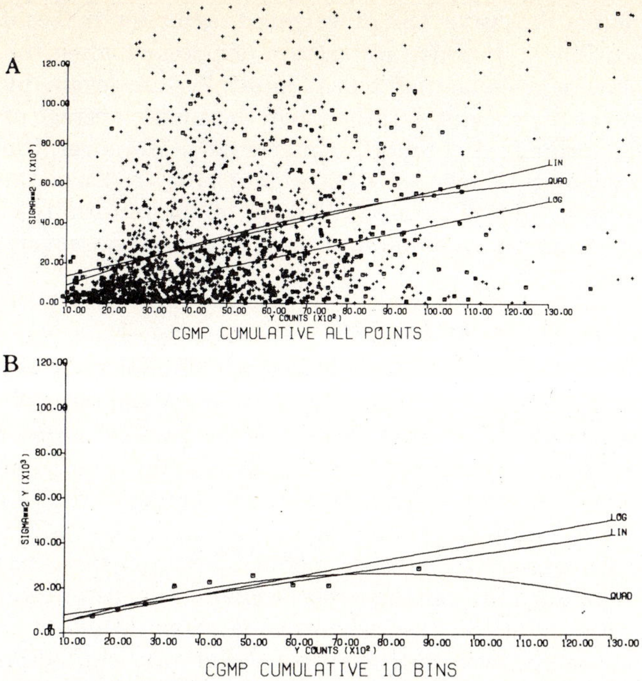

Fig. 3 *A*. Relationship between $s_{\bar{Y}}^2$ and $\bar{Y}$ for a cyclic GMP assay, on pooling data over assays containing 2000 points altogether

Although at first inspection, this appears to be a random scattergram, utilization of linear, quadratic, or log-log regression indicates a clear-cut relationship, such that $s_{\bar{Y}}^2$ varies systematically with $\bar{Y}$

B. The data of Figure 3*A* has been clustered into 10 bins containing 200 observations per bin. The median variance within each "bin" is determined

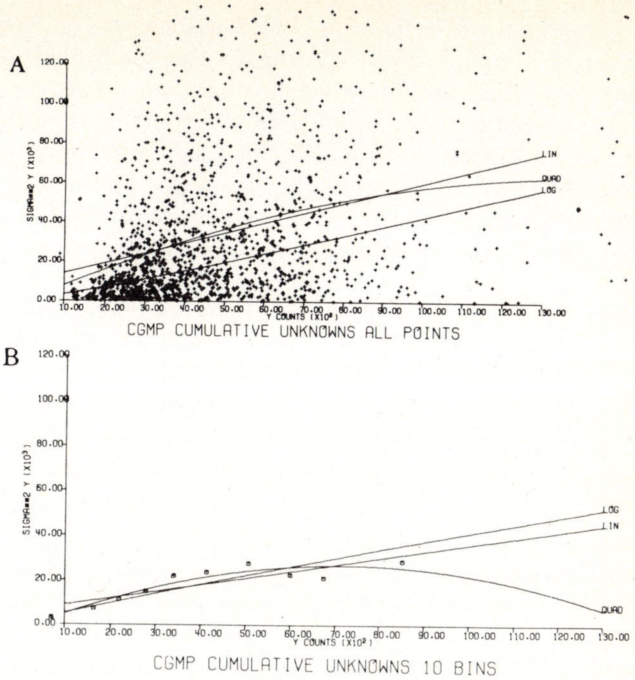

Fig. 5. *A*. Relationship between the $s_{\bar{Y}}^2$ and $\bar{Y}$ for data from "unknowns" only, excluding data from standards

B. Same data, after binning and finding the local median

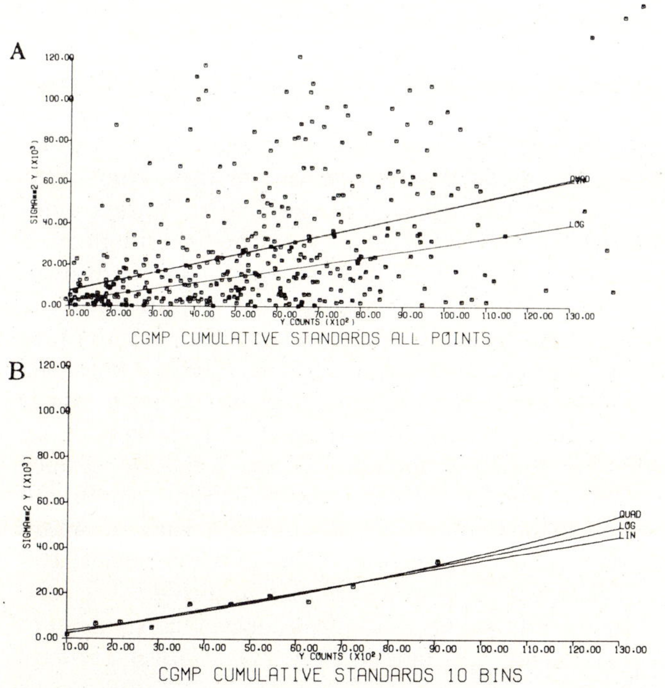

Fig. 4 *A*. Relationship between $s_{\bar{Y}}^2$ and $\bar{Y}$ for the cyclic GMP RIA, on pooling over 22 assays but utilizing data for "standards" alone and excluding data from "unknowns"

B. Data of Figure 4*A*, after clustering into bins and finding the median variance within each bin. There is marked nonuniformity of variance, and any of the three models used is adequate to describe the data

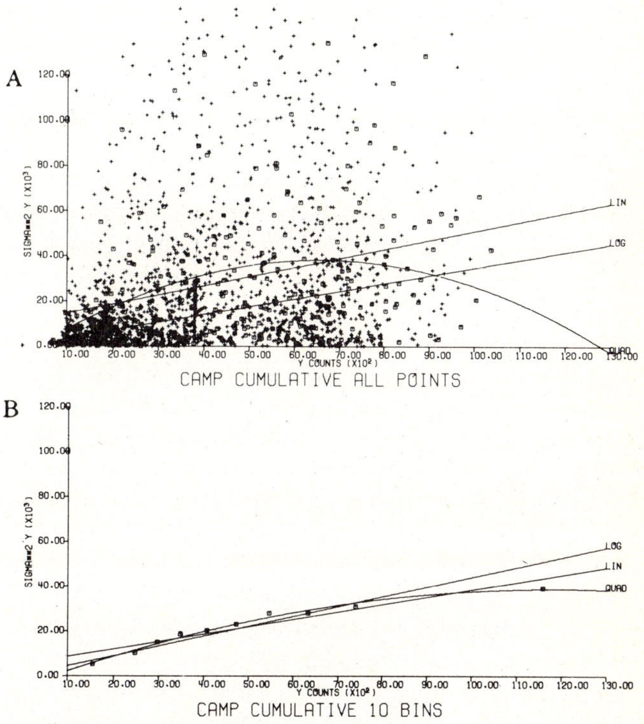

Fig. 6 *A*. $s_{\bar{Y}}^2$ vs. $\bar{Y}$ for RIA for cyclic AMP, on combining data from both standards and unknowns over 23 assays, including 2000 points

B. Some data as Figure 6*A*, after pooling data into 10 bins with 200 observations per bin

Again, there is marked nonuniformity of variance, which might have escaped detection if one utilized only casual perusal of Figure 6 *A* of freedom and reliability. For instance, we do not "weight" each point according to the reciprocal of any one "dot" in Figure 2*A*; instead, we weight according to the value of σ_Y^2 predicted by the smooth curve in Figures 2 to 6. By "pooling" information from all dose levels, from standards and unknowns, and from many assays, we have drastically reduced the effect of sampling error and extracted information about the underlying nature of the error in the response variable. Other methods of pooling or smoothing could be used. For purposes of estimating parameters for a given model, the "binning" of points (Figures 2*B*–6*B*) is unnecessary. We obtained very similar parameter estimates when using curve fitting based on all of the points (Table 2). However, the use of "binning" makes it possible to see the underlying relationship more clearly. This is even more important when individual estimates of s_Y^2 are based on duplicates, and hence have only one degree of freedom.

Having established the relationship between σ_Y^2 and Y, one can now weight each of the points (X,Y) in a least-squares regression according to the inverse of the *predicted* (rather than the observed) variance for that point. Because the variances are calculated on the basis of the response variable rather than on the basis of the dose or X variable, we should readjust the weights after each iteration, recalculating the weights on the basis of the response level predicted for that dose level on the basis of the previous iteration. In this manner, the weights become an implicit function of the dose level, and all replicates for a given dose are given the same weight. This technique has been used in the methods given in references *1–4* and is analogous to what is commonly done in probit or logit analysis with use of quantal response variables (*24*). This approach to weighting is also applicable to *all* other methods of least-squares curve fitting, including multiple polynomials, spline-fitting, mass-action law models, etc. With computerized calculations no additional effort is required on the part of the user.

The present results confirm previous findings of significant nonuniformity of variance for RIAs. Hence, in the assays for cGMP and cAMP and in general, unless proven otherwise, it is desirable to utilize weighted regression. Failure to do so will not necessarily result in serious error in the estimate of the curve (*9, 17, 19, 23*), but it invalidates attempts to calculate the 95% confidence limits or the coefficient of variation for the potency estimate based on the scatter of the points around the standard curve. Use of a nonweighted logit-log regression and the assumption of uniformity of variance will result in serious underestimation of the error at certain positions (the extremes) of the dose–response curve and overestimation of the error at other portions (the center) of the curve [see Table 2 in (*17*)]. Use of a nonweighted four-parameter logistic (*4*) will (usually) result in underestimation of the error in the low-dose region and overestimation of the error in the high-dose region of the curve. Use of weighted regression makes it possible to improve estimation of potency when the same sample is analyzed at multiple dose levels, by use of the weighted, rather than the simple average of the individual potency estimates (*26*). Moreover, the present findings, on a large data base, confirm the theoretical predictions (*1, 18, 19*) of nonuniformity of variance for radioimmunoassay dose–response variables.

Choice between Models

In the cAMP and cGMP assays analyzed here, any of the models 1–5 would have been satisfactory. We expect that for other assay systems one or more of these models will fail [e.g., see (*3*)]. Indeed, for some assays, a "best" model may clearly emerge. Model 1 has the simplicity of a linear model and involves two parameters. In contrast, model 2 involves three parameters and is slightly more general; for instance, it can handle the case where σ_Y is proportional to Y (i.e., a constant coefficient of variation) (*4*). This is quite important in some applications (*3*), particularly immunoradiometric assays. Model 2 can handle the case where Y is a binomial variate, and thus can be applied to quantal assays. However, in model 2, the parameters are very unstable from assay to assay, and it becomes much more difficult, if not impossible, to pool results (coefficients) from several successive assays (Table 2). Equation 2 also has the undesirable property of frequently predicting a zero or negative variance. To circumvent this, Equation 2 could be "fit" subject to the nonlinear constraint that σ_Y^2 must be positive over the range of Y observed in the assay.

Model 3 is "linear" after log transforms of both axes. This model is not directly applicable to linearly transformed response variables such as B/T or B/B_0 when the mean nonspecific counts ($\bar{N}$) is not zero. This model has the advantages that it confers a degree of uniformity of variance to the dependent variable, $\log(s_Y^2)$, which is quite important for analysis of results from a single assay (before "binning"). Also, model 3 (or 5) avoids the problem of having the predicted σ_Y^2 becoming negative. Model 3 has a potential problem when the observed sample variance (s_Y^2) is zero. This is readily remedied by use of $\log(s^2 + c)$, where c is a small constant. Model 5 has the serious problem that for limited data of the type usually obtained for a single assay it is very difficult to obtain convergence of a non-linear curve-fitting routine, and (or) estimates of a_0 and j are very unstable.[4]

In our laboratory, we have adopted the strategy of always using the model with the smallest residual

[4] A reviewer suggested another model that may be appropriate for the present data:

$$\sigma_Y^2 = \frac{a_0 Y}{a_1 + a_2 Y}$$

Indeed, any simple model may be used. We prefer equations 1–3 to this hyperbolic model, especially because upward rather than downward curvature is expected in most RIA systems.

variance provided it predicts a positive σ_Y^2 over the observable range. There are advantages and disadvantages to each of the models. It is essential that the final model that is selected fits the data characteristic for each assay system in each laboratory. The methods described above allow an investigator to evaluate his assay for an appropriate model. Our current programs for analysis of RIA results allows the user to select the model he prefers (*26*). These programs should be useful for a wide variety of analyses in the clinical chemistry laboratory, in addition to RIAs.[3]

Conclusions

The radioimmunoassays for cAMP and cGMP analyzed here show nonuniformity of variance for the response variable. Accordingly, weighting should be used for optimal data processing. Several models are available to describe the relationship between the variance of the response and the response level. Parameters of these models should be obtained by objective, least-squares regression methods. It is desirable to compare the results from the standards and the unknowns and to pool the data from these two sources, if appropriate. Further, data can be pooled over several assays in a stable assay system. Then, parameters for the model (e.g., a_0, a_1, a_2) can be used for curve-fitting in subsequent asssays if the assay remains in satisfactory quality control. These parameters can then be updated periodically, for example, after every 10 assays. With an automated, computerized approach, these parameters can be estimated and updated after each assay. Direct inspection of the error in the response variable facilitates quality-control programs because this error, together with the slope of the dose–response curve, completely determines the precision of an estimate at any point on the dose–response curve.

D. M. Hutt of the Standard Information Systems, McLean, Va., assisted with computer programming for a prototype of this program. V. B. Faden provided equations 12 and 13. R. Sheats provided expert assistance with the computations involving the MLAB system of the DEC-10 computer. T. Sellner prepared the manuscript on the WYLBUR text-editing system of the NIH Division of Computer Research and Technology. A. Guirguis expertly performed the assays. D. Tang critically reviewed the manuscript. D. J. Finney provided many helpful suggestions and access to unpublished material.

Appendix

The present analyses have been performed on the original response variable or raw data, i.e., counts bound. This appears to be the most efficient approach when subsequent data processing is by a method such as the four-parameter logistic (*3, 4, 6*) or others (*7, 10, 12, 15*) that also make use of the raw counts. The present program may also be used when subsequent processing makes use of a linear transform of the response (e.g., B/T, B/B_0) or a nonlinear transform, e.g., logit (B/B_0). For instance, if Y and a_0, a_1, a_2 apply to "raw counts", and

$$Y' = \text{“}B/B_0\text{”} = \frac{(Y - \bar{N})}{(\bar{B}_0 - \bar{N})} \qquad (10)$$

where $\bar{B}_0$, $\bar{N}$ are constants, then

$$\mathrm{Var}(Y') = c_0 + c_1Y' + c_2(Y')^2 \qquad (11)$$

where

$$c_0 = (a_0 + a_1\bar{N} + a_2\bar{N}^2)/(\bar{B}_0 - \bar{N})^2$$
$$c_1 = (a_1 + 2a_2\bar{N})/(\bar{B}_0 - \bar{N})$$
$$c_2 = a_2 \qquad (12)$$

Alternatively:

$$a_0 = (B_0 - \bar{N})^2c_0 - \bar{N}(\bar{B}_0 - \bar{N})c_1 + \bar{N}^2c_2$$
$$a_1 = (\bar{B}_0 - \bar{N})c_1 - 2\bar{N}c_2$$
$$a_2 = c_2 \qquad (13)$$

Thus, determination of the coefficients for models 1–5 allows one to calculate the variance for any linearly transformed variable.

Note that models 1, 2, and 4 can be applied to linearly transformed variables (e.g., B/T, B/B_0) directly. Equations 3 or 5 can be applied to variables transformed by a constant multiplicative factor, but cannot be applied directly to variables involving a translation of the axes.

It is possible to combine results over assays only when the curves are stable with regard to their position, in terms of both the X and Y axis, and with regard to the magnitude of the scatter and the dependence of the scatter on the position on the dose response curve. In the present studies, we have "pooled" results over assays, on the basis of the original response variable (Y). Alternatively, one could pool the results over assays based on the dose levels (*25, 19*). Under certain assumptions the method used here is superior, although in practice either of these methods should be satisfactory. It is a moot point as to whether it is better to pool results over assays (e.g., Figures 3–6) and use analyses in terms of raw counts or to use B/B_0. Certainly if total counts, $(B/T)_0$, or $\bar{B}_0$ changes appreciably between assays, then it is highly doubtful that one can pool results over assays (either in terms of s^2, $\bar{Y}$, or in terms of a_0, a_1, a_2). Likewise, if one is to pool results over assays when using B/B_0 as the response variable, the assay system should be "stable". However, analyses in terms of B/B_0 should be less affected by changes in total counts, counting time, or specific activity of the tracer.

References

1. Rodbard, D., and Lewald, J. E., Computer analysis of radioligand assay and radioimmunoassay data. *Karolinska Symposia, Research Methods in Reproductive Endocrinology* (Geneva, March 1970). *Acta Endocrinol.* (Copenhagen) **64,** *Suppl. 147,* 79–103 (1970).

2. Rodbard, D., and Frazier, G. R., *Radioimmunoassay Data Processing,* 2nd ed. National Technical Information Service, Springfield, Va. 22151. (PB 217366 for magnetic tape, PB 217367 for printed listings), 224 pp, 1973.

3. Rodbard, D., and Hutt, D. M., Statistical analysis of radioimmunoassays and immunoradiometric (labeled antibody) assays: A generalized weighted, iterative, least-squares method for logistic curve fitting. In *Symposium on RIA and Related Procedures in Medicine,* **Vol. 1.** Int. Atomic Energy Agency, Vienna, Austria (available from Unipub, Box 433, Murray Hill Station, New York, N. Y. 10016), pp 165–192, 1974.

4. Rodbard, D., Statistical quality control and routine data processing for radioimmunoassays (RIA) and immunoradiometric assays (IRMA). *Clin. Chem.* **20,** 1255 (1974).

5. Midgley, A. R., Niswender, G. D., and Rebar, R. W., Principles for the assessment of the reliability of radioimmunoassay methods (precision, accuracy, sensitivity, specificity). In *Immunoassay of Gonadotropins: Karolinska Symposium on Research Methods,* E. Diczfalusy and A. Diczfalusy, Eds., (No. 1), *Acta Endocrinol.* (Copenhagen) *Suppl. 142,* Stockholm, p 163, 1969.

6. Healy, M. J. R., Statistical analysis of radioimmunoassay data. *Biochem. J.* **130,** 207 (1972).

7. Burger, H. G., Lee, V. W. K., and Rennie, G. C., A generalized computer system for the treatment of data from competitive protein-binding assays including radioimmunoassays. *J. Lab. Clin. Med.* **80,** 302 (1972).

8. Leclerq, R., Taljedal, L-B., and Wold, S., Evaluation of radioisotope data in steroid assays based on competitive protein binding. *Clin. Chim. Acta* **36,** 257 (1971).

9. Vivian, S. R., and La Bella, F. S., Classic bioassay statistical procedures applied to radioimmunoassay of bovine thyrotropin, growth hormone and prolactin. *J. Clin. Endocrinol. Med.* **33,** 225 (1971).

10. Arrigucci, A., Porti, G., Fiorelli, G., et al., Mathematical analysis of the results of competitive binding methods. In *The Endocrine Function of the Human Testis* **I,** V. H. T. James, M. Serio, and L. Martini, Eds. Academic Press, New York, N. Y., 1973.

11. Meinert, C. L., and McHugh, R. B., The biometry of an isotope displacement immunological microassay. *Math. Biosci.* **2,** 319 (1968).

12. Gilman, A. G., A protein binding assay for adenosine 3′:5′-cyclic monophosphate. *Proc. Nat. Acad. Sci. USA* **67,** 305 (1970).

13. Bliss, C. I., Dose response curves for radioimmunoassay. In *Statistics in Endocrinology,* J. W. McArthur and T. Colton, Eds. MIT Press, Cambridge, Mass., 1970, pp 431–452.

14. Duddleson, W. G., Midgley, A. R., and Niswender, G. D., Computer program sequence for analysis and summary of radioimmunoassay data. *Comput. Biomed. Res.* **5,** 205 (1972).

15. Spona, J., Rapid assay for luteinizing hormone and evaluation of data by new computer program. In *Radioimmunoassay and Related Procedures in Medicine* **I,** Int. Atomic Energy Agency, Vienna, 1974, pp 123–130.

16. Rodbard, D., Bridson, W., and Rayford, P. L., Rapid calculation of radioimmunoassay results. *J. Lab. Clin. Med.* **74,** 770 (1969).

17. Chang, P. C., Rubin, R. T., and Yu, M., Optimal statistical design of radioimmunoassays and competitive protein-binding assays. *Endocrinology* **96,** 973 (1975).

18. Rodbard, D., and Cooper, J. A., A model for prediction of confidence limits in radioimmunoassays and competitive protein binding assays. *Proceedings, Symposium on Radioisotopes in Medicine: In Vitro Studies.* Int. Atomic Energy Agency, Vienna, 1970, pp 659–674.

19. Rodbard, D., Statistical aspects of radioimmunoassay. In *Competitive Protein Binding Assays,* W. Odell and W. Daughaday, Eds. J. B. Lippincott Co., Philadelphia, Pa., 1971, chap. 8, pp 204–259.

20. Steiner, A. L., Parker, C. W., and Kipnis, D. M., Radioimmunoassay for cyclic nucleotides. *J. Biol. Chem.* **247,** 1106 (1972).

21. Steel, R. G. D., and Torrey, J. H., *Principles and Procedures of Statistics,* McGraw-Hill, New York, N. Y., 1960.

22. Knott, G. D., and Reece, D. K., *Proceedings, On Line '72 Symposium,* Brunel University, Uxbridge, Middlesex, England, Brunel U. Press, 1973.

23. Jacquez, J. A., and Norusis, M., Sampling experiments on the estimation of parameters in heteroscedastic linear regression. *Biometrics* **29,** 771 (1973).

24. Finney, D. J., *Statistical Method in Biological Assay.* Griffin, London, 1964.

25. Hunter, W. M., and Greenwood, F. C., A radioimmunoelectrophoretic assay for human growth hormone. *Biochem. J.* **91,** 43 (1964).

26. Rodbard, D., and Faden, V. B., *Radioimmunoassay Data Processing,* 3rd ed., National Technical Information Service, Springfield, Va. 22151, 1975. (PB 246222 for magnetic tape, and PB 246223-4 for printed listings).

CLIN. CHEM. 22/3, 359-363 (1976)

Nonchromatographic Radioimmunoassay of Unconjugated Estriol in Plasma, with Polyethylene Glycol as Precipitant

Harvey S. Schiller and Margaret A. Brammall

We describe a rapid, reliable radioimmunoassay for unconjugated estriol in plasma. Polyethylene glycol (Carbowax 6000) is used to separate antibody-bound and free steroid. The assay is sensitive (25 pg for standards), precise, and accurate. At high and low concentrations of estriol, intra-assay coefficients of variation were 7.1% and 7.6%, respectively, and inter-assay coefficients of variation were 7.2% and 10.0%, respectively. Free [^{3}H]estriol is not precipitated by polyethylene glycol. This radioimmunoassay of estriol, with a highly specific antiserum and with polyethylene glycol as the antibody precipitant, is a reliable one-day assay that is practical both for the clinical laboratory and the obstetrician.

Additional Keyphrases: *monitoring fetal well-being* • *normal values*

A critical facet in radioimmunoassays is the separation of antibody-bound and free ligand. The original observation (*1*) that polyethylene glycol (PEG) was useful for this separation procedure in polypeptide hormone assays induced us to study this precipitant for steroid radioimmunoassays. Subsequently we demonstrated that use of PEG was practical for a radioimmunoassay of estradiol-17β[1] and suggested that this method might have general applicability for steroid radioimmunoassays (*2*). We developed other steroid radioimmunoassays in which PEG was used to separate antibody-bound and free steroids (*3, 4*).

The present report demonstrates the practicability of PEG in a rapid, nonchromatographic radioimmunoassay of unconjugated estriol in plasma.

Departments of Laboratory Medicine and Obstetrics and Gynecology, University of Washington School of Medicine, SB-10, Seattle, Wash. 98195.

[1] Trivial names and abbreviations used: estradiol-17β, 1,3,5(10)-estratriene-3,17β-diol; estriol, 1,3,5(10)-estratriene-3,16α,17β-triol; 16-epiestriol, 1,3,5(10)-estratriene-3,16β,17β-triol; 17-epiestriol, 1,3,5(10)-estratriene-3,16α,17α-triol; 16,17-epiestriol, 1,3,5(10)-estratriene-3,16β,17α-triol; estrone, 3-hydroxy-1,3,5(10)-estratriene-17-one; 6-oxoestradiol, 3,17β-dihydroxy-1,3,6(10)estratriene-6-one; 6-oxoestriol, 3,16α,17β-trihydroxy-1,3,5(10)estratriene-6-one; 11-deoxycortisol, 17α,21-dihydroxy-4-pregnene-3,20-dione; testosterone, 17β-hydroxy-4-androsten-3-one; and PEG, polyethylene glycol.

Received Nov. 4, 1975; accepted Jan. 2, 1976.

Materials and Methods

Materials

Antiserum: The specific antibody to estriol used for the assay was raised in an ewe against estriol-6-carboxymethyl-oxime/bovine serum albumin and was a gift from Dr. Uwe Goebelsmann, Department of Obstetrics and Gynecology, University of Southern California. The lyophilized antiserum (UG-R2-09) was reconstituted in distilled water and small aliquots were frozen at −45 °C. Each month, an aliquot was diluted 2000-fold with barbital/acetate/gelatin buffer (see below) and stored at 4 °C.

Steroids and estriol standards: The purity of estriol (Sigma Chemical Co., St. Louis, Mo. 63178) was assessed from its melting point. The stock solution was prepared twice a year in benzene/ethanol (9/1). From this, a working standard solution was prepared monthly containing 5 ng of estriol per milliter of the barbital/acetate buffer. All other radio-inert steroids were obtained from Steraloids, Inc., Pawling, N.Y. 12564, and from Sigma Chemical Co.

[6,7-^{3}H]Estriol (spec. activity 53.1 kCi/mol) was purchased from New England Nuclear Corp., Boston, Mass. 02118. Its purity was tested every three to six months by chromatography on Celite, and it was used when the purity exceeded 95%.

Buffers: The stock sodium barbital/acetate was prepared by dissolving 7.357 g of sodium barbital and 4.857 g of anhydrous sodium acetate in 250 ml of distilled water. The working buffer, used in all instances except for preparing the antiserum dilution, was prepared by mixing 50 ml of this stock solution with 900 ml of sodium chloride solution (8.5 g of NaCl per liter) and adjusting the pH with hydrochloric acid (6 mol/liter) to pH 7.0. The working barbital/acetate/gelatin buffer, used for diluting the antiserum, was prepared similarly except that 3.5 g of reagent-grade gelatin (Mallinckrodt Chemical Works, St. Louis, Mo. 63160) was added per liter.

Solvents: Ethyl acetate (Mallinckrodt), *n*-hexane (Fisher Scientific Co., Pittsburgh, Pa. 15219), and benzene (Fisher Scientific Co.) were redistilled before use. Freshly opened diethyl ether (Mallinckrodt) and absolute ethanol (U.S. Industrial Chemicals, Anaheim, Calif. 92805) were used without distillation.

Bovine γ-globulin, fraction II, was obtained from Miles Laboratory, Elkhart, Ind. 46514.

The *polyethylene glycol* reagent, used as a precipitant, was prepared as a 300 g/kg solution of polyethylene glycol ("Carbowax 6000"; Union Carbide Corp., San Francisco, Calif. 94138) in the buffer.

Radioactivity was determined by using a modified Bray's solution (*5*), lacking methanol and ethylene glycol.

Procedure

Plasma extraction: Duplicate 0.5-ml aliquots of plasma were incubated for 30 min at room temperature with 1000 dpm (2.5 pg) of [6,7-^{3}H]estriol and then extracted with 3 ml of ethyl acetate in *n*-hexane (10/90 by vol). The organic phase was discarded, and the aqueous phase was extracted with 3 ml of ethyl acetate in *n*-hexane (40/60 by vol). The organic phase was evaporated under nitrogen and the residue was dissolved in 0.5 ml of buffer. For estimating recoveries, 0.15-ml aliquots were transferred to scintillation vials to which 10 ml of Bray's solution was added. For assay purposes, 0.15-ml sample aliquots were used.

Radioimmunoassay: The standard curve was prepared in triplicate by adding 0, 10, 20, 40, 70, 120, 200, 300, and 400 μl of the 5 ng/ml estriol standard. After adding buffer to all samples to give a total volume of 0.4 ml, 40 000 dpm (100 pg) of [6,7-^{3}H]estriol in 0.1 ml of buffer was added to all tubes, which were shaken gently. Then 0.2 ml of the antiserum, diluted 2000-fold to produce an initial 70% antibody-binding of [^{3}H]estriol in the absence of standard, was added to all tubes except those used to calculate the total radioactivity. The contents of the tubes were gently mixed and allowed to equilibrate for 2 h at 0 °C.

After the addition of 1 mg of bovine γ-globulin in 50 μl of buffer and 0.75 ml of the polyethylene glycol solution, the contents of the tubes were mixed on a vortex-type stirrer, returned to an ice-water bath, and centrifuged (1750 × *g*, 30 min, 4 °C). The supernate was decanted into scintillation vials, 10 ml of Bray's solution added, and the radioactivity in the mixture was then counted.

Estriol concentrations in the analyzed samples were determined from the constructed standard curves, and plasma concentrations were calculated as follows:

$$\text{Estriol } (\mu g/\text{liter}) = (100 \times X \times V)/(R \times P \times B)$$

where X = pg from standard curve, V = total volume of buffer used for redissolving residue (ml), R = % recovery, P = volume of plasma assayed (ml), and B = volume of buffer aliquot assayed (ml). When 0.5 ml of plasma is extracted, 0.5 ml of buffer is used to redissolve the residue, and 0.15 ml of this solution is assayed and counted for recovery (as is described for our typical assay), then the calculations are further simplified as follows:

$$\text{Estriol } (\mu g/\text{liter}) = X/r$$

where r = (cpm in 0.15 ml aliquot)/(total cpm added to the sample for recovery).

Results

Separation of Antibody-Bound and Free Estriol

Polyethylene glycol concentration: Figure 1 illustrates the complete solubility of [^{3}H]estriol. Even at 200 g/kg concentrations of PEG the [^{3}H]estriol remains in the supernate. The concentration of PEG is important for achieving maximum precipitation of antibody-bound estriol, but the optimum range for maximum precipitation is very wide. We used 150 g of PEG per kilogram for all subsequent work.

Protein concentration: In the absence of antibody the [^{3}H]estriol was not precipitated nonspecifically by the bovine γ-globulin (Figure 2). The presence of γ-globulin, however, did facilitate the precipitation of antibody-bound [^{3}H]estriol, because less antibody-bound [^{3}H]estriol precipitated in its absence. About 0.6 mg of γ-globulin was necessary for maximum precipitation; we chose to use 1 mg of γ-globulin, to ensure optimum conditions.

Precipitation time: We studied two timing requirements for the separation of antibody-bound and free estriol. First, standard curves were set up as usual, and, after the incubation at 0 °C, PEG was

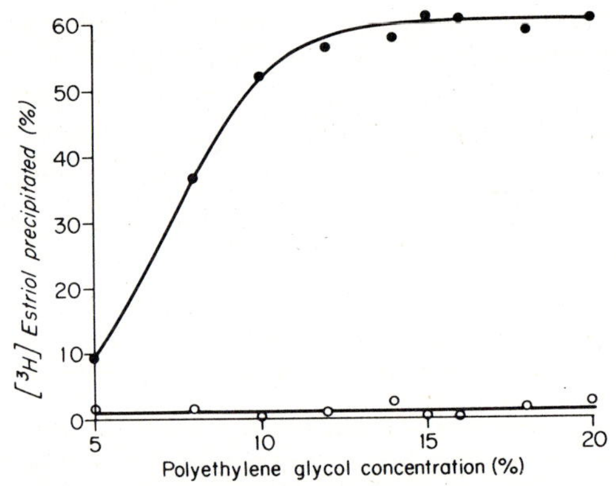

Fig. 1. Solubility of [^{3}H]estriol with various final concentrations (g/100 g) of polyethylene glycol in buffer
Open symbols, without antibody; *closed symbols,* with antibody

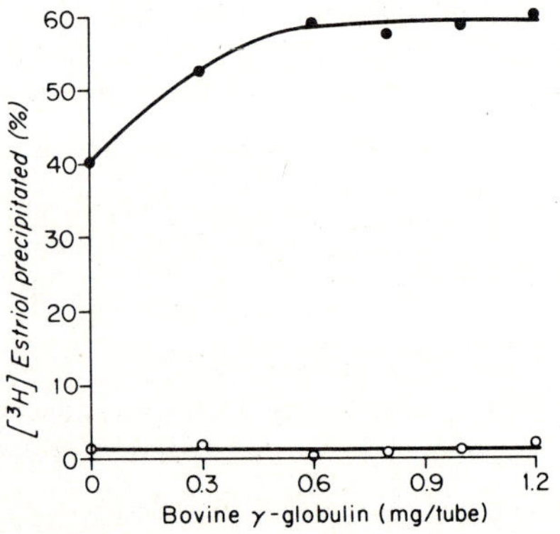

Fig. 2. Precipitation of antibody-bound estriol as a function of protein concentration
Open circles, without antibody; *closed circles,* with antibody

Table 1. Initial Percent of Estriol Antibody Bound as a Function of Time in PEG Separation Procedure

Time (h)	<0.1	0.25	0.5	1	2	4
Delayed centrifugation	74.8	73.3	69.1	66.8	63.2	57.6
Delayed decantation	68.9	68.3	70.1	68.7	69.8	68.4

added in the usual manner. Then the tubes were centrifuged after various time intervals. A decrease of the initial percent of antibody-bound estriol was observed when centrifugation was delayed (Table 1). This decrease has not been observed in our previously reported steroid hormone assays (*2, 3*). Therefore, a prolonged delay in centrifugation after adding PEG could result in erroneously low values. To eliminate this possibility, we investigated the timing for our routine assay. Less than 10 min is required for complete addition of PEG to 50–60 tubes. During this period we could not detect a significant change in the standard curve. To magnify the effect, we centrifuged the tubes for three standard curves at 10-min intervals, 1 h after adding PEG. A slight decline in the standard curve could be detected after 20 min, but not after 10 min, indicating that under the prescribed conditions of our assay, the separation procedure is valid. To further ensure the validity of this method, the assays should be set up such that PEG is added in the following order: standard curve, patents' samples and controls, standard curve, patients' samples and controls, standard curve. Any significant decline in the percent bound caused by an inadvertent delay will then be recognized.

The second time period studied was the time delay after centrifugation and before decantation. There was no time dependence in this step; the initial percent bound remained constant for 6 h (Table 1).

Analytical Variables

Sensitivity, blank, recovery, and precision: The lowest amount of estriol that routinely was significantly different from zero (no standard estriol present) was 25 pg. Sensitivity could be improved by increasing the antiserum dilution, but the range of the standard curve was narrowed and the increased sensitivity was not considered advantageous. The blank ranged from 0–70 pg for 17 assays and was not subtracted from the sample values, because it represented less than 3% of the standard-curve range (*13*). Since 55 to 65% of the estriol was recovered in the ethyl acetate/hexane extract, the lowest measurable dosage, in the absence of blank, is 0.3 μg/liter. Because plasma concentrations are vastly higher in serum during pregnancy, this sensitivity is more than adequate, even with the small blank.

The precision of the method was studied by performing repetitive determinations on pooled plasma from pregnant women with high and low concentrations of estriol, in replicate and from day to day. The means (±SD) for two samples, assayed in replicate (n = 10), were 16.9 ± 1.2 μg/liter and 4.6 ± 0.35 μg/liter, respectively, with corresponding coefficients of variation of 7.1% and 7.6%. The means (±SD) for two different samples assayed from day to day were 14.4 ± 1.04 μg/liter (n = 17) and 4.44 ± 0.44 μg/liter (n = 14), with respective coefficients of variation of 7.2% and 10.0%.

Table 2. Antiserum Cross Reactivity of Steroids

Steroid	Relative cross reactivity (%)
Estriol	100
6-Oxoestriol	100
6-Oxoestradiol-17β	10
16-Epiestriol	8
Estradiol-17β	0.8
17-Epiestriol	0.1
Estrone	<0.01
16,17-Epiestriol	<0.01

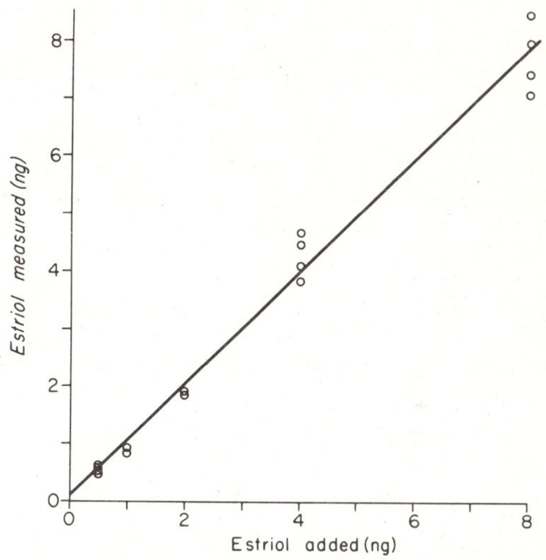

Fig. 3. Recovery of estriol added to plasma

Accuracy. The accuracy of the method was studied in three ways. The cross-reactivity of steroids with the antiserum was determined by the method of Abraham (*6*). With this antiserum the 6-oxo-derivative of estriol and estradiol-17β demonstrated 100% and 10% cross reactivity, respectively (Table 2). The 16-epiestriol, but not the 17-epiestriol, also demonstrated significant cross reactivity. Less than 1% cross reactivity was observed for the other steroids.

For the second method of assessing accuracy, we added various amounts of radio-inert estriol to plasma from men, and the plasma was subsequently assayed. The amount of estriol observed was close to the expected results (Figure 3) and ranged from 94 to 106% of that added.

Finally, various volumes of pooled plasma from women were assayed. Linear regression analysis calculated by the least-squares method resulted in a

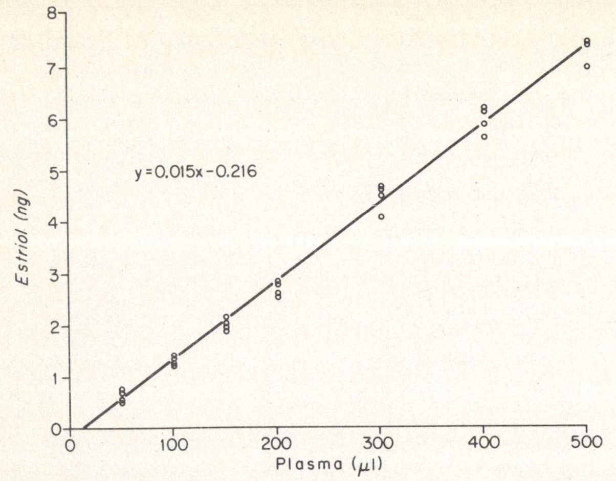

Fig. 4. Estriol concentration measured as a function of sample plasma volume

straight line with a correlation coefficient of 0.996 and *y*-intercept of −0.216 ng (Figure 4).

Normal Values

One hundred twenty-two samples were obtained from healthy women at various times in the last trimester of pregnancy (Table 3). The values are similar to those reported by other investigators (*7–11*).

Discussion

We have demonstrated for the first time that PEG can be used in a sensitive, precise, and accurate radioimmunoassay of unconjugated estriol in plasma. Other reported radioimmunoassays have utilized solid-phase (*6*), dextran-coated charcoal (*7–14*), gel filtration (*15*), and ammonium sulfate (*16–18*) techniques for separating antibody-bound and free estriol.

We have shown that PEG is a useful and convenient method of separating antibody-bound and free steroid for other radioimmunoassays (*2–4*). When we described those steroid radioimmunoassays in which PEG is used, we suggested that the method might be applicable for all steroid radioimmunoassays, but it would be necessary to demonstrate this for each new assay. Our original method for estradiol-17β (*2*) and subsequent assay for a less polar steroid, testosterone (*3*), had the significant advantage over the commonly used dextran/charcoal method in that there was complete lack of time dependence in the separation procedure. This was not observed for the estriol radioimmunoassay described here.

The conditions of the different assays were quite similar. Therefore, the explanation for this phenomenon appeared related to either the antisera or the steroid characteristics. Our present data (unpublished) suggest that the apparent time-dependent dissociation of the antibody–estriol complex is due, at least in part, to the characteristics of the antiserum.

Using PEG, we have found sensitivities for a variety of antisteroid antisera that agree with those reported by other investigators using dextran-coated charcoal for separation. In addition, our precision for several radioimmunoassays, including that for estriol, has consistently equaled or bettered that reported by other investigators. Although we cannot conclude that PEG separation technique improves the precision of the method, we have demonstrated that with this method we consistently achieve a between-day coefficient of variation between 5 and 10%. This includes radioimmunoassays of estradiol-17β (*2*), testosterone (*3*), and estriol. We have previously pointed out that gelatin did improve the precision of our assay for estradiol-17β with use of PEG (*2*), and we have continued to use gelatin in all our steroid radioimmunoassays.

Table 3. Plasma Estriol in Last Trimester of Pregnancy

Weeks of pregnancy	No. determinations	Mean (μg/liter)	Range (μg/liter)
28–32	20	6.3	3.4–13.9
33–36	23	10.0	6.2–21.5
37–40	57	13.1	4.5–21.0
41–42	22	17.0	7.5–33.0

The measurement of urinary estriol is a well-accepted procedure for monitoring fetal well-being during the last trimester of pregnancy (*19–21*). Both gas-chromatographic (*22*) and fluorometric (*23*) assays were originally used. However, a 24-h urine specimen is required and the difficulties in accurate collection and the 24-h delay have prompted several investigators to develop plasma assays to avoid these disadvantages.

Recently radio receptor assays (*24, 25*) and radioimmunoassays have been developed for measuring plasma estriol. An unspecific antiserum for estriol and its conjugates was originally used by Gurpide et al. (*16*). High specificity for unconjugated estriol in plasma when moderately specific antisera are used has been achieved with either column chromatography on Celite (*7, 11, 13*) or LH-20 Sephadex (*8, 12, 14*).

Recently, highly specific antisera have been prepared against estriol conjugated to a protein via either the A (*10, 26–28*) or the B (*9, 10, 29–33*) ring. The antiserum produced from the latter antigen (the 6-carboxymethyloxime protein derivative) has had higher cross reactivity with the estriol sulfate and glucuronide conjugates. These conjugates obviously do not interfere in an assay with a simple solvent-extraction step. The 6-oxo derivatives also significantly cross react with the latter antisera, but the concentrations of these steroids are too low for significant interference (*10*). Using either type of antiserum, accurate and rapid radioimmunoassay of unconjugated estriol is now possible (*9, 10, 28*). The method is therefore attractive for routine use in clinical laboratories.

The clinical utility of plasma estriol assays in various conditions of pregnancy is presently under investigation in several laboratories. By developing the nonchromatographic method with PEG described here, we have been able to analyze hundreds of samples in a practical manner at relatively low cost. The results of our study comparing plasma and urinary estriol concentrations are presently being evaluated.

The high specificity of the antiserum permitted us to eliminate an additional separation procedure to remove interfering steroids. Unfortunately, antisera prepared against the 6-carboxymethyloxime or the 4-carboxyphenylazo derivatives of estriol have not been made generally available commercially. However, if the plasma estriol assay proves to be as valid clinically as the urinary estriol procedure, then commercial companies will be strongly encouraged to make these highly specific antisera available for all clinical laboratories.

This project was supported in part by a grant to the Department of Obstetrics and Gynecology from The Ford Foundation and by NIH grant No. 5T01HD00272-10. We thank Drs. Paul E. Strandjord, Alex Kaplan, and Walter L. Herrmann for their advice and encouragement, and Dr. Uwe Goebelsmann for his generous gift of the antiestriol antiserum.

References

1. Desbuquois, B., and Aurbach, G. D., Use of polyethylene glycol to separate free and antibody-bound peptide hormones in radioimmunoassays. *J. Clin. Endocrinol. Metab.* **33,** 732 (1971).

2. Schiller, H. S., and Brammall, M. A., A radioimmunoassay of plasma estradiol-17β with the use of polyethylene glycol to separate free and antibody-bound hormone. *Steroids* **24,** 665 (1974).

3. Anderson, P. H., Fukushima, K., and Schiller, H. S., Radioimmunoassay of plasma testosterone with use of polyethylene glycol to separate antibody-bound and free hormone. *Clin. Chem.* **21,** 708 (1975).

4. Lee, L. M. Y., and Schiller, H. S., Nonchromatographic radioimmunoassay of plasma 11-deoxycortisol, for use in the metyrapone test, with polyethylene glycol as the precipitant. *Clin. Chem.* **21,** 719 (1975).

5. Bray, G. A., A simple efficient liquid scintillator for counting aqueous solutions in a liquid scintillation counter. *Anal. Biochem.* **1,** 279 (1960).

6. Abraham, G. E., Solid-phase radioimmunoassay of estradiol-17β. *J. Clin. Endocrinol. Metab.* **29,** 866 (1969).

7. Tulchinsky, D., and Abraham, G. E., Radioimmunoassay of plasma estriol. *J. Clin. Endocrinol. Metab.* **33,** 775 (1971).

8. Wu, C. H., and Lundy, L. E., Radioimmunoassay of plasma estrogens. *Steroids* **18,** 91 (1971).

9. Den, K., Fujii, K., Yoshida, T., and Takagi, S., A simplified radioimmunoassay of human gravid plasma estriol. *Endocrinol. Jpn.* **20,** 315 (1973).

10. Katagiri, H., Stanczyk, F. Z., and Goebelsmann, U., Estriol in pregnancy. III. Development, comparison and use of a specific antisera for rapid radioimmunoassay of unconjugated estriol in pregnancy plasma. *Steroids* **24,** 225 (1974).

11. Cohen, M., and Cohen, H., A radioimmunoassay of plasma unconjugated estrogens in normal pregnancy. *Am. J. Obstet. Gynecol.* **118,** 200 (1974).

12. Powell, J. E., and Stevens, V. C., Simple radioimmunoassay of five unconjugated ovarian steroids in a single sample of serum or plasma. *Clin. Chem.* **19,** 210 (1973).

13. Abraham, G. E., Radioimmunoassay of steroids in biological materials. *Acta Endocrinol.* (Copenhagen) *Suppl.* **183,** 7 (1974).

14. Loriaux, D. L., Ruder, H. J., Knab, D. R., and Lipsett, M. B., Estrone sulfate, estrone, estradiol and estriol plasma levels in human pregnancy. *J. Clin. Endocrinol. Metab.* **35,** 887 (1972).

15. Christner, J. E., and Fetter, M. C., A sephadex column radioimmunoassay of unconjugated estriol in pregnancy plasma. *Steroids* **24,** 327 (1974).

16. Gurpide, E., Giebenhain, M. E., Tseng, L., and Kelly, W. G., Radioimmunoassay for estrogens in human pregnancy urine, plasma, and amniotic fluid. *Am. J. Obstet. Gynecol.* **109,** 897 (1971).

17. Wilson, G. R., Radioimmunoassay of oestriol in pregnancy plasma. *Clin. Chim. Acta* **46,** 297 (1973).

18. Lindberg, B. S., Lindberg, P., Martinsson, K., and Johansson, E. D. B., Radioimmunological methods for the estimation of oestrone, oestradiol-17β and oestriol in pregnancy plasma. *Acta Obstet. Gynecol. Scand., Suppl.* **32,** 5 (1974).

19. Grune, J. W., and Touchstone, J. C., Urinary estriol as an index of placental function. *Am. J. Obstet. Gynecol.* **85,** 1 (1963).

20. Taylor, E. S., Burns, P. D., and Drose, V. E., Estriol excretion in normal and complicated pregnancies. *Clin. Obstet. Gynecol.* **8,** 550 (1965).

21. Beischer, N. A., and Brown, J. B., Current status of estrogen assays in obstetrics and gynecology. Part 2: Estrogen assays in late pregnancy. *Obstet. Gynecol. Surv.* **27,** 303 (1972).

22. Schindler, A. E., and Herrmann, W. L., Determination of steroids by gas-liquid chromatography. I. The measurement of estriol in pregnancy urine. *Gynecologia* **161,** 446 (1966).

23. Natchigall, L., Bassett, M., Hogsander, U., et al., A rapid method for the assay of plasma estriol in pregnancy. *J. Clin. Endocrinol. Metab.* **26,** 941 (1966).

24. Tulchinsky, D., Hobel, C. J., and Korenman, S. G., A radioligand assay for plasma unconjugated estriol in normal and abnormal pregnancies. *Am. J. Obstet. Gynecol.* **111,** 311 (1971).

25. Corker, C. S., and Naftolin, F., A rapid method for the measurement of oestriol in pregnancy plasma by competitive protein binding analysis. *J. Obstet. Gynaecol. Br. Commonw.* **78,** 330 (1971).

26. Cross, S. J., Campbell, D. H., and Wectall, H. H., Production of antisera to steroids coupled to proteins directly through the phenolic A ring. *Immunochemistry* **5,** 55 (1968).

27. Gross, S. J., Grant, J. D., Bennett, R., et al., Estriol-specific antibody for steroid assays. *Steroids* **18,** 555 (1971).

28. Soares, J. R., Gross, S. R., and Bashore, R. A., Evaluation ot azoestriol antisera for estriol measurement in pregnancy plasma directly after extraction. *J. Clin. Endocrinol. Metab.* **40,** 970 (1975).

29. Lindner, H. R., Perel, E., Friedlander, A., and Zeitlin, A., Specificity of antibodies to ovarian hormones in relation to the site of attachment of the steroid hapten to the peptide carrier. *Steroids* **19,** 357 (1971).

30. Kuss, E., and Goebel, R., Determination of estrogens by radioimmunoassay with antibodies to estrogen-C6-conjugates. I. Synthesis of estrone-, estradiol-17β-, and estriol-6-albumin conjugates. *Steroids* **19,** 509 (1971).

31. Wright, K., Collins, D. C., and Preedy, J. R. K., Comparative specificity of antisera raised against estrone, estradiol-17β and estriol using 6-O-carboxymethyloxime bovine serum albumin derivatives. *Steroids* **21,** 755 (1973).

32. Walker, C. S., Clark, S. J., and Wotiz, H. H., Factors involved in the production of specific antibodies to estriol and estradiol. *Steroids* **21,** 259 (1973).

33. De Lauzon, S., Cittanova, N., Defosses, B., and Jayle, M. F., A new approach for quantitative evaluation of cross-reactivity of steroids with an antiserum by radioimmunoassay: Application to a highly specific antiestriol. *Steroids* **22,** 747 (1973).

CLIN. CHEM. 22/3, 364–368 (1976)

Measurement of 25-Hydroxyvitamin D_3 in Serum

Roger Bouillon,[1] Piet Van Kerkhove,[2] and Pieter De Moor

We describe a method for measuring 25-hydroxyvitamin D_3 in serum. Extraction with dichloromethane/methanol (2/1 by vol), followed by chromatography on a column of Sephadex LH-20, resulted in an overall analytical recovery of 82% ± 3.5% (SD). Diluted normal rat serum was used as binding protein because it contains a transport protein that has both a high affinity (K_a = 2 × 10^{10} liter/mol) and a high capacity (3 × 10^{-6} mol/liter) for 25-hydroxyvitamin D_3. There is no advantage in using more complex binding proteins derived either from rachitic animals or from cytosol preparations. Concentrations of 25-hydroxyvitamin D_3 (13.4 ± 4 μg/liter) in the serum of apparently normal Belgian subjects are lower than those reported for North Americans, but resemble those reported for the United Kingdom.

Additional Keyphrases: *binding protein for 25-hydroxyvitamin D • competitive protein-binding assay • reference values • assessing vitamin D status • rickets*

Measurement in serum of 25-hydroxyvitamin D_3, the principal circulating metabolite of vitamin D_3 (*1*), is a relatively good index to overall vitamin D status if renal 25-hydroxyvitamin D-1-hydroxylase activity is normal. Indeed, values are high during vitamin D intoxication (*2*) and low during vitamin D deficiency (*3*). All present methods (*3–8*) are based on the competitive protein-binding principle (*9*). Basically, they involve a preliminary extraction and purification, to eliminate the interfering binding protein for 25-hydroxyvitamin D_3 that is present in serum and to remove related substances (mainly vitamin D_3 itself) that cross react with the 25-hydroxyvitamin D_3 binding protein. Secondly, an incubation allows measurement of the competition between labeled and unlabeled 25-hydroxyvitamin D_3 for a limited amount of binding protein. The traditional source of this binding protein has been either serum from rachitic rat (*3, 6–8*) or rachitic man (*5*), or kidney cytosol from rachitic rats (*4*). Some authors have claimed that partially purified 25-hydroxyvitamin D_3 binding protein from rat serum is more sensitive than whole diluted serum (*6*). It is not yet clear (*7*) whether a purification step—with use of either silicic acid (*3, 4, 8*), Sephadex LH-20 (*6*), or thin-layer chomatography (*5*)—is needed.

We describe our efforts to optimize the analytical procedure and to evaluate its clinical usefulness.

Laboratorium voor Experimentele Geneeskunde, Katholieke Universiteit Leuven, Rega Instituut, Minderbroedersstraat 10, B-3000 Leuven, Belgium.

[1] Aangesteld navorser.

[2] Aspirant N.F.W.O.

Received Oct. 15, 1975, accepted Jan. 6, 1976.

Materials

Unlabeled vitamin D_3 and D_2 were obtained from Merck (Darmstadt). Unlabeled 25-hydroxyvitamin D_3 was either a gift from Roussel (France) or from Philips-Duphar (The Netherlands). The quantity of steroid was assessed from the ultraviolet absorbance at 265 nm.

[26(27)-*Methyl*-^{3}H]-25-hydroxyvitamin D_3 was obtained from Amersham (specific activity, 2.9 kCi/mol) or New England Nuclear (specific activity, 9.5 kCi/mol).

Rachitic chicks and rats were reared in a windowless room illuminated with incandescent light bulbs. They were fed a rachitogenic diet containing 1.03 g of calcium, and 0.78 g of phosphorus per 100 g (from Hope Farms, Wourden, The Netherlands).

Radioactivity was counted in a liquid-scintillation counter (Packard Tri-Carb 2425) with use of a toluene scintillator [8 g of naphthalene, 4 g of 2,5-diphenyloxazole, and 50 mg of 2,2-*p*-phenylene-bis(4-methyl-5-phenyl-oxazolol) in 600 ml of toluene and

400 ml of ethylene glycol monomethylether]. Quenching was estimated for each sample by an external-standard method.

Methods

Extraction of 25-hydroxyvitamin D_3. We tried different methods for extracting radiolabeled 25-hydroxyvitamin D_3 from serum. A modification of the total lipid extraction according to Bligh and Dyer (*10*) proved to be largely superior on simple or repetitive extraction with diethyl ether or dichloromethane. The final method chosen consisted of extracting 0.2 ml of serum mixed successively with 10 μl of tritiated 25-hydroxyvitamin D_3 (0.25 pmol), 1 ml of water, 2.5 ml of methanol, and 5 ml of dichloromethane. Four milliliters of the dichloromethane layer obtained after vigorous mixing (5 min) and centrifugation (5 min, 3000 rpm) is removed with a syringe and replaced by the same amount of dichloromethane. After repeating the same procedure the combined (8 ml) dichloromethane layer is evaporated under a stream of nitrogen in a water bath at 40 °C.

Purification of 25-hydroxyvitamin D_3. The extracted 25-hydroxyvitamin D_3, dissolved in two successive 0.3-ml portions of chloroform/hexane (1/1 by vol) is applied on a Sephadex LH-20 (Pharmacia) column (21 × 1 cm) and eluted with the same mixture. Each column was calibrated with 25-hydroxyvitamin D_3 and radiolabeled vitamin D_3 tracer before use. By extensive washing of the columns they could be re-used at least 20 times.

For routine assays, only the peak fraction of the 25-hydroxyvitamin D_3 eluate (12 ml) is collected and evaporated. The evaporated 25-hydroxyvitamin D_3 is dissolved in 0.3 ml of ethanol; 150 μl is used for counting the recovery and 40 μl or less is used, in duplicate, for the competitive protein-binding assay.

Competitive protein-binding assay. The total volume of 0.98 ml consisted of 0.2 ml of binding protein (usually normal rat serum diluted 2000-fold or other proteins as specified further); 0.7 ml of lipoproteins extracted from whole serum (*3*) diluted 400-fold in diethylbarbiturate buffer, 0.1 mol/liter, pH 8.6; 40 μl of ethanol containing either standard 25-hydroxyvitamin D_3 (0, 100, 200, 300, 400, 500, or 50 000 pg) or the unknown extracted and purified sample; and 40 μl of ethanol containing 1 pmol of tritiated 25-hydroxyvitamin D_3.

After incubation at 0 °C (usually for 1 h unless specified otherwise) the bound and free 25-hydroxyvitamin D_3 are separated by adding 1 ml of cold dextran-coated charcoal [1.6 mg charcoal (Norit A) and 0.16 mg of dextran (Dextran 70, Pharmacia)]. After mixing a total contact time of 30 min at 0 °C, the tubes are centrifuged (3000 rpm, 10 min, 4 °C) and all the supernate is transferred with a disposable pipette to the counting vial, containing 10-ml scintillation liquid, and counted for 10 min.

Measurement of the association constant and the binding capacity of the binding proteins was performed as described elsewhere (*11*) and calculated according to Rosenthal (*12*).

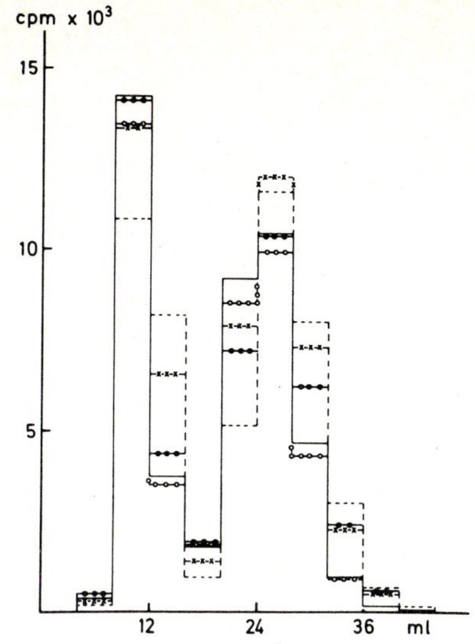

Fig. 1. Relation between radioactivity in eluate and volume eluted

Chromatography of a mixture of [³H]-vitamin D_3 and [³H]-25-hydroxyvitamin D_3 applied to five different 21 × 1 cm columns containing Sephadex LH-20 (as indicated by five different symbols), and eluted at room temperature with a mixture of chloroform/hexane (50/50, by vol). Fractions of 2 ml collected, evaporated under nitrogen, dissolved in toluene, and counted for 10 min

Results

Extraction of 25-Hydroxyvitamin D_3

The total analytical recovery of tritiated 25-hydroxyvitamin D_3 added to the serum before the extraction was 94.8% ± 1.29% (mean ± SD; n = 5), with a theoretical maximum of 96%. When dichloromethane was replaced by chloroform in the same procedure, the total extraction was only 91.9% ± 1.27% (n = 5). Repetitive extractions with either dichloromethane or diethylether alone resulted in less than 80% recovery.

Purification of 25-Hydroxyvitamin D_3

The separation between vitamin D_3 and 25-hydroxyvitamin D_3, as assessed by the elution pattern of the tritiated vitamins, was nearly complete (Figure 1). If all fractions containing 25-hydroxyvitamin D_3 were collected, more than 90% was recovered. Overall recovery after both extraction and purification on Sephadex LH-20, collecting only the peak elution of 25-hydroxyvitamin D_3, was 82% ± 3.5% (SD) (n = 50).

Optimal Conditions for the Competitive Protein-Binding Assay

Choice of binding protein for 25-hydroxyvitamin D_3: Binding proteins for 25-hydroxyvitamin D_3 were sought in the serum of three different species (human, rat, and chicken), both normal and rachitic. The cytosol prepared from liver, kidney, intestine, and muscle of both the rat and the chicken were also examined. The affinity constant of the binding pro-

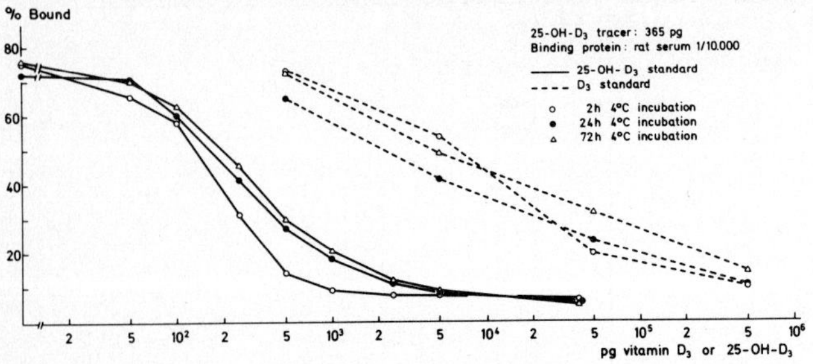

Fig. 2. Influence of total incubation time (at 4 °C) on the assay of 25-hydroxyvitamin D_3, and its interference with vitamin D_3

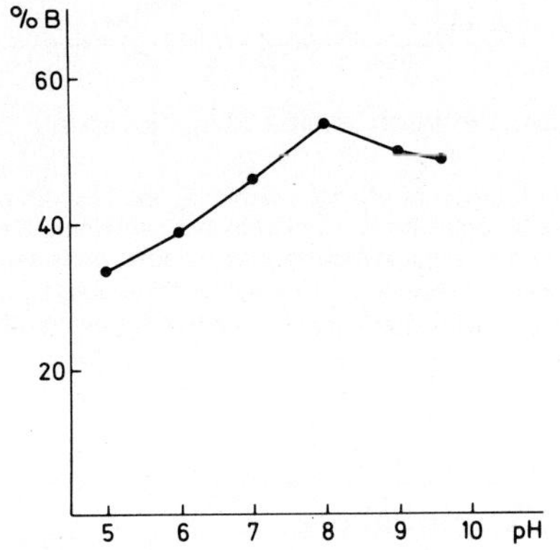

Fig. 3. Influence of pH on the binding of 25-hydroxyvitamin D_3 to its serum binding protein (from the rat)
Binding protein and tracer concentration are constant

tein present in all rat preparations was nearly identical to the one found in human serum (about 2×10^{10} liter/mol) and 10-fold higher than the one found in the chicken serum (6.2×10^8 liter/mol) or chicken cytosols (about 3×10^9 liter/mol). There was no important difference between the K_a of the binding protein found in tissues from rachitic or normal men or animals. In view of the high capacity (10^{-6} mol/liter) of rat and human serum, which permits ample dilution, there is no need to use more complex binding systems.

Temperature and duration of incubation: The association constant was about five-fold higher at 0 °C than at 37 °C. The association rate constant, even at 0 °C, was very high (*11*). From this, one may predict that a short incubation at 0 °C is the best choice for optimal sensitivity. This was confirmed experimentally (Figure 2).

pH: The optimal pH for binding of 25-hydroxyvitamin D_3 was between 8 and 9 (Figure 3).

Tracer concentration: The influence of different tracer concentrations was extremely important (Figure 4). However, because the concentration of 25-hydroxyvitamin D_3 in serum is usually high, there was no need to use the most sensitive procedure, which would have necessitated a longer counting time.

Other aspects: The presence of a small amount of lipoproteins resulted in a small increase in the binding of 25-hydroxyvitamin D_3 without increase in the nonspecific binding of 25-hydroxyvitamin D_3, probably because of the better solubility of the tracer.

The presence of more than 10% ethanol in the incubation volume progressively decreased the binding of 25-hydroxyvitamin D_3. A specific binding of labeled 25-hydroxyvitamin D_3 to dextran-coated charcoal in the presence of an excess of nonlabeled 25-hydroxyvitamin D_3 was 5.1% ± 1% (SD). The "water blank" (the amount of 25-hydroxyvitamin D_3 measured when water was extracted instead of serum) was 1.3 ± 1 (SD) ng/ml (n = 25).

Variation and Sensitivity

Between-assay variation was 13% for a sample containing a mean concentration of 17.7 μg/liter (n = 5) and 16% for another sample with 17.8 μg/liter (n = 5). Within-assay variation was 8.8% for a sample containing 4.9 μg/liter (n = 5). The coefficient of variation, calculated from the standard deviation for 42 samples run in duplicate, was 10%.

The sensitivity of the system—defined as the point two standard deviations below the B_0 (50.9% of total radioactivity)—was 20 pg. In five samples, 25-hydroxyvitamin D_3 was measured the same day after extraction from 0.2 and 0.1 ml. In the 0.1-ml samples the calculated concentration was 99.5% ± 7% of the values obtained when 0.2 ml was used for extraction.

Interference by Vitamins D_2 and D_3

The displacement of labeled 25-hydroxyvitamin D_3 from its binding protein by vitamin D_2 and D_3 was identical; no displacement was found on adding cholesterol. The relative potency of vitamin D_3 is difficult to express exactly, because its curve does not parallel the one obtained for 25-hydroxyvitamin D_3 and because the interference increases with duration of incubation (Figure 2). At the point of 50% inhibition during a 2-h incubation at 0 °C, the relative potency of vitamin D_3 was 1%.

Clinical Results

Normal values obtained for 51 apparently healthy volunteers during a survey of serum cholesterol values in the normal Belgian population (May 1974) were 13.4 ± 4.1 (SD) μg/liter. The correlation between serum 25-hydroxyvitamin D_3 and serum calcium was 0.25 ($0.1 < P < 0.05$).

In *rachitic persons and animals* the concentrations of 25-hydroxyvitamin D_3 were below 4 μg/liter. In a North African family that had lived in Belgium for two years, we found two children with radiologically manifest rickets and 25-hydroxyvitamin D_3 values of 1.7 and 3.1 μg/liter (*13*).

Institutionalized persons. The 25-hydroxyvitamin D_3 concentrations in 20 patients living in a psychiatric institution were subnormal, 8.6 ± 3.2 μg/liter. In 20 other patients treated with anticonvulsant drugs

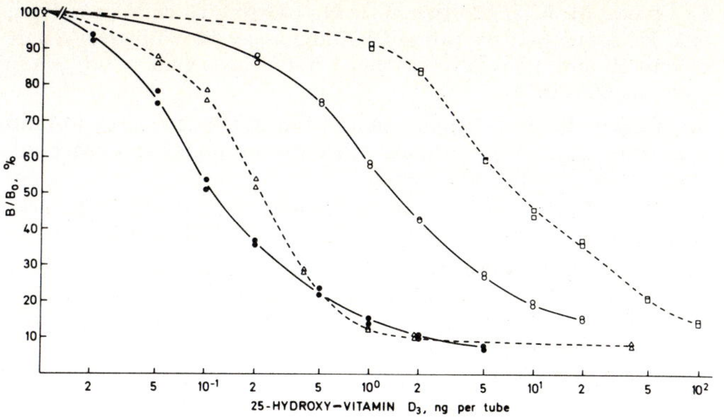

Fig. 4. Influence of substrate concentrations on the assay of 25-hydroxyvitamin D_3 (4 °C, 24-h incubation)

Final rat serum dilution and amount of [^{3}H] 25-hydroxyvitamin D_3 per tube are, respectively: ● — ●, 20 000-fold and 60 pg; △ . . . △, 10 000-fold and 365 pg; ○ — ○, 5000-fold and 1100 pg; □ . . . □, 500-fold and 6000 pg

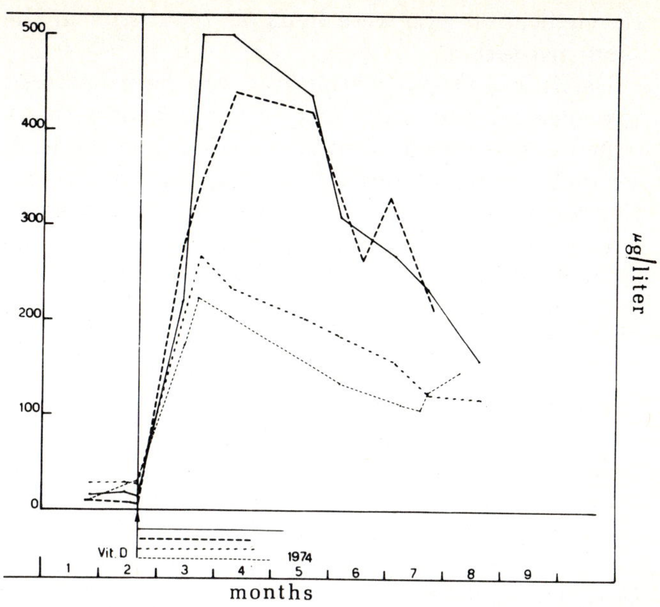

Fig. 5. 25-Hydroxyvitamin D_3 concns. in sera of four patients with chronic renal failure who were being treated with pharmacological doses of vitamin D_3 (15 mg/week)

Lines under abscissa indicate when treatment was stopped for each patient

during a mean period of 12 years and living in the same institution, the values were still lower, 6.4 ± 3.4 µg/liter (*14*).

Effect of dosage with vitamin D_3. During treatment of four patients with renal osteodystrophy with pharmacological doses of vitamin D_3 (15 mg weekly), very high values were obtained (*15*), ranging from 220 to 500 µg/liter. After interruption of therapy their 25-hydroxyvitamin D_3 values remained very high for several months (Figure 5).

Discussion

Extraction of 25-hydroxyvitamin D_3: A total lipid extraction proved to be superior to simple ether or dichloromethane extraction. Use of a dichloromethane/methanol mixture resulted in a slightly higher recovery than did a chloroform/methanol mixture, and the dichloromethane layer is more easily evaporated.

The purification on Sephadex LH-20 is relatively simple, but is the rate-limiting step in the assay. However, for serum samples obtained from patients treated with pharmacological doses of vitamin D_3 much lower values were obtained when a LH-20 separation step was used, as compared to the values obtained by a direct assay (*7*) without purification. Indeed, Belsey et al. (*7*) found values for 25-hydroxyvitamin D_3 that much exceeded 1000 µg/liter after treatment with pharmacological doses of vitamin D_3, whereas our values are only between 200 and 500 µg/liter. Moreover, their values are higher than the maximum binding capacity of the specific transport protein present in human serum (*11*). Therefore we conclude that without prior elimination of vitamin D_3, measurement of 25-hydroxyvitamin D_3 can be interfered with in samples obtained after treatment with pharmacological doses of vitamin D_3.

Some other factors. The binding protein was chosen very carefully. High association constant (K_a = 10^{10} at 0 °C) were found for the binding proteins present in human and rat serum (whether rachitic or not) or in different cytosol preparations from rachitic rats. Differences between the association constants of all these preparations were small. These values are higher than those reported previously (*2*), but correspond theoretically (*16, 17*) to the high assay sensitivity we and others (*8*) have found. For serum and cytosol preparations of rachitic chicks the affinity constants at 0 °C were much lower. The capacity of the binding proteins, present in all sera, is extremely high (10^{-6} mol/liter), so that a high dilution can be used in the assay. Although the binding capacity of rachitic sera is somewhat higher than those of nonrachitic origin, the advantage of using this kind of serum is negligible. Moreover, the residual endogenous (stable) 25-hydroxyvitamin D_3 present in the assay tube is extremely small (1–3 pg) compared to the amount of labeled 25-hydroxyvitamin D_3 (400 pg).

Owing to the rapid association at 0 °C, a 1-h incubation is sufficient.

Clinical results. These confirm the presence of near-blank values in rachitic persons (*7, 8, 18*).

Normal values in North America—27 µg/liter (*3*) and 35 µg/liter (*7*)—are much higher than those found in European countries—15 µg/liter (*6*) and 12 µg/liter (*8*) in the U.K., 15 µg/liter in France (*5*) and 14 µ/liter (our data) in Belgium—although one group (*18*) has found higher values in a London population (18 to 36 µg/liter).

As found by others (*19–21*), we noted low 25-hydroxyvitamin D_3 concentrations in the serum of patients being treated with antiepileptic drugs. This is due both to the antiepileptic drugs and to the living circumstances, because lower than normal values were also found in control people without antiepileptic medication who were living as inpatients in the same institution.

Between 100 and 500 μg/liter can be considered toxicological values, as found in one patient with accidental overdosage (serum calcium, 190 mg/liter; serum 25-hydroxyvitamin D_3, 114 μg/liter) and in patients with renal insufficiency who have been treated with pharmacological doses of vitamin D_3 (220 to 500 g/liter). These values are much lower than those found by a direct assay (without prior purification of 25-hydroxyvitamin D_3) (7) probably because the high concentrations of vitamin D_3 interfere with the 25-hydroxyvitamin D_3 assay (Figure 2).

In conclusion, 25-hydroxyvitamin D_3 concentrations can be measured rapidly and conveniently, and seem to reflect the overall vitamin D status except in cases of absence of the kidney 25-hydroxyvitamin D_3-1-hydroxylase (*22*).

The excellent technical assistance of Mr. Tan Biauw Keng and Mrs. M. P. Janssens-Quintens is gratefully acknowledged.

References

1. Blunt, J. W., De Luca, H. F., and Schnoes, H. K., 25-Hydroxycholecalciferol. A biologically active metabolite of vitamin D_3. *Biochemistry* **7,** 3317 (1968).
2. Haddad, J. G., and Stamp, T. C. B., Circulating 25-hydroxyvitamin D. *Am. J. Med.* **57,** 57 (1974).
3. Belsey, R., De Luca, H. F., and Potts, J. T., Jr., Competitive binding assay for vitamin D and 25-hydroxyvitamin D. *J. Clin Endocrinol.* **33,** 554 (1971).
4. Haddad, J. G., and Chyu, K. J., Competitive protein-binding radioassay for 25-hydroxycholecalciferol. *J. Clin. Endocrinol.* **33,** 992 (1971).
5. Bayard, F., Bec, P., and Louvet, J. P., Measurement of plasma 25-hydroxycholecalciferol in man. *Eur. J. Clin. Invest.* **2,** 195 (1972).
6. Edelstein, S., Charman, M., Lawson, D. E. M., and Kodicek, E., Competitive protein-binding assay for 25-hydroxycholecalciferol. *Clin. Sci. Mol. Med* . **46,** 231 (1974).
7. Belsey, R. E., De Luca, H. F., and Potts, J. T., Jr., A rapid assay for 25-hydroxyvitamin D_3 without preparative chromatography. *J. Clin. Endocrinol.* **38,** 1046 (1974).
8. Preece, M. A., O'Riordan, J. L. H., Lawson, D. E. M., and Kodicek, E., A competitive protein-binding assay for 25-hydroxycholecalciferol and 25-hydroxycholecalciferol in serum. *Clin. Chim. Acta* **54,** 235 (1974).
9. Murphy, B. E. P., Application of the property of protein-binding to the assay of minute quantities of hormones and other substances. *Nature* **201,** 679 (1964).
10. Bligh, E. G., and Dyer, W. J., A rapid method of total lipid extraction and purification. *Can. J. Biochem.* **37,** 911 (1959).
11. Bouillon, R., Van Kerkhove, P., and De Moor, P., Characteristics of the vitamin D binding proteins in different species. Presented at the "XI European Symposium on Calcified Tissues." *Calcified Tissue Research,* in press.
12. Rosenthal, H. E., A graphic method for the determination and presentation of binding parameters in a complex system. *Anal. Biochem.* **20,** 525 (1967).
13. Corbeel, L., Bouillon, R., Dechamps, L., and Geussens, L., Vitamin D sensitive rickets in adolescents. *Acta Paediatr. Belg.,* in press.
14. Bouillon, R., Reynaert, J., Claes, J. H., et al., The effect of anticonvulsant therapy on serum levels of 25-hydroxyvitamin D, calcium and parathyroid hormone. *J. Clin. Endocrinol.,* 1975, in press.
15. Verberckmoes, R., and Bouillon, R., Influence of vitamin D treatment on serum levels of parathyroid hormone in patients with chronic renal failure. In *Vitamin D and Problems to Uremic Bone Disease,* Walter de Gruyter & Co, Berlin, New York, 1975, p 629.
16. Heyns, W., and De Moor, P., Use of specific plasma proteins for determination of steroids. *Res. Steroids* **4,** 269 (1970).
17. Ekins, R. P., Newman, G. B., and O'Riordan, J. L. H., Theoretical aspects of "saturation" and radioimmunoassay. In *Radioisotopes in Medicine: In Vitro Studies.* R. L. Hayes, F. A. Goswitz, and B. E. P. Murphy, Eds. U. S. Atomic Energy Commission, 1968, p 59.
18. Mc Laughlin, M., Ragatt, P. R., Faviney, A., et al., Seasonal variations in serum 25-hydroxycholecalciferol in healthy people. *Lancet* **ii,** 536 (1974).
19. Stamp, T. C. B., Round, J. M., Rowe, D. J. F., and Haddad, J. C., Plasma levels and therapeutic effect of 25-hydroxycholecalciferol in epileptic patients taking anticonvulsant drugs. *Br. Med. J.* **iv,** 9 (1972).
20. Hahn, T. J., Hendin, B. A., Sharp, C. R., and Haddad, J. G., Effect of chronic anticonvulsant therapy on serum 25-hydroxycholecalciferol levels in adults. *New Engl. J. Med.* **287,** 900 (1972).
21. Baud, L., Paunier, L., Preece, M. A., et al., Concentrations plasmatiques de 25-hydroxycholécalciferol et traitement anticonvulsant. *Schweiz. Med. Wochenshr.* **104,** 1908 (1974).
22. Fraser, D. R., and Kodicek, E., Unique biosynthesis by kidney of a biologically active vitamin D metabolite. *Nature* **228,** 764 (1970).

CLIN. CHEM. 22/3, 369–372 (1976)

Simple Fluorometric Determination of Aldosterone in Urine without Use of Isotopes or Chromatography

William R. Whigham

Aldosterone 18-glucuronide in urine is hydrolyzed by adjusting the pH to 1.0 and allowing the mixture to stand overnight at room temperature. The free aldosterone is then extracted into dichloromethane, which is washed with carbonate to remove acidic compounds and evaporated. The residue is partitioned between a nonpolar organic phase and an aqueous phase, and the aldosterone oxidized to the 13-carboxylic acid derivative with Benedict's qualitative glucose reagent. Neutral compounds are extracted from this oxidation mixture with dichloromethane at pH 7.5, the mixture is acidified, and the oxidized aldosterone extracted into dichloromethane. After washing with pH 3.5 buffer, this extract is evaporated and the oxidized aldosterone determined fluorometrically via a two-stage reaction with sulfuric acid/water (85/15 by vol) and methanol containing ferric chloride.

Many clinical laboratories routinely determine 17-ketosteroids, 17-hydroxycorticosteroids, serum cortisol, and perhaps other steroids. To offer a more complete service in steroids, it is desirable for them to also offer measurements of urinary aldosterone. However, most methods for doing so require a liquid-scintillation counter and expertise in chromatography. Recently, simple nonchromatographic radioimmunoassays have appeared for aldosterone determination (*1–4*), but these methods also require a liquid-scintillation counter and must depend on the purchase of expensive kits or antibody.

The method presented here requires no isotopes or chromatography, and multiple specimens may be run in one day (after overnight hydrolysis).

Pathologists Service Professional Associates, Inc., P.O. Box 50122, Federal Annex, Atlanta, Ga. 30302.

Received Oct. 10, 1975; accepted Dec. 3, 1975.

Materials and Methods

Apparatus

This includes screw-cap vials, 40 ml, such as Kimble No. 60957; polyethylene-lined caps for these vials, such as Poly-Seal 24-400; a Kahn shaker such as the two-speed model of Eberbach with utility carrier; an air-blowing apparatus constructed of copper tubing to fit vial supports such as Scientific Products S9215, and a compressed-air source; and a spectrofluorometer such as the Perkin-Elmer Model 204.

Reagents

All reagents are reagent grade, used without further purification, De-ionized water is used for all aqueous reagents.

Dichloromethane. Reagent grade is acceptable.

Anhydrous sodium sulfate, granular.

Sodium carbonate, 50 g/liter. Dissolve 10 g of anhydrous Na_2CO_3 in 200 ml of water.

Ethyl acetate. Reagent grade is acceptable.

Ethanol/water, 10 ml of absolute ethanol plus 90 ml of water.

Benedict's reagent. Dissolve 3.5 g of $CuSO_4{\cdot}5H_2O$ in 20 ml water in a flask (may require a little heat). Dissolve 35 g of sodium citrate dihydrate and 20 g of anhydrous sodium carbonate in 160 ml of water (may also require warming). Cool the two solutions and combine them.

Glycine buffer, pH 3.5. Dissolve 7.5 g of glycine in water, add 1.4 ml of HCl (6 mol/liter), and dilute to 250 ml. Check the pH and adjust if necessary.

Sulfuric acid, dilute. Mix cautiously, in an ice bath, 85 ml of concentrated H_2SO_4 and 15 ml of water.

Methanol containing $FeCl_3{\cdot}6H_2O$. Dissolve 100 mg of $FeCl_3{\cdot}6H_2O$ in 100 ml of methanol. Dilute 5 ml of this with 95 ml of methanol.

Standards: d-Aldosterone (Sigma Chemical Co. St. Louis, Mo. 63178; cat. No. A6628) is stored overnight in a desiccator before weighing.

"A" standard, 0.4 g/liter. Dissolve 40 mg of aldosterone in isopropanol and dilute to 100 ml. Store in a dark bottle in the refrigerator. The solution is stable longer than six months.

"B" standard, 4 mg/liter. Dilute 1.0 ml of "A" standard to 100 ml with isopropanol. Store in a dark bottle in the refrigerator. The solution is stable longer than six months.

Procedure

Place 20 ml of urine into a 40-ml screw-capped vial, adjust the pH to 1 with HCl (6 mol/liter), cap, and let stand for 20 h or more at room temperature in the dark. Add 20 ml of dichloromethane, shake slowly for 10 min or longer, centrifuge (1500 rpm) for 2 min or longer, and aspirate the urine (upper) phase, leaving behind any emulsion that may have formed.

Add about 2 g of anhydrous Na_2SO_4 to each vial and shake to break up the emulsion, centrifuge, and pour the dichloromethane into clean vials, leaving the Na_2SO_4 behind. Add 5 ml of the Na_2CO_3 solution to the dichloromethane, shake vigorously for 2 min, centrifuge, aspirate the carbonate (upper) phase, and wash the dichloromethane with 3 ml of water.

Transfer 17 ml of the dichloromethane into a clean vial, add a boiling chip, and evaporate at 56 °C in a water bath under a gentle stream of air.

Evaporate 0.2 ml (0.8 μg) of aldosterone "B" standard in each of two tubes, for duplicate standards. Label a clean tube "B" for blank. Treat standards and blank exactly like unknowns from this point on.

Add 3 ml of ethyl acetate to all tubes, mix to dissolve the residue, add 2 ml of the ethanol/water mixture and 20 ml of *n*-heptane, and shake the mixture for 3 min. Centrifuge, and aspirate as much of the heptane (upper) layer as possible without removing any of the aqueous layer.

Add 2 ml of Benedict's reagent, mix well, cap, and incubate for 30 min at 56 °C. This oxidizes aldosterone to its 13-carboxylic acid derivative.

Add 3 ml of $NaH_2PO_4 \cdot H_2O$ (100 g/liter), mix, add 20 ml of dichloromethane, shake the mixture for 3 min, centrifuge, and carefully aspirate the dichloromethane (lower) layer.

Add 1 ml of HCl (6 mol/liter) to each tube dropwise with vigorous mixing, to remove CO_2. Add 20 ml of dichloromethane, shake for 3 min, centrifuge, and aspirate the aqueous (upper) layer as completely as possible.

Add 5 ml of the glycine buffer to the organic phase, shake for 2 min, centrifuge, and aspirate the aqueous (upper) layer as completely as possible. Repeat this wash with glycine buffer one more time.

Transfer 17 ml of the dichloromethane to clean tubes and evaporate it at 56 °C in a water bath, under a gentle stream of air. Add 2 ml of the dilute H_2SO_4 to each tube and mix vigorously to dissolve the steroid, cap, and heat for exactly 15 min at 56 °C. Place the tubes in an ice bath for 5 min. When the tubes are cold, add 2 ml of the methanol/$FeCl_3 \cdot 6H_2O$ to each and mix vigorously for 5 s. Return to the ice bath. (It is best to do just two tubes at a time, adding the methanol, mixing immediately, and returning to the ice bath.) After methanol has been added and mixed, cap the tubes and place them in water at room temperature for 2 min, then in the dark at room temperature for exactly 25 min.

Read the fluorescence within the next 5 min, because it reaches a peak and then fades rapidly. The excitation wavelength is 580 nm, the fluorescence wavelength is 610 nm. Average the readings for the two standards.

Calculation

(Unknown fluorescence − blank fluorescence/standard fluorescence − blank fluorescence) × 47 = aldosterone, μg/liter

To correct for an average 6% loss of aldosterone in the first extraction with dichloromethane and its washing, the factor (μg/liter)/.94 is used. Then: (μg/liter (corr.)) × (liters/24 h) = μg/24 h.

The 24-h urines used were collected without preservative (refrigerated during collection) or contained either 10 ml of glacial acetic acid or 10 ml of toluene that had been put into the collection jug. They were refrigerated soon after collection.

Results and Discussion

Method Development

Pre-extraction. Pre-extraction as described by Drewes et al. (*1*) did not alter values significantly, so was not done.

Hydrolysis. The specimens are hydrolyzed in the usual manner (*1, 5*) by incubation overnight at pH 1 and room temperature, which hydrolyzes aldosterone 18-glucuronide. Incubation at 56 °C for 2 h at pH 1 gave similar values, but pigment formation was increased considerably, so the overnight hydrolysis was preferred.

Initial extraction. At first, we washed the original dichloromethane extract with 0.1 mol/liter NaOH. The resulting analytical recovery of aldosterone was poor and inconsistent. This problem was corrected by substituting the Na_2CO_3 solution for the NaOH solution. Analytical recovery averaged 94% through these steps, and is corrected for in the calculations. After this correction, analytical recovery for urine taken through the entire procedure averaged very nearly 100%.

Water taken through the entire procedure gave a blank identical to the blank started after the initial dichloromethane evaporation. Thus, introduction of the blank at this stage is acceptable. Introduction of the standard at this stage is compensated for by the recovery correction factor.

Partition between ethyl acetate/heptane and water/ethanol. Running the procedure without this partition results in values that are about 65% higher than with this partition. In addition, the final fluorescent solution has a faint brown color, which varies from specimen to specimen. Experiments were done to study aldosterone partition between 20 ml of *n*-heptane containing various amounts of ethyl acetate and 2 ml of water containing 0, 10, 20, or 30 ml of ethanol per deciliter. Those conditions chosen give good recovery of aldosterone in the aqueous phase and remove considerable interfering material.

Oxidation. Oxidation of aldosterone is essentially complete in 20 min at 56 °C with half-strength Benedict's reagent. Routinely, 30-min incubation was used.

Addition of $Na_2HPO_4 \cdot H_2O$ (100 g/liter) after oxidation lowers the pH to about 7.5, still well above the expected pK_a of the aldosterone oxidation product, which is retained in the aqueous phase at this step.

Wash with pH 3.5 glycine buffer. Cortisol standards were run through the entire procedure initially without this wash. It was found that there was no fluorescence when I omitted heating of the Benedict's reagent. However, when heating was included, cortisol gave a fluorescence equivalent to 2% that of an equal amount of aldosterone in the method. A reasonable explanation is that cortisol is being oxidized to some extent by the Benedict's solution; most likely to the 17-carboxylic acid derivative. Because this derivative would be expected to have a pK_a near 3.5, while that of aldosterone derivative should be near 5, a double wash with pH 3.5 buffer was included in the procedure. This diminished the interference of cortisol from 2% to about 0.2% without causing undue loss of aldosterone oxidation product.

Development of fluorescence. I thought that, after optimization of the oxidation step, a one-stage reaction to develop fluorescence similar to that of cortisol used by Clark and Rubin (*6*) or perhaps a two-stage reaction similar to that for dehydroisoandrosterone used by Allen et al. (*7*) might be satisfactory for the aldosterone oxidation product. Thus sulfuric acid concentrations, amounts of methanol or ethanol, and heating times were varied in one-stage and two-stage reactions to obtain maximum color (assuming that the colored product would fluoresce). Initially, the reaction was optimized without including iron in the methanol. A yellow product was formed with absorbance and excitation peaks at 480 nm and a fluorescence peak at 525 nm. I attempted to intensify the color by adding Fe^{3+} to the methanol, because it is used in some sensitive cholesterol methods (*8*). When this was done, the second-stage reaction occurred rapidly at room temperature, but instead of a more intense yellow color, the yellow color was decreased by about half and a red color was formed with absorbance and excitation peak at 586 nm and a fluorescence emission peak at 610 nm. I found that the red fluor gave a relatively lower blank than did the yellow fluor (although the fluorescence was not as great) and that the red fluor gave lower values with partially purified urine extracts than did the yellow fluor, so I considered the red fluor the better of the two for measurement in the procedure.

Analytical Variables

Standardization. Aldosterone standards from 0.4 to 4.0 μg, representing 25 to 250 μg of aldosterone per liter of urine, were taken through the procedure. There was no significant deviation from linearity over this range.

Blank. The blank value averaged the equivalent of about 2.5 μg of aldosterone per liter, but was very consistent, so that blank-corrected aldosterone concentrations even lower than this can probably be considered significantly different from zero (see *sensitivity*).

Day-to-day precision. Ten control urines run on different days by the same technologist gave values ranging from 5.0 to 6.7 μg/liter, with a mean of 5.87 μg/liter and a standard deviation of 0.58 μg/liter.

Sensitivity. A value two standard deviations above zero could be considered significantly different from zero, such that the sensitivity could be considered to be 1.16 μg/liter. This assumes that the method standard deviation is the same at zero aldosterone concentration as at 5.87 μg/liter (the control value). Actually, the method may be a little more sensitive than this.

Accuracy and specificity. A manual scan of excitation and fluorescence peaks at 5-nm intervals of the standard and of control urine from 565 to 590 nm and from 610 to 635 nm indicated that after subtracting the blank, the control spectra were essentially identical to those of the standard over these wavelengths. The values for urine have been corrected to yield an apparent 100% recovery through the entire procedure. The mean obtained for 25 randomly selected urine specimens (11.1 μg/24 h) was not significantly different from that obtained by other accepted procedures for aldosterone (*1, 2, 5*).

Ten steroids and the drug spironolactone were tested for interference when run through the entire assay. The percent fluorescence compared to aldosterone is shown in Table 1.

Table 1. Fluorescence Produced by Some Other Steroids Relative to That Produced by Aldosterone

Steroid	Fluorescence
Aldosterone	100.00
Cortisol	0.18
Cortisone	0.00
Corticosterone	1.40
11-Deoxycorticosterone	0.10
11-Deoxycortisol	0.33
Tetrahydrocortisol	0.02
Tetrahydrocortisone	0.00
Tetrahydro 11-deoxycortisol	0.02
β-Cortol	0.02
β-Cortolone	0.06
Spironolactone	0.00

The method has been used routinely for several months in this laboratory. During this time, three specimens have had abnormally high aldosterone values: 32, 46, and 48 μg/24 h. All three were from patients hospitalized with severe hypertension. On the last two of these plasma renin values were above normal at about the same time as the urines were collected, confirming a diagnosis of secondary hyperaldosteronism.

Additional clinical studies still remain to be done, as well as comparisons with other methods. It may be that the fluorescence reaction can be improved. In all probability though, the method is acceptable for clinical use, and the suggestion of Cope and Loizou (*5*) that aldosterone excretions exceeding 30 μg/24 h be considered strong evidence for a diagnosis of hyperaldosteronism can be applied to this procedure, because 30 μg/24 h is nearly three standard deviations above the mean of 11.1 μg/24 h I found for 25 normal specimens.

A technologist can conveniently run one blank, two standards, a control, and four unknown specimens in about 6 h, with actual bench time a little less than this. Thus, this is a very economical assay for aldosterone.

Normal Range

Twenty-five 24-h urines for which a normal 17-hydroxycorticosteroid value had been obtained were assayed for aldosterone by this method. They ranged from 0 to 22 μg/24 h, with a mean of 11.1 μg/24 h and a standard deviation of 6.8 μg/24 h. A statistical normal range of 0–25 μg/24 h therefore was accepted for patients whose diets and activity are not being controlled.

I thank Trini Addis for assaying the normal specimens and the patients' specimens and Dr. Dale Nabb for allowing ample time from regular duties for development of this method.

References

1. Drewes, P. A., Demetriou, J. A., and Pilegg,, V. J., Measurement of urinary aldosterone by a simplified radioimmunoassay procedure. *Clin. Biochem.* **6,** 88 (1973).

2. Farmer, R. W., Roup, W. G., Jr., Pellizzari, E. D., and Fabre, L. F., Jr., A rapid aldosterone radioimmunoassay. *J. Clin. Endocrinol. Metab.* **34,** 18 (1972).

3. Jowett, T. P., Slater, J. D. H., Piyasena, R. D., and Ekins, R. P., Radioimmunoassay of aldosterone in plasma and urine: Validation of a novel separation technique and a rapid urine assay. *Clin. Sci. Mol. Med.* **45,** 607 (1973).

4. Stuart, J., Keane, P. M., Viol, G., and Gupta, R. N., A rapid method for the radioimmunoassay of urinary aldosterone. *Clin. Biochem.* **6,** 285 (1973).

5. Cope, C. L., and Loizou, S., Simplification of urinary aldosterone measurement by radioimmunoassay. *J. Clin. Pathol.* **26,** 628 (1973).

6. Clark, B. R., and Rubin, R. T., New fluorometric method for the determination of cortisol in serum. *Anal. Biochem.* **29,** 31 (1969).

7. Allen, W. M., Hayward, S. J., and Pinto, A., A color test for dehydroisoandrosterone and closely related steroids, of use in the diagnosis of adrenocortical tumors. *J. Clin. Endocrinol. Metab.* **10,** 54 (1950).

8. Henry, R. J., *Clinical Chemistry: Principles and Techniques,* 2nd ed., Harper and Row, Hagerstown, Md., 1974, p 1433.

CLIN. CHEM. 22/3, 372–374 (1976)

Glucose Oxidase Chemiluminescence Measurement of Glucose in Urine Compared with the Hexokinase Method

David C. Williams,[1] Glenn F. Huff, and W. Rudolf Seitz

This method is more sensitive and specific than an enzymatic (hexokinase) technique with which it was compared, has a greater range of linearity, and presents no problems of background correction.

Because of the presence of other reducing substances in urine (primarily uric acid), it is difficult to quantitate the glucose in urine. These reducing substances interfere with nonenzymatic methods for glucose, making them unsuitable for quantitation of glucose in urine samples. The hexokinase (EC 2.7.1.1) method requires that three measurements of absorbance be made because there is a significant absorbance by both the reagents and the sample (*1*). Bostick and Hercules reported a chemiluminescent (CL) method for glucose in blood, but they were unable to apply the method to urine samples because uric acid interfered by reducing the peroxide (*2–4*). We have developed and evaluated a method for removing the interferences from urine by using the Somogyi precipitate obtained by adding equimolar portions of $Ba(OH)_2$ and $ZnSO_4$. The centrifugate from the above mixture reportedly is free of reducing substances other than glucose (*5*).

Materials and Methods

Instrumentation

The apparatus we used was very similar to that reported by Bostick and Hercules (*2–4*). An infusion pump drives three flow lines containing 10^{-2} mol/liter $K_3Fe(CN)_6$, 2×10^{-4} mol/liter luminol in 0.1 mol/liter KOH/H_3BO_3 buffer, and 10^{-3} mol/liter pH 5.6 acetate buffer, respectively. The ferricyanide and luminol are mixed before they enter the CL cell. The acetate line flows over a column of immobilized glucose oxidase before entering the CL cell. A sampling valve is used to introduce the glucose sample to the acetate flow line. As the glucose passes over the enzyme column it is converted to H_2O_2, which then mixes directly with the $Fe(CN)_6^{-3}$/luminol in the CL cell. The CL cell is positioned directly in front of a photomultiplier that measures CL intensity. For more detail, see reference *2*.

One major change from the previous study was to use glucose oxidase (EC 1.1.3.4) immobilized on porous glass rather than on the Sepharose support used in the previous study. The glass (CPG-10-500, 200–400 mesh; Electro-Nucleonics, Inc., Fairfield, N. J. 07006) was aminated by the procedure of Robinson et al. (*6*). The aminated glass was then coupled to the enzyme by a standard procedure for azo linkage (*7*). This change substantially reduced the back pressure of the enzyme column, making it possible to use a Model 975 infusion pump (Harvard Apparatus Co., Inc., Millis, Mass. 02054) to drive the flow system rather than the more powerful pump required in the previous study. Sensitivity and linear range were not affected by changing the enzyme support.

Procedures

To remove the interfering substances from urine, we added 1 ml of 0.1 mol/liter $Ba(OH)_2$ and 1 ml of 0.1 mol/liter $ZnSO_4$ to 0.1 ml of urine. A 0.25 ml aliquot of the centrifugate from this solution was diluted with 4.0 ml of the acetate buffer (*8*). One milliliter of the diluted sample was then aspirated into the sample loop of the CL flow system.

Hexokinase kits (cat. No. UV15-10; Sigma Chemical Co., St. Louis, Mo. 63178) were used in a correlation study. The reagent was diluted according to the manufacturer's directions. A 3.0-ml aliquot of the reagent was used to determine reagent blank absorbance at 340 nm. The urine blank absorbance was determined by diluting 0.1 ml of urine with 3.0 ml of NaCl solution (8.5 g/liter). The absorbance of the reaction mixture was determined after about 10 min of incubation, and the glucose concentration was determined from standard curves.

For the correlation study, 100 μl of each urine sample was added to three different test tubes: one containing the hexokinase reagent, another containing NaCl solution, and a third in which the precipitation was done for the CL

Department of Chemistry, University of Georgia, Athens, Georgia 30602.

[1] Present address: Hartford Hospital, Hartford, Conn. 06119.

Received Feb. 17, 1975; accepted Dec. 5, 1975.

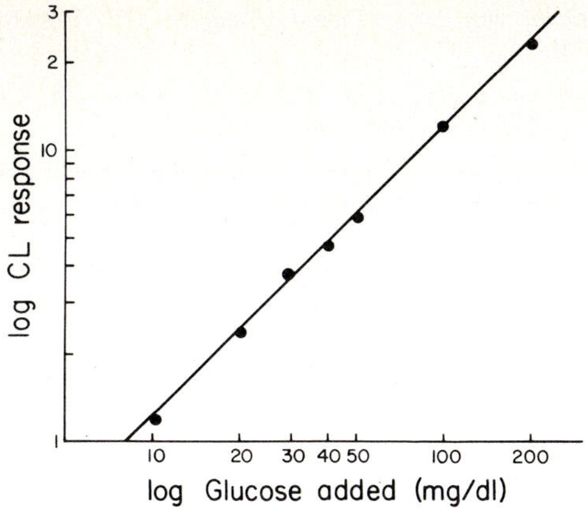

Fig. 1. Log of chemiluminescence intensity as a function of log of concentration of added glucose

Table 1. Glucose Recovery Study

Added	Determined	Recovery, %
mg/liter		
—	78	—
—	78	—
50	130	104
50	130	104
100	178	100
100	178	100
500	550	94
500	570	98
1000	1080	100
1000	1120	104
	av	100.5 ± 3.3%

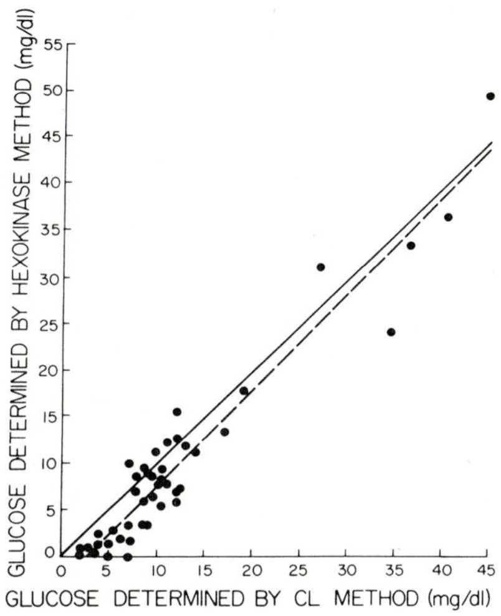

Fig. 2. Glucose determined by the chemiluminescent (*CL*) method vs. glucose determined by hexokinase method

Concentrations indicated are those in the original sample. Perfect correlation is indicated by the *solid* line, for comparison with the *broken line* obtained by linear regression analysis (*10*) of these data

method. Absorbances were measured with a Bausch & Lomb Spectronic 88, with use of 1-cm square quartz cuvettes.

Standards were prepared by diluting aqueous standard (1 g/liter) obtained from Sigma. The standards were then treated as the samples. In the correlation study all glucose concentrations were determined from standard curves, which eliminates the need for the bandpass correction in the hexokinase method (*1*).

Results and Discussion

To show that the precipitation technique removes the interfering substances, we prepared aqueous samples containing, per deciliter, 0, 8, 16, 24, 32, and 40 mg of potassium urate and 2.5 mg of glucose. After precipitation and dilution as described, the resulting solutions were free of any interference from the uric acid; each of the samples caused identical CL response.

Figure 1 relates CL intensity and glucose concentration for added glucose in a 24-h urine specimen that was itself glucose-free as judged by dipstick test. These analyses were performed after adding the appropriate amounts of glucose to 2.0-ml samples of urine. After precipitation and dilution, the samples were introduced into the flow system and analyzed.

Further to check the performance of the precipitation procedure, we made a recovery study. For this study pooled urine was obtained from a local hospital. The amounts of glucose added and found are shown in Table 1. The average recovery (100.5 ± 3.3%) is an improvement over the recoveries reported for the hexokinase method (109.4 ± 7.3%) (*8*).

A correlation study was next performed to show the relation between glucose values obtained with the CL method and the hexokinase method. For this study we used 45 urine samples obtained from the university's infirmary. Because the population from which the samples were obtained was expected to have normal urinary glucose values, samples selected without conscious bias had glucose added and their glucose concentrations were determined by the two methods (Figure 2). The slope of the correlation line is 1.05, the hexokinase intercept −3.0, and the correlation coefficient 0.96 (*10*). Clearly, results by the two methods correlate, but a paired t-test indicates that the hexokinase method gives consistently lower glucose values than does the CL method (*10*). We attribute this to the blank corrections in the hexokinase method, which are greater than the change of absorbance observed for the low concentrations of glucose found in most urines. Errors in determining the blanks, which might easily occur with cloudy samples, are believed to be responsible for the lower concentration determined by the hexokinase method. We did encounter samples that gave a negative net change of absorbance with the hexokinase method (i.e., an apparent glucose concentration of less than zero), a fact that supports the hypothesis that at low concentrations, at least, there is a systematic error in the hexokinase method. Further investigation with hospital-patient urine specimens is necessary in order to verify the usefulness of the method in a clinical setting.

This work was supported in part by funds provided to the University of Georgia by NIH Research Grant No. 17913-01. G. F. H. was supported by NSF Grant No. EPP-750-4665.

References

1. Sigma Technical Bulletin, No. 15-UV: The quantitative enzymatic determination of glucose in serum, plasma, cerebrospinal fluid or urine at 340 nm. Sigma Chemical Co., St. Louis, Mo., 1974.

2. Bostick, D. T., Enzyme induced chemiluminescence determination of blood glucose using luminol. Thesis, University of Georgia, Athens, Ga., 1974.

3. Bostick, D. T., and Hercules, D. M., The quantitative determination of blood glucose using enzyme induced chemiluminescence of luminol. *Anal. Chem.* **47,** 447 (1975).

4. Bostick, D. T., and Hercules, D. M., Enzyme induced chemiluminescence-determination of blood glucose using luminol. *Anal. Lett.* **7,** 347 (1974).

5. Levinson, S. A, and Mac Fate, R. P., *Clinical Laboratory Diagnosis,* 7th ed., Lea and Febiger, Philadelphia, Pa., 1969, p 359.

6. Robinson, P. J., Dunnill, P., and Lilly, M. D., Porous glass as a solid support for immobilization or affinity chromatography of enzymes. *Biochim. Biophys. Acta* **242,** 659 (1971).

7. *Biomaterial Supports,* Pierce Chemical Co., Rockford, Ill. 61105 (1973).

8. *Handbook of Biochemistry,* 2nd ed., H. Sober, Ed., Chemical Rubber Co., Cleveland, Ohio., 1966, p J234.

9. Peterson, J. I., and Young, D. S., Evaluation of the hexokinase/glucose-6-phosphate dehydrogenase method of determination of glucose in urine. *Anal. Biochem.* **23,** 301 (1968).

10. Natrella, M. G., *Experimental Statistics,* N. B. S. Handbook 91, U.S. Government Printing Office, Washington, D.C., 1966, pp 5–10.

CLIN. CHEM. 22/3, 374–378 (1976)

Evaluation of Contemporary Methods for Serum CO_2

Jack A. Lustgarten, Ronald J. Creno, Charles G. Byrd, and Robert E. Wenk

We evaluated and inter-compared several newer methods for CO_2 analysis—titrimetric (Van Slyke), automatic titrator, continuous-flow/indicator, and coupled-enzyme procedures—with respect to accuracy, precision, specificity, interferences, and management criteria. All methods studied appeared to be clinically acceptable; but precision decreased (standard deviations increased) for the last two methods in above-normal ranges.

Additional Keyphrases: *carbon dioxide content, bicarbonate, and total CO_2 • titrimetry • continuous-flow analysis • enzymatic analysis • analysis of variance*

Reliable measurements for total CO_2 in serum (*1*) were developed years ago (*2*), and many laboratories still use these classical titrimetric, volumetric, or manometric methods successfully. In general, cumbersome equipment has yielded to microgasometric analyzers, semiautomatic and automatic titrators that incorporate either glass electrodes or photodetectors, but these devices require constant operator attention and analyses are relatively slow. Faster systems are required in laboratories with high volume; continuous-flow analysis of CO_2 content is one of the most commonly used procedures.

Here, we compare several contemporary methods and comment on their relative merits in our laboratory.

Methods

We directly compared four methods that are or will be used in many laboratories:

Automatic photometric titrimetry (Stat/Ion; Technicon Instruments Corp., Tarrytown, N.Y. 10591). In this method, serum bicarbonate (not dissolved CO_2, H_2CO_3, or carbamino compounds) is measured by Van Slyke's principle, in which excess acid (in fixed volume and concentration) is used to drive off CO_2 gas. Excess acid is back-titrated by coulometric generation of hydroxyl ions to a change in indicator color (phenol red) at pH 7.55. Bicarbonate concentration is proportional to titration time × current.

Coupled enzymatic method (Automatic Clinical Analyzer, *aca;* Du Pont Instrument Products, Wilmington, Del. 19898). In this method, serum is made alkaline to convert gaseous and acid forms of CO_2 to bicarbonate and carbonate. Phospho*enol*pyruvate, catalyzed by phospho*enol*pyruvate carboxylase (EC 4.1.1.31) in the presence of Mg^{2+}, yields oxalacetate and inorganic phosphate. Oxalacetate + NADH is catalyzed in acid medium by malate dehydrogenase (EC 1.1.1.37) to yield NAD^+ and malate. The decrease in absorbance of NADH at 340 nm is proportional to CO_2 concentration.

Continuous-flow analysis (Technicon, method N-8b I/II). In this method, CO_2 gas is released into alkaline phenolphthalein. The resulting decrease in pH decreases the red indicator color in proportion to CO_2 content.

Manual titration (Oxford Laboratories, Foster City, Calif. 94904). An Oxford Titrator is used to titrate to a visual endpoint, according to the procedure of Van Slyke (*2*) as modified by Oxford Laboratories.

Results

Comparisons with Patients' Specimens

Serum total CO_2 and bicarbonate concentrations were determined by the four methods in 60 serum specimens collected without conscious bias on several different occasions from various clinical services. The specimens were analyzed and the results from low, normal, and elevated CO_2 and bicarbonate ranges were compared statistically by an analysis of variance (*3*) and several regression analyses (*3, 4*). Analysis of variance (Table 1) indicated that variability of the error among the methods is greater than variability of the random error. The *F* value was calculated and judged to be significant. Scattergrams are illustrated in Figure 1 and regression data is shown in Table 2. Where the regression data for slope are compared with the slope data from Table 3, it can be seen that they are similar in magnitude and direction.

Department of Pathology, Sinai Hospital, Baltimore, Md. 21215.
Address reprints to R.E.W.
Received Nov. 5, 1975; accepted Dec. 5, 1975.

Table 1. Analysis of Variance for Bicarbonate and Carbon Dioxide Method

Source of error	Sum of squares	Degrees of freedom	Mean squares	*Fa*
Between-individuals	15625.730	59	264.843	127.588
Between-methods	156.540	3	52.180	25.138
Residual	367.412	177	2.076	—
Total	16149.682	239	67.572	—

[a] *F* value, critical value of *F* at the 1% level of probability is 3.78. The methods are behaving differently ($P < .01$) when compared to the random error pooled within the methods.

Table 2. Comparison of Bicarbonate and CO_2 in Patients' Specimens[a]

Methods compared *X vs. Y*	Slope	Intercept	*r*	SE of estimate
AutoAnalyzer vs. Stat/Ion	1.026	−1.15	0.975	0.932
AutoAnalyzer vs. Oxford	0.947	2.941	0.971	1.883
AutoAnalyzer vs. *aca*	0.937	1.617	0.969	1.962

[a] Regression data are calculated by the least-squares method.

Table 3. Statistics for Comparative Analysis of Primary Aqueous Bicarbonate Standards (10–35 mmol/liter)

	Method			
	Stat/Ion	AutoAnalyzer	*aca*	Titrator
Slope	0.9249	0.9457	1.009	0.9560
Intercept	1.561	−0.6808	−0.83550	0.5757
Corr. coeff., *r*	0.999	0.999	0.998	0.997
SE of estimate	0.2965	0.3758	0.4344	0.6490

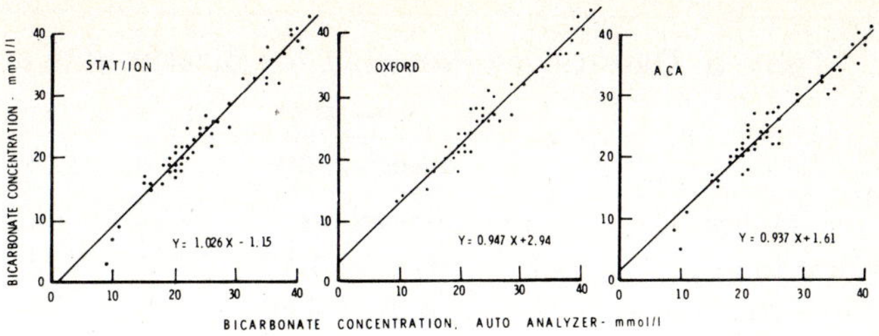

Fig. 1. Serum bicarbonate determinations by continuous-flow analysis compared with three other methods

Representative patients' specimens in low, normal, and high clinical range were analyzed by all four methods, and the regression line calculated by the method of least squares

Analytical Variables

Recovery studies. Mixtures of freshly reconstituted lyophilized control materials (Monitrol, from Dade Division, American Hospital Supply Corp., Miami, Fla. 33152; and Versatol, from Warner-Chilcott Laboratories, Morris Plains, N.J. 07950) were prepared to yield concentrations of bicarbonate between 9 and 48 mmol/liter. The mixtures were analyzed in triplicate by the test methods and results were compared with the expected values. To assure ourselves that the reconstituted sera actually contained a manufacturer's stated amount, we calibrated our instruments with freshly prepared primary standards, analyzed the water or diluent buffer used to reconstitute the control sera, and then analyzed the reconstituted material itself. Values averaged 96% of stated values for the manufacturer's serum controls. Recovery studies are summarized in Table 4. Three of the four methods showed low recovery values at low bicarbonate concentrations. Analytical recovery was poorest in the case of the manual procedure.

Linearity. A stock primary aqueous bicarbonate standard was diluted with water to yield solutions with concentrations ranging from 15 to 35 mmol/liter. Each method was calibrated according to the manufacturer's suggested procedures by using standards supplied with the method. The primary standard solutions were analyzed and the measured bicarbonate concentrations were plotted vs. the theoretical bicarbonate concentrations, and intercepts, slopes, and standard errors of estimate of the lines were tabulated.

All methods appeared to be linear between 15 and 35 mmol HCO_3^- per liter, in the measurement of both aqueous solutions and protein-based materials. A comparison of slope and intercept data (Table 3) indicates that the Stat/Ion performed differently in both magnitude and direction from the other three methods. The data also indicate that

Table 4. Comparison of Analytical Recoveries of Bicarbonate and CO_2 in Mixtures of Different Commercial Control Sera[a]

	Recovery, %							
	Stat/Ion		AutoAnalyzer		*aca*		Titrator	
HCO_3^- concn, mmol/liter	Mean	± Range	Mean	± Range	Mean	± Range	Mean	± Range
12.5	109.6	0.0	94.9	5.0	96.4	11.9	88.5	13.3
16.2	96.3	0.6	98.3	3.5	101.8	3.0	90.2	6.7
20.4	96.8	1.5	97.8	0.0	104.6	6.9	94.4	0.0
26.0	103.6	1.5	99.3	0.0	100.3	1.6	95.9	3.2
30.0	102.7	0.8	101.1	0.0	98.5	2.8	94.5	3.1

[a] All experiments done in triplicate.

Table 5. Day-to-Day Precision for Bicarbonate and CO_2 in Control Sera of Various Clinical Ranges[a]

	Low range				Normal range				High range			
		Mean	SD			Mean	SD			Mean	SD	
Method	n	(mmol/liter)		CV, %	n	(mmol/liter)		CV, %	n	(mmol/liter)		CV, %
Stat/Ion	23	16.1	1.43	8.8	22	26.4	1.31	4.9	22	34.9	1.44	4.1
AutoAnalyzer	21	16.0	0.86	5.4	21	24.9	1.14	4.6	21	34.9	1.33	3.8
aca		—	—		21	25.3	1.45	5.7	20	43.4	1.80	4.1
Oxford		—	—		32	26.2	1.43	5.5	30	41.1	0.88	2.2

[a] Identical control pools were used for Stat/Ion and AutoAnalyzer, different identical pools for *aca* and Titrator.

Table 6. Effect on Bicarbonate Results of Various Chemical Abnormalities of Serum

	Apparent bicarbonate concn, mmol/liter			
Constituent, concn	AutoAnalyzer	Stat/Ion	*aca*	Titration
Glucose				
3180, mg/liter	29	33	34	32
4580, mg/liter	24	25	29	26
3320, mg/liter	26	28	30	27
Hemolysis				
slight	23	29	28	25
moderate	16	19	19	17
gross	18	22	25	22
Lipemia				
slight	19	22	22	25
moderate	23	25	27	22
gross	19	18	22	20
BUN				
1010 mg/liter	8	6	7	5
1560, mg/liter	15	15	—	—
BSP				
40% retention	20	23	24	21
35% retention	23	25	28	23
40% retention	25	26	—	—
Total bilirubin				
330, mg/liter	19	20	22	21
200, mg/liter	23	22	—	—
Direct 113 mg/liter				
Lactate dehydrogenase, 3400 U/liter	23	25	—	—
Alk. phosphatase, 436 U/liter	27	29	—	—
BUN 2930 mg/liter, creatinine 168 mg/liter	8	7	—	—

there were constant systematic differences among the methods.

Precision. Day-to-day precision, expressed as coefficient of variation, was calculated from daily analytical values obtained for reconstituted, lyophilized control sera (low, intermediate, and high clinical ranges).

The precision in terms of standard deviation for the Stat/Ion is acceptable and nearly constant in all ranges of bicarbonate concentrations. However, the precision of the AutoAnalyzer and *aca* worsened with increasing CO_2 content. The precision of the Oxford method improved as the bicarbonate concentration of serum increased (Table 5). Long-term evaluation of the several methods tended to corroborate the data shown.

Interference and specificity studies. During several months we collected serum from several hundred patients with increased glucose, urea, bilirubin, or lipids, and hemolyzed sera. The sera were analyzed by at least two of the four methods (about 100 by all four), as we looked for possible interference. Sera from patients admitted without gross abnormality were run simultaneously to detect more subtle interferences and method biases. We saw no system-

Table 7. Convenience Features or Practical Aspects of HCO_3-Methods

Feature/Condition	Stat/Ion	AutoAnalyzer	Du Pont *aca*	Titration
Start-up, min				
1. From cold	27	60	Immediate (standby)	20
2. During run	6	12	8	5
3. For emergency	1	7	8	2
Samples/hour (unknowns, not standards)	48	60	53	30
Serum sample volume, μl	100 μl	104 μl	20 μl	50 μl
Reagent				
1. Volume consumed, ml/test	4.5	7.9	prepackaged	0.9
2. Preparation time	purchased, add surfactant 5 min	20 min/day	none	purchased
Costs				
1. Reagents	inexpensive	inexpensive	$1.48/test	inexpensive
2. Instrument	$16 000 to $19 900	$15 000	$75 000	$265 + $46/ pkg of 600 cups & solution
3. Personnel time/100 tests (min)	45	120	50	250
Downtime, scheduled				
1. Preventive maintenance	30 min/w rotate Na^+ electrode	1/2 h/w	seldom	little or none
Downtime, unscheduled	10%	1%	rare	—
1. Common problems	printer, reagent deterioration, electronic, mechanical,	aspiration of acid into trap, dialyzer		broken tips bad reagents controls
2. Trouble shooting	simple	simple or complex	simple or complex	simple
Operation	simple	simple to more complex	simple	simple
Shutdown time	press off	wash 20 min	none	none
Calibration				
1. linearity	manual	standard curve required	set when new lot numbers arrive	manual
2. calibration	automatic			manual

atic error that could be attributed to variables such as hemolysis, lipemia, uremia, hyperglycemia, or jaundice in any of the methods (Table 6). Protein affected three methods (Stat/Ion, *aca,* AutoAnalyzer); each gram of protein per deciliter decreased apparent bicarbonate by 0.6 mmol/liter. In the Oxford method (Figure 2), by comparison, for each gram of protein increase per deciliter there was an increase in apparent bicarbonate of 0.4 mmol/liter.

Convenience features. The widespread demand for high-volume and emergency analyses for bicarbonate prompted us to compare criteria of management such as start-up time, samples per unit time, sample requirements, reagent preparation, costs, maintenance, and operator involvement. These data appear in Table 7.

Discussion

The differences among the methods do not seriously detract from their clinical usefulness.

The Stat/Ion method (Tables 3 and 2) apparently responds differently from other procedures; the effect of protein on the measurement of total CO_2 and bicarbonate needs to be investigated further. Mechanized equipment offers many advantages and convenience, but its complexity makes it subject to breakdown. In our experience, downtime for the Stat/Ion bicarbonate method has been inordinate and completely unacceptable in its present state; with the two instruments in our laboratory, problems relating to chemical (deteriorated reagents), electronic, and mechani-

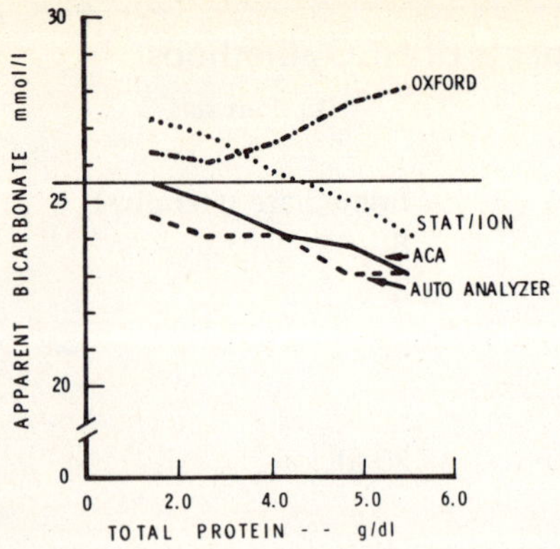

Fig. 2. Effect of protein concentration on the various bicarbonate methods

The mean bicarbonate value of a serum pool was established by analysis in triplicate. A primary bicarbonate standard was prepared at the mean serum pool concentration value and was used as a diluent for the serum pool, thereby altering the protein concentration while maintaining the bicarbonate value at a fixed value

cal functions have all been observed. We believe, however, that with proper instruction and training from the vendor, downtime could be decreased considerably. The Stat/Ion makes use of an automated version of the classical Van Slyke titrimetric method, with two important advances: a precise dual-wavelength log-ratio photometer provides for a more reproducible end-point and minimizes interference from various pigments, and coulometric generation of hydroxyl ions yields a more reliable titration and obviates the need to prepare standard (and unstable) alkali.

With the titration method, one determines only HCO_3^-; therefore, as the manufacturer says (*5*), the method is not subject to loss of CO_2 in sample because of improper storage or handling. Thus the colorimetric endpoint has been set at a color corresponding to pH 7.55 (which is equivalent to pH 7.4 at 37 °C). Because the amount of OH^- generated is inversely related to the HCO_3^- concentration, the lower the pH at which the titration is terminated (i.e., the less OH^- generated), the higher the HCO_3^- value obtained. This in effect, is a blanket correction factor for the possible loss from serum of any CO_2 (and HCO_3^-) that might have occurred upon standing.

On the other hand, a fixed endpoint corresponding to pH 7.4 would tend to result in an overestimation of HCO_3^- in alkalotic patients, and an underestimation of HCO_3^- in acidotic patients.

The effect of protein on the HCO_3^- concentration determined by Stat/Ion and Oxford titration methods was noted to be opposite in effect, which might reflect differences in the reactivity of the various reagents with serum proteins.

We gratefully acknowledge the technical assistance of Barbara Hall, B.S., and the statistical assistance of John Kennedy, M.S.

References

1. Bittner, D. L., and Hall, S. G., The titration of bicarbonate in plasma: Clinical factors. *Am. J. Clin. Pathol.* **42,** 522 (1964).

2. Van Slyke, D. D., Studies of acidosis: Determination of bicarbonate concentration of blood and plasma. *J. Biol. Chem.* **52,** 495 (1922).

3. Steel, R. G., and Torie, J. H., *Principles and Procedures of Statistics.* McGraw Hill, New York, N.Y., 1960, pp 99–106, 171, 173, and 179.

4. Westgard, J. O., and Hunt, M. R., Use and interpretation of common statistical tests in method-comparison studies. *Clin. Chem.* **19,** 49 (1973).

5. Method Number SK-4-000 2 P L 4, Technicon Instruments Corp., Tarrytown, N.Y. 10591.

CLIN. CHEM. 22/3, 379–380 (1976)

Modified Colorimetric Method for Procainamide in Plasma

Daniel S. Sitar,[1,3,4,5] Donald N. Graham,[1] Robert E. Rangno,[1,3,4] Louis R. Dusfresne,[2,3] and Richard I. Ogilvie[1,3,4]

We describe a modified colorimetric method for determining procainamide in plasma by use of a diazotization and coupling reaction with *N*-(1-naphthyl)-ethylenediamine dihydrochloride (Marshall's reagent). The sensitivity of the assay is increased twofold over the originally reported colorimetric method, and the lower limit of detection for the assay of a 1.0-ml plasma sample has been decreased to 0.5 mg/liter.

The original colorimetric assay for plasma procainamide, which utilized a diazotization step in the production of a colored product for spectrophotometric analysis (*1*), is characterized only between 5 and 40 mg/liter (*2*). In our hands, the assay as originally described gave highly variable results below 5 mg of procainamide per liter. A fluorometric assay for this drug is not specific, in that *N*-acetylprocainamide, a metabolite of the drug, interferes in the analysis (*3*). Significant concentrations of *N*-acetylprocainamide in plasma can result after doses of procainamide to man (*4, 5*). The reproducibility or precision of the fluorometric method is not indicated. However, a recently reported fluorometric method for both procainamide and its *N*-acetyl metabolite appears to have overcome these difficulties (*6*). A gas–liquid chromatographic method has also been reported for procainamide (*7*), but we encountered inadequate reproducibility of this method at concentrations in plasma of less than 4 mg/liter.

We have modified the colorimetric method of Mark et al. (*2*) to develop an assay for procainamide that can be used to investigate the disposition of this drug in patients with chronic renal failure, as it has been recently demonstrated that good agreement exists between the colorimetric and gas–liquid chromatographic methods for determination of this drug (*8*). Here, we report the results of this modified assay, and compare them with results by the original colorimetric method (*2*).

Divisions of Clinical Pharmacology[1] and Nephrology,[2] Montreal General Hospital; and Departments of Medicine[3] and Pharmacology and Therapeutics,[4] McGill University, Montreal, Quebec, H3G 1A4, Canada.

[5] Monat Scholar, McGill University.

Address correspondence to: D. S. S. at the Clinical Pharmacology Division, Montreal General Hospital, Montreal, Quebec H3G 1A4 Canada.

Received Mar. 24, 1975; accepted Dec. 12, 1975.

Materials and Methods

Reagents. Procainamide hydrochloride was supplied by E. R. Squibb and Sons Ltd., Montreal, P.Q. *N*-Acetylprocainamide hydrochloride was supplied by Dr. D. Drayer (Temple University, Philadelphia, Pa.). Both chemicals were used as received. Hydrochloric acid ("Baker Analyzed Reagent") was obtained from Canadian Laboratory Supplies Ltd., Montreal, P.Q. Sodium nitrite, sodium hydroxide, and sodium chloride ("Analar" grade) were obtained from British Drug Houses Ltd., Montreal, P.Q. Ammonium sulfamate ("Certified") and *N*-(1-napthyl)-ethylenediamine dihydrochloride (Marshall's reagent; N-30) were obtained from Fisher Scientific Co., Montreal, P.Q. All chemicals were dissolved in doubly distilled water.

Solutions. Hydrochloric acid (1 mol/liter), sodium hydroxide (5 mol/liter), sodium nitrite (1 g/liter), ammonium sulfamate (5 g/liter), and Marshall's reagent were stored in glass containers at 2–4 °C until used. Procainamide hydrochloride (5.77 g/liter) was dissolved in distilled water to give a stock solution of 5 g/liter with respect to procainamide. The nitrite and sulfamate solutions were stable for at least two weeks. All other solutions were stable for at least one month. Prepared plasma standards kept frozen at −20 °C were stable for at least three months.

Procainamide assay. Pipette 1.0 ml of plasma into a 12-ml test tube containing 0.25 g of sodium chloride, 0.2 ml of sodium hydroxide, and 0.5 ml of water. Stir the contents on a vortex-type mixer. Pipette 10 ml of dichloromethane into the tube. Cap the tube and shake it for 20 min. Centrifuge the tube (10 min, 1000 × *g*), remove 8.0 ml of the organic (lower) layer, and evaporate it at 40 °C under a stream of nitrogen (we used a Brinkman SC/48 Sample Concentrator; Brinkman Instruments Canada Ltd., Toronto, Ont.). Place the containers in an ice bath, add 2.0 ml of hydrochloric acid, mix the contents with a vortex-type mixer, and return the container to the ice bath for 10 min. Add 1.0 ml of the ammonium sulfamate solution, mix, and add 1.0 ml of Marshall's reagent. Remove the sample from the ice bath, stir, and allow to stand at room temperature for 15 min. Determine the absorbance of the solution vs. a plasma blank at 550 nm.

Calibration curve. Pipette procainamide standard solution into a known volume of plasma to give a solution that contains 25 mg of procainamide per liter. Use this plasma standard to prepare other plasma standards that contain

Table 1. Comparison of the Colorimetric Assay for Procainamide Reported Herein with the Method of Mark et al.[a]

	Mark et al.	Sitar et al.
Extraction efficiency	98 ± 2%	101 ± 1%
Aliquot for dye coupling	56%	80%
Plasma volume extracted, ml	1.5	1.0
Slope of regression for standard curve	0.0172 ± 0.0026	0.0345 ± 0.0009
Intercept	−0.0003 ± 0.0002	−0.0017 ± 0.0008

[a] The comparison is made for concentrations of 0.5 to 25 mg of procainamide per liter of plasma. ± values represent ± SE.

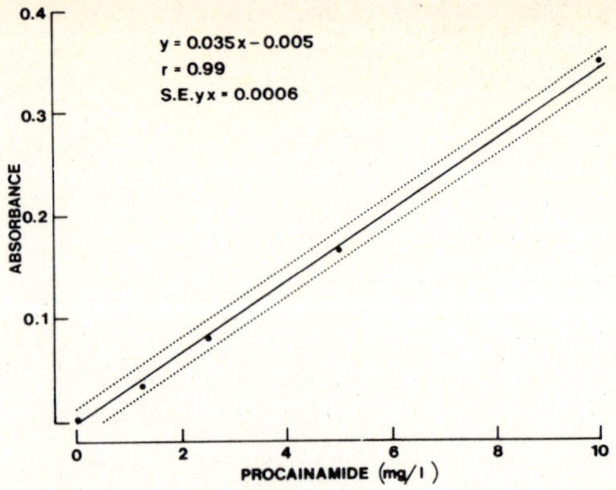

Fig. 1. Representative calibration curve for the analysis of procainamide in plasma samples

Each point represents the mean of duplicate determinations. The *dotted lines* represent the 95% confidence interval for the determinations

from 0.5 to 25 mg procainamide per liter. Analyze these standards in duplicate as described above.

Statistics. The calibration-curve data were analyzed by a least-squares regression method. This regression analysis was then subjected to analysis of variance, and the 95% confidence limits were determined (*9*).

Results and Discussion

Figure 1 shows a representative calibration curve, with its 95% confidence limits, derived from data generated by the method just described. Although the curve represents only concentrations to 10 mg/liter procainamide, the slope and accuracy are the same from 0.5 to 25 mg/liter (Table 1). Repetition of this assay on 10 separate days between the concentrations of 0.5 to 25 mg of procainamide per liter gave a slope of 0.0343 ± 0.0006 (mean ± SE). Repetitive analysis of a 5 mg/liter standard resulted in a mean (± SE) concentration of 4.97 ± 0.07 mg/liter for procainamide (n = 10). These determinations were made over a six-month period.

Although mean values are indicated for each concentration in Figure 1, all values were used in the determination of variance and calculation of confidence limits. The analysis indicated a significant regression with insignificant variation owing to multiple determinations for any given drug concentration. Therapeutic concentrations of lidocaine, digoxin, hydrochlorothiazide, triamterene, furosemide, or warfarin in plasma do not interfere. Whole blood, plasma, or erythrocytes from the blood bank gave no absorbance at 550 nm; i.e., we have found no interference with this assay attributable to storage of blood samples or to endogenous components of blood. However, one must bear in mind that Marshall's reagent can react with other primary aromatic amines that might be present, such as sulfonamides. We have not encountered such problems commonly. Added *N*-acetylprocainamide did not alter results for procainamide in plasma by this method. Hemolyzed or lipemic samples did not interfere with the assay. Either plasma, packed erythrocytes, or whole blood could be used as the sample; all give similar values. The least variance was encountered with plasma samples.

Table 1 compares our assay and that of Mark et al. (*2*). Analytical recovery is quantitative for both methods, but variance is less and sensitivity greater by the modified procedure we report here.

One of the most important factors affecting consistency in this assay is temperature control (0–2 °C) during the diazotization procedure. Use of an ice bath to stabilize the diazo intermediate until the coupling dye is added is essential. It results in increased coupling owing to stabilization of the intermediate and also prevents hydrolysis of *N*-acetylprocainamide back to procainamide in the acid medium. The increased sensitivity of our method allows more accurate determinations of procainamide concentrations of less than 4 mg/liter; this is important for accurate investigation of the kinetic disposition of the drug after a therapeutic dose. The smaller blood sample required for these determinations in renal-failure patients is important. The assay requires less solvent for the extraction step, so there is a substantial cost-saving when many assays are required. We estimate that it is possible to derive a calibration curve and analyze more than 40 samples per day in duplicate by this method.

This investigation was supported by the Kidney Foundation of Canada and the Canadian Foundation for the Advancement of Therapeutics. We acknowledge the excellent technical assistance of Mr. D. Shaw and Mrs. M. Perry.

References

1. Bratton, A. C., and Marshall, E. K., Jr., A new coupling component for sulfanilamide determination. *J. Biol. Chem.* **128,** 537 (1939).

2. Mark, L. C., Kayden, H. J., Steele, J. M., et al., The physiological disposition and cardiac effects of procaine amide. *J. Pharmacol. Exp. Ther.* **102,** 5 (1951).

3. Koch-Weser, J., and Klein, S. W., Procainamide dosage schedules, plasma concentrations and clinical effects. *J. Am. Med. Assoc.* **215,** 1454 (1971).

4. Giardina, E-G. V., Dreyfuss, J., Bigger, J. T., Jr., and Schreiber, E. C., *N*-Acetyl procaine amide after procaine amide^{14}C treatment. *Circulation* **49–50,** *Suppl. 3,* 899 (1974).

5. Karlsson, E., Molin, L., Norlander, B., and Sjoqvist, F., Acetylation of procaine amide in man studied with a new gas chromatographic method. *Br. J. Clin. Pharmacol.* **1,** 467 (1974).

6. Matusik, E., and Gibson, T. P., Fluorometric assay for *N*-acetylprocainamide. *Clin. Chem.* **21,** 1899 (1975).

7. Atkinson, A. J., Jr., Parker, M., and Strong, J., Rapid gas chromatographic measurement of plasma procainamide concentration. *Clin. Chem.* **18,** 643 (1972).

8. Sterling, J., Cox, S., and Haney, W. G., Comparison of procainamide analyses in plasma by spectrophotofluorometry, colorimetry and GLC. *J. Pharm. Sci.* **63,** 1744 (1974).

9. Goldstein, A., *Biostatistics: An Introductory Text,* Macmillan, New York, N.Y., 1964, p 63.

CLIN. CHEM. 22/3, 381-383 (1976)

Improved Method for Measuring Fibrinogen in Plasma, with Use of a Plasmin Inhibitor

Loren W. Steffen and Barbara W. Steffen

We describe a modified procedure for quantitating plasma fibrinogen by use of the thrombin-clottable protein technique. The method is accurate and requires about 30 min to complete. During its formation and isolation, the clot is protected from the degradative action of plasmin by an inhibitor, ε-aminocaproic acid.

Because a quantitative fibrinogen determination is frequently requested in an emergency situation, the ideal method is one that not only is accurate, but also rapid.

The procedure of Ware et al. (*1*) as presented by Henry (*2*) meets the first requirement but is too time consuming for emergency use. Furthermore, if the patient's fibrinolytic system has been activated, the clot formed in vitro would be degraded and a falsely low result obtained.

We have significantly modified the method of Henry (*2*). Like other authors (*3, 4*), we use ε-aminocaproic acid as a plasmin (EC 3.4.21.7) inhibitor. Time-saving steps have been introduced for dissolving the clot and quantitating the protein. The net result is a procedure that can be performed in about 30 min with no apparent loss of accuracy.

Materials and Methods

Instrumentation

All spectrophotometric readings were made with a Coleman, Jr. Spectrophotometer at 545 nm, with 19 × 150 mm cuvettes.

Reagents

The thrombin and biuret reagents have been described previously (*2*).

Clotting buffer. The directions given below should be followed exactly if precipitation of $Ca_3(PO_4)_2$ is to be avoided. With the aid of a magnetic stirrer, dissolve 0.91 g of KH_2PO_4 and 0.47 g of Na_2HPO_4 in about 850 ml of de-ionized water (phosphate concentration is 10 mmol/liter, pH 6.4). Dissolve 0.20 g of $CaCl_2$ in about 100 ml of de-ionized water. Reduce the speed of the stirrer to only that needed for adequate agitation and add the $CaCl_2$ solution. After about 30 s add 5.0 g of ε-aminocaproic acid (Sigma Chemical Co., St. Louis, Mo. 63178), 1.0 g of NaN_3, and 9.0 g of NaCl. Stir only long enough to dissolve the solid chemicals. If necessary, adjust the pH to 6.4 with dilute HCl or NaOH. Transfer, with rinsing, to a 1-liter volumetric flask and bring to volume. The reagent can be stored at room temperature and appears to be stable indefinitely.

Fibrinogen protein standard. This can be prepared by diluting the standard used for total protein determinations with saline (NaCl, 9.0 g/liter). A standard equivalent to a 3.0 g/liter fibrinogen concentration is considered ideal. Since 2.5 ml is used in the procedure, the stock protein standard is diluted to 1.20 g/liter. Stored at 4 °C, the solution is stable for at least six months.

Alkaline saline solution. Mix equal volumes of saline and a 60 g/liter NaOH solution.

Streptokinase solution, approximately 100 units/ml. A 10 000 unit "Varidase" oral tablet (Lederle Laboratories, Pearl River, N. Y. 10965) was ground up and mixed with 100 ml of saline. The mixture was allowed to stand at room temperature for about 2 h before use.

Fibrinogen reference plasma. "Q-Pack" Fibrinogen Reference Plasma, Human Dried, Hyland Laboratories, Costa Mesa, Calif. 92626.

Pooled plasma. Blood that had been drawn into 5-ml "Vacutainer" tubes containing tripotassium ethylenediaminetetraacetate (Becton, Dickinson, and Co., Rutherford, N. J. 07070) was centrifuged at 2100 × *g* for 10 min. The plasma was aspirated, pooled, and either used within 1 h or divided into aliquots and frozen at −20 °C.

Procedure

Plasma anticoagulated with oxalate, citrate, or ethylenediaminetetraacetate may be used (*2*).

While the blood is being centrifuged, add 30 ml of clotting buffer to the required number of 50-ml Ehrlenmeyer flasks. Pipet 1.0 ml of plasma (or 2.0 ml, if a low value is expected) into the appropriate flask and mix by swirling the flask. Add 0.20 ml of the thrombin reagent and mix throughly but gently. Allow the flask(s) to stand undisturbed for 15 min at room temperature.

During this time, warm about 3 ml of the protein standard to room temperature. Label 15-ml conical centrifuge tubes for the reagent blank, standard, control, and each patient. To the standard tube, add 2.5 ml of the protein standard and 2.5 ml of the 60 g/liter NaOH solution. Add 5.0 ml of the alkaline saline solution to the other tubes.

At the end of 15 min, the clots are isolated as follows. Tip the flask at about a 45 degree angle and lay a glass stirring rod onto the clot. Turn the rod slowly and move it down through the clot to wind the clot around it. Simultaneously, slowly decant the reaction solution into a 50-ml beaker. Decanting shortens the time required to wind the clot. Inspect the solution in the beaker to be certain that all the clot was isolated. Wash the glass rod and clot with a gentle stream of de-ionized water, and blot dry with a paper towel or filter paper. Insert the rod into the appropriate centrifuge tube.

St. Peter Hospital Laboratory, 413 N. Lilly Rd., Olympia, Wash. 98506.

Received Oct. 6, 1975; accepted Dec. 28, 1975.

Table 1. Inhibition of Fibrinolytic Activity by ε-Aminocaproic Acid

Reagents added	Fibrinogen concn,[a] g/liter
1. (*a*) 50 mg of ε-aminocaproic acid/liter	4.12
(*b*) 50 units of streptokinase[b]	
2. (*a*) No ε-aminocaproic acid	0
(*b*) 50 units of streptokinase	
3. (*a*) 50 mg of ε-aminocaproic acid/liter	4.03
(*b*) No streptokinase	

[a] Av of three determinations.
[b] Added to reaction solution before thrombin.

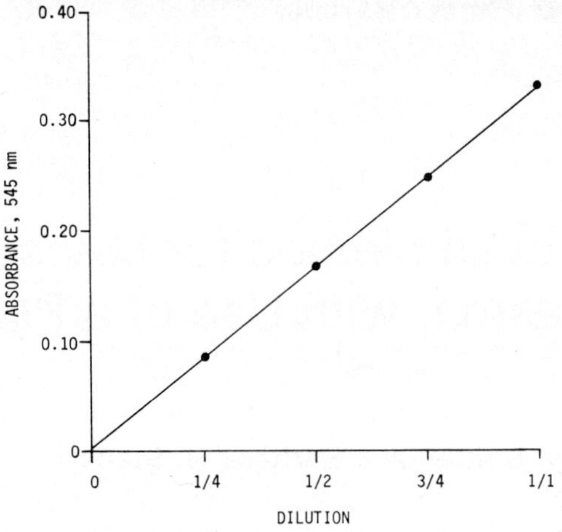

Fig. 1. Linearity of the procedure

When all the clots have been isolated, turn off the heat under a boiling water bath (this is essential, because superheating at the bottom of the tube results in turbid solutions of badly denatured protein) and place *all* the centrifuge tubes into the water bath. Rotate the glass rods a couple of times during a 5-min warming, then remove the tubes from the water bath. Carefully tilt the sample tubes so that the solution runs toward the mouth, and rotate the glass rod briefly. This ensures that all fibrin is removed from the rod. Touch the bottom of the rod against the top inside wall of the tube for a few seconds to minimize fluid loss. Remove the rod from the tube. Add 1.0 ml of the biuret reagent to all the tubes and mix on a vortex-type mixer. Pour the solutions into appropriately labeled 19 × 150 mm Coleman cuvettes. This step shortens cooling time. After 5 min, zero the instrument with the blank at 545 nm and record the absorbance (A) of the standard and test solutions. The fibrinogen concentration is calculated as follows:

$$\text{Concn (g/liter)} = \frac{A\ \text{(unknown)}}{A\ \text{(standard)}} \times \text{standard value (g/liter)}$$

If 2 ml of plasma were used, divide the final answer by 2.

Analytical Variables

Concentration of ε-aminocaproic acid. After reviewing the work cited in references (*3*) and (*4*), we arbitrarily decided to include 5 mg of ε-aminocaproic acid per milliliter of clotting buffer. To be certain that this concentration would inhibit fibrinolytic activity in human plasma, the procedure was performed in triplicate on pooled plasma under the conditions shown below. Streptokinase (no EC no. assigned) was added to activate plasminogen in the sample.

1. The buffer solution contained 5 mg of ε-aminocaproic acid per milliliter, and 50 units of streptokinase was added before the thrombin reagent.

2. The buffer solution contained no ε-aminocaproic acid, and 50 units of streptokinase was added before the thrombin solution.

3. The buffer solution contained 5 mg of ε-aminocaproic acid per milliliter; no streptokinase was added.

The results are shown in Table 1.

Color development and linearity of the biuret reaction. The absorbance of the protein standard, treated as indicated above, was followed as a function of time after it was removed from the water bath and biuret reagent added. We found no significant increase in absorbance after the first 5 min.

Standard solutions ranging in concentration from 750 to 6000 mg/liter were prepared and run in triplicate through the procedure. Absorbance and concentration were linearly related.

Linearity of the procedure. To see if dilution and absorbance were linearly related, we diluted pooled plasma with saline (serum cannot be used, owing to the presence of thrombin and calcium) to produce ¾, ½, and ¼ dilutions. The procedure was performed in triplicate on these dilutions. The results are shown in Figure 1. The concentration range was from about 1.0 to 4.0 g/liter.

Modification for measuring extremely low fibrinogen concentrations. At extremely low fibrinogen concentrations, the clot formed from 1.0 ml of plasma is generally not isolated completely, because it lacks cohesiveness and tends to disintegrate when one tries to wind it around the glass rod. To establish experimental conditions under which extremely low fibrinogen concentrations could be quantitated, we assayed a plasma pool and then diluted it with saline to produce a fibrinogen concentration of about 1000 mg/liter. We then assayed this diluted plasma in triplicate, using 1.0 ml of plasma to establish the value. The plasma was then further diluted with saline to ¾, ½, and ¼ of this concentration. The minimum volume necessary to produce a well-formed clot was determined for these three dilutions. Using these minimum volumes, the diluted plasmas were assayed in triplicate. The values calculated based on dilution factor, the values actually obtained, and the minimum volumes necessary are shown in Table 2.

Within-run precision. The assay procedure was performed approximately 20 times on two plasma pools. One pool was diluted with saline to establish precision at the lower end of the normal range. The undiluted pool gave a mean value of 4.33 g/liter, a standard deviation of 64 mg/liter, and a coefficient of variation of 1.5%. The diluted pool gave a mean value of 1.74 g/liter, a standard deviation of 40 mg/liter, and a coefficient of variation of 2.9%.

Between-run precision. For routine quality control, an aliquot of a plasma pool is run with each analysis. The pool usually contains about 20 aliquots and lasts about three months. Results for one such pool, containing 17 samples and considered representative of the between-run precision of the method, were: mean value, 3.70 g/liter; standard deviation, 82 mg/liter; and coefficient of variation, 2.2%.

Accuracy of the method. We used a commercial fibrinogen standard (Hyland Laboratories, Costa Mesa, Calif. 92626) to assess the accuracy of the method. Sixteen vials

Table 2. Plasma Volume Increases to Quantitate Abnormally Low Fibrinogen Levels

Value expected[a]	Value found[b]	Minimum plasma
mg/liter		volume, ml
—	1100	1.0
820	780	2.0
550	550	2.0
270	280	4.0

[a] Calculated values based on dilution of plasma pool.
[b] Av of three determinations.

from the same lot were analyzed during three months. The manufacturer's stated value was 3.30 g/liter. The mean value we obtained by our method was 3.25 g/liter.

Results and Discussion

The effect of plasmin on the fibrin clot unprotected by the presence of ε-aminocaproic acid was quite dramatic. At the end of the 15-min incubation period, only a few stringy pieces of gelatinous material could be seen in the flask. A 5 g/liter concentration of ε-aminocaproic acid is considered sufficient to inhibit plasmin and protect the clot.

The alkaline saline reagent was developed during the study of the linearity of the biuret reaction. Absorbance at zero dilution was closer to zero when the NaCl concentration was about the same in the protein standards and reagent blank, and the clot dissolves faster in this reagent than in 30 g/liter NaOH.

Henry (*2*) indicates that using ethylenediaminetetraacetate as an anticoagulant results in friable clots with poor tensile strength. In our experience, the quality of the clot obtained in this procedure was not influenced by the anticoagulant. It is also stated that adding the biuret reagent after dissolving the clot yields lower results. In this procedure the biuret reagent must be added after the tubes are removed from the water bath to avoid the appearance of a variable amount of CuO precipitate. The value obtained for the Hyland reference plasma argues against falsely low results caused by this change in technique. The fact that the standard and blank are subjected to the same conditions as the fibrin clot probably accounts for the elimination of this problem.

Trapping of plasma proteins in the clot has been discussed as a source of positive error (*2*). In theory, the greater the plasma dilution, the less trapping there should be. If a much larger volume of clotting buffer was used, the clot tended to fragment when we attempted to isolate it. If the volume was decreased to much less than 20 ml, the apparent fibrinogen concentration increased, as compared to values obtained when 30 ml of clotting buffer was used.

Foster et al. (*5*) reported turbidity in the final solution. They believed that this was produced by impurities in the thrombin reagent. We have not encountered this problem with patients' samples. Turbidity has developed during the assay of lyophilized material such as some lots of the Hyland product and the survey samples from the College of American Pathologists (also produced by Hyland). Extracting the solutions with diethyl ether significantly decreases the turbidity. We found that optimum results were obtained by extracting the standard and blank also.

Normal range. It seemed desirable to compare the normal range estimated by this method with the generally accepted range of 2.0 to 4.0 g/liter. Our normal-value studies were far from ideal because our hospital obtains blood extramurally from a regional blood bank and outpatient services are provided by another laboratory. Thus we used blood samples from patients being admitted for elective minor surgery, if review of the clinical history did not indicate any condition thought to influence fibrinogen concentrations. The samples were assayed only by our method. The mean value ($n = 45$) was 3.18 g/liter, and the standard deviation was 740 mg/liter. The most significant result is the fact that the mean value did lie near 3.0 g/liter.

The method presented was developed because a rapid method for quantitating fibrinogen was needed by clinicians in our institution, but we did not wish to sacrifice analytical capabilities for speed. Every attempt was made to keep the technique as simple as possible. The procedure has been in use over a year in our laboratory, and we find it to be simple, rapid, and reliable.

References

1. Ware, A. G., Guest, M. M., and Seegers, W. H., Fibrinogen—with special reference to its preparation and certain properties of the product. *Arch. Biochem.* **13,** 231 (1947).
2. Henry, R. J., *Clinical Chemistry: Principles and Techniques.* Harper and Row, New York, N. Y., 1964, p 228.
3. Rosenberg, A. A., and Peabody, R. A., Rapid estimation of fibrinogen in fibrinolytic and nonfibrinolytic states. *Clin. Chem.* **18,** 666 (1972).
4. Bottema, J. K., and Vervoort, H. J. P., A rapid screening method for demonstrating fibrinolysis during surgical operations. *Clin. Chim. Acta* **9,** 179 (1964).
5. Foster, L. B., Frings, C. S., and Hochholzer, J. M., Fibrinogen assay during heparin therapy of disseminated intravascular coagulation. *Clin. Chem.* **17,** 1216 (1971).

special report

The International Federation of Clinical Chemistry[1][2]

IFCC Section no. 2

Editor: Nils-Erik Saris

Dept. of Med. Chemistry University of Helsinki, Siltavuorenpenger 10, SF-00170 Helsinki 17, Finland

INTERNATIONAL FEDERATION OF CLINICAL CHEMISTRY

Committee on Standards

Expert Panel on Enzymes

G. N. Bowers, Jr, Hartford, Ct (U.S.A.), Chairman, H. U. Bergmeyer, Tutzing (G.F.R.), *D. W. Moss,* London (U.K.)

PROVISIONAL RECOMMENDATION (1974) ON IFCC METHODS FOR THE MEASUREMENT OF CATALYTIC CONCENTRATION OF ENZYMES

This Provisional[3]) Recommendation of the International Federation of Clinical Chemistry has been prepared by the Expert Panel on Enzymes and accepted by the Committee on Standards. It has been reviewed by other Expert Panels. In this process the Expert Panel on Quantities and Units has criticized the choice of quantities and units, i.e. *catalytic activity* and *catalytic concentration* with the corresponding units *Moles per sesond*, and *moles per second and litre*, respectively. Instead it suggests that the quantities *catalytic amount* and *catalytic concentration* with the units *katal* and *katal per litre* should be recommended. However, the Expert Panel on Enzymes has not found it possible to change its choice of quantities and units. The Committee on Standards has decided in favour of the view held by the Expert Panel on Quantities and Units. Nevertheless it decided that both viewpoints should be expressed in the Provisional Recommendation and formed the undersigned 'ad hoc' committee for the editing. Finally the Executive Board decided to present the Provisional Recommendation to the National Representatives in the Council in the form suggested by the Committee on Standards. In this Recommendation the controversial sections are numbered 1.2.7 and 1.2.8. The version of the Expert Panel on Enzymes is designated 'A' while 'B' is the version submitted by the Expert Panel on Quantities and Units in accordance with its own submitted Definitive[3]) Recommendation 1973 [2,3], to be acted upon by the Council 1975.

Comments on this Provisional Recommendation may be sent before the end of 1975 to Dr. D. W. Moss, Royal Postgraduate Medical School, London W12 OHS. (U.K.).

R. Dybkaer, Copenhagen (Denmark)
D. W. Moss, London (U.K.)
N.-E. Saris[4]), Helsinki (Finland)

1. General considerations concerning the determination of the catalytic concentration of an enzyme in the blood serum or plasma of man

Introduction

The members of the Expert Panel on Enzymes (EPE) of the Committee on Standards (CS) of the International Federation of Clinical Chemistry (IFCC) believe

[1]) Reprinted from Clin. Chim. Acta (1975) Vol. 61, pp. F 11–24, following p. 238 with the authorization of the Executive Board of the IFCC and the permission of the Editor.

[3]) The terms 'provisional' and 'definitive' refer to stages in the development of IFCC Recommendations.

[4]) To whom reprint requests should be addressed.

that the selection of a method which is to serve as an internationally agreed method of reference to measure the catalytic activity of an enzyme must rest upon experimental observations which have been verified in many laboratories. These methods are to be called *IFCC Methods* in the remainder of this paper.

The problem of reaching agreements through the detailed definition of a method is considered here, in contrast to the alternative but complementary route of defining the specifications for reference enzyme materials. Since wide acceptance of *IFCC Methods* is desired, the goals of this international effort in clinical enzymology must be set out early in the programme for review and comment. Furthermore, the definition of terms used must be clear and unambiguous in order to avoid confusion and misunderstanding.

After the initial period of time needed to develop this document within the Expert Panel, the proposals have been reviewed and commented upon by the Associate Members (AM). After further revision as a result of the comments by AMs, the recommendations were sent to the Chairmen of other panels, then to the CS and when accepted by the CS to the Executive Board of IFCC for final approval by vote of the National Representatives. It is the view of the present members of the EPE that the EPE should not, as a group, engage in experimental data brought to light during discussions within the EPE or between the EPE, its AMs and the CS should be conveyed to the scientific community so that appropriate research is stimulated, with publication of results in the usual way.

1.1. The goals

The central consideration in these efforts to define an IFCC Method should be to achieve a blend of maximum reliability and optimum conditions. Any mechanism which establishes an IFCC Method in clinical enzymology should also include a means for change so that further research is not inhibited.

1.1.1. The diagnostic value of determining the catalytic activity of an enzyme in serum which has made it important in medicine should be maintained or enhanced. Each method should contribute to differentiating healthy persons from individuals with diseases known to be associated with an elevation (or depression) of the catalytic activity. The effect on total activity of alterations in the proportions of multiple molecular forms of a particular enzyme found in human serum must also be considered.

1.1.2. The major aim of an IFCC Method is to achieve maximum reproducibility of analysis both within each laboratory and between laboratories throughout the world. Therefore, the sensitivity, precision, specificity and accuracy of the analytical measuring system must be of primary importance.

It is not anticipated that these methods will immediately receive wide acceptance for use in service laboratories. Therefore, the constraint that they initially be 'routine' methods, compatible with existing mechanized analytical equipment, was dismissed since such a limitation might jeopardize their longterm suitability as IFCC Methods.

1.1.3. The need to reach agreement on and to establish a broad acceptance of IFCC Methods must not impair innovative efforts and systematic research to improve enzyme measurements. The scientific demonstration of new conditions which are recognized as significant improvements should lead to adoption of a new modified IFCC Method after suitable review. Once accepted, the newer method becomes the official IFCC Method and the older method is no longer endorsed.

1.2 Definition of terms

Whenever possible, the recommendations on nomenclature, classification and symbols of the Report fo the Commission on Biochemical Nomenclature of the International Union of Biochemistry should be followed [1]. Recent changes and proposals by other IFCC Expert Panels and the IUPAC Commission on Quantities and Units in Clinical Chemistry [2,3] should be noted. The following terms need further clarification of their use in this document and subsequent EPE draft proposals or recommendations:

1.2.1. Nomenclature of IFCC Methods. (This must evolve and be consistent with recommendations of the IFCC Reference Materials and Methods Office).

1.2.2. In the previous sections or those which follow, the term 'optimum conditions' means those conditions supporting maximum catalytic effect at the selected temperature in respect to each of the following:

(a) the identity and concentrations of substrate, cofactors, activators, buffer and allosteric factors;
(b) the catalytic concentration of indicator enzyme(s) and of auxiliary enzyme(s) (see 1.2.5);
(c) the pH and ionic strength of the reaction mixture, and
(d) other variables (e.g. exclusion of known inhibitors).

An optimized method embodies the concept of optimum conditions being modified only to that extent required to achieve maximum reproducibility of the final measuring system. Therefore, a method must first be 'optimized' before it is recommended for consideration as an IFCC Method.

1.2.3. The term 'serum enzyme' is to be avoided since what is meant is 'an enzyme occurring in serum', e.g. one may say aspartate aminotransferase in serum; but should not say serum aspartate aminotransferase.

1.2.4. The term 'kinetic technique (or method)' should be avoided when what is meant is the continuous monitoring of the progress of the reaction. Instead of 'kinetic method' the term 'continuous (monitoring) method' is recommended. Ambiguity may result from the fact that kinetic techniques are also employed to determine the concentration of many metabolites.

1.2.5. The terms to describe the two or more single reaction steps of a coupled test system to measure enzyme activity are: (a) the 'primary reaction', (b) the 'indicator reaction' and, if present, (c) the 'auxiliary reaction(s)'. The source of the enzyme catalyzing the primary reaction is serum or other biological material while the indicator and auxiliary enzyme(s) are incorporated as reagents.

1.2.6. The terms describing an IFCC Method should not contain eponyms or acronyms other than those accepted by the Commission on Biochemical Nomenclature.

1.2.7.A. Catalytic activity. *Symbol:* z.
Unit: moles per second (mol s^{-1} or mol/s).

kmol s^{-1}	kmol/s
mol s^{-1}	mol/s
mmol s^{-1}	mmol/s
μmol s^{-1}	μmol/s
nmol s^{-1}	nmol/s

Notes

1. In the Recommendations (1972) of the Commission on Biochemical Nomenclature (CBN) on the Nomenclature and Classification of Enzymes together with their Units and the Symbols of Enzyme Kinetics [1] it is recommended that:

"a. the concept of 'enzyme unit' as a physically undefined 'amount of enzyme' be abandoned;"
"b. enzymic activity (alternatively 'catalytic activity') be defined as the rate of reaction of substrate that may be attributed to catalysis by an enzyme."

2. The coherent (S.I.) unit is 'mole per second' because the kind of quantity is defined as a reaction rate. CBN has given this unit the name 'katal'; however, a new special name for a simple derived unit is against the present international trend and cannot be recommended.
3. The use of the 'enzyme unit' (symbolized U) corresponding to a reaction rate of 1 μmol/min should be discouraged progressively so that it may eventually be abandoned.
4. For a given method 1 μmol/min corresponds to 10^{-6} mol/60 s = 16,67 × 10^{-9} mol/s = 16,67 nmol/s.
5. If the method employed precludes the use of this kind of quantity and its unit, an arbitrary kind of quantity and unit should be defined.

Rationale

For most practical purposes, the enzyme contents of different solutions of an enzyme (e.g. different samples of serum) can only be compared quantitatively in terms of their respective catalytic activities; i.e. by their relative effects on the rate of the specific reaction catalyzed by that enzyme. Although catalytic activity is related directly to the number of active enzyme molecules present in the system, numerical factors expressing this relationship are known for only a few enzymes, under appropriate reaction conditions. IFCC Methods in clinical enzymology consist of closely specified methods for determining the rate of reaction in the presence of a known volume of the enzyme sample. It is therefore necessary to report the results given by these methods in units appropriate to the measurement of reaction rates. The appropriate derived coherent S.I. unit measures rate of chemical change in terms of moles of substrate transformed during one second. Multiples and sub-multiples of this unit, with their symbols, are given above.

The catalytic activity of an enzyme can only exist and be measured in the presence of the substrate and under conditions which support catalysis. Furthermore, the magnitude of the observed activity of a given enzyme sample will vary with alterations in reaction conditions. Measurements of enzyme activity are therefore entirely method dependent. When solutions of highly purified and characterized enzymes are under consideration (as is rarely the case in clinical chemistry) it is possible to measure enzymes as substances, rather than as catalysts. In these circumstances the appropriate unit is that for amount of substance, i.e. the mole.

1.2.7.B. Catalytic amount. Symbol: *z*.
Unit: katal (kat).
kkat
kat
mkat
μkat
nkat

Notes

1. The provisionally base unit 'katal' is defined as the catalytic amount of any catalyst (including any enzyme) that catalyses a reaction rate of one mole per second in an assay system (IUPAC Recommendations 1973, Section 4.7, [2]).
2. The catalyzed reaction can be symbolized

$$\nu \cdot S \xrightarrow{\text{catalyst}} P$$

where S is substrate, P is product(s), and ν is the stoichiometric number of S (the number of entities of substrate converted in one 'elementary transformation'); ν is usually one. The mean reaction rate during a certain time is the amount of substance (in moles) of (elementary entities of) substrate converted, divided by its stoichiometric number ν and by time. The special quantity to be measured in the assay system is the reaction rate of a zero-order reaction according to the reaction scheme. (The term initial rate is often used, however, any 'lag-phase' must be excluded.)

3. Any quantity (i.e. a measurable property) using the kind of quantity 'catalytic amount' is named by stating the system (e.g. serum), the functional component (e.g. aspartate aminotransferase), and the kind of quantity (catalytic amount). Further the quantity name must cite a source for details of the assay method including the assay system with its components (pH), temperature, etc.
4. The unit 'katal', which corresponds to a certain reaction rate, does not depend on the assay method. However, the same volume of a given system, measured by different assay methods, may (and probably will) give different results (numberical value × katal) because the quantities are different by definition owing to the different methodology.
5. Comparisons between values obtained by one method and those obtained by another should be treated with extreme caution, since unknown accelerators and inhibitors, and their effects on different forms of the enzyme may preclude a single conversion factor.
6. The conceptual basis of the 'katal' is identical with that of the 'enzyme unit', symbolized U, as defined by the International Union of Biochemistry (IUB, 1964). They are both provisional base units but differ in magnitude, since 1 U corresponds to a reaction rate of 1 μmol/min and 1 kat to a reaction rate of 1 mol/s. For a given assay method, 1 U ≡ 1 μmol/min = 10^{-6} mol/min = 16,67 nmol/s ≙ 16,67 nkat.
7. The use of 'enzyme unit' (symbolized U) should be progressively discouraged (IUB, 1972).

Rationale

In 1972, IUB recommended a new unit for the *derived* kind of quantity 'enzymic activity' and defined the derived unit 'one katal' as *equal* to a reaction rate of one mole per second. The Expert Panel on Quantities and Units (EPQU) (and the IUPAC Commission on Quantities and Units in Clinical Chemistry) has chosen to recommend a *provisionally base* kind of quantity and unit, mainly in order to avoid dimensional problems. The unit should express an extensive property of the original specimen, not a reaction rate in a special assay mixture with conditions that are not obtainable in the original system. The term 'amount' in the name of the kind of quantity reflects the extensive nature of the quantity, whereas 'activity' is used in chemistry for intensive properties. The provisionally base approach creates no problems when derived kinds of quantities and units are created, whereas the derived concept does because the properties of the assay system and original system become mixed (see Section 1.2.8.B). In either case the numerical values are identical.

1.2.8.A. Catalytic concentration. Symbol: *b*.
Unit: mole per second and litre (mol s^{-1} l^{-1} or mol/(s l)).

kmol s^{-1} l^{-1}	kmol/(s l)
mol s^{-1} l^{-1}	mol/(s l)
mmol s^{-1} l^{-1}	mmol/(s l)
μmol s^{-1} l^{-1}	μmol/(s l)
nmol s^{-1} l^{-1}	nmol/(s l)

Notes

1. This kind of quantity is the catalytic activity of the component divided by the volume of the system. The numerical value depends on the temperature and other method parameters apart from *thermal inactivation* of the catalyst. The system mentioned in the definition is the original system containing the enzyme (e.g. serum), *not* the reaction mixture specified by the method of determination.
2. The use of 'enzyme unit per millilitre' (symbolized U/ml) and 'enzyme unit per litre' (symbolized U/l) should be progressively discouraged.
3. For a given method 1 U/l corresponds to 16,67 nmol s^{-1} l^{-1}.

1.2.8.B. Catalytic concentration. Symbol: *b*.
Unit: katal per litre (kat/l).

kkat/l	μkat/l
kat/l	nkat/l
mkat/l	

Notes

1. This kind of quantity is the catalytic amount of the component (enzyme) divided by the volume of the system. The numerical value depends on the temperature and pressure of the system through their effects on volume (IUPAC Recommendations 1973, Section 4,16 in ref. 2).
2. The system mentioned in the definition is the original system containing enzyme, *not* the reaction mixture specified by the method of determination.
3. The derived coherent unit is 'katal per cubic metre', but in accordance with chemical practice the 'katal per liter' is preferred for clinical chemistry.
4. The use of 'enzyme unit per millilitre' (symbolized U/ml) and 'enzyme unit per litre' (U/l) should be progressively discouraged (IUB, 1972).
5. For a given quantity (specified by a given method) 1 U/ml = 16,67 μkat/l.

Rationale

In 1972, IUB recommended the name 'enzymic activity concentration' and the derived unit 'katal per litre' equal to mol s^{-1} l^{-1}. EPQU maintains that this unit is dimensionally incorrect, because the 'mol/s' refers to the assay mixture whereas the 'l' applies to the original (specimen) system. Such problems are avoided by using a (provisionally) base unit where both the katal and the litre refer to the original system, even if the measurement of the number of katals is made in a special assay system. Whichever definition is chosen the numerical values are identical.

2. Reaction temperature

The set point in degrees Celsius of the reaction temperature is to be assigned as a part of the method. Only one temperature should be endorsed for each method and its choice fully documented in the appendage. It is recommended that with as few exceptions as possible, the IFCC Methods be carried out at a uniform temperature of 30,00 °C.

2.1. Temperature control specifications

The methods, procedures and equipment used for controlling temperature, in mixing specimens with reagents, and in inserting them into the measuring device shall be such that during the entire actual time of observation of the reaction mixture, the recorded temperature of the liquid near its centre varies by less than ± 0,05 °C from the nominal set-point temperature, expressed as the standard deviation of at least 16 measurements made following exactly the same procedures and using the same reagents as used in determining the catalytic activity.

2.2. Temperature sensor specification

The temperature sensing element used shall have the following characteristics:

2.2.1. Accuracy. The mean value of the reaction temperature shall be traceable to the International Practical Temperature Scale of 1968 [4,5].

2.2.2. Thermal mass, self heat and conductance. The immersion element plus its leads shall have a heat capacity relative to that of the heat capacity of the volume of liquid reaction mixture into which it is immersed of less than 0,01 (1 %).

The thermal conductance of the immersion element at the most extreme external environmental temperature difference from that of the liquid in the cuvette, and the self-heat generated, if any, shall be such that the change of temperature caused thereby shall be less than ± 0,05 °C during the specified observation time.

2.2.3. Speed of response. To ensure that significant short-term transient temperature changes are observed, the time constant of the exponential response of the immersion element and its recording system shall be less than 0,1 (10 %) of the specified observation time during which the determination of the catalytic concentration is made.

3. Method selection

In addition to some of the broad generalizations stated under Goals (Section 1.1) and in the Definition of terms (Section 1.2), the following criteria are to be considered:

3.1

A recommended method should be specific enough to be of diagnostic value and this must be taken in account when optimum conditions are evaluated. For example, tosyl arginine methyl ester is hydrolyzed at high rate by thrombin and could thus be considered as an optimum substrate; however, it is also hydrolyzed by many other proteases and esterases and is therefore not recommended for a reference assay of thrombin in plasma. Such considerations will apply for the choice of recommended substrates for the acid phosphatase of prostate, lipase, aminopeptidase (arylamidase, EC 3.4.11.2), cholinesterase (EC 3.1.1.8), and other hydrolases.

3.2

Measurement techniques which follow the progress of the reaction directly and continuously are to be preferred over sampling techniques requiring additional manipulations. However, regardless of the technique employed, multiple points sufficient in number to define clearly the progress curve of each test are essential [6,7].

3.3

Calculations of the catalytic activity should be based upon that portion of the progress curve which is zero-order with respect to concentration of substrate(s); i.e. the initial, linear portion of the curve after allowing for mixing effects or lag-phases which cannot be eliminated by changes in the reaction conditions.

3.4

The number and types of operational steps should be reduced whenever possible to avoid excessive errors from multiple pipettings and contact with numerous container surfaces. If possible, combined reagent mixtures should be utilized [8].

3.5

The description of the method should include an Appendix giving the important experimental data needed to establish its blend of reliability and optimum conditions.

3.5.1. Graphic and tabular format should be used to document the conditions chosen, e.g. plots allowing the evaluation of Michaelis constants (K_m), and results of other relevant studies comparing such factors as alternative buffers and substrates should be given.

3.5.2. The sample volume should constitute a fixed volume fraction of the total reaction mixture. The ratio of sample volume to total volume must be such that any effects due to buffering capacity of the sample are eliminated and the effects of inhibitors, cofactors, metabolites and other enzymes are reduced.

Although the initial rate of reaction theoretically increases with enzyme concentration without limit, providing that the substrate is present in saturating concentrations, in practice a limit is imposed by the finite time required to establish the shape of the progress curve. The design of an IFCC Method should maximize the range of enzyme activity which can be measured without the need for special treatment of the sample, such as dilution. Since it is impossible to recommend a universally satisfactory dilution procedure for enzyme samples, it should be recognized that, for each method, a range of enzyme activity will exist beyond which the results obtained must be regarded as less reliable, even though a specific sample-dilution procedure may be recommended for use with a particular method.

3.5.3. The establishment of the reproducibility of the method should be with a clearly characterized human enzyme(s) of the type found in serum, preferably at a catalytic concentration which best separates healthy individuals from those persons known to have enzyme activity changes due to a concurrent active disease process.

3.6. Outline for write-up

In the title give the EC 'recommended name' (formerly the 'trivial' name) and follow with the number and systematic name both in parenthesis. The date should also be easily seen. For example:

IFCC Method (1974) for
Alkaline phosphatase in human serum (EC 3.1.3.1, orthophosphoric-monoester phosphohydrolase, alkaline optimum)

Introduction and method selection. Give brief description of the enzyme(s) and any other information which is necessary for clarity.

Principle. Give the reaction formula(e) in such a way as to show the direction of measurement and a brief statement concerning the measuring technique.

Optimal conditions for measurement
Instrumentation and equipment
Reagents
Specimen procurement, transportation and storage
Measurement procedures
Interpretation
Appendices and references

4. Instrumentation and equipment

The instruments and equipment employed should meet clearly stated specifications to reduce measurement errors from laboratory to laboratory.

4.1

Spectrometers must meet spectral purity (wavelength, band pass and stray light) and spectrometric accuracy specifications which are to be stated for each method. Similar specifications should be given for other types of instruments not involving spectrometry. Photometric errors are often neglected, but can readily introduce systematic relative differences in absorbance of 0,01 to 0,05 [9,10]. Errors due to fluorescent effects can be especially troublesome in measurements with reduced NAD.

4.2

Cuvettes should have parallel faces of optical glass or quartz which transmit light without significantly reducing the light intensity due to absorption, reflections or other scattering effects. The light beam should in no way be influenced by the walls of the cuvette or events on the wall's surfaces, and the internal pathlength should be 10,00 mm and deviate less than ± 0,01 mm [11]. If cuvettes with other dimensions are used, the performance specifications must be equal to those above.

4.3

pH meters should be calibrated at the reaction temperature with reference buffers from an authoritative source (e.g. IUPAC or NBS). When the final pH must be adjusted with measurements from a pH meter, specifications to avoid slope errors, sodium-ion errors at high pH and junction potential errors should be given.

4.4

All volumetric glassware should meet stated specifications (BSI or NBS class A or other national equivalents) or should be calibrated by the user. Corrections for cubic expansion of liquids must be made if the glassware were calibrated at a temperature different from the reaction temperature.

4.5

Surfaces in contact with any part of the sample, reagents, or reaction mixture must be chemically clean and free from traces of acids, metals or detergents or other compounds known to interfere with enzyme activity measurements.

5. Reagents

Specifications for reagent chemicals, water and enzymes should refer to an authoritative source. If these are not available or are found to be inadequate to insure the method's success, the needed additional specifications should be included.

5.1 Reagent chemicals

These reagents must be of a known purity and free of impurities known to influence the reaction rates. For example the need for added specifications to guard against the 'lactate dehydrogenase inhibitor' in reduced NAD used to measure the catalytic concentration of lactate dehydrogenase in serum has been shown [12,13]. The following sources have been considered to be 'authoritative'.

5.1.1 Reagent Chemicals, 4th edn (1968) American Chemical Society, Washington, D.C. [14].

5.1.2. Specifications and Criteria for Biochemical Compounds, 3rd edn (1972) Publ. 1344, Natl. Acad. Sci.-Natl. Res. Council, Washington, D.C. [15].

5.1.3. Bergmeyer, H. U. (1974) Methods of Enzymatic Analysis, pp. 417–556, Academic Press, New York [16].

5.2. Reagent water

Water specifications must meet the requirements of an authoritative source [17]. In addition, known inhibitors of the enzyme in question must, if present, be below the minimum inhibitory concentration. (These minimum levels should be given.) Sterile water (free of any additives) may be required for reagent solutions which are to be stored for any length of time.

5.3. Reagent enzymes

Enzymes employed as reagents (indicator and auxiliary enzymes of Section 1.2.5) must be of stated quality [18] and meet specifications of authoritative sources. These reagent enzymes must be essentially free from contamination with other enzymes, metabolites and impurities which might alter the rate of the primary or secondary reaction being followed. If contaminants or side activities are unavoidable, they should be described.

5.4. Comparison material ('standard')

The composition and purity of the comparison material (usually a substrate, product or coenzyme, but not an enzyme material) must receive additional specifications which go beyond Section 5.1. The molar (linear) absorption coefficient [8] of the comparison material must be determined at increasing concentrations under the conditions which prevail in the final reaction mixture.

5.5. Buffers

Buffers should be prepared by using an explicitly stated, easily reproduced technique with clearly defined reagents of specified purity. The buffer capacity should be adequate to hold the pH of the reaction mixture to within pre-established limits. These limits should be such that the change in pH, from any source, during the period of measurement should not introduce relative changes in the measurements of catalytic activity exceeding 0,005 (0,5 %). Storage time limits for the buffer should be established such that changes in pH or production of rate influencing decomposition products arising from storage will not introduce relative changes in catalytic activity measurements exceeding 0,005 (0,5 %). Buffer substances should not react with any compound of the analytical system unless such a reaction is specifically described (e.g. transphosphorylation with some amino alcohol buffers in alkaline phosphatase methods).

6. Specimen procurement, transportation and storage

6.1. Preparation of the individual and obtaining specimen

The catalytic concentration of an enzyme in human serum (or other biological materials) may vary physiologically for a number of reasons. Differences may relate to age, sex, body habits, weight, food or beverage intake, fasting, dietary habits, exercise or diurnal rhythms (e.g. the catalytic concentrations of creatine kinase, aspartate aminotransferase and lactate dehydrogenase in blood serum increase in individuals after heavy muscular exercise). Variations have also been observed from race to race and from occupational, geographic, climatic and other environmental factors. Therefore, even under well-defined conditions of patient preparation and the use of internationally agreed IFCC Methods to measure the catalytic concentration of an enzyme in large groups of the world's population, it will still be necessary in the future to study the individuals within each group in great detail.

6.2. Serum or plasma specimens

If plasma rather than serum is to be used, the type and concentration of anticoagulant employed must be stated and shown not to alter the enzyme activity. Serum or plasma showing visible evidence of haemolysis, lipaemia or excessive colour (pigments) may well interfere with activity measurements and appropriate precautions should be described as a part of the method.

6.3. Specimen stability

Information regarding the stability of enzymes in the freshly drawn blood and separated serum with the passage of time at various storage temperatures should be included as a part of the method. Frozen serum or reconstituted lyophilized enzyme control and calibration materials may show rather extreme variations in activity with time which should be noted [19].

6.4. Other body fluids or tissues – (optional)

Special instructions about patient preparation, details of collection or biopsy procedures as well as handling and storage precautions must be given.

7. Measurement procedure

All manipulatory operations to determine the catalytic concentration of an enzyme should be given in detail.

7.1. *Instrumental*

Give the nominal wavelength setting (e.g. 402 nm) and the tolerance limits of the band width (e.g. ± 2 nm at half peak height). Explicit details for blank correction, timing of readings and the control of non-enzymatic changes are also required. The temperature control and equilibration for the cuvette, its holder, and transfer of solutions should be also given in detail.

7.2. *Analytical system*

Give these instructions in tabular format as follows:

Pipette	Volume (ml)	Final substance concentrations in reaction mixture
(I) Buffer/reagent mixture	....	.... mol/l
(II) Serum (Sample)	....	volume fraction = ...
Incubate at 30,00 °C for *x* minutes		
(III) Initiating reagent	....	.... mol/l

Mix well and record the changing absorbance at .... nm for .... seconds. Calculate $\Delta A/\Delta t$, the avarage change of absorbance with time (in s^{-1}). Correct for blank reactions.

7.3. *Calculations*

$$\text{Catalytic concentration} = \frac{\Delta A}{\epsilon l \Delta t} \cdot \frac{V}{v} \, (\text{mol s}^{-1}\ \text{m}^{-3})$$

where V is reaction volume (in m^3);
ΔA is absorbance change (in the unit 1);
Δt is the time increment (in s);
l is pathlength of cuvette (in m);
v is serum volume (in m^3);
ϵ is molar (linear) absorption coefficient (in $mol^{-1}\ m^2$).
Inserting V and v in l, l in m, ϵ in $mol^{-1}\ m^2$).
Δt in s, and dividing by 1000 gives values in $mol\ s^{-1}\ l^{-1}$.

8. Interpretation

8.1. *Variability of the method*

The proper evaluation of any draft proposal, recommendation, or final IFCC Methods requires a sound statistical-experimental design which ties together the efforts of several laboratories. Each laboratory must receive and handle or collect the specimen(s) in an identical manner if bias is to be reduced. Similarly, replicate analyses on each specimen should be performed according to such a stated design that between-days and within-run variation can be evaluated. The tissue or blood source of any reference enzyme material as well as its solvent matrix must be given in detail [20].

8.2. *Observation in health and disease*

Data on the catalytic concentration of an enzyme found in body fluids or tissues of apparently healthy individuals and patients are the consequence of the application of a method and, therefore *should not constitute a part of the method* (experience with an IFCC Method can be given in an appendix).

8.3. *Sources of error*

Give a listing of known drug and other interferences including pharmacologic (in vivo) and measurement (in vitro) effects in the appendix.

9. Appendices and references

9.1

Appendices should be used to give greater detail concerning background studies, relevant historical information (e.g., the EPE deliberation and instrumental and reagent specification).

References

1. Enzyme Nomenclature. Recommendations (1972) of the Commission on Biochemical Nomenclature on the Nomenclature and Classification of Enzymes together with their Units and the Symbols of Enzyme Kinetics. Prepared by the Commission on Biochemical Nomenclature and approved by I.U.P.A.C. & I.U.B., Elsevier, Amsterdam.
2. I.U.P.A.C. & I.F.C.C. (1974) Quantities and Units in Clinical Chemistry. Recommendation 1973, Pure Appl. Chem. *37*, 519–546.
3. I.U.P.A.C. & I.F.C.C. (1974). List of Quantities and Units in Clinical Chemistry. Recommendation 1973, Pure Appl. Chem. *37*, 549–572.
4. The International Practical Temperature Scale of 1968 (1969), Metrologia *5*, 35–44.
5. Mangum, B. W., (1974). Clin. Chem. *20*, 670–672.
6. Dixon, M. & Webb, E. C., (1934). Enzymes, pp. 10–11, Academic Press, New York.
7. Moss, D. W., (1972). Clin. Chem. *18*, 1449–1454.
8. Englhardt, A. & Noetges, A., (1970). Aerztl. Lab. *16*, 42–49.
9. Rand, R. N., (1969). Clin. Chem. *15*, 839–863.
10. Burnett, R. W., (1972). J. Res. Natl. Bur. Stand. Sect. A 76A, No. 5
11. Mavrodineanu, R. & Lazar, J. W. (1973). Clin. Chem. *19*, 1053–1057.
12. McComb, R. B. & Gay, R. J., (1968). Clin. Chem. *14*, 754–763.
13. Gerhardt, W., Kofoed, B., Westlund, L. & Pavlu, B., (1974). Scand. J. Clin. Lab. Invest. *33*, Suppl. 139.
14. Reagent Chemicals, 4th edn (1968). American Chemical Society, Washington, D.C.
15. Specifications and Criteria for Biochemical Compounds, 3rd edn (1972) Natl. Acad. Sci. – Natl. Res. Council Public. 1344, Washington, D.C.
16. Bergmeyer, H. U., (1974). Methods of Enzymatic Analysis, pp. 417–556 Academic Press, New York.
17. Winstead, M., (1967). Reagent Grade Water: How, When and Why? Publication of Am. Soc. Med. Technologists. The Stech. Co., Austin, Texas.
18. Bergmeyer, H. U., (1972). Scand. J. Clin. Lab. Invest. *29*, Suppl. 126, Abstract 12.2.
19. Brojer, B. & Moss, D. W., (1971). Clin. Chim. Acta *35*, 511–513.
20. Bowers, Jr, G. N., Kelley, M. L. & McComb, R. B., (1967). Clin. Chem. *13*, 595–607.

AMERICAN ASSOCIATION FOR CLINICAL CHEMISTRY

The purpose for which the Association is formed is to further the public interest by encouraging the study, advancing the science, and improving the practice of clinical chemistry. To achieve these objectives the Association shall:

1. Establish standards for education and training in the field of clinical chemistry.
2. Encourage the creation, promotion and maintenance of standards for certification of individuals in the field of clinical chemistry.
3. Encourage individuals in the field to pursue advanced studies and to engage in scientific investigations.
4. Promote scientific knowledge of clinical chemistry through meetings, seminars, discussions, reports and publications.
5. Initiate and participate in programs related to clinical chemistry that are in the interest of the public.
6. Promote programs for the recognition of the profession of clinical chemistry.

—from Article II, revised (1976) Constitution

OFFICERS, 1976

President: Dr. Royden N. Rand, Rochester, NY

Secretary: Dr. Samuel Meites, Columbus, OH

President-Elect: Dr. Norbert W. Tietz, Chicago, IL

Treasurer: Mr. Joseph S. Annino, Boston, MA

For information concerning the Association, membership application blanks, etc., write: American Association for Clinical Chemistry, 1725 K St., NW, Washington, D. C. 20006 (tel: 202/833-3590)

SECRETARIES, LOCAL SECTIONS

CAPITAL
Thomas R. Koch, *Secretary,* 280 Stanmore Road, Baltimore, MD 21212

CHICAGO
Barbara Phee, *Secretary,* 2900 Maple Ave., No. 24 C, Downers Grove, IL 60515

CLEVELAND
Marvin C. Hallberg, *Secretary,* St. Luke's Hospital, Chem., 11311 Shaker Blvd., Cleveland, OH 44104

CONNECTICUT VALLEY
Charles L. Woronick, *Secretary,* Med. Research Labs., Hartford Hospital, 80 Seymour St., Hartford, CT 06115

FLORIDA
Priscilla Stevens, *Secretary,* 18530 Caribbean Blvd., Miami, FL 33157

MICHIGAN
Donald K. Soules, *Secretary,* Oakwood Hospital, 18101 Oakwood Blvd., Dearborn, MI 48124

MIDWEST
Virginia P. Cook, *Secretary,* Wesley Medical Center, Dept. of Labs., 550 North Hillside, Wichita, KS 67208

NEW JERSEY
Elsie J. Shrawder, *Secretary,* Clay Adams, 18 Woodland Ave., Denville, NJ 97834

NEW YORK METRO
Susanna A. Levy, *Secretary,* Laboratory, St. Barnabas Hospital, 184th & 3rd Ave., Bronx, NY 10457

NEW YORK UPSTATE
Mary Bellinger Sloan, *Secretary,* 17 Parkhurst Blvd., Buffalo, NY 14223

NORTH CAROLINA
Peter H. Anderson, *Secretary,* Director of Chemistry, VA Hospital, 508 Fulton St., Durham, NC 27705

NORTHEAST
Louis Amoruso, *Secretary,* Boston Medical Laboratory, 15 Lunda Street, Waltham, MA 02154

NORTHERN CALIFORNIA
Harold J. Drews, *Secretary,* 5868 Sierra Ave., Richmond, CA 94805

OHIO VALLEY
John A. Lott, *Secretary,* Ohio State University, Dept. of Pathology, Rm 342, Columbus, OH 43210

PACIFIC NORTHWEST
John E. Thompson, *Secretary,* 1629 Harvard Ave., No. 504, Seattle, WA 98122

PHILADELPHIA
Robert F. Foery, *Secretary,* W. Chester State College, Chemistry, West Chester, PA 19380

PITTSBURGH
John J. Moore, *Secretary,* Pathology Dept., Western Pa. Hospital, 4800 Friendship Ave., Pittsburgh, PA 15224

ROCKY MOUNTAIN
Kent Painter, *Secretary,* Box 1826, Fort Collins, CO 80522

SOUTHEAST
Thomas C. Stewart, *Secretary,* Earl K. Long Memorial Hosp., Dept. of Pathology, 5825 Airline Highway, Baton Rouge, LA 70812

SOUTHERN CALIFORNIA
Denis O. Rodgerson, *Secretary,* Dept. of Pathology, Ctr. for Health Sciences, UCLA, Los Angeles, CA 90024

TEXAS
Mabelle E. Adams-Mayne, *Secretary,* 3310 Aberdeen Way, Houston, TX 77025

letters

Drug Screening for Employment Purposes: The Importance of Telling It Like It Is

To the Editor:

Each positive result of a drug-screening program is vitally important to the person whose sample is being studied. During a routine physical examination, a professional individual was "found" to be using morphine and cocaine, and this analysis report was placed in this person's employment files. After an official protest and being left with little other recourse, the person asked Delaware State College to find out what, if anything, was causing the false positives. Two substances found in the subject's urine sample were isolated and identified. Thin-layer chromatography, ultraviolet spectrophotometry, gas chromatography, spectrofluorometry, and infrared spectrophotometry were used to show that the positive morphine and cocaine were in fact quinine and its metabolite formed by the hydroxylation of the quinuclidine nucleus. The details can be summarized as follows.

A careful review of the woman's daily eating and drinking habits disclosed that she frequently drank tonic water and bitter lemon, both of which contain quinine. Results were negative when a urine sample was examined after the beverages had not been consumed, but after resuming them the urine gave a positive for quinine and some unknown substance, which we set out to identify.

The first and second urine samples submitted to us by the woman were analyzed by the Gelman thin-layer chromatography drug-analysis procedure. As mentioned before, the first sample was negative, but the second was positive for quinine and some unknown substance. The spot in the second (positive) urine sample was tentatively identified from its R_F (0.68) and its characteristic bluish-purple color under ultraviolet (375 nm) light. The unknown spot had a smaller R_F value (0.36) and was green under ultraviolet light.

Each of the two spots was eluted from the chromatogram with methanol, evaporated, and the residue dissolved in H_2SO_4 (50 mmol/liter). The solution showed ultraviolet maxima at 247 nm (R_F 0.68 spot) and 225 nm (R_F 0.36 spot). Quinine in 50 mmol/liter H_2SO_4 has an absorption maximum at 250 (*1*).

Similarly prepared solutions of the two spots were examined by gas chromatography (SP-2250 packing, flame-ionization detector, column temperature 220 °C). The spot with R_F 0.68 had the same retention time as the quinine standard. The substance represented by the spot with R_F 0.36 had a retention time 99.3% that of the quinine control.

Similar methanol solutions of the two spots were evaporated, and the residue was dissolved in acetic acid. They were then examined with a fluorometer with the following results:

R_F 0.68 spot	
Excitation:	419 nm
Emission:	554 nm
R_F 0.36 spot	
Excitation:	422 nm
Emission:	550 nm
Quinine reference	
Excitation:	420 nm
Emission:	550 nm

Similar methanol solutions of the two spots were evaporated and redissolved in CCl_4. This solution was dropped onto a heated KBr pellet, leaving a residue of the spot material. The following infrared maxima were observed:

R_F 0.68 spot	
3400 cm^{-1}	OH str
2900	OH str
2850	aromatic CH str
1600	pyridine ring
R_F 0.36 spot	
2910 cm^{-1}	CH str
2850	aromatic CH str
2350	NC=O str
1600	pyridine ring

The compound represented by the spot with R_F 0.36 had a structure similar to quinine. We think it is the keto form of the most frequently occurring quinine metabolite (*2*).

This study shows the importance of confirming all positive drug reports by other analytical procedures. In this case it would appear that quinine was mistakenly identified as morphine and the metabolite of quinine as cocaine. Such cases emphasize the need for constantly monitoring the efficiency of laboratories involved in this type of work. They also remind us that we are influencing the lives of people and must continuously guard against treating such analysis as routine. Only then can we truly "tell it like it is."

References

1. Williams, R., *Detoxication Mechanisms*, Wiley, New York, N. Y., 1959, pp 655–657.

2. Clark, E. G. C., *Isolation and Identification of Drugs,* Pharmaceutical Press, London, 1969, pp 532–533.

Donald R. Wilkinson
Patricia Jensen
Doris Winsley

Department of Chemistry
Delaware State College
Dover, Del. 19901

Further on Light Scatter vs. Turbidimetry

To the Editor:

The Letter of Blom and Hjørne (*1*) makes a valid point with regard to the use of turbidimetric measurements for specific protein determination by immunochemical reactions. Their recent paper (2) demonstrates that human serum albumin can be determined by turbidimetric measurements with an unmodified centrifugal analyzer and with a final albumin reaction concentration of 0–4 mg/liter. This albumin reaction concentration represents a final serum dilution of 21/600. Our reference to turbidimetric measurements was made in the first paragraph of the *Discussion* section (3), in our attempt to point out the difference in the terms "turbidimetric measurement" and "light-scatter measurement," and it was directed in particular to the miniature Fast Analyzer, in which a rotor with a 0.5-cm pathlength cuvette is used. We intended no reference to turbidimetric measurements made with other instruments, but obviously it can be so inferred.

However, I cannot agree with the remainder of the Letter, which attempts to explain why turbidimetric measurements are more sensitive than light-scatter measurements. Blom and Hjørne demonstrated a maximum absorbance change to 0.060 *A* for their highest albumin standard under their reaction conditions (e.g., 0–4 mg of albumin per liter of final reaction mixture). Under the reaction conditions used the for light-scatter measurements, they used similar specific protein concentrations in the reaction, with full-scale sensitivity being achieved at reasonably low photomultiplier voltages (400–600 V). They further refer to the total measurement of ΔI change (in turbidimetric measurements) as opposed to a part (in light-scatter measurements) as a logical physical justification for the greater sensitivity of turbidimetric measurements. ΔI for turbidimetric measurements is a loss in intensity of the impinging light source because of light scatter, not because of increase or decrease in absorbance, and it represents a small change in a large signal. ΔI for light scatter (a different entity), although a measurement of only a fraction of the total 360° light scatter as seen by the detector, is a measurement of a significant signal over a small background signal.

The discussion of which method is more sensitive is a minor point, however, in the realization that clinically useful procedures have been set up that may speed up the analysis process, that can provide test economy, and that provide a convenient means of determining several specific proteins in human serum and plasma.

References

1. Blom, M., and Hjørne, N., Specific protein analysis by light-scatter measurement with a miniature Centrifugal Fast Analyzer. *Clin. Chem.* **21**, 1691 (1975). Letter to the Editor.

2. Blom, M., and Hjørne, N., Immunochemical determination of serum albumin with a centrifugal analyzer. *Clin. Chem.* **21**, 195 (1975).

3. Tiffany, T. O., Parrella, J. M., Johnson, W. F., and Burtis, C. A., Specific protein analysis by light-scatter measurement with a miniature centrifugal analyzer. *Clin. Chem.* **20**, 1055 (1974).

T. O. Tiffany

Pathology Associates, Inc.
Spokane, Wash. 99220

Instrument Control by Computer an Improvement?

To the Editor:

The recent paper by Davis and Lewis [*Clin. Chem.* **21**, 1221 (1975)] illustrates an important pitfall in the conventional approaches to laboratory computerization. These authors have undertaken to design a computer interface for the SMA 12/60, so as to increase its productivity. After expenditure of $25,000 in direct costs and a much larger amount in labor costs, what have they produced? A reduction in useful channels from 12 to 8, and an increase in rate from 60 to 120 samples per hour—a net gain of 33%. The resulting assemblage is more complex, hence more unreliable. If the system goes down, you lose 120 specimens per hour instead of 60. No technologist time is saved, not all malfunctions are observed—indeed, there are some that clearly no computer interface can observe. Once it is set up, the equipment locks in the laboratory to the existing methodology: alterations are likely to be as expensive as the original development.

But is there any alternative? Yes: first, spend the money for a second 12/60 to get redundancy in the most unreliable component, and then design your operation to use the efficiencies of keypunching. A full hour's output on a 12/60 can be keypunched in 15 min; the delay is insignificant in the overall laboratory report cycle, but the operation significantly improves the chances of detecting errors in overall laboratory processing of the specimens. Build into the system features that facilitate checking of results by technologist and professional staff; this cannot be overlooked if we are to meet our professional responsibilities to the patient.

A system of this kind has been running successfully for five years in our laboratory.

Samuel Raymond

William Pepper Laboratory
Hospital of the University of Pennsylvania
Philadelphia, Pa. 19104

The authors of the paper in question respond:

To the Editor:

Dr. Raymond appears to have some misconceptions about our device, and we appreciate this opportunity to reply to them. Our paper reported preliminary results from a feasibility study. Since that report was submitted, however, the prototype has operated successfully on all channels of the SMA-12 at 120 samples per hour. Contrary to Dr. Raymond's inference, the microprocessor controller is physically *less* complex than the original controller it replaces. There are no cams or mechanical relays. We have changed methodologies on our instrument, and the controller parameter table was modified in a matter of minutes to accommodate the changes. No program modifications were required.

We feel that one of the most significant contributions of microprocessor technology to clinical instrumentation will be in instrument reliability and data integrity. A large proportion of the software in our controller is dedicated to checking both the instrument and the controller itself to assure proper operation.

At least two firms have announced computerized replacement controllers, and data will soon be available from which to judge whether we or Dr. Raymond are correct.

Our paper concerned dedicated computer control of a single instrument, not the laboratory data-handling task implied by the phrase "laboratory computerization." It has been 3½ years since we abandoned a keypunch reporting system (similar to Dr. Raymond's) for a computerized on-line laboratory system. We have no regrets. Furthermore, a recent study from our laboratories [*Clin. Chem.* **21**, 1648 (1975)] shows manual keyboard entry to have a higher error rate than on-line data collection.

James E. Davis
John W. Lewis

Barnes Hospital
St. Louis, Mo. 63110

Laboratory Computers: On- or Off-line?

To the Editor:

The issue raised by Drs. Davis and Lewis in their reply (this issue) is possibly the most significant one facing our profession today. If they are right and their view is widely accepted, we shall see a change in the practice of clinical chemistry (and of clinical pathology generally) that will equal or exceed the effects of automated analysis itself. If they are wrong but their view still succeeds in dominating (which seems likely, since it is supported by the computer industry, government granting agencies, and most of the active workers in this field), laboratories everywhere will spend untold amounts unnecessarily, the practice of laboratory medicine will be seriously impeded by inept applications of computer technology, and the physicians using laboratory data will be inadequately served.

What is the issue? It is, most simply, whether the laboratory computer should be on-line or off-line. Drs. Davis and Lewis believe it should be on-line, and so they devote large sums of money and much professional effort to an on-line interface. I believe it should be off-line, and so our effort has been directed to a reliable and efficient off-line system, with two primary functions: get it right, and get it to the doctor.

I, as well as they, want to see the "best" system in the laboratory. In whatever way we make this value judgment, it surely should rest upon objective facts and logical analysis, free from bias. It is not clear that such facts and such analysis are currently available. It is clear that laboratory computerization had a bad reputation in the vast majority of the nation's laboratories, presumably because the facts and the analysis are poorly understood or are in dispute. This gap should be filled.

I suggest, therefore, that we join in an effort to ascertain what are the facts about computerization, and what are the principles we can derive from them to help us in designing our computer systems. It may be that there are no principles applicable to all laboratories, or that the area of personal preference or arbitrary judgment is decisive. It would be most unusual if this were so, but at least we should recognize that much, and stop writing papers about it.

The response to this suggestion may be that the answers are already well known and firmly established. I should therefore provide at least a reasonable case against the established doctrine:

1. Our laboratory has operated effectively without on-line computing for five years. During this time our workload has doubled, and our workforce has actually decreased, using an off-line computer.

2. The total cost of our off-line computer system (equipment, rental, supplies, operating personnel, *plus all research and development*) has been very much less than the rental alone of the conventional on-line system.

3. Our overall reliability, off-line, appears to be better than that reported in the Barnes Hospital study referred to by Drs. Davis and Lewis. (I intend to analyze this study in another place.)

4. Our system enjoys overwhelming support among the medical staff, sufficient, for example, to maintain it against recommendations by three outside consulting groups to replace it with conventional on-line systems.

How can this issue be finally decided? I appeal to the profession as a whole: full publicity, no coverup by established interests, no evasions of objective facts and logic, and informed decision by every clinical chemist on his professional responsibility. Our professional responsibilities demand no less.

Samuel Raymond

William Pepper Laboratory
Hospital of the University of Pennsylvania
Philadelphia, Pa. 19104

Determination of Salicylate and Its Metabolites in Urine

To the Editor:

The note by Farid et al. (*1*) claims, based on the results of an experiment with one human subject, that our method of total salicylate determination in the urine (*2*) leads to recovery of 120.3% of the dose (which would make the method useless). They then imply that our reported recoveries of 95 to 100% were obtained because we chose to collect urine until we had obtained this extent of recovery! Had Farid et al. examined the full publication by Levy and Tsuchiya (*3*) of the 1969 abstract that they cited, they would have found the "accuracy" data that they claim do not exist: a recovery from urine 99.7 ± 2.1% (mean ±SD, n = 5) of a 1-g dose of aspirin when urine was collected until salicylate (above blank values) could no longer be detected. The latter practice is obviously followed routinely, as evident not only in the paper by Levy and Tsuchiya, but even in a report that we published as early as 1964 (*4*). Our method for total salicylate determination in urine is being used in several laboratories and has consistently yielded close to 100% recovery when aspirin was administered to human subjects in solution or in rapidly dissolving tablets.

References

1. Farid, H. A., Born, G. S., Kessler, W. V., et al., Improved colorimetric determination of salicylic acid and its metabolites in urine. *Clin. Chem.* **21**, 1167 (1975).

2. Levy, G., and Procknal, J. A., Drug biotransformation interactions in man. I. Mutual inhibition in glucuronide formation of salicylic acid and salicylamide in man. *J. Pharm. Sci.* **57**, 1330 (1968).

3. Levy, G., and Tsuchiya, T., Effect of activated charcoal on aspirin absorption in man. Part I. *Clin. Pharmacol. Ther.* **13**, 317 (1972).

4. Levy, G., and Hollister, L. E., Failure of U.S.P. disintegration test to assess physiologic availability of enteric coated tablets. *N. Y. Med. J.* **64**, 3002 (1964).

Gerhard Levy
Josephine Procknal

Department of Pharmaceutics
School of Pharmacy
State University of New York at Buffalo
Buffalo, N. Y. 14214

Ed. note: The authors of the paper in question were invited to comment, but no response was received.

Improved Detection of Morphine on TLC Plates

To the Editor:

Detection of morphine at low concentrations in urine is very important to laboratories that use thin-layer chromatography (TLC) as a major screening procedure and to those that use hydrolysis followed by TLC for analysis of the drug. It is also important when TLC is used in conjunction with an immunoassay as an initial screening procedure.

Detection of free morphine by TLC very often depends on the experience that a technician has had in interpreting chromatography plates. Even experienced technicians can miss concentrations of 0.5 to 1.5 mg/liter if a plate has been oversprayed or otherwise altered by any one of the many "lab accidents" that almost every toxicology lab has experienced with TLC plates.

We find transmitted high-intensity light to be indispensable for the visualization of morphine. It is used routinely for every plate and is especially useful for hydrolyzed samples. We hold the plates about six inches from the light source so that light shines through the layer. We find the procedure to be most effective when the layer is on top. The light intensifies the blue color of morphine so that interfering compounds at the same R_F may be differentiated.

This procedure has saved countless hours of confirmation time; it is reliable and is sensitive to at least 0.5 mg of free morphine per liter.

Joyce A. McIntyre
Arlene E. Armandi

Laboratory Service
Veterans Administration Hospital
Sepulveda, Calif. 91343

Triiodothyronine Radioimmunoassay: Incubation Time, Temperature, and Antisera

To the Editor:

Various reaction conditions have been proposed for assay of triiodothyronine (T_3) in serum. Chopra et al. (*1*) suggested a single incubation at 4 °C for 24 h, Larson (*2*) proposed a sequential assay with incubation at 4 °C for 2–3 days, and Sekadde et al. (*3*) recommended a sequential incubation of 37 °C for 30 min, then 4–6 °C for 10 min. More recently, Lenz et al. (*4*) have suggested uniform incubation times and temperatures for eight radioimmunoassays, including T_3, and found that binding of T_3 was optimum after an initial incubation of 30 min at 37 °C followed by a 60-min incubation at 6–8 °C.

Table 1. Time Required to Reach Equilibrium in T_3 Assay at Different Incubation Temperatures

Time, min	Percent bound (B/T) at 4 °C	25 °C	27 °C
1	11.5	30.2	33.2
5	13.7	41.0	43.5
15	19.0	58.5	61.0
30	24.2	64.0	67.3
45	30.0	70.0	73.0
60	36.2	71.0	72.5

Our experience indicates that equilibrium in the T_3 reaction mixture is more than 90% complete after a 30-min incubation at either 25 or 37 °C, but not at 6 °C (Table 1). Furthermore, a sequential incubation—in which there is an initial incubation of 15 min, then I-125 labeled T_3 is added and then a second 30-min incubation—will generate adequate standard curves when the incubations are at 25 and 37 °C (Table 2). This sequential incubation at 4 °C results in a standard curve with lower binding and less total displacement (Table 2).

Attaining equilibrium in this assay in 30 min at 37 °C agrees with the report of Lenz et al. (*4*). However, these workers reported that equilibrium binding was lower at 37 °C (15%) than at 6 °C (25%). The reason for this discrepancy is not clear, but could be related to differences in the nature of the T_3 antibodies used in the respective assays. We use a T_3 antiserum obtained from Rocky Mountain Biologicals, Lakewood, Colo. 80226, and an assay protocol as described by Sekadde et al. (*3*), except that (*a*) the 15- and 30-min sequential incubations are at 25 °C as described here, and (*b*) we add 100 μl of goat anti-rabbit serum (diluted 40-fold) immediately before the Carbowax 6000, to promote the bound/free separation. A logit conversion of a typical standard curve of 0 to 5000 μg/liter obtained in our assay yields a slope of −1.408, Y intercept of 6.99, and a correlation coefficient of 0.994. The mean value of our nonspecific binding or blank values is 9.4 ± 1.2%, and typical B_0/B_t values are between 65–70%.

Table 2. T_3 Assay Standard Curves Obtained with a 4, 25, or 37 °C 45-min Sequential Incubation

T_3 μg/liter	4 °C	25 °C	37 °C
0	47.5	69.0	67.5
310	43.0	61.4	59.5
620	37.0	54.5	52.5
1250	31.5	42.7	44.5
2500	24.5	33.5	35.0
5000	18.7	27.5	27.0

With use of the method of calculation described by Lenz et al. (*4*), a typical standard curve from our assay yields: slope 86; Y intercept of B/B_0 curve 103; coefficient of correlation 0.986; B_0/B_t 66.5; and blank 9.8%.

From the preceding data and that in other reports, I conclude that a 30-min incubation at either 37 or 25 °C will establish equilibrium conditions and that a 15-min initial incubation at 25 °C followed by addition of radiolabeled T_3 and a 30-min incubation at 25 °C leads to a relatively rapid, convenient, and precise T_3 assay.

References

1. Chopra, I. J., Ho, R. S., and Lam, R., An improved radioimmunoassay of triiodothyronine in serum: Its application to clinical and physiological studies. *J. Lab. Clin. Med.* **80,** 729 (1972).
2. Larsen, P. R., Direct immunoassay of triiodothyronine in human serum. *J. Clin. Invest.* **51,** 1939 (1972).
3. Sekadde, C. B., Slaunwhite, W. R., Jr., and Aceto, T., Jr., Rapid radioimmunoassay of triiodothyronine. *Clin. Chem.* **19,** 1016 (1973).
4. Lenz, P. H., Wien, G. H., and Toth, T. M., Standardization of incubation time and temperature for eight radioimmunoassays. *Clin. Chem.* **21,** 1169 (1975).

J. C. Standefer

Radioimmunoassay Laboratory
Bernalillo County Medical Center
Albuquerque, N. Mex. 87106

Dr. Lenz and his associates respond:

To the Editor:

Previously, we reported the optimal incubation time and temperature for triiodothyronine (T_3) radioimmunoassay to be 30 min at 37 °C and 60 min at 6–8 °C (*1*) when the reagents and procedure developed by Wien Laboratories, Inc. are used (*2*). When we incubated the reaction mixture at a single temperature, the percent binding was maximum at 6–8 °C after 120 min of incubation; these data are reproduced from the earlier paper in Table 3, lot No. 00193N. Similar data were obtained for seven other radioimmunoassay procedures. Standefer (*above*) obtained similar results when he used the same combination of incubation times and temperatures in a different T_3 radioimmunoassay system, but demonstrated maximum percent binding at 37 °C after 60 min of incubation when he used a single incubation temperature. He suggests the discrepancy between his data and ours was due possibly to the use of different antibodies.

Table 3. Influence of Incubation Time and Temperature on the Binding of T_3 to Antisera from Three Different Rabbits

Time, min	Percent bound (*B/T*) at 6–8 °C	25 °C	37 °C
Lot No. 00218E			
10	13.6	13.2	15.5
20	14.8	18.0	21.1
30	15.5	22.8	22.5
60	18.4	28.4	28.4
120	25.1	35.8	33.8
Lot No. 00663			
10	11.4	14.4	14.3
20	13.4	20.4	20.2
30	14.5	22.7	20.4
60	18.8	31.4	23.2
120	27.2	38.6	25.3
Lot No. 00193N[a]			
10	19.5	19.0	11.0
20	19.5	20.5	11.5
30	24.0	22.5	12.5
60	25.5	23.5	13.5
120	28.5	22.5	14.5

[a] The data for lot No. 00193N were originally published in Lenz et al. (*1*)

To ascertain whether the difference in avidity was in fact attributable to such differences, we repeated our study with use of two other lots of antiserum produced by different rabbits (Table 3). Maximum percent binding was obtained at 25 °C after 120 min of incubation for both lot No. 00218E and lot No. 00663. Comparing the data obtained by the two laboratories for four different T_3 antisera, one may conclude that different antibodies to the same antigen do require different incubation times and temperatures for maximum binding. Different antisera to the same antigen are known to vary in their avidity for the antigen owing to differences in each antibody's affinity for a given antigen, or the number of sets of antibodies in each antisera for a particular antigen, or the number of binding sites (divalent vs. polyvalent) available for binding to the antigen (*3*). The variation in these characteristics from one antiserum to another may help to explain why the optimal incubation time and temperature may vary whenever a new lot of antiserum is used.

T_3 standard curves were determined at different incubation times and temperatures with use of antibody lots No. 00218E and 00663 (Table 4). The slope of the standard curve increased with incubation time at all temperatures for the two lots of T_3 antiserum tested, with few exceptions. The slopes were lowest at 6–8 °C for both lots of antisera. The slopes were highest at 25 °C after 120 min for antiserum lot No. 00663 and at 37 °C after 120 min for antiserum lot No. 00218E. Therefore, the later incubation times and temperatures would be preferred when these respective lots of T_3 antisera are used with the Wien Laboratories procedure. These data indicate that the optimal incubation time and temperature needed to obtain the best standard curve (highest slope) vary with the antisera from different rabbits.

Similar studies are being conducted for other radioimmunoassay procedures. At present, the optimal incubation time and temperature for aldosterone remains at 30–60 min and 6–8 °C, respectively, for two different lots of antisera, confirming our earlier report (*1*).

Table 4. Linear Regression Curves[a] Obtained for T_3 Radioimmunoassay with Various Incubation Times and Temperatures

Time, min	Antisera lot no. 00218E	00663
6–8 °C		
10	$y = 0.00030x + 0.97$	—
20	$y = 0.00030x + 1.16$	$y = 0.00004x + 1.05$
30	$y = 0.00026x + 1.10$	—
60	$y = 0.00014x + 1.04$	$y = 0.00035x + 1.07$
120	$y = 0.00030x + 1.06$	$y = 0.00073x + 1.24$
25 °C		
10	$y = 0.00017x + 0.98$	$y = 0.00043x + 1.03$
20	$y = 0.00035x + 1.00$	$y = 0.00074x + 1.04$
30	$y = 0.00032x + 1.16$	$y = 0.00099x + 1.03$
60	$y = 0.00072x + 1.04$	$y = 0.00133x + 1.22$
120	$y = 0.00105x + 1.09$	$y = 0.00173x + 1.20$
37 °C		
10	$y = 0.00070x + 1.04$	$y = 0.00061x + 1.11$
20	$y = 0.00089x + 1.02$	$y = 0.00042x + 1.19$
30	$y = 0.00068x + 1.11$	$y = 0.00089x + 1.24$
60	$y = 0.00100x + 1.17$	$y = 0.00118x + 1.10$
120	$y = 0.00136x + 1.20$	$y = 0.00117x + 1.16$

[a] The standard curve is obtained by plotting the ratio of zero standard cpm/standard cpm, *y* axis, vs. T_3 concn in picograms per tube, *x* axis.

References

1. Lenz, P. H., Wien, G. H., and Toth, J. M., Standardization of incubation time and temperature for eight radioimmunoassays. *Clin. Chem.* **21**, 1169 (1975).

2. Lenz, P. H., Wien, G. H., and Toth, J. M., Circulating Triiodothyronine (T_3-I^{125}) Test Set, package insert. Catalog No. TS-555, Wien Laboratories, Inc., P. O. Box 227, Succasunna, N. J. 07876 (January 1975).

3. Eisen, H. N., *Immunology. An Introduction to Molecular and Cellular Principles of the Immune Response,* Harper and Row, New York, N. Y., 1974, pp 384–385.

Paul H. Lenz[1]
George H. Wien[2]
Janice M. Toth[2]

[1] *Department of Biological Sciences Fairleigh Dickinson University Madison, N. J. 07940*
[2] *Wien Laboratories, Inc. P. O. Box 227 Succasunna, N. J. 07876*

Effective Quality Control

To the Editor:

I enjoyed reading Dr. Eilers' comprehensive survey of quality control (*1*). "Effectiveness" is a concept that I would like to see included in future considerations. An *effective* quality-control procedure *discriminates* unusual events from the inherently characteristic fluctuations of data among all runs (*2*).

Much attention has been given to the sensitivity of quality-control procedures to variation. Procedures that do not detect variation are useless. However, there are many ways of observing variation. The key to success is not to pick up variation, but to distinguish an unexpected deviation from the usual random fluctuations. For example, time-series methods may be the most effective when drift is a significant source of error (*3*).

The concept of effectiveness becomes especially useful when one is trying to select a control method to be introduced as a standard operating procedure. Two methods of control may be quite sensitive to variation, but one of these may be the more effective. For example, we have found that within-run and between-run variations for determinations of calcium may be readily observed by either the use of a reference serum or use of the patient mean. However, in a hospital population, the reference serum was more effective. It more readily picked up unusual shifts. On the other hand, in an out-patient population the patient mean was the more effective quality-control parameter.

In the following, I have outlined one type of technique that is useful in selecting the most effective quality-control procedure when a variety of sensitive parameters is available. This quantitative technique is not a substitute for the subjective judgments that one must make in supervising an overall quality-control program (*4*). Probably the best way to manage quality control is to view the traditional charts. However, visual inspection of charts is not an adequate method for selecting at the outset the most effective protocol.

The key step in the technique is one that calibrates the candidate control protocols to a common sensitivity under characteristic conditions (step 4 below). After calibration, sensitivity to different types of unusual variations can be compared.

Example

1. Select two control parameters for comparison of their effectiveness: (*a*) the mean R of calcium values for two reference samples ($n_R = 2$) measured in a run [a reference sample method (*5*)]; and (*b*) the mean P of calcium values collected on n_P patients in the same run [akin to the average-of-normals method (*6*)].

2. Accumulate production data: Data on hospitalized patients' values were accumulated for 30 consecutive operating days. Determinations of two types of controls were made on 29 of those days (nominal values, 91 mg/liter and 101 mg/liter). Laboratory procedures were the same as described previously (*2*).

Given a few simple characteristics of the production data, we can make some predictions about the outcome of the actual comparison technique. From the 30 days' patient data, the standard deviation was estimated as $\sigma_P = 12.1$ mg/liter (d.f. = 688). From the determinations on two types of controls during 29 of those days, the standard deviation owing to method error was estimated as $\sigma_R = 2.06$ mg/liter (d.f. = 28). For the mean of patients' values to have the same standard deviation as a mean of two control values, the patient sample size would have to be $n_P = n_R\ (\sigma_P/\sigma_R)^2 = 68$. This number greatly exceeded the average number of daily determinations actually made (about 24) at the time of the study. We predict, therefore, that the mean of controls is the more effective quality-control procedure.

3. Select the type of action limits: (*a*) for each run a signal is generated when the mean of controls is outside a boundary $\pm d$, defined by the nominal mean (100.8 mg/liter) $\pm d$; and (*b*) in the second protocol under consideration, a signal is generated when the daily patients' mean departs from a nominal value (90.7 mg/liter) as determined by a one-sample *t*-test (*7*). A *t*-value exceeding 2 is taken as the signal. This latter signal would occur with probability 5–6% if the values were gaussian distributed with true mean 90.7 and common standard deviation. In fact, signals of the latter type were produced on two of the 30 days (7%).

4. Calibrate the action limits: The comparison of methods is calibrated empirically at 7% by setting $d = 2.5$ (Table 1). To hit upon the calibration value of *d* requires a trial-and-error procedure. Warnings are counted for various values of *d*, until the selected frequency of 7% is achieved.

The value of 7% is not arbitrary, but represents a realistic cut-off for error signals generated under the usual everyday operation. We use a value of 5–7%, so that warning signals are limited to roughly one analytical run out of 20 when no unusual events are occurring.

5. Calculate the probability of detecting error: As a test of shift or drift, we add ±4 mg/liter (nominally two standard deviations of the laboratory method) to all data (both reference and patients' samples). (Other methods to simulate errors could be used, including methods that account for gradual accumulation of error. The magnitude of error should be representative of borderline control situations.) After the shift is added, a count is taken of the number of runs for which the action limit is exceeded. In method *a* the shift produces 79% warnings, while in *b* it is 38% (Table 1). As expected, the mean of patients' values (numbering 15 to 45 per day, standard deviation 12 mg/liter for the distribution) provided a less effective signal than the mean of reference samples (two per day, standard deviation 2 mg/liter).

This technique illustrates that "effectiveness" is a practical concept. It helps one decide which quantitative protocol to select for controlling the release of patient data obtained on a particular run. Also "effectiveness" provides a basis for evaluating procedures empirically when they are thought to incorporate theoretical advantages.

Table 1.

Warning method	Action limit	Occurrence of warning signals (%) with simulated error (mg/liter) of 0 (calibration level)	4[a]
A. Mean of reference samples (R)	$d \geq 2.5$	7	79
B. Patient mean (P)	$t \geq 2$	7	38

[a] We have taken the average for shifts of +4 and −4 mg/liter.

References

1. Eilers, R. J., Quality assurance in health care: Missions, goals, activities. *Clin. Chem.* **21,** 1357 (1975).

2. Heilbron, D. C., Eastman, J. W., and Kelly, D., Warning methods for quality control in determinations of serum calcium. *Clin. Chem.* **20,** 1416 (1974).

3. Harris, E. K., Some theory of reference values. I. Stratified (categorized) normal ranges and a method for following an individual's clinical laboratory values. *Clin. Chem.* **21,** 1457 (1975). See p 1462 (a computer-generated example).

4. Boutwell, J. H., *Quality Control—Clinical Chemistry.* U.S. Dept. of HEW, Center for Disease Control, Atlanta, Ga. (1968).

5. Amenta, J. S., Analysis of variance, control charts, and the clinical laboratory. *Am. J. Clin. Pathol.* **49,** 842 (1968).

6. Hoffmann, R. G., and Waid, M. E., The average of normals method of quality control. *Am. J. Clin. Pathol.* **43,** 134 (1965).

7. Barnett, R. N., *Clinical Laboratory Statistics,* Little, Brown, and Co., Boston, Mass., 1971.

John W. Eastman

Western Pathology Laboratories
2945 Webster St.
Oakland, Calif. 94609

Volatiles and Osmometry

To the Editor:

In a recent report on the increase in serum osmolality caused by ethanol, the authors warned against measuring osmolality by vapor-pressure osmometry (*1*). However, in a letter to the editor Weisberg pointed out that the Wescor Vapor Pressure Osmometer (Wescor, Inc., Logan, Utah 84321) does not detect volatiles because it is a dew-point osmometer (*2*).

Because this laboratory has both a freezing-point osmometer and the Wescor dew-point osmometer, an experiment was set up to demonstrate the increase in osmolality caused by various volatiles as measured by the two instruments.

From a single lot of a lyophilized pool serum I prepared specimens containing different amounts of ethanol, isopropanol, methanol, or acetone (final volume for all specimens, with or without additive, was 10.0 ml). The specimens were run on both instruments and the osmolality of the same pooled serum, diluted similarly with pure distilled water, was subtracted from each observed value, to calculate the increase in osmolality caused by the different volatiles. The expected increase caused by each of the volatiles was taken from Glasser et al. (*3*). Both instruments were calibrated according to the manufacturer's instructions and standardized against the same sodium chloride standards, and all specimens were run on the same day by the same technician. The results (Table 1) show that the dew-point osmometer does not detect volatiles, although this may not be true for vapor-pressure instruments (*4*). It is important to note that the instrument manual that accompanies the Wescor osmometer does not warn about this potential problem.

References

1. Champion, H. R., et al., Alcohol intoxication and serum osmolality. *Lancet* **i,** 1402 (1975).

2. Weisberg, H. F., Osmolality—calculated, "delta," and more formulas. *Clin. Chem.* **21,** 1182 (1975). Letter to the Editor.

3. Glasser, L., Sternglanz, P. D., Combie, J., and Robinson, A., Serum osmolality and its applicability to drug overdose. *Am. J. Clin. Pathol.* **60,** 695 (1973).

4. Dorwart, W. V., and Chalmers, L., Response to ref. *2*. *Clin. Chem.* **21,** 1185 (1975).

Richard M. Rocco

Chemistry Laboratory
Cardinal Cushing General Hospital
Brockton, Mass. 02401

Table 1. Increased Osmolality Caused by Four Volatiles Added to Serum, as Measured by a Freezing-Point and Dew-Point Osmometer[a]

Substance	Concn., mg/liter	Expected increase mOsm/kg	Measured increase, Freezing point (mOsm/kg)	Measured increase, Dew point (mOsm/kg)
Ethanol	3500	80	80	2
Isopropanol	3400	60	61	4
Methanol	800	27	26	3
Acetone	550	10	11	5

[a] All determinations done in duplicate. The variation within either instrument was <2 mOsm/kg. Osmolality was underestimated by the dew-point osmometry at ethanol concns. of 100–300 mg/dl.

book reviews

Biochemical Fluorescence Concepts, 1. R. F. Chen and H. Edelhoch, Eds. Marcel Dekker, Inc., New York, N. Y. 10016, 1975, xii + 408 pp. $29.50.

This book, the first of a two-volume series, consists of a discussion of seven selected topics of special interest in biochemistry, written by prominent authorities in the field. The topics discussed, and their authors, are: (1) Decay of Fluorescence Anisotropy, by Philippe Wahl of C.N.R.S. in France; (2) Time Decay Fluorometry by Photon Counting, by Irving Isenberg at Oregon State University; (3) Fluorescence Polarization: Some Trends and Problems, by I. Steinberg of the Weizmann Institute, Israel; (4) Polarized Excitation Energy Transfer, by Robert Dale of Johns Hopkins University and J. Eisinger of Bell Labs.; (5) Measurement of Intramolecular Distances by Energy Transfer, by Peter Schiller of the Clinical Research Institute of Montreal; (6) Fluorimetric Kinetic Techniques: Chemical Relaxation and Stopped Flow, by T. M. Jovin of the Max Planck Institute, Goettingen, West German; and (7) Fluorescence Polarization Kinetic Studies of Macromolecular Reactions, by S. Levinson of Scripps Clinic and Research Foundation, La Jolla, California. The second volume of the series will consist of 16 more contributions, including two by the editors of the series, Ray Chen and Harold Edelhoch of the National Institutes of Health, Bethesda, who have done an above-average job of ensuring continuity of style and content throughout this first volume.

The potential reader should realize that this series is not a fundamental one for novices, such as the Udenfriend series, in which the basics of fluorescence are presented and a survey of methods for a variety of biochemical compounds is given. Rather, it is an assembly of important research on selected subjects of significance to scientists who work with the luminescence and photochemistry of biologically important molecules. Between the two volumes, a wide variety of such subjects is covered, and the series is highly recommended.

George G. Guilbault

Dept. of Chemistry
University of New Orleans
New Orleans, La. 70122

Cantarow and Trumper Clinical Biochemistry, 7th ed. A. L. Latner. W. B. Saunders Co., Philadelphia, Pa. 19106, 1975, xxxix + 918 pp. $27.50.

Clinical Biochemistry, a now-classic text originally written by Abraham Cantarow and Max Trumper, was first published in 1932. Six previous editions were prepared by the original authors, and this, the seventh, has been completely revised by Professor Albert L. Latner, with a chapter on hormone assay and endocrine function by Reginald Hall and Gordon M. Besser. This edition maintains the clarity and detail of the original text with considerable updating and in many instances completely new sections. The book combines basic discussions of biochemistry with practical considerations of its relationship to disease. For example, the chapter on carbohydrate metabolism contains the traditional explication of the metabolism of carbohydrates, recent information about hormonal control of carbohydrate metabolism, and extensive information vital for the clinical chemist concerning the performance and interpretation of tolerance tests and the clinical biochemistry of the many inborn metabolic errors of carbohydrate metabolism (such as von Gierke's disease, Pompe's disease, limit dextrinosis, amylopectinosis, and McArdle's disease).

The chapter on lipid metabolism is detailed and filled with information valuable to clinical chemists, including outlines of sterol and cholesterol biosynthesis, lipid transport, classification of fatty liver, and the many lipid-storage diseases, as well as an easily understood description of the Fredrickson classification of hyperlipoproteinemia. Surprisingly, the chapter on protein metabolism still includes a discussion of little-used cephalin-flocculation and other flocculation tests, but also a great deal of new and well-written information concerning immunoglobulin structure, as well as the biochemistry, pathology, and clinical chemistry of this group of compounds. The chapter on nucleic acids is excellent, and includes a complete description of the role of nucleic acids in protein synthesis and theory of conventional cancer chemotherapy.

Although the book in general is complete, there are some omissions: the chapter on calcium metabolism does not include recent information on the role of parathyroid hormone in calcium homeostasis, the chapter on trace elements is scanty, the one on enzymes disappointing. Chapter references are few and mostly from the older literature. These defects are more than compensated for by the excellent chapters on acid–base balance, gas exchange, and fluid balance. The 118-p chapter on endocrine function is a book within the book, and will be of considerable value to the clinical chemists. The last chapter details the history of clinical chemistry as well as a prospectus of its future. Included is a lucid consideration of SI units. The book contains a detailed index. The seventh edition of *Clinical Biochemistry* will be a valuable addition to the library of all clinical chemists and is enthusiastically recommended to all who need a textbook in this field as well as those wanting a reference book for answering the kinds of questions that arise each day in a busy clinical laboratory.

Morton K. Schwartz

Memorial Hospital
444 E 68th St.
New York, N.Y. 10021

Books Received

Review of Laboratory Medicine, 2nd ed. J. S. Meyer, L. S. Steinberg, L. A. Sherman. C. V. Mosby Co., St. Louis, Mo. 63103. ix + 341 pp (paperback). $10.95. Pub. Aug. 1975. A question-and-answer type of review of all areas of the subject, including 47 pp on clinical chemistry, 15 pp on closely related subjects.

Chromatographic Analysis of the Environment. R. L. Grob. Marcel Dekker, Inc., New York, N. Y. 10016. x + 734 pp. $49.50. Pub. Sept. 1975.

Progress in Chemical Fibrinolysis and Thrombolysis, 1. Proceedings of the Second International Conference on Synthetic Fibrinolytic-Thrombolytic Agents. J. F. Davidson, M. M. Samama, and P. C. Desnoyers, Eds. Raven Press, New York, 10036. xv + 435 pp. $26.00. Pub. Sept. 1975.

Diagnostische Laboratoriumsmethoden, VII. Lieferung. 3046/DL/VII. Akademie-Verlag, Berlin. Dm.-M. Unpaginated.

Physicians' Desk Reference for Radiology and Nuclear Medicine. 5th ed. L. M. Freeman and M. D. Blaufox, Editorial Consultants. Medical Economics Co., Oradel, N. J. 07649. 308 pp. $9.50. Pub. 1975.

the clinical chemist

Compiled by J. S. King, Executive Editor

Journal Progress: A Report to Our Readers

The Institute for Scientific Information (Philadelphia, Pa. 19106) informs us that the "impact factor" for *Clinical Chemistry* in 1974, the latest year for which data are available, was 3.19, up from 2.701 in 1972 and 0.683 in 1969. This factor is a measure of the average number of citations per paper during 1974, adjusted for journal size and frequency so that various journals may more accurately be inter-compared [*cf. Clin. Chem.* **21,** 179 (1975)]. In 1974, by this criterion, *Clinical Chemistry* was clearly the leader in its field (the factor for *Clin. Chim. Acta,* e.g., was 1.66). Of the practicable ways of assessing the real value of a journal, this certainly is one of the best. In any event, the "impact" of *Clinical Chemistry* is now comparable with that for such acknowledged leaders in scientific and medical journalism as *Analytical Chemistry,* the *British Medical Journal,* the *Biochemical Journal,* the *Journal of the American Medical Association,* and *Nature.*

A second development during recent years is the increasing number of submissions from abroad, and the corresponding increase in non-U. S. papers appearing in *Clinical Chemistry.* Foreign authors of important work for whom English is not the first language are reminded that this Editorial Office offers help in putting papers in their best linguistic light, and such authors are encouraged to allow us the opportunity of assessing such work solely on its scientific merits.

Our circulation abroad has shown a parallel increase, and we are especially pleased that this is true of the Orient; for example, 360 copies now go to Japan each month (vs. 14 to the U.S.S.R.)

11 557 copies of our February 1976 issue were mailed, as compared with (e.g.) 6680 copies of the February 1970 issue.

Necessarily, our declination rate has gradually increased (for 1975 it was about 40%) as contributions of regular papers and Notes have increased from 166 in 1969 to 472 in 1975. We expect that economic considerations will limit the number of regular text pages printed in 1976 to about 2100—which is to say, the same as for 1975.

We regretfully report the obvious—that promised improvements in postal service [*Clin. Chem.* **20,** 1489 (1974)] have not materialized. An editorial in TIME magazine (Feb. 2, 1976) points up some other problems of increased postal rates that all periodicals share.

We are glad, however, to learn that the paper shortage has apparently abated, even if paper prices have not. Beginning with the January 1976 issue we have made our first sacrifice of esthetic quality: a lighter-weight paper is being used for text pages, because of the substantial savings on both paper costs and postage.

—**J.S.K.**

Symposia Program for the 28th National Meeting, AACC

Tuesday, August 3, 9:00 a.m.: **The Clinical Chemist—Identity and Roles**

Chairperson: Max M. Friedman, Ph.D.

The Clinical Chemist—A Historical Perspective, Wendell T. Caraway, Ph.D.

The Clinical Chemist as a Member of the Health Care Team, Donald C. Cannon, M.D., Ph.D.

Intermission

The Clinical Chemist in Industry, Richard G. Nadeau, Ph.D.

The Clinical Chemist—A Government Perception, Joseph H. Boutwell, Ph.D., M.D.

New Horizons in Clinical Chemistry—I

Chairperson: William D. O'Dell, M.D., Ph.D.

Receptor Assays, William L. McGuire, M.D.

Some Clinical Applications of Cyclic Nucleotides, Ferid Murad, M.D., Ph.D.

Intermission

Tissue Enzymes, Dante G. Scarpelli, M.D., Ph.D.

Non-isotopic Immunoassays, John Landon, M.D.

Wednesday, August 4, 9:00 a.m.: **Toxicology**

Chairperson: Irving Sunshine, Ph.D.

Laboratory Response to the Toxicological Emergency, Robert V. Blanke, Ph.D.

Use of Drug Interference Data in Clinical Chemistry, Donald S. Young, M.B., Ph.D.

Intermission

Trace Metals and Metal Metabolism, Walter Mertz, M.D.

Antenatal Toxicology, Reba M. Hill, M.D.

Education in Clinical Chemistry

Chairperson: Norman D. Lee, Ph.D.

Education Programs for Clinical Chemists—A Historical Perspective, Alex Kaplan, Ph.D.

Education Programs for Clinical Chemists—Relevant Objectives, Edward W. Bermes, Ph.D.

Intermission

Education Programs for Clinical Chemists—A Government View, Robert S. Melville, Ph.D.

Education of Clinical Chemists; One Physician's View, Theodore L. Goodfriend, M.D.

Thursday, August 5, 9:00 a.m.: **Enzymes**

Chairperson: Norbert W. Tietz, Ph.D.

Standardization Efforts in Clinical Enzymology, George N. Bowers, Jr., M.D.

Enzymatic Analysis, Donald W. Moss, Ph.D.

Intermission

Selection of Enzyme Profiles for Clinical Diagnosis, Arthur Karmen, M.D.

Antenatal Diagnosis of Enzyme Defects, William E. Bucknall, M.D.

Research in Clinical Chemistry

Chairperson: Jocelyn M. Hicks, Ph.D.

Necessary Resources for Research in Clinical Chemistry, Max E. Chilcotte, Ph.D.

Impact of Government Support on Medical Research, George Z. Williams, M.D.

Intermission

Research in Industry, Royden N. Rand, Ph.D.

Evaluation of Data, Alvan R. Feinstein, M. D.

Friday, August 6, 9:00 a.m.: **Administration and Management**

Chairperson: Jesse F. Goodwin, Ph.D.

Financial Management Considerations of a Hospital Clinical Labo-

Selected Methods—Closing Vol. 8

Readers are reminded that the Selected Methods that have appeared in this journal were presented for your critical appraisal before being collected into a bound volume [see editorial in *Clin. Chem.* **19**, 1207 (1973)]. All comments or criticisms must be in the hands of the Editor-in-Chief no later than mid-April. Methods that have appeared are listed below:

Authors	*Method for*	*Clin. Chem.*
Cali et al.	Calcium	**19**, 1208 (1973)
Fleisher et al.	Carcinoembryonic Antigen	**19**, 1214
Dietz et al.	Cholinesterase	**19**, 1309
Ratliff and Hall	Cortisol (fluorometric)	**19**, 1400
Cameron and Scarisbrick	Progesterone	**19**, 1403
Dietz et al.	α_1-Antitrypsin	**20**, 396 (1974)
Ambrose	Tyrosine	**20**, 505
Lash and Fleischer	Angiotensin	**20**, 620
Nichoalds	Riboflavin	**20**, 624
Velasco et al.	Insulin	**20**, 700
Coch et al.	Lecithin/Sphingomyelin Ratio	**20**, 1366
de la Pena and Goldzieher	Cortisol (competitive protein binding)	**20**, 1376
Juselius and Barnhart	Cortisol (competitive protein binding)	**20**, 1470
Auletta et al.	Prostaglandins E, F, and A	**20**, 1580
Warnock	Transketolase (thiamine deficiency)	**21**, 432 (1975)
Biggs et al.	Triglycerides	**21**, 437
Doetsch and Gadsden	Urinary Total Protein	**21**, 778
Jung et al.	Serum Cholesterol	**21**, 1526
Chisolm and Brown	Porphyrin	**21**, 1669
Besch and Watanabe	Digoxin and Digitoxin	**21**, 1815
Bowers et al.	Serum Control Materials	**21**, 1830
Bowers and McComb	Alkaline Phosphatase	**21**, 1988
Sauberlich et al.	Ascorbic Acid	**22**, 105 (1976)

The bound volume should be released in the late fall of 1976. Please help us make it as useful as possible. The address of the Editor-in-Chief, Dr. Gerald Cooper, is: Chamblee Center for Disease Control, Building 8, Lipid Section, Atlanta, Ga. 30333.

ratory Department—A Hospital Administrator's Perspective, Richard J. Oszustowicz

OSHA Requirements and Laboratory Safety, Michael H. Sulak, M.D.

Intermission

Clinical Laboratories—Malpractice Claims, Risks, and Problems, Raymond R. Kravetz

Federal Government Clinical Laboratory Legislation, David J. Sencer, M.D.

New Horizons in Clinical Chemistry II

Chairperson: Eloise Eavenson, Ph.D.

Asbestos, Silicates, and Tissue Particulate Materials, Keith Griffiths, Ph.D.

Is Molecular Pathology an Endless Frontier?, Norman G. Anderson, Ph.D.

Intermission

Evaluation of Fetal Well-Being, Richard Dickey, M.D., Ph.D.

High Performance Liquid Chromatography, Robert H. McCluer, Ph.D.

Pine Mountain Conference on Drug Monitoring

At deadline, we are informed that the limited quota for this meeting [details in "The Clinical Chemist," *Clin. Chem.* **21**, 1696 (1975)] is not yet full and that registrations will be accepted until it is filled or "well into March," whichever comes first. Write: Pine Mountain Conference, AACC, P. O. Box 29134, Atlanta, Ga. 30327.

Awards Nominations Solicited

Nominations are now being solicited for all AACC Awards. Each member has the privilege of nominating someone for each of the four awards. The nominations may be made by individuals, by a group of members, or by the local section as a unit.

The AACC Awards are bestowed by the AACC membership. Consequently, recipients of these awards are recognized as outstanding in the field of clinical chemistry and as representative of the clinical chemist. It behooves all members to make an effort to place in nomination the names of those persons they feel represent the best in clinical chemistry.

A letter describing the activities that qualify the nominee for a particular award should be sent to the Business Office before May 1, 1976. The *Handbook and Directory* lists all past recipients.

The 1976 Awards are:

• The AACC Award for Outstanding Contributions to Clinical Chemistry, sponsored by Ames Division of Miles Laboratories.

• The AACC Award for Outstanding Contributions through Service to

Clinical Chemistry as a Profession, sponsored by the Fisher Scientific Company.

- The AACC Award for Outstanding Contributions to Clinical Chemistry through Education, sponsored by SmithKline Corp.
- The AACC Award for Outstanding Contributions to Clinical Chemistry in a Selected Area, sponsored by Boehringer Mannheim Corp. Nominations in any area of specialization in clinical chemistry may be submitted.

Miriam Reiner
Chairman, Committee on Awards

Seminar on Thyroid Function

The Capital Section, AACC, will present this seminar at the Holiday Inn, Route 198, Laurel, Md. (between Washington, D. C. and Baltimore), on May 8, 1976. Fee of $20 includes coffee, lunch, and social hour.

8:50 AM Opening Announcements

9:00 AM The Biosynthesis of Thyroid Hormones
Jan Wolff, M.D., Ph.D., National Institute of Arthritis and Metabolic Diseases, National Institutes of Health, Bethesda, Maryland

9:30 AM The Peripheral Action of Thyroid Hormones
Jack H. Oppenheimer, M.D., Professor of Medicine, Albert Einstein College of Medicine & Head, Division of Endocrinology, Montefiore Hospital and Medical Center, Bronx, New York

10:00 AM Thyroid Function in the Child and Adolescent
Gilbert P. August, M.D., Associate Professor of Child Health, George Washington University & Associate Endocrinologist, Children's Hospital National Medical Center, Washington, D.C.

10:30 AM Coffee

10:45 AM The Clinical Aspects of Hypothyroidism
Kenneth D. Burman, M.D., Division of Endocrinology, Walter Reed Army Institute of Research, Washington, D.C.

11:15 AM The Clinical Aspects of Hyperthyroidism
John J. Canary, M.D., Professor of Medicine, Georgetown University Medical School, Washington, D.C.

12:00 NOON Thyroid Function in Non-thyroidal Disease
Robert I. Gregerman, M.D., Associate Professor of Medicine, John Hopkins University; Chief, Endocrinology Section, National Institute on Aging; and Head, Endocrinology Division, Baltimore City Hospitals; Baltimore, Maryland

12:30 PM Lunch

1:30 PM The Assessment of Thyroid Status with *In vivo* Tests
Richard C. Reba, M.D., Chairman, Nuclear Medicine Department, Washington Hospital Center, Washington, D.C.

2:00 PM *In vitro* Radiometric Tests for Thyroid Function
Albert E. Herner, Ph.D., Herner Laboratories, Rockville, Maryland

2:30 PM Quality Control of Radio Assay Tests
George F. Johnson, Ph.D., Assistant Professor, Department of Laboratory Medicine, Division of Clinical Chemistry, Johns Hopkins Hospital, Baltimore, Maryland

3:00 PM Coffee

3:30 PM Influence of Drugs on Thyroid Function Tests
Donald S. Young, M.D., Ph.D., Chief, Clinical Chemistry Service, National Institutes of Health, Bethesda, Maryland

4:00 PM The Rational Diagnosis of Thyroid Dysfunction
Kenneth Sterling, M.D., Veterans Administration Hospital, Bronx, New York

4:45 PM Social Hour

Make check payable to "Capital Section, AACC, Conference," and mail to W. L. Ruff, Ph.D., Clinical Laboratories, Howard Univ. Hosp., Washington, D. C. 20010 (Tel. 202/745-1352).

Other Meetings

Conference on Biomedical Role of Trace Elements in Aging, April, 28–30, 1976, St. Petersburg, Fla. (Write: Dr. Richard W. Neithamer, Eckerd College Gerontology Center, Eckerd College, St. Petersburg, Fla. 33733).

10th Miles Internat. Symp., on "Impact of Recombinant Molecules on Science and Society," at Kresge Auditorium, Mass. Institute of Technol., June 8–10, 1976 (write: Ed. G. Bassett, Symposium Coordinator, Miles Laboratories, Elkhart, Ind. 46514; Tel. 219/264-8460).

Can. Soc. Clin. Chemists, 20th Annual Meeting, July 12–16, 1976, Skyline Hotel, Ottawa. Includes symposia on RIA, SI units, monitoring drug concentrations, releasing hormones. (Write: J. E. Logan, 151 Slater St., Suite 906, Ottawa, Canada K1P 2H3).

MIT Summer School Program on "Enzymes and Their Use in Analysis and Clinical Diagnosis," July 12–16, 1976. (Write: Director of the Summer Session, Rm. E19-356, Mass. Institute of Technology, Cambridge, Mass. 02139).

Internat. Symposium on Toxic Metals, to be held Mar. 3–5, 1977, at the International Conference Center, Monaco. IFCC/IUPAC sponsored. (Write: F. W. Sunderman, Jr., Dept. Lab. Med., Univ. Conn. School Med., Farmington, Conn. 06032).

International Symposium of Microchemical Techniques, May 22–27, 1977. Davos, Switzerland. IFCC sponsored. (Write: Dr. W. Merz, Chairman of Organizing Committee, International Symposium on Microchemical Techniques, Untersuchungslaboratorium, BASF Aktiengesellschaft, D-6700 Ludwigshafen/Rhein, Federal Republic of Germany).

International Symposium on Inborn Errors of Metabolism in Man, Tel Aviv, Israel, June 19–25, 1977. (Write: Scientific Secretariat, Dr. O. Sperling, P. O. Box 16271, Tel Aviv, Israel).

Knavery

The CBS television program "60 Minutes" devoted its first segment on February 15 to exposing some unsavory practices of certain independent clinical laboratories in Chicago: variously disguised kickbacks by laboratories to referring physicians, rip-offs of Medicaid dollars, questionable (to put it mildly) laboratory performance, and the like. An item on NBC News the following evening reported further on this.

The present climate of erosion of integrity; state-federal buck passing with respect to inspection, audit, and control; and the temptations of taxpayer-supplied megabucks—all these have combined to put the conscientious independent or hospital laboratory— to say nothing of the conscientious physician, pharmacist, et al.—at a clear disadvantage in competing with those whose ideas of propriety are more elastic. Indeed, one laboratory representative on the CBS program stated that without fee-splitting with his clients' physicians he would be out of business overnight.

The unmistakable implication was left with the viewer that such nauseous practices are the rule rather than the exception among independent laboratories in the U.S.

One can only hope that the shadow cast over the profession by this presentation will be counterbalanced by action to correct these abuses.

—J. S. K.

Useful Literature

Unlike most catalogs, the 1976–1977 general catalog of Pierce Chemical Co., P.O. Box 117, Rockford, Ill.

61105, contains much ancillary handy technical information on matters related to chromatography, such as thumbnail reviews—one with 68 references—and a tabulation of molecular weights of, and 14 references on, amino acid derivatives.

The Numbers Game

A Letter to the Editor in the January 15 issue of *The New England Journal of Medicine* (p 174) discusses analytical error, frequency of incorrectly reported results, and the resulting impressions of clinicians on laboratory reliability.

Science Graduate Enrollment

Complete results of an NSF survey of 1300 graduate science departments will be released in mid-April. (Write: National Science Foundation, 1800 G Street, N.W., Washington, D. C. 20550.)

Forthcoming Papers

Expression of Random Analytical Error as a Percentage of the Range of Clinical Interest
John H. Glick, Jr.

Serum Iron Determination in Patients Receiving Therapy with Iron Dextram ("Imferon")
Max E. McIntosh, Jerry K. Lynn, Norma Meyerriecks, and Irene Contant

Automated Separation and Measurement of Lactate Dehydrogenase Isoenzymes
Michael G. Busby, Paul J. Kudirka, R. Neill Carey, and E. Clifford Toren, Jr.

High-Pressure Liquid-Chromatographic Separation of Lactate Dehydrogenase Isoenzymes
Paul J. Kudirka, Ronald R. Schroeder, Thomas E. Hewitt, and E. Clifford Toren, Jr.

Evaluation of a New Enzymatic Kit for Serum Triglycerides
Timothy Carter, Paul J. Martin, Peter Wilding, and David M. Goldberg

Preparation of Optically Clear Lyophilized Human Serum for Use in Preparing Control Material
Gary J. Proksch and Dean P. Bonderman

Fluorometry of Plasma Amino Nitrogen, with Use of Fluorescamine
Bernard Klein and Fontaine Standaert

γ-Glutamyltransferase: Substrate Inhibition, Kinetic Mechanism, and Assay Conditions
Johan H. Stromme and Liv Theodorsen

Electrophoretic Pattern of Amylase Isoenzymes in Serum and Urine of Normal Persons
Makoto Otsuki, Susumu Saeki, Hosai Yuu, Mitsuo Maeda, and Shigeaki Baba

Stability of Fatty Acids in Hyperlipoproteinemic Plasma during Long-Term Storage
Eugene Z. Hirsch, Sandra Slivka, and Austin P. Gibbons

Method for Monitoring Plasma Progesterone Concentrations in Pregnancy
Per Winkel, Preben Gaede, and Jorgen Lyngbye

Development of an Aqueous Temperature-Indicating Technique and its Application to Clinical Laboratory Instrumentation
Lemuel Bowie, Fred Esters, Jeffrey Bolin, and Nathan Gochman

Fast, Economical Technique for Separating Serum from Blood Samples
Gurjit S. Ahluwalia, Z. Jerry Kuczala, and Lanny R. Carlson

Clinical Laboratory Evaluation of the Perkin-Elmer KA-150 Enzyme Analyzer
Eugene Hardin, Richard B. Passey, Ronald L. Gillum, John B. Fuller, and Debbie Lawrence

CLIN. CHEM. 22/4, 413-416 (1976)

Fluorometry of Plasma Amino Nitrogen, with Use of Fluorescamine

Bernard Klein and Fontaine Standaert

We describe a fluorometric procedure, with use of fluorescamine, for determining plasma amino nitrogen in a 10-μl sample of deproteinized plasma. Values for apparently healthy human subjects agree well with those obtained by spectrophotometry. The simplicity and speed of the assay recommends it as a screening procedure for detecting aminoacidopathies.

Additional Keyphrases: *inherited aminoacidopathies • reaction with primary amines • free amino acids in plasma • normal values • screening*

It is important to identify cases of hereditary aminoacidopathies (*1*). To do so, one usually examines plasma and urine qualitatively by thin-layer chromatography (*2*), or, for more quantitative definition, by cation ion-exchange chromatography (see *3* for review of the latter). Both procedures are time-consuming. Ion-exchange chromatography, depending on the degree of resolution desired, requires 2 to 6 h. Existing spectrophotometric assays of plasma for amino nitrogen content, though less time-consuming, each have shortcomings. That of Frame et al. (*4*) is nonspecific, and the colored reaction product formed with the β-naphthoquinone-4-sulfonate reagent does not adhere to Beer's law. In other procedures, unstable reagents are used—e.g., dinitrofluorobenzene (*5*, *6*), 2,4,6-trinitrobenzenesulfonate (*7*), or ninhydrin (*8*).

Department of Diagnostic Research, Hoffmann-La Roche Inc., Nutley, N. J. 07110.

Received Nov. 26, 1975; accepted Jan. 8, 1976.

Fluorescamine, 4-phenylspiro-{furan-2-(3H), 1′-phthalan}-3,3′-dione, which forms highly fluorescent pyrrolinone derivatives with primary amines, is a more sensitive reagent than ninhydrin for detecting amino acids that have been separated by ion-exchange chromatography (*9*, *10*). This prompted us to apply it to the determination of plasma amino nitrogen content. We developed a rapid, quantitative assay of free amino acids in a 10-μl sample of deproteinized plasma. The simplicity and speed of the procedure suggests its use as a presumptive or screening test for hyperaminoacidemia.

Materials and Methods

Sodium tungstate solution. Dissolve 100.0 g of sodium tungstate in a liter of de-ionized water.

Sulfuric acid solution, 1.32 mol/liter.

Tungstic acid reagent. To 80 ml of de-ionized water add 5.0 ml of the sodium tungstate solution and 5.0 ml of the sulfuric acid solution. This solution will keep for several days at room temperature.

Borate buffer, pH 9.5 (25 °C), 0.2 mol/liter. With a sodium hydroxide solution (1.0 mol/liter), titrate to pH 9.5 a solution of 12.37 g of boric acid in 500 ml of de-ionized water and dilute to 1 liter.

Fluorescamine reagent. Dissolve 10.0 mg of fluorescamine ("Fluram"; Roche Diagnostics, Division of Hoffmann-La Roche Inc., Nutley, N. J. 07110) in 100 ml of reagent-grade acetone.

Amino nitrogen standards. For a stock solution, 0.2 g of amino nitrogen/liter, dissolve oven-dried (at

100 °C) glycine, 0.268 g (7.14 mmol/liter), and glutamic acid, 0.525 g (7.13 mmol/liter), in 200 ml of deionized water containing 1.0 g of sodium benzoate. Add 4.0 ml of concentrated hydrochloric acid and dilute the solution to 500 ml with water.

Prepare a working standard (5.0 ng of amino nitrogen per liter) by diluting 250 μl of the stock solution to 10.0 ml with the dilute tungstic acid solution. Dilute this solution appropriately to give solutions with amino nitrogen concentrations of 0.5 to 2.5 ng amino nitrogen/liter.

Procedure

To 10.0 ml of tungstic acid reagent, add 100 μl of plasma and, after vortex mixing, centrifuge for 5 min at 3000 × *g*. To a 1.0-ml aliquot of the supernate add 2.0 ml of the borate buffer, with vortex mixing, followed by 1.0 ml of the fluorescamine reagent. Measure the fluorescent response of the well-mixed solution, with the instrument set on a reagent blank prepared by mixing 1.0 ml of dilute tungstic acid solution with the same volumes of buffer and reagent.

Also measure the fluorescence of 1.0-ml duplicates of each of the standard solution treated as above.

We used a Model 111 fluorometer (Turner Associates, Palo Alto, Calif. 94303) fitted with a Corning 7-51 (390 nm) primary filter and a Wratten 4 (465 nm) secondary filter. For most readings a 1 slit and a 3× aperture was used. Some measurements were also made with a microphotofluorometer (American Instrument Co., Silver Spring, Md. 20910) with the same filters. Water at 25 °C was circulated around the cuvettes. The fluorometer was calibrated daily with a quinine standard (1 μg of quinine sulfate per milliliter of 0.1 mol/liter sulfuric acid).

Table 1. Precision and Reproducibility of Amino Nitrogen Analysis with Fluorescamine

	Within-run[a]				
Standards, ng/liter	0.5	1.0	1.5	2.0	2.5
$\bar{X}$	14.0	25.1	35.9	46.1	55.7
SD	0.6	1.5	0.7	0.9	1.5
CV, %	4.3	6.0	2.0	2.0	2.7
	Day-to-day reproducibility[b]				
$\bar{X}$	22	43	60	76	90
SD	1.9	2.6	3.2	4.7	6.8
CV, %	8.6	6.0	5.3	6.1	7.6
	Reproducibility of results for calibration sera				
Serum, mg/liter	A	B	C	D	
$\bar{X}$	8.9	12.2	14.6	11.7	
SD	0.4	0.4	0.4	0.3	
CV, %	4.4	2.4	2.7	2.6	

[a] Fluorescence in arbitrary units; Aminco fluorometer.
[b] Fluorescence in arbitrary units; Turner fluorometer.

Calculation

Prepare a calibration curve by plotting mean fluorescence (in arbitrary units) of each duplicate pair of standards vs. amino nitrogen concentration (mg/dl). The amino nitrogen content of the plasma specimens is obtained by reference to this plot. Alternatively, if a single-point reference is used (e.g., the 2.0 ng/liter amino nitrogen standard), the calculation would be: (fluorescence plasma/fluorescence standard) × 20 = plasma amino nitrogen, in milligrams per liter.

Results

Calibration curves plotted with data obtained with both fluorometers showed that the fluorescence of the reaction product is linearly related to amino nitrogen concentration over a range of 0.5 to 2.5 ng/liter, but with different slopes. Table 1 shows (*a*) the within-run precision of ten replicate analyses of a series of amino acid standards; (*b*) the day-to-day reproducibility of these standards measured daily for 15 days; and (*c*) the amino nitrogen content of four commercial calibration sera, each analyzed 10 times. The mean coefficients of variation were: (*a*) 3.4% (range, 2.06–6.0%); (*b*) 6.72% (range, 5.3–8.6%); and (*c*) 3.2% (range, 2.4–4.4%), respectively.

Recovery Study

The mean analytical recovery of amino nitrogen standards added to aliquots of several pools of calibration sera was 105.6% (range: 94–120%).

Plasma Analysis

Plasma specimens, obtained from 18 healthy adults of both sexes, analyzed by the fluorometric procedure, had a mean amino nitrogen content of 49 ± 6 (1 SD) mg/liter of plasma (range, 39 to 58 mg/liter). This is consistent with mean plasma amino nitrogen values measured by other methods (*6*).[1]

Discussion

The Fluorescamine Reaction

The fluorometric assay for plasma amino nitrogen described here embodies several advantageous features. Firstly, the reagent, specific for primary amines, does not react with the major nonprotein nitrogenous substances commonly present in plasma—i.e., urea, creatinine, urate, or ammonia. However, the reagent also does not react with proline, the secondary amino acid that usually constitutes approximately 5–7% of normal human plasma (*2, 5*). Nevertheless, plasma amino nitrogen values determined by the present procedure agree with previously published data. Recent studies have demonstrated that proline and other secondary amino acids can be measured with fluorescamine after oxidation with *N*-

[1] In this feasibility study, we were not prepared to undertake a study of clinical samples, but we will be happy to discuss the procedure with investigators who wish to evaluate and apply the technique to clinical problems.

chlorosuccinimide (*11–14*). This reaction is currently under investigation for application to the present procedure.

Secondly, the reagent solution, in contrast to ninhydrin and fluorodinitrobenzene, is remarkably stable. In the present study, a fluorescamine solution was used for one month without any detectable alteration; a 12-week stability has been reported (*15*). Furthermore, solutions of the product of the reaction between fluorescamine and plasma filtrates are also stable. For example, 1.0 ml of the 2 ng/liter standard was treated with buffer and the fluorescamine reagent, mixed, the tube was placed in the cuvette compartment and the resulting fluorescence was recorded for 45 min. No change in fluorescence was observed for the first 25 min. During the next 20 min, a change of three fluorescence units (3.7%) occurred.

Thirdly, the procedure is simple. In contrast to other such procedures for primary amines, neither incubation at an elevated temperature nor solubilizing solvents are required. The reaction between primary amino acids and fluorescamine occurs in milliseconds at 23 °C (*16*). Unreacted reagent is rapidly destroyed, as well, producing no fluorescent interfering by-products (*15*).

Fourthly, the reaction is manyfold more sensitive than the analogous spectrophotometric ninhydrin reaction (*10*). In our procedure, 100 μl of plasma is required. This and the volume of precipitant can be proportionately decreased while maintaining a 100-fold dilution of the plasma and affording the equivalent of 10 μl of deproteinized plasma for reaction with the reagent.

When the fluorescence of the test solution, prepared as described, was off-scale, smaller aliquots of the deproteinized plasma taken through the procedure gave results that were identical with those obtained by deproteinizing diluted plasma and repeating the test.

We found that 10 mg of fluorescamine per deciliter of solvent is sufficient to give quantitative conversion of the plasma amino acids to their fluorescent pyrrolinone derivatives (*15*), although other workers have used up to 50 mg/dl of solvent.

Standardization of the Assay

The reaction of fluorescamine with individual amino acids gives products with differing fluorescence intensities (*9, 10*). Thus, standardization of the assay with a single amino acid would afford results that would be different from those based on calibration with another amino acid. For example, results based on a calibration curve prepared with glutamic acid solutions only, in the same concentration as the mixed standard, gave values that averaged 40% higher than those obtained with the mixed standard. Moreover, in the example cited, at concentrations exceeding 1.5 ng of glutamic acid per liter a nonlinear fluorescent response was apparent (quenching?), which restricts the range of measurement. For these reasons we used the accepted and customary calibration mixture containing both glycine and glutamic acid (*6*).

Amino nitrogen standards prepared in aqueous solution gave fluorescent responses that averaged 40% higher than the corresponding standards prepared in diluted tungstic acid. The decrease in fluorescence was probably caused by the tungstate. Because plasma samples were deproteinized by dilute tungstic acid, amino nitrogen standards were also prepared in tungstic acid, thereby eliminating a possible error.

Deproteinization

Deproteinization is necessary because fluorescamine reacts with proteins (*17*). Criteria for choosing a deproteinizing agent were: (*a*) noninterference with the fluorescamine reaction, (*b*) convenient adjustment of the pH of the deproteinized plasma to the optimum for the fluorescamine reaction, and (*c*) a single solution of reasonable stability yielding clear, nonfluorescent protein-free fluids and contributing minimal reagent blank. Sulfosalicylic (*18*), picric (*19*), and trichloroacetic acids were eliminated because the deproteinized filtrates produced were too acid and gave high reagent blanks. Heating with dilute acetic acid (*8*) was too cumbersome. Membrane ultrafiltration (*20*) gave erratic and nonreproducible results. Diluted tungstic acid produced deproteinized plasma solutions, pH about 3. Adding pH 9.5 borate buffer to aliquots of supernatant fluid, as described here, brought the pH to 9, suitable for the reaction with fluorescamine.

Plasma Analyses

The results of plasma amino nitrogen analyses of apparently healthy adult subjects in the limited study presented here agree well with published values. Goodwin (*6*) found a mean of 55.6 ± 8.43 mg/liter of plasma (range, 36–70 mg/liter) among 20 normal adults. Similar values reported by other investigators using other techniques and reagents were included in the same report. We found a mean of 49 ± 6 (1 SD) mg/liter of plasma (range, 39 to 58 mg/liter).

Saifer et al. (*2, 8*) reported *serum* amino nitrogen values for normal humans ranging from 42 to 62 mg/liter. We found that, by the present technique, serum amino nitrogen content averaged 6 mg/liter higher than the corresponding values for plasma. This, too, is in agreement with published studies (*6, 21*) and is explained by the release of amino acids during clotting.

Our efforts to adapt this assay to a conventional continuous-flow automated procedure were unsuccessful.

References

1. Scriver, C. R., Clow, C. L., and Lamm, P., On the screening, diagnosis, and investigation of hereditary aminoacidopathies. *Clin. Biochem.* **6**, 142 (1973).

2. Saifer, A., Rapid screening methods for the detection of inherited and acquired aminoacidopathies. *Adv. Clin. Chem.* **14,** 145 (1971).

3. Peters, J. H., and Berridge, B. J., The determination of amino acids in plasma and urine by ion-exchange chromatography. *Chromatogr. Rev.* **12,** 157 (1970).

4. Frame, E. G., Russell, J. A., and Wilhelmi, A. E., The colorimetric estimation of amino nitrogen in blood. *J. Biol. Chem.* **149,** 255 (1943).

5. Goodwin, J. F., The colorimetric estimation of plasma amino nitrogen with DNFB. *Clin. Chem.* **14,** 1080 (1968).

6. Goodwin, J. F., Spectrophotometric quantitation of plasma and urinary amino nitrogen with fluorodinitrobenzene. *Stand. Methods Clin. Chem.* **6,** 89 (1970).

7. Palmer, D. W., and Peters, T., Automated determination of free amino groups in serum and plasma using 2,4,6-trinitrobenzene sulfonate. *Clin. Chem.* **15,** 891 (1969).

8. Saifer, A., Gerstenfeld, S., and Harris, A. F., Photometric microdetermination of amino acids in biological fluids with the ninhydrin reaction. *Clin. Chim. Acta* **5,** 131 (1960).

9. Udenfriend, S., Stein, S., Bohlen, P., et al., Fluorescamine: A reagent for assay of amino acids, peptides, proteins and primary amines in the picomole range. *Science* **178,** 871 (1972).

10. Stein, S., Bohlen, P., Stone, J., et al., Amino acid analysis with fluorescamine at the picomole level. *Arch. Biochem. Biophys.* **155,** 203 (1973).

11. Weigele, M., DeBernardo, S., and Leimgruber, W., Fluorometric assay of secondary amino acids. *Biochem. Biophys. Res. Commun.* **50,** 352 (1973).

12. Felix, A. M., and Terkelsen, G., Fluorometric analysis of *N*-methyl-amino acids using fluorescamine. *Anal. Biochem.* **60,** 78 (1974).

13. Felix, A. M., and Terkelsen, G., Total fluorometric amino acid analysis using fluorescamine. *Arch. Biochem. Biophys.* **157,** 177 (1973).

14. Felix, A. M., and Terkelsen, G., Determination of hydroxyproline in fluorometric amino acid analysis with fluorescamine. *Anal. Biochem.* **56,** 610 (1973).

15. DeBernardo, S., Weigele, M., Toome, V., et al., Studies on the reaction of fluorescamine with primary amines. *Arch. Biochem. Biophys.* **163,** 390 (1974).

16. Stein, S., Bohlen, P., and Udenfriend, S., Studies on the kinetics of reaction and hydrolysis of fluorescamine. *Arch. Biochem. Biophys.* **163,** 400 (1974).

17. Bohlen, P., Stein, S., Dairman, W., and Udenfriend, S., Fluorometric assay of proteins in the nanogram range. *Arch. Biochem. Biophys.* **155,** 213 (1973).

18. Oddy, V. H., A semiautomated method for the determination of plasma alpha amino nitrogen. *Clin. Chim. Acta* **51,** 151 (1974).

19. Moore, S., and Stein, W. H., Procedures for the chromatographic determination of amino acids on four percent cross-linked sulfonated polystyrene resins. *J. Biol. Chem.* **211,** 893 (1954).

20. Farese, G., Mayer, M., and Blatt, W. F., A membrane ultrafiltration procedure for determining diffusible calcium in serum. *Clin. Chem.* **16,** 226 (1970).

21. MacFadyen, D. A., Determination of amino acids in plasma by the ninhydrin carbon dioxide reaction without removal of proteins. *J. Biol. Chem.* **145,** 387 (1942).

CLIN. CHEM. 22/4, 417–421 (1976)

γ-Glutamyltransferase: Substrate Inhibition, Kinetic Mechanism, and Assay Conditions

Johan H. Strømme and Liv Theodorsen

γ-Glutamyltransferase activity in serum is shown to be competitively inhibited by the two substrates γ-glutamyl-4-nitroanilide and glycylglycine. Awareness of this is of importance when one is choosing final reaction conditions for the assay of the enzyme. γ-Glutamyltransferase probably acts by a "ping-pong bi-bi" kinetic mechanism, which fits with the double competitive substrate inhibition demonstrated. The product, 4-nitro-aniline, appears to be an uncompetitive dead-end inhibitor of both substrates. Various amino acids, particularly glycine and L-alanine, inhibit the enzyme. Their inhibition patterns are uncompetitive with glycylglycine and competitive with γ-glutamyl-4-nitroanilide. On the basis of the present and other studies, the Scandinavian Society for Clinical Chemistry and Clinical Physiology is going to recommend for routine use a γ-glutamyltransferase method in which the final concentrations of γ-glutamyl-4-nitroanilide and glycylglycine are 4 and 75 mmol/liter, respectively.

Additional Keyphrase: *enzyme activity*

During the last few years the activity of γ-glutamyltransferase (GT, EC 2.3.2.2) has become one of the most frequently measured serum enzyme activities in many clinical chemical laboratories, for reasons dealt with in several recent reviews (*1–3*).

GT shows a low degree of substrate specificity. Various natural (*4, 5*) and synthetic substrates (*6–8*) have been used in determining its activity. However, most of the present methods in daily use in clinical chemical laboratories (*3*) are based on the donor substrate γ-glutamyl-4-nitroanilide (glu-4-NA) (*7*) and the acceptor substrate glycylglycine (glygly) (*9*), as for example the procedures proposed by Szasz (*10*) and by Rosalki and Tarlow (*11*). Several kits based on this principle are commercially available.

Division of Clinical Chemistry, Institute of Medical Biology, University of Tromsø, 9000 Tromsø; and Clinical Laboratory, The Norwegian Radium Hospital, Oslo 3, Norway.

Received Nov. 14, 1975; accepted Jan. 13, 1976.

In an attempt to improve the precision and the comparability of the enzyme determinations performed in hospital laboratories, the Scandinavian Society for Clinical Chemistry and Clinical Physiology has recently recommended methods for alanine aminotransferase, aspartate aminotransferase, lactate dehydrogenase, and alkaline phosphatase (*12*). Recommendations on a method for GT will soon be published (*13*). However, the choice of the final reaction conditions to be recommended for the GT method, which will be based on use of the two aforementioned substrates, has been complicated by the fact that both these substrates may inhibit the enzyme. Although glu-4-NA in high concentrations has previously been shown to inhibit GT (*11*), no kinetic studies on the double substrate inhibitory effect have been reported.

The present report shows that the inhibition of GT by glu-4-NA and glygly is double competitive. The inhibition is easily explained by the fact that GT seems to act according to a "ping-pong bi-bi" kinetic mechanism [Cleland's nomenclature (*14*)]. In addition, we examined the inhibition of the enzyme by various amino acids, especially glycine and L-alanine. Such compounds serve as relatively poor acceptor substrates for the enzyme, and their inhibition patterns are uncompetitive with glygly and competitive with glu-4-NA.

Materials and Methods

L-γ-Glutamyl-4-nitroanilide (glu-4-NA), glycylglycine (glygly), glycine, L-alanine, L-lysine, L-serine, L-leucine, L-aspartate, and L-glutamate were obtained from Sigma Chemical Co., St. Louis, Mo. 63178, and L-glutamine from Nutritional Biochemicals Corp., Cleveland, Ohio 44128. 4-Nitroaniline was purchased from BDH Chemicals Ltd., Poole, BH12 4NN, England. *N*-Carbamylglycylglycine [in which the free amino-group of glygly is blocked (*15*)] was synthesized by reacting 0.75 mol/liter potassium cyanate with 1 mol/liter glygly in water (pH about 7.0) for 2 h at room temperature. The product was precipitated by cooling, after adjustment of the pH to 2.9 with 4 mol/liter HCl. The precipitate was washed in 10 mmol/liter HCl and twice recrystallized from hot water. The final product was dried in a desiccator under reduced pressure. It did not show evidence of impurities; in particular, no glygly was found by thin-layer chromatography. Pooled human sera with final GT activities at 37 °C ranging from 30–350 U/liter (normal values for adult men, <35 U/liter) were used as the source of the enzyme.

GT was assayed at 37 °C, with glu-4-NA and glygly as substrates. The rate of formation of 4-nitroaniline during the first 1–2 min was monitored photometrically at 407 nm. The standard final reaction mixture contained, per liter: Tris/HCl, 100 mmol, pH 7.6 (37 °C); $MgCl_2$, 10 mmol; glu-4-NA, 4 mmol; and glygly, 50 mmol. The assay was done either in an LKB 7600 Enzyme Analyzer, with use of 100 μl of glu-4-NA in 0.15 mol/liter HCl as starting reagent (final volume, 1.2 ml with a volume fraction of serum of 0.083), or in a GEMSAEC centrifugal analyzer (initial reading 15 s, reading interval 20 s, number of readings 4–8), with serum as start reagent and a final volume of 0.65 ml with a volume fraction of serum of 0.07. Deviations from the standard conditions are stated in the figure legends.

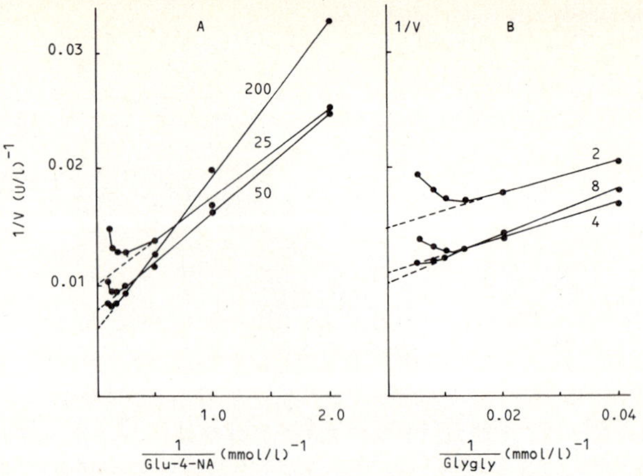

Fig. 1A. Effect on GT-activity of various glu-4-NA concentrations (0.5–10 mmol/liter) at three concentrations (25, 50, and 200 mmol/liter) of glygly

Serum with GT activity 104 U/liter (standard conditions) was used as the source of enzyme. The reaction was started with glu-4-NA dissolved in diluted HCl. The final pH of the medium was 7.6 (37 °C). Each result is the mean of four parallel determinations

Fig. 1B. Effect on GT-activity of various glygly concentrations (25–200 mmol/liter) at three concentrations (2, 4, and 8 mmol/liter) of glu-4-NA

Serum with GT activity 72.5 U/liter (standard conditions) was used as the source of enzyme. The enzyme reaction was started with glu-4-NA dissolved in diluted HCl. The final pH of the medium was 7.6 (37 °C). Each result is the mean of four parallel determinations

Results

Figure 1*A* shows the double-reciprocal plots of GT-activity vs. glu-4-NA concentrations in the range 0.50–10 mmol/liter at three fixed concentrations (25, 50, and 200 mmol/liter) of the second substrate, glygly. Figure 1*B* shows the double-reciprocal plots when glygly was varied in the range 25–200 mmol/liter at three fixed concentrations of glu-4-NA (2, 4, and 8 mmol/liter). In both situations approximately linear curves were obtained in the lower concentration range. However, at the higher concentrations of the variable substrate a marked inhibition was found, as shown by the upward deviation of the curves. It is apparent that the inhibitory effect of the variable substrate is more marked at lower concentrations of the nonvariable substrate.

Figures 1*A* and 1*B*, moreover, show that the slope of the curves increases with increasing concentrations of the nonvariable substrate. This implies that the apparent K_m for the variable substrate will increase markedly as the concentration of the fixed substrate is increased. This effect of the nonvariable substrate on the slope is opposite to the one seen in a straightforward sequential mechanism of enzyme action. The approximately linear curves at the lower concentration range of the variable substrate show by extrapolation (stippled curves of Figures 1*A* and 1*B*) a progressively lower vertical intercept by increasing concentrations of the fixed substrate. In fact, the Lineweaver–Burk plots presented in Figure 1 represent a characteristic pattern for competitive substrate inhibition by both substrates of an enzyme acting according to a ping-pong mechanism (*16*).

Because the complex pattern of the reciprocal plots in Figures 1*A* and 1*B* most likely arises from double competitive substrate inhibition effects, it can be avoided by using much lower substrate concentrations (Figures 2*A* and 2*B*). Under these highly suboptimized conditions, the double-reciprocal plots show families of apparently parallel straight lines, consistent with a ping-pong mechanism. Replots of the slopes and intercepts of these lines vs. the reciprocal concentration of the nonvariable substrate are shown in insets of Figures 2*A* and 2*B*. From these plots, the true K_m of GT for glu-4-NA was calculated to be 1.05 mmol/liter (Figure 2*A*, *inset*) and 1.13 mmol/liter (Figure 2*B*, *inset*), and for glygly 15.6 mmol/liter (Figure 2*A*, *inset*) and 16.0 mmol/liter (Figure 2*B*, *inset*).

Seemingly parallel lines in double-reciprocal plots do not represent unequivocal proof of a ping-pong mechanism (*16*). Kinetic studies of product inhibition were therefore done with the product 4-nitroaniline, a known inhibitor of GT (*17*). The results (Figures 3*A* and 3*B*) suggest that 4-nitroaniline is an uncompetitive inhibitor for both substrates over a wide range of substrate concentrations. Thus, the inhibition still appeared uncompetitive when the concentration of the nonvariable substrate was lowered, e.g., from 4 to 1 mmol/liter in the case of glu-4-NA, and from 50 to 15 mmol/liter in the case of glygly (results not shown). Admittedly we are unable to explain the

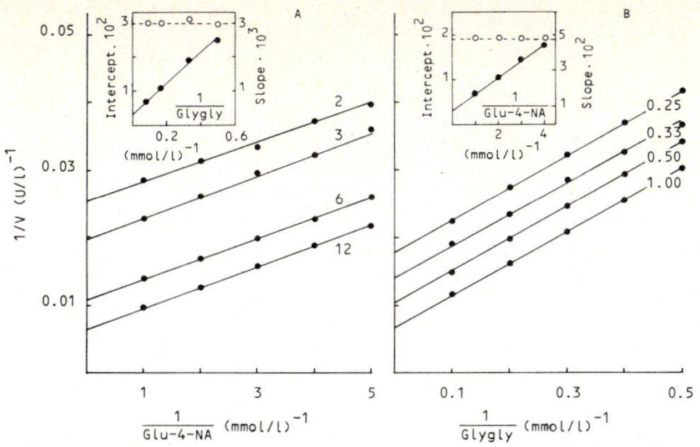

Fig. 2A. Effect on GT-activity of various glu-4-NA concentrations (0.2–1.0 mmol/liter) at four concentrations (2, 3, 6, and 12 mmol/liter) of glygly

Serum with GT activity of 256 U/liter (standard conditions) was used as the source of enzyme. The activities were measured in triplets in a centrifugal analyzer. *Inset* shows the replots of the slopes (*stippled curve*) and the intercepts vs. the reciprocal glygly concentrations

Fig. 2B. Effect on GT-activity of various glygly concentrations (2–10 mmol/liter) at four different concentrations (0.25, 0.33, 0.50, and 1.00 mmol/liter) of gly-4-NA

Serum with GT activity of 246 U/liter (standard conditions) was used as the source of enzyme. Activities measured in triplicate in a centrifugal analyzer. *Inset* shows the replots of the slopes (*stippled curve*) and intercepts vs. the reciprocal glu-4-NA concentrations

Table 1. Inhibition of GT by Various Amino Acids[a]

Amino acid	GT-activity, % Serum 1	Serum 2	Serum 3	Mean
None	100	100	100	100
Glycine	63.0	60.7	61.9	61.9
L-Alanine	68.5	68.9	72.2	69.9
L-Glutamate	76.7	77.0	77.8	77.1
L-Glutamine	76.7	78.7	77.8	77.3
L-Serine	82.2	82.0	83.3	82.5
L-Aspartate	82.2	86.1	85.7	84.7
L-Asparagine	95.9	95.1	100.0	97.0
L-Leucine	97.3	96.7	100.0	98.0
L-Lysine	95.9	99.2	100.8	98.6

[a] The GT was assayed according to the standard conditions in the presence or absence of 10 mmol of the respective amino acids per liter. The results (mean of two parallels) are expressed as percentage of the GT-activity without amino acids (Serum 1: 37 U/liter; serum 2: 61 U/liter; serum 3: 63 U/liter).

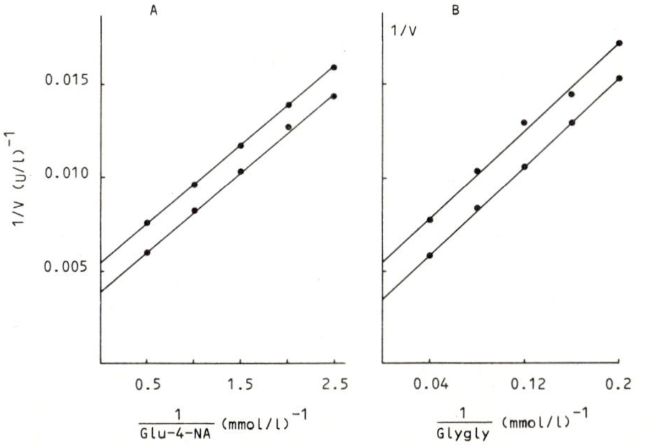

Fig. 3. Inhibition of GT by 0.15 mmol/liter 4-nitroaniline

Serum with GT activity of 194 U/liter (standard conditions) was used as the source of enzyme. Activities measured in triplets in a centrifugal analyzer. *A*: Glu-4-NA was varied (0.4–2 mmol/liter) at a fixed concentration of glygly (50 mmol/liter). *B*: Glygly was varied (5–25 mmol/liter) at a fixed concentration of glu-4-NA (4 mmol/liter). The assays were done with (*upper curves*) and without (*lower curves*) 4-nitroaniline

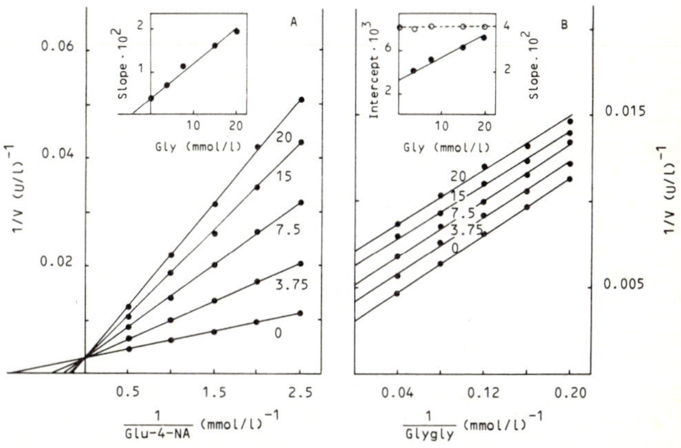

Fig. 4. Inhibition of GT by glycine

Serum with GT-activity of 253 U/liter (standard condition) was used as enzyme. The final concentrations of glycine were measured in triplets in a centrifugal analyzer. *A*: Glu-4-NA was varied (0.4–2.0 mmol/liter) at a fixed concentration of glygly (50 mmol/liter). *B*: Glygly was varied (5–25 mmol/liter) at a fixed concentration of glu-4-NA (4 mmol/liter). *Inset* shows the slopes (*stippled curves*) and intercepts of the respective figures vs. glycine concentrations

apparent parallel lines obtained in these experiments. Such inhibition patterns are not consistent with a sequential or a ping-pong mechanism, and suggest that 4-nitroaniline is not acting as a single-product inhibitor, but probably forms some kind of dead-end complexes with the enzyme, a common problem in product inhibition studies (*16*). In accordance with this, the product 4-nitroaniline inhibits significantly at concentrations (0.15 mmol/liter), which are low as compared to the substrate concentrations used (Figure 3), in spite of the fact that the equilibrium constant of this reaction most likely exceeds one (*18*).

Table 1 shows that various amino acids inhibit GT, glycine and alanine being the most potent of the amino acids tested. It would be reasonable to expect that these amino acids could serve as binding analogs of glu-4-NA and (or) glygly, and thus act as dead-end inhibitors of the enzyme. Figure 4*A* shows that glycine gives a pure competitive inhibition pattern with glu-4-NA as the variable substrate. A replot of the slopes vs. the glycine concentrations shows a linear competitive inhibition (*inset* of Figure 4*A*), the K_i for glycine being about 4 mmol/liter. Consequently, glycine appears to act as a binding analog of glu-4-NA. On the other hand, glycine with glygly as the variable substrate gives a clear uncompetitive inhibition pattern (Figure 4*B*). Quite similar inhibition patterns were found with alanine (results not shown), K_i in this case being about 7 mmol/liter. A competitive pattern with glu-4-NA and an uncompetitive pattern with glygly are consistent with the view that the GT acts according to a ping-pong mechanism. The other mechanism compatible with these inhibition patterns is an ordered sequential mechanism, in which glygly is the first and glu-4-NA the second substrate bound. However, this mechanism does not fit with the results in Figures 1 and 2.

In an attempt to study a binding analog to glygly, we synthesized a carbamide derivative of glygly in which the free amino-group of glygly is blocked. Unexpectedly, however, this derivative did not show any significant inhibition of GT when it was present in the incubation medium in a concentration as high as 40 mmol/liter.

Discussion

The present kinetic data indicate that when glu-4-NA and glygly are used as substrates, serum GT acts by a ping-pong bi-bi mechanism. A glutamyl enzyme complex is evidently formed as an intermediate, a conclusion consistent with recently reported kinetic data on purified rat kidney GT assayed with other substrates (*5, 19*). The likely sequence of reactions taking place is shown in modified Cleland notation (*14*) in Figure 5.

GT is able to act upon a variety of substrates, the acceptor site being relatively less specific than the γ-glutamyl site. Thus, Tate and Meister (*5*), when using glu-4-NA as donor substrate and highly purified rat kidney preparations as enzyme, observed considerable acceptor function of many different amino acids (including glycine and alanine) and of dipeptides. With serum as enzyme we found the acceptor function of amino acids to be far less pronounced. Thus, the GT activity with alanine (20 mmol/liter) was 8% of that with 50 mmol/liter glygly, and with glycine (20 mmol/liter) as well as with no acceptor substrate it was 6%. Relative to the activity found with 20 mmol/liter glygly, the respective values were 12% and 8%. The lack of acceptor activity of glycine is in agreement with results of Goldbarg et al. (*20*), who also used serum as source of enzyme. On the other hand, the present report demonstrates that various amino acids, particularly glycine and alanine, are inhibitors of GT, giving a pure competitive inhibition pattern with glu-4-NA and a pure uncompetitive pattern with glygly. Previously serine in the presence of borate (*21*) and glutamate (*22*) have been shown to inhibit GT. The most likely site of action of these amino acids is schematically indicated in Figure 5.

The present inhibition studies would lead one to predict that amino acids like glycine and alanine would indeed be poor acceptors. When such compounds are tested for their acceptor activities, their apparent ability to act as binding analogs of the donor results in the formation of dead-end complexes. It may thus be impossible clearly to separate the acceptor function from the inhibitory effect of such amino acids.

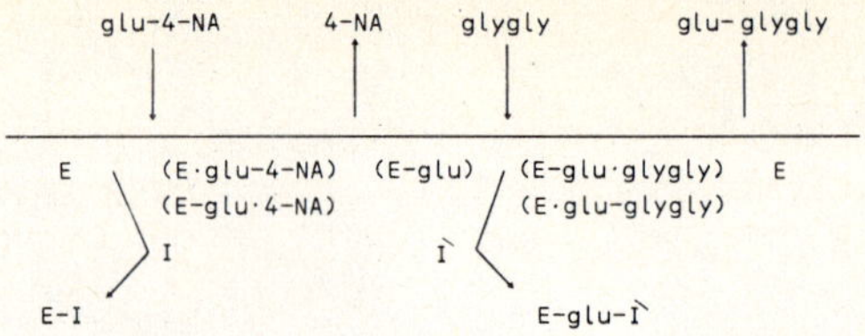

Fig. 5. Schematic illustration, in Cleland notation (*14*), of the most likely reactions

I = glygly, or amino acids (e.g., glycine or alanine), *I'* = glu-4-NA

Glycine and alanine are present in serum in far too low concentrations (normally about 0.2 and 0.3 mmol/liter, respectively) to influence the results of the GT measurements. The alanine inhibition, however, may represent a practical problem in clinical chemical laboratories, because the GT-incubation medium may be contaminated with alanine if the same enzyme analyzer with automatic pipetting of the second substrate is used to assay both alanine aminotransferase and GT.

The double competitive substrate inhibition here demonstrated is characteristic of a ping-pong mechanism to the extent that it is in itself an argument for such a mechanism (*16*). This means that glu-4-NA, besides reacting with the free enzyme, may combine in dead-end fashion with the glutamyl-enzyme complex, whereas glygly, besides reacting with the latter complex, also forms a dead-end complex with the free enzyme (Figure 5).

The double inhibitory substrate effect implies that the choice of concentration in the assay medium for the one substrate must entirely depend on the concentration chosen for the second substrate, and vice versa. Rosalki and Tarlow (*11*) have recently described an "optimized" method (37 °C) for GT in which the final concentration for glu-4-NA and glygly were 9 mmol/liter and 120 mmol/liter, respectively. However, it may be deduced from the curves in Figure 1*A* that under these conditions there must be a significant inhibition by glu-4-NA of the enzyme activity (deviation from a linear curve). Perhaps more severe shortcomings of the proposed modification come from practical considerations. The method requires that the reaction be started by glu-4-NA, which must be dissolved in 0.5 mmol/liter HCl because of its low solubility at neutral pH. Moreover, at this pH the glu-4-NA undergoes rapid hydrolysis, making the starting reagent unsuitable within a few hours on the bench (*13*). Thus, the spontaneous formation of 4-nitroaniline will not only increase the initial optical density of the incubation medium but may also inhibit the enzyme (Figure 3).

In our opinion, the concentration of glu-4-NA in the incubation medium should for practical reasons not exceed 4 mmol/liter. Figure 1*B* shows that under these conditions maximum activities will be obtained with a final concentration of glygly between 75 and 100 mmol/liter (the inflection of the curve). Accordingly, the Scandinavian Society for Clinical Chemistry and Clinical Physiology has recommended a method with final concentrations of 4 and 75 mmol/liter for glu-4-NA and glygly, respectively (*13*). It may be estimated from Figure 1*B* that this method, which offers important practical advantages, will give activities that are only 5 to 10% lower than those by the method proposed by Rosalki and Tarlow (*11*).

The excellent technical assistance of Oddvar Gamst and Anne Marie Sauren is gratefully acknowledged. We also want to express our sincere thanks to Clive Little, Ph.D., for valuable suggestions and discussions.

References

1. Schmidt, E., and Schmidt, F. W., γ-Glutamyl transpeptidase. *Dtsch. Med. Wochenschr.* **98,** 1572 (1973).

2. Kokot, F., and Sledzinski, Z., Die γ-Glutamyltransferase (γ-GT). *Z. Clin. Chem. Klin. Biochem.* **12,** 374 (1974).

3. Rosalki, S. B., Gamma-glutamyl transpeptidase. *Adv. Clin. Chem.* **17,** 53 (1975).

4. Ball, E. G. Revel, J. B., and Cooper, O., The quantitative measurement of γ-glutamyl transpeptidase activity. *J. Biol. Chem.* **221,** 895 (1956).

5. Tate, S. S., and Meister, A., Interaction of γ-glutamyl transpeptidase with amino acids, dipeptides, and derivatives and analogs of glutathione. *J. Biol. Chem.* **249,** 7593 (1974).

6. Orlowski, M., and Szewezuk, A., Determination of γ-glutamyl transpeptidase activity in human serum and urine. *Clin. Chim. Acta* **7,** 755 (1962).

7. Orlowski, M., and Meister, A., γ-Glutamyl-*p*-nitroanilide: A new convenient substrate for determination and study of L- and D-γ-glutamyl transpeptidase activities. *Biochim. Biophys. Acta* **73,** 679 (1963).

8. Szasz, G., Weimann, G., Stähler, F., et al., New substrates for measuring γ-glutamyl transpeptidase activity. *Z. Klin. Chem. Klin. Biochem.* **12,** 228 (1974).

9. Dimov, D. M., and Kulhánek, V., Comparison of four methods for the estimation of γ-glutamyl transpeptidase activity in biological fluids. *Clin. Chim. Acta* **16,** 271 (1967).

10. Szasz, G., A kinetic photometric method for serum γ-glutamyl transpeptidase. *Clin. Chem.* **15,** 124 (1969).

11. Rosalki, S. B., and Tarlow D., Optimized determination of γ-glutamyltransferase by reaction rate analysis. *Clin. Chem.* **20,** 1121 (1974).

12. Recommended methods for the determination of four enzymes in blood. *Scand. J. Clin. Lab. Invest.* **33,** 291 (1974).

13. Recommended method for the determination of γ-glutamyl transferase in blood. *Scand. J. Clin. Lab. Invest,* in press.

14. Cleland, W. W., The kinetics of enzyme-catalyzed reactions with two or more substrates or products. *Biochim. Biophys. Acta* **67,** 104 (1963).

15. Stark, G. R., Modification of proteins with cyanate. In *Methods in Enzymology,* **25,** S. P. Colowick and N. O. Kaplan, Eds. Academic Press, New York, N. Y., 1972, pp 579–584.

16. Cleland, W. W., Steady state kinetics. In *The Enzymes,* **II,** P. D. Boyer, Ed. Academic Press, New York, N. Y., 1970, pp 1–65.

17. Huseby, N. E., and Strømme, J. H., Practical points regarding routine determination of γ-glutamyl transferase (γ-GT) in serum with a kinetic method at 37 °C. *Scand. J. Clin. Lab. Invest.* **34,** 357 (1974).

18. Leibach, F. H., and Binkly, F., γ-Glutamyl transferase of swine kidney. *Arch. Biochem. Biophys.* **127,** 292 (1968).

19. Elce, J. S., Bryson, J., and McGirr, L. G., γ-Glutamyl transpeptidase of rat kidney. Some properties and kinetic constants. *Can. J. Biochem.* **52,** 33 (1974).

20. Goldbarg, J. A., Pineda, E. P., Smith, E. E., et al., A method for the colorimetric determination of γ-glutamyl transpeptidase in human serum; enzymatic activity in health and disease. *Gastroenterology* **44,** 127 (1963).

21. Taniguchi, N., Purification and some properties of γ-glutamyl transpeptidase from azo dye-induced hepatoma. *J. Biochem.* **75,** 473 (1974).

22. Bondar, R. J. L., and Moss, G. A., Enhancing effect of glutamate on apparent serum γ-glutamyltranspeptidase activity. *Clin. Chem.* **20,** 317 (1974).

CLIN. CHEM. 22/4, 422–428 (1976)

Method for Monitoring Plasma Progesterone Concentrations in Pregnancy

Per Winkel, Preben Gaede, and Jørgen Lyngbye

We present a time-series model for monitoring concentrations in plasma of hormones produced in the placenta, progesterone being chosen as an example. The model, which is based on the assumption that variations in plasma progesterone concentration in pregnant subjects mainly reflect variations in the growth rate of the placenta, was applied to eight series of progesterone values measured during pregnancy in eight subjects. In the model, which was found to fit the data, it is assumed that progesterone concentration is proportional to the size of the placenta and that the growth rate of the placenta varies at random, with a mean value α. The variation of α was of the same magnitude among and within the subjects. If the average of many subjects' α values is used, a single subject may be used as her own reference, based on only one previous observation. When two observations are available, an individual's own α value may be estimated and used for the prediction. The predictive power of the new method was found to be far superior to the conventional method in which a single sample reference material is used. Furthermore, one need not know the gestational age in order to use the method.

Additional Keyphrases: *monitoring and predicting values for hormones in plasma • pregnancy, changes during • placental growth • fetal status*

In evaluating the result of a laboratory test a reference interval based on data from an appropriate group of healthy subjects is often used.

For monitoring purposes (e.g.) much is gained by using the subject as his or her own reference, to eliminate inter-individual variation from the comparison. This requires the presence of one or more previous observations, obtained during a period when it was known that the subject was in a stable state, e.g., in "good health." But it is also necessary to know how to use these observations to predict what the values for future observations should be if the former stable state still exists. Thus a study of a chronological series of biological data is necessary before we can use the subject as his (or her) own reference.

Departments of Clinical Chemistry A and B, Rigshospitalet, University of Copenhagen, Copenhagen 2100; and Department of Clinical Chemistry, Central Hospital, Hillerod 3400, Denmark; and Institute of Mathematical Statistics, University of Copenhagen, Denmark.

Address correspondence to P.W., at the Department of Clinical Chemistry A, Rigshospitalet, 9 Blegdamsvej, University of Copenhagen, DK 2100, Copenhagen 0, Denmark.

Received June 25, 1975; accepted Jan. 15, 1976.

In the present investigation we used such a time-series model to analyze intra-individual changes in plasma progesterone concentration during pregnancy in a group of healthy subjects. For comparison, we computed the average time course of plasma progesterone concentrations during pregnancy, by using values for single samples obtained from healthy subjects at various stages of pregnancy.

Material and Methods

Materials

Plasma samples from each of 324 pregnant women with reliable menstrual data were used as the basis for calculating the nonparametric reference interval.

Plasma was sampled from eight pregnant women with reliable menstrual data at one- to three-week intervals during their pregnancy. A total of 72 samples were used in the consecutive series study (Figure 1).

All blood samples were drawn from the antecubital vein into heparinized glass tubes.

In all cases, pregnancy and the neonatal period were uncomplicated and birth took place in week 38 to 42. The infants' birth weights all exceeded 2500 g.

Analytical Method

Progesterone in plasma was estimated by a competitive protein-binding method (*1*), which we slightly modified: after extraction with petroleum ether (Mallinckrodt, "Nanograde") we took an aliquot (1500 μl) instead of the whole petroleum ether fraction (2000 μl) to improve the precision.

As binding protein, we used serum taken from the antecubital venous blood of postmenopausal women treated with high doses of estrogen (4 mg of estradiol, perorally, each day for eight days).

Statistical Methods

The subject as her own reference: We first examined if a simple exponential growth curve could fit the data obtained from the same subject. With this model the following assumptions are made:

(*a*) During later pregnancy—i.e., after the 12th week of pregnancy—the plasma progesterone value reflects the size of the placenta except for biological and analytical variation.

(*b*) At any given time (*t*) after the 12th week the growth rate of the placenta is proportional to the size it has already attained.

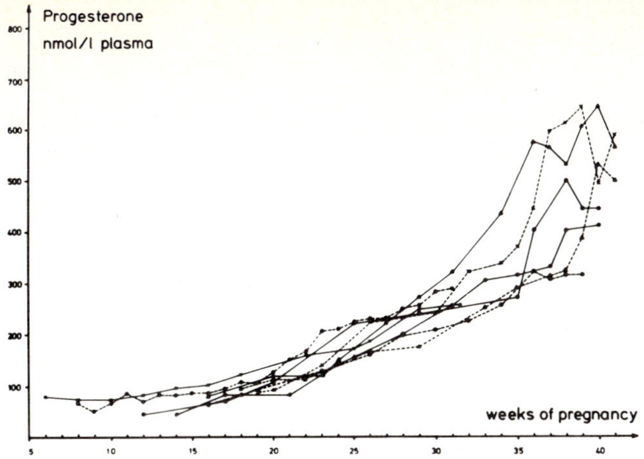

Fig. 1. Consecutive plasma progesterone values in eight pregnant women

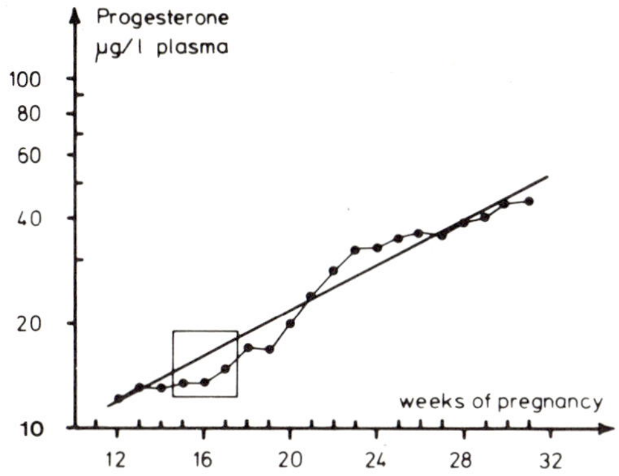

Fig. 2. Plasma progesterone values of a healthy pregnant subject as a function of duration of pregnancy

The regression line depicting the logarithm of the plasma progesterone value as a function of time is also shown. Note that the scale of the ordinate is logarithmic. The framed part of the figure is reproduced in Figure 3

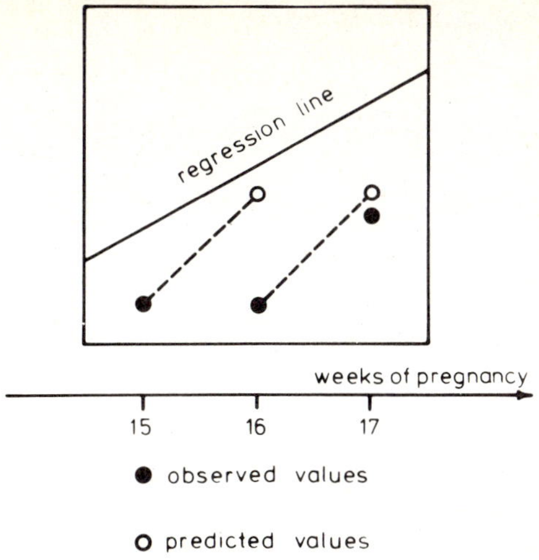

Fig. 3. A comparison of the prediction of plasma progesterone values in a pregnant subject by use of the regression line of Figure 2 and the method of the present study

The segment of the regression line and the corresponding observed values are taken from Figure 2

If the plasma progesterone value is proportional to the size of placenta, we have the following differential equation where $X(t)$ signifies the plasma progesterone level at time t: $\mathrm{d}X(t)/\mathrm{d}t = kX(t)$. The solution of this equation is $X(t) = A\mathrm{e}^{kt}$. This implies that the log of $X(t)$ is a linear function of time. Figure 2 shows the log of the plasma progesterone as a function of time for one of the eight healthy pregnant subjects. The regression line corresponding to the data is also shown. Note that the data points are not scattered at random around the regression line and that the slope between consecutive progesterone values varies considerably. Thus the model did not fit the data. We therefore choose another model that is based on the following assumptions:

(*a*) The plasma progesterone concentration reflects the size of placenta.

(*b*) The growth rate of the placenta is proportional to the size it has already attained; however, the proportionality constant varies at random over time, a growth model first studied by Lewontin and Cohen in 1969 (*2*). The model implies that the slope of the log of plasma progesterone depicted as a function of time will vary with time.

(*c*) The slope between consecutive progesterone values in such a semilogarithmic system reflects the growth rate over that period; i.e., we assume that the remaining biological and analytical variation is negligible in this context.

It should be noted that the model is only assumed to be valid between the 12th and 36th week of pregnancy. We may now compute an average of all slopes between consecutive progesterone values and use this average slope to predict a new progesterone value from the one previously observed. Let us focus on a smaller segment of the curve shown in Figure 2 and see how this type of prediction behaves as compared to that of the regression line. In Figure 3 we have computed the average of all the slopes of the previous curve. The prediction from one data point to the following is done as follows. Starting from one data point, one draws a line having the average slope that we just mentioned. The predicted value is found on this line. It is seen that the predicted points are much closer to the observed points than is the regression line. This is true for almost all the points shown on Figure 2.[1] Figure 4 shows how the average slope is computed. It appears that we are only using the first and the last observation. This means that the further apart the observations are in time, the better we are able to estimate the average slope. This is an important quality of the model in that it implies that if one observation is obtained during early pregnancy one can always get the best possible estimate of the average slope. The slopes then vary at random around a

[1] We submit that our comparison between the regression model and the present model does not allow us to draw any definite conclusions, because it was only based on one example where the sample size was sufficiently large for the performance of a detailed comparison between the two models. However, our main reason for choosing the present model is that we think that the assumptions upon which this model is based are more realistic than those upon which the regression model is based.

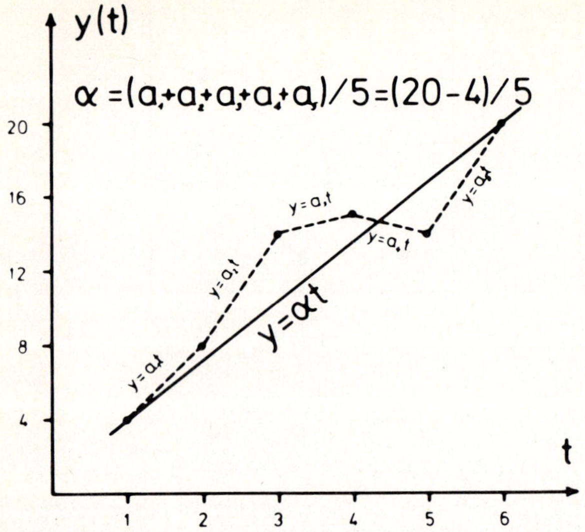

Fig. 4. A constructed example where $Y(t)$ symbolizes the log of the plasma progesterone value and t symbolizes the duration of pregnancy

The example illustrates the computation of the average value (α) of the slopes of the lines connecting consecutive Y-values. It is noted that the net result of the computations may be obtained as the difference between the last and the first Y-value divided by the difference between the corresponding t-values

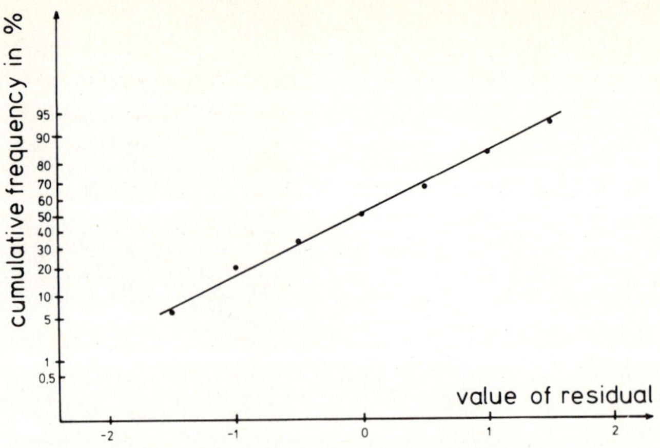

Fig. 5. Empirical distribution of the normalized residuals in the consecutive plasma progesterone series

The figure was drawn on normal-probability paper

mean value, α. The estimate of α is $\hat{\alpha} = (Y_n - Y_1)/t_n - t_1$, where Y_n denotes the log of the nth or last observation of the plasma progesterone value and Y_1 the first one, t_n is the last observation time and t_1 the first observation time. The variance of the slopes (σ^2) may also be estimated from the data (see the Appendix). We emphasize that although only the first and last observation are used when α is estimated, all observations are used in estimating σ^2. The change in the log of the plasma progesterone value over the time period $\Delta t = (t_{i+1} - t_i)$ may be predicted by the model as $\hat{\alpha} \times \Delta t$, and the deviation from the observed change $(Y_{i+1} - Y_i)$ computed as $r_i = (Y_{i+1} - Y_i) - (\hat{\alpha} \times \Delta t)$. For each subject and for all pairs of consecutive values we computed r_i and divided by its variance (see Appendix) to obtain a normalized deviation from the model. To examine the validity of the model we compared the common distribution of all normalized residuals to a normal distribution with mean zero and variance one (see Figure 5).

Single-sample analysis: We analyzed the data from the single samples observations from the 324 pregnant women by a nonparametric method previously published by one of us (*3*).

Results

The analysis of the empirical distribution of the normalized residuals showed that the model adopted for the eight subjects for whom consecutive progesterone values were available adequately described the data; that is to say, the empirical distribution based on all the 72 normalized residuals did not differ significantly from the theoretical. The two distributions are depicted in Figure 5. Evidently there is very good correspondence between the distributions. Table 1 shows the estimates of α_i and σ_i^2 for each of the eight females. The autocorrelation coefficients in those cases where we were able to calculate them did not differ significantly from zero.[2]

Table 1. Estimates of α_i and σ_i^2 for Eight Pregnant Women

Patient no.	Gestation, weeks	$n_i - 2$	$\hat{\alpha}_i \times 10^2$	$\hat{\sigma}_i^2 \times 10^4$
1	21	6	4.02	35
2	18	7	4.02	18
3	24	5	3.96	61
4	17	6	2.81	6
5	23	7	2.86	16
6	20	7	4.26	14
7	19	7	2.57	4
8	19	18	3.02	9
Weighted averages			3.46	17.1

The comparison of the variances for the eight women showed that they were significantly different ($\chi^2_{(7)} = 36.5$, $P < 0.01$), mainly owing to the large variances observed in subjects 1 and 3. The variation of α_i among the subjects was 9×10^{-4}, which is of the same order of magnitude as within the subjects. The common estimates of σ^2 and α were 17.1×10^{-4} and 3.46×10^{-2}, respectively.

Based on these two estimates, two tables were constructed. The first (Table 2) relates the minimal percentage increase in the plasma progesterone concentration to the number of weeks elapsed since the first

[2] The estimate obtained by pooling the individual $R_i(1)$ values (for nomenclature see Appendix) is −0.27, which is significantly different from zero. By contrast the estimate obtained by pooling the $R_i(2)$ values is 0.04, which is not significantly different from zero. Thus it appears that the differences are statistically interdependent on account of measurement error.

Table 2. Minimum Relative Increase of Concentration When Only One Earlier Observation Is Available

Gestation, weeks	Minimum increase, in percent of observed value	Lower limit, in percent of observed value
1/7	−4.7	95.3
1/2	−6.9	93.1
1	−7.5	92.5
2	−6	94
3	−3	97
4	0	100
5	5	105
10	35	135
15	80	180
20	144	244

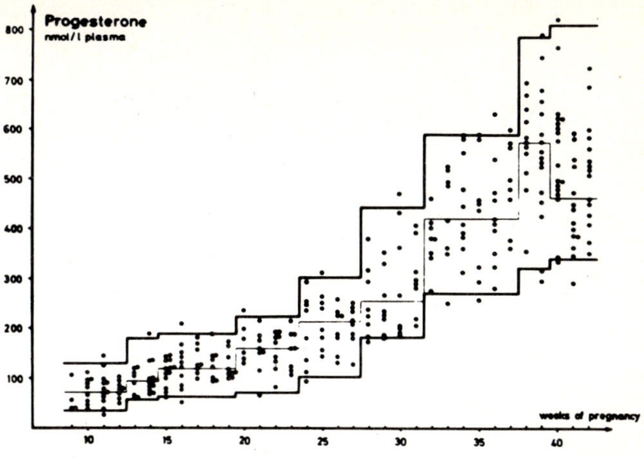

Fig. 6. The single-sample plasma progesterone values together with the 0.05, 0.50, and 0.95 fractiles corresponding to the sets of observations, with use of a nonparametric method

observation; i.e., this table is applicable if only one previous observation is available. The second table (Table 3) gives the lowest probable values of the observations (in percent of the predicted values) that is allowable at the 5% level of significance. The tolerance depends on the number of weeks elapsed since the first and the last measurements (see Appendix). This table may be used when more than one observation is available.

The single-sample plasma progesterone values are depicted in Figure 6 as a function of the duration of pregnancy together with the 0.05, 0.50, and 0.95 fractiles corresponding to the sets of observations delimited by the nonparametric method.

Figure 7 shows progesterone values observed in a patient who had an abortion during the 21st week of pregnancy. None of the values is abnormal in the sense that it is lower than the lower normal limit computed from the single sample values. However, when Table 2 is used to compute the lower 5% limit for observation number 2—i.e., when the subject is used as her own reference—it is seen that this obser-

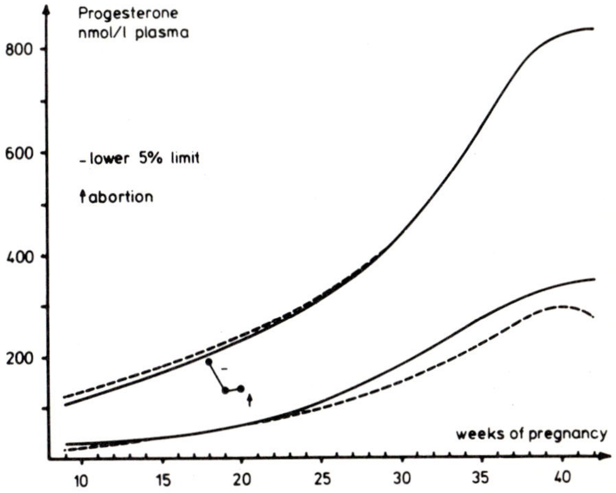

Fig. 7. Three plasma progesterone values for a patient who had an abortion during the 21st week of pregnancy

Smooth curves of the nonparametric reference interval (0.05 and 0.95 fractiles, *solid lines, cf.* Figure 3), and the reference interval determined by an ordinary parametric method (mean ±2 SD) on the same set of observations (*dotted lines*)

Table 3. Minimum Concentration, in Percent of Predicted Value, in Case of More Than One Observation

No. weeks since last observation / No. weeks since first observation	1/7	1/2	1	2	3	4	5	10
1	93.8	85.5						
2	94.0	88.0	80.1					
3	94.1	88.5	82.5	68.1				
4	94.1	88.8	83.4	73.0	58.0			
5	94.2	88.9	83.9	75.1	65.0	49.5		
10	94.2	89.2	84.7	78.0	72.2	66.7	60.8	
15	94.2	89.3	85.0	78.8	73.8	69.3	65.0	42.3
∞	94.2	89.5	85.5	80.1	76.2	73.0	70.5	60.8

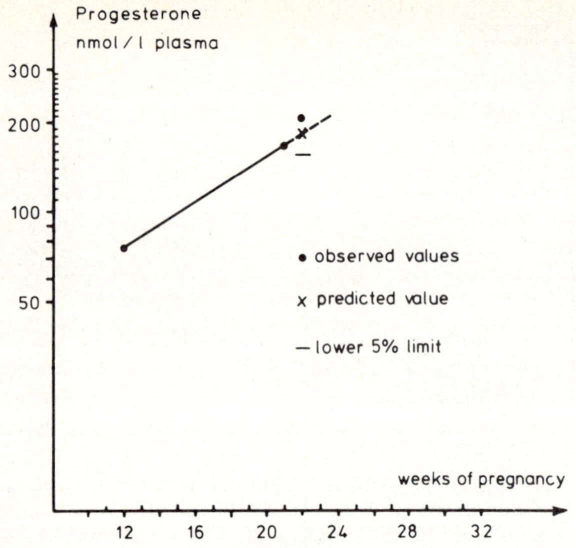

Fig. 8. Three observed plasma progesterone values in subject No. 8, plotted on semilogarithmic paper

The first and second values are connected by a straight line to obtain the predicted value at the time of the third observation; the lower 5% limit is obtained by using Table 4

vation is highly abnormal. Figure 8 illustrates that the method is also easy to use when two observations are available. The values observed in subject No. 8 are used as an example. If we want to find the value predicted for week 22 based on the two values observed during the 12th and 21st week, respectively, the latter two values are plotted on semilogarithmic paper and connected by a straight line. The predicted value is read from this line and the lower 5% value is computed by using Table 3. It is seen that the value observed during the 22nd week is well above the 5% limit.

Discussion

In the present study we have compared a method for using an individual as her own reference and compared this procedure with the use of a conventional reference interval based on single-sample values.

By comparison with earlier investigations in which comparable analytical techniques were used (competitive protein-binding, radioimmunoassay) it appears that between the 15th and 25th week of pregnancy the lower limit of the single-sample reference interval is a little lower than that found by other workers (*4–6*). This difference may not be attributed to our use of nonparametric statistics, because we obtained nearly the same lower limit in this period of pregnancy by using an ordinary parametric method (mean ±2 SD; see Figure 7).

In late pregnancy (week 27–36), however, we found the lower limit to be about 30% higher by using nonparametric statistics compared to the ordinary parametric method applied to the same progesterone values.

An important aspect of the model in which a subject is used as her own reference is that the growth rate of the placenta is not assumed to be related to the size of placenta by a fixed proportionality factor. The model allows the latter factor to vary at random, which in our opinion is a more realistic concept. It should be noted, however, that the production and elimination of progesterone is assumed to be in equilibrium at time t, so that $X(t)$ only reflects the size of placenta. While the growth rate is allowed to vary at random in the model, the production of progesterone is assumed to be related to the size of placenta by an unknown but constant proportionality factor. This concept is not realistic when the placenta is small, because the production of progesterone will probably vary from cell to cell and also within the same cell from time to time, and a considerable part of the progesterone will still come from the persisting corpus luteum. The model is not applied before the 12th week of pregnancy. Later in pregnancy, as an approximation, the assumption is a realistic one in that the number of placental cells now is so large that the law of large numbers should apply.

Nevertheless, we want to emphasize that in all probability the model only represents a very crude approximation to the biological mechanisms regulating plasma progesterone. Thus for a given population of cells the total production of progesterone may vary over time. Also it should be remembered that progesterone is stored in the fatty tissue and the transport of progesterone between water and fat may be slow and subject to the influence of many varying factors. It is also assumed in the model that the analytical error is negligible, although there are some indications that this assumption may be incorrect.[3] However, our purpose was not to study the biological mechanisms regulating the progesterone concentration, but rather to devise a method that, although based on crude assumptions, is of value for predictive purposes.

The application of the model implies that the gestational age is between 12 and 36 weeks, but no further assumptions are made. Thus it is not necessary to know the exact gestational age to apply the model. Therefore, in cases where the gestational age is uncertain the model might be used to predict the time of birth, in that the model should not apply just before birth.

We found a statistically significant variation among the intra-individual variances, but this does not preclude that an estimate of the common variance may be used. This approach is probably better

[3] The assumption that the differences between consecutive observations are independent was not valid, because the measurement error was not negligible. In the present study we ignored this violation. Alternative approaches would be to include this dependency in the model or to decrease the measurement error. The former approach is very complicated even if measurements are obtained at equidistant times, and almost untractable if they are not. Thus, to impose this restriction severely limits the practical applicability of the model. Therefore we would recommend that either the measurement error be decreased or that one ignore the dependency as we did. But some clinical experience with the model is needed before it is possible to decide this issue.

than to estimate the variance separately for each subject, because such an estimate usually tends to be very poor, owing to the small number of samples. Furthermore, with this method it is necessary to have at least two observations before a prediction can be made.

However, we want to emphasize that our estimate of the common variance, which is based only on data from eight subjects, may be unreliable. Therefore Tables 2 and 3, which we used for the predictions, should only be taken as an illustrative example.

The method presented here is useful in practice, and in our opinion it is based on assumptions that are more realistic than those of the regression analysis.

We emphasize that the present work is a methodological study. Human placental lactogen and estriol (or its derivatives) are probably more valuable quantities in the clinical context than is progesterone (7). Because the production of estriol involves both the fetus and the placenta, the present model may not apply. However, placental lactogen is produced solely in the placenta and may therefore follow the same model as progesterone. We now are exploring this possibility.

References

1. Johansson, E. D. B., Progesterone levels in peripheral plasma during the luteal phase of the normal human menstrual cycle measured by a rapid competitive protein binding technique. *Acta Endocrinol.* (Copenhagen) **61,** 592 (1969).
2. Lewontin, R. C., and Cohen, D., On population growth in a randomly varying environment. *Proc. Nat. Acad. Sci. USA* **62,** 1056 (1969).
3. Winkel, P., and Jorgensen, K., A method for the computation of age-dependent reference intervals. *Scand. J. Clin. Lab. Invest.* **31,** 481 (1973).
4. Abraham, G. E., Swerdloff, R., Tulchinsky, D., and Odell, W. D., Radioimmunoassay of plasma progesterone. *J. Clin. Endocrinol.* **32,** 619 (1971).
5. Johansson, E. D. B., Plasma levels of progesterone in pregnancy measured by a rapid competitive protein binding technique. *Acta Endocrinol.* (Copenhagen) **61,** 607 (1969).
6. Luisi, M., Levanti, S., and Franchi, F., The description and evaluation of a competitive protein-binding radioassay of plasma progesterone in pregnancy. *Fert. Steril.* **22,** 435 (1971).
7. Braunstein, G. D., Grodin, J. M., Vaitukaitis, J., and Ross, G. T., Secretory rate of human chorionic gonadotropin by normal trophoblast. *Am. J. Obstet. Gynecol.* **115,** 447 (1973).

Appendix

Stephen L. Lauritzen

Stochastic Model

As the stochastic model we choose an approximation to a model for cell growth in a random environment, suitable when the total number of cells is large. The model was first studied by Lewontin and Cohen (*A1*). See also Capocelli and Ricciardi (*A2*), Keiding and Nielsen (*A3*) and Keiding (*A4*).

We assume that the concentration $X(t)$ of plasma progesterone at time t is a stochastic process satisfying the differential equation

$$\frac{dX(t)}{dt} = a(t)X(t),$$

where $a(t)$ is "white noise," i.e., all $a(t)$'s are independent and identically normally distributed. Let $Y(t) = \log X(t)$. It follows that $Y(t)$ is a Wiener process with linear drift; in other words, the $Y(t)$'s are normally distributed with mean and variance proportional to t and with increments over disjoint time-intervals independent.

Statistical Model

For patient i, let $t_{i1}, \ldots, t_{in_i}$ denote the points in time at which measurements were made, and let $Y(t_{i1}), \ldots, Y(t_{in_i})$ denote these measurements. Let, for $i = 1, \ldots, 8$, $j = 1, \ldots, n_i - 1$, $\Delta_{ij} = Y(t_{i,j+1}) - Y(t_{ij})$ and $d_{ij} = t_{i,j+1} - t_{ij}$.

If we assume that the measurement error is negligible as compared to the random variations of the concentrations themselves, then Δ_{ij}, $i = 1, \ldots, 8$, $j = 1, \ldots, n_i - 1$ are independent normally distributed with mean $E\{\Delta_{ij}\} = \alpha_i d_{ij}$ and variance $V\{\Delta_{ij}\} = \sigma_i^2 d_{ij}$, where $\sigma_i^2 > 0$ and $-\infty < \alpha_i < \infty$ are unknown.

Analysis of the Model

By standard linear methods (*A5*) we get the estimates

$$\hat{\sigma}_i = \frac{\sum_{i=1}^{n_i-1} \Delta_{ij}}{\sum_{j=1}^{n_i-1} d_{ij}} = \frac{Y(t_{in_i}) - Y(t_{i1})}{t_{in_i} - t_{i1}}$$

$$\hat{\sigma}_i^2 = \frac{1}{n_i - 2} \sum_{j=1}^{n_i-1} \frac{\Delta_{ij}^2}{d_{ij}} - \frac{\left(\sum_{j=1}^{n_i-1} \Delta_{ij}\right)^2}{\sum_{j=1}^{n_i-1} d_{ij}}$$

the α_i's, and $\hat{\sigma}_i^2$ being statistically independent, $\hat{\alpha}_i$ normally distributed with mean α_i and variance $\sigma_i^2/(t_{in_i} - t_{i1})$, and $\hat{\sigma}_i^2$ following and χ^2/f distribution with $f = n_i - 2$ degrees of freedom.

Under the hypothesis that $\sigma_1^2 = \sigma_2^2 = \ldots = \sigma_8^2 = \sigma^2$ (which is tested by Bartlett's test), the common estimate of σ^2 is

$$\hat{\sigma}^2 = \frac{\sum_{i=1}^{8} (n_i - 2])\hat{\sigma}_i^2}{\sum_{i=1}^{8} n_i - 16} \qquad (1)$$

Under the assumption of identical variances and of

$$\alpha_1 = \alpha_2 = \ldots = \alpha_8 = \alpha \qquad (2)$$

the common estimate of α is

$$\hat{\hat{\alpha}} = \frac{\sum_{i=1}^{8} \hat{\alpha}_i (t_{in_i} - t_{i1})}{\sum_{i=1}^{8} (t_{in_i} - t_{i1})} = \frac{\sum_{i=1}^{8} \sum_{j=1}^{n_i-1} \Delta_{ij}}{\sum_{i=1}^{8} \sum_{j=1}^{n_i-1} d_{ij}}$$

The hypothesis (2) is tested by an F-test comparing the estimate (1) of σ^2 with

$$\hat{\hat{\sigma}}^2 = \frac{1}{7}\sum_{i=1}^{8} (\hat{\alpha}_i - \hat{\alpha})^2 (t_{in_i} - t_{i1})$$

Under (2), σ^2 is estimated by

$$\tilde{\sigma}^2 = \frac{\left(\sum_{i=1}^{8} n_i - 16\right)\hat{\sigma}^2 + 7\hat{\hat{\sigma}}^2}{\sum_{i=1}^{8} n_i - 9}$$

Control of the Model

Let

$$r_{ij} = \frac{\Delta_{ij} - \hat{\alpha}_i d_{ij}}{\hat{\sigma}_i \sqrt{d_{ij}}}$$

be the normalized residuals. Under the assumption that the Δ_{ij}'s are independent, the autocorrelations

$$R_i(k) = \sum_{j=1}^{n_i-k} r_{ij} r_{i,j+k}$$

follow a distribution with mean approximately zero and variance approximately equal to $1/(n_i - k + 1)$. It follows that

$$R(k) = \frac{\sum_{i=1}^{8} (n_i - k - 1) R_i(k)}{\sum_{i=1}^{8} n_i - 8(k+1)}$$

is approximately normal, with mean zero and variance $1/\sum_{i=1}^{8} n_i - 8((k+1)$.

An alternative to the Δ_{ij}'s being independent could be caused by a nonnegligible measurement error; i.e., suppose that we instead of $Y(t)$ observe $Y^*(t) = Y(t) + \epsilon(t)$, where the ϵ's are independent of the Y's, the $\epsilon(t)$'s being i.i.d.r.v. following a normal distribution with mean 0 and variance τ^2. In that case we should have

$$R_i(1) \approx \frac{-\tau^2}{\alpha_i^2 + \tau^2} = \frac{E(\Delta_{ij} - \alpha_i d_{ij})(\Delta_{i,j+1} - \alpha_i d_{i,j+1})}{\sqrt{E(\Delta_{ij} - \alpha_i d_{ij})^2 E(\Delta_{i,j+1} - \alpha_i d_{ij})^2}}$$

and analogous here to

$$R_i(k) \approx 0 \text{ for } k \geq 2.$$

Prediction

One observation available: Assuming equal known variance σ^2, and drift α, we get, if $Y(t_0)$ is observed, the predicted value at time t to be

$$Y(t) = Y(t_0) + \alpha(t - t_0)$$

and the prediction error

$$\epsilon(t) = Y(t) - \hat{Y}(t) = Y(t) - Y(t_0) - \alpha(t - t_0)$$

which has a normal distribution with mean 0 and variance $\sigma^2(t - t_0)$. Hence a lower β-confidence limit for $Y(t)$ based on $Y(t_0)$ is

$$Y(t_0) + \alpha(t - t_0) - u_\beta \sigma \sqrt{t - t_0}$$

where u_β is the β-fractile in the U-distribution. For the original observation we then have that $X(t)$ should be *at least*

$$10^{Y(t_0)} + \alpha(t - t_0) - u_\beta \sigma \sqrt{t - t_0}$$

which is a relative increase of at least

$$100 \times (10^{\alpha(t-t_0)} - u_\beta \sigma \sqrt{t - t_0} - 1)\,\% \qquad (3)$$

Expression (3) is computed in Table 3 for $\sigma^2 = 17.1 \times 10^{-4}$, $\beta = 95\%$, $\alpha = .0346$.

More than one observation available: Under the assumption of σ^2 being known and fixed for all patients, we get the predicted value $\hat{Y}(t+h)$ from observations $Y(t_1), Y(t_2), \ldots, Y(t)$, where $t_1 < t_2 < \ldots < t < t + h$, because

$$\hat{Y}(t+h) = Y(t_1) + (Y(t) - Y(t_1))\frac{t - t_1 + h}{t - t_1}$$

Note that only the end-point observations $Y(t_1)$ and $Y(t)$ are required to compute $\hat{Y}(t+h)$.

We have the prediction error

$$\epsilon(t,t+h) = Y(t+h) - \hat{Y}(t+h) = (Y(t+h) - Y(t)) - \frac{h}{t - t_1}(Y(t) - Y(t_1))$$

which is normal with mean zero and variance

$$\sigma^2\left(h + \frac{h^2}{t - t_1}\right)$$

A lower β-confidence limit for $Y(t+h)$ is then

$$Y(t) - Y(t_1)\frac{t - t_1 + h}{t - t_1} + Y(t_1) - \sigma u_\beta \sqrt{h\frac{t + h - t_1}{t - t_1}}$$

i.e., $Y(t+h)$ has to be *at least*

$$100 \times 10^{-\sigma u_\beta \sqrt{h \times t + h - t_1/t - t_1}}\,\% \qquad (4)$$

of its predicted value. This expression has been computed in Table 4 for $\beta = 95\%$ and $\sigma^2 = 17.1 \times 10^{-2}$.

References to the Appendix

A1. Lewontin, R. C., and Cohen, D., On population growth in a randomly varying environment. *Proc. Nat. Acad. Sci. USA* **62,** 1056 (1969).

A2. Capocelli, R. M., and Ricciardi, L. M., A diffusion model for population growth in random environment. *Theor. Popul. Biol.* **5,** 28 (1974).

A3. Keiding, N., and Nielsen, J. E., The growth of supercritical branching processes with random environments. *Ann. Probability* **1,** 1065 (1973).

A4. Keiding, N., Extinction and exponential growth in random environments. *Theor. Popul. Biol.* 8 (1975) (to appear).

A5. Rao, C. R., *Linear Statistical Inference and its Applications.* Wiley, New York, N.Y., 1965.

CLIN. CHEM. 22/4, 429–433 (1976)

Adaptation of Blank-Corrected Methods for Measurement of Total and Conjugated Bilirubin and Uric Acid to the Centrifugal Analyzer

Robert E. Cross, M. Geraldine Heintges, John Savory, and Peter W. Wentz

The blank-corrected determination in serum of total and conjugated bilirubin and of uric acid has been adapted to the centrifugal analyzer. Bilirubin is measured by a modified Jendrassik and Grof procedure; uric acid is determined kinetically by using a reaction based on reduction of ferric ion, including a uricase-treated blank. Sensitivity and precision of both methods are excellent, and results compare well with those obtained by commonly used procedures.

Interferences with spectrophotometric determinations generally fall into one of two categories. In the "static" type of interferences, those involving interferants that do not undergo chemical change during the analytical reaction, the blank correction consists of a simple subtraction. In the other ("kinetic") type of interference, the interfering substance(s) chemically reacts with some component of the analytical mixture, so that the relative importance of its contribution is time-dependent as well as concentration-dependent. If the interfering material reacts appreciably faster than the analyte, its presence may be effectively corrected for by a kinetic analysis, with prudent choice of the time interval selected for measurement. On the other hand, if the interferant reacts at about the same rate as the analyte, then it is corrected for by doing the determination with the analyte present and absent. Again, the correction is a simple subtraction.

Here, we exemplify blank corrections for each of these two types of interferences when the centrifugal analyzer is used.

In developing centrifugal analyzer methods for measuring total and conjugated bilirubin by the procedure of Jendrassik and Grof (*1*), we saw that two types of static interference would be encountered. Because of the relatively large sample/reagent volume ratio necessary to attain the desired sensitivity, certain sera, especially if lipemic or hemolytic, gave rise to rather large sample blanks. Furthermore, the reagent blank itself was not only significant, but also varied somewhat with time. The methods we report correct for both of these static interferences.

The methods for the measurement of total and conjugated bilirubin are based on the Jendrassik and Grof procedure (*1*). The procedure for uric acid involves treating serum with a reagent containing Fe^{3+} and 2,4,6-tri-(2-pyridyl)-*s*-triazine. Uric acid reduces Fe^{3+} to Fe^{2+}, and an intensely purple chelate is concomitantly formed with the ligand; this chelate is monitored kinetically at 600 nm in the centrifugal analyzer by use of a two-point fixed-time rate program. Calculations are based on comparing reagent blank-corrected absorbance changes of samples and standard between 30 and 180 s after the reaction is begun. Because serum contains non-uric acid reducing substances, a blank is run for each serum sample by pre-incubating an aliquot of serum with uricase (urate oxidase, EC 1.7.3.3) before the analytical reaction.

Division of Clinical Chemistry, Departments of Medicine, Pathology, Biochemistry, and Hospital Laboratories, The University of North Carolina at Chapel Hill, Chapel Hill, N. C. 27514.

Received Nov. 11, 1975; accepted Jan. 15, 1976.

Materials and Methods

Apparatus

The centrifugal analyzer we used was an Aminco Rotochem II (American Instrument Co., Silver Spring, Md. 20901) that is under complete computer control and has a 15-place transfer disc. We used an automatic dispensing device (Rotofill II, American Instrument Co.) that can load a transfer disc in 84 s. Eppendorf microliter pipets (Brinkmann Instruments, Inc., Westbury, N. Y. 11590) were used for all manual pipetting functions.

Reagents

For total and conjugated bilirubin.

Caffeine. Dissolve 50 g of caffeine, 75 g of sodium benzoate, and 125 g of sodium acetate in water at 60 °C, and dilute to 1.00 liter when cool. This reagent is stable for six months at room temperature.

Sulfanilic acid. Dissolve 10 g of sulfanilic acid in water containing 15 ml of concentrated HC1 and dilute to 1.00 liter. This reagent is stable for six months at room temperature.

Sodium nitrite. Dissolve 0.5 g of sodium nitrite in 100 ml of water. This reagent is stable for a week when stored at 4 °C.

Diazo reagent. Mix 10 ml of sulfanilic acid reagent with 0.25 ml of sodium nitrite reagent. Prepare just before use.

Standard. In the absence of direct light, dilute lyophilized control serum (Versatol Pediatric; General Diagnostics, Morris Plains, N. J. 07950) with physiological saline to about 50 mg of bilirubin per liter, based on the manufacturer's assay value. The calculated value for each new batch of this secondary standard should be confirmed before use by running it as a sample against a dimethyl sulfoxide solution of bilirubin Standard Reference Material (National Bureau of Standards, Washington, D. C. 20234) in a phosphate-buffered solution of albumin, prepared according to Gadd (*2*), as the primary standard. Alternatively, the solution of reference material itself may be used for standardization. Rapidly dispense 2-ml aliquots into plastic vials, seal, and store in the dark at −20 °C. Thaw and mix thoroughly just before use. This standard is stable for one month at −20 °C.

For uric acid.

Acetate buffer, pH 4.95. To 800 ml of distilled water add 12 g of sodium hydroxide, 29 ml of glacial acetic acid and 2 ml of "Triton X-100" surfactant. Adjust the pH to 4.95 with concentrated hydrochloric acid, and dilute to 1.00 liter with distilled water. Prepare freshly each month.

2,4,6,-Tri-(2-pyridyl)-s-triazine, 24 mmol/liter. Dissolve 1.878 g of 2,4,6,-tri-(2-pyridyl)-*s*-triazine (Aldrich Chemical Co., Inc., Milwaukee, Wis. 53233) in an acid-washed 250-ml volumetric flask to which 200 ml of water and 4 ml of concentrated hydrochloric acid have been added. Mix thoroughly and dilute to 250 ml. Prepare freshly each month.

Ferric chloride, 40 mmol/liter. To a 100-ml volumetric flask containing 0.16 ml of concentrated hydrochloric acid in distilled de-ionized water, add 1.08 g of $FeCl_3 \cdot 6H_2O$ and dilute to volume. The reagent is stable for one month at room temperature.

Bovine albumin, 300 g/liter (Pentex, Miles Laboratories, Kankakee, Ill. 60901).

2-Propanol, Certified ACS "Spectranalyzed" (Fisher Scientific Co., Fair Lawn, N. J. 07410).

1-Butanol, ACS reagent grade.

Working reagent. To a 100-ml graduated cylinder add 50 ml of acetate buffer, 20 ml of 2-propanol, 13 ml of 1-butanol, 16 ml of 2,4,6,-tri-(2-pyridyl)-*s*-triazine solution, and 3.2 ml of the ferric chloride solution. Mix after each addition and allow to stand for 5 min before use. Prepare this reagent immediately before use.

Uricase, approximately 18 000 U/liter, in glycerol/water (equal volumes) (Boehringer Mannheim Corp. New York, N. Y. 10017). New batches of this reagent must be checked for adequate activity before use. This is done by running a uricase blank on the 100 mg/liter uric acid standard by the procedure described for serum blanks. Incubation of this standard for 2–5 min with 5 μl of uricase should eliminate all uric acid activity, so that a final reading of 0–4.0 mg/liter is printed out for the cuvette containing the standard blank.

Bovine albumin, 60 g/liter. Dilute 20 ml of bovine albumin (300 g/liter) to 100 ml with distilled de-ionized water. Stable for one month.

Stock uric acid standard, 1 g/liter. Add exactly 1.000 g of uric acid Standard Reference Material (National Bureau of Standards, Washington, D. C. 20234) and 600 mg of lithium carbonate to 800 ml of distilled de-ionized water in a 1-liter volumetric flask. Sonicate the flask in an ultrasonic bath until the contents have dissolved, and dilute to 1.00 liter. Keep refrigerated and make freshly each month.

Working uric acid standard, 100 mg/liter. Pipet 10 ml of stock uric acid standard into a 100-ml volumetric flask to which 50 ml of distilled de-ionized water and 20 ml of bovine albumin (300 g/liter) have been added. Mix carefully, dilute to volume, and store at 4 °C. Prepare fresh working standard weekly.

Table 1. Protocol for Transfer-Disc Loading for Bilirubin Measurements

Cuvette no.	Sample well	Reagent well
Bilirubin, blank		
0	—	H_2O, 500 μl
1	H_2O, 50 μl	Sample,[a] 50 μl Saline flush, 200 μl H_2O, 200 μl
2–14	H_2O, 50 μl	Sample,[a] 50 μl Saline flush, 200 μl H_2O, 200 μl
Bilirubin, total		
0	—	H_2O, 500 μl
1–14	Diazo reagent, 50 μl	Sample,[a] 50 μl Saline flush, 200 μl Caffeine reagent, 200 μl
Bilirubin, conjugated		
0	—	H_2O, 500 μl
2	Diazo reagent, 50 μl	Sample,[a] 50 μl Saline flush, 200 μl Caffeine reagent, 200 μl
1, 3–14	Diazo reagent, 50 μl	Sample,[a] 50 μl Saline flush, 200 μl HCl, 200 μl

[a] Water is contained in sample well at position 1, standard in position 2, test sera in positions 3–14.

Procedures

For bilirubin. The analyses are performed in the following sequence. A transfer disc is loaded for the blank measurements (Table 1) and analyzed by use of a Cuvette Calibration program, which stores the blank absorbance values. The determinations of total and conjugated bilirubin in these same samples are then performed in sequential transfer discs by use of an Endpoint II program (Table 1). Note that the standards in those transfer discs used for the measurement of conjugated bilirubin are run under the same conditions used for the total assay, because this material contains only unconjugated bilirubin.

All measurements are made at 550 nm, after an initial 10-s mixing of sample and reagents. The computer is programmed to take a final absorbance reading after 60 s for the samples and 30 s for the blanks. The loading sequence of samples and reagents into the transfer disc is given in Table 1.

Calculations are performed automatically by the computer as follows: $C_u = C_s \times [A_u - (A_{RB} + A_{UB})]/[A_s - (A_{RB} + A_{SB})]$, where C_u = concentration of bilirubin in serum sample; C_s = concentration of standard; A_u = absorbance of serum reaction; A_{RB} = absorbance of reagent blank; A_{UB} = absorbance of serum blank (stored during the blank measurements); A_s = absorbance of standard; and A_{SB} = absorbance of standard blank.

For uric acid. In the uric acid procedure, blank corrections are made from the blanks that occupy positions of the transfer disc adjacent to their respective test samples.

Deliver 10 μl of uricase reagent to the sample wells of the serum blank positions (positions 4, 6, 8, 10, 12, 14) of the transfer disc. In sample position 1, which serves as a reagent blank, is bovine albumin solution (60 g/liter); standard is in position 2, sample 1 in position 3, the blank for sample 1 in position 4, etc. The conditions for the test are given in Table 2. Before any measurements are made in the centrifugal analyzer, the transfer disc is allowed to stand for 5 min at room temperature to allow the uricase to completely destroy the uric acid in the sample blanks. The program is initiated and results are calculated by the computer with use of a Kinetic Rate III program, which provides for a reagent-blank correction.

Table 2. Conditions for Measurement of Serum Uric Acid

Sample vol, μl	20
Flush vol, μl	120
Reagent vol, μl	500
Computer program[a]	Kinetic rate III
Temperature, °C	30
Wavelength, nm	600
Time of initial reading, s	30
Time of final reading, s	180

[a] The computer programs mentioned in this paper are all routinely supplied with the computerized centrifugal analyzer we used.

Correlation Studies

The comparison method for total and conjugated bilirubin was the continuous-flow adaptation (*3*) of the Jendrassik and Grof technique for the SMA 6/60 AutoAnalyzer (Technicon Instrument Corp., Tarrytown, N. Y. 10591). The reference method for serum uric acid was based on the decrease in absorbance at 293 nm caused by oxidation of uric acid in the presence of uricase. The reagents for the procedure, based on that described by Praetorius and Paulsen (*4*), were obtained in a kit from a commercial source (Boehringer Mannheim).

Results and Discussion

Bilirubin Standard

The standard we used during the initial stages of this work was a solution of bilirubin Standard Reference Material (National Bureau of Standards, Washington, D. C. 20234) in dimethyl sulfoxide/phosphate buffer containing albumin, prepared as described by Gadd (*2*). The use of Pediatric Versatol as a secondary standard was adopted only after the manufacturer's assay value for several lots of this material was found to be accurate when measured against this primary standard. We have adopted this approach in order to simplify preparation of the standard and to minimize exposure of laboratory personnel to dimethyl sulfoxide. The validity of the manufacturer's assay value is checked each time a new batch of secondary standard is prepared, either against the primary standard, or by overlapping for a period of one week with a previously prepared batch of secondary standard which itself has been checked against the primary standard. A separate commercial lyophilized serum (Hyland, "Level II") is included as a control with each routine run. As previously mentioned, because the standard contains only unconjugated bilirubin, it is run under the conditions for the total assay (caffeine instead of HCl), for the assay of conjugated as well as total bilirubin.

Analytical Variables

Linearity and sensitivity. In the bilirubin procedures, concentration and absorbance are linearly related to at least 200 mg/liter, with excellent sensitivity—giving 8 milliabsorbance units change per milligram of bilirubin per liter. In the uric acid procedure this relation is linear to 150 mg/liter, with 1 mg/liter of uric acid giving an absorbance change of 5 milliabsorbance units.

Precision. The precision of the bilirubin determinations was evaluated in two ways. Within-run precision was estimated from replicate analyses of a serum sample containing abnormally high concentrations of both unconjugated and conjugated bilirubin. Day-to-day precision was evaluated by using a lyophilized

Table 3. Precision of Bilirubin and Uric Acid Procedures

Test	No. analyses	Mean mg/liter	SD mg/liter	CV, %
Total bilirubin				
Within-run precision	24	67	0.8	1.2
	24	3.6	0.2	6.3
Day-to-day precision	70	43.9	1.5	3.3
Conjugated bilirubin				
Within-run-precision	24	49.2	1.8	3.6
	24	4.3	0.4	10.2
Uric acid				
Within-run precision	60	28	1.3	4.7
	60	109	2.4	2.2
Day-to-day precision	70	82.5	2.0	2.4

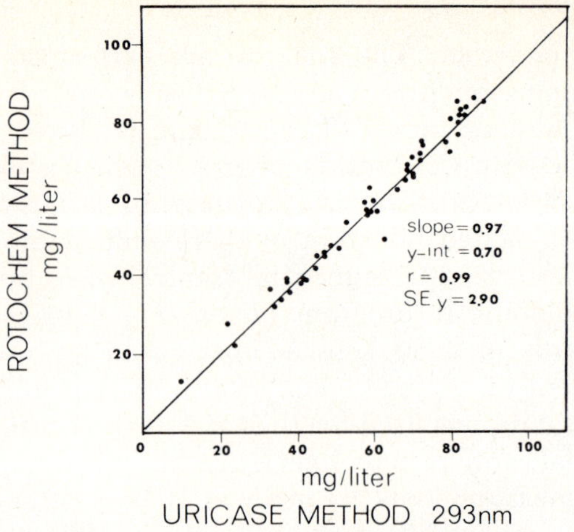

Fig. 1. Comparison of results of centrifugal analyzer procedure and manual uricase procedure for serum uric acid

control serum (Hyland, "Level II") that contained only unconjugated bilirubin, and thus only results for total bilirubin are reported. The precision of the uric acid method was evaluated by within-run and day-to-day replicate analyses of two lyophilized control sera spanning the normal and abnormal ranges. The precision data (Table 3) attest to the excellent reproducibilities of the methods, which in large part can be attributed to the high degree of sensitivity inherent in each of the procedures.

Correlation Studies

The procedures for total and conjugated bilirubin were compared to a continuous-flow technique based on the Jendrassik and Grof method (*3*), for sera from 63 patients. The regression equation for total bilirubin was $y = 0.93x - 1.9$ mg/liter, $r = 0.98$, $SE_y = \pm 1.6$ mg/liter, with a range of 2.0 to 42 mg/liter. For conjugated bilirubin, the regression equation was $y = 0.78x - 0.1$ mg/liter, $r = 0.93$, $SE_y = \pm 2.1$ mg/liter, based on a range of 1.0 to 32 mg/liter. The values obtained with the centrifugal analyzer were always lower than the corresponding continuous-flow values. This is reflected by negative y-intercepts and slopes of less than unity, and is most probably accounted for by the lack of application of true sample/reagent blank corrections in the continuous-flow method. The uric acid method was compared to a manual uricase technique by 59 human sera. The results (Figure 1) demonstrate acceptable agreement.

Measurement Conditions

The conditions for the measurement of bilirubin with the Jendrassik and Grof procedure are well established. The present method involves measurements of total and conjugated bilirubin after a 60-s reaction period, because we found in the initial development of the method that both reactions were essentially complete after this time. This time study was performed directly in the centrifugal analyzer by using an Absorbance Print program, which enables the investigator to obtain printed absorbance values for all cuvettes at selected times. The Jendrassik and Grof procedures usually include addition of base after the bilirubin-diazo reagent reaction, to change the absorbance maximum of the product from 550 nm to 600 nm. At 600 nm, non-bilirubin yellow pigments and other red and brown pigments have negligible absorbances, and the need for blank correction becomes minimized. However, commercially available centrifugal analyzers now have no means of introducing additional reagents during the course of the reaction. The present method involves a final measurement at 550 nm and uses a sample-blank correction for all samples.

Uric acid posed a more complicated problem, and initially a procedure was investigated for using the reagent described, but without uricase. The basis of the original method was a procedure described by Morin (*5*), which, in common with the present method, involved oxidation of uric acid by Fe^{3+}. It was necessary to alter the composition of the reagent from that described by Morin, because the 2,4,6-tri-(2-pyridyl)-*s*-triazine consistently precipitated from solution, and nonlinearity was also observed. The modifications involved increasing the Fe^{3+} concentration twofold and the 2,4,6-tri-(2-pyridyl)-*s*-triazine concentration threefold over the original reagent described by Morin. To prevent precipitation of these reagents, we used an aqueous 2-propanol/1-butanol solvent system in place of the acetone/methanol used by Morin. It is advisable to prepare all reagents in acid-washed flasks, to prevent contamination by ferrous ion. The working reagent is prepared directly before use and appears to be stable for as long as 4 h. The need to incorporate albumin into the standards because of its profound, although apparently concentration-independent, effect on the stoichiometry of the reaction has already been pointed out by Morin.

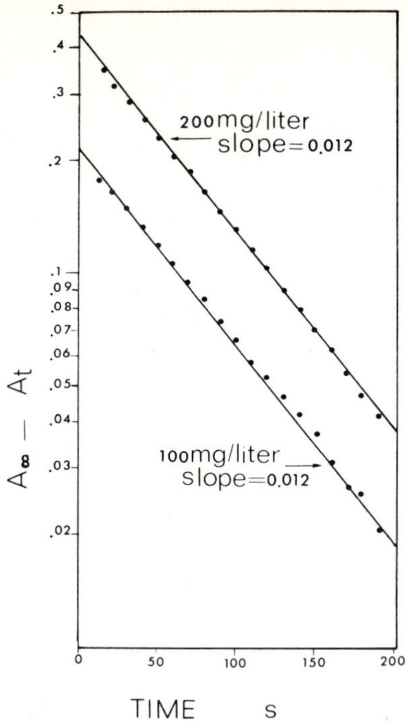

Fig. 2. First order [$\log (A_\infty - A_t) = -kt/2.303 + \log A_\infty$] rate plot for 100 and 200 mg/liter urate standard solutions

In developing the kinetic method, we at first assumed that the reaction might follow first-order kinetics when the described reagent concentrations were used. Under these conditions, reaction rate would then be directly proportional to the concentration of uric acid. Because the difference between the absorbance of the reaction mixture at any time and the absorbance of the reaction mixture at completion is directly proportional to the uric acid concentration at that time, and because the initial absorbance is effectively zero, the rate law can be stated in terms of absorbance, which predicts that a linear relationship should exist between $\log (A_\infty - A_t)$ and time. We decided to test our system, and Figure 2 shows the results. We followed the absorbance changes of 100 and 200 mg/liter urate standards with time and plotted the appropriate absorbance change vs. time on semilogarithmic paper. As anticipated, two straight lines with equal slopes were obtained. Furthermore, the antilog of the y-intercept for the 200 mg/liter standard is twice that of the 100 mg/liter standard. These results are consistent with the first-order rate expression.

Because a pseudo-first-order rate scheme had now been demonstrated, it was valid to use a two-point fixed-time kinetic assay. However, the reagent itself was observed to change slowly with time, so that a reagent-blank correction was applied to the fixed-time absorbance changes. The use of kinetic assays such as this one not only completely eliminates static interferences, but also serves to correct for the kinetic type of interference if reactivity differences are appreciable.

When we compared results by this method with those by a 293-nm uricase method, we saw that—although most of the samples investigated demonstrated excellent agreement—several samples, notably icteric specimens, gave significantly higher values with the present method. Evidently, certain samples contained kinetic interferants that reduced Fe^{3+} at about the same rate as did urate.

To ensure accuracy, we decided to modify the method by running uricase-incubated sample blanks as described in the *Procedures* section. The 5-min uricase incubation at room temperature was demonstrably more than adequate for the complete destruction of uric acid in concentrations up to 250 mg/liter. The method is not interfered with by abnormally high concentrations of creatinine, glucose, salicylate, ascorbic acid, albumin, or bilirubin. Analytical recoveries were essentially quantitative.

Too often, the tedium and technical difficulty associated with performing blank corrections—together with the possibility of compounding errors when two or more spectrophotometric measurements must be made in order to obtain a single answer—have resulted in not applying these corrections, even when it can be demonstrated that serious errors in accuracy may result. We have found, however, that the centrifugal analyzer system, with its double-beam-in-time spectrophotometric characteristics, its ultimate control of the time variable, and its computer system that allows considerable versatility in the customized accumulation, storage, and processing of data, is ideally suited to this task.

References

1. Jendrassik, L., and Grof, P., Vereinfachte photometrische Methoden zur Bestimmung des Blutbilirubins. *Biochem. Z.* **297,** 81 (1938).

2. Gadd, K. G., Preparation of bilirubin standards. *J. Clin. Pathol.* **19,** 300 (1966).

3. Gambino, S. R., and Freda, V. J., The measurement of amniotic fluid bilirubin by the method of Jendrassik and Grof. *Am. J. Clin. Pathol.* **46,** 198 (1966).

4. Praetorius, E., and Paulsen, H., Enzymatic determination of uric acid, with detailed directions. *Scand. J. Clin. Lab. Invest.* **5,** 273 (1953).

5. Morin, L. G., Determination of serum urate by direct acid Fe^{3+} reduction or by absorbance change (at 293 nm) on oxidation of urate with alkaline ferricyanide. *Clin. Chem.* **20,** 51 (1974).

CLIN. CHEM. 22/4, 434–438 (1976)

Clinical Laboratory Evaluation of the Perkin-Elmer KA-150 Enzyme Analyzer

Eugene Hardin, Richard B. Passey,[1] Ronald L. Gillum,[2] John B. Fuller, and Debbie Lawrence

We evaluated the Perkin-Elmer KA-150 Enzyme Analyzer in a clinical laboratory situation according to a rigid evaluation protocol. The factors evaluated for five commonly assayed enzymes were as follows: (*a*) rate of analysis of patient samples, (*b*) analytical linearity, (*c*) overall precision (within-run and between-day), (*d*) carry-over from a sample with activity near 1000 U/liter, (*e*) error detection at low and high concentrations, (*f*) correlation of values with those obtained by methods used in our laboratory, and (*g*) normal-value ranges. We find the KA-150 to be an effective and rapid enzyme analyzer.

We have evaluated the Perkin-Elmer KA-150 Enzyme Analyzer (*1*) and its reagents for the clinical assay of lactate dehydrogenase (EC 1.1.1.27), creatine kinase (EC 2.7.3.2), aspartate aminotransferase (EC 2.6.1.1), alanine aminotransferase (EC 2.6.1.2), and alkaline phosphatase (EC 3.1.3.1).

The KA-150 is a rapid enzyme analyzer in which the classic two-reagent determinations are used. An automated pipetting system delivers 10 μl of sample and 90 μl of diluent to 50 μl of reagent R_1. This is followed by a preincubation of 6 min and then 50 μl of the second activating reagent, R_2, is added, whereupon the kinetic reaction is monitored by a silicon diode detector with use of a light source from one of two hollow-cathode tubes for the generation of 340- or 404-nm monochromatic light. All reactions are done in sample magazines, the location of which during the pipetting, incubation, and aspiration phases is constantly monitored by a fiber-optic detection system. Reactions are at 30 °C. The temperature is monitored by a thermistor that is in contact with an aluminum block surrounding the cuvette. A thermoelectric pump receives signals from the thermistor to regulate the temperature. There is both internal and external washing of the sample pickup probe, to eliminate carry-over. It also has an error-detection system that responds to four types of errors, to add validity to the printed answers.

Department of Pathology, University of Texas Medical Branch, Galveston, Tex. 77550.

[1] Address communications to R. B. P.

[2] Current address: Department of Pathology, University of Texas Health Science Center, Houston, Tex. 77025.

Received Nov. 20, 1975; accepted Jan. 16, 1976.

With the increasing number of "sophisticated" instruments introduced for use in the clinical laboratory, there is an increasingly important need for thorough independent evaluation of these instruments in the clinical laboratory situation. The criteria for evaluation we used here were very similar to those used in the evaluation of the Beckman TR Enzyme Analyzer (*2*). The only involvement of the Perkin-Elmer Corporation in this study was that they furnished reagents.

Materials and Methods

Instrument and Controls

A KA-150 Enzyme Analyzer (serial no. 102200) was purchased from Perkin-Elmer Corp., Norwalk, Conn. 06856. The manufacturer slightly modified the instrument during the study: changed the transfer probe movements from a hydraulic drive to a mechanical drive and added a fan and shield near the central light source to decrease the instrument temperature. These changes are irrelevant to the data reported here. The reagents we used were those produced and supplied by Perkin-Elmer Corp. We used lyophilized commercially supplied control materials: Hyland A, B, C, I, and II (Hyland Laboratories, Inc., Costa Mesa, Calif. 92626) and Monitrol II (Dade Division, American Hospital Supply Corp., Miami, Fla. 33152). Hyland controls A, B, and C are specifically enzyme controls and are clear; the others are general-purpose controls.

In all assays the volumes used were: 10 μl of sample, 90 μl of diluent, and 100 μl of reagent—a total reaction volume of 200 μl. Two wavelengths were generated by a cobalt (340 nm) and a manganese (404 nm) hollow-cathode lamps.

Reagents for Use with the KA-150

The reagents used, and their final concentrations, were as follows (activating substances are in boldface type):

Lactate dehydrogenase reagent, containing, per liter, sodium phosphate buffer, 115 mmol, pH 7.4; **sodium pyruvate,** 1.0 mmol; NADH, 0.195 mmol; mannitol, 34 g; dextran, 1.5 g; glycine, 9 g; and "Triton X-100" surfactant, 90 ng.

Aspartate aminotransferase reagent, containing, per liter, sodium phosphate buffer, 50 mmol, pH 7.5; **L-aspartate,** 150 mmol; **2-oxoglutarate,** 10.25 mmol; NADH, 0.19 mmol; malate dehydrogenase, 2.5 kU; lactate dehydrogenase, 1.25 kU; mannitol, 34 g; dextran, 3 g; sodium hydroxide, 7.4 g; and Triton X-100, 90 g.

Alkaline phosphatase reagent containing, per liter, AMP buffer, 0.5 mmol, pH 10.10; $MgCl_2$, 0.1 mmol; ***p*-nitrophenyl phosphate,** 14.0 mmol; mannitol, 5.6 g; Triton X-100, 90 mg; and HCl, 4 g.

Creatine kinase reagent containing, per liter, piperazine-*N,N'*-bis(2-ethane sulfonic acid) buffer, 100 mmol, pH 6.8, magnesium aspartate, 14 mmol; dithiothreitol, 8 mmol; D-glucose, 17 mmol; ADP, 1.25 mmol; AMP, 10 mmol; NAD^+, 2.25 mmol; hexokinase (yeast) 8 U, glucose-6-phosphate dehydrogenase, 4 kU; glycine, 7 g; dextran, 1 g; and **creatine phosphate** 21 mmol.

Alanine aminotransferase reagent containing, per liter, sodium phosphate buffer, 55 mmol, pH 7.5; **L-alanine,** 175 mmol; **2-oxoglutarate,** 14 mmol; β-NADH (yeast), 0.16 mmol; lactate dehydrogenase, 4 kU; mannitol, 34 g; dextran, 1.5 g; Triton X-100, 90 mg; and sodium hydroxide, 1.2 g.

Comparison Methods

The instruments and reagents for the comparison methods (those routinely used in our laboratory) were all for single-reagent determinations and are as follows:

Lactate dehydrogenase reagent. Assays were performed with the Model 3401 System (Gilford Instruments, Oberlin, Ohio 44074) at 30 °C, with reagents from Boehringer-Mannheim Corp., New York, N. Y. 10017 (kit No. 15948).

Alkaline phosphatase reagent. Our reagents contained, per liter, 4.2 mmol of *p*-nitrophenyl phosphate, 1.0 mmol of magnesium chloride, and 625 mmol of 2-methyl-2-amino-1-propanol buffer (pH 10.25) for use with the Model 3401 at 37 °C.

Aspartate aminotransferase, alanine aminotransferase and creatine kinase were assayed with kits No. 15791, 15792, and 12926, respectively, used with a centrifugal analyzer (CentrifiChem; Union Carbide Corp., Tarrytown, N. Y. 10591) at 30 °C.

Procedure

The loading sequence for an enzyme run on the KA-150 is five water blanks, to check instrument reagent zero, followed by patients' samples and controls. Many of the operating variables such as temperature, dilutions, and photometry can be checked as one functioning unit by using the calibration check procedure specified by the manufacturer. The calibration check procedure requires five calibration solutions (*p*-nitrophenyl phosphate for 404 nm or sodium pyruvate for 340 nm) followed by five water blanks. These solutions either have a known absorptivity, such as *p*-nitrophenyl (absorbance at 404 nm), or a reaction is used in which a known quantity of substance is converted to give a known absorbance—for example, the lactate dehydrogenase-catalyzed conversion of sodium pyruvate and NADH to lactate and NAD^+, as measured at 340 nm. The mean value obtained for the five blanks is subtracted from the mean value of the five solutions, to give an assay absorbance value that must be within 2% of the expected value. This procedure is unique because it avoids the use of enzymes as standards, and each calibration check procedure simultaneously evaluates the instrument's operating variables. However, this procedure obviously gives no information about individual component malfunction or warning of any mutally offsetting errors that could result in an artifactually correct value for the absorbance calibration.

Results

Analytical Variables

Rate of analysis. We could measure 125 samples per hour for either alanine aminotransferase, aspartate aminotransferase, alkaline phosphatase, or lactate dehydrogenase, beginning with sample pickup. Because of the 12-min lag time for creatine kinase, the rate for it was slightly slower, 122 samples per hour. The lag time (time required to obtain the first result) is 10 min for the other enzymes. To assay a full tray of samples (35 samples and five blanks) through all five enzyme assays required 96 minutes.

Linear range. We calculated the range within which concentration and readings were linearly related by using dilutions of three above-normal patients' sera or patients' sera with human-organ extracts of enzymes added. The ranges of linearity (Table 1, Figure 1) were: for lactate dehydrogenase, up to 1593 U/liter; for aspartate aminotransferase, up to 3277 U/liter; for alanine aminotransferase, up to 2118 U/liter; for creatine kinase, up to 2493 U/liter; and for alkaline phosphatase, up to 1891 U/liter. Those data that did not fall on the regression line are symbolized in Figure 1 by filled dots, and are included to show the curvature, but were not used in the calculations of the statistical data in Table 1. The limit of linearity was calculated after first selectively eliminating data points and then iteratively calculating the regression line until the smallest y-intercept and $S_{y \cdot x}$ were found. The limit of linearity was designated acceptable if the observed limit value was within ±2 CV (based on the within-run precision data obtained with use of Hyland C, Table 2) of the expected value determined by solving the best regression equation for y (the equation with the smallest y-intercept and $S_{y \cdot x}$). (The statistic $S_{y \cdot x}$ is the standard deviation of y about x.)

Precision. Within-run precision was very good (Table 2), with CV's generally less than 3%; the only exception was alanine aminotransferase samples with low mean values. The maximum standard deviation for any enzyme was 4.4 U/liter (alkaline phosphatase).

Table 1 LINEARITY[a] OF THE KA-150 ENZYME ANALYZER

U/liter	Lactate Dehydrogenase	Aspartate Amino-transferase	Alanine Amino-transferase	Creatine Kinase	Alkaline Phosphatase
Serum #1					
y-Intercept[b]	4.4	2.9	10.9	-7.9	13.9
Slope[b]	2996	3159	2144	8513	2849
Sy·x[b]	26.8	16.2	10.4	6.3	4.6
r	.9988	.9999	.9998	1.000	1.000
Linear to	1203	3140	2118	2060	1829
Serum #2					
y-Intercept[b]	18.2	24.8	10.7	27.4	15.6
Slope[b]	3189	3223	1672	6319	2832
Sy·x	24.8	40.5	17.4	12.1	21.5
r	.9986	.9994	.9995	.9997	.9994
Linear to	1593	3277	1684	1037	1891
Serum #3					
y-Intercept[b]	25.1	12.8	8.2	24.6	10.5
Slope[b]	3173	3020	1672	8475	2915
Sy·x[b]	9.7	19.6	12.5	48.5	13.2
r	.9999	.9997	.9998	.9972	.9995
Linear to	1561	2975	1684	2493	1816

[a]Patient sera, spiked with tissue extract and diluted in saline. Activity ranged from 60-3,000 U/liter using 9 dilutions over the entire range.

[b]U/liter

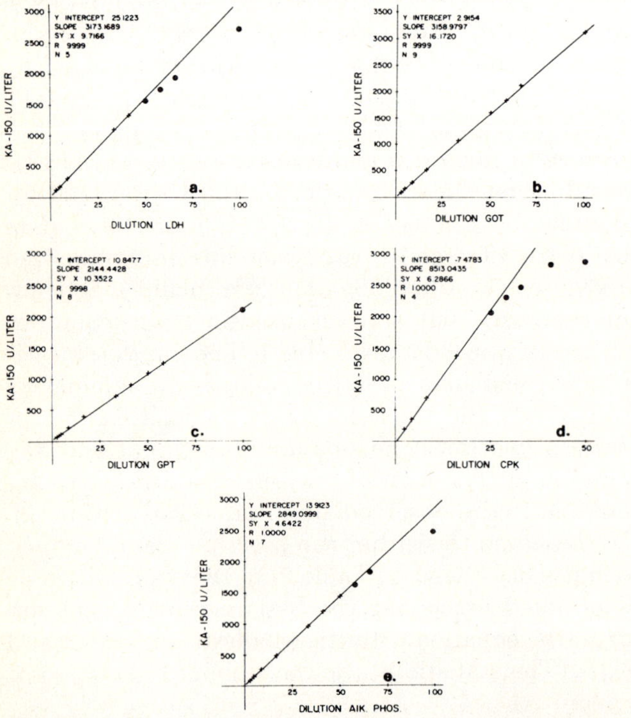

Fig. 1. Linearity of respective enzyme assays on the Perkin-Elmer KA-150, for high-activity sera or sera supplemented with either high-activity sera or with high-activity extracts from tissue

All dilutions of sera were with physiological saline. (*a*) lactate dehydrogenase, (*b*) aspartate aminotransferase, (*c*) alanine aminotransferase, (*d*) creatine kinase, and (*e*) alkaline phosphatase

Table 2 AVERAGE[a] WITHIN-RUN PRECISION ON THE KA-150

Enzyme	U/liter	Hyland A	Hyland B	Hyland C
Lactate dehydrog-enase	Mean	138	281	355
	SD[b]	3.9	2.3	2.4
	CV, %[c]	2.8	0.84	0.66
Aspartate amino-transferase	Mean	57	94	115
	SD[b]	1.8	2.1	2.5
	CV, %[c]	3.14	2.23	2.17
Alanine amino-transferase	Mean	8.8	80	174
	SD[b]	2.3	1.7	2.3
	CV, %[c]	26.14	2.15	1.32
Creatine kinase	Mean	73	295	333
	SD[b]	1.7	2.7	3.3
	CV, %[c]	2.33	0.92	0.99
Alkaline phos-phatase	Mean	47	90	154
	SD[b]	.89	1.4	4.4
	CV, %[c]	1.89	1.56	2.86

[a]The mean in the table is the overall average of 20 assays repeated on three separate days

[b]Av. SD = $\sqrt{\frac{\Sigma SD^2}{N}}$

[c]Av. CV = $\frac{\sqrt{\frac{\Sigma SD^2}{N}}}{\text{mean}} \times 100$

Table 3 DAY-TO-DAY[a] PRECISION ON THE KA-150

Mean (U/liter)	SD (U/liter)	CV, %	Mean (U/liter)	SD (U/liter)	CV, %
Lactate dehydrogenase			Creatine kinase		
124	5.8	4.6	71	4.3	6.0
256	9.0	3.5	301	16.0	5.4
331	10.7	3.2	322	28.0	8.7
116	4.3	3.7	* 15	3.6	24.3
*298	11.7	3.9	*853	54.9	6.4
*491	21.5	4.4	*188	26.9	14.3
205[b]	7.5	3.7	63[b]	6.0	9.5
Aspartate aminotransferase			Alkaline phosphatase		
55	3.2	5.8	47	3.8	8.1
90	3.6	4.0	97	5.7	5.8
111	6.1	5.6	154	10.2	6.6
13	2.8	22.2	37	2.0	5.4
67	5.7	8.5	130	4.7	3.6
*57	7.1	12.5	*187	5.0	2.7
17[b]	0.5	2.5	75[b]	4.7	6.2
Alanine aminotransferase					
7	2.2	31.7			
80	4.0	5.1			
170	5.1	3.0			
4	2.3	58.0			
24	3.5	14.4			
*77	5.1	6.6			
19[b]	2.3	11.5			

[a] n = 30 days except where noted with * (29 days). The first 3 values are the clear controls Hyland A, B, C and the last 3 are the more turbid controls Hyland I, II and Monitrol II, respectively.

[b] SD and CV are estimated at upper limit of the normal range using data from the clear controls

Table 4 CARRY-OVER ON THE KA-150

		Day 1	Day 2	Day 3	Average
Lactate dehydrogenase	(a)	1.0	-1.0	6.5	2.5
carry-over U/liter	(b)	3.0	0.5	10.0	4.5
	(c)	-5.0	1.5	3.0	-0.2
overall average carry-over					2.3
Aspartate aminotransferase	(a)	1.0	0.5	-6.5	-1.5
carry-over U/liter	(b)	0.5	-3.0	5.5	1.0
	(c)	3.0	0.0	3.0	2.0
overall average carry-over					0.5
Alanine aminotransferase	(a)	1.0	2.0	1.0	1.3
carry-over U/liter	(b)	1.0	1.5	2.5	1.7
	(c)	4.0	3.0	3.0	3.3
overall average carry-over					2.1
Creatine kinase	(a)	1.0	-1.0	4.5	1.5
carry-over U/liter	(b)	1.0	2.0	5.0	2.7
	(c)	-0.5	2.0	3.0	1.5
overall average carry-over					1.9
Alkaline phosphatase	(a)	5.0	1.0	3.5	3.2
carry-over U/liter	(b)	3.5	3.5	6.0	4.3
	(c)	4.0	0.0	6.5	3.5
overall average carry-over					3.7

(a) and (b) represent carry-over from high patient (HP) to normal patient (NP)

(c) represents carry-over from HP to water

A 30-day quality-control experiment was performed by using six lyophilized control sera, assayed daily for each enzyme (Table 3). The resulting CV's were generally less than 15%, except for alanine aminotransferase, aspartate aminotransferase, and creatine kinase, all with low mean values.

The day-to-day CV at the upper limit of normal, calculated according to the method of Passey et al. (2), was less than 10% for the clear Hyland A, B, and C controls, except for alanine aminotransferase with a low upper limit (Table 3). The turbid controls Hyland I and II and Monitrol in several instances gave much higher CV's, presumably because of their turbidity.

Freezing the reconstituted clear enzyme controls for longer than 10 days decreased creatine kinase activity, as the following experiment showed. Aliquots of the clear enzyme control were frozen, after reconstitution, and one sample was analyzed each day for 30 days. Results showed expected distributions for the first 10 days, then activity decreased steadily during the remaining 20 days of the experiment.

Carry-over. Carry-over (Table 4) was evaluated by using three aliquots of a high-activity (near 1000 U/liter) patient's serum followed by three aliquots of a normal patient's serum. This sequence was repeated, followed by three aliquots of the same high-activity serum and three samples of water. Any carry-over shows up as an increased activity in the first aliquot of the normal patient's serum (or water) in the sequence. The second and third aliquots of the normal patient's serum in a sequence are used to establish an average value for the sera. Carry-over was calculated by $NP_1-[(NP_2 + NP_3)/2]$. Carry-over was evaluated for all five enzymes on three different days, with different normal and high-activity sera being used each day. For all five enzymes it was very small, the largest average carry-over into the normal sera being 4.5 U/liter and into water 3.5 U/liter (Table 4). The average standard deviation from the within-run precision study on Hyland A (Table 2) was, except for alkaline phosphatase, larger than the carry-over. Therefore, the carry-over for the other four enzymes was not significant and for alkaline phosphatase it was negligible.

Error messages. The KA-150 incorporates four error-detection devices. The high-error message (HI) denotes either a highly absorbing serum (>1.5 absorbance units, *A*) or a high-activity serum the absorbance of which is increasing at the time it is being measured. The low-error message (LO) shows an activity that has exhausted the substrate to give absorbance readings of less than 0.5 for decreasing absorbance reactions. AC and DC refer to the accelerating or decelerating curvatures of the data points used by the KA-150 to calculate the enzyme activity; if the curvature varies either way from the slope of the line by more than 5%, the value is flagged (i.e., the result is printed in red along with the appropriate error code).

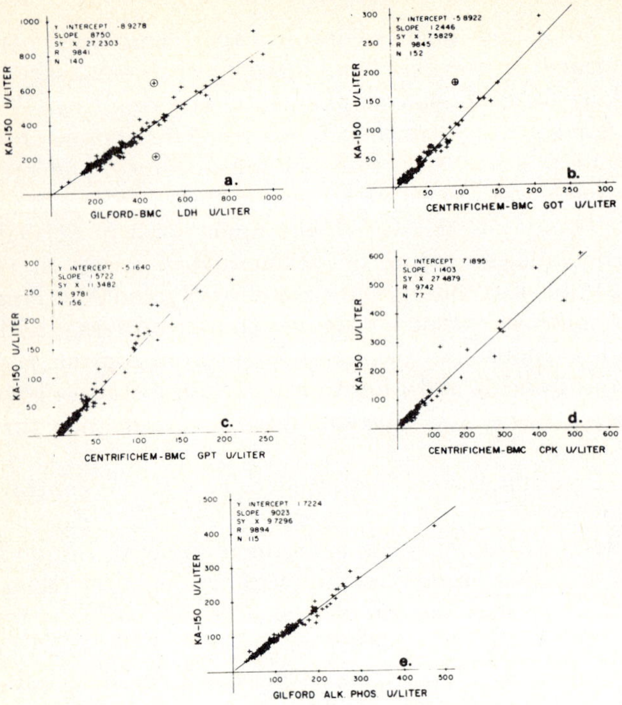

Fig. 2. Enzyme assay comparisons between the method used in our laboratory (x) and the Perkin-Elmer KA-150 (y)
Patients' sera were used for the comparisons. (a) lactate dehydrogenase, (b) aspartate aminotransferase, (c) alanine aminotransferase, (d) creatine kinase, and (e) alkaline phosphatase

Solutions of NADH for the LO error message, and p-nitrophenyl for the HI error message were diluted through the error message range to find the exact triggering point. Dilutions for the LO message encompassed A from 0.48–0.53, in increments of 0.01; HI was diluted from 1.45–1.53, in increments of 0.01. The LO code for decreasing absorbance reactions came on between .50 and .51 A. The HI error code for high absorbance reactions was activated between 1.48 and 1.49 A.

Comparisons of patients' sera. Enzyme assay values obtained by the above indicated methods were compared with values from the KA-150 for duplicate aliquots of patient samples (Figure 2). All such comparisons were done on the same day within 1 or 2 h of each other, 77 to 156 samples being used for each enzyme comparison. The constant bias for all assays was small, 8.9 U/liter being the largest y-intercept. The slope deviations from unity are due to different methodologies and ranged from .87 to 1.6. Correlation coefficients were between .974 and .989. The few outliers (circled in Figure 2), those values further than three standard deviations from the regression line, were not used in the calculations. None of the comparisons were corrected for temperature differences.

Normal Values

Normal values were established for the KA-150 by analyzing samples from apparently healthy individuals, in duplicate. A single specimen was drawn from each of 50 laboratory personnel during five days and were analyzed in duplicate the same day collected. We calculated the normal ranges (Table 5), using the mean ±2 SD as well as a central 95 percentile group. The standard deviations in Table 5 were calculated for the duplicate values. These standard deviations were all less than 5.0 U/liter; accordingly, the SD's are well within those obtained in the between-day precision study.

Table 5 NORMAL VALUES[a] ON THE KA-150

	Range Mean ±2 SD	Range 95 Percentile	SD[b] Duplicates
Lactate dehydrogenase	95 - 203	100 - 205	4.7
Aspartate aminotransferase	<20	2 - 17	3.2
Alanine aminotransferase	<20	2 - 19	3.1
Creatine kinase	<130	17 - 63	2.3
Alkaline phosphatase	14 - 98	25 - 75	0.9

[a] $n = 50$

[b] $SD = \left[\frac{\Sigma(x - \bar{x})^2}{2n}\right]^{\frac{1}{2}}$

Discussion

During our evaluation of the KA-150, troubles made it necessary to stop for 8 to 10 h of a total of 600 operating hours. We found the instrument easy to use and its operation simple to teach. It can accommodate a large workload, with linearity up to at least 1500 U/liter for all five enzymes (Figure 1).

For these five enzymes the KA-150 has a maximum within-run standard deviation of 4.4 U/liter. Day-to-day precision was good and can be improved by using the clear enzyme controls. However, these controls should be divided into aliquots and frozen for no longer than 10 days if values for creatine kinase activity are to be valid. Carry-over for the KA-150 is negligible for analytical purposes. The error-detection system for low and high error messages shows good monitoring of these factors. Results of inter-method comparisons (Figure 2) were excellent. The highest $S_{y \cdot x}$ that we saw was 27.5 U/liter for a range up to 1000 U/liter. There was a small but constant bias between methods; the largest y-intercept was −8.9 U/liter.

We conclude that the Perkin-Elmer KA-150 enzyme analyzer is a dependable, rapid, and precise instrument.

References

1. Atwood, J. G., and DiCesare, J. L., Making enzymatic methods optimum for measuring compounds with a kinetic analyzer. *Clin. Chem.* **21**, 1263 (1975).

2. Passey, R., Gillum, R. L., Giles, M. L., and Fuller, J. B., Evaluation of the Beckman "System TR Enzyme Analyzer". *Clin. Chem.* **21**, 1107 (1975).

CLIN. CHEM. 22/4, 439–444 (1976)

Electrophoretic Pattern of Amylase Isoenzymes in Serum and Urine of Normal Persons

Makoto Otsuki, Susumu Saeki, Hosai Yuu, Mitsuo Maeda, and Shigeaki Baba

We separated and measured amylase isoenzymes in the serum and urine of 3036 normal persons by electrophoresis on a thin layer of polyacrylamide gel. We wished to establish the normal pattern of these isoenzymes and to evaluate the usefulness of this method of electrophoresis in clinical diagnosis. Results for patients with hyper- or hypofunctioning pancreas and salivary glands suggested that essentially all the isoamylases in human serum and urine are derived from the salivary glands and the pancreas, and revealed that isoamylases of more than 98% of normal persons consisted of two major isoenzymes and two to three minor ones. Although these observations indicate that data on changes in the proportion of amylase activity of each isoenzyme can be useful in clinical medicine, the following points should be remembered: (*a*) quantitative differences in the isoenzyme pattern were observed, depending upon the condition of the samples; (*b*) because the proportion of isoamylase activity in serum of different normal persons differs, seriatim determination of amylase isoenzymes is necessary; and (*c*) because five different genetically controlled types of isoamylases were observed in normal persons, genetic investigations are also necessary.

Additional Keyphrases: *electrophoresis on polyacrylamide gel* • *normal values* • *origin of serum amylase* • *diagnosis of pancreatitis* • *genetics* • *isoenzyme pattern in infants* • *interindividual variation*

Measurement of total serum amylase activity is used in the diagnosis of acute pancreatitis, the first enzymatic method to be used in clinical medicine (*1*). Abnormally high amylase activities in serum have been reported in a large variety of conditions (*2–5*), and thus a more accurate diagnosis should result if one separates the amylase isoenzymes, identifies the source of each, and ascertains which isoenzymes are related to which disease.

Such a separation is now possible as one of the routine tests in many laboratories (*6–22*), but the normal pattern of amylase isoenzymes in serum and urine has not yet been established.

We determined amylase isoenzymes in serum and urine of 3036 normal persons by electrophoresis on polyacrylamide gel, in an attempt to establish the normal pattern of amylase isoenzymes. Furthermore, the usefulness of this method in clinical medicine was investigated.

The Second Department of Internal Medicine, Kobe University School of Medicine, Kusunoki-cho, Ikuta-ku, Kobe, Japan.

Received Oct. 9, 1975; accepted Jan. 20, 1976.

Materials and Methods

Samples

The types of samples we examined included saliva, pancreatic juice, urine, serum, and homogenates of human pancreas, parotid glands, and liver. Whole human saliva was collected sublingually, without preliminary stimulation, by continuous aspiration into a collecting tube, and centrifuged to remove particulates. Pancreatic juice was obtained at surgery by intubation of the pancreatic duct. The urine used was the first morning specimen, collected from 3036 students, 20 to 25 years old and without known diseases. Serum was collected before breakfast from 750 students 22–25 years old and 150 additional samples from apparently normal children 0–13 years old. The samples from patients included five cases of mumps, 10 of acute pancreatitis, three cases of decreased amylase activity of saliva, a case of complete pancreatectomy, and a case of chronic relapsing pancreatitis. Specimens of pancreas, parotid glands, and liver were obtained within 3 h after death of patients who had died of myocardial infarction. The tissues were freed of connective tissue, washed with distilled water, and homogenized at 4 °C in three volumes of a sucrose solution (0.25 mol/liter) containing $CaCl_2$ (20 mmol/liter), in a Potter–Elvenhjem homogenizer with Teflon pestle. The homogenates were centrifuged (27 000 × *g*, 30 min, 4 °C) and the supernates used for electrophoresis.

Amylase isoenzymes were separated and measured within 48 h of specimen collection; storage was at 4 °C for urine, −20 °C for serum.

Procedures

Amylase Isoenzyme Determination

A discontinuous buffer system was used; the gel buffer consisted of 0.19 mol/liter Tris [tris(hydroxymethyl)aminomethane], pH 8.8, the electrode buffer of 0.3 mol/liter borate, pH 8.2.

The monomer-mixture solution was prepared by dissolving acrylamide and bis(*N,N'*-methylethylenebisacrylamide) in a proportion by weight of 95 to 5 in gel buffer. As the catalyst, we used ammonium persulfate (1.2 g/liter) and TEMED (*N,N'*-tetramethylethylene diamine, 70 mmol/liter). Two parts of monomer mixture solution and one part of each of the two catalyst solutions were mixed and poured into the gel mold to make a gel 1 mm in thickness. Four microliters of the sample was applied in the sample groove of the gel with a micropipet and horizontal electrophoresis was done at 4 °C for 2.5 h at 0.8 mA per centimeter (Toyo Immunoelectrophoresis System, Toyo AE-2; Toyo Electrophoresis Stabilizer, PS-310; Toyo Kagaku Sangyo Co. Ltd., Osaka).

After electrophoresis, the gel plate was incubated for 30 min at 37 °C in soluble-starch solution (10 g/liter) containing NaCl (2 g/liter), followed by incubation of the gel plate alone at 37 °C for 15 to 120 min, depending on the amylase activity of the sample. The gel plate was soaked in dilute acetic acid (50 ml/liter) for 5 min and then stained with an iodine/potassium iodide solution (30 g of KI and 13 g of I_2 per liter). The area in which amylase activity was present was identified as a light yellow or transparent band against a dark-blue background. The preparations were scanned with a densitometer (Toyo Digital Densitrol, DMU-33C, Toyo Kagaku Sangyo Co.) and the gel plate was printed on a printing paper to get a replica transfer of the electropherogram.

Fundamental Studies on Measurement of Amylase Isoenzymes

Pre-electrophoresis: We tested the effect of ammonium persulfate on amylase isoenzymes by removing it by pre-electrophoresis of the polyacrylamide gel before samples were applied.

Colum chromatography: Column-chromatographic investigations were performed to find out whether or not there were changes in molecular weight during electrophoresis on polyacrylamide gel. The columns for gel filtration were packed according to the instructions of the suppliers of the materials, and all experiments were done at 4 °C. We passed the fresh sample before electrophoresis and the eluates from the gel plate after electrophoresis through a column (2.6 × 90 cm) packed with Sephadex G-75, Superfine (Pharmacia, Uppsala, Sweden). The column was equilibrated and eluted with Tris/maleate buffer (50 mmol/liter, pH 7.0) containing $CaCl_2$ (20 mmol/liter) and NaCl (20 mmol/liter). We collected 4.0-ml fractions and assayed them by a chromogenic method (*23*) with use of a blue-dyed starch polymer (Pharmacia-Shionogi, Osaka, Japan).

Comparison of two methods for measuring amylase isoenzymes: After performing the electrophoresis, we cut the polyacrylamide gel plate into thin slices of 1 mm width, and separately suspended them in 1 ml of phosphate buffer (50 mmol/liter, pH 6.8) at 4 °C for 24 h. Amylase activity so extracted from each slice was measured by both the chromogenic method and the iodometric method.

Measurement of Total Amylase Activity

Total amylase activity was measured by a chromogenic method (*23*) with use of the blue-dyed starch polymer (Pharmacia). Results were expressed as Somogyi units per 100 ml for serum and Somogyi units per hour for urine.

Results and Discussion

Our results essentially accord with the findings of others (*6–9, 11–22, 24, 25*) and confirm the presence of two principal amylase isoenzymes in human serum and urine. However, our methods appear to be more sensitive, because two to three additional isoenzymes were identified. Although Robyt et al. (*26*) reported that during electrophoresis amylase was decomposed into subunits by ammonium persulfate, the strong oxidizing agent used in preparing polyacrylamide gel, the same pattern of amylase isoenzymes was observed whether or not the gel-plate had been pre-electrophoresed. Column chromatographic investigations (Sephadex G-75 gel filtration) revealed no changes in molecular weight during electrophoresis on polyacrylamide gel, though peak 1 was no longer detectable in eluates from the gel after electrophoresis of human pancreatic amylase (Figure 1). This peak accounted for less than 5% of the total pancreatic amylase activity (*24*) even in the original sample, and no relative corresponding increase in peak 2 was observed; thus, the disappearance of peak 1 from the eluates of the gel after electrophoresis may simply be a reflection of low recovery of total amylase activity.

The possibility of mistaking the amyloclastic activity of other serum proteins as amylase activity (*27, 28*) was obviated by soaking the gel plate in an acetic acid solution before staining. Furthermore, we satisfied ourselves as to the suitableness of our iodometric assay method by the agreement between patterns obtained with the iodine/starch reaction and those by the chromogenic method (Figure 2). We concluded that the transparent or light-yellow bands against the dark-blue background surely indicate the presence of amylase activity.

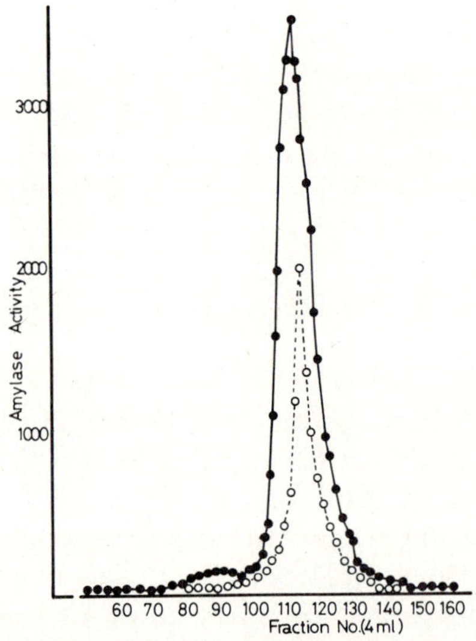

Fig. 1. Results of gel filtration of human pancreatic amylase on a column of Sephadex G-75 (2.6 × 90 cm)

We used a Tris/maleate buffer (50 mmol/liter, pH 7.0) containing $CaCl_2$ (20 mmol/liter) and NaCl (20 mmol/liter). 4.0-ml fractions were collected. *Closed circles:* elution pattern of unelectrophoresed human pancreatic amylase; *open circles:* elution pattern of eluates from the gel after electrophoresis of human pancreatic amylase

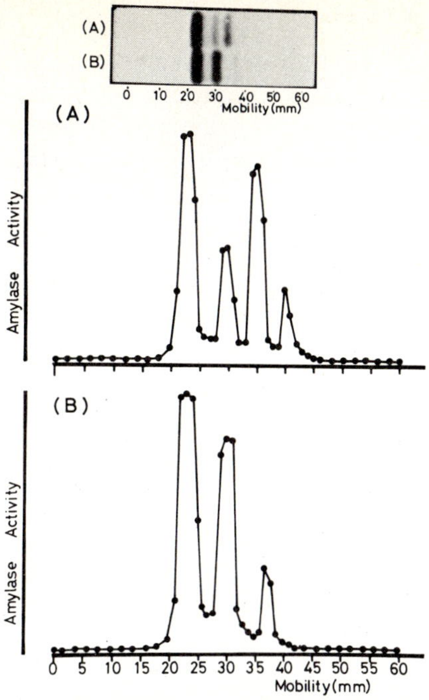

Fig. 2. Amylase isoenzymes detected in urine of a normal person (*A*) and a patient with acute pancreatitis (*B*)

Direct photocopy of the gel plate after staining with starch/iodine (*top*) and densitometry of amylase activity as measured by the chromogenic method (*bottom*) in the eluates of gel-segments sectioned after electrophoresis are shown

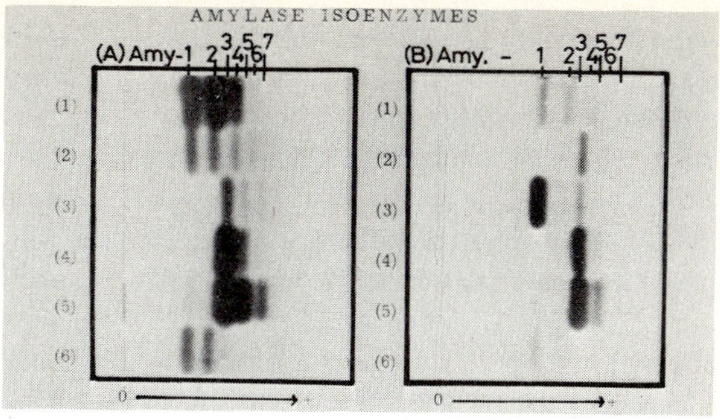

Fig. 3. Amylase isoenzymes in pancreatic (part *A*, row *1*) and parotid gland (*A-4*) extracts, in saliva (*B-4*), in serum of patients with acute pancreatitis (*A-2, B-1*), pancreatectomy (*A-3, B-2*), mumps (*A-5, B-5*), and decreased amylase activity of saliva (*A-3, B-2*), and in serum of a normal adult person (*B-3*)

Amylase isoenzymes (*numbered at the top*) in pancreatic extracts and in serum from patients with acute pancreatitis are the same in mobility, and those in parotid gland extracts, saliva, and serum from a patient with pancreatectomy are the same. Amylase-1 and -2 in normal persons have mobilities indistinguishable from those of pancreatic isoamylases; amylase-3 and -5 have mobilities similar to those of salivary isoamylases

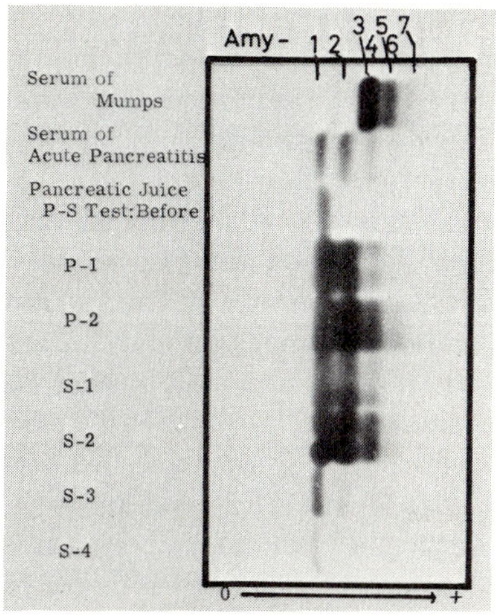

Fig. 4. Amylase isoenzymes in serum of patients with mumps and acute pancreatitis, and in pancreatic juice obtained during pancreozymin/secretin test

P-1 and *P-2* were sampled 10 and 20 min, respectively, after injection of pancreozymin and *S-1, S-2, S-3,* and *S-4* were obtained 10, 20, 40, and 60 min, respectively, after secretin injection. Amylase isoenzymes in serum of a patient with acute pancreatitis have the same mobilities as those in pancreatic juice. Note the increase of the number of isoenzymes toward the anode side in pancreatic juice obtained after stimulation of pancreozymin and secretin

Amylase isoenzymes were then evaluated on the basis of the above studies. Figure 3 shows the results of electrophoretic studies of unmodified serum from the patients mentioned above and of extracts of pancreatic and parotid gland. The patterns of amylase isoenzymes from pancreas and for serum of patients with acute pancreatitis and decreased amylase activity in saliva were the same, but differed from those for saliva and serum of patients with mumps or who had undergone total pancreatectomy. These observations of amylase isoenzyme patterns in hyper- or hypofunctioning states of pancreas or salivary glands would seem to make it possible to specify the origin of the amylase isoenzymes that appear in human serum and urine. However, the existence of extrapancreatic and extrasalivary sources of serum and urinary amylase is still a moot question. Although we could not find any amylase activity in extracts of human liver, Joseph et al. (*10*) identified an amylase that differed electrophoretically from pancreatic and salivary amylase and proposed its hepatic origin, a hypothesis supported by the observation that amylase activities are decreased in liver diseases (*29, 30*). Fridhandler et al. (*31*) reported that amylase activity in liver extracts is too low for it to be a significant source of human serum and urine amylase, and found no isoamylase component peculiar to liver extracts in serum or urine. Finding some differences between serum or urinary amylase and salivary or pancreatic amylase in the degree of inactivation of their activity on heating at 65 °C for 15 min or by trypsin, Warshaw (*32*) concluded that most amylase activity in normal serum and urine did not originate in either pancreas or salivary glands. Although there were some differences with respect to rate of inactivation of amylase activity by heat at 65 °C for 15 min between serum or urinary amylase and salivary or pancreatic amylase, amylases in all these samples were completely destroyed within 90 min (*33*). Electrophoretic analysis of heat-treated serum or urine of normal persons revealed (*34*) that the amylase activity of pancreatic isoenzyme was decreased faster than that of saliva, in agreement with the previous report. From these observations, it seems difficult to confirm the hypothesis that circulating amylase is neither of pancreatic nor salivary origin.

We attempted, therefore, to make use of the differences in mobility of pancreatic and salivary amylase isoenzymes for diagnosis. It becomes necessary to identify each isoenzyme. Although there are recommendations for the nomenclature of isoenzymes from the IUPAC/IUB International Commission on Enzymes, they seem to us to be unsuitable for amylase isoenzymes because the anodal end of the amylase isoenzyme pattern changes depending upon the amylase activity of the samples, reaction time, or conditions of samples. For example, Figure 4 demonstrates the changes of amylase isoenzymes toward the anode side depending on total amylase activity or on the concentration of bicarbonate in pancreatic juice obtained during pancreozymin/secretin test. The same changes in amylase isoenzymes were observed in serum of patients with acute pancreatitis. Quantitative changes in the isoenzyme pattern have been observed in stored samples (*25, 33*). Similar changes in the isoenzyme pattern were found in pleural fluids and ascites. Such observations move us to propose that the bands be numbered from cathode to anode, as already is being done by some authors (*13, 43, 46*). That is, "amylase-1" indicates the amylase isoenzyme with the slowest anodic mobility. It is also premature to designate these isoenzymes as P1, P2 or S1, S2 on the basis of their principal origin (*12, 15, 22, 24*), because increased amylase activity of the salivary type has been found not only in patients with diseases of salivary glands but also in cases of lung cancer, pneumonia, diabetic coma, and postoperative hyperamylasemia (*21, 31, 35–37*). With respect to their electrophoretic mobility, amylase isoenzymes 1, 2, 4, and 6, found in serum and urine, showed the same mobility as pancreatic isoamylases, and amylase-3, 5, and 7 the same as salivary isoamylases. Thus, the isoenzymes of the former group are considered the "pancreatic type" and the latter the "salivary type," for the present. The difference in mobility between pancreatic and salivary amylase isoenzymes is slight. Therefore, in case of inadequate separation or of comparative study of different electrophoretic strips as in previous studies, amylase-2 and amylase-3 are apt to be taken as one constitutent, although they differ from each other and originate from the pancreas and the salivary gland, respectively. The inadequate methodology for separating these isoenzymes may cause important errors in interpretation of the data obtained and the results. For these reasons, we believe that the densitometric method is incompletely satisfactory.

Total serum and urinary amylase activity of normal infants up to 4 months was below the so-called normal range. Densitometric analysis revealed that pancreatic isoamylase activity, both in serum and urine of newborn infants, was quite low and increased gradually with age (Figure 5). This may reflect the postnatal development of exocrine function in the pancreas (*38–40*).

Serum and urinary isoamylases of normal adult persons consist of two major isoenzymes (amylase-1 and -3) with high amylase activity and two to three minor ones with low amylase activity. One of the major isoenzymes (amylase-1) has the same electrophoretic mobility as does pancreatic isoamylase; the mobility of the other (amylase-3) is the same as for salivary isoamylase. The pattern of serum amylase isoenzymes was classified into three densitometric types: (*a*) amylase activity of the pancreatic type is higher than that of salivary type, (*b*) amylase activity of pancreatic and salivary type is the same, or (*c*) amylase activity of salivary type is higher than that of pancreatic type. For normal adults, the activity of the pancreatic-type isoenzyme averaged 52.3% of the total. Although the isoenzyme *patterns* in serum and urine were qualitatively the same, the *proportion* of amylase activities of isoenzymes in serum and urine from the same person differed: amylase activity of pancreatic-type isoamylases was always higher than that of the salivary type in the urine of almost all of normal adults. This may be the result of higher renal clearance of pancreatic type amylase, as shown by Kamaryt (*41*) and Duane et al. (*42*), but the same results were obtained even in patients with renal failure. From these findings, it could be said that the smaller proportion of pancreatic isoenzyme in urine may indicate an insufficiency of pancreatic exocrine function when the value for total urinary amylase activity is normal. However, because the proportion of

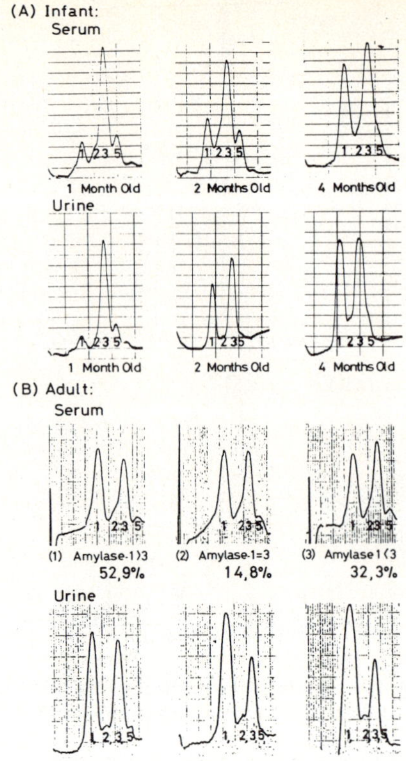

Fig. 5. Densitometric analysis of serum and urinary amylase isoenzymes of normal infants (*A*) and normal adult persons (*B*)

The origin is at the left. Total serum and urinary amylase activity is also low in infants. The proportion of amylase activity of pancreatic isoamylase-(amylase-1) is low in the infants, but increases with age

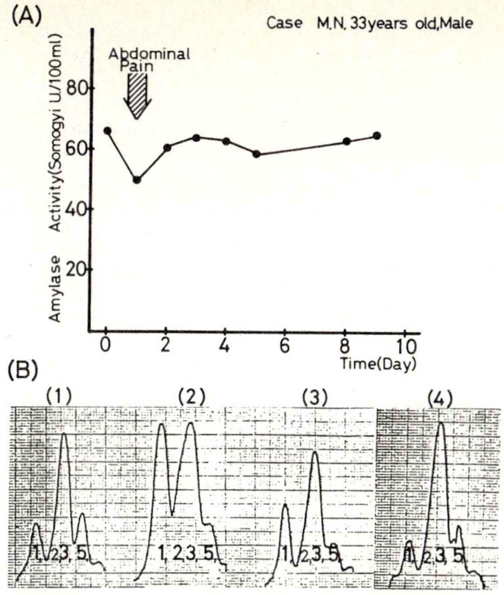

Fig. 6. Activities of total serum amylase (*A*) and of amylase isoenzymes (*B*) in serum of a patient with chronic relapsing pancreatitis

The origin is at the left. *B-1:* Amylase isoenzymes in serum before the attack of abdominal pain. The proportion of amylase activity of pancreatic-type isoenzyme is 17%, indicating pancreatic exocrine insufficiency. *B-2:* Amylase isoenzymes in serum during the attack. The proportion of pancreatic-type isoamylase increased up to 50%. The pattern of amylase isoenzymes and the proportion of amylase activity of each isoamylase are now normal. *B-3, 4:* Amylase isoenzymes in serum sampled four and nine days after the attack. The proportion of pancreatic-type isoamylase gradually decreased to the pre-attack levels. The relapse of pancreatitis can be diagnosed only by means of such serial determinations of serum amylase isoenzymes

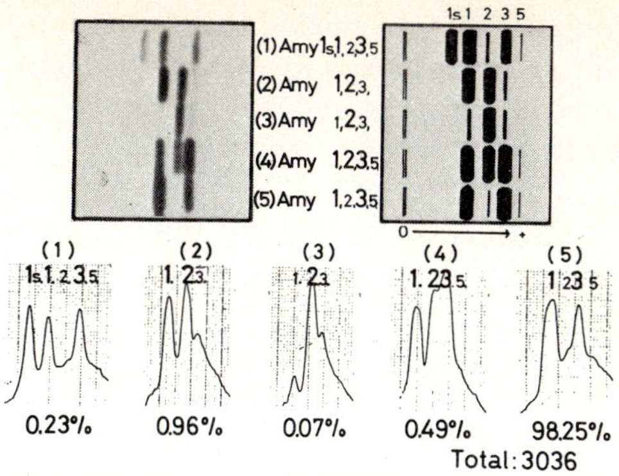

Fig. 7. Various representative patterns of amylase isoenzymes found in 3036 supposedly normal adult persons, and the corresponding densitometric tracings

There was no difference between the isoenzyme patterns in urine and serum of normal adult persons in whom both were examined. The prevalence of each pattern of amylase isoenzymes is shown at the bottom of the figure

amylase isoenzyme activity in the serum of normal persons differs among individuals, serial examinations of serum amylase isoenzymes are necessary in clinical practice. The importance of serial determination of serum amylase isoenzymes is shown by data for a patient (Figure 6). Total serum amylase activity was at the low normal level and did not change during the period of observations, although the patient complained of severe abdominal pain (Figure 6*A*). Analysis of serum amylase isoenzymes revealed that pancreatic-type isoamylase, which accounted for only 17% of the total serum amylase activity before the attack of abdominal pain (Figure 6*B*-1), had increased by as much as 50% during the attack (Figure 6*B*-2). From these changes in the proportion of pancreatic-type isoamylases, the patient was diagnosed as having suffered a relapse of chronic pancreatitis. Because the pattern of amylase isoenzymes in serum obtained during the attack (Figure 6*B*-2) showed the same pattern as in normal persons (Figure 5*B*), one might well have overlooked the relapse of pancreatitis if serial determinations of serum amylase isoenzymes had not been undertaken.

Although the serum and urinary amylase isoenzymes of more than 98% of normal persons consisted of two major isoenzymes and two to three minor ones, four different patterns of amylase isoenzymes were observed, as exemplified in Figure 7. Of normal persons, 0.23% had an isoenzyme with slower mobility than amylase-1. We call this rare isoenzyme "amylase-1_s" for the present. In the next three patterns, amylase activity of amylase-2, one of the minor components, was increased up to the same levels as amylase-1 or -3; 0.96% of these normal subjects showed decreased amylase activity of amylase-3, 0.07% showed decreased activity of both amylase-1 and -3, and 0.49% showed high activity of amylase-1 -2, and -3. It is not clear whether amylase-1_s is the same one as those called "Amy SE-1" by Boettcher and De La Lande (*43*), or "duplicated pancreatic amylase isoenzyme" by Kamaryt and Laxova (*7, 44*) and Vacikova and Blochova (*45*), or "Amy_2 B and C" by Merritt et al. (*46*), or "P_1" by Benjamin and Kenny (*22*). The prevalence of amylase-1_s is 0.23%, which is very low as compared with the 16.1% prevalence of duplicated P reported by Kamaryt and Laxova (*7, 44*), the 10.5% in Caucasian-Americans by Merritt et al. (*46*), the 10% by Boettcher and De La Lande (*43*), or the 5.3% reported by Vacikova and Blochova (*45*). Are these differences in prevalence due to racial differences or to the method of electrophoresis? Kamaryt and Laxova (*7, 44*) and Vacikova and Blochova (*45*) found the duplicated P isoenzyme by use of agar gel electrophoresis. Boettcher and De La Lande (*43*) and Merritt et al. (*46*) used polyacrylamide gel slab electrophoresis, whereas our amylase-1_s was found by electrophoresis on thin layers of polyacrylamide. We tentatively conclude that the difference in prevalence of this rare isoamylase is not attributable to the method of electrophoresis but is racial in origin.

Results of family studies (*47*) indicate that all of the four patterns of amylase isoenzymes shown in Figure 7 are under genetic control, so it is important to consider not only diseases but also genetic background before coming to a conclusion when amylase isoenzymes are used for clinical medicine.

In summary, we could separate the isoenzymes of amylase in serum, urine, and extracts of tissue homogenates by simple electrophoresis on thin-layer polyacrylamide gel. Such analysis of amylase isoenzyme is useful as a diagnostic tool for various diseases. However, it is always necessary to consider the conditions of samples and the genetic background carefully before coming to a conclusion.

References

1. Wohlgemuth, J., Über eine neue Methode zur quantitative Bestimmung des diastatischen Ferments. *Biochem. Z.* **9**, 1 (1908).

2. Weiss, M. J., Edmondson, H. A., and Wertman, M., Elevated serum amylase associated with bronchogenic carcinoma. *Am. J. Clin. Pathol.* **21**, 1057 (1951).

3. Kellev. M. L., Elevated serum amylase level associated with ruptured ectopic pregnancy. *J. Am. Med. Assoc.* **164**, 406 (1957).

4. Janowitz, H. D., and Dreiling, D. A., The plasma amylase; source, regulation and diagnostic significance. *Am. J. Med.* **27**, 924 (1959).

5. Hanafy, H. M., Gursel, E. O., and Veenema, R. L., Increased serum amylase levels in prostatic disease. *Urology* **1**, 372 (1973).

6. Berk, J. E., Searcy, R. L., Hayashi, S. and Ujihira, I., Distribution of serum amylase in man and animals. *J. Am. Med. Assoc.* **192**, 129 (1965).

7. Kamaryt, J., and Laxová, R., Amylase heterogeneity, some genetic and clinical aspects. *Humangenetik* **1**, 579 (1965).

8. Oger, A., and Bischops, L., Les iso-enzymes de l'amylase. *Clin. Chim. Acta* **13**, 670 (1966).

9. Afonso, E., On human serum amylase. *Clin. Chim. Acta* **14**, 195 (1966).

10. Joseph, R. R., Olivera, E., and Ressler, N., Electrophoretic study of human isoamylase. *Gastroenterology* **51**, 377 (1966).

11. Götz, H., Wüst, H., and Raies, F., Agar electrophoretische Studien zur Frage von Isoenzymen der Amylase. *Clin. Chim. Acta* **19**, 235 (1968).

12. Aw, S. E., Hobbs, J. R., and Wootton, I. D. P., Chromatographic purification of isoenzymes of human α-amylase. *Biochim. Biophys. Acta* **168**, 362 (1968).

13. De La Lande, F. A., and Boettcher, B., Electrophoretic examination of human serum amylase isoenzymes. *Enzymology* **37**, 335 (1969).

14. Skude, G., Combined electrophoretic and immunological methods in the study of human amylase. *Hereditas* **65**, 277 (1970).

15. Rosalki, S. B., A direct staining technique for amylase isoenzyme determination. *J. Clin. Pathol.* **23**, 373 (1970).

16. Meites, S., and Rogols, S., Amylase isoenzymes. *CRC Crit. Rev. Clin. Lab. Sci.* **2**, 103 (1971).

17. Davis, T. J., A fast technique for the separation and detection of amylase isoenzymes using a chromogenic substrate. *J. Clin. Pathol.* **25**, 266 (1972).

18. Straus, B., Mladinic, N., and Vujinovac, A., Electrophoretic separation of amylase isoenzymes. *Acta Pharm. Jugosl.* **22**, 83 (1972).

19. Taussig, L. M., Wolf, R. O., Woods, R. E., and Deckelbaum, R. J., Use of serum amylase isoenzymes in evalustion of pancreatic function. *Pediatrics* **54**, 229 (1974).

20. Otsuki, M., Sakoyama, Y., Park, K. A., et al., Electrophoretic examination of human serum amylase isoenzymes by using a simple thin layer polyacrylamide gel electrophoresis. *Physico-Chem. Biol.* **18**, 129 (1974).

21. Harada, K., Kitamura, M., and Ikenaga, T., Isoamylase study of postoperative transient hyperamylasemia. *Am. J. Gastroenterol.* **61**, 212 (1974).

22. Benjamin, D. R., and Kenny, M. A., Clinical value of amylase isoenzymes determination. *Am. J. Clin. Pathol.* **62**, 752 (1974).

23. Ceska, M., Birath, K., and Brown, B., A new and rapid method for the clinical determination of α-amylase activities in human serum and urine. *Clin. Chim. Acta* **26**, 437 (1969).

24. Fridhandler, L., Berk, J. E., Montgomery, K. A., and Wong, D., Column-chromatographic studies of isoamylases in human serum, urine, and milk. *Clin. Chem.* **20**, 457 (1974).

25. Kauffman, D. L., Zager, N. I., Cohen, E., and Keller, P. J., The isoenzymes of human parotid amylase. *Arch. Biochem. Biophys.* **137**, 325 (1979).

26. Robyt, J. F., Chittenden, C. G., and Lee, C. T., Structure and function of amylase; I. The subunit structure of porcine pancreatic α-amylase. *Arch. Biochem. Biophys.* **144**, 160 (1971).

27. McGeachin, R. L., and Lewis, J. P., Electrophoretic behavior of serum amylase. *J. Biol. Chem.* **234**, 795 (1959).

28. Dreiling, D. A., Janowitz, H. D., and Josephberg, L. J., An electrophoretic study of the blood amylase and the patterns observed in pancreatic disease. *Ann. Intern. Med.* **58**, 235 (1963).

29. Kumar, S., Gupta, M. C., and Tyagi, S. P., A study of serum amylase in infective hepatitis. *J. Indian Med. Assoc.* **55**, 194 (1970).

30. Bhutta, I. H., and Rahman, M. A., Serum amylase activity in liver disease. *Clin. Chem.* **17**, 1147 (1971).

31. Fridhandler, L., Berk, J. E., and Ueda, M., Isolation and measurement of pancreatic amylase in human serum and urine. *Clin. Chem.* **18**, 1493 (1972).

32. Warshaw, A. L., Studies on isoenzymes of human amylase; evidence for a circulating amylase not of pancreatic or salivary origin. *J. Surg. Res.* **16**, 360 (1974).

33. Otsuki, M., Saeki, S., Yuu, H., et al., Electrophoretic studies on human urinary amylase isoenzymes by using a simple thin layer polyacrylamide gel electrophoresis. *Physico-Chem. Biol.* **19**, 139 (1975).

34. Stiefel, D. J., and Keller, P. J., Preparation and some properties of human pancreatic amylase, including a comparison with human parotid amylase. *Biochim. Biophys. Acta* **302**, 345 (1973).

35. Ammann, R. W., Berk, J. E., Fridhandler, L., et al., Hyperamylasemia with carcinoma of the lung. *Ann. Intern. Med.* **78**, 521 (1973).

36. Otsuki, M., Saeki, S., Yuu, H., et al., Reassesment of clinical significance of amylase isoenzymes. *Clin. Chem.* **21**, 948 (1975). Abstract.

37. Otsuki, M., Saeki, S., Yuu, H., and Baba, S., Amylase and the lung. *Excerpta Med. Int. Congr. Ser.* **369**, 67 (1975).

38. Burt, R. L., and McAlister, J. A., Serum amylase in pregnancy and the puerperium, and in fetal blood. *Obstet. Gynecol.* **28**, 351 (1966).

39. Hadorn, B., Zoppi, G., Shmerling, D. H., et al., Quantitative assessment of exocrine pancreatic function in infants and children. *J. Pediat.* **73**, 39 (1968).

40. Lilibridge, C. B., and Townes, P. L., Physiologic deficiency of pancreatic amylase in infancy. *J. Pediat.* **82**, 279 (1973).

41. Kamaryt, J., Nieren-clearance der Isoamylasen beim Menschen. *Z. Klin. Chem. Klin. Biochem.* **7**, 51 (1969).

42. Duane, W. C., Frerichs, R., and Levitt, M.D., Distribution, turnover and mechanism of renal excretion of amylase in the baboon. *J. Clin. Invest.* **50**, 156 (1971).

43. Boettcher, B., and De La Lande, F. A., Unusual salivary and serum amylase isoenzymes in a man. *Enzymology* **40**, 234 (1970).

44. Kamaryt, J., and Laxova, R., Amylase heterogeneity variants in man. *Humangenetik* **3**, 41 (1966).

45. Vacikova, A., and Blochova, L., Isoamylase in blood donors. *Humangenetik* **8**, 162 (1969).

46. Merritt, A. D., Rivas, M. L., Biller, D., and Newell, F., Salivary and pancreatic amylase: electrophoretic characterizations and genetic studies. *Am. J. Hum. Genet.* **25**, 510 (1973).

47. Otsuki, M., Genetical investigation and clinical evaluation of amylase isoenzymes. *Physico-Chem. Biol.*, in press.

CLIN. CHEM. 22/4, 445–448 (1976)

Stability of Fatty Acids in Hyperlipoproteinemic Plasma During Long-Term Storage

Eugene Z. Hirsch, Sandra Slivka, and Austin P. Gibbons

Aliquots of hyperlipoproteinemic plasma were stored at −20 °C in a nitrogen atmosphere with added disodium ethylenediaminetetraacetate for up to one year, to determine the stability of fatty acids in the four major lipid classes under these conditions. Assays were performed at zero time and at 2, 5, and 12 months. No uniform fatty acid change was found. Minor statistically significant changes were found in total triglyceride fatty acids and in some of the individual fatty acids in cholesterol esters, phospholipid, and free fatty acids. These minor changes could not be accounted for by plasma lipid concentrations, lipolysis, or fatty acid peroxidation. Evidently, plasma can be stored in this manner for as long as a year without substantial change in fatty acids in any of the four major lipid classes.

In spite of the general belief that plasma lipid fatty acids should be separated and assayed promptly (*1*), there are few published data documenting the consequence of delay or verifying stability under appropriate conditions of storage. Whether in research or in clinical studies that may require the monitoring of adherence to a dietary regimen (*2, 3*), practical considerations encourage the serial accumulation of a number of samples of plasma, which are all analyzed at the same time, as convenient. The present study was undertaken to determine the stability of fatty acids, whether TGFA, CEFA, PLFA, or FFA[1] when plasma was stored frozen for up to one year. Only minor changes were encountered during the special conditions of storage.

Methods

Patients included in this study (Table 1) were diagnosed as having hyperlipoproteinemia on the basis of serial values for serum cholesterol and plasma triglyceride, determined by routine continuous-flow techniques, and for lipoprotein, as evaluated by electrophoresis (Pol-E-Film system; Pfizer Diagnostics Div., New York, N. Y. 10017). Some patients were being treated with diet and hypolipidemic agents.

Venous blood samples were drawn into chilled test tubes containing disodium EDTA, 1 mg/ml. Plasma was immediately centrifuged at 4 °C and filtered. An excess of EDTA was added and the insoluble portion allowed to settle. Four separate aliquots were removed from the supernate. One was extracted within 1 h and processing begun the same day. The other three (2.0–2.5 ml) were placed in screw-top tubes for analysis in sequence at 2, 5, and 12 months. Pure nitrogen was bubbled through each sample for 1 to 2 min, carefully, to avoid frothing. The tubes were capped, sealed with tape, and stored in a freezer at −20 °C. Each sample was frozen only once.

Plasma, 0.25 ml, was extracted in duplicate or triplicate with 9 ml of chloroform/methanol (2/1 by vol) (*4*). Internal standards were added to the extraction mixture for subsequent calculation of TGFA, CEFA, and FFA content. The mixture was shaken every 15 min. After 1 h, 20 ml of dilute H_2SO_4 (0.5 ml/liter) was added. The mixture was stored overnight at 4 °C. The lower phase was removed and evaporated under nitrogen. Thin-layer chromatography was done in hexane/diethyl ether/glacial acetic acid (90/10/1 by vol) on silica gel C plates, 250 μm thickness, from Analtech Inc., Newark, Del. 19711. Index spots of plasma extracts were stained in an iodine chamber. Methyl esters were prepared from unstained spots by heating silica gel scrapings with 1–2 ml of dilute H_2SO_4 (20 ml/liter) in methanol at 70 °C for 2 h (*5*); the esters were then extracted with hexane and the extract was washed with distilled water.

Gas-liquid chromatography was done on a Hewlett-Packard Model 402 flame-ionization chromatograph with a 185 cm (six foot) column containing 6% diethylene glycol succinate on 80–100 mesh Diatoport S (Hewlett-Packard, Avondale, Pa. 19311) at an oven temperature of 185 °C, with helium as the carrier gas. Chromatograms resolved long-chain fatty acids up to and including C20:4. The insignificant amounts of higher fatty acids that are present are not of clinical importance and could not have been measured accurately by our system.

Areas under the following chromatographic peaks were measured by triangulation: C16:0, C16:1, C18:0, C18:1, C18:2, and C20:4.[2] By comparison with areas

Veterans Administration Hospital, and the Department of Medicine, Case-Western Reserve University, Cleveland, Ohio 44106.

[1] Nonstandard abbreviations used: TGFA, triglyceride fatty acids; CEFA, cholesterol ester fatty acids; PLFA, phospholipid fatty acids; FFA, "free" fatty acids; and EDTA, ethylenediaminetetraacetate.

Received Oct. 14, 1975; accepted Jan. 21, 1976.

[2] The conventional symbolism; e.g., C16:1 signifies a 16-carbon fatty acid with one double bond.

Table 1. Pertinent Clinical Data

Sample no.	Patient[a]	Age	Serum cholesterol[b] (mg/liter)	Plasma triglyceride[b] (mg/liter)	Hyperlipoproteinemia type
1	F.T.	49	2500	6000	IV
2	R.J.	53	2460	2220	IV
3	W.T.	63	3280	1980	IIa
4[c]	J.D.	43	3430	11000	IV
5	S.M.	33	1950	2000	IV
6	S.S.	59	1600	4410	IV
7[c]	J.D.	43	3180	2160	IV
8	L.M.	36	2570	2530	IV
9	L.K.	47	3350	1200	IIa

[a] Patients fasted for 14–16 h before sample collection.
[b] Continuous-flow analysis within several days of blood collection for fatty acid determinations.
[c] Blood sampled at different times from the same patient.

given by the respective internal standards for TGFA, CEFA, and FFA, the content of each of these was calculated. The total of the six was called 100%, and was considered to represent total fatty acid content. Each separate category then was expressed as percentage of the total. With no internal standard available for PLFA, the individual components were expressed simply as percentage of the total as based on area measurements alone. Fatty acids were identified by comparison with National Institutes of Health standards. With each daily series of determinations the NIH standard mixture KD (from Applied Science Laboratories, State College, Pa. 16801) was reproducible within limits of 5% for major fatty acids and 10% for minor fatty acids.

Because the value determined in freshly drawn blood was subject to the same analytical errors as were the succeeding three values after storage, all four values were used to construct a regression line by least-squares fit (*6*). Regression lines were constructed for total TGFA, CEFA, and FFA values (Figure 1) and for percentage of individual fatty acid in the four major lipid classes of each patient's plasma. The intercept of each line at zero time (y_0) was taken as the best approximation of a starting value, and the point on the line at 12 months (y_{12}) was compared to y_0 in terms of percentage change ($(y_{12} - y_0/y_0) \times 100$). A mean value for percentage change was then calculated, and its significance was determined by Student's *t*-test.

Because all assays were performed in duplicate or triplicate, the technical precision of fatty acid measurements in each of the lipid classes could be compared with each other by calculating the dispersion shown in the respective replicates. Thus, analytical error of replicate extraction and assay was judged on the basis of the root-mean-square of the percent deviations of members of replicate groups from their mean. Table 2 shows the technical standard error of

Table 2. Technical Standard Error of Measurement of Total and Two Major Fatty Acids (SD Expressed as Percent of Total Fatty Acids) in Four Categories of Lipids

	Total	C18:1	C18:2
TGFA	3.8	1.15	0.66
CEFA	4.4	0.87	1.34
PLFA	—	0.55	0.79
FFA	12.4	1.36	1.32

Table 3. Mean Fatty Acid Composition at Zero Time (y_0), and Change at 12 Months

	TGFA		CEFA		PLFA		FFA	
Fatty acid	Initial %	% Change[a]	Initial %	% Change	Initial %	% Change	Initial %	% Change
C16:0	25.9	+1.2 ± 2.1	12.7	−0.3 ± 0.7	29.3	+0.9[b] ± 0.8	28.8	+0.9 ± 2.5
C16:1	3.6	−0.1 ± 1.3	3.0	−0.2 ± 1.5	1.5	−1.0 ± 1.4	1.9	+0.4 ± 1.1
C18:0	3.9	−0.4 ± 0.6	1.4	−0.3[b] ± 0.2	15.3	+0.1 ± 0.9	12.6	−1.6[b] ± 0.8
C18:1	44.4	+0.6 ± 1.7	22.4	+0.01 ± 2.0	13.5	+1.2[b] ± 0.8	38.5	−0.6 ± 2.5
C18:2	20.9	−0.1 ± 1.5	52.3	+0.2 ± 2.6	24.1	−0.5 ± 0.8	17.5	+1.7 ± 2.5
[c]	*	*	*	*	4.4	−0.7[b] ± 0.3	*	*
C20:4	1.8	−0.2 ± 0.9	8.9	−0.9 ± 2.2	12.8	−1.2[b] ± 0.8	*	*

[a] ± values are SD
[b] $P \leq 0.01$ by *t*-test
[c] Unidentified peak
* No peak

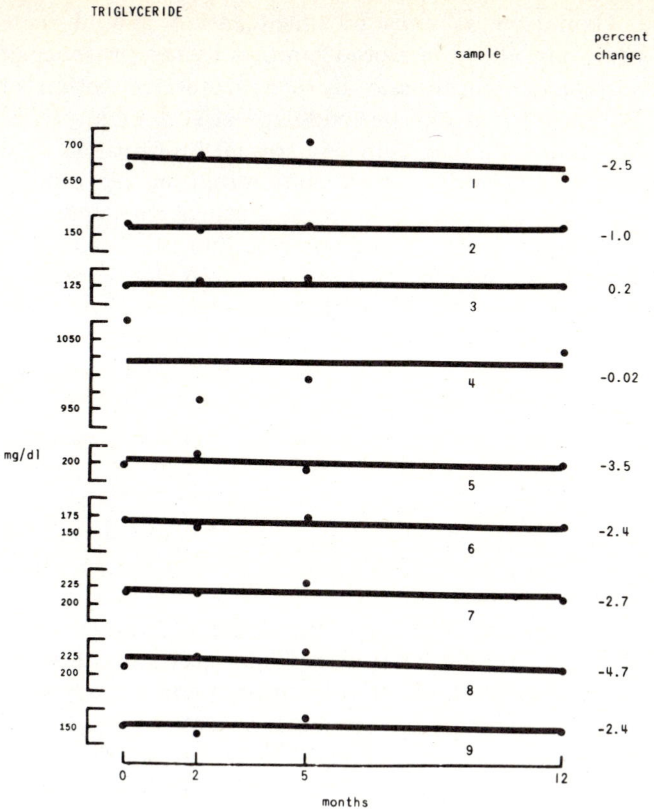

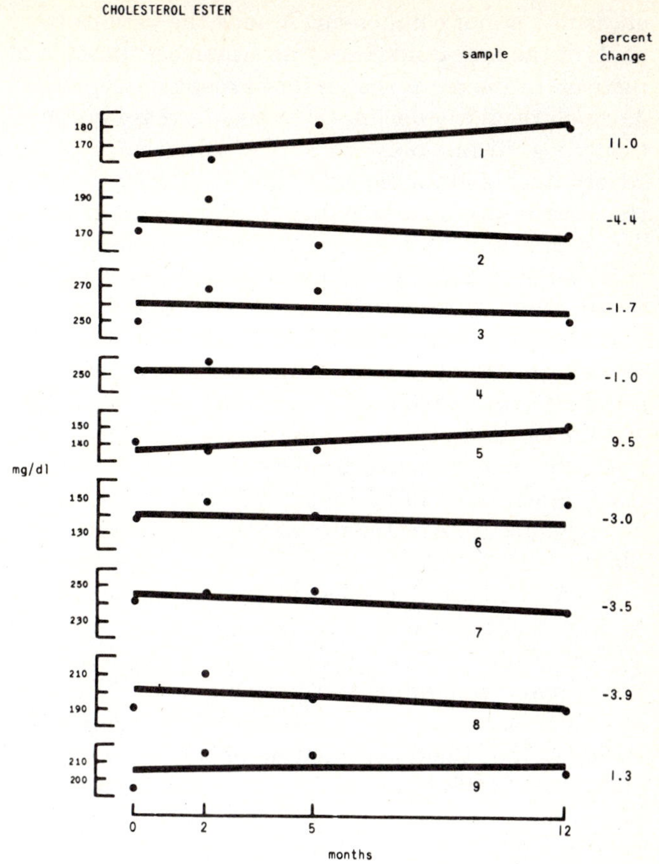

the measurement of total and two major individual fatty acids in each lipid class. By expressing variation in percentage units it was possible to calculate the standard deviation for a series of measurements performed on plasma with widely differing lipid concentration. Thus, SD = $\sqrt{d^2/n}$, where d is percent deviation of a replicate number from its associated mean, and n >72 with 36 plasma samples.

Results

Figure 1 shows data points and regressions for total fatty acids of TGFA, CEFA, and FFA at 0, 2, 5, and 12 months, as obtained for each of the nine samples. On the right is the percentage change for each sample, based on the intercepts of these lines at zero time and 12 months. The mean change for TGFA in 12 months was −2.1% ± 1.49% SD, that for CEFA was +0.5% ± 5.5% SD, and for FFA, −4.8% ± 12.7% SD. The mean decline for TGFA is significantly different from zero by the t-test (P <0.005), but the change in the other two lipids is not significant. Lacking a suitable gas-chromatographic standard for PLFA, we could not calculate the total concentration of this fraction.

In Table 3 the initial percent contribution of each class of fatty acids to the group as a whole is given for all four categories of lipids. Few significant changes are apparent at 12 months. The greatest proportional change relative to starting value is for C18:0 fatty acid of CEFA, which declined from 1.4% of total to 1.1%. Likewise, C18:0 declined in TGFA (P <0.05) and in FFA. Although these changes are statistically significant, they represent small numerical differ-

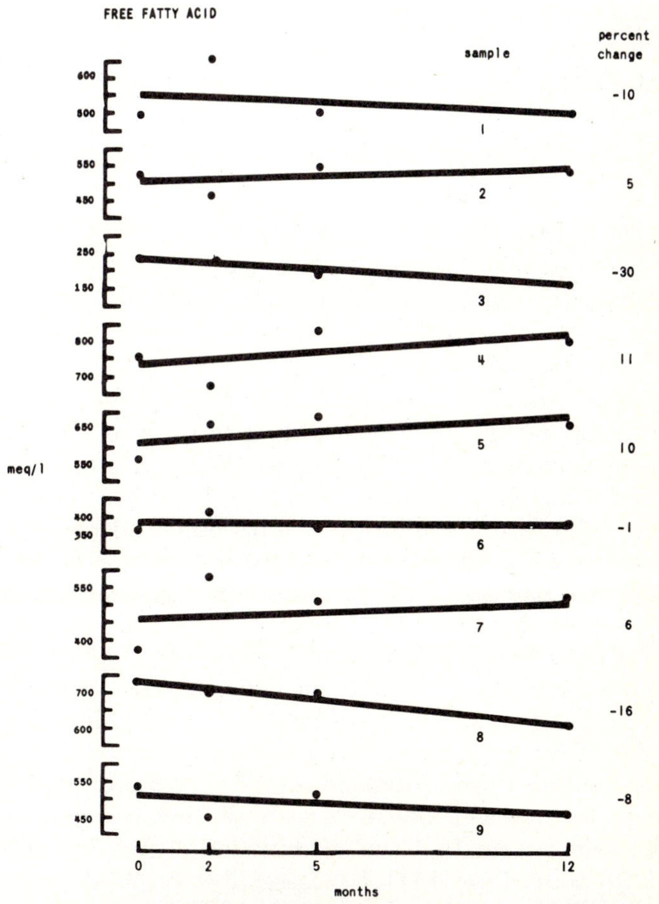

Fig. 1. Triglyceride, cholesterol ester, and free fatty acid total fatty acid values, least-squares regression lines, and individual twelve month percent change for each sample

ences in a minor component. Among the various fatty acids of the four lipid classes no systematic pattern of increase or decrease is apparent except for type C20: 4, which regularly declines, but the decrease is statistically significant only for PLFA. Differences in recovery during extraction should not affect change in the distribution of individual fatty acids as given in Table 3. Such differences should be randomly distributed at 0, 2, 5, and 12 months, and hence not introduce any systematic effect on trend with time.

It should be pointed out that chloroform/methanol extraction, although a favorable procedure for recovering esterified lipids, is not ideal for FFA. We added H_2SO_4 to the extraction mixture to maximize FFA recovery. Nevertheless, total FFA values calculated from constituent fatty acids cannot be taken as an entirely accurate estimate of its concentration in plasma.

Table 2 shows that there is greater variability in measurement of total fatty acids in FFA than in TGFA or CEFA. In contrast, variability of representative major individual fatty acids of FFA (Table 2) is similar to that of the other lipid fatty acids. This indicates that the determination of the percentage of individual fatty acids in FFA, as we did, is an appropriate basis on which to judge change in percentage of individual FFA fatty acids during storage.

The severity of hyperlipoproteinemia (from Table 1) shows no correlation with 12-month changes in total TGFA, CEFA, or FFA, or with changes in individual fatty acid constituents. Likewise, total TGFA, CEFA, and FFA values at y_0 show no correlation with changes in individual fatty acids. Thus, plasma lipid concentrations do not influence stability of fatty acids.

Discussion

There is no question that serum cholesterol is stable with refrigeration (*3*). Likewise, there is no question that lipoproteins are altered rapidly by freezing and storage (*7*). However, we have not found evidence to support suggestions that triglycerides, phospholipids, and presumably their fatty acids are invariably unstable with storage. With titrimetric or colorimetric determination of total FFA, two studies showed FFA instability over a period of several days (*8, 9*), while others demonstrated stability for as long as five months (*10, 11*). No uniform conditions have been used that would allow for a critical comparison of these divergent results.

A possible mechanism for deterioration of esterified lipids would be hydrolysis leading to an increase in FFA accompanied by a decrease of fatty acids in esterified form. Although TGFA decreased by 2% during storage, total free acids did not increase. It would appear that the combination of freezing and the addition of EDTA successfully prevents appreciable cleavage by plasma lipases. EDTA is known to inhibit lipoprotein lipase (*12*) and to effectively inhibit in vitro lipid peroxidation.

Oxidation at sites of unsaturation should have been minimized in stored samples by the presence of ambient nitrogen and by the protective action of EDTA against the peroxidative effects of any contaminating hemoglobin. No special precautions were taken to avoid plasma contamination by minute amounts of hemoglobin from erythrocytes they may have lysed during blood drawing and plasma separation. The approximate 10% decline in the percentage contribution by C20:4 fatty acids in the three lipid classes of Table 3 suggest that oxidative change might not have been completely prevented. However, only for PLFA was the decrease statistically significant, and the C18:2 acids, a major component of all lipids, showed no significant tendency to decrease.

In our subjects the contributions of fatty acid types within TGFA, CEFA, and PLFA (Table 3) are similar to those reported by Dayton et al. (*2*), albeit their values for C18:2 fatty acids were slightly lower in a general population receiving a "conventional diet." In the National Diet–Heart Study (*3*) the C18: 2/C18:1 ratio (linoleate/oleate) in a similar series averaged 2.65–2.70, as compared to 4.44 for subjects on lipid-lowering diets. In the present study this mean ratio was 2.24. These differences appear to be relatively small compared with differences in patient selection and sampling size.

Variability was independent of plasma lipid concentration. Presumably normo-lipoproteinemic plasma would respond similarly.

References

1. Messerschmidt, H. G. M., Lipid screening and lipoprotein electrophoresis by Collegel. *Clin. Chim. Acta* **36,** 51 (1971).
2. Dayton, S., Hashimoto, S., Dixon, W., and Pearce, M. L., Composition of lipids in human serum and adipose tissue during prolonged feeding of a diet high in unsaturated fat. *J. Lipid Res.* **7,** 103 (1966).
3. The National Diet–Heart Study Final Report. *Am. Heart Assoc. Monograph No. 18,* 1968; American Heart Association, Inc., 44 E. 23rd St., New York, N. Y. 10010.
4. Folch, J., Lees, M., and Sloane-Stanley, G. H., A simple method for preparation of total pure lipide extracts from brain. *Fed. Proc.* **13,** 209 (1954).
5. Havel, R. J., Felts, J. M., and VanSluyne, C. M., Formation and fate of endogenous triglycerides in blood plasma of rabbits. *J. Lipid Res.* **3,** 297 (1962).
6. Mendenhall, W., *Introduction to Statistics.* Wadsworth Pub. Co., Belmont, Calif., 1964.
7. Hatch, F. T., and Lees, R. S., Practical methods for plasma lipoprotein analysis. In *Advances in Lipid Research* **6,** R. Paoletti and D. Kritchevsky, Eds. Academic Press, New York, N. Y., 1968, p 30.
8. Forbes, A. L., and Camlin, J. A., Effects of storage on serum nonesterified fatty acid concentrations. *Proc. Soc. Exp. Biol. Med.* **102,** 709 (1959).
9. Fairweather, D. V. I., and Layton, R., Observations on the collection and handling of blood samples for N.E.F.A. estimation. *J. Clin. Pathol.* **20,** 665 (1967).
10. Broechoven, C., and Parijs, J., Effects of storage on plasma non-esterified fatty acid concentration. *Clin. Chim. Acta* **20,** 530 (1968).
11. Pehrson, B., Studies of the blood lipid pattern in healthy dairy cows. *Acta Vet. Scand.* **12,** 230 (1971).
12. Korn, E. D., and Quigley, T. W., Lipoprotein lipase of chicken adipose tissue. *J. Biol. Chem.* **226,** 833 (1957).

CLIN. CHEM. 22/4, 449–455 (1976)

Development of an Aqueous Temperature-Indicating Technique and Its Application to Clinical Laboratory Instrumentation

Lemuel Bowie, Fred Esters, Jeffrey Bolin, and Nathan Gochman

We describe a new technique for monitoring intra-cuvette temperatures in temperature-controlled spectrophotometric cells by use of two solutions, one for which absorbance is highly sensitive to temperature and one for which absorbance is insensitive to temperature. The first solution, cresol red in tris(hydroxymethyl)aminomethane buffer, is used to construct an absorbance-vs.-temperature calibration curve. The second solution, cresol red in sodium hydroxide, is used for optical calibration of the spectrophotometric system to be tested. The combination of these two procedures allows accurate estimation of temperature. We show how this technique is applied to temperature measurement in several types of laboratory instrumentation.

Additional Keyphrases: *temperature-equilibrium times for samples in various automated instruments • temperatures of solutions in cuvettes during analysis • change in pH with temperature of various buffers*

With the advent of sophisticated automated instrumentation and the increasing use of enzyme activity measurements in the laboratory, the need for accurate temperature calibration and regulation is becoming increasingly more important. It is well known, for instance, that the rate of enzymatic reactions may change by 10% or more per degree Celsius change in temperature (*1*). Therefore, for accurate and reproducible results, the temperature should be known and regulatable to within ±0.1 °C or less. In fact, the Expert Panel on Enzymes of the International Federation of Clinical Chemistry recommends (*2*) that temperature be known and maintained to ±0.05 °C.

Currently most automated and manual systems make use of external probes (usually thermistors) to monitor temperature. These devices all suffer a major drawback: they cannot be readily inserted into the fluid that is to be analyzed, or even into the wall of the reaction vessel.

We believed it would be desirable to have an aqueous temperature-indicating system, which could be subjected to the same conditions as reaction mixtures to be analyzed and which would respond to temperature changes by changes in absorbance. Therefore, we decided to couple the well-known temperature–pH dependency of certain alkaline buffers to the pH dependency of the absorbance of certain organic chromophores.

Independent of our investigations, a method was developed for measuring temperature-equilibration times in the centrifugal analyzer by use of a buffered phenolphthalein solution (*3*). The aqueous temperature-indicating technique that we propose here can be used to monitor both thermal-equilibration times and actual intra-cuvette temperature. The latter objective is achieved by uniquely providing a dual measuring technique, to compensate for optical differences between the calibrating spectrophotometer and the test system.

Materials and Methods

Instrumentation

Model 118C Recording Spectrophotometer (Varian Instrument Division/Cary Products, Monrovia, Calif. 91016). This instrument was used for all scans of absorption spectra and also in preparing calibration curves (absorbance vs. temperature.) All scanned spectra were recorded at 25 °C with use of the double-beam and auto-slit modes, with a gain of 2.5 and a scan rate of 1.0 nm/s. The instrument was

Laboratory Service, VA Hospital, San Diego, Calif. 92161.
Received Dec. 1, 1975; accepted Jan. 23, 1976.
Presented in part at the 9th International Congress on Clinical Chemistry, Toronto, Canada, July 13–18, 1975 [paper 159; *Clin. Chem.* **21**, 971 (1975)].

equipped with a Model 01-644200-00 thermostattable cell holder and a Model 01-640150-00 thermostattable cell compartment. Unless otherwise noted, all measurements were made with a 3-ml volume, in 1-cm pathlength quartz cells equipped with Teflon stoppers to prevent evaporation. In preparing calibration curves, we introduced 3-ml aliquots into the cells, stoppered them, and allowed them to equilibrate for at least 20 min at each temperature. Temperature was controlled by use of a Lauda Model K-2/R circulating bath connected to the thermostattable cell holder.

To check the accuracy of temperature control, we placed a National Bureau of Standards (NBS) calibrated thermistor in the cuvette that contained 3-ml of CR-T[1] and sealed the top with Parafilm. Voltages across the thermistor as a function of temperature were recorded and the corresponding resistances calculated. The temperature of the fluid inside the cuvette could then be read with an accuracy of ±0.01 °C from a resistance-vs.-temperature calibration curve that was supplied with the thermistor. An NBS constant-current source was used to generate a constant current (about 10 μA) that was independent of the resistance value of the thermistor. Voltages were read (from 180.00 mV to 70.00 mV) on a Model 3465A Digital Multimeter (Hewlett-Packard, Palo Alto, Calif. 94304).

Absorbances were measured at 575 nm, with water in the reference path. In those experiments to determine thermal equilibration times in the Cary spectrophotometer, we incubated reagents and pipettes for at least 30 min at 4 °C or 25 °C before introducing the indicator solution into an empty cuvette, which had also been thermally regulated for at least 20 min at either 30 °C or 37 °C.

Model 300-N Spectrophotometer (Gilford Instrument Laboratories, Inc., Oberlin, Ohio 44074). The Gilford 300-N equipped with a Model 3017 (flow through) thermo-cuvette was electronically maintained at 30 or 37 °C, and the equilibration times and equilibrium temperatures were determined. The instrument was zeroed against water, followed by two 3-s purges with air. CR-T, which had been equilibrated for 30 min at room temperature (26.5 °C) or in an ice bath, was then aspirated into the spectrophotometer. Again, all measurements were made at 575 nm.

GEMSAEC *centrifugal analyzer* (Electro-Nucleonics, Inc. Fairfield, N. J. 07006). This instrument was thermally regulated at 30 °C or 37 °C (±0.01 °C) with a Lauda K-2/R circulating bath. In this system, temperature was controlled by passing the temperature-control fluid through a cowl that surrounds (but is not in contact with) the rotor that contains the spinning cells. Reagent and pipettes were equilibrated for 30 min at 4 °C or at 25 °C and 0.5-ml aliquots were rapidly transferred into the "C" positions of the transfer disc, which had been in position in the analyzer for at least 5 min. The instrument was started immediately and the changes in absorbance were monitored. This modified procedure permitted measurement of the initial changes in absorbance during temperature equilibration, which would not be observed with the usual sample-loading steps. About 45 s elapsed between the time of aspiration and the time the "READ" light came on. The instrument was programmed to take the first reading at 10 s (setting IR = 10), after initiation of the READ sequence followed by 20 readings (NR = 20), 60 s apart (RI = 60). Readings were taken at 575 nm, with water in the reference cuvette (position 1).

Du Pont Automatic Clinical Analyzer (*aca;* E. I. du Pont De Nemours & Co., Inc., Wilmington, Del. 19898). The *aca* incorporates a combination of air heaters/circulators and contact heaters for temperature control at 37 °C. Reagents (5 ml) were introduced into "ABS" packs that were modified to code for an unused channel (in our case, channel 28).[2] The unused channel was then programmed to take absorbance readings at 583 nm (filter No. 10) and subtract the absorbances at 600 nm (filter No. 12). A calibration curve of absorbance vs. temperature (data from the Cary 118C), prepared by subtraction of readings at 600 nm from those obtained at 583 nm, was used to determine *aca* temperature from these readings. CR-N was also read at 583 nm and 600 nm, and the readings were used to correct absorbance differences to absorbance differences on the Cary 118C (see *Procedure for temperature estimation*).

Temperature-controlled pH measurements were made with a Radiometer Model pHM26 pH meter, with use of a combination electrode and internal temperature compensation. The system was calibrated at 30 °C against pH 7.0 phosphate buffer. The buffer (5 ml) was placed in a standard 28 mm × 61 mm scintillation vial with a screw cap to prevent evaporation. The closed vial was placed in a custom-prepared, temperature-controlled brass vial holder, which was connected to a Lauda K-2/R circulator and allowed to equilibrate for 30 min at the appropriate temperatures. The cap was then removed and the electrode was placed in the solution until a stable reading was obtained. The temperature of the solution in the vial was then measured with an NBS thermometer (Standard Reference Material No. 934). The vial was then recapped and equilibrated at the next temperature, after which the operation was repeated.

Reagents

Cresol red (*o*-cresol sulfonphthalein) was obtained from Aldrich Chemical Co., Inc., Milwaukee, Wis. 53233. Tris buffer was prepared from "Trizma" base (Sigma Chemical Co., St. Louis, Mo. 63178) and ad-

[1] Nonstandard abbreviations used: CR-T, cresol red in Tris (0.1 mol/liter, pH 7.5); Tris, tris(hydroxymethyl)aminomethane; CR-N, cresol red in NaOH (1 mol/liter); and NBS, National Bureau of Standards.

[2] Contact the authors for additional details regarding modification of pack coding and photometer method switching-board parameters.

justed to the proper pH with concentrated hydrochloric acid. A stock solution of cresol red (10 g/liter) in methanol, stored at 4 °C, was used to prepare the working solutions of cresol red, CR-T and CR-N.[1]

Procedure for Temperature Estimation

1. A calibration curve for temperature vs. absorbance at 575 nm is prepared for CR-T on a suitable spectrophotometer as described under *Instrumentation: Cary 118C*. A wide-range calibration curve is obtained by monitoring the absorbance change in 2 °C increments over a range of about 20 °C (e.g., 20–40 °C). For increased accuracy about a single temperature, a narrow-range calibration curve can be prepared that brackets the temperature of interest by ±2–5 °C and is generated in 0.5 °C increments. Because the absorbance vs. temperature relation for CR-T exponential in character,[3] it can be described by the following equation:

$$A_{\text{corrected}} = a e^{-bT} \tag{1}$$

where the coefficients a and b are determined experimentally for each batch of CR-T working solution, and T is the temperature in °C.

2. The absorbance at 575 nm of the solution of CR-N is then measured on the same spectrophotometer at about the temperature of the spectrophotometric system of interest. Because the absorbance change per degree change in temperature is almost negligible for this solution, this temperature setting is not critical.

3. The CR-T solution is introduced into the spectrophotometric test system and the absorbance at 575 nm is allowed to stabilize for a length of time that depends on the system and may vary from less than 1 min to longer than 30 min. The value of this stabilized absorbance is noted.

4. The system's cuvette is thoroughly rinsed, the CR-N solution is introduced, and the absorbance of this solution is noted.

5. The absorbance of CR-T on the test system ($A_{\text{CRT-Test}}$) is then normalized to that of the calibrating system by multiplying by the ratio of the absorbance of CR-N on the calibrating spectrophotometer ($A_{\text{CRN-CAL}}$) to the absorbance of CR-N on the test system ($A_{\text{CRN-Test}}$):

$$A_{\text{corrected}} = (A_{\text{CRN-CAL}}/A_{\text{CRN-Test}}) \times A_{\text{CRT-Test}}$$

6. The temperature of the test system is then determined by using this corrected absorbance to read the temperature from the absorbance-vs.-temperature calibration curve. Alternatively, the temperature of CR-T can also be directly calculated from the corrected absorbance by this equation, which follows from equation 1:

$$T = (\ln A_{\text{corrected}} - \ln a)/-b \tag{2}$$

In typical experiments, a is found to equal 2.732 and b is equal to 0.0351, which gives a calculated curve with a correlation coefficient of 0.998 with the experimentally determined points.

[3]The data have also been analyzed by regression analysis for goodness of fit to a parabolic model ($A_{\text{corrected}} = a + b\,T + c\,T^2$) and a power model ($A_{\text{corrected}} = aT^b$). Between 20 and 40 °C, the parabolic model gives essentially the same correlation coefficient as does the exponential model (0.998–0.999). However, the exponential model is theoretically more appropriate, because it is well known that the relation between temperature and reaction rates and equilibria is (within relevant limits) exponential in character. The correlation coefficient for the data analyzed by the power model was 0.986.

Table 1. Temperature Coefficients of Aqueous Buffers[a]

Buffer	Concn, mol/liter	Coefficient ($\Delta pH/\Delta T$) $\times 10^3$
Citrate	0.05	−2.2
Tartrate	0.0341	−1.4
Phthalate	0.05	+1.2
Phosphate	0.025	−2.8
Tris	0.167	−15.0
Borax	0.01	−8.2
Sodium carbonate	0.025	−9.6
Calcium hydroxide	0.0203	−33.0

[a] Adapted from references *4* and *5*.

Results

Table 1 lists the temperature coefficients of several aqueous buffers. Note that, in general, the alkaline buffers give higher temperature coefficients (i.e., large $\Delta pH/\Delta T$). In particular, calcium hydroxide, which has maximum buffer capacity in the range between pH 11 and 13, and Tris, which has maximum buffer capacity in the range between pH 7 and 9, give large changes in pH with temperature. Calcium hydroxide has the disadvantage, however, that it can absorb carbon dioxide from the atmosphere and in time form insoluble calcium carbonate and concomitant turbidity.

For this reason, we selected Tris as the best buffer system for the temperature-sensitive component of the system. Figure 1 shows the actual variation in pH as a function of temperature of a solution of 0.1 mol/liter Tris. Under our conditions the average change in pH is about 0.03 pH units per degree Celsius. It should also be noted that pH change per degree is somewhat greater at low than at higher temperatures.

A number of aromatic compounds with ionizable groups have absorption spectra that are sensitive to the pH of the solvent. Perhaps some of the most well-known and useful ones (those with high molar absorptivities) are the classical acid–base indicators. Of a number of indicators tried (including phenol red, neutral red, *p*-nitrophenol, thymol blue, and phenolphthalein), cresol red was found to be the best chromophore with regard to solubility, stability, and

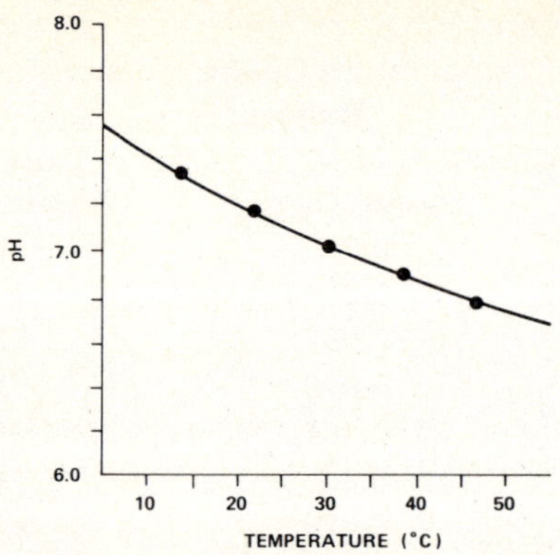

Fig. 1. Variation in pH of Tris buffer, 0.1 mol/liter, as a function of temperature

Buffer volume was 5 ml and the vial containing the buffer was thermally regulated as described in *Materials and Methods*

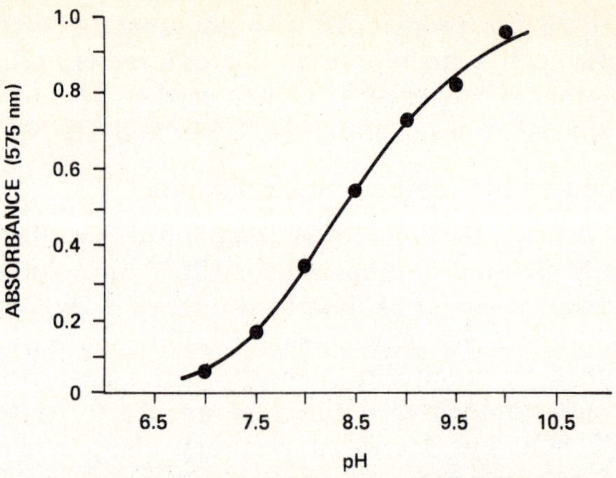

Fig. 3. Variation in the absorbance at 575 nm of cresol red (4.3 mg/liter) in Tris, 0.1 mol/liter, as a function of pH

Absorbance measured with a Cary 118C. The results indicate a pK of 8.45 for the ionization of cresol red

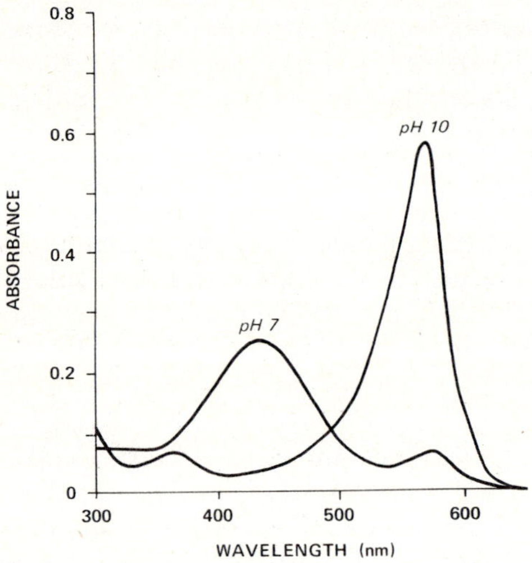

Fig. 2. Absorption spectra of cresol red at 25 °C in 0.1 mol/liter Tris at pH 7.0 and at pH 10.0

Spectra recorded with a Cary 118C; cresol red concentration, 4.3 mg/liter

spectral properties when used in combination with Tris buffer solutions at selected pH's. The absorption spectra of this chromophore at neutral and alkaline pH's are shown in Figure 2. Maximum absorption occurs at 435 nm at neutral pH, but the absorption maximum shifts to 575 nm when the chromophore becomes ionized in alkaline buffer. Although not shown in this figure, as pH is slowly increased from pH 7 to pH 10, absorption at 435 nm progressively decreases while the absorption at 575 nm continually increases. The change in absorbance is about 2.5-fold greater at 575 nm than at 435 nm. Therefore the anionic form of the chromophore at 575 nm is much more sensitive to pH changes than the un-ionized chromophore, whose major visible absorption is at 435 nm. Figure 3 shows the pH dependence of the absorption of cresol red at 575 nm in 0.1 mol/liter Tris. The shape is typical of a titration curve for an ionizing group with a pK of 8.4. A similar curve, obtained by plotting the decrease in absorbance at 435 nm, as a function of pH, also gives a pK of about 8.4.

The combination of the temperature-dependent pH change of Tris buffer with the pH-dependent absorbance change of cresol red results in a solution for which the light-absorbing properties are highly temperature-sensitive. Although the change in absorbance with pH is greatest near pH 8.4 (Figure 3), we found that the change in absorbance vs. temperature continually increased as the pH was decreased from pH 9.5 (0.007 *A* per °C) to pH 7.0 (0.03 *A* per °C). Owing to the poor buffering capacity of Tris below pH 7.0 and because of the importance of pH stability of the system, we chose pH 7.5 as the most appropriate pH for the system. The upper curve in Figure 4 shows the absorbance at 575 nm as a function of intra-cuvette temperature of 30 mg of CR-T per liter, pH 7.5. The curve is exponential, giving rise to slightly higher absorbance changes per degree at lower temperatures than at higher temperatures. At temperatures far above ambient (e.g., 40 °C) the intra-cuvette temperature can differ by as much as 2 °C from the temperature of the fluid in the circulatory bath, as determined by the use of an NBS calibrated thermistor. These heat losses between the circulating bath and the thermostatted cell can be minimized by insulating the connecting tubing, or shortening the length of tubing between the bath and cell, or both. The intra-cuvette temperature was measured in 5 °C increments between 20 and 40 °C with the NBS thermistor. The absorbance change in CR-T bath temperature was then measured in 2 °C increments and corrected by using the data from the thermistor-derived temperatures to correct for heat losses at higher temperatures. As can be seen, the absorbance change per degree near 30 °C is about 0.033. The sensitivity of the CR-T solution, however, is more accurately described in terms of the percentage change of the total absorbance per degree (approximately 3.3% per degree). Therefore, to increase the sensitivity

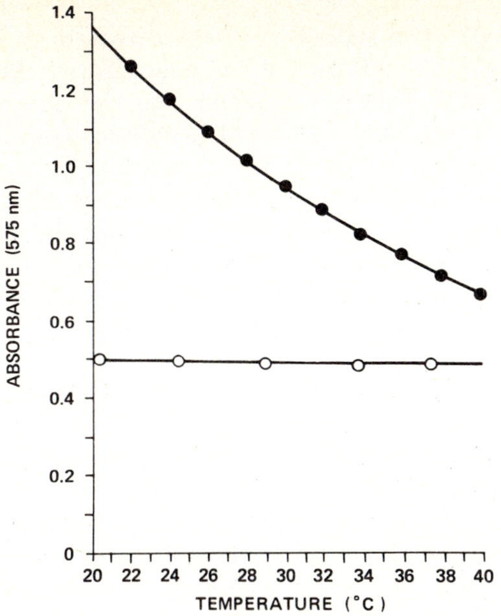

Fig. 4. Variation of absorbance at 575 nm of cresol red (30 mg/liter) in Tris (0.1 mol/liter) pH 7.5 (●) and cresol red (10 mg/liter) in 1.0 mol/liter NaOH (○) as a function of temperature

These results were obtained with the Cary 118C, with a 3-ml volume of the above solutions in a temperature-controlled rectangular cell. Temperatures represent intra-cuvette temperatures, as determined by an NBS thermistor

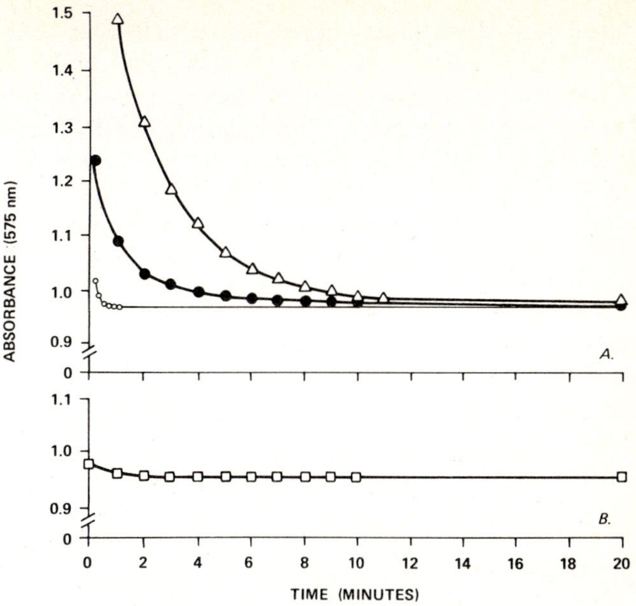

Fig. 5. *A*. Variation in the absorbance at 575 nm of cresol red (30 mg/liter) in Tris (0.1 mol/liter, pH 7.5) as a function of time as determined with the Cary 118C (△), the GEMSAEC centrifugal analyzer (●), and the Gilford 300-N equipped with a thermocuvette (○)

In all cases the samples were introduced into the systems after preincubation for 30 min at 4 °C. Each of the instruments was thermally regulated at 30 °C

B. Variation in the absorbance at 575 nm of this same solution as a function of time for the GEMSAEC analyzer thermostatted at 30 °C (□)

In this case the sample was introduced into the instrument after preincubation at room temperature (24.6 °C) for 30 min

2.5-fold to 0.083 *A* per degree, the solution of cresol red in Tris is simply made 2.5-fold more concentrated, so that it gives a total absorbance at 575 nm of 2.5 *A* at 30 °C. Ultimate sensitivity is therefore limited to the highest absorbance that any spectrophotometric system can measure reliably.

The lower curve in Figure 4 shows the absorption of a CR-N solution (10 mg/liter) as a function of temperature. Note that the absorption of this solution is virtually independent of temperature. This is because, in a strongly alkaline medium, the equilibrium is shifted far in the direction of the anionic form of the chromophore, and so any small changes in pH as a function of temperature still have little or no perceptible effect on the equilibrium between ionized and un-ionized forms of the dye and, therefore, on absorption at 575 nm. Thus this solution can be used as a calibrator to correct for slight differences between spectrophotometers and is absolutely required for accurate temperature estimation. The absorption spectrum of CR-N has the same wavelength maximum (575 nm) and the same natural bandwidth as CR-T. For this reason, it can be used to correct absorbance readings on spectrophotometric systems that have different spectral bandwidths, percentages of stray light, or even slight errors in wavelength calibration as compared to the instrument on which the absorbance-vs.-temperature calibration curve prepared with CR-T was obtained. An alternative calibrating system can be prepared by taking advantage of certain buffers for which pH is relatively insensitive to temperature. For example, we have prepared cresol red (30 mg/liter) in phosphate buffer (0.1 mol/liter, pH 7.5) because phosphate buffer has a very low temperature coefficient (Table 1). This solution has the advantage that it gives exactly the same absorption spectrum as does CR-T and is therefore slightly more desirable from a spectral point of view. However, it does give a small, but measurable change in absorbance vs. temperature, about 0.7% of the total absorbance per degree as compared to 0.2% per degree for CR-N. Other techniques—such as use of the isosbestic points of indicators at wavelengths where the absorbance is independent of pH and, therefore, of temperature, or of other organic or inorganic solutions such as potassium dichromate for which absorbance is relatively temperature independent—all have the disadvantage that neither the appropriate wavelengths nor the bandwidths approximate that of the CR-T solution.

Figure 5 shows our results obtained when CR-T was used to monitor equilibration times and equilibrium temperatures in a number of spectrophotometric systems commonly used in clinical laboratories. Figure 5*A* shows the time dependence of thermal equilibration of CR-T in three analytical systems that require different sample volumes and have different temperature-control mechanisms. The CR-T solution was incubated at 4 °C for 30 min and introduced into the systems described, which were thermally regulated at 30 °C.

The Cary 118C spectrophotometer, as used in this experiment, contained a 3.0-ml aliquot of CR-T in a stoppered rectangular cuvette, which was thermally regulated by passing water at 30 °C through a cell holder that was in direct contact with the walls of the cuvette on two sides and in partial contact with the cuvette on the faces perpendicular to the incident and emerging beams. Obviously, even 15 min later the solution has not reached thermal equilibrium. This can be attributed in part to the large sample volume (3 ml) and in part to the geometry of the thermostattable cell holder.

The GEMSAEC *centrifugal analyzer* includes an external bath to regulate the temperature of a cowl, which surrounds, but is not in contact with, the cuvette-containing rotor assembly. The temperature of the cowl can be read from the instrument's thermistor located in the cowl. When 0.5 ml of CR-T at 4 °C was introduced into each of the cuvettes in the rotor, the time required for thermal equilibration to within 0.5 °C of the equilibrium temperature was about 10 min, although the actual cowl temperature as indicated by the thermistor is relatively constant over this whole time period. In addition, the actual value of the intra-cuvette temperature as indicated by the CR-T system comes to within 0.2 °C of the cowl temperature only after about 20 min.

The Gilford 300-N Spectrophotometer, equipped with a flow-through thermocuvette, also requires a sample volume of about 0.5 ml. However, as seen in the bottom-most curve of Figure 5*A*, the equilibration time of CR-T aspirated at 4 °C is about 30 s. This difference in equilibration times between the Gilford System and the GEMSAEC system is primarily a result of the direct thermoelectric regulation of the sample compartment in the Gilford system and of the smaller intra-cuvette sample volume (<50 μl).

That equilibration time is also a function of sample temperature is indicated by the curve in Figure 5*B*. These data demonstrate that it takes about 3 min to come within 0.2 °C of the equilibrium temperature when the sample is aspirated at *room temperature* (in this case, 24.6 °C) in the GEMSAEC system.

If the CR-T solution at 4 or 24.6 °C is introduced into these three systems thermally regulated at 37 °C, all systems require an even longer time for equilibration, except for the Gilford system, which still takes about 30 s to come within 0.2 °C of the equilibrium value. Even when the CR-T solution is introduced at room temperature into the GEMSAEC system, the intra-cuvette temperature differs by more than 1 °C from the cowl temperature (37 °C) after 20 min.

Du Pont aca. Although not shown in the figure, we also checked thermal equilibration times for the Du Pont *aca*. In this discrete system each reagent pack is totally enclosed, and the optical measurement is made directly in the analytical pack. The system incorporates two successive contact heaters to rapidly bring the temperature of the analytical packs up to 37 °C until they are indexed into the photometer, where absorbances are read. Analytical packs were filled with 5.0 ml of the CR-T solution, incubated at room temperature or at 4 °C, and introduced into the instrument. It takes about 5 min for the pack to reach the photometer where the absorbance is measured. Our results indicate that, even when the solution is incubated at 4 °C, the analytical pack still equilibrates at 37 °C by the time it reaches the photometer.

To demonstrate the usefulness of the aqueous temperature-indicating technique on a day-to-day basis in the clinical laboratory, we checked the precision and accuracy of temperature regulation on the GEMSAEC system at 30 °C during 15 days. The CR-T working solution was dispensed at room temperature by the GEMSAEC automatic pipetting system into the "C" well of the transfer disc. The disc was placed into the analyzer and absorbances measured after 10 min. The within-run cuvette-to-cuvette temperature had a mean value of 29.7 °C (0.9627 *A*) and a coefficient of variation of 0.22% (0.06 °C). The day-to-day mean was 29.9 °C (0.9563 *A*), with a coefficient of variation of 0.95% (0.91 °C). Because the precision of the analyzer optical system as demonstrated by similar readings on potassium dichromate indicated a coefficient of variation of 0.08% (at 0.85 *A*), the CR-T solution is able to readily detect changes of 0.1 °C on this system.

As a check on the stability of the CR-T working solution when it is stored at 4 °C, we prepared and repeated temperature calibration curves after five months. The results indicated less than a 1% difference in absorbance at 575 nm over the range of 20 to 40 °C. CR-N working solutions were usually freshly prepared.

Discussion

Our results indicate the usefulness of an aqueous temperature-indicating technique in the clinical laboratory. This technique can give information about thermal equilibration times, but, more importantly, it can also be used to obtain an accurate estimate of the temperature of an aqueous reaction solution inside the cuvette of a spectrophotometric system. For it to do so, however, an accurate calibrating system is required. Therefore, we emphasize the absolute necessity of using a calibrator—in this case, cresol red in strong base—to correct for optical differences between the calibrating instrument and the system of interest.

The usefulness of this kind of aqueous temperature probe is particularly evident from our results for the GEMSAEC centrifugal analyzer and the Du Pont *aca*, both of which have cells that are virtually inaccessible by conventional thermistor probes. In centrifugal analyzers the cuvettes actually spin in front of the optical system, and preclude the insertion of conventional thermistors. Some of these analyzers now have a permanently enclosed thermistor in one of the cuvette walls. The cells of the Du Pont *aca* represent an even more formidable problem for temperature estimation. The spectrophotometric cells in this system are formed from the transparent plastic walls of a totally sealed reagent pack. However, because the CR-T solution can be introduced into the packs just as any sample–reagent mixture would be, it can monitor the environment inside the pack directly. The use of CR-N in the *aca* as a calibrating solution also demonstrates the usefulness of this kind of calibrator. Because the *aca* is a single-beam, dual-wavelength filter instrument, and the Cary 118C is a double-beam, single-wavelength grating instrument, measurement of the 583–600 nm changes in absorbances in both systems demonstrates how easy it is to correct for optical differences in widely different systems.

We therefore propose the use of this aqueous temperature-indicating technique in almost any photometric system, from manual and automated clinical analyzers to special-purpose instrumentation such as stopped-flow and temperature-jump instruments, for the accurate estimation of intra-cuvette temperatures.

We thank Mr. Thomas Leech for his assistance in performing the precision studies on the GEMSAEC analyzer. We are also grateful to Dr. B. W. Mangum of the NBS for the use of the calibrated thermistors and constant current source and to Dr. R. F. Lie for the use of the temperature-controlled scintillation-vial holder for the pH-vs.-temperature measurements.

References

1. Bergmeyer, H. U., Principles of enzymatic analysis. In *Methods of Enzymatic Analysis,* section A, H. U. Bergmeyer, Ed. Academic Press, New York, N. Y., 1965, p 9.

2. Bowers, G. N., Jr., Bergmeyer, H. U., and Moss, D. W., Draft proposal (No. 8) for IFCC reference methods for enzymes. *Clin. Chem.* **19,** 268 (1973).

3. Blume, P., Experiences with the GEMSAEC Fast Analyzer at the University of Minnesota. In *Enzymology in the Practice of Laboratory Medicine,* P. Blume and E. F. Freier, Eds. Academic Press, New York, N. Y., 1974, pp 246–249.

4. *Handbook of Chemistry and Physics,* R. C. Weast, Ed. Chemical Rubber Company, Cleveland, Ohio, 53rd ed., 1973, p D-103.

5. Buffers for accurate pH measurements. In *Industrial Applications Research Data Sheet,* Beckman Scientific Instruments Division, Fullerton, Calif.

CLIN. CHEM. 22/4, 456–460 (1976)

Preparation of Optically Clear Lyophilized Human Serum for Use in Preparing Control Material

Gary J. Proksch and Dean P. Bonderman

We describe a simple, rapid process—which includes the specific precipitation of pre-beta and beta-lipoproteins with dextran sulfate and divalent metal ions—for preparing an optically clear human serum that retains its clarity upon reconstitution with water after having been frozen and lyophilized. Such serum contains the normal constituents of human serum, except for the removed lipoproteins. The process causes no apparent interference with results of analyses for 22 of the more commonly measured constituents. Fresh or aged pooled serum or blood-bank plasma containing acid-citrate-dextrose or citrate–phosphate–dextrose are equally suitable as raw materials. This stabilized serum is an excellent matrix for use in preparing standards and quality-control material for assay of components of human serum.

Human plasma or serum are commonly used in preparing chemical standards and quality-control materials in the clinical laboratory; routinely, they are preserved by freezing or lyophilization. These procedures, particularly lyophilization, increase the turbidity of the reconstituted serum because serum lipid constituents become insoluble (*1*). This in turn increases the absorbance of the material throughout most of the visible spectrum (*2*), for which a blank may be needed to compensate. Several methods for decreasing this turbidity have been reported (*3, 4*), but none we tried resulted in a truly clear solution.

Polysulfated polymers—such as heparin, dextran sulfate, sulfated polygalacturonic acid methyl ester methyl glycoside, polyanetholsulfonate, sulfate amylopectin, and polyvinyl sulfate—combined with divalent metal cations form insoluble complexes with human serum lipoproteins (*5*), and these techniques have been used for purifying lipoproteins. We observed that when human serum was so treated, a stable and optically clear serum resulted, which retained its clarity upon lyophilization and reconstitution. We describe here the preparation, properties, and advantages of this processed human serum as a base matrix for calibration standards.

Department of Clinical Pathology, Indiana University Medical Center, Indianapolis, Ind. 46202.

Received Nov. 6, 1975; accepted Jan. 23, 1976.

Materials and Methods

Analytical Methods

Sodium, potassium, chloride, CO_2, blood urea nitrogen, glucose by glucose oxidase, aspartate aminotransferase (EC 2.6.1.1), lactate dehydrogenase (EC 1.1.1.27), alkaline phosphatase (EC 3.1.3.1), creatine kinase (EC 2.7.3.2), "direct" bilirubin, total bilirubin, creatinine, uric acid, phosphate, calcium, albumin, and total protein were determined with Technicon SMA 6/60 and Technicon SMA 12/60 continuous-flow analyzers (*10*). Aspartate aminotransferase and lactate dehydrogenase were measured by monitoring absorbance change at 340 nm. Protein and lipoprotein were electrophoresed on cellulose acetate strips (*11*). Total lipids (*12*), cholesterol (*13*), triglycerides (*14*), and amylase activity (*15*) were measured by manual techniques.

Variables Tested

Dextran sulfate concentration: A pool of outdated acid-citrate–phosphate preserved blood-bank plasma from normal persons was dialyzed against an NaCl solution (7.0 g/liter) to remove the calcium chelators. After dialysis, the calcium concentration was increased to 12.5 mmol/liter by adding $CaCl_2$ and the pH was adjusted to 7.4 with an NaOH solution (6 mol/liter). The plasma was defibrinogenated with 1 ml of topical bovine thrombin (1000 NIH units/ml; Parke-Davis, Detroit, Mich. 48232) per liter, and the serum was expressed from the clot. The serum was divided into 100-ml aliquots and various amounts of dextran sulfate (Type 500-S; Sigma Chemical Co., St. Louis, Mo. 63178) were added to each. After 2 h at 25 °C, the mixtures were centrifuged (35000 × *g*, 10 °C, 15 min) and the clear supernates decanted.

Table 1 shows the effect of various concentrations of dextran sulfate on cholesterol and triglyceride content. In our experience with outdated acid-citrate–phosphate and acid-citrate–dextrose plasma pools, 300 mg of dextran sulfate per liter was sufficient. If an occasional pool is encountered that has an abnormally high lipid content, the dextran sulfate concentration should be increased at the rate of 1 mg of dex-

Table 1. Effect of Dextran Sulfate on Human Serum Cholesterol and Triglyceride Concentrations

Dextran sulfate, mg/liter	Cholesterol		Triglyceride	
	mg/liter	% removed	mg/liter	% removed
0	1780	0	830	0
50	1730	3	780	6
100	1200	33	510	38
150	530	70	230	72
200	430	76	120	86
250	410	77	180	78
300	390	78	150	82

tran sulfate per 6 mg/liter that the cholesterol value exceeds 1800 mg/liter.

Calcium concentration: A pool of fresh acid-citrate-phosphate plasma was dialyzed as in the previous experiment. The pH of the dialysate was adjusted to 7.4, and 75 mg of calcium chloride was added per liter. The plasma clotted spontaneously, indicating that the calcium-binding agents had been effectively removed. The serum was expressed from the clot and divided into 100-ml aliquots, to which various further amounts of calcium were added. Then 30 mg of dextran sulfate was added to each sample. After 2 h at 25 °C the fractions were centrifuged as before, the clear supernates were decanted, and each sample was divided into two equal parts. One set of samples was frozen for two days at −60 °C, then thawed for analysis. The other was frozen, lyophilized, and reconstituted with water to the original volume.

Table 2 shows the effect of various calcium concentrations on the resulting serum turbidity, measured at 710 nm. The minimum concentration of calcium required for the lipid insolubilization appears to be about 10.3 mmol/liter. Increasing the calcium concentration to 14.7 and 19.2 mmol/liter neither precipitated the residual triglyceride or cholesterol nor significantly increased the optical clarity upon freezing, lyophilization, and reconstitution. Interestingly, although calcium ions are required to precipitate the lipoprotein/dextran sulfate complex, only a small fraction of the available calcium (about 0.5 mmol/liter) is removed in the precipitate. Apparently, calcium is only loosely bound by the complex.

Divalent magnesium and manganese ions are as effective as calcium in facilitating the precipitation of lipoproteins with dextran sulfate. We used calcium because of the ease with which physiological concentrations could be restored by use of ion-exchange chromatography, precipitation of calcium as the insoluble oxalate salt, or dialysis. The calcium also aided in the coagulation of fibrinogen. Blood-bank plasma, such as acid-citrate–dextrose plasma, contains a sufficient amount of citrate to complex about 20 mmol of calcium per liter. To ensure that calcium was in excess, in various plasma pools, we used a calcium concentration of 50 mmol/liter for anticoagulated plasma.

Recommended Procedure

To 1 liter of plasma (free of hepatitis-associated antigen by radioimmunoassay) add 5.55 g (50 mmol/liter) of calcium chloride and adjust the pH to 7.4 with NaOH solution (6 mol/liter). Incubate the solution at 37 °C and add 1.0 ml of bovine topical thrombin (1000 NIH units per milliliter; Parke-Davis). Allow the plasma to coagulate and express the serum from the clot. Dissolve dextran sulfate (300 mg/liter) in a minimum volume of water and add it to the serum at 25 °C. A flocculent lipoprotein/dextran sulfate precipitate forms immediately. After 30 min, centrifuge the mixture (4500 × *g*, 20 min, 10 °C), decant the clear supernate and dialyze it against a saline solution, 6.5 g of NaCl per liter, until the calcium ion concentration is decreased to the desired value. The clear yellow supernate is now ready to be used as a protein base for augmentation by anions, cations, enzymes, or other constituents, after which the material is aliquoted and lyophilized.

Results

Optical Clarity

The absorbance spectra from 800 to 525 nm of untreated and dextran sulfate treated aliquots of a serum pool were scanned before and after lyophilization. The treated sample was still optically clear after

Table 2. Effect of Calcium on Removal of Cholesterol and Triglyceride from Serum with Dextran Sulfate

Dextran sulfate, mg/liter	Calcium before DS	Calcium after DS	Triglyceride	Cholesterol	A_{710nm}	
	mmol/liter		mg/liter		Frozen	Lyophilized
00	1.1		1070	1250	0.14	0.68
300	1.1	1.1	760	650	0.88	1.60
300	5.7	5.4	540	390	0.50	0.66
300	10.3	9.8	120	250	0.50	0.06
300	14.7	13.9	130	220	0.08	0.08
300	19.2	18.8	120	230	0.03	0.03

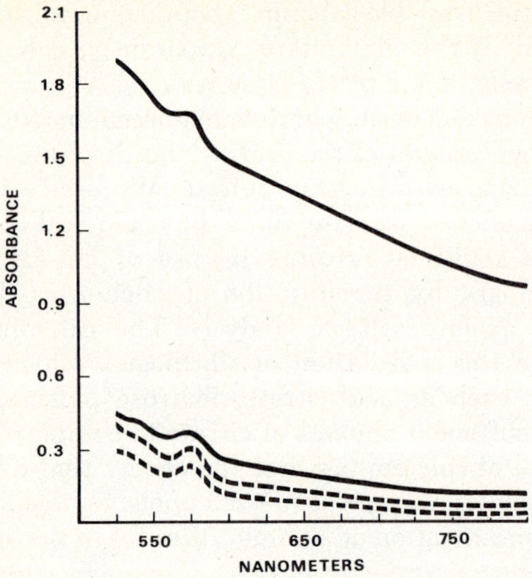

Fig. 1. Absorbance spectra of untreated and dextran sulfate-treated serum before and after lyophilization

Lower dotted line, DS-treated serum before lyophilization; *upper dotted line*, DS-treated serum after lyophilization; *lower solid line*, untreated serum before lyophilization; *upper solid line*, untreated serum after lyophilization

lyophilization and reconstitution, whereas the untreated fractions exhibited a much increased absorbance at all wavelengths (Figure 1).

Effect of Dextran Sulfate on Serum Proteins and Lipoproteins

The effects of dextran sulfate treatment on total serum lipids and protein are given in Table 3. Cholesterol and triglyceride are evidently the major lipid constituents affected. Total protein concentration was only slightly decreased, from 58 to 57 g/liter.

Figure 2 shows densitometer tracings after lipoprotein electrophoresis of treated and untreated serum. The untreated serum produced a lipoprotein pattern with normal lipid proportions; the dextran sulfate-treated serum contained primarily alpha-lipoproteins. Densitometer recordings of the serum proteins, electrophoresed at pH 8.6 on cellulose acetate, showed only minor differences between untreated and treated serum: the untreated serum showed a major and a minor peak in the beta zone; the treated sample yielded only a single symmetrical peak. These results indicate that dextran sulfate treatment removes only pre-beta- and beta-lipoproteins, leaving the other proteins in solution.

Effect of Dextran Sulfate on Serum Constituents

Sera selected for high enzyme activities were pooled and frozen. When a sufficient sample was obtained, the pooled serum was thawed and divided into two 250-ml fractions, I and II, and 0.6 g (15 mmol/liter) of calcium acetate was added to each. The divalent ion concentration was reduced from the previously recommended values to keep the ionic strength of the final product as close to that of the

Table 3. Effect of Dextran Sulfate Concentration on Serum Lipids and Protein

	Total lipid	Cholesterol	Triglyceride	Total protein
		mg/liter		g/liter
Untreated serum	4500	1460	750	58
Treated serum	2700	400	200	57

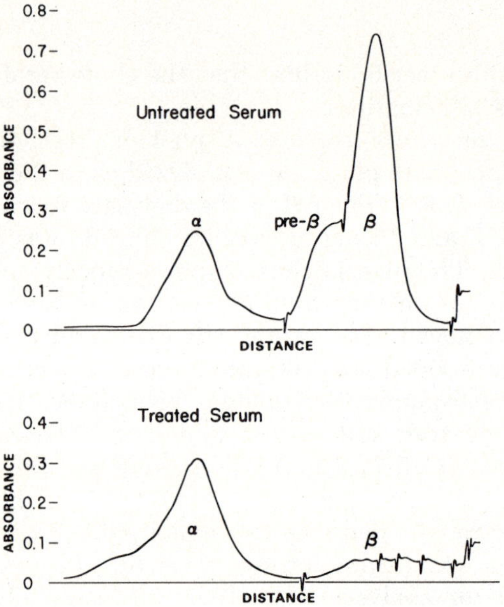

Fig. 2. Lipoprotein electrophoresis of untreated and dextran sulfate-treated serum

starting serum as possible so that no dialysis would be required. Experiments described above show that this concentration of calcium is sufficient. Dextran sulfate (75 mg) was added to fraction II. The preparations were centrifuged at 30 000 × *g* for 15 min, and to 200 ml of the clear supernates of both fractions we added 0.425 g (15 mol/liter) of ammonium oxalate monohydrate to remove excess calcium ions. The two solutions were stored for 12 h at 5 °C, to allow for the complete precipitation of calcium oxalate, then centrifuged (4500 × *g*) to remove the calcium oxalate, the clear supernates were decanted, and aliquots of each were lyophilized.

The lyophilized samples were reconstituted to their original volume and allowed to stand for 3 h at 25 °C before analysis, then analyzed for 22 chemical constituents. Eleven of the constituents—glucose, blood urea nitrogen, chloride, potassium, sodium, lactate dehydrogenase, "direct" bilirubin, total bilirubin, creatinine, uric acid, and albumin—produced the same values for all fractions; i.e., neither dextran sulfate treatment nor lyophilization affected the assay results. Table 4 lists the results in which differ-

Table 4. Effect of Dextran Sulfate on Serum Constituents

Constituent	Serum	Fract. I	Fract. II	Oxalate Fract. I	Oxalate Fract. II	Lyophilized Fract. I	Lyophilized Fract. II
CO_2, mmol/l	21	20	19	17	16	4	6
Aspartate aminotransferase, U/l	95	96	96	98	101	87	87
Creatine kinase, U/l	805	616	629	811	861	617	646
Alkaline phosphatase, U/l	179	174	170	167	163	153	152
Phos., mg/l	39	38	19	38	19	38	19
Ca, mg/l	86	>161[a]	>161[a]	75	21	76	19
Tot. prot., g/l	69	69	67	67	68	67	67
Amylase, U/l	1930	1940	2000	1970	1900	2270	1940
Cholest., mg/l	2070	2080	700	2150	710	2080	730
Trigly., mg/l	1490	1450	340	1510	320	1620	310
Tot. lipid, mg/l	4600	—	—	—	—	4600	2250

[a] Represents full-scale deflection of instrument. Actual values for calcium exceed this.

ences were observed. The total protein value for fraction II is slightly lower than for the serum base and fraction I, as would be expected because of the removal of lipoproteins. Bicarbonate concentration varied with the different fractions, probably associated with CO_2 losses from exposure to atmospheric conditions and lyophilization. An 8% loss of aspartate aminotransferase activity occurred on lyophilization of either fraction I or II. Fraction I showed a 10% increase in amylase activity after lyophilization and reconstitution, but the amylase activity of fraction II was unchanged throughout the process. The increase in amylase activity of lyophilized fraction I might have been due to the failure to include a blank to correct for the increased turbidity of the sample. Creatine kinase activities were inhibited by about 20% by the excess calcium. Removal of the added calcium restored activity to original values. Lyophilization of fractions I and II again produced a similar 20% inactivation for both samples. The loss of creatine kinase activity appears to be independent of the lipoprotein precipitation. The phosphate concentration of the dextran sulfate-treated fraction is about half that of the untreated fraction. Apparently some phosphate is co-precipitated with either the lipoproteins or as $CaHPO_4$. Because of the addition and removal of calcium, values for it varied throughout the various steps. The lower calcium concentrations of the dextran sulfate-treated fractions probably reflect the inclusion of some calcium in the lipoprotein precipitate or the precipitation of $CaHPO_4$. As discussed previously, total lipid, cholesterol, and triglyceride concentrations were lower in the dextran sulfate-treated fraction. Alkaline phosphatase activity was about 4% less in fractions containing 15 mmol of calcium per liter. Removal of the calcium with oxalate did not restore the activity, but instead resulted in an additional decrease. The alkaline phosphatase activity of both fraction I and II was decreased by about 6% during lyophilization for an overall loss of 15% for each aliquot during the total process. A solution of dextran sulfate (300 mg/liter) was free of glucose reacting material when assayed by a manual *o*-toluidine procedure (*16*).

Variability of Reconstituted Sera

Twenty duplicate samples of lyophilized fractions I and II, prepared as in the previous section, were each reconstituted with 5.0 ml of water. (The original serum was divided into 5.0-ml aliquots, and the addition of 5.0 ml of diluent, owing to the partial specific volumes of the components, was observed to result in approximately a 6% dilution.) After 3 h at 25 °C, to allow for the stabilization of alkaline phosphatase activity (see following section), the samples were analyzed for 18 chemical constituents by continuous-flow analysis with the SMA 6/60 and SMA 12/60 instruments. The resulting data for the two serum fractions yielded comparable coefficients of variation for all the constituents analyzed. The removal of lipoproteins with dextran sulfate apparently did not affect the vial-to-vial precision of the reconstituted serum, as described.

Stability of Reconstituted Serum

Lyophilized samples of fraction I and II, prepared as in the previous section, were reconstituted at various times and stored at 5 °C. The rate of reconstitution of the constituents of both sets appeared to be similar. Values for total protein, albumin, calcium, phosphate, uric acid, creatinine, total bilirubin, aspartate aminotransferase, and creatine kinase were consistent for 12 days for both fractions. The values for lactate dehydrogenase activity in both fraction I and II were consistent at 420 U/liter for about 24 h, followed by a gradual loss of activity in each sample, amounting to about 25% after 12 days. Alkaline phosphatase activity (initially 125 U/liter) in both samples gradually increased by 13 to 15% after reconstitution; in both untreated and treated serum nearly half of this increase occurred within the first 24 h, the remainder during the next 11 days.

Discussion

This technique is simple, requiring little specialized equipment, and is easily adapted for use with large-scale pools. Insoluble material may be removed by centrifugation, or, alternatively, it will settle out on standing overnight, and about 70% of the treated serum can be decanted off.

After the calcium ion concentrations are adjusted to physiological values, the serum is optically clear and may be augmented with additional desired constituents. It may be used immediately, stored frozen and used in a quality-control frozen-pool program (*17*), or lyophilized. When reconstituted, the powder dissolves readily (typically within 10 min) and remains clear. Except for the lipid constituents and a lowered phosphate concentration (phosphate may be added back to attain desired concentrations after dextran sulfate treatment without affecting the serum), the process did not produce any change in the values or affect the stability of the constituents to lyophilization. The analytical precision and stability of the measured constituents in the reconstituted treated serum was similar to that obtained with the untreated fractions.

The processed serum will be useful as a base material for the preparation of calibration materials or quality-control materials for many procedures, including protein electrophoresis. This product has a particular advantage over other lyophilized materials used in the laboratory in preparing "blind" quality-control samples: the optical clarity of the product allows it to be unrecognized by the technologist as a quality-control specimen.

The starting material most frequently used in our laboratory has been out-dated acid-citrate–dextrose plasma, because it is readily available from the blood bank. However, virtually any source of human plasma, such as out-dated acid-citrate–phosphate plasma or fresh heparinized acid-citrate–dextrose or acid-citrate–phosphate plasma are equally satisfactory. Even plasmapheresis material from a patient with multiple myeloma that had been stored frozen for four years yielded an optically clear product for use as an abnormal (IgG) protein-electrophoresis control.

Lipid analysis of dextran sulfate-treated serum indicates that cholesterol and triglyceride concentrations are decreased to about 25% of original values. These constituents are of course important in diagnosis. We are now evaluating methods for restoring cholesterol and triglyceride to normal or abnormal high values without affecting the optical clarity of the product.

References

1. Oncley, J. L., Gurd, F. R. N., and Melin, M., Preparation and properties of serum and plasma proteins. XXV. Composition and properties of human serum, beta-lipoproteins. *J. Am. Chem. Soc.* **72,** 458 (1950).

2. Atwood, J. G., and Marshall, H. W., Factors in serum that limit speed and precision of ultramicro enzyme rate measurements. *Lab. Med. Newsl.* **5,** 6 (1973).

3. Louderback, A. L., Liquid blood serum control standard. U.S. Patent No. 3,682,835; August 8, 1972.

4. Rush, R. L., and Vlastelica, D. L., Turbidity reduction in serum and plasma samples using polyoxyethylated lauric acid compounds. U.S. Patent No. 3,853,465; December 10, 1974.

5. Burstein, M., and Samaiele, J., Sur la clarification du serum lipemique par l'heparine in vitro. *C. R. Acad. Sci.* **241,** 664 (1955).

6. Burstein, M., Scholnick, H. R., and Morfix, R., Rapid method for the isolation of lipoproteins from human serum by precipitation with polyanions. *J. Lipid Res.* **11,** 583 (1970).

7. Burstein, M., and Samaiele, J., Sur la precipitation selective des beta-lipoproteins du serum par l'heparine et heparinoides de synthese en presence du calcium chloride. *J. Physiol.* (Paris) **49,** 83 (1957).

8. Bernfeld, P., Donahue, V. M., and Berkowitz, M. E., Interaction of human serum beta-lipoglobulin with polyanions. *J. Biol. Chem.* **226,** 51 (1957).

9. Bernfeld, P. Bonner, C. D., and Berkeley, B. J., Serum beta-lipoprotein levels in health and disease, as determined by the nephelometric method with amylopectin sulfate as reagent. *J. Clin. Invest.* **39,** 1864 (1960).

10. Technicon Pub. No. UA4-0160-00. Installation and operation manual for the Technicon SMA 12/60 Multichannel Biomedical Analyzer, **I, II,** and **III;** Technicon Instrument Corp., Tarrytown, N.Y. 10591, 1974.

11. Golias, T. L., Helena Laboratories Electrophoresis Manual, **IV,** 1974.

12. Frings, C. S., Fendley, T. W., Dunn, R. T., and Queen, C. A., Improved determination of total serum lipids by the sulfo-phospho-vanillin reaction. *Clin. Chem.* **18,** 673 (1972).

13. Parekh, A. C., and Jung, D., Cholesterol determination with ferric acetate-uranium acetate and sulfuric acid-ferrous sulfate reagents. *Anal. Chem.* **42,** 1423 (1970).

14. Levy, A. L., and Keyloun, C., A colorimetric assay for triglycerides: Automated and manual. *Clin. Chem.* **17,** 640 (1971).

15. Klein, B., Foreman, J. A., and Searcy, R. L., New chromogenic substrate for determination of serum amylase. *Clin. Chem.* **16,** 32 (1970).

16. Hultman, E., Rapid method for determination of aldosaccharides in body fluids. *Nature* **183,** 108 (1959).

17. Bowers, G. N., Burnett, R. W., Jr., and McComb, R. B., Preparation and use of human serum control materials for monitoring precision in clinical chemistry. *Clin. Chem.* **21,** 1830 (1975).

New Techniques for Ion-Selective Measurements of Ionized Calcium in Serum after pH Adjustment of Aerobically Handled Sera

H. Donald Schwartz

I report further experience in measuring ionized calcium (Ca^{2+}) with the AMT Electrion System and its serum standards and solid-state, dip, calcium-selective electrodes. With this system, serum pH can be adjusted with CO_2 gas and Ca^{2+} and pH simultaneously measured; when 5.2% CO_2 (40 mm p_{CO_2}) is used for sample equilibration, the standard bicarbonate concentration is also provided. I measured serum Ca^{2+} as a function of pH between pH 7.0 and 9.0 and found the relationship to be reproducible, with no evidence of irreversible complexing of Ca^{2+}. When the pH of aerobically exposed, mailed sera was restored to the original values, their values for Ca^{2+} were the same as for the fresh sera. Measurement of Ca^{2+} in routinely (aerobically) handled sera after pH restoration with CO_2 gas was therefore validated, both samples from within an institution and mailed specimens. Standardization to pH 7.40 is recommended for routine measurements, is generally more accurate than use of heparin or quasi-anaerobic techniques, and is a practical approach. In patients with possible uncompensated acid-base disturbance (which may be indicated by an abnormal standard bicarbonate concentration if not suspected clinically), patient pH should be measured independently as part of the usual strict, anaerobic blood-gas-analysis procedures. Abnormal patient pH must be considered in the interpretation of Ca^{2+} results determined at pH 7.40 which are borderline or slightly abnormal; most accurately, Ca^{2+} may be measured in the separated sera at the previously determined patient pH value. Studies of aqueous solutions with the currently used Ca^{2+} electrodes showed a selectivity coefficient (the constant which relates the activity of an interfering ion to the activity of calcium that would contribute the same emf) $K_{Na} = 0.0031 \pm 0.0003$ (SE) and $K_{Mg} = 0.046 \pm 0.004$ (SE). At physiological concentrations of Ca^{2+}, physiologically encountered variation in Na^+ is of no significance in resulting Ca^{2+}, but extreme variation in Mg^{2+} may cause an error of approximately 1%.

Additional Keyphrases: *electrolytes • blood gases • variation, source of • Electrion System*

Ever since the classic work of McLean and Hastings in 1934 (*1*) it has become increasingly evident that the ionized fraction is the physiologically active and clinically meaningful portion of the serum total calcium concentration (*2*). Major technological advances in calcium-selective electrode technology were noted with the important work of Ross in 1967 (*3*) and in subsequent advances by Orion Research Inc. (Cambridge, Mass. 02139). Unfortunately, these techniques, based mainly on membrane electrodes, flow-through configuration, and aqueous calibrating solutions, have generally not been practical or reliable enough for routine use with serum (*4, 5*). The reasons, complex and frustrating, include limitations in the electrodes and lack of an adequate supporting electro-mechanical and calibration system.

In a recent publication (*6*), I reported fundamental performance characteristics of the new Electrion System. Here, I report experience in applying the adjustment of serum pH with CO_2 gas provided by the system to the measurement of Ca^{2+} in routinely (aerobically) handled sera, and the selectivity of the present electrodes for Ca^{2+}.

Materials and Methods

Equipment and Reagents

I measured ionized calcium (Ca^{2+}) at 37 °C with the Electrion System and its serum standards and solid-state, dip, calcium-selective electrodes (Applied Medical Technology, Box 689, Menlo Park, Calif. 94025). Some performance characteristics of the system are reported in a recent publication (*6*), but the entire working system used, including the components utilized for pH adjustment, is shown in Figure 1. A tank containing CO_2/O_2 (10/90 by volume) and a tank of pure O_2 were used for pH adjustment. All measurements of sera were done by calibration with reconstituted normal-range (1.01 mmol/liter) and high-range (1.91 mmol/liter) lyophilized sera Ca^{2+} standards (Applied Medical Technology) (*6*). Aqueous solutions used for the selectivity studies were prepared from stock solutions of reagent-grade chemicals in demineralized water, as described by Ladenson and Bowers (*7*), of the following compositions (in mmol/liter): NaCl, 1400; KCl, 50; $MgCl_2{\cdot}6H_2O$, 10.0; $CaCl_2$, 23.

Definitions and Equations

The selectivity coefficient *K* is used in the expanded Nernst equation to include the contributions to the net emf made by Mg^{2+} and Na^+ as well as by Ca^{2+}:

Division of Oncology and Ion-Specific Laboratory, Room M-011A, Stanford University Medical Center, Stanford, Calif. 94305.
Received Nov. 17, 1975; accepted Jan. 25, 1976.

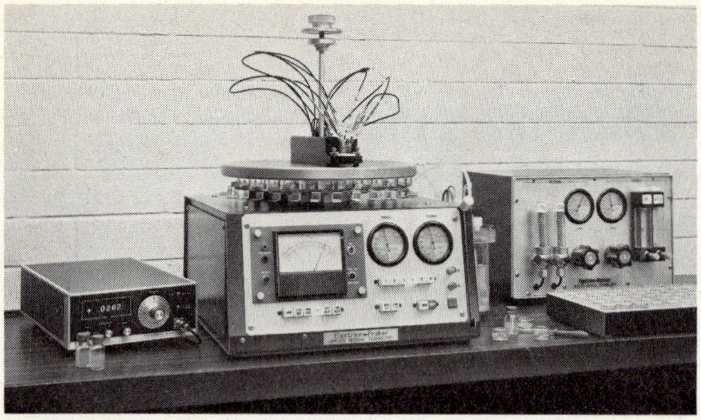

Fig. 1. Laboratory arrangement of working components of Electrion System

Samples are initially placed in pre-warmed, disposable cups in cup-warmer (*far right*) and transferred to the Electrion Prober. Gas jets from holes in the Prober plenum above the cups permit continuous pH control with CO_2; the gas mixture may be determined independently for the probe station and 29 carrier stations by the two pairs of flowmeters in the gas-blender (*far right*). In the probe holder, the two calcium electrodes are in front; the other electrodes are pH, reference, Na^+, K^+, and Cl^- electrodes. Emf from the electrodes in the sample at the probe station is sampled during 1 min. 30 sample cups are automatically indexed and sampled sequentially. Values in mV are displayed digitally (*far left*) with the Model Cam I shown, or calculated results are printed out with the Model Auto I (not shown)

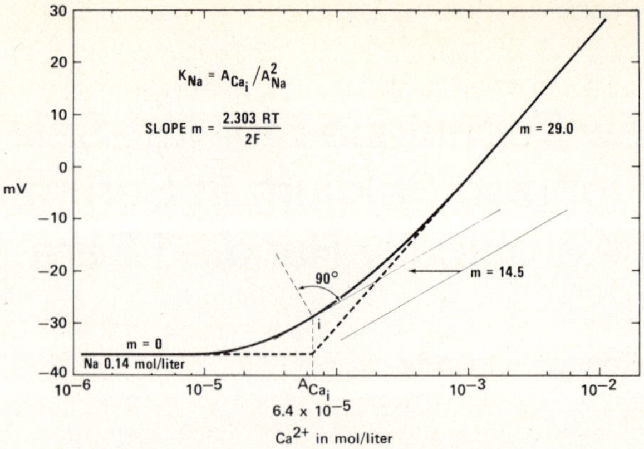

Fig. 2. Calculation of selectivity coefficient K_{Na}

Either Ca^{2+} or Na^+ concentration may be held constant and the other varied. The figure shows a common procedure in which Na^+ is held constant at the normal serum Na^+ concentration and Ca^{2+} is varied. The straight Nernstian slope for the higher Ca^{2+} concentrations and the horizontal plateau at extremely low Ca^{2+} concentrations, where the system is nonresponsive to changes in Ca^{2+} and there is zero functional slope, are extrapolated to intersect. A vertical line through this intersection defines the intersection with the emf curve, point "i," and the Ca^{2+} activity A_{Ca_i}. A line tangent to the potential curve at point "i" demonstrates that the functional slope is exactly half its Nernstian value, which means that the A_{Ca_i} and A_{Na} are contributing equally to the emf. An easier and equivalent way to define A_{Ca_i} is therefore to draw a line at the right that has a slope equal to half the Nernstian slope and then displace this line to the left until it touches the emf curve, defining point "i" and A_{Ca_i}

$$E = E_0 + \frac{2.303RT}{2F} \cdot \log\,[A_{Ca} + K_{Mg}A_{Mg} + K_{Na}A_{Na}{}^2] \qquad (1)$$

E is the potential (emf) recorded; E_0 is a constant which reflects, among other things, the reference system used; 2.303 $RT/2F$ is the electrode slope, m, which at 37 °C is 30.07 for an ideal calcium electrode; and A is the activity of the ion[1] (*8, 9*).

K_{Mg} may be conveniently determined from a pure Ca^{2+} solution and a pure Mg^{2+} solution in which $A_{Ca} = A_{Mg}$ (*10*):

$$K_{Mg} = \text{antilog}\left[\frac{E_{Mg} - E_{Ca}}{\text{m}}\right], \qquad (2)$$

where E_{Mg} is the emf from the pure Mg^{2+} solution and E_{Ca} is the emf from the pure Ca^{2+} solution.

Alternatively, K_{Mg} is commonly determined from a pure CA^{2+} solution and a solution containing the same A_{Ca} but also Mg^{2+} (*10*):

$$K_{Mg} = \frac{\text{antilog}\left[\dfrac{E_{CaMg} - E_{Ca} + \text{m}\log A_{Ca}}{\text{m}}\right] - A_{Ca}}{A_{Mg}} \qquad (3)$$

where E_{CaMg} is the emf from the mixed solution.

K_{Na} is usually determined from:

$$K_{Na} = A_{Ca_i}/A_{Na}{}^2, \qquad (4)$$

where A_{Ca_i} and A_{Na} are activities of Ca^{2+} and Na^+ that contribute equally to the emf and are conveniently determined by a graphical technique (Figure 2).

"Selectivity" for calcium over an interfering cation is operationally defined (*11*) as the ratio of the activity of the interfering cation to Ca^{2+} activity required for the two cations to contribute equally to measured emf under otherwise identical conditions.

Performance Characteristics

The performance characteristics with respect to Ca^{2+} activity reported were all obtained with the Electrion System and its current solid-state calcium electrodes and, as noted previously (*6*), may not be obtained with the isolated electrode.

Results and Discussion

Applications of Adjustment of Serum pH with CO_2 Gas

Serum pH was varied, by utilizing the appropriate blend of CO_2 and O_2 (Figure 1), between pH 7.0 and 9.0. This was done many times, with both normal and pathological sera. The inverse relationship between Ca^{2+} and pH in each serum studied was reproducible and reversible, confirming that there is no irreversible complexing of Ca^{2+} in this pH range. In normal sera, in the range of physiologically encountered pH and normal Ca^{2+} concentration, a pH difference of

[1] Although measurement of ionized calcium concentration, C, is a major advance over the conventionally used total calcium concentration, only ionized calcium activity, A, is physiologically active and sensed by calcium-selective electrodes. Activity is related to concentration by the activity coefficient γ as follows: $A = \gamma C$. γ has been calculated as a function of solution ionic strength (*8, 9*), but γ varies only slightly and is close to 0.54 over the range of ionic strength encountered physiologically and in aqueous calibrating solutions prepared to have physiological ionic strength, such as normal saline (*8, 9*). Because activity and concentration are therefore related by a constant, γ is generally ignored and the ionized calcium activity is expressed as the corresponding concentration. In this paper I follow this convention.

Table 1. Ionized Calcium in 15 Sera after Exposure to the Atmosphere, Mailing,[a] and Restoration of pH

Days in refrigerator and mail[b]	Initial [Ca^{2+}]	[Ca^{2+}] after mailing and pH restoration
	mg/100 ml	
R1-M4-R3	4.45	4.40
R4-M4-R3	4.01	3.96
R4-M4-R3	7.13	7.37
R3-M3-R3	4.57	4.50
R1-M4-R3	5.72	5.64
R1-M8	4.85	4.75
R1-M8	5.77	5.82
R3-M3	5.59	5.56
R3-M3	4.55	4.48
R3-M3	5.42	5.29
R2-M14	4.00	3.99
R2-M14	4.18	4.08
R2-M14	4.11	4.11
R2-M14	4.07	4.05
R2-M14	3.24	3.03

[a] For each sample, [Ca^{2+}], the concentration of ionized calcium, was measured at the same pH initially and after mailing and pH restoration.

[b] M is the total no. of days the sample was in the mail or at ambient temperature, R the no. of days refrigerated.

0.1 corresponded to a difference in Ca^{2+} of about 60 μmol/liter (0.25 mg/100 ml), a useful figure for quick estimation of the effect of pH change on Ca^{2+}. In pathological sera, however, the magnitude of the inverse relationship between Ca^{2+} and pH varied substantially.[2] In another series of experiments, pH change was induced rapidly and cyclically over a narrow H^+ mV range in order to see how quickly the system responded to the rapidly changing activity of Ca^{2+} that was expected to result. I previously did this over a 10 mV H^+ activity range, reading H^+ mV and Ca^{2+} mV digitally to the nearest 0.1 mV. The Ca^{2+} activity responded to within 0.1 mV in ≤15 s (*6*). To assess response speed more accurately, I repeated this experiment but induced more rapid cyclic changes over a narrower H^+ activity range of 4 mV, and used an analog chart recording of the emf measured by the Ca^{2+} and pH electrodes simultaneously to record mV changes of about 0.02 mV. The Ca^{2+} activity responded rapidly and changed direction at the H^+ mV inflection points, tracking to ≤0.02 mV within a few seconds. The essentially instantaneous change in Ca^{2+} with change in pH emphasizes the importance of knowing the pH of a sample at the time the Ca^{2+} is measured.[3]

In 15 unselected sera for which Ca^{2+} assay had been ordered from the Clinical Laboratory, a separate aliquot of serum was left at ambient temperature and exposed to the atmosphere for a few days, permitting the pH to increase (generally to above pH 8.3). The sera were then placed in small plastic cups and mailed in padded envelopes to San Francisco (40 miles), where the envelopes were re-addressed and mailed back to me. When the samples were received, Ca^{2+} was measured in each sample at the same pH at which it was measured originally, which in a few cases was actual patient pH and in most was a standardized pH of 7.40. Results are shown in Table 1. In Table 1, there was no significant difference between Ca^{2+} initially and after mailing and pH restoration ($P > 0.05$, 2-tailed paired *t*-test). Also, linear regression of Ca^{2+} after mailing and pH restoration as a function of initial Ca^{2+} yielded a slope and correlation coefficient that do not differ significantly from unity and a *y*-intercept that does not differ significantly from zero. This confirms that control over pH with CO_2 gas is a key to valid measurement of Ca^{2+} in routinely (aerobically) handled and mailed sera (*12, 13*). It is possible, however, that in sera of pathological types not studied, or with exposure to more extreme climatic variation, Ca^{2+} values might change.[4]

Because serum Ca^{2+} can readily be measured at a standardized pH as well as at the patient's pH (*6*), the effect of pH standardization was studied in normal subjects.[5]

In Table 2, the SD for Ca^{2+} in the series measured at standardized pH 7.37 is not different from the SD in the series measured at fresh venous pH. Also, graphical analysis on probability paper revealed that the Ca^{2+} values in the series at fresh venous pH had a normal (gaussian) distribution, and that performing the measurements at the standardized pH of 7.37 did

[2] The factors influencing the magnitude of the inverse relationship between Ca^{2+} and pH in sera are not known. The effect of protein has been given some attention, and data on the influence of other calcium-binding substances such as citrate and various anions are largely lacking. Nomographic efforts to correct Ca^{2+} values in pathological sera from the pH of aerobically handled sera to a normal pH entail considerable error. Elucidation of the quantitative influence of various substances on the pH/Ca^{2+} slope might well be of only academic interest, however, because the onus of having to measure these variables in each pathological sera in order to make a nomographic correction would probably make this an impractical if not inaccurate approach.

[3] Measuring the pH of a sample and then transferring it to a system for measurement of Ca^{2+} and assuming that the pH at the time of Ca^{2+} measurement has not changed may entail considerable error. We found that the act of transferring serum to a tuberculin syringe by careful technique, which appeared to be anaerobic, could result in a substantial pH increase (*12*).

[4] Similar experiments show that Ca^{2+} may be validly measured even after several days of refrigeration, or freezing. However, I have had some indication that speed and temperature of freezing and possibly intrinsic variables in certain pathological sera may affect results, and therefore I withhold a definite opinion on effects of freezing pending further studies of these variables. These findings agree with previous reports (*7, 12, 13*).

[5] Standardization at a normal pH value should be more valid than standardization at a normal p_{CO_2}, such as after equilibration with 5.2% CO_2 as has been practiced by some. The physiological reason is that blood Ca^{2+} is believed to be primarily a function of pH, and influenced by p_{CO_2} only insofar as p_{CO_2} influences pH. For example, in primary metabolic acid-base disturbance, effective respiratory compensation may require abnormal p_{CO_2} to maintain normal pH, and the abnormal p_{CO_2} would not be expected to change the Ca^{2+} activity.

Table 2. Serum $[Ca^{2+}]$[a] in Normal Subjects[b] Measured with the Electrion System at Fresh Venous pH[c] and at Standardized pH

	Mean	SD	SE	CV[d]	Mean − 2 SD	Mean + 2 SD
Fresh venous pH[c]	7.37	0.029	0.005	0.39%	7.31	7.43
Ca^{2+} @ fresh venous pH	1.07	0.040	0.008	3.69%	0.99	1.15
	(4.27)	(0.160)	(0.030)	3.69%	(3.95)	(4.59)
Ca^{2+} @ standardized pH 7.37	1.07	0.035	0.007	3.23%	1.00	1.14
	(4.27)	(0.140)	(0.026)	3.23%	(3.99)	(4.55)
Ca^{2+} @ standardized pH 7.40	1.05	0.034	0.006	3.20%	0.98	1.12
	(4.19)	(0.136)	(0.025)	3.20%	(3.92)	(4.45)

[a] $[Ca^{2+}]$ in mmol/liter, with value in mg/100 ml below in parentheses.
[b] 29 adult blood donors without known disease or medications.
[c] The pH of fresh venous sera separated anaerobically from fresh venous blood.
[d] CV = coefficient of variation = relative SD.

not alter this pattern. Thus, if one establishes a normal subject series by measuring Ca^{2+} in routinely and aerobically handled sera at a standardized pH of 7.37, the mean Ca^{2+} value, range, and distribution are the same as those obtained by measuring Ca^{2+} in anaerobically handled sera. Further, when the sera measurements were standardized at the normal pH of whole blood, 7.40, the mean Ca^{2+} was lower, as expected, but the SD and normal (gaussian) distribution were likewise not altered. An identical study previously performed on 30 normal subjects at 27 °C likewise revealed that pH standardization caused no significant change in either SD or distribution pattern. Because of its greater simplicity, we therefore favor the pH-standardized technique for establishing normal series, and at this institution standardize to pH 7.40, which yields a normal range of 1.05 mmol/liter (0.98–1.12), or 4.19 mg/100 ml (3.92–4.46).[6]

The inevitable question is whether this convenient pH-standardized technique can also be validly applied to measurement of Ca^{2+} in individual patients. The pH dependence of Ca^{2+} makes it axiomatic that Ca^{2+} measured at an individual patient's pH reflects most precisely the in vivo situation. However, pH is very narrowly regulated in most people, even in disease. The pH error from assuming a normal pH of 7.40 is unlikely to exceed 0.05 pH units, and the Ca^{2+} difference resulting from this is therefore unlikely to exceed 0.12 mg/100 ml (30 μmol/liter), but this does exceed the precision now available and may determine whether a Ca^{2+} result that is at the borderline of normality (or within 0.1 mg/100 ml of the normal limits) is considered to be normal or not. Larger pH alterations (>0.1 pH unit) occur in conditions where Ca^{2+} is important such as renal insufficiency, parathyroid disease, and cancer; however if such pH abnormality is not suspected clinically it will in most cases be revealed by a standard bicarbonate concentration that is more than 3.5 mEq/liter from the normal mean value (when 5.2% CO_2 (40 mm p_{CO_2}) is used for sample equilibration, the standard bicarbonate is readily provided from the p_{CO_2} of 40 mm and the measured pH by means of the Astrup calculation).

The procedure that has therefore been found very satisfactory at this institution is as follows. All routinely ordered sera Ca^{2+} measurements for which there is no information about patient pH are performed at pH 7.40. A result for Ca^{2}+ which is slightly abnormal or borderline, such as within 0.15 mg/100 ml of the normal limits, may be due to the patient's blood pH being abnormal as indicated by an abnormal standard bicarbonate concentration. In such cases, pH and possibly other blood gases should be directly measured by the usual strict, anaerobic blood-gas-analsysis techniques; if the patient's pH is found to be abnormal, then this can be considered in the interpretation of the Ca^{2+} result or a repeat Ca^{2+} made at this pH. Alternatively, if the patients actual pH value is initially provided to the laboratory along with the separated sera the Ca^{2+} measurement is performed at this pH; in most cases, however, such measurement of patient pH is not necessary.

The alternative approach is to measure Ca^{2+} in anaerobically handled samples. Unfortunately, strict anaerobic techniques, necessary for precise pH and blood gas analysis, require use of anticoagulants, commonly heparin, which is well known to bind Ca^{2+} and introduce error (*7, 14–16*). With very careful control over both the quality of heparin and the ratio of heparin to sample used, it may be possible to keep the heparin error low or possibly consistent enough to correct the result for it (*7*). However, in common experience, the heparin error generally exceeds that caused by standardizing to pH 7.40. It also should be borne in mind that unexpected and variable complexing of Ca^{2+} by various substances has plagued Ca^{2+} measurements and generally turned out to be a more significant problem than initially suspected (*5,*

[6] The Ca^{2+} values reported in this paper for normal persons are 2% lower than I previously reported (*6*). The effect of normal serum Mg^{2+} concentration on emf at normal Ca^{2+} concentration is small (about 0.18 mV), and in the previous preliminary studies was not statistically significant. The selectivity studies detailed in this paper, however, indicate that this difference is real.

12). I therefore agree with Ladenson and Bowers (7) that heparin should generally be avoided. Obligatory speedy measurement of anaerobically handled, heparinized samples is therefore a poor approach to most routine Ca^{2+} measurements if speedy Ca^{2+} results are not needed and if an accurate value for Ca^{2+}, with proper consideration to pH, is the object.

When samples are collected by various quasi-anaerobic techniques that seek to circumvent the heparin error—such as with variable delays before separation of sera from clot, with conventional syringes with oil, or in Vacutainers that are not permitted to fill quite to capacity (*7, 12, 15*)—and when samples are handled by nonspecialized personnel, the pH is frequently likewise in error by more than that involved in standardizing at pH 7.40. Also, the act of transferring sera to a syringe, even by careful and apparently anaerobic techniques, may result in an unexplained pH increase (*12*). I therefore believe that it is more reliable to measure the pH of a sample at the time that the Ca^{2+} is being measured, by measuring the pH and Ca^{2+} in the same sample essentially simultaneously (*6*).

The commonest need for speedy Ca^{2+} results is during rapid transfusion with citrated blood. Studies at this institution and elsewhere have demonstrated an extreme decrease in Ca^{2+} and resulting depression of myocardial contractility during rapid transfusion, and fast Ca^{2+} measurements are needed to monitor the administration of calcium to prevent or correct this. However, the Ca^{2+} derangements during rapid transfusion are of such major degree and change so rapidly that the refinement of a Ca^{2+} value at the actual pH rather than at the standardized pH of 7.40 is of no clinical advantage, and in this most important and common situation where speedy results are required pH refinement in Ca^{2+} measurement is therefore ironically least important. Errors from heparin, required for whole-blood measurement in flow-through electrodes, may also be of less clinical significance in the setting of rapid transfusion. When solid-state electrodes that dip directly into samples in individual disposable containers are used, as with the system reported, an alternative to heparin when an immediate Ca^{2+} measurement is needed is immediate measurement of whole blood without addition of heparin or any anticoagulant. The measurement is completed in less than 90 s after the sample is taken, before the blood has time to clot: the sample clots later, after it has been indexed away from the measuring station, and is simply discarded (*6*). Because the solid-state electrodes dip and sample directly in the blood specimen, there is no tubing or transport system to be clogged. If measurement of such a sample is delayed and there is clotting around the electrode tips, the clot can be readily rinsed or wiped off with no apparent damage to the electrodes (*6*). Preliminary experience with this approach indicates that it may work well in critical speed-demanding situations when the equipment can be in the room with the patient, such as in the operating room during rapid transfusion.

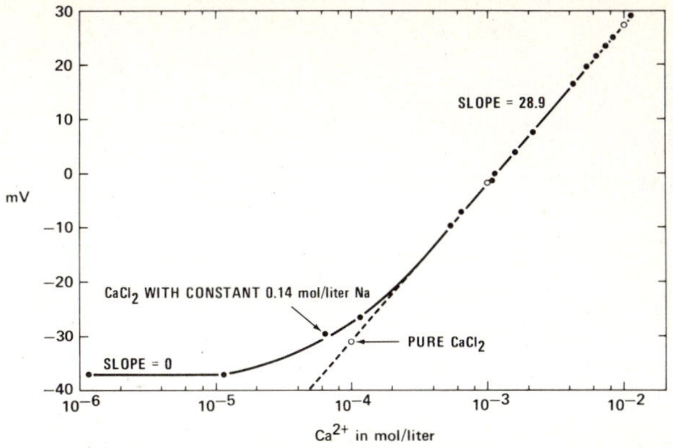

Fig. 3. Emf generated by Electrion System, with use of a typical solid-state calcium-selective electrode

In pure $CaCl_2$ solutions (*open* circles), emf is linearly proportional to log A_{Ca}, in accord with Nernstian electrode behavior, and $E = E_0 + 2.303RT/2F \log A_{Ca}$. In the presence of a normal serum Na^+ concentration (*filled circles*) the potential at lower Ca^{2+} concentrations curves away from Nernstian linearity and slope decreases, and $E = E_0 + 2.303RT/2F \log [A_{Ca} + K_{Na}A_{Na}{}^2]$

Clearly, the procedure and techniques for handling the pH question in Ca^{2+} measurements are open to individual and institutional preference. However, we have made approximately 8000 measurements of Ca^{2+} in about 3000 subjects and tried several approaches to the handling of pH, and in our experience the procedure described is preferable to others from the point of view of accuracy, practicality, and cost.

Selectivity Studies in Aqueous Solutions

Figure 3 shows that at physiological Na^+ concentrations, emf is significantly influenced by Na^+ only at Ca^{2+} concentrations below the physiological serum Ca^{2+} range. The extreme is seen for Ca^{2+} concentration $<10^{-5}$ mol/liter, where Na^+ concentration is $>$10 000-fold that of Ca^{2+} and there is nonresponsiveness to change in Ca^{2+} concentration.

The experiment of Figure 3 was repeated at seven different calcium concentrations in the range 10^{-6} to 10^{-2} mol/liter, with five calcium-selective electrodes, in media of four different concentrations (in mmol/liter): Na^+ only (Na^+ 140); Na and Mg^{2+} (Na^+ 140, Mg^{2+} 0.50); Na^+ and K^+ (Na^+ 140, K^+ 5.0); and Na^+, Mg^{2+}, and K^+ (Na^+ 140, Mg^{2+} 0.50, K^+ 5.0). The effect of K^+ was insignificant at all Ca^{2+} concentrations and is therefore omitted from further discussion. Results are shown in Figure 4.

Figure 4 shows that in the presence of normal serum Ca^{2+} and Na^+ concentration, a normal serum Mg^{2+} concentration contributes about 0.18 mV to the measured emf, a 1.7% effect. At an Ca^{2+} concentration of 6×10^{-4} mol/liter, about half the normal value, the concentration is 5 mV, an 8% contribution to the measured emf. This experiment was repeated,

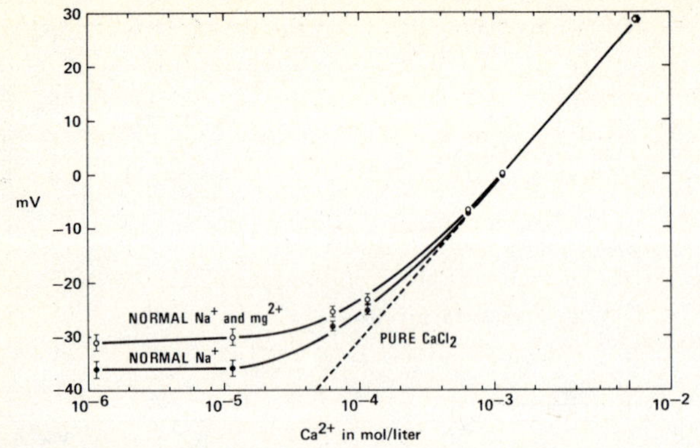

Fig. 4. Effect of normal background Mg^{2+} on emf in the presence of normal background Na^+

Values are the mean ± SE of 5 solid-state calcium electrodes. (*Open circles* are for 140 mmol/liter Na^+ and 0.5 mmol/liter Mg^{2+}. *Filled circles* is 140 mmol/liter Na^+. - - - - is a pure $CaCl_2$ solution.) The emf is given by $E = E_0 + 2.303RT/2F \log [A_{Ca} + K_{Mg}A_{Mg} + K_{Na}A_{Na}^2]$

with the same five calcium electrodes, with Mg^{2+} absent or present at 1.1 mmol/liter, at the four different calcium concentrations (0.115, 0.575, 1.15, and 2.30 mmol/liter). The selectivity coefficient K_{Mg} for the five calcium electrodes at the eight different calcium concentrations between 6.3×10^{-5} and 2.3×10^{-3} mol/liter[7] was calculated by equation 3, and K_{Mg} was 0.044 ± 0.004 (SE); K_{Mg} was independent of Ca^{2+} concentration within the range studied. Thirteen other calcium electrodes were used to measure solutions containing only Ca^{2+} or Mg^{2+}, both 10^{-2} mol/liter; K_{Mg}, calculated from equation 2, was 0.046 ± 0.006 (SE). K_{Mg} as calculated by these two different techniques is therefore the same and close to 0.045 for the 18 calcium electrodes.[8] Since selectivity over Mg^{2+} is the reciprocal of K_{Mg}, the system is therefore 22-fold as selective for Ca^{2+} as for Mg^{2+} on a molar ratio basis.

The contribution to the apparent Ca^{2+} activity made by the Mg^{2+} in a physiological solution[9] is therefore $= 0.045 \times A_{Mg}$. If a sample containing Mg^{2+} is measured against a standard that contains a different concentration of Mg^{2+} the error is:

$$\text{Error in apparent } Ca^{2+} \text{ activity of sample} = 0.045\,(A_{Mg\text{ in sample}} - A_{Mg\text{ in standard}}) \quad (5)$$

In normal serum with Ca^{2+} of 1 mmol/liter and Mg^{2+} of 0.5 mmol/liter the Mg^{2+} therefore contributes the equivalent of $0.045 \times 0.5 = 22$ μmol of Ca^{2+} per liter to the apparent Ca^{2+} activity. If such sera were measured against magnesium-free standards this would constitute a 2% error.[6] For measuring serum or blood we use serum standards (*6*) that contain a normal Mg^{2+} concentration of about 0.5 mmol/liter. Calculated against these standards, a sample with a Mg^{2+} concentration that is extremely high (0.75 mmol/liter) or extremely low (0.25 mmol/liter) would therefore have an apparent Ca^{2+} value that is 1% falsely high or falsely low, respectively. In routine clinical applications with the system reported, therefore, the Mg^{2+} error should be of no clinical significance. If the Mg^{2+} in a sample is extreme, then its concentration in the sample may be estimated and a correction made by use of equation 5.

To calculate the selectivity coefficient of sodium, K_{Na} (equation 4), concentrations of Ca^{2+} and Na^+ that contribute equally to emf are conveniently determined by the graphical technique shown in Figure 2. Determined independently, K_{Na} for five calcium electrodes was 0.0031 ± 0.0003 (SE). At the Na concentration of 0.140 mol/liter studied, A_{Ca_i} was 6.4×10^{-5} mol/liter; thus the selectivity[10] for Ca^{2+} over $Na^+ = 2200$.

The effect on emf and apparent A_{Ca} of physiologically encountered variation in Na^+, however, is due not only to the selectivity effect but also to the effect on solution ionic strength. Unlike in the simpler case of physiologic variation in A_{Mg},[9] physiologically encountered changes in Na^+ may have a substantial effect on the ionic strength of extracellular fluids; a higher Na^+ concentration will increase the ionic strength of the solution and thereby decrease the activity coefficient, γ, thus decreasing the emf[1] (*8, 9*). This influence on ionic strength of change in Na^+ concentration is therefore opposite in direction to the influence of selectivity. Excellent treatment was given the resulting effect of these two opposing influences by Ladenson and Bowers (*7*). I did a similar experiment, and prepared solutions at calcium concentrations 0.115, 0.575, 1.15, and 2.30 mmol/liter, in which Na^+ concentration was either 112 or 168 mmol/liter. At the lowest Ca^{2+} concentration the selectivity influence dominated, and the high-concentration Na^+ solution had increased emf and an apparent A_{Ca} greater by 6% than in the low Na^+ solution. At the other three Ca^{2+} concentrations, which are physiologically encountered, however, there was

[7] K_{Mg} was not calculated for Ca^{2+} concentrations $<1.15 \times 10^{-5}$ mol/liter because Figure 4 showed that with the normal background Na^+ concentration the system is not responsive to change in A_{Ca} below this value. Also, a constant background concentration of Na^+ cancels out in the derivation of equation 3 and can therefore be ignored in calculating K_{Mg}.

[8] These two techniques (equations 2 and 3) are both commonly used, and the agreement in results obtained is expected. The conceptually clearest way to calculate K would be to find the activity of Mg^{2+} that yields the same emf as a particular Ca^{2+} activity. K_{Mg} would then be simply $A_{Mg^{2+}}/A_{Ca^{2+}}$ (*11* and *Methods*). This is more trouble to do, however, and the techniques of equations 2 and 3 appear simplest.

[9] Ionic strength of a physiological extracellular fluid is determined predominantly by the Na^+ concentration, which is about 280-fold, on a molar basis, that of serum Mg^{2+}. Physiologically encountered changes in Mg^{2+} concentration therefore have no significant effect on ionic strength in such a solution (*8, 9*), and physiological Mg^{2+} changes should therefore affect measured emf only by the selectivity effect.

[10] It should be appreciated that the selectivity over Na^+ is not the simple reciprocal of the selectivity coefficient, as is the case for Mg^{2+} but, rather, that selectivity over Na^+ may be calculated as a function of the Na^+ concentration. Selectivity over Na^+ by the operative definition (see *Methods*) $= A_{Na}/A_{Ca_i} = A_{Na}/K_{Na}A_{Na}^2$. Within the range of physiological Na^+ variation the difference in selectivity over Na^+ is small.

no significant difference in emf in the high and low Na^+ solutions, even though the selectivity effect based on K_{Na} would predict a significant positive influence in the high Na^+ solution. At the normal Ca^{2+} concentration of 1.15 mmol/liter, the solution with 168 mmol of Na^+ per liter had a nonsignificant increase of 0.13 mV with respect to the 112 mmol/liter Na^+ solution, corresponding to a nonsignificant increase of 1.3% in apparent Ca^{2+} activity. The selectivity effect would predict that the high Na^+ solution would have an apparent Ca^{2+} activity 4.1% greater than that for the low Na^+ solution. The net observed apparent A_{Ca} in 168 mmol/liter Na^+ was therefore 2.8% lower than that predicted from selectivity considerations alone. The explanation for the discrepancy appears to reside in the ionic strength effect. Ladenson and Bowers (*7*) calculated that at a normal A_{Ca} a solution with 168 mmol/liter Na^+ should, on ionic strength considerations alone, have an apparent Ca^{2+} activity about 3% lower than with 112 mmol/liter Na^+, which is almost exactly the discrepancy I found. Thus, at physiologically encountered Ca^{2+} concentrations, physiological variation in Na^+ appears to cause a selectivity effect and an ionic strength effect that fortuitously almost exactly cancel each other. The net pragmatic "sodium effect" on apparent Ca^{2+} concentration measured with the system reported therefore appears to be insignificant for clinically encountered situations.

Variability in selectivity characteristics in previously available calcium-selective electrode technology has been noted (*7*), and although I have found close agreement in the selectivity characteristics of the new solid-state electrodes of the Electrion System, there is no assurance that these may not be variable. Although it appears unlikely that significant clinical error could result, particularly if there is good agreement in results from two simultaneously used calcium electrodes as I have recommended (*6*), it would seem prudent, at least until further and extensive experience with this new system shows it unnecessary, to maintain an ongoing check on selectivity.

With the techniques described, the Ca^{2+} test has been found particularly revealing at this institution in renal insufficiency, transfusion vs. cardiac activity, proteinopathies, and hypercalcemia of malignancy—situations in which it is well known that values for total calcium frequently give no indication of the Ca^{2+} concentration. These areas will be covered in detail in forthcoming publications. With reliable techniques for measuring Ca^{2+} now available, I agree with Gordan and Vaughan (*17*) that "it is thus highly probable that eventually calcium ion determinations will replace total calcium measurements, since the two yield disparate values in many clinically important situations."

I thank Rutlandra Hodges, Alysen Clark, John R. Daniels, Rupert Miller, Eva A. Fisch, Harold M. Malkin and the MML/Solano Laboratories in Palo Alto, Calif. Aided by American Cancer Society grant CI-106.

References

1. McLean, F. C., and Hastings, A. B., A biological method for the estimation of calcium ion concentration. *J. Biol. Chem.* **107,** 337 (1934).

2. Neuman, W. F., and Neuman, M. W., *The Chemical Dynamics of Bone Mineral,* University of Chicago Press, Chicago, Ill., 1958, pp 1–22.

3. Ross, J. W., Calcium-selective electrode with liquid ion exchanger. *Science* **156,** 1378 (1967).

4. Sachs, C., Selective electrodes for the measurement of blood ionized calcium. Present state and future perspectives. *Presse Med.* **78,** 1547 (1970).

5. Burr, R. G., A source of error with the calcium-specific ion electrode. Solvent effects in aqueous solution. *Clin. Chim. Acta* **43,** 311 (1973).

6. Schwartz, H. D., Serum ionized calcium by electrodes: New technology and methodology. *Clin. Chim. Acta* **64,** 227 (1975).

7. Ladenson, J. H., and Bowers, G. N., Free calcium in serum. I. Determination with the ion-specific electrode, and factors affecting the results. *Clin. Chem.* **19,** 565 (1973).

8. Shatkay, A., Activity coefficients of calcium ions in mixed solutions. *J. Phys. Chem.* **71,** 3858 (1967).

9. Moore, E. W., and Ross, J. W., NaCl and $CaCl_2$ activity coefficients in mixed aqueous solutions. *J. Appl. Phys.* **20,** 1332 (1965).

10. Srinivasan, K., and Rechnitz, G. A., Selectivity studies on liquid membrane, ion-selective electrodes. *Anal. Chem.* **41,** 1205 (1969).

11. Rechnitz, G. A., Kresz, M. R., and Zamochnick, S. B., Analytical study of an iodide-sensitive membrane electrode. *Anal. Chem.* **38,** 973 (1966).

12. Schwartz, H. D., McConville, B. C., and Christopherson, E., Serum ionized calcium by specific ion electrode. *Clin. Chim. Acta* **28,** 97 (1971).

13. Subryan, V. J., Popovtzer, M. D., Parks, S. D., and Reeve, E. B., Measurement of serum ionized calcium with the ion-exchange electrode. *Clin. Chem.* **18,** 1459 (1972).

14. Moore, E. W., Studies with ion-exchange calcium electrodes in biological fluids: Some applications in biomedical research and clinical medicine. In *Ion-selective Electrodes.* R. A. Durst, Ed., *Nat. Bur. Stand. Spec. Publ. 314,* U. S. Government Printing Office, Washington, D. C., 1969, pp 215–285.

15. Li, T. K., and Piechocki, J. T., Determination of serum ionic calcium with an ion-selective electrode: Evaluation of methodology and normal values. *Clin. Chem.* **17,** 411 (1971).

16. Pedersen, K. O., Determination of calcium fractions of serum. III. Ionized calcium in ultrafiltrates of normal and examination of pertinent variables. *Scand. J. Clin. Lab. Invest.* **25,** 223 (1970).

17. Gordan, G. S., and Vaughan, C., *Clinical Management of the Osteoporoses.* Publishing Sciences Group, Acton, Mass., 1976, p 54.

Note added in proof: Using these techniques an inverse correlation between serum Ca^{2+} and parathyroid hormone has been demonstrated: Schwartz, H. D., Serum ionized calcium (Ca^{2+}) and parathyroid hormone (PTH) in renal insufficiency. Program/Abstracts book, Endocrine Society, June 1976. Also, a quantitative linear dependence of myocardial contractility on serum Ca^{2+} has been demonstrated over a wide range, in intact humans and in dogs: Schwartz, H. D., Bristow, M. R., and Goldman, R. H., Myocardial contractility as a function of serum ionized calcium (Ca^{2+}) in vivo. Clin. Res., *April 1976.*

CLIN. CHEM. 22/4, 468–470 (1976)

Automated Separation and Measurement of Lactate Dehydrogenase Isoenzymes

Michael G. Busby, Paul J. Kudirka, R. Neill Carey, and E. Clifford Toren, Jr.[1]

We describe a totally automated, computer-controlled system for separating and measuring the activity of lactate dehydrogenase (EC 1.1.1.27) isoenzymes. These isoenzymes in tissue extracts were separated on disposable DEAE-cellulose mini-columns. Resolution was complete except that LD-1 was not resolved from LD-2.

The determination of isoenzymes has, until recently, been frequently characterized by poor accuracy and precision. The most commonly used techniques are (*a*) electrophoresis and (*b*) kinetic enzymatic analyses wherein isoenzymes are differentiated on the basis of heat stabilities, inhibitors, activators, and (or) different substrates. Although ion-exchange column procedures have been available for quite some time, these procedures have been too time-consuming for routine clinical application. Hicks and Nalevac (*1*) automated a column method for assay of lactate dehydrogenase (LD, EC 1.1.1.27); however, the large column used caused retention times to be relatively long. Recently, Mercer (*2*) described a manual mini-column procedure for creatine kinase (CK, EC 2.7.3.2). Later, he (*3*) described a similar mini-column procedure for simultaneously separating CK-MB and LD isoenzymes 1 and 2 from CK-MM and LD-3, 4, and 5. In this work, we describe a prototype of an automated mini-column method.

The computer-controlled automation for sequential chemical testing has been described (*4*), evaluated (*5*), and later improved by the development of a thermostatted reaction cuvette (*6*). This system was designed for further follow-up tests based on prior test results and demographic information. The follow-up tests may show the need for additional tests, etc., until the analytical potential of the specimen is exhausted (*4*). Because the follow-up tests may be other than simple end-point or kinetic spectrophotometric methods—e.g., radioimmunoassay, column chromatography, or ion-selective potentiometry—much flexibility and versatility has been designed into the system. The capability for radioimmunoassay has been described (*7*). For example, the need for an insulin radioimmunoassay may be indicated by a low result for serum glucose, and an isoenzyme determination may be indicated by an elevated abnormally high result for LD or CK, or both, on routine screening. This paper describes the further application of this system to both the separation, on disposable DEAE-cellulose mini-columns, and quantitation of LD isoenzymes. Control of chromatography, measurement of enzyme activity, calculations, and data presentation were all done automatically by the computer-controlled system.

Departments of Pathology and Medicine, University of Wisconsin, Center for Health Sciences, Madison, Wis. 53706.

This paper is number V in a series. Preceding papers (I, II, and IV) are references *4*, *5*, and *6*; III is in preparation.

[1] Author to whom correspondence should be addressed.

Received Sept. 9, 1975; accepted Jan. 24, 1976.

Materials and Methods

Sample Preparation

Samples of human heart and spleen, obtained at autopsy, were frozen immediately. The samples were cut into small cubes, 2 ml of phosphate buffer (0.10 mol/liter, pH 7.80) was added per gram of tissue, and the mixture was homogenized for 5 min (Model 700B Blendor; Waring Products Corp., Winsted, Conn. 06098). The homogenate was filtered through cheesecloth, and the filtrate was centrifuged (19 620 × *g*, 45 min, 4 °C). The supernates were decanted, and 4-ml aliquots were frozen until analysis. During several weeks, we did not observe any significant decreases in LD activities of tissue extracts attributable to freezing and thawing.

Eluent Preparation

The primary eluent was a 50 mmol/liter tris(hydroxymethyl)aminomethane ("Tris"; Sigma grade 7–9, crystalline, 99–99.5% pure, Sigma Chemical Co., St. Louis, Mo. 63178) buffer adjusted to pH 8.40 with HCl. Secondary eluents 1, 2, 3, and 4 contained, respectively, 0.10, 0.13, 0.175, and 0.50 mol of NaCl per liter, along with 50 mmol/liter Tris buffer that had been adjusted to pH 8.40 with HCl.

Column Preparation

DEAE-cellulose (DE-23; Whatman Biochemicals, Ltd., Maidstone, England) was pretreated by the procedure given in the Whatman Laboratory Manual

(*8*), but followed by an equilibration in primary eluent overnight and for 2 h just before introduction into the columns.

A 12 cm × 5 mm (i.d.) glass column (made to specifications by Norman Erway, Inc., Oregon, Wis. 53575) was prepared by first inserting a plug of glass wool into the bottom of the column. The column was packed by adding a suspension of exchanger (one part of pre-equilibrated DEAE-cellulose to five parts of primary eluent) to a bed height, after settling, of about 8 cm. The column was then washed with 25 ml of primary eluent.

Column Elution Sequence

The elution sequence was a stepwise NaCl gradient, which was found to provide maximum resolution in the shortest time. This sequence was: 5.4 ml of primary eluent, 10.8 ml of secondary eluent No. 1, 10.8 ml of secondary eluent No. 2, 10.8 ml of secondary eluent No. 3, and 12.6 ml of secondary eluent No. 4.

Analysis of Effluents

LD activity measurements were based on the enzymatic oxidation of NADH to NAD^+. The concentration of NADH was monitored at 340 nm and 25 °C. The reagents were obtained from Calbiochem, La Jolla, Calif. 92037 ("LDH-P" kits).

Automation

Column chromatography and effluent analysis were mechanized with the system described by Toren et al. (*4–6*). A new software ratemeter (*9*) was used to provide better accuracy with reaction rates that result in absorbance changes of less than 20 milliabsorbance units/min. The system configuration is shown in Figure 1. The computer controlled the elution process by delivering 1.8-ml portions of eluent to the top of the column. The eluents were aspirated through the column in six 0.3-ml aliquots. A 5-s pause was used between aliquots, to relieve back-pressure. Effluents were collected and mixed in a sampler cup in 1.8-ml fractions. Once 1.8 ml of effluent was collected, another 1.8 ml of eluent was added to the top of the column. This process was repeated until all isoenzymes were eluted.

Each 1.8-ml effluent fraction was analyzed for LD activity after all isoenzymes were eluted from the column. First, 2.80 ml of analytical reagents was delivered to the spectrophotometric cuvette. Then 800 μl of sample was removed from a sampler cup, and 200 μl of it was also delivered to the cuvette. The reaction rate was read by the computer. Finally, the sample was discarded, and the cuvette was washed successively with methanol and distilled water. This sequence was repeated until all effluent fractions were analyzed.

In summary, the computer-controlled system delivered the eluents, collected the effluents, performed multipoint kinetic analyses on the effluent fractions, stored the data (fraction number vs. LD activity), and presented the data both as a chromatogram via a

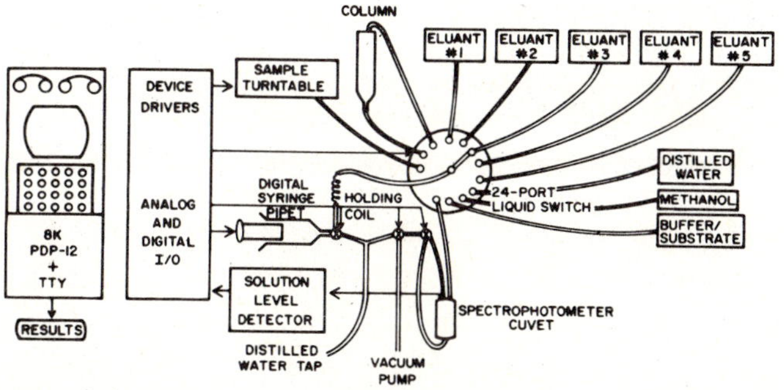

Fig. 1. Diagram of the automated isoenzyme separation system

The computer, through the interface, controls the digital pipet, the sample turntable, the 24-port liquid switch, and the solenoid valves used to wash the cuvette and holding coil. The computer monitors the reaction rate of the sample by measuring the rate of change of absorption at 340 nm, and presents these data via the teletype. Containers of methanol, distilled water, buffer/substrate, and eluents are connected to the liquid switch by Tygon tubing

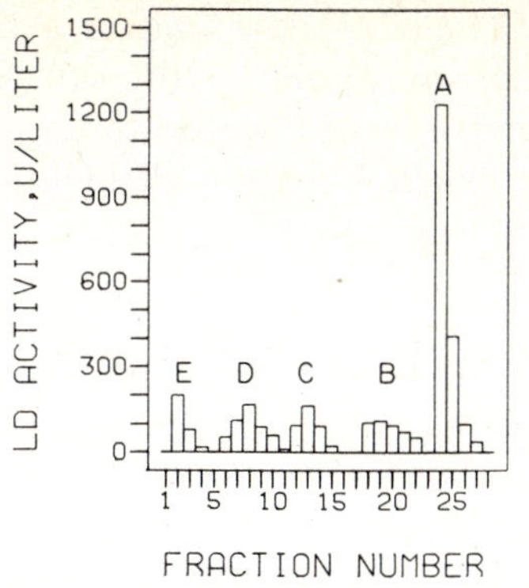

Fig. 2. Automated separation of LD isoenzymes in extract of human tissue (three parts heart + two parts spleen) on a DEAE-cellulose mini-column

Sample size = 1.0 ml. Elution gradient described in text. 28 1.8-ml effluent fractions were collected and analyzed for LD activity. Peak *E* is LD-5, *D* is LD-4, *C* is LD-3, *B* is LD-2, and *A* consists of about equal amounts of LD-2 and LD-1

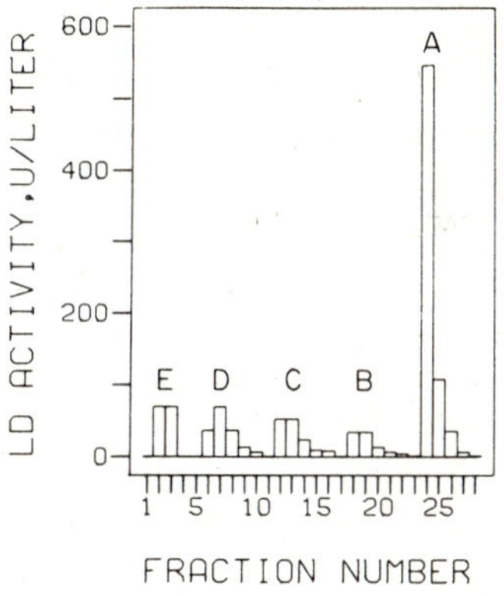

Fig. 3. Manual separation of LD isoenzymes in an extract of human tissue (equal parts of heart and spleen) on a DEAE-cellulose mini-column

Sample size = 1.0 ml. Elution gradient; 6.0 ml of primary eluent, and 12.0 ml, 12.0 ml, 12.0 ml, and 14.0 ml of the respective secondary eluents. 28 2.0-ml effluent fractions were collected and analyzed for LD activity. Peaks identified as in Figure 2 computer-controlled plotter and as a teletypewriter printout. Only application of the sample to the column, the starting variables for column elution, and the plotting variables for the chromatogram needed to be entered by the operator.

Electrophoresis

Electrophoresis was done with Gelman high-resolution buffer (Prod. No. 51104; Gelman Instrument Co., Ann Arbor, Mich. 48106), an electrophoresis cell and general purpose electrophoresis plates (both from Analytical Chemists, Inc., 490 San Antonio Rd., Palo Alto, Calif. 94306), the electrophoresis cell being powered by a Model IP-17 high voltage power supply (Heath Corp., Benton Harbor, Mich. 49022). The samples were electrophoresed for 50 min at 100 V d.c. Then we applied 2 ml of a solution consisting of 18.7 ml of sodium lactate (600 g/liter) plus 81.3 ml of pH 7.4 Tris buffer plus 5 mg of NAD^+ per milliliter. The plate was incubated for 30 min at 37 °C, dried, and read visually under a 340-nm ultraviolet light (UV-21; Ultraviolet Products, Inc., 5114 Walnut Grove Ave., San Gabriel, Calif. 91776).

Results and Discussion

Figure 2 shows a typical chromatogram of an automated separation and analysis of LD isoenzymes, and Figure 3 shows the similar typical results of a manual separation done as a check on the automated separation. These mini-columns containing DEAE-cellulose gave 85 ± 10% recovery of total LD activity with either the automated or manual elution procedure.

Chromatographic peak identities were verified by electrophoresis. Several of the highest LD activity fractions of each chromatographic peak were electrophoresed with the original sample on the same electrophoresis film. The results shown in Figures 2 and 3 illustrate the complete resolution of all LD isoenzymes, except that peak A consists of about equal amounts of LD-1 and -2. Several unsuccessful attempts were made to effect better resolution of LD-2 from LD-1 by varying both the pH and NaCl concentration of the eluents. It appears that the complete separation of LD-2 from LD-1 on DEAE-cellulose mini-columns is impractical. Apparently one would have to use either relatively large columns of classical DEAE ion-exchangers (*1*) or modern high-pressure liquid chromatography (*10*) to completely resolve all LD isoenzymes.

In summary, our automated system is very versatile in that it can be used to separate and measure LD isoenzymes, as well as for sequential chemical clinical testing and radioimmunoassay, which have been described previously (*4, 5, 7*). This automated system was not designed to supplant the use of techniques such as electrophoresis for doing large numbers of LD isoenzyme assays, but our work does demonstrate the feasibility of a completely mechanized system for isoenzyme assays.

This work was supported by grant GP-43624X from the NSF and grant GM 10978 from the NIH. One of us (M.G.B.) was a predoctoral trainee in the Pathology Department in a program supported by grant 5-T01-GM 00130 from the NIH.

References

1. Hicks, G. P., and Nalevac, G. N., Rapid separation and continuous monitoring of enzyme activity in chromatographic column effluents. *Anal. Biochem.* **13,** 199 (1965).

2. Mercer, D. W., Separation of tissue and serum creatine kinase isoenzymes by ion-exchange column chromatography. *Clin. Chem.* **20,** 36 (1974).

3. Mercer, D. W., Simultaneous separation of serum creatine kinase and lactate dehydrogenase isoenzymes by ion-exchange column chromatography. *Clin. Chem.* **21,** 1102 (1975).

4. Toren, E. C., Jr., Carey, R. N., Cembrowski, G. S., and Schirmer, J. A., Computer controlled instrument system for sequential clinical chemical testing. I. Description of instrumentation and system features. *Clin. Chem.* **19,** 1114 (1973).

5. Toren, E. C., Jr., Mohr, S. A., Busby, M. G., and Cembrowski, G. S., Computer controlled instrument system for sequential clinical chemical testing. II. Evaluation of instrumental performance. *Clin. Chem.* **19,** 1122 (1973).

6. Busby, M. G., Cottrell, D. B., Cembrowski, G. S., and Toren, E. C., Jr., A versatile temperature controlled reaction cuvet. *Clin. Chem.* **21,** 1175, (1975).

7. Cottrell, D. B., Toren, E. C., Jr., Magnuson, J. A., and Updike, S. J., Computer controlled automation of radioimmunoassay based on gel entrapment of antibody. *Clin. Chem.* **21,** 829 (1975).

8. *Whatman Advanced Ion-Exchange Celluloses Laboratory Manual,* Whatman Biochemical, Ltd., Maidstone, England.

9. Cembrowski, G. S., Cottrell, D. B., and Toren, C. E., Jr., POLAC, A *P*roblem *O*riented *L*anguage for *A*nalytical *C*hemistry. *Comput. Chem.* **7,** 45 (1976).

10. Kudirka, P. J., Schroeder, R. R., Hewitt, T. E., and Toren, E. C., Jr., High-pressure liquid-chromatographic separation of lactate dehydrogenase isoenzymes. *Clin. Chem.* **22,** 471 (1976).

High-Pressure Liquid-Chromatographic Separation of Lactate Dehydrogenase Isoenzymes

Paul J. Kudirka, Ronald R. Schroeder,[1] Thomas E. Hewitt,[2] and E. Clifford Toren, Jr.[3]

The isoenzymes of lactate dehydrogenase (EC 1.1.1.27) were separated with excellent resolution in less than 1 h by high-pressure anion-exchange chromatography. These isoenzymes were determined in some tissue extracts and high-activity serum samples by this technique.

The complete separation of lactate dehydrogenase (LD, EC 1.1.1.27) isoenzymes by use of ion-exchange column chromatography is a well-established technique (*1*). However, classical ion-exchangers that permit the exchange of isoenzymes (e.g., cellulose, dextrans, or polyacrylamide gels) collapse under high pressure (*2–4*). Hence low pressures, with resulting low flow rates and long separation times, are required to completely resolve all LD isoenzymes (*1*). Other classical ion-exchangers, those with ion-exchange groups bound to highly crosslinked styrene/divinylbenzene polymers, are relatively incompressible and are presently widely used for separations by high-pressure liquid chromatography (*2, 4, 5*). However, these highly cross-linked polymers have relatively small (<1 nm diameter) pore sizes, which exclude large solutes.

We have studied the use of modern ion-exchangers for isoenzyme separations and have previously described the use of high-pressure liquid chromatography in separating creatine kinase isoenzymes (*6*). Here we describe the rapid and complete separation of LD isoenzymes by high-pressure liquid chromatography.

Departments on Pathology and Medicine, University of Wisconsin, Center for Health Sciences, Madison, Wis. 53706.

[1] On leave from Department of Chemistry, Wayne State University.

[2] Division of Biochemistry, Jewish Hospital, St. Louis, Mo. 63110.

[3] To whom correspondence should be addressed.

Received Dec. 23, 1975; accepted Jan. 24, 1976.

Materials and Methods

Sample Preparation

Samples of serum obtained from our clinical laboratory were subjected to high-pressure liquid chromatography without any additional sample preparation. Tissue samples, obtained at autopsy, were either frozen or processed immediately. The samples were cut into small cubes, 2 ml of phosphate buffer (0.10 mol/liter, pH 7.80) was added per gram of tissue, and then homogenized for 5 min in a Model 700B Blendor (Waring Products Corp., Winsted, Conn. 06098). The homogenate was centrifuged (4920 × *g*, 30 min, 5 °C), and the supernate was filtered through Whatman No. 1 filter paper and either used immediately, frozen, or refrigerated (4 °C) until analysis.

LD homopolymers (LD-5, A_4, cat. No. L2875, and LD-1, B_4, cat. No. L0377) were obtained commercially as suspensions in ammonium sulfate solutions (Sigma Chemical Co., St. Louis, Mo. 63178). Solutions of these homopolymers were diluted with phosphate buffer to a concentration of 5 mg of protein per deciliter of the phosphate buffer and refrigerated at 4 °C.

High-Pressure Liquid Chromatographic Instrumentation

We used two different high-pressure liquid chromatographs in this work; a Model 820 liquid chromatograph (E.I. du Pont de Nemours & Co., Inc., Instrument Products Division, Wilmington, Del. 19898) was used at first and later an instrument we assembled from discrete components here in our laboratory (Figure 1).

The heart of the system diagrammed in Figure 1 is the 16-port valve (No. ASCD-16-HPa-C20; Valvco Instruments Co., Houston, Tex. 77024) with which a

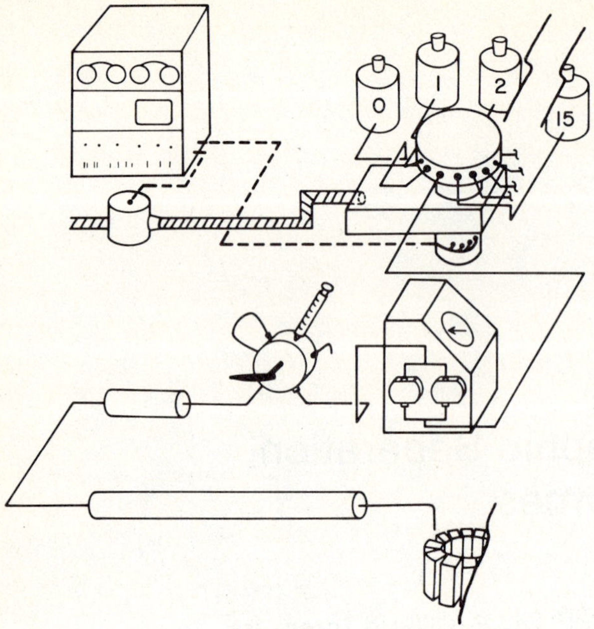

Fig. 1. Diagram of the high-pressure liquid chromatograph
Electrical connections (*dashed lines*), air connections (*crosshatched lines*), and liquid connections (*solid lines*) are shown

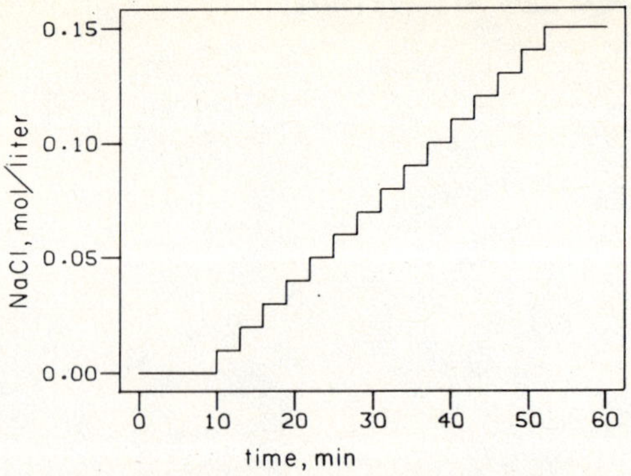

Fig. 2. 16-step elution gradient, with each succeeding step being a 10 mmol/liter increase in NaCl concentration
All eluents were identical (20 mmol/liter Tris, brought to pH 7.80 with acetic acid) except for NaCl concentration. Each elution step represents a discrete solution, selected by the 16-port valve

multistep gradient can be generated such as that shown in Figure 2. This 16-port valve can be operated by a programmable timer (*7*). However, in this laboratory it was most convenient to operate the valve by use of a modification of the laboratory computer system described previously (*8*).

A controlled flow-rate was obtained by use of a reciprocating piston pump (Model No. 721-31 Solvent Delivery System, 16-320 ml/h capacity; Laboratory Data Control, a Division of Milton Roy Co., Riviera Beach, Fla. 33404). Sample, 100 μl, was injected with a Model 204590 six-port sample-loop valve (Du Pont).

Columns

All chromatographic separations were made at room temperature with either a 21.6 cm × 7 mm (i.d.) or a 40 cm × 7 mm (i.d.) No. 316 stainless-steel column packed with DEAE-Glycophase/CPG-250, 5-10 μm particles (Corning Glass Works, Corning Biological Products Department, Medfield, Mass. 02052). "Glycophase" is a glycerol monolayer that is covalently bound to the glass support material. Certain components of these samples became irreversibly bound to the ion-exchange material under our elution conditions. Hence, we used precolumns containing similar ion-exchange material [4.0 cm × 4.6 mm (i.d.) No. 316 stainless-steel packed with DEAE-Glycophase/CPG-250, 120/200 mesh particles; Corning] to trap these components and prevent fouling of the analytical columns. The contents of the precolumns were changed after about every six runs. Columns and precolumns were both fitted at each end with stainless-steel filter discs (2 μm av. pore diameter; Whatman, Inc., Clifton, N. J. 07014), and were equilibrated after each experiment by elution with 15 to 20 column volumes of primary eluent.

Eluents

The primary eluent, except where noted, was a 20 mmol/liter tris(hydroxymethyl)aminomethane (Tris, "Trizma base," reagent grade; Sigma) buffer adjusted to pH 7.80 with acetic acid. Secondary eluents, except where noted, contained from 10 to 150 mmol of NaCl per liter of the Tris buffer, adjusted to pH 7.80 after addition of NaCl.

Analysis of Effluents

Effluents were collected in a fraction collector and analyzed for LD activity with an AutoAnalyzer II single-channel colorimeter (Technicon Instruments Corp., Tarrytown, N. Y. 10591). LD activity was measured by the enzymatic reduction of NAD^+ to NADH, monitored at 340 nm (*9*). Except for the electrophoresis buffer (0.10 mol/liter Tris buffer adjusted to pH 7.80 with HCl), the samples were electrophoresed, stained, and the separation made visible as reported previously (*10*).

Results and Discussion

Several dozen samples were separated by high-pressure liquid chromatography. Typical chromatograms for serum samples are shown in Figures 3 and 4, for tissue samples in Figures 5 and 6. The elution sequence of LD isoenzymes with DEAE-Glycophase/CPG-250 is identical to that obtained with analogous ion-exchangers such as DEAE-cellulose or DEAE-Sephadex. However, additional LD peaks appeared in most of our high-pressure liquid chromatograms. LD-3 was usually at least partly resolved into either two or three peaks. Furthermore, some spleen extracts (e.g., Figure 5) showed yet another peak; one eluting just after, and incompletely resolved from,

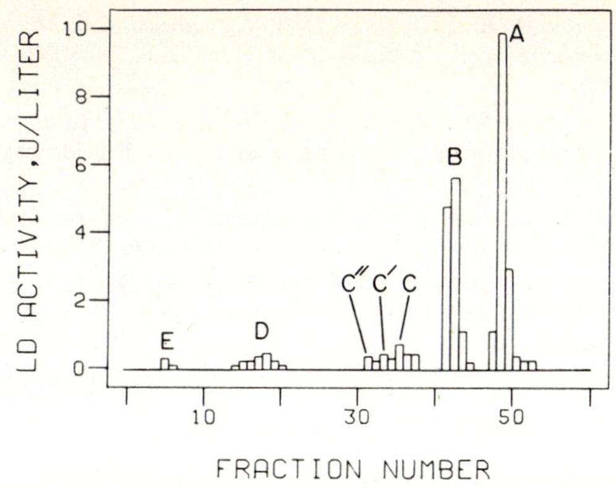

Fig. 3. Chromatographic separation of LD isoenzymes in serum

100-μl sample, total LD = 648 U/liter. Run on instrument shown in Figure 1; gradient of Figure 2; 40 cm column; flow rate, 2.0 ml/min. Sixty 2.0-ml fractions collected and analyzed for LD activity. Peak *E* is LD-5, *D* is LD-4, *C* is LD-3, *B* is LD-2, *A* is LD-1. Undetermined LD peaks are designated by letters marked with primes

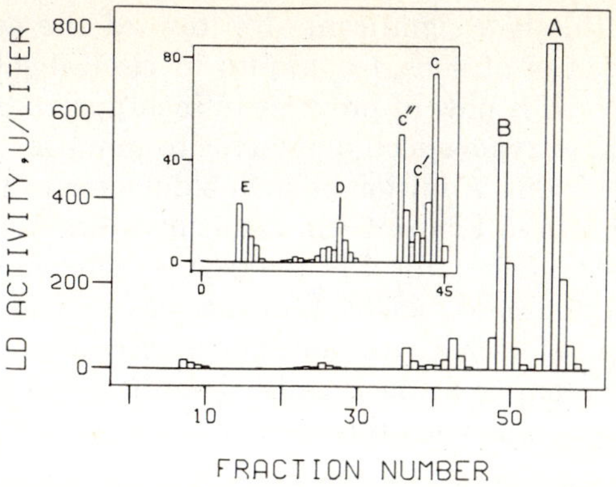

Fig. 6. Chromatographic separation of LD isoenzymes in a heart extract

100-μl sample, sample frozen and thawed once. Run using Du Pont Mode 820 chromatograph with the following gradient: primary eluent, 20 mmol/liter Tris, brought to pH 7.80 with acetic acid, for fractions 1–5; a 2%/min linear change from 100% primary to 100% secondary eluent (same as primary eluent plus 0.12 mol/liter NaCl) for fractions 6–50, and 100% secondary eluent for fractions 51–60. 21.6-cm column; flow rate, about 1.0 ml/min. 60 1.0-ml fractions collected and analyzed for LD activity. Peak identities as in Figure 3. No electrophoretic data obtained for the small unlabeled peaks between peaks *E* and *D*

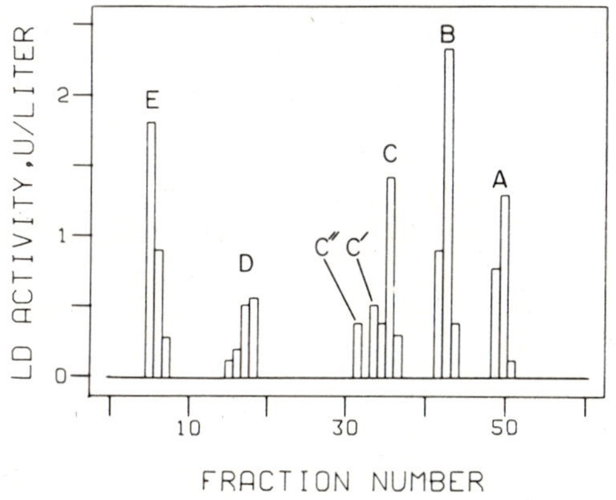

Fig. 4. Chromatographic separation of LD isoenzymes in serum

100-μl sample, total LD = 442 U/liter. Experimental conditions and peak identities as in Figure 3

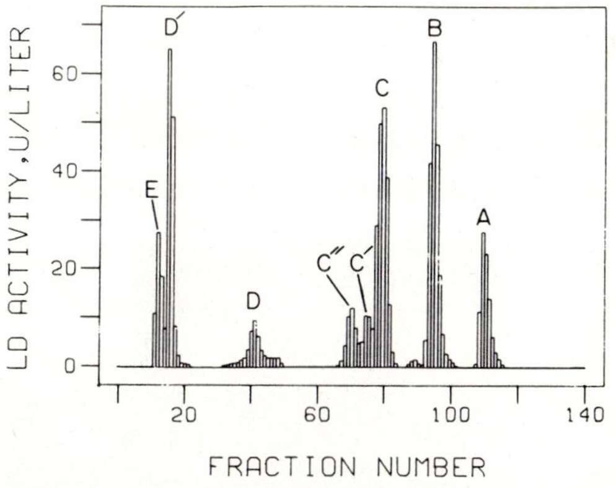

Fig. 5. Chromatographic separation of LD isoenzymes in a spleen extract

100-μl sample, never frozen. Run on instrument shown in Figure 1; gradient of Figure 2; 40-cm column; flow rate, 2.0-ml/min. 140 0.86-ml fractions collected and analyzed for LD activity. Peak identities as in Figure 3. No electrophoretic data obtained for the small unlabeled peak between peaks *C* and *B*

LD-5. This behavior does not appear to be an artifact of either the sample preparation or the high-pressure liquid chromatographic separation, because such peaks did not always appear. These additional peaks remind us of the recently reported electrophoretic data of Papadopoulos (*11*), who observed three extra LD isoenzyme bands, two located between LD-3 and LD-4 and one between LD-4 and LD-5.

The identities of these chromatographic peaks were verified by electrophoresis. Several of the most active fractions of each chromatographic peak were co-electrophoresed with the original sample on the same electrophoresis film. On electrophoresis, none of our samples showed more than five LD isoenzyme bands. We did not try to improve the resolution of the electrophoresis. Thus we were unable to determine whether the additional chromatographic peaks that we observed had any relationship to the three extra LD isoenzyme bands reported by Papadopoulos (*11*). The significance of these additional chromatographic peaks is now under investigation.

To test whether the LD homopolymers retain their tetrameric integrity under the chromatographic conditions we used, we chromatographed solutions of the homopolymers under conditions identical to those used to obtain the results shown in Figures 3 and 4, and found one peak for each of these homopolymers when they were chromatographed individually; A_4 (LD-5) was eluted at the position of the first peak in Figures 3 and 4, and B_4 (LD-1) was eluted near the position of the last peak. When co-chromatographed, the chromatogram showed only two peaks, one corresponding to the A_4 peak and the other to the B_4 peak.

High-pressure liquid chromatographic techniques speed separations. Thus we could separate LD isoenzymes with excellent resolution in less than 1 h. We think this is a significant step toward the eventual routine use of such techniques in clinical laboratories. Work is now in progress in incorporating an instream, enzyme-specific detector to monitor the column effluent. Addition of such a detector to the system shown in Figure 1 will result in a completely automated system for LD isoenzyme determinations. Furthermore, we believe that the column and elution gradient of such a system can be modified so as to enable the entire analysis to be done in a quantitative fashion in much less than 30 min.

We wish to thank E. I. du Pont de Nemours & Co. and Technicon Instruments for some of the instrumentation and Corning Glass Works, Biological Products Department for the column packing materials used in this work. This work was supported by grant No. GP-43624X from the NSF and grant No. GM 21752 from the NIH.

References

1. Hicks, G. P., and Nalevac, G. N., Rapid separation and continuous monitoring of enzyme activity in chromatographic column effluents. *Anal. Biochem.* **13,** 199 (1965).

2. Snyder, L. R., and Kirkland, J. J., *Introduction to Modern Liquid Chromatography,* John Wiley & Sons, Inc., New York, N. Y., 1974, chap. 9.

3. *Sephadex Ion Exchangers, A Guide to Ion Exchange Chromatography.* Pharmacia Fine Chemicals, Inc., Piscataway, N. J. 08854, 1970.

4. Khym, J. X., *Analytical Ion-Exchange Procedures in Chemistry and Biology; Theory, Equipment, Techniques,* Prentice-Hall, Inc., Englewood Cliffs, N. J., 1974, chap. 3.

5. Scott, C. D., High pressure ion exchange chromatography. *Science* **186,** 226 (1974).

6. Kudirka, P. J., Busby, M. G., Carey, R. N., and Toren, E. C., Jr., Separation of creatine kinase isoenzymes by high-pressure liquid chromatography. *Clin. Chem.* **21,** 450 (1975).

7. Scott, R. P. W., *Analabs, Inc., Research Notes, Vol 14, No. 1,* Analabs, Inc., North Haven, Conn. 06473, Mar., 1973.

8. Toren, E. C., Jr., Carey, R. N., Cembrowski, G. S., and Schirmer, J. A., Computer-controlled instrument system for sequential clinical chemical testing. I. Instrumentation and system features. *Clin. Chem.* **19,** 1114 (1973).

9. *Technicon Method No. SE4-0021FJ4,* Technicon Instruments Corp., Tarrytown, N. Y. 10591, Sept., 1974.

10. Busby, M. G., Kudirka, P. J., Carey, R. N., and Toren, E. C., Jr., Automated separation and measurement of lactate dehydrogenase isoenzymes. *Clin. Chem.* **22,** 468 (1976).

11. Papadopoulos, N. M., Electrophoretic demonstration of three extra lactate dehydrogenase isoenzymes in the serum of a "normal" individual. *Clin. Chem.* **20,** 841 (1974).

CLIN. CHEM. 22/4, 475–483 (1976)

Expression of Random Analytical Error as a Percentage of the Range of Clinical Interest

John H. Glick, Jr.

I propose that random method error be expressed as a percentage of the range(s) of clinical interest (upper range limit minus lower range limit), in addition to its usual forms of presentation. The interpretation of this percent random error is simple because a given percentage error implies the same reliability, regardless of test or range of clinical interest. Two different upper limits for percent random analytical error are suggested, based on the medical application of the test and the statistical properties of various amounts of error. When the purpose of the test is to distinguish an upper medically defined limit from a lower medically defined limit, a maximum random error equivalent to 60% of the difference between the limits is proposed. If the purpose of the test is to monitor values in the neighborhood of a normal range or therapeutic range, an upper limit for random error equal to 20% of the difference between the limits of the range is suggested.

Additional Keyphrases: *statistics • systematic error • more informative reporting of results*

The maximum acceptable random analytical error for a method is related to the range or interval of values for which the method is used. Various criteria are used to define acceptable random error. Barnett (*1*) used the consensus standard deviations of clinicians and laboratory specialists. Tonks (*2*) suggested that the allowable error should be equal to one-fourth of the normal range. Cotlove et al. (*3*) recommended that the "tolerable analytic variability" equal $0.5S_B$, where S_B is the total biological standard deviation.[1] Lindberg and Watson (*7*) pointed out that disease prevalence and importance of diagnosis must be considered in deciding the beneficial effect of increasing the precision of a particular test. Most authors use one of these approaches in defining the acceptable limit of analytical error (*5, 8–9*).

The units for expression of random or systematic analytical error are commonly given as test units (*1–3, 5, 8*). In the case of random analytical error, the coefficient of variation is also frequently used (*1–3, 8–9*). The presentation of observed random analytical error in these units requires that a consideration be made of the range(s) of clinical interest of the test, before the medical usefulness of the method can be decided.

Department of Pathology, Division of Clinical Laboratories, University of Kansas Medical Center, Kansas City, Kan. 66103.
Received Nov. 7, 1975; accepted Jan. 28, 1976.

[1] Terminology used: S_A, after Harris et al. (*4*), is the observed total analytical standard deviation of a method, including within-run arnd run-to-run components; S_{AU} is the 95% upper limit for repeated measurements of S_A; $\bar{x}_A$ is the observed mean value that corresponds to a particular S_A; F_U is the factor for the upper 95% limit for a standard deviation, as given by Westgard et al. (*5*); μ_A and σ_A are the population parameters of which $\bar{x}_A$ and S_A are estimates.

ρ_{BA} is a normal range or a therapeutic range that corresponds to 95% confidence limits of a population of test values (ρ_{BA} = 97.5% limit–2.5% limit), where the limits are measured in an appropriate manner (*6*). No particular distribution is assumed unless specifically stated; σ_{BA} is the standard deviation of a single value in this population of test values. This standard deviation includes biological and random analytical components, σ_B and σ_A, respectively. The range factor, F_R is a ratio, ${}_{\%RE1}\sigma_{BA}/{}_{\%RE2}\sigma_{BA}$, where ${}_{\%RE1}\sigma_{BA}$ and ${}_{\%RE2}\sigma_{BA}$ are standard deviations, σ_{BA}, that contain the same biological component, σ_B, but different amounts of random analytical component, σ_A (and consequently different percentages of random error, RE1 and RE2).

ρ_M, a medically defined range, is the difference between upper and lower medically specified test values. No confidence limits are implied in this range.

The formulation of laboratory data in relative terms has been used for several applications. Hoffman (*10*) and Burns et al. (*11*) have expressed patients' results relative to the normal range. Acland and Lipton (*12, 13*) have presented random analytical error as a ratio, σ_1/σ_2, where σ_1 is the standard deviation of repeated determinations on a single sample and σ_2 is the standard deviation of accurately determined values in a population of healthy subjects. Although the relative form of presentation, if given alone, suffers from the loss of absolute values, it makes the identification of abnormal results a more rapid process.

The subject of the present report is the formulation of random analytical error in relative terms, as a percentage of the interval or range of clinical interest. Several properties of different percentages of random analytical error are given, and upper limits for the percent random error for two types of clinical application are proposed. The two clinical applications are: (*a*) the upper limit of a specified medical decision range, ρ_M, must be distinguished from the lower limit; and (*b*) values within a specified normal range or therapeutic range, ρ_{BA}, must be monitored within, or adjacent to, the range. For these two applications, several criteria are used to formulate acceptable upper limits of random analytic error. The criteria are: (*a*) that a repeat analysis, in a different run, of the same specimen will be acceptably close to the first analysis (*14*); (*b*) that an observed absolute difference, equivalent to the range, between two different specimens in different runs will not be the result of analytical error, in most cases (*15*); (*c*) that false-positive and false-negative results owing to imprecision are tolerable (*12, 13*); and (*d*) that the imprecision does not excessively widen the biological range (*3*). Criteria *a* and *b* are applied to the use of range ρ_M; criteria *a*, *c*, and *d* to the use of range ρ_{BA}.

Materials and Methods

The 95% normal ranges and the measured total analytical standard deviations for 13 tests were obtained from Roberts (*16*). Suggested standard deviations for acceptable performance at several medical decision points were obtained from Barnett (*1*).

Random analytical error, expressed as a percentage of the range of clinical interest, is calculated as follows: the 95% upper limit for observed percent random error, calculated from measured values, is $(100)(1.96)(F_U)(S_A)/(\text{range})$, where the range is ρ_{BA} or ρ_M; the theoretical percent random error from population parameters is $(100)(1.96)(\sigma_A)/(\text{range})$, where the range is ρ_{BA} or ρ_M. For these calculations, it is assumed that the 95% range, ρ_{BA}, includes the amount of random analytical error represented by σ_A or S_A. Values for the 95% upper limit of the observed standard deviation, S_A, and for the population standard deviation, σ_A, can be calculated by rearrangement of the above formulas, provided the percent random error is given (see Appendix).

Terms used in the paper are defined in a footnote[1]. The derivation of the data in Tables 1 and 2 is presented in the Appendix.

Results

Table 1 summarizes some properties of random analytical error as a function of the range of clinical interest. Methods for calculating the data in this table are given in the Appendix. The range and the random error are given in σ_A units, and the error is also expressed as a percentage of the range. One of two types of range apply in this table, depending on the amount of error and the consequent probable application of the test. For errors of 50% or less,[2] the range is considered to be ρ_{BA}, the difference between the 97.5 and the 2.5 percentiles of a set of values that might, for example, correspond to a normal range for a test or a therapeutic range for a drug. For errors greater than 50%, the range is considered to be ρ_M, the difference between two medically defined limits. These limits do not describe a confidence interval for a population. Instead, they can be thought of as an upper point at or beyond which one type of action is taken, and a lower point at or below which another type of action is taken. A point within the range would indicate further tests.

Table 1 gives the upper confidence limits for the absolute difference between two analyses of the same sample in different runs, as a multiple of the range of clinical interest. These data were obtained from Pearson (*14*). For example, if the random error is 60% of the range, the absolute difference between two analyses of the same sample in different runs would exceed (0.85)(range) in 5% of cases.[3] For a 20% error, the corresponding value is (0.28)(range). This property of random error is presented because it relates to the manner in which a questionable result is usually handled in the laboratory, i.e., the analysis is repeated on the same specimen but in another run. These data assume that the random analytical error follows a gaussian distribution. There are no restrictions in regard to the population of values included within the range.

Table 1 also lists the chance (%) that an absolute difference equal to the range between two different samples in different runs is due to analytical error. This information, derived from Campbell and Owen (*15*), is useful for deciding whether a method is sufficiently precise for medical decision applications related to ρ_M. The values for random errors less than 40% are insignificant and are not given. For a random method error equivalent to 60% of the range, the probability is 2.1% that an absolute difference equal to the range is the result of method error. The corre-

[2] When the error equals 50%, the standard deviation of the method, σ_A, is equal to the standard deviation of the population σ_{BA} that is described by the range ρ_{BA}. This assumes that the error distribution and the population distribution are both gaussian distributions.

[3] The first result would differ from the second result in a specified direction by more than (0.85)(range) in 2.5% of cases.

Table 1. Properties of Different Amounts of Random Analytical Error as a Function of the Range of Clinical Interest[a]

Range		Random error		Statistical properties of random error											
				Pearson (14) Upper confidence limits[c]						Campbell and Owen (15)	Acland and Lipton (12, 13)				Cotlove et al. (3)
													False classifications[f]		
Type	Value σ_A units	σ_A units	% of range	95%	90%	80%	70%	60%	50%	Chance,[d] %	Ratio, σ_A/σ_{BA}	Normal samples,[e] %	Limit ± range/4, %	Limit ± range/8, %	Increase,[g] %
ρ_M	1.96	1.96	100	1.41	1.19	0.92	0.75	0.61	0.48	16.5	2.0				
ρ_M	2.18	1.96	90	1.27	1.07	0.83	0.67	0.55	0.44	12.4	1.8				
ρ_M	2.45	1.96	80	1.13	0.95	0.74	0.60	0.49	0.39	8.4	1.6				
ρ_M	2.80	1.96	70	0.99	0.83	0.65	0.52	0.42	0.34	4.8	1.4				
ρ_M	3.27	1.96	60	0.85	0.71	0.55	0.45	0.36	0.29	2.1	1.2				
ρ_{BA}	3.92	1.96	50	0.71	0.59	0.46	0.38	0.30	0.24	0.6	1.0	14	16	31	
ρ_{BA}	4.90	1.96	40	0.57	0.48	0.37	0.30	0.24	0.19	0.1	0.8	10	11	27	66.7
ρ_{BA}	5.60	1.96	35	0.49	0.42	0.32	0.26	0.21	0.17		0.7	*b*	8	24	40.0
ρ_{BA}	6.53	1.96	30	0.42	0.36	0.28	0.23	0.18	0.15		0.6	6	5	21	25.0
ρ_{BA}	7.84	1.96	25	0.35	0.30	0.23	0.19	0.15	0.12		0.5	5	2	16	15.5
ρ_{BA}	9.80	1.96	20	0.28	0.24	0.18	0.15	0.12	0.10		0.4	3	1	11	9.1
ρ_{BA}	13.07	1.96	15	0.21	0.18	0.14	0.11	0.09	0.07		0.3	2		5	4.8
ρ_{BA}	19.60	1.96	10	0.14	0.12	0.09	0.08	0.06	0.05		0.2	1		1	2.1
ρ_{BA}	39.20	1.96	5	0.07	0.06	0.05	0.04	0.03	0.02		0.1	1			0.5

[a] The terminology is given in footnote[1]. The calculations are discussed in the text and described in the Appendix.
[b] Value not given.
[c] For absolute difference between two analyses of same sample in different runs, as multiple of range.
[d] That absolute difference equal to range between two different samples in different runs is due to error.
[e] That give abnormal results, owing to error.
[f] Near-range limits owing to error.
[g] In biological range owing to error.

sponding probability for a difference of this magnitude with a specified sign (+ or −) is 2.1/2 = 1.05%. These results assume that the random analytical error follows a gaussian distribution. There are no assumptions about the population of values included within the limits of the range.

Some properties of random error in relation to false-positive and false-negative results are also shown in Table 1. These data, derived from Acland and Lipton (*12, 13*), assume that both the random error and the population of results (of which the range ρ_{BA} is a part) follow gaussian distributions. The data include the ratio σ_A/σ_{BA}, similar to Acland and Lipton's σ_1/σ_2, and probabilities (%) of false-positive and false-negative errors that are related to random analytical error. For example, in the case of a 25% random error, 5% of a normally distributed group of "true" within-range samples will actually give results outside of the range, because of analytical error (*13*). For the same amount of error, and for specimens with "true" values at distances of ± (range/4) or ± (range/8) from either the upper or lower limit of the range, the percentages of analyses that give false results (on the opposite side of the limit) are 2% and 16%, respectively (*12*). These false classifications are attributable to analytical error. They should be distinguished from the 5% of normal persons whose "true" values are outside of a 95% normal range.

The last column of Table 1 gives the approximate percent artifactual increase in the biological range owing to analytical error. The data are derived from the formula of Cotlove et al. (*3*) as outlined in the Appendix. To compute the figures for this column, I have assumed in this report that the population of results of which the range ρ_{BA} is a part follows a gaussian distribution.

Based upon the data of Table 1, upper limits for random analytical error of approximately 60% and 20% are suggested for medical decision applications (range is ρ_M), and monitoring in the neighborhood of ranges (range is ρ_{BA}), respectively. This is considered in more detail in the *Discussion*.

Table 2 gives values for the 95% upper limit of method standard deviation that correspond to several values of random analytical error. The derivation of the data is described in the Appendix. The standard deviations are expressed as multiples of $\rho_{BA}F_R$ or ρ_M. The range factor F_R is used when the selected percent random error, column 1, is different from the percent random error that is involved in the estimation of the range ρ_{BA} that is used as the multiplier. The factor is equal to (100 + percent increase in biological range for selected error)/(100 + percent increase in biological range for error involved in the estimation of ρ_{BA}). The percentage increases in biological range are obtained from the last column of Table 1. The derivation of F_R is described in the Appendix.

Table 2 is useful for calculating the required standard deviation that corresponds to a given percent error and range. For example, if the upper limit of error for a medical decision application is specified as 60%, and the range ρ_M is defined as (20–19) = 1 mg/100 ml, the measured run-to-run standard deviation (30 degrees of freedom) should be no greater that 0.24 ρ_M = 0.24 mg/100 ml, in 95% of trials. As another example of the use of this table, suppose that, for reasons of efficiency, a change in methodology of a test is contemplated. A published method is selected, and the desired upper limit of random error is specified as 20% of the adult 95% normal range. The published 97.5% and 2.5% confidence limits for normal adults by the proposed method are 140 and 130 mmol/liter, respectively. The random error associated with the estimation of the range, calculated from the published data as described in *Materials and Methods*, is 30%. The required 95% upper limit for the measured run-to-run standard deviation, for 30 degrees of freedom, is 0.080 $\rho_{BA}F_R$ = (0.080)(140 − 130)(109.1)/(125.0) = 0.7 mmol/liter.

As explained in the Appendix, the factors given in Table 2 are conservative. The calculated standard deviations in this table are considered to be the 95% upper limit for the observed standard deviation, in replicate experiments. If used in this way, the calculated standard deviations of Table 2 will yield 95% upper limits of random error that are equal to or less than the stated errors in the table, in 95% of cases.

Table 3 lists the 95% normal ranges and the measured run-to-run random analytical error for 13 tests as reported by Roberts (*16*). The measured analytical error is presented in three ways: (*a*) standard deviation, S_A; (*b*) coefficient of variation (usually relative to a point in the normal range); and (*c*) random error, as a percentage of the range of normal values, ρ_{BA}, calculated as described in *Materials and Methods*. In calculating the random error from the reported standard deviation, S_A, 100 degrees of freedom are assumed.

Table 2. Values for Observed Method Standard Deviation That Correspond to Several Percentages of Random Analytical Error[a]

Error[b]	Degrees of freedom[c]	95% upper limit[d]
70	20	0.263
70	30	0.280
60	20	0.225
60	30	0.240
25	20	0.094
25	30	0.100
20	20	0.075
20	30	0.080

[a] The terminology is given in footnote[1]. The calculations are discussed in the text and described in the Appendix.
[b] As percent of range ρ_{BA} or ρ_M.
[c] For calculation of observed value, S_A.
[d] For observed value, as multiple of $\rho_{BA}F_R$ or ρ_M.

Table 3. Random Analytical Error in the Normal Range for 13 Clinical Chemical Methods for Serum[a]

Test		95% Normal range for males, ρ_{BA}			Random analytical error		
Name	Units	97.5% limit[b]	2.5 limit[b]	Range[b]	S_A[b]	CV, %	% of range
Alkaline phosphatase	King-Armstrong/100 ml	13	4	9	1	5.9	24.7
Amylase	Somogyi units/100 ml	117	31	86	7	4.1	18.1
Bilirubin	mg/100 ml	0.9	0.1	0.8	0.075	8.3	20.8
Calcium	mg/100 ml	10.4	9.0	1.4	0.15	1.2	23.8
Chloride	mmol/liter	107	98	9	1.25	1.3	30.8
Creatinine	mg/100 ml	1.4	0.8	0.6	0.1	7.1	37.0
Inorganic phosphorus	mg/100 ml	4.2	2.2	2.0	0.2	6.7	22.2
Potassium	mmol/liter	4.8	3.6	1.2	0.075	1.9	13.9
Total protein	g/100 ml	7.4	6.1	1.3	0.1	1.6	17.1
Albumin	g/100 ml	4.8	3.7	1.1	0.1	4.8	20.2
Seromucoids	mg/100 ml	134	51	83	5	10.6	13.4
Sodium	mmol/liter	143	134	9	1.25	1.0	30.8
Urea	mg/100 ml	43	21	22	1.5	4.3	15.1

[a] Data from Roberts (*16*). The terminology is given in footnote[1]; calculations described in *Materials and Methods.*
[b] Concentration expressed in the units given in column two.

Table 4. Random Analytical Error at Several Medical-decision Values for Serum Glucose and Bilirubin[a]

Test		Medical-decision	Arbitrary	Random analytical error		
Name	Units	value[b]	range[b]	σ_A[b]	CV, %	% of range
Glucose	mg/100 ml	50	10	5.0	10.0	98
Glucose	mg/100 ml	50	20	5.0	10.0	49
Glucose	mg/100 ml	50	30	5.0	10.0	33
Glucose	mg/100 ml	50	40	5.0	10.0	25
Glucose	mg/100 ml	120	10	5.0	4.2	98
Glucose	mg/100 ml	120	20	5.0	4.2	49
Glucose	mg/100 ml	120	30	5.0	4.2	33
Glucose	mg/100 ml	120	40	5.0	4.2	25
Bilirubin	mg/100 ml	1.00	0.20	0.2	20.0	196
Bilirubin	mg/100 ml	1.00	0.40	0.2	20.0	98
Bilirubin	mg/100 ml	1.00	0.60	0.2	20.0	65
Bilirubin	mg/100 ml	1.00	0.80	0.2	20.0	49
Bilirubin	mg/100 ml	20.0	2.0	1.5	7.5	147
Bilirubin	mg/100 ml	20.0	4.0	1.5	7.5	73
Bilirubin	mg/100 ml	20.0	6.0	1.5	7.5	49
Bilirubin	mg/100 ml	20.0	8.0	1.5	7.5	37

[a] The decision values and suggested standard deviations, σ_A, are from Barnett (*1*). The ranges are arbitrarily chosen.
[b] Concentration expressed in the units given in column two.

The tests in Table 3 that are least efficient for monitoring values in the neighborhood of the normal range can be most easily identified by reference to the random analytical error expressed as a percentage of the normal range. Chloride, creatinine, and sodium are least efficient. On the other hand, potassium, seromucoids, and urea are the three tests that are most efficient for this medical application, based upon the criteria of Table 1.

Table 4 illustrates the calculation of random analytical error for several medical decision ranges or intervals, ρ_M. One of the limits[4] for these ranges is a "medical-decision level" of Barnett (*1*). The ranges are arbitrary intervals, chosen to illustrate the effect of range on the percent random analytical error. The standard deviations are the desirable upper limits recommended by Barnett for medical significance (*1*). For calculation of the percent random error in Table 4, the recommended standard deviations are treated as population parameters, σ_A, instead of measured values, S_A. Therefore a confidence factor (*5*) is not used to calculate the percent error.

In the case of glucose, and for ranges of 20 mg/100 ml or greater, the recommended upper limit of standard deviation of Barnett, 5 mg/100 ml, gives percent errors that are less than 60% and adequate to ensure that the upper limit of the range can be distinguished from the lower limit, by the criteria of Table 1.

[4] Upper limit, if increases in the level are medically critical; lower limit, if decreases in the level are critical.

For the bilirubin data of Table 4, at the medical decision level of 20 mg/100 ml and an interval of 2 mg/100 ml, a method standard deviation σ_A equal to 1.5 mg/100 ml gives a percent random error of 147%. According to the criteria of Table 1, this amount of error would not permit one to distinguish the upper limit from the lower limit of the 2 mg/100 ml range with reasonable assurance.

For the random error to be 60% for a 2 mg/100 ml interval, the run-to-run standard deviation of the method, σ_A, should be 0.6 ρ_M/1.96 = 0.6 mg/100 ml. If a decision range of 1 mg/100 ml is required, the upper limit for σ_A would be 0.3 mg/100 ml. The corresponding 95% upper limits for the observed standard deviations, S_A, as obtained from Table 2 (30 degrees of freedom) are 0.48 and 0.24 mg/100 ml, respectively.

Discussion

I propose in this report that random analytical error be expressed as a percentage of the range(s) of clinical interest, in addition to its usual forms of presentation, method standard deviation and (or) coefficient of variation. Expression of random analytical error as a percentage of the range of clinical interest enables one to determine readily whether the error is sufficiently low for the proposed use of the method (Table 1). Upper limits for random error are suggested in terms of the percentage expression. One of two upper limits for the percent random error is proposed, depending upon the application of the test.

If the method is used to monitor values in the neighborhood of a 95% normal range or a therapeutic range, an upper limit for run-to-run random method error equal to 20% of the range is suggested. This would assure that the absolute difference between a first result and a repeat analysis of the same specimen in another run exceeds (0.28)(range) in only about 5% of cases (Table 1). Also, only 3% of "true" within-range specimens from a gaussian-distributed population would fall outside the range, because of analytical error. Values at ± (range/4) and ± (range/8) of either limit would be falsely reported on the opposite side of the limit in 1% and 11% of cases, respectively. And, finally, for a 20% random error, a biological range would be artifically expanded by about 9%.

An upper limit for random method error equal to 20% of the range of clinical interest demands more precision than several recent proposals. Tonks (*2*) recommended an upper limit equal to 25% of the normal range, and Cotlove et al. (*3*) suggested a limit for the analytical standard deviation equivalent to (0.5)(biological standard deviation). In terms of the present report, random error corresponding to this latter criterion is equal to about 22.5% of a range, ρ_{BA}, that includes biological and total analytical variation (σ_B and σ_A). As a minimal target value, it is suggested that the random method error should not exceed 20% of a 95% normal adult range or "reference interval" that has been determined in a reliable manner (*6*). A smaller run-to-run method standard deviation would be required to achieve the same 20% error if the range of clinical use is narrower. This would be the case, for example, if an individual normal range or reference interval was the range of clinical interest (*3*). The same 20% upper limit of random error is suggested for any range in which the purpose is monitoring of values in the neighborhood of the range. For instance, a 95% upper limit for run-to-run method standard deviation, S_A, corresponding to 20% error, could be derived for lithium or digoxin analyses, provided the therapeutic ranges, ρ_{BA}, are specified (Table 2).

Although the 20% upper limit of random error for the monitoring application is somewhat arbitrary, the performance criteria for a 20% error (Table 1) are good by current standards. They are not, however, more demanding than necessary (*17*). In fact, by restricting the artificial expansion of the biological range and by providing good precision, an upper limit of 20% for random analytical error might improve the usefulness of laboratory tests in the diagnostic process (*18, 19*).

When a method is used to distinguish between medically defined upper and lower limits of a decision range, an upper limit for random analytical error equal to 60% of the range is recommended. For this amount of random error, the probability is 2.1% that an absolute difference equal to the range between two different specimens is due to analytical error (Table 1). The probability is about 1% for the same difference in a specified direction. For instance, if analyses show that the first specimen is equal to the lower limit and the second specimen, in another run, is equal to the upper limit, the chance that this is the result of analytical error is about 1%.

From Table 1, and assuming a 60% error, it is also seen that two analyses of the same specimen in different runs will have an absolute difference that exceeds (0.85)(range) in 5% of cases. This same difference will be exceeded in a specified direction in 2.5% of cases. For example, if a result is near the lower limit, a repeat analysis of the same specimen in another run will differ from the first analysis in the direction of the upper limit by more than (0.85)(range) in only 2.5% of trials.

Although the recommendation of an upper limit for random analytical error equal to 60% of the medical decision range is also somewhat arbitrary, the data of Table 1 suggest that it would be acceptable for even critical medical decisions. Specifically: (*a*) two successive specimens from different runs with values at opposite limits of the range will be truly different, in the indicated direction, in about 99% of cases; and (*b*) a single specimen with a first analysis at one limit will give a second analysis in another run that is closer to the first limit than to the opposite limit in more than 70% of cases. For most of the remaining cases, the second analysis is unlikely to exceed the opposite limit.

In this paper, the use of a medically defined decision range, ρ_M, and a 60% limit for random error is suggested as a means for calculating the 95% upper limit of method standard deviation, S_A, for medical-decision applications in general (Table 2). On the other hand, much of the current literature in this field is related to a decision value or point (*1, 6, 7*) and not to a set of limits. The value by itself is not sufficient for medical decisions, however. In addition, the physician must have an idea of the analytical error of the method. Upper limits of random error have been suggested on a case-by-case basis for medical decisions (*1*).

The range and the value or point concepts for medical decisions can be combined if the decision value (*1, 6, 7*) is designated as the critical limit of a decision range, ρ_M (the limit at which decisive action is taken). The opposite limit would be a second medically defined value that must be clearly differentiated from the critical limit. A value at this second limit would indicate no action or a less critical activity. A value within the range would suggest further testing or additional information, after the manner of Zieve (*20*).

The present paper suggests the use of a single upper limit for random analytical error as applied to medical decisions. This 60% limit of error would have the same statistical implications, in terms of the limits, for all medical decisions. The limits themselves would be selected on the basis of medical needs. This would include the proper positioning of the critical limit, depending on several factors, including the consequences to the patient of a false-positive versus a false-negative result (*6, 7*).

It is generally agreed that a decrease in the random analytical error of a test is desirable (*7, 17*). However, Lindberg and Watson (*7*) suggested that the decision to decrease the random analytical error, which is perhaps a costly or otherwise impracticable process, should include consideration of factors such as the medical use of the test. This is a valid argument, and it raises the question of whether a single upper limit for random analytical error, such as 20% or 60% of the range of clinical interest (depending on the application), is useful. I feel that it is useful in the sense that it indicates the approximate upper limit of random error for "good" performance (Table 1). For various reasons (*7*), this level of performance will probably not be attained in some tests. Nevertheless, this is not a reason for defining additional error limits for "fair" performance, which might be misinterpreted or misapplied. It should suffice to present the measured random error of the "fair" test, including the calculation of error as a percentage of the range of clinical interest.

Although this paper is mainly concerned with random analytical error, systematic errors (*5, 21*) could also be expressed as a percentage of a range. I have not done this in the present report because of problems related to terminology and interpretation. Furthermore, long-term systematic errors do not usually cause a problem in regard to the interpretation of laboratory data by the physician.

If it is desirable to express systematic errors as percentages, several differences from random error should be noted and allowance made for them. First, systematic error is, of necessity, related to a reference method or material, and, in specifying this type of error, it is necessary to identify the reference method, the sign of the error (+ or −), and the level at which the error applies. This is required, of course, regardless of the units in which the systematic error is expressed. Second, if a systematic error is given as a percentage of a range of clinical interest, it is also necessary to specify whether the range is given in terms of the new method or the reference method. This would be important if the ranges (upper limit minus lower limit) for the new method and the reference method were different. In order to avoid confusion, and because a range for the reference method might not be available, it seems preferable to use a range(s) associated with the new method, if systematic errors are expressed in percentage form. This choice would also be compatible with the range that is used for random error.

Finally, a systematic error expressed as a percentage of a range would not have the same statistical implication as an equal percentage of random error. For example, a test with a random analytical error equal to 40% of an adult 95% normal range would be undesirable for monitoring values within the range. On the other hand, a test with a constant systematic error equal to 40% of an adult 95% normal range might be completely acceptable, provided the precision was good and the systematic error was allowed for by physicians in their interpretation of the results.

For the above reasons, and because systematic error can be theoretically eliminated (*21*), it does not seem advantageous to express systematic error as a percentage of a range of clinical interest.

Appendix

Table 1. Calculations from Pearson (*14*). During the quality control of an analytical method, values for run-to-run analyses of aliquots of the same material are accumulated. Assume that the population of these results follows a gaussian distribution with mean and standard deviation μ_A and σ_A, respectively. Then the total random analytical error at level μ_A for a single value (includes within-run and run-to-run variability), expressed as a two-sided 95% confidence interval, is $\pm 1.96\ \sigma_A$.

Assume that pairs of values are randomly selected from this population of run-to-run values. In the long run, only 5% of these pairs should have an absolute difference greater that 2.77 σ_A, and only 10% should have an absolute difference greater than 2.33 σ_A, etc. (*14*).

If the range(s) of clinical interest, ρ_{BA} or ρ_M, for the test is expressed in σ_A units (and assuming σ_A

applies to values for the range in question), the total random error and the upper confidence limits for the absolute difference between run-to-run duplicates can be expressed in terms of the range(s). For example, if the range of clinical interest, ρ_{BA}, is equivalent to 9.80 σ_A, the total random error is equal to (1.96 σ_A)(100)/9.80 σ_A, or 20.0% of the range ρ_{BA}. The 95% upper confidence limit for the absolute difference between run-to-run duplicates, expressed as a multiple of the range ρ_{BA}, is 2.77 σ_A/9.80 σ_A = 0.28. The 90% upper confidence limit for the same situation is 2.33 σ_A/9.80 σ_A = 0.24. The percent random errors and the confidence limits for the analysis of the same specimen in two different runs were derived in this manner.

Table 1. Calculations from Campbell and Owen (15). The column in Table 1 "chance that an absolute difference equal to the range between two different samples in different runs is due to error" is derived as for Campbell and Owen's Table 2, column B (*15*). For example, in the case of 60% random error, where the range (and the assumed difference between two different samples in two different runs) is 3.27 σ_A, the calculations are: difference/standard error of difference = 3.27 $\sigma_A/(\sigma_A^2/1 + \sigma_A^2/1)^{1/2}$ = 3.27/(2)$^{1/2}$ = 2.31. This corresponds to an area under one side of the standard normal curve of 0.48956. The probability that the difference $|3.27\ \sigma_A|$ is due to analytical error is 1.00000 − 2(0.48956) = 0.02088, or approximately 2.1%.

Table 1. Calculations from Acland and Lipton (12, 13). In Table 1, the data in the column "normal samples that give abnormal results due to error" were taken from Acland and Lipton (*13*). The data are the percentages of a normal healthy population for whom the "true" results fall within a 95% gaussian normal range, but for whom the actual observations are outside the range because of random analytical error. In using Acland and Lipton's Table I (*13*), their term r = σ_1/σ_2 is replaced by σ_A/σ_{BA}. Although σ_2 is mainly biological variability whereas σ_{BA} is biological plus analytical variability, the term σ_{BA} was used (instead of σ_B) for calculation of the ratio so that the probabilities of error would be in terms of the actual range ρ_{BA} (which includes analytical variation). Probabilities for values of the ratio greater than 1.0 are not given. For these calculations, it is assumed that both the 95% normal range ρ_{BA} and the random analytical error are from gaussian distributions.

The two columns of Table 1 labeled "false classifications" were calculated from the probability formulas of Acland and Lipton (*12*). These columns give the percentages of observed results that are outside or inside of a 95% normal range, ρ_{BA}, when the "true" values are inside or outside, respectively, of the upper or lower range limits at distances equal to $\rho_{BA}/4$ and $\rho_{BA}/8$. It is assumed that both the 95% normal range and the random analytical error are from gaussian distributions. Calculations were not done for ratios of σ_A/σ_{BA} greater than 1.0.

Table 1. Calculations from Cotlove et al. (3). The normal range or the therapeutic range, ρ_{BA}, includes biological variation and random analytical variation. In Table 1, the calculation of the artifactual increase in the biological range due to analytical error is based upon the following relation (*3*): $\sigma_{BA}^2 = \sigma_B^2 + \sigma_A^2$. In order to estimate σ_{BA}, it is assumed for this calculation that the range, ρ_{BA}, follows a gaussian distribution and expresses the two-sided 95% confidence limits. Under these circumstances, $\sigma_{BA} = \rho_{BA}/3.92$ = 0.255 ρ_{BA}. For the case in which the random analytical error is equal to 20% of the range, ρ_{BA}, the calculations are as follows:

$$\begin{aligned}\sigma_A &= (0.20)(\rho_{BA})/1.96\\ &= 0.102\ \rho_{BA}\\ \sigma_B^2 &= \sigma_{BA}^2 - \sigma_A^2\\ &= (0.255\ \rho_{BA})^2 - (0.102\ \rho_{BA})^2\\ &= 0.05462\ \rho_{BA}^2\\ \sigma_B &= 0.2337\ \rho_{BA}\end{aligned}$$

The percent increase in σ_B, owing to σ_A, is $(100)(\sigma_{BA} - \sigma_B)/\sigma_B$ = (100)(0.2550-0.2337) ρ_{BA}/0.2337 ρ_{BA} = 9.1%

Because the assumption of normality is probably not true for most ranges, the estimates of artifactual increase in the biological range given in Table 1 are only approximate for a real situation. Values were not calculated for random errors greater than 40% of the range.

Table 2. Calculations from Westgard et al. (5). The value for the 95% upper limit of a standard deviation is equal to $(F_U)(S_A)$, where S_A is the observed value and F_U is the appropriate factor for the upper limit (*5*). Consider the case in which it is required to calculate the 95% upper limit for the standard deviation that corresponds to a random error equal to 60% of a specified medical decision range, ρ_M. For 30 degrees of freedom in the determination of S_A, the 95% upper limit for the measured value of S_A, S_{AU}, is calculated as follows:

$$\begin{aligned}\text{Random error} = 0.60\ \rho_M &= 1.96(F_U)(S_{AU})\\ &= (1.96)(1.274)(S_{AU})\\ S_{AU} &= 0.60\ \rho_M/(1.96)(1.274)\\ &= 0.240\ \rho_M\end{aligned}$$

If, as a result of replicate experiments, the observed values of S_A have a 95% upper limit, S_{AU}, as calculated above, the method will yield 95% upper limits of random analytical errors that are equal to or less than the percent errors given in Table 2, in 95% of cases.

If a similar calculation is done for an observed 95% normal range or therapeutic range, ρ_{BA}, and the selected percent random error is different from the percent random error associated with the estimation of ρ_{BA}, a range factor, F_R, should be included in the formula (Table 2). This will allow for a change in the size of the range ρ_{BA}, owing to the change in the random error. For example, assume that the selected error is 20%, and the range is estimated under conditions of 30% random error. The factor, F_R, which expresses the contraction of the range in going from 30% error to 20% error, is ${}_{20}\sigma_{BA}/{}_{30}\sigma_{BA}$. The standard deviations, ${}_{20}\sigma_{BA}$ and ${}_{30}\sigma_{BA}$, are the biological plus random analytical variability for the 20% and 30% errors, respectively. The ratio, $F_R = {}_{20}\sigma_{BA}/{}_{30}\sigma_{BA}$, is equal to (100 + 9.1)/(100 + 25.0). This can be demonstrated by rearrangement of the formula $(100)(\sigma_{BA} - \sigma_B)/\sigma_B$, above, for each of the two percentage errors, and substitution of the appropriate values from the last column of Table 1. In this paper, the derivation of the factor F_R via the formula from Cotlove et al. (*3*) assumes that the 95% normal or therapeutic range is from a gaussian distribution.

References

1. Barnett, R. N., Medical significance of laboratory results. *Am. J. Clin. Pathol.* **50,** 671 (1968).

2. Tonks, D. B., A study of the accuracy and precision of clinical chemistry determinations in 170 Canadian laboratories. *Clin. Chem.* **9,** 217 (1963).

3. Cotlove, E., Harris, E. K., and Williams, G. Z., Biological and analytic components of variation in long-term studies of serum constituents in normal subjects. III. Physiological and medical implications. *Clin. Chem.* **16,** 1028 (1970).

4. Harris, E. K., Kanofsky, P., Shakarji, G., and Cotlove, E., Biological and analytic components of variation in long-term studies of serum constituents in normal subjects. II. Estimating biological components of variation. *Clin. Chem.* **16,** 1022 (1970).

5. Westgard, J. O., Carey, R. N., and Wold, S., Criteria for judging precision and accuracy in method development and evaluation. *Clin. Chem.* **20,** 825 (1974).

6. Sunderman, F. W., Jr., Current concepts of "normal values", "reference values", and "discrimination values" in clinical chemistry. *Clin. Chem.* **21,** 1873 (1975).

7. Lindberg, D. A. B., and Watson, Fr. R., Imprecision of laboratory determinations and diagnostic accuracy: Theoretical considerations. *Method. Inf. Med.* **13,** 151 (1974).

8. Gilbert, R. K., The size and the source of analytic error in clinical chemistry. *Am. J. Clin. Pathol.* **61,** 904 (1974).

9. Logan, J. E., Evaluation of commercial kits. *CRC Crit. Rev. Clin. Lab. Sci.* **3,** 271 (1972).

10. Hoffman, R. G., Statistics in the practice of medicine. *J. Am. Med. Assoc.* **185,** 864 (1963).

11. Burns, E. L., Hanson, D. J., Schoen, I., et al., Communication of laboratory data to the clinician. *Am. J. Clin. Pathol.* **61,** 900 (1974).

12. Acland, J. D., and Lipton, S., Precision in a clinical chemistry laboratory. *J. Clin. Pathol.* **20,** 780 (1967).

13. Acland, J. D., and Lipton, S., Laboratory precision and diagnostic errors. *J. Clin. Pathol.* **24,** 369 (1971).

14. Pearson, E. S., The probability integral of the range in samples of n observations from a normal population. I. Foreword and tables. *Biometrika* **32,** 301 (1942).

15. Campbell, D. G., and Owen, J. A., Clinical laboratory error in perspective. *Clin. Biochem.* **1,** 3 (1967).

16. Roberts, L. B., The normal ranges, with statistical analysis for seventeen blood constituents. *Clin. Chim. Acta* **16,** 69 (1967).

17. Henry, R. J., Cannon, D. C., and Winkelman, J. W., *Clinical Chemistry; Principles and Technics,* 2nd ed., Harper and Row, Hagerstown, Md., 1974, p 298.

18. Korvin, C. C., Pearce, R. H., and Stanley, J., Admissions screening: Clinical benefits. *Ann. Intern. Med.* **83,** 197 (1975).

19. Wilson, J. M. G., Current trends and problems in health screening. *Scand. J. Clin. Lab. Invest.* **29** (*Suppl. 126*), 21.1 (1972).

20. Zieve, L., Misinterpretation and abuse of laboratory tests by clinicians. *Ann. N. Y. Acad. Sci.* **134,** 563 (1966).

21. Westgard, J. O., and Hunt, M. R., Use and interpretation of common statistical tests in method-comparison studies. *Clin. Chem.* **19,** 49 (1973).

CLIN. CHEM. 22/4, 484–488 (1976)

Direct Radioimmunoassay for Serum Estriol during Pregnancy

Jim Standefer

I describe an assay for serum estriol during pregnancy, which does not require prior extraction or chromatography of the serum. Fifty microliters of 20-fold diluted serum can be assayed to detect as little as 20 pg of estriol. For a 20 μg/liter serum estriol concentration the CV was 16%; for 100 μg/liter concentration it was 5%. There was no significant interference by serum "binding" proteins. The assay measures unconjugated estriol, estriol conjugated with either sulfate or glucuronide at the 3′ position, and a portion of the estriol 16α-(β-D-glucuronide). Serum estriol concentrations increase during gestation from a low at 20 weeks of <10 μg/liter to a high of 100–150 μg/liter at term. Serum estriol values correlate well with those for urinary total estrogens and with values for human placental lactogen in serum at various gestational ages.

Additional Keyphrases: *fetal status* • *changes during pregnancy* • *human placental lactogen* • *urinary estrogens* • *cesarean section*

Determination of total urinary estrogens has been used in evaluating fetal stress during the third trimester of pregnancy; the amount of estrogens in the urine continually increases during normal gestation; declining values indicate fetal stress. Problems of collecting accurate serial 24-h urines have prompted the development of assays for serum estrogens during gestation, particularly since the usefulness of such information in predicting fetal stress has been demonstrated (*1–3*). Apparently all estrogens of fetal and placental origin (including estrone, estrone sulfate, estradiol, and estriol) increase during gestation (*1, 4*) and the concentrations of any or all (*5*) of these in serum could be measured to monitor fetal status.

The methods used to measure plasma estrogens during pregnancy have included extraction followed by gas chromatography (*6, 7*); extraction and column chromatography followed by a competitive protein-binding technique, with a "rabbit uterine cytosol" as the binding agent (*8, 9*); and extraction and column chromatography followed by radioimmunoassay, with use of specific antibodies raised against estrogen/albumin conjugates (*10*). All of these methods require considerable sample preparation and laboratory analysis time. Owing to the serious clinical implications of low and declining estriol values, there is a need for a relatively rapid and sensitive serum estrogen assay.

This report describes an assay for serum estriol that does not require extraction, is relatively rapid, is specific for estriol and its conjugates, and provides information that is useful for monitoring fetal stress during the third trimester of gestation.

Department of Pathology, University of New Mexico School of Medicine, Albuquerque, N. Mex. 87110.

Received Oct. 29, 1975; accepted Feb. 4, 1976.

Materials

Phosphate buffer, pH 7.4, 10 mmol/liter. Dissolve 1.39 g of K_2HPO4, 0.28 g of NaH_2O, 7.9 g of NaCl, 5.0 g of bovine serum albumin, and 3.8 g of disodium ethylenediaminetetraacetate in 900 ml of de-ionized water. Adjust the pH to 7.4 and the volume to 1 liter.

Glutamate buffer, pH 3.3, 40 mmol/liter. Dissolve 1.2 g of L-glutamic acid and 0.4 mg of KCN in 180 ml of de-ionized water, adjust the pH to 3.3 and the final volume to 200 ml. Stable for one month at 4 °C.

Buffered dextran-coated charcoal. Dissolve 1.47 g of sodium barbital, 0.97 g of sodium acetate, and 7.9 g of NaCl in 900 ml of de-ionized water. Adjust the pH to 7.4 with 1 mmol/liter HCl and the volume to 1 liter with water. To 100 ml of this barbital buffer, add and dissolve 0.5 g of dextran (No. D-4751, clinical grade; Sigma Chemical Co., St. Louis, Mo. 63178). To a separate 100-ml portion, add and mix 5.0 g of activated charcoal (No. C-5385, Sigma). Add the charcoal suspension to the dextran solution and mix well. This suspension is stable at 4 °C for one month and must be mixed well to resuspend the charcoal immediately before each use.

Antiserum. An estriol antiserum, produced in rabbits from an estriol-6-oxime/bovine serum albumin conjugate, was purchased in lyophilized form (Endocrine Sciences, Tarzana, Calif. 91356). Reconstitute this antiserum according to the supplied instructions, and store 100-μl portions at −20 °C. Dilute each aliquot 50-fold with phosphate buffer; this can be stored at 4 °C as a "working" antibody solution for at least two months. The final dilution of the reconstituted antiserum in the reaction mix is 150-fold, and at this dilution about 60–80 pg of estriol is bound. The affinity constant of this antiserum for estriol is about 8×10^9 mol^{-1}.

Radiolabeled estriol. [2,4-H^3]Estriol (38 kCi/mol) was purchased from Amersham/Searle Corp., Arlington Heights, Ill. 60006, divided into 20-μl portions, and is stable at −20 °C for at least six months. For the assay, dilute aliquots with phosphate buffer to a concentration of about 1500 pg/ml, a mixture that is stable at 4 °C for at least four months.

Standards. Dissolve estriol, estriol-3-sulfate, estriol-3-(β-d-glucuronide), estriol-16α-(β-d-glucuronide), estriol-17β-(β-d-glucuronide), estrone, estrone-3-sulfate, and estradiol (Sigma Chemical Co.) in ethanol and store at −20 °C. Prepare dilutions of the estriol standard in pooled serum from men to produce concentrations ranging from 0 to 200 μg/liter. Similarly dilute the other estrogen standards to produce concentrations ranging from 0 to 2000 μg/liter. The dilutions of these standards in serum are stable at −20 °C for at least six months.

Methods

Human placental lactogen assay. We assayed human placental lactogen according to the instructions included in the kit by the manufacturer (Amersham/Searle).

Urinary total estrogen assay. We assayed urinary estrogens according to the instructions included with the reagents supplied by the manufacturer (Stanbio Laboratory, Inc., San Antonio, Tex. 78202).

Estriol assay. Dilute all sera (standards and patients) 20-fold with phosphate buffer and pipet 50-μl aliquots of the dilutions into 12 × 75 glass disposable test tubes. Add phosphate buffer (100 μl), antiserum (100 μl), and H^3-labeled estriol (100 μl, 20000 cpm/150 pg). Nonspecific binding is measured by including tubes that contain buffer and H^3-labeled estriol, but no antisera. Mix all ingredients on a vortex-type mixer and place the tubes in an ice bath for 15 min. Add dextran-coated charcoal (250 μl) and, after 5 min in the ice bath, centrifuge the tubes at 1000 × *g* and 4 °C. Decant the supernate into scintillation vials containing 10 ml of scintillation fluid (Amersham/Searle) and measure the radioactivity in a liquid-scintillation counter (we used one supplied by Searle Analytic Inc., Des Plaines, Ill. 60018).

Incubation with β-glucuronidase. Dilute sera 20-fold with phosphate buffer containing 50 U of β-glucuronidase (Sigma) per milliter and incubate at 37 °C for 18 h. Then assay the diluted sera for estriol by the described procedure.

Results

Precision. I assessed the precision of this assay by averaging and converting to a logit plot the data from five separate standard curves generated by this assay protocol (Figure 1). The resulting standard curve had a slope of −1.335, intercept of 2.707, and the precision coefficient, λ (*11*), ranged from 0.028 to 0.084, which compares well with those reported for other radioimmunoassays (*12*). Figure 1 also shows results obtained for assays of dilutions of serum containing 110 μg of estriol per liter; the resulting curve does not differ significantly from the standard curve.

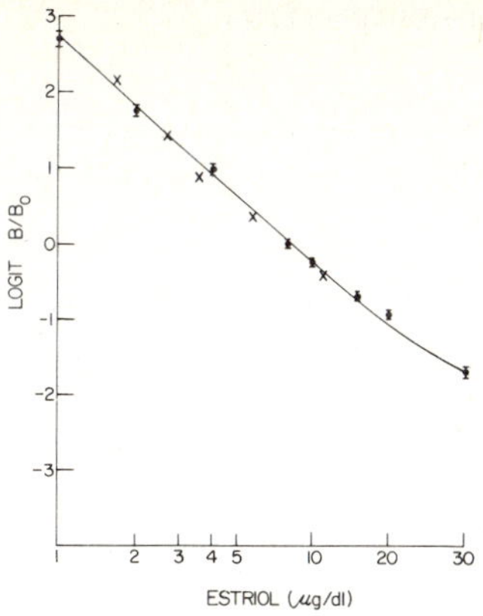

Fig. 1. Standard curve and serum dilution curve
Filled circles: mean ± 1 SD for five separate standard curves. *Crosses:* a serum containing 110 μg/liter was diluted and analyzed according to the described protocol

Table 1. Precision of Direct Serum Assay

	n	Mean	SD	CV,%
		μg/liter		
Day-to-day [a]				
Serum, 20 μg/liter	20	19.9	3.2	16.1
Serum, 100 μg/liter	20	101.9	6.2	6.1
Within-day				
Serum, 20 μg/liter	20	19.5	3.0	15.4
Serum, 100 μg/liter	20	101.7	4.7	4.6

[a] Estriol was added to a pool of serum from men, to produce the indicated concentrations and then assayed once each day for 20 consecutive days (day-to-day) and 20 times in one assay (within-day).

The precision of this assay was also evaluated by multiple analyses of two estriol-supplemented sera (Table 1). The precision for low and high estriol concentrations compares well with that reported for a direct radioimmunoassay of estradiol in serum (*13*).

Sensitivity. The sensitivity of this assay is expressed by using criteria recently suggested by Boutwell (*14*). The mean and standard deviation for 20 sera negative for estriol was 0 ± 3.8 μg/liter. With twice the SD as a "noise" level, the least detectable concentration in undiluted serum would be about 8.0 μg/liter, or 20 pg per 50 μl of serum diluted 20-fold for assay. The within-run "analytical standard deviation" (*14*) for the assay is expressed (Table 1) by the mean ± 1 SD for 20 assays at low and high estriol concentrations.

The incubation time and temperature necessary to achieve equilibrium are indicated in Figure 2. The reaction reaches equilibrium quickly at room temperature or at 4 °C; however, the binding is about 10–15% higher at 25 °C.

Serum estriol determined by this assay was compared to total urinary estrogens in 10 patients sampled at various times during the third trimester. This comparison (Figure 3) yields a regression equation of $y = 0.287x + 1.2$, with a sample correlation coefficient of 0.871.

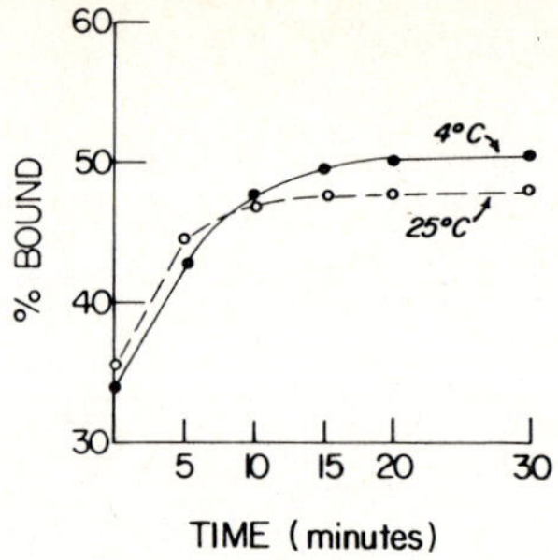

Fig. 2. Percent of bound [H^3]estriol vs. time of incubation at 4 °C (*filled circles*) and 25 °C (*open circles*)

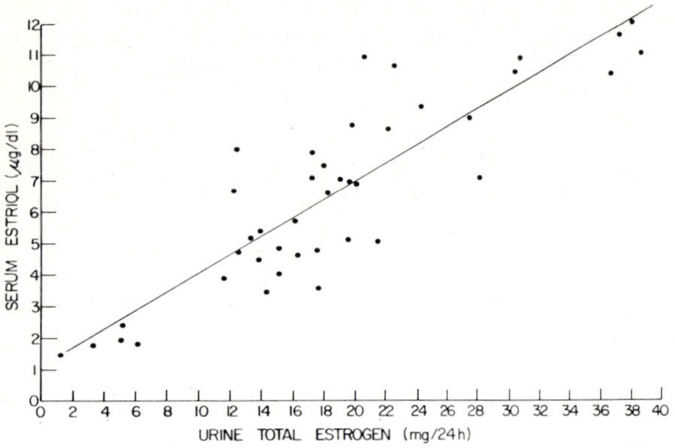

Fig. 3. Serum and 24-h urine samples were collected on the same day from 10 patients, during the third trimester, and analyzed for serum estriol and total urinary estrogens

In directly assaying serum for estriol, one must exclude interference by serum proteins that may compete with the antibody during estriol binding. One approach to eliminating such "serum binding" is to heat the serum at low pH to denature and thus inactivate the binding protein (*15*). Serum was diluted 20-fold with glutamate buffer, heated at 90 °C for 15 min, and assayed for estriol. There was no significant difference ($P = .01$) between estriol values for the samples that were heated and duplicate sera that were analyzed directly.

In another test of interference by "serum binding" proteins, 20 pregnancy sera were assayed for estriol before and after adding 100 μl of serum from either men or women to the assay tubes. There was no significant differences in the values ($P < .05$).

The reactivity of the estriol antibody with estrone, estrone-3-sulfate and estradiol is shown in Figure 4. There is about 2% cross-reaction with each of these estrogens (measured at $B/B_0 = .5$). Because the total concentration of estrone and estradiol in pregnancy serum is about half that of total estriol (*1*), the contribution of these estrogens to estriol assayed by this method would be 1% or less.

Several other estriol conjugates that are present in pregnancy serum also react with this estriol antibody (Figure 5). The approximate cross-reactivity for the 3-glucuronide derivative is 100%; for the 3-sulfate conjugate, 70%; for the 16α-(β-D-glucuronide), 20%; and for the synthetic derivative, 17-β-(β-D-glucuronide), 5%. Because this method does not measure total serum estriol, it is important to establish (*a*) that estriol determined by this assay is proportional to total serum estriol and (*b*) that the measured serum estriol reflects fetal status.

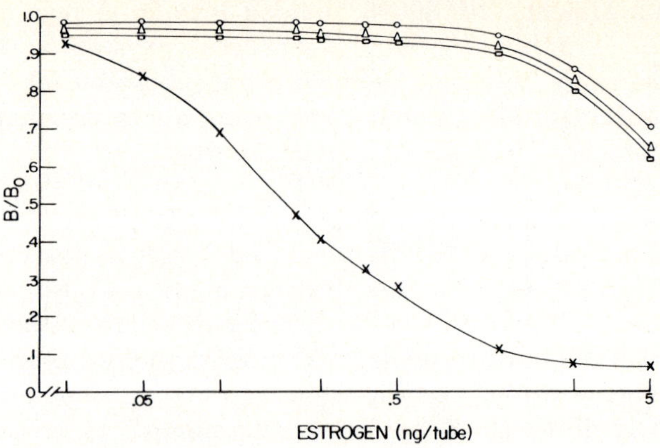

Fig. 4. Cross-reaction with the estriol antibody of estrone, □—□; estrone-3-sulfate, Δ—Δ; and estrone sulfate, O—O; compared to estriol, X—X

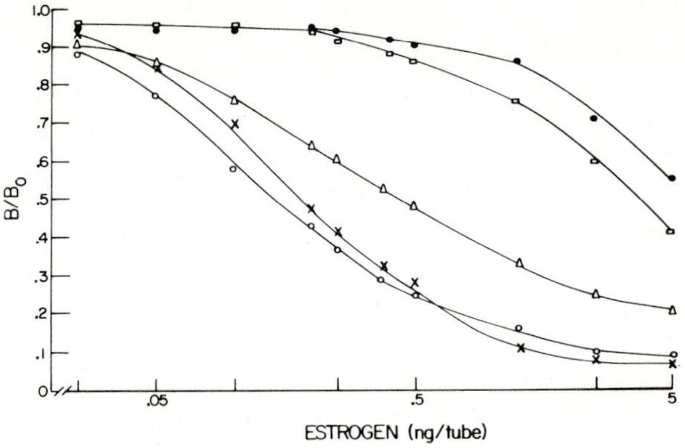

Fig. 5. Cross-reaction of conjugated estriol derivatives with the estriol antibody
estriol 16-α-(β-D-glucuronide), □—□; estriol 17-β-(β-D-glucuronide), ●—●; estriol 3-sulfate, Δ—Δ; estriol 3-(β-D-glucuronide), O—O; and estriol, X—X

Estriol values from sera assayed before and after incubation with β-glucuronidase (EC 3.2.1.31) at 37 °C for 18 h show a correlation coefficient of 0.75 for direct values greater than 6 μg/dl (Figure 6). For estriol values smaller than 6 μg/dl the nature of the correlation changes, and the total estriol is about twofold higher than the directly measured estriol. Figure 7 illustrates another indication of the relationship between the directly assayed and total serum estriol; assays of serum from a pre-eclamptic patient who was sampled daily showed similar changes in both the directly assayed and total serum estriol.

Evidence that this direct serum estriol assay reflects fetal status is shown in Figure 8. Serum estriol values increase during gestation, and values for one patient who delivered a stillbirth progressively decline until they are below those for normal pregnancies.

There is correlation between directly measured serum estriol levels and the serum placental lactogen

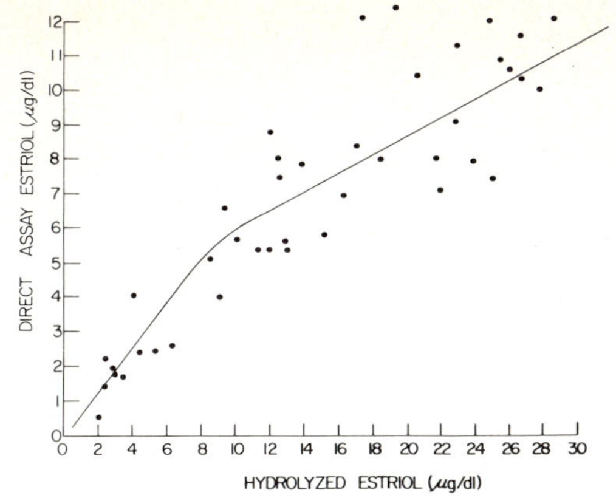

Fig. 6. Serum estriol values obtained before (*direct*) and after (*hydrolyzed*) treatment with β-glucuronidase for 18 h at 37 °C

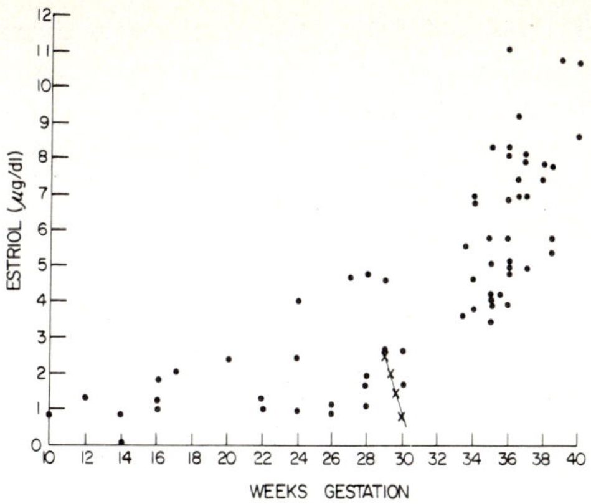

Fig. 8. Serum estriol assayed at various gestational ages
Serial determinations from stillbirth pregnancy, X—X

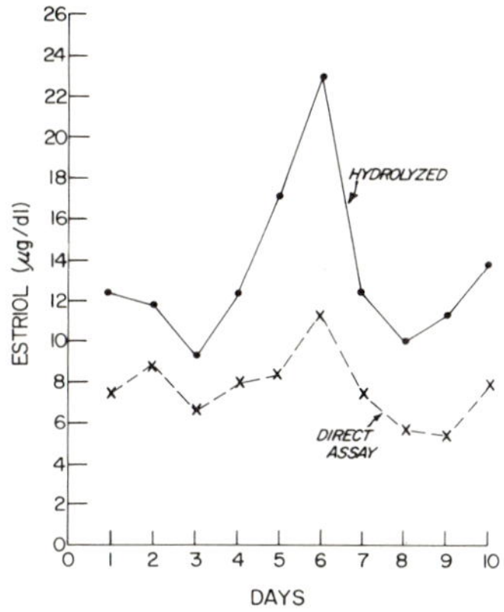

Fig. 7. Daily serum estriol values from one patient diagnosed as pre-eclamptic at 36 weeks gestation
Sera were analyzed before and after hydrolysis with β-glucuronidase at 37 °C for 18 h

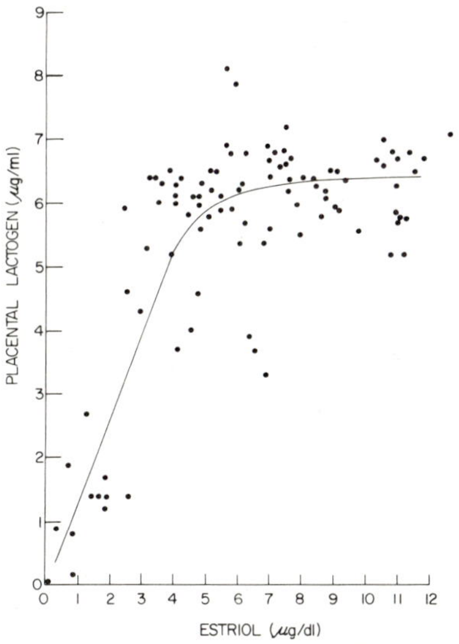

Fig. 9. Serum estriol and human placental lactogen concentrations in sera at various gestational ages

concentrations in sera taken at various times during gestation (Figure 9). Values for both lactogen and estriol increase until placental lactogen values of 6 to 7 mg/liter are reached at gestational ages of 34–36 weeks. At later gestational ages it does not increase significantly, but the increase in estriol continues, resulting in the nonlinear relationship as shown.

Discussion

Most reported assays for estrogens in pregnancy serum have involved relatively long sample-preparation steps in order to isolate and purify estrogens before assay. The data presented here indicate that these initial steps are not necessary for accurate measurements of serum estriol. The usual reasons for such purification and concentration steps before the assay are to increase both the selectivity and sensitivity of the assay. Because all estrogens of fetal and placental origin increase in serum during gestation (*1, 4*) and the use of an antibody confers some degree of specificity to the estrogen assay, high selectivity is not necessarily the prime consideration in designing a direct serum estrogen assay.

The selectivity of this assay depends on the antibody specificity, which in turn is related to the nature of the pregnancy serum estriol conjugates. Goebelsmann et al. (*16*) reported that half of serum estriol is present as the 16α-(β-D-glucuronide) and 3-sulfate-16α-(β-D-glucuronide) conjugates, the other half being unconjugated estriol, estriol 3-sulfate, and estriol 3-(β-D-glucuronide). Using this information, together with the observations that (*a*) the concentration of serum estriol measured by this direct assay is approximately half that reported for total serum estriol (*16*), (*b*) both the 3-sulfate and 3-glucuronide derivatives react well with the estriol antibody, while the 16α derivative reacts to a lesser degree, and (*c*) there is a two- to threefold increase in assayed serum estriol after hydrolysis, one may conclude that this assay primarily measures "free" estriol and estriol conjugated at the 3-position. Because the concentration of conjugated estriol is 20-fold higher than "free" estriol during the third trimester (*1*) and the free estriol concentration is about 10 µg/liter (*1, 9*), one must assume that most of the estriol being measured in this assay is conjugated at the 3′ position.

However, since 30–40% of the estriol is conjugated at the 16α position (*16*), this derivative also contributes to the directly measured estriol.

The values for directly assayed estriol do correlate well with gestational age and show the expected agreement with the serum placental lactogen values. Also, there is good correlation (r = 0.87) between values for serum estriol and for total estrogens in urine during the third trimester.

An additional observation that supports the clinical validity of this assay is the 10-fold increase in the directly assayed serum estriol values between 20 and 40 weeks of gestation. The magnitude of this increase agrees well with that reported for unconjugated serum estriol during the same gestational period (*1*, *9*). Also, the directly assayed estriol values are proportional to the total serum estriol values in one patient analyzed daily, and in several patients analyzed throughout gestation. This parallelism indicates that the values obtained by this assay reflect both the "free" and conjugated serum estriol, and that they provide a valid estimate of serum estriol concentrations during gestation.

The nonlinear relationship between placental lactogen and estriol is consistent with a proportionally smaller increase in placental lactogen as compared to estriol after 34–36 weeks of gestation. After about 34 weeks of gestation, serum placental lactogen concentrations reportedly increase very little (*17*) or actually decrease (*18*). This leveling off of placental lactogen values contrasts with the continuous increase in serum estriol that is even greater after 30 weeks of gestation (*4*).

The sensitivity of the assay, expressed as the detection limit in undiluted serum containing 8 μg of estriol per liter, is such that abnormally low serum estriol concentrations can be detected beyond 26–28 weeks gestation. Because the clinical alternative to delivery by cesarian section becomes feasible only after about 26 weeks, the sensitivity of this direct assay is sufficient to support that clinical determination. The sensitivity, when expressed as the precision of assaying low and high estriol concentrations, is sufficient to detect a shift of greater than 32% (±2 SD) in low values and 12% (±SD) in high values assayed in daily serum samples. Based on one example of a patient who delivered a stillbirth, a decrease of greater than 100% might be expected in serial serum samples during fetal distress.

To conclude, my data support the use of a direct serum estriol assay as an indication of fetal well-being. This method provides an alternative to the more time-consuming extraction assays and allows for relatively rapid and simple daily serum estriol determinations.

References

1. Loriaux, D. L., Ruder, H. J., Knab, D. R., and Lipsett, M. B., Estrone sulfate, estrone, estradiol and estriol plasma levels in human pregnancy. *J. Clin. Endocrinol. Metab.* **35,** 887 (1972).

2. Masson, G. M., Plasma estriol in normal and preeclamptic multiple pregnancies. *Obstet. Gynecol.* **42,** 568 (1973).

3. Cleary, R. E., and Young, P. C. M., Serum unconjugated estriol in normal and abnormal pregnancy. *Am. J. Obstet. Gynecol.* **118,** 18 (1974).

4. DeHertogh, R., Thomas, K., Bietloy, Y., et al., Plasma levels of unconjugated estrone, estradiol and estriol and of HCS throughout pregnancy in normal women. *J. Clin. Endocrinol. Metab.* **40,** 93 (1975).

5. YoungLai, E. V., Two-hour plasma estrogen assay. *Am. J. Obstet. Gynecol.* **117,** 584 (1973).

6. Wotiz, H. H., Charransol, G., and Smith, I. N., Gas chromatographic measurement of plasma estrogens using an electron capture detector. *Steroids* **10,** 127 (1967).

7. Fischer-Rasmussen, W., A gas-liquid chromatographic method for the measurement of oestradiol-17β in human plasma during the second half of pregnancy. *J. Steroid Biochem.* **2,** 251 (1971).

8. Korenman, S. G., Radioligand binding assay of specific estrogens using a soluble uterine macromolecule. *J. Clin. Endocrinol. Metab.* **28,** 127 (1968).

9. Tulchinsky, D., and Korenman, S. G., The plasma estradiol as an index of fetoplacental function. *J. Clin. Invest.* **50,** 1490 (1971).

10. Tulchinsky, D., and Abraham, G. E., Radioimmunoassay of plasma estriol. *J. Clin. Endocrinol. Metab.* **33,** 775 (1971).

11. Bliss, C. I., *Statistics in Biology,* **I,** McGraw-Hill Inc., New York, N. Y., 1967, p 421.

12. Skelley, D. S., Brown, L. P., and Besch, P. K., Radioimmunoassay. *Clin. Chem.* **19,** 146 (1973).

13. Jurjens, H., Pratt, J. J., and Woldring, M. G., Radioimmunoassay of plasma estradiol without extraction and chromatography. *J. Clin. Endocrinol.* **40,** 19 (1975).

14. Boutwell, J. H., Jr., A modest proposal, specifying sensitivity. *Clin. Chem.* **21,** 1542 (1975). Letter to the Editor.

15. Foster, L. B., and Dunn, R. T., Single antibody technique for radioimmunoassay of cortisol in unextracted serum or plasma. *Clin. Chem.* **20,** 365 (1974).

16. Goebelsmann, V., Chen, L. C., Saga, M., et al., Plasma concentration and protein binding of estriol and its conjugates in pregnancy. *Acta Endocrinol.* (Copenhagen) **74,** 592 (1973).

17. Letchworth, A. T., Boardman, R. J., Bristor, R. J., et al., A rapid semi-automated method for the measurement of human chorionic somatomammotropin. The normal range in the third trimester and its relation to foetal weight. *J. Obstet. Gynaecol. Br. Commonw.* **78,** 542 (1971).

18. Teoh, E. S., Spellacy, W. N., and Buhl, W. C., Human chorionic somatomammotropin (HCS): A new index of placental function, *J. Obstet. Gynaecol. Br. Commonw.* **78,** 673 (1971).

CLIN. CHEM. 22/4, 489–496 (1976)

Performance Studies on the Technicon "SMAC" Analyzer: Precision and Comparison of Values with Methods in Routine Laboratory Service

James O. Westgard, R. Neill Carey, Donald H. Feldbruegge, and Lola M. Jenkins

We present performance studies on the Technicon "SMAC" analyzer. Precision was estimated from control data during routine operation and from blind duplicates of sera from patients. Patients' specimens were analyzed with the SMAC and the SMA 12/60 during initial evaluation studies. Comparisons were also made with the Du Pont *aca* and other methods during routine service. Performance is judged relative to medical usefulness requirements, by using previously developed criteria and recommendations for decision levels and allowable errors.

Additional Keyphrases: *quality-control • inter-method comparison • mechanized analysis • analytical systems*

Schwartz et al. (*1*) reported results of performance studies on a prototype "SMAC" [1] analyzer. Here, we present results of similar studies on a production-model instrument. Results in this report are from initial evaluation experiments as well as performance studies conducted during the first six months of 1975, when the SMAC was in routine service operation.

Departments of Medicine, Pathology, and Clinical Laboratories, University of Wisconsin-Center for Health Sciences, Madison, Wis. 53706.

[1] Nonstandard abbreviations used: SMAC, Technicon *S*equential *M*ultiple *A*nalyzer with *C*omputer; 12/60 or SMA 12/60, Technicon *S*equential *M*ultiple *A*nalyzer; *aca*, Du Pont *A*utomatic *C*linical *A*nalyzer; AST, aspartate aminotransferase (L-aspartate: 2-oxoglutarate aminotransferase, EC 2.6.1.1); LD, lactate dehydrogenase (L-lactate:NAD oxidoreductase, EC 1.1.1.27); and ALP, alkaline phosphatase (orthophosphoric acid monester phosphohydrolase, EC 3.1.3.1).

For least-squares statistics: B, slope; SD_B, standard deviation of the slope; A, *y*-intercept; SD_A, standard deviation of the intercept; $S_{y/x}$, standard error about the regression line; SD_x, standard deviation of the population of *x* values; and *r*, correlation coefficient.

For paired t-test statistics: $\bar{X}$, mean of the values by the comparison method; bias, difference between average values by the two methods; SD_d, standard deviation of the paired differences; and *t*, *t*-values.

For error decision: X_C, medical decision concentration; CV, coefficient of variation; E_A, medically allowable error; TE, total analytical error; TE_l, lower 95% confidence limit of TE; TE_u, upper 95% confidence limit of TE; RE, random error; RE_l, lower 95% confidence limit of RE; RE_u, upper 95% confidence limit of RE; SE, systematic error; SE_l, lower 95% confidence limit of SE; SE_u, upper 95% confidence limit of SE.

Received Oct. 29, 1975; accepted Feb. 4, 1976.

We reported previously a comparison of the Technicon SMA 12/60 with the Du Pont *aca* and the need for comparability of results if these instruments are to be used together in the same laboratory (*2*). The integration of SMAC into a service laboratory presents a similar situation. If results are not identified by instrument in the final reporting, then comparability must be assured. In our laboratory, most of the determinations available on SMAC may also be performed by different methods, depending on whether they are ordered as a screening panel, a routine single request, or as an emergency request. To determine whether SMAC would be compatible with this mode of laboratory operation, we made comparisons with methods in routine service.

Materials and Methods

SMAC (Technicon Instruments Corp., Tarrytown, N. Y. 10591). A conventional production model (serial No. 113) was used. The chemical methods have been described by Schwartz et al. (*1*) and include glucose by glucose oxidase/peroxidase-MBTH (3-methyl-2-benzothiazolinone-*N,N*-dimethylaniline), inorganic phosphorus by phosphomolybdate at 340 nm, albumin by bromcresol green, LD by a two-point rate reaction measuring NADH at 340 nm, AST by a three-point rate reaction measuring NADH at 340 nm, sodium and potassium by ion-selective electrodes (*3*), chloride by mercuric thiocyanate, and carbon dioxide by phenolphthalein. Other methods reported here were the same as for the SMA 12/60. All parts, reagents, and services were provided under a Technicon rental contract. Technicon lyophilized calibration materials (lots No. B4J143 and B4F940) were used for calibration. Initially, we assigned set-point values for calcium by assaying the calibration material by atomic absorption spectroscopy, for albumin by assaying the calibration material with the *aca* (bromcresol green method), and glucose by assaying the calibration material on the *aca* (hexokinase method). Other set-point values were those recommended by Technicon. In later studies, enzyme set-points were adjusted on SMAC to provide better comparability with other methods in routine service.

The routine data presented here were obtained primarily with version "six and one-half" of the SMAC computer software. Version "seven" has since been introduced and contains several system modifications, most importantly, changes in the AST methodology. In this laboratory, SMAC is interfaced with the laboratory PDP-12 digital computer (Digital Equipment Corp., Maynard, Mass. 10754), using the basic LABCOM software (Laboratory Computing, Inc., Madison, Wis. 53704) with the interface developed by Eggert and Westgard (*4*).

SMA 12/60 (Technicon). The instrument used was a conventional survey model up-dated with LD and AST ultraviolet methods, albumin by bromcresol green (*5*), and glucose by glucose oxidase (*6*). A slight flow system change was made for cholesterol by using a separate sample probe to reduce interaction. Reagents were purchased from Simmler and Son, Inc., St. Louis, Mo. 63108 and glass parts from Acculab, Norwood, N. Y. 07648. Lyophilized SMA 12/60 calibration material from Technicon was used with set points established in our laboratory (*2*).

aca *discrete analyzer* (E.I. du Pont de Nemours and Co., Inc., Wilmington, Del. 19898). All methods were as described elsewhere (*2*) except for the following revised methods: calcium by cresolphthalein complexone, uric acid by uricase, blood (serum) urea nitrogen by the urease glutamate dehydrogenase (EC 1.4.1.3) end-point method, and total bilirubin by *p*-nitrobenzene diazonium tetrafluoroborate. The *aca* has operated under a continuous maintenance contract with Du Pont. Primary standards were used to standardize glucose, urea nitrogen, uric acid, creatinine, and calcium. Albumin was calibrated with fresh patients' sera that had values determined by electrophoresis on cellulose acetate. For bilirubin, the stock standard was prepared as recommended by the joint committee on bilirubin standardization (*7*). Dilutions of this stock standard were prepared with a 50 g/liter albumin solution.

AutoAnalyzer I (Technicon). Creatinine was measured with an AutoAnalyzer I by a micro adaptation of the Jaffé reaction (*8*). Aqueous primary standards and reagents were purchased from Simmler and Son. Routine service was transferred to an AutoAnalyzer II on January 24, 1975.

AutoAnalyzer II (Technicon). Creatinine was measured by the Jaffé reaction (*9*). Aqueous primary standards and reagents were obtained from Simmler and Son.

Atomic absorption spectrophotometer (Instrumentation Laboratory, Inc., Lexington, Mass. 02173). Calcium was measured with an IL 153 Atomic Absorption Spectrophotometer. A 50-μl sample was diluted to 2.5 ml with a lanthanum oxide diluent (5.85 g/liter in 0.3 mol/liter HCl), with use of a Micromedic Automatic Pipette (Micromedic Systems, Inc., Rohm and Haas, Co., Philadelphia, Pa. 19105). Stock aqueous standards were purchased from Fisher Scientific Co., Pittsburgh, Pa. 15219, and diluted with Na/K (140/5 mmol/liter) viscosity-adjusted standard from IL.

Flame photometer (Instrumentation Laboratory). Sodium and potassium were measured by use of an IL 343 flame photometer, a 1/200 automatic dilutor, and a lithium internal standard. Viscosity-adjusted standards were obtained from IL.

AutoAnalyzer I (Technicon). With AutoAnalyzer I, chloride was measured by a mercuric thiocyanate method and carbon dioxide by use of cresol red indicator. Aqueous primary standards were obtained from Sigma Chemical Co., St. Louis, Mo. 63178. Reagents were purchased from Simmler and Son.

Cotlove Chloride Titrator (American Instrument Co., Silver Spring, Md. 20910). Chloride was measured by coulometric titration. Primary aqueous standards were prepared in our laboratory.

Natelson Microgasometer (Scientific Industries, Inc., Bohemia, N. Y. 11716). Carbon dioxide was measured manometrically with a Model 650 Natelson Microgasometer.

Refractometer (American Optical Co., Buffalo, N. Y. 14215). A temperature-compensated refractometer was used to measure total serum protein. The refractometer is used routinely when analyzing emergency and single requests, about 20–40 determinations per month.

Statistical calculations. The statistical procedures and calculations as applied in this report are described elsewhere (*10, 11*).

All comparison instruments operated under routine service protocol during this study. Regular laboratory staff performed all determinations. An extensive quality-control program, in which many control and commercial calibration materials are used, was in effect on all methodologies.

Results

Precision

SMAC precision estimates are summarized in Tables 1 and 2. Table 1 presents estimates obtained from lyophilized control sera that were analyzed during six months of routine operation, beginning January 1975. Here, N is the average number of determinations per month. Our protocol called for analyzing one control per rack of seven samples and recalibrating every 40 samples. At a rate of 200–600 samples per day, 6–20 values were measured per control per day, and about 1500 determinations for each control during the six month period. The standard deviation presented here is that for the six months, as obtained by pooling the monthly variances, dividing by the number of months, then extracting the square root. Table 2 presents estimates from blind duplicates, i.e., analyses performed on fresh patients' sera from two different blood-drawing tubes, on different calibration runs, but within a day. These blind duplicates were collected over a period of 53 working days.

Table 1. Precision as Estimated from Six Months' Routine Operation

Test		N	Mean	SD	CV, %
Glucose	(1)	237	83[c] mg/dl	1.62	2.0
	(2)	234	87[a]	2.23	2.6
	(3)	226	212[b]	4.78	2.2
	(4)	227	354[d]	5.59	1.6
Urea Nitrogen	(5)	311	12[c] mg/dl	0.373	3.1
	(6)	278	21[a]	0.447	2.1
	(7)	265	58[b]	0.988	1.7
	(8)	302	90[d]	1.11	1.2
Creatinine	(9)	234	1.1[c] mg/dl	0.0805	7.3
	(10)	203	2.0[a]	0.084	4.2
	(11)	195	5.5[b]	0.110	2.0
	(12)	225	7.4[d]	0.114	1.5
Calcium	(13)	292	7.1[c] mg/dl	0.150	2.1
	(14)	262	8.9[a]	0.166	1.9
	(15)	253	11.2[b]	0.203	1.8
	(16)	274	11.8[d]	0.212	1.8
Phosphorus	(17)	309	2.6[c] mg/dl	0.0623	2.4
	(18)	278	4.2[a]	0.0727	1.7
	(19)	294	6.9[d]	0.104	1.5
	(20)	265	7.1[b]	0.111	1.6
Uric Acid	(21)	308	3.8[c] mg/dl	0.0794	2.1
	(22)	276	6.8[a]	0.107	1.6
	(23)	293	9.0[d]	0.132	1.5
	(24)	266	9.2[b]	0.143	1.6
Cholesterol	(25)	266	134[b] mg/dl	3.11	2.3
	(26)	307	147[c]	3.53	2.4
	(27)	274	154[a]	2.82	1.8
	(28)	292	283[d]	4.90	1.7
Total Protein	(29)	296	4.8[c] g/dl	0.0909	1.9
	(30)	274	6.3[b]	0.095	1.5
	(31)	276	7.2[a]	0.103	1.4
	(32)	290	8.1[d]	0.114	1.4
Albumin	(33)	283	2.9[c] g/dl	0.0669	2.3
	(34)	260	3.0[b]	0.0786	2.6
	(35)	276	4.0[a]	0.0843	2.1
	(36)	292	4.6[d]	0.100	2.2
Bilirubin	(37)	291	0.78[c] mg/dl	0.0417	5.3
	(38)	270	2.59[a]	0.0727	2.8
	(39)	270	5.29[b]	0.137	2.6
	(40)	285	7.30[d]	0.156	2.1
Alkaline Phosphatase	(41)	222	63.32[c] U/l	2.20	3.5
	(42)	242	84.70[a]	2.60	3.1
	(43)	252	141.6 [d]	3.21	2.3
	(44)	255	215.6 [b]	6.36	2.9
Lactic Dehydrogenase	(45)	294	127[c] U/l	5.11	4.0
	(46)	264	202[a]	5.78	2.9
	(47)	288	368[d]	7.83	2.1
	(48)	255	446[b]	10.2	2.3
Aspartate Aminotransferase	(49)	190	43[c] U/l	3.78	8.8
	(50)	253	47[a]	2.73	5.8
	(51)	215	118[b]	3.14	2.7
	(52)	185	152[d]	7.01	4.6
Sodium	(53)	178	118[c] mmol/l	1.43	1.2
	(54)	194	128[b]	1.61	1.2
	(55)	206	142[a]	1.62	1.1
	(56)	198	149[d]	2.04	1.4
Potassium	(57)	236	2.8[c] mmol/l	0.132	4.7
	(58)	226	3.6[b]	0.125	3.5
	(59)	229	6.0[a]	0.154	2.6
	(60)	226	8.9[d]	0.309	3.5
Chloride	(61)	270	86[c] mmol/l	1.64	1.9
	(62)	247	104[b]	1.55	1.5
	(63)	255	113[d]	1.59	1.4
	(64)	257	114[a]	1.55	1.4
CO_2	(65)	294	15[c] mmol/l	0.704	4.7
	(66)	268	25[a]	0.834	3.3
	(67)	286	31[d]	1.02	3.3
	(68)	261	35[b]	1.00	2.8

[a] Dade normal, lot number SPXL 342
[b] Dade abnormal, lot number SPXP 539
[c] Technicon Scale 1, lot number B4M249
[d] Technicon Scale 2, lot number B4K175

Table 2. Precision as Estimated from Blind Patient Duplicates. (Between-run, Within-day Duplicates over 53-day Period)

Test		N	Mean	SD	CV, %
Glucose	(1)	107	129 mg/dl	2.13	1.6
Urea Nitrogen	(2)	121	23 mg/dl	0.498	2.2
Creatinine	(3)		Not evaluated		
Calcium	(4)	101	9.2 mg/dl	0.132	1.4
Phosphorus	(5)	118	3.5 mg/dl	0.076	2.2
Uric Acid	(6)	122	5.5 mg/dl	0.092	1.7
Cholesterol	(7)	112	183 mg/dl	4.106	2.2
Total Protein	(8)	120	6.4 g/dl	0.104	1.6
Albumin	(9)	120	3.4 g/dl	0.057	1.7
Bilirubin	(10)	107	1.3 mg/dl	0.054	4.2
Alkaline Phosphatase	(11)	107	113 U/l	1.84	1.6
Lactic Dehydrogenase	(12)	94	195 U/l	15.03	7.7
Aspartate Aminotransferase	(13)	102	37 U/l	3.01	8.1
Sodium	(14)	103	138 mmol/l	1.12	0.8
Potassium	(15)	110	4.3 mmol/l	0.106	2.5
Chloride	(16)	112	102 mmol/l	1.12	1.1
CO_2	(17)	118	27 mmol/l	0.889	3.3

Comparison of Values

Initially we compared the SMAC with the SMA 12/60, because we wanted to know if we could validly substitute the SMAC for the SMA 12/60. Additionally, we compared results for calcium with those by atomic absorption spectroscopy, enzyme results with those obtained with the Du Pont *aca*, creatinine results with those from an AutoAnalyzer I, sodium and potassium values with those from a flame photometer, and values for chloride and CO_2 with those from an AutoAnalyzer I.

Before statistical analysis of these results, the data were plotted (SMAC as y, routine method as x) and visually inspected for presence of nonlinearity and outliers. When necessary, data sets were restricted to the linear range and no more than one outlier per 100 data points was excluded. Data were analyzed statistically using regression and paired t-test calculations (*11*). These results are presented in Table 3. Columns 1–3 describe the comparison experiment by listing the test channel, the comparison method, and the number of patients' specimens compared. Columns 4–10 list the regression statistics: the slope (B), the standard deviation of the slope (SD_B), the y-intercept (A), the standard deviation of the intercept (SD_A), the standard error about the regression line ($S_{y/x}$), the standard deviation of the x values or the population studied (SD_x), and the correlation coefficient (r). The last columns (*11–14*) give the t-test statistics: the mean of the values by the comparison method ($\bar{x}$), the bias between the two methods, the standard deviation of the paired differences (SD_d), and the t-value.

Because comparability in enzyme results was desired for routine service application, some proportional adjustments of SMAC results were made by

Table 3. Statistical Analysis of Patient-comparison Data Collected during Initial Evaluation Studies (SMAC vs. Method Listed)

TEST		EXPERIMENT: COMPARISON METHOD	N	REGRESSION STATISTICS: SLOPE B	SD_B	INTERCEPT A	SD_A	$S_{y/x}$	SD_x	r	t-TEST STATISTICS: $\bar{X}$	BIAS	SD_d	t
Glucose	(1)	12/60 Oxidase	309	1.039	0.003	−4.35	0.42	3.07	52.1	0.998	114.7	0.08	3.67	0.39
Urea Nitrogen	(2)	12/60	292	0.963	0.003	0.006	0.07	0.76	13.9	0.998	18.1	0.66	0.92	12.32
Creatinine	(3)	AA I	181	0.989	0.004	0.002	0.01	0.11	2.2	0.998	2.0	0.02	0.11	2.42
Calcium	(4)	12/60	308	0.982[a]	0.011	0.28	0.10	0.17	0.90	0.982	9.21	0.117	0.17	11.95
	(5)	Atomic Absorp.	214	0.999[a]	0.013	0.10	0.12	0.19	1.00	0.983	9.07	0.084	0.19	6.60
Phosphorus	(6)	12/60	243	0.985[a]	0.007	0.01	0.03	0.10	0.92	0.994	3.53	0.050	0.10	7.69
Uric Acid	(7)	12/60	247	1.018	0.004	−0.04	0.02	0.12	1.86	0.998	5.45	0.055	0.13	6.97
Cholesterol	(8)	12/60	220	1.027	0.013	−11.8	2.59	8.21	43.3	0.983	197.7	6.38	8.28	11.43
Total Protein	(9)	12/60	246	1.103[a]	0.017	−0.74	0.11	0.16	0.6	0.972	6.7	0.05	0.17	4.32
Albumin	(10)	12/60 BCG	229	1.002	0.014	0.07	0.05	0.12	0.6	0.978	3.8	0.08	0.12	9.80
Bilirubin	(11)	12/60	227	0.986	0.006	−0.05	0.01	0.08	0.85	0.995	0.7	0.06	0.08	11.65
Alkaline Phosphatase	(12)	12/60	221	1.036	0.013	0.07	1.30	9.61	50.7	0.968	88.4	3.24	9.76	4.65
Lactate Dehydrogenase	(13)	12/60 UV	232	1.113	0.013	−7.89	2.43	12.47	61.7	0.984	171.6	11.6	14.27	12.32
Asparate Aminotransferase	(14)	12/60 UV	239	0.975	0.027	3.70	0.96	6.82	16.5	0.920	31.6	2.9	6.82	6.59
Alanine Aminotransferase	(15)	aca	112	0.876	0.040	2.26	1.08	7.79	18.4	0.903	20.1	0.2	8.09	0.29
Sodium	(16)	IL Flame	197	1.011[a]	0.020	−1.57	2.75	1.33	4.8	0.962	138.3	0.25	1.32	2.74
Potassium	(17)	IL Flame	180	1.080[a]	0.014	−0.24	0.06	0.11	0.6	0.986	4.2	0.10	0.12	11.23
Chloride	(18)	AA I	209	1.142[a]	0.015	−14.41	1.51	1.28	5.9	0.981	100.9	0.11	1.37	1.10
CO_2	(19)	AA I	217	1.045[a]	0.022	−1.06	0.58	1.12	3.5	0.954	26.6	0.14	1.12	1.82

[a] Slope calculated by equation, $B = \dfrac{S_{xy}}{S_{xx} - (N-1)\sigma_x^2}$ which corrects for random error in the x variable (*15*).

changing the set-point values for the SMAC calibration material. Table 4 shows the statistical summary of the comparison data with the *aca*, collected before and after the calibration adjustments on SMAC.

Comparison data were also collected under conditions of routine operation. In these studies, two serum pools, each comprised of 3–6 fresh specimens from patients, were both analyzed each day for six months. For electrolytes, individual patient's samples were analyzed concurrently. Results were compared to those obtained by other methods that are in continuing service and are statistically summarized in Table 5.

Summary of Observed Analytical Errors

Table 6 summarizes the random and systematic components of error as well as the total analytical error. The concentrations for which these errors are estimated are the medical decision concentrations (X_C) recommended by Barnett (*12*) and are given in column 2. In the case of the enzymes, we selected a value near the upper limit of the expected range of activity for normal persons. Column 3 lists a 95% limit for allowable analytical error, derived by multiplying Barnett's maximum allowable standard deviations by two. This format for judging performance

Table 4. Statistical Analysis of Enzyme Patient Comparison Data before and after Calibration Adjustments (SMAC vs. *aca*)

TEST		EXPERIMENT: COMPARISON METHOD	N	REGRESSION STATISTICS: SLOPE B	SD_B	INTERCEPT A	SD_A	$S_{y/x}$	SD_x	r	t-TEST STATISTICS: $\bar{X}$	BIAS	SD_d	t
Alkaline Phosphatase	(1)	aca	117	8.066	0.142	2.70	1.98	13.25	8.6	0.983	10.9	---	---	---
adjusted	(2)	aca	75	1.082	0.011	−4.8	0.13	6.80	70.9	0.996	95.4	3.0	8.9	2.92
Lactate Dehydrogenase	(3)	aca	118	1.009	0.012	22.2	2.44	12.11	92.6	0.991	179.2	23.9	12.09	21.43
adjusted	(4)	aca	103	0.900	0.014	24.0	2.65	11.64	84.8	0.989	175.8	6.5	14.35	4.57
Asparate Aminotransferase	(5)	aca	118	0.920	0.019	−1.90	0.69	3.81	18.2	0.975	31.0	4.4	4.06	11.66
adjusted	(6)	aca	46	1.008	0.060	0.93	0.45	7.40	18.4	0.930	30.0	1.2	7.32	1.07

Table 5. Statistical Analysis of Patient Comparison Data Collected during Routine Operation (SMAC vs. *aca*)

		EXPERIMENT		REGRESSION STATISTICS							t-TEST STATISTICS			
				SLOPE		INTERCEPT								
TEST		COMPARISON METHOD	N	B	SD_B	A	SD_A	$S_{y/x}$	SD_x	r	$\bar{X}$	BIAS	SD_d	t
Glucose	(1)	aca	545	0.998	0.006	3.46	0.83	3.80	60.8	0.998	129.7	3.01	3.91	18.00
Urea Nitrogen	(2)	aca	316	1.032	0.009	−0.31	0.23	0.97	13.2	0.997	21.1	0.40	1.08	6.50
Creatinine	(3)	Auto II	304	0.959	0.031	0.04	0.04	0.12	1.2	0.974	1.6	0.14	0.13	18.7
	(4)	aca	222	1.012	0.005	0.02	0.01	0.10	1.3	0.994	1.39	0.04	0.11	5.22
Calcium	(5)	Atomic Absorp.	328	1.007	0.038	−0.02	0.35	0.17	0.69	0.959	9.28	0.059	0.17	6.18
	(6)	aca	299	0.938	0.017	0.66	0.16	0.19	0.64	0.909	9.32	0.082	0.19	7.32
Uric Acid	(7)	aca	310	0.971	0.027	0.31	0.15	0.26	1.19	0.973	5.37	0.172	0.26	11.39
Total Protein	(8)	Refractometer	246	0.912	0.045	0.52	0.31	0.16	0.45	0.925	6.8	0.08	0.17	8.12
Albumin	(9)	aca	312	0.999	0.049	−0.09	0.20	0.14	0.35	0.929	4.0	0.09	0.14	11.84
Bilirubin	(10)	aca	329	1.076	0.028	−0.24	0.03	0.12	0.93	0.976	1.0	0.16	0.15	19.80
Alkaline Phosphatase	(11)	aca	342	1.153	0.013	−0.02	0.16	0.59	5.5	0.995	11.1	1.7	1.01	30.72
Lactate Dehydrogenase	(12)	aca	332	0.924	0.014	18.7	2.92	8.92	81.0	0.991	189.6	4.8	10.96	8.03
Asparate Aminotransferase	(13)	aca	324	1.095	0.023	−4.14	0.97	3.96	19.7	0.981	37.5	1.06	4.46	4.27
Sodium	(14)	IL Flame	239	0.987	0.027	1.99	3.72	1.80	5.4	0.955	137.6	0.19	1.63	1.85
Potassium	(15)	IL Flame	243	0.994	0.019	0.05	0.08	0.14	0.6	0.978	4.3	0.02	0.14	2.61
Chloride	(16)	Chloridometer	83	1.104	0.044	−8.69	4.29	1.89	6.8	0.970	97.2	1.75	2.00	7.96
CO_2	(17)	Natelson	81	0.879	0.040	2.53	1.10	1.14	4.6	0.962	27.2	0.72	1.25	5.17

has been discussed previously (*10*). Table 6 gives the observed analytical errors (RE, SE, TE in columns 4, 8, 13, respectively) along with their 90% confidence interval (or lower and upper 95% one-sided confidence limits). The "source of data" columns indicate the table number and line number for the data we used in the calculations. The random errors are calculated from precision data in Table 1, which represents performance under routine operating conditions. The coefficient of variation (CV) for the control product whose concentration was closest to the decision concentration was used to calculate random error, except where the decision concentration was between control concentrations. In that case, the CV's of controls which bracketed the decision value were averaged to give a CV representative of the decision concentration. The estimates of systematic error are calculated from the comparison data in Tables 3–5 and tabulated with the "data sources" and the comparison methods. Estimates of total analytical error are based on the random and systematic components in that same line of Table 6. The last column gives the number of the figure, which graphically presents the error estimates.

Discussion

The acceptability of performance can be judged by comparing the observed analytical errors with some specified limit of allowable error (E_A). We have used Barnett's recommendations for allowable error (*12*) because they most closely represent medical usefulness requirements. Barnett lists the important medical decision concentrations (X_C) and the allowable maximum standard deviations. We define allowable error as a 95% limit and therefore must multiply Barnett's allowable SD's by 2 to obtain E_A. For enzymes, Barnett provides no recommendations; therefore, we considered Tonks' recommendation that the maximum error (total) should be from 10 to 20% (*13, 14*). We adopted a rather stringent 10% limit for ALP and LD and 15% for AST. Recommendations for enzyme performance are especially lacking and our chosen limits may be subject to debate.

Figure 1 shows the comparison between the observed total analytical error and the specified limit for allowable error for the studies comparing SMAC and the SMA 12/60. The length of the bar represents total error, which is the TE_u estimate in Table 6. The hatched portion is random error, as given by RE_u in Table 6. The remaining plain portion of the bar represents systematic error, together with a small amount of uncertainty in its estimate. Whenever the length of the bar is less than the limit for allowable error as represented by the solid vertical line (E_A), the measurements by the two analyzers are within limits of acceptable performance. All tests except the enzymes show acceptable agreement. In the case of the enzymes, the systematic differences between SMAC and the SMA 12/60 are due in part to differences in calibration and methodology. These systematic differences could be effectively reduced by calibration adjustments.

Figure 2 summarizes SMAC performance for enzyme activity in comparison with the Du Pont *aca*. The differences are large, especially for ALP, which is reported in U/dl on the *aca* and U/liter on SMAC.[2] The random error was acceptable in all cases; it is the

[2] We initially changed the ALP units on SMAC to U/dl, to agree with those on the *aca* because the *aca* was in routine service. On completion of these studies, which assured us that we could maintain the SMAC in routine service, we changed to U/liter on both SMAC and *aca*.

Table 6. Summary of Performance Standards (Specifications for Allowable Error, E_A, Medically Important Decision Concentrations, X_C) vs. Observed Performance (Estimates of Random, Systematic, and Total Analytical Errors)

TEST	PERFORMANCE STANDARD X_C	PERFORMANCE STANDARD E_A	RANDOM ERROR[a] RE	RE_1	RE_u	Data Source Table-Line	SYSTEMATIC ERROR[b] SE	SE_1	SE_u	Data Source Table-Line	COMPARISON METHOD	TOTAL ANALYTIC ERROR TE	TE_1	TE_u	Figure
Glucose	50 mg/dl	10.0	2.0	1.9	2.0	1 1	2.4	1.8	2.9	3 1	SMA 12/60 Oxidase	4.4	4.4	4.5	1
	120 mg/dl	10.0	6.1	5.9	6.3	1 2	0.3	0.0	0.7	3 1	SMA 12/60 Oxidase	6.4	6.2	6.6	1
	50 mg/dl	10.0	2.0	1.9	2.0	1 1	3.4	2.8	3.9	5 1	aca	5.4	5.3	5.4	3
	120 mg/dl	10.0	6.1	5.9	6.3	1 2	3.2	2.9	3.5	5 1	aca	9.3	9.2	9.5	3
Urea Nitrogen	27 mg/dl	4.0	1.1	1.1	1.1	1 6	1.0	0.9	1.1	3 2	SMA 12/60	2.1	2.1	2.1	1
	27 mg/dl	4.0	1.1	1.1	1.1	1 6	0.6	0.4	0.7	5 2	aca	1.7	1.6	1.7	3
Creatinine	2.0 mg/dl	0.4	0.16	0.16	0.17	1 10	0.02	0.00	0.04	3 3	AA I	0.18	0.18	0.19	– –
	2.0 mg/dl	0.4	0.16	0.16	0.17	1 10	0.04	0.03	0.06	5 3	AA II	0.20	0.20	0.21	4
	2.0 mg/dl	0.4	0.16	0.16	0.17	1 10	0.04	0.03	0.06	5 4	aca	0.20	0.20	0.21	3
Calcium	11.0 mg/dl	0.5	0.39	0.38	0.40	1 15	0.08	0.04	0.12	3 4	SMA 12/60	0.47	0.46	0.48	1
	11.0 mg/dl	0.5	0.39	0.38	0.40	1 15	0.06	0.01	0.11	5 5	Atomic Absorption	0.45	0.44	0.46	4
	11.0 mg/dl	0.5	0.39	0.38	0.40	1 15	0.02	−0.04	0.28	5 6	aca	0.41	0.40	0.43	3
Phosphorus	4.5 mg/dl	0.5	0.15	0.14	0.15	1 18	0.06	0.04	0.08	3 6	SMA 12/60	0.21	0.20	0.21	1
Uric Acid	6.0 mg/dl	1.0	0.19	0.18	0.19	1 22	0.34	0.33	0.36	3 7	SMA 12/60	0.53	0.52	0.54	1
	6.0 mg/dl	1.0	0.19	0.18	0.19	1 22	0.14	0.10	0.17	5 7	aca	0.32	0.32	0.33	3
Cholesterol	250 mg/dl	40	8.3	8.1	8.6	1 28	5.0	3.3	6.8	3 8	SMA 12/60	13.4	13.3	13.8	1
Total Protein	7.0 g/dl	0.6	0.19	0.19	0.20	1 31	0.02	0.00	0.04	3 9	SMA 12/60	0.21	0.21	0.22	1
	7.0 g/dl	0.6	0.19	0.19	0.20	1 31	0.10	0.07	0.12	5 8	Refractometer	0.29	0.28	0.29	4
Albumin	3.5 g/dl	0.5	0.16	0.16	0.16	1 34, 35	0.06	0.04	0.08	3 10	SMA 12/60 BCG	0.22	0.22	0.23	1
	3.5 g/dl	0.5	0.16	0.16	0.16	1 34, 35	0.09	0.07	0.12	5 9	aca	0.25	0.25	0.26	3
Bilirubin	1.0 mg/dl	0.4	0.10	0.10	0.11	1 37	0.06	0.05	0.08	3 11	SMA 12/60	0.16	0.16	0.17	1
	1.0 mg/dl	0.4	0.10	0.10	0.11	1 37	0.16	0.15	0.18	5 10	aca	0.26	0.26	0.27	3
Alkaline Phosphatase	100 U/l	10	6.1	5.9	6.3	1 42	3.7	2.4	5.0	3 12	SMA 12/60	9.8	9.7	10.1	1
	100 U/l	10	6.1	5.9	6.3	1 42	709	684	734	4 1	aca	715	705	735	2
	100 U/l	10	6.1	5.9	6.3	1 42	3.4	1.8	5.0	4 2	aca	9.5	9.5	9.8	2
	100 U/l	10	6.1	5.9	6.3	1 42	15.3	14.3	16.3	5 11	aca	21.4	21.3	21.6	3
Lactate Dehydrogenase	200 U/l	20	11.4	11.0	11.7	1 46	14.7	12.9	16.5	3 13	SMA 12/60 UV	26.1	25.9	26.6	1
	200 U/l	20	11.4	11.0	11.7	1 46	24.0	22.0	26.0	4 3	aca	35.4	35.3	35.9	2
	200 U/l	20	11.4	11.0	11.7	1 46	4.0	2.0	6.0	4 4	aca	15.4	15.3	16.0	2
	200 U/l	20	11.4	11.0	11.7	1 46	3.5	2.5	4.5	5 12	aca	14.9	14.6	15.3	3
Asparate Aminotransferase	50 U/l	7.5	5.7	5.5	5.8	1 50	2.4	1.1	3.8	3 14	SMA 12/60 UV	8.1	8.1	8.4	1
	50 U/l	7.5	5.7	5.5	5.8	1 50	5.9	4.9	6.9	4 5	aca	11.6	11.5	11.8	2
	50 U/l	7.5	5.7	5.5	5.8	1 50	1.3	−1.9	4.5	4 6	aca	7.0	6.7	8.0	2
	50 U/l	7.5	5.7	5.5	5.8	1 50	0.6	0.0	1.1	5 13	aca	6.3	6.2	6.5	3
Sodium	130 mmol/l	4.0	3.1	3.0	3.2	1 54	0.3	−0.1	0.7	5 14	IL Flame Photo.	3.4	3.3	3.5	4
	150 mmol/l	4.0	4.1	4.0	4.3	1 56	0.0	−0.5	0.6	5 14	IL Flame Photo.	4.1	4.1	4.3	4
Potassium	3.0 mmol/l	0.5	0.24	0.23	0.24	1 57, 58	0.03	−0.01	0.07	5 15	IL Flame Photo.	0.27	0.26	0.28	4
	6.0 mmol/l	0.5	0.31	0.30	0.32	1 59	0.01	−0.04	0.07	5 15	IL Flame Photo.	0.32	0.32	0.33	4
Chloride	90 mmol/l	4.0	3.4	3.2	3.4	1 61	0.7	0.1	1.3	5 16	Coul. Titrator	4.1	4.0	4.2	4
	110 mmol/l	4.0	3.0	2.9	3.1	1 63	2.8	1.9	3.6	5 16	Coul. Titrator	5.8	5.8	6.0	4
CO_2	20 mmol/l	2.0	1.6	1.5	1.6	1 65, 66	0.1	−0.4	0.6	5 17	Natelson	1.7	1.5	1.7	4
	30 mmol/l	2.0	1.9	1.9	2.0	1 67	1.1	0.8	1.4	5 17	Natelson	3.0	3.0	3.1	4

[a] t factors for calculating one-sided 95% confidence limits for a standard deviation are taken from Natrella (*16*).
[b] $t_{1-\alpha/2}$ for calculation of ω for systematic error upper and lower limits are taken from Natrella (*17*).

addition of systematic error that limits acceptability. When calibration adjustments were made for all three enzymes, the systematic components of error were decreased and the observed errors were within the limits specified as allowable.

Figure 3 summarizes the performance of SMAC vs. the *aca* while under routine operation and with adjusted enzyme-calibration set points. All methods except that for ALP gave results that meet the performance standard for allowable error. ALP results shifted during routine operation; continual monitoring of enzyme methods is evidently necessary to maintain good comparison. Because of the long-term performance stability of the *aca*, it serves as a practical in-house reference for controlling methodologies for which calibration is less stable. While this approach to maintaining comparability is not analytically satisfying, it does provide a practical solution to a difficult problem.

Figure 4 summarizes SMAC performance vs. the

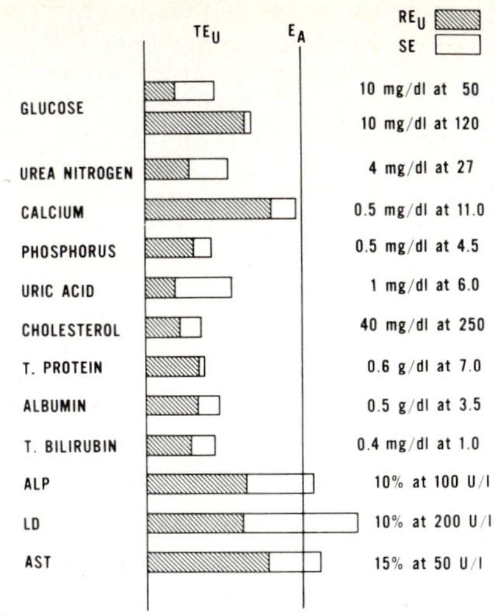

Fig. 1. Comparison of total analytical error (TE_u) with medically allowable error (E_A)
SMAC vs. SMA 12/60 comparison methods

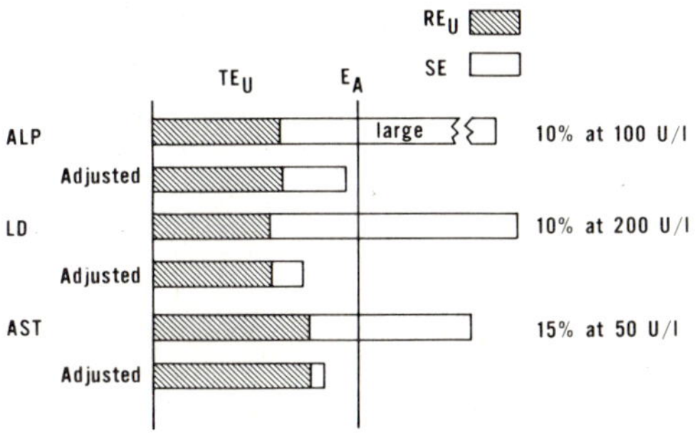

Fig. 2. Comparison of total analytical error (TE_u) with medically allowable error (E_A) for enzyme channels
SMAC vs. Du Pont *aca* as comparison method, before and after calibration adjustments during initial evaluation period

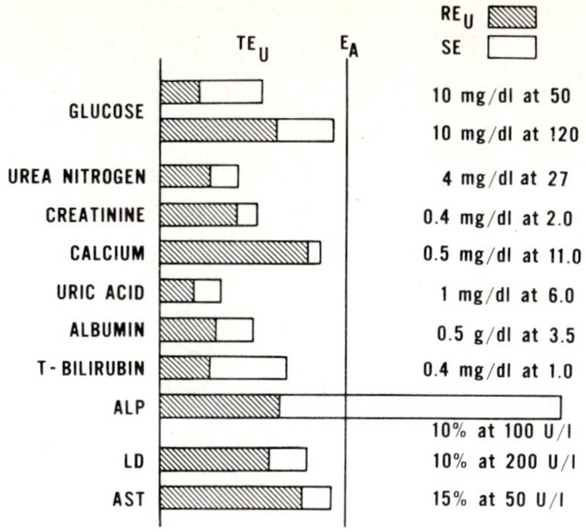

Fig. 3. Comparison of total analytical error (TE_u) with medically allowable error (E_A)
SMAC vs. Du Pont *aca* as comparison methods during routine service operation

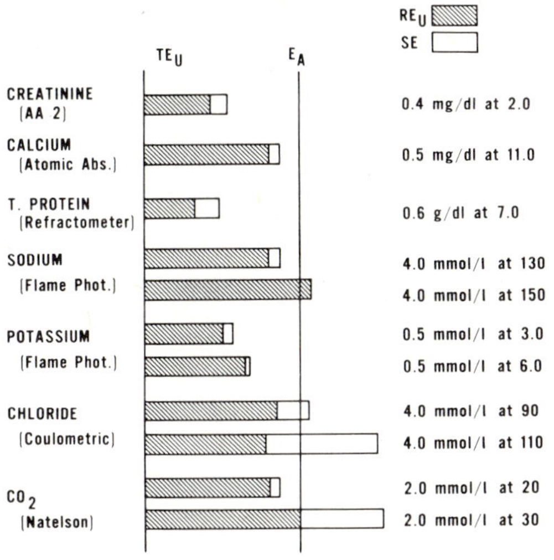

Fig. 4. Comparison of total analytical error (TE_u) with medically allowable error (E_A)
SMAC vs. routine service methods

other routine methods. Although systematic error is small, the random error for sodium is at the upper limit of acceptability. The performance of the sodium ion selective electrode is acceptable only if systematic error is maintained at a very low level. Random errors for chloride and CO_2 are also near the upper limit, and systematic errors must likewise be reduced or eliminated. The systematic error for chloride presents an interesting problem. SMAC control materials, assayed daily with a coulometric titrator for one month, gave mean values that were identical to the manufacturer's recommendations for SMAC set-point values. Yet use of those set-point values gave a systematic error of 0.7 mmol/liter at 90 mmol/liter and 2.8 at 110 mmol/liter. We have not been able to eliminate the source of this error and have found it necessary to compensate for it by calibration adjustments, at least until such time as we are able to isolate the cause and make appropriate correction. For CO_2, inconsistencies in sample handling contribute to the observed systematic error, as well as the rounding to the whole integer when measurements are reported by SMAC. Improved performance may be desirable, though the present performance meets the practical demand in our laboratory.

It is apparent in all of these graphical summaries that the extent of random error itself is acceptable, the only borderline cases being sodium, chloride, and CO_2. The presence of systematic differences when comparing methodologies is not unexpected; however, the differences are too large to permit the interchangeable use (inter-instrument) of enzyme-activity values unless some calibration adjustments are made. In interpreting the systematic difference, it should be remembered that our studies permit only an estimate of the differences between methods and not which method gives the more nearly correct results. Our objective is to maintain performance consistent with our present routine techniques; therefore we assume those routine values as our baseline for comparison purposes.

Finally, it is readily apparent that all the decisions on acceptability depend on the specification for allowable error. Rigorous specifications are lacking at present; therefore, the user must make some judgment as to what specifications he thinks are appropriate. We have referred to Barnett's and Tonks' recommendations; however, another user may wish to substitute different limits for allowable error. To determine acceptability based on the data here, he would then compare the estimates of observed error in Table 6 with his specifications for allowable error.

The assistance of the Clinical Chemistry Laboratory staff is gratefully acknowledged. Their goodwill and cooperation through the year of this study are greatly appreciated. We thank Ms. Marian Hunt for her careful review of the manuscript and Ms. Peggy Hintzman for cheerfully typing the drafts of the manuscript and tables.

References

1. Schwartz, M. K., Bethune, V. G., Fleischer, M., et al., Chemical and clinical evaluation of the continuous flow analyzer "SMAC". *Clin. Chem.* **20,** 1060 (1974).

2. Westgard, J. O., and Lahmeyer, B. L., Comparison of results from the Du Pont *"aca"* and Technicon "SMA 12/60". *Clin. Chem.* **18,** 340 (1972).

3. Rao, J., Pelavin, M. H., and Morgenstern, S., SMAC: High-speed, continuous flow, ion-selective electrode for sodium and potassium: Theory and design. In *Advances in Automated Analysis, Technicon International Congress 1972,* **1:** *Clinical Chemistry Methods,* Mediad Inc., Tarrytown, N. Y., 1973, pp 33–36.

4. Eggert, A. A., and Westgard, J. O., The integration of the SMAC™ into a clinical laboratory computer system. *Clin. Chem.* **21,** 1005 (1975). Abstract.

5. Westgard, J. O., and Poquette, M. A., Determination of serum albumin with the "SMA 12/60" by a bromcresol green dye-binding method. *Clin. Chem.* **18,** 647 (1972).

6. Carey, R. N., Feldbruegge, D., and Westgard, J. O., Evaluation of the adaptation of the glucose oxidase/peroxidase-3-methyl-2-benzothiazolinone-*N,N*-dimethylaniline procedure to the Technicon "SMA 12/60", and comparison with other automated methods for glucose. *Clin. Chem.* **20,** 5 (1974).

7. Representatives of the American Academy of Pediatrics, the College of American Pathologists, the American Association of Clinical Chemists, and the National Institutes of Health: Recommendation on a uniform bilirubin standard. *Stand. Methods Clin. Chem.* **5,** 75 (1965).

8. Westgard, J. O., and Lehane D. P., Micro autoanalyzer systems. In *Microtechniques for the Clinical Laboratory: Concepts and Applications,* chap. 21, Mario Werner, Ed. John Wiley and Sons, Inc., New York, N. Y., in press.

9. *Technical Publication No. UA4-0170-00,* Technicon Method No. SE 4-0011FH4. Technicon Instruments Corp., Tarrytown, N. Y. 10591, August, 1974.

10. Westgard, J. O., Carey, R. N., and Wold, S., Criteria for judging precision and accuracy in method development and evaluation. *Clin. Chem.* **20,** 825 (1974).

11. Westgard, J. O., and Hunt, M. R., Use and interpretation of common statistical tests in method-comparison studies. *Clin. Chem.* **19,** 49 (1973).

12. Barnett, R. N., Medical significance of laboratory results. *Am. J. Clin. Pathol.* **50,** 671 (1968).

13. Tonks, D. B., A study of the accuracy and precision of clinical chemistry determinations in 170 Canadian laboratories. *Clin. Chem.* **9,** 217 (1963).

14. Tonks, D. B., A quality control program for quantitative clinical chemistry estimation. *Can. J. Med. Technol.* **30,** 38 (1968).

15. Davies O. L., and Goldsmith, P. L., *Statistical Methods in Research and Production.* Hafner Pub. Co., New York, N. Y., 1972, pp 208–209.

16. Natrella, M. G., *Experimental Statistics. Nat. Bur. Stand. Handb.* **91,** U. S. Government Printing Office, Washington, D. C., 1963, pp 4-1 to 4-7 and Table A-21, p T-36.

17. *Ibid.* pp 5-14 to 5-19 and Table A-4, p T-5.

CLIN. CHEM. 22/4, 497–499 (1976)

Immunofixation. I. General Principles and Application to Agarose Gel Electrophoresis

Robert F. Ritchie and Rosemary Smith

Immunofixation offers the worker an economical means of physically locating a protein in an electrophoretic strip and is ideally suited to forensic medicine, genetic studies, or research. The method is as simple and economical as the commonly used one- or two-dimensional immunoelectrophoresis, yet yields considerably more information.

Many plasma proteins display molecular heterogeneity when viewed with special procedures. Perhaps the most direct and frequently used method is electrophoresis, in which the isoelectric points (IP) of the various polymorphic forms of an individual protein species is what principally dictates their locations within a strip of gel or on a separatory column in systems that do not also involve molecular sieving. Both molecular alteration and genetic variation affect a protein's carbohydrate and peptide content, which, in turn, alters the IP of a given species, subspecies, or fraction. Therefore, electrophoresis inherently is a technique for demonstrating microheterogeneity, but because of the nonspecific means used to make visible the protein in the gel matrix (staining), resolution is poor.

Ordinarily, serum protein electrophoresis resolves six to eight major fractions that contain about a dozen major species and more than 100 minor fractions (Figure 1). The IP of many are close, hence the small number of fractions that are resolved in even the best agarose or membrane systems. Because of the many minor fractions that often represent degradation products or variants of completely unrelated species, high-resolution gels make identification even more confusing. Immunological identification offers the only sure means of detecting protein fractions that move in unusual positions because of genetic variation or biochemical alteration. Alper and Johnson (*1*) described a technique called "immunofixation," which allows the worker to anchor, in situ, proteins of a single immunologic species by exposing the protein-containing gel to specific antibody after electrophoresis. Afonso (*2*) described a forerunner of true quantitative immunoelectrophoresis that was to be described two years later by Laurell (*3*). Afonso's description made use of the basic concept of immunofixation, but with a polyspecific antiserum overlaid on microimmunoelectrophoresis films. The results were as difficult to interpret as the usual microimmunoelectrophoresis developed with polyspecific antiserum.

The purpose of this paper is to describe the easy application of a modified immunofixation method to two unmodified agarose electrophoresis systems that are in wide use (*4*).

Materials and Methods

Electrophoretic systems: System A, consisting of agarose gel bonded to plastic film, was obtained from Millipore Biomedica, Acton, Mass. 01720. The buffer system at pH 8.6 is used as supplied by the manufacturer. System B is a water-cooled, agarose ("Seakem

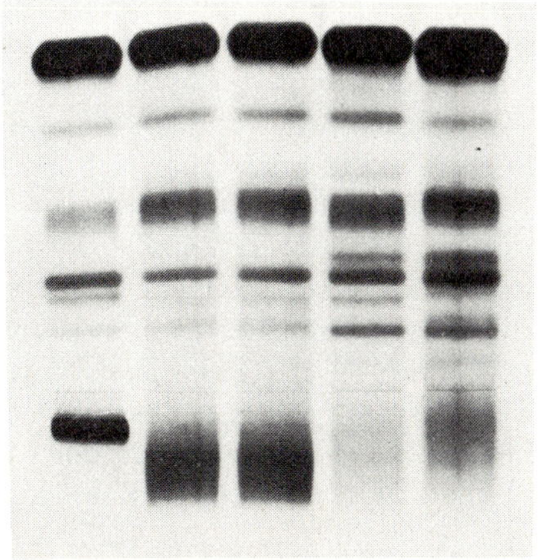

Fig. 1. Agarose gel electrophoresis (system A) of unselected human serum samples

Resolution is sufficient to resolve 18 to 22 fractions in the original. Good separation of the major electrophoretic zones is important to immunofixation

Rheumatic Disease Laboratory, Maine Medical Center, Portland, Maine 04102.

Received Dec. 24, 1975; accepted Feb. 5, 1976.

Agarose"; Marine Colloids, Inc., Rockland, Maine 04841) electrophoresis system as described by Laurell (*3*), without modification except that in casting the gel film no sample pockets are included.

Gel preparation: For system A, the plastic mask for sample application supplied by the manufacturer is stripped completely from the gel surface, in contrast to the recommended procedure. For both systems, a 2.5-cm wide strip of cellulose acetate membrane (supplier not critical) is applied smoothly over the application area for 10 to 15 s. Filter paper or blotter is *not* suitable for absorbing surface moisture. The slotted mask is then applied to the gel surface. Bubbles should be excluded carefully.

Sample preparation and application: Whole serum, plasma, other body fluids, or protein fractions are applied directly to the slotted mask, without mixing samples.

The amount of protein that diffuses into the gel can be controlled by either varying the duration of application, or by previously diluting the sample appropriately. Application time can vary from 30 s to 10 min, with a shorter time being used for samples with high protein concentration, longer times for those of low concentration.

If the dilution technique is used, a final concentration of 0.15–0.3 g/liter is desirable for discretely banded proteins and 2 g/liter for the heterogeneous immunoglobulins. Depending on the potency and avidity of the antiserum used, adjustment by trial and error may improve the final results.

Electrophoresis. Voltage is maintained at 300 V for system B, but because of manufacturer's engineering limitations, only 200 V can be applied to System A. Electrophoresis time is 10 to 20 min and 45 min, respectively. For proteins that have several closely migrating fractions, a relatively prolonged electrophoresis may be desirable.

Immunofixation. Cellulose acetate strips, 1 × 4 cm, are dipped into antiserum (Nephelometric grade; Atlantic Antibodies, Westbrook, Maine 04092) of the appropriate concentration, drained against the side of the container, and applied to the gel surface immediately after removal from the electrophoresis chamber. The strips are placed to cover the zone known to be occupied by the protein under study (Figure 2). Care should be taken to remove air bubbles from beneath the strips and to ensure that the adjacent strips containing different antibodies do not touch. In this approach, several different antisera can be used on a single gel film. If one protein is being studied in several samples, the strips can be wider and longer to cover as many samples as desired (Figure 2). The gel is incubated in a moist chamber for about 1 h. (The incubation temperature is not critical.)

Processing. At completion, the acetate strips are removed and discarded. Smooth filter paper of any variety is moistened with physiological saline and applied directly to the entire gel film. This is overlaid with 3 to 5 dry absorbent paper towels and covered

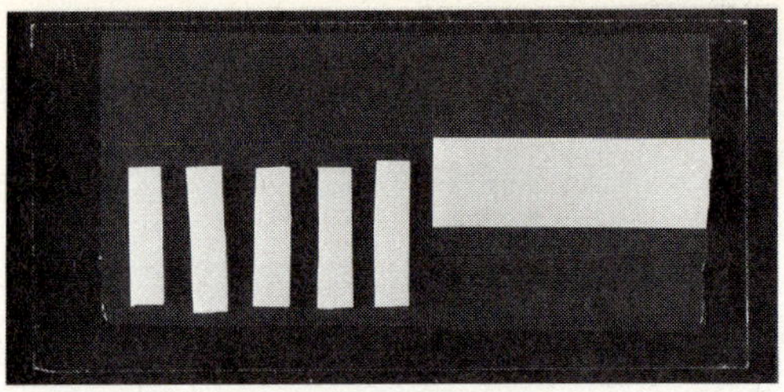

Fig. 2. Application of antiserum to the completed electrophoretic gel

At *left* are several strips, each containing individual antisera. At *right*, a large film for the study of several samples simultaneously with the same antiserum

Table 1. Optimal Conditions for Immunofixation of Some Serum Proteins

	Normal serum dilution	Antibody dilution
α_1-Antitrypsin	1:6	1:1
α_2-Macroglobulin	1:5	1:2
Cls	1:1	1:1
C3 (C3b, C3c)	1:5	1:1
C4	1:1	1:1
Gc Globulin	1:2	1:1
IgA	1:2	1:1
IgG	1:5	1:1
IgM	1:1	1:1
Properdin factor B	1:2	1:2
Transferrin	1:8	1:2

with a plastic plate that will bear and distribute a weight of 5 kg over a 10 × 20 cm area. The plate is kept under this pressure for 10 min. After careful removal of the absorbent pads, the thinned gel is washed in a 1-liter agitated-saline bath overnight, dried in a stream of cool air, and stained with Amido Black or Coomassie Brillant Blue in dilute acetic acid (50 ml/liter) exactly as for conventional protein electrophoresis.

Results

The improved resolution obtained with high-quality monospecific antiserum in this system presents convincing evidence that a given band or series of bands are a specific protein, regardless of the isoelectric point. The method described is easily applied to any protein present in a concentration exceeding 50 mg/liter. In the system described, similar results can be attained by adjusting the protein content by dilution of the sample and exposure of each dilution for a set period of time, or by exposure of each sample for periods of time ranging from 30 s to 10 min.

Electrophoresing excessive amounts of antigen decreases resolution and requires higher concentrations of antibody. If insufficient antibody is available the central portion of a protein band may remain unfixed through the process of antigen excess. For optimum

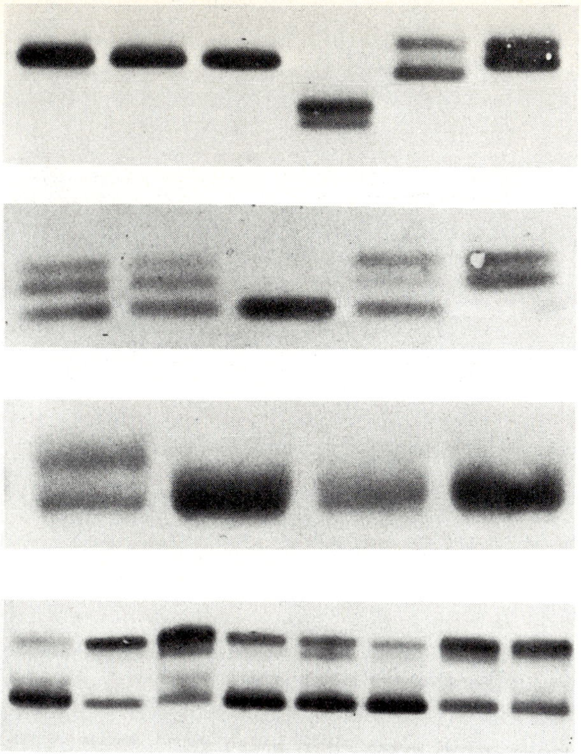

Fig. 3. Results of immunofixation studies of four different proteins that demonstrate genetic variation or different isoelectric points as the result of molecular degradation

Top to bottom: A, serum transferrin with three normals (*left*) and three genetic variants. *B,* serum Gc globulin showing the three normally encountered genetic variants. *C,* serum properdin Factor B, showing one variant. *D,* serum C3 studied with an antibody possessing activity against native C3 (*lower band*) and degraded C3c (*upper band*). Several lesser bands are present that represent activity against intermediate forms and products of C3 breakdown. Anode at the top. (Figures cropped to show only zone in which protein appears)

separation and sufficient intensity for visual detection or photometric recording, care must be taken in adjusting antibody content, sample concentration, time, and voltage. Table 1 lists conditions we found by trial and error to be optimal for several human serum proteins. Some final results are illustrated in Figure 3.

Consumption of high-quality antisera suitable for this technique is about 25 μl per square centimeter of cellulose acetate membrane, or, at the most, 100 μl per sample. With experience this can be decreased to 30 μl (by comparison, conventional immunoelectrophoresis requires 60 to 100 μl of antiserum).

Discussion

Microimmunoelectrophoresis and two-dimensional, crossed antigen-antibody electrophoresis have both been extensively used to study the microheterogeneity of human plasma proteins. Both have a common drawback not shared by immunofixation: long migration time with resulting low resolution. Immunofixation in the method described here combines excellent resolution produced by an extremely narrow application zone, rapid electrophoresis in a very thin gel, and anchoring of the protein by specific antibody within minutes after electrophoresis. The technique has the added value of allowing the worker to compare a band, as seen on immunofixation, with a band or zone seen with conventional protein electrophoresis in exactly the same system.

In the original technique (*1*), liquid antiserum was applied to the gel surface. In our experience, resolution was enhanced by the use of the membrane strip, which prevented diffusion of antigen upward and laterally in the liquid film. The membrane strips, also, considerably reduced the consumption of antiserum and prevented leakage of the material away from the desired area.

I thank Miss Karen Lee Tompson for assistance in preparation of the manuscript and the Department of Audiovisual Aids for illustrative material.

References

1. Alper, C. A., and Johnson, A. M., Immunofixation electrophoresis: A technique for the study of protein polymorphism. *Vox Sang.* **17,** 445 (1969).

2. Afonso, E., Quantitative immunoelectrophoresis of serum proteins. *Clin. Chim. Acta* **10,** 114 (1964).

3. Laurell, C-B., Antigen-antibody crossed electrophoresis. *Anal. Biochem.* **10,** 358 (1965).

4. Ritchie, R. F., Specific protein assay. *Fed. Proc.* **34,** 2139 (1975).

CLIN. CHEM. 22/4, 500–512 (1976)

On the Design of Clinical Chemistry Quality-Control Sera

George F. Grannis and W. Greg Miller[1]

Quality-control specimens having quantitative inter-specimen relationships were prepared by (*a*) making admixtures of two serum pools and (*b*) making various dilutions of the admixtures. The specimens were analyzed for many constituents to illustrate how the data obtained could be manipulated and used. The inter-related specimens permit the reduction of quality-control data to a few target values and should be particularly useful for the evaluation of multi-channel analyzers, and for use in inter-laboratory proficiency surveys. Aspects of the design of quality control and proficiency test specimens are also discussed.

Additional Keyphrases: *proficiency testing and proficiency test specimens • use of inter-related control specimens • variation, source of • biases • statistics*

Serum-based solutions of analytes (i.e., quality-control sera, proficiency-testing sera, and reference or calibration sera) have multiple uses in clinical chemistry. Quality-control sera are used extensively by laboratories to aid in the detection of analytical problems and to help assure the reliability of their analyses (*1–3*). Similar sera are used as proficiency testing specimens in inter-laboratory surveys (*4–6*). Such surveys are a valuable mechanism for establishing performance standards for groups of laboratories, for evaluating each laboratory with respect to its peers, and for comparing methods, instruments, and kits as they are used in the field (*7*). Serum-based solutions of analytes are also increasingly used as reference or calibration sera, particularly with multi-channel analyzers, and thus are used essentially as working standards for the routine analysis of clinical specimens (*8, 9*).

Division of Clinical Chemistry, Department of Pathology, Ohio State University, 410 W. 10th Ave. Columbus, Ohio 43210.

A preliminary report was presented at the 1974 National Meeting of the AACC, Las Vegas, Nevada. [*Clin. Chem.* **20**, 875 (1974)] Abstract.

[1] Dr. Miller was a postdoctoral trainee in clinical chemistry at Ohio State University 1973–75. His current address is: William T. Haebler Memorial Laboratory, New Rochelle Hospital Medical Center, New Rochelle, N. Y. 10802.

Received Sept. 15, 1975; accepted Feb. 9, 1976.

Most currently available quality-control, proficiency-testing, and reference sera are prepared from single, large pools of serum so that all specimens prepared from the pool are virtually identical, and are unrelated to specimens derived from other pools. Analyses of such specimens provide information that necessarily is restricted to a single concentration of each analyte. In addition, the use of these identical specimens has led to "systems" of quality control and proficiency testing that are based almost exclusively on replicative analyses, with periodic summarization of the data as the mean, and standard deviation or coefficient of variation (relative standard deviation) for each separate specimen.

Sera that have had quantitative inter-specimen relationships established during their preparation have been shown to offer alternative approaches to quality control and proficiency testing (*3, 10–14*). The advantages of inter-related specimens derive in part from the fact that the data from sets of such specimens can be combined in a variety of ways, even though the specimens are analytically unique, to provide information over a range of analyte concentration, and the data can be condensed to a few basic parameters.

The purpose of the present report is to describe and illustrate some concepts that underlie the design of serum-based solutions of analytes that have a variety of quantitative inter-specimen relationships.

Some Basic Considerations in the Design of Quality-Control and Proficiency-Testing Sera

(*a*) *Classes of analytical errors:* In general, quantitative analytical procedures involve the establishment of the relationship between some instrumental response and the concentration of an analyte. A specimen is then assayed by converting the instrumental response that it generates when carried through the analytical procedure to the equivalent concentration of standard analyte. Although there are numerous ways to accomplish each analysis, quality-control specimens are used primarily to assess the accept-

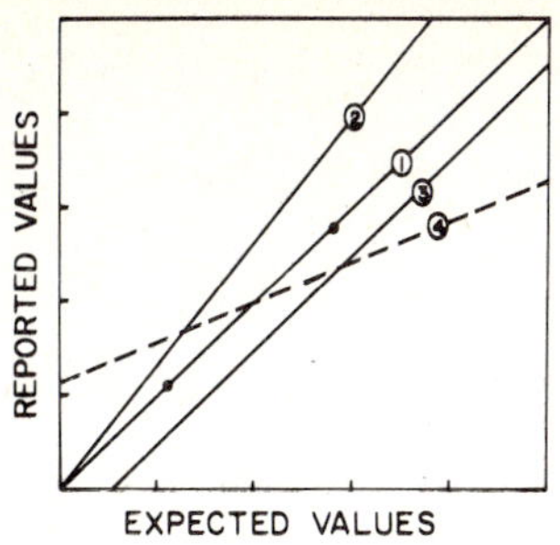

Fig. 1. Illustration of how analytic biases may affect the correlation of reported and expected results
See text for details

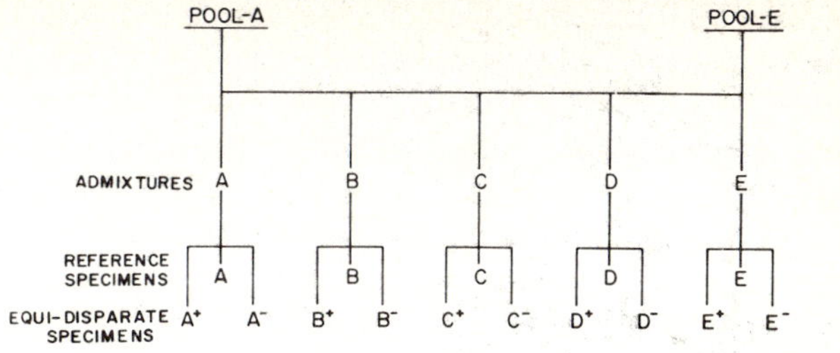

Fig. 2. Flow chart illustrating how quantitative inter-specimen relationships could be established
Master pools A and E are prepared with low and high concentrations of each analyte, and several admixtures are made. Specimens prepared from the admixtures with a nominal dispensing volume serve as reference specimens, while specimens prepared by dispensing more, or less, than the nominal volume provide high-low specimen pairs

ability of the final results obtained each time the procedure is performed, and to detect emergent problems of accuracy and precision (*3*). Similarly, proficiency surveys are conducted to assess the acceptability of final results obtained by various laboratories that use a variety of analytical procedures.

In this very general perspective of quality control and proficiency testing, the reported values for some analyte ideally should correspond exactly with the expected values and, when plotted as in Figure 1, the data should fall along the line of slope 1.0 (line 1). Analytical errors, or biases, can affect either the slope or intercept of line 1. Biases that affect only the slope of the line may be termed "Class I biases," and cause all reported results to be increased (line 2) (or decreased) by an amount that is *proportional* to analyte concentration. An example of an error that results in Class I bias is faulty method standardization caused by a too-concentrated or too-dilute standard solution.

Biases that affect only the intercept of line 1 may be termed "Class II biases," and cause all results to be shifted (increased or decreased) by a *constant* amount (line 3). An example of Class II bias might be an inappropriate "blank" or "baseline" correction. Line 4 illustrates the effects of a combination of Class I and II biases.

One reason that specimens having linear inter-relationships should be useful for quality control and proficiency testing is the fact that such specimens make it possible to assess with certainty the linear relationships between reported and expected values, and these relationships provide important clues to the nature of particular analytical problems. Similar specimens should be helpful for calibration purposes, wherever serum calibrators are appropriate, because the known relationships enhance the certainty of the calibration set-points and check-points, and thereby should facilitate the verification of proper method calibration at the time analyses are performed.

Other design considerations, such as the number of specimens necessary to evaluate these linear relationships, and the selection of appropriate analyte concentrations, are discussed in Appendix II of this report.

(*b*) *Technical considerations:* Although some liquid control sera are available (*12*), most commercial quality-control sera are lyophilized products, manufactured by preparing a large volume (hundreds or thousands of liters) of pooled sera, adjusting the pool to the desired constituent concentrations, and then dispensing it into small vials, which are lyophilized and sealed. These specimens are reconstituted by the user with distilled water or a prepared diluent.

There are many ways by which quantitative inter-specimen relationships could be established in the final product.[2] However, in practice a manufacturer is limited to a few simple operations, because time for processing the large volume pool must be kept to a minimum to avoid pool deterioration. Probably the simplest and most reliable operations (i.e., the most easily controlled and least subject to error) are: (1) on-line admixture of serum pools by use of an automatic proportioning device, and (2) controlled variation of the volumes dispensed into the final specimen vials. The following discussion will pertain to lyophilized specimens ostensibly prepared by a combination of these procedures, but either procedure alone probably could be adapted to achieve a similar result.

(*c*) *Establishing inter-specimen relationships, and their graphical representation:* A flow chart showing how a set of control sera might be prepared by these two techniques (admixtures, and variable dispensing volumes) is shown in Figure 2. Two serum pools, A and E, having analyte concentrations at the lower and upper parts of their analytical ranges, respectively, are prepared. Three admixtures of pools A and E are also prepared (pools B, C, D, Figure 2). Now, from each of the five pools pairs of specimens are dispensed by a technique that is best described as "equi-disparate" dispensing. In this technique a constant total volume is proportioned between two vials. For example, if the total volume, say 20 ml, were proportioned equally between the two vials each would

[2] We reject at the outset the notion (*11*) that laboratorians should routinely establish inter-specimen relationships for themselves—it is uneconomical for thousands of users to prepare and process multiple small batches of serum when a few manufacturers could more easily and reliably make these preparations on a large scale for all.

receive 10.0 ml. However, if the volume delivered to one vial were decreased, say to 9.0 ml, then the remaining 11.0 ml would be delivered to the second vial. When these vials are lyophilized and then reconstituted to the same final volume (e.g., 10.0 ml each), the concentration of each analyte will differ from that in the original admixture by amounts that are equal, but opposite in direction (Table 1).[3] These equi-disparate specimens will be referred to as high-low specimen pairs.

The interspecimen relationships that are established by this mode of preparation are illustrated in Figure 3, in which the analytical values for some analyte are graphed against the known percentage composition of the admixture pools. The values for the reference specimens should fall along a straight line that is described by its X-intercept and slope. Similarly, when all of the high-low specimen pairs are prepared with the same dispensing ratio, the values for the "high" and "low" members of the equi-disparate pairs fall along lines that have the same X-intercept as the reference line. The slopes of the latter two lines are greater or less than the slope of the reference line by a constant fraction that was fixed by the disparity in the volumes dispensed in the preparation of the specimens.

Several characteristics of the three sets of specimens illustrated in Figure 3 are noteworthy: (1) linear regression analysis of the analytical values on the corresponding percentage composition should yield three lines that have the same X-intercept and have slopes that differ by known proportions. Deviations of the slopes from expected values should usually be indicative of Class I biases, and deviations of the X-intercepts should usually be indicative of Class II biases. (2) The slope of the reference line has the dimensions concentration of analyte per percent of Pool E in the admixture. Hence the slope multiplied by 100 is a measure of the concentration of analyte in Pool E that is in excess of the analyte concentration in Pool A.[4] If the excess was caused by the addition of a known amount of analyte to pool E, then the recovery of added analyte may be calculated (*13*). (3) The ratio of the slope of the line on which the data from the "high" specimens fall to that of the "low" specimens is a constant, which is calculable from the known disparity in the volumes dispensed in the preparation of the specimens. (4) *All* analytes should demonstrate this *same* constant ratio of slopes. This fact is important because it means that when deviations from expected values are observed for one analyte, the results from other analytes may be examined to confirm that the deviation was in fact attributable to the analytical procedure and not to mistakes in the preparation or reconstitution of the specimens.

Table 1. The Concept of Equi-Disparate Dispensing

Specimen	Dispensed vol/specimen	Total vol/ specimen pair
	ml	
1a	10.0	20.0
1b	10.0	
2a	9.7	20.0
2b	10.3	
3a	9.0	20.0
3b	11.0	

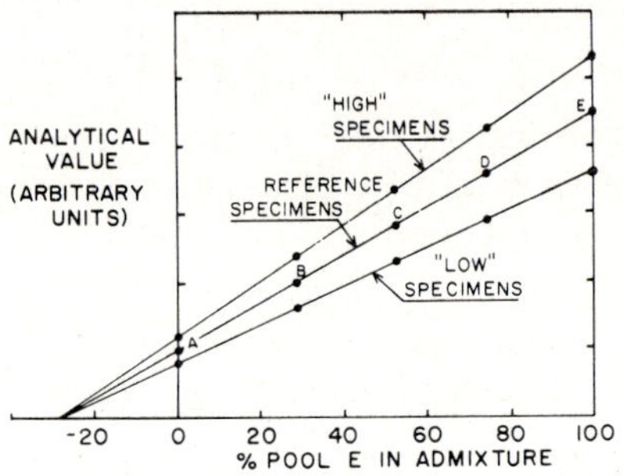

Fig. 3. When the results of analyses of control specimens prepared as illustrated in Figure 2 are plotted vs. the known percentage composition of the specimens, three straight lines should be obtained

The lines have a common origin, and their slopes differ by known proportions

(*d*) *An alternative graphical representation of the inter-specimen relationships.* The interspecimen relationships that are established by the procedure illustrated above (Figure 2) can also be presented as in Figure 4, in which the analytical values for some constituent in pools A, B, C, D, and E are plotted vs. their expected values, and should fall along the control line of slope 1.00. The analyte concentration in the "high" member of each specimen pair is plotted against that of the "low" member, and the data should fall along a line of constant slope. In this perspective, the constituent concentrations of pools A and E establish two *primary* reference points (Figure 4).

The constituent concentrations of the admixture pools B, C, and D may be calculated (rather than determined by independent analysis) from knowledge

[3] When lyophilized specimens are reconstituted, the final volume is somewhat greater than the volume of reconstitution fluid. The effect of this volume change on the inter-specimen relationships is discussed in Appendix I.

[4] This statement can be expressed mathematically: The equation of a straight line (e.g. the line of the "reference" specimens, Figure 3) is:

$$y = mx + b$$

in which m is the slope of the line and b is the Y-intercept. Rearranging,

$$(y - b) = mx$$

Let y be the total amount of analyte in Pool *E* (i.e., corresponding to 100% Pool *E*, Figure 3), and b the amount of analyte in Pool *A* (i.e., 0% Pool *E*, Figure 3). Then $(y - b)$ is the amount of analyte in Pool *E* in excess of that in Pool *A*. As x has a value of 100%,

$$(y - b) = 100\ m. \quad (1)$$

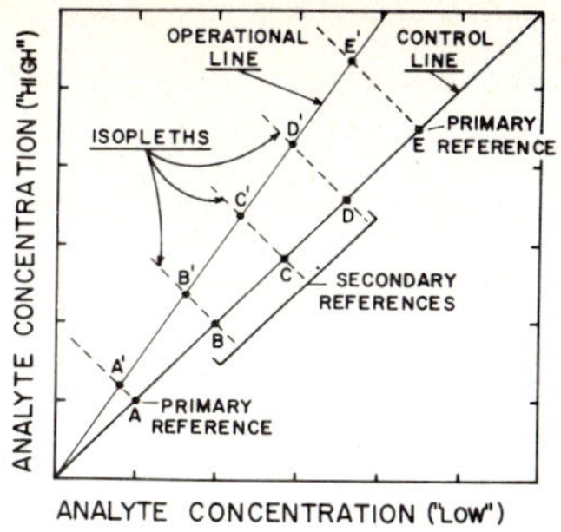

Fig. 4. Illustration of the inter-specimen relationships established by the procedure outlined in Figure 2

Specimens prepared from master pools A and E with a nominal dispensing volume provide primary reference points, and those from admixture pools B, C, and D provide secondary reference points. The references fall on the control line, and the intervals between the reference points are fixed by the admixture ratios used in the preparation of the specimens. The analyte concentrations in equi-disparate specimens prepared from the master and admixture pools provide points that fall along an operational line, the slope of which was fixed by the ratio of volumes dispensed in the preparation of the specimens. In addition, the latter points fall on the isopleth corresponding to each reference specimen. See text for details

of the constituent concentration of pools A and E and their relative proportions in each admixture.[5] Pools B, C, and D provide *secondary* reference points (Figure 4). The intervals on the control line between the primary and secondary reference points are fixed by the particular admixture ratios that were used in the preparation of the specimens. The intervals correspond to the percentage composition intervals illustrated in Figure 3.

When the constituent concentrations of the high members of each specimen pair are graphed vs. those of the low member (Figure 4, points A′, B′, C′, D′, and E′) each point will fall on an isopleth[6] that passes through the corresponding reference point. The displacement of each point from its reference value is fixed by the ratio of the volumes that were dispensed during the preparation of the specimen pair. Furthermore, because *all* specimen pairs were prepared with the *same* dispensing volume ratios, then the points A′, B′, C′, D′, and E′ should all fall along a line of constant slope, which is termed the *operational line* (Figure 4). The slope of the operational line is fixed by the ratio of the volumes that were dispensed in the preparation of the specimen pairs.

To summarize, the constituent concentrations of all of the specimens described in Figures 2, 3, and 4 are based on: (1) the constituent concentrations of the master pools A and E, which establish primary reference points, (2) the admixture ratios selected for the preparation of secondary pools B, C, and D, and (3) the dispensing ratios used in the preparation of the high-low specimen pairs. The admixture ratio fixes the isopleth intervals along the control line, and the dispensing ratio fixes the slope of the operational line.

Materials and Methods

As it was not practicable in our particular situation to prepare lyophilized specimens, we used an alternative approach to prepare sets of liquid specimens having relationships analogous to those described above, as follows.

Preparation of Master Pools

A pool having low values of each analyte (Pool A) was prepared by reconstituting a commercial lyophilized serum (Hyland QPAK-Chemistry Level 1)[7] with 0.6 the usual volume of water, and dialyzing briefly (20 min) against 10 volumes of water (0.0010-inch wall dialysis tubing; A. H. Thomas Co., Philadelphia, Pa. 19104). This brief dialysis was necessary to decrease the concentrations of urea, glucose, uric acid, creatinine, calcium, phosphorus and iron to the lower portion of their analytical ranges. The dialyzed serum was analyzed, the concentrations of Na^+, K^+, and Cl^- were adjusted to desired values with NaCl and KCl, and the serum was diluted to 0.8 of the reconstitution volume specified by the supplier.

A pool having high concentrations of analytes (Pool E) was prepared by reconstituting commercial lyophilized serum (Versatol A and Versatol A Alternate)[7] with 0.6 the specified usual reconstitution volume. We made additions of NaCl, KCl, $MgCl_2$, $CaCl_2$, $FeCl_3$, NaH_2PO_4, ferric ammonium citrate, urea, creatinine, creatine kinase (EC 2.7.3.2; Sigma rabbit muscle), alkaline phosphatase (EC 3.1.3.1; Sigma type I, calf intestinal mucosa), lactate dehydrogenase (EC 1.1.1.27; Sigma Type III, beef heart), and aspartate aminotransferase (EC 2.6.1.1; Sigma Type I, pig heart), thereby adjusting the analyte concentrations to the high portion of their analytical ranges, and the pool was then diluted to 0.8 of the reconstitution volume specified by the supplier.

Preparation of Admixtures

Three admixtures of Pools A and E were prepared as shown in Table 2 (Pools B, C, D). Thus, we produced five reference pools having constituent concentrations distributed over their analytical ranges. Portions of these five concentrated pools were diluted to the volume of the original lyophilized serum, and aliquots were frozen. These pools provide the primary and secondary reference points described in Figure 4.

[5] The capability for establishing reliable constituent values is being developed by the College of American Pathologists, with their "well-assayed" Survey Sera (*15*), and by various members of the National Committee for Clinical Laboratory Standards and other organizations with their studies of definitive and reference methods. Also, the kind of specimen described in the present report should facilitate the establishment of reliable constituent concentrations in multiple lots of quality-control sera.

[6] An isopleth is a line through points of constant value. The use of "equi-disparate" dispensing (or an equivalent procedure) in the preparation of the specimens causes the data points to fall on the isopleths of the reference points. The points on the isopleth represent specimen pairs for which the combined concentrations of each analyte are constant.

[7] Ideally, the same serum base material would be used in Pools A and E; however, this constraint is unimportant for the purpose of the present demonstration, and so we used these commerical materials, which happened to be readily available to us.

Table 2. Composition of Reference Pools

Pool	A	B	C	D	E
% Pool A	100	90	70	40	0
% Pool E	0	10	30	60	100
Admixture ratio[a]	0.000	0.100	0.300	0.600	1.000

[a] Admixture ratio = volume of pool E/total volume.

Preparation of Equi-disparate Specimen Pairs

The remainder of each of the concentrated pools A–E was used to prepare sets of high-low specimen pairs. For example, for one set, two portions of 36.0 ml and 44.0 ml were dispensed, each was diluted with water to the nominal reconstitution volume of 50.0 ml, and 5-ml aliquots were frozen. The dispensing ratio (D.R.) of these paired specimens is the ratio of the volume of reference pool, $V_{R,H}$, dispensed in the preparation of the high specimen to the volume, $V_{R,L}$, dispensed for the low specimen, as shown in equation (2):

$$\text{D.R.} = \frac{V_{R,H}}{V_{R,L}} \quad (2)$$

In this way, paired specimens having dispensing ratios of 1.11, 1.22, and 1.35 (i.e., ±5, 10, and 15% of the concentrations of the reference pools) were prepared. These specimens provide a variety of points along three operational lines.

Analysis of the Specimens

The specimens were submitted to the Ohio State University Clinical Chemistry Laboratory, and in one instance to another laboratory, for analysis. Details of the analytical methods are unimportant for the purpose of this study, which was simply to acquire real data to illustrate some of the theoretical concepts described above.

Results

Confirmation of the Inter-specimen Relationships

Results of four analyses for four analytes (determined simultaneously on a 4-channel AutoAnalyzer (Technicon Corp.) are presented in Figure 5 (*A–D*). The solid lines in these figures were calculated from (1) the initial analyses of master pools A and E, (2) the admixture ratios, and (3) the dispensing ratios used in the preparation of the specimens. In general, the analytical results are distributed as expected. That the exact relationships we believed to have been established in the preparation of the specimens had in fact been established was confirmed by calculating, from the analytical data for the four separate analyses, the apparent admixture and dispensing ratios, and comparing these determined values with the known ratios. The apparent admixture ratio (A.R.) was calculated for each analyte in each specimen pair from the equation:

$$\text{A.R.} = \frac{\tfrac{1}{2}(C_H + C_L) - C_A}{(C_E - C_A)} \quad (3)$$

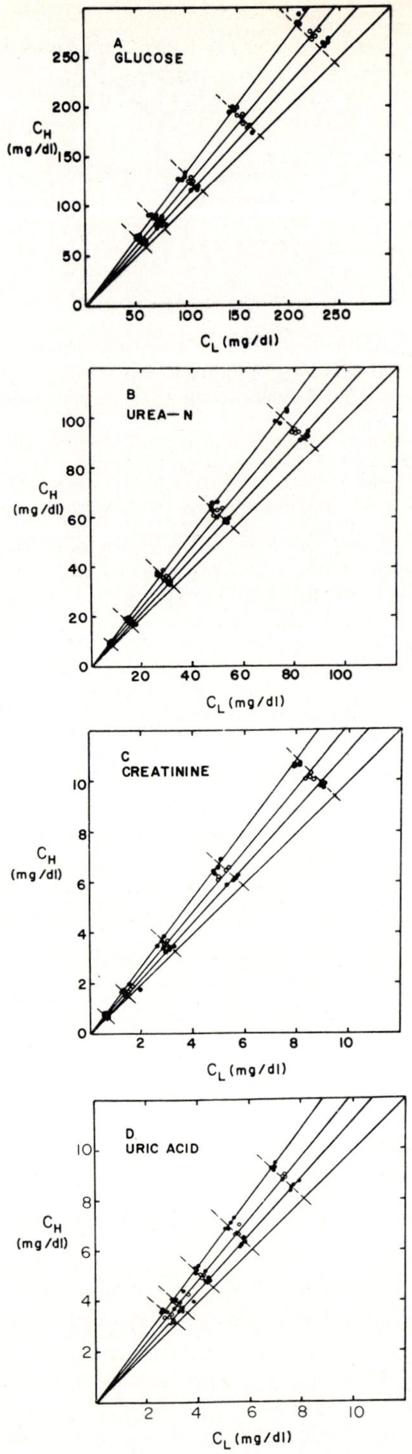

Fig. 5. (*A–D*) Results of four analyses, for four analytes, in three sets of specimens each set representing five concentration levels of each analyte

Each chart shows the control line of slope 1.00, three operational lines having slopes of 1.11, 1.22, and 1.35, and isopleths representing five concentration levels. These lines were established by the admixture and dispensing ratios used in the preparation of the specimens. The isopleths were positioned on the concentration scale by initial analyses of the master pools A and E. Analyses for glucose (*A*), urea nitrogen (*B*), creatinine (*C*), and uric acid (*D*) were performed on a four-channel AutoAnalyzer

Table 3. Comparison of the Determined Admixture (A.R.) and Dispensing (D.R.) Ratios with the Known Ratios

A.R. Expected	A.R. Found	D.R. Expected	D.R. Found
0.000	0.003	1.11	1.11
0.100	0.103	1.22	1.23
0.300	0.297	1.35	1.35
0.600	0.596		
1.000	1.008		

in which C_H and C_L are the analyte concentrations of the high and low members of each specimen pair, and C_A and C_E are the analyte concentrations in the master pools A and E. The slope (D.R.) of each operational line was determined by weighted linear regression analysis of the paired data (*15*). The weighting factor was the inverse of the variance of the analytical procedure at each concentration of analyte. The change in variance with concentration for each analytical procedure was available from routine quality-control data (*3*). The average values for A.R. and D.R. are compared with the theoretical values in Table 3, and demonstrate excellent agreement.

It should be noted that the data in Table 3 are based on only four analyses of each specimen pair, for four analytes. With ordinary control materials this amount of data (four values for each specimen) would be insufficient for a valid statistical analysis. However, because these specimens have quantitative interrelationships, the data from *all* of the specimens and for *all* analytes can be combined. Thus, for each of the five concentration levels there are 48 pieces of data (four analyses × three specimen pairs × four analytes) to evaluate each isopleth (A.R.), and there are 80 pieces of data (four analyses × five concentration levels × four analytes) available to evaluate the slope of each operational line (D.R.).

Evaluation of Accuracy

In most clinical chemical analyses, it is difficult to be certain of the true (i.e., the accurate) concentration of a particular analyte. However, *changes* in accuracy can easily be determined once a reference standard has been selected. In the present illustration the standard of reference is the analyte concentration initially established in master pools A and E. From these values the expected concentrations (C_e) in each reference admixture is calculated. The percentage difference between the analytically determined concentration and the expected concentration is given by the equation:

$$\% \text{ Difference} = [\tfrac{1}{2}(C_H + C_L) - C_e]/C_e \times (100) \quad (4)$$

in which C_H and C_L are the results of analyses of the high and low members of a specimen pair and C_e is the previously calculated expected, or reference, concentration. It is because the specimen pairs are prepared as equi-disparate specimens that the averages of the analyte concentrations should equal the concentration in the reference specimens.

Table 4. Percentage Difference Between Expected and Observed Concentrations in a Typical Analysis

Specimens: Admixture ratio	Specimens: Dispensing ratio	Urea nitrogen	Glucose	Uric acid	Creatinine
		Differences, %			
0.0	1.11	1.19	1.04	1.04	−1.52
	1.22	2.68	2.08	0.23	−7.27
	1.35	5.65	2.71	1.04	0.30
0.1	1.11	2.71	−0.88	0.06	2.45
	1.22	3.48	0.71	0.42	0.06
	1.35	3.48	0.39	0.42	−0.77
0.3	1.11	0.45	−2.46	0.89	−2.70
	1.22	0.45	−1.55	0.89	−2.67
	1.35	1.22	−2.89	0.89	−3.06
0.6	1.11	0.34	−0.88	−0.82	−2.62
	1.22	0.11	0.23	0.41	−3.02
	1.35	1.00	0.41	0.41	−3.02
1.0	1.11	1.08	1.87	0.97	−0.26
	1.22	−0.33	1.81	0.52	−1.29
	1.35	0.54	1.97	0.82	−1.31

Table 4 lists the percentage differences between the observed and expected concentrations in a typical analysis. In general, the values range between ±3%, as might be expected.

Accuracy can also be assessed by examining the data from each set of specimens, as was illustrated in Figure 3, and by calculating the X-intercept and slope for each set of specimens. These parameters, calculated from a single analysis of the specimens for the four analytes, are compared with the reference values in Table 5. The results show that the X-intercepts of all sets of specimens are very similar for each analyte, and that the slopes of the various sets bear the expected relationships to one another. That is, the ratio of slopes of the sets of high-low specimen pairs are in close agreement with the expected values. As was noted earlier and is documented in another report (*13*), the slope, multiplied by 100, is an estimate of the amount of analyte in Pool E that is in excess of that in Pool A and can be used to estimate percentage recovery of added analyte, or changes in recovery.

Evaluation of Precision

The precision of each test procedure can be measured as the coefficient of variation (relative standard deviation; CV) of the slope of the operational line. The coefficient of variation of the slope is calculated as the square root of the variance of the slope, expressed as a percentage of the slope (*15*).

Table 5. X-Intercepts, Slopes, and Ratio of Slopes of Three Sets of High-Low Specimen Pairs, Analyzed for Four Analytes

Specimen set	X-intercept Theoret.	X-intercept Observed	Slope Theoret.	Slope Observed	Ratio of slopes (H/L) Theoret.	Ratio of slopes (H/L) Observed
			Glucose			
1.11 H	−32.70	−30.0	1.944	2.011	1.11	1.12
L	−32.70	−30.9	1.759	1.797		
1.22 H	−32.70	−31.4	2.037	2.079	1.22	1.22
L	−32.70	−31.6	1.666	1.709		
1.35 H	−32.70	−30.6	2.129	2.194	1.35	1.37
L	−32.70	−31.3	1.574	1.597		
			Urea nitrogen			
1.11 H	−10.63	−10.1	0.840	0.853	1.11	1.11
L	−10.63	−10.5	0.760	0.767		
1.22 H	−10.63	−11.7	0.880	0.864	1.22	1.20
L	−10.63	−11.0	0.720	0.721		
1.35 H	−10.63	−11.6	0.920	0.917	1.35	1.34
L	−10.63	−10.8	0.680	0.685		
			Creatinine			
1.11 H	−7.17	−7.3	0.0939	0.0918	1.11	1.09
L	−7.17	−7.0	0.0850	0.0842		
1.22 H	−7.17	−7.5	0.0984	0.0956	1.22	1.20
L	−7.17	−7.0	0.0805	0.0796		
1.35 H	−7.17	−7.9	0.1029	0.0989	1.35	1.31
L	−7.17	−6.7	0.0760	0.0753		
			Uric acid			
1.11 H	−60.48	−60.1	0.0533	0.0536	1.11	1.09
L	−60.48	−59.1	0.0482	0.0492		
1.22 H	−60.48	−59.4	0.0558	0.0565	1.22	1.25
L	−60.48	−61.9	0.0457	0.0452		
1.35 H	−60.48	−57.5	0.0584	0.0588	1.35	1.35
L	−60.48	−59.9	0.0431	0.0436		

Table 6. Values Obtained for Four Analyses for Four Analytes

Slope of operational line D.R.	Coefficient of variation of slope of operational lines, %			
	Urea nitrogen	Glucose	Uric acid	Creatinine
1.11	1.45	1.37	1.35	1.11
1.22	1.18	1.28	1.00	0.90
1.35	1.04	1.25	1.44	0.79

There is analytical error in the determination of both variates, C_H and C_L. However, the actual concentrations of an analyte in a given specimen pair are within ±15% of the reference pool value because the dispensing ratios used in the preparation of the specimen were within these limits. Consequently, the variance of C_H is essentially the same as that of C_L, and regression of C_H on C_L yields a CV for the slope that accurately reflects the precision of the analytical method monitored. The coefficient of variation of the slope should be a sensitive measure of analytic variability caused by random errors (rather than systematic errors) because, if both specimens of a pair are treated identically in an analytical procedure, the resulting point on a graph such as Figure 4 or 5 should fall on the operational line, even though the method may be improperly standardized (i.e., inaccurate). Thus, the scatter of data about the operational line is due to random differences in the treatment of the two specimens and is reflected in the value of CV of the slope of the line. The values calculated from the four analyses for four analytes are listed in Table 6, and range to about 1.5%.

Method Evaluation by Inter-Constituent Relationships

To illustrate the use of these specimens for extended monitoring of a large number of laboratory procedures, pairs of specimens having an operational line slope (D.R.) of 1.22 were analyzed for 16 analytes on a random basis over a period of several weeks. The admixture ratios and slopes of the operational lines were calculated as before. The determined admixture ratios agreed closely with the theoretical ratios. However, the slopes revealed that two procedures, those for sodium and chloride, were subject to analytical bias. The slopes and the coefficient of variation of the

Table 7. Slope and Precision of Operational Lines

Analyte	Slope	CV for slope, %[a]
Urea nitrogen	1.22	0.78
Glucose	1.26	1.83
Uric acid	1.23	1.20
Creatinine	1.25	0.96
Sodium	0.93[b]	15.5
Potassium	1.21	0.73
Chloride	1.05[b]	6.44
Calcium	1.21	2.06
Magnesium	1.15	2.89
Inorganic phosphorus	1.20	4.10
Iron	1.25	0.85
Creatine phosphokinase	1.19	0.87
Lactate dehydrogenase	1.13	2.27
Aspartate aminotransferase	1.21	0.68
Alkaline phosphatase	1.24	2.04
LDH heart isoenzyme	1.28	5.12
Av	1.22	
Theoretical	1.22	

[a] Coefficient of variation of slope.
[b] Not included in average.

slopes for the 16 procedures are listed in Table 7. With the exception of sodium and chloride analyses, the slopes are in close agreement with the theoretical value; indeed, the average slope for the 14 methods having acceptable slopes is identical to the expected value. The fact that the analyses for 14 constituents confirm the theoretical ratio establishes unequivocally that the control materials had been prepared properly. Thus, it is clear that during this monitoring period both sodium and chloride analyses were noticeably biased.

The actual analytical data for sodium and chloride are graphed in Figure 6 (A and B) and for comparison the corresponding data for calcium, inorganic phosphorus, and blood urea nitrogen are given in Figure 6 (C, D, and E). It is clear that sodium and chloride analyses were subject to a systematic, concentration-dependent bias (combination of Class I and Class II biases) during the period of observation. This bias was not clearly evident from the results of analyses of the usual controls that were in routine use at the time. The cause of this bias will be discussed in a later report.

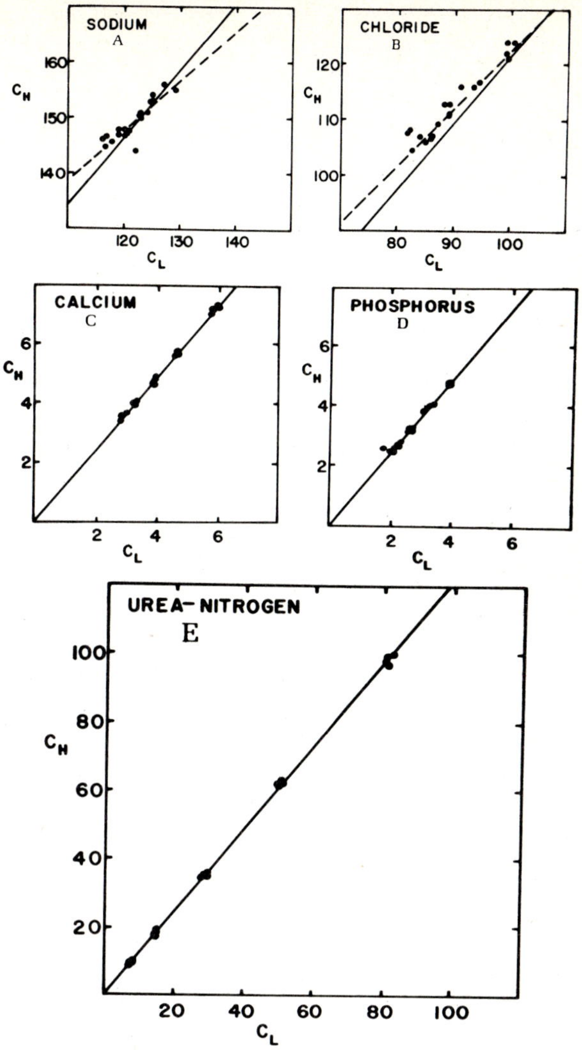

Fig. 6. (*A–E*). Results of repeated analyses of one set of specimens during several weeks

In each chart the expected operational line of slope 1.22 is shown by the *solid line,* and for sodium and chloride the best line calculated by linear regression analysis of the data is shown by the *dashed line.* Results for calcium, phosphorus, and urea nitrogen agree well with the expected relationship, which confirms that the specimens had been properly prepared, and that these analyses were well controlled during the period of observation. The results for sodium and chloride demonstrate concentration-dependent analytical bias

Use of Control Specimens for Performance Evaluation of Multichannel Analyzers

Specimens having quantitative relationships should have special relevance for the evaluation of multi-channel analyzers, which are often routinely standardized at a single concentration of each analyte. To illustrate how such specimens might be used, we asked another laboratory to analyze a single set of three specimen pairs (DR = 1.11; AR = 0.00, 0.300, 1.00) one time only, on each of their two SMA 12/60 (Technicon Corp.) analyzers. The results obtained for blood urea nitrogen on both instruments are illustrated in Figure 7, and the results for 12 constituents, analyzed on one instrument, are illustrated in Figure 8.

In Figure 7 the target values (i.e., the intersection of the isopleths with the operational line of slope 1.11) were determined in our laboratory. The analytical values were determined on the two SMA 12/60 analyzers. The figure shows (1) generally good agreement of both laboratories over the full analytical range, and (2) a small difference in the two SMA 12/60 analyzers, which is concentration dependent. The discrepancy is probably attributable to a small difference in the calibration of the two instruments (Class I bias).

In Figure 8 all of the data points fall close to the

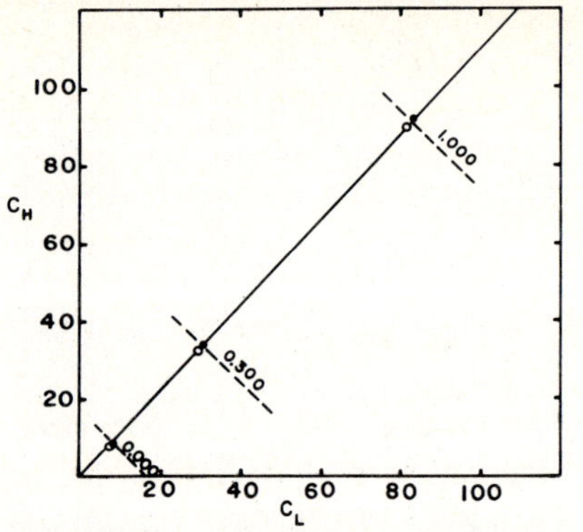

Fig. 7. Comparison of urea-nitrogen determinations by three instruments in two laboratories

The slope of the operational line (*solid line*) and the isopleth (*dashed lines*) intervals were established in the preparation of the specimens. The position of the isopleths on the concentration scale was established in Laboratory No. 1, which used an AutoAnalyzer. The data points are the results of analyses by Laboratory No. 2, which used two SMA 12/60 analyzers. (The *open circles* and *dots* represent SMA No. 1 and No. 2, respectively.) The results show that the AutoAnalyzer and SMA No. 2 were in nearly exact agreement over a large concentration range, but that SMA No. 1 was apparently subject to concentration-dependent bias

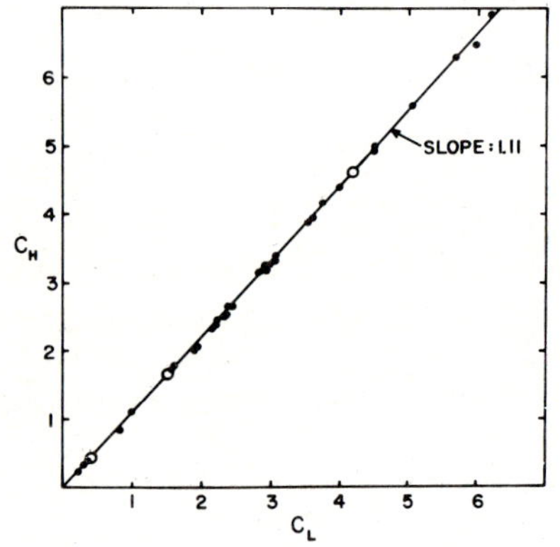

Fig. 8. Results of a single analysis of three specimen pairs for 12 analytes with use of an SMA 12/60

All data were placed on a single chart by using the following scale factors: Bilirubin, inorganic phosphorus, albumin: X1; creatinine, uric acid, calcium and total protein: X2; urea-nitrogen, alkaline phosphatase: X20; cholesterol, lactate dehydrogenase, and aspartate aminotransferase: X50. The data fall along the expected operational line of slope 1.11. The *open circles* indicate the urea-nitrogen analyses. The isopleths for each constituent are not shown as they (a total of 36 lines) would obscure the data. However, see Figure 9 for further evaluation of these data

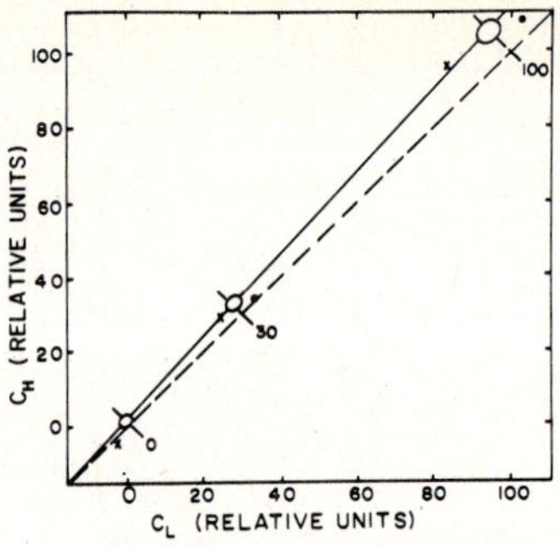

Fig. 9. Illustration of the massive data reduction made possible by use of specimens having quantitative inter-relationships

The data of Figure 6 (i.e., 72 analyses: three specimen pairs, 12 analytes) have been converted to relative units and re-graphed. The relative units represent the percentage composition of the reference pools. Reference points for all analytes occur where the isopleths labeled 0, 30, and 100 intersect the control line (*dashed line*). The reference points correspond to master pool A (0% E), an admixture of pools A and E which contains 30% E, and master pool E (100% E). The expected, or target, points occur where the isopleths intersect the operational line of slope 1.11. For each analyte, the concentrations of pool A and E, as determined by one SMA 12/60, were assigned relative values of 0 and 10. The analyses from the other SMA 12/60 were then converted to these relative units and graphed. With the exception of two analytes, all data fell within the ovals surrounding the target values. Bilirubin analysis (X) was clearly out of limits, and cholesterol (O) analyses deviated noticeably from the target values

theoretical operational line, and to the appropriate isopleths (the individual isopleths are not shown in Figure 8).

The data of Figure 8, which represent 72 analytic values (12 analytes, 6 specimens) can be condensed in several ways. For example, the data may be converted to relative units and regraphed as shown in Figure 9. The operational line and isopleth intervals shown in the figure are those that were introduced in the preparation of the specimens. A scale of relative units (which relates each analyte concentration to the % composition of the admixtures) was established from the data from one SMA 12/60, and the data from the other SMA 12/60 were read from this scale. The results for 10 of the 12 analytes fell within the limits indicated for each target value. The values for one analyte (bilirubin) were clearly out of these limits and the values for another analyte (cholesterol) also deviated noticeably from the target values. The reason for these deviations was that these analytes were present in similar concentrations in all of the specimens. Consequently, small changes in analytical values resulted in large percentage changes when expressed as relative units. Nevertheless, Figure 9 illustrates how the data from multiple specimens and multiple analytical procedures can be reduced to a very few common target values.

Alternatively, the data of Figure 7 could also be summarized as the X-intercept and slope for each set of specimens (see Figure 3 and Table 5).

Discussion

Significance of Results

Effective quality control in the clinical chemistry laboratory involves the collaborative efforts of all laboratory personnel—analysts, supervisors, and chemistry laboratory director—with frequent and open communication concerning various laboratory problems. Thus, quality-control data are used by various individuals who have differing perspectives of the laboratory operation. The specimens described in this report are designed to yield data that can be examined selectively in various formats that are most appropriate for each level of interest.

Analysts. For example, the analysts, at any one time, are interested primarily in the most recent quality-control data relevant to those specific analyses for which they are individually responsible. All analytical procedures are attended by a host of potential sources of error, and control specimens are used to detect emergent or unanticipated problems or to document the absence of such problems. The format illustrated by Figures 3 or 4 should be particularly useful for routine monitoring of individual analytical procedures. The data points illustrated might be acquired one by one in successive analytical runs, but results could be monitored either graphically, as shown, or by tabulation of the apparent X-intercept, slope, and (or) apparent recovery (Table 5). The latter variables should be particularly helpful in assuring reproducible standardization of each method, and when a problem is indicated a full set of linear specimens could be analyzed to help identify the nature of the problem.

Laboratory supervisors are interested in a larger number of procedures, performed by several analysts, and over a longer period of time. The format illustrated in Figures 7 and 8 should be helpful in the simultaneous evaluation of groups of related tests, such as those performed in each supervisorial area, or those performed on multi-channel analyzers. The cumulative data from such analyses can be summarized in terms of the means and standard deviations of the admixture and dispensing ratios (Table 3), or in terms of the X-intercept and slope of the operational lines (Table 7). These data provide a very concise summary because all constituents have the same target values. That is, all Y-intercepts should have a value of 0.0 and the slopes (D.R.) should all have the same values. Table 7 and Figure 6 (*A–E*) illustrate how problems can be readily detected by examination of these data.

The chemistry laboratory director is interested in the quality of total laboratory performance in relation to past performance, and in relation to the performance of other laboratories and to other analytical methods. The format illustrated in Figure 9, or a tabulation of basic data as illustrated in Table 3 should be useful for rapidly assessing overall laboratory performance and identifying apparent problem areas.

Rationale Underlying the Design of Inter-related Specimens

Quality-control and proficiency-testing data can be viewed in either graphical or tabular format, and the data may be processed manually or by computer with peripheral visual display or printing devices. Specimens having quantitative inter-relationships yield data that can be processed and displayed in many different ways in addition to those described in this report. To aid in the development of these various approaches it may be helpful to consider in more detail the rationale underlying the design of the specimens. Figure 1 shows how inter-related specimens may be prepared from two serum pools simply by varying (1) the admixture proportions of the pools, and (2) the volumes dispensed from the admixtures in the preparation of specimen pairs. Figures 3 and 4 illustrate the relationships established by this preparative procedure.

Any point on a graph such as Figure 4 can be specified in two coordinate systems. For example, point C' in Figure 4 has the rectilinear coordinates (C_2,C_1), in which C_2 and C_1 represent the analyte concentrations in the high and low members of a pair of specimens. Point C' can also be specified as the intersection of the operational line, for which the slope is the dispensing ratio used in the preparation of the specimens, and of the isopleth, the relative position of which along the control line is the admixture ratio used in the preparation of the specimens. This dual-coordinate system means that a manufacturer might vary target values of a set of control specimens in a very predictable manner simply by varying the admixture and dispensing ratios, while the user, functioning on the usual rectilinear coordinate system is expected to "hit" the appropriate targets.

Although there are several possible ways to evaluate these relationships, we used the concept of the operational line and iospleth because *all* constituents in a set of specimens prepared in this manner should have the *same* operational lines and isopleths. This means that all analytical results may be displayed in a common graphical format. *Each* constituent may be examined over its full analytical range (e.g., on a graph such as Figure 3 or 7), or *all* constituents may be examined simultaneously at selected concentrations, as in Figure 8 or 9. Charts such as Figures 3, 7, 8, and 9 might be termed "universal" control charts, because data from all areas of a laboratory could be displayed in a consistent, concise, and easily interpretable format. In addition, all data could be summarized statistically in terms of the variability of the slope and Y-intercept of the operational line, and of the isopleth values—values that should be respectively identical for all constituents.

Other Considerations in the Design of Serum-based Specimens

The specimens described above are deficient for some purposes, such as "blind" controls or for proficiency surveys, in which ideally the analyst should be unaware that inter-specimen relationships exist, because a knowledgeable analyst could deduce the inter-specimen relationships from the results of assays for a few analytes. This deficiency could be overcome by preparing the specimens from admixtures of three master pools, rather than two. For example, suppose that specimens similar to those for which the analyses are illustrated in Figure 8 had been prepared as described except that a constant amount of a third pool had been added to each initial admixture. The effect would be to displace each target value from the common operational line; the magnitude of the displacement would vary from constituent to constituent, depending on their concentrations in the third master pool. The target's inter-relationships could be obscured to the user but would be readily calculable from knowledge of the exact details of the specimen preparation.

This concept of using triple admixtures has other implications. Suppose that several lots or batches of specimens were to be manufactured sequentially. The introduction of a small, constant amount of a third pool into each batch could provide a common quantitative element that could be used to firmly establish the inter-lot consistency or reproducibility of target values.

Although we have not implemented the use of these control materials in our routine quality-control program, because of the impracticality of manufacturing the large volumes required for routine quality control, we do use such specimens for investigating problems brought to light in our routine quality-control program. We believe the various concepts discussed herein may be helpful to others, particularly manufacturers of control sera, in developing further applications of such sera.

We are grateful to Drs. H.-D. Gruemer and J. A. Lott for helpful advice in the course of our studies, and to Mrs. Kay Cook for secretarial assistance. We are especially appreciative of the aid of many technologists in the Ohio State University Hospital Clinical Chemistry Laboratory. The Instructional and Research Computing Center of Ohio State University provided facilities and assistance in the analysis of our data.

References

1. Levey, S., and Jennings, E. R., Use of control charts in the clinical laboratory. *Am. J. Clin. Pathol.* **20,** 1059 (1950).

2. Copeland, B. E., Ed., *Quality Control Manual.* The American Society of Clinical Pathologists, Chicago, Ill., 1960.

3. Grannis, G. F., Gruemer, H.-D., Lott, J. A., et al., Proficiency evaluation of clinical chemistry laboratories. *Clin. Chem.* **18,** 222 (1972).

4. *Quality Evaluation Program, 1975 Survey Manual,* College of American Pathologists, Skokie, Ill.

5. *Guide to Proficiency Testing. Proficiency Testing, Dec., 1972* Center for Disease Control, Atlanta, Ga.

6. Laessig, R. H., Schwartz, T. H., and Paskey, T. A., Cooperative survey of "SMA" Analyzers in Wisconsin—A method of improving interlaboratory performance. *Clin. Chem.* **19,** 62 (1973).

7. *Participant Summary: Chemical Procedures, and Chemistry Kits Data.* College of American Pathologists, 1975.

8. Technicon SMA Reference Serum. *Technical Data Bulletin,* Technicon Instruments Corp., Tarrytown, N. Y. 10591, 1972.

9. Calibrate Automated Lock-in. *Technical Bulletin 901G530* General Diagnostics, Division Warner-Lambert Co., Morris Plains, N. J. 07950, 1974.

10. Grannis, G. F., An optimum system of quality control. *Clin. Chem.* **19,** 649 (1973). Abstract.

11. Bowers, G. N., Jr., Burnett, R. W., and McComb, R. B., Preparation and use of human serum control materials for monitoring precision in clinical chemistry. *Clin. Chem.* **21,** 1830 (1975).

12. Frajola, W. J., A stable liquid human reference serum. *Health Lab. Sci.* (1976). In press.

13. Grannis, G. F., Interlaboratory survey of enzyme analyses I. Preliminary studies. *Am. J. Clin. Pathol.* (1976). In press.

14. Grannis, G. F., Studies of the reliability of consensus target values obtained in inter-laboratory surveys. *Clin. Chem.* (1976). In press.

15. *Surveys/75 Manual,* p *xi,* College of American Pathologists, Skokie, Ill., 1975.

16. Steel, R. G. D., and Torrie, J. H., *Principles and Procedures of Statistics,* McGraw-Hill, New York, N.Y., 1960, pp 161–182.

Appendix I. Inter-Specimen Relationships in Lyophilized Specimens

Although our studies were conducted with liquid specimens, most commercial sera are lyophilized products. The process of lyophilization and reconstitution is associated with volume changes which, although minor, may alter some constituent inter-relationships, and should be discussed.

Suppose that a series of specimens were prepared as was proposed—by dispensing various volumes (e.g., 10.6, 10.0, or 9.4 ml) from a reference pool and lyophilizing. When these specimens are later reconstituted by dissolving in a constant volume (e.g., 10.0 ml) of water, the final volume will be greater than 10.0 ml owing to the "solution volume" of the total solids of the specimen. The solution volume is primarily a function of the total protein concentration, and for various sera should range from about 5 to 8% of the dispensed volumes. Equations for calculating the essential parameters in lyophilized specimens are derived as follows:

1. Slope of the operational line: Let: Cp represent a constituent concentration in a reference pool. V_D^H, V_D^N, V_D^L represent the *v*olumes *d*ispensed in the preparation of *H*igh, *N*ormal, and *L*ow specimens, respectively. C_H, C_N, C_L represent the constituent *c*oncentration in the reconstituted High, Normal, and Low specimens. V_R^H, V_R^N, V_R^L represent the volumes of the *r*econstituted high, normal, and low specimens, respectively. Then the following equalities exist:

$$C_P \times V_D^H = C_H \times V_R^H \quad (5)$$

$$C_P \times V_D^N = C_N \times V_R^N \quad (6)$$

$$C_P \times V_D^L = C_L \times V_R^L \quad (7)$$

Rearranging:

$$C^H = \frac{C_P \times V_D^H}{V_R^H} \quad (8)$$

$$C_N = \frac{C_P \times V_D^N}{V_R^N} \quad (9)$$

$$C_L = \frac{C_P \times V_D^L}{V_R^L} \quad (10)$$

The slope of the operational line is then:

$$\frac{C_H}{C_L} = \frac{C_P \times V_D^H}{V_R^H} \times \frac{V_R^L}{C_P \times V_D^L} \quad (11)$$

$$= \frac{V_D^H}{V_D^L} \times \frac{V_R^L}{V_R^H} \quad (12)$$

The reconstituted volumes are calculated from the relations:

$$V_R^H = (V_0 + k \cdot V_D^H) \quad (13)$$

$$V_R^N = (V_0 + k \cdot V_D^N) \quad (14)$$

$$V_R^L = (V_0 + k \cdot V_D^L) \quad (15)$$

in which V_0 is the volume of water added to reconstitute the specimen, and k is the fraction of the dispensed volume that will contribute to the reconstituted volume. Equation 12 is then expanded to:

$$\frac{C_H}{C_L} = \frac{V_D^H}{V_D^L} \times \frac{(V_0 + k \cdot V_D^L)}{(V_0 + k \cdot V_D^H)} \qquad (16)$$

Thus, the slope of the operational line is calculated from the volumes dispensed during the preparation and reconstitution of the specimens, with correction for the solids content of the reference pool.

2. Slope of the isopleth: The slope of the isopleth is given by the relation:

$$\text{slope} = \frac{C_H - C_N}{C_L - C_N} \qquad (17)$$

Substituting from equations 8, 9 and 10:

$$\text{slope} = \frac{\dfrac{C_P \times V_D^H}{V_R^H} - \dfrac{C_P \times V_D^N}{V_R^N}}{\dfrac{C_P \times V_D^L}{V_R^L} - \dfrac{C_P \times V_D^N}{V_R^N}} \qquad (18)$$

Rearranging and simplifying,

$$\text{slope} = \frac{V_R^L}{V_R^H} \times \frac{V_D^H \times V_R^N - V_D^N \times V_R^H}{V_D^L \times V_R^N - V_D^N \times V_R^L} \qquad (19)$$

As the volumes are known, or can be calculated (equations 13, 14, 15), the isopleth slope can be calculated.

3. Calculation of the constituent concentrations expected in the high and low specimens, when the concentration in the "normal" specimen is known: Rearranging equation 9:

$$C_P = C_N \times \frac{V_R^N}{V_D^N} \qquad (20)$$

Substituting this equality for C_P in equation 8 and rearranging:

$$C_H = C_N \times \frac{V_R^N}{V_R^H} \times \frac{V_D^H}{V_D^N} \qquad (21)$$

Similarly:

$$C_L = C_N \times \frac{V_R^N}{V_R^H} \times \frac{V_D^L}{V_D^N} \qquad (22)$$

Thus, the expected concentrations in the high and low specimens can be calculated (equations 21, 22) from the values determined for the calibration specimen (C_N) and from the volumes dispensed in the manufacture of the specimens and the volumes of the reconstituted specimens.

4. Inverse relationships: The above equations are applicable to any constituent for which the unit reported is directly proportional to analyte concentration (e.g., glucose and most other constituents). The equations must be modified for determinations such as T_3 uptake, in which an *increase* in the critical analyte (thyroid binding globulin) results in a *decreased* unit of measure. The modification simply involves interchanging the values for the high-low specimens or, alternatively, calculating as for the other constituents in which case the predicted operational line will have a slope less than, rather than greater than, 1.0.

Appendix II. Aspects of the Compositional Design of Quality-Control Specimens

Quality-control and proficiency-testing specimens are used to assess the analytical reliability of results, and to ascertain whether medically useful results are being produced by a laboratory. The constituent concentrations of such specimens should therefore be adjusted to permit (*a*) evaluation of accuracy over the full analytical range of each analyte and (*b*) routine monitoring of precision at clinically critical concentrations of analytes—i.e., at those concentrations at which clinical decisions are made.

A rationale for selecting appropriate constituent concentrations can be developed as follows:

When the determined values for a constituent of control specimens are plotted against the expected values, a straight line of slope 1.0 and intercept 0.0 *should* be obtained. Various factors can cause this line to have a slope other than 1.0 and an intercept other than 0.0, and these parameters can fluctuate from day to day (*3*).

One purpose of quality-control specimens is to evaluate the slope, intercept and variability of this line for each constituent. To make this evaluation valid at least five points along the line should be determined. Thus, there should be at least five control specimens available that cover the full analytical range of each constituent.

Figure 10 shows the frequency distribution of glucose values observed in a typical hospital population. Quality-control specimens, particularly those introduced into the laboratory as "blinds", should have glucose concentrations that are near clinical decision levels (i.e., those values used as cut-off values in evaluating borderline hypo- and hyper-glycemia, and the peak of the glucose tolerance curve), but that are not

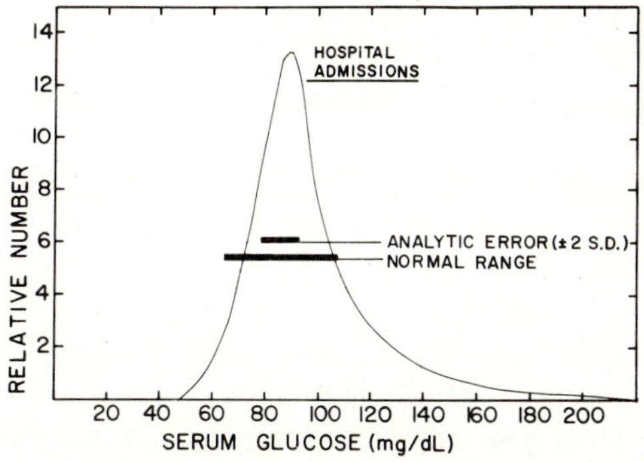

Fig. 10. Frequency distribution of glucose analyses performed on 650 consecutive patients admitted to a hospital
The normal range, and the range of the laboratory's long-term analytical error is indicated. These data provide a basis for deciding the analyte concentrations at which the glucose method ought to be monitored

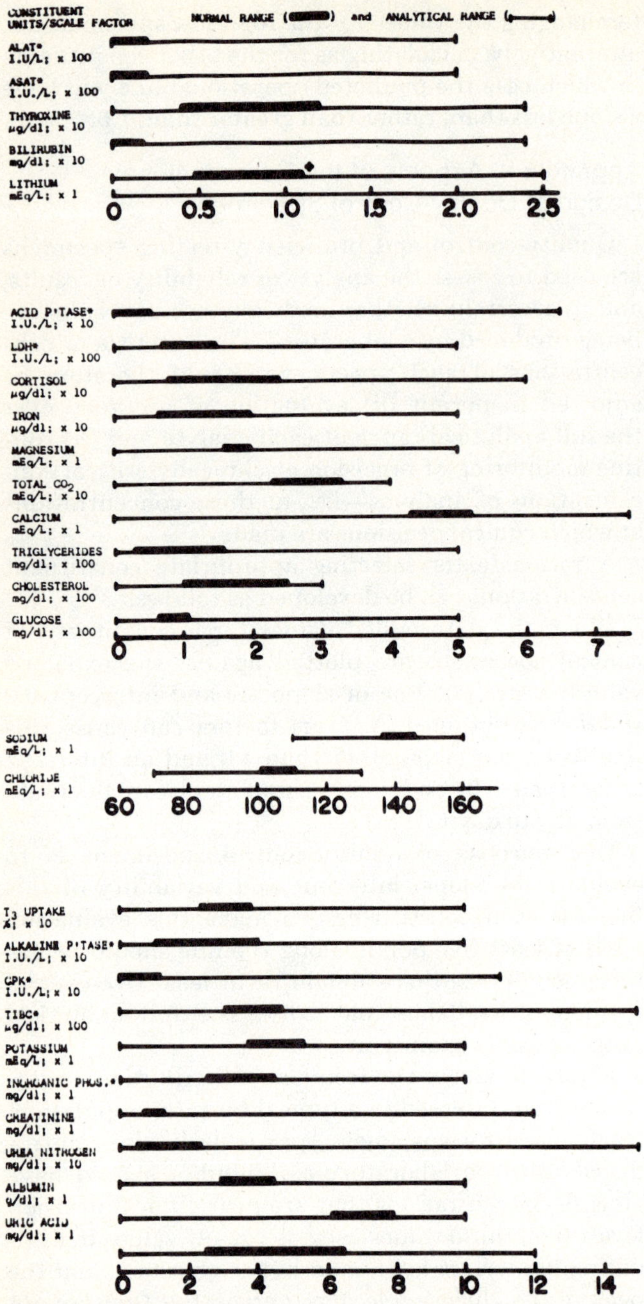

Fig. 11. Graphical summary of the analytical and normal ranges of 28 analytes

For each analyte, the indicated scale factor should be applied. The range indicated for lithium is the therapeutic range. Abbreviations are:

ALAT:	Alanine aminotransferase
ASAT:	Aspartate aminotransferase
P'TASE:	Phosphatase
LDH:	Lactate dehydrogenase
CPK:	Creatine phosphokinase
TIBC:	Total iron-binding capacity
PHOS:	Phosphorus

so extreme as to be obvious. Thus, control sera should include glucose concentrations of about 60, 130, and 160 mg/dl. Similarly, for each constituent, those concentrations most appropriate for clinical monitoring can be defined so as to be compatible with the routine clinical specimens.

As a generalization, then, the constituent concentrations of controls should range from about 10% to 90% of the analytical range for most analytes, and should include the clinically critical concentrations. The latter concentrations for many analytes will be around the 10th and 90th percentiles of the distribution of values observed in a healthy population. Thus, for glucose, which for many methods has an analytical range of about 300 mg/dl, a set of control specimens should have the approximate concentrations: 60, 120, 160, 220, and 280 mg/dl.

Because serum-based specimens are used primarily to assure the analytical and clinical reliability of laboratory analyses, there is no compelling reason why *all* constituents should be at either above- or below-normal concentrations, or all at normal or abnormal concentrations. Rather, analytes should be combined in patterns that yield the greatest amount of useful information with the least amount of redundant information.

As an aid in approaching the compositional design of specimens, we have prepared Figure 11, which presents the analytical range and the normal range for 28 procedures performed in our laboratory. Assuming that five different concentrations of each analyte are to be monitored, the two master pools A and E would have their concentrations of each analyte adjusted to near the lower and upper limits of the analytical range. Then various admixture ratios must be selected to provide specimens having analyte concentrations at the clinical decision levels, as well as to provide specimens for monitoring the remainder of each analytical range.

Although the formulation of such specimens appears to be rather complex, the problem can be simplified by having certain constituents elevated in Master pool A, and other constituents elevated in Master pool E. By judicious selection of the combination of analytes in the master pools, and careful choice of admixture ratios, it should be possible to prepare a variety of serum-based specimens that are designed specifically to fulfill their several important functions in clinical chemistry.

CLIN. CHEM. 22/4, 513–518 (1976)

Comparison of Three Procedures for Isolating Human Ferritin, for Use as a Standard in an Immunoradiometric Assay

Lorraine M. Gonyea, Colleen M. Lamb, R. Dorothy Sundberg, and Amos S. Deinard

We evaluated three methods for isolating ferritin, for use as a standard, with respect to purity of the products, ease of preparation, and yield. Examination of the respective products by gel filtration on Sephadex G-200 and Sepharose 6B suggested that the preparations isolated by ammonium sulfate and cadmium sulfate precipitation (Method 1) and by ultracentrifugation (Method 2) were homogeneous, while the product of a procedure including precipitation with ammonium sulfate (Method 3) contained significant amounts of nonferritin protein. The ratios of ferritin as measured by immunoradiometric assay to the amount of protein in the product indicated the ferritin prepared by Method 1 to be the most highly purified. Methods 1 and 2 were both comparatively simple. Although the yield from Method 1 was lowest, it is probably the method of choice, on the basis of the ease of obtaining a highly purified product. The most appropriate method for estimating protein in the isolated preparations appears to be that of Lowry et al.

Immunoradiometric analysis (IRMA) (*1*) has made it possible to measure ferritin in serum at normal and decreased concentrations as well as at increased concentrations. Clinical studies have shown that estimation of serum ferritin by this technique is useful (*2–4*).[1] At the present time the biological reagents required for this assay are not available commercially, and the methods for preparing them are therefore of interest to clinical laboratories that are considering offering this assay.

Departments of Laboratory Medicine and Pathology, and Pediatrics, University of Minnesota Hospitals, Minneapolis, Minn. 55455.

[1] *Ed. note:* Readers should be alerted to an important paper that casts serious doubt on serum ferritin values as an index to iron stores in precirrhotic familial hemochromatosis [*New Engl. J. Med* **294,** 302 (Feb. 5, 1976), and editorial, p 333].

Received Dec. 8, 1975; accepted Feb. 9, 1976.

Ferritin can be isolated from tissue in a highly purified state with relative ease. Properties of ferritin that have been exploited for this purpose include water solubility, stability up to 80 °C, insolubility in half-saturated $(NH_4)_2SO_4$ and in $CdSO_4$, and its large molecular weight (> 450 000). The purity of the standard for measuring ferritin in serum is the main criterion in choosing a method for isolation, although the ease with which it can be prepared and the yield have practical significance as well.

Estimation of the protein content of the purified preparations is the basis for standardization of the IRMA. Because the ferric component of ferritin greatly increases the absorptivity from the apoprotein at 210, 280, and 310 nm, the method for measuring the protein must be selected with care.

The following is a report of our observations with respect to these considerations. We compared the classical method of Granick (*5*) with two more-recent methods (*6, 7*) for the isolation of ferritin from human spleens. Results for ferritin, apoferritin, and bovine serum albumin were compared by the Lowry et al. (*8*), biuret (*9*), and Tombs et al. (*10*) methods for estimating protein concentration.

Materials and Methods

Isolation and Purification of Ferritin

Spleens obtained at surgery or autopsy were processed within 24 h or after storage at −70 °C. Some were assumed to be rich in ferritin because of the patients' histories, while others were unknown in this respect. The three methods used for purification were based on studies of Granick (*5*), Penders et al. (*6*), and Linder and Munro (*7*).

The procedures were done at room temperature, except where indicated. All centrifuging was done at 4 °C.

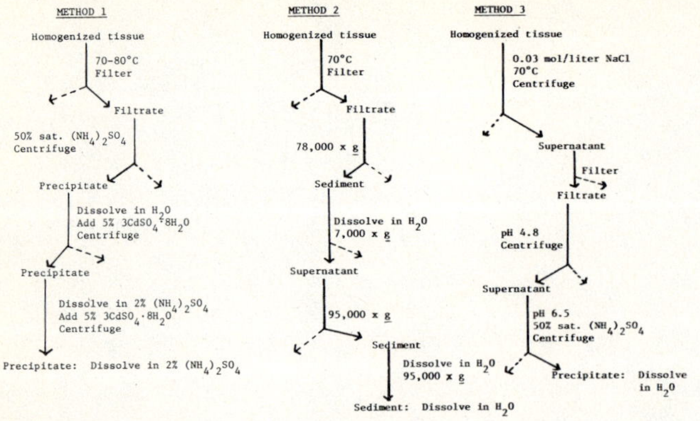

Fig. 1. Flow diagram for three methods for isolating ferritin from human spleen
The broken arrows indicate discarded fractions

Method 1 (Granick, *5*) (Figure 1). The spleen was sliced, homogenized in a Waring Blendor with a volume of distilled water equivalent to 1.5-fold the weight of the tissue, and brought to 70–80 °C for 10 min. The coagulated protein was removed by filtration (Schleicher and Schuell No. 520-B), and $(NH_4)_2SO_4$ was added to the filtrate to half-saturation (2.4 mol/liter). After 18 h at 4 °C, the insoluble fraction was collected by centrifugation and redissolved in a minimal volume of distilled water. Five grams of $3CdSO_4 \cdot 8H_2O$ per 100 ml of solution was added (final concn, 194 mmol/liter). After the mixture had stood overnight at 4 °C, the resulting crystals were collected by centrifugation and dissolved in a minimal volume of $(NH_4)_2SO_4$ (20 g/liter). Five preparations were made by this method.

Method 2 (Penders et al., *6*). The spleen was homogenized, heated, and filtered as in Method 1. The filtrate was ultracentrifuged at 78 000 × *g* for 3 h. The pellet was suspended in a minimal volume of water and centrifuged at 7000 × *g* for 1 h. The supernatant fraction was ultracentrifuged at 95 000 × *g* for 1 h. The sedimented material was resuspended in a minimal volume of water and ultracentrifuged again at 95 000 × *g* for 1 h. The sedimented ferritin was resuspended in a minimal volume of water. Three preparations were made by this method.

Method 3 (Linder and Munro, *7*). The spleen was homogenized in a volume of water equivalent to the weight of the tissue. An equal volume of 30 mmol/liter NaCl was added, the homogenate was heated at 70 °C for 10 min, cooled in iced water to room temperature, centrifuged, and the supernatant fraction filtered. The pH of the filtrate was adjusted to 4.8 with 0.2 mol/liter sodium acetate. After 30 min in an ice bath and ultracentrifugation at 12 000 × *g* for 10 min, the pH of the supernatant fraction was adjusted to 6.5 with 0.2 mol/liter K_2HPO_4. Ammonium sulfate was then added to half-saturation. After precipitation overnight at 4 °C, the insoluble ferritin was collected by centrifugation and redissolved in the smallest necessary volume of water. Four preparations were made by this method.

Gel filtration. The ferritin preparations were stored at either 4 °C or −20 °C until gel filtration on Sephadex G-200 (Pharmacia Fine Chemicals, Piscataway, N. J. 08854), which was the final purification step. The gel was equilibrated in, and the samples were run with, 0.15 mol/liter NaCl. Columns measuring 2.5 × 60 cm and 3.2 × 90 cm were used, and gel filtration was done at room temperature. The protein peak containing ferritin was concentrated by ultracentrifugation at 105 000 × *g* for 3 h. After centrifugation, the pellet was resuspended in the smallest necessary volume of 0.15 mol/liter NaCl.

Protein in the preparations was estimated by the method of Lowry et al. (*8*), by the microbiuret method of Itzhaki and Gill (*9*), and by absorbance at 210 nm (*10*) and at 280 nm. Bovine serum albumin (Metrix protein standard solution; Armour Pharmaceutical Co., Chicago, Ill. 60690) was also measured, for comparison.

Apoferritin was prepared from ferritin by reduction with sodium mercaptoacetate (thioglycolate) of the Fe^{3+} in ferritin to Fe^{2+}, followed by removal of Fe^{2+} by dialysis (*7*).

Immunoradiometric assay (IRMA) for ferritin was done as described by Miles et al. (*11*). The preparation used as a standard was isolated by Method 1, chromatographed on Sephadex G-200, concentrated by ultracentrifugation, and the protein concentration measured by the method of Lowry et al. (*8*).

Antiserum. Anti-ferritin antibodies were raised in rabbits by using ferritin isolated by Method 1 as the antigen. Each animal was injected subcutaneously with 0.5 mg of ferritin, emulsified in an equal volume of Freund's complete adjuvant. A second subcutaneous injection of 0.1–0.2 mg ferritin in twice the volume of Freund's complete adjuvant was given three weeks later, and a usable antiserum was obtained six weeks after the initial immunizing dose. Antibody titer was maintained in the rabbits by repeating the second immunizing dose at three- to four-week intervals.

Purity of the isolated preparations was assessed by electrophoresis on cellulose acetate ("Microzone" apparatus; Beckman Instruments Inc., Fullerton, Calif. 92634), by immunoelectrophoresis and double immunodiffusion (Immunoelectrophoresis and Immunodiffusion Kits; Gelman Instrument Co., Ann Arbor, Mich. 48106), and by gel filtration on Sepharose 6B (Pharmacia Fine Chemicals). Columns measuring 1 × 60 cm were used with the Sepharose 6B, and the samples were run with 0.15 mol/liter NaCl at room temperature.

On electrophoresis, immunoelectrophoresis, and immunodiffusion, the separated protein band was assumed to contain ferritin when it stained for ferric iron with the ferric ferrocyanide reaction (Prussian blue). Samples were always run in duplicate, one of which was stained for protein by immersion in a solution of Ponceau S (cellulose acetate electrophoresis) or Amido Black (immunoelectrophoresis and immunodiffusion). The other was immersed in the Prussian blue reagent, a mixture of one volume of potassium ferrocyanide (20 g/liter) and three volumes of 5 ml/liter HCl.

The yield of ferritin was calculated for each method, before gel filtration on Sephadex G-200, in terms of milligrams of ferritin protein (method of Lowry et al.) and milligrams of ferritin (IRMA) per gram of spleen.

Results

Gel filtration. Preparations isolated by Methods 1 and 2 and filtered through Sephadex G-200 gave a single symmetrical protein peak, which appeared close to the gel-excluded volume (Figure 2, *A* and *B*). Effluent corresponding to this peak had the characteristic amber color of ferritin. The product of Method 3 contained an additional protein (Figure 2*C*), which emerged from the Sephadex column in a volume comparable to that of serum albumin. Refiltration of the ferritin peaks on a Sephadex G-200 column (3.2 × 90 cm) did not resolve additional protein from any of the preparations. Use of Sepharose 6B for gel filtration revealed heterogeneity of the unchromatographed preparations that was not seen with Sephadex G-200. By IRMA, only the protein in the main symmetrical peak from Sepharose 6B contained ferritin. For the Method 3 preparations, Sepharose 6B after Sephadex G-200 filtration also revealed some heterogeneity, while the Sephadex G-200 peaks from preparations 1 and 2 appeared to be essentially homogeneous (Figure 3).

Analysis of protein content. The absorbance spectra of ferritin and apoferritin, compared with that of bovine serum albumin, were of use in evaluating the methods for measuring protein. Absorbance of apoferritin in the ultraviolet region was similar to, but much lower than, that of ferritin (Figure 4*a*). There is no prominent peak for either of these proteins near 280 nm, as there is for bovine serum albumin. After color development with the biuret method, the spectrum for apoferritin was the same as that for bovine serum albumin, while the spectrum for ferritin was markedly different (Figure 4*b*). In contrast to these observations, with the method of Lowry et al. the spectrum for the reaction product from ferritin appeared essentially identical to that from apoferritin and from bovine serum albumin (Figure 4*c*). The concentrations of protein in the ferritin preparations as measured by the biuret method were approximately 20% higher than those determined by the method of Lowry et al.

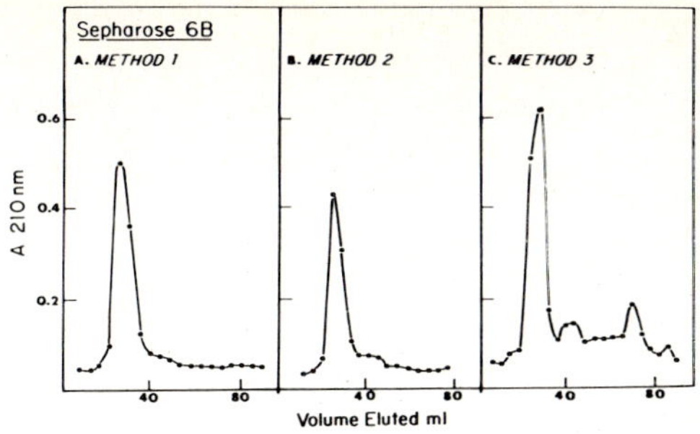

Fig. 3. Pattern of gel chromatography (Sepharose 6B) of the ferritin peaks of Figure 2

Column size, 1 × 60 cm. Five-tenths ml samples were applied. Flow rate was 5.5 ml/cm²/h, and 4.5 ml fractions were collected

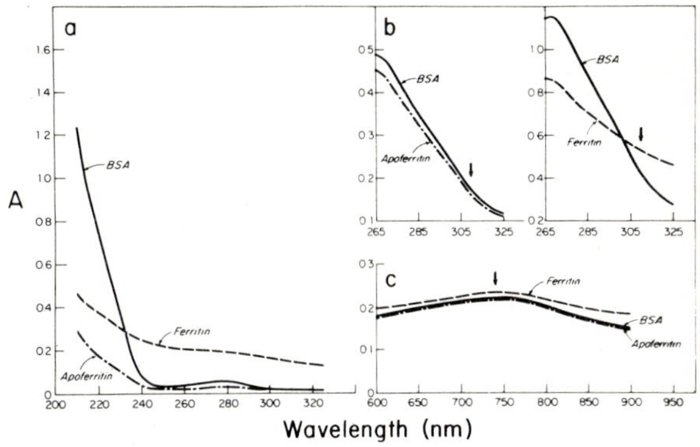

Fig. 4. Absorbance spectra for ferritin, apoferritin, and bovine serum albumin

a, Solutions of proteins in 0.15 mol/liter NaCl; *b*, After color development, biuret method (*9*); *c*, After color development, method of Lowry et al. (*8*). In *b* and *c*, the vertical arrows indicate the wavelengths used for estimating protein concentrations with those methods

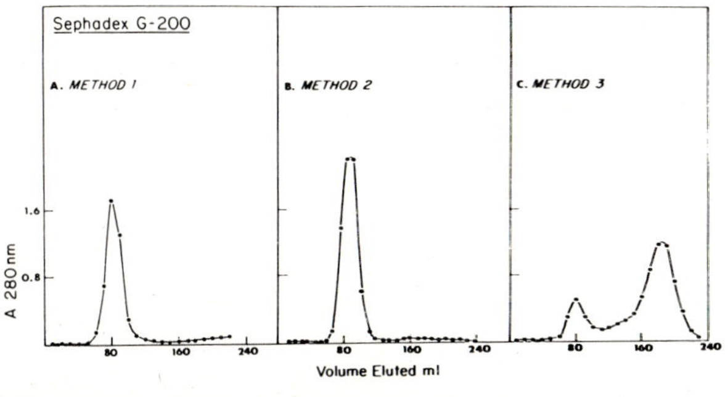

Fig. 2. Pattern of gel chromatography (Sephadex G-200) of preparations from Methods 1, 2, and 3

Column size, 2.5 × 60 cm. Six ml samples were applied. Flow rate was 6.5 ml/cm²/h, and 8 ml fractions were collected

The apparent protein content of the ferritin preparations was significantly different according to the methods of isolation. Protein values were in reasonable agreement as measured by the Lowry and the micro-biuret methods for the Sephadex G-200 purified samples from two different Method 1 preparations, although results by the biuret method were consistently higher (Table 1). Using protein values obtained by the Lowry method, absorptivity (a) for the two samples of ferritin was calculated to be 60 liter $g^{-1}cm^{-1}$ at 210 nm and 25 liter $g^{-1}cm^{-1}$ at 280 nm. When these a values were applied to the other preparations, protein concentrations calculated from the absorbances (A) at 210 nm and at 280 nm were in

Table 1. Results of Protein and Immunoreactive Ferritin Analysis of Various Preparations by Method 1

Spleen no.	Protein: Lowry method	Protein: Biuret method	Ferritin IRMA
	g/liter		g/liter
3	0.50	0.60	0.50[a]
1	0.38	0.44	0.38
1[b]	0.37	0.46	0.38

Each sample was isolated by Method 1, and the product then purified on Sephadex G-200.

[a] This preparation was used as the standard in the IRMA, the indicated value being defined by the protein concentration as measured by the method of Lowry et al.

[b] This sample was converted to apoferritin.

Table 2. Absorptivity Values for Ferritin, Apoferritin, and, for Comparison, Bovine Serum Albumin

	a, liter g^{-1} cm^{-1} At 280 nm	At 210 nm
Ferritin	24.8	59.9
Apoferritin	2.5	24.6
Bovine serum albumin	0.9	20.0

Ferritin was prepared from spleen 1 by Method 1 plus gel filtration on Sephadex G-200. Apoferritin was then prepared from this same ferritin sample.

agreement for all samples except the unchromatographed preparation from Method 3, suggesting that it is a mixture of proteins having markedly different absorptivities at these wavelengths (Table 2). Some nonferritin protein is present in the preparation by Method 3 before G-200 filtration, as shown by the ratio of IRMA-measured ferritin to ferritin protein (Table 3). The ratio of immunoreactive ferritin to protein was consistently higher for the preparations by Method 1, both before and after gel filtration, than for either of the other methods.

Apoferritin was prepared from the purest material available (Method 1 plus Sephadex G-200 filtration) by reduction of Fe^{3+} and removal of Fe^{2+}. Neither the protein value (Lowry method) nor the ferritin value (IRMA) was altered by this procedure (Table 1).

The absorbances of sample blanks were also of interest with respect to measuring ferritin protein. With the Lowry method, we detected no contribution to the absorbance of the assay sample from a sample blank for bovine serum albumin, apoferritin, or ferritin. With the biuret method, sample blanks showed slight absorbance in the case of bovine serum albumin and apoferritin, but the ferritin blank showed an absorbance equal to 85–90% of the absorbance of the assay sample, with a relatively small net absorbance from the apoprotein.

After electrophoresis on cellulose acetate, the preparations from Methods 1 and 2, both before and after Sephadex G-200 chromatography, showed a single sharp band of protein that migrated between the α_1- and α_2-globulins of serum. This band stained for Fe^{3+} with the Prussian blue reagent. The unchromatographed preparation from Method 3 showed, in addition to this band of ferritin, a diffuse zone of protein, which did not stain for Fe^{3+}, trailing between ferritin and the γ-globulin region. After gel filtration on Sephadex G-200 the gel-excluded peak from preparation 3 was identical with the ferritin band while the retarded peak was identical with the diffuse band.

Immunoelectrophoresis of all preparations, versus anti-human ferritin antiserum, showed a single arc of immunoprecipitation, which contained Fe^{3+} and remained close to the site of application. We saw no reaction of ferritin with antiserum to whole human serum. The low-molecular-weight protein isolated with Method 3 gave no detectable reaction with antisera to human ferritin, human serum, transferrin, prealbumin, haptoglobulin, or α_2-macroglobulin. With the more sensitive technique of double diffusion, a very faint line of precipitation was seen between the wells containing antiserum to whole human serum and this unidentified protein, but no reaction was evident with this technique between anti-ferritin and human serum.

Yield. Because the amount of ferritin isolated from any given specimen can be expected to vary with the condition of iron storage in that specimen, results were compared by different methods of isolation with a single spleen (Table 4). Methods 1 and 2 were compared with the use of a single, presumably iron-laden spleen. Method 2 yielded about threefold as much ferritin as Method 1, although the ratio of immunospecific ferritin to protein of the product of Method 1

Table 3. Comparison of Ferritin Concentrations as Measured by Protein Content (*8*) and by Immunoradiometric Assay

Spleen no.	Method of isolation	A Protein (*8*)	B Ferritin, by IRMA	Ratio, B/A
		g/liter		
3	1[a]	0.50[c]		
1	1[a]	0.38	0.38	1.0
6	2[a]	0.28	0.19	0.68
6	3[a]	0.50	0.30	0.60
7	1[a]	0.035	0.033	0.94
6	2[b]	3.0	1.13	0.38
6	3[b]	3.85	0.35	0.09
7	1[b]	0.85	0.61	0.72
7	2[b]	5.12	3.23	0.63

[a] The isolated product was further purified on Sephadex G-200.

[b] The isolated product was *not* purified by gel filtration.

[c] This preparation was used as the standard in the IRMA.

Table 4. Yield of Ferritin Isolated from Spleen by Three Methods

Method of isolation	Wet wt of tissue, g	Yield, per gram of spleen: Ferritin protein, mg	Immunoreactive ferritin, mg
Spleen No. 7			
1	82	0.08	0.06
2	111	0.32	0.20
Spleen No. 6			
2	68	0.35	0.13
3	72	4.28	0.39

indicated it to be somewhat more nearly pure. Methods 2 and 3 were compared by using a spleen with unknown iron content. Method 3 yielded more ferritin, but the product was considerably less pure. Freezing the spleen before ferritin was isolated did not affect the quality or the yield of ferritin with any of the methods.

After gel filtration on Sephadex G-200, 79–90% of the protein applied (assessed from absorbance at 280 nm) was recovered from preparations by Methods 1 or 2 in the single peak containing ferritin. With Method 3, 20–40% of the protein applied was recovered in the ferritin-containing peak, while 16–75% of the protein applied was recovered in the nonferritin peak. The relative amount of nonferritin protein in these preparations was presumably characteristic of the spleen, because it was consistent for all chromatograms from a single preparation but varied with the spleen.

Discussion

Isolation of ferritin either by precipitation with $(NH_4)_2SO_4$ and $CdSO_4$ (*5*) or by ultracentrifugation (*6*) is highly efficient in terms of simplicity of procedure and purity of the product, even before a further gel-filtration step.

A method based on a report by Linder and Munro (*7*) but omitting the step of precipitation of ferritin by antibody (because no antibody was available until ferritin was isolated) is more cumbersome in that it involves multiple centrifugations of large volumes, and the product, before gel filtration, was markedly less pure than the products of the first two methods.

The choice between Methods 1 and 2 would probably be dictated by available facilities, because Method 2 requires an ultracentrifuge. The product of Method 1, both before and after gel filtration on Sephadex G-200, seems to be more nearly pure than the product of either of the other two methods, as judged by the ratio of immunoreactive ferritin to protein. Gel filtration of the products on either Sephadex G-200 or Sepharose 6B, or both, revealed no detectable differences in purity between the products of Methods 1 and 2 to explain the lower ferritin-to-protein ratio of the product obtained with Method 2. Because ferritin emerges from the Sephadex G-200 column approximately with the excluded volume, other high-molecular-weight proteins may also be present. Refiltration of the Sephadex G-200 peaks on Sepharose 6B gave no evidence that this was the case, at least for the products of Methods 1 and 2.

The yield of ferritin for use as a standard is of less importance than the purity of the final product. Even with the relatively low yields with Method 1, a 200-g spleen containing a moderate amount of iron yielded 10–20 mg of ferritin after gel filtration on Sephadex G-200, an amount sufficient for hundreds of ferritin assays; about 5 μg is required for preparation of standards for a single run. The relatively low yields with Method 1 might be explained by incomplete precipitation of ferritin in the $CdSO_4$ solution. Fineberg and Greenberg (*12*) found that the relative concentrations of $CdSO_4$ and $(NH_4)_2SO_4$ were critical for optimal crystallization of ferritin from guinea pig spleens. The yield from human tissue might be improved by altering the concentration of $CdSO_4$ used after precipitation by $(NH_4)_2SO_4$.

The accuracy of the method chosen for estimating ferritin protein in a preparation to be used as a standard in the immunoradiometric assay is particularly important. The absorptivities of purified ferritin at 210 nm and at 280 nm are markedly higher than those of most other proteins, at least in part because of the presence of ferric hydroxide, which gives ferritin its characteristic amber color (*5*). There is also an apparent interference with the biuret reaction, presumably owing to the Fe^{3+} in ferritin. If apoferritin is formed by reducing the Fe^{3+} and removing the Fe^{2+}, the amber color is no longer present and there is a large decrease in absorptivity in the ultraviolet region and no longer any interference with the biuret reaction. If both ferritin protein and nonferritin protein are present in a sample such as the unchromatographed preparations from Method 3, protein values calculated from absorbances at 210 and 280 nm, based on the respective absorptivities for purified ferritin at those wavelengths, are not in agreement. The biuret method is also of questionable validity because of the divergent absorbance spectra of ferritin and bovine serum albumin and because of the high absorbance of ferritin blanks. The biuret method is primarily a measure of peptide bonds, which react with Cu^{2+} in alkaline solution to form a colored complex. The method of Lowry et al. (*8*) is largely a measure of tyrosine groups—which react with a complex phosphotungstomolybdic acid reagent—and, to some extent, of peptide bonds because of the presence in the reagent of alkaline Cu^{2+}. It seems likely that the difference in the behavior of ferritin with these two methods for measuring protein is due to absorbance by ferric hydroxide at 310 nm but not at 750 nm. Most investigators have used the method of Lowry et al. to determine the protein content of ferritin preparations. The absorbance spectra for ferritin and for bovine serum albumin with this method coincide and there is no significant absorbance by sample blanks, and so there appears to be no interference because of the presence of iron. For these reasons, it is probably the best method for establishing the protein content of ferritin preparations. Until standardized preparations are readily available from reliable sources, exchange of samples among laboratories is advisable.

A portion of this study was done in partial fulfillment for a Master of Science degree (C.M.L.). This work was supported in part by grant MC-R-Z70179 from the Bureau of Community Health Services, USPHS, DHEW. We acknowledge with gratitude the technical assistance of Miss Colleen Handevidt and the invaluable technical advice of Dr. Peter Dallman in developing the immunoradiometric assay for ferritin.

References

1. Addison, G. M., Beamish, M. R., Hales, C. N., et al., An immunoradiometric assay for ferritin in the serum of normal subjects and patients with iron deficiency and iron overload. *J. Clin. Pathol.* **25,** 326 (1972).

2. Lipschitz, D. A., Cook, J. D., and Finch, C. A., A clinical evaluation of serum ferritin as an index of iron stores. *New Engl. J. Med.* **290,** 1213 (1974).

3. Siimes, M. A., Addiego, J. E., and Dallman, P. R., Ferritin in serum: Diagnosis of iron deficiency and iron overload in infants and children. *Blood* **43,** 581 (1974).

4. Jacobs, A., and Worwood, M., Ferritin in serum. Clinical and biochemical implications. *New Engl. J. Med.* **292,** 951 (1975).

5. Granick, S., Ferritin. Its properties and significance for iron metabolism. *Chem. Rev.* **38,** 379 (1946).

6. Penders, T. J., De Dooij-Dijk, H. H., and Leijnse, B., Rapid isolation of ferritin by means of ultracentrifugation. *Biochim. Biophys. Acta* **168,** 588 (1968).

7. Linder, M. C., and Munro, H. N., Assay of tissue ferritin. *Anal. Biochem.* **48,** 266 (1972).

8. Lowry, O. H., Rosebrough, N. J., Farr, A. L., and Randall, R. J., Protein measurement with the Folin phenol reagent. *J. Biol. Chem.* **193,** 265 (1951).

9. Itzhaki, R. F., and Gill, D. M., A micro-biuret method for estimating proteins. *Anal. Biochem.* **9,** 401 (1964).

10. Tombs, M. P., Souter, F., and Maclagan, N. F., The spectrophotometric determination of protein at 210 mu. *Biochem. J.* **73,** 167 (1959).

11. Miles, L. E. M., Lipschitz, D. A., Bieber, C. P. and Cook, J. D., Measurement of serum ferritin by a 2-site immunoradiometric assay. *Anal. Biochem.* **61,** 209 (1974).

12. Fineberg, R. A., and Greenberg, D. M., Ferritin biosynthesis. I. Crystallization of guinea pig ferritin. *J. Biol. Chem.* **214,** 91 (1955).

CLIN. CHEM. 22/4, 519–520 (1976)

Fast, Economical Technique for Separating Serum from Blood Samples

Gurjit S. Ahluwalia, Z. Jerry Kuczala, and Lanny R. Carlson

We evaluated the effectiveness with which polystyrene beads separate serum from blood. Paired blood samples were analyzed for 23 different serum constituents. One specimen of each pair was processed by the conventional separation method, the other by a single centrifugation with the polystyrene beads. Differences between the assay means were evaluated by the *z*-test, and the data pairs were compared by regression analysis. No statistically significant differences were found.

The conventional method for separating serum from blood accounts for a substantial portion of technician time and effort. Two sample centrifugations and transfers are usually involved. Recently, various devices have been marketed to facilitate this process and to increase the yield of serum. Evaluation of these devices has indicated their usefulness (*1, 2*). However, for many laboratories, especially smaller facilities, the cost may preclude their use. We therefore evaluated in detail an inexpensive procedure, in which polystyrene beads are used to rapidly separate serum from blood and assessed what effect, if any, this process has on various methods and instruments routinely used in a clinical laboratory.

Such use of polystyrene granules, on an experimental basis, has been briefly reported (*3*). This procedure required that the granules be soaked overnight, rinsed, and dried before use. It was stated, without documentation, that the granules were inert.

The polystyrene beads we used in this study (Walter Sarstedt, Inc., Princeton, N. J. 08540) are about 4 mm long, 2 mm in diameter, and have a relative density of 1.04. Consequently, they form an interface between serum and cells on centrifugation. These beads are used directly, with no pretreatment. They are delivered with a semi-automatic plunger-like device (Walter Sarstedt, Inc.), which dispenses about 0.75 g of the polystyrene beads in one stroke.

Department of Laboratory Medicine, Binghamton General Hospital, Binghamton, N. Y. 13903.

Received Nov. 29, 1975; accepted Jan. 13, 1976.

Materials and Methods

Specimens: Duplicate tubes of blood were drawn from hospitalized patients into Vacutainer tubes (Becton Dickinson and Co., Rutherford, N. J. 07070). Specimens were chosen without conscious bias and processed for serum, one tube of each pair being processed by the conventional (two-centrifugation) separation method while the second specimen was treated with the polystyrene beads. The beads were dispensed into the tubes after allowing the specimen to clot for 15–30 min, and the serum was decanted after a single centrifugation. Samples were centrifuged for 10 min at 1100 × *g*. Sera were assayed for various analytes within 24 h, except those for radioimmunoassay, which were stored at −30 °C until assayed.

Methods: An SMA 12/60 continuous-flow analyzer (Technicon Instruments Corp., Tarrytown, N. Y. 10591) was used to determine concentrations of calcium, phosphorus, glucose (neocuproine method), urea nitrogen, uric acid, cholesterol, total protein, albumin, and total bilirubin, and alkaline phosphatase (EC 3.1.3.1), lactate dehydrogenase (EC 1.1.1.27), and aspartate aminotransferase activities (EC 2.6.1.1) (*4*). The last two enzymes were assayed by ultraviolet methodology. An ABA-100 (Abbott Laboratories, So. Pasadena, Calif. 91030) was used to assay kinetically the enzymic activity of lactate dehydrogenase, and α-hydroxybutyrate dehydrogenase (EC 1.1.1.30), and aspartate aminotransferase, with use of A-Gent test kits (Abbott Laboratories). Test kits were also used to measure creatine kinase (EC 2.7.3.2) activity (Worthington Biochemical Corp., Freehold, N. J. 07728) and triglycerides (Calbiochem, La Jolla, Calif. 92037). A Model 343-01 flame photometer with an automatic diluter (Instrumentation Laboratories, Inc., Lexington, Mass. 02173) was used to determine sodium and potassium, and a CMT chloride titrator (London Co., Westlake, Ohio 44145) was used for chloride ion measurement. Carbon dioxide was assayed with the Technicon single-channel AutoAnalyzer (N-86 methodology, general operating instrument manual, Technicon Instruments, Inc.). Radioimmunoassays were done with the Immuno T_4 and T_3 kits (Pantex, Malibu, Calif. 90265), The

GammaCoat cortisol kit (Clinical Assays, Inc., Cambridge, Mass. 02142), and the Phadebas insulin kit (Pharmacia Laboratories, Inc., Piscataway, N. J. 08854). All reagents were used according to manufacturer's instructions.

Results

Data sets for each analyte were statistically analyzed for significant ($P \leq 0.05$) differences between the two means by the z-test (*5*), which is similar to Student's t-test and is used when the number of specimens is greater than 30 (*5*). Both z and P were not significant in all instances. The data pairs were compared by regression analysis and the correlation coefficient in all cases was greater than 0.940, except 0.879 for cortisol.[1]

Discussion

The polystyrene beads effectively separated serum from whole blood on a single centrifugation, and the packing action of the beads increased the volume of supernatant serum. However, the beads did not always pack tightly, causing some of them to dislodge on decantation, resulting in a slight loss of recoverable serum. It was therefore essential to decant carefully to maximize serum recovery. We conclude that the final volume of serum obtained with use of the polystyrene beads at best equals that obtained with the conventional separation technique, but the need for only a single centrifugation is a major advantage.

As we have stated, various efficient serum separation devices are available, but for many laboratories their cost is prohibitive. The current cost of the beads as dispensed with the semi-automatic dispenser in our study is about 0.4¢ per tube, as compared with 10 or 20¢ per tube for two other separation devices.

We now use the beads routinely in our laboratory, with a resulting decrease in blood-processing time and risk of disease-transmission via serum contact. The procedure has also significantly decreased the incidence of sample misidentification.

[1] The authors or the Editorial Office will supply interested readers with the statistical details.

We gratefully acknowledge the technical assistance of Misses Charlotte L. Holdrege and Linda M. Vavra.

References

1. Mathies, J. C., Evaluation of a new device for rapidly separating serum or plasma from blood. *Clin. Chem.* **20**, 1573 (1974).

2. Corvac Performance Data—clinical tests, Corning Glass Works, Corning, N. Y. 14830, 1975.

3. Nishi, H. H., A rapid technique for the preparation of cell-free blood serum and plasma. *Clin. Chim. Acta* **11**, 290 (1965).

4. *Technical Publication No. UA4-0160B00,* Technicon Instruments, Inc., Tarrytown, N. Y. 10591, 1974.

5. Averill, E. W., *Elements of Statistics,* John Wiley & Sons, Inc., New York, N. Y., 1972, pp 119–143.

CLIN. CHEM. 22/4, 520–524 (1976)

Evaluation of a New Enzymatic Kit for Serum Triglycerides

Timothy Carter, Paul J. Martin, Peter Wilding, and David M. Goldberg

We evaluated a new enzymatic kit for serum triglycerides (triacylglycerols) in two laboratories. The procedure involved both enzymatic hydrolysis of the triglycerides and conversion of the glycerol, which was linked to an indicator reaction. There was excellent agreement with the mechanized procedure of Kessler and Lederer and with a manual method. The test requires 50 μl of serum and can be completed in about 50 min. Inter- and intra-laboratory variation, linearity, accuracy, and specimen storage were studied.

Additional Keyphrases: *inter-laboratory performance • continuous-flow, manual, enzymatic methods compared • quality control*

Wolfson Research Laboratories, Queen Elizabeth Medical Centre, Edgbaston, Birmingham B15 2TH, U.K. (T.C. and P.W.); and the Department of Chemical Pathology, Royal Hospital, West St., Sheffield S1 3SR, U.K. (P.J.M. and D.M.G.)

Address for reprints: Dr. D. M. Goldberg, Department of Biochemistry, Hospital for Sick Children, Toronto, Ontario M5G 1X8, Canada.

Received Dec. 8, 1975; accepted Jan. 24, 1976.

Serum triglycerides (triacylglycerols) have been measured by various manual or mechanized colorimetric methods (*1–5*), but these are tedious and some are less specific than the more recently described enzymatic methods. Early enzymatic methods, such as that of Wieland (*6*), for estimating glycerol made use of glycerol kinase (EC 2.7.1.30) to produce glycerol 3-phosphate. This reaction was monitored by measuring the appearance of NADH when glycerol 3-phosphate was oxidized by its specific dehydrogenase.

$$\text{Glycerol} + \text{ATP} \rightarrow \alpha\text{-glycerol 3-phosphate} + \text{ADP}$$

$$\alpha\text{-Glycerol 3-phosphate} + \text{NAD}^+ \rightleftharpoons \text{dihydroxyacetonephosphate} + \text{NADH} + \text{H}^+$$

Hagen and Hagen (*7*) reported a method with use of glycerol dehydrogenase (EC 1.1.1.6), which directly generated NADH. This was later improved by Davidson and Karjala (*8*), who detected the NADH fluorometrically in a method that was capable of handling more specimens, yet was still slow. More recently, the ADP formed when glycerol kinase acts on glycerol and ATP has been measured by the following indicator reaction:

Phospho*enol*pyruvate + ADP → pyruvate ± ATP

Pyruvate + NADH + H^+ ⇌ lactate + NAD^+

A stoichiometric relationship exists between the glycerol present and NADH utilized. A further refinement is the use of a bacterial lipase to achieve the initial hydrolysis of triglyceride to free glycerol and fatty acids (*9*), in place of chemical saponification. The method has been adapted in kit form by Boehringer Mannheim Corporation, and we evaluate the kit in this paper by an inter-laboratory study, because the growing use of serum triglyceride assays in population screening renders it important for results and reference values to be reproducible among laboratories.

Materials and Methods

Enzymatic Assay Procedures

A study was done in Sheffield (Lab. S) and Birmingham (Lab. B) to evaluate the most satisfactory form of the assay for routine purposes. Both laboratories were provided with reagents from the Boehringer Mannheim Corporation, Bilton House, Uxbridge Road, London, made up in the following kit:

Solution 1: 50 mmol/liter phosphate buffer, pH 7.0, containing 2 mmol of magnesium sulfate per liter.

Solution 2, per liter: 10 mmol of NADH, 25 mmol of ATP, 19 mmol of phosphoenol pyruvate, 300 kU of lactate dehydrogenase (EC 1.1.1.27), and 50 kU of pyruvate kinase (EC 2.7.1.40).

Solution 3, per liter: 5000 kU of lipase (EC 3.1.1.3) and 400 kU of esterase (from porcine liver, EC 3.1.1.1).

Solution 4: 150 kU of glycerol kinase per liter.

Both hospitals prepared the reaction mixture in the same proportions and used it within 4 h when kept at 20–25 °C, or within 8 h if kept at 4 °C. Its composition was

Solutions 1, 2, and 3: 100/2/2 by volume.

We studied three forms of the assay as suggested by the manufacturer:

Form A (serum blank method): Reaction mixture, 5 ml, was mixed with 10 μl of serum in a test tube and incubated for 20–30 min at 37 °C. Then 2.50 ml was pipetted into a 10-mm lightpath cuvette and 10 μl of Solution 4 was added. The rest of the solution was poured into another cuvette, and served as the blank. The absorbance at 340 nm was measured vs. air after a further 10-min incubation, and the difference of absorbance between test and blank was noted.

Form B (10-min method): Reaction mixture 2.50 ml, was mixed with 50 μl of serum in a test tube and incubated for 20–30 min at 37 °C. The contents of the tube were then poured into a cuvette (10-mm lightpath) and the absorbance at 340 nm was measured. Solution 4, 10 μl, was added to the cuvette and mixed. The absorbance was again measured after 10 min at room temperature, and the difference in absorbance noted.

Form C (extrapolation method): This procedure was the same as *B* except that a third absorbance reading was taken after a further 10-min incubation, and this small additional absorbance difference was subtracted from the absorbance difference obtained in *B*.

Blanks

On each occasion a "water blank" was determined by measuring the absorbance difference when water was substituted for serum in the assay. The manufacturers recommend that this difference be subtracted from the final absorbance in all three forms, but it is due to spontaneous NADH destruction, which is already taken into account in forms *A* and *C*, and so this step is actually necessary only in form *B*.

Method Comparison

Results by the enzymatic method were compared with those by the mechanized fluorometric triglyceride method (*2*). Laboratory B adsorbed the phospholipids onto neutral alumina during 15 min, whereas Laboratory S used zeolite for 60 min, as in the original procedure. Laboratory S also compared the enzymatic method with a manual colorimetric procedure involving solvent extraction (*10*). Analyses on the same specimen were done by all methods within the same 24-h period.

Interlaboratory Study

Fifty sera were collected in each laboratory, divided into two aliquots, and stored at −20 °C. These were transported between the two laboratories without thawing, re-stored, and analyzed by both laboratories by the continuous-flow and enzymatic procedures. All sera were analyzed on identical days by both laboratories.

Linearity

This was assessed by each laboratory by use of sera with high and low triglyceride values, mixed in the following respective proportions: 3/1 (4/1 in the case of Laboratory B), 2/1, 1/1, 1/2, 1/3, (1/4 in the case of Laboratory B).

Results

Choice of Procedure

Table 1 shows the precision obtained with the three forms *A, B,* and *C*. Both laboratories agree that the coefficient of variation was lowest with form *B*. Because it was also the simplest (and cheapest), it was adopted for the remainder of the study.

Table 1. Precision Obtained with Three Forms of Enzymatic Triglyceride Assay

Lab.	Mean, mmol/liter	n	CV, %	Range, mmol/liter
Form A (serum-blank)				
S	0.85	20	10.60	0.70–0.97
B	0.78	20	7.99	0.64–0.89
S	2.29	20	3.05	2.14–2.42
B	1.74	20	4.38	1.62–1.89
S	3.49	20	2.87	3.30–3.66
B	3.12	20	2.12	3.04–3.28
Form B (10 min)				
S	0.59	20	5.40	0.53–0.63
B	0.81	20	2.95	0.77–0.85
S	1.71	20	4.10	1.61–1.88
B	1.83	20	2.16	1.75–1.90
S	3.14	22	2.54	3.02–3.39
B	3.16	20	1.90	3.07–3.25
Form C (extrapolation)				
S	0.52	21	7.05	0.46–0.59
B	0.73	20	4.61	0.67–0.78
S	1.59	20	3.76	1.53–1.68
B	1.78	20	3.12	1.68–1.89
S	3.07	23	3.60	2.89–3.35
B	3.08	20	3.04	2.89–3.21

Table 2. Comparison of Methods for Triglyceride Assay

Comparison	Lab.	No. samples	Slope	Intercept	Correl. coeff.
AutoAnalyzer vs. enzymatic	B	97	1.071	0.158	0.979
AutoAnalyzer vs. enzymatic	S	84	0.943	0.028	0.974
Manual vs. enzymatic	S	84	0.990	0.036	0.991

Table 3. Interlaboratory Comparison for 100 Sera[a]

	Intercept	Slope	Correl. coeff.
Comparison of enzyme method. (Birmingham value (x), Sheffield value (y))	−0.08	0.942	0.989
Comparison of enzyme and AutoAnalyzer method. (Enzymatic value (x), AutoAnalyzer (y))			
Birmingham results	0.128	1.137	0.966
Sheffield results	0.143	0.898	0.981
Comparison of AutoAnalyzer method			
Birmingham (x) Sheffield (y)	0.089	0.723	0.975

[a] 50 sera prepared in Sheffield, 50 in Birmingham

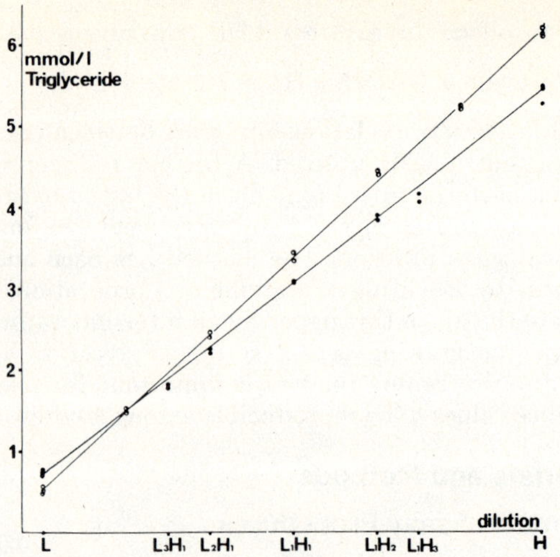

Fig. 1. Linearity of enzymatic triglyceride method with increasing concentration

The abscissa denotes the proportion of a high concentration serum (H) and a low concentration serum (L) present in the mixture analyzed

■, Sheffield experiment; □, Birmingham experiment

Table 4. Between-Batch Variation of Three Pooled Sera[a]

	Low	Medium	High
Lab. S			
$\bar{x}$, mmol/liter	0.48	1.02	4.37
SD, mmol/liter	0.04	0.08	0.24
CV, %	8.33	7.84	5.49
Lab. B			
$\bar{x}$, mmol/liter	0.77	1.79	2.68
SD, mmol/liter	0.04	0.05	0.08
CV, %	5.60	2.79	2.98

[a] Each pool was held at −20 °C in aliquots, which were assayed individually on 10 different days by the enzymatic method

Intermethod Comparison

As seen from Table 2, there was very good correlation between the continuous-flow and enzymatic methods and also between the manual and enzymatic methods.

Interlaboratory Comparisons (Table 3)

Both laboratories obtained good results with the enzymatic method, which gave an excellent correlation (0.989) for the Sheffield and Birmingham specimens combined. A comparison of the continuous-flow procedure in both laboratories showed that the Birmingham results were higher, but in spite of this the enzymatic and continuous-flow results in both laboratories correlated well.

In three instances, Laboratory S discarded the initial result obtained because it was obviously erroneous. The source of these discrepancies was traced to glycerol contamination of the pipette used to add serum.

Correlation was independent of the laboratory from which the sera originated. However, a small but statistically significant difference, detectable only when the paired t-test was done on the data ($t = 5.915$; $P < 0.001$), revealed that Laboratory S systematically produced slightly lower results than did Laboratory B. This was ultimately traced to failure of the micropipette used to add serum by Laboratory S to deliver the full volume, although its precision was better than 1%.

Linearity

These experiments demonstrated that over the range of triglyceride values 0.5–6.0 mmol/liter, there is excellent linearity (Figure 1).

Long-term Precision and Accuracy

Between-batch variation on unassayed sera gave coefficients of variation ranging from 2.79%–8.33% (Table 4).

Laboratory B assayed five different control sera twice on each of 10 days (Table 5). Laboratory S also assayed two control sera once only on each of 10 days. Laboratory B estimated four of the control sera by three different methods and the mean value is included in the table. Some of the differences between the results may be attributed to varying levels of free glycerol in sera. In the present method 0.11 mmol/liter is subtracted from all results (to allow for free glycerol), and of course this does not allow for variation among individual sera.

Storage

Laboratory S kept some control sera at 7–8 °C in a cold room and noted a decline in triglyceride values as determined enzymatically during one month, with decreases of 2.77 to 1.71, 0.45 to 0.22, and 1.01 to 0.50 mmol/liter. However, no decline could be detected by either the manual method or the Kessler and Lederer procedure (*2*) over this time. Studies by Laboratory S on six patients' sera kept at room temperature over two weeks revealed a tendency for

Table 5. Results Obtained in Birmingham and Sheffield[a]

	Quality Assurance Serum Level 1	Lipitrol	Precilip	Validate	Hyland Elevated
Manufacturer's value, mmol/liter	—	2.44[b]	1.26[c]	1.06[d] 1.60[e]	3.8[f]
Birmingham (n = 20)					
$\bar{x}$, mmol/liter	0.37	2.74	1.21	1.56	3.30
SD, mmol/liter	0.028	0.08	0.14	0.05	0.11
CV, %	7.64	2.91	11.6	3.20	3.33
Sheffield (n = 10)					
$\bar{x}$, mmol/liter	—	2.72	1.16	—	—
SD, mmol/liter	—	0.10	0.10	—	—
CV, %	—	3.67	8.62	—	—
Mean of 20 estimations by method in ref. no.					
11	0.46	2.04	—	1.14	2.90
2	0.91	3.02	—	1.59	3.67
12	0.59	2.59	—	1.32	3.39

[a] Sera stored at −20 °C, assayed on 10 separate days. Lab. B estimated each aliquot twice and Lab. S only once on each occasion.
[b] Dade Tri-25
[c] Eggstein
[d] AutoAnalyzer
[e] Kessler
[f] Carlson and Wadstrom: Kessler

values as measured with the enzymatic method to increase—occasionally by more than half. This phenomenon was also confirmed by Laboratory B, which found values to be stable when patients' sera were stored at 4 °C or at −20 °C.

Discussion

Since the publication of the first enzymatic triglyceride assay in which the present reaction sequence is used (*9*), many modifications have been proposed. Mechanization procedures have been described for continous-flow analysis (*13*), for centrifugal analysis (*14, 15*), and for other instruments (*16, 17*). Alterations to the chemistry of the assay include initiation with lipase (*16*) and extending the range of pseudo-first-order kinetics by increasing ATP concentration (*15*). We have used the method in its simplest form, appropriate for inexpensive equipment, and obtained satisfactory results. Twenty specimens can be analyzed in about 50 min. The manufacturers expect the cost to be about 20 p (25¢) per test when the quantities quoted in this communication are used, but this may be reduced dramatically by using smaller volumes.

The AutoAnalyzer technique was stated by Kessler and Lederer (*2*) to give a coefficient of variation of 2% when a pooled serum with a triglyceride value of 1.35 mmol/liter was assayed during 20 days. This is much better than can be achieved by most routine laboratories. Because of the extreme simplicity of the enzymatic method it is likely that the coefficients of variation obtained, which ranged from 1.90% in a within-batch analysis to 11.6% in a between-batch analysis, give a much better representation of what is to be expected for a routine laboratory. The superior precision attained by Laboratory B probably reflects the fact that their data were obtained by scientific staff spending a high proportion of time at the bench whereas the data from Laboratory S were provided by medical staff. Not unexpectedly, form B gave the best precision, because the number of readings and manipulative steps were minimized in this procedure.

The reliability of the enzymatic test was compared with that of the continuous-flow (*2*) and manual (*10*) procedures by Laboratory S as an adjunct to the intermethod comparison but without biasing the correlation study. Results differing by greater than 20%, or 0.2 mmol/liter at concentrations <1.0 mmol/liter, were repeated by each method. Error was assigned to a method if the result of the repeat analysis differed by >15% of the first value and lay within 10% of the mean given by the alternative method (provided these assays were within 10% of each other). Faulty results were given three times more frequently by the AutoAnalyzer than by the enzymatic or manual methods; the manual method was slightly less reliable than the enzymatic. All tests were performed on a single production batch; the reliability of production has thus not been tested.

The accuracy study (Table 5) is not easy to interpret because appropriate standards are lacking. Values given by the enzymatic method were closest to the manufacturer's value for a control material ("Precilip"), suggesting that this would be the best quality-control material for use with the test. With the other commerical sera assayed, the enzymatic method gave values between the extremes obtained with the remaining three methods, indicating that it might approach a consensus value.

The stability study yielded unexpected results. Further work is planned to determine why the commercial sera showed decreasing and the patients' sera increasing triglyceride values (as determined enzymatically) when stored at temperatures above 4 °C. From the practical point of view, both may be stored at −20 °C if preservation is necessary.

The usefulness of an inter-laboratory study in evaluating commerical enzyme tests has previously been demonstrated (*18, 19*). In our case, random errors (glycerol contamination) and systematic errors (faulty pipette calibration) came to light that may not otherwise have done. It is a precaution against limitations in laboratory performance being assigned to the test under evaluation. The satisfactory agreement obtained with the enzyme test contrasts with the large systematic difference between the two laboratories with the widely used AutoAnalyzer method and suggests that results with the former from different centers should be more reproducible. This could be a desirable feature in monitoring patients under therapy for lipid disorders in view of population mobility and the life-long requirements for treatment.

References

1. Van Handel, E., and Zilversmit, P. B., Micromethod for the direct determination of serum triglycerides. *J. Lab. Clin. Med.* **50**, 152 (1957).

2. Kessler, G., and Lederer, H., Fluorimetric measurement of triglycerides. In *Automation in Analytical Chemistry, Technicon Symposia 1965;* L. T. Skeggs, et al., Eds. Mediad, New York, N. Y., 1966, p 341.

3. Levy, A. L., Measurement of triglycerides using nonane extraction and colorimetry. *Ann. Clin. Lab. Sci.* **2**, 474 (1972).

4. Roger, M. E., and Ko, H., A simplified semi-automated assay for plasma triglycerides. *Anal. Biochem.* **29**, 405 (1969).

5. Lofland, H. B., A semi-automated procedure for the determination of triglycerides in serum. *Anal. Biochem.* **9**, 383 (1964).

6. Wieland, O., Eine enzymatische Methode zur Bestimmung von Glycerin. *Biochem. Z.* **329**, 313 (1957).

7. Hagen, H. J., and Hagen, P. B., An enzymatic method for the estimation of glycerol in blood and its use to determine the effect of noradrenaline on the concentration of glycerol in blood. *Can. J. Biochem. Physiol.* **40**, 1129 (1962).

8. Davidson, M. B., and Karjala, R., Simplified fluorimetric method for the determination of plasma glycerol. *J. Lipid Res.* **11**, 609 (1970).

9. Bucolo, G., and David, H., Quantitative determination of serum triglycerides by the use of enzymes. *Clin. Chem.* **19**, 476 (1973).

10. Martin, P. J., A quick inexpensive method for serum triglycerides. *Clin. Chim. Acta* **62**, 79 (1975).

11. Soloni, F. G., Simplified manual micromethod for determination of serum triglycerides. *Clin. Chem.* **17**, 529 (1971).

12. Eggstein, M., and Kreutz, F. H., Eine neue Bestimmung der Neutralfette im Blutserum und Gewebe. *Klin. Wochenschr.* **44**, 262 (1966).

13. Bucolo, G., Yabut, J., and Chang, T. Y., Mechanized enzymatic determination of triglycerides in serum. *Clin. Chem.* **21**, 420 (1975).

14. Tiffany, T. O., Morton, J. M., Hall, E. M., and Garrett, A. S., Jr., Clinical evaluation of kinetic enzymatic fixed-time and integral analysis of serum triglycerides. *Clin. Chem.* **20**, 476 (1974).

15. Ziegenhorn, J., Improved method for enzymatic determination of serum triglycerides. *Clin. Chem.* 21, 1627 (1975).

16. Bucolo, G., McCroskey, R., and Whittaker, N., Lipase-triggered kinetic assay of serum triglycerides. *Clin. Chem.* **21**, 424 (1975).

17. DiCesare, J. L., Optimum kinetic enzymatic procedures for glucose and triglycerides in plasma and serum. *Clin. Chem.* **21**, 1448 (1975).

18. Wilkinson, J. H., Boutwell, J. H., and Winsten, S., Evaluation of a new system for the kinetic measurement of serum alkaline phosphatase. *Clin. Chem.* **15**, 487 (1969).

19. Winsten, S., Wilkinson, J. H., and Boutwell, J. H., Evaluation of a new system for the kinetic measurement of serum glutamic oxalacetic transaminase. An interlaboratory study. *Clin. Chem.* **15**, 496 (1969).

CLIN. CHEM. 22/4, 524–527 (1976)

Serum Iron Determination in Patients Receiving Therapy with Iron Dextran ("Imferon")

Max E. McIntosh,[1] Jerry K. Lynn,[1] Norma Meyerriecks, and Irene Contant

Imferon (Lakeside Labs., Inc.), an iron dextran complex, is widely used for parenteral therapy with iron. Colorimetry and atomic absorption spectroscopy give different values for serum iron concentration in patients receiving such therapy. Values determined by atomic absorption spectroscopy were usually much higher than those obtained by either a manual or an automated colorimetric procedure, and also were higher than the total serum iron-binding capacity of the same sera. This difference is attributed to circulating iron being present both as iron dextran as as transferrin-bound iron. We conclude that atomic absorption spectroscopy should be used to determine serum iron in patients receiving Imferon.

Additional Keyphrases: *colorimetry (bathophenanthroline) vs. atomic absorption spectroscopy • total iron-binding capacity • anemia • transferrin-bound iron*

"Imferon" (Lakeside), an iron dextran complex, was introduced in 1954 as the first parenteral iron preparation that could be given intramuscularly (*1*). Subsequently, intramuscular or, under certain circumstances, intravenous administration of iron dextran has become an established technique in treatment of iron-deficiency anemia. The intravenous route allows introduction of 2 to 3 g of iron into the blood stream (*2*). Iron dextran is cleared slowly after such infusion, with a half-time of 2.5 to 3 days (*3*). Body-

Department of Pathology, University of South Florida, School of Medicine; and Laboratory Service, Veterans Administration Hospital, Tampa, Fla. 33620.

[1] Present address: VA Hospital, Laboratory Service, 16111 Plummer St., Sepulveda, Calif. 91343. Address reprint requests to M. E. McI. at this address.

Received Sept. 1, 1975; accepted Jan. 27, 1976.

surface scintillation counting after administration of radiolabeled iron dextran showed radioactivity in the body for longer than three weeks (*4*).

Serum iron and total iron-binding capacity (TIBC) of serum can be determined either by colorimetry or by atomic absorption spectroscopy. When both procedures were applied in our laboratory, patients receiving iron dextran therapy presented a special problem. During routine analysis for serum iron and TIBC by atomic absorption spectroscopy, we noticed that some patients, mostly those in the hemodialysis unit, had abnormally high values for both. In these patients the serum iron concentration often exceeded the TIBC, indicating that the excess iron was present in some form other than iron–transferrin complex. When iron was determined in the same samples with the *aca*, the results fell within the physiological range. Upon inquiry, all such patients were found to have received Imferon intravenously three to 12 days before the blood was sampled. To explain these discrepant results we did the following studies.

Materials and Methods

Reagents

All reagents were prepared from AR grade chemicals (Fisher Scientific Co.) with de-ionized water. A colorimetric procedure (American Monitor, Indianapolis, Ind. 46240) was used with reagents supplied by the manufacturer. Imferon containing 50 mg of elemental iron per milliliter was obtained from the distributor (Lakeside Laboratories, Inc., Milwaukee, Wis. 53201; manufactured by Fisons Limited, Holmes Chapel, England).

Equipment

A Coleman Jr. II spectrophotometer (Coleman Instruments, Maywood, Ill. 60153) was used to prepare a calibration curve for determination of iron concentration by the colorimetric procedure. Wavelength calibration was ascertained with a didymium filter at 585 ± 1 nm and linearity checked with a ammonium cobaltous sulfate solution, 45 g/liter of dilute sulfuric acid (Spectro Chek; Oxford Laboratories, Foster City, Calif. 94404).

Atomic absorption spectroscopic assays were done with a Model 403 spectrophotometer equipped with a three-slot burner head and used with an air/acetylene flame (Instrument Division, Perkin-Elmer Corp., Norwalk, Conn. 06856). Analyses were made at a wavelength of 248.3 nm with a single-element hollow-cathode lamp supplied by the manufacturer and a spectral slit width of 0.2 nm.

An Automatic Clinical Analyzer (*aca;* E. I. du Pont de Nemours and Co., Inc., Instrument Products Division, Wilmington, Del. 19898) was used for the automated measurement of serum iron and TIBC, based on colorimetric procedures. Wavelength calibration was checked according to the manufacturer's instructions, i.e., filter balancing followed by linearity certification with cobalt (II) sulfate in sulfuric acid, 10 ml/liter (cat. No. 00938000, lot No. 3480).

Corning disposable glassware was used wherever possible in the procedures. Corning disposable pipettes were used to transfer serum samples. All other glassware was treated with dilute nitric acid (200 ml/liter) followed by five successive rinses with de-ionized water, and air dried.

Procedures

The range of linearity for the *aca* and atomic absorption spectrophotometer was determined by using aqueous ferric chloride standards (Fisher) and assayed serum controls (General Diagnostics). A linear range of 0–10.00 mg/liter was established for both instruments. Manual assays of serum iron and TIBC were done by a colorimetric procedure, modified from the original method by the manufacturer, obtained commercially in kit form from American Monitor (*5*). Atomic absorption spectroscopic analysis of specimens was routinely done after protein precipitation with trichloroacetic acid (200 g/liter) to avoid potential interference from hemoglobin iron (*6*).

Serum iron and TIBC were also determined with an *aca* that had been calibrated with aqueous iron standards (Technical Bulletin, *aca*, Iron; Du Pont) (*7*). This procedure is an end-point reaction, done at an acid pH at which the iron–transferrin complex dissociates. The free iron, reduced to the ferrous state (Fe^{2+}) by hydroxylamine (NH_2OH), forms a complex with bathophenanthroline, the color of which, measured at 540 nm, is directly proportional to the iron concentration in the sample. Sodium dodecyl sulfate is incorporated into the reaction mixture to prevent precipitation of protein.

Results

Analytical Recovery Studies

A pool of patients' sera was prepared, and increasing amounts of ferric chloride were added to different aliquots of it. The iron concentration of each aliquot and that of the original pool was determined by atomic absorption spectroscopy, with the *aca*, and by the manual method.

The serum pool iron content was found to be 800, 530, and 610 μg/liter, respectively, by the three methods. Recovery of added iron ranged from 72 to 114% by the three methods. At each concentration of serum iron, each of the three methods gave about the same percentage recovery; for example, when the iron concentration was adjusted to 2 mg/liter plus its original serum pool value, respective recoveries were 114, 102, and 100%. Resulting curves for all three methods showed a good linear relationship and close parallelism to each other up to 10 mg/liter, when the measured concentration was plotted vs. added iron (Figure 1).

Next, we added various known amounts of iron dextran instead of ferric chloride to aliquots of the same serum pool and repeated the above recovery studies (Table 1). Analytical recovery of the added iron by atomic absorption spectroscopy ranged from 60 to 37%, gradually decreasing with increasing iron dextran concentration. In contrast, we ob-

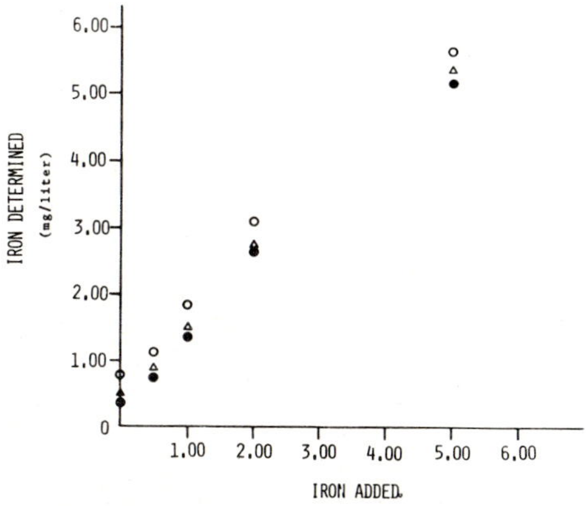

Fig. 1. Comparative analytical recovery of aqueous ferric chloride in a serum pool by atomic absorption spectroscopy (O), Automatic Clinical Analyzer (●), and a manual method (Δ)

Each point is the average of five determinations

Table 1. Analytical Recovery of Imferon-Iron Added to Serum

	Method					
	AAS[a]		*aca*		Manual	
Iron added	Iron recovered	Recovery, %	Iron recovered	Recovery, %	Iron recovered	Recovery, %
mg/liter			mg/liter		mg/liter	
0.40	0.24	60	0.01	2.5	0	0.0
1.00	0.48	48	0.01	1.0	0.02	2.0
2.00	0.90	45	0.02	1.0	0.04	2.0
5.00	2.18	44	0.09	1.8	0.15	3.0
10.00	3.66	37	0.16	1.6	0.27	2.7

[a] Atomic absorption spectroscopy. Specimens were deproteinized with trichloroacetic acid (200 g/liter) before analysis.

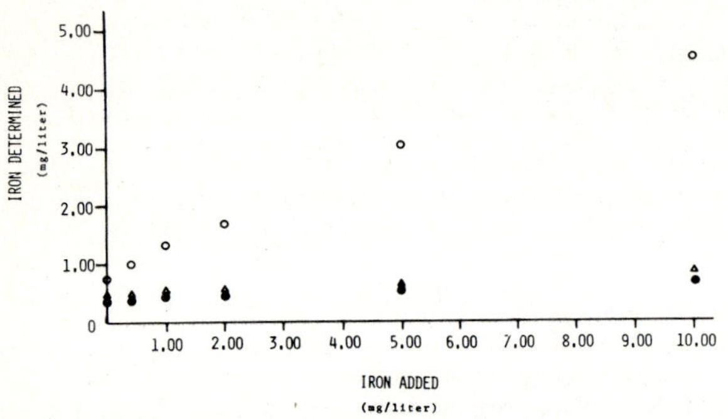

Fig. 2. Comparative analytical recovery of Imferon-iron in a serum pool by atomic absorption spectroscopy (O), Automatic Clinical Analyzer (●), and a manual method (△)
Each point is the average of five determinations

Table 2. Analytical Recovery, by Atomic Absorption Spectroscopy, of Imferon-Iron Added to Serum Without Prior Removal of Serum Proteins

Added	Recovered	Recovery, %
mg/liter		
0.40	0.38	90
1.00	0.88	88
2.00	1.72	86
5.00	4.64	93
10.00	9.39	94

Table 3. Apparent Serum Iron Concentrations in Five Patients Receiving Imferon Therapy, as Determined by Atomic Absorption Spectroscopy (AAS) and Automatic Clinical Analyzer (*aca*)

AAS		
Aqueous dilutions of serum	TCA filtrates of serum	*aca*
Iron, mg/liter		
25.60	6.42	0.68
10.20	4.20	0.96
32.64	10.16	1.37
53.76	13.10	1.80
35.20	10.56	1.00

served very poor (0–3%) recovery of iron dextran by either the *aca* or manual method for all concentrations of added iron. Recoveries of iron in the form of iron dextran in a serum pool diverged strikingly (Figure 2) when results by these three methods were plotted.

We routinely used protein-free filtrates for determination of iron by atomic absorption spectroscopy. Recovery of added iron dextran by this procedure varied but never exceeded 60%. When samples were simply diluted with distilled water and their iron concentrations determined by atomic absorption spectroscopy, recovery approached 100% (Table 2). When the iron in five patients' sera which contained injected Imferon were determined by atomic absorption spectroscopy after dilution with water, much higher iron concentrations were obtained than by using protein-free filtrates (Table 3). Clearly, a portion of the iron dextran complex in serum, whether injected or added in vitro, is removed along with serum proteins by trichloroacetic acid treatment and thus escapes detection by atomic absorption spectroscopy.

Discussion

Imferon is used extensively for treatment of iron-deficiency anemia by intravenous injection. Reported studies concerning the structure of the preparation, which contains 50 mg of elemental iron and 20 mg of dextran per milliliter (*8*), indicate that the iron is complexed at the terminal glucose units of the dextran chains, which have been converted into metasaccharinic acid. In solution, the dextran chains can be visualized as radiating randomly from the ferric oxyhydroxide (FeOOH) "core" and are attached to it via the terminal metasaccharinic acid units (*9*).

Our results show that intravenous injection of this iron dextran complex will give rise to a form of circulating serum iron that is detectable by atomic absorption spectroscopy but not by the bathophenanthroline procedure on which both the *aca* and colorimetric manual methods are based. This is apparently because the iron in the iron dextran complex is in the "core" of it. The iron dextran attachment is probably firm enough to resist dissociation with acid and subsequent complex formation between the iron and bathophenanthroline reagent (*10*).

Our results also indicate that the circulating iron dextran complex is only partly removed from serum by trichloroacetic acid treatment (Table 3) and that its presence interferes with determination of transferrin-bound iron in protein-free filtrates by atomic absorption spectroscopy. Therefore, water-diluted serum samples should be used to measure total circulating iron. Furthermore, a small proportion of iron dextran (up to 3%, as seen in Table 1) present in a given serum sample may react unaccountably in the colorimetric procedures, becoming significant in patients with exceedingly high concentrations of circulating iron dextran (Table 3). Thus, the use of the *aca* or manual colorimetric methods involving the bathophenanthroline procedure becomes unreliable for serum iron determination for patients receiving Imferon therapy. Atomic absorption spectroscopy measures total circulating iron, both transferrin- and dextran-bound; colorimetric methods measure a little of the dextran-bound iron, enough to prevent accurate measurement of transferrin-bound iron in some patients. Determination of transferrin-bound iron in these patients is a difficult problem for which we have no solution at the present.

When one wishes to monitor total circulating iron, the best laboratory procedure would be to determine serum iron by atomic absorption spectroscopy on water-diluted serum, as demonstrated in this paper. But in doing so one should be aware of potential error caused by hemoglobin in the serum. Webster (*11*) has described a modified bathophenanthroline procedure that supposedly measures total circulating iron, i.e., both transferrin- and dextran-bound iron. It may be of interest to compare results by this method with those by atomic absorption spectroscopy, which also measures both.

There are several published studies of rates of clearance of iron dextran from plasma (*3, 4, 12–14*). These studies and our own experience show that patients who have received iron dextran within the preceding three weeks will show an abnormally high serum iron content. Such patients should be identified and a proper procedure such as the one described in this paper should be used for determining the total circulating iron concentration.

References

1. *Imferon in Clinical Medicine,* Fisons Pharmaceuticals Limited, Loughborough, Leicestershire, England, 1966.

2. Dawson, D. W., Goldthorp, W. O., and Spencer, D., Parenteral iron therapy in pregnancy. *J. Obstet. Gynaecol. Br. Commonw.* **72,** 89 (1965).

3. Will, G., and Groden, B. M., The treatment of iron deficiency anaemia by iron dextran infusion: A radio-isotope study. *Br. J. Haematol.* **14,** 61 (1968).

4. Wood, J. K., Milner, P. F. R., and Pathak, U. N., The metabolism of iron dextran given as a total-dose infusion to iron deficient Jamaican subjects. *Br. J. Haematol.* **14,** 119 (1968).

5. Goodwin, J. F., Murphy, B., and Guillemette, M., Direct measurement of serum iron and binding capacity. *Clin. Chem.* **12,** 47 (1966).

6. Olson, A. D., and Hamlin, W. B., A new method for serum iron and total iron-binding capacity by atomic absorption spectrophotometry. *Clin. Chem.* **15,** 438 (1969).

7. Jung, D. H., and Parekh, A. C., A semi-micromethod for the determination of serum iron and iron-binding capacity without deproteinization. *Am. J. Clin. Pathol.* **54,** 813 (1970).

8. Cox, J. S. G., King, R. E., and Reynolds, G. F., Valency investigations of iron dextran (Imferon). *Nature* (London) **207,** 1202 (1965).

9. Cox, J. S. G., Kennedy, G. R., King, J., et al., Structure of an iron dextran complex. *J. Pharm. Pharmacol.* **24,** 513 (1972).

10. Fielding, J., Intravenous iron dextran in iron-deficiency anaemia. *Br. Med. J.* **ii,** 279 (1961).

11. Webster, D., The determination of serum iron after the intravenous injection of iron dextran. *J. Clin. Pathol.* **13,** 246 (1960).

12. Cox, J. S. G., Moss, G. F., Bremner, I. and Reason, J., Intravenous iron dextran: Studies on unsaturated iron-binding capacity. *J. Clin. Pathol.* **21,** 611 (1968).

13. Henderson, P. A., and Hillman, R. S., Characteristics of iron dextran utilization in man. *Blood* **34,** 357 (1969).

14. Wallerstein, R. O., Intravenous administration of large doses of iron dextran. *Clin. Res.* **13,** 105 (1960).

case report

Effect of Tobramycin on Urinary γ-Glutamyltransferase Activity: Studies in a Case of Renal Carcinoma

Peter Richard Beck, M.Sc., M.B., Ch.B., and Ajay K. R. Chaudhuri

γ-Glutamyltransferase activity was studied in a man presenting with recurrent septicemia owing to pyonephrosis and renal carcinoma. Increased activity in the urine was ascribable to administration of the aminoglycoside antibiotic, tobramycin. That the renal carcinoma did not contribute to the increased values was confirmed by homogenization and enzyme histochemistry of the tumor. Although the activity of this enzyme in serum was greater than normal, this persisted postoperatively, and thus was not related to the renal carcinoma.

Studies of the activity of urinary γ-glutamyltransferase [γ-GT; (γ-glutamyl)-peptide:amino-acid γ-glutamyltransferase, EC 2.3.2.2] in renal disease are scanty. Recent German papers (*1–3*) have shown that urinary γ-GT activity may increase in inflammatory renal disease and decrease in chronic noninflammatory disease. These papers have also shown the important relationship between urinary γ-GT and creatinine clearance.

Here, we describe results of our various γ-GT investigations in a patient with renal carcinoma, and emphasize the importance of the aminoglycoside antibiotic, tobramycin, in altering urinary γ-GT activity.

Case Summary

The patient, a 75-year-old man, was admitted on December 15, 1974, with *Escherichia coli* septicemia, which was treated with tobramycin. He was anemic (80 g of hemoglobin per liter of blood) and had a persistently elevated erythrocyte sedimentation rate of about 130 mm/h. A double-dose intravenous pyelogram at this time demonstrated splayed midcalyces in the left kidney, caused by either a cyst or a tumor. He was readmitted on February 20, 1975, with recurrence of *E. coli* septicemia, again treated with tobramycin. He improved and his tobramycin was stopped on March 11. *E. coli* persisted in his urine, and this infection was treated with nalidixic acid.

On April 15, 1975, a left nephrectomy was performed. The specimen consisted of a shell of normal renal tissues that surrounded a pyonephrosis, enclosing a renal carcinoma, about 1.5 cm in diameter. Histological examination showed a well-differentiated clear-cell carcinoma with large areas of hemorrhage. His postoperative course was uneventful and he was discharged home well at the end of April 1975.

Methods

γ-GT assay. γ-GT was assayed at 37 °C, pH 8.1, and 410 nm, with use of an LKB 8600 reaction-rate analyzer. Buffered substrate was freshly prepared by heating to 70 °C L-γ-glutamyl-p-nitroanilide (Boehringer), 4.6 mmol/liter in 230 mmol/liter tris(hydroxymethyl)aminomethane buffer, pH 8.1.

To 1.4 ml of buffered substrate, 0.1 ml of serum or urine was added, and the reaction was initiated with 0.1 ml glycylglycine (640 mmol/liter; 40 mmol/liter in the final reaction mixture). The results were expressed as U/liter by using the following equation: γ-GT activity, U/liter = [(absorbance change/min) $\times$ 1000 $\times$ V]/($E \times v$) = absorbance change/min $\times$ 1882, where V = total volume in tube, 1.6 ml; v = serum (urine) volume, 0.1 ml; and E = millimolar absorptivity of p-nitroaniline at 410 nm and pH 8.1, 8.502 (*4*).

Urine specimens were complete 24-h collections, without preservative, stored at 4 °C, and were well-mixed before assay. The enzyme is stable under such

Department of Biochemistry, Royal Infirmary, and Department of Infectious Diseases, Belvidere Hospital, Glasgow, G4 OSF, Scotland.

Received Nov. 24, 1975; accepted Jan. 8, 1976.

conditions (5). Creatinine was measured with the Jaffé reaction in a Technicon AutoAnalyzer I system. A highly significant positive correlation, $r = 0.855$, $P < 0.001$, exists between urinary γ-GT and creatinine clearance in normal individuals (6), and the regression equation for this, $y = 20.4x + 8.13$, has been used to calculate a γ-GT/creatinine clearance ratio (γ-GT/ml):

$$\gamma\text{-GT/ml} = \frac{\gamma\text{-GT(U/24 h)} - 8.13}{\text{creatinine clearance (ml/s)}}$$

Homogenization. About 1 g of tissue was homogenized in 20 ml of cold 230 mmol/liter tris(hydroxymethyl)aminomethane buffer, pH 8.1, with a mechanically driven Teflon-and-glass homogenizer. The homogenates were centrifuged for 1 h at 4 °C and 2000 × *g*, and the supernates used for γ-GT assays. Protein contents were estimated by the technique of Lowry et al. (7).

The histochemical technique, that of Albert et al. (8), was used on acetone-fixed tissues. γ-GT in tissue sections reacts with γ-glutamyl-α-naphthylamide to release α-naphthylamine. This latter combines with Fast Garnet GBC Salt to give an insoluble red-brown diazo complex, which indicates the site of enzyme activity.

Results

Blood and Urine

The first γ-GT assays were done on March 5, during the patient's second admission, and when he had been receiving tobramycin for 13 days. Relevant results were:

Serum creatinine, 140 μmol/liter (normal, 35–115 μmol/liter). Creatinine clearance, 0.17 ml/s (normal, 1.42–2.33 ml/s). Serum γ-GT, 78 U/liter (normal, 1–35 U/liter). Urinary γ-GT, 67 U/24-h specimen (normal, 22–55. U/24-h specimen). γ-GT/CC, 325.8 (normal, 10.2–31.2) (CC = creatinine clearance).

We thought the abnormally high γ-GT values were attributable to the renal tumor, but serial measurements showed clearly that the urinary γ-GT values decreased almost to normal within one week after tobramycin injections were stopped (Figure 1). The urinary γ-GT activities of 25–30 U/24 h that were found pre-operatively fell slightly to 18–23 U/24 h in the early postoperative period.

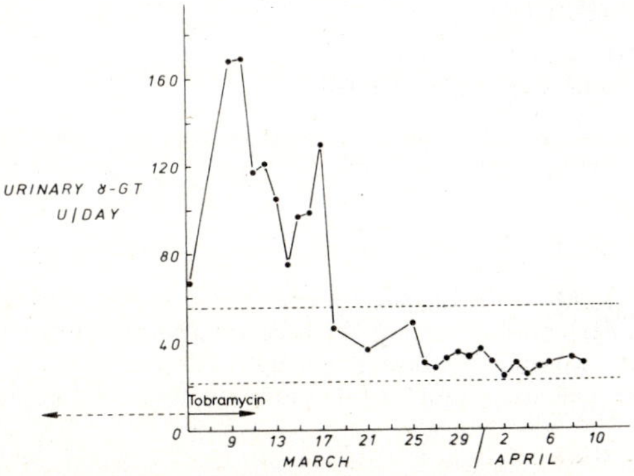

Fig. 1. Urinary γ-GT excretion during and after treatment with tobramycin
Dotted lines indicate the normal range

Table 1. γ-GT/Creatinine Clearance at Various Times during the Study of the Patient

Date and situation	Urinary γ-GT, U/24-h spec. (normal 22–55)	γ-GT/CC ratio (normal 10.2–31.2)
03-05-75 (admission; on tobramycin)	67	325.8
03-11-75 (end of tobramycin therapy)	117	427.2
03-25-75 (2 weeks post-tobramycin)	48	71.4
04-09-75 (6 days pre-op.)	30	43.2
04-27-75 (12 days postop.)	23	29.4

Table 2. γ-GT Activities of Homogenates of Normal Renal Tissue and of Renal Carcinoma

Tissue examined	γ-GT activity, U/g fresh tissue	γ-GT activity, U/g protein
Superficial renal cortex	17.8	310
Deep renal cortex	20.4	562
Renal medulla	6.0	196
Renal carcinoma	4.0	—

The high γ-GT/CC ratios found during tobramycin therapy (Table 1) had returned almost to normal preoperatively, and became so postoperatively.

Serum γ-GT activity was persistently increased to between 55 and 90 U/liter at all times pre-operatively, but did not decrease postoperatively, a sample taken on April 29 giving a result of 79 U/liter.

γ-GT activities of homogenized tissues taken from the nephrectomy specimen are given in Table 2. The protein concentration of the tumor tissue could not be estimated satisfactorily because of the large amount of blood present. It can be seen that the activity of γ-GT (expressed as U/g fresh tissue) in the carcinomatous tissue is a quarter to a fifth that of normal renal cortical tissue, and is also less than that of renal medulla.

Histochemistry. Figures 2–4 show respectively the γ-GT activity in renal cortex, renal medulla, and renal carcinoma. In Figure 2 the very high γ-GT activity is seen as dark staining in proximal tubules, particularly the "brush borders." In medulla (Figure 3) the γ-GT activity is entirely confined to "casts" within the tubules. Many bacteria are visible. The carcinoma itself (Figure 4) shows small amounts of activity, mainly in the periphery of the cells.

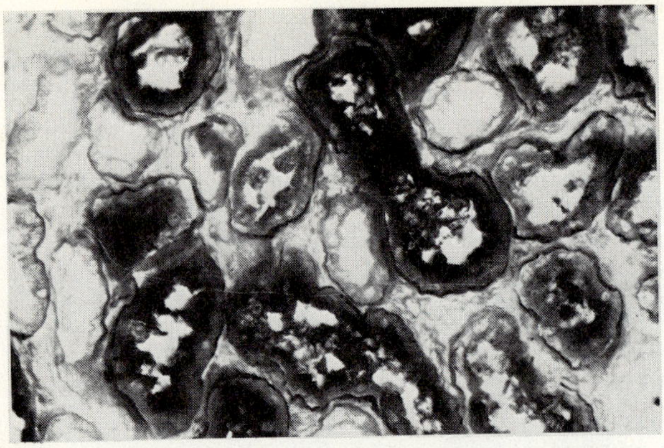

Fig. 2. γ-GT activity of normal renal cortex
Dark areas of staining are seen particularly in the "brush borders" of proximal tubular cells (× 800)

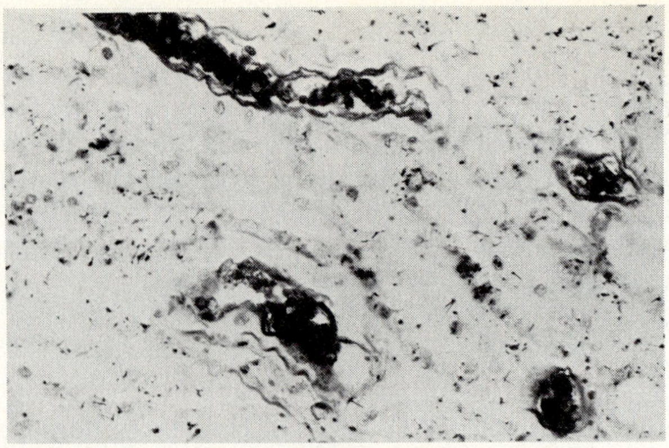

Fig. 3. γ-GT activity of normal renal medulla
Staining is confined to "casts" within tubules (× 800)

Discussion

Serum. Only three studies (*9–11*) have specifically mentioned an increased γ-GT activity in the serum in cases of renal tumor. None of them gives a detailed analysis of their findings. The present case, although showing an increased serum γ-GT, lends no support to the idea that renal carcinoma is accompanied by an increase, because γ-GT activity remained constant for a considerable period postoperatively. Although the cause of the increase is unknown, it may be related to repair processes, as has been suggested (*12*) for heart disease.

Urine. Kley et al. (*2*) are the only authors to mention urinary γ-GT in renal tumor, but they give no details, and their results are difficult to interpret. We at first attributed the increased values for urinary γ-GT in the present case to the renal carcinoma. The presence of *E. coli* does not affect urinary γ-GT activity (*6*). The γ-GT activity that we found in the homogenized carcinoma might be low because of contamination by a considerable quantity of blood. However, the histochemistry confirmed that the γ-GT activity of the carcinoma was low, and was considerably less than that of normal renal cortex. The carcinoma, therefore, would contribute little to the urinary γ-GT activity.

The urinary γ-GT values returned to normal after treatment with tobramycin was stopped. The slight decrease in urinary γ-GT activity that occurred postoperatively would be expected with removal of a partly functioning kidney. We have shown that tobramycin does not affect the γ-GT assay in vitro.

The increase in urinary γ-GT values that results from administration of tobramycin is both interesting and important, in view of the doubt concerning nephrotoxicity of aminoglycoside antibiotics (*13*). The change in γ-GT (two- to three-fold the upper limit of normal) was even greater (10- to 15-fold normal) when the γ-GT/CC ratio was calculated, illustrating that the calculation of such a ratio provides a more useful index for the interpretation of the urinary γ-GT values than does excretion rate alone.

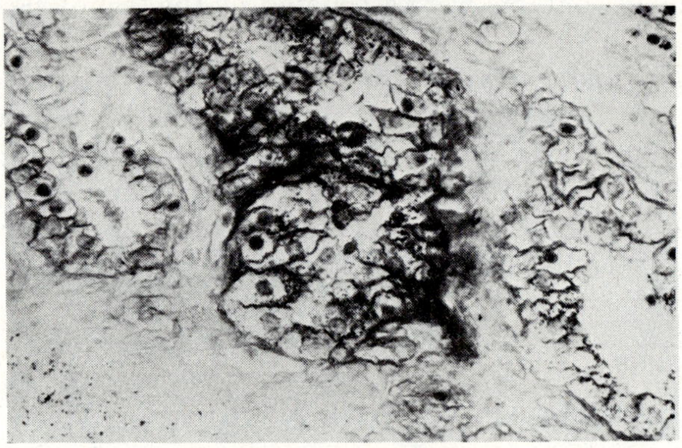

Fig. 4. γ-GT activity of renal carcinoma
Note the much lower intensity of staining as compared to normal renal cortex illustrated in Figure 2 (× 800)

The change in urinary γ-GT was not associated with other evidence of renal dysfunction; serum creatinine and creatinine clearance remained constant, and proteinuria was insignificant. We do not know whether the change in urinary γ-GT was the result of renal damage or of enzyme induction. In view of the propensity of the liver to respond to drug administration by inducing γ-GT (*14*), such induction is a distinct possibility.

Kanamycin similarly increases urinary γ-GT (*6*), and a more extensive study of the effect of the aminoglycoside antibiotics on urinary γ-GT is in progress.

We thank Mr. R. Scott for allowing access to the patient while under his care during surgery. Thanks are also due to the Department of Histopathology, Royal Infirmary, for preparing the tissues before histochemistry and for taking the photomicrographs.

References

1. Lévy, A., and Dubach, U. C., γ-Glutamyltranspeptidase-Aktivität im Urin bei urorenalen Krankheiten. *Klin. Wochenschr.* **50,** 438 (1972).

2. Kley, V. R., Bahre, G., and Holzhüter, H., Die Bestimmung der γ-glutamyl transpeptidase im Urin von nierengesunden und nierenkranken Personen mit einer automatischen kinetischen Methode. *Z. Klin. Chem. Klin. Biochem.* **11,** 537 (1970).

3. Thiele, K. G., γ-Glutamyltranspeptidase Aktivität im Urin bei Gesunden und Nierenkranken. *Klin. Wochenschr.* **51,** 339. (1973).

4. O'Meara, J., M.Sc. thesis, University of Birmingham, 1975.

5. Beck, P. R., and Sammons, H. G., A stabilising factor for γ-glutamyl transpeptidase in urine. *Clin. Chim. Acta,* in press.

6. Beck, P.R., A study of urinary gamma-glutamyl transpeptidase with special reference to renal disease. M.Sc. thesis, University of Birmingham, 1974.

7. Lowry, O. H., Rosebrough, N. S., Farr, A. L., and Randall, R. J., Protein measurement with the Folin phenol reagent. *J. Biol. Chem.* **193,** 265 (1951).

8. Albert, Z., Orlowski, M., and Szewczuk, A., Histochemical demonstration of gamma-glutamyl transpeptidase. *Nature* **191,** 767 (1961).

9. Szewczuk, A., and Orlowski, M., The use of (N-γ-DL-glutamyl)-aminoproprionitriles for the colorimetric determination of a specific peptidase in blood serum. *Clin. Chim. Acta* **5,** 680 (1960).

10. Kokot, F., Kuska, J., Grzybek, H., and Cekanski, A., γ-Glutamyl transpeptidase in tumor diseases. *Arch. Immunol. Ther. Exp.* **13,** 586 (1965).

11. Kotlarek-Haus, S., Aktywność gammaglutamylotranspeptidazy surowicy krwi w scharzeniach nowotworowych. *Pol. Tyg. Lek.* **17,** 1365 (1962) [quoted in Zein, M., and Discombe, G., *Lancet* **ii,** 748 (1970)].

12. Szczeklik, A., Szewczuk, A., Nowosad, H., and Kolaczkowska, B., Serum peptidases in myocardial infarction. *Br. Heart J.* **34,** 232 (1972).

13. Scottish Gentamicin Symposium. *Scott. Med. J.* **20,** 141 (1975).

14. Davidson, D. C., McIntosh, W. B., and Ford, J. A., Assessment of plasma glutamyl transpeptidase activity and urinary D-glucaric acid excretion as indices of enzyme induction. *Clin. Sci. Mol. Med.* **47,** 279 (1974).

special report

The International Federation of Clinical Chemistry[1][2]

IFCC Section no. 3

Editor: Nils-Erik Saris

Dept. of Med. Chemistry, University of Helsinki, Siltavuorenpenger 10, SF-00170 Helsinki 17, Finland

INTERNATIONAL FEDERATION OF CLINICAL CHEMISTRY

Committee on Standards

Expert Panel on Nomenclature and Principles of Quality Control in Clinical Chemistry

J. Büttner, Hannover (G.F.R.), Chairman, *R. Borth*, Toronto (Canada), *J. H. Boutwell*, Atlanta, Ga. (U.S.A.), *P.M.G. Broughton*, Leeds (U.K.)

PROVISIONAL RECOMMENDATION ON QUALITY CONTROL IN CLINICAL CHEMISTRY

Part 1. General Principles and Terminology

(Stage 2, Draft 2[3])

This paper is the first of a series of recommendations on quality control, and has been prepared by the Expert Panel after consideration of comments on earlier drafts made by National Societies of clinical chemistry.

Subsequent papers will deal with:

Part 2. Assessment of analytical methods for routine use.
Part 3. Calibration and control materials.
Part 4. Internal quality control.
Part 5. External quality control.
Part 6. Quality requirements from the point of view of health care.

Comments on these Provisional Recommendations are invited and should be received not later than 1975-12-31 by

Prof. J. Büttner,
Medizinische Hochschule,
D-3000 Hannover-Kleefeld,
Karl-Wiechert-Allee 9.

After revision, the Provisional Recommendations will eventually be submitted as Definitive Recommendations for acceptance by the Council of the International Federation of Clinical Chemistry.

Contents

1. General
2. Precision
3. Accuracy
4. Statistical methods
5. Terminology
6. References

---

[1]) Reprinted from Clin. Chim. Acta (1975) Vol. 63, pp. F 25–38, following p. 108 with the authorization of the Executive Board of the IFCC and the permission of the Editor.

[3]) Part 1 was drafted for the EP-NPQC Meeting Copenhagen 1972–06. Stage 1, draft 2: Copenhagen 1972–06. Stage 1, draft 3: Geneva 1972–12. Stage 1, draft 4: by correspondence. Stage 1, draft 5: Munich 1973-08. Stage 2, draft 1: by correspondence 1973-12 (to Associate members 1974-01). Stage 2, draft 2: Hannover 1974-12.

1. General

1.1

Communities provide funds for clinical chemistry (CC) as a part of health care. The most important purpose of CC is to measure, in body fluids and tissues of individual patients, those substances which are relevant for the understanding, prevention, diagnosis, or treatment of disease.

1.2

This purpose requires many diverse activities. Scope and relevance change as medical knowledge is growing. Measurements, whether of concentration or of any other type of quantity, need a yardstick (standard), a system of units, and a method, as well as personnel and facilities. Interpretation of analytical results must take into account their reliability as well as the variation known to exist in health and disease. Administration, organization, and handling of information are involved at all stages.

1.3

Analytical methods (whether in CC or other fields) are fully described by their performance characteristics: specificity, accuracy, precison, and sensitivity (Jointly referred to as reliability criteria); and speed, cost, technical skill requirements, dependability[4]), and laboratory safety (jointly referred to as practicability criteria). These performance characteristics are both necessary and sufficient: all of them must be considered, and any other considerations one might wish to include as relevant to analytical performance can in fact be shown to be covered implicitly by this set of concepts. If the degree of reliability achievable with a method is less than required for a stated purpose, the method should be declared unsuitable.

1.4

The definition of the term Quality Control (QC) in CC deserves careful consideration because of the special technical meaning involved.

1.4.1. In its widest sense, QC would have to be concerned with the reliability of laboratory information about patients. This information would include not only laboratory results, but also the background data which are needed to interpret results correctly, such as circadian and other intra-human variation, the effect of drugs, and knowledge of the appropriate normal range or reference values. However, most of these factors are outside the control of the laboratory.

1.4.2. Therefore, QC in CC is defined (see Section 5 for definitions of technical terms) as the study of those errors which are the responsibility of the laboratory, and of the procedures used to recognize and minimize them, including all errors (such as random variation and bias) which arise within the laboratory between the receipt of the specimen and the despatch of the report. The responsibility of the laboratory may extend to the collection of the specimen from the patient, and the provision of a suitable container. Crude errors or mistakes (e.g. wrong sample identification, incorrect transcription), although they cannot be controlled by the usual statistical QC methods, are nevertheless the concern of the laboratory.

1.4.3. In a narrower sense, the term QC in CC refers mainly to the monitoring of precision and accuracy of the performance of analytical methods.

1.4.4. It must be made clear to laboratory personnel that QC is an obligation to the patient, that it is designed to give analysts confidence in the methods used, and that its purpose is not to find scapegoats or to punish mistakes. There should be clear instructions and assignments of responsibility for remedial action when the performance of an analytical method deteriorates.

1.5

Different authors have adopted different basic philosophical positions (different models of reality) in discussing the "true meaning" of the terms and concepts used in QC. It can be argued, for example, that there is no single true value for a quantity, but rather a distribution of true values. Others consider that the true value is unknowable. The choice of a particular position, although endlessly debatable, is essentially arbitrary. Certain basic assumptions are implicit in any treatment of the subject, and the following premises are adopted in this document:

(1) Concentration and other types of quantity in CC are continuous variates in the mathematical sense.
(2) Specimen quantities have true values.
(3) The purpose of measurements is to obtain results which are useful estimates of true values.
(4) Precision and accuracy refer to a set of results obtained under stated conditions, not to single results.
(5) Probability is a relative frequency of chance occurrence derived from stated assumptions.

1.6

For important practical reasons, such as problems of operation and experimental design, it is convenient to make a distinction between internal QC (within a laboratory), and external QC (involving at least two laboratories). The theoretical basis is the same.

1.7

Essentially, both precision and accuracy are assessed by doing replicate assays on samples of the same specimen which are assumed to be stable and identical regarding the quantity investigated. In statistical terminology, the replicate results used are considered a random sample from a hypothetical population of replicates; the mean (as well as other measures of location or central tendency) of this sample reflects the performance of the

---

[4]) This concept refers to the risk or frequency of breakdowns.

method with respect to accuracy, and the standard deviation (S.D.) (as well as other measures of dispersion) with respect to precision.

1.8
Both precision and accuracy are conventionally measured in terms of quantities which decrease in value as the reliability is increased or improved: more precise methods have smaller standard deviations between replicate results; more accuracy is reflected in a smaller deviation of results from the true value. There is some linguistic awkwardness in this inverse relationship. In the past, this has been dealt with in three ways:

(1) Most authors have ignored it.
(2) Others have defined new parameters which are reciprocals of the conventional ones; e.g. the inverse value of the S.D. has been called "precision".
(3) Still others have used the dictionary words "imprecision" and "inaccuracy" in their respective ordinary meaning to rename the conventional parameters, that is, the S.D. has been called *imprecision* and the deviation from the true value *inaccuracy.*

In this document, the third approach has been selected as the preferred compromise between linguistic consistency and current usage. The exact definitions are given in Section 5. It is realized that the compromise may satisfy neither the advocates of the two other possibilities nor those who would prefer other terms for the same concepts.

1.9
This part of the recommendations is an attempt to produce consistency and unification of concepts and terms through selection from the literature combined with some innovation. To achieve wide acceptability and rapid general adoption in practice, it was thought mandatory that innovations should be limited in scope, easily comprehensible, and recognizably derived from tradition and current practice.

2. Precision

2.1
As stated in Section 1.8 and in the definitions in Section 5, precision should be understood to have no numerical value, and the measured parameter corresponding to this performance characteristic should be referred to as *imprecision*; roughly equivalent terms sometimes used in the past include "scatter" and "analytical variability". Imprecision is determined by making replicate assays of the same specimen, or of each of a set of specimens, according to a stated replication design (e.g. between-days, within-series, etc.), and then calculating the S.D. of replicate results per specimen. The specimens used may be patients' specimens received for analysis, or they may be control specimens. The only assumption, whether tested or tacit, is that the replicate samples of a specimen have the same true value.

2.2
The S.D. obtained in this way may reflect only unattributed random variation, or it may include identifiable sources of variation arising from the use of different specimens, concentrations, series, reagents, instruments, analysts, days (or other periods of time), methods, and laboratories. Each of these may be of methodological interest, and each requires an adequate experimental design and statistical analysis for its determination. These factors can contribute to imprecision and, very important, can also produce inaccuracy. In reporting estimates of imprecision, it should always be clearly stated which sources of variation have been included in the experimental design used.

2.3
In the absence of recognized criteria for cost-benefit analysis, recommendations regarding the frequency and design of replicate assays for QC purposes have to be based on the intuitive assessment, by experienced workers, of minimum requirements and maximum feasibility. Since assay results within a laboratory will usually be subject to most of the sources of variation listed in 2.2, it seems reasonable to include them all in the QC estimation of precision.

2.4
Precision is said to be under control as long as the replicate variation (imprecision) remains below a limit predicted from probability considerations and previous performance. The probability level chosen is the permissible frequency of values exceeding this limit.

2.5
The precision of results obtained by an analytical method may be under control as defined in 2.4 without being satisfactory for certain purposes. No simple rigorous criterion for acceptability of a method is likely to cover even values, of a treatment effect, or of a time trend. The usefulness of an analytical method in CC is established through a slow process of trial and error, and the relation between achievable precision, biological variation, and the magnitude of changes to be detected is part of this empirical assessment. Consequently, there are at present three schools of thought. One school regards imprecision as a descriptive parameter reflecting the state of the art, which is subject to almost limitless improvement. Another school recommends that imprecision should in some way be related to biological variation such as that between and within healthy individuals. The third school stipulates pragmatically that the precision of an analytical method should be assessed in terms of its clinical usefulness.

3. Accuracy

3.1

The accuracy of analytical results will be affected by the same identifiable sources of variation which contribute to imprecision (Section 2.2). Each may be of methodological interest, and each can be investigated using an adequate experimental design and statistical analysis. In addition, the calibration process and calibration standards can be important sources of inaccuracy. This problem requires careful consideration before methods of monitoring inaccuracy can be discussed usefully.

3.2. Calibration standards in clinical chemistry

3.2.1. In some contexts, the use of the word standard, without additional explanation, may be ambiguous, e.g. standards for instruments (which could refer to calibration standards or to performance requirements), standardization of methods (which could refer to their calibration or their uniformity). The specific term *calibration standard* should be used for the standards discussed in this section, whenever necessary to avoid such ambiguity.

3.2.2. It is customary to set up one or more calibration standards with each run or series of samples, and to calculate the assay results from the calibration readings. This approach has several important limitations.

3.2.2.1. The method may not be specific: the sample then generates an unwanted signal which does not arise with a pure substance. In an attempt to overcome this, the substance may be incorporated into a biological matrix so that the calibration standard resembles the sample. However, the non-specific components may be different in the standards and samples and may varying inaccuracies with different samples which cannot be corrected by changing the calibration material.

3.2.2.2. With some analyses, it may be impossible to put a calibration standard through all stages in the analytical procedure.

(i) Sometimes aqueous standards cannot be treated in exactly the same manner as specimens (e.g. in methods involving protein precipitation or enzymic degradation of conjugates).

(ii) The calibration standard may be unstable, expensive, or inadequate for other reasons, and therefore not easily used in daily routine analysis. In these cases, the specimen concentration may be calculated by using some characteristic of the standard (e.g. molar absorption coefficient) or by comparison with some other material which has a known relationship with the standard (e.g. the methyl red standard used in some bilirubin methods).

(iii) Calibration standards for the component determined may not exist (e.g. enzymes). In such cases, the result is calculated partly or solely from instrument readings of time, temperature, mass, volume, pressure, etc.

3.2.3. IUPAC has classified standards into 5 grades:

Grade A: atomic weight standard.
Grade B: ultimate standard.
Grade C: primary standard, a commercially available substance of purity 100 ± 0,02%.
Grade D: working standard, a commercially available substance of purity 100 ± 0,05%.
Grade E: secondary standard, a substance of lower purity, which can be standardized against primary (Grade C) material.

At present this classification is inadequate for the standards used in clinical chemistry for the following reasons:

(i) The statements of purity are not given in a form useful in practice. The nature as well the content of the impurities may be important.

(ii) Most commercial specifications state only the maximum limits of impurities, and the actual content of impurities may vary with each batch. Consequently, it may be impossible to categorize the standard in terms of the IUPAC classifications.

(iii) Most standards used in CC are less pure than Grade D, but often these cannot be standardized against Grade C material because a suitable standard of this grade does not exist.

(iv) Many standards used in CC (mixtures, arbitrary standards) are completely outside the IUPAC classification.

3.2.4. In this document a pragmatic approach is used, and standards are classified into two easily recognizable groups. Solutions only are considered here, but the approach is valid for gases and solids as well.

(i) A primary standard solution is one in which the concentration is determined solely by dissolving a weighed amount of standard material in an appropriate solvent and making to a stated volume or weight. The accuracy of a primary standard solution depends solely on the purity of the standard material and other components, and the accuracy with which the solution is prepared.

(ii) A secondary standard solution is one in which the concentration or other quantity is determined by an analytical method of stated reliability. The accuracy of a secondary standard therefore depends on the accuracy of the analysis, which in turn will involve a standard: ultimately this must be a primary standard. With this classification, both potassium permanganate solution and serum can function as secondary standards. In this document, no attempt is made to distinguish between them by use of terms such as calibration material, reference material, or standard specimen.

3.2.5. The concentration or other type of quantity of the standard must be stated in units which are approved by IFCC and IUPAC. This value may be a stated value, reference method value, or certified value (see Section 5).

3.2.6. In CC a wide variety of calibration standards may be used, and these may be classified by using the following additional descriptive terms as appropriate:

(i) Composition, e.g. nature and purity of constituents and of any solvent or matrix.
(ii) Physical state, e.g. solid, solid after lyophilisation, liquid, solution, suspension, gas.
(iii) Origin, e.g. name of manufacturer, batch number, species, tissue.
(iv) Quantification, e.g. determined by weighing (primary standard) or analysis (secondary standard), together with a statement of confidence limits. For secondary standards, the method by which the value is obtained must be stated, together with any assumptions made.
(v) Stability, e.g. shelf life under stated storage conditions, nature and amount of any preservatives.
(vi) Application, e.g. the type of analysis for which the standard is intended.
(vii) Additional terms: in some instances it may useful to add additional terms, such as international, arbitrary, internal, etc. These must always be defined.

3.3

Various methods have been proposed to monitor accuracy: the use of control specimens, recovery experiments, calculation of the daily mean, and the assay of specimens obtained from healthy subjects. The methods differ considerably in their theoretical basis and applicability.

3.3.1. Inaccuracy can be monitored by assaying control samples assumed to have the same true values, namely, that of the control specimen from which they are taken. If the true value in the control material is not known, the procedure will detect only changes in accuracy. If the true value is known, the procedure will, in addition, measure the inaccuracy, i.e. the mean deviation from the true value in a set of replicate results. Calibration and blank readings should be monitored along with results of control assays, as accuracy changes detected by the control system can often be traced to changes in the calibration process.

3.3.2. In recovery experiments, assays are made on a pair of samples of a specimen, a known amount of substance having been added to one of the two samples. The difference between results within the pair is the amount recovered, and the deviation of this from the amount added is a measure of the inaccuracy in the range covered and for the sample used.

3.3.3. According to the daily mean method, the mean is calculated from results obtained during a day, or other suitable period of time. Within such a period, either all results are used, or only those which fall within a suitable defined range; the definition of the latter may be quite arbitrary. Changes in this mean are taken to reflect changes in accuracy. This claim is based on the premise that day-to-day changes in the set of specimens received for analysis are negligible in their effect on the mean. Whether this is true or not will depend on local conditions and their change with time. It is not surprising, therefore, that confirmatory as well as refuting evidence on the usefulness of this method has been published. It should be noted that the alleged stability of the hospital population mean can be properly investigated only by an independent method of detecting inaccuracy, and that apparent stability of this mean may possibly mask true changes in accuracy. On the other hand, it is noteworthy that the daily mean method is the only QC method which takes into account sources of variation which might affect specimens before they arrive in the laboratory.

3.3.4. When introducing a new method, the laboratory will usually determine a series of reference values in healthy subjects ("normal range"). Any subsequent alteration in the accuracy of the method will produce a change in reference values. If the range of reference values in healthy subjects is small, one or more reference specimens (e.g. from laboratory staff) can be used as control specimens to monitor changes in accuracy. This method of QC is particularly useful for components which are absent or unstable in other types of control specimen.

3.4

There are no agreed criteria for cost-benefit analysis, and the frequency and design of control assays will be decided on the basis of an intuitive assessment of requirements and feasibility (as in Section 2.3). If these assays are done in replicate, they will provide data on precision as well as accuracy.

3.5

Inaccuracy should be zero within the error of the estimate. If it is not, remedial steps should be taken to make it so. Circumstances, including the state of the art, may make inevitable the temporary use of a method which is performing with a consistent bias. But continued toleration of inaccuracy is definitely not acceptable in CC.

3.6

Assay results can be numerically corrected for known inaccuracy. However, it should be emphasized that this procedure is valid only under the assumptions that the inaccuracy (i) has been reliably determined, and (ii) is known to vary no more than negligibly between specimens. Unless these assumptions are verified, routine numerical correction may produce a deceptive impression of good accuracy not warranted by fact.

4. Statistical methods

4.1

Statistical methods are an essential part of QC. Specimens of control material are included in a run of patients' specimens, and the results found for the control specimens are regarded as representative of all of the patients' specimens in that run. Consequently, there is always the implicit assumption and intent that the control specimens behave and are treated in the same way as patients' specimens. The results of the control specimens undergo statistical tests which are intended to show whether the analytical method is "under control". Before using a statistical test, the applicability of the mathematical model from which it is derived should be examined; for example, the distribution of the data should be approximately Gaussian if the test requires this for its validity. From past experience it seems likely that means and standard deviations will be adequately applicable to most QC problems in CC, and that recourse to other parameters (e.g. median, mode, mean deviation) or to nonparametric statistical methods will seldom be of significant advantage.

4.2

The main statistical tool employed in QC is the control chart. This is a graph in which the quantity or statistic to be controlled is plotted against time of observation. The time variation of the quantity or statistic is estimated, preferably with at least 20–30 degrees of freedom, during an initial period in which the performance of the analytical method was regarded as satisfactory, either intuitively, or by comparison with objective criteria where these exist. From the observed distribution, control limits are calculated within which most (customarily, 95 or 99 percent) of the values are likely to fall, and these limits are also plotted on the graph. The method is said to be under control as long as values outside the control limits occur less frequently than once in 20 or 100 times, depending upon the chosen probability of chance occurrence. The calculation of control limits is repeated at suitable intervals, based on the performance data which accumulate over months and years of satisfactory operation. Control charts should be kept up to date and displayed.

4.3

Occasionally, an observed change may be just large enough to be significant in terms of the statistical test used, while being at the same time so small that it can be disregarded for all practical purposes. Statistical test should not be applied mechanically: while a statistically significant change is, in terms of the statistical model used, unlikely to have occurred by chance, it remains nevertheless the analyst's (not the statistician's) responsibility to decide what is relevant in the practical context. This general rule applies to QC as it does to all other uses of statistical tests.

4.4

Conversely, from a mechanical use of the control chart, the risk of committing an "error of the second kind", i.e. of failing to detect a real change in performance, may seem to be of little importance in QC, since it is the logical basis of the control chart method that fluctuations, whether real or random, are negligible as long as they remain within the control limits. In practice, however, a consistent trend or permanent change should, of course, not be ignored by the analyst merely because control limits fail to be crossed.

4.5

If markedly discrepant results, so called outliers, are discarded and replicates averaged, variation is, of course, reduced, and the control chart will look better (despite the fact that calculated limits will also be narrower). Some authors seem to imply that this is an end in itself, and they advocate these procedures as if they were means to improve performance. Needless to say this is not so, and the frequency of outliers and the magnitude of run-to-run variation must not be ignored in assessing performance.

4.6

The quantity plotted may be a single result on a control sample or a mean (inaccuracy), a standard deviation or range (imprecision). The underlying distribution may or may not be approximately Gaussian, and the statistical methods required to calculate the percentiles used as control limits must be chosen accordingly.

4.7

A useful refinement in plotting accuracy data is the so called cumulative sum ("cusum") chart, which enhances the visibility of changes and trends. The statistic plotted is the accumulating algebraic sum of signed, i.e. positive or negative deviations of the results from their expected value. Accuracy is said to be under control as long as the plotted points scatter randomly about a line of constant slope. This is assessed by testing randomness or slope variation. It should be emphasized that the slope of the plotted line cannot be zero unless the expected value used is exactly equal to the mean value found.

4.8

Appropriate designs and analysis of variance techniques will provide information on the relative importance of sources of variation. The calculation of variance components may be of interest, but a single component should, of course, not be used to predict variation which in reality is bound to include several components.

5. Terminology

Terms are listed in alphabetical order. Cross references to terms which are defined elsewhere in the list are indicated by underlining. Undefined terms are used in their ordinary dictionary meanings which are assumed to be obvious from the context. The list includes some terms which will be used in subsequent parts of the Recommendations.

Accuracy. Agreement between the best estimate of a quantity and its true value. It has no numerical value. See inaccuracy.

Aliquot. Measured portion of a whole having the same composition. General term referring to any solution, sample, mixture, etc.

Analyte. The component to be measured.

Analytical method. See method, analytical.

Analytical range. See range, analytical.

Assigned value. See value.

Bias. Same as inaccuracy.

Calibration. Process of relating the reading to the quantity required to be measured.

Carryover. The influence of a sample upon a following

Certified value. See value, certified.

Control material. Material used for quality control purposes.

Control specimens, control solution. Specimen or solution which is analyzed solely for quality control purposes, not for calibration.

Definitive method. See method, definitive.

Definitive value. See value, definitive.

Detection limit. The smallest single result which, with a stated probability (commonly 95%), can be distinguished from a suitable blank. The limit may be a concentration or an amount and defines the point at which the analysis becomes just feasible.

Error. Difference between the estimated value of a quantity and its true value. This difference (positive or negative) may be expressed either in the units in which the quantity is measured, or as a percentage of the true value.

External quality control. Procedure of utilizing, for quality control purposes, the results of several laboratories which analyze the same specimen(s).

Imprecision. Standard deviation or coefficient of variation of the results in a set of replicate measurements. The mean value and number of replicates must be stated, and the design used must be described in such a way that other workers can repeat it. This is particularly important whenever a specific term is used to denote a particular type of imprecision, such as between-laboratory, within-day, or between-day.

Inaccuracy. Numerical difference between the mean of a set of replicate measurements and the true value. This difference (positive or negative) may be expressed in the units in which the quantity is measured, or as a percentage of the true value.

Interference. The effect of a component, which does not by itself produce a reading, on the accuracy of measurement of another component.

Internal quality control. Procedure of utilizing the results of only one laboratory for quality control purposes.

Method, analytical. Set of written instructions which describe the procedure, materials, and equipment, which are necessary for the analyst to obtain a result.

Method, definitive. A method which after exhaustive investigation is found to have no known source of inaccuracy or ambiguity.

Method, reference. A method which after exhaustive investigation has been shown to have negligible inaccuracy in comparison with its imprecision.

Method of known bias. An analytical method in which the amount of bias has been established (the amount may be zero).

Method of unknown bias. An analytical method of unknown accuracy.

Precision. Agreement between replicate measurements. It has no numerical value. See imprecision.

Quality control in clinical chemistry. The study of those errors which are the responsibility of the laboratory, and the procedures used to recognize and minimize them. This study includes all errors arising within the laboratory between the receipt of the specimen and the dispatch of the report. On some occasions, the responsibility of the laboratory may extend to the collection of the specimen from the patient, and the provision of a suitable container. See external and internal quality control.

Random. Due to unattributed causes; not affected by any kind of systematic selection or arrangement.

Range, analytical. The range of concentration or other quantity in the specimen over which the method is applicable without modification.

Reading. The value indicated on the scale of an instrument or analytical device.

Reference method. See method, reference.

Reference method value. See value, reference method.

Result. Final value obtained for a measured quantity after performing a measuring procedure including all sub-procedures and laboratory evaluations.

Run. This usually refers to a set of consecutive assays performed without interruption. The results are usually calculated from the same set of calibration standard readings. However, this definition may not be universally applicable, and in these cases the word series should be used after defining it.

Sample. The appropriately representative part of a specimen which is used in the analysis. This sample should be called a test sample when it is necessary to avoid confusion with the statistical term "random sample from a population".

Sensitivity. The ability of an analytical method to detect small quantities of the measured component. It has no numerical value. See detection limit.

Specificity. The ability of an analytical method to determine solely the component(s) it purports to measure. It has no numerical value. It is assessed on the evidence available on the components which contribute to the result, and on the extent to which they do.

Specimen. Material available for analysis.

Standard. Material or solution with which the sample is compared in order to determine the concentration or other quantity. The compound term calibration standard should be used whenever needed to avoid confusion

with other technical or colloquial meanings of the word standard.
Standard, arbitrary. Calibration standard containing an unknown quantity of specified substance. The content is assigned by convention, and expressed in arbitrary units defined by convention for the material concerned. Examples: international biological standards, immunoglobulin standards.
Standard, internal. A substance, not normally present in the specimen and clearly distinguishable from the substance to be analyzed, which is added in known amount to the sample, or to both the standard and the sample, for the purpose of correcting results for inaccuracy.
Standard material, primary. Substance of known chemical composition and sufficient purity to be used in preparing a primary standard solution.
Standard solution, primary. Solution used as calibration standard in which the concentration is determined solely by dissolving a weighed amount of primary standard material in an appropriate solvent, and making a stated volume or weight.
Standard solution, secondary. Solution used as a calibration standard in which the concentration or other quantity has been determined by an analytical method of stated reliability.
Stated value. See value, stated.
Systematic error. Same as inaccuracy.
Value. (of concentration or other types of quantity in calibration standards, control specimens, etc., used in the following compound terms). The method by which the value is obtained must always be stated.
Value, assigned. Value assigned either arbitrarily (e.g. by convention), or from preliminary evidence (e.g. in the absence of a recognized reference method).
Value, certified. Value certified by some official body subject to conditions established by that body.
Value, definitive. A value given by a definitive method.
Value, reference. Those quantities with which an observed value is compared for interpretative purposes[5]).
Value, reference method. Best available estimate of the true value; most probable value derived from a set of results obtained by the most reliable reference methods available.
Value, stated. Value without official certification.
Value, true. Term considered to have a self-evident meaning requiring no definition. In practice, true values are approximated by reference method values.

Comment: The definitions given for value correspond to the definitions of methods as follow:

Method	Value
–	True value
Definitive method	Definitive value
Reference method	Reference method value (stated or certified)*
Method with known bias Method with unknown bias	Assigned value (stated or certified)*

* These four definitions reflect two independent classifications and are, therefore, not exclusive: reference method values as well as assigned values may at the same time be either certified or stated values.

[5]) This definition has been proposed by the IFCC Expert Panel on Theory of Reference Values.

Selected bibliography

1. Anido, G., van Kampen, E. J. & Rosalki, S. B., (1973), Progress in Quality Control in Clinical Chemistry, Transactions of the 5th International Symposium, Geneva, April 10–11, 1973. H. Huber
2. Bergmeyer, H. U. (1974), Methods of Enzymatic Analysis. Vol 1: Statistical Analysis, Control, and Assessment of Experimental Results. Academic Press and Verlag Chemie
3. Broughton, P. M. G. & Annan, W. (1971), Measurement of Analytical Precision in Clinical Chemistry, Clin. Chim. Acta *32*, 433–441.
4. Broughton, P. M. G. & Raine, D. N. (1969), Quality Control in Clinical Biochemistry, Ann. Clin. Biochem. *6*, 89–148.
5. Cali, J. P., Bowers, G. N. and Young, D. S. (1973), A Referee Method for the Determination of Total Calcium in Serum, Clin. Chem. *19*, 1208–1213.
6. Cooper, G. R. (1969), Quality Performance in Clinical Pathology, Progr. Clin. Pathol. *3*, 1–71.
7. Cotlove, E., Harris, E. K. & Williams, G. Z. (1970), Biological and Analytic Components of Variation in Long-Term Studies of Serum Constituents in Normal Subjects. III. Physiological and Medical Implications, Clin. Chem. *16*, 1028–1032.
8. Dixon, K. & Northam, B. E. (1970), Quality Control Using the Daily Mean, Clin. Chim. Acta *30*, 453–461.
9. Eisenhart, C. (1968), Expression of the Uncertainties of Final Results, Science *160*, 1201–1204.
10. Harris, E. K., Kanofsky, P., Shaker, G. & Cotlove, E. (1970), Biological and Analytic Components of Variation in Long-Term Studies of Serum Constituents in Normal Subjects. II. Estimating Biological Components of Variation, Clin. Chem. *16*, 1022–1027.
11. Ingle, J. D. (1974), Sensitivity and Limit of Detection in Quantitative Spectrometric Methods, J. Chem. Educ. *51*, 100–105.
12. International Symposium on Statistical Quality Control in the Analytical Laboratory (1968), Z. Anal. Chem. *243*, 751–825.
13. Lang, H., Rick, W. & Róka, L. (1973), Optimierung der Diagnostik (Merck-Symposium 1973 of the German Society of Clinical Chemistry). Springer-Verlag, Berlin
14. Meinke, W. W. (1971), Standard Reference Materials for Clinical Measurements, Anal. Chem. *43*, 28 A–47 A.
15. Proceedings: International Conference on Standardization of Diagnostic Materials. June 5–8, 1973. U.S. Department of Health, Education and Welfare (Oct. 1974). (Obtainable from Centre for Disease Control, Atlanta, Georgia, U.S.A.)

16. Rappoport, A. E. (1972), Quality Control in Clinical Chemistry. Transactions of the 4th International Symposium, Geneva, May 12–14, 1971, H. Huber
17. Stamm, D. (1974), Calibration and quality control materials, this j. *12*, 137–145.
18. Stevens, J. F. (1973), Control Materials for Clinical Biochemistry. Tech. Bull. No. 29, Ann. Clin. Biochem. *10*, 133–145.
19. Tonks, D. B. (1963), A Study of the Accuracy and Precision of Clinical Chemistry Determinations in 170 Canadian Laboratories. Clin. Chem. *9*, 217–233.
20. Westgard, J. O., Carey, R. N. & Wold, S. (1974), Criteria for Judging Precision and Accuracy in Method Development and Evaluation, Clin. Chem. *20*, 825–833.
21. Whitby, L. G., Mitchell, F. L. and Moss, D. W. (1967), Quality Control in Routine Clinical Chemistry, Adv. Clin. Chem. *10*, 65–156.
22. Williams, G. Z., Young, D. S., Stein, M. R. & Cotlove, E. (1970), Biological and Analytic Components of Variation in Long-Term Studies of Serum Constituents in Normal Subjects. I. Objectives, Subject Selection, Laboratory Procedures and Estimation of Analytic Deviation, Clin. Chem. *16*, 1016–1021.
23. Wilson, A. L. (1970), The performance characteristics of analytical methods. 1, Talanta *17*, 21–29.
24. Wilson, A. L. (1970), The performance characteristics of analytical methods. 2, Talanta *17*, 31–34.
25. Young, D. S., Harris, E. K. & Cotlove, E. (1971), Biological and Analytic Components of Variation in Long-Term Studies of Serum Constituents in Normal Subjects. IV. Results of a Study Designed to Eliminate Long-Term Analytic Deviations, Clin. Chem. *17*, 403–410.
26. Young, D. S. & Mears, T. W. (1968), Measurement and Standard Reference Materials in Clinical Chemistry, Clin. Chem. *14*, 929–943.

special report

Report of the Second Conference on Education in Clinical Chemistry

The first conference on education in clinical chemistry was held in Columbus, Ohio, March 29–30, 1973 and reported in *Clinical Chemistry* **19**, 1419–22 (1973). The site of the second conference sponsored by the AACC Committee on Education was the Howard Johnson O'Hare International Motor Hotel, Schiller Park, Illinois, a suburb of Chicago. Loyola University of Chicago served as the host institution. The conference, which was held on September 19–20, 1975, was attended by 75 people representing approximately 50 institutions.

The first morning of the conference was opened with a brief introduction by Dr. Paige K. Besch, Chairman of the Committee on Education. This was followed by an address of welcome from Dr. Raymond P. Mariella, Dean, The Graduate School, Loyola University of Chicago. The subject of "Accreditation and Certification of Chemists" was then discussed by Gene A. Zerlaut, who has been active in the American Institute of Chemists program for the certification of chemists and chemical engineers [*Chem. Eng. News* **53,** No. 13, 18–27 (1975)]. Dr. Morton K. Schwartz, then President of the AACC, spoke on the AACC position on accreditation and certification. This was followed by a talk on the role of the Council on Medical Education of the American Medical Association in the accreditation of pre- and post-doctoral programs in clinical chemistry. The talk, which was given by Dr. John E. Beckley, concluded the first morning's session.

In the afternoon, individual group sessions were organized to review guidelines for training in B.S., M.S., Ph.D., and postdoctoral programs. An additional session consisting of clinical chemists who are now in training or have recently completed their training was also formed. Each committee was to develop position papers to be reported to the conference on the following morning.

In the evening session, two talks were presented. Dr. Robert S. Melville, National Institutes of Health, spoke on "The Future Role of the National Registry in Clinical Chemistry in the Field of Clinical Chemistry." This was followed by a talk on "The Future Role of the American Board of Clinical Chemistry in the Field of Clinical Chemistry," by Dr. Kurt M. Dubowski, University of Oklahoma.

Bachelor's Degree Programs

Committee Chairman: Gary A. Zimmerman, Seattle University, Seattle, Washington 98122. Ten representatives from eight educational institutions and one hospital clinical laboratory attended the baccalaureate-level discussions. Only four had programs in actual operation: two having graduates of their program, another with several last-minute defections from the senior class, and one with its first enrollments this fall. Two additional programs anticipate administrative approval for initial enrollment by fall, 1976. The others were considering proposals in various stages of readiness. This mix forced a shift away from a discussion of experiences with the Columbus guidelines to a more general exchange of program-planning ideas.

It was agreed that some review of the Columbus statement regarding bachelor's degree programs would be needed in the near future, especially to allow the Association to respond in greater detail to inquiries about the essentials of a good program, and to form a more explicit basis for accreditation evaluations. It was suggested that all known program directors at this level be given an opportunity to review proposed modifications to the statement should it require alteration before the group meets again. Several points for consideration in such a review were raised, but no consensus was reached. The purpose of practical training and its duration might be expanded. An expansion of specified areas of biology to be included in recommended curricula should be considered. The level of competency to be achieved in biochemistry might be made more explicit. The level of training of faculty personnel associated with the program is not stated in the Columbus document but considerable attention was paid to the competency appropriate to the program director. While certification may not be an absolute necessity for a competent faculty program-director, it appears that at least the practical portion of the training should be under the supervision of a person with such recognition. The use of adjunct professors to furnish needed technical expertise may be particularly helpful to programs on smaller campuses.

There was unanimous agreement that accreditation at the baccalaureate level was desirable and that the parent institutions would actively seek this recognition when it becomes available. Such accreditation would give the discipline sharper focus on the campus, enhance the graduates' appeal to potential employers, and aid the program director in seeking continued support from the administration. There was concern expressed that baccalaureate accreditation not be divorced from that process used for the recognition of other levels of clinical chemistry training. Consigning B.S. programs to one route, the other three to another would be a serious blow to the continued identity of the discipline at this level.

Identity is still a problem for baccalaureate programs. A better publicity job needs to be done, perhaps with Association help, to underscore the theoretical and practical basis of this level of training, that would give the graduate the potential for a faster rate of advancement and a greater flexibility in the face of continuing technical advances than that of a medical technologist at a comparable baccalaureate level. A better definition of job identity for this kind of training will aid both the graduate and the potential employer.

The group felt it was important to maintain strong ties to the *chemistry* department. Proposed transfers of clinical chemistry training into newly formed Allied Health Sciences Departments probably should be resisted if the fundamental ties to the chemistry faculty would be weakened or eliminated by the transfer.

Membership in AACC for all training program personnel was strongly urged. It is proposed that the Directors meet regularly, at each AACC national meeting. The lack of communication among program personnel between these biannual meetings was noted with chagrin; the national meeting gatherings would not need to replace this kind of workshop, but they could bridge the communications gap. The national Committee on Education should formalize the collection of graduation statistics from each level of training and publish these data each year.

Master of Science Programs

Committee Chairman: Norbert W. Tietz, Mount Sinai Hospital Medical Center of Chicago, Chicago, Ill. 60605.[1] The committee felt that educational programs on the masters degree level are important to advance the professional competency of individuals and to fill the need for clinical laboratory supervisors.

Objectives

It is intended that graduates of this program have the theoretical and practical knowledge to perform and evaluate routine and advanced clinical chemical techniques and to establish as well as maintain proper quality-control programs. The graduate should be able to participate in the teaching, research, and administrative functions of the laboratory.

[1] Present address: University of Kentucky Medical Center, Lexington, Ky. 40506.

Prerequisites

Two types of entrants to masters degree programs can be identified. (*a*) baccalaureate graduates with a major in chemistry or in a closely related discipline having at least 32 semester hours of chemistry with training in general chemistry, quantitative analysis, organic chemistry, biology, mathematics, and physics; and (*b*) graduates with a bachelors degree in medical technology.

In all cases persons awarded a masters degree in clinical chemistry should acquire credits for a total of at least 32 semester hours in chemistry in addition to the requirements listed below.

Requirements

The student shall receive instructions in principles of modern clinical chemistry including pathophysiological chemistry, physical chemical principles, instrumentation, statistics, and quality control. It is also recommended that students develop skills in management, supervision, and teaching. A clinical chemistry service laboratory component including advanced and specialized techniques must be an integral part of the program. A candidate must also demonstrate the capability for individual investigation by a thesis dealing with a project related to clinical chemistry. A research project resulting in a published paper that includes a literature search may be accepted in lieu of a written thesis. It is anticipated that about two academic years of full-time study will be required to complete the curriculum.

It is recommended by this committee that the AACC introduce a system of accreditation of the masters degree program.

Doctorate Programs

Committee Chairman: Max E. Chilcote, Erie County Laboratories, State University of New York at Buffalo, Buffalo, N. Y. 14215.

Introduction

The committee recognizes that this training is now carried out within one of four different academic departments (or combination of departments):

(1) university chemistry department
 (a) analytical division
 (b) biochemistry division
 (c) chemistry and biology departments
(2) school of medicine, biochemistry department
(3) school of medicine, pathology department
(4) school of medicine, biochemistry and pathology departments

The committee also recognizes that the education and training of a clinical chemist to the awarding of the doctoral degree cannot of itself produce a completely trained clinical chemist. Further seasoning will be necessary for this graduate to qualify for a senior position in clinical chemistry. Prior experience of the doctoral graduate, depth of experience provided during the doctoral training period, and the indi-

The committee consisted of individuals who are in training or who have recently completed training programs. They were to give their views on their experiences with the respective pre- and postdoctoral programs to the program directors. The committee was composed of one predoctoral student, two postdoctoral fellows, three individuals who have been through postdoctoral training programs, and one individual who had been through a training program in a commercial laboratory. The following is not considered simply as criticism but rather in the nature of suggestions or recommendations that will alert program directors to some needs which are not now being sufficiently stressed in the training of clinical chemists.

The group was of the opinion that people who go through a predoctoral program in clinical chemistry, while they may benefit from many advantages, could not consider themselves sufficiently experienced to direct a clinical laboratory upon receipt of the Ph.D. degree. One advantage which redounds to a person going through a predoctoral program in clinical chemistry is that the postdoctoral training may be of shorter duration, i.e., one year instead of the two years which might be the case for an individual who has received his Ph.D. degree in biological chemistry or in chemistry. Most of the committee's members, having been trained in academic programs, were of the opinion that the postdoctoral training should take place in a major center of medical care where a person could be exposed to both research in clinical chemistry and the broad application of a clinical chemistry service group in an actual operating clinical laboratory. One person disagreed with this view; he had been trained in a commercial laboratory. He felt that there are actually some advantages to being trained outside the university hospital laboratory setting. A combination of training in a major medical center, a commercial laboratory, and as an apprentice clinical chemist would contribute toward the making of a well-rounded clinical chemist. However, it was generally appreciated that arranging a program that would encompass all three areas is not always possible. The group agreed that there should be, in addition to the normal clinical laboratory services, a reasonably active research program, with guidelines for people who have had no previous clinical research experience.

At this point the presentation is divided into three areas, all of which are related only to postdoctoral programs. They are:

I. The technical training area
II. The administrative area
III. Legal aspects

Technical Training

Clinical laboratory procedures and data handling: In the technical area, the group felt that one of the first steps in the postdoctoral training program should be experience in performing procedures that are in use in the clinical laboratory and orientation to the day-to-day "sample and data-handling processes" that occur in a hospital or commercial laboratory. It was the opinion of the group that this experience was being obtained in all training programs.

Clinical correlations: The postdoctoral trainee, if he is to communicate with residents and clinicians and learn the technical jargon and clinical correlations, should be involved in active interplay. He should not only learn the clinical correlations for clinical chemistry but should also learn enough about hematology, serology, and immunohematology to permit him to maintain a practical interchange of information with residents, clinicians, and pathologists. This lack of exposure to clinical correlations was regarded as one of the serious defects in a training program in a commercial laboratory.

Applied research and development: Experience in this area should be such that the trainee is able to evaluate methods, to know whether they are based on sound scientific principles, and be able to evaluate laboratory instrumentation.

The trainee should be made aware at this point of the practical facts of life concerning expenditures for setting up new procedures and for instruments. He must learn to think in a practical manner—that is, what is the best return on an investment, in terms of profit or service, even if he's not in an institution that must make a profit. The trainee should learn systematic approaches to trouble-shooting, even in a hectic laboratory situation.

Quality control: In the opinion of the group, this area is poorly covered in most training programs. The individual needs to be aware of the philosophical reasons for maintaining a quality-control system, and to have practical experience in setting up and maintaining a quality-control program.

The group feels that experience in quality control should be emphasized much more than it is at the present time. However, the emphasis should not be the usual academic approach of simply having trainees take another course in statistics.

Scope of programs: It was the consensus of the group that in the university hospital situation the programs were not always sufficiently well-rounded. There is some tendency, for example, either to overemphasize or underemphasize endocrinology or toxicology.

The reason offered for the lack of a well-rounded program in the university hospital is the fragmentation of laboratory services. In the usual situation, the endocrinology laboratory services (e.g.) are not under the control of the clinical chemistry program director. Quite often the trainee does not get adequate experience in one of the largest growing areas of clinical chemistry, namely, radioimmunoassay procedures.

Administrative Training

Supervisory experience: The group feels that an essential part of the training of the clinical chemist, one which should be in the last half of the program, is actual supervisory experience in running several sections clinical laboratory where there is *real* responsibility for the work being performed and *real* authority over the technologists performing this work. While receiving this experience the trainee should be directly confronted with any mistakes by the clinician, the pathologist, or the program director, whoever first becomes aware of the mistakes.

Management techniques: In the opinion of the group, the most serious deficiency in the academic training programs is the almost complete lack of training in management techniques. The trainee needs to be made aware of management techniques from the standpoint of planning, organizing, setting up priorities, preparing budgets, and delegation of authority. The most important area under this management training is delegation of authority and responsibility. The consensus of the group is that the program directors, even though they are managers, do not adequately delegate responsibility and authority.

Screening and hiring of personnel: The trainee should receive experience in screening and hiring technical and nontechnical personnel. The trainee should be able to judge whether a person is technically competent and whether he or she has the personality to fit in with the rest of the laboratory staff.

Performance evaluation systems: The trainee needs to receive an understanding of, and practice in, performance evaluation systems and the problems involved in a working laboratory, such as the poor worker and the excellent-but-unmotivated worker. A trainee also needs to have an understanding of salary systems and the basis for the salary system. It should be noted that in most of the academic settings there is usually a School of Business Administration available, which should be utilized as a resource by the program director. The program director should be aware of the pertinence of the management training which may be available.

Since computers are so widely available nowadays, the students should have some contact with data-processing systems in order to be able to use this tool effectively in a laboratory setting.

The question was raised as to what is the optimal size for a postdoctoral training group. At the present time, they vary in size from two to about 10 trainees. The number should be governed by the amount of time the program director can devote to the training program and be consistent with the production of a quality product.

Legal Aspects

The group felt that the legal aspects of running a clinical laboratory, both for a hospital and as a commercial laboratory, have not been effectively dealt with in the academic situation. Some areas that are not considered sufficiently are: (*a*) the personal liability of the laboratory director; (*b*) the legislative regulations, both on a state and federal level, that are often ignored because in the academic situation the university hospital laboratory is exempt from these regulations.

The trainee should be conversant with CLIA 76 at the end of his program and be aware of pending legislation that will affect his future.

Closing Statement

The postdoctoral trainee should leave the program with quality technical training and administrative experience, including management training. The trainee should be exposed to and have access to the area of laboratory management. Trainees in commercial laboratories should receive hospital experience as part of their training, because this is regarded as a serious deficiency in training programs based in commercial laboratories.

Accreditation

It was the consensus of those in attendance at this conference that accreditation of training programs is essential to ensure quality and to provide standardization in the educational effort. Accreditation should set minimum standards in the educational programs and ensure that the clinical aspects of training are in laboratories of the highest possible quality. All subcommittees recommended that until such time as the newly-created Accreditation Commission is organized in a manner sufficient to perform the tasks satisfactorily, accreditation should be made by appropriate committees of the AACC in consultation with the American Board of Clinical Chemistry and the National Registry in Clinical Chemistry.

Conclusion

An important issue raised at the conference was the continued need for communication among educators in clinical chemistry. Yearly meetings of program directors are desirable, to allow for exchange of ideas, to maintain a census of programs and students and to consider problems related to greater standardization of curricula. Permanent subcommittees of the Committee on Education should be established to prepare curriculum guides for each level of training and to provide guidance to those who wish to initiate programs or who require assistance in upgrading their activities.

Paige K. Besch
Baylor College of Medicine
Houston, Texas 77025
Edward W. Bermes, Jr.
Hugh J. McDonald
The Medical Center
Loyola University of Chicago
Maywood, Illinois 60153

Appendix 1: Training Programs

The following institutions have been reported to the American Association for Clinical Chemistry as offering training programs in clinical chemistry. This listing does not imply AACC approval. Correction, deletions, or additions to this list should be communicated to the AACC National Office, 1725 K St., NW, Washington, D.C. 20006.

Institution	*Level*	*Responsible individual*
Albany State College Chemistry Department Albany, Ga. 31707	B.S.*	Dr. Jack Steele
Auburn University Auburn, Ala. 36830	M.S.	Dr. Herbert H. Kohl
Baylor College of Medicine Dept. of Ob. & Gyn. Houston, Tex. 77025	Postdoctoral	Dr. Paige K. Besch
Bronx-Lebanon Hospital Ctr. Chemistry Division Grand Concourse Bronx, N. Y. 10457	Postdoctoral	Dr. Max Friedman
Buffalo General Hospital Buffalo, N. Y. 14203	Postdoctoral	Dr. Charles Bishop
City of Hope National Med. Ctr. Dept. of Clinical Pathology 1500 E. Duarte Road Duarte, Calif. 91010	Postdoctoral	Dr. Peter Dewhurst
Cleveland State University Dept. of Chemistry Cleveland, Ohio 44115	M.S., Ph.D., Postdoctoral*	Dr. Julius Kerkay
Erie County Lab State University of New York at Buffalo 462 Grider Street Buffalo, N. Y. 14215	Ph.D., Postdoctoral	Dr. Max E. Chilcote
Georgetown University Georgetown Univ. Hospital 3800 Reservoir Rd., N.W. Washington, D.C. 20007	Postdoctoral	Dr. Martin Rubin
Georgia State University Dept. of Chemistry Atlanta, Ga. 30303	B.S., M.S., Ph.D.*	Dr. William G. Trawick
Hahnemann Medical College Dept. of Biological Chem. 230 N. Broad Street Philadelphia, Pa. 19102	M.S., Ph.D., Postdoctoral, B.S.*	Dr. Thomas M. Devlin
Hartford Hospital Hartford, Conn. 06115	Postdoctoral	Dr. Robert W. Burnett
Harvard Medical School Dept. of Biological Chem. Biophysics Research Lab. 721 Huntington Avenue Boston, Mass. 02115	Postdoctoral	Dr. Bert L. Vallee
Henry Ford Hospital 2799 W. Grand Blvd. Detroit, Mich. 48202	Postdoctoral	Dr. Daniel H. Basinski
Louisiana State University Dept. of Pathology 1542 Tulane Avenue New Orleans, La. 70112	M.S., Ph.D., Postdoctoral	Dr. Myrton F. Beeler Dr. H. Peter Lehmann
Loyola Univ. Medical Center 2160 So. First Avenue Maywood, Ill. 60153	M.S., Ph.D., Postdoctoral	Dr. Hugh J. McDonald Dr. Edward W. Bermes
Medical College of Pennsylvania Philadelphia, Pa.	Postdoctoral	Dr. George J. Kaldor
Medical College of Virginia Dept. of Pathology 12th & Marshall Sts. Richmond, A. 23219	M.S., Ph.D., Postdoctoral	Dr. Seymour Bakerman

Institution	*Level*	*Responsible individual*
Medical Laboratory Assoc. 1025 So. 18th Street Birmingham, Ala. 35205	Postdoctoral	Dr. Christopher Frings
Michael Reese Medical Ctr. Dept. of Biochemistry Chicago, Ill. 60616	Postdoctoral	Dr. Samuel Natelson
Mt. Sinai Hospital Med. Ctr. Chicago, Ill. 60608	M.S., Ph.D.	Dr. Norbert W. Tietz
Mt. Sinai School of Medicine Dept. of Chemistry Fifth Ave. and 100th St. New York, N. Y. 10029	Postdoctoral	Dr. F. Hutterer
HIGMS-NIH Automation Section— Biomedical Engineering Program 5333 Westbard Avenue Bethesda, Md. 20014	Ph.D., Postdoctoral	Dr. Robert S. Melville
North Carolina Mem. Hospital Clinical Chemistry Lab. Chapel Hill, N. C. 27514	Ph.D., Postdoctoral	Dr. John Savory
Northeastern University College of Pharmacy & Allied Health Professions Boston, Mass. 02115	M.S.	Dr. Robert W. Giese
Ohio State University College of Medicine Columbus, Ohio 43210	M.S., Ph.D., Postdoctoral	Dr. Hanns-Dieter Gruemer
Quinnipiac College Mount Carmel Avenue, Box 131 Hamden, Conn. 06518	B.S.	Dr. Kent S. Marshall
Richmond College of the City University of New York 130 Stuyvesant Place Staten Island, N. Y. 10301	B.S.	Dr. George Odian
Royal Columbian Hospital New Westminister British Columbia, Can.	Postdoctoral	Dr. Ralph Spitzer
Rush Medical College Dept. of Biochemistry Chicago, Ill.	M.S.,* Ph.D.,* Postdoctoral*	Dr. Howard H. Sky-Peck
Seattle University Seattle, Wash. 98122	B.S.	Dr. Gary A. Zimmerman
Simon Fraser University Dept. of Chemistry Burnaby, B. C., Can.	B.S.*	Dr. R. A. Rockerbie
State Univ. of New York at Buffalo Dept. of Medical Technology 462 Grider Street Buffalo, N. Y. 14215	M.S.	Dr. Helen Lees
Suffolk University 41 Temple Street Boston Mass. 02114	B.S.	Dr. Maria Bonaventura
Univ. of Arkansas for Medical Sciences Dept. of Biochemistry 4301 W. Markham Little Rock, Ark. 72201	M.S., Ph.D., Postdoctoral*	Dr. Marge A. Brewster
Univ. of Calif. at San Diego Dept. of Chemistry LaJolla, Calif.	Postdoctoral, M.S.,* Ph.D.*	Dr. Nathan Gochman
University of Colorado 1100 14th Street Denver, Colo. 80202	Ph.D.*	Dr. John A. Lanning
University of Connecticut School of Medicine Drawer B Newington, Conn. 06111	Postdoctoral	Dr. William Sunderman, Jr.

Institution	*Level*	*Responsible individual*
University of Dayton Dept. of Chemistry Dayton, Ohio 45469	M.S.	Dr. S. L. Eveslage
University of Delaware Dept. of Chemistry Newark, Del. 19711	Ph.D.*	Dr. Robert Curry
University of Florida Gainesville, Fla. 32601	B.S., M.S., Ph.D., Postdoctoral	—
Univ. of South Florida Dept. of Chemistry Tampa, Fla. 33620	B.S.	Dr. Eugene D. Olsen
University of Iowa Dept. of Biochemistry Iowa City, Iowa 52242	M.S., Postdoctoral	Dr. J. I. Routh
University of Kentucky Med. Ctr. Lexington, Ky. 40506	Ph.D.*	Dr. Norbert W. Tietz
Univ. of Maryland Hospital 22 S. Greene St. Baltimore, Md.	M.S., Ph.D., Postdoctoral	Col. Edward C. Knoblock
Univ. of Minnesota Med. Ctr. Dept. of Lab Medicine & Path. Minneapolis, Minn. 55455	M.S.	Dr. Esther F. Freier
Univ. of Oklahoma Health Sciences Ctr. Dept. of Biochemistry and Molecular Biology P. O. Box 26901 Oklahoma City, Okla. 73190	Ph.D.	Dr. Kurt M. Dubowski
Univ. of Oregon Health Sciences Ctr. Dept. of Clinical Pathology Portland, Ore. 97201	M.S., Postdoctoral	Dr. J. Robert Swanson
Univ. of Pennsylvania Philadelphia, Pa. 19104	Postdoctoral	Dr. Dean A. Arvan
Univ. of Tennessee Dept. of Pathology Clinical Chemistry 800 Madison Avenue Memphis, Tenn. 38103	M.S., Ph.D.	Dr. Charles H. Smith
Univ. of Texas Medical Branch Clinical Laboratory Galveston, Tex.	M.S., Ph.D.*	Dr. Richard B. Passey
University of Toronto Dept. of Clin. Biochemistry Banting Institute Toronto, Can.	M.S., Ph.D., Postdoctoral	Dr. A. G. Gornall
University of Washington Dept. of Lab Medicine SB10 Seattle, Wash. 98195	Postdoctoral	Dr. Alex Kaplan
University of Windsor Dept. of Chemistry Windsor 11, Ontario, Can.	M.S., Ph.D.	Dr. R. J. Thibert
Univ. of Wisconsin-Madison 300 University Ave. Madison, Wis. 53706	M.S.	Dr. Merle Evenson
Washington Univ. School of Medicine and Barnes Hospital Division of Laboratory Med. St. Louis, Mo. 63110	Postdoctoral	Dr. Jack Ladenson
West Chester State College Dept. of Chemistry West Chester, Pa. 19380	B.S.	Dr. Robert F. Foery
Youngstown State Univ. Dept. of Chemistry Youngstown, Ohio 44555	M.S., B.S.,* Ph.D.*	Dr. Thomas Dobbelstein

* Programs now being planned.

Plasma P_i and Erythrocyte 2,3-Diphosphoglycerate Concentrations of Non-Acidotic Diabetics in Various Degrees of Metabolic Control

To the Editor:

Recently Kalofoutis et al. (*1*) suggested that erythrocyte 2,3-diphosphoglycerate (2,3-DPG) concentration in diabetics is the same as in normal persons. However, others find that in diabetics it fluctuates in relation to the state of metabolic control, not only during ketoacidosis and recovery when initially the erythrocyte 2,3-DPG content is markedly depressed (*2, 3*), but also in non-acidotic patients (*4, 5*). We have attempted to assess whether variation of plasma inorganic phosphate (P_i) affects the erythrocyte 2,3-DPG concentration in non-acidotic diabetics as it does in patients recovering from severe ketoacidosis (*3*).

Table 1 presents results for P_i and erythrocyte 2,3-DPG measured in a group of 10 non-acidotic, newly diagnosed, and otherwise healthy youth-onset type diabetics (8 males, 2 females; age range, 15 to 40 years) on the day of hospital admission, before insulin treatment (Group I); on the day after insulin therapy had been started (Group II); and on the day of best metabolic control (Group III), usually about a week after hospital admission. Group IV consisted of 15 apparently healthy nonsmoking volunteers, whose glucose-tolerance tests were normal. No significant differences were found among the four groups in arterial pH, p_{CO_2}, standard bicarbonate, and oxyhemoglobin saturation. (For methods, see ref. *3*.)

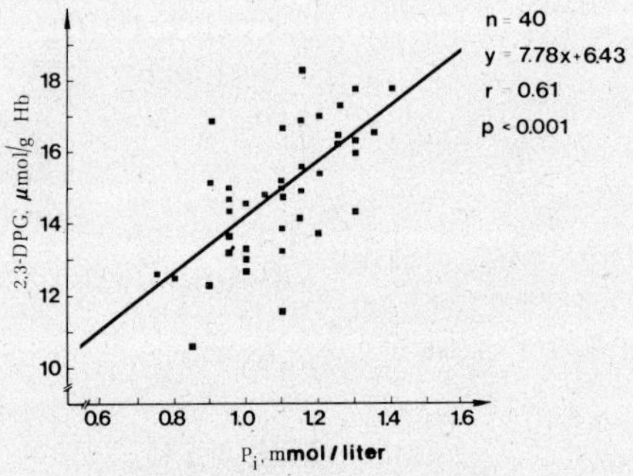

Fig. 1. Relation between erythrocyte 2,3-diphosphoglycerate and plasma inorganic phosphate concentrations

As Table 1 shows, P_i fluctuated in the diabetics, starting at an almost normal value on admission (Group I) to a lower range on the day after insulin treatment had been initiated (Group II), and rose again to slightly above-normal concentrations on the day of best metabolic control (Group III). 2,3-DPG exhibited the same fluctuating pattern as P_i, and in fact was correlated with P_i for all measurements performed in the diabetics on a total of 40 days (Figure 1).

Altered P_i in diabetic subjects may originate from several mechanisms: hemoconcentration and hemodilution, variation in urinary loss according to the degree of glycosuria, and (or) changes in cellular uptake of P_i in relation to glucose, especially by insulin-sensitive tissues. For all these reasons diabetics are highly susceptible to variations in the phosphate pool available for the erythrocytes. In the erythrocyte itself P_i is likely to influence 2,3-DPG concentration by its effect on 6-phosphofructokinase (EC 2.7.1.11) (*6*) and glyceraldehyde-phosphate dehydrogenase (EC 1.2.1.12) (*7*).

Hence, and as our results indicate, during changing metabolic conditions of diabetes P_i seems to be a strong determinant of erythrocyte 2,3-DPG content. Obviously the metabolic state of diabetes has to be considered, even in non-acidotic patients, before a reliable statement can be made on the amount of 2,3-DPG in diabetics. Depending on our selection criteria for patients, we could have reported 2,3-DPG values to be normal, decreased, or increased in diabetics. The conflict of data in the literature concerning erythrocyte 2,3-DPG concentration in non-acidotic diabetics (*1, 4, 5, 8–10*) therefore, seems likely to be attributable to differences in metabolic control.

Apparently it is important that erythrocyte 2,3-DPG concentrations can be low in non-acidotic diabetics in some metabolic states and that the oxygen-delivering capacity of erythrocytes is probably concurrently impaired in such patients.

Table 1. Some Clinical Chemical Values in 10 Newly Detected, Non-acidotic Diabetics at Various Stages of Metabolic Control and in 15 Normal Controls

Group	n	Hemoglobin, g/100 ml	Blood glucose, mmol/liter	P_i, mmol/liter	2,3-DPG, μmol/g Hb
Diabetics					
I	7	15.5 ±1.4	16.1 ±4.4	1.08 ±0.11	14.94 ±1.40
II	10	15.1 ±1.5	11.9 ±1.9	0.98 ±0.14	13.10 ±1.46
III	10	14.3 ±1.2	6.1 ±1.4	1.20 ±0.10	16.53 ±1.19
Normal controls					
IV	15	14.2 ±1.1	5.1 ±0.9	1.13 ±0.10	14.40 ±1.28

Significance (*P*-values) between groups

Group	P_i I	P_i II	P_i III	P_i IV	2,3-DPG I	2,3-DPG II	2,3-DPG III	2,3-DPG IV
I	—	<0.005	<0.05	N.S.[a]	—	<0.02	<0.01	N.S.
II		—	<0.005	<0.01		—	<0.001	<0.05
III			—	N.S.			—	<0.001

[a] N.S., nonsignificant.

References

1. Kalofoutis, A., Jullien, G., Koutselinis, A., and Miras, C., Erythrocyte 2,3-diphosphoglycerate as related to diabetes and obesity. *Clin. Chem.* **21**, 1414 (1975).

2. Alberti, K. G. M. M., Darley, J. H., Emerson, P. M., and Hockaday, T. D. R., 2,3-Diphosphoglycerate and tissue oxygenation in noncontrolled diabetes mellitus. *Lancet* **ii**, 391 (1972).

3. Ditzel, J., and Standl, E., The oxygen transport system of red blood cells during diabetic ketoacidosis and recovery. *Diabetologia* **11**, 255 (1975).

4. Standl, E., and Kolb, H. J., 2,3-Diphos-

phoglycerate fluctuations in erythrocytes reflecting pronounced blood glucose variation. In-vivo and in-vitro studies in normal, diabetic and hypoglycemic subjects. *Diabetologia* **9,** 461 (1973).

5. Ditzel, J., and Standl, E., The problem of tissue oxygenation in diabetes mellitus. II. Evidence of disordered oxygen release from the erythrocytes of diabetics in various conditions of metabolic control. *Acta Med. Scand., Suppl.* **578,** 59 (1975).

6. Kühn, B., Jacobasch, G., Gerth, C., and Rapoport, S. M., Kinetic properties of phosphofructokinase from erythrocytes of rats and rabbits. 1. The influence of potassium and ammonium ions and of inorganic phosphate. *Eur. J. Biochem.* **43,** 437 (1974).

7. Rapoport, S. M., Maretzki, D., and Schewe, C., In *Oxygen Affinity of Hemoglobin and Red Cell Acid Base Status,* M. Rørth, and P. Astrup, Eds., Munksgaard, Copenhagen; Academic Press, New York, N.Y., 1972, p 527.

8. Alberti, K. G. M. M., Emerson, P. M., Darley, J. H., and Hockaday, T. D. R., Red cell 2,3-diphosphoglycerate and diabetes. *Lancet* **i,** 843 (1972).

9. Rørth, M., Parving, H. H., and Munksgaard, S., Red-cell oxygen affinity and 2,3-diphosphoglycerate in diabetes. *Lancet* **i,** 1179, (1972).

10. Ditzel, J., Andersen, H., and Daugaard, P. N., Increased hemoglobin A_{1c} and 2,3-diphosphoglycerate in diabetes and their effects on red cell oxygen-releasing capacity. *Lancet* **ii,** 1034 (1973).

Jørn Ditzel

Section of Endocrinology
Department of Medicine
Aalborg Regional Hospital
9000 Aalborg, Denmark

Eberhard Standl

Diabetes Research Unit
City Hospital Schwabing
8000 Munich, Germany (FRG)

Thyroid-function Tests in Diphenylhydantoin-treated Patients

To the Editor:

A recent article in your journal (*1*) made two important points: that therapeutic concentrations of diphenylhydantoin in serum do not affect the binding of thyroxine to serum proteins, and that a free-thyroxine index may not be a valid indicator of thyroid status in diphenylhydantoin-treated patients. The authors found that by the Ames method 21% of patients tested had free-thyroxine indices that were within the hypothyroid range, and that by the Murphy–Pattee method the mean free-thyroxine index was significantly lower than in normal controls, although none of the individual values were within the hypothyroid range.

We believe that the true results are more striking than this, because the authors have not used their own reference ranges, but rather those of the manufacturer of the kits and of a distant laboratory. If one assumes the distributions of serum total thyroxine concentration and free-thyroxine index to be gaussian and uses the authors' data, the 95% reference ranges (±2 SD) for these two measurements are respectively 44–84 μg/liter and 44–84 for the Ames and 54–94 μg/liter and 53–90 for the Murphy–Pattee method. With these reference ranges, about 40–50% of diphenylhydantoin-treated patients have low serum total thyroxine concentrations and free-thyroxine indices by both techniques.

This illustrates the necessity to use reference ranges that have been determined in the population from which the tested patients are drawn. Perhaps laboratories performing tests on specimens received from a distance should point out that their own quoted reference ranges may not necessarily apply to the specimens tested. We know of one study in which specimens were sent to a laboratory 2500 miles away for serum total thyroxine assay and the use of the laboratory's quoted reference range led to incorrect conclusions (*2*); we have written to the authors to this effect.

In the original report on the effect of diphenylhydantoin on thyroxine binding to serum proteins (*3*), pharmacological drug concentrations were used, and if one extrapolates the data to a therapeutic diphenylhydantoin concentration of 15 mg/liter in the serum tested, the mean effect on erythrocyte triiodothyronine uptake was less than 6%.

In the study under discussion, in the Ames method, therapeutic concentrations of diphenylhydantoin in serum added to the Sephadex column did not affect triiodothyronine uptake. However, if an equivalent amount of the drug was first added to the column and serum then tested, triiodothyronine uptake was increased by 35%. We were puzzled by these apparently conflicting observations.

Other workers (*4*) have found high serum thyrotropin hormone and low serum total triiodothyronine concentrations in diphenylhydantoin-treated patients, whereas the authors of this study found normal serum thyrotropin hormone concentrations and would presumably predict high serum total triiodothyronine concentrations because of increased peripheral conversion of thyroxine to triiodothyronine. The reasons for these discrepancies are not clear.

The major finding of this study is obviously of great importance: nearly half of apparently euthyroid diphenylhydantoin-treated patients will have "hypothyroid" serum total thyroxine concentrations and free-thyroxine indices when compared to nontreated controls. Thus, alternative measurements (e.g., of serum thyrotropin hormone concentration) are necessary to evaluate thyroid status. We await with interest further reports on the effects of diphenylhydantoin on thyroid-function tests.

References

1. Stjernholm, M. R., Alsever, R. N., and Rudolph, M. C., Thyroid-function tests in diphenylhydantoin-treated patients. *Clin. Chem.* **21,** 1388 (1975).

2. Stock, J. M., Surks, M. I., and Oppenheimer, J. H., Replacement dosage of L-thyroxine in hypothyroidism. A re-evaluation. *New Engl. J. Med.* **290,** 529 (1974).

3. Oppenheimer, J. H., Fisher, L. V., Nelson, K. M., and Jailer, J. W., Depression of the serum protein-bound iodine level by diphenylhydantoin. *J. Clin. Endocrinol. Metab.* **21,** 252 (1961).

4. Hansen, J. R., Skovsted, L., Lauridsen, U. B., et al., The effect of diphenylhydantoin on thyroid function. *J. Clin. Endocrinol. Metab.* **39,** 785 (1974).

P. J. Phillips
R. W. Pain

Division of Clinical Chemistry
Institute of Medical & Veterinary Science
Adelaide, South Australia, 5000

The authors of the paper in question respond:

To the Editor:

We thank Drs. Phillips and Pain for their critical observations, which are in accord with our stated views regarding the "'hypothyroid' total thyroxine concentration and free thyroxine indices" in diphenylhydantoin-treated patients. We agree that the comparison between our controls and the patients is even more striking if the 95% reference ranges (±2 SD) are used. We elected not to do this because of the small number of normal controls. Instead, we used the manufacturer's range to emphasize that such a range is not valid for patients being treated with diphenylhydantoin.

Therapeutic concentrations of diphenylhydantoin in serum have no practical effect upon the triiodothyronine uptake test. In the experiment in which diphenylhydantoin was preloaded on Sephadex columns, the conditions differed from those of the routine assay. Some of the labeled diphenylhydantoin was eluted from the Sephadex column by the serum, presumably because of protein binding, when the column had been preloaded with diphenylhydantoin. Whether the amount of diphenylhydantoin displaced from the Sephadex is accessible to samples of serum and becomes "more free" to displace labeled triiodothyronine than the diphenylhydantoin already in sera of treated patients is a matter of conjecture.

The explanation for the normal serum thyrotropin concentrations in our patients as compared to the elevation reported by Molholm-Hansen et al. [*J. Clin. Endocrinol. Metab.* **39**, 785 (1974)] is as obscure to us as to others. The methods of assay were different. Moreover, they showed that the more sensitive thyrotropin-releasing factor (thyroliberin) stimulation test was not altered by diphenylhydantoin treatment.

We are pleased to see that Drs. Phillips and Pain agree that, in lieu of alternative thyroid tests, "determination of serum thyrotropin concentration may be the best single test of thyroid status during diphenylhydantoin therapy" (*1*).

Melvin R. Stjernholm
Robert N. Alsever
Merritt C. Rudolph

Univ. of Colorado Med. Center
Denver, Colo. 80220

Table 1. Effect of Two Kinds of Gloves on Apparent Radioactivity

Time after cap placed on vial, min	Empty vial: Vinyl gloves	Empty vial: Latex gloves	Vial + scintillation fluid: Latex gloves	Vial + scintillation fluid: Vinyl gloves
	cpm			
1	6 (>20%)	43209 (2%)	1120 (7%)	13 (>20%)
11	19 (>20%)	2567 (5%)	1050 (7%)	8 (>20%)
21	6 (>20%)	676 (10%)	15946 (2%)	6 (>20%)
31	12 (>20%)	929 (7%)	33 (>20%)	6 (>20%)
71	9 (>20%)	466 (10%)	6 (>20%)	13 (>20%)
101	10 (>20%)	8 (>20%)	60 (>20%)	8 (>20%)

Parenthetic percentages are maximum counting errors, in this Table and Table 2.

Table 2. Transfer of Charge to Empty Vials

Time after cap placed on vial, min	A Latex gloves	B Latex–Vinyl gloves	C Latex gloves; no external std.	D Latex gloves; external std.
	cpm			
1	85642 (2%)	760 (10%)	5607 (3%)	1083 (7%)
11	40520 (2%)	350 (15%)	3486 (5%)	526 (10%)
21	10410 (2%)	150 (>20%)	1311 (7%)	225 (15%)
31	5010 (3%)	50 (>20%)	238 (15%)	900 (7%)
71	580 (10%)	20 (>20%)	161 (>20%)	50 (>20%)
101	860 (7%)	40 (>20%)	17 (>20%)	30 (>20%)

"The Case of the Latex Gloves" in Scintillation Counting

To the Editor:

We think Holmes and Watson would approve of our detective work on a problem that baffled us recently. We had observed that when particular individuals in the laboratory performed procedures involving scintillation "cocktails" in the counting of radioactivity, they not only could increase the blank values, but could also obtain counts for the cocktails that far exceeded the total counts used in the assay. The following data (with 2.0% counting error) illustrate the point.

True blank cpm	16	18	16	14
Observed blank cpm	54000	15000	5280	120642
True cpm placed in tube	2500	2550	2490	2510
Observed total cpm in tube	150861	220156	5880	80000

We are familiar with other problems previously encountered in radioisotopic techniques such as quenching in scintillation counting and the problems of talc from gloves acting as adsorbents in radioimmunoassay procedures, and with the effect of nylon in build-up of static, but we were unaware of such problems ascribable to latex gloves. The error that could be so introduced into radioimmunoassay involving liquid-scintillation counting ranged from 0.2 to 9000% or even higher if we really tried! This fiendish ploy of our employees has been traced to latex gloves worn by particular ones while they were manipulating tracers. As we discovered, the problem arises from the static electricity generated by the friction associated with placing the screw caps in position on the counting vials (glass or polypropylene) while the operator is wearing latex gloves. The resulting charge is detected by the photomultiplier. The discharge of the charge was time-dependent (Table 1, columns B and C), and we have seen the charge remain on the tubes for as long as 24 h. Vinyl gloves cause no such problems. It should be pointed out, however, that if one wears latex gloves while placing the screw caps in position and changes to vinyl gloves without an intervening hand washing, the charge may be transferred to the vinyl gloves and then to successive counting vials (Table 2, columns A and B). The charge cannot be removed from the vials simply by precounting the tubes in the presence of an external standard (gamma emitter) in the scintillation counter (Table 2, columns C and D). The problem is not attributable to radioactivity on the gloves, because placing the gloves in the scintillation fluid in the vial does not contribute to the background counts if latex gloves are not used when the lids are placed on the vials. Our data show that charge can be generated on the vials independent of scintillation fluid and independent of activity or scintillation fluid in the vial.

For those wishing to repeat this Professor Moriarty ploy, we list the conditions we used: Scintillation counter: Beckman LS-150; Channel used: Tritium; Counting efficiency: 51.6% for tritium; Gloves: Becton-Dickinson, Rutherford, N. J. 07070 Featherweight vinyl examination gloves; Gloves: Pharmaseal Laboratories, Glendale, Calif. 91201 Flexam Floor/Examination latex gloves No. 8851; Counting vials: Beckman Poly-Q vials or Beckman glass vials. Relative humidity in laboratory: 10–15%.

Should the increase in counts be within the range expected of the assay, it may go undetected, particularly as we have observed that on duplicate samples we can induce approximately equal counts.

P. B. Dewhurst
J. C. Travis

City of Hope National Medical Center
Duarte, Calif. 91010

Poor Separation of Creatine Kinase Isoenzymes with Column-chromatographic Kits

To the Editor:

Since the introduction of the "mini-column" ion-exchange chromatographic technique for detecting the three isoenzymes of creatine kinase (CK; EC 2.7.3.2) MM, MB, and BB (*1*), commercial adaptations of this technique have been attempted. I report here a comparison between my original column method and the Worthington kit method (Worthington Biochemical Corp., Freehold, N.J. 07728). As the data in Table 1 demonstrate, there is significant carryover of MM and MB isoenzymes in the Worthington procedure.

MM isoenzyme carryover in the Worthington kit is best demonstrated in sera of patients without myocardial infarction but with elevated CK activity as a result of various noncardiac disorders (Table 1). In samples of this type, electrophoretic analysis (fluorometric agarose system) of the Worthington column MB fraction confirmed the suspected MM carryover; an electrophoretic band of MM activity was present in the MB fraction. The magnitude of MM carryover is demonstrated by CK activity in Worthington's MB fraction four- to 13-fold the Mercer values (Table 1). When MB values are expressed as percent of total CK, Mercer MB values ranging from 0.3 to 1.1% are within normal limits (less than 2%) previously established for MB isoenzyme in healthy laboratory technicians and in hospitalized patients with various noncardiac conditions (*2, 3*). However, Worthington %MB values in patients with no evidence for myocardial infarction are markedly above normal (4 to 11%) and similar to %MB values observed in five patients reported in Table 1 with myocardial infarction (6 to 12%). Thus, the carryover of MM is significant enough to change a normal MB activity into a falsely increased abnormal value. Obviously, when CK isoenzymes are measured in a sample with increased total CK, the MB test as performed by Worthington is of no clinical value, because MB values will overlap and provide no real distinction between cardiac and noncardiac conditions.

MB isoenzyme carryover into Worthington's BB fraction is best demonstrated in patients with myocardial infarction and increased MB activity. Electrophoretic analysis of the BB fraction confirmed the suspected MB carryover: a single MB electrophoretic band was present and no trace of BB isoenzyme. The magnitude of MB carryover is exhibited by CK activity in the BB fraction 23- to 31-fold the Mercer values (Table 1). Considering the significant amounts of MM and MB carryover in the Worthington system, it is surprising that a close comparison exists between Worthington and Mercer MB values. Apparently the MB activity that is eluted and lost to the BB fraction is replaced by a nearly equal amount of MM carryover into the MB fraction.

The reason for isoenzyme carryover is undoubtedly related to the experimental conditions prescribed by Worthington for eluting CK isoenzymes from the ion-exchange column. Although Worthington's kit method is an adaptation of my original column procedure (stepwise elution on a mini-column filled with DEAE-Sephadex), column conditions such as flow rate, pH, and sodium chloride concentrations of eluents differ markedly from those I described. Rather, Worthington follows the column conditions of Takahashi et al. (*4*), which were designed to separate tissue CK isoenzymes by gradient elution on a macro-column, not to separate serum CK isoenzymes by stepwise elution on a mini-column. Another column CK isoenzyme kit, from E-C Apparatus Corp., St. Petersburg, Fla. 33709, was not tested, but kit directions reveal eluate sodium chloride concentrations that are markedly different from mine. My column conditions (*1, 2*) were carefully chosen to provide rapid and uncontaminated separations of serum CK isoenzymes. Deviation from these conditions, as demonstrated in Table 1, can lead to poor separations and inaccurate determinations of CK isoenzymes.

References

1. Mercer, D. W., Separation of tissue and serum creatine kinase isoenzymes by ion-exchange column chromatography. *Clin. Chem.* **20,** 36 (1974).

Table 1. Comparison of Worthington[a] and Mercer[b] Column Procedures for Separation of MB and BB Isoenzymes

	Total CK	Worthington MB	Mercer MB	Worthington MB	Mercer MB	Worthington BB	Mercer BB
	U/liter			% of total CK		U/liter	
Patients without myocardial infarction							
Hypothyroidism	778	85	8.0	10.9	1.0	36	0.5
Intramuscular injection	616	26	2.4	4.2	0.3	10	1.5
Alcoholism	328	17	3.5	5.1	1.1	7	0.8
Acute renal failure	965	64	6.0	6.6	0.6	29	1.3
Alcoholism	225	20	2.2	8.9	0.9	10	0.9
Postoperative recovery	416	19	2.6	4.6	0.6	19	0.7
Postoperative recovery	921	44	6.4	4.8	0.6	14	0.6
Patients with myocardial infarction							
	611	73	50	11.9	8.1	52	2.2
	742	70	54	9.4	7.3	55	1.8
	1965	160	140	8.1	7.1	112	3.6
	1905	156	176	8.2	9.2	128	4.1
	613	35	11	5.7	3.6	17	0.6

[a] Sample volume applied to the column, 0.250 ml. Worthington MB and BB fractions collected and assayed according to kit directions. MB fraction (3 ml pool of 50 mmol/liter Tris-HCl, pH 7.5, with 150 millimolar NaCl), BB fraction (3 ml pool of 50 mmol/liter Tris-HCl, pH 7.5, with 300 millimolar NaCl).

[b] Sample volume applied to the column, 0.500 ml. Mercer MB fraction collected and assayed as described previously (*1, 2*). MB fraction (3 ml pool of Tris-HCl, 50 mmol/liter, pH 8.0, with 200 millimolar NaCl). Mercer BB fraction was collected and assayed after an additional 4 ml of 200 millimolar NaCl buffer. BB fraction (3 ml pool of 50 mmol/liter, Tris-HCl, pH 7.0, with 300 millimolar NaCl).

2. Mercer, D. W., and Varat, M. A., Detection of cardiac-specific creatine kinase isoenzyme in sera with normal or slightly increased total creatine kinase activity. *Clin. Chem.* **21**, 1088 (1975).

3. Varat, M. A., and Mercer, D. W., Cardiac specific creatine phosphokinase isoenzyme in the diagnosis of acute myocardial infarction. *Circulation* **51**, 855 (1975).

4. Takahashi, K., Ushikubo, S., Oimoni, M., and Shinko, T., Creatine phosphokinase isoenzymes of human heart muscle and skeletal muscle. *Clin. Chim. Acta* **38**, 285 (1972).

Donald Mercer

Department of Pathology
The Montefiore Hospital
Pittsburgh, Pa. 15213

Worthington Biochemical Corp. was invited to respond, and did so as follows:

To the Editor:

The report by Dr. Mercer of excessive carryover of the CK isoenzymes with the Worthington column procedure is greatly at variance with our data and that of several independent investigators. When good techniques are employed there is negligible MM isoenzyme in the MB fraction. Some carryover of MB into the BB fraction can be observed when the MB activity exceeds 40 U/liter, but recent improvements in our procedure alleviate this problem.

Table 1 typifies data collected at Worthington. The experiment was designed specifically to evaluate MM to MB carryover by following the usual 5-ml MM fraction (MM eluent is 50 mmol/liter Tris-HCl, pH 7.5) with a 0.5-ml aliquot of MB buffer (50 mmol/liter Tris-HCl, pH 7.5, containing 150 mmol of NaCl per liter). This is similar in concept to the "carryover" fraction described by Varat and Mercer (*1*). The resulting column eluate was assayed. Subsequent elution of the MB fraction followed the prescribed procedure. As Table 1 indicates, the MB values obtained by the regular procedure are not significantly different from the MB values obtained after the additional MB buffer (modified procedure). The MM fractions also compare quite favorably. The extra 0.5-ml aliquots were assayed for CK activity and for isoenzyme content by electrophoresis after a 20-fold concentration. Traces of MM isoenzyme were seen in the aliquots from samples 2, 3, and 8 (Table 1). Back-calculating the aliquot activity as related to the total MM content, there was 98% or greater removal of the MM fraction in the prescribed volume. The general trend was no more than 1% carryover of MM to MB, a percentage that, in our opinion, appears to be clinically insignificant. The remaining aliquots showed no observable bands or enzymatic activity.

A recently published paper also implies virtually no MM to MB carryover with Worthington columns (*2*). These authors were concerned with misinterpretation of isoenzyme data obtained by ion-exchange chromatography because of an electrophoretically "abnormal" band (specifically one migrating anodically and appearing between MM and MB). Electrophoresis of the column fractions collected by these authors showed "a normally migrating band for the MM eluate, the abnormally migrating band for the MB eluate . . . ." Clearly, no carryover of MM to MB was indicated. Furthermore, distinct separation of two electrophoretically *less* different species than are MM and MB appears to have been accomplished.

An evaluator (*3*) addressed himself to the question of MM to MB carryover. A patient's serum with a total CK activity of 1220 U/liter was fractionated on a Worthington column. The MB fraction was found to contain an activity of 83 U/liter (6.8%). After fractionation the

> MB fraction was reduced to a sample capable of being electrophoresed. A single band was observed on the strip, suggesting minor, if any, contamination [with CK-MM] of the CK-MB fraction eluted from the column.

This finding was consistent with eight additional sera.

Table 1. Evaluation of MM to MB Carryover

		MM, U/l[b]		MB, U/l	
Sample	Total CK, U/l	Normal procedure	Modified procedure	Normal procedure	Modified procedure
1	87	76	75	5	3
2[a]	431	393	472	26	21
3[a]	246	232	208	15	13
4	100	72	88	4	4
5[a]	250	266	251	15	16
6[a]	172	170	186	10	9
7[a]	324	285	396	8	7
8[a]	175	242	226	24	21
9[a]	187	207	185	10	9
10[a]	224	229	227	13	15

[a] Samples from known myocardial infarct patients.
[b] The combined values of MM and MB are higher, at times, than the total CK value, probably because of the dilution effect on CK. The CK value reported is that present in the 5-ml fraction only.

Table 2. Isoenzyme Distribution in Patients' Sera

A, Patients without myocardial infarction

Diagnosis	Total CK, U/liter	MB[a], U/liter	% MB
Renal failure	548	12	2.2
Postoperative recovery	409	0	0
Angina pectoris	996	24	2.4
Multiple fractures	1194	36	3
Chemical bronchitis	829	10	1.2
Coronary insufficiency	892	20	2.2

B, Patients with myocardial infarction

Site of infarct	Total CK, U/liter	MB[b], U/liter	% MB
Anterior	2060	309	15
Inferior	688	48	7
Anterior	417	24	6
Anterolateral	1296	77	6
Inferior	1975	187	9.5
Inferior	1220	83	6.8
Inferior	727	84	12

[a] MB values for these patients remained fairly consistent (±1%) over 72-h period.
[b] MB values shown are peak values, generally seen 12—24 h after onset of chest pain.

Table 3. Comparison of MM Values Obtained by Electrophoresis and Worthington Column Procedure

Fraction activity, U/liter	
Electrophoresis[a]	Worthington column
40	38
142*	152
390*	441
104*	98
72	76
840*	913
67	77
100	97
638*	638
3587*	3624
1258*	1415
77	75
183*	187
1038	1049

[a] Beckman agarose gel at 4 °C.
* Samples from patients with a diagnosed myocardial infarction.

Table 2*A* shows the isoenzyme distribution, determined with the Worthington procedure, of sera from patients without myocardial infarction (*4, 5*). A number of points must be considered: first, the MB values are always ≤3% of the total CK value and, second, the MB value either remained constant over a three-day period or fluctuated without any identifiable peak. This is in agreement with the findings of Varat and Mercer (*1*), which suggest the necessity of observing an identifiable MB peak (generally within the first 12–24 h after onset of chest pain) and that the peak MB activity be ≥4% of total CK for the diagnosis to be myocardial infarction. The peak MB values obtained on patients with a myocardial infarction by the Worthington procedure (Table 2*B*) have consistently been ≥5% of total.

The data presented in Dr. Mercer's letter are quite perplexing. In the patients without a myocardial infarction he shows nearly an order-of-magnitude difference between the MB fractions by his procedure as compared to that obtained by the Worthington procedure. The MB fractions from the patients with a diagnosed myocardial infarct, however, are reasonably comparable. Certainly, if carryover exists, one should see it whether or not there has been an infarction. Also, it would have been interesting to see the MM values obtained. With a nearly 10-fold difference in MB fractions one might expect to see significantly different MM values, with the Worthington values being lower if MM is being carried over to the MB fraction. Table 3 shows data comparing the MM values an outside evaluator (*6*) obtained by the Worthington column procedure and by Beckman agarose-gel electrophoresis. The electrophoretic results were calculated by planimetry of the peak areas observed after fluorescent scanning. The MM activities in U/liter were calculated by relating the peak area to the total CK activity of the sample. The excellent correlation (r = 0.999; $y = 0.98x - 11.9$, where the electrophoretic data were on the y-axis) obtained suggests little likelihood of incomplete MM isoenzyme removal with the column procedure. The equality of the MM to MB carryover to the MB to BB carryover suggested is difficult to accept.

Table 4. Fractionation of Four Samples of Human Muscle Extract on Worthington Columns

Total CK	MM	MB	BB
	U/liter		
1500	1497	0	0
950	996	19	0
610	620	0	0
274	285	8	0

Table 4 contains data obtained with the Worthington column after fractionating human muscle extract diluted in heat-denatured serum. A normal (up to 3% MB) isoenzyme distribution was observed.

We are highly aware of the importance of following good technique when using the isoenzyme columns. If the sample is abruptly added to the column and if complete drainage is not allowed (we have been recommending the application of slight positive pressure to the column subsequent to fraction drainage), excessive carryover may occur. Additionally, if each fraction is not thoroughly mixed after collection and before assay, erroneous results may be obtained. It should be noted, with reference to procedure, that Dr. Mercer refers to his previous papers (*1, 7*), but here uses a third procedure (0.5 ml of sample instead of the previously prescribed 1 ml and the Mercer BB fraction here was collected after a *total* of 7 ml of Mercer MB buffer had been applied, of which only 3 ml was used for assay purposes; the original procedures called for a maximum of 4 ml of MB eluate).

With regard to the MB-to-BB carryover, we, too, as well as an evaluator (*6*), have observed this phenomenon with Worthington columns. Table 5 shows typical data collected at Worthington in order to evaluate this carryover. After elution of the MM fraction, the MB fraction was eluted either with the normal MB buffer (50 mmol/liter Tris-HCl, pH 7.5 containing 150 mmol of NaCl per liter) or with a modified (NaCl increased to 200 mmol/liter) MB buffer. The BB fractions were collected with the usual

Table 5. Eight-Sample Evaluation of the MB-to-BB Carryover[a]

Normal MM	Modified MM	Normal MB	Modified MB	Normal BB	Modified BB
		U/liter			
362	365	35	50	30	10
81	81	8	8	1	1
680	690	25	57	60	20
522	526	23	26	5	4
83	82	0	0	0	0
1130	1140	37	35	10	12
156	172	2	2	0	0
0	0	178	200	40	5

[a] Last sample is partly purified MB from heart.

Table 6. Comparison of Worthington Procedure to the Yasmineh–Hanson Procedure

Sample	Total CK, U/liter	Worthington procedure[a] % MM	% MB	% BB	Y.–H. procedure % MM	% MB	% BB
1[b]	450	83	16	1	82	17	1
2	105	100	0	0	100	0	0
3	186	92	7	1	93	7	0
4[c]	1875	59	15	26	63	14	23

[a] MB buffer modified to contain 200 mmol/liter NaCl.
[b] Baboon heart extract in saline/albumin base.
[c] Helena Isoenzyme Control: Expected values MM: 58%, MB: 17%, BB: 25%.

buffer (50 mmol/liter Tris-HCl, pH 7.5, containing 300 mmol of NaCl per liter). The BB values are significantly different in samples 1, 3, and 8, where the true MB activity is >40 U/liter. The remaining samples with <40 U of MB per liter do not show any significant carryover of MB to BB. We are in the process of changing the MB buffer-salt content; this will essentially eliminate the MB to BB carryover at high MB values.

Mercer implies that a system designed to separate CK isoenzymes by gradient elution on macro-columns will not work on micro-columns with a discontinuous gradient. Yasmineh and Hanson (*8*), however, showed excellent correlation between gradient elution on macro-columns and discontinuous elution on micro-columns. To date, comparison of isoenzyme data obtained by Worthington's procedure and that of Yasmineh and Hanson has been limited. Table 6 shows four representative samples of our initial data; the values are quite comparable.

We feel our isoenzyme procedure is the best available and has a performance in numerous laboratories far superior to that found by Mercer.

References

1. Varat, M. A., and Mercer, D. W., Cardiac specific creatine phosphokinase isoenzyme in the diagnosis of acute myocardial infarction. *Circulation* **51**, 855 (1975).
2. Velletri, K., Griffiths, W. C., and Diamond, I., Abnormal electrophoretic mobility of a creatine kinase MM isoenzyme. *Clin. Chem.* **21**, 1837 (1975).
3. Hoag, G., personal communication (1975).
4. Paul, K., personal communication (1975).
5. deSilva, J., personal communication (1975).
6. Mastrofrancesco, P., personal communication (1975).
7. Mercer, D. W., Separation of tissue and serum creatine kinase isoenzymes by ion-exchange chromatography. *Clin. Chem.* **20**, 36 (1974).
8. Yasmineh, W. G., and Hanson, N. Q., Electrophoresis on cellulose acetate and chromatography on DEAE-Sephadex A-50 compared in the estimation of creatine kinase isoenzymes. *Clin. Chem.* **21**, 381 (1975).

Richard J. L. Bondar
Gerald A. Moss

Worthington Biochemical Corp.
Freehold, N. J. 07728

Turbidimetry vs. Light Scattering in Immunochemistry

To the Editor:

A recent Letter (*1*) comparing the efficacy of light scattering to turbidimetry for the monitoring of immunochemical reactions in solution has prompted this reply.

M. Blom and N. Hjørne consider turbidimetry to be a more sensitive measure of changes in particle size and concentration than light scattering measurement, because turbidimetry, which measures the decrease in transmittance per centimeter, is a measure of the sum total of light scatter from the solution. In turbidimetry, one measures the decrease in transmittance per centimeter owing to scattering and absorption of radiation minus the light scattered within the arc observed by the detector. For the measurement of light scattering from antigen/antibody complexes, the most intense scattering occurs at smaller angles (<90°), thereby minimizing the total decrease in transmittance that would be observed theoretically (*2*).

The inherent advantage of light-scattering measurement over turbidimetry measurement is that with the former one can accurately discern small incremental changes in intensity, an advantage attributable to the fact that the background intensity is very low or zero compared to the background intensity against which the same measurement must be made if a turbidimetric mode is used.

Blom and Hjørne overlooked a crucial difference in the apparent equilibrium turbidimetric method they described for serum albumin measurement (*3*) and the kinetic methods presented by others (*4, 5*). For a kinetic measurement of the reaction, small changes in intensity are observed, because of the short time-interval examined as compared to an equilibrium measurement, which in the case of the albumin procedure mentioned requires 5 min for completion. If the data given by Blom and Hjørne were presented within a 2-min time interval, the total absorbance change for a 45 g/liter and a 15 g/liter sample would be decreased from about 0.041 to 0.017 and from approximately 0.015 to 0.006, respectively. Measurement of such small absorbance changes as would be encountered in the kinetic measurement could be best performed against the small background signal present when a light-scattering approach is used.

Both methods of monitoring immunochemical reactions have positive features and certainly overlap in application. However, the arguments presented by the authors for turbidimetry with a centrifugal analyzer for specific protein analysis are as biased as that opinion to which they respond.

References

1. Blom, M., and Hjørne, N., Specific protein analysis by light scatter measurement with a miniature centrifugal fast analyzer. *Clin. Chem.* **21**, 1691 (1975). Letter to the Editor.
2. Buffone, G. J., Savory, J., and Hermans, J., Evaluation of kinetic light scattering as an approach to the measurement of specific proteins with the centrifugal analyzer. II. Theoretical considerations. *Clin. Chem.* **21**, 1735 (1975).
3. Blom, M., and Hjørne, N., Immunochemical determination of serum albumin with a centrifugal analyzer. *Clin. Chem.* **21**, 195 (1975).
4. Tiffany, T. O., Parella, J. M., Johnson, W. F., and Burtis, C. A., Specific protein analysis by light-scatter measurement with a miniature centrifugal analyzer. *Clin. Chem.* **20**, 1055 (1974).
5. Buffone, G. J., Heintges, M. G., Savory, J., and Killingsworth, L., The kinetic nephelometric measurement of IgG and albumin in serum and CSF using a laser modified Aminco Rotochem centrifugal fast analyzer. *Clin. Chem.* **21**, 943 (1975). Abstract.

Gregory J. Buffone

Clinical Chemistry Department
George Washington University
School of Medicine and
Children's Hospital
National Medical Center
Washington, D. C. 20009

Interbatch Variability in Measurement of Urinary Amylase with a Commercial Kit

To the Editor:

Ceska et al. (*1–3*) reported the use of a colored (with Cibacron blau F 3GA) cross-linked starch substrate for determination of α-amylase (EC 3.2.1.1) activity. This is the basis of a convenient and widely used commercial kit (Phadebas Alpha-Amylase Test; Pharmacia AB, Uppsala, Sweden). Irie et al. (*4*) showed that adding pure albumin to the incubation mixture enhanced the α-amylase activity of low-protein samples such as normal urine and recommended the use of a 50 mg/liter albumin solution instead of distilled water in the dilution step of the kit method. Recently the same group (*5*) proposed the use of polyvinylpyrrolidone as a cheaper and equally effective substitute for albumin. Neither of these recommendations have been incorporated into the "Directions for Use" accompanying each kit.

We have used the Phadebas Amylase test for a number of years and have found it reproducible and convenient. However, in the course of an investigation into the amylase/creatinine clearance ratios we were struck by the low values obtained with a particular batch. This observation was investigated further as follows:

1. We compared α-amylase activity of a commercial serum, patients' sera, and normal and abnormal urine samples, using the "defective" batch (batch No. AC6892) and an apparently "normal" batch (No. 263666). In all

Table 1. Amylase Activity in Different Samples, as Measured with the "Defective" and a "Normal" Amylase Kit

Sample		Amylase activity, U/liter	
		"Defective" kit	"Normal" kit
Commercial serum		160	160
Patients' sera	(1)	190	190
	(2)	100	90
Patients' urine samples[a]	(1)	192	353
	(2)	54	115
	(3)	3800	7400
	(4)	1240	2920

[a] All urine samples diluted with 4 ml of a 50 mg/liter albumin solution instead of distilled water in step 2 of Phadebas method.

experiments, unless stated otherwise, urine samples were diluted with a 50 mg/liter solution of albumin (Bovine Albumin, crystallized; Miles Laboratories, code 82-001) instead of distilled water in step 2 of the prescribed method. The results (Table 1) indicate that both batches gave equivalent values with serum samples but that for urines the "defective" batch yielded values half as large as the "normal" batch.

2. We examined the effect of increasing the albumin concentration in the diluting fluid, for both the "defective" and the "normal" batches. In both cases, concentrations exceeding 50 mg/liter resulted in an increased α-amylase activity; this was more marked with the "defective" batch, but even at 2.0 g/liter the values were only about 75% of "normal." With use of the "normal" batch, the values for α-amylase activity leveled at an albumin concentration of 100 mg/liter.

3. We obtained essentially similar results when we used polyvinylpyrrolidone in concentrations of 25 to 100 mg/liter in the diluting fluid. Again, a 50 mg/liter concentration yielded maximum α-amylase activity with the "normal" batch while the activity continued to increase with the "defective" batch. However, at a concentration of 100 mg/liter the activity obtained with the use of the "defective" batch was only 75% of normal.

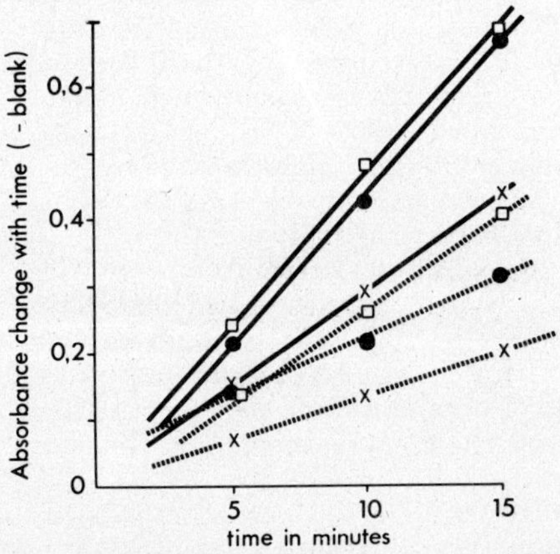

Fig. 1. Linearity of relation between soluble product formation and time with Phadebas Amylase test, with use of a "normal" (*solid lines*) and the "defective" batch (*broken lines*) to measure α-amylase in urine

X, no additions; ●, 200 mg/liter albumin; and □, 100 mg/liter PVP

4. The linearity of the reaction during the 15-min incubation was checked with both batches in the absence of added albumin or polyvinylpyrrolidone and in the presence of various concentrations of both compounds. In each case the reaction was linear. Representative graphs are shown in Figure 1. Incubations of less than 5-min duration were not tested, and the possibility of nonlinearity between 0 and 5 min cannot be excluded.

5. If two substrate tablets instead of one were added to the incubation mixture, both batches gave increased α-amylase activity, the increase observed with the "normal" batch being somewhat the greater.

6. Extra calcium and sodium chloride did not increase the α-amylase activity of urine with the "defective" or a "normal" batch.

7. The pH of the solution formed by dissolving a tablet from the "defective" kit in water was approximately 7 when tested with pH indicator paper.

These observations establish that urinary amylase values obtained with the Phadebas Amylase test, batch No. AC6892, are too low, though the reason is obscure. We are unable to obtain samples from a variety of different batches from the local representative of Pharmacia AB to ascertain the extent and degree of interbatch variability. However, in view of these findings, users of the Phadebas Amylase test kit should include a low-protein, amylase-containing solution as a control in addition to serum controls.

References

1. Ceska, M., Hultman, E., and Ingelman, B. G. A., A new method for determination of α-amylase. *Experientia* **25**, 555 (1969).

2. Ceska, M., Birath K., and Brown, B., A new and rapid method for the clinical determination of α-amylase activities in human serum and urine. Optimal conditions. *Clin. Chim. Acta* **26**, 437 (1969).

3. Ceska, M., Brown, B., and Birath, K., Ranges of α-amylase activities in human serum and urine and correlations with some other α-amylase methods. *Clin. Chim. Acta* **26**, 445 (1969).

4. Irie, A., Hunaki, M., Bando, K., and Kawai, K., Determination of α-amylase activity in serum and urine using blue starch substrate. *Clin. Chim. Acta* **42**, 63 (1972).

5. Irie, A., Hunaki, M., Bando, K., and Kawai, K., Activation of α-amylase in urine. *Clin. Chim. Acta* **51**, 241 (1974).

G. M. B. Berger
W. Liesching

Department of Pathology (Chemical)
Red Cross War Memorial
Children's Hospital
Cape Town, R.S.A.

Pharmacia Laboratories was asked to respond, and did so as follows:

To the Editor:

We thank you for allowing us to respond to the interesting views expressed by Dr. Berger and his associates regarding our Alpha-Amylase Test.

We would like to make the following clarifications:

1. Batch Number AC6892 of the Alpha-Amylase Test reported in Dr. Berger's letter has been tested against previous and later batches in our laboratories on a total of 40 fresh urine samples. Urinary amylase values obtained for most of these urine samples ranged from 91 to 93% of the values obtained with other batches. This is acceptable for diagnostic purposes considering the wide range of "normal" values for urinary amylase (100 to 1600 U/liter) (ref. *3* above) and the known difficulties and variabilities associated with other routine urinary amylase methods (Melnychuk, A., *Can. J. Med. Technol.* **35**, 9, 1973). The greater variability reported in Dr. Berger's letter, however, may be due to the relatively few samples tested in their report and possibly to inadequate storage and shipping conditions of both urine and reagents.

2. Improper shaking of the tubes after addition of the tablets may contribute to lack of accuracy and reproducibility of the results.

3. It has been our experience that the best way to check interbatch reproducibility in urinary amylase determination with the Alpha-Amylase Test is to use a *panel* of freshly collected normal samples rather than only one urine sample or a low-protein control specimen.

4. Pharmacia Research Group fully evaluates the rationale and practicability of all new and suggested modifications to an established procedure such as the Alpha-Amylase test before it is finally recommended in our package insert. The effect of adding bovine serum albumin or PVP to the incubation mixture is currently the subject of intensive investigation in our research organization. Our findings on this subject will soon be ready for release.

In the meantime, we appreciate the suggestion by Dr. Berger and his associates and all other concerned groups to add bovine serum albumin or PVP to our reagents mixture for urinary amylase. However, similar studies are also needed on other available α-amylase methods in order to establish the merits of proposing this additional step.

Rida M. Ali

Pharmacia Laboratories, Inc.
Piscataway, N.J. 08854

Eva Cederberg

Pharmacia AB, Sweden

Faster Continuous-flow Analysis for Triglycerides and Cholesterol

To the Editor:

Increasing requests for triglycerides (TG) and cholesterol (CHOL) reflect the recognized diagnostic importance of cardiovascular risk factors. For this reason our laboratory has changed during the last two years from manual performance of these two tests to a partly mechanized simultaneous method on the AutoAnalyzer II. CHOL is determined according to Technicon Method No. 24a and TG are fluorometrically determined after Kessler and Lederer (*1*). With this original method we have a CV of 3.79% day to day and 1.44% within a series for CHOL. A CV of 3.41% from day to day and 2.35% within a series was found for TG. Furthermore we are no longer satisfied with a total of 50 tests per hour, which is recommended by Technicon in the method description. Use of the 50/1 cam is recommended by Technicon to avoid carryover. To increase the test rate we used the 80/1 cam instead the 50/1 cam and found no appreciable carryover. The CHOL-channel was left completely as in the original Technicon description. The heating-bath manifold, pump configuration, and fluorometer remain the same for the TG-channel in our 80/h method as in the 50/h method. The only modifications are simple, between the metal sample needle and the pump. Technicon recommends a Kel-F probe connection for TG to be not longer than 51 cm. We used in place of the Kel-F for a connection an orange-yellow pump tube (0.02″ i.d.) of Solvaflex, cut to a length of 20 cm. The thin metal needle can be directly inserted into one end of this 20-cm Solvaflex connecting tubing; the other end is connected to the pump by a metal nipple. We found excellent correlation between results by the Technicon original procedure and our modifications. Our modifications have two advantages:

1. Quality of the tests is identical and carryover is not greater.

2. The modifications are simple and inexpensive. We can therefore save reagents and at the same time run 1.6-fold as many tests.

Reference

1. Kessler, G., and Lederer, H., In *Automation in Analytical Chemistry, Technicon Symposia 1965;* L. T. Skeggs et al., Eds. Mediad, New York, N. Y., 1966, pp 341 *ff.*

Hillard Zyman
Franz Gabl
Peter M. Bayer

I. Med. Dept.
Univ. of Vienna
Dept. Clin. Chem.
Lazarettgasse 14
Vienna, Austria

Ed. note: These authors supplied documentation, which is available on request from the Editorial Office or from the authors.

A Lipase Problem in an Enzymatic Procedure for Serum Triglycerides

To the Editor:

We recently described a single reagent enzymatic procedure for serum triglyceride determination [*Clin. Chem.* **21,** 1983 (1975)] which may be used with the Abbott Bichromatic Analyzer (Abbott Labs., Diagnostics Division, Pasadena, Calif. 91030). The reagent was prepared by combining the contents of the Triglyceride-Glycerol (3-vial) reagent (Calbiochem, La Jolla, Calif. 92037) into one reagent.

Recently we received a new lot number of triglyceride reagent and found the method did not perform as we described. Investigation revealed that vial C (lipase) did not display the activity in the combined reagent we reported previously. Instead of quantitatively hydrolyzing the triglycerides in serum samples with elevated values in less than 4 min, 10 to 15 min was required. The same reagents appeared to work satisfactorily in the Abbott recommended procedure, because the lipase is incubated with the sample 30 min prior to the final reading. We therefore caution laboratories using this procedure to compare the results obtained on several control sera and patients' samples against the Abbott recommended procedure on the ABA-100 with each new lot number of Calbiochem triglyceride reagent.

Eric J. Sampson
Laurence M. Demers
Arthur F. Krieg

Division of Clinical Pathology
The Milton S. Hershey Medical Center
The Pennsylvania State University
Hershey, Pa. 17033

Effect of Glutamate on γ-Glutamyltransferase Activity

To the Editor:

Bondar and Moss (*1*) produced data based on two patients' sera that showed a stimulation of γ-glutamyltransferase activity (γGT, EC 2.3.2.2) in the presence of glutamate. Rock and Slickers (*2*) attempted to confirm the findings of Bondar and Moss, using nine patients' sera of normal and abnormal activity, assayed in triplicate, and found no activation of γGT such as was originally indicated by Bondar and Moss, either in any individual specimen or in the nine sera collectively.

In reply to the work of Rock and Slickers, Bondar and Moss (*3*) repeated their initial experiment on four additional sera and again demonstrated an increase in γGT activity in all sera within a range of glutamate concentration 60–80 nmol/liter. They could not repeat their initial claim of 100% activation but showed an average activation of 44%. The activation peak at 1 mmol/liter concentration of glutamate, described in their original paper, could not be confirmed. Bondar and Moss also used Student's *t*-test to reevaluate the data presented by Rock and Slickers and suggested that an activation was actually present.

In addition, a recent paper by Gerhardt et al. (*4*) has shown that no increase in γGT activity could be demonstrated when L(+)-glutamate (0.01 to 5.0 mmol/liter) was incorporated into the reaction media and the assay done at 25, 30, or 37 °C.

In the light of the conflicting situation regarding activation of γGT by L-glutamate, we attempted to repeat the work of Rock and Slickers and also to ascertain the effect of L-glutamate on the γGT assay currently used in this laboratory.

We selected ten patients' sera of various γGT activity to be assayed in triplicate by two methods in the pres-

Table 1. γGT Activity vs. Glutamate Concentration for 10 Plasmas, Two Methods

Final added glutamate concentration, mmol/liter

0.00	0.02	0.04	0.06	0.08	0.10	0.50	1.00	0.00[a]
				γGT activity, U/liter				
Method 1								
12.0	11.9	12.0	11.5	12.0	13.0	11.2	11.3	11.1
37.2	37.1	37.6	38.1	37.2	38.2	35.3	32.6	37.6
45.4	45.3	44.6	43.9	43.9	43.8	42.0	40.5	44.5
9.0	9.3	8.7	9.3	9.1	9.0	8.3	7.8	9.5
9.7	9.5	9.1	9.4	10.4	9.8	9.4	8.6	10.0
36.7	36.3	37.6	37.8	37.5	36.0	35.0	33.0	36.8
18.0	18.4	18.6	18.7	19.4	19.5	18.0	16.0	19.2
31.0	31.8	31.8	32.2	31.6	31.9	31.1	29.2	31.5
13.8	14.2	14.5	13.8	14.0	14.6	13.8	12.4	13.9
27.5	27.7	27.3	27.8	27.0	28.4	26.6	24.8	26.6
Method 2								
31.8	31.2	31.5	30.3	31.0	31.5	31.8	31.6	31.7
105	107	106	106	106	105	106	105	105
121	126	124	123	123	123	120	123	120
23.3	23.2	23.5	23.6	23.5	23.7	22.4	23.2	22.9
28.1	29.1	27.7	28.2	27.8	28.1	27.6	28.2	26.9
98.2	98.2	96.8	96.8	96.8	96.8	96.8	96.8	98.2
49.4	48.6	49.4	48.6	48.0	48.1	48.4	49.5	49.0
81.8	83.2	85.9	81.8	84.6	80.5	83.2	84.6	82.5
33.4	34.9	33.8	34.0	34.6	34.1	34.4	34.6	32.9
72.3	72.3	70.9	70.9	71.0	72.3	72.3	69.6	72.3

[a] Assay with no added glutamate repeated at end of experiment.

ence of increasing concentrations of L-glutamate. The final reaction mixture for the first method approximates the method used by Rock and Slickers, but was done at 37 °C and contained, per liter, 4 mmol of γ-glutamyl-*p*-nitroanilide (Sigma), 40 mmol of glycylglycine, and 185 mmol of tris (hydroxymethyl) aminomethane buffer (pH 8.25). L-Glutamic acid (Sigma) was added to the buffer to give a final concentration in the reaction mixture ranging from 0 to 1.0 mmol/liter. The final reaction mixture had a sample/volume ratio of 1/29. The reaction was measured by measuring the rate of change of absorbance at 410 nm at 37 °C, by use of an LKB Model 8600 reaction rate analyzer, and the activity was calculated in U/liter.

The final reaction mixture for the second method (*5*)—a method currently in use in this laboratory—contained, per liter, 8 mmol of γ glutamyl-*p*-nitroanilide (Sigma), 67 mmol of glycylglycine, and 100 mmol of 2-amino-2-methylpropane-1,3-diol buffer (pH 8.30). The final reaction mixture had a sample/volume ratio of 1/12. Identical concentrations of L-glutamate were used as in the first method.

Data collected during this study showed good precision, similar to that described previously (*5*), and a similar precision for both the first and second methods.

Table 1 shows the mean results of triplicate determinations. The assays were performed in the order shown left to right in the Table, each set of results for a given patient being obtained within the same analytical batch. A zero concentration of L-glutamate was analyzed at the beginning and end of each patient batch. These results are reported to one decimal place, but one should not infer that single γGT determinations are this precise. The precision of these results is about 0.5 to 1.0 standard deviation units as a result of their being the mean of triplicate determinations.

Comparison of activities with Student's *t*-test for paired observations did not show any significant activation ($P > 0.1$) by either of the two methods at any concentration of added glutamate. The first method showed a decrease in γGT activity at 0.5 mmol/liter concentration of L-glutamate ($0.05 < P > 0.02$) and a highly significant ($P < 0.001$) decrease at 1.0 mmol/liter L-glutamate concentration. This is possibly the result of product inhibition at the lower (and suboptimal) substrate concentration used in this method.

References

1. Bondar, R., and Moss, G., Enhancing effect of glutamate on apparent serum γ-glutamyltranspeptidase activity. *Clin. Chem.* **20,** 317 (1974).
2. Rock, R., and Slickers, K., Glutamate and γ-glutamyltranspeptidase activity. *Clin. Chem.* **21,** 166 (1975). Letter to the Editor.
3. Bondar, R., and Moss, G., *Clin. Chem.* **21,** 167 (1975). Response to ref. *2*.
4. Gerhardt, W., Persijn, P., and Rosalki, S. B., Lack of significant effect of L(+)-glutamate on serum γ-glutamyltransferase activity determined in the presence of glycylglycine. *Clin. Chem.* **21,** 1515 (1975).
5. Farrance, I., Krauja, V. W., and Dennis, P. M., The determination of γ-glutamyltranspeptidase by reaction rate assay at 37 °C. *Pathology* **7,** 237 (1975).

B. J. Gibson
I. Farrance
P. M. Dennis

Department of Chemical Pathology
Prince Henry's Hospital
St. Kilda Road
Melbourne, 3004
Australia

Bichromatic Analyses with the ABA-100—A Critical Assumption

To the Editor:

A bichromatic analyzer measures the difference in absorbance at two preselected wavelengths ($A_d = A_{\lambda_1} - A_{\lambda_2}$). An underlying assumption is that the absorbance at the blanking wavelength (λ_2) relative to the test wavelength (λ_1) is the same for all standards and samples. Said another way, if standards and samples were appropriately diluted, their absorbance spectra would be superimposable. If a sample absorbed relatively more at the blank wavelength than at the test wavelength, a falsely low result would be obtained. Conversely, if a particular sample absorbed relatively more at the test wavelength than at the blank wavelength, a falsely high result would be obtained.

We evaluated the Hycel procedure for serum (and plasma) phosphorus measurements on the ABA-100 bichromatic analyzer (Abbott Scientific Products Division, South Pasadena, Calif. 81030). During the first month of running the ABA-100 procedure in parallel with our routine procedure (Technicon N-39 on an AutoAnalyzer I system), we found that about 4% of the samples (8 of 184) gave results that differed by more than 10 mg/liter. A few months later, when we were running in parallel again as part of a program to train medical technol-

Table 1. Absorbance Differences and Results for Phosphorus Obtained for Three Selected Samples

Sample	$A_{650} - A_{550}$	Phosphorus, mg/liter: Auto-Analyzer I	Phosphorus, mg/liter: ABA-100
Serum	−0.004	35	30
Heparinized plasma	−0.091	26	0
Serum	−0.013	29	0

ogists on the ABA-100, we found that about 13% of the samples (22 of 169) gave results which differed by more than 10 mg/liter.

This prompted us to test the assumption concerning the effectiveness of the blanking wavelength. The test wavelength is 650 nm and the blank wavelength is 550 nm for the phosphorus procedure on the ABA-100. We selected two patients' samples that had given discrepant results and one that had not, and diluted them 26-fold with physiological saline. These solutions were scanned (vs. saline) from 700 to 400 nm with a ratio-recording spectrophotometer (DK-2A; Beckman Instruments, Fullerton, Calif. 92634). Table 1 shows the absorbance differences for these samples. The patients' diagnoses were, respectively, cervical carcinoma, gunshot wound, and leukemia. All of these samples absorbed more at the blank wavelength than at the test wavelength and the absorbance difference varied with the patient. Results for phosphorus assays performed on these samples are also shown in the Table. These three examples serve to warn that extreme caution may have to be exercised whenever a bichromatic analyzer is used for endpoint measurements. It may not be readily apparent how much comparison work is needed before a new procedure can be used with confidence. Rather, the amount of comparison work appears to be a function of the source(s) of samples that are being assayed by the particular laboratory; that is, of whether the patient population is relatively normal or is a combination of patients who are relatively normal and those who are receiving tertiary care.

Another point also worth considering is that most of the method interferences documented to date are for procedures in which the blank and test mixtures are read at the same wavelength, information that may not be directly transferable to a bichromatic procedure.

J. Richard Pearson
Thurston Matsuura

Central Laboratory
University of Colorado Medical Center
Denver, Colo. 80220

"Albumin-Titratable Bilirubin" as an Index to Bilirubin Binding

To the Editor:

McCluskey et al. (*1*) reported a modification of the Roth fluorometric method for the determination of bilirubin (*2*). Krasner et al. (*3, 4*) had previously reported their use of the method to directly titrate neonatal serum with bilirubin. The present authors emphasized that the physiological significance of "albumin-titratable bilirubin" was unknown. However, they suggested that it represented that fraction of the total bilirubin that was not tightly bound to albumin—i.e., that it represented the fraction bound to the lower-affinity site of albumin and to other components of blood (*5, 6*). The authors proposed that clinical management could be based on this "albumin-titratable bilirubin": "... infants with albumin-titratable bilirubin >50 mg/liter should be considered for exchange transfusion."

I believe there is adequate data in the literature to show that the Roth fluorometric method does not measure the binding of bilirubin to the high-affinity site of albumin. Saturation of the site is believed to increase greatly the risk of kernicterus. Since the proposed method does not provide a measure of saturation of that site, it should not be utilized in the clinical management of hyperbilirubinemia.

That the high-affinity site on albumin has the capacity to bind an equimolar concentration of bilirubin has been established by the peroxidase method (*5*), by circular dichroism (*7*), and by quenching of ultraviolet fluorescence (*6*). However, the fluorescence yield of a bilirubin/albumin mixture is linear through a bilirubin/albumin molar ratio of at least 2.0 (*3, 6*), implying that such fluorescence does not reflect binding to the high-affinity site.

In his original report Roth emphasized that the fluorescence remained unchanged even when the bilirubin had been photoöxidized (*2*). He concluded that photoöxidation products were equally as reactive as native bilirubin. This might be advantageous in the clinical determination of total bilirubin, but again leads to the conclusion that the method does not measure the binding of bilirubin to the high-affinity site of albumin.

Further, Krasner et al. (*3, 4*) examined the effect of added drugs on the fluorescence in the Roth method. Sulfisoxazole had been shown to increase the risk of kernicterus in premature infants (*8*). Brodersen utilized the peroxidase method to directly demonstrate the displacement of bilirubin by sulfisoxazole in vitro (*9*). If the Roth method were dependent on binding at the high-affinity site, one should have seen a similar effect when sulfisoxazole was added. No effect could be demonstrated, even at rather high concentrations of drug (*3, 4*).

The authors emphasized the correlation between "albumin-titratable bilirubin" and the bilirubin/albumin ratio as evidence that their method measured a clinically significant entity. However, such a correlation would be of clinical significance only if it resulted from a dependence of bilirubin fluorescence on binding to the high-affinity site. The evidence cited above shows that this is not the case.

The observed correlation could be the result of other physical interactions. Bilirubin fluorescence appears dependent on a hydrophobic environment (*10*). It may be that the albumin-mediated enhancement of fluorescence results from orientation in such an environment (*10, 11*).

In any event, the method does not measure bilirubin binding to the high-affinity site. It should therefore not be utilized in the clinical management of hyperbilirubinemia in the newborn.

References

1. McCluskey, S. B., Storey, G. N. B., Brown, G. K., et al., Fluorometric determination of "albumin-titratable bilirubin" in the jaundiced neonate. *Clin. Chem.* **21**, 1638 (1975).
2. Roth, M., Dosage fluorimétrique de la bilirubin. *Clin. Chim. Acta* **17**, 487 (1967).
3. Krasner, J., Giacoia, G. P., and Yaffe, S. J., Drug-protein binding in the newborn infant. *Ann. N. Y. Acad. Sci.* **226**, 101 (1973).
4. Krasner, J., Fluorescent properties of bovine serum albumin-bilirubin complex. *Biochem. Med.* **7**, 135 (1973).
5. Jacobsen, J., Binding of bilirubin to human serum albumin—determination of the dissociation constants. *FEBS Lett.* **5**, 112 (1969).
6. Chen, R. F., The fluorescence of bilirubin-albumin complexes. In *Fluorescence Techniques in Cell Biology*, A. A. Thaer and M. Sernetz, Eds. Springer-Verlag, New York, N. Y., 1973, pp 273–282.
7. Beaven, G. H., d'Albis, A., and Gratzer, W. B., The interaction of bilirubin with human serum albumin. *Eur. J. Biochem.* **33**, 500 (1973).
8. Silverman, W. A., Andersen, D. H., Blane, W. A., and Crozier, D. N., A difference in mortality rate and incidence of kernicterus among premature infants allotted to two prophylactic antibacterial regimens. *Pediatrics* **18**, 614 (1956).

9. Brodersen, R., Competitive binding of bilirubin and drugs to human serum albumin studied by enzymatic oxidation. *J. Clin. Invest.* **54,** 1353 (1974).

10. Cu, A., Bellah, G., and Lightner, D. A., On the fluorescence of bilirubin. *J. Am. Chem. Soc.* **97,** 2579 (1975).

11. Brodersen, R., Funding, L., Pedersen, A. O., and Röigaard-Petersen, H., Binding of bilirubin to low-affinity sites of human serum albumin in vitro followed by co-crystallization. *Scand. J. Clin. Lab. Invest.* **29,** 433 (1972).

Rodney L. Levine

Division of Perinatal Medicine
University of Colorado
Medical Center
and
Department of Perinatology
The Children's Hospital
1056 E. 19th Ave.
Denver, Colo. 80206

The authors of the paper in question respond (Mrs. McCluskey is deceased):

To the Editor:

Dr. Levine has correctly drawn attention to potential theoretical weaknesses in the technique developed in our laboratories. We believe, however, that his criticisms somewhat misrepresent our findings and may not be completely warranted. The following points might be made:

(*a*) There appears to be some confusion in the basis for Dr. Levine's critique. He equates Roth's (*1*) method, as used by us, with that of Krasner et al. (*2, 3*). Though both are fluorescent techniques, with similar (but not identical) spectral characteristics, there are substantive differences. Krasner et al. did experiments under approximately physiological conditions while our experiments were in the presence of high concentrations of phosphoric acid. Under the latter conditions, it is almost certain that the properties of the binding site have altered significantly. Thus, we do not see how it is possible for Levine to extrapolate from results reported by Krasner et al. concerning both the fluorescence yield and the results of competition experiments (with particular respect to sulfisoxazole) in order to repudiate our results.

(*b*) Our method also differs slightly from that of Roth in that we used human serum albumin rather than bovine serum albumin and there are distinctive differences in the mode of binding of bilirubin to these two protein molecules (*4*). Further, a titration of a constant concentration of bilirubin with variable albumin by our technique gives a curve very similar to the curve in Figure 2A of Beaven et al. (*5*), viz. a sharp inflexion at 1:1, followed by a much more gradual rise in fluorescence intensity.

(*c*) We would emphasize that Levine's criticisms of our work are based on results reported from experiments designed to determine the reserve binding capacity of albumin. We have felt it more important to try and assess the excess bilirubin beyond that tightly bound to albumin, as this is the problem in the jaundiced neonate.

(*d*) We do not believe that any meaningful statement can be made about the properties of photoöxidation products of bilirubin (which could remain bound to albumin) in the absence of knowledge of their identity.

(*e*) The correlation between "albumin-titratable bilirubin" and the bilirubin/albumin ratio was only considered as supportive evidence that a clinically significant value was being observed. The more important correlation was considered to be with the saturation index of Odell et al. (*6*). This appears to measure a similar biological function by an independent method and has proved of predictive value (*7*).

(*f*) Finally, we consider it unfortunate that Dr. Levine feels that our results should be dismissed on theoretical grounds, without advancing supportive experimental evidence for his views. We have advanced the method as a possible clinical test, and follow-up studies of the patients involved is the only way of establishing its usefulness.

References

1. Roth, M., Dosage fluorimetrique de la bilirubine. *Clin. Chim. Acta* **17,** 487 (1967).

2. Krasner, J., Giacoia, G. P., and Yaffe, S. J., Drug-protein binding in the newborn infant. *Ann. N. Y. Acad. Sci.* **226,** 101 (1973).

3. Krasner, J., Fluorescent properties of bovine serum albumin-bilirubin complex. *Biochem. Med.* **7,** 135 (1973).

4. Chen, R. F., The fluorescence of bilirubin-albumin complexes. In *Fluorescence Techniques in Cell Biology,* A. A. Thaer and M. Sernetz, Eds., Springer-Verlag, New York, N. Y., 1973, pp 273–282.

5. Beaven, G. H., d'Albis, A., and Gratzer, W. B., The interaction of bilirubin with human serum albumin. *Eur. J. Biochem.* **33,** 500 (1973).

6. Odell, G. B., Cohen, S. N., and Kelly, P. C., Studies in kernicterus II. The determination of the saturation of serum albumin. *J. Pediatr.* **74,** 214 (1969).

7. Odell, G. B., Storey, G. N. B., and Rosenberg, L. A., Studies in kernicterus. III. The saturation of serum proteins with bilirubin during neonatal life and its relationship to brain damage at five years. *J. Pediatr.* **76,** 12 (1970).

W. J. O'Sullivan

School of Biochemistry
University of New South Wales
Kensington, N. S. W., Australia

G. K. Brown

Department of Medicine
University of Sydney
Sydney, N. S. W., Australia

G. N. B. Storey

Department of Pediatrics
Royal Prince Alfred Hospital
Camperdown, N. S. W. 2050
Australia

Misuse of Calibration Sera in Automated Laboratory Testing Instruments

To the Editor:

A common practice in the operation of automated biochemical testing instruments is to test a single sample of "calibration serum" after every 10th or 20th patients' sample. Results for each such control are used immediately to "adjust" (recalibrate) the instrument for the constituent involved. Unless the constituent can be tested with perfect precision (zero variance of the results), this practice is certain to *increase the testing error,* just the opposite of what is intended.

The truth of this statement is illustrated with a hypothetical example. For instance, consider glucose assay. (In the following discussion, all values are in mg/100 ml.)

Assume that an instrument was initially calibrated perfectly, and then samples from a serum pool with a "true concentration" of 100 were tested many times without adjusting the instrument. A distribution of the results like that shown at the top of Figure 1 might be obtained. Their average would be 100, but the results would vary. This variation is the "indeterminate error" (random variation) of the biochemical method, instrument, and variation of the aliquots. The vertical lines identify the ±2 SD (95%) range of the results. Each test is independent of all others, i.e., there is no "drift" or correlation of any kind among results.

In the above example, if the instrument were calibrated accurately, and left alone, it would produce the most accurate and precise results possible. But consider what happens if small, immediate adjustments are made with results of tests of single calibration samples interspersed among the patients' samples.

When the first calibration sample came along, suppose a reading of 97 was observed, and the analyst adjusted the scale to obtain 100 (first adjustment). This has the effect of adding 3 to all following results, as is illustrated. When the second calibration

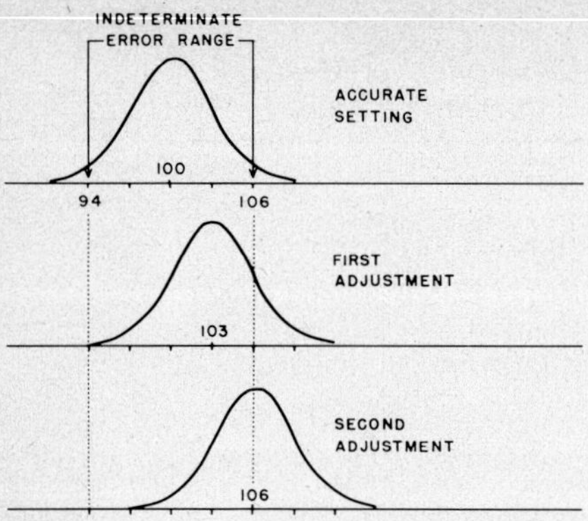

Fig. 1.

sample came along, again a reading of 97 was observed, and again the scale was adjusted to add 3 (second adjustment). The second adjustment adds to the first, and the instrument is now yielding results 6 mg too high. The results for the "true concentration" of 100 are now being reported, on the average, as 106 mg. All patients' samples are affected by the adjustments too.

The erroneous adjustments were made because the analyst failed to realize that the observed 3 mg departures from what he expected were indeterminate error. Theoretically, the minimum indeterminate error variance is about doubled with such erroneous adjustments. The only possibility for reducing indeterminate error is to average the results of several tests of aliquots.

In the example given above, the discussion was limited to adjustments made within a testing run, but the same problem is present in the initial calibration. In the initial calibration, if the analyst relies on close agreement between two successive tests of calibration serum, he is also in trouble. He is selecting two results on the basis of their indeterminate error, and the calibration is based on his selection. It cannot be emphasized enough that an unknown amount of error is present in every test, and the only correct way to reduce the error is to average the results of several calibration sample tests. This *average* is the best estimate of the point at which the instrument is set during their tests. The average should then be used as the basis for making any adjustment.

Everything has been discussed in terms of an analyst making the adjustments, but there are now instruments on the market with built-in computers. The source of an "adjusting signal" is immaterial, and so the same remarks are true for the computer-controlled instruments. Laboratories with them should assure themselves that the computers are correctly programmed. The problems are also the same with the manual methods.

The 3 mg standard deviation for glucose assay in the above example was taken from results of a survey of medical-school hospital laboratories by Straumfjord and Copeland (*1*). They reported 3.2 mg/100 ml as the average standard deviation for 27 laboratories. They also reported the range of the standard deviations as 0.5 to 7.6. Something is obviously wrong with the values at the ends of the range.

One wonders where in the training of some laboratory personnel, the erroneous practices arose. In an old textbook on quantitative analysis, the authors describe indeterminate errors, and state that several determinations (tests of aliquots) should be averaged for the "most probable result" (*2*). Judging from this bit of information, the source of current misinformation is not in the teaching of analytical chemistry.

I think the matters raised in this letter deserve careful study in all laboratories where they are not well understood. Since the problems are complex, it is best not to do too much at one time. The first thing that might be done is to estimate the indeterminate error within a single testing run. All that is required is the following:

1. On one occasion, test at least 40 aliquots of a calibration serum, reference samples, or a pool of sera, *without adjusting the process.*

2. In the same order in which the specimens were tested, plot each result on a "control chart" type of graph. Any substantial drifts will be apparent; otherwise only indeterminate error will be observed.

The above results will provide the basis for further study. This is an unavoidably vague statement, because the above results must be known before making any reasonable decisions about further studies.

For those who write to me, I will be glad to help a few laboratories to study the accuracy and precision of their testing procedures.

References

1. Straumfjord, J., and Copeland, B. E., Clinical chemistry quality control values in 33 medical school hospitals. *Am. J. Clin. Pathol.* **44**, 252 (1965).

2. Pierce, W. C., and Haenisch, E. L., *Quantitative Analysis.* John Wiley & Sons, Inc., New York, N. Y., 1940.

Robert G. Hoffmann

1321 Blue Road
Coral Gables, Fla. 33146

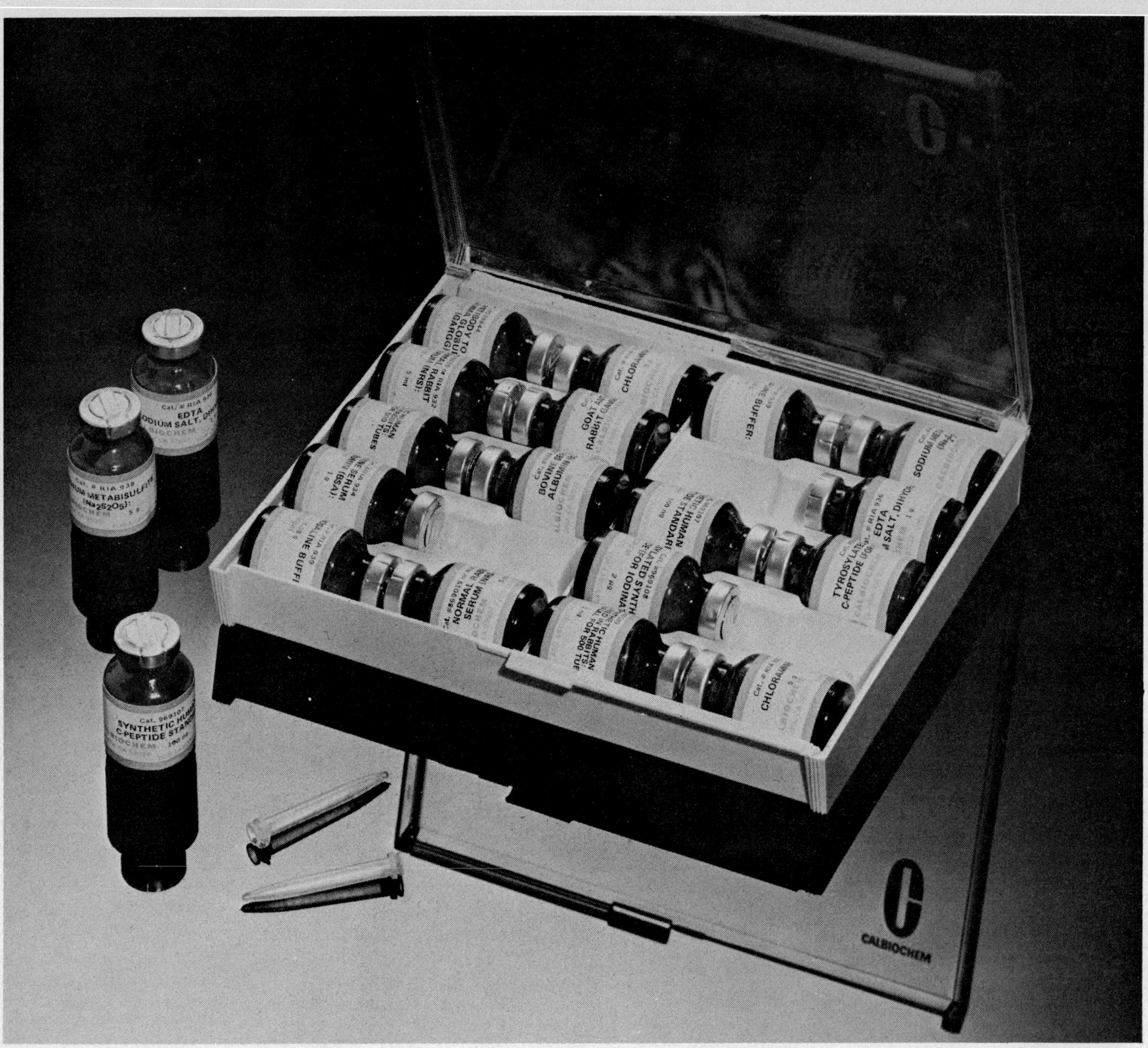

C-Peptide RIA Set from Calbiochem...$150.

Proinsulin is enzymatically degraded in the β-cells of the pancreas, yielding equimolar quantities of insulin and C-peptide (connecting peptide), as well as two pairs of basic aminoacids. Insulin and C-peptide are secreted into the peripheral circulation where they have been found in approximately equimolar quantities, along with some proinsulin and proinsulin-like components.

Radioimmunoassay of C-peptide is now possible with the C-Peptide RIA kit from Calbiochem, exclusive U.S. manufacturers. When used as instructed, the material listed below will permit the processing of approximately 500 assay tubes. Price of the kit is $150.00.

Reagents provided:

Synthetic human C-peptide standard, 100ng
Tyrosylated synthetic C-peptide (for iodination), 2μg
Rabbit Antiserum to synthetic human C-peptide, 1ml, sufficient material for 500 tubes
Bovine Serum Albumin (BSA), 1g
Normal Rabbit Serum (NRS), 5ml
Goat Antibody to Rabbit Gamma Globulin (GARGG), 5ml
EDTA (disodium salt, dihydrate), 1g
Sodium Metabisulfite ($Na_2S_2O_5$), 5g
Chloramine-T, 5g
Phosphosaline Buffer, 5.58g

Send for free protocol "Guide for the radioimmunoassay of Human C-Peptide" or order the set now: **Cat. No. 969111,** $150. CALL RIA HOTLINE (714) 453-4680, or WRITE, LOUIS DILTS, P.O. Box 12087, San Diego, Ca. 92112.

CALBIOCHEM

Circle No. 296 on Reader's Service Card

the clinical chemist

Compiled by J. S. King, Executive Editor

AACC 28th National Meeting, Houston, August 1–6

Persons wishing to attend this meeting—and nonmembers are most welcome—may obtain particulars on special events, workshops (nine of them), roundtable discussions (46 of them), events for youngsters, side trips, registration forms and hotel registration forms from either (preferably) Scherago Associates, P. O. Box 874, Montclair, N. J. 07043, or from AACC National Meeting, P. O. Box 20661, Astrodome Station, Houston, Tex. 77025 (or pp 573–576, this issue).

Scientific program and abstracts will appear in our July issue. All signs are that this meeting will be AACC's biggest and best.

Travel Grants

The National Education Committee has budgeted $1500 for 1976 to assist pre- and post-doctoral students to travel to the annual National Meeting of the American Association for Clinical Chemistry. This amount has been designated by the Education Committee to provide 15 one-hundred dollar travel grants. Directors of pre- and post-doctoral programs are requested to submit the names of students in their program desiring to receive these grants on a priority basis (i.e., first, second, third, etc., recommendation). The students are then required to request such grants by writing to the Chairman of the Subcommittee on Continuing Education. The names of 15 of these students receiving a first priority recommendation will then be drawn by lot from a pool containing all their names. The first 15 chosen will be awarded the travel grants.

Students eligible for the travel grants must either be members or student members of the Association. Directors of the academic program must also be members of AACC. Only one travel grant will be given to a program unless there are fewer than 15 programs requesting this assistance. The deadline of May 1, 1976, has been set for receiving applications for these grants to assist in travel to the National Meeting of the AACC in Houston, Texas, on August 1–6, 1976.

Program directors are requested to submit their recommendations for their graduate students, and graduate students are requested to submit their written request for travel grant to: Herndon G. Shepherd, Ph.D., Chairman of Subcommittee on Continuing Education, National AACC Education Committee, Mason-Barron Laboratories, Inc., 4720 West Montrose Ave., Chicago, Ill. 60641, (312) 282-9500.

Awards and Honors

Nominations are now being solicited for all AACC Awards. Each member has the privilege of nominating someone for each of the four awards. The nominations may be made by individuals, by a group of members, or by the local section as a unit.

The AACC Awards are bestowed by the AACC membership. Consequently, recipients of these awards are recognized as outstanding in the field of clinical chemistry and as representative of the clinical chemist. It behooves all members to make an effort to place in nomination the names of those persons they feel represent the best in clinical chemistry.

A letter describing the activities that qualify the nominee for a particular award should be sent to the Business Office before May 1, 1976. The *Handbook and Directory* lists all past recipients.

The 1976 Awards are:

- The AACC Award for Outstanding Contributions to Clinical Chemistry, sponsored by Ames Division of Miles Laboratories.
- The AACC Award for Outstanding Contributions through Service to Clinical Chemistry as a Profession, sponsored by the Fisher Scientific Company.
- The AACC Award for Outstanding Contributions to Clinical Chemistry through Education, sponsored by SmithKline Corp.
- The AACC Award for Outstanding Contributions to Clinical Chemistry in a Selected Area, sponsored by Boehringer Mannheim Corp. Nominations in any area of specialization in clinical chemistry may be submitted.

At its March 20 meeting, the New Jersey Section presented the Gerulat Award to Dr. Martin Rubin, a certificate of honor to Dr. Richard J. Henry, and a Distinguished Service Award to Dr. Paul Lenz.

Nominations are solicited from anyone (including the authors) for the 1977 Pittsburgh Applied Analytical Chemistry Award ($1000) for the outstanding paper published in the previous five years (Jan. 1, 1971–Dec. 31, 1975) in this field. Send five copies of the nominated paper, no later than June 1, 1976, to Eleanor L. Saier, Department of Laboratory Medicine, Singer Memorial Laboratory, 320 East North Ave., Pittsburgh, Pa. 15212.

Dr. Nathan Gochman, a member of the editorial board of this journal, has been appointed to the Instrumentation Advisory Panel of *Analytical Chemistry*.

Welcome, Gentlemen, to the Wonderful World of SI Units

Our friends and colleagues over at the *American Journal of Clinical Pathology* have announced [**65,** 19 (1976)] that they are going to make a real effort to use SI units in that journal. To encourage this, they feature a lead article by H. P. Lehmann in which ranges of normal values are given in the traditional units and in SI units, with the corresponding conversion factors—an exercise that essentially repeats that of *Clinical Chemistry* Board of Editors Chairman Donald Young, in *The New England Journal of Medicine* **292,** 795 (April 10, 1975), except that Dr. Lehmann's normal values are those appearing in the 15th (1974) edition of Davidson and Henry's *Clinical Diagnosis by Laboratory Methods* and Dr. Young's are those of the Massachusetts General Hospital [*New Engl. J. Med.* **290,** 39 (1974)].

The introductory editorial concludes "... it has clearly become our responsibility to take the lead in reuniting the presently separated halves of the world's medical literature [that is, European and Australian authors, who have more readily adopted SI units, and American, who have not], and we accept the responsibility."

We are glad to see these inspiring words, and we offer two comments to our friends.

First, you have your work cut out for you. We predict that you will not find such a transition to be easy, even taking into account that there usually are only one or two articles of a chemical nature in any given issue of *Am. J. Clin. Pathol.*, which leads me to the second comment.

Way back in 1969 [*Clin. Chem.* **15,** 427] our people decided to implement the use of SI units in this journal "in a fashion which would encourage smooth transition from the existing to the preferred useage [*sic*]." Since then we have striven manfully to do so, and, indeed, the transition is now perhaps 95% complete. Believers in gradualism, we try to keep our strictures within reason and do not at present insist, for example, that figures submitted for publication be redrawn because the units depicted are mg/dl rather than mg/liter. Nor do we now insist on (e.g.) the international spelling of "litre" and "metre," or the use of the "katal." This would be the sort of thing that drives away good contributors. We still use the terms "pH" and "osmol." Old and new units are both given in cases where the derived SI unit is likely to be unintelligible to most of our readers—for example the pascal. Because almost all of the papers in this journal involve SI units, we must spend a total of perhaps 12 hours or so a month in making such changes in manuscripts, a tedious and expensive business.

So it has been a lonely struggle, in which we are now encouraged to persevere with the entry at last of another influential U. S. journal.

Not the least of our problems has been the lack of agreement among authorities as to certain derived SI units. For example, is μg/ml as acceptable as μg/liter, and is μmol/liter more acceptable than μg/liter? Some approve M as a symbol for mol/liter; we do not, nor does the official U. S. bible for SI units, NBS Special Publication 330 (for sale by the Superintendent of Documents, U. S. Govt. Printing Office, Washington, D. C. 20402; SD cat. No. C 13.10:330/2, Stock No. 0303-0970). We do not have a current price at hand, but the 1972 edition cost thirty cents. More and more, our readers are going to need to have a copy.

—J.S.K.

Agree or Disagree?

"... proficiency testing, as it is usually conducted, generally tends to rate laboratories well above the rank they would earn were the rating based on the quality of the actual daily routine work."

—Dr. Morris Schaeffer

Report from Japan

To the Editor:

On November 28th, 1975, the undersigned presented a paper, by invitation, at the National Meeting of The Japan Society of Clinical Chemistry in Tokyo. The title of my presentation was, "The Application of Modern Concepts of Acid Base Balance to the Management of the Neonate."

While I was in Japan, I had an opportunity to visit a number of hospitals and medical institutions throughout Japan and inspect their laboratories of clinical chemistry. I suggest that it would be of interest to American readers to find out how clinical chemistry is practiced in Japan.

The Japan Society of Clinical Chemistry has 400 members, approximately equally divided between Doctors of Medicine and Philosophy. There are a few members who have their Master's or Bachelor's Degree. The Society is managed by a Board of Directors, headed by Yuichi Yamamura, M.D. The Board is concerned with two different disciplines. There is a Biochemistry and an Analytical Division of the Board of Directors. The Board also serves to review papers presented for the *Japan Journal of Clinical Chemistry* and for their Annual Meeting.

The Japan Society of Clinical Chemistry is a member of the IUPAC. There is one Annual National Meeting. For 1975, the meeting occupied two full days, November 28th and 29th. This was the fifteenth Annual Meeting of the Society. The Chairman of this Meeting was Dr. Masayuki Saito of Kitasato University Hospital.

The analytical papers presented at the meeting were typical of what one would expect at a clinical chemistry symposium. For example, Akira Takasaka of Nagoya University presented a paper on the use of an enzyme bound to the inside of a tube, for continuous-flow analysis.

Emiko Takano (National Hospital, Kyoto) presented a paper on the estimation of the peroxide generated by the action of oxidases on glucose and cholesterol, respectively, by its reaction in oxidizing homovanillic acid to a fluorescent substance. Very small amounts of serum could be used for these tests. Novel radioimmunoassay techniques were also presented. Typical are procedures for estriol and corticosteroids by Mitzuteru Numazawa (Tohoku Univ.) and Hokei Nishina (Toranomon Hosp.).

Mechanisms for several analytical procedures were also explored. Examples were the study of the mechanism of the Jaffé reaction, by Juro Takahashi (Osaka Univ.), and the effect of various ions on the activity of lipase, by Katsusuke Kobayashi (Wakayama Med. College).

Much stress in the program was placed on the isolation and purification of biologically active materials from natural sources. Isolation and purification studies were made for disphosphoglyceromutase from erythrocytes (Takashi Nishikawa, Kitasato Univ.), phosphofructokinase (Keizi Ueda, Osaka Univ.), prostaglandin endoperoxide isomerase from bovine seminal vesicles (Seishu Ogino, Kyoto Univ.), angiotensin from placenta (Edahiko Murakami, Aichi College), phosphatase from bovine nasal epidermis (Toshihiro Hitaka, Kurume Univ.), and others.

In general, there was a different balance between analytical clinical chemistry and what is referred to now as clinical biochemistry than is now seen at our national meetings in the United States. Of a total of approximately sixty presentations, only thirteen concerned themselves with methodology. The others were reports on fundamental studies in clinical biochemistry. Many papers were presented, the likes of which are now rare at our national meetings. For example, Masayuki Saito (Ehime Univ.) reported on the mechanism of absorption of disaccharides from the small intestine. Sadamichi Tamura (Tokushima Univ.) studied the activation of the C1 component of the complement system.

Of major interest was a symposium on hormone receptor sites. Aberrations in disease and the use of the receptor site as an analytical tool were stressed. The role of receptor sites in membrane permeability, action of adrenaline, insulin and other hormones was also explored.

The clinical chemistry laboratories are under the direction of either a doctorate with a medical degree or a Ph.D biochemist. Both are usually also members of The Japan Society of Clinical Pathology. Description of the laboratories at Kitasato University Hospital, under the directorship of Masayuki Sato, M.D. is representative of the better laboratories in Japan.

The laboratories, including research laboratories, are housed in a separate building. All laboratory work is performed there, including Microbiology, Chemistry, Hematology, BMR, EEG, and EKG scans. Equipment for radioisotope scanning for thyroid disorders are also housed in this building.

The chemistry laboratories are packed with equipment designed and built in the United States, but also much of which was constructed in Japan. The Technicon AutoAnalyzer II is used routinely. For emergency work the Du Pont *aca* Analyzer is used.

Clinical chemistry is under the directorship of Sȩiya Sato, Ph.D. Dr. Sato was originally trained at Michael Reese Medical Center in Chicago. He runs a highly sophisticated operation. For example, catecholamines are fractionated routinely by automated high-pressure liquid chromatography.

Some of the laboratories are automated and computerized. The Clinical Laboratory at Kawasaki Hospital in Okayama uses the computer not only to present the results to the physician but also to indicate whether the findings are compatible with the diagnosis presented. In addition, suggestions are made by the computer as to what further tests could be done to clarify the diagnosis. In this respect, the Japanese are attempting to apply computerization to the area of diagnosis as well as the accumulation and recording of data.

The training programs for medical technologists in Japan are very impressive. Typical of these is the Kawasaki Paramedical School in Kurashiki. This program is supervised by Masahide Sasaki, M.D. The technicians, mainly girls, live in dormitories and spend a long day which may extend from 8:00 in the morning to 5:00 in the evening. They are first introduced to clinical chemistry by the handling of tools. Projects are carried out which require the use of electric drills and other electrical equipment. This basic training is designed because of the need of the technologist to cope with the automated equipment used in the laboratory. The medical technology course is a four-year course, similar to our college course in medical technology.

In contrast to the training at Kawasaki Paramedical School in Kurashiki is the training at the Kanagawa Pref. Med. Tech. School, in Yokohama, which is supervised by Kihachiro Takahara, M.D. Here, the training is more formal and more like the training one obtains in an American university. However, since the students are in residence, it is practicable to program projects for them which go beyond the regular school day. It is not unusual for the students to have their evening meal and return to finish a project. These projects are in the nature of the development of new procedures or to study or improve a particular procedure.

In order to obtain an idea as the operation of clinical chemistry in hospitals not in large cities, I visited a laboratory at Tenri, which is approximately 25 miles from Kyoto. This is a religious institution run by a Buddhist sect. The laboratory was directed by Hiroshi Takahashi, M.D., who operates a fairly sophisticated system of analysis, with a minimum of automation. Methodology chosen, was in each case, internationally acceptable methodology. Very little compromise was made in substituting approximate methods for precise and accurate methods of analysis. The instrumentation used (e.g., colorimeters and spectrophotometers) were of excellent quality. They were made in Japan for the most part. The precision with which the technicians worked was impressive.

Overall, one can safely state that the analytical laboratories of clinical chemistry in Japan are well run. However, automation is used to a significantly lesser extent than in the United States. This is compensated for by the high quality of technical personnel doing the analyses, supported by an effective system of technician training schools attached to the university hospitals and medical schools.

As far as the direction of the laboratories are concerned, the directors are thoroughly conversant with American instrumentation, as well as their own. Their thinking is oriented toward the application of the data obtained and research in clinical biochemistry.

An interesting observation is that there are many instruments used in Japan which, more or less, are duplicates of instruments made in the United States, but are not sold outside of Japan. When inquiry was made, it was pointed out that there was a market for about 700 instruments, if generally accepted. Since these instruments are expensive, the initial sale and service makes a practical market for a smaller company. These smaller companies are able to service the instrument effectively because of the compact nature of Japanese geography.

In summary, while on a smaller scale the clinical chemistry practiced in Japan compares very favorably with that of the United States, it is my impression that the Japanese Medical Technology is equal to the best that the United States has to offer.

Samuel Natelson, Ph.D.
Director
Department of Biochemistry
Michael Reese Medical Center
Chicago, Ill. 60616

Supplement 1 to Enzyme Nomenclature

Enzyme Nomenclature: Recommendations (1972) of the International Union of Pure and Applied Chemistry and the International Union of Biochemistry. Supplement 1: Corrections and Additions (1975) will be published in vol. **429** of *Biochimica et Biophysica Acta,* pp 1–45, appearing in March, 1976.

Reprints may be purchased from Elsevier Scientific Publishing Co., P. O. Box 1345, Amsterdam, The Netherlands, at the following rates (prices include postage): 1 or more copies: Dfl. 15.00 each, 10 or more copies: Dfl. 14.00 each, 50 or more copies: Dfl. 12.00 each, 100 or more copies: Dfl. 11.00 each.

Developments in Industry

Bio-Rad's "Quantitative Immunoelectrophoresis" (Bulletin 1035) outlines theory, applications, and seven specific techniques.

Dow Diagnostics announces the availability of a new family of latexes: Dow Carboxylate-Modified Uniform Latex Particles. These latexes are the result of many requests for particles that would permit covalent (chemical) bonding of antigens, antibodies, enzymes, etc., to the surface of latex particles. The new latexes should permit attachments by amide bonds—amino groups on the biochemical species reacted with the carboxylic acid groups on the latex particle surface. These carboxylate-modified particles have surfaces whose adsorption characteristics also should be different from polystyrene latex surfaces. Dow Diagnostics plans to offer other diameters and functional groups in their new family of latex particles in the near future.

Synthesis and Natural Product Notes is a new publication providing answers to the isolation, purification, and analysis problems of the organic chemist. The current issue of this newsletter briefly discusses the preparation of pure cannabinol metabolites for biological research, the separation of optically active diastereomers, and the purification of synthesis reaction mixtures. In addition, this issue contains an announcement of a new preparative liquid chromatograph that can isolate gram quantities of ultrapure organic compounds from complex matrices in minutes. For a free copy of this publication, write Waters Associates, Inc., Maple Street, Milford, Mass. 01757.

Pharmacia Laboratories Inc. and Pharmacia Fine Chemicals Inc. have been consolidated into one corporation: Pharmacia, Inc., Piscataway, N. J. 08854. Effective January, 1976, Pharmacia Inc. consists of three divisions: Pharmacia Laboratories, the pharmaceutical products division; Pharmacia Diagnostics, the clinical laboratory products division; and Pharmacia Fine Chemicals, the separation products division.

Applied Science Laboratories, Inc., State College, Pa. 16801, now has available a series of well-characterized major metabolites of morphine, heroin, cocain, codeine, and methadone that should be welcome for use as standards.

SRM: pH

NBS Special Publication 260-53 is a 48-p booklet on *Standard Reference Materials: Standardization of pH Measurements,* by Richard A. Durst, of the National Bureau of Standards. A useful reference for all clinical chemists. For sale ($1.05, +25% for non-U. S. mailings) from the Supt. of Documents, U. S. Govt. Printing Office, Washington, D. C. 20412. (Order by SD cat. No. C 13.10:260-53.)

Meetings and Continuing Education

The Pharmacological, Biochemical and Clinical Relationships of Drug Therapy is the title of the joint spring Symposium of the Pacific Northwest Section of AACC and the British Columbia Section of CSCC. The symposium will feature as keynote speaker, the current AACC tour speaker, Dr. E. J. Ariens (University of Nijmegen, the Netherlands) as well as presentations by Dr. Donald Young (NIH) and Dr. Marjorie Horning (Baylor College of Medicine). The symposium will be held April 28, 29, and May 1, 1976 at the Sacred Heart Medical Center and the Sheraton Hotel, Spokane, Washington. Details from Dr. Thomas O. Tiffany, Symposium Chairman, Pathology Associates Inc., P.S., Terminal Annex Box 2687, Spokane, Wash. 99220.

Clinical Laboratory Programs at UCLA Extension. Two programs for laboratory technologists, clinical chemists and students in the health and life sciences will be offered by

UCLA Extension's Department of Continuing Education in Health Sciences and the UCLA School of Medicine for the Spring Quarter.

"Current Topics in the Biochemistry of Diseases: Why Am I Doing This Test?" is scheduled for Wednesdays, April 7 to May 12, 7:30 p.m., in the auditorium of the Hospital of the Good Samaritan Medical Center, 634 South Lucas, Los Angeles.

A panel of distinguished guest lecturers will focus on integrating the clinical aspects of various diseases and the biochemical tests performed to diagnose and monitor those diseases.

Course chairman is Denis O. Rodgerson, Ph.D., head of clinical chemistry and associate professor of pathology, UCLA Hospital and Clinics, and course coordinator is Solomon Notrica, Ph.D., general manager, Laboratory Procedures, Inc., Woodland Hills.

The fee is $65 and one unit of credit is available.

"Clinical Immunology" is scheduled for Thursdays, April 1 to June 17, 7 to 10 p.m., in Room 43-105 of UCLA's Center for the Health Sciences.

The course will feature five major areas; a review of modern immunobiology, antigen-antibody reactions, pathogenesis of auto-immune diseases; immunodeficiencies, and tumor and transplantation immunology.

The instructor is U. Blachman, Ph.D., Department of Pathology, Olive View Medical Center, Sylmar.

The fee is $75 and three units of credit may be earned.

For additional information write Health Sciences, UCLA Extension, P. O. Box 24902, Los Angeles, Calif 90024 or call (213) 825-8421.

The Academy of Clinical Laboratory Physicians and Scientists is holding its annual meeting at the International Inn, Washington, D. C., on June 3 and 4, 1976. The program includes sessions on recent advances in laboratory medicine, reviews of selected topics in each of the major areas of clinical pathology, selection and interpretation of clinical laboratory tests, as well as submitted papers from young investigators. Further details may be obtained from Dr. D. S. Young, Bldg. 10, Rm. 4N-309, National Institutes of Health, Bethesda, Md. 20014.

The Second International Symposium on Column Liquid Chromatography will be held May 17–19 in Wilmington, Del. This state-of-the-art meeting on high performance liquid chromatography will bring together many experts in the field. A program of invited papers on original research and informal discussion periods is planned. Participants are invited to propose short (5–10 min) presentations of their recent research for the informal sessions.

The symposium is being organized by the Chromatography Forum of the Delaware Valley and Du Pont Instruments' Scientific and Process Division. It will be co-chaired by Dr. J. J. Kirkland of the Central Research and Development Department, Du Pont Company; Professor John H. Knox of the University of Edinburgh, Scotland; and Professor J. F. K. Huber of the University of Vienna, Austria.

Attendance at the symposium will be limited to 350. For more details, contact Dr. Paul F. Levy, Du Pont Instruments, Scientific and Process Division, Wilmington, Del. 19898.

Simplex Optimization in Research and Development is the title of a short course sponsored by the Department of Chemistry, College of Natural Sciences and Mathematics, University of Houston, in two sessions, May 3 to May 5, 1976, and July 29 to July 31, 1976. The course is designed to provide a sound introduction to the use of sequential simplex designs in research and development. Three days of intensive lectures will deal with developmental strategies, optimization techniques, and the use of planned experimental designs in the region of the optimum. Real chemical examples will be presented. In addition, several laboratory sessions employing models of experimental systems will allow participants to become facile with the calculations and logic of the various simplex methods. Academic, industrial, and governmental scientists engaged in research and/or development may apply. No previous experience with response surface methodology or statistics is necessary. The total tuition-laboratory fee is $250 and should be made payable to "Simplex Optimization Short Course." An application form is obtainable from Department of Chemistry, University of Houston, Houston, Tex. 77004.

Gordon Research Conferences, 1976: Those of interest to clinical chemists include those on hemostasis, lipid metabolism, molecular pathology, drug metabolism, medicinal chemistry, analytical chemistry, food and nutrition, and enzymes, coenzymes and metabolic pathways. Conferences are in New England (except the last mentioned, which is in Santa Barbara). Scheduled June through August. Write for details to Alexander M. Cruickshank, Director, Pastore Chemical Laboratory, University of Rhode Island, Kingston, Rhode Island 02881.

J. Lloyd Johnson Associates will hold meetings on *Laboratory Management* (June 7–10), *Laboratory Medicine for Management* (June 8–10), *Emerging Capital Approval Requirements Under PL 92-603 and PL 93-641* (June 11), and *The Computer and Laboratory Medicine* (June 12–13) at the Ambassador West Hotel, Chicago. Contact Mrs. Betty Fisher, Clinical Sciences Division, J. Lloyd Johnson Associates, 778 Frontage Road-Suite 118, Northfield, Ill. 60093, (312) 441-7060.

Points to Ponder

From *Thinking About the Future 1/2*, Dec. 1975 (a publication of Alexander & Alexander Inc., New York, N. Y. 10036):

- It took ten thousand years for the number of people in this world to grow from a handful to the present four billions. The next four billions will arrive in only thirty or thirty-five years.
- One-quarter of the persons who ever lived on this planet are alive today. There were 1.6 billions of people in the world in 1900, 3.6 billions in 1970, 4 billions now, and indications point to 6.5 or 7 billions by the year 2000, and 8 billions only a few years after that.
- . . . the rate of exponential growth has now speeded up to 2.1% a year, with a doubling time of only 30 years.
- This shift in tempo of growth has arisen not so much from an increase in births as from the conquest in the last thirty years of infectious and childhood diseases (more survivors per 100 births) and the recently improved survival rates at all ages. Life expectancies in the Western world have increased from 18 years in the days of the pharaohs to 22 years at the beginning of the Christian era, to 33 years in the year 1200, 41 years in 1850, 49 years in 1900, 67 years in 1946, and 71 years now. But birth rates have been falling in the Western world for many decades; the main problem of population growth does not lie here.
- Today two-thirds of the world's people live in the equatorial hunger belt, producing only one-fifth of the food, but having four-fifths of the babies.
- 94 percent of the increase from 1970 to 2025 will have arisen in the less-developed regions.

Forthcoming Papers

Improved Determination of Prostatic Acid Phosphatase (Sodium Thymolphthalein Monophosphate Substrate)
Lilian M. Ewen and Ralph W. Spitzer

Diagnostic Use of Pancreatic Lipase Determination by Radial Enzyme Diffusion and Design of a Routine Pancreatic Profile
Jack M. Goldberg

Decreased Radioassay Values for Folate after Serum Extraction when Pteroylglutamic Acid Standards Are Used

Gary A. Mitchell, Sharon P. Pochron, Philip V. Smutny, and Rogelia Guity

The Anion Gap: Its Use in Quality Control
David L. Witte, John L. Rogers, David A. Barrett, II

Improved Specificity of Serum Albumin Determination and Estimation of "Acute Phase Reactants" by Use of the Bromcresol Green Reaction
Jan E. C. Gustafsson

Gas-Liquid Chromatographic Profile of Neutral and Acidic Metabolites in Cerebrospinal Fluid from Newborns and Infants
Richard D. Malcolm and Richard Leonards

Rapid Radioimmunoassay of Total Urinary Estriol
Dennis W. Anderson and Uwe Goebelsmann

Chemistry of the Kober Reaction
Ronald W. A. Oliver, Soren B. Jensen, and Gordon Crossley

Radioimmunoassay of Bile Acids in Serum
Laurence M. Demers and Gershon Hepner

Kinetic Determination of Serum Lipase Activity with the Abbott ABA-100
Ronald D. Feld, David L. Witte, and David A. Barrett II

Standardization in Principle and Practice
D. R. Bangham

Comparison of Three Procedures for Isolating Human Ferritin, for Use as a Standard in an Immunoradiometric Assay
Lorraine M. Gonyea, Colleen M. Lamb, R. Dorothy Sundberg, and Amos S. Dienard

Specificity and Reproducibility of Acetone Precipitation in Identifying Surface-active Phosphatidylcholine in Amniotic Fluid
L. L. Penney, Dwain D. Hagerman, and Catherine A. Sei

Normative Values of Serum Immunoglobulins by Single Radial Immunodiffusion: A Review
Shirley E. Maddison and Charles B. Reimer

Standardization of Human Immunoglobulin Quantitation: A Review
Charles B. Reimer, and Shirley E. Maddison

AMERICAN ASSOCIATION OF CLINICAL CHEMISTS
28th National Meeting
Astrohall, August 1-6, 1976, Houston, Texas

Registration # ____________

★ADVANCE REGISTRATION FORM★

Please Type or Print Heavily:

Name ____
(last) (first) (initial)

Institution ______________________ Department ______________________

Address ____

City ______________________ State ______________ Zip ______________

Pre-Registration Fees: Check appropriate space with number of persons

____ Member AACC $35.00 ($50.00 after April 1) ____ One Day Registration $10.00
____ Spouse $ 5.00 ____ Students $15.00
____ Each Child $ 5.00 ____ Non Member $50.00

All Pre-Registrants will participate in Bonus Drawing for trip to Mexico City or alternate site.

TOTAL REGISTRATION FEES ____________
(Enter pre-registration total at bottom of page also)

Special Events Registration

	No. of Tickets	Fee	Amount Enclosed
Sunday, August 1			
AACC Mixer, 7-11 PM		gratis	
Monday, August 2			
Fashion Show & Luncheon at Galleria, 10 AM - 2 PM		$ 14.00	
Wine Tasting, 2 - 5 PM		8.50	
Medical Center Tour, 10 AM		gratis	
Tuesday, August 3			
NASA Tour, 8:30 AM - 12:30 PM		6.50	
Medical Center Tour, 10 AM		gratis	
Houston City Tour, 1 - 3 PM		5.00	
Medical Center Tour, 2 PM		gratis	
President's Reception — Bar-B-Que. Rodeo. Dance. 5 PM,		10.00	
7 PM		10.00	
Wednesday, August 4			
Mini City & Heritage Home Tour, 9 AM - 12:30 PM		6.50	
Medical Center Tour, 10 AM		gratis	
Mini City & Heritage Homes Tour & Mystery Luncheon, 9:30 AM - 2:30 PM		14.50	
Continental Cuisine			
Gulf Seafood			
Mexican Food			
Mini City Tour & Mystery Luncheon, 10:30 AM - 2:30 PM		12.50	
Continental Cuisine			
Gulf Seafood			
Mexican Food			
NASA Tour, 1 - 5 PM		6.50	
NASA Tour & San Jacinto Inn Seafood Dinner, 1 - 9 PM		19.00	
San Jacinto Seafood Dinner, 5 - 9 PM		15.50	
Thursday, August 5			
Galveston Tour & Luncheon, 10 AM - 5 PM		19.00	
Mini City & Heritage Homes Tours & Mystery Luncheon, 9:30 AM - 2:30 PM		14.50	
Continental Cuisine			
Gulf Seafood			
Mexican Food			
Mini City Tour & Mystery Luncheon, 10:30 AM - 2:30 PM		12.50	
Continental Cuisine			
Gulf Seafood			
Mexican Food			
Pre-Banquet Reception, 7 - 8 PM		gratis	
Awards Banquet, 8 PM		15.00	
Friday, August 6			
San Antonio, Texas Trip (prices per person) Double		55.00	
Single		74.00	
Triple		50.00	
Mexico City Trip Double		214.00	
Single		244.00	
Triple		209.00	
Thursday, August 12			
Acapulco Extension of Mexico City Trip Double		81.50	
Single		99.50	
Triple		79.00	

SUB TOTALS
SPECIAL EVENTS ____________
PRE-REGISTRATION ____________
YOUTH PROGRAM ____________
WORKSHOPS ____________
ROUNDTABLES ____________
★TOTAL AMOUNT ENCLOSED ____________

★ BABYSITTING SERVICE ★

Registration # ____________

Children Attending:

Name ______________________ Age ________ Name ______________________ Age ________

Name ______________________ Age ________ Name ______________________ Age ________

Number of Children on: (Gratis Group-Sitting in Daytime)

	Monday	Tuesday	Wednesday	Thursday	Friday
AM	____	____	____	____	____
AFT	____	____	____	____	
PM	____	____	____	____	

★ YOUNG PEOPLE'S PROGRAM ★

	No. of Tickets	Fee	Amount Enclosed
Sunday, August 1			
Teen Mixer and Children's Program, 7 - 10 PM		gratis	
Monday, August 2			
Port Tour & Visit to Busch Bird Park & Box Lunch, 9 AM - 1 PM		$ 10.75	
Tuesday, August 3			
Day at Hermann Park & Box Lunch, 9 AM - 2 PM		11.50	
In-House Program, 2 - 4 PM		3.00	
Wednesday, August 4			
Botanical Gardens & Galleria, 9 AM - 2 PM		7.00	
Thursday, August 5			
Galveston, All Day, 10 AM - 9 PM		25.00	
Special Program to Include All of the Above Items		55.00	
★ YOUNG PEOPLE'S OPTIONAL EVENTS ★			
Monday, August 2			
Evening at Astroworld, 6 PM - Midnight		15.00	
Tuesday, August 3			
Bar-B-Que & Rodeo, 5 PM		10.00	
(Children under 12)		5.00	
Wednesday, August 4			
NASA Tour & San Jacinto Inn Seafood Dinner, 1 PM - 9 PM		19.00	
(Children under 12)		10.00	
San Jacinto Inn Seafood Dinner, 5 - 9 PM		15.50	
(Children under 12)		6.00	
		★ TOTAL	

(Enter in space at bottom of main registration form)

NOTE: Admission Tickets to Astroworld (no transportation, no supervision) Will be Available

★ NOTICE:

NO REFUNDS will be made during the meeting

ALL CANCELLATIONS for any event must be made by mail (only), 10 days prior to meeting.

NOTIFICATION on refunds from any oversubscription to any event will be made as soon as possible.

★ MAKE OUT CHECK OR DRAFT TO:

28th National Meeting A.A.C.C.

★ RETURN WITH REGISTRATION FORM TO:

Scherago Associates
P.O. Box 874
Montclair, New Jersey 07043
(NO LATER THAN MAY 1, 1976)

★ BREAKFAST ROUNDTABLE DISCUSSIONS ★ Registration # ____________

Fee: $10.00 each which includes breakfast. *Limit:* 9 per table. *Time:* 7:30-8:40 a.m. — Please indicate your first, second, and third choice for each day in the area below. Locations will be announced later.

Please Type or Print Heavily:

Your Name ____
(last) (first)

Address ____

City, State, Zip ____

Tuesday, August 3 and Thursday, August 5

No.	Roundtable	Tuesday	Thursday
1.	George N. Bowers, Jr., "Total Alkaline Phosphatase: Laboratory Management and Clinical Interpretation".		
2.	Evan C. Horning, "Gas Chromatography: Mass Spectrometry of Endogenous Substances".		
3.	Reba M. Hill, "Monitoring of Drugs: Clinical Utility in Pediatric Patients".		
4.	Leo P. Cawley, "Application of RIA and EIA to Autoimmune Diseases".		
5.	F.W. Sunderman, Jr., "Electro-Thermal Atomic Absorption of Trace Metals".		
6.	Paul A. Van Dreal, "The Use of Computers in Laboratory Medicine".		
7.	Richard P. Dickey or Clark Hinkley, "Evaluation of Fetal Well-Being".		
8.	Adrian Hainline, Jr., or Anne Yobs, "Basic Quality Control".		
9.	Peter Jatlow, "Emergency Toxicology".		
10.	Edward W. Bermes, Jr., "Operation of a Clinical Chemistry Training Program".		
11.	Robert Farmer, "Steroid Radioassay".		
12.	Charles Roe, "Infarct Size Estimation by Serial Enzyme Analysis".		
13.	Robert S. Melville, "Government Supported Research in Clinical Chemistry".		
14.	Donald S. Young, "Using Drug Interference Data".		
15.	Kurt M. Dubowski, "Research Support for Clinical Toxicology".		
16.	Paul E. Strandjord, "The Current Status of Diagnostic Enzymology".		
17.	Edward C. Knoblock, "New Applications of Centrifugal Analyzers".		
18.	Robert Schaffer, "Standards in Clinical Chemistry".		
19.	Henry R. Besch, Jr., "Mechanism of Action of Digitalis".		
20.	Jack E. Wallace, "Current Trends in the Analytical Toxicology Laboratory".		
21.	Harry L. Pardue or Stanley Deming, "Analog and Digital Electronics for Clinical Scientists".		
22.	William D. Odell, "Where is RIA Heading?".		
23.	Alvin R. Feinstein, "Evaluation of Data".		

Wednesday, August 4 and Friday, August 6

No.	Roundtable	Wednesday	Friday
24.	Marjorie G. Horning, "Gas Chromatography: Mass Spectrometry of Exogenous Substances".		
25.	Irving Sunshine, "Monitoring of Drugs: Analytical Methods".		
26.	Keith Griffiths, "Analytical Methods for Silicates/Asbestos".		
27.	Wendell T. Caraway, "The Scientific Development of Clinical Chemistry".		
28.	Graham M. Widdowson, "Normal Values".		
29.	Jocelyn M. Hicks, "Pediatric Microchemistry".		
30.	Donald C. Cannon, "Principles of Laboratory Management".		
31.	Alex Kaplan, "Accreditation of Clinical Chemistry Training Programs".		
32.	Norman D. Lee, "Continuing Education Programs (ACCENT)		
33.	Joseph H. Boutwell, Jr., "Current Federal Legislation of Clinical Laboratories".		
34.	J. Stanton King, Jr., "Preparation of Papers for Journal Publication".		
35.	Martin Fleisher, "Tumor Associated Antigens in Human Cancer".		
36.	Judith A. Hopkins, "Survey of Commercial RIA Products".		
37.	Bruno Jirgensons, "Protein Structure from Physical Measurements".		
38.	William E. Bucknall, "Analytical Methods in Genetic Disorders".		
39.	Max E. Chilcote, "Laboratory Design and Construction".		
40.	Roger E. Juselius, "Adrenocortical Function: What to Use?".		
41.	Theodore Peters, Jr., "Serum Albumin—Assays and Uses".		
42.	Gerald Cooper, "Suggested Procedure for the Determination of Serum Lipoprotein Patterns".		
43.	William E. Neely, "Micro-Analysis".		
44.	August Watanabe, "Autonomic Nervous System Modulation of Cardiac Performance".		
45.	Harry F. Weisberg, "Acid Base Balance and Blood Gases".		
46.	Robert H. McCluer, "High Pressure Liquid Chromatography in the Clinical Laboratory".		

Number of Roundtables selected ____________

★ TOTAL $ ____________

(Enter on main registration form)

★ REGISTRATION FOR WORKSHOPS ★

Registration # ______________

All workshops will be held from 1:30 p.m. to 5:00 p.m. in the *Astrohall* and on the days indicated.

Workshops No. 4 and 6 consist of three (3) parts—one part each on Monday (August 2), Wednesday (August 4), and Thursday (August 5).

Workshop No. 5 consists of two (2) parts—one part on Monday and the other part on Thursday.

The remaining workshops repeat on the days indicated.

Please indicate your choice of workshops in the area below. Every attempt will be made to assign your first choice if possible.

Your Name ______________________________ (last) ______________________________ (first)

Address ______________________________

City, State, Zip ______________________________

Workshops:	Limit	Fee	Days Given
1. "Combined Isoenzyme Analysis in the Diagnosis of Myocardial Injury" Charles Roe, M.D.	75	$35.00	Weds. Thurs. ________ or ________
2. "Laboratory and Clinical Management of the Patient on Digitalis Medication" H.R. Besch, Jr., Ph.D., and August Watanabe, M.D.	75	$35.00	Mon. Weds. ________ or ________
3. "Pediatric Clinical Chemistry" Jocelyn Hicks, Ph.D.	40	$35.00	Mon. Thurs. ________ or ________
4. "Application of Gas-Liquid Chromatography in the Clinical Laboratory" Jack E. Wallace, Ph.D.	40	$75.00 (all three parts)	Mon., Weds., & Thurs. ________
5. "Common Sense Approach to Basic Quality Control" Adrian Hainline, Jr., Ph.D.	100	$35.00 (both parts)	Mon., & Thurs. ________
6. "Analog and Digital Electronics for the Clinical Scientist" Harry L. Pardue, Ph.D.	35	$50.00 (all three parts)	Mon., Weds., & Thurs. ________
7. "Evaluation of Fetal Well-Being: Clinical and Analytical Considerations" Richard Dickey, M.D., Ph.D.	50	$35.00	Weds. Thurs. ________ or ________
8. "Acid Base Balance and Blood Gases" Harry F. Weisberg, M.D.	50	$35.00	Mon. Weds. ________ or ________
9. "Fundamentals of Steroid Radioassay" Robert Farmer, Ph.D.	50	$35.00	Weds. Thurs. ________ or ________

★TOTAL $ ______________

(Enter on main registration form)

guest editorial

Standardization of Human Immunoglobulin Quantitation: A Review of Current Status and Problems

Charles B. Reimer and Shirley E. Maddison

Extreme molecular heterogeneity of the immunoglobulins creates persistent problems of their accurate quantitation. A future solution of these problems demands a more careful consideration of calibrators, antisera, and methodology.

Of all the serum proteins, the immunoglobulins (Ig's), functionally and structurally, are probably the most heterogeneous. Every second each of us may be synthesizing a million different kinds of Ig molecules. Depending on our unique genetic constitution and environmental and immunologic exposure, the heterogeneity of each of our individual antibody populations reflects our personal "nature and nurture." Although the Ig's are antibodies, they are not quantified as such by immunoprecipitin analysis. First, antibodies are raised in animals against highly purified subsets of the human Ig's. One hopes that these antisera are made specific to the molecules of interest by absorptions, and then some form of a precipitin test is used to quantify the different subpopulations of Ig's as antigens. Currently, immunoprecipitin analysis is most frequently performed by single radial immunodiffusion either to quasi-equilibrium, as suggested by Mancini et al. (*1*), or by the kinetic modification of Fahey and McKelvey (*2*). Also, one sees increasing use of variations of quantitative electroimmunoassay (*3*) and manual or automated immunonephelometric analysis (*4*), the latter technique now capable of giving analytical precision of between 1 and 2% (coefficient of variation).

To properly standardize immunoprecipitin analysis, not only must we consider methodology but we must deal with the complexity of the human specimen as a heterogeneous molecular population of Ig antigens dispersed in the complex milieu called serum, and we certainly must contend with the complex nature of our analytical reagents. Is the human reference serum that is used as a standard for comparison similar to the unknown serum specimen or is it made up of a different heterogeneous molecular population? What do we really know of the actual molecular specificity of an animal antiserum we use as our principal analytical reactant? It, too, is a heterogeneous antibody population.

Immunoglobulin complexity. Meaningful measurement requires that the specific quality of interest be selectively measured and all varieties of it be measured without bias. There are four immunologically characterized subclasses of IgG, two of IgA; subclasses of IgM have been described but are not well characterized. In normal human serum, the relative amounts of the IgG subclasses 1, 2, 3, and 4 have been reported respectively as 61, 30, 5, and 4% (*5*). There is little if any good information regarding changes in these ratios with infectious or other diseases other than in the malignant transformation of antibody-forming cells, such as in multiple myeloma. IgG subclass 1 and 3 fix complement well, therefore they must be especially important in infectious and autoimmune disease. Subclass 2 fixes complement poorly, and subclass 4 not at all. Generally, antibody to polysaccharide is IgG subclass 2. Rh antibodies are never subclass 2. Antibodies to human blood-clotting factor VIII are limited to subclass 4. Genetic polymorphism produces IgG subclasses containing specific antigenic allotypes that have different distributions in different racial groups (*6*). Perhaps the persistence of different Ig allotypes in different human subpopulations in part reflects the unique geographic history in the evolution of the races of man with respect to different infectious diseases and man's present disease susceptibility or resistance, as the case may be. Ig heterogeneity caused by genetic factors must eventually be quantitatively considered in a proper analytical system.

Physical-chemical heterogeneity of the sample gives additional measurement problems. IgM is usu-

Biological Products and Parasitology Divisions, Bureau of Laboratories, Center for Disease Control, USPHS, U. S. Dept. of HEW, Atlanta, Ga. 30333.

Based on a paper presented at the first AACC Pine Mountain (Ga.) Conference (on Diagnostic Immunochemistry), March 3, 1975; and at the Symposium on "Immunology—Interrelations with Clinical Chemistry," Ninth International Congress on Clinical Chemistry, Toronto, July 17, 1975.

Received Feb. 20, 1976; accepted Feb. 21, 1976 (reviewed before receipt).

ally present as the stable 19 *s* pentamer of 7 *s* subunits, which, however, occasionally are found free in a 7 *s* form. In serum, one finds 7 *s* monomeric IgA and an 11 *s* dimeric IgA. In secretions, a further complication occurs in that dimeric IgA contains a disulfide-linked glycoprotein, or "secretory piece," which also occurs in somewhat altered conformational form as "free secretory piece." Because the diffusion rate depends on the molecular weight, polymeric forms of an Ig will give different disc diameters in single radial immunodiffusion, particularly during the kinetic phase of the precipitin reaction, before quasi-equilibration occurs and the disc of precipitation stops growing. Antigen valence is different in the mono- and polymeric forms. Occasionally, 19 *s* IgM and, rarely, other Ig classes have rheumatoid factor activity; that is, they act as antibody to IgG and, as such, they may exist as soluble immune complexes with other Ig's and with serum complement components as mixed cryoprecipitates. Human rheumatoid factors may precipitate with the animal reagent IgG, particularly if the latter has been heat-aggregated, as in the preparation of a single radial immunodiffusion plate. Obviously, such a situation can give spurious analytical results.

IgD occurs in low concentrations in human serum, a few milligrams per liter. The role of IgD as a lymphocyte surface membrane receptor (*7, 8*), as well as the standardization of tests and reagents used to evaluate immunoglobulins bound to the surface of B-lymphocytes presents special methodological and standardization problems (*9, 10*) and will not be further discussed in this brief review.

The IgE immunoglobulins are the reaginic antibodies that result in immediate hypersensitivity and manifestations of allergy. The low concentrations of IgE in serum necessitate the use of a quantitative technique such as radioimmunoassay, of greater sensitivity than that available with simple gel techniques. This Ig subset has been recently reviewed elsewhere (*11*).

Specificity problems of reagent antisera. As a practical matter, manufacturers of immunological products are expected to produce uniform diagnostic reagents year after year. They confront very difficult standardization problems. Figure 1, taken from a publication by Haber et al. (*12*), shows diagrammatically the complex, three-dimensional folding of the polypeptide backbone of pancreatic ribonuclease, a relatively small, homogeneous protein, less than one-tenth the molecular weight of human IgG. The dotted and dashed rectangles represent the size of two of many hypothetically different antibody-combining sites, 1.1 × 2.5 nm, having overlapping specificity to the same dinitrophenol hapten epitope attached to the epsilon amino lysine at position 41. Depending on the evolutionary or genetic differences between this protein when it is used as an immunogen and the homologous protein from the animal species or individual animal which is immunized to produce diagnostic

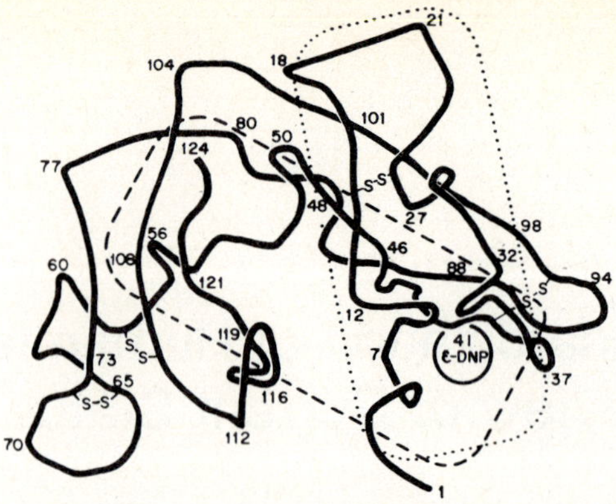

Fig. 1. Three-dimensional structure of bovine pancreatic ribonuclease

Based on an illustration by Harker et al. [*Chem. Eng. News* **45** 7, 60 (1967)]. The heavy circle, *ε-DNP*, represents a haptene on the lysine group at position 41, used by Eisen et al. [*Biochemistry* **3**, 996 (1964)]. The *dotted* and the *dashed* outlines are the size of the hypothetical antibody combining sites, 2.5 × 1.1 nm. [Reprinted with permission from the publishers and Haber, E., Richards, F. F., Spragg, J., Austen, K. F., Vallotton, M., and Page, L. B., Modifications in the heterogeneity of the antibody response. *Cold Spring Harbor Symp. Quant. Biol.* **32,** 301 (1967)]

antisera, different regions of this foreign protein surface might appear as self or as non-self. If the molecule folded up differently, a new subset of antibodies to this hapten could be elicited to the new conformational determinants produced as a result of the altered tertiary structure. It is easy to understand that if one uses a much larger and more complex immunogen, such as an individual Ig molecule from another species, one usually will obtain a very heterogeneous antibody response. During the course of animal immunizations, the antibody population changes. Certain lymphocytes, prepossessing on their surfaces specific recognition molecules for non-self determinants, are selected by the best-fitting antigens to be preferentially stimulated to divide and eventually to establish clones of plasma cells that produce antibody molecules of the same specificity as the recognition molecules on the lymphocytes that were stimulated. Depending on the continued availability of antigen and the goodness of fit between antibody-binding sites and antigenic determinants, continuing competition for limited amounts of antigen will usually select those clones of cells that will produce antibody with the highest binding affinity. Philosophers have said that we never step in the same river twice. In view of the facts of antigen heterogeneity, changing immunogen and antibody concentrations, the changing population of antibody-producing cells, and antibody turnover rates, one probably should rarely speak of antibody specificity in the singular.

Several years ago, we decided to examine the immunological specificity of commercially available antisera to human IgG, IgA, and IgM at the level of sensitivity appropriate for immunoprecipitin analysis in gels (*13–16*). At that time we examined almost 200 commercial reagents and found that only one of every three or four antisera to IgA or IgM was class specific. More than 95% of antisera to IgG precipitated inappropriately with Ig's other than IgG. Three years ago only one of six firms selling single radial immunodiffusion plates to measure the concentrations of human Ig was consistently producing kits that were specific for each of the three major Ig classes—IgG, IgM, and IgA—although two firms produced class-specific IgM plates. Recently we re-tested the specificity of single radial immunodiffusion plates from these six suppliers, all of whom were found to produce plates that were class specific for measuring IgA and IgM. In addition, three of these six firms supplied plates that were specific for human IgG as well, giving easily-read single discs—a decided improvement in quality control in three years.

Morell et al. (*17*) found IgG subclass bias for eight of 10 IgG class-specific antisera they studied. Recently, using a panel of highly purified IgG myeloma proteins of known subclass, we looked for the presence of IgG subclass bias in currently available commercial IgG single radial immunodiffusion plates and in our own IgG specific antisera. Generally, we confirmed the findings of the aforementioned authors. Currently available IgG class-specific antisera tend to have relatively more antibody molecules that precipitate with IgG subclass 1 or 2 than with subclass 3 or 4. With some antisera, equal masses of the latter two subclasses may, at equilibrium, form single radial immunodiffusion discs with 150% of the disc area produced by an equal mass of IgG subclass 1.

Problems with the calibrator. Given good antisera, the other very important variable reagent of any Ig quantitation system is the calibrator, or comparison reference standard, from which the base units and quantity are derived. Ig concentrations have been most frequently expressed as a ratio of mass to volume in familiar units common to physics and chemistry, e.g., milligrams per deciliter. However, in a 1970 cooperative effort, Rowe et al. (*18, 19*) found that the means of Ig concentrations of six coded serum samples gave unacceptably wide ranges between the lowest and the highest values obtained by experts when each independently used his own standard calibration sera and antisera. For the same samples, they got a between-lab range of 2.2-fold for IgG, 3.2-fold for IgA, and 5.0-fold for IgM! To improve agreement among laboratories, the organizers of this effort asked the British National Institutes of Biological Standards and Control to process and freeze-dry a pool of human serum. They then assigned arbitrary potency units to this pool to represent the unknown concentrations of IgG, IgA, and IgM, and distributed it as a comparison material to each of the cooperating investigators. When all laboratories used this preparation as a common arbitrary reference standard, the ranges of relative means between the lowest and the highest values obtained were greatly improved: 1.36-fold for IgG, 1.17-fold for IgA, and 1.31-fold for IgM. Encouraged by this result, the authors of the study, supported by an expert committee (*20, 21*), made this freeze-dried human serum pool available generally as the World Health Organization International Reference Preparation of Human Immunoglobulins IgG, IgA, and IgM, each vial containing 100 (arbitrary) international units of each of these three Ig's. Recommendations were made for the gradual but exclusive adoption of these arbitrary units—i.e., int. units—for all measurements of these human serum Ig's; milligram values were not assigned to this preparation.

Since these recommendations were made, a problem of general acceptance of these units instead of more familiar measures has given rise to some controversy (*22–24*). Some investigators have advocated reporting Ig concentrations as "percentage of the mean normal value" by comparison with the values obtained with a serum pool made from the sera of "normal" adults that one encounters in his own laboratory practice (*25*). The dependence of Ig concentration on age, sex, and race factors (*26–32*) creates inherent problems when reporting results as percent of mean normal or in attempting to produce reference preparations that represent the "normal" population. Either one must have human serum pools representing each of the normal subpopulations of interest or one must try to make a single serum pool to represent the hypothetical "average" patient and accept the intrinsic greater variability of "normal" values.

Some believe that fundamental units of biological measurement should not be redefined apart from the basic units of physics and chemistry. Some say we do not yet have enough reliable normative data in the newer unfamiliar unitage to make valid comparisons between health and disease or to interpret differences caused by age, sex, and race. Most clinicians have become accustomed to the more familiar mass per unit volume dimensions, and some even believe that they know true normative ranges in these units, thereby making any change difficult. Recognizing these problems, another expert committee (*23*) authorized use of conversion factors obtained from the published data of Rowe et al. (*19*) to relate the two systems of measurement: 80.4 μg IgG, 14.2 μg of IgA, or 8.47 μg of IgM are equivalent to 1.00 international unit.

Categorically, the Ig content of the WHO International Reference Preparation is accurately—that is, truly—defined in international units with a between-vial CV of less than 1%, reflecting the ease of reproducibility in filling vials. However, the conversion factors to mass units are subject to much uncertainty and probably will change with further efforts to improve both precision and accuracy. At present, so that comparisons of results obtained from different geographic areas, at different times, or from different investigators will be valid irrespective of the units used, Ig should always be measured by comparison with the WHO International Reference Preparation or a secondary standard carefully calibrated relative to it. Manufacturers usually supply secondary standards calibrated against the WHO preparation (in arbitrary international units) and the same secondary standard also calibrated with a weighed or otherwise quantified mass of each class of purified Ig using the more familiar units of the *Système International d'Unites* (SI). Many errors can arise in the calibration of mass units. The mass of Ig may have been incorrectly determined because the preparation was not completely pure, or, commonly, it may not immunologically represent all subsets of a heterogeneous Ig class. The purified preparation may have become antigenically altered during purification or may have become aggregated, or, for some other reason, may behave differently in the calibration system than does the native molecule in a serum matrix. If the manufacturer used the same purified monoclonal protein for calibration that he used as an immunogen to produce his antiserum, the presence of antibody to idiotypic determinants would make calibration bias likely. Bias could also arise if class-specific antisera had subclass selectivity, as already discussed. These and other reasons can explain why reagent suppliers usually give somewhat different conversion factors relating international units to mass-per-unit volume in each of their calibration materials, as shown in Table 1.

In May 1973, the U. S. CDC Licensure and Proficiency Testing Branch evaluated the performance of 125 laboratories performing quantitative Ig tests (*33*). Three samples were sent; two were coded duplicates of the same normal human serum and one was a coded macroglobulinemic serum with greatly supranormal concentration of IgM and subnormal IgG and IgA. Almost all tested laboratories used commercial reference standards and purchased single radial immunodiffusion plates that would have permitted these laboratories to report their results in either dimensional system, international (arbitrary) units or SI (mass units). Less than 5% of these laboratories chose to use the WHO international units, which with normal sera gave an 11% CV for IgG, a 7% CV for IgA, and a 20% CV for IgM. The corresponding variation of results from the majority of independent laboratories reporting in SI units and using a variety of methods and materials was 17% CV for IgG, 21% CV for IgA, and 32% CV for IgM. Somewhat more variability was found for the macroglobulinemic serum. Ig proficiency testing by the College of American Pathologists has recently given concordant CV's (personal communication, Pierre W. Keitges). The results from these laboratories, which were generally concerned with providing ordinary routine diagnostic service, were in much better agreement than were the previously mentioned results of the world experts obtained three years earlier, in 1970, before the WHO Reference Preparation was available. Regardless of general acceptance or nonacceptance of international units for Ig measurement, this case history of effective technology transfer to produce more uniform clinical results clearly demonstrates the value of a commonly available reference preparation, the WHO preparation, here used by reagent manufacturers as a common, arbitrary calibrator to adjust their "in house" reference preparations which, in turn, are distributed to clinical users.

Table 1. Number of Micrograms of Immunoglobulins Corresponding to 1.00 International Unit

Source of information	IgG	IgA	IgM
Rowe et al. (*19, 23*)	80.4 (CV 7.5%)	14.2 (CV 7.9%)	8.47 (CV 9.2%)
Buckley and Dorsey (*27*)	59.5	·43.1	3.06
Cejka et al. (*29*)	85.0	16.5	8.30
Pilgrim et al. (*36*)	94.0	10.0	6.00
Behringwerke[a]	86.8	16.8	8.70
Helena[a]	75.2	11.3	8.68
Hyland[a]	86.8	20.9	7.74
Kallestad[a]	87.0	18.0	5.65
Meloy[a]	81.9	15.0	7.70
Miles[a]	81.6	—	—
Pfizer[a]	87.0	17.3	8.56
Technicon[a]	87.1	16.8	8.67

[a] Data from manufacturers' package literature.

Considerations for future research. About 2 years ago, J. Paul Cali of our National Bureau of Standards wrote an editorial in *Clinical Chemistry* entitled: "An Idea Whose Time Has Come," wherein he suggested that we are now able to reach an era of more meaningful measurements in clinical chemistry (*34*). Although traditionally our National Bureau of Standards has dealt with much simpler phenomena than are usually encountered in biology and medicine, they have been able effectively to generalize the intellectual process that they use for standardizing physical and chemical analytical systems. Table 2 lists Cali's requirements for a standardization process leading to meaningful measurement. The first requirement, acceptance of base units, is one that most of us tend to neglect. Actually there has been a great deal of discussion recently about which base units should be used for immunoglobulin measurement—that is, whether we should use the SI units that, as chemists, we are comfortable with or the arbitrary international units recommended by the WHO Expert Committee on Biological Standardization. Those who feel comfortable, perhaps even secure, with the base units customary to the physical sciences, should recall that most measurements consist of two parts: a number that expresses quantity and the associated base unit that provides the dimensions for that number. There is some subtle psychology involved in our preference for the dimensions of physics and chemistry. We feel comfortable with the notion of the unity of science, and, as chemists, we prefer base units that

Table 2. Standardization Requirements for Meaningful Measurements (*34*)

1. A rational system of BASE UNITS for measurements
2. Certified STANDARD REFERENCE MATERIALS
3. Accurate REFERENCE METHODS of analysis
4. Practical FIELD METHODS and tests
5. Periodic PROFICIENCY TESTING for continued control of quality

fundamentally relate to the analytical balance and volume measurements that reduce to operations that are performed with metric scales. However, we must not delude ourselves by our desire for familiar terms and operations. Because we intuitively accept the dimensional units of the SI, we cannot uncritically accept as correct the numbers that are associated with these units. If we had a way to stoichiometrically extract all of the IgG from a unit volume of serum, free it from other components, and, without loss, put it on a balance to weigh it, we would have the correct answer. Instead, we must use the comparison methods of immunoprecipitin analysis that we discussed earlier—hence the need for arbitrary base units.

Probably the crux of most biological standardization problems is the general unavailability of adequate standard reference materials, Cali's second requirement. Note his use of the word "certified" here, which implies a consensus by some authoritative group of experts who establish adequate reference materials that are quantitatively described in appropriate base units acceptable to most of us. Also notice that the word "standard" is reserved here for designating a material preparation for use as a reference. This is quite different from using the word "standard" as a synonym for "specification" which, unfortunately, is often done when attempting to standardize diagnostic tests by formulating legalistically worded documents called "Performance Standards." When certifying a standard reference material, biological systems of standardization generally try to select a native preparation that is as analytically similar to the thing of interest as is possible. Of course, the *sine qua non* for any material standard is stability—stability during storage and, particularly, stability during shipment. It is impossible to consider as native a whole serum that has been frozen and thawed, or freeze-dried; however, the molecules of interest must be undenatured. As previously mentioned, great improvement was made in precision (reproducibility) and in accuracy (conformity to a standard) by use of this simple process for Ig quantitation. Unfortunately, there has not been universal acceptance of the base units (int. units) proposed by the WHO Expert Committee on Biological Standards for the WHO Reference Preparation of Human Immunoglobulins IgG, IgA, and IgM. A possible solution for this type of biological standardization problem is to use two systems of base units for each complex reference preparation. One system would use an arbitrary unitage; by decree or definition there would be, say, 100 arbitrary (or international) units of activity in each vial; the confidence interval for this unitage could be represented by the coefficient of variation obtained for vial filling, which would be quite small. The second unitage would use the base units of the SI to give the best mean estimate of each component of interest and its standard deviation as derived from experiment and consensus. The indeterminacy here might be quite large. If a user felt compelled to use the mean value in SI units for anything other than a conversion factor, he should be aware that a large error may accompany this value. It is to be hoped that, in time, we would approach the "true" value of this mean with improved confidence, although the value of the mean in international units would always be 100, by definition.

In Cali's third requirement, note the use of the word "accurate"—denoting validity or truth—rather than the word "precise"—denoting mere reproducibility—to characterize reference methods of analysis. Knowledge of the biochemical specificity of any method is crucial to assessment of its accuracy. Immunoprecipitin analysis is capable of great specificity which, nevertheless, must be proven in each situation. Characterization of the molecular specificity of analytical antisera used for quantitation is itself a difficult standardization problem. Unfortunately, in biology there are few, if any, "absolute" or "definitive" methods of analysis such as the isotope dilution mass spectrometry method for calcium (*35*), which is proposed as a model for the standardization of many chemical analyses. Rarely, if ever, will it be possible to specify accurate Reference Methods for analysis of biological substances without also providing stable certified Reference Materials. Hopefully, use of a proper Standard Reference Material will allow us to obtain the same (valid) results by several methods. But what is one to do if two apparently useful methods (say single radial immunodiffusion and immunonephelometric analysis), with use of the same antisera, reference preparations, and base units, give significantly different results with the same specimens? A practical solution would be to experimentally determine and authoritatively select the most precise of these methods as the arbitrary reference method and develop appropriate correction factors to bring the mean values obtained with the less precise method into agreement.

Cali's first three requirements are best met by the compulsive, perfectionist type of scientist. Pertinence of results for the clinical patient is most indirect. In fact, the patient is almost an annoyance at this level of development of standards. The essence of the first three requirements is operationally to define the correct numbers to be associated with the proper units. With the fourth requirement, we approach the practical clinical situation. Generally, practical field methods must be economical, rapid, adequately sensitive, and accessible to laboratories. With field methods, we can cut corners sometimes, but only if we have the reference preparations and methods to back them up and reference laboratories that are competent to look objectively at field methods and say what really is being measured. In an evaluation of field methods, we seek the scientific consensus of experts, guided by referee methodology and reference standards, not necessarily a democratic consensus of everyone who might have an interest in a certain test. Finally, we have a fifth requirement, which includes good manufacturing practice, quality-control assurance, and periodic proficiency testing designed to control drift and prevent system degeneration. Currently, we tend to put most of our strength here. Proficiency testing is a kind of democratic vote to determine truth; truth is considered to be the consensus of what everybody says it is. The trouble with this approach is that disagreement rather than consensus is often the result, and this is poor for good diagnosis and for uniform patient treatment. Perhaps if we worked more diligently with Cali's first three requirements, particularly the second one, and supplied appropriate and acceptable standard reference materials, we would have much less variance and controversy with the control of quality as measured by proficiency testing results.

References

1. Mancini, G., Carbonara, A. O., and Heremans, J. F., Immunochemical quantitation of antigens by single radial immunodiffusion. *Immunochemistry* **2**, 235 (1965).

2. Fahey, J. L., and McKelvey, E. M., Quantitative determination of serum immunoglobulins in antibody agar plates. *J. Immunol.* **94**, 84 (1965).

3. *A Manual of Quantitative Immunoelectrophoresis*, N. H. Axelsen, J. Kroll, and B. Weeks, Eds., *Scand. J. Immunol.* **2**, *Suppl.* 1 (1973).

4. Ritchie, R. F., Theory and practice of automated nephelometry. In *Protides of Biological Fluids*, 21st Colloquium, Brugge (1973), H. Peeters, Ed., Pergamon Press, New York, N. Y., 1974.

5. Morell, A., Skvaril, F., Steinberg, A. G., et al., Correlations between the concentrations of the four subclasses of IgG and Gm allotypes in normal human sera. *J. Immunol.* **108**, 195 (1972).

6. Grubb, R., *The Genetic Markers of Human Immunoglobulins*. Springer-Verlag, New York, Heidelberg, Berlin, 1970.

7. Rowe, D. S., Hug, K., Faulk, W. P., et al., IgD on the surface of peripheral blood lymphocytes of the human newborn. *Nature, New Biol.* **242**, 155 (1973).

8. Rowe, D. S., Hug, K., Forni, L., and Pernis, B., Immunoglobulin D as a lymphocyte receptor. *J. Exp. Med.* **138**, 965 (1973).

9. Aiuti, F., et al., Identification, enumeration, and isolation of B and T lymphocytes from human peripheral blood. *Scand. J. Immunol.* **3**, 521 (1974).

10. Kunkel, H. G., Surface markers of human lymphocytes. *Johns Hopkins Med. J.* **138**, 216 (1975).

11. General Discussion of Session II: Structure, function and quantitation of IgE. In *The Biological Role of the Immunoglobulin E System*, K. Ishizaka and D. H. Dayton, Eds. U. S. Dept. of HEW Publication No. (NIH) 73-502, 1973, p 2.

12. Haber, E., Richards, F. F., Spragg, J., et al., Modifications in the heterogeneity of antibody response. *Cold Spring Harbor Symp. Quant. Biol.* **32**, 301 (1967).

13. Reimer, C. B., Phillips, D. J., Maddison, S. E., and Shore, S. L., Comparative evaluation of commercial precipitating antisera against human IgM and IgG. *J. Lab. Clin. Med.* **76**, 949 (1970).

14. Phillips, D. J., Shore, S. L., Maddison, S. E., et al., Comparative evaluation of commercial precipitating antisera against human IgA. *J. Lab. Clin. Med.* **77**, 639 (1971).

15. Shore, S. L., Phillips, D. J., and Reimer, C. B., Umbrella effect: Pitfall in analysis of specificity of antisera to immunoglobulins. *Immunochemistry* **8**, 562 (1971).

16. Reimer, C. B., Standardization of immunoglobulin reagents. *Health Lab. Sci.* **9**, 178 (1972).

17. Morell, A., Skvaril, F., and Barandun, S., Qualitative and quantitative investigations on the reactions of normal and myeloma IgG with antisera to IgG. *Clin. Exp. Immunol.* **13**, 293 (1973).

18. Rowe, D. S., Anderson, S. G., and Grab, B., A research standard for human serum immunoglobulins IgG, IgA and IgM. *Bull. WHO* **42**, 535 (1970).

19. Rowe, D. S., Grab, B., Anderson, S. G., An international reference preparation for human serum immunoglobulins G, A, and M, content of immunoglobulins by weight. *Bull. WHO* **46**, 67 (1972).

20. Anderson, S. G., Bangham, D. R., Batty, I., et al., Measurements of the concentrations of human serum immunoglobulins. *J. Immunol.* **107**, 1798 (1971).

21. WHO Expert Committee on Biological Standardization: 23rd Report. *WHO Tech. Rep. Ser. No.* **463**, 20 (1971).

22. Reimer, C. B., *Proceedings: WHO/CDC International Conference on Standardization of Diagnostic Materials*, General Discussion—Sessions VIII–XII, p 277, Center for Disease Control, Atlanta, Ga., 1974.

23. Humphrey, J. H., and Batty, I., International reference preparation for human serum IgG, IgA, and IgM. *Clin. Exp. Immunol.* **17**, 708 (1974).

24. Soothill, J. F., Immunoglobulin standards. *Lancet* **i**, 39 (1975).

25. Heremans, J. F., and Masson, P. L., Specific analysis of immunoglobulins, techniques and clinical value. *Clin. Chem.* **19**, 294 (1973).

26. Hobbs, T. R., Immunoglobulins in clinical chemistry. *Adv. Clin. Chem.* **14**, 291 (1971).

27. Buckley, C. E., and Dorsey, F. C., Serum immunoglobulin levels throughout the lifespan of healthy man. *Ann. Intern. Med.* **75**, 679 (1971).

28. Rowe, D. S., Concentration of serum immunoglobulins in healthy young adult males estimated by assay against the international reference preparation. *Lancet* **ii**, 1232 (1972).

29. Cejka, J., Mood, D. W., and Kim, C. S., Immunoglobulin concentrations in sera of normal children: Quantitation against an international reference preparation. *Clin. Chem.* **20**, 656 (1974).

30. Becker, W., Variations in immunoglobulins in disease. *J. Clin. Pathol.*, in press, 1976.

31. Maddison, S. E., Stewart, C. C., Farshy, C. E., and Reimer, C. B., The relationship of race, sex and age to concentrations of serum immunoglobulins expressed in international units in healthy adult U. S. residents. *Bull. WHO* **52**, 179 (1976).

32. Maddison, S. E., and Reimer, C. B., Normative values of serum immunoglobulins by single radial immunodiffusion: A review. *Clin. Chem.* **22**, 594 (1976).

33. *Proficiency Testing: Non-syphilis Serology, Quantitative Immunoglobulins*. Center for Disease Control, USPHS, U. S. Department of HEW, Atlanta, Ga. 30333, 1973.

34. Cali, J. P., An idea whose time has come. *Clin. Chem.* **19**, 291 (1973). Editorial.

35. Cali, J. P., Moore, L. J., and Young, D. S., A referee method for determination of total calcium in serum. *Clin. Chem.* **19**, 1208 (1973).

36. Pilgrim, U., Fontanellaz, H. P., Evers, G., and Hitzig, W. H., Normal values of immunoglobulins in premature and full-term infants, calculated in percentiles. *Helv. Paediatr. Acta* **30**, 121 (1975).

CLIN. CHEM. 22/5, 583–593 (1976)

review

Theoretical Approaches to Estimation of Plasma Renin Activity: A Review and Some Original Observations

Suzanne Oparil

Performance of accurate, reproducible, and interpretable assays for plasma renin activity and other components of the renin/angiotensin system in the clinical setting requires a clear understanding of the various reactions in the renin/angiotensin cascade and the nature of their interactions. Plasma renin activity, the rate of angiotensin generation from plasma incubated in vitro, is the most commonly used clinical index of function in the renin/angiotensin system. Renin activity is measured by radioimmunoassay of angiotensin I generated in vitro under carefully controlled conditions. The value obtained for plasma renin activity depends on pH and duration of incubation and on the method used to protect the angiotensin I generated. We recommend incubation at neutral pH in buffered plasma for three hours in the presence of either ethylenediaminetetraacetate + 8-hydroxyquinoline + dimercaprol or ethylenediaminetetraacetate + phenylmethylsulfonylfluoride. Addition of a standard preparation of human renin to the plasma incubation step of the renin activity assay serves the dual purpose of permitting measurement of renin activity and furnishing an internal standard for comparison of assay procedures. The many variables among renin assay methods can be cancelled by referring to a common internal renin standard.

Introduction

Measurements of plasma renin (EC 3.4.99.19) activity are widely used in the clinical evaluation of hypertensive patients. Since systemic hypertension is the most common chronic disease treated by physicians in the United States, afflicting 15% of the population, appropriate diagnosis and treatment of these patients is an important health issue (*1, 2*). Effective drug treatment for hypertension is available and has been shown to reduce the incidence of strokes, heart failure, and renal failure in hypertensive populations (*3, 4*). Unfortunately, long-term medical treatment of hypertension is often unsuccessful because of excessive cost, inconvenience, and side effects of drugs. For this reason it is desirable to identify potentially curable secondary causes of hypertension when the patient's condition is first evaluated. Many of these secondary causes can be defined by abnormalities in the renin/angiotensin system. Further, recent studies suggest that it may be possible to subclassify "essential" hypertensive patients on the basis of their plasma renin activity and aldosterone excretion, in an attempt to individualize antihypertensive treatment (*5, 6*). Rational drug therapy based on defined pathophysiological mechanisms is expected to be more effective and free of side effects than existing empirical regimens.

Mechanism of Renin Action

A clear understanding of the clinical importance of plasma renin activity presupposes familiarity with the biochemistry and physiology of the renin/angiotensin system (*7*). The renin/angiotensin system is an important regulator of blood pressure and volume homeostasis in normal and hypertensive man. Figure 1 summarizes the biochemical events related to the action of renin. Renin is a highly specific proteolytic enzyme produced in specially modified cells in the afferent arteriole of the kidney near the glomerulus, the "juxtaglomerular cells." Renin cleaves its substrate, an α_2-globulin synthesized by the liver, to produce the decapeptide angiotensin I. Converting enzyme (no EC no. assigned), a dipeptidylcarboxypeptidase found mainly in lung but also in circulating plasma and in peripheral capillary beds, removes the carboxyl terminal His-Leu from angiotensin I to produce the octapeptide angiotensin II. Angiotensin II, the most potent vasoconstrictor hormone known, also stimulates adrenal aldosterone production and thereby extracellular fluid

Pritzker School of Medicine, University of Chicago, Chicago, Ill. 60637.

This paper was presented at the first Pine Mountain Conference sponsored by the AACC, this one being on "Diagnostic Immunochemistry," March 2–6, 1975, at Callaway Gardens, Pine Mountain, Ga.

Received and accepted Feb. 7, 1976 (prereviewed).

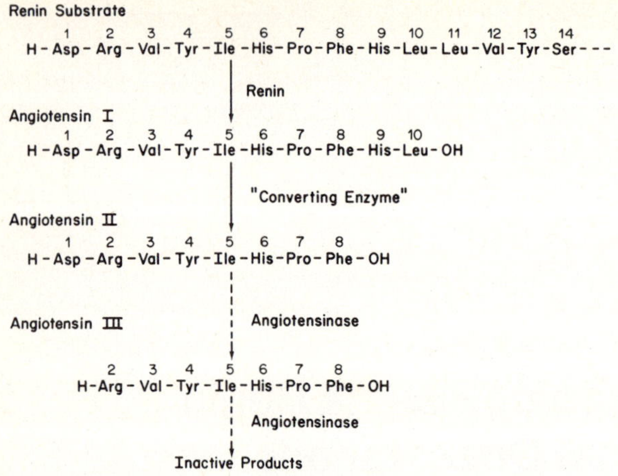

Fig. 1. Biochemistry of the renin/angiotensin system

volume expansion. Thus angiotensin II acts to increase blood pressure by two independent mechanisms. Angiotensin II is rapidly metabolized in peripheral capillary beds by a number of enzymes (angiotensinases). One of its metabolites, the des-Asp[1] heptapeptide, has recently been shown to produce vasoconstrictor and positive inotropic effects similar to angiotensin II (*8, 9*) and to stimulate aldosterone synthesis in adrenal cell suspensions in vitro (*10–12*) and in the intact animal (*13*). The des-Asp[1] heptapeptide, recently named "angiotensin III," has been postulated as the final mediator of the aldosterone-stimulating effects of the renin/angiotensin system (*14*). Administration of a competitive inhibitor of angiotensin III has been shown to reduce the increase in circulating aldosterone induced by sodium restriction in the conscious rat (*15*). These data suggest that naturally occurring angiotensin III may play a role in the regulation of aldosterone production in vivo. Further studies are needed to determine whether angiotensin III is normally present in the arterial circulation and whether it plays a major role in circulatory homeostasis. The other metabolic products of angiotensin II have little biological activity and are rapidly removed from the circulation.

Renin release is thought to be the rate-limiting step in the control of blood pressure and volume homeostasis by the renin/angiotensin system, although regulation at subsequent steps in the sequence of reactions has not been fully evaluated. Better understanding of the kinetics of these reactions and the nature of their interactions will be needed before the role of renin in normal pressure and volume homeostasis and in the pathogenesis of hypertension can be fully appreciated. The rest of this discussion will focus on an analysis of these reactions in relation to the clinical measurement of plasma renin activity and other components of the renin/angiotensin system. [The control of renin release was discussed by Dr. Goodfriend in another part of this symposium.]

[1] Nonstandard abbreviations are spelled out in Table 1.

Renin Activity

Plasma renin activity, the rate of angiotensin generation from plasma incubated in vitro, is the most commonly used clinical index of function in the renin/angiotensin system. Plasma renin activity correlates well with circulating angiotensin II concentration, but is much easier to measure because of the 50- to 100-fold increase in plasma peptide concentration after the in vitro incubation step. Renin activity can be measured by either bioassay or radioimmunoassay of the generated angiotensin.

Bioassay. Sensitive and reproducible methods for estimating renin activity by bioassay have been and are still being used for both investigative and clinical purposes in many laboratories. Most of the bioassays depend on the ability of angiotensin II, generated under standardized conditions in vitro, to cause smooth-muscle contraction. Preparations that have been used include isolated strips of rabbit aorta (*16*), rat uterus (*17*), and rat colon (*18*); intact, nephrectomized rats (*19*); and nephrectomized and ganglion-blocked rats (*20*). The measured biological response is smooth-muscle contraction in the in vitro preparations and systemic pressor effect in the intact animals. Responses are related to control injections of standard angiotensin II. The reason that bioassays for renin activity have not been widely used in clinical laboratories relates to problems of inconsistent standardization and reproducibility, the time-consuming sample processing, and the frequent lack of sensitivity and specificity.

Radioimmunoassay. Plasma renin activity is most commonly measured by radioimmunoassay of angiotensin I, generated in vitro as the product of the reaction of endogenous renin with endogenous substrate in the patient's plasma, under carefully controlled conditions. After the initial incubation step, the reaction is stopped, usually by freezing. In a second step, ^{125}I-labeled angiotensin I and anti-angiotensin I antiserum are added and allowed to equilibrate with the generated angiotensin I. Bound and free ^{125}I-labeled angiotensin I are separated by conventional techniques and quantified by gamma counting. The amount of angiotensin I present is determined by comparison with a standard curve.

Failure to take into account the complexity of chemical events occurring during the incubation of plasma has contributed to the difficulty of developing accurate and reproducible assays for renin activity. The activities of renin, converting enzyme, and a number of other angiotensinases, as well as the availability of substrate and the possible presence of plasma proteases other than renin must be considered when selecting conditions for the initial incubation step (*21*). In addition, inhibitors and facilitators of the renin–substrate reaction have been described which may play a role in angiotensin generation in man (*22–25*).

Renin–Substrate Reaction

Renin reacts with substrate in circulating blood and in blood-vessel walls (*26, 27*) and isolated tissues (*28,*

29) to generate angiotensin I. The pH optimum and cofactor requirements for the reaction are species dependent. The reaction of human renin with human substrate in plasma or buffer appears to have a pH optimum between 5.5 and 6.5 (*30, 31*). Because there are several molecular forms of both renin and substrate (*32, 33*), the data are only approximate, and the shape of the pH optimum curve may vary considerably. In normal human plasma, the enzyme kinetics appear to be first order in that the velocity of the renin–substrate reaction depends on the substrate concentration (*34*).

Renin substrate is a glycoprotein synthesized by the liver; several molecular species of it have been described (*33, 35*). Substrate concentrations vary with the state of hepatic function, glucocorticoid secretion, and estrogen production. Severe parenchymal liver disease in man is associated with depressed substrate concentrations and secondarily depressed plasma renin activity (*36*). Substrate concentration is decreased after bilateral adrenalectomy (*37*) and in Addison's disease (*38*), increased after administration of exogenous glucocorticoid (*39*) or corticotropin (*40*) and in Cushing's syndrome (*41*). In contrast, mineralocorticoid administration and the syndromes of mineralocorticoid excess are not associated with increased substrate concentrations (*42*). Estrogen administration and pregnancy stimulate substrate production (*37, 43, 44*). Glucocorticoids and exogenous estrogen in the form of oral contraceptives can enhance substrate synthesis sufficiently to increase renin activity in vitro. Bilateral nephrectomy also stimulates increased renin substrate concentrations because of rapid inactivation of endogenous renin by the liver, with consequent failure to consume substrate, and because of increased substrate synthesis (*45*). The renin–substrate reaction rate is increased in nephrectomized and estrogen-treated animals (*46–49*). This has been attributed simply to increased circulating substrate concentration (*50, 51*). Alternatively, changes in the kinetics of the renin–substrate reaction have been described in plasma after bilateral nephrectomy or estrogen treatment (*52–54*), which could be related to changes in substrate or renin structure, the disappearance of a renin inhibitor, or the appearance of an activator. An analysis of the molecular radius, net charge, or isoelectric point of plasma renin substrate by use of polyacrylamide-gel electrophoresis and iso-electric focusing has shown that these do not change after bilateral nephrectomy or estrogen treatment (*55*). More extensive molecular characterization of renin substrate and more rigorous studies of renin–substrate kinetics under conditions of increased substrate production are needed before the increased velocity of the renin–substrate reaction after nephrectomy or estrogen administration can be fully explained.

Chemical alteration of the substrate molecule in vitro affects renin activity. For example, acidification of human plasma to pH 3.9 in an attempt to inhibit angiotensinases before angiotensin generation at pH 5.5 produced a 20% decrease in renin activity (*16*). Similarly, selective denaturation of human-derived substrate has been demonstrated on warming plasma to 32 °C for 1 h at pH 3.3 (*56*). In another study, the progressive acidification of human substrate (either in plasma or partially purified) before incubation with renin led to an irreversible loss of activity proportional to the pH decrease (*57*). Activity was decreased below pH 5.0; the decrease amounted to 40% at pH 4.0 and 80% at pH 3.0. The effect seemed to be greater when strong acids were used to lower pH than when buffer was used. Porcine renin and the purified tetradecapeptide substrate were less sensitive to acid denaturation. Acidification of renin alone produced no change in activity until the pH was less than 3.0. These studies emphasize the importance of substrate configuration in determining renin activity and the importance of the method of pH adjustment in preparation of plasma for radioimmunoassay.

Most current evidence indicates that renin attacks all forms of substrate at similar rates to produce the same angiotensin I. The amino terminal tetradecapeptide portion of the molecule is an adequate substrate for renin, which specifically hydrolyzes the Leu^{10}-Leu^{11} bond in the substrate. A number of peptide analogs of portions of the tetradecapeptide sequence have been synthesized and shown to competitively inhibit the renin–substrate reaction (*58*). These are being used to explore in greater detail the structural requirements for renin action and the role of the renin/angiotensin system in maintaining pressure and volume homeostasis in vivo. Their potential use as reagents in in-vitro assays of components of the renin/angiotensin system has not yet been exploited.

Angiotensin I Metabolism in Plasma

The product of the renin–substrate reaction, angiotensin I, is rapidly removed from plasma by the combined action of converting enzyme and angiotensinases. The half-life of tracer amounts of ^{125}I-labeled angiotensin I in heparin-treated plasma incubated at 37 °C in the absence of enzyme inhibitors is 3–5 min. The in vivo half-life of ^{125}I-labeled angiotensin or native angiotensin I is even shorter—about one circulation time (15 s). Angiotensin I has little or no biological activity when circulating at physiological concentrations. It may be thought of as a circulating prohormone that is converted to angiotensin II by converting enzyme, which is found in highest concentration in the pulmonary capillary bed and in lesser concentrations in circulating blood, kidney, and various other systemic capillary beds (*59–61*). The production site of the converting enzyme in plasma is not yet certain, but it is assumed to be released into the circulation from lung and other tissues in which it is present in large quantities. Physiological regulation of its activity has not been described in man. Plasma converting enzyme activity is reportedly increased in patients with untreated active sarcoidosis and decreased in other forms of chronic lung disease (*62*), but the decrease was not quantitatively related to the severity of the lung disease, and steroid treatment of sarcoidosis restored activity to normal. Presumably these phenomena relate to alterations in quantity or function of pulmonary converting enzyme, which is found in association with endothelial cell membranes (*63*). It is not known whether these alterations in converting enzyme activity cause changes in circulating angiotensin II concentration or circulatory homeostasis.

The substrate specificity and cofactor requirements of converting enzyme have been determined in considerable detail, both in vivo (*64, 65*) and in vitro (*66–69*). The kinetic properties of the enzyme partially purified from plasma and from mammalian lung are similar (*70*), but it is not certain whether the enzyme from the two sources is the same. The pH optimum for converting enzyme acting on angiotensin I is about 7.5. The reaction is chloride dependent (optimal Cl^- concentration, 0.1 mol/liter) and divalent-cation dependent. Converting enzyme is stable to repeated freezing and thawing, but enzyme activity is lost if the pH of the medium is decreased to less than 4.5 (*69*). The enzyme is inhibited by a variety of peptides derived from the venoms of several species of snakes (*71*). One of these, the nonapeptide pyr-Trp-Pro-Arg-Pro-Gln-Ile-Pro-Pro (pyr = pyrrolidone carboxylic acid), a long-lasting competitive inhibitor of converting enzyme, has been used in studies of the role of the renin/angiotensin system in blood pressure and volume homeostasis and as a diagnostic and therapeutic agent in angiotensin-dependent hypertension (*72*).

Angiotensin I is destroyed in plasma by a variety of proteolytic enzymes, the angiotensinases (EC 3.4.99.3). The best characterized of these are an aminopeptidase (angiotensinase A) with a pH optimum of 7.5 (*73*) and an endopeptidase (angiotensinase B) with a specificity similar to that of chymotrypsin (EC 3.4.21.1) and a pH optimum of 5.5 (*30*). The aminopeptidase is the predominant angiotensinase in plasma under physiological conditions. Its specificity is the same as that of aminopeptidase A (*74*), and it requires protein-bound calcium ion for activation. Angiotensinase A is blocked by modifications of the amino terminus of angiotensin I, such as substitution of D-aspartic acid, succinic acid, or sarcosine, or β-rearrangement of aspartic acid.

Enzyme Inhibitors

Generated angiotensin I must be protected from converting enzyme and angiotensinases if the concentration of the decapeptide is to accurately reflect renin activity. This cannot be done for angiotensin II, because conditions favorable for in vitro conversion also permit extensive angiotensinase action, causing simultaneous generation and destruction of angiotensin II. Despite the use of internal standards, this makes the assay of generated angiotensin II a cumbersome and nonreproducible measure of plasma renin activity. When plasma renin activity is assayed as generated angiotensin I, chemical inhibitors of both angiotensinases and converting enzyme are added to the incubation mixture to maximize recovery of the angiotensin I generated. Table 1 lists the most commonly used inhibitors of angiotensinases and converting enzyme and their mechanisms of action. Dimercaprol (BAL),[1] 8-quinolinol sulfate, and ethylenediaminetetraacetate (EDTA) act as chelating agents. They are potent inhibitors of plasma angiotensinase A, which is Ca^{2+} dependent, and of converting enzyme, which appears to be Ca^{2+}, Zn^{2+}, and Co^{2+} dependent, because these ions—but not Fe^{2+}, Co^{2+}, and Mn^{2+}—reverse EDTA inhibition (*75*). Diisopropylfluorophosphate (DFP) acts as a phosphorylating agent and phenylmethylsulfonylfluoride (PMSF) as a sulfating agent, both binding covalently to enzyme serine. DFP is a potent inhibitor of angiotensinase B (*30*) but is ineffective against angiotensinase A and the converting enzyme in plasma (*76*). PMSF has a mechanism of action similar to DFP (*77*), so presumably has a similar enzyme specificity. It has recently been substituted for DFP in a number of plasma renin activity assay protocols because of its relative lack of toxicity. None of these enzyme inhibitors is known to interfere with the renin–substrate reaction or with the radioimmunoassay for angiotensin I, so all are acceptable reagents in the plasma renin-activity assay.

Table 1. Renin Inhibitors

Inhibitor	Abbreviation	Mechanism
Dimercaprol	BAL	Chelating agent
8-Quinolinol sulfate	8-HQ	Chelating agent
Ethylenediaminetetra-acetate	EDTA	Chelating agent
Diisopropylfluoro-phosphate	DFP	Phosphorylating agent[a]
Phenylmethylsulfonyl-fluoride	PMSF	Sulfonating agent[a]

[a] Covalently bound to serine.

Alternatively, nonenzymatic methods of protecting generated angiotensin I have been used successfully in renin assays. Prior acidification of plasma to pH 3.5–4.0 destroys angiotensinases but also denatures substrate, and so exogenous substrate must be added (*56*). Adsorption of angiotensin to a solid support with a large surface area—such as Dowex 50, fuller's earth, or charcoal—affords effective protection against angiotensinases and converting enzyme. The angiotensin I must then be eluted from the solid support with appropriate reagents, concentrated, and bioassayed or radioimmunoassayed. The anti-angiotensin I antibody molecule is used both for protection against enzymatic conversion and degradation and for quantitation of angiotensin I in the trapping method (*78*) for analysis of renin activity. This rapid and versatile method can also be used to determine renin and substrate concentration.

Angiotensin I Survival in Plasma

The efficacy of angiotensinase and converting enzyme inhibitors in immunoassay can best be evaluated by testing the survival of angiotensin I in plasma treated

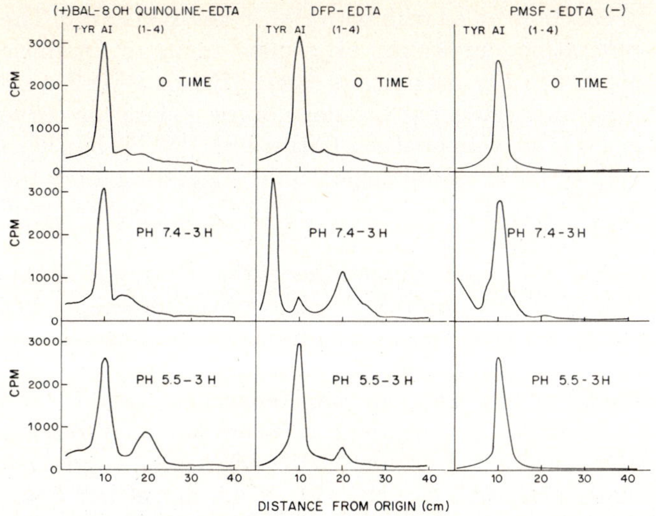

Fig. 2. Survival of ^{125}I-labeled angiotensin I in plasma containing BAL/8HQ/EDTA, DFP/EDTA, or PMSF/EDTA

High-voltage paper electrophoretic separation of plasma samples incubated with ^{125}I-labeled angiotensin I for the periods of time specified. The position to which standards migrated are indicated at the top of the diagram. *Tyr* = ^{125}I-labeled tyrosine, *AI* = ^{125}I-labeled angiotensin I, (*1–4*) = the peptide Asp-Arg-Val- [^{125}I] Tyr

with the inhibitors and incubated under assay conditions. To maximize the sensitivity of this kind of evaluation, we prepared singly labeled ^{125}I-labeled angiotensin I by the method of Nielsen et al. (*79*). The specific activity of the material was sufficiently high (estimated 750 kCi/mol) to permit its use as a tracer in femtomole quantities. Plasma from male anephric patients that was shown to contain no intrinsic renin activity was treated with EDTA (2.6 mmol/liter final concentration) and adjusted either to pH 5.5 with 0.5 mol/liter HCl or to 7.4 with 4 mol/liter Tris HCl. We used three inhibitor combinations, BAL (1.6 mmol/liter final concentration), 8HQ (3.4 mmol/liter final concentration), and EDTA (*80*); DFP (1.09 mmol/liter final concentration), neomycin sulfate (2.0 g/liter final concentration) and EDTA (*81*); and PMSF (15 mmol/liter final concentration) and EDTA. Monoiodinated angiotensin I, 2.0×10^5 cpm, or approximately 0.15 pmol, was added to each milliliter of treated plasma and the mixture was incubated at 37 °C for 3 h. Aliquots of the reaction mixture were spotted on Whatman 3 MM paper and electrophoresed at 4000 V for 1 h in pyridine acetate buffer, pH 3.55. The paper was dried, cut into 1-cm strips, and their radioactivity was counted in a gamma counter.

Figure 2 summarizes the results. The BAL/8HQ/EDTA combination resulted in preservation of 90% of ^{125}I-labeled angiotensin I after 3 h at pH 7.4, but was less effective at pH 5.5. In contrast, DFP/neomycin/EDTA resulted in 85% preservation of ^{125}I-labeled angiotensin I after incubation at pH 5.5 and only 10% preservation at pH 7.4. The PMSF/EDTA was nearly 100% effective at pH 5.5 and 85% effective at pH 7.4. Thus, selection of enzyme inhibitors for assay of plasma renin activity depends on the conditions of incubation: BAL and 8HQ are more effective at neutral than at acid pH; DFP is effective only at acid pH; PMSF is effective at both, but is slightly better at pH 5.5 than pH 7.4. These results are consistent with the known enzyme specificities of the inhibitors. It is important to consider the variability of inhibitor effectiveness when comparing the quantity of angiotensin I generated at different pH's in plasma.

Angiotensin I Generation Studies

Inhibitors. The pH/enzyme-inhibitor relationship was further explored by examining the effects of various inhibitor combinations on the shape of the pH "optimum" curves for the renin–substrate reaction in human plasma. Pooled EDTA-treated plasma from male anephric patients was divided into 1.0-ml aliquots and the pH adjusted at intervals of 0.5 pH unit between 4.5 and 9.0 with 0.5 mol/liter HCl or 0.5 mol/liter NaOH. Plasma was treated with the three combinations of enzyme inhibitors in concentrations described previously. After addition of partially purified human renin, 0.2 mU, (sample No. 13; kindly donated by Dr. Erwin Haas, Mt. Sinai Hospital, Cleveland, Ohio) to each tube, the mixture was incubated for 3 h at 37 °C and radioimmunoassayed for angiotensin I (*80*). Figure 3 shows the angiotensin I generation curves. The apparent pH optimum for the reaction was 6.0 in the presence of all three sets of inhibitors. The quantity of angiotensin I generated at optimal pH was greater for PMSF than for DFP or BAL-8HQ. The curves for DFP and PMSF were steeper at high pH values than was the curve for BAL-8HQ, so that at physiological pH, generation of angiotensin I was 40% of maximum in the presence of DFP, 40% of maximum in the presence of PMSF, and 70% of maximum in the presence of BAL-8HQ. The variation in shape of angiotensin I generation curves with choice of enzyme inhibitor suggests that the curves reflect a titration of inhibitor effectiveness as well as a measure of renin activity. The apparent pH optimum was 6.0 with all three sets of inhibitors, confirming several previous studies in human plasma (*30, 31, 83*). The

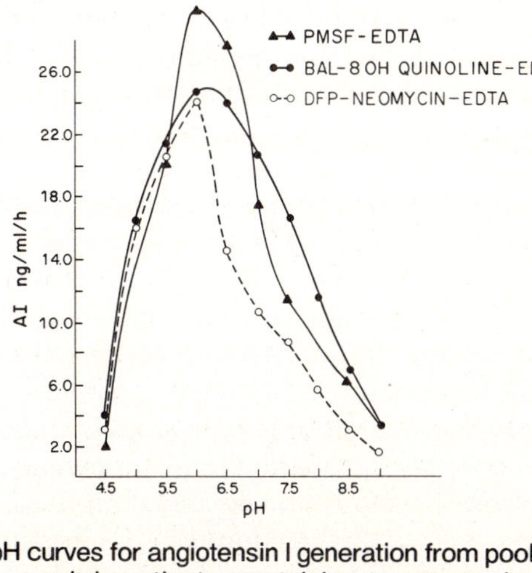

Fig. 3. pH curves for angiotensin I generation from pooled plasma of male anephric patients, containing exogenous human renin

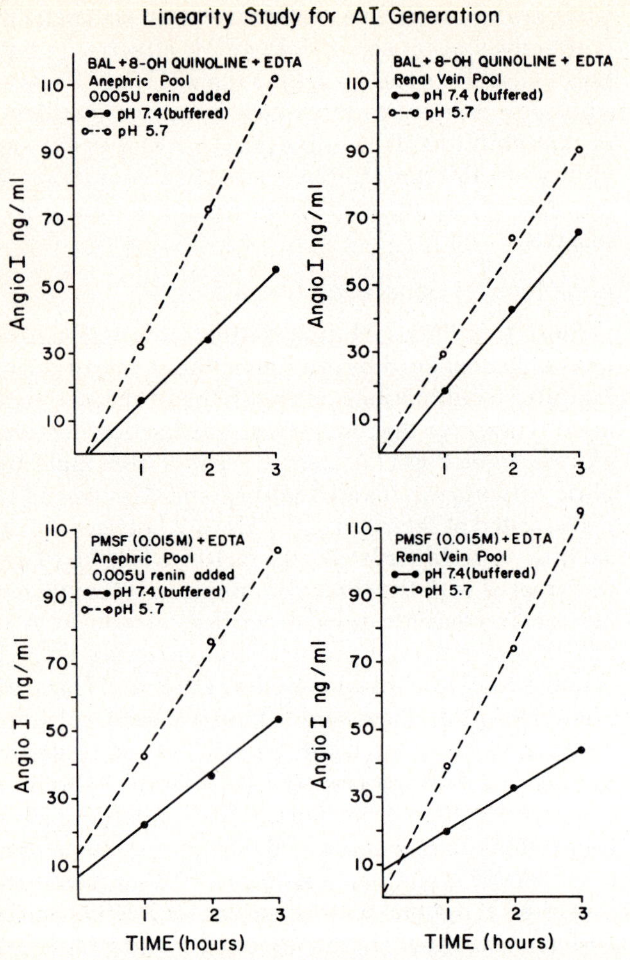

Fig. 4. Angiotensin I generation from exogenous human renin reacting in pooled anephric plasma and from endogenous renin in pooled renal vein samples in the presence of BAL/8HQ/EDTA and PMSF/EDTA

amount of angiotensin I generated at optimal pH was 20% higher with PMSF-EDTA than with the other combinations; this presumably reflects its superior inhibitor effectiveness at acid pH under the conditions of this experiment.

To evaluate the effects of the various enzyme inhibitors on the apparent generation of angiotensin I from endogenous renin and endogenous substrate in clinical samples, we performed two kinds of experiments.

In the first studies, we pooled samples of EDTA-treated renal venous plasma from three patients with renovascular hypertension who had high endogenous plasma renin activity, and adjusted the pH to 5.7 or 7.4. The plasma was treated with BAL/8HQ or PMSF in the concentrations previously described, (plus EDTA), incubated at 37 °C for 3 h, and radioimmunoassayed for angiotensin I. An anephric plasma pool containing exogenous human renin, 5 U/liter, was processed similarly for comparison. Figure 4 shows that generation of angiotensin I was linear at both pH values with both sets of inhibitors. When incubation time was extended to 18 h, generation became nonlinear under all these conditions. The quantity of angiotensin I measured was greater and the slope of the generation curve steeper at pH 5.7 than at 7.4 with both PMSF and BAL/8HQ. The generation curves for exogenous renin in anephric plasma in the presence of BAL/8HQ or PMSF were superimposable, but the slope of the generation curve in the renal vein pool was flatter with PMSF than with BAL/8HQ at physiological pH, suggesting that the former inhibitor was less effective in the pooled renal venous plasma.

In a second set of experiments the efficacy of inhibition by PMSF and BAL/8HQ at physiological pH was compared in 48 successive unselected plasma samples submitted to our laboratory for renin assay. Incubation was for 18 h, and aliquots were removed at 3 and 18 h for renin activity determination. There was no difference in renin activity between the PMSF (2.8 ± 2.2 ng/ml per hour) and BAL + 8HQ (3.0 ± 2.8 ng/ml per hour) treated samples. During the 18-h incubations generation of angiotensin I was linear for low renin samples treated with PMSF but not for those treated with BAL/8HQ. Generation was not linear for normal- or high-renin samples treated with either inhibitor.

pH. Because the renin-substrate reaction takes place at pH 7.4 in vivo and because of concern about the effects of lowering pH on substrate reactivity and about artifactual generation of angiotensin I from substrate at low pH by action of acid proteases circulating in plasma (*84, 85*), pH 7.4 has been selected for the initial incubation step in many assays of renin activity (*78, 80, 86*). Other laboratories have used a pH of 5.5 to 6 for the renin–substrate reaction, based on the belief that this was closer to the pH optimum of the enzyme (*81, 87–89*). The concentrations of angiotensin I generated under these conditions were two- to fourfold those generated at pH 7.4 (*81, 87*). The interpretation of these data is complex, because both the apparent pH optimum of the reaction and the amount of angiotensin generated at any pH depends profoundly on the efficacy of inhibitors of angiotensin degradation, the reactivity of substrate, and, to a lesser extent, the contribution of enzymes other than renal renin to the generation of peptides that react with angiotensin I antibody.

To examine the question of whether plasma proteases other than renin contribute to the increased generation of angiotensin I at pH 5.5, we divided plasma samples from seven anephric patients into aliquots, adjusted either to pH 5.5 with 0.5 mol/liter HCl (*81*) or pH 7.4 with 4 mol/liter Tris HCl (*80*), and incubated at 37 °C for 18 h with appropriate enzyme inhibitors for each pH as previously discussed. Results are summarized in Figure 5. At pH 5.5, all seven samples generated substantial quantities of angiotensin I in the absence of added renin. At pH 7.4, no angiotensin I was detected in any of the samples. Survival of labeled angiotensin I under both sets of incubation conditions was identical. Thus, enzymes other than renal renin contribute to the generation of angiotensin I in plasma incubated at acid pH. These may be renin isoenzymes produced by other tissues or completely unrelated proteases. Their physiological significance is uncertain. In plasmas containing low concentrations of renin, the non-renin-related

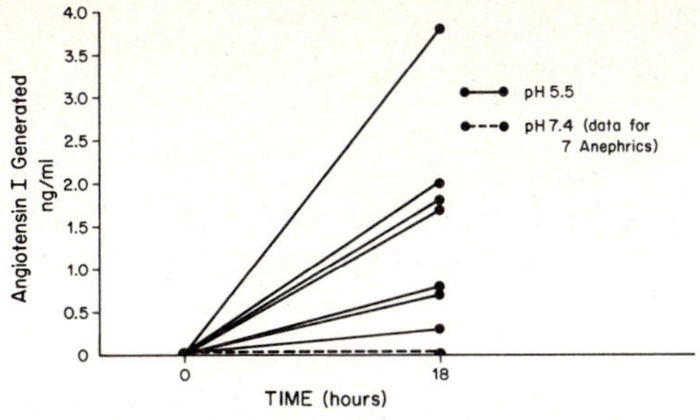

Fig. 5. Angiotensin I generation in anephric plasma
Reproduced from Oparil et al. (*21*) with the permission of the publishers

generation of angiotensin I could make a significant contribution to total "renin activity."

To evaluate the effect of pH on endogenous renin activity in clinical samples containing optimal enzyme inhibitors, we subjected to radioimmunoassay plasma from 99 successive unselected EDTA-treated samples submitted to our laboratory for renin determination, with use of three different conditions: (*a*) pH 7.4, unbuffered, containing BAL/8HQ/EDTA; (*b*) pH 7.4, buffered with 4 mol/liter Tris HCl, containing BAL/8HQ/EDTA; and (*c*) pH 5.5, in the presence of DFP/neomycin/EDTA. There was a consistent increase in generation of angiotensin I on buffering the plasma at pH 7.4. This is compatible with the observation that plasma pH can increase by as much as one unit during a 3-h incubation at 37 °C, resulting in conditions unfavorable for the renin–substrate reaction (*51*). Use of the concentrated Tris buffer minimized the dilution of plasma, which decreases the rate of angiotensin I generation. The mean renin activity of samples incubated at pH 5.5 (7.4 ± 1.2 ng/ml per hour) was significantly ($P < 0.001$) greater than for samples incubated at neutral pH (5.2 ± 0.8 ng/ml per hour). The greatest increases were seen in those samples with high renin activity. Low-renin samples frequently showed no change or a decrease in renin activity on adjusting the pH to 5.5 (*21*). Thus, although lowering the pH tended to increase apparent angiotensin I generation, there was considerable sample-to-sample variation in magnitude of the response. To the extent that this may represent variable sensitivity of substrate configuration to acid treatment or variable activation of plasma proteases other than renal renin, determination of renin activity in an acidic medium may represent an unphysiological measurement. Downward adjustment of plasma pH offers little advantage in terms of assay sensitivity, because low-renin samples show the smallest increases in apparent angiotensin generation. For these reasons, our laboratory prefers incubation at physiological pH. As long as appropriate enzyme inhibitors or an angiotensin-capture technique is used, incubation at acid pH is acceptable if care is taken not to lower the pH much below 5.0 and thus denature the substrate. A comparison of the most commonly used methods and detailed description of procedures can be found elsewhere (*7, 90*) and are beyond the scope of this discussion.

Comparison of Bioassay with Radioimmunoassay

It is difficult to compare results obtained by bioassay with those obtained by radioimmunoassay of plasma renin activity because of variability in incubation conditions for generating angiotensin and in angiotensin standards. Dr. Bangham will address the problem of standardization in greater detail elsewhere in this symposium (Ed. note: This paper will also appear in *Clin. Chem.*) Normal values for renin concentration obtained by radioimmunoassay in a number of laboratories are reportedly lower than bioassay values, both based on an international renin standard (*91*). Other studies have given values for renin activity by radioimmunoassay that are higher than (*81, 87, 92*), comparable to (*93, 94*), or lower than (*95*) bioassay values. Critical comparison of procedures will require measurement of angiotensin generated under identical conditions by both bioassay and radioimmunoassay in the absence of toxic enzyme inhibitors with use of the same angiotensin standard (*7*).

Plasma Renin Concentration

Plasma renin concentration is the total quantity of renin present per milliliter of plasma. By reference to an internationally acceptable standard preparation of renin, it is possible to calculate the concentration of endogenous renin in serum or plasma (PRC) in terms of Goldblatt units (GU/ml of plasma). The plasma renin concentration is measured indirectly by adding graded amounts of renin to the first incubation step of the renin activity assay and determining the increase in reaction rate caused by the exogenous renin (*78, 91, 97, 98*). Concentration measured in this way correlates well with plasma renin activity in most clinical situations. Homologous, endogenous substrate, normally present in plasma, was used in some of these studies, while in others purified substrate was added in high concentration to enhance the rate of angiotensin generation and thereby to improve the precision of the assay. Under these conditions the angiotensin generation rate becomes independent of the substrate concentration and proportional to the renin concentration [zero-order kinetics (*57, 78, 96*)].

Excess ovine substrate has been used in the measurement of plasma renin concentration in man because at comparable substrate concentrations human renin reacts fivefold faster with ovine than with human substrate (*56, 96*). The incubation of human renin/ovine substrate is done at pH 7.4, the pH optimum for this combination. Potential interference from endogenous human substrate has been eliminated by preincubation of plasma at pH 3.3 to denature substrate (*56*). The most recent demonstration that addition of plasma from an anephric subject (high endogenous substrate) did not alter the rate of formation of angiotensin I from standard human renin reacting with sheep substrate suggests that the acid-inactivation step may be unnecessary (*96*). Because several times as much angiotensin I is generated after incubation with exogenous (ovine) substrate, the procedure has been applied to patients

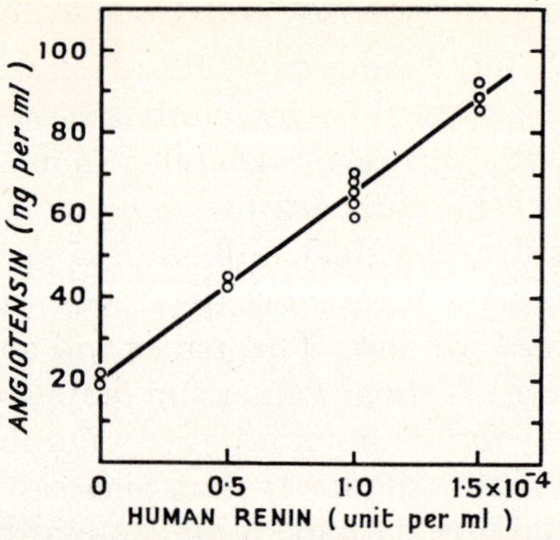

Fig. 6. Assay of renin in 0.5 ml of pooled, normal human serum (rat blood-pressure bioassay)

Slope (method of least squares) = 44.5 × 10^4 ng of angiotensin per Goldblatt unit of renin. Intercept (method of least squares) = 21.4 ng of angiotensin per 0.5 ml of serum. Concentration of endogenous renin = 0.96 × 10^{-4} Goldblatt unit per milliliter of serum (Reprinted from Haas et al. (*97*), with the permission of the publishers)

with low plasma renin activity, particularly the syndromes of mineralocorticoid excess, to increase the sensitivity of renin measurement (*96*).

Addition of a standard preparation of human renin to the first incubation step of the renin activity assay serves the dual purpose of permitting measurement of renin concentration and furnishing an internal standard for comparison of assay procedures. The many variables among renin assay methods can be cancelled by referring to a common internal renin standard. The principle of this renin-addition method is that under conditions of complete angiotensinase and converting enzyme inhibition, generated angiotensin I increases linearly with the amount of renin added. The concentration of endogenous plasma renin can be calculated from the slope of the line, which represents the quantity of angiotensin I produced per Goldblatt unit (see below) of added renin, and the intercept, which represents the amount of angiotensin I produced with no added renin (Figure 6). The human renin standard currently in use for this method is a moderately purified, angiotensinase-free preparation purified by Dr. Erwin Haas and associates (*99*) and distributed by the British Medical Research Council. The renin standard has been calibrated in Goldblatt units (G.U.) (1 G.U. = the quantity of renin or angiotensin which, when injected intravenously into a conscious, trained dog, raises the direct mean femoral arterial blood pressure by 4kPa [30 mmHg]) (*100*); 1 G.U. of standard renin generated angiotensin at a rate of 0.56 μg/min during incubation in vitro with isologous substrate in angiotensinase-free human serum (*101*). 1 G.U. is equivalent to 1 IUB unit (Dr. Erwin Haas, personal communication). A sample calculation of endogenous renin concentration as units of renin in reference to Figure 6 follows:

$$\frac{\text{Endog. renin acty. (= ng of angiotensin/ml of serum)}}{\text{Slope (= ng of angiotensin/G.U. of renin)}} =$$

$$\frac{42.8}{44.5 \times 10^4} = 0.96 \times 10^{-4} \text{ G.U. of renin/ml of serum}$$

Assuming that angiotensin I generation from endogenous renin is linear with time, for a 16-h incubation:

$$\text{Renin activity} = \frac{42.8}{16} =$$

$$2.68 \text{ ng of angiotensin/ml per hour}$$

For routine purposes, assays can be done with only two samples (no added renin and a single concentration of added renin). The slope then becomes the difference between the two angiotensin concentrations divided by the concentration of added renin (*97*). If standard human renin can be supplied in adequate quantity, the use of an internal renin standard is recommended for general use in quality control of renin assays and in standardization of investigative results (*91*).

In general, plasma renin activity and plasma renin concentration are very highly correlated, so it is not necessary to measure both for clinical purposes. There are some exceptions. Conditions of estrogen excess such as oral contraceptive pill administration are associated with increases in substrate concentration sufficient to cause elevations in plasma renin activity. Plasma renin concentration remains normal under these circumstances, presumably due to feedback suppression of renin release by angiotensin II (*102–104*). Renin concentration far in excess of renin activity has been reported in the plasma of a hypertensive child with Wilm's tumor (*105*). The tumor was shown to produce a high-molecular-weight form of renin, which was activated in the acidification step of the renin concentration assay. The "big renin" secreted by the tumor was considered to be a possible renin prohormone. Substantial increases in renin activity and content over time in frozen stored plasma have recently been reported and attributed to activation of a circulating prorenin (*106*). Further investigation is needed before the status of renin prohormone(s) can be assessed.

Circulating Angiotensin I, Angiotensin II, and Renin Substrate Concentrations

Assay procedures with sufficient sensitivity to measure circulating concentrations of angiotensin I (*107*) and angiotensin II (*108–114*) in normal man, if plasma-extraction procedures are used, are available for general use. Values for angiotensin II correlate well with those for renin activity (*80, 81*), but the assay for angiotensin II is seldom performed in clinical practice because the extraction procedures required are time consuming and nonreproducible. Development of a satisfactory method for circulating angiotensin I was delayed by inability to stop the renin–substrate reaction in vitro. Collection of blood into cold ethanol provided a satisfactory solution to that problem (*107*), but has not eliminated the tedious concentration steps. For that reason, neither circulating angiotensin I nor angiotensin II is commonly measured in the clinical setting.

Renin substrate can be measured indirectly by quantifying the angiotensin generated from the renin–substrate reaction done in the presence of excess homologous renin. Many techniques are available for measurement of generated angiotensin I and II, (*16, 30, 115–117*), angiotensin II (*118*), or angiotensin I (*41, 119*) from such reactions. Plasma renin substrate determinations are not useful clinically. Nevertheless, the availability of sensitive and specific assays for substrate, as well as other components of the renin–angiotensin system, has increased our understanding of blood-pressure control in normal and hypertensive man.

I wish to acknowledge the contribution of Terry J. Koerner, University of Chicago, Pritzker School of Medicine, to this work.

This work was supported by grants HL-14982 and RR-55 from the NIH and by The Louis Block Fund of The University of Chicago. Dr. Oparil is an Established Investigator of the American Heart Association.

References

1. U.S. Department of Health, Education and Welfare: Blood pressure of adults by race and area, United States, 1960–1962. National Health Survey, National Center for Health Statistics Series 11: Number 5, 1964.

2. U.S. Department of Health, Education and Welfare: Blood pressure of adults by age and sex, United States, 1960–1962. National Health Survey, National Center for Health Statistics Series 11: Number 4, 1964.

3. Veterans Administration Cooperative Study Group on Antihypertensive Agents. Effects of treatment on morbidity and mortality: Results in patients with diastolic blood pressures averaging 115 through 129 mm Hg. *J. Am. Med. Assoc.* **202,** 1028–1034 (1967).

4. Veterans Administration Cooperative Study Group on Antihypertensive Agents. Effects of treatment on morbidity and mortality: results in patients with diastolic blood pressure averaging 90 through 114 mm Hg. *J. Am. Med. Assoc.* **213,**1143–1152 (1970).

5. Brunner, H. R., Laragh, J. H., Baer, L., et al., Essential hypertension: Renin and aldosterone, heart attack and stroke. *New Engl. J. Med.* **286,** 441–449 (1972).

6. Koch-Weser, J., Correlation of pathophysiology and pharmacotherapy in primary hypertension. In *Hypertension Manual,* J. H. Laragh, Ed. Dun Donnelley Pub. Corp., New York, N.Y., 1973, pp 759–785.

7. Oparil, S., and Haber, E., The renin-angiotensin system. *New Engl. J. Med.* **291,** 389–401 (1974).

8. Kent, K. M., Goodfriend, T. L., McCallum, Z. T., et al., Inotropic agents in hypoxic cat myocardium. *Circ. Res.* **30,** 196–204 (1972).

9. Schwyzer, R., and Turrian, H., The chemistry and pharmacology of angiotensin. *Vitam. Horm.* **18,** 237–268 (1960).

10. Blair-West J. R., Coghlan, J. P., Denton, D. A., et al., The effect of the heptapeptide (2–8) and hexapeptide (3–8) fragments of angiotensin II on aldosterone secretion. *J. Clin. Endocrinol. Metab.* **32,** 575–578 (1971).

11. Peach, M. J., and Chiu, A. T., Stimulation and inhibition of aldosterone biosynthesis in vitro by angiotensin II and analogs. *Circ. Res.* **34,** *Suppl 1,* 7–113 (1974).

12. Goodfriend, T., Allmann, D., Kent, K., et al., Angiotensin's inotropic and mitochondrial effects. *Clin Res.* **19,** 316 (1971).

13. Campbell, W. B., Brooks, S. N., and Pettinger, W. A., Angiotensin II and angiotensin III-induced aldosterone release in vivo in the rat. *Science* **184,** 994–996 (1974).

14. Goodfriend, T. L., and Peach, M., Angiotensin III: (des-aspartic acid[1])-angiotensin II: Evidence and speculation for its role as an important agonist in the renin-angiotensin system. *Circ. Res.* **36,** *Suppl. I,* 38–48 (1975).

15. Sarstedt, C. A., Vaughan, E. D., Jr., and Peach, M. J., Angiotensin antagonists on aldosterone excretion in conscious rats. *Pharmacologist* **16,** 296 (1974).

16. Helmer, O. M., and Judson, W. E., The quantitative determination of renin in the plasma of patients with arterial hypertension. *Circulation* **27,** 1050–1060 (1963).

17. Needleman, P., Johnson, E. M., Jr., Vine, W., et al., Pharmacology of antagonists of angiotensin I and II. *Circ. Res.* **31,** 862–867 (1972).

18. Regoli, D., and Vane, J. R., A sensitive method for the assay of angiotensin. *Br. J. Pharmacol.* **23,** 351–359 (1964).

19. Boucher, R., Biron, P., Genest, J., et al., Procedure for isolation and determination of human blood angiotensin. *Can. J. Biochem.* **39,** 581–590 (1961).

20. Gunnels, J. C., Jr., Grim, C. E., Robinson, R. R., et al., Plasma renin activity in healthy subjects and patients with hypertension. *Arch. Intern. Med.* **119,** 232–240 (1967).

21. Oparil, S., Koerner, T. J., and Haber, E., Effects of pH and enzyme inhibitors on apparent generation of angiotensin I in human plasma. *J. Clin. Endocrinol. Metab.* **39,** 965–968 (1974).

22. Maebashi, M., Miura, Y., and Yoshinaga, K., Renin inhibitor in plasma of uremic patients. *Lancet* **ii,** 1408–1409 (1968).

23. Kotchen, T. A., Rice, T. W., and Walters, D. R., Renin reactivity in normal, hypertensive and uremic plasma. *J. Clin. Endocrinol.* **34,** 928–937 (1972).

24. Sambhi, M. P., and Wiedman, C. E., Renin activation in the venous plasma from the involved kidney in the patient with renal hypertension. *J. Clin. Invest.* **51,** 22–30 (1972).

25. Kotchen, T. A., Hedrick, J. L., Miller, M. C., et al., Effect of prostaglandins on the velocity of the reaction between human renin and homologous renin substrate. *J. Clin. Endocrinol.* **39,** 530–535 (1974).

26. Gould, A. B., Skeggs, L. T., Jr., and Kahn, J. R., The presence of renin activity in blood vessel walls. *J. Exp. Med.* **119,** 389–399 (1964).

27. Rosenthal, J., Boucher, R., Rojo-Ortega, J. M., et al., Renin activity in aortic tissue of rats. *Can. J. Physiol. Pharmacol.* **47,** 53–56 (1969).

28. Granger, P., Dahlheim, H., and Thurau, K., Enzyme activities of the single juxtaglomeruler apparatus in rat kidney. *Kidney Int.* **1,** 78–88 (1972).

29. Ganten, D., Marquez-Julio, A., Granger, P., et al., Renin in dog brain. *Am. J. Physiol.* **221,** 1733–1737 (1971).

30. Pickens, P. T., Bumpus. F. M., and Lloyd, A. M. Measurement of renin activity in human plasma. *Circ. Res.* **17,** 438–448 (1965).

31. Rosenthal, J., Wolff, H. P., Weber, P., et al., Enzyme kinetic studies on human renin and its purified homologous substrate. *Am. J. Physiol.* **221,** 1292–1296 (1971).

32. Skeggs, L. T., Lentz, K. E., Kahn, J. R., et al., Studies on the preparation and properties of renin. *Circ. Res.* **21,** *Suppl.* II, 91–100 (1967).

33. Skeggs, L. T., Jr., Lentz, K. E., Hochstrasser, H., et al., The chemistry of renin substrate. *Can. Med. Assoc. J.* **90,** 185–189 (1964).

34. Gould, A. B., Skeggs, L. T., and Kahn, J. R., Measurement of renin and substrate concentration in human serum. *Lab. Invest.* **15,** 1802–1813 (1966).

35. Skeggs, L. T., Lentz, K. E., Hochstrasser, H., et al., The purification and characterization of several forms of hog renin substrate. *J. Exp. Med.* **118,** 73–98 (1963).

36. Ayers, C. R., Plasma renin activity and renin-substrate concentration in patients with liver disease. *Circ. Res.* **20,** 594–598 (1967).

37. Helmer, O. M., and Griffith, R. S., Biological activity of steroids as determined by assay of renin-substrate (hypertensinogen). *Endocrinology* **49,** 154–161 (1951).

38. Brown, J. J., Fraser, R., Lever, A. F., et al., Renin, angiotensin, corticosteroids, and electrolyte balance in Addison's disease. *Q. J. Med.* **37,** 97–118 (1968).

39. Lazer, J., and Hoobler, S. W., Studies on the role of the adrenal in renin kinetics. *Proc. Soc. Exp. Biol. Med.* **138,** 614–618 (1971).

40. Haynes, F. W., Forsham, P. H., and Hume, D. M., Effects of ACTH, cortisone, desoxycorticosterone and epinephrine on the plasma hypertensinogen and renin concentration of dogs. *Am. J. Physiol.* **172,** 265–275 (1953).

41. Krakoff, L. R., Measurement of plasma renin substrate by radioimmunoassay of angiotensin I: Concentration in syndromes associated with steroid excess. *J. Clin. Endocrinol. Metab.* **37,** 110–117 (1973).

42. Reid, I. A., Tu, W. H., Otsuka, K., et al., Studies concerning the regulation and importance of plasma angiotensinogen concentration in the dog. *Endocrinology* **93,** 107–114 (1973).

43. Crane, M. G., Heitsch, J., Harris, J. J., et al., Effect of ethinyl estradiol (Estinyl) on plasma renin activity. *J. Clin. Endocrinol. Metab.* **26,** 1403–1406 (1966).

44. Helmer, O. M., and Judson, W. E., Influence of high renin substrate levels on renin-angiotensin system in pregnancy. *Am. J. Obstet. Gynecol.* **99,** 9–17 (1967).

45. Nasjletti, A., and Masson, G. M. C., Hepatic origin of renin substrate. *Can. J. Physiol. Pharmacol.* **49,** 931–932 (1971).

46. Bing, J., and Magill, F., Potentiation of sensitivity to renin in normal rats by cross circulation with nephrectomized rats. *Acta Pathol. Microbiol. Scand.* **59,** 485–490 (1963).

47. Blaquier, P., Hoobler, S. W., Schroeder, J., et al., Effect of bilateral nephrectomy on pressor response to renin. *Am. J. Physiol.* **203,** 339–343 (1962).

48. Carretero, O., and Gross, F., Renin substrate in plasma under various experimental conditions in the rat. *Am. J. Physiol.* **213,** 695–700 (1967).

49. Catt, K. J., Cain, M. D., and Menard, J.. Radioimmunoassay studies of the renin-angiotensin system in human hypertension and during estrogen treatment. In *Hypertension '72.* J. Genest, and E. Koiw, Eds. Springer-Verlag, New York, 1972, pp 591–604.

50. Blaquier, P., Kinetic studies on renin-angiotensinogen reaction after nephrectomy. *Am. J. Physiol.* **208,** 1083–1086 (1965).

51. Poulsen, K., No evidence of active renin inhibitors in plasma. The kinetics of the reaction between renin and substrate in non-pretreated plasma. *Scand. J. Clin. Lab. Invest.* **27,** 37–46 (1971).

52. Montague, D., Kinetics of the renin-angiotensinogen reaction in plasma of normal rats and nephrectomized rats. *Am. J. Physiol.* **215,** 78–83 (1968).

53. Romero, J. C., and Hoobler, S. W., Changes in renin kinetics induced by nephrectomy. *Am. J. Physiol.* **223,** 1076–1080 (1972).

54. Rieger, D., Romero, J. C., Lazer, J., et al., Definition and use of renin reaction velocity in the study of human hypertension. *J. Lab. Clin. Med.* **80,** 342–350 (1972).

55. Menard, J., Breminer, J., and Corvol, P., Physicochemical properties of plasma renin substrate in normal, binephrectomized, and estrogen-treated rats. *Am. J. Physiol.* **226,** 1434–1437 (1974).

56. Skinner, S. L., Improved assay methods for renin "concentration" and "activity" in human plasma. *Circ. Res.* **20,** 391–402 (1967).

57. Favre, L., Roussel-Deruyck, R., and Vallotton, M. B., Influence of pH on human renin activity with different substrates: Role of substrate denaturation. *Biochim. Biophys. Acta* **302,** 102–109 (1973).

58. Poulsen, K., Burton, J., and Haber, E., Competitive inhibitors of renin. *Biochemistry* **12,** 3877–3882 (1973).

59. Oparil, S., Sanders, C. A., and Haber, E., In vivo and in vitro conversion of angiotensin I to angiotensin II in dog blood. *Circ. Res.* **26,** 591–599 (1970).

60. Ryan, J. W., Stewart, J. M., Leary, W. P., et al., Metabolism of angiotensin I in the pulmonary circulation. *Biochem. J.* **120,** 221–223 (1970).

61. Aiken, J. W., and Vane, J. R., The renin-angiotensin system: Inhibition of converting enzyme in isolated tissues. *Nature* **228,** 30–34 (1970).

62. Lieberman, J., A new confirmatory test for sarcoidosis. Serum angiotensin converting enzyme: Effect of steroids and chronic lung disease. *Am. Rev. Respir. Dis.* **109,** 743 (1974).

63. Soffer, R. L., Reza, R., and Caldwell, P. R. B., Angiotensin-converting enzyme from rabbit pulmonary particles. *Proc. Nat. Acad. Sci. U.S.A.* **71,** 1720–1724 (1974).

64. Oparil, S., Tregear, G. W., Koerner, T., et al., Mechanism of pulmonary conversion of angiotensin I to angiotensin II in the dog. *Circ. Res.* **29,** 682–690 (1971).

65. Oparil, S., Koerner, T., and O'Donoghue, J. K., Structural requirements for substrates and inhibitors of angiotensin I-converting enzyme in vivo and in vitro. *Circ. Res.* **34,** 19–26 (1974).

66. Lentz, K. E., Skeggs, L. T., Woods, K. R., et al., Amino acid composition of hypertensin II and its biochemical relationship to hypertension. I. *J. Exp. Med.* **104,** 183–191 (1956).

67. Cheung, H. S., and Cushman, D. W., Inhibition of homogeneous angiotensin-converting enzyme of rabbit lung by synthetic venom peptides of *Bothrops jararaca. Biochim. Biophys. Acta* **293,** 451–463 (1973).

68. Yang, H. Y. T., Erdos, E. G., and Levin, Y., A depeptidylcarboxypeptidase that converts angiotensin I and inactivates bradykinin. *Biochim. Biophys. Acta* **214,** 374–376 (1970).

69. Dorer, F. E., Kahn, J. R., Lentz, K. E., et al., Purification and properties of angiotensin-converting enzyme from hog lung. *Circ. Res.* **31,** 356–365 (1972).

70. Huggins, C. G., Corcoran, R. J., Gordon, J. S., et al., Kinetics of the plasma and lung angiotensin I converting enzymes. *Circ. Res.* **27,** *Suppl I,* 93–101 (1970).

71. Sander, G. E., West, D. W., and Huggins, C. G., Inhibitors of the pulmonary angiotensin I-converting enzyme. *Biochim. Biophys. Acta* **289,** 392–400 (1972).

72. Gavras, H., Brunner, H. R., Laragh, J. H., et al., An angiotensin converting-enzyme inhibitor to identify and treat vasoconstrictor and volume factors in hypertensive patients. *New Engl. J. Med.* **291,** 817–821 (1974).

73. Khairallah, P. A., Bumpus, F. M., Page, I. H., et al., Angiotensinase with a high degree of specificity in plasma and red cells. *Science* **140,** 672–674 (1963).

74. Glenner, G. G., McMillan, P. J., and Folk, J. E., A mammalian peptidase specific for the hydrolysis of *N*-terminal α-L-glutamyl and aspartyl residues. *Nature* **194,** 867 (1962).

75. Fitz, A., Boyd, G. W., Peart, W. S., Converting enzyme activity in human plasma. *Circ. Res.* **28,** 246–253 (1971).

76. Bumpus, F. M., Smeby, R. R., and Page, I. H., Angiotensin, the renal pressor hormone. *Circ. Res.* **9,** 762–767 (1961).

77. Fahrney, D. E., and Gold, A. M., Sulfonyl fluorides as inhibitors of esterases. I. Rates of reaction with acetylcholinesterase, α-chymotrypsin, and trypsin. *J. Am. Chem. Soc.* **85,** 997–1000 (1963).

78. Poulsen, K., and Jorgensen, J., An easy radioimmunological microassay of renin activity, concentration and substrate in human and animal plasma and tissues based on angiotensin I trapping by antibody. *J. Clin. Endocrinol. Metab.* **39,** 816–825 (1974).

79. Nielsen, M. D., Jorgensen, M., and Giese, J., ^{125}I-labelling of angiotensin I and II. *Acta Endocrinol.* **67,** 104–116 (1971).

80. Haber, E., Koerner, T., Page, L. B., et al., Application of a radioimmunoassay for angiotensin I to the physiologic measurements of plasma renin activity in normal human subjects: Renin activity by angiotensin I radioimmunoassay. *J. Clin. Endocrinol.* **29,** 1349–1355 (1969).

81. Sealey, J. E., Gerten-Banes, J., and Laragh, J. H., The renin system: Variations in man measured by radioimmunoassay or bioassay. *Kidney Int.* **1,** 240–253 (1972).

82. Kodish, M. E., and Katz, F. H., Plasma renin concentration: Comparison of angiotensinase inhibitors and correlation with plasma renin activity and aldosterone. *J. Lab. Clin. Med.* **83,** 705–715 (1974).

83. Boucher, R., Veyrat, R., DeChamplain, J., et al., New procedures for measurements of human plasma angiotensin and renin activity levels. *Can. Med. Assoc. J.* **90,** 194–201 (1964).

84. Croxatto, H., and Croxatto, R., "Pepsitensin," a hypertensin-like substance produced by peptic digestion of proteins. *Science* **95,** 101–103 (1942).

85. Fernandez M. T. F., Paladini, A. C., and Delius, A. E., Isolation and identification of a pepsitensin. *Biochem. J.* **97,** 540–546 (1965).

86. Boyd, G. W., Adamson, A. R., Fitz, A., et al., Radioimmunoassay determination of plasma-renin activity. *Lancet* **i,** 213–218 (1969).

87. Cohen, E. L., Grim, C. E., Conn, J. W., et al., Accurate and rapid measurement of plasma renin activity by radioimmunoassay. *J. Lab. Clin. Med.* **77,** 1025–1038 (1971).

88. Lehfeldt, D. C., and Hutchens, T. T., A kinetic method for determination of plasma renin activity using radioassay of angiotensin I. *Am. J. Clin. Pathol.* **55,** 513–522 (1971).

89. Katz, F. H., and Smith, J. A., Radioimmunoassay of angiotensin I: Comparison of two renin activity methods and use for other measurements of the renin system. *Clin. Chem.* **18,** 528–533 (1972).

90. Freedlender, A. E., Fyhrquist, F. Y., and Hollemans, H. J. G., Renin and the angiotensins. In *Methods of Hormone Radioimmunoassay.* B. M. Jaffe, and H. R. Behrman, Eds. Academic Press, New York, N.Y., 1974, pp 455–469.

91. Haas, E., and Goldblatt, H., Indirect assay of plasma renin. *Lancet* **i,** 1330–1332 (1972).

92. Menard, J., and Catt, K. J., Measurement of renin activity, concentration and substrate in rat plasma by radioimmunoassay of angiotensin I. *Endocrinology* **90,** 422–430 (1972).

93. Kotchen, T. A., Flamenbaum, W., Cirksena, W., et al., Comparison of a biological and an immunological assay for the measurement of plasma renin activity. *J. Clin. Endocrinol. Metab.* **36,** 804–810 (1973).

94. Fukachi, S., Takeuchi, T., and Torikai, T., Determination of plasma renin activity by radioimmunoassay of angiotensin I. *Clin. Sci.* **44,** 43–54 (1973).

95. Hollemans, H. J. G., Van Der Meer, J., and Kloosterziel, W., Measurement of renin activity in plasma by a radioimmunoassay for angiotensin I. *Clin. Chim. Acta* **24,** 353–357 (1969).

96. Stockigt, J. R., Collins, R. D., and Biglieri, E. G., Determination of plasma renin concentration by angiotensin I immunoassay. *Circ. Res.* **28,** *Suppl II,* 175–191 (1971).

97. Haas, E., Gould, A. B., and Goldblatt, H., Estimation of endogenous renin in human blood. *Lancet* **i,** 657–660 (1968).

98. Giese, J., Jorgensen, M., Nielsen, M. D., et al., Plasma renin concentration measured by use of radioimmunoassay for angiotensin I. *Scand. J. Lab. Invest.* **26,** 355–367 (1970).

99. Haas, E., Goldblatt, H., Gipson, E. C., et al., Extraction, purification and assay of human renin free angiotensinase. *Circ. Res.* **19,** 739–749 (1966).

100. Goldblatt, H., Katz, Y. J., Lewis, H. A., et al., Studies on experimental hypertension; bioassay of renin. *J. Exp. Med.* **77,** 309–313 (1943).

101. Haas, E., and Goldblatt, H., Kinetic constants of the human renin and human angiotensin reaction. *Circ. Res.* **20,** 45–55 (1967).

102. Beckerhoff, R., Luetscher, J. A., Wilkinson, R., et al., Plasma renin concentration, activity and substrate in hypertension induced by oral contraceptives. *J. Clin. Endocrinol. Metab.* **34,** 1067–1073 (1972).

103. Cain, M. C., Walters, W. A., and Catt, K. J., Effects of oral contraceptive therapy on the renin-angiotensin system. *J. Clin. Endocrinol. Metab.* **33,** 671–676 (1971).

104. Low, J., and Oparil, S., Oral contraceptive pill hypertension. *J. Reprod. Med.* **15,** 201–208 (1975).

105. Day, R. P., and Luetscher, J. A., Big renin; a possible prohormone in kidney and plasma of a patient with Wilms' tumor. *J. Clin. Endocrinol. Metab.* **38,** 923–926 (1974).

106. Sealey, J. E., and Laragh, J. H., Prorenin in human plasma: Methodological and physiological implications. *Circ. Res.* **36,** *Suppl. I,* 10–16 (1975).

107. Waite, M. A., Measurement of concentrations of angiotensin I in human blood by radioimmunoassay. *Clin. Sci. Mol. Med.* **45,** 51–64 (1973).

108. Boyd, G. W., Landon, J., and Peart, W. S., Radioimmunoassay for determining plasma-levels of angiotensin II in man. *Lancet* **ii,** 1002–1005 (1967).

109. Catt, K. J., Cain, M. C., and Coghlan, J. P., Measurement of angiotensin II in blood. *Lancet* **ii,** 1005–1007 (1967).

110. Gocke, D. J., Gerten, J., Sherwood, L. M., et al., Physiological and pathological variations of plasma angiotensin II in man: Correlation with renin activity and sodium balance. *Circ. Res.* **24,** *Suppl. I,* 131–146 (1969).

111. Sundsfjord, J. A., Radioimmunoassay of angiotensin II in plasma. *Acta Endocrinol.* (Copenhagen) **64,** 181–192 (1970).

112. Goodfriend T. L., Ball, D. L., and Farley, D. B., Radioimmunoassay of angiotensin. *J. Lab. Clin. Med* **72,** 648–662 (1968).

113. Page, L. B., Haber, E., Kimura, A. Y., et al., Studies with the radioimmunoassay for angiotensin II, and its application to measurement of renin activity. *J. Clin. Endocrinol. Metab.* **29,** 200–206 (1969).

114. Moore, M. A., Horvath, J. S., and Walker, W. G., Angiotensin II and renin responses to Na restriction and Na depletion in normal subject. *Circulation* **48,** *Suppl. 4,* 70 (1973).

115. Bing, J. L., Mechanism of increased sensitivity to renin in nephrectomized animals. *Acta Pathol. Microbiol. Scand.* **60,** 311–333 (1964).

116. Gould, A. B., Skeggs, L. T., and Kahn, J. R., Measurement of renin and substrate concentration in human serum. *Lab. Invest.* **15,** 1802–1813 (1966).

117. Boucher, R., Menard, J., and Genest, J., A micromethod for measurement of renin in the plasma and kidneys of rats. *Can. J. Physiol. Pharmacol.* **45,** 881–890 (1967).

118. Poulsen, K., Estimation of plasma renin concentration using radioimmunoassay of angiotensin II. *Scand. J. Clin. Lab. Invest.* **24,** 291–300 (1969).

119. Ryan, J. W., and McKenzie, J. K., Properties of renin substrate in rabbit plasma with a note on its assay. *Biochem. J.* **108,** 687–692 (1968).

CLIN. CHEM. 22/5, 594–601 (1976)

Normative Values of Serum Immunoglobulins by Single Radial Immunodiffusion: A Review

Shirley E. Maddison and Charles B. Reimer

Many previous studies of normative values in adults have suggested that race, age, sex, and environment all have significant effects on the mean values for IgG, IgA, IgM, and IgE in various groups of individuals. Single radial immunodiffusion is the technique most widely used to quantitate immunoglobulins of the three major classes (IgG, IgM, and IgA) in sera. Measurements have been expressed in terms of mass concentration, as percentages of the mean normal adult value, and in arbitrary international units. To improve agreement among laboratories, the WHO has supported the distribution of an International Reference Preparation for the Human Immunoglobulins IgG, IgA, and IgM, and similar (separate) preparations for IgD and IgE.

Additional Keyphrases: *factors affecting concentrations • reference materials • techniques • reference values*

This survey will largely be directed to a review and discussion of normative values of IgG, IgA, and IgM in human serum from adults, with only brief comments on the findings in children and on the present status of normative values for IgD and IgE. Reviews on the subject include those by Kalff (*1*), Hobbs (*2*), McFarlane (*3*), Bradley (*4*), and Becker (*5*).

IgG, IgA, and IgM are quantitated by means of three techniques, all of which are based on the fundamental principles of immunoprecipitation as defined by Heidelberger and Kendall (*6*). The most commonly used quantitative assay is single radial immunodiffusion, which is performed according to either the original technique of Mancini et al. (*7*) or its modification described by Fahey and McKelvey (*8*). Another quantitative immunoprecipitation assay is electroimmunoassay or "rocket electrophoresis," the method of Laurell (*9*). The third method is nephelometric immunoassay (*10–12*).

Because of its simplicity, single radial immunodiffusion is the most frequently used means of quantitating immunoglobulins. Not only is this method used as a research tool by a large number of investigators but agarose-antibody plates and reference sera are obtainable as kits in the U.S.A. from at least nine commercial houses. Quantities as low as 10 mg/liter can be precisely measured, and this degree of sensitivity can be increased 20-fold to about 500 μg/liter by procedures such as DL-3,4-dihydroxyphenylalanine (DOPA) treatment (*13*), which intensify the precipitin ring or 250-fold (to 40 μg/liter) by the radioactive double-antibody method (*14*).

The results of immunoglobulin quantitation have been expressed in familiar units of mass concentration (g/liter), as percentages of mean values for the normal adult population, or in terms of arbitrary international units (arb. units/liter). In early studies of normative values investigators each used their own standard sera and antisera, leading to great variability between laboratories. In an attempt to standardize immunoglobulin quantitation, a cooperative study by expert laboratories showed that use of individual reagents and standards gave unacceptably wide ranges of immunoglobulin values for six coded serum samples (*15*). Agreement was considerably improved when a single reference preparation was used by the collaborating laboratories. As a result of these studies, a freeze-dried pool of human serum has been prepared and distributed on a worldwide basis under the aegis of the World Health Organization (WHO) (*16–19*). This International Reference Preparation of Human Immunoglobin contains 100 int. units each of

The Parasitology and Biological Products Divisions, Bureau of Laboratories, Center for Disease Control, Public Health Service, U. S. Department of Health, Education, and Welfare, Atlanta, Ga. 30333.

Based on a paper presented at the first AACC Pine Mountain (Ga.) Conference (on Diagnostic Immunochemistry), March 3, 1975.

Received and accepted February 20, 1976 (reviewed before receipt).

IgG, IgA, and IgM. We have discussed the problem of standardization in greater depth in our accompanying paper (*20*).

Only comparatively few studies of normative values related to the WHO Reference Preparation have been reported (*5, 21–26, 55*). Previous studies in adults have most frequently used milligram values. The results of some of these investigations of normative values may contain bias because of the selection of the samples studied. In some instances the sera were drawn largely from hospital personnel. In other studies age, sex, or race were not defined for the sample. Screening for monoclonal proteins in individuals with a high concentration of one or more of the immunoglobulins was not done in all investigations. Nevertheless, these earlier studies indicate that a number of factors—including race, age, and sex—significantly affect the mean values for IgG, IgA, and IgM observed in various groups of individuals tested.

In a given normal subject the individual variation of immunoglobulins over periods of five months appears to be very low (*27, 28*). In a study (*29*) in Gambia, the immunoglobulin concentrations observed in individual subjects were relatively stable during a year in spite of infectious disease and climatic conditions. According to Hobbs (*2*), the individual variation usually remains within ±20% over a period of years.

The question of genetic vs. environmental influence on immunoglobulin concentrations is an interesting one. Striking examples of familial incidence of selective immunoglobulin deficiency, particularly of IgA, suggest a genetic influence. However, a study of monozygotic and dizygotic twins by Rowe et al. (*30*) showed that the genetic effect is small. The results of family studies of immunoglobulin concentrations in Gambia (*31*) indicate that genetics plays a greater role in the regulation of IgG and IgE than of IgM. In contrast the genetic influence on IgA and IgD concentrations appeared to be very low or negligible.

The concept that environment and antigenic challenge plays the major roles in stimulating immunoglobulin production and maintaining concentrations of the immunoglobulins is strongly supported by results of experiments with germ-free animals. Such animals have very low concentrations of immunoglobulins, which increase when the animal is exposed to environmental antigens.

In a study of children and adults in the U.S.A., Stiehm and Fudenberg (*32*) did not observe differences owing to race. Hobbs (*2*) noted that natives of underdeveloped countries have higher IgG and IgM concentrations than do subjects in Britain. These abnormally high immunoglobulin values may reflect environmental differences such as increased infectious diseases; individuals from such underdeveloped countries showed a decrease in immunoglobulin concentrations to 140% of mean adult value in the U.K. after living in Britain for some years. Hobbs (*2*) suggests that this residual elevation may reflect the genetic survival value of such subjects in their countries of origin. Caution, however, must be used in interpreting the immunoglobulin concentrations of subjects who move from underdeveloped countries to countries such as Britain. These individuals may also reflect advanced economic opportunity in their country of origin. No report could be found in which immunoglobulin concentrations of such groups or individuals were measured before or soon after arrival in Britain and again some months or years later. Cohen et al. (*33*) observed that West Africans who had lived in Britain for several years synthesized γ-globulin at almost twice the daily rate observed in healthy Europeans. Mohammed et al. (*34*) observed significant differences in the IgG, IgA, and IgM values in healthy individuals from a Nigerian village and from the Old City of Zaria in Nigeria. It was noted that the pattern of parasitic infections differs in these two communities.

In a study of American Indians in Surinam (*35*), the IgG, IgM, and IgA values were significantly higher than those of a control group of Dutch subjects. Mean IgG and IgA values for normal adult Indians in Bombay, India, were found to be significantly higher than reported values for Europeans and English (*36*). A combination of hygienic and climatic conditions the net result of which was an increased antigenic stimulus was considered as a possible explanation. In contrast to the immunoglobulin pattern observed in India, Yadav and Shah (*37*) found that IgG, IgA, and IgM values for Malaysians fell within the range reported for Caucasians, and below those observed in West Africans.

In the U.S.A., Buckley and Dorsey (*21*) observed that the mean IgG and IgA concentrations were higher in black males than in white males, while IgM values in these two groups were not significantly different. Karayalcin et al. (*38*), in New York, reported that both black males and females had higher values for IgG, IgA, and IgM than did white males and females. These authors did not examine environmental factors and therefore concluded that their results did not necessarily reflect a genetic cause.

Sex appears to be a factor influencing immunoglobulin concentrations, particularly IgM. Rhodes et al. (*39*) found that women with XXX or XXXY chromosomes had higher concentrations of IgM than did normal women (XX chromosomes). Normal women, in turn, had higher IgM values than those for men (XY chromosomes). These findings suggest that IgM concentrations are influenced by genes located on the X chromosomes. This role of the X chromosome is substantiated by the observations of Wood et al. (*40*) that IgM concentrations in normal females are greater than in women with XO chromosomes. The family studies by Grundbacher (*41*) showed that the correlation in terms of IgM values was much closer between boys and their mothers than between boys and their fathers. The IgM concentrations in girls were more closely correlated with those of their fathers than

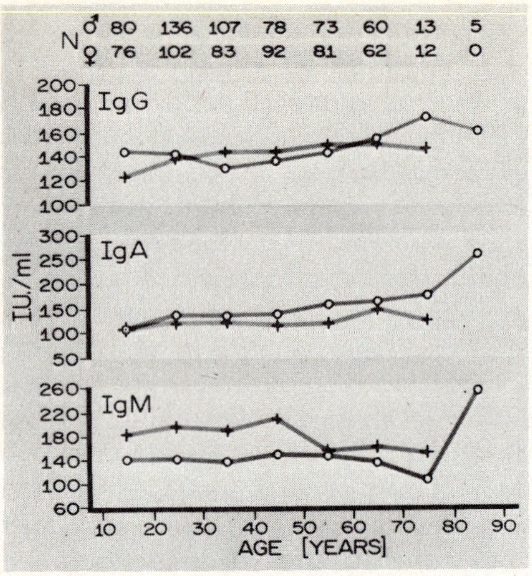

Fig. 1. Normal immunoglobulin concentrations in relation to age
(From W. Becker 1974, courtesy of the author and Charles C Thomas, publisher). O - - O Male; x - - x Female

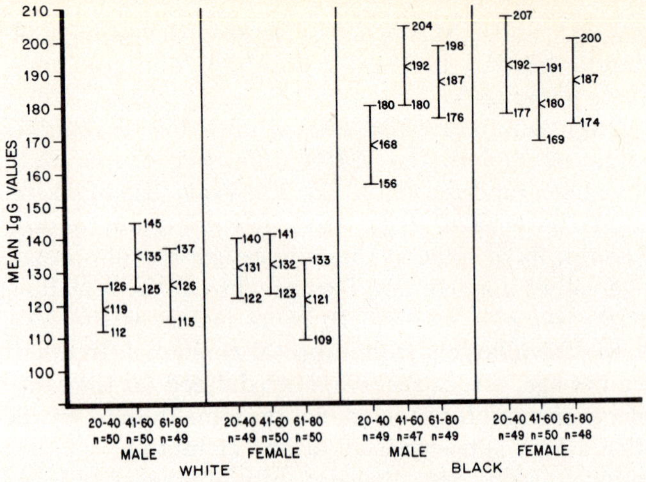

Fig. 2. Mean IgG values plus and minus two standard errors of the mean for race, sex, and age groups

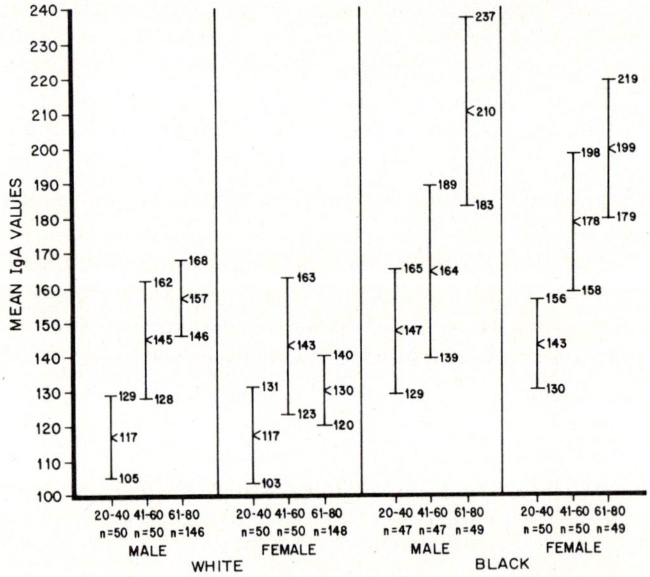

Fig. 3. Mean IgA values plus and minus two standard errors of the mean for race, sex, and age groups

with those of their mothers. These observations plus the observed higher mean values of IgM in both black and white females support the hypothesis that in humans the X chromosome carries genes that control IgM concentrations.

Stoop et al. (*42*), in a study on children, found higher concentrations of both IgG and IgM in girls than in boys; they questioned whether these observations reflected either genetic or other influencing factors. The sex-related difference in IgM concentrations is observed as early as four to five years of age (*29, 42*). No sex-related difference in IgG or IgM values was reported in two other studies involving children (*32, 43*). In studies of adults, differences in IgG values between males and females have not usually been observed.

The pattern of adult immunoglobulin concentrations in relation to age is not clear cut. The age groups used in the analysis of various studies have frequently differed, making comparisons difficult. Increased concentrations of IgG and IgA were found to be associated with senility in a study by Haferkamp et al. (*44*), but not by Hobbs (*2*). Becker (*5*) summarizes the effect of age as a continuous increase of IgG and IgA in adults up to senility, whereas highest IgM values, particularly in females, are observed during the 5th decade. Becker's own results (*5*) on a total of 960 sera are shown in Figure 1. There is a gradual increase in the immunoglobulins with age. A sharp increase in IgA and IgM is observed in males between the ages of 75 and 85 years but IgG reaches a peak a decade earlier. The highest age of the females in this study was a decade lower than that of the males; it therefore is not known whether females also show an increase in IgA and IgM after the 75th year of age.

In a study of 800 U.S. residents (*25*), we attempted to establish normal adult values for IgG, IgA, and IgM in terms of int. units. All sera were obtained from the Center for Disease Control Serum Bank. The sera were collected over a 10-year period in five states during epidemiological surveys for specific antibodies after viral outbreaks. The sera were stored at −20 °C and were not thawed more than twice during the investigation. The original design of the study required groups of 50 sera from black and white males and females in each of the following age groups: 20–40 years, 41–60 years, and 61–80 years. After the initial study was completed we decided that more reliable estimates of population variables were needed for IgG and IgM data on white men between 61 and 80 years of age, and for IgA data on white women in this same age group. We therefore tested an additional 100 sera in each of these groups.

The measurements were made according to the original technique of Mancini et al. (*7*) with goat antisera prepared in our laboratories. A secondary standard was calibrated against the WHO Reference Preparation. Four dilutions of the standard and, in addition, one or two internal control sera were included with the nine unknown sera in each plate.

Figure 2 shows the IgG values plus and minus two standard errors of the mean which we obtained according to race, age, and sex. For all age groups the mean IgG concentration was higher in blacks than in whites. A more modest elevation of IgA in blacks as compared with whites is seen in Figure 3. In addition, except for white females there was a significant increase in mean IgA with age for both races. In the younger adults (age 20 to 40 years) mean IgM values were markedly higher in females than in males (Figure 4). A decrease of IgM with age was observed particularly in the females of both races; however, this did not occur in white males.

There appears to be general agreement between the int. unit values for the adult white U.S. residents in our study and the int. unit values reported for adults by Cejka et al. (*24*) for U.S. males of unstated race, by Rowe (*22*) for European males, by Sinkov et al. (*23*) for Bulgarian males and females, and by

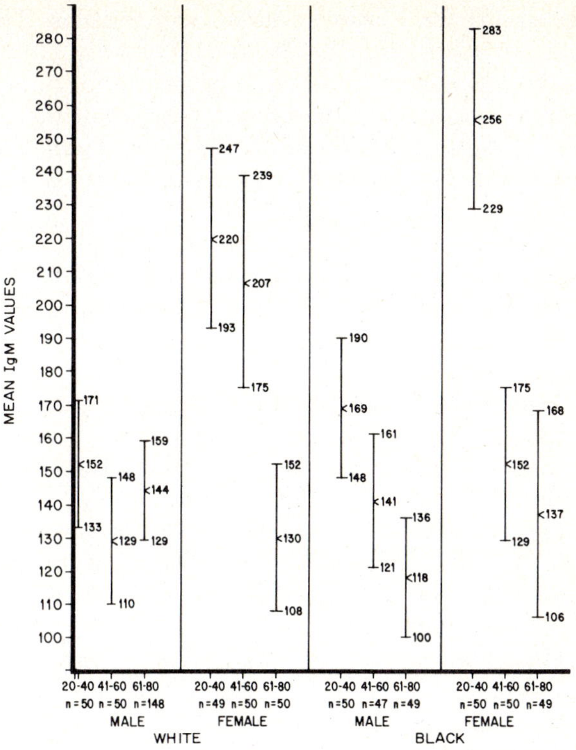

Fig. 4. Mean IgM values (int. units/ml) plus and minus two standard errors of the mean for race, sex, and age groups

Table 1. Serum Immunoglobulin Concentrations of Healthy Adult U.S. Whites and Europeans

Investigator	Country (race)	Age	Sex	Mean immunoglobulin concn, int. units/ml: IgG	IgA	IgM
Maddison et al. 1976	U.S. (white)	20–40	♂	119(72–166)[a]	117(59–209)	152(58–299)
	U.S. (white)	20–80	♂	127	138	142
	U.S. (white)	20–80	♀	128	130	188
Cejka et al. 1974	U.S. (unknown)	Adult	♂	137(82–229)	113(50–254)	157(48–310)
Rowe 1972	European	20–29	♂	125	116	141
Becker 1972	Germany/ Switzerland	15–80	♂ and ♀	141(90–200)[b]	132(50–250)	M 145) F 180) (60–300)
Sinkov et al. 1973	Bulgaria	21–50	♂ and ♀	129(64–180)[b]	114(48–240)	M 115 (60–295) F 147 (90–220)
Becker 1972	Germany	15–64	♂ and ♀	144(92–207)[b]	125(54–268)	M 144) F 184) (69–322)

[a] Empirical 5th and 95th percentiles
[b] Range

Note: To convert to milligrams per liter, multiply these values by 80.4 for IgG, 14.2 for IgA, and 8.47 for IgM (See reference *19*).

Table 2. Serum Immunoglobulin Concentrations of Healthy Young Adult Black Males in the U.S. and Nigeria

Investigator	Country (race)	Age	Sex	Mean immunoglobulin concn, int. units/ml: IgG	IgA	IgM
Maddison et al. 1976	U.S. (black)	20–40	Male	168(100–250)[a]	147(53–274)	169(79–321)
Rowe 1972	Nigeria	20–29	Male	287(146–567)[b]	80(31–207)	211(32–1413)

[a] Empirical 5th and 95th percentile
[b] 95% confidence limits

Becker (*5*) for European males and females. These data are summarized in Table 1. The only group of blacks with which comparison of any of our data appeared possible was the group of Nigerian males in Rowe's report (*22*). These are shown in Table 2. Because of environmental differences, it was not surprising to find that the IgG and IgM concentrations were higher in the Nigerians than in the U.S. black residents. The low IgA values in the Nigerians is not so readily explained. However, Turner and Voller (*45*), in a study done in Nigeria, observed IgA values similar to those for persons living in the U.K.: the IgG and IgM values for the Nigerians were significantly higher than those for the British. Shulman et al. (*26*) did not show data on each of the three immunoglobulin classes studied in respect to the age groups of their South African subjects. However, they also observed higher values in blacks than in whites; in addition, they noted influences of age and sex on immunoglobulin concentrations.

The results of our study show that one cannot conclude that the mean IgG concentrations are affected by age if sex is ignored, or by sex if age is ignored. Except for white women between the ages of 61 and 80 years, there was a significant increase in mean IgA with age for both races. This exception indicates that there is a significant interaction between race and age in relation to IgA values in white women. Lamy et al. (*46*) observed increased values for IgA in black males and females with age and that IgA values were significantly higher in men than in women between the ages of 45 and 65 years. Except in white males, we observed a marked decrease in IgM levels with age in all subjects, particularly females of both races. A less pronounced decrease occurred in black males. While our results do not parallel those of Cassidy et al. (*47*) in that we observed decreased concentrations of IgM with age in all groups except white males, and of IgA in white females, we concur with these investigators in our observation of statistically significant interactions between race, age, and sex factors for all three immunoglobulin classes. We suggest that a much larger population study is needed to provide true normative limits.

The apparent effect of seasonal change on immunoglobulin values was observed by McFarlane (*48*) but not by McGregor et al. (*29*) in West Africa where the wet season parallels an increased rate of transmission of parasitic and other infectious diseases and, therefore, increased antigenic stimulus. The data reported by Rowe (*22*) show that healthy young adult males in Mexico City have lower mean IgA and IgM concentrations than do similar groups in most other geographic areas. In the same study, IgG and IgM concentrations in natives of Algiers (Algeria) and Perth (Australia) were shown to be almost identical, but were higher than those in most other areas. However, the IgA values for Perth are considerably lower than those for Algiers. Such factors as altitude, mass vaccinations, and protein intake may constitute persistent environmental differences that affect the immunoglobulin concentrations.

The question of immunoglobulin levels in pregnancy also requires consideration. Cohen et al. (*33*) found that considerably less γ-globulin was synthesized by a woman who was three months pregnant at the time of testing than was synthesized by the comparable general population in the study. McGregor et al. (*29*) found mean IgG and IgA values to be significantly lower during pregnancy. The same authors did a longitudinal study on a cross-sectional group; IgG appeared to decrease progressively throughout pregnancy, and reached the lowest values in the last 10 weeks of gestation. IgA also decreased in the first and second trimester, but increased in the third trimester. Maroulis et al. (*49*) also observed significant decrease of IgG during the second and third trimester and postpartum. Lower IgA values were not observed until postpartum.

Immunoglobulin concentrations of the mother may markedly affect the subsequent values for the neonate (*2*). Normal full-term infants have IgG concentrations that are nearly the same as those of their respective mothers; such infants have low IgM concentrations and undetectable or only trace amounts of IgA. The upper limit of normality for IgM is usually considered to be 200 mg/liter, but Yeager (*50*) observed that the cord-blood IgM value varies with birth weight. She suggests that in high-weight babies normal values may exceed 200 mg/liter. However, no such correlation between high weight and IgM values was observed by Winsten (*51*), nor did Logie et al. (*52*) find a consistent relationship between IgG and birth weight although they observed a low mean IgG value in infants with lowest birth weight. Postmature infants with prolonged gestational periods have detectable amounts of IgA but their IgM concentrations are not abnormally high (*53, 54*). Some investigators observed slightly supranormal values for IgG in postmature infants (*53*); others found that prolonged gestation resulted in decreased concentrations of IgG in maternal-blood and cord-blood (*54*).

Up to 4% of full-term infants fail to replace the maternal IgG in time and may suffer from agammaglobulinemia (*2*). This may be, but is not usually, due to the mother having subnormal concentrations of IgG. In rare instances the cause has been defined as maternal antibodies reacting against the infant's allotype of IgG, or as maternal paraprotein influencing the infant's synthesis and catabolism of IgG. In premature infants the amount of placentally transmitted maternal IgG is considerably less than in full-term infants (*55*). Most of the infants who fail to replace the maternal IgG on time, however, appear merely to be "slow starters" (*2*), and catch up within a year; serum IgM and IgA concentrations are normal.

It is important that these factors just discussed be taken into consideration in the selection of cord bloods and sera from infants up to one year of age for studies of normative immunoglobulin values.

Studies of immunoglobulin concentrations in children have resulted in some discrepancies (*24*). Present knowledge suggests that adult values of IgG are reached between six and 10 years of age (*24, 42, 43, 56*). Some studies suggest that adult IgM values are attained between one and two years of age (*27, 43, 56*); others suggest they are not reached until about 16 years of age (*24, 38*). The numbers of samples investigated between birth and age 16 years have usually been small, and various results related to age and sex have been reported. Because of this and because of the probable interrelationships of these and other factors in adults, we suggest that further studies on adequate samples of different populations of children are needed.

A WHO Research Standard for Human Serum IgD is available (*57*), but few reports of normative values of IgD appear in the literature. Probably the small number of such studies reflects the fact that the functional activity of this immunoglobulin has not yet been defined. Hobbs (*2*) states that his measurements of IgD in over 2000 sera have provided no clinically useful information. IgD is not usually detectable in cord serum (*58, 59*), but wide ranges are demonstrable in children and adults. The recent observations of IgD on the surface of peripheral blood lymphocytes of the human newborn (*60*) and its possible role as a lymphocyte receptor (*61*) have rekindled interest in this immunoglobulin.

The IgE immunoglobulins are the reaginic antibodies which give immediate hypersensitivity and manifestations of allergy (*62*). The low concentrations of IgE in serum necessitate the use of quantitative technique of greater sensitivity than simple single radial immunodiffusion. By intensifying the precipitate ring with DOPA (*13*), Sieber and Becker (*63*) were able to use the single radial immunodiffusion technique in IgE determinations. Both radioactive radial immunodiffusion and competitive protein binding radioimmunoassays have been used by several investigators.

WHO has made available a Research Standard for Human Serum IgE (*64*) to which international units have been assigned. When the Reference Preparation was used in a collaborative study by five laboratories (*65*), fairly good agreement between participant results was obtained irrespective of the techniques and antisera used. However, a number of investigators have encountered problems in attempting to compare measurement, particularly of low concentrations of IgE, by different techniques (*66*).

When one attempts to compare normative IgE values reported in several studies, it becomes obvious that, to date, not only have most investigators used their own individual reference preparations, but also there are a great many modifications of the basic technique. Nevertheless, some basic information on IgE levels is now available. Although maternal IgE is said not to cross the placenta, low concentrations of IgE were demonstrable in all of 37 cord sera examined by Johansson (*67*). His study indicated that adult values for IgE are reached before seven years of age. A wide range of values was found in healthy adults and children (*67–71*). In a study of 4700 blood donors, Orren and Dowdle (*72*) observed a significant decrease in IgE concentrations with age, and females had significantly lower levels of IgE than males. These investigators (*73*) also showed that IgE values varied in three ethnic groups in South Africa. Higher values were observed in black Africans, intermediate in "coloreds," and lowest in whites. In studies of Swedish and Ethiopian children (*74*) and of adults (*75*) no sex-related differences were found. The higher values for IgE in Nigerian blood donors compared with those in expatriates living in Nigeria and with Swiss blood donors probably reflect the high prevalence of parasitic infections (other than malaria) in Africa, rather than racial differences (*76*). The results of a family study in Canada (*71*) suggest that low IgE concentrations are controlled by two dominant genes and that high values occur if one of these genes is absent.

The use of single radial immunodiffusion for quantitating immunoglobulins has been extended to the subclasses of IgG (*77, 78*). As yet, close agreement has not been obtained by investigators. However, in this new application of the technique the difficulties associated with obtaining representative anti-subclass antisera have been well documented (*79*). Nevertheless, van der Giessen et al. (*77*) observed that IgG2 increased slowly with age, with adult values not yet reached at the age of 12 years. IgG4 shows a similar rise but in a lesser degree. In contrast, the IgG1 and IgG3 values of children did not vary significantly from those of adults.

In conclusion, it becomes apparent from this brief review that the effects of environment, race, sex, and age and their interactions have not been fully defined for any of the five classes of immunoglobulins. It is anticipated that the true normal ranges of the various immunoglobulins will vary significantly in subpopulations of man. It is essential that these normal ranges be accurately established if the patient's immunoglobulin data are to be of the greatest possible diagnostic aid to the clinician.

The question of sample selection for further studies of immunoglobulin concentrations in normal individuals is extremely important. Because of the interaction of race, age, sex, and environment, Kalff (*1*) challenges the concept of "normal" human immunoglobulin values, and suggests that in a given individual the observed values can only be interpreted in terms of the values for a control group matched for age, sex, race, and changing and persistent environmental factors.

We suggest that in the U.S.A., a large, truly randomized, and fully documented probability sample of the nation's population, somewhat similar to the Health and Nutrition Examination Survey (HANES) collection of sera, should be studied in order to define more clearly the interaction of the various factors which regulate immunoglobulin levels. The use of the WHO Reference Preparations for the various immunoglobulin classes will facilitate the comparison of data between laboratories.

References

1. Kalff, M. W., A population study on serum immunoglobulin levels. *Clin. Chim. Acta* **28,** 277 (1970).

2. Hobbs, J. R., Immunoglobulins in clinical chemistry. *Adv. Clin. Chem.* **14,** 291 (1971).

3. McFarlane, H., Immunoglobulins in populations of subtropical and tropical countries. *Adv. Clin. Chem.* **16,** 153 (1973).

4. Bradley, J., Immunoglobulins. *J. Med. Genet.* **11,** 60 (1974).

5. Becker, W., Variations of immunoglobulins in disease. *J. Clin. Pathol.* in press.

6. Heidelberger, M., and Kendall, F. E., Quantitative studies on the precipitin reaction. The determination of small amounts of a specific polysaccharide. *J. Exp. Med.* **55,** 555 (1935).

7. Mancini, G., Carbonara, A. O., and Heremans, J. F., Immunochemical quantitation of antigens by single radial immunodiffusion. *Immunochemistry* **2,** 235 (1965).

8. Fahey, J. L., and McKelvey, E. M., Quantitative determination of serum immunoglobulins in antibody-agar plates. *J. Immunol.* **94,** 84 (1965).

9. Laurell, C., Quantitative estimation of proteins by electrophoresis in agarose gel containing antibodies. *Anal. Biochem.* **15,** 45 (1966).

10. Schultz, H. E., and Schwick, H. G., Quantitative immunologische Bestimmung von Plasmaproteinen. *Clin. Chim. Acta* **4,** 15 (1959).

11. Killingsworth, L. M., and Savory, J., Manual nephelometric methods for immunochemical determination of immunoglobulins IgG, IgA, and IgM in human serum. *Clin. Chem.* **18,** 335 (1972).

12. Ritchie, R. F., Theory and practice of automated nephelometry. In *Protides of Biological Fluids,* **21.** Colloquium Brugge (1973). H. Peeters, Ed., Pergamon Press, New York, N. Y., 1974, p 569.

13. Madhosingh, C., and Wood, I. M., Dopa stain for precipitins in gel. *Anal. Biochem.* **44,** 523 (1971).

14. Rowe, D. S., Radioactive single radial diffusion: A method for increasing the sensitivity of immunochemical quantification of proteins in agar gels. *Bull. WHO* **40,** 613 (1969).

15. Rowe, D. S., Anderson, S. G., and Grab, B., A research standard for human serum immunoglobulins IgG, IgA, and IgM. *Bull. WHO* **42,** 535 (1970).

16. WHO Expert Committee on Biological Standardization: 23rd Report. *WHO Tech. Rep. Ser. No.* **463,** 20 (1971).

17. Anderson, S. G., Bangham, D. R., Batty, I., et al., Measurements of concentrations of human serum immunoglobulins. *Clin. Chim. Acta* **36,** 276 (1972).

18. Rowe, D. S., Grab, B., and Anderson, S. G., An international reference preparation for human serum immunoglobulins G, A, and M: Content of immunoglobulins by weight. *Bull. WHO* **46,** 67 (1972).

19. Humphrey, J. H., and Batty, I., International reference preparation for human sera IgG, IgA, and IgM. *Clin. Exp. Immunol.* **17,** 708 (1974).

20. Reimer, C. B., and Maddison, S. E., Standardization of human immunoglobulin quantitation: A review of current status and problems. *Clin. Chem.* **22,** 577 (1976).

21. Buckley, C. E., and Dorsey, F. C., Serum immunoglobulin levels throughout the life-span of healthy man. *Ann. Intern. Med.* **75,** 673 (1971).

22. Rowe, D. S., Concentrations of serum immunoglobulins in healthy young adult males estimated by assay against the international reference preparation. *Lancet* **ii,** 1232 (1972).

23. Sinkov, D., Toleve, T., and Stereva, T., Concentrations of IgG, IgA, and IgM in terms of international units in the sera of healthy individuals. *Bull. WHO* **49,** 217 (1973).

24. Cejka, J., Wood, D. W., and Kim, C. S., Immunoglobulin concentrations in sera of normal children: Quantitation against an international reference preparation. *Clin. Chem.* **20,** 656 (1974).

25. Maddison, S. E., Stewart, C. C., Farshy, C. E., and Reimer, C. B., The relationship of race, sex, and age to concentrations of serum immunoglobulins expressed in international units in healthy adult U.S. residents. *Bull. WHO* **52,** 179 (1976).

26. Shulman, G., Gilich, G. C., and Andrews, M. J. A., Serum immunoglobulins G, A, and M in white and black adults on the Witwatersrand. *S. Afr. Med. J.* **49,** 1160 (1975).

27. Allansmith, M., McClennan, B., and Butterworth, M., Stability of human immunoglobulin levels. *Proc. Soc. Exp. Biol.* **125,** 404 (1967).

28. Mondorf, W., and Kollmar, M., Das quantitative Verhalten von IgG, IgA and IgM, sowie des Transferrins, Coeruloplasmins, α_1-Antitrypsins and des β_1A-Globulins bei normal Personen im Verlaufe von 5 Monaten. *Klin. Wochenschr.* **47,** 1055 (1969).

29. McGregor, I. A., Rowe, D. S., Wilson, M. E., and Billewicz, W. Z., Plasma immunoglobulin concentrations in an African (Gambian) community in relation to season, malaria and other infections and pregnancy. *Clin. Exp. Immunol.* **7,** 51 (1970).

30. Rowe, D. S., Boyle, J. A., and Buchanan, W. W., Plasma in immunoglobulin concentrations in twins. *Clin. Exp. Immunol.* **3,** 233 (1968).

31. Billewicz, W. Z., McGregor, I. A., Roberts, D. F., et al., Family studies on immunoglobulin levels. *Clin. Exp. Immunol.* **16,** 13 (1974).

32. Stiehm, E. R., and Fudenberg, H. H., Serum levels of immune globulins in health and disease: A survey. *Pediatrics* **37,** 715 (1966).

33. Cohen, S., McGregor, I. A., and Carrington, S., Gamma-globulin and acquired immunity to human malaria. *Nature* **192,** 733 (1961).

34. Mohammed, I., Tomkins, A. M., and Greenwood, B. M., Normal immunoglobulins in the tropics. *Lancet* **i,** 481 (1973).

35. Zegers, B. J. M., Geerdink, R. A., and Sanders, P. C., Serum immunoglobulin levels in Trio and Wajana Indians in Surinam. *Vox Sang.* **24,** 457 (1973).

36. Samuel, A. M., Deshparde, U. R., and Singh, B., Immunoglobulins in normal adult Indians. *Indian J. Med. Res.* **58,** 56 (1970).

37. Yadav, M., and Shah, F. H., Normal plasma-immunoglobulin levels in Malaysians. *Lancet* **ii,** 450 (1973).

38. Karayalcin, G., Rosher, F., and Sawitsky, A., Quantitative serum immunoglobulins in healthy negroes. *N. Y. State J. Med.* **73,** 751 (1973).

39. Rhodes, K., Markham, R. L., Raxwell, P. M., and Monk-Jones, M. E., Immunoglobins and the X-chromosome. *Br. Med. J.* **iii,** 439 (1969).

40. Wood, C. S., Martin, W., Adinolfi, M., and Polani, P. E., Immunoglobulins and the X-chromosome. *Br. Med. J.* **iv,** 110 (1969).

41. Grundbacher, F. J., Human X chromosome carrier quantitative genes for immunoglobulin M. *Science* **176,** 311 (1972).

42. Stoop, J. W., Zegers, B. J., Sander, P. C., and Ballieux, R. E., Serum immunoglobulin levels in healthy children and adults. *Clin. Exp. Immunol.* **4,** 101 (1969).

43. Buckley, R. H., Dees, S. C., and O'Fallon, W. M., Serum immunoglobulins: 1. Levels in normal children and in uncomplicated childhood allergy. *Pediatrics* **41,** 600 (1968).

44. Haferkamp, O., Schlettsein-Gsell, D., Schwick, H. G., and Storiko, K., Serum protein in an aging population with particular reference to evaluation of immune globulins and antibodies. *Gerontologia* **12,** 30 (1966).

45. Turner, M. W., and Voller, A., Studies on immunoglobulins of Nigerians 1. The immunoglobulin levels of a Nigerian population. *J. Trop. Med. Hyg.* **69,** 99 (1966).

46. Lamy, J., Titeca, C., and Weill, J., Valeurs de référence des IgA sériques humaines. *Ann. Biol. Clin.* **32,** 529 (1974).

47. Cassidy, J. T., Nordby, G. L., and Dodge, H. J., Biologic variation of human serum immunoglobulin concentrations: Sex-age specific effects. *J. Chronic Dis.* **27,** 507 (1974).

48. McFarlane, H., Immunoglobulins in Nigerians. *Lancet* **ii,** 445 (1966).

49. Maroulis, G. B., Buckley, R. H., and Younger, J. J., Serum immunoglobulin concentration during normal pregnancy. *Am. J. Obstet. Gynecol.* **109,** 971 (1971).

50. Yeager, A. S., Variation in cord IgM level with birth weight. *Pediatrics* **51,** 616 (1973).

51. Winsten, S., Personal communication.

52. Logie, D. E., McGregor, I. A., Rowe, D. S., and Billewicz, W. Z., Plasma immunoglobulin concentrations in mothers and newborn children with special reference to placental malaria. *Bull. WHO* **49,** 547 (1973).

53. Ackerman, B. D., Taylor, W. F., and O'Loughlin, B. J., Serum immunoglobulin levels in postmature infants. *Pediatrics* **43,** 956 (1969).

54. Papadatos, C., Alexiou, D., Papaevangelou, H., et al., Serum levels of immune globulins in postmaturity. *Arch. Dis. Child.* **49,** 222 (1974).

55. Pilgrim, U., Fonanellaz, H. P., Evers, G., and Hitzig, W. H., Normal values of immunoglobulins in premature and in full-term infants, calculated as percentiles. *Helv. Paediatr. Acta* **30,** 121 (1974).

56. Uffelman, J. A., Engelhard, W. E., and Jolliff, C. R., Quantitation of immunoglobulins in normal children. *Clin. Chim. Acta* **28,** 185 (1970).

57. Rowe, D. S., Anderson, S. G., and Tackett, L., A Research Standard for human sera immunoglobulin D. *Bull. WHO* **43,** 607 (1970).

58. Rowe, D. S., Crabbé, P. A., and Turner, M. W., Immunoglobulin D in serum, body fluids and lymphoid tissues. *Clin. Exp. Immunol.* **3,** 477 (1968).

59. Rowe, D. S., McGregor, I. A., Smith, S. J., et al., Plasma immunoglobulin concentrations in a West African (Gambian) community and in a group of healthy British adults. *Clin. Exp. Immunol.* **3,** 63 (1968).

60. Rowe, D. S., Hug, K., Faulk, W. P., et al., IgD on the surface of peripheral blood lymphocytes of the human newborn. *Nature, New Biol.* **242,** 155 (1973).

61. Rowe, D. S., Hug, K., Forni, L., and Pernis, B., Immunoglobulin D as a lymphocyte receptor. *J. Exp. Med.* **138,** 965 (1973).

62. Ishizaka, K., and Ishizaka, T., Reversed type allergic skin reactions by anti-gamma E-globulin antibodies in humans and monkeys. *J. Immunol.* **110,** 556 (1968).

63. Sieber, A., and Becker, W., Quantitative determination of IgE by single radial immunodiffusion, a comparison of three different methods for intensification of precipitates. *Clin. Chim. Acta* **50,** 153 (1974).

64. Rowe, D. S., Grab, B., and Anderson, S. G., An International Reference Preparation for Human Serum Immunoglobulin E. *Bull. WHO* **49,** 320 (1973).

65. Rowe, D. S., Quantitation of IgE in human serum. In *The Biological Role of the Immunoglobulin E System.* K. Ishizaka and D. H. Dayton, Eds., U. S. Dept. HEW Publication No. (NIH) 73-502, 1973, p 47.

66. General Discussion of Session II: Structure, Function, and Quantitation of IgE. In *The Biological Role of the Immunoglobulin E System.* K. Ishizaka and D. H. Dayton, Eds. U. S. Dept. of HEW Publication No. (NIH) 73-502, 1973, p 56.

67. Johansson, S. G. O., Serum IgND levels in healthy children and adults. *Int. Arch. Allergy* **34,** 1 (1968).

68. Rowe, D. S., and Wood, C. B. S., The measurement of serum immunoglobulin E levels in healthy adults and children and in children with allergic asthma. *Int. Arch. Allergy* **39,** 1 (1970).

69. Gleich, G. J., Averbeck, A. K., and Swedlund, H. A., Measurement of IgE in normal and allergic serum by radioimmunoassay. *J. Lab. Clin. Med.* **77,** 690 (1971).

70. Arbesman, C. E., Iro, K., Wypych, J. I., and Wicher, K., Measurement of serum IgE by a one-step single radial radiodiffusion method. *J. Allergy Clin. Immunol.* **49,** 72 (1972).

71. Gerrard, J. W., Horne, S., Vickers, P., et al., Serum IgE levels in parents and children. *J. Pediatr.* **85,** 660 (1974).

72. Orren, A., and Dowdle, E. B., IgE-analysis of serum level in 4700 blood donors with special reference to effect of age and sex. *S. Afr. Med. J.* **47,** 967 (1973).

73. Orren, A., and Dowdle, E. B., The effects of sex and age on serum IgE concentrations in three ethnic groups. *Int. Arch. Allergy Appl. Immunol.* **48,** 824 (1975).

74. Johansson, S. G. O., Mellbin, T., and Vahlquist, B., Immunoglobulin levels in Ethiopian preschool children with special reference to high concentrations of immunoglobulin E (IgND). *Lancet* **i,** 1118 (1968).

75. Nye, L., Merrett, T. G., Landon, J., and White, R. J., A detailed investigation of circulating IgE levels in a normal population. *Clin. Allergy* **1,** 13 (1975).

76. Houba, V., and Rowe, D. S., A comparison of African and European serum levels of immunoglobulin E. *Bull. WHO* **49,** 539 (1973).

77. Van der Giessen, M., Rossouw, E., Algra-van Veen, T., et al., Quantification of IgG subclasses in sera of normal adults and healthy children between 4 and 14 years of age. *Clin. Exp. Immunol.* **21,** 501 (1975).

78. Shakib, F., Stanworth, D. R., Drew, R., and Catty, D., A quantitative study of the distribution of IgG sub-classes in a group of normal human sera. *J. Immunol. Methods* **8,** 17 (1975).

79. Bokhout, B. A., Divergent results in radial immunodiffusion with antisera differing in precipitation properties with respect to individual immunoglobulin substances. II The antiserum factor. *J. Immunol. Methods* **7,** 199 (1975).

CLIN. CHEM. 22/5, 602-606 (1976)

Radioimmunoassay of Bile Acids in Serum

Laurence M. Demers and Gershon Hepner

We developed four radioimmunoassay procedures for the determination of glycine-conjugated bile acids in serum. Antibodies to two primary bile acids, cholylglycine and chenodeoxycholylglycine, and to two secondary bile acids, sulfolithocholylglycine and deoxycholylglycine, were raised in rabbits after the acids were covalently linked to albumin by use of the carbodiimide reaction. Assay sensitivity for each of these bile acids is in the picomole range with the standard curve extending from 10-80 pmol. The concentration of bile acids in serum is increased in various states of liver disease and its measurement appears to be an extremely sensitive indicator of liver function.

Additional Keyphrases: *liver function test • diagnostic differentiation of hepatic disease • normal values • cancer • antibody specificity*

Sherlock and Walshe (*1*) first showed that bile acids are increased in the serum of patients with hepatobiliary disease. Since then it has been established that the concentration of bile acids in serum can reflect states of liver function and the integrity of the biliary system (*2-11*). Makino et al. (*5*), using gas chromatography, measured serum bile acids in patients with various liver diseases and found significant correlations with the status of liver function. More recently, Simmonds et al. (*8*) developed the radioimmunoassay approach to serum bile acid measurement and successfully raised antibodies to conjugates of cholic acid. They used this assay to study concentrations of cholate conjugates in patients with chronic active hepatitis and anicteric viral hepatitis (*11*).

Departments of Pathology and Medicine, The M. S. Hershey Medical Center, The Pennsylvania State University, Hershey, Pa. 17033.

Presented in part at the 9th International Congress of Clinical Chemistry, Toronto, Canada, July 1975.

Received Nov. 14, 1975; accepted Feb. 11, 1976.

Since that report, we have developed a highly specific radioimmunoassay for four glycine-conjugated bile acids, two primary and two secondary bile acids: cholic (3α,7α,12α-trihydroxy-5β-cholanoic acid), chenodeoxycholic (3α,7α-dihydroxy-5β-cholanoic acid), deoxycholic (3α,12α-dihydroxy-5β-cholanoic acid), and sulfolithocholic acid (3α-hydroxy-5β-cholanoic acid sulfate). This radioimmunoassay is detailed here.

Materials and Methods

Preparation and Characterization of Antibodies

Preparation of immunogen. We prepared bile acid/albumin conjugates by covalently coupling bovine serum albumin to bile acids, by using the carbodiimide reaction. Bile acids (Maybridge Chemical Company, Tintagel, Cornwall, England) were purified by thin-layer chromatography on silicic acid plates in the solvent system isoamyl acetate/propionic acid/*n*-propanol/water (40/30/40/10 by vol). We combined 10 mg of purified bile acid in 0.8 ml of ethanol with 16 mg of fatty acid-free bovine serum albumin in 7.2 ml of distilled de-ionized water. With constant stirring, 8 mg of carbodiimide [1-ethyl-3-(3-dimethyl-amino propyl)-carbodiimide hydrochloride] was added. The total mixture was then vortex-mixed and allowed to stand at −20 °C for 24 h. After equilibration at room temperature, the mixture was extensively dialyzed against phosphate-buffered physiological saline (10 mol of phosphate per liter, pH 7.4) at 4 °C for 72 h. Use of radiolabeled bile acids in the original reaction mixture indicated that a consistent 30-35% of the bile acid had become conjugated to bovine serum albumin. We stored 0.5-ml aliquots of the dialyzed conjugate at −20 °C for subsequent injection.

Immunization. Adult New Zealand rabbits were

Table 1. Cholylglycine Antiserum Specificity

Compound	Relative cross reaction, %
Cholylglycine	100
Cholyltaurine	18
Cholic acid	8
Chenodeoxycholylglycine	4
Chenodeoxycholic acid	4
Deoxycholylglycine	1
Deoxycholic acid	<0.1
Lithocholic acid	<0.1
Lithocholylglycine	3
Sulfolithocholylglycine	1
Chenodeoxycholyltaurine	<0.2
Deoxycholyltaurine	<0.1
Lithocholyltaurine	<0.1
Cortisol	<0.1
Cholesterol	<0.1
Estrogen	<0.1
Testosterone	<0.3
Progesterone	<0.3

Table 2. Chenodeoxycholylglycine Antiserum Specificity

Compound	Relative cross reaction, %
Chenodeoxycholylglycine	100
Chenodeoxycholyltaurine	8
Chenodeoxycholic acid	1
Lithocholyltaurine	0.3
Lithocholylglycine	0.3
Cholyltaurine	<0.1
Lithocholic acid	<0.1
Deoxycholylglycine	<0.1
Deoxycholic acid	<0.1
Deoxycholyltaurine	<0.1

injected with 0.5 ml of the conjugate preparation that had been emulsified with 0.5 ml of complete Freund adjuvant. The injections were made at four or five different sites once a week for four weeks and then a booster injection monthly. Rabbits were bled from the marginal ear vein after one month and then 10 days after the monthly booster injection. The resulting antiserum was lyophilized and subsequently characterized for specificity for each of the four bile acids. The highest titers were those for antisera collected about six months after the initial conjugate injection.

Specificity of antisera. The relative specificity of each bile acid antiserum is shown in Tables 1–4. Relative cross reactivity is expressed in percentage, as the mass required to displace 50% of bound radiolabeled bile acid from its respective antibody. There was no significant cross reactivity with any of the compounds tested.

Table 3. Deoxycholylglycine Antiserum Specificity

Compound	Relative cross reaction, %
Deoxycholylglycine	100
Deoxycholic acid	16
Deoxycholyltaurine	3
Lithocholic acid	<0.1
Lithocholylglycine	<0.1
Sulfolithocholylglycine	<0.1
Chenodeoxycholic acid	<0.1

Table 4. Sulfolithocholylglycine Antiserum Specificity

Compound	Relative cross reaction, %
Sulfolithocholylglycine	100
Lithocholylglycine	6
Chenodeoxycholylglycine	0.4
Cholylglycine	<0.1
Deoxycholylglycine	<0.1
Lithocholic acid	<0.1
Sulfodeoxycholic	5
Sulfochenodeoxycholylglycine	1

Radioimmunoassay Procedure

Radioimmunoassays were done in duplicate, in 12 × 75 mm acid-washed disposable test tubes. Standards of cholylglycine, chenodeoxycholylglycine, deoxycholylglycine, and sulfolithocholylglycine were dissolved in the phosphate-buffered saline, and used in amounts ranging from 5 to 80 pmol to prepare the radioimmunoassay standard curve.

Standards and patients' sera in dilutions ranging from threefold to 20-fold, depending on serum bile acid concentrations, were added to each tube in 0.1-ml aliquots. This was followed by 0.1 ml of antiserum, diluted in buffer to a concentration at which 50% of the radiolabeled bile acid was bound. Then 0.1 ml of radiolabeled bile acids (New England Nuclear, Worcester, Mass. 01608) with radioactivity equivalent to about 10 000 cpm was added to each tube, including the blank and total count tubes.

The tubes were then gently shaken by vortex-type mixing and allowed to equilibrate, first for 60 min at 42 °C, then at 4 °C for 18–24 h.

After this equilibration, 0.1 ml of twofold diluted normal rabbit serum, free of bile acids, was added to each tube. The bile acid-free serum was prepared by charcoal extraction, the charcoal was removed by centrifugation, and the serum was aspirated through a 45-mm diameter Millipore filter (Millipore Corp., Bedford, Mass. 01730).

Antibody-bound and free bile acids were then separated by adding 1 ml of ammonium sulfate (600 g/liter). The mixture was vortex-mixed, allowed to stand on ice for 10 min, and then centrifuged at 2000 rpm for 20 min.

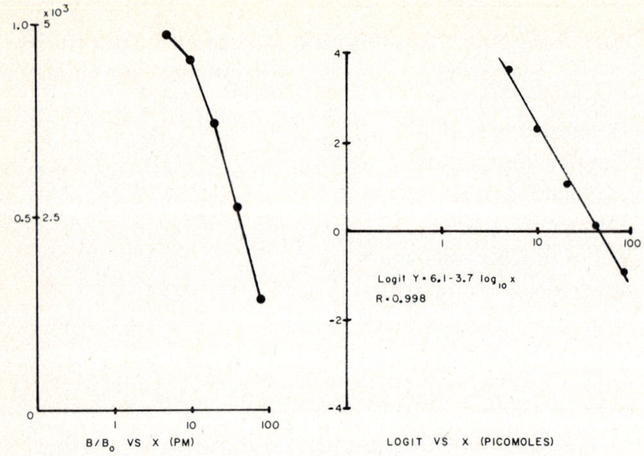

Fig. 1.

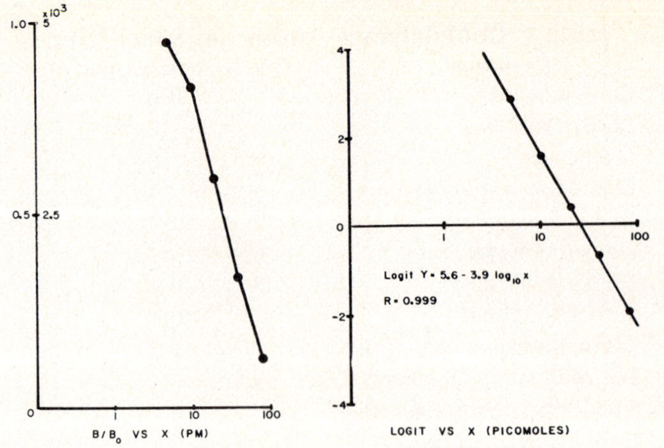

Fig. 2.

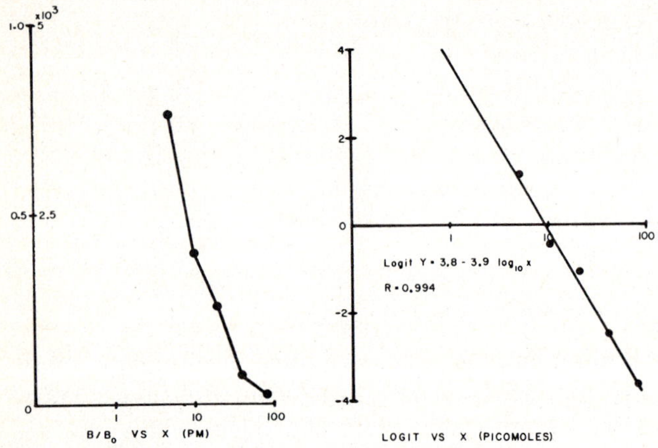

Fig. 3.

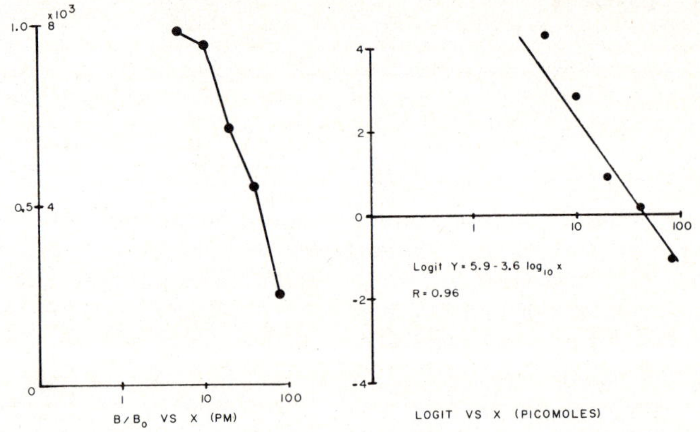

Fig. 4.

Fig. 1–4. Standard curves for radiommunoassay of glycocholic acid, glycochenodexoycholic acid, sulfolithocholylglycine, and glycodexoxycholic acid, respectively

In each Figure, curve on *left* represent B/B_0 plotted vs. log dose concentration. Curve on *right* reflects a logit transformation of B/B_0 vs. log dose concentration

The supernate was then decanted directly into scintillation vials containing 10 ml of "Aquasol" (New England Nuclear, Worcester, Mass. 01608) scintillation fluid.

Radioactivity was determined with an Analytic Isocap 300 Liquid Scintillation Counter (Searle Analytic Inc., Des Plaines, Ill. 60018). Data appeared on paper punch tape and were automatically reduced by using Rodbard (*12*) statistics of logit plot analysis with weighted linear regression. Figures 1 to 4 show characteristic standard curves of B/B_0 (counts bound for an arbitrary dose relative to that for zero dose) and logit transformation for each of the four bile acids studied.

Assay Sensitivity and Accuracy

Sensitivity. As shown by the data for the standard curve, as little as 10 pmol of standard bile acid can displace significant amounts of tracer at an antibody titer binding 50% of labeled hormone. Thus the standard curve range was set at 10–80 pmol.

Accuracy. To validate the individual bile acid radioimmunoassays, recovery and parallelism studies were performed with each assay.

(*a*) Recovery Studies. The accuracy of the different bile acid assays was reflected in the analytical recovery of the four individual bile acids added to bile acid-free serum. Figures 5 and 6 show representative recovery studies for two of the bile acid radioimmunoassays. Measured and expected bile acid values agreed well for each of the four bile acids determined, with the linear relationship between amount added and amount found that extended to 10 nmol.

(*b*) Parallelism. A necessary condition for assay specificity is parallelism. As shown in Figures 7 and 8, we assayed serial dilutions of a pool of serum with an abnormally high bile acid and found that the relation between bile acid concentrations measured and

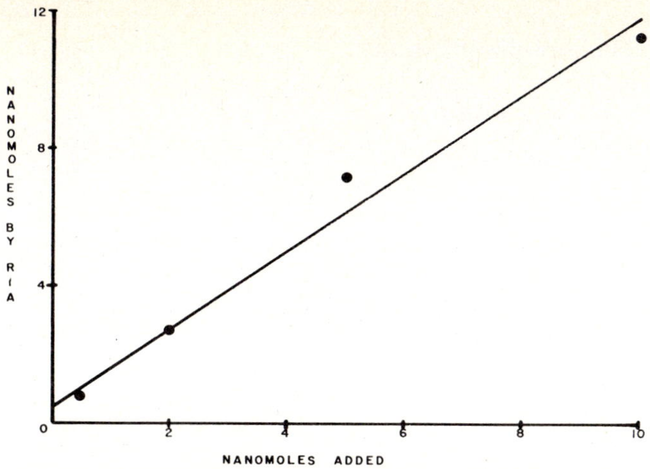

Fig. 5. Glycochenodeoxycholic acid recovery study
Indicated amounts of this acid were added to bile acid-free serum and the samples assayed for it. $r = 0.9903$

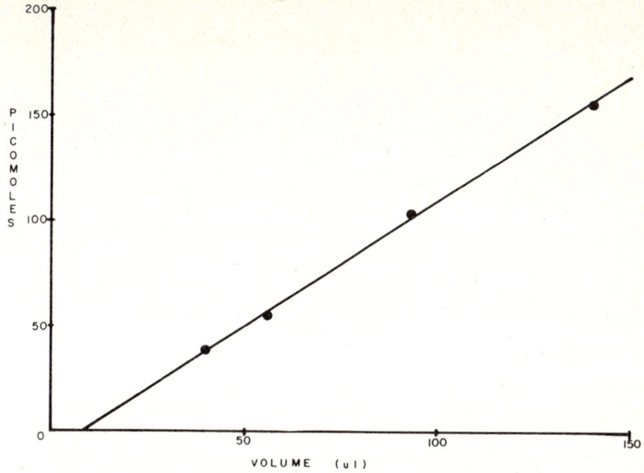

Fig. 7. Glycochenodeoxycholic acid parallel study
Different concentrations of a high-value patient's sample were radioimmunoassayed for this acid serum volume and plotted vs. the concentration determined

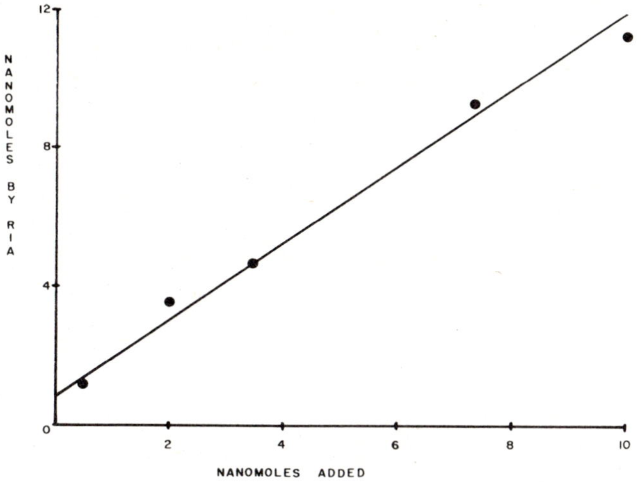

Fig. 6. Sulfolithocholylglycine recovery study
Different amounts of this acid were added to bile acid-free serum and the samples assayed for it. $r = 0.9986$

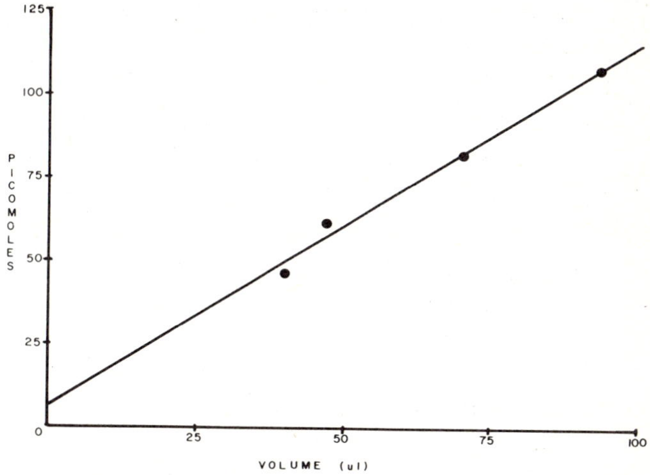

Fig. 8. Glycocholic acid parallel study
Done as described in legend to Figure 7

the concentrations used in the assay was linear for each of the four bile acids determined.

Normal Values and Concentrations of the Individual Bile Acids in Serum in Various States of Hepatobiliary Disease

To establish the clinical relevance of these individual bile acids in health and disease, we determined the individual bile acids in the serum of 25 control subjects with no evidence of liver disease, of 40 patients with known hepatic malignancy confirmed by liver biopsy, of 22 patients with cholestasis, of 14 patients with diagnosed hepatitis, and of 34 patients with portal cirrhosis (Table 5). The control values were consistent with values previously reported by other investigators, who used gas chromatography. In hepatobiliary disease the concentration of bile acids is significantly higher than in controls, with several-hundred-fold increases seen in certain bile acids in cases of liver cancer and hepatitis.

Discussion

The antisera produced against the bile acids were highly specific, with negligible cross reactivity between different structurally related forms of bile acids. The sensitivity of these radioimmunoassays is such that picomole amounts can be determined in serum. Because bile acids are present in nanomole concentrations, these assays are convenient for measuring basal values as well as pathologically increased values.

As shown by Hofmann et al. (*10, 11*), serum bile acids as determined by radioimmunoassay proved to be a more sensitive index to liver disease than other conventional indexes of liver function such as aspartase aminotransferase, bilirubin, sodium sulfobromo-

Table 5. Serum Bile Acids in Hepatobiliary Disease

Patients	No.	CG[a]	CDG	DG	SLCG
		μmol/liter[b]			
Controls	25	0.27 ± 0.03[c]	0.20 ± 0.03	0.06 ± 0.01	0.06 ± 0.01
Cirrhosis	34	57.2 ± 19.4	1.56 ± 0.09	0.33 ± 0.05	1.26 ± 0.20
Hepatitis	14	120.6 ± 51.1	0.88 ± 0.08	0.20 ± 0.04	1.15 ± 0.25
Cholestasis	22	24.6 ± 1.2	15.20 ± 1.50	0.12 ± 0.67	1.76 ± 1.23
Liver cancer	40	94.1 ± 44.2	0.91 ± 0.11	0.16 ± 0.04	1.92 ± 0.63

[a] Abbreviations: CG, cholylglycine; CDG, chenodeoxycholylglycine; DG, deoxycholylglycine; and SLCG, sulfolithocholylglycine.
[b] Results are expressed in micromoles of glycine-conjugated bile acids per liter of serum.
[c] Mean ± SD.

phthalein (Bromsulphalein) retention, alkaline phosphatase activity, or total protein, in that increased concentrations of bile acids in the serum preceded any change in these other liver-function tests in patients who relapsed into liver dysfunction. Because of the convenience and simplicity of the radioimmunoassay, this technique promises to be of major use in the detection of biochemically "silent" liver disease (*10*). Moreover, the relative production of the various bile acids may be of diagnostic value in differentiating various forms of liver disease (*3*).

We acknowledge financial support from the Pharmaceutical Manufacturers Research Association and the technical assistance of Kathy Smith, Rick Roberts, Naomi Cole, and Marie Miller.

References

1. Sherlock, S., and Walshe, V., Blood cholates in normal subjects and in liver disease. *Clin. Sci.* **6,** 223 (1948).

2. Rudman, D., and Kendall, R. E., Bile acid content of human serum. I. Serum bile acids in patients with hepatic disease. *J. Clin. Invest.* **36,** 530 (1957).

3. Carey, J. B., The serum trihydroxy-dihydroxy bile acid ratio in liver and biliary tract disease. *J. Clin. Invest.* **37,** 1494 (1958).

4. Osborn, E. C., Wootton, I. D. P., DaSilva, L. C., and Sherlock, S., Serum bile acids in liver disease. *Lancet* **ii,** 1049 (1959).

5. Makino, I., Nakagawa, S., and Maskimo, K., Conjugated and unconjugated serum bile acid levels in patients with heptobiliary diseases. *Gastroenterology* **56,** 1033 (1969).

6. Neale, G., Lewis, B., Weaver, V., and Panveliwalla, D., Serum bile acids in liver disease. *Gut* **12,** 145 (1971).

7. Kaplowitz, N., Kok, E., and Javitt, M. B., Postprandial serum bile acid for the detection of hepatobiliary disease. *J. Am. Med. Assoc.* **225,** 292 (1973).

8. Simmonds, W. J., Korman, M. G., Go, V. W. L., and Hofmann, A. F., Radioimmunoassay of conjugated cholyl bile acids in serum. *Gastroenterology* **65,** 705 (1973).

9. Van Berge Henegouwen, G. P., Ruben, A., and Brandt, K. H., Quantitative analysis of bile acids in serum and bile using gas-liquid chromatography. *Clin. Chim. Acta* **54,** 249 (1974).

10. Korman, M. C., Hofmann, A. F., and Summerskill, W. H. J., Assessment of activity of chronic active liver disease: Serum bile acids compared with conventional test and histology. *New Engl. J. Med.* **290,** 1399 (1974).

11. Hofmann, A. F., Korman, M. G., and Krugman, S., Sensitivity of serum bile acid assay for detection of liver damage in viral hepatitis Type B. Prospective study in five patients. *Am. J. Dig. Dis.* **19,** 908 (1974).

12. Rodbard, D., Statistical quality control and routine data processing for radioimmunoassays and immunoradiometric assays. *Clin. Chem.* **20,** 1255 (1974).

13. Demers, L. M., and Hepner, G., Serum bile acids in hepatobiliary disease. Submitted to *Am. J. Dig. Dis.*

CLIN. CHEM. 22/5, 607–610 (1976)

Kinetic Determination of Serum Lipase Activity with the Abbott ABA-100

Ronald D. Feld, David L. Witte, and David A. Barrett II

A turbidimetric procedure for lipase has been adapted for use on the Abbott Bichromatic Analyzer (ABA-100). The method is rapid and results compare well with those by the more traditional method of Cherry and Crandall [*Am. J. Physiol.* **100,** 266 (1932)]. Advantages of this method include shorter incubation time (2 min), smaller sample size (50 μl), neglible interference from bilirubin, and greater dynamic range (to eightfold normal).

An abnormally high activity of α-amylase (EC 3.2.1.1) in serum or urine confirms the clinical diagnosis of acute pancreatitis. However, serum lipase (triacylglycerol acyl-hydrolase, EC 3.1.1.3) activity may increase earlier and remain elevated longer than does amylase activity in acute pancreatitis (*1, 2*). Lifton et al. (*3*) showed that pancreatitis can be detected more frequently when both serum amylase and lipase are determined at the time of a patient's admission.

The traditional Cherry–Crandall titrimetric method for the determination of serum lipase activity has many disadvantages (*4*). The original method required 24 h but subsequent modifications of the method have shortened the incubation time to 6 h. However, this long incubation period makes the determination of serum lipase of limited usefulness in emergency situations. In addition, a relatively large volume of serum (2 ml) is required, the endpoint of the colorimetric titration is highly subjective, and icteric samples affect the color at the endpoint. The need for a serum blank and the lack of a linear relation between titer and enzyme activity (*5*) leaves the accuracy and usefulness of this assay method open to question.

Department of Pathology, University of Iowa, Iowa City, Iowa 52242.

Presented in part at the Ninth International Congress on Clinical Chemistry, Toronto, Ontario, July 1975.

Received Nov. 24, 1975; accepted Feb. 10, 1976.

Shihabi and Bishop (*6*) introduced a turbidimetric method for the determination of serum lipase that overcomes many of the disadvantages of even the modified Cherry–Crandall method. Assay time was decreased so that the test can be offered on an emergency basis. In addition micro samples (50 μl) may be used.

We have adapted the method of Shihabi and Bishop (*6*) for use with the Abbott ABA-100 (Abbott Bichromatic Analyzer; Abbott Labs., Pasadena, Calif. 91030) Commercial quality-control sera is easily used, a serum blank is not necessary, and interference from bilirubin has been eliminated.

Materials and Methods

Methods

Amylase activity was determined by the "Amylochrome" method (Roche Diagnostics, Nutley, N. J. 07110). Enzyme activity in this method is related to the amount of dye-starch complex that is solubilized. Lipase was also determined by the modified Cherry–Crandall method, with use of a substrate supplied by Sigma Chemical Co., St. Louis, Mo. 63178. The incubation time was 6 h at 37 °C. Lyophilized serum containing increased amounts of bilirubin ("Bilirubin Control") was purchased from Dade, Miami, Fla. 33152.

Reagents

Mix 50 ml of olive oil (Fisher Scientific Co.) with 10 g of aluminum oxide for 60 min, allow to settle, and filter. Dissolve 1 g of freshly purified olive oil in 100 ml of absolute ethanol. Dissolve 3.0 g of tris(hydroxymethyl)aminomethane and 6.0 g of sodium deoxycholate[1] in 1 liter of water. Adjust the pH to 8.8

[1] Enzyme activity is slightly greater at a sodium deoxycholic acid concentration of 3 g/liter, but it is less linear than with a 6 g/liter concentration (reviewer's comment).

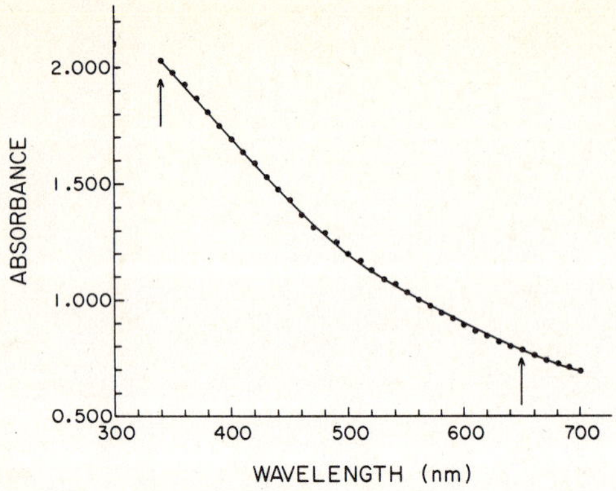

Fig. 1. Absorption spectrum of the olive oil substrate

with concentrated HCl. Add 4 ml of the ethanolic olive oil solution slowly to 100 ml of the Tris buffer, with stirring.

Procedure

The ABA-100 measures the absorbance of a chromogen at two wavelengths. The absorbances at these two wavelengths are then subtracted, resulting in an absorbance difference (A_d). For example, the olive oil substrate used in this procedure has absorbances of 2.030 and 0.790 at 340 nm and 650 nm, respectively (Figure 1). For these two absorbances A_d is 1.240. The instrument has a range of linear response from 0 to about 1.400 A_d. A change with time of the A_d is a rate change and is represented by ΔA_d/time. To observe a positive ΔA_d/time in this reaction, which involves a decrease in ΔA_d/time, program the instrument with the Reaction Direction Switch in the DOWN position. The instrument then subtracts the absorbance at 340 nm from that at 650 nm. This setting gives A_d readings such as 8760 (10 000–1240) and also allows ΔA_d per unit of time to be a positive number.

The ABA-100 is programmed as follows:

Control	*Setting*
Mode	Fast-Kinetic 30′
Position Block Locating Pin	2nd hole
Temperature	37 °C
Operating Mode Selector	Endpoint
Reaction Direction	Down
Decimal Point	0000.
Zero	0000 (air in cuvette)
Calibration Factor	0500
Filter	340/650

Lipase substrate, 1 ml, is manually pipetted into cuvette position No. 2 and succeeding cuvette positions depending on the number of samples to be analyzed. No substrate is added to position No. 1. Empty sample cups are inserted for position No. 1 and for each filled cuvette position to activate the ABA-100 reading system. Substrate is equilibrated at 37 °C for

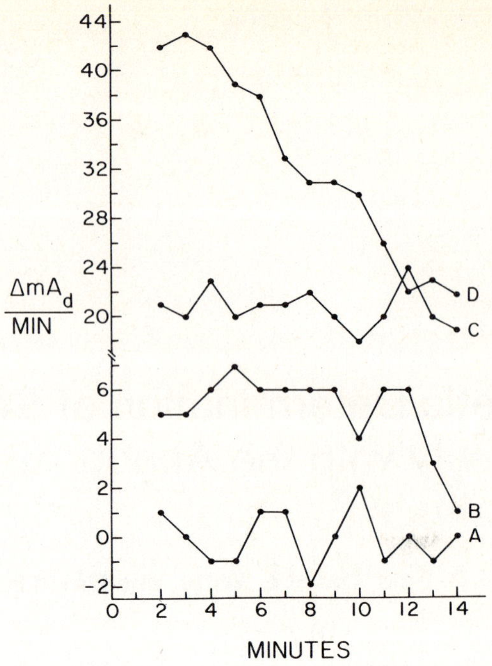

Fig. 2. Reaction rate vs. time for (*A*) substrate alone, (*B*) serum with normal lipase activity, (*C*) serum with twofold normal lipase activity, and (*D*) serum with fourfold normal lipase activity

Table 1. Relation between Initial Absorbance of the Substrate and Change in Absorbance Difference

Initial A_d of the substrate	ΔmA_d/min: Normal patient	ΔmA_d/min: Abnormal patient
8953	6, 6, 6	26, 24, 26
8718	9, 8, 9	30, 31, 30
8573	13, 13, 12	37, 36, 37

5 min. The analysis is initiated by depressing the STOP and then the RUN buttons. Position 1, which contains air, will serve as blank and should read near zero. Position 2, which contains only substrate, will serve as a reagent blank to monitor reagent absorbance and drift (see *Discussion*). Positions 3 to 31 are used for samples. The use of calibration factor 0500 allows readings to be obtained in terms of absorbance difference (A_d). The first reading is stored and the subsequent three readings are taken at 30-s intervals and printed out.

No sample is added to cuvette positions 1 and 2. As cuvette position No. 3 enters the light path, 50 µl of sample is added directly into the cuvette and quickly mixed. The first printed A_d measurement (at 1 min) is subtracted from the third and final measurement (at 2 min) to give a Δ mA_d/min (change, in milliabsorbance units per minute). After the final A_d is printed, the carousel advances one position and the next sample may be added. All measurements are in units of Δ mA_d/min. These units can be converted

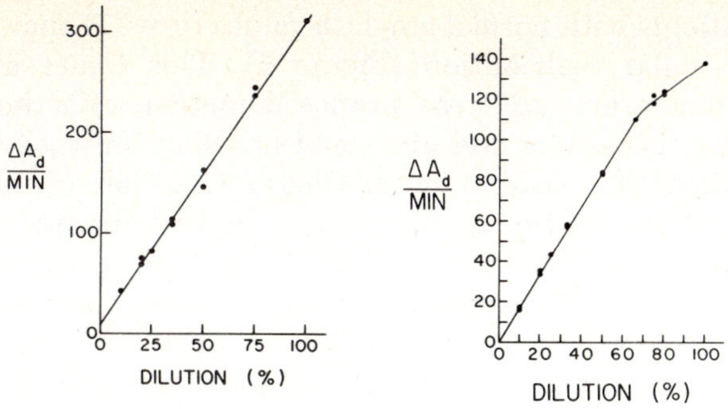

Fig. 3. Linearity of observed lipase activity, as assessed with peritoneal fluid (*left*) and serum (*right*)

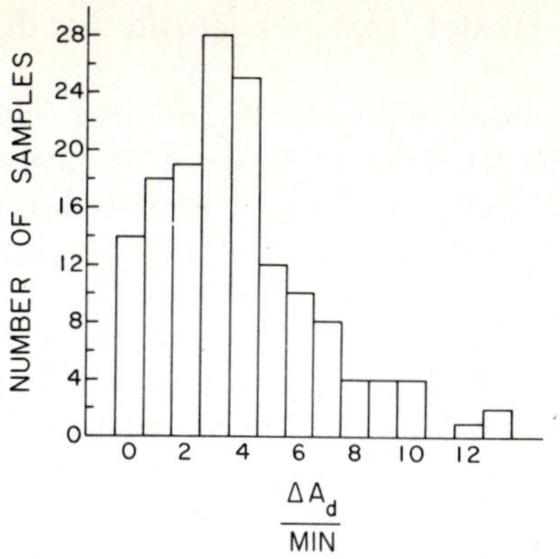

Fig. 4. Lipase activity of serum of 149 persons whose values were normal for routine screening (SMA 12/60)

Table 2. Between-Day and Within-Run Precision of Lipase Assay

	Mean	SD	
	ΔA_d/min		CV, %
Between-day [a]			
Frozen serum pool	7.6	1.3	17.0
Lyophilized serum control	23.3	3.0	13.0
Within-run [b]			
Frozen serum pool	7.3	0.44	6.0
Lyophilized serum control	22.1	0.56	2.5

[a] n = 10 days
[b] n = 28

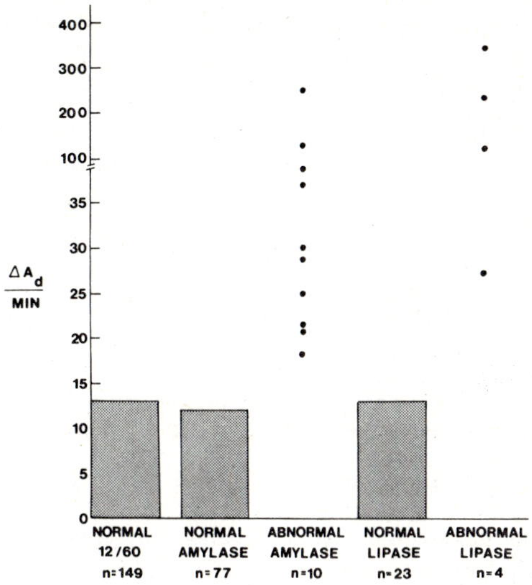

Fig. 5. Range of observed serum lipase activities of (*left to right*) patients with normal values for routine screening (SMA 12/60), normal and above-normal amylase activities by the Amylochrome procedure, and normal and above-normal lipase activities by the Cherry-Crandall procedure

into international (IUB) units (*7*), but it is operationally simpler to use Δ mA_d/min.

Results and Discussion

Figure 1 shows the absorption spectrum of the olive oil emulsion as determined with a Gilford Spectrophotometer (Model 240). A 340 nm/650 nm filter pair produced the greatest adsorbance difference (A_d) and hence the increased sensitivity. Figure 2 shows the kinetics of the reaction. Curve *A* demonstrates the small fluctuation around a rate of 0 Δ mA_d/min of the substrate alone. Curve *B* is a serum from a patient with normal serum lipase activity as determined by the Cherry–Crandall method (*4*). The reaction rate is nearly constant (variance of only 2 Δ mA_d/min) and the Δ mA_d/min is always positive. Curves *C* and *D* represent serum from patients with two- and fourfold the normal serum lipase activity. Curve *C* is almost linear; i.e., the reaction rate is almost constant. Curve *D*, however, has a constant rate for only the first 4 min, in agreement with the findings of others (*6*). In our analysis, rate measurements are made between the first and second minute. This ensures measurement of the initial rate of the reaction.

Table 1 shows the relation of observed lipase activity to initial absorbance of the substrate. Substrates with various initial A_d's were prepared by varying the amounts of ethanolic olive oil solution added to the Tris buffer. Quality-control ranges and normal values should be determined by each individual laboratory by using a substrate with a carefully controlled starting absorbance. We recommend that an initial absorbance for a substrate be maintained within ±50 mA_d units. We routinely use an initial A_d of 8750 ± 50. This provides adequate substrate concentration without exceeding the range of linear response of the instrument.

Figure 3 demonstrates the linearity of the reaction. We used dilutions of a peritoneal fluid and serum from a patient with a high serum lipase activity. Although the readings for the peritoneal fluid are linearly related to activity to 300 Δ mA_d/min units, this relationship is true for the serum to only about 100 Δ mA_d/min units. We think that sera with an initial Δ

mA_d/min greater than 80 should be diluted and rerun.

Table 2 shows between-day and intra-run precision obtained by replicate analysis for 10 days of a frozen serum pool that was stored frozen and a lyophilized control serum with an abnormally high lipase activity.

The presence of high concentrations of bilirubin in a serum makes the determination of lipase by the Cherry–Crandall method more difficult because of the ambiguity in the endpoint indicator color. Bilirubin was added to a serum at various concentrations up to 200 mg/liter and no interference with the lipase determination was noted in the proposed method. Highly lipemic samples may be difficult to analyze by our method because the combined turbidity of sample and substrate may exceed the range of linear response of the instrument. As noted by other authors (*7*), the proposed method is unsuitable for measurement of lipase activity in urine. However, it is uncertain whether there is any lipase activity in urine (*7*).

Figure 4 shows the distribution of data on 149 patients whose SMA 12/60 profiles were normal. The histogram shows a nongaussian distribution, as observed by others (*8*). The central 98% of this population had a range of values from 0 to 10 Δ mA_d/min.[2]

[2] The manufacturer indicates that the variability between filters should be small (much less than 10%); therefore, this procedure should be transferable to another instrument and filter system. However, we suggest that the normal range should be checked with other 340/650 filters.

Ed. note added in proof: In Figures 3–5, "ΔA_d" should read "$\Delta_m A_d$."

Patients with normal amylase values (n = 77) showed a similar distribution (Figure 5). This figure also demonstrates that the proposed method effectively predicts normal and abnormal lipase or amylase activities as measured by the Cherry–Crandall or Amylochrome method, respectively. The turbidimetric lipase method overcomes many of the disadvantages of traditional lipase methods and is faster and more convenient. The sensitivity of the ABA-100 to small changes in absorbance makes it particularly suitable for these measurements.

References

1. Bockus, H. L., and Raffensperger, E. C., Acute pancreatitis. *N. Y. State J. Med.* **48,** 2252 (1948).
2. Song, H., Tietz, N. W., and Tan, C., Usefulness of serum lipase, esterase, and amylase estimation in the diagnosis of pancreatitis: A comparison. *Clin. Chem.* **16,** 264 (1970).
3. Lifton, L. J., Slickers, K. A., Pragay, D. A., and Katz, L. A., Pancreatitis and lipase. *J. Am. Med. Assoc.* **229,** 47 (1974).
4. Cherry, I. S., and Crandall, L. A., Specificity of pancreatic lipase: Its appearance in blood after pancreatic injury. *Am. J. Physiol.* **100,** 266 (1932).
5. Seligson, D., Some thoughts on enzyme measurement. In *Enzymology in the Practice of Laboratory Medicine.* P. Blume and E. Freier, Eds., Academic Press, New York and London, 1974, pp 149–152.
6. Shihabi, Z. K., and Bishop, C., Simplified turbidimetric assay for lipase activity. *Clin. Chem.* **17,** 1150 (1971).
7. Kreutzer, H. H., Penningo, A. W., Punt, J. M., and Verdiun, P. A., Further studies on the determination of lipase activity. *Clin. Chim. Acta* **60,** 273 (1975).
8. Verndiun, P. A., Punt, M. H., and Kreutzer, H. H., Studies on the determination of lipase activity. *Clin. Chim. Acta* **46,** 11 (1973).

CLIN. CHEM. 22/5, 611–615 (1976)

Rapid Radioimmunoassay of Total Urinary Estriol

Dennis W. Anderson and Uwe Goebelsmann

We describe a radioimmunoassay for total urinary estriol in pregnancy. A 25-μl aliquot of the urine specimen is acid hydrolyzed, neutralized, and diluted before assay. We use rabbit antisera against estriol-6-(*O*-carboxymethyl)oxime/bovine serum albumin and ammonium sulfate precipitation at room temperature. Results are unaffected by glucose or methenamine mandelate, a urinary tract antiseptic. Using semi-automatic pipetting equipment, one laboratory technologist can complete 50 assays within 8 h. This technique is both reliable and convenient and should decrease the expense of routine estriol assays.

Additional Keyphrases: *fetal status* • *normal values*

For about 15 years, maternal urinary estriol (E_3) assays have been used as an indicator of fetal status in a variety of high-risk pregnancies (*1*). Although reliable and convenient plasma E_3 radioimmunoassays (RIA's) have been described (*2*), it is still unclear whether plasma E_3 measurements are clinically as useful as urinary E_3 determinations (*3*). Until it has been established which plasma E_3 concentrations or patterns of change indicate fetal distress requiring delivery of a potentially premature infant, many obstetricians will continue to rely upon urinary E_3 assays, for which many procedures have been published.

The few reliable methods are time consuming and costly, and the more numerous "rapid" techniques are insufficiently accurate to be of clinical value. Therefore, we have attempted to develop a rapid RIA for urinary E_3 in pregnancy that would be as reliable as the best conventional methods presently available.

This paper describes a specific RIA for E_3 in highly diluted, unextracted aliquots of urine after hot-acid hydrolysis and neutralization. In this RIA, we used rabbit antiserum to estriol-6-(*O*-carboxymethyl)oxime/bovine serum albumin and ammonium sulfate precipitation.

Department of Pathology and Obstetrics and Gynecology, University of Southern California School of Medicine and Los Angeles County-University of Southern California Medical Center, 1240 N. Mission Road, Los Angeles, Calif. 90033.

Received Sept. 3, 1975; accepted Feb. 20, 1976.

Materials and Methods

Equipment

Centrifuge, nonrefrigerated (Model V-2, equipped with Model IEC-266 horizontal head and six Model IEC-1028, 28-place carriers; International Equipment Co., Needham Heights, Mass. 02194).

Liquid scintillation counter (Model LS 250; Beckman Instruments, Inc., Fullerton, Calif. 92634).

Microburet (Syringe Microburet, Model SB2; Micro-Metric Instrument Co., Cleveland, Ohio 44122).

Pipettor/Dilutor (Beckman).

Reagents

All reagents were of analytical grade, except gelatin. The water used in this assay was demineralized, charcoal-filtered, and doubly glass-distilled.

Phosphate/gelatin buffer, 0.1 mol/liter, pH 6.8 ± 0.1. Prepare by dissolving 4.68 g of NaH_2PO_4, 8.66 g of $NaHPO_4$, 9.0 g of NaCl, 1.0 g of sodium azide, and 1.0 g of Knox unflavored gelatin in 1 liter of water.

Bicarbonate buffer, 1.7 mol/liter, pH 10.0 ± 0.5. Dissolve 80 g of $NaHCO_3$ in 800 ml of water and add 150 ml of NaOH (5 mol/liter), and dilute with water to 1 liter.

Saturated ammonium sulfate solution. Dissolve 300 g of $(NH_4)_2SO_4$ in 1 liter of water in an Erlenmeyer flask at 60 °C and allow to cool to room temperature. Use the supernatant solution.

Radioimmunoassay Components

[6,7-^{3}H]Estriol, listed specific activity of 50 mCi/mol, was purchased from New England Nuclear, Boston, Mass. 02118. Dissolve an amount equivalent to 250 μCi of this compound in 5 ml of ethanol/benzene (7/3 by vol). Check it for radiochemical purity by chromatographing an aliquot, together with authentic E_3 (R_F = 0.09), on paper in benzene/methanol/water (2/1/1 by vol). Store the rest at 4 °C. As needed, dilute 0.5 ml of this solution containing 25 μCi of tritiated E_3 with 4.5 ml of ethanol/water (7/3 by vol) and store the resulting diluted tritiated E_3 stock solution at 4 °C. To prepare a solution of 12 500 cpm of tritiated E_3 per 50 μl of phosphate/gelatin buffer, dilute 0.5 ml of the diluted tritiated E_3 stock solution with 10.0 ml of phosphate/gelatin buffer at the beginning of each RIA.

Authentic estriol was purchased from Steraloids, Wilton, N. H. 03086, and recrystallized twice before use. Prepare a stock solution of 10 mg of estriol in 100 ml of absolute ethanol and store it at −15 °C.

Antiserum. Rabbit anti-estriol-6-(*O*-carboxymethyl)oxime/bovine serum albumin serum was obtained as previously described (*4*). The batch used in this study (R2-09) cross-reacted 68% with 6-oxo-estriol, 6.8% with 16-epi-estriol, 2.7% with 2-hydroxyestriol, 0.2% with estradiol-17β, and <0.01% with estrone, 16α-hydroxyestrone, 16β-hydroxyestrone, or 16-oxo-estradiol-17β. The antiserum was stored undiluted in 0.5-ml aliquots at −15 °C. One 0.5-ml aliquot was thawed as needed, diluted 100-fold by adding 49.5 ml of phosphate/gelatin buffer, divided into ten 5-ml aliquots and stored at −15 °C. One 5-ml aliquot of the 100-fold diluted antiserum was thawed as needed and divided into fifteen 300-μl aliquots, which were stored in liquid-scintillation counting vials at −15 °C. At the beginning of each RIA, one 300-μl aliquot of the 100-fold diluted antiserum was further diluted by adding 15.6 ml of phosphate/gelatin buffer, to give a final 5300-fold dilution. This dilution was used in all assays. The unused portion of this diluted antiserum was discarded each day because it was noted that freezing and thawing of diluted antiserum resulted in rapidly decreasing titers.

Scintillation fluid. Forty-two milliliters of "Liquifluor" (a 2,5-diphenyloxazole/p-bis-[2-(5-phenyloxazoyl)]benzene/toluene mixture, available from New England Nuclear, Boston, Mass. 02118) was added to 1 liter of toluene. The counting efficiency was 55.3% of the tritiated E_3 present in 1.1 ml of the mixture of phosphate/gelatin buffer–ammonium sulfate solution decanted after completion of the RIA into 10 ml of scintillation fluid and extracted into the latter by mixing with a vortex-type mixer.

Procedure

Dispense 25-μl aliquots of urine, together with 0.50 ml of distilled water, with the pipettor/dilutor, and add 1.0 ml of HCl (3.0 mol/liter) to the diluted urine aliquots. Mix with a vortex-type mixer. Cover each of the 16 × 150 mm tubes with a clean glass marble, place them for 30 min in a metal-block heater at 110 °C, and then chill them in ice water. Add 2.0 ml of bicarbonate buffer to neutralize the hydrolysates to pH 6.8–7.0. Dispense 50 μl of each hydrolysate with a third pipettor/dilutor, together with 200 μl of distilled water, into 13 × 100 mm disposable test tubes. To this, add 800 μl of absolute ethanol and mix the contents on a vortex-type mixer.

Dispense 25-μl aliquots of this hydrolyzed, neutralized, and ethanol-diluted urine, together with 200 μl of phosphate/gelatin buffer, in triplicate, into 10 × 75 mm disposable test tubes for RIA. Mix the contents of the 10 × 75 mm RIA tubes on a vortex-type mixer. With a microburet, add 50 μl of phosphate/gelatin buffer containing 12 500 cpm of tritiated E_3 and 100 μl of appropriately diluted antiserum.

Mix the contents of all RIA tubes on a vortex-type mixer and incubate the tubes for 60 min in a water bath at 32 °C. Add 0.80 ml of a saturated $(NH_4)_2SO_4$ solution to all RIA tubes at room temperature, allow the tubes to stand for 2 to 5 min, and then gently agitate the tubes and centrifuge them for 10 min at 3600 × *g*. Decant the supernatant fluid into scintillation vials containing 10 ml of scintillation fluid. Mix the contents of each scintillation vial for 5 s on a vortex-type mixer and allow the scintillation vials to equilibrate for 30 min in the liquid scintillation counter before counting is begun.

Run a standard curve with each assay. Dispense, in triplicate, 25-μl aliquots of standard solutions containing 0, 0.78, 1.56, 3.13, 6.25, 12.5, 25, and 50 ng of E_3 per milliliter of ethanol/water (7/3 by vol) into 10 × 75 mm RIA tubes. Add 200 μl of phosphate/gelatin buffer, 12 500 cpm of tritiated E_3 dissolved in 50 μl of phosphate/gelatin buffer, and 100 μl appropriate diluted antiserum to all tubes and mix the contents on a vortex-type mixer. The total number of cpm of tritiated E_3 present in the supernate after ammonium sulfate precipitation in the absence of antiserum (T), representing total cpm of tritiated E_3 that is not subject to unspecific precipitation by ammonium sulfate, is determined as follows: dispense, in triplicate, 25 μl of ethanol/water (7/3 by vol), 300 μl of phosphate/gelatin buffer and 12 500 cpm of tritiated E_3 dissolved in 50 μl of phosphate/gelatin buffer into 10 × 75 mm RIA tubes. Mix the contents of all tubes on a vortex-type mixer. Do the incubation, ammonium sulfate precipitation, centrifugation, and liquid scintillation counting of all standard curve samples together with and in the same way as that of all unknown samples.

Calculation of Results

The cpm of tritiated E_3 present in the total tubes (T) to which no antiserum was added, and the cpm of free (F) tritiated E_3 were measured in the supernate of all standard and unknown sample tubes. The ratio of free (F) to bound (B) tritiated E_3 was calculated according to the formula $F/B = F/(T\text{-}F)$. Plotting F/B ratios vs. concentrations of E_3 standards, linear standard curves were obtained between 0.78 ng/ml and 50 ng/ml, with correlation coefficients that invariably exceeded 0.99. With a Compucorp Model 265E electronic calculator, the linear regression line for the standard curve was calculated and used to determine the E_3 concentration in all unknown samples. The difference between the results for the zero-tube (no E_3 added to the tritiated E_3/antiserum incubation mixture) and the water blank (25 μl of distilled water processed instead of urine) was subtracted from each unknown sample. The raw values thus obtained for the unknown samples, read as nanograms of E_3 per milliliter, were converted to milligrams of E_3 per milliliter of urine by multiplying the raw values with the factor of 2.961×10^{-3} by which we accounted for sample volume as well as dilutions. Multiplication by the total 24-h urine volume (in milliliters) yielded the entire 24-h urinary E_3 excretion in mg per 24 h. Three 24-h control urines obtained from pregnant women containing 10, 25, and 50 mg of E_3, respectively, as determined by our colorimetric urinary E_3 assay, were analyzed in each RIA. The results for all unknown samples in each RIA were normalized by multiplication with a correction factor determined by dividing the expected control urine values by their actual results observed in that particular RIA. The average correction factor was 1.

Results

Standard Curve

About 60 to 65% of the tritiated E_3 incubated was bound to the antibody when no unlabeled E_3 was added to the tritiated E_3/antiserum incubation mixture (B_0) and about 10% of the tritiated E_3 was bound when 25 μl of an E_3 standard solution was added that contained 50 ng of E_3 per milliliter. Standard curves were prepared by plotting the ratio of F/B vs. E_3 concentration (Figure 1). All standard curves were linear between 0.78 and 50 ng of E_3 per milliliter with correlation coefficients greater than 0.99. When logit transformation (*5*) was used to construct standard curves, plots of logit B/B_0 vs. log E_3 concentration were also linear between 0.78 and 50 ng of E_3 per milliliter (Figure 2). At the dilutions used in this procedure, E_3 concentrations ranging from 2.3 to 148 mg/liter of urine can be measured without altering the urine aliquot used for hydrolysis.

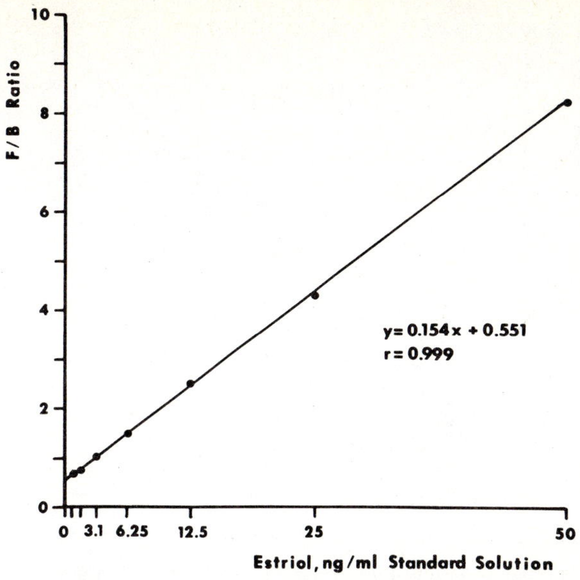

Fig. 1. Standard curve for estriol (E_3) radioimmunoassay (RIA)
The ratio of unbound ("free," F) to antibody-bound (B) [^{3}H]-E_3 is plotted vs. the E_3 concentrations in the standard solutions, of which 25 μl was added to each RIA tube. When no E_3 was added, 62% of the [^{3}H]-E_3 was bound

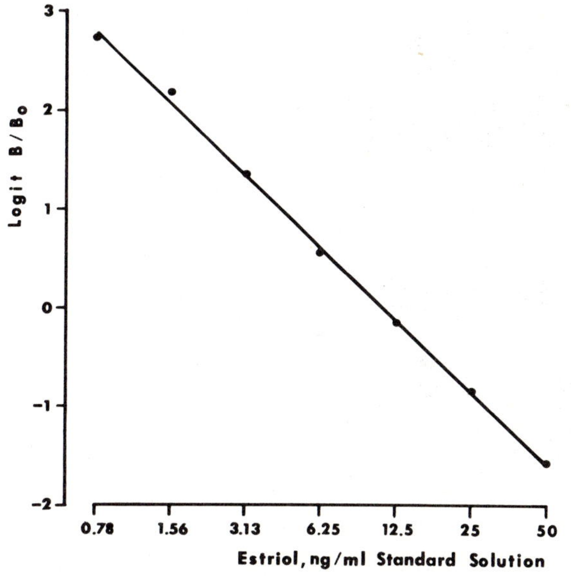

Fig. 2. Logit B/B_0 vs. log estriol (E_3) concentration (*5*)
B represents the amount of [^{3}H]-E_3 bound to the antibody at any given E_3 concentration, B_0 the [^{3}H]-E_3 bound when no E_3 was added, and the E_3 concentrations are those of the standard solutions of which 25 μl was added to each radioimmunoassay (RIA) tube. B was calculated as the difference between the total [^{3}H]-E_3 present in all RIA tubes and the [^{3}H]-E_3 not bound to the antibody

Analytical Variables

Precision. The intra-assay coefficient of variation was determined by assaying 10 aliquots from each of three urine samples averaging 7.1, 27.6, and 49.9 mg of E_3 per liter. The intra-assay coefficients of variation calculated from the results of these determinations were 8.2, 6.2, and 6.7%, respectively. Day-to-day precision was assessed by assaying, on each of two days, aliquots of 100 different urines from women found to excrete 6.2 to 81 mg of E_3 per 24 h. The inter-assay coefficient of variation for these 100 duplicate measurements, done in 17 different RIA's by four different technologists, was 9.98%.

Accuracy. This was assessed by assaying 100 urine samples containing between 5 and 65 mg per 24 h volume by this RIA procedure as well as by our colorimetric procedure, which was shown to be highly accurate (*6*). Comparison of urinary E_3 determined by colorimetry (x) with that assayed by RIA (y) yielded the regression equation $y = 0.992x + 1.28$ and a correlation coefficient $r = 0.953$ (Figure 3). These data indicate that the results obtained with this RIA for urinary E_3 are virtually identical with those measured by our colorimetric technique.

Specificity. The specificity of this RIA depends on the specificity of the antiserum used; ours cross-reacted as described under *Antiserum.* We saw no cross-reaction with neutral steroids. As both estriol-3-sulfate and estriol-3-glucosiduronate are hydrolyzed to E_3, neither one of these two cross-reacting E_3 conjugates will interfere.

Sensitivity. Using the 25-μl urine aliquot and the subsequent dilutions suggested in this RIA procedure, we could measure 2.3 mg of E_3 per liter of urine reliably. Owing to the relative and absolute abun-

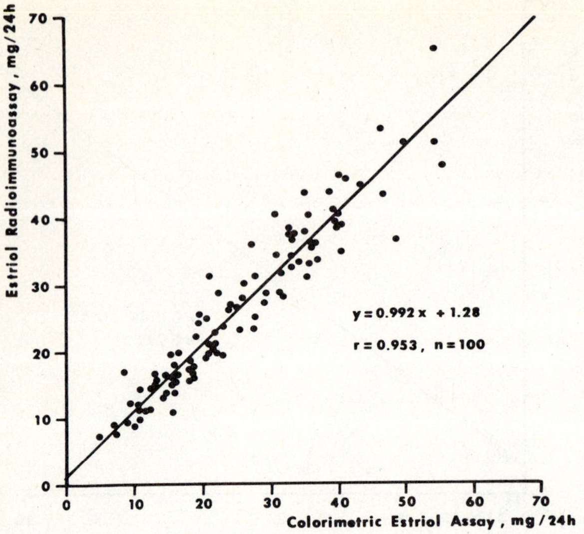

Fig. 3. Correlation between results for 24-hour urinary estriol, as obtained by an accurate colorimetric procedure (*x*) and by the radioimmunoassay technique (*y*) described here

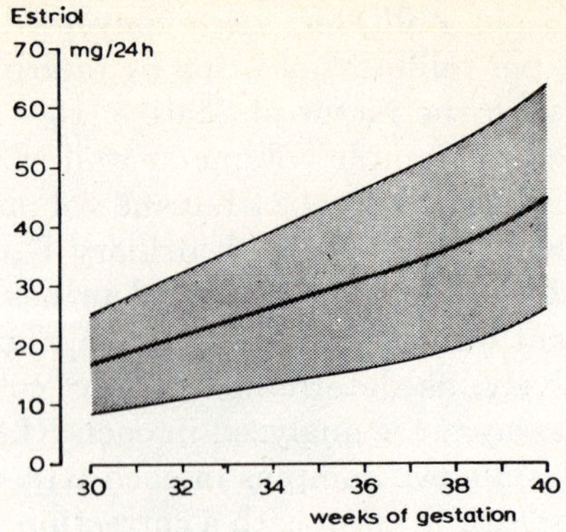

Fig. 4. Means (±2 SD) for 24-h urinary estriol excretion, as measured by our colorimetric method (*6*) during the last 10 weeks of uncomplicated pregnancies

These normal values are found by this RIA as well. [From Goebelsmann et al., *Am. J. Obstet. Gynecol.* **112,** 802 (1972), by permission]

Table 1. Effect of Methenamine Mandelate (MM) on Urinary Estriol Assays for Seven Subjects[a]

Colorimetric assay	Radioimmunoassay	
Without MM[b]	Without MM	With MM
12.8	10.4	11.2
15.5	15.6	15.2
8.6	8.5	7.4
17.7	20.4	17.2
43.9	41.3	34.1
11.2	11.4	11.1
4.6	4.5	4.5

[a] Figures are mg estriol per 24-h urine.

[b] With MM, there was no color and virtually 0% recovery of tritiated estriol-16-glucosiduronate used as internal standard.

dance of E_3 in pregnancy urine, sensitivity does not appear to be at all a limiting factor.

Interfering substances. Glucose added to urine aliquots to concentrations of 20 g per liter had no influence on results of this RIA.

The effect of methenamine mandelate, a urinary tract antiseptic, on this procedure was assessed as follows. A male volunteer ingested 8 g of methenamine mandelate daily (twice the recommended dose) for three days and collected urine during the third day. Urine aliquots from seven women in late pregnancy were diluted with equal volumes of urine collected from the male volunteer before and on the third day of methenamine mandelate intake. All samples were assayed by RIA as well as by our colorimetric procedure. As depicted in Table 1, the RIA results were essentially unchanged whether or not the added male volunteer's urine contained methenamine mandelate. However, colorimetric E_3 determination produced virtually zero readings and 0% recovery of the tritiated estriol-16-glucosiduronate used as internal standard (*6*) when the urinary tract antiseptic was present. These data indicate that methenamine mandelate does not interfere in this RIA.

Normal Values

We conclude from the agreement between the results measured by our colorimetric E_3 assay and by this RIA that the normal values obtained with this method agree with those determined by our colorimetric procedure in uncomplicated pregnancies (Figure 4).

Discussion

The method presented in this paper has been shown to be specific, precise, and accurate. One technician using appropriate semi-automatic pipetting equipment can easily complete 50 triplicate urinary E_3 determinations in 8 h.

Extraction has been eliminated, but acid hydrolysis is still required, because virtually all the E_3 excreted in the urine is conjugated, predominantly as estriol-16-glucosiduronate and estriol-3-glucosiduronate but also as estriol-3-sulfate and estriol-3-sulfate-16-glucosiduronate (*7*). Only estriol-3-sulfate and estriol-3-glucosiduronate cross-react with the antiserum (*4*), but all four E_3 conjugates are readily hydrolyzed to unconjugated E_3 and quantitated by RIA after neutralization of the acid hydrolysate.

Davis and Loriaux (*8*) recently described a simple RIA for urinary E_3 in highly diluted, unhydrolyzed pregnancy urine. This assay is more convenient than the one described in this paper because acid hydrolysis and neutralization are eliminated. Their procedure, however, measures almost exclusively estriol-16-glucosiduronate instead of the sum of all urinary estriol conjugates determined in our assay. About two-thirds of the E_3 produced is excreted as estriol-16-glucosiduronate (*7*). The ratio of urinary estriol-16-glucosiduronate to the sum of all urinary estriol conjugates depends upon estriol metabolism and excretion. It may vary between patients, and from day-to-day in any one patient. We concluded that urinary

E_3 results might vary less if total urinary E_3 was measured instead of estriol-16-glucosiduronate.

Glucose and methenamine mandelate, which are known to interfere with acid hydrolysis in conventional urinary E_3 assays (*9*), have no effect in this procedure, most likely because the 25-μl urine aliquot is diluted 60-fold before acid hydrolysis. Comparison of results for urinary E_3 obtained by our RIA procedure with those observed by our colorimetric technique—in which tritiated estriol-16-glucosiduronate is used as internal standard and solvent partitions, methylation, and chromatography are used for specificity (*6*)—indicate that this urinary E_3 RIA is virtually accurate without correcting for losses that might occur during acid hydrolysis. This may be explained by the possibility that other estrogens present in the hydrolysate, particularly 6-oxo-estriol, may increase the RIA estimate of E_3, compensating for such losses.

In contrast to the dextran-coated charcoal separation procedure, the ammonium sulfate technique is not particularly affected by time or temperature, eliminating the need for low-temperature equilibrium, a refrigerated centrifuge, and rapid centrifugation to separate supernate and precipitate. Statistically accurate counts are obtained more rapidly when unbound tritiated E_3 in the ammonium sulfate supernate is counted instead of antibody-bound tritiated E_3 present in the supernatant fluid after dextran-coated charcoal separation. Furthermore, unbound tritiated E_3 is easily extracted from the ammonium sulfate supernate by the toluene scintillation fluid. Expensive solubilizers used to dissolve aqueous material in toluene, and which reduce counting efficiency, are not required. Under the conditions described in this paper, counting time for a ±3% counting error averaged 1 min per vial.

Utilization of ^{125}I-labeled instead of tritiated E_3 as radioligand would further decrease the cost of this RIA by eliminating expenses for liquid scintillation counting vials and liquid. Many laboratories which have gamma counters but no liquid scintillation counter could perform this technique if ^{125}I-labeled E_3 were used.

As described in this paper, calculation can be done without electronic data-handling equipment. However, use of such equipment in combination with appropriate programs utilizing logit transformation (*5*) would save time and eliminate miscalculation caused by human error or use of inappropriate standard curves or parts thereof. We consider it essential to use in each assay a low, medium, and high urinary E_3 pool that has been standardized by a reliable method. Deficiencies in any part of the assay, including hydrolysis and data handling, will be reflected by a deviation of the results for the pools. Normalizing all assay results by multiplication by the average actual pool result and division by the average expected pool result provided clinically reliable data in some 4500 individual urinary E_3 RIA's performed during the past 12 months.

In summary, this method is an accurate, precise, specific, convenient and economical technique for measuring urinary E_3 in pregnancy. It is a considerable improvement of our previous urinary RIA procedure for E_3, which, because of the use of an unspecific antiserum, had to include ether extraction and solvent partition before RIA (*10*).

We gratefully acknowledge the expert technical assistance of Misses K. M. Hullett, M. Acero, M. C. Clark and P. Mak. This work was supported, in part, by Grant HD 05932 from the National Institute of Child Health and Human Development, USPHS, Bethesda, Md.

References

1. Beischer, N. A., and Brown, J. B., Current status of estrogen assays in obstetrics and gynecology. Part 2: Estrogen assays in late pregnancy. *Obstet. Gynecol. Surv.* **27,** 303 (1972).

2. Goebelsmann, U., Katagiri, H, Stanczyk, F. Z., et al., Estriol assays in obstetrics. *J. Steroid Biochem.* **6,** 703 (1975).

3. Katagiri, H., Distler, W., Freeman, R. K., a Goebelsmann, U., Estriol in pregnancy. IV. Normal concentrations, diurnal and/or episodic variations and day-to-day changes of unconjugated and total estriol in late pregnancy plasma. *Am. J. Obstet. Gynecol.* **124,** 272 (1976).

4. Katagiri, H., Stanczyk, F. Z., and Goebelsmann, U., Estriol in pregnancy. III. Development, comparison and use of specific antisera for rapid radioimmunoassay of unconjugated estriol in pregnancy plasma. *Steroids* **24,** 225 (1974).

5. Feldman, H., and Rodbard, D., Mathematical theory of radioimmunoassay. In *Principles of Competitive Protein-Binding Assays,* W. D. Odell, and W. H. Daughaday, Eds., J. B. Lippincott, Philadelphia, Pa., 1971, p 158.

6. Goebelsmann, U., A reliable method for the determination of urinary estriol in pregnancy. *Clin. Chim. Acta* **23,** 469 (1969).

7. Goebelsmann, U., and Jaffe, R. B., Oestriol metabolism in pregnant women. *Acta Endocrinol.* (Copenhagen) **66,** 679 (1971).

8. Davis, S. E., and Loriaux, D. L., A simple specific assay for estriol in maternal urine. *J. Clin. Endocrinol. Metab.* **40,** 895 (1975).

9. Bolognese, R. J., Corson, S. L., and Touchstone, J. C., Factors affecting the yield of urinary estriol. *Obstet. Gynecol.* **39,** 683 (1972).

10. Goebelsmann, U., Thorneycroft, I. H., Nakamura, R. M., and Mishell, D. R., Jr., Estriol in pregnancy. I. A radioimmunoassay for urinary estriol. *Am. J. Obstet. Gynecol.* **112,** 802 (1972).

CLIN. CHEM. 22/5, 616-622 (1976)

Improved Specificity of Serum Albumin Determination and Estimation of "Acute Phase Reactants" by Use of the Bromcresol Green Reaction

Jan E. C. Gustafsson

The reaction of serum samples with bromcresol green proceeds in two steps. Albumin is responsible for the faster (<1 min) reaction; the slower (30-min) reaction is a measure of "acute phase reactant(s)" in serum. Serum is simply mixed with bromcresol green reagent and the absorbance is measured twice, immediately and at 60 min. Albumin concentrations, determined from the absorbance at 0 min, correlate well with those determined by Laurell "rocket" immunoelectrophoresis; $r = 0.95$ with no certain deviation from unity for the slope and with a negligible difference at zero concentration. The slow reaction was expressed as $\Delta A\% = 100\ (\Delta A_s/\Delta A_v)$ where ΔA_s and ΔA_v are the changes in absorbance between 60 and 0 min for the sample and a commercial control serum, respectively. The value for $\Delta A\%$ correlates well with the percentage of α_2-fraction as determined by electrophoresis on cellulose acetate, as well as with orosomucoid and ceruloplasmin, all of which are acute phase reactant(s). Whether these proteins or other acute phase reactant(s) actually cause the slow reaction has not yet been established.

Many methods have been described for determining albumin in serum (*1–17*), among them various dye-binding methods such as 2-(4′-hydroxyazobenzene)-benzoic acid (HABA) (*6–8*), methyl orange (*9, 10*) and bromcresol green (BCG) (*11–17*).

The dye-binding methods are simple, rapid, suitable for automation, and can be routinely used for many samples in the ordinary clinical laboratory. The reagents are easy to prepare, inexpensive, and stable. However, it has been claimed that they are not very specific. The bromcresol green method has been investigated by several authors, and although its specificity is better than that of another commonly used method (*13*), for example, it has only been recommended as a screening method (*14–16*). Results by the bromcresol green method do not compare well with more specific methods for albumin determination, especially in the clinically important lower concentration range (*15, 17*), the BCG method giving artifactually high values for such sera. In contrast, agreement is good for albumin concentrations near 40 g/liter.

Our own experience with different BCG methods suggests that the method described by Doumas et al. (*12*) is superior. The standard curve is linear, with suitable absorbances of the final solutions over the desired concentration range. Moreover, these authors evaluated the susceptibility of the method to possible interfering substances.

We made the fundamental observations reported here during an attempt to standardize the BCG method within a laboratory group in Sweden. The aim of our studies was to optimize the standardization and to improve the performance of the method.[1] We demonstrate here that the reaction of BCG with serum samples proceeds in two stages, one fast and one slow; albumin causes the fast reaction and the slow reaction is with other serum proteins.

Materials and Methods

BCG method

Reagents. The reagents were those for the manual method described by Doumas et al. (*12*). Bromcresol green from Hopkin & Williams Ltd (Romford RM1 1HA Essex, England) was used.

Kabi protein standard (KABI AB, S-104 25 Stockholm, Sweden) was used. This standard is a 100 g/liter solution of at least 98% pure human serum albumin, pH 7.3, containing no stabilizers or preservatives. This standard was diluted with distilled water to contain 20, 40, and 60 g/liter.

Department of Clinical Chemistry, Central Hospital, S - 721 89 Västerås, Sweden.
Received Jan. 1, 1976; accepted Feb. 24, 1976.

[1] Some of the results were presented at the XV Nordic Congress on Clinical Chemistry in Aarhus, Denmark, 25–27 June 1975.

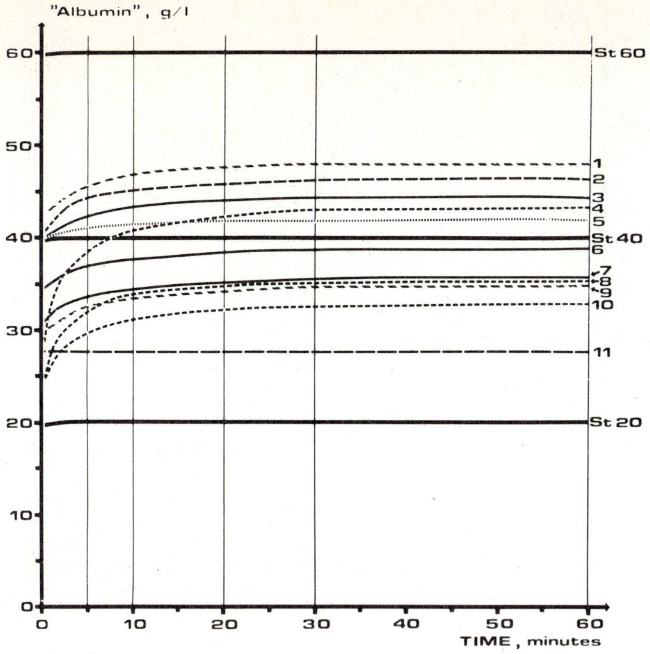

Fig. 1. The time course of color development with BCG for different samples

Apparent "albumin" values (g/liter) on the ordinate. *St20, St40*, and *St60* are pure human albumin standards, 20, 40, and 60 g/liter, respectively. *11*, albumin fraction from preparative electrophoresis; *3, 6, 7*, normal patients' sera; *2*, patient serum with a slight inflammatory response; *10*, patient serum with a moderate degree of inflammatory response; *4, 8*, patient sera with intense inflammatory response; *5*, newborn; *1*, human control serum (Versatol); and *9*, horse control serum (Seronorm)

The commercial lyophilized human control serum we used was "Versatol" (General Diagnostics, Morris Plains, N. J. 07950) and the commercial lyophilized equine control serum used was "Seronorm" (Nyegaard & Co AS, Oslo, Norway).

Apparatus. Absorbances were measured at 629 nm with a Model 124 spectrophotometer (Coleman Instruments Division, Maywood, Ill. 60153) equipped with an original water-thermostatted sample cell assembly set at 25 °C, and a recorder with a balancing time of less than 0.5 s/250 mm.

Procedure. Pipet 2.0 ml of dye solution[2] into a measuring cuvette and into a blank cuvette. Add 10 μl of the serum sample or standard to the measuring cuvette with a disposable capillary micro pipette and stir immediately. Note the exact time of mixing. Follow the increase in absorbance for 2–3 min on the recorder before the next sample is measured. After 60 min at room temperature, again measure the absorbances of all standards and sera.

Electroimmunoassay (EIA)

We used the Laurell (*4, 18*) "rocket" technique. We added antihuman albumin antiserum to a 10 g/liter solution of buffered Induboise A37 Agarose (L'Industrie Biologique Francaise S.A., Gennevilliers, Seine, France) at 53–54 °C.

The rabbit antihuman albumin serum was obtained from Dr. B. G. Johansson, Department of Clinical Chemistry, University Hospital, S-221 85 Lund, Sweden. The specificity of the antiserum was tested by crossed immunoelectrophoresis with intermediate gel (*18, 19*). The intermediate gel contained the antiserum to be tested and the rest of the plate was covered with antihuman (polyvalent) serum (Dakopatt A/S, DK 2900 Hellerup, Denmark). When a human serum sample was run, only trace amounts of impurities were found in the anti-albumin serum, and its specificity against human albumin had been clearly shown.

Standards (Kabi, 20 to 60 g/liter) and sera were diluted 200-fold with the electrophoresis buffer, a barbital/sodium barbital buffer (75 mmol/liter, pH 8.6, containing 2 mmol of calcium lactate per liter) as described elsewhere (*18, 19*).

Of the diluted samples, 5 μl was applied to each of the 2.5-mm-diameter wells with a Hamilton syringe, and electrophoresed at 10 V/cm for 3 h. The subsequent drying and staining procedures were carried out according to Axelsen et al. (*19*). Peak heights were measured and plotted and the resulting standard curve was used to ascertain albumin concentration in the samples.

The other proteins were similarly determined, rabbit antihuman serum against orosomucoid (from Dr. B. G. Johansson), ceruloplasmin, haptoglobin, and hemopexin (Dakopatt A/S) being used.

Electrophoresis on Cellulose Acetate (CA)

We followed the manufacturer's prescribed technique for "Microzone" electrophoresis (Beckman Instruments Inc., Fullerton, Calif. 92634), with the following exceptions. "Sepraphore III" membranes were used (Gelman Instrument Co., Ann Arbor, Mich. 48106) and the fixation, staining, clearing, and drying procedures were changed accordingly. The protein fractions were quantitated with an automatic scanner (Camag, CH-4132 Homburger Strasse 24, Switzerland) equipped with an electronic integrator, printer, and recorder.

Total protein concentration in the samples was determined by a biuret method on an AutoAnalyzer I system (Technicon Instrument Corp., Tarrytown, N. Y. 10591; method no N-14b) with Seronorm (Nyegaard & Co A/S) as the calibration material.

Preparative Agarose Electrophoresis

This was done as described by Johansson (*20*). About 0.8 ml serum or plasma could be processed in each run. The purity of the albumin fraction was controlled by means of analytical separation by electrophoresis on agarose according to Johansson (*20*).

Results

Some Analytical Variables

Rate of the serum/bromcresol green reaction. Figure 1 illustrates the time course of the increase in absorbance seen with various standards and serum samples. All curves were followed on the recorder from about 5

[2] Per liter, 0.15 mmol of BCG, 75 mmol of sodium succinate, and 4.0 ml. of "Brij 35" surfactant (300 g/liter); pH 4.20 ± 0.05.

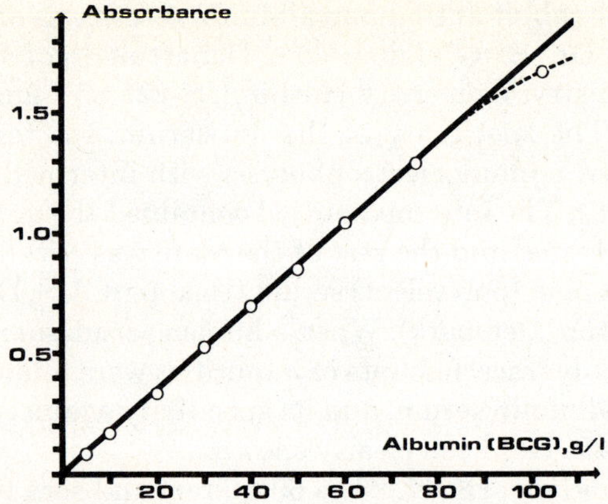

Fig. 2. Standard curve of albumin determination by the BCG reaction at 0 min

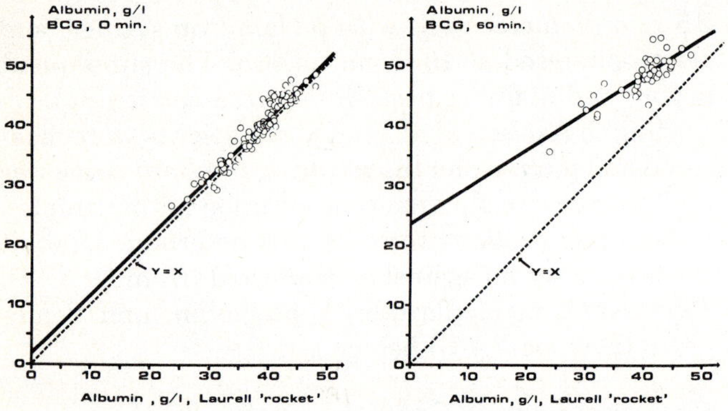

Fig. 3. Results by the BCG method at 0 (*left*) and 60 min (*right*) reaction times are compared to results by "rocket" immunoelectrophoresis
(*left*) $y = 1.83 + 0.98\,x$ ($n = 90$; $r = 0.95$)
(*right*) $y = 23.56 + 0.62\,x$ ($n = 42$; $r = 0.84$)

s after mixing. The values on the y-axis are the values obtained with albumin as standard. Thus the values that would have been obtained at a given time by conventional methods of standardization can be seen.

Pure albumin standards and the albumin fraction obtained from preparative electrophoresis (Figure 1, no. 11) reach their final value in less than 1 min. In contrast, sera both of human and animal origin showed not only this fast reaction but also a much slower one, which reaches a steady value within 30 min at room temperature, although there is a considerable variation in the contribution to the total absorbance from the slow-reacting component(s) with different sera. Sera from patients with acute illness tended to show a more pronounced slow-reacting phase.

Estimation of fast- and slow-reacting components. The contribution to the absorbances from the fast reaction were estimated by extrapolating the recorder curve to the time of mixing, 0 min. The absorbance difference between 0 and 60 min was calculated and called ΔA.

An arbitrary unit of the slow-reacting component is calculated from $\Delta A\% = 100(\Delta A_{\text{sample}}/\Delta A_{\text{v}})$ where ΔA_{v} is the ΔA for Versatol. Versatol was chosen for convenience as the value for the batch we used agreed well with that found for a serum pool from healthy blood donors.

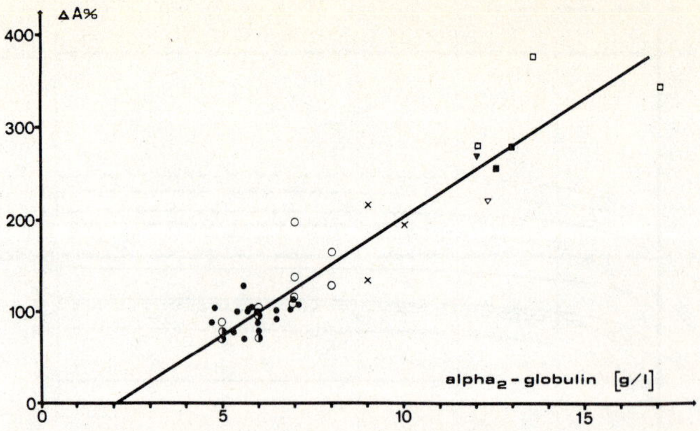

Fig. 4. Comparison of the slow reaction of the BCG method, expressed as $\Delta A\%$, and the α_2-globulin fraction from cellulose acetate electrophoresis
The regression line was: $y = -51.7 + 25.7\,x$ ($n = 39$; $r = 0.94$). ● = normals (blood donors); ○ = normals from routine electrophoresis; ×* = patients with a slight inflammatory reaction; ▽ ▼* = patients with a moderate inflammatory reaction; □ ■* = patients with intense inflammatory reaction; ◑ = newborns
* indicates chronic inflammatory reaction of corresponding degree

Linearity and sensitivity of the BCG method. A standard curve with albumin read at 0 reaction time (Figure 2) is linear up to 75 g of albumin per liter, with a sensitivity suitable for most photometers.

Comparison with Other Methods

Figure 3 shows results obtained with different patients' sera by the BCG method at 0 and 60 min, respectively, as compared with corresponding results by "rocket" immunoelectrophoresis. The linear regression curves and correlation coefficients (r) calculated by classical technique assuming no variability in x or reference measurement were: y (BCG, 0 min) = $1.83 + 0.98\,x$ (in g/liter; $n = 90$; $r = 0.95$) and y (BCG, 60 min) = $23.56 + 0.62\,x$ (in g/liter; $n = 42$; $r = 0.84$).

The slope and intercept were recalculated by Deming's procedure as described by Wakkers et al. (*21*). Assuming $\lambda = 1$ (equal standard deviations of the methods) the regression curve is modified to: y (BCG, 0 min) = $-0.04 + 1.03\,x$ (in g/liter; $n = 90$). Results were similar when the BCG method at 0 and 60 min was compared with cellulose acetate electrophoresis. The following equations describe this comparison: y (BCG, 0 min) = $2.31 + 1.01\,x$ (in g/liter; $n = 110$; $r = 0.91$); y (BCG, 60 min) = $21.71 + 0.60\,x$ (in g/liter; $n = 57$; $r = 0.84$).

Recalculation by Deming's procedure (as above) will give: y (BCG, 0 min) = $-2.01 + 1.13\,x$ (in g/liter; $n = 110$).

Results by the BCG method compare well with those by more specific methods for albumin determination when zero-minute values are estimated. Considerably higher values are obtained at 60 min, especially for patients' sera of subnormal albumin concentration. With a reaction time between these two extremes, intermediate results are obtained.

Table 1. Comparison of $\Delta A\%$ with Concentrations of Some Proteins in Human Serum Samples[a]

Code[b]	$\Delta A\%$ (%)	Orosomucoid (%)	Ceruloplasmin (%)	C3 β_{1A}-β_{1C} (%)	Haptoglobin (%)	Hemopexin (%)
N	71	64		103	44	
Nb	72				15	
Nb	72	69			24	
Nb	73	36	80	155	23	54
N	78	66			67	
N	78	84			39	
N	88	89			79	
N	88	109			97	
αN	89	117			17	
N	92	114			79	
Nb	98	73	93	217	21	68
N	100	97		105	73	
N	100	110			99	
N	101	116			129	
N	102	100	113	136	79	110
N	102	100			109	
αLC	102		93	93	18	92
N	103	77	93	116	147	82
N	104	86			80	
N	105	93		127	121	
N	105	107			144	
N	109	141		134	126	
N	114	109			147	
N	114				156	
N	117				165	
N	118				162	
N	128	114			120	
LC	134		139	161		101
Control	137	143	131	126		100
P	138			165		
L	139				116	
L	165		151	147	111	100
LC	172		136	139		59
LC	196		163	228	165	136
L	198	210	140	140	215	148
IC	217	257				
LC	218		160	141		123
IC	220	193		187		
M	221	230	115	180	164	100
IC	281	307			263	
I	281	383		174	256	
MC	292	380	191	188		122
I	345	360	317	241		136
I	378	427	260	241		151
n[c]	—	32	16	23	34	16
A[d]	—	24.2	−10.6	−55.5	47.2	−48.8
B[d]	—	.79	1.31	1.44	.68	2.21
r[e]	—	.97	.91	.71	.82	.73
$c_{100\%}$[f]	5.1	.90	.45	.35	.95	.90

[a] To simplify this comparison all proteins are expressed in an arbitrary unit defined as the percentage concentration ratio between the actual sample and a serum pool of healthy blood donors.

[b] Code: N = normals; Nb = newborns; L = low (or slight) inflammatory reaction; M = moderate degree of inflammatory reaction; I = intense inflammatory reaction; P = pregnant woman; α = hemolytic disease (consumption of haptoglobin); C = chronic disease.

[c] n = no. determinations.

[d] $\Delta A\% = A + B\,x$, where x is the concentration of the different proteins.

[e] r = Correlation coefficient.

[f] $c_{100\%}$ is the actual concentration in g/liter corresponding to the serum pool used which is defined as being 100%. (For $\Delta A\%$: "Apparent albumin reactants" in g/liter is given).

Studies on the Slow Reaction Step

Figure 4 compares the earlier-defined ΔA% with values for α_2-globulin obtained by cellulose acetate electrophoresis for sera from newborns, blood donors, and from patients for whom routine electrophoresis was done in the laboratory. The latter were classified by an independent interpreter. They were interpreted as being normal or showing slight, moderate, or intense acute inflammatory reaction on the basis of decrease in albumin and elevation of α_1- and α_2-globulin, or as chronic inflammatory reaction, based on elevation of γ-globulin.

We compared ΔA% for five proteins: orosomucoid, ceruloplasmin, complement C3($= \beta_{1A} - \beta_{1C}$), haptoglobin, and hemopexin. Haptoglobin was determined according to Tarukoski (*22*); the other proteins were evaluated by the Laurell "rocket" technique.

As Table 1 shows, ΔA% correlated well with orosomucoid and ceruloplasmin. These two proteins are accepted as acute phase reactants. Of the other proteins investigated, reasonable correlation exists between ΔA% and haptoglobin concentration, whereas the correlation with complement C3 and hemopexin is rather poor.

Table 1 includes the codes for different patient groups, to show some examples of the variations in ΔA% for these groups.

Discrepancies from the general pattern in Table 1 include the low haptoglobin values for newborns and for patients with hemolytic disease, and the high complement C3 values for newborns.

Factors Influencing the Reaction

pH. Table 2 shows the influence of pH (3.9 to 4.5) on the fast and slow reaction. Two patients' sera and one standard (40 g of albumin per liter) were tested. The sera were read against a blank solution of corresponding pH. The results for albumin and ΔA% were constant in this pH range, but there was a slight increase in the corresponding absorbances up to pH 4.4. Because all measurements were made with an appropriate blank solution, the influence of pH on the blank value is not considered here.

Temperature. The influence of temperature on the fast and slow reaction is shown in Table 3. The temperature was increased stepwise in the thermostatted cell. Two patients' sera (not the same as above) and one standard (40 g of albumin per liter) were tested. Sample and blank solutions were at the same temperature. The absorbance and final result for the fast reaction (albumin) was constant between 20 and 45 °C. For the slow reaction the absorbance differences increased with increasing temperature above 30 °C, but the results, expressed as ΔA%, were constant between 20 and 35 °C. An increase was noted for sample 1 at 40 and 45 °C. The second (slow) reaction showed a slightly increased reaction rate, presented in Table 3 as the absorbance difference between 1.5 and 0 min.

Information Obtained by the BCG Method

Figure 5 shows an example of a combination of the information from the fast (albumin) and the slow (ΔA%) reaction step. Two sloping (dotted) lines were drawn to effect the best separation of the patient groups. The four solid lines represent the normal concentration range for albumin and ΔA%. The vertical and horizontal dotted lines separate different patient groups according to the intensity of their inflammatory reaction. Orosomucoid values indicate that the results represented by the four uppermost unfilled circles ("normal" patients from routine electrophoresis) should be designated "slight inflammatory response".

We could categorize the results for the different subjects into four groups: normals, newborns, and patients with slight and those with a more intense inflammatory reaction.

Discussion

We have demonstrated that normal and abnormal serum albumin concentrations can be reliably determined if the absorbance of the albumin/BCG complex is read at the time of mixing, 0 min. The experiments in which pure albumin standard or albumin prepared electrophoretically were used showed that the fast phase of the BCG reaction is attributable to albumin. By ex-

Table 2. Influence of pH on the Fast (Albumin) and the Slow ("Acute Phase Reactant") Phases of the BCG Reaction

	Albumin (0 min)						ΔA%			
	Standard		Sample 1		Sample 2		Sample 1		Sample 2	
pH	$A \times 10^3$	Concn, g/liter	$A \times 10^3$	Concn, g/liter	$A \times 10^3$	Concn, g/liter	$\Delta A^a \times 10^3$	ΔA%, %	$\Delta A^a \times 10^3$	ΔA%, %
3.9	497	40	507	40.8	460	37.0	080	137	128	220
4.0	515	40	532	41.3	483	37.5	084	139	137	227
4.1	564	40	579	41.1	526	37.3	091	139	149	227
4.2	609	40	627	41.2	564	37.0	097	137	158	223
4.3	625	40	641	41.0	578	37.0	101	139	161	220
4.4	631	40	644	40.8	579	36.7	099	135	162	220
4.5	644	40	621	38.6	557	34.6	105	139	145	193

[a] $\Delta A = A$(at 60 min) $- A$(at 0 min).

Table 3. Influence of Temperature on the Fast (Albumin) and the Slow ("Acute Phase Reactant") Phases of the BCG Reaction

	Albumin (0 min)						ΔA%					
	Standard		Sample 1		Sample 2		Sample 1			Sample 2		
Temp, °C	$A \times 10^3$	Concn, g/liter	$A \times 10^3$	Concn, g/liter	$A \times 10^3$	Concn, g/liter	$\Delta A_{1.5}$ [a] $\times 10^3$	ΔA [b] $\times 10^3$	ΔA%, %	$\Delta A_{1.5}$ [a] $\times 10^3$	ΔA [b] $\times 10^3$	ΔA%, %
20	602	40	579	38.5	715	47.5	017	084	112	019	075	100
25	600	40	585	38.7	717	47.5	021	087	115	021	074	98
30	600	40	574	38.3	709	47.3	035	084	112	029	075	100
35	601	40	571	38.0	715	47.6	054	103	114	037	090	100
40	602	40	575	38.2	712	47.3	072	148	148	053	099	99
45	602	40	583	38.7	710	47.2	077	170	131	056	131	101

[a] $\Delta A_{1.5} = A$(at 1.5 min) − A(at 0 min) is included in the table to demonstrate the increase in reaction rate with increasing temperature.
[b] $\Delta A = A$(at 60 min) − A(at 0 min).

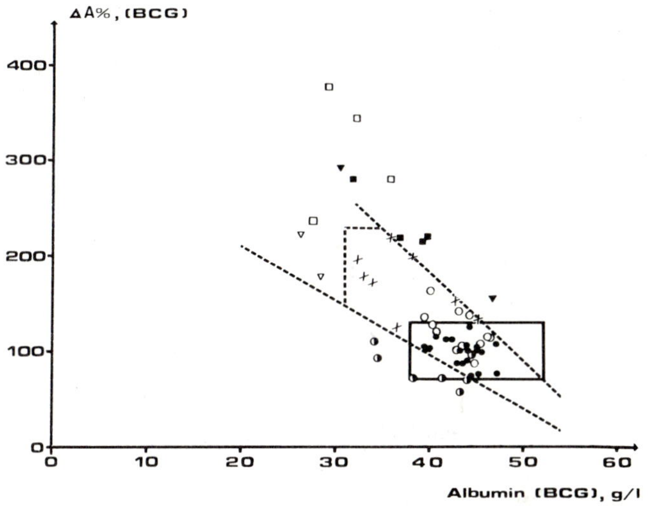

Fig. 5. Relation between values for albumin and ΔA%, obtained by the BCG method

Symbols same as in Figure 4. The four *solid* lines represent the normal concentration range for albumin and ΔA%

trapolating the recorder registration to zero time, a reliable albumin value was obtained. As can be seen in Figure 3, results for the BCG method compare well with those for the Laurell "rocket" technique and, as shown above, with those for cellulose acetate electrophoresis. The use of two different statistical procedures gives a good correlation with no detectable systematic difference between the results from these method of albumin determination.

In contrast, values obtained with the BCG method after 60 min reaction time differ considerably from albumin values determined by more specific methods (Figure 3). Reaction times of 5 to 30 min have been used in all work published so far. The resulting values thus are higher than the true albumin values because the value includes other components, which react more slowly. As can be seen in Figure 1, most of the slow-reacting components react with BCG during the first 5 min, and after 30 min the slow reaction is complete.

As an example the albumin concentration in one sample was found to be 27 g/liter at 0 min, while at 60 min the value was 43 g/liter. The value by the "rocket" technique was 28.5 g/liter.

The problems discussed above arise especially in the lower concentration range, where the diagnostic and prognostic value of accurate albumin determinations is particularly great. The problem of the poor comparison of the BCG method with more specific methods have been shown, among others, by Webster et al. (*15*) and Schirardin and Ney (*17*).

Figure 2 shows an albumin standard curve as determined by the BCG method. It is linear up to about 75 g of albumin per liter, and it passes through the origin. Thus only one standard, 40 g of albumin per liter, is needed for routine analyses.

The results for albumin were unaffected by changing the reaction temperature between 20 and 45 °C. An increase in absorbance of the albumin/BCG complex was seen when the pH was increased from 3.9 to 4.5, but nevertheless the serum albumin values were constant between pH 3.9–4.4.

As defined above, the measure of the slow-reacting component is called ΔA%. In accordance with the practice in common use of expressing the concentration of proteins in serum, an arbitrary unit of ΔA% is defined as the ratio between the value for the actual sample and a pooled specimen of serum from apparently healthy blood donors. (This ratio is multiplied by 100 to give %.)

Others (*15, 16*) have shown that globulin fractions are responsible for the overestimation of albumin in sera with low albumin concentrations. We soon found that the contribution from the slow reaction varied considerably with sera from different patients.

Newborns showed low values (Figure 1) despite a high serum bilirubin content (35–70 μmol/liter). Serum samples from patients with intense inflammatory reaction patterns showed a very marked increase in the slow-reacting component, up to about 400% of the normal.

ΔA% and the α_2-globulin fraction from cellulose acetate electrophoresis can be compared in Figure 4. The correlation is good and the patients are grouped along the regression line in order of increasing degree of inflammatory reaction. High concentrations of γ-globulin, characteristic of chronic inflammatory reaction, did not affect the results.

As Table 1 shows, ΔA% seems to be correlated to the intensity of the inflammatory reaction; we found a good correlation between ΔA% and orosomucoid and between ΔA% and ceruloplasmin.

The haptoglobin concentration determined, according to Tarukoski (*22*), was also compared with ΔA%. Discrepancies were found in the case of sera from newborns and patients with hemolytic disease. Haptoglobin measured by "rocket" immunoelectrophoresis showed essentially the same pattern except that newborns and patients with hemolytic disease showed even lower values.

Both complement C3 [we measured the inactive form, β_{1A} (*23, 24*) in most samples because the serum samples were not quite fresh] and hemopexin correlated poorly with ΔA%.

In a number of serum samples from pregnant women ΔA% was increased (130–170% of normal), suggesting that estrogen positively affects ΔA%.

We found a good correlation between the second (slow) reaction, ΔA%, and orosomucoid and ceruloplasmin values, which indicates that ΔA% can be used as a measure of "acute phase reactants," although we have not yet established which component(s) actually cause the slow reaction. This problem is currently being investigated.

Figure 5 shows the information from the two available measures of the BCG reaction, albumin and ΔA%. This diagram exemplifies how the two pieces of information obtained by this method can be combined. Although the lines in this figure are rather arbitrary and not intended to be definitive borderlines for different patient groups, it can be seen that it is possible to classify patients according to the degree of their inflammatory reaction. It is also apparent from this figure that attempts to calculate an "index" between albumin and ΔA% will result in loss of information, and the various patient groups will be intermixed.

References

1. Watson, D., Albumin and "total globulin" fractions from blood. *Adv. Clin. Chem.* **8**, 237 (1965).
2. Webster, D., A simple method of serum protein fractionation on cellulose acetate and a comparison of the albumin levels with a method of sodium sulphite fractionation. *Clin. Chim. Acta* **11**, 101 (1965).
3. Mancini, G., Carbonara, A. O., and Heremans, J. F., Immunochemical quantitation of antigens by single radial immunodiffusion. *Immunochemistry* **2**, 235 (1965).
4. Laurell, C.-B., Quantitative estimation of proteins by electrophoresis in agarose gel containing antibodies. *Anal. Biochem.* **15**, 45 (1966).
5. Schulze, H. E., and Schwick, G., Quantitative immunologische Bestimmung von Plasmaproteinen. *Clin. Chim. Acta* **4**, 15 (1959).
6. Martinek, R. G., Evaluation of a dye-binding method for determination of serum albumin. *Clin. Chem.* **11**, 441 (1965).
7. Ness, A. T., Dickerson, H. C., and Pastewka, J. V., The determination of human serum albumin by its specific binding of the anionic dye, 2-(4′-hydroxybenzeneazo)-benzoic acid. *Clin. Chim. Acta* **12**, 532 (1965).
8. Rutstein, D. D., Ingenito, E. F., and Reynolds, W. E., The determination of albumin in human blood plasma and serum. A method based on the interaction of albumin with an anionic dye 2-(4′-hydroxybenzeneazo) benzoic acid. *J. Clin. Invest.* **33**, 211 (1954).
9. Keyser, J. W., Determination of serum albumin. *Clin. Chem.* **14**, 360 (1968).
10. Crowley, L. V., An evaluation of serum protein fractionation using a methyl orange method for determination of albumin. *Clin. Chem.* **10**, 1131 (1964).
11. Rodkey, F. L., Direct spectrophotometric determination of albumin in human serum. *Clin. Chem.* **11**, 478 (1965).
12. Doumas, B. T., Watson, W. A., and Biggs, H. G., Albumin standards and the measurement of serum albumin with bromcresol green. *Clin. Chim. Acta* **31**, 87 (1971).
13. Leonard, P. J., Persaud, J., and Motwani, R., The estimation of plasma albumin by BCG dye binding on the Technicon SMA 12/60 analyser and a comparison with the HABA dye binding technique. *Clin. Chim. Acta* **35**, 409 (1971).
14. Ferreria, P., and Price, C. P., A comparison of bromocresol green and immunoprecipitation methods for the determination of serum albumin. *Clin. Chim. Acta* **55**, 259 (1974).
15. Webster, D., Bignell, A. H. C., and Attwood, E. C., An assessment of the suitability of bromocresol green for the determination of serum albumin. *Clin. Chim. Acta* **53**, 101 (1974).
16. Webster, D., A study of the interaction of bromocresol green with isolated serum globulin fractions. *Clin. Chim. Acta* **53**, 109 (1974).
17. Schirardin, Von H., and Ney, J., Eine vereinfachte Micromethode zur Bestimmung von Serumalbumin mit Hilfe von Bromkresolgrün. *Z. Klin. Chem. Klin. Biochem.* **10**, 338 (1972).
18. Laurell, C.-B., Electroimmuno assay. *Scand. J. Clin. Lab. Invest.* **29**, *Suppl. 124*, 21 (1972).
19. Axelsen, N. H., Kroll, J., and Weeke, B., A manual of quantitative immunoelectrophoresis, methods and applications, Universitetsforlaget, Oslo, 1973.
20. Johansson, B. G., Agarose gel electrophoresis. *Scand. J. Clin. Lab. Invest.* **29**, *Suppl. 124*, 7 (1972).
21. Wakkers, P. J. M., Hellendoorn, H. B. A., op de Weegh, G. J., and Heerspink, W., Applications of statistics in clinical chemistry. A critical evaluation of regression lines. *Clin. Chim. Acta* **64**, 173 (1975).
22. Tarukoski, P. H., Quantitative spectrophotometric determination of haptoglobin. *Scand. J. Clin. Lab. Invest.* **18**, 80 (1966).
23. Schultze, H. E., and Heremans, J. F., *Molecular Biology of Human Proteins with Special Reference to Plasma Proteins*, Vol. 1, Elsevier Publ. Co., Amsterdam, 1966, p 214.
24. Burtin, P., and Grabar, P., Nomenclature and identification of the normal human serum proteins. In *Electrophoresis, Theory, Methods and Applications*, **II**, M. Bier, Ed., Academic Press, New York, N. Y., 1967, pp 131–134.

CLIN. CHEM. 22/5, 623-626 (1976)

Gas–Liquid Chromatographic Profile of Neutral and Acidic Metabolites in Cerebrospinal Fluid from Newborns and Infants

Richard D. Malcolm and Richard Leonards

A profile (chromatographic pattern) of the neutral and acidic metabolites present in cerebrospinal fluid from newborns and infants was obtained by gas–liquid chromatography. The metabolites are those extracted with ethyl acetate and diethyl ether. They are converted to trimethylsilyl ether derivatives, and chromatographed on a column containing 5% silicone OV-101 (methyl) packed on Chromosorb W. Several substances were tentatively identified from their methylene unit values. We established a control profile for infants, and compared profiles for infants and adults. Noteworthy qualitative and quantitative differences from the control were seen for cerebrospinal fluid from subjects with neurological disorders or infections. The technique may be of use in neurological diagnosis.

Additional Keyphrases: *newborns • pediatric chemistry • diagnostic aid • neurological disorders • screening*

CSF[1] from adults has been examined by GLC for neutral and acidic metabolites (*1*), fatty acid composition (*2–4*), and metabolic products of cerebral metabolism that are associated with neurological disorders (*5–7*). There is no information about the GLC profiles of CSF from newborns and infants younger than three months. However, the composition of their CSF is known to differ in some respects from that of adults (*8–10*); therefore the GLC patterns may also differ.

Department of Pediatrics, Children's Hospital of San Francisco, San Francisco, Calif. 94119.

[1] Nonstandard abbreviations used: CSF, cerebrospinal fluid; GLC, gas–liquid chromatography (-ic); and MU, methylene unit (a measure of retention time).

Received Nov. 14, 1975; accepted Feb. 23, 1976.

Here, we report the metabolic profile of neutral and acidic components of CSF from newborns and infants. Sub-milliliter amounts of the CSF are extracted, derivatives are formed, and the product is chromatographed. We show that the resulting profiles may be of value in the diagnosis of neurological disorders and infections.

Materials and Methods

Subjects

A total of 37 samples were obtained from 33 babies, 26 of whom were males, admitted to the Neonatal Intensive Care Unit at Children's Hospital of San Francisco. Their ages ranged from 1 to 84 days, with 28 younger than 30 days. Their various diagnoses included suspected sepsis, ventriculitis, meningitis, hydrocephalus, and intracranial hemorrhage.

Reagents

Reagents and chemicals were: ethyl acetate, diethyl ether, and methanol (all "Nanograde"; Mallinckrodt Chemical Works, St. Louis, Mo. 63160); and bis(trimethylsilyl)-trifluoroacetamide in glass ampules, with 10 ml of trimethychlorosilane added per liter; and glass-distilled pyridine (both from Regis Chemical Co., Morton Grove, Ill. 60053).

Standards

Hydrocarbon standards and fatty acid standards were obtained from Applied Science Laboratories, State College, Pa. 16802. Homovanillic acid, 3,4-dihydroxyphenylacetic acid, 5-hydroxyindoleacetic acid, 3-methoxy-4-hydroxyphenethyleneglycol, and 3-methoxy-

4-hydroxyphenylethanol were obtained from Calbiochem, San Diego, Calif. 92112. Lactic acid, succinic acid, maleic acid, and citric acid were obtained from Arthur Thomas Co., Philadelphia, Pa. 19105.

Sample Treatment

CSF, obtained by lumbar puncture from newborns and infants with suspected sepsis or neurological disorder, was centrifuged at 1000 × *g* for 5 min and the supernate was stored at −40 °C until use. We saw no changes in the chromatographic profile after three months of storage at −40 °C.

The CSF was extracted with ethyl acetate and diethyl ether (*11*). Half-milliliter samples of CSF were diluted to 20 ml with de-ionized water, saturated with sodium chloride, acidified to pH 1.0 with a few drops of dilute hydrochloric acid (6 mol/liter), and the mixture was placed in a separatory funnel. The diluted sample was extracted three times with 30-ml portions of ethyl acetate and three times with 30-ml portions of diethyl ether. The extracts were pooled, dehydrated over anhydrous sodium sulfate, and filtered. The solvent was evaporated under reduced pressure and the residue transferred in about 3 ml of methanol to a Teflon-lined mini-reaction vial with a screw cap (Regis Chemical Co.). The methanol was evaporated in a stream of dry nitrogen at room temperature.

The residue containing the extracted substances was redissolved in 25 μl of pyridine. Trimethylsilyl ether derivatives were prepared by adding 25 μl of bis(trimethylsilyl)-trifluoroacetamide and allowing the silylation reaction to proceed overnight at room temperature before GLC analysis.

Gas Chromatography

We used a Model 1440 chromatograph (Varian Aerograph, Walnut Creek, Calif. 94598), equipped with a hydrogen-flame ionization detector and a 25.5-cm potentiometric recorder (Beckman Instruments, Fullerton, Calif. 92634). Glass columns, 1.83 m long, 2 mm i.d., and 6.35 mm o.d. were silanized with dimethyldichlorosilane and packed with 5% silicone OV-101 (methyl) coated on Chromosorb W, 80/100 mesh, AW, DMCS (Applied Science Laboratories). A small amount of silanized glass wool held the packing in place. The injection-port temperature was 210 ± 15 °C (190–240 °C), and we used an injection-port extender.

Detector temperature was 280 ± 15 °C (270–320 °C), and nitrogen ("zero" grade; Liquid Carbonic Corp., Chicago, Ill. 60603) was used as the carrier gas. Gas-flow rates (ml/min) were: hydrogen 30, air 300, and nitrogen 30.

A total of 6.0 μl was injected (12% of total sample volume). The column was immediately temperature-programmed at a rate of 2 °C/min from 65 to 260 °C, and then held at 260 °C for 20 min. The range setting was 10^{-11} A/mV. Attenuation was reduced from 128 to 16 after succinic acid emerged. All samples were analyzed in duplicate.

A de-ionized water blank was extracted and analyzed

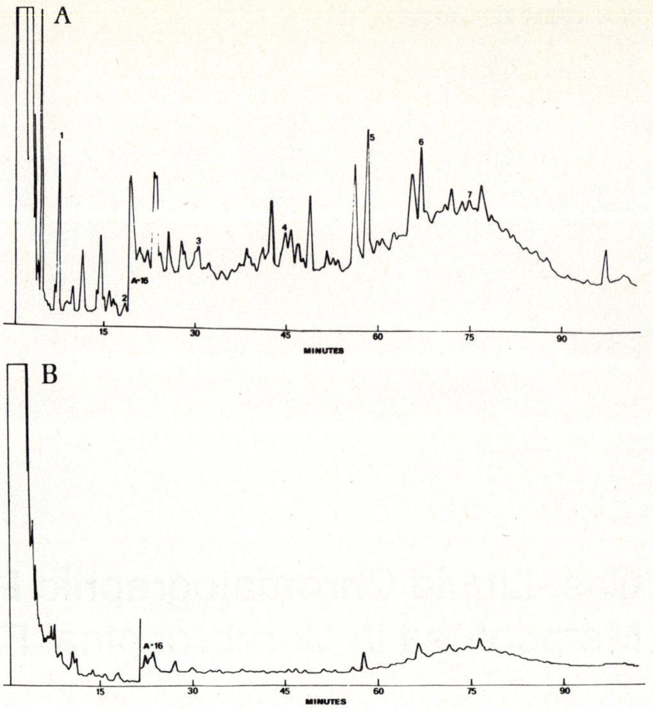

Fig. 1. *A*. Control profile for cerebrospinal fluid from a 6-day-old boy with hepatic and renal failure, but no nervous system disorder

1, lactic acid; *2*, succinic acid; *3*, maleic acid; *4*, homovanillic acid; *5*, palmitic acid; *6*, stearic acid; *7*, arachidic acid

B. Blank chromatogram for de-ionized water that was extracted, derivatized, and analyzed identically to the CSF samples

as a control for each batch of CSF samples. Trace amounts of organic compounds, which we believe to be from the de-ionized water, gave some very small peaks (Figure 1).

Results

If the infants without metabolic or neurological disorders had normal CSF values (*8*) as shown in Table 1, and the results of the Gram stain and bacteriological culture were negative, their profiles were considered controls. Twenty such control profiles were examined. Figure 1 shows a typical one.

Despite the variety of the clinical disorders, all not directly affecting the central nervous system, their profiles demonstrated a consistent pattern. Two large peaks and three small peaks were present in all profiles. They were tentatively identified as palmitic, stearic, lauric, myristic, and arachidic acids, respectively. Peaks consistent with the other fatty acids were seen in small amounts in some profiles. The peaks corresponding to lactic, succinic, and homovanillic acids varied in size but appeared consistently for all samples. A peak consistent with 3-methoxy-4-hydroxyphenylethanol was seen in 25 of the 37 samples we analyzed. Other peaks in the profiles corresponded in their chromatographic behavior to 3,4-dihydroxyphenylacetic acid, 3-methoxy-4-hydroxyphenethyleneglycol and 5-hydroxyindoleacetic acid.

Table 1. Values for Leukocyte Count, and Glucose and Protein Concentration in CSF from Control Infants

	Range	Mean	SD
Leukocytes per μl	0–25	6.76	±6.35
Protein, g/liter	0.38–1.82	0.934	±0.345
Glucose, g/liter	0.27–0.82	0.548	±0.135

Table 2. MU Values on Three Chromatographic Stationary Phases for Compounds in CSF from Newborns and Infants[a]

Compounds	OV-101	OV-17	OV-25
		MU values	
Lactic acid	10.63	11.20	12.08
Succinic acid	13.03	14.10	14.50
Maleic acid	14.88	16.69	17.14
3-Methoxy-4-hydroxyphenylethanol	17.04	18.21	19.90
Homovanillic acid	17.58	19.31	18.80
3,4-Dihydroxyphenylacetic acid	18.32	19.31	20.00
Citric acid	18.33	19.02	19.44
Myristic acid	18.46	19.02	19.46
3-Methoxy-4-hydroxyphenethyleneglycol	18.52	18.21	19.80
Palmitic acid	20.44	20.99	21.21
5-Hydroxyindoleacetic acid	22.03	24.23	25.26
Stearic acid	22.42	22.97	23.24
Arachidic acid	24.45	24.91	25.15

[a] Compounds were chromatographed as trimethylsilyl ether derivatives. All stationary phases are 5% liquid phase on Chromosorb W 80/100 mesh, AW, DMCS: OV-101 (liquid methyl silicone), OV-17 (methyl phenyl silicone), and OV-25 (phenyl silicone).

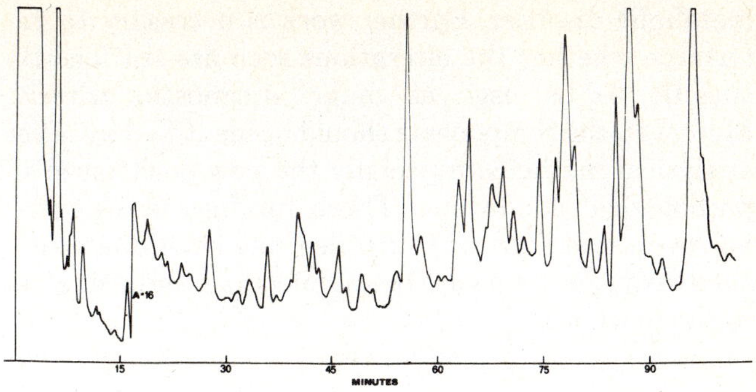

Fig. 2. Profile for cerebrospinal fluid from a 1-day-old premature female infant with an intracranial hemorrhage

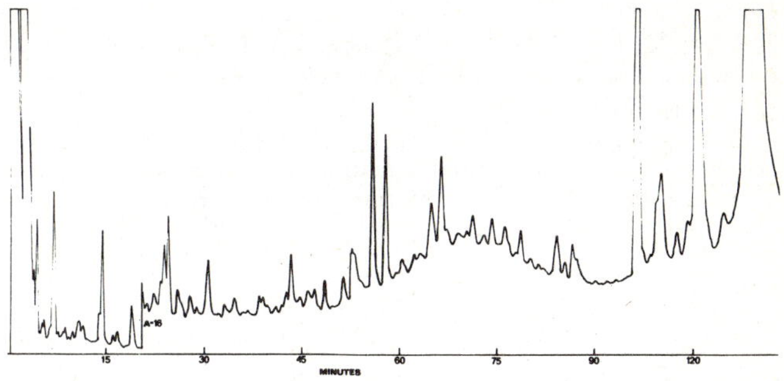

Fig. 3. Profile for cerebrospinal fluid from a 72-day-old premature male infant with ventriculitis

Metabolites present in the extracts of the CSF were tentatively identified on the basis of their MU values (*11*). MU values for standards and substances in the profile were systematically determined by using three columns with different liquid phases (5% OV-101, 5% OV-17, 5% OV-25). Table 2 shows MU values for metabolites in the CSF of newborns and infants.

Profiles of CSF from newborns with neurological disorders had patterns that differed from those for the controls. Figure 2 demonstrates the gross alterations seen in a case of intracranial hemorrhage. Several additional peaks are present in the later portion of the profile. In another example of neurological disorder, a baby with hydrocephalus secondary to toxoplasmosis, the profile had a high 5-hydroxyindoleacetic acid peak and two additional peaks in the later portion of the chromatogram.

Certain peaks in the profiles for newborns and infants with neurological infections rather than neurological disorders, also differed qualitatively from the controls. The pattern for an infant with ventriculitis (Figure 3) had additional peaks at the end of the profile. All of the meningitis samples examined showed a series of six peaks that were absent in all other profiles. The peaks were regularly spaced, suggesting that they may represent homologs.

Discussion

A profile of the neutral and acidic metabolites in the CSF from newborns and infants has been obtained by a method that allows measurement to be made on very small samples. A number of substances in the profiles have been provisionally identified. Although many of these were previously reported as components of CSF from adults (*1–3, 5–7, 12, 13*), no quantitative or qualitative studies have been made on infants.

3-Methoxy-4-hydroxyphenylethanol is inconsistently present in infants' CSF, as was the case for adults (*1*). However, stearic acid, a relatively minor component of CSF from adults (*1*), is a major component in CSF from infants.

We found that the profile for newborns was reproducible enough that we could establish a control profile, which can be compared with profiles from adults (*1*) and from infants with neurological disorders and infections.

Quantitative changes in the existing peaks or the appearance of new peaks may reflect neurological or metabolic disorder. Further work is necessary to determine whether the alterations seen are sufficiently specific to be used as major diagnostic criteria. Moreover, the components should be identified by other analytical methods, especially the new peaks seen in pathological conditions. These findings do suggest, however, that such GLC profiles may be of diagnostic value in suspected neurological infections and disorders in the newborn.

We thank Drs. June P. Brady and A. T. Shulgin for their helpful discussions and review of the manuscript, and Ms. Jewel Valentine for her assistance in its preparation. The study was supported by a grant from the Charles Merrill Trust.

References

1. Waterbury, L. D., and Pearce, L. A., Separation and identification of neutral and acidic metabolites in cerebrospinal fluid. *Clin. Chem.* **18,** 258 (1972).

2. Tuna, N., Logothetis, J., and Kammereck, R., The fatty acids of the human cerebrospinal fluid: Their relation to the serum fatty acids. *Neurology* **13,** 331 (1963).

3. Pazzagli, A., Arnetoli, G., Pepeu, I., and Amaducci, L. A., Fatty acid changes of cerebrospinal fluid in neurological disorders as an index of changes in the blood-brain barrier. *Neurology* **20,** 783 (1970).

4. Berry, J. F., Logothetis, J., and Bovis, M., Determination of the fatty acid composition of cerebrospinal fluid by gas-liquid chromatography. *Neurology* **15,** 1089 (1965).

5. Wilk, S., Davis, K. L., and Thacker, S. B., Determination of 3-methoxy-4-hydroxyphenethyleneglycol (MHPG) in cerebrospinal fluid. *Anal. Biochem.* **39,** 498 (1971).

6. Gottfries, C. G., Gottfries, I., and Ross, B. E., Homovanillic acid and 5-hydroxyindoleacetic acid in the cerebrospinal fluid of patients with senile dementia, presenile dementia and Parkinsonism. *J. Neurochem.* **16,** 1341 (1969).

7. Mann, D. C., Pearce, L. A., and Waterbury, L. D., Amantadine for Parkinson's disease. *Neurology* **21,** 958 (1971).

8. Naidoo, B. T., The cerebrospinal fluid in the healthy newborn infant. *S. Afr. Med. J.* **9,** 953 (1968).

9. Otila, E., Studies on the cerebrospinal fluid in premature infants. *Acta Paediatr. Scand., Suppl 8,* 3 (1948).

10. Widell, S., On the cerebrospinal fluid in normal children and in patients with acute abacterial meningoencephalitis. *Acta Paediatr. Scand., Suppl 115,* 5, (1958).

11. Dalgliesh, C. E., Horning, E. C., Horning, M. G., et al., A gas-liquid chromatographic procedure for separating a wide range of metabolites in urine or tissue extracts. *Biochem. J.* **101,** 792 (1966).

12. Ashcroft, G. W., Crawford, T. B. B., Eccelston, D., et al., 5-Hydroxyindole compounds in the cerebrospinal fluid of patients with psychiatric or neurological diseases. *Lancet* **ii,** 1049 (1966).

13. Waterbury, L. D., and Pearce, L. A., Gas-liquid chromatographic analysis of cerebrospinal fluid metabolites. *Fed. Proc.* **30,** 426 (1971).

CLIN. CHEM. 22/5, 627–632 (1976)

Improved Determination of Prostatic Acid Phosphatase (Sodium Thymolphthalein Monophosphate Substrate)

Lilian M. Ewen and Ralph W. Spitzer

We have modified a previously described method for determining acid phosphatase, with thymolphthalein monophosphate as substrate, to increase its sensitivity. We assessed effects of serum on variables influencing acid phosphatase activity as measured by this method. The method is shown to be not completely specific for prostatic acid phosphatase. The importance of standardizing methodology in measurement of enzyme activities is demonstrated.

A method for measuring acid phosphatase [orthophosphoric-monoester phosphohydrolase (acid optimum), EC 3.1.3.2] activity in serum, with thymolphthalein monophosphate as substrate, was described by Roy et al. (*1*) and is the basis of a "kit" method (Worthington Biochemical Corp., Freehold, N.J. 07728) and the method used in the "SMAC" (Technicon Instruments Corp., Tarrytown, N. Y. 10591) system. The method is described as having "good sensitivity over a wide range of activity" and almost complete specificity for prostatic acid phosphatase.

Daily use of the method in our laboratory has shown the method to be extremely insensitive, whether we used kit reagents or reagents that we prepared as described by Roy et al. (*1*). Activities at the upper limit of the normal range gave changes in absorbance under the conditions of assay of only 0.02 with a reagent blank of 0.07 and a serum-in-reagent blank that may exceed 0.10 with turbid sera. Patients whose acid phosphatase activity in serum gave a change in absorbance under the conditions of the method only 0.005 above the upper limit of the normal range were occasionally found to have cancer of the prostate gland. Such small absorbance differences between normal and abnormal activities fall almost within the error tolerance of commonly used laboratory spectrophotometers such as the Gilford-300-N instrument, and decrease confidence in the reliability of results.

Department of Biochemistry, Royal Columbian Hospital, New Westminster, B. C., Canada.

Received June 4, 1974; accepted Feb. 11, 1976.

We examined factors influencing acid phosphatase activity, in an attempt to increase the sensitivity of the method. Here, we describe modifications that improve the sensitivity while at the same time decreasing the volume of specimen required, and we also describe the effects of the serum/final reaction-mixture volume ratio on results for prostatic acid phosphatase determined by this method. Nonspecificity of the method for prostatic acid phosphatase is noted and the importance of reagent and methodology standardization is illustrated. The modified method we describe has been in routine use in our laboratory for two years.

Materials and Methods

Reagents

Sources. Thymolphthalein monophosphate, disodium salt, was obtained from Regis Chemical Co., Morton Grove, Ill. 60053; from Sigma Chemical Co., St. Louis, Mo. 63178; and from Worthington Biochemical Corp. Formula weights for the product from the three sources were given as: Regis, 671 (17.7% H_2O); Sigma, 625.5 ($4H_2O$); and Worthington, 606 ($4H_2O$). Reagents in kit form were also obtained from Worthington Biochemical Corp. The surfactant Brij-35 (300 g/liter solution) was obtained from BDH Chemicals, Montreal Canada. All other chemicals were of the highest purity available.

Acetate buffer, 5 mol/liter, pH 5.4 (25 °C). Dissolve 68.0 g of sodium acetate trihydrate in distilled water and dilute to 100 ml with distilled water. Measure 28.87 ml of glacial acetic acid into a 100-ml volumetric flask and dilute to the mark with distilled water. To this solution add the sodium acetate solution until the pH of the mixture is 5.4 at 25 °C.

Substrate/buffer reagent. Dilute the Brij-35 solution with distilled water to a concentration of 3.24 g/liter, and dissolve 74.7 mg of disodium thymolphthalein monophosphate (17.7% H_2O) in 50 ml of it. Add 1.92 g of sodium acetate trihydrate to the solution, mix until dissolved, and adjust the pH of the solution to 5.4 (25

°C) with 0.1 mol/liter HCl. Bring the total volume to 100 ml with distilled water. Store refrigerated and discard after one month or when blank values become unacceptable.

Alkaline solution for color development (Na_2CO_3, 1.0 mol/liter in NaOH, 1.0 mol/liter). Dissolve 53 g of anhydrous Na_2CO_3 and 20 g of NaOH in distilled water and dilute to 500 ml. Dilute this solution 10-fold before use (working solution).

Thymolphthalein stock standard solution, 3 mmol/liter. Dissolve 129.0 mg of thymolphthalein (mol wt, 431) in sufficient *n*-propanol/water (70/30 by vol) to make a total volume of 100 ml.

Procedures

Preparation of prostatic extract. Fresh prostatic tissue was finely chopped and ground in acetate buffer (0.25 mol/liter, pH 5.4) with a pestle and mortar. The resulting slurry was centrifuged to sediment debris and the clear supernatant fluid was further diluted with acetate buffer as required, for assay of prostatic acid phosphatase activity.

Preparation of tubes for serum preservation. Pipette 25 µl of the acetate buffer (5 mol/liter, pH 5.4) into tubes. Evaporate in an oven at 60 °C. Stopper and store until required.

Preservation of serum. Immediately after the blood samples are centrifuged, add 0.5 ml of the serum to tubes containing the dry acetate buffer. Agitate gently to dissolve the acetate salts, then store the specimens frozen if they are not to be assayed on the same day.

Measurement of acid phosphatase activity in serum. Concentrations of reagents in the final reaction mixture are: acetate buffer, 0.15 mol/liter; thymolphthalein monophosphate, 1.0 mmol/liter; and Brij-35, 1.5 g/liter.

For each specimen to be assayed two tubes are used (control and test). Pipette into each 550 µl of buffered substrate. Bring the "test" solutions to 37 °C in a water bath and at convenient intervals (e.g., 30 s) add 50 µl of each specimen to the appropriate "test" tube, mix gently and allow to incubate at 37 °C for exactly 30 min. Add 1.0 ml of the working alkaline solution to each "test" tube and mix.

While the "test" samples are incubating, add 1.0 ml of the working alkaline solution to each of the "control" tubes, followed by 50 µl of the appropriate serum, and mix.

Read the absorbances of test and control solutions at 590 nm, subtract control from test absorbances and determine acid phosphatase activity from a standard curve prepared as described below.

For specimens with acid phosphatase activity yielding a color exceeding the limits of the spectrophotometer (up to an absorbance of 3.0) either dilute the specimen and re-assay or repeat the assay, with use of a 5-min incubation, read the absorbance at 590 nm, subtract the absorbance of the control, read the activity from the standard curve and multiply the answer by six.

Preparation of standard curve; standardization to 80 U/liter. Dilute stock thymolphthalein solution by

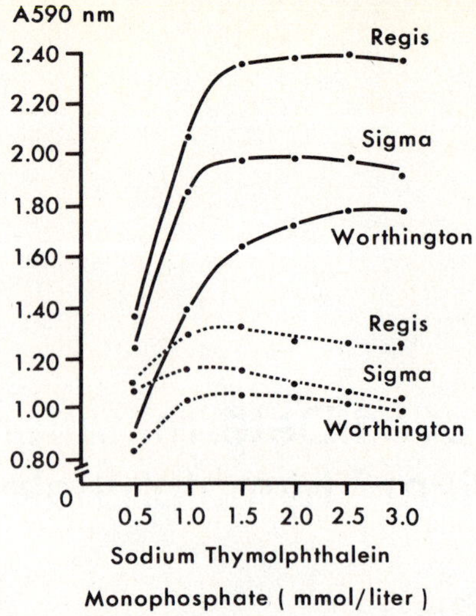

Fig. 1. Optimum substrate concentration for acid phosphatase activity as determined with thymolphthalein monophosphate from three suppliers

Reaction mixture, 0.6 ml citrate buffer (0.1 mol/liter, pH 6.0, containing Brij-35, 1.5 g/liter) and (●- - - -●) 50 µl and (●—●) 100 µl of serum containing prostatic extract

adding enough of the propanol/water mixture to 0.1, 0.2, 0.3, 0.4, 0.5, 0.6, 0.7, and 0.8 ml of thymolphthalein stock standard solution to make 1.0 ml in each case. Into a set of nine tubes dispense 550 µl of buffered substrate reagent and 1.0 ml of the working alkaline solution. Pipette 50 µl of distilled water into the first of these tubes and 50 µl of each diluted standard solution into subsequent tubes. Mix well and read the absorbances of these solutions at 590 nm, using the first of the tubes as blank.

The absorbances obtained will be equivalent to those obtained by the action of 10, 20, 30, 40, 50, 60, 70, and 80 U of acid phosphatase per liter of serum. Plot absorbances vs. U/liter on linear graph paper.

Results

Effect of Source of Substrate

Roy et al. (*1*) found that under the conditions of their method, prostatic acid phosphatase activity was maximal with a substrate concentration of 2.2–2.4 mmol/liter. Morin (*2*), using ammonium thymolphthalein monophosphate, also found the optimal substrate concentration to be 2–3 mmol/liter. Using thymolphthalein monophosphate supplied by Regis Chemical Co. and the method described by Roy et al. (*1*), we found that a substrate concentration half that obtained by these workers gave maximal activity. When we compared substrate concentration optima for thymolphthalein monophosphate from the three sources listed above, we found that optimal concentration for maximum prostatic acid phosphatase activity varied with the source of thymolphthalein used, as did also the values for activities of prostatic acid phosphatase—the activity was greatest when substrate from Regis Chemical Co. was used, followed by those from Sigma and Worthington (Figure 1).

Two different lot numbers of thymolphthalein monophosphate from Regis Chemical Co., one purchased

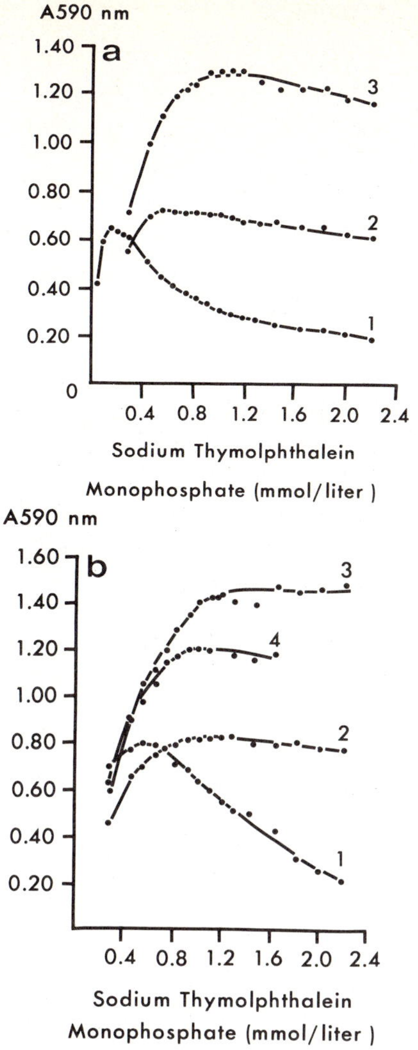

Fig. 2. (*a*) Effect of s/r ratio on optimum substrate concentration for prostatic acid phosphatase activity

Reaction mixture, 0.6 ml buffer described in Figure 1, and (*1*) 50 μl of diluted prostatic extract, (*2*) 50 μl of serum containing prostatic extract, or (*3*) 100 μl of serum containing prostatic extract

(*b*) Effect of s/r ratio on optimum substrate concentration for prostatic acid phosphatase activity

Reaction mixture, 0.6 ml acetate buffer (150 mmol/liter, pH 5.4, containing Brij-35, 1.5 g/liter) and (*1*) 50 μl of diluted prostatic extract, (*2*) 50 μl of serum containing prostatic extract, (*3*) 100 μl of serum containing prostatic extract, or (*4*) 50 μl of serum from patient with prostatic carcinoma

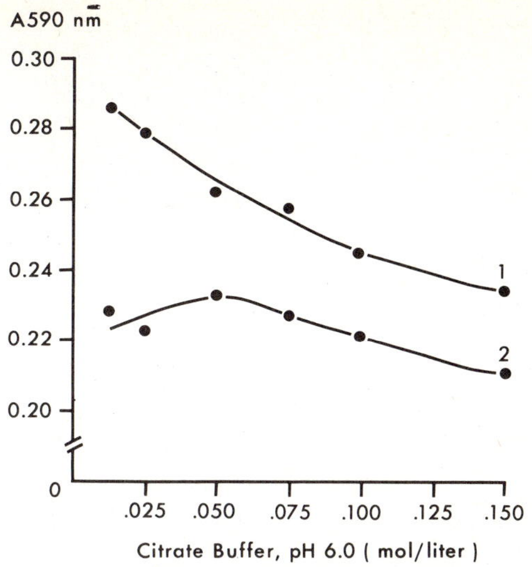

Fig. 3. Effect of citrate concentration on acid phosphatase activity with use of thymolphthalein monophosphate from Regis Chemical Co.

Reaction mixture, 0.6 ml citrate buffer (pH 6.0, containing Brij-35, 1.5 g/liter) thymolphthalein monophosphate, 1 mmol/liter; and 100 μl of serum. (*1*) prostatic extract in serum containing 20 μl of acetate buffer (5 mol/liter, pH 5.0) per milliliter of serum. (*2*) prostatic extract in serum containing no added acetate as preservative

a year earlier and stored at room temperature and the second purchased three months earlier and stored at −20 °C, gave identical acid phosphatase activities, although blank values were about 40% smaller with the product stored at −20 °C. We used thymolphthalein monophosphate from Regis for the rest of the work reported here, except as specifically noted.

Effect of S/R Volume Ratio[1]

Roy et al. (*1*) used an s/r ratio of 1/6 and Morin (*2*) used a ratio of 1/3.5. We found that optimum substrate concentration was influenced by this ratio, decreasing as the ratio was decreased; for prostatic extract alone the optimum substrate concentration was as low as 0.15 mmol/liter, when we used the buffer conditions of Roy et al. (*1*)—i.e., citrate buffer, 0.1 mol/liter, pH 6.0 (Figure 2*a*). The ratio also influenced substrate concentration giving maximal activity in the modified method described herein, although less markedly in this acetate buffer medium than in the citrate buffer of Roy et al. (*1*). The optimum substrate concentration by our method (s/r ratio, 1/12) was 1.0–1.2 mmol/liter. With a ratio of 1/6, similar to that of Roy et al. (*1*), activity was greatest with a substrate concentration of 1.2–1.4 mmol/liter, and with prostatic extract alone optimum substrate concentration was 0.6 mmol/liter (Figure 2*b*).

Effect of Buffer

Citrate buffer. Roy et al. (*1*) states that prostatic acid phosphatase activity was maximal with a 0.1 mol/liter concentration of citrate buffer (80 mmol/liter when dilution by sample is considered). We observed no peak activity for acid phosphatase in citrate buffer, pH 6.0 in concentrations ranging from 10 mmol/liter to 200 mmol/liter as long as the pH of the serum or extract used was preadjusted to reaction pH by addition of acetate buffer; increasing citrate concentrations resulted in decreasing acid phosphatase activities. We confirmed these results by use of thymolphthalein monophosphate from the three suppliers. When serum was not acidified buffer concentrations with substrate from all three sources, but under these conditions the pH of the reaction medium deviated from the original pH. Data illustrating this are shown in Figure 3 for substrate from Regis Chemical Co.

Acetate buffer. With serum containing prostatic extract and an s/r ratio of 1/12, the optimal acetate

[1] The "s/r ratio" is the ratio of the volume of serum sample to the volume of the final reaction mixture.

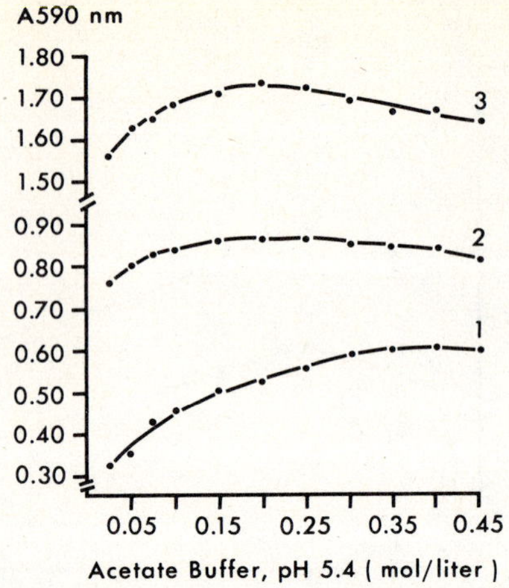

Fig. 4. Effect of acetate buffer concentration on acid phosphatase activity
Reaction mixture, 0.6 ml thymolphthalein monophosphate (1.0 mmol/liter, in acetate buffer, 0.15 mol/liter, pH 5.4, containing Brij-35, 1.5 g/liter) and (*1*) 50 μl of diluted prostatic extract, (*2*) 50 μl serum containing prostatic extract (2 μl), or (*3*) 50 μl of serum containing prostatic extract (4 μl)

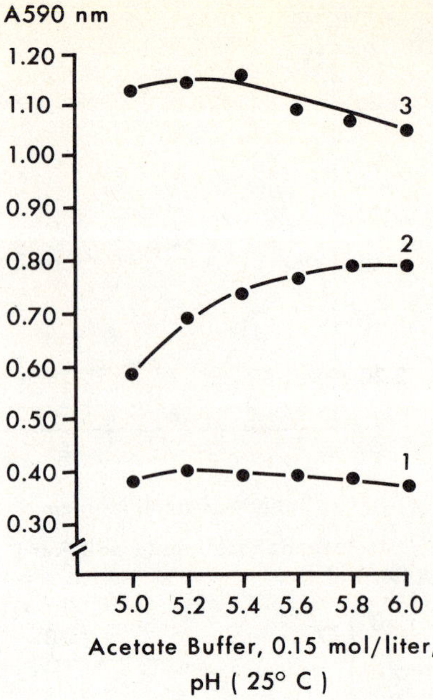

Fig. 5. Effect of pH on acid phosphatase activity
Reaction mixture, 0.6 ml: substrate described in Figure 4 and (*1*) and (*3*), 50 μl of serum containing aliquots of prostatic extract or (*2*) 50 μl of diluted prostatic extract

buffer concentration was 150–200 mmol/liter at pH 5.4. In the absence of serum a buffer concentration of 350–400 mmol/liter was required for maximal prostatic acid phosphatase activity (Figure 4). The optimal pH with acetate buffer 150 mmol/liter was 5.2–5.4 with an s/r ratio of 1/12, and 5.8–6.0 for prostatic extract alone (Figure 5).

Effect of Surfactant

The concentration of Brij-35 optimal for hydrolysis of substrate by prostatic acid phosphatase in our method was determined. In the presence of serum (s/r ratio, 1/12) a concentration in the final reaction mixture of 1.5 g/liter was found to be optimal. In the absence of serum a concentration of 5 g of Brij-35 per liter was required to give maximal activity, and in the absence of both serum and Brij-35, the activity of prostatic acid phosphatase was negligible (Figure 6). Roy et al. (*1*) used Brij-35 (5 g/liter) in their reaction mixture to stabilize the substrate in the buffer solution. In the absence of the surfactant we, too, noticed that precipitation occurred in the substrate/buffer reagent on refrigeration, but inclusion of Brij-35 at the concentration giving maximal activity under our conditions (1.5 g/liter) prevented this.

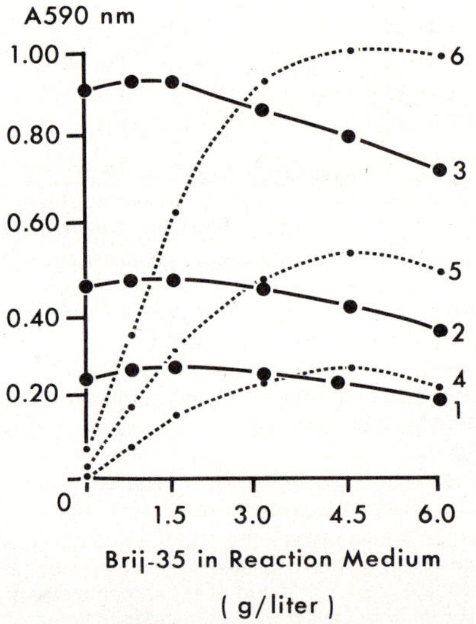

Fig. 6. Effect of Brij-35 surfactant on prostatic acid phosphatase activity
Reaction mixture, 0.6 ml thymolphthalein monophosphate, 1.0 mmol/liter in acetate buffer, 0.15 mol/liter, pH 5.4 and (●- - - -●) prostatic extract alone or (●—●) prostatic extract in 50 μl of normal serum

Linearity

Prostatic acid phosphatase activity is linearly related to time of incubation for at least 30 min in the presence of a constant concentration of serum and of saturating substrate conditions. Linearity with concentration extends to an absorbance of 6.0 in the kit method and to an absorbance of 10.0 in the method described herein (determined in each case by dilution of the final colored solutions with working alkali color developer solution to bring the absorbance into a readable range) in the absence of serum but addition of normal serum decreased the range of linearity in both the kit and modified methods (Figure 7). Activities first increased and then decreased with increasing s/r ratio when the medium contained a constant concentration of prostatic extract (Figure 7). With an s/r ratio of 1/12 linearity with concentration of prostatic acid phosphatase extended to an absorbance of 3.5. When the s/r ratio exceeded 1/12, activity became nonlinear with concentration of enzyme (Figure 8).

Termination of Reaction, and Color Development

Roy et al. (*1*) used 5 ml of Na_2CO_3 (50 mmol/liter) and NaOH (50 mmol/liter) solution per 1.2 ml of reac-

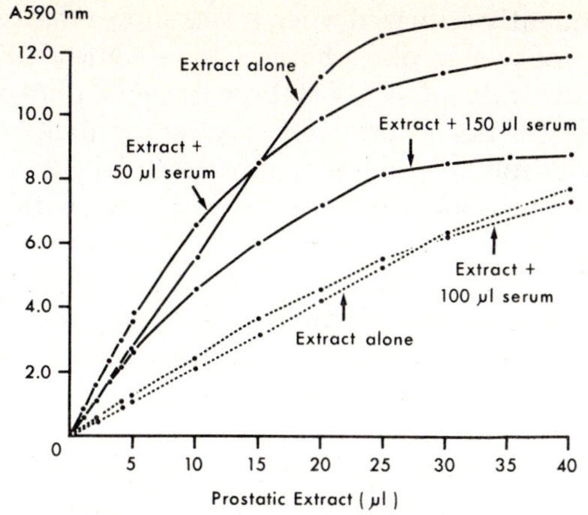

Fig. 7. Effect of serum on linearity of acid phosphatase activity in a prostatic extract

(*a*) ●- - - -●, activities found by use of the kit method (half specified volumes, 0.6 ml total reaction mixture). (*b*) ●—●, activities found by our modified method (0.6 ml total reaction mixture). Absorbance of 3.5 equivalent to 100 U/liter

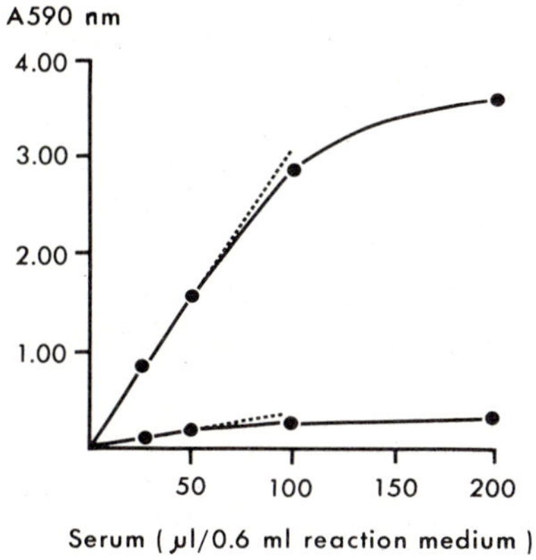

Fig. 8. Linearity of acid phosphatase with increasing concentrations of serum containing prostatic acid phosphatase

Reaction mixture: that of the present method, 0.6 ml. Absorbance of 1.75 equivalent to 50 U/liter

tion mixture (a final concentration of 40 mmol/liter) to terminate acid phosphatase activity and develop the color. This resulted in more than fivefold dilution of thymolphthalein liberated by enzyme activity. We reduced the volume of alkali to 1.0 ml per 0.6 ml of reaction mixture, so that liberated thymolphthalein was diluted only half as much and final absorbances were thus doubled. A solution of Na_2CO_3, 0.1 mol/liter, and NaOH, 0.1 mol/liter, (equivalent to a final concentration of 60 mmol/liter) was found to be adequate for color development and pH change.

Serum Preservative

Roy et al. (*1*) recommended use of 20 µl of acetate buffer (5 mol/liter, pH 5.0) per milliliter of serum as preservative. Because acetate buffer, 0.15 mol/liter, pH 5.4 (25 °C), is used in the final reaction medium of the modified method, we used 50 µl of acetate buffer, 5 mol/liter, pH 5.4, per milliliter of serum to bring the pH to that required and adjusted the concentration of acetate in the buffer substrate reagent to allow for this.

Table 1. Activities of Prostatic Acid Phosphatase as Measured by Our Modified Method (I), the Method of Roy et al. (II)[a] and the Worthington Kit Method (III)

Activity (U/liter)			Increase in sensitivity	
I[b]	II	III	I/II	I/III
17.9	2.8		6.3	
17.7	2.7		6.5	
7.7	1.7		4.5	
23.7	7.3		3.2	
22.6	8.8		2.6	
22.6	7.9		2.9	
19.3	6.6		2.9	
19.0	7.3		2.6	
18.8	6.2		3.0	
18.7	7.3		2.6	
15.1	5.4		2.8	
13.6	5.2		2.6	
11.9	4.4		2.7	
10.6	4.0	3.2	2.6	3.3
10.5	3.9	3.3	2.7	3.9
10.5	4.9	3.3	2.6	3.2
10.0	4.1	3.2	2.4	3.1
8.5	3.0	2.4	2.8	3.5
2.5	0.8		3.1	

[a] But containing Brij-35 surfactant, 1.5 g/liter.

[b] First three data are for prostatic extract; remaining 16 are for serum samples containing prostatic extract.

Comparison of Acid Phosphatase Activities by Our Modified Method, the Method of Roy et al. (*1*), and the Worthington Kit Method

Table 1 compares acid phosphatase activities obtained by the modified method described herein; the method of Roy et al. (*1*), but using thymolphthalein monophosphate from Regis Chemical Co.; and the Worthington kit method. An about threefold increased sensitivity is apparent in the modified method when prostatic extract is added to normal serum. Absence of serum from the reaction medium, shown above to affect optimum substrate and buffer concentration, results in greater increase in activity of prostatic acid phosphatase under the conditions of the modified method compared with the other procedures.

Acid Phosphatase Activity in Normal Serum

By either the unmodified kit method or our modified method described above, acid phosphatase activities were similar in sera of both male and female hospital patients. The normal range of activities in individuals without prostatic disease ranged from 0.5 to 1.9 U/liter ($\bar{X} \pm 2$ SD) by our modified method as compared to a normal range of up to 0.53 U/liter for the kit method.

Acid Phosphatase Activity in Urine

Acid phosphatase activities in undialyzed urines of female children ranged up to 20-fold the activities in sera of normal men.

Discussion

The modifications we have introduced into the method of Roy et al. (*1*) include reduction in substrate concentration; change in buffer type, ionic strength and pH; reduction in s/r ratio; reduction in concentration of Brij-35; reduction in total reaction volume and in volume of alkaline color developer; and a change in the pH and final concentration of acetate buffer used as acid phosphatase preservative in serum. These modifications increase the sensitivity of the method by a factor of three, enabling use of one-quarter the volume of serum (50 μl) used previously (0.2 ml). Linearity of the reaction under the modified conditions extends to an absorbance of about 3.5, 100 U/liter. Variations in the optimum concentration of buffer and surfactant that occur on addition of serum to the reaction medium and on changing the s/r ratio could be related to an effect of the protein or Brij-35 in complexing with the thymolphthalein monophosphate and providing a more readily available substrate for the enzyme.

The work reemphasizes the already well known but often neglected importance of standardization in clinical enzyme methodology. The observed effects of the s/r ratio on prostatic acid phosphatase activity, together with the differences found on using thymolphthalein monophosphate from different manufacturers, illustrates the necessity for absolute definition of methods, even to source of reagents. The complexity of phosphatase reactions, well-documented with respect to alkaline phosphatase, where changing buffer ion markedly alters enzyme activity, applies also to acid phosphatases. Discrepant results and much confusion can arise as a result of even the most minor modification in methodology. Our point of view about the importance of standardization has previously been expressed (*3*).

While Roy et al. (*1*) have shown that thymolphthalein monophosphate provides a substrate with greater specificity for prostatic acid phosphatase than some other substrates commonly used, it is apparent from the acid phosphatase activities found in urines of female children that the substrate is not completely specific for the prostatic form of the enzyme. This is confirmed by the similarities in the ranges of acid phosphatase activities found in the serum of males and females. The latter observation agrees with the inference of other workers (*4, 5*) that the acid phosphatase normally found in serum is not of prostatic origin.

A method involving an alternative substrate, α-naphthyl phosphate, shown previously to have relatively high specificity for prostatic acid phosphatase (*6*), was subsequently criticized when it was shown that platelet and urinary acid phosphatases have some affinity for this substrate (*4*, 7). Erythrocyte acid phosphatase apparently has a lower affinity for thymolphthalein monophosphate than other substrates considered to be relatively specific for prostatic acid phosphatase, such as α-naphthyl phosphate, but the relative activity of platelet to prostatic acid phosphatase with thymolphthalein monophosphate as determined by Roy et al. (*1*) indicates only a small increase in specificity—a ratio of 1.5 for α-naphthyl phosphate as compared with 1.0 for thymolphthalein monophosphate (*1*, Table 3). During routine use of our method here we have observed that acid phosphatase activities more than twice the upper limit of the normal range may be found in patients with lymphoproliferative disorders and markedly elevated platelet counts. Platelets can be differentiated from prostate as a source of acid phosphatase in specimens from such patients by comparing the acid phosphatase activity in platelet-free heparinized plasma with that of serum; if the elevated activity in serum is of blood-cell origin, the activity falls within the normal range in the platelet-free plasma.

In summary, we have increased approximately threefold the sensitivity of the method for determination of acid phosphatase with thymolphthalein monophosphate as substrate, and have shown that serum affects critical variables for determination of prostatic acid phosphatase activity, and that the source of substrate affects the activities obtained. The work reemphasizes the importance of standardization of methodology for determination of enzyme activities in clinical laboratories.

References

1. Roy, A. V., Brower, M. E., and Hayden, J. E., Sodium thymolphthalein monophosphate: A new acid phosphatase substrate with greater specificity for the prostatic enzyme in serum. *Clin. Chem.* **17,** 1093 (1971).

2. Morin, L. G., Ammonium thymolphthalein monophosphate as a new substrate for alkaline and acid phosphatase determinations in serum. *Clin. Chem.* **18,** 1135 (1973).

3. Spitzer, R., and Ewen, L., Enzyme standardisation—Reference Methods or Official Methods? *Clin. Biochem.* **6,** 63 (1973).

4. Amador, E., Price, J. W., and Marshall, G., Serum acid α-naphthyl phosphatase activity. *Am. J. Clin. Pathol.* **51,** 202 (1968).

5. Zucher, M. B., and Borrelli, J., Platelets as a source of serum acid nitrophenyl phosphatase. *J. Clin. Invest.* **38,** 148 (1959).

6. Babson, A. L., Read, P. A., and Phillips, G. E., The importance of the substrate in assays of acid phosphatase in serum. *Am. J. Clin. Pathol.* **32,** 83 (1959).

7. Amador, E., and Price, J. W., Serum acid α-naphthylphosphatase activity. *Clin. Chem.* **14,** 185 (1968).

CLIN. CHEM. 22/5, 633–637 (1976)

Evaluation of Lipase Activity in Serum by Radial Enzyme Diffusion

Jack M. Goldberg and Peter Pagast

Results of determination of serum lipase by radial enzyme diffusion correlate well with those by a titrimetric reference method in the abnormal range. The specificity of the diffusion assay allows the differentiation of patients with pancreatic disease, even when the lipase activity of the serum is within the normal limits of the titrimetric assay. Pancreatic lipase is not detectable by the diffusion assay in the serum of individuals who are free from pancreatic disease.

Additional Keyphrases: *pancreatic disease • titrimetry compared • tissue lipases • urinary lipase • enzyme-binding inhibitor*

Determination of lipase activity in serum is useful in the evaluation of diseases of the pancreas (*1*). Several procedures in routine use for measurement of lipase activity are based on the Cherry and Crandall method (*2, 3*) in which olive oil is hydrolyzed and the fatty acids formed are measured titrimetrically. Alternatively, the fatty acids liberated have been determined by the formation of their copper soaps (*4*). Other tests of lipase activity are based on the clearing of very dilute emulsions of olive oil (*5, 6*).

The assay we describe here depends on measurement of the zones of clearing of a turbid emulsion of olive oil immobilized in buffered agarose by radial enzyme diffusion of lipase in the gel. The zone of clearing is shown to be proportional to the enzyme activity in the serum. The method is rapid, requires only a small sample, is easily performed, and is adequately sensitive. The results are compared with those obtained by the titrimetric assay of Tietz and Fiereck (*3*).

Departments of Biochemistry, Biophysics and Pathology, Stritch School of Medicine, Loyola University of Chicago, Maywood, Ill. 60153; and Department of Pathology, Resurrection Hospital, Chicago, Ill. 60631.

Received Dec. 11, 1975; accepted Feb. 24, 1976.

Materials and Methods

We purchased materials for the titrimetric assay of lipase in kit form from Sigma Chemical Co., St. Louis, Mo. 63178. Lipase diffusion plates were purchased in kit form from Advanced Biomedical Methods, Inc., Niles, Ill. 60648. The kit (Diffuzyme Lipase) contains 10 10-well plates of the Petri dish type, 50 mm in diameter. According to the manufacturer, they contain 4 ml of a mixture of 40 mg of olive oil, 2 g of sodium deoxycholate, 1 g of sodium azide, and 10 g of agarose, all in 1 liter of tris(hydroxymethyl)aminomethane HCl buffer (pH 9.1, 50 mmol/liter). A detailed description of the manufacture of the plates has been published (*7*).

Titrimetric Assay of Lipase

We used the Sigma kit ingredients for the assay of Tietz and Fiereck (*3*), except that half volumes were used. We modified the preparation of the blank for each specimen as follows. Olive oil emulsion, 5 ml, in one tube, and 1.25 ml of water, 0.5 ml of buffer, and 0.5 ml of serum in another tube were incubated for 3 h at 37 °C. The contents of the two tubes were then combined and used for the assay of the specimen blank.

Measurement of Lipase by Diffusion

A commercial control serum (Enzatrol, Lot No. ET241A; Dade, Div. American Hospital Supply Co., Miami, Fla. 33512) was used as a secondary standard; it gave a value of 806 U/liter by the titrimetric assay. Successive double dilutions of this standard serum with a pool of normal (blood donors) serum yielded a set of standards with pancreatic lipase activities of 806, 403, 202, 101, 50, and 25 U/liter. (A "normal" pool of serum is designated as one having no activity in the assay described below and is assigned zero activity.) Ten microliters of each of these standards was placed into wells

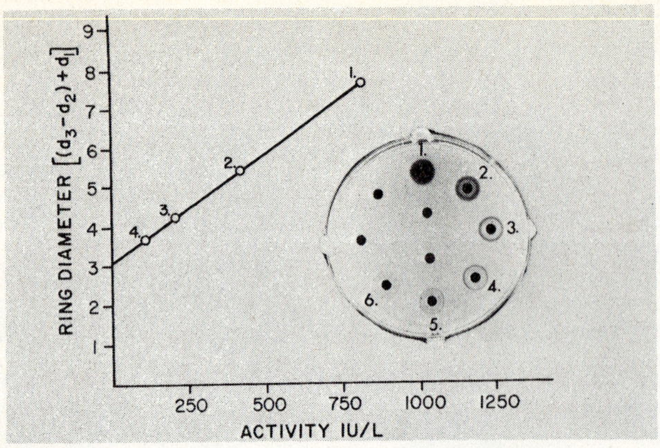

Fig. 1. Typical standard curve for serial dilutions of control serum in pooled normal serum. (Inset: photo of actual plate)
Dark zones represent cleared substrate. Values (U/liter) are: *1*, 806; *2*, 403; *3*, 202; *4*, 101; *5*, 50; *6*, 25

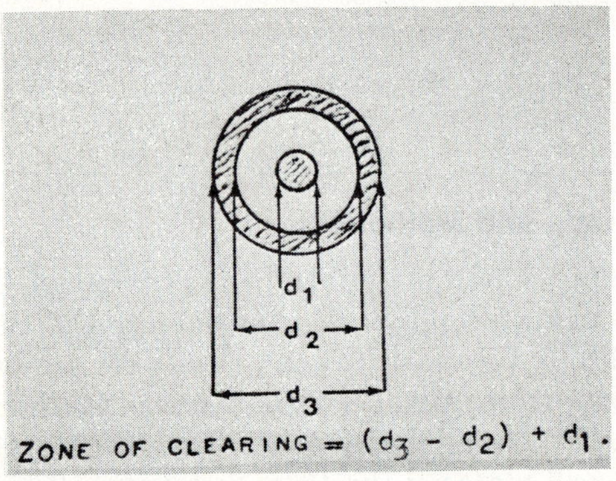

Fig. 2. Diagrammatic representation of "bulls-eye" phenomenon and calculation of diameter of clearing zone

1–6 (3-mm wells) and 10-μl portions of patients' sera were placed in the remaining wells. The plate was covered with its tightly fitting lid and incubated for 2 h by floating the plate in a water bath set at 37 °C. After incubation, the plate was opened, observed by transmitted light from a bright incandescent lamp, and a Polaroid photograph taken. In latter experiments, only three standard dilutions were run per plate. As shown in Figure 1, the undiluted Enzatrol shows a zone of clearing (dark zone) from the edge of the sample well. However, subsequent dilutions in pooled normal serum exhibit a zone of uncleared substrate around the sample well surrounded by a zone of clearing. This is shown diagrammatically in Figure 2. Measurements of the cleared zones in these cases were used as follows. The outer diameter of the clear zone (d_3), inner diameter of the cleared zone (d_2) and the diameter of the sample well (d_1) were measured and the zone of clearing expressed according to the formula $(d_3 - d_2) + d_1$. A standard curve was obtained by plotting, on normal graph paper, lipase activity on the abscissa against the diameter of the cleared zones on the ordinate. Lipase activity of each patient's serum was estimated from this standard curve. Sera with activity >800 U/liter were diluted with the pooled normal serum and reassayed.

Table 1. Statistical Comparisons of Two Procedures for Estimating Lipase Activity

	Titration		Diffusion	
	Intra-day	Between-day	Intra-day	Between-day
Mean, U/liter	539	534	639	630
SD, U/liter	42	44	14	20
CV %	7.8	8.3	2.2	3.2
n	20	20	20	20

Assay of Tissue Lipases

Extracts of various human organs obtained from autopsy were analyzed by both diffusion and titration. The extracts were prepared by homogenizing 10 g of tissue in 100 ml of physiological saline. The homogenates were centrifuged (1000 × *g*, 5 min) to remove coarse material and the supernates centrifuged (40 000 × *g*, 20 min). These final supernates were used for evaluation of lipase activity.

Assay of Urinary Lipase

One hundred random urines and six urines from patients with acute pancreatitis were assayed for lipase activity on the diffusion plates. Successive doubling dilutions of Enzatrol (806 U/liter) with pooled urine as diluent was used for standard curve generation.

Results

Table 1 summarizes our evaluations of 20 Monitrol 11 control serum samples by both methods. These results are within-lot data. However, we have not found any significant lot-to-lot variation in the three lots we have tried. Shelf life on the plates is excellent (we have used one lot for nine months) if the plates are stored in their polyethylene bag in the refrigerator. Failure to store properly has resulted in some plates deteriorating because of evaporation and consequent shrinking and drying of the gels.

Sera suspected of containing abnormal lipase activity (from patients suspected of having pancreatic disease) were investigated, and the results are summarized in Table 2. Of 45 patients with serum lipase estimated within the "normal" range by the titrimetric assay, 30 (67%) showed no activity by the diffusion method and were assigned 0 activity. The remaining 15 samples did show activity, although the highest activity observed was 220 U/liter, and of these patients three were diagnosed as having pancreatitis at laparotomy, two had common-duct stones, with abnormally high concentrations of bilirubin in the serum, one had traumatic pancreatitis, one had hepatic coma, and three had malignancies with no primary site found. Of 25 samples abnormal by the titrimetric assay only three showed no activity by diffusion analysis. However, the value for all three fell within 3 SD of the mean of the "normal" values of the titrimetric assay, and normal values were obtained for serum amylase activities.

Table 2. Serum Lipase Activity Evaluated by Two Techniques for Patients' Sera Suspected of Elevated Activity

Titration		Diffusion	
No. patients	Activity, U/liter	No. patients	Activity, U/liter
45	0–278	30	0
		5	28
		5	83
		3	139
		1	167
		1	222
19	279–556	3	0
		9	28–139
		4	140–278
		3	279–556
1	834	1	1557
1	917	1	1835
1	1027	1	389
1	1223	1	556
1	1696	1	2760
1	4000	1	3670

Table 3. Lipase Activities of Organ Extracts,[a] as Assessed by Two Techniques

	Titration	Diffusion
Organ	U/liter of extract	
Small intestine	167	0
Stomach	139	0
Heart	56	0
Liver	56	0
Kidney	167	0
Spleen	28	0
Pancreas	6950	5560

[a] 100 g of tissue was extracted per liter of saline. Activity expressed per gram wet wt is therefore 1% of the above values.

Table 3 summarizes our results for extracts of various tissues obtained at autopsy.

Urine showed no lipase activity by diffusion analysis, even when the patient had acute pancreatitis.

The limit of sensitivity of the diffusion assay, defined as the lowest activity detectable after 2 h at 37 °C, was assessed by diluting two samples of a serum with very high lipase activity (3892 U/liter, measured titrimetrically). The first sample we diluted with pooled normal serum and observed activity at 256-fold dilution (15 U/liter); the second sample, diluted with physiological saline, did not exhibit the double zone "bulls-eye" effect and activity was observed at 1/128 dilution (30 U/liter).

Discussion

This study suggests that determination of lipase activity in serum by radial enzyme diffusion is a simple and reliable procedure. Correlation with the titrimetric assay is difficult to assess, because the two procedures appear to measure different variables. However, if one determines the relationship on an abnormal/normal basis, correlation of the diffusion assay is excellent when the titrimetric assay is abnormal. One-third of the patients judged to be "normal lipase" patients by the titration method were classed as pancreatic disease patients by the diffusion assay; of these, two-thirds were otherwise established as true cases of pancreatic inflammation. Hence the diffusion assay is as reliable as the titrimetric assay in cases of acute pancreatitis, but owing to its apparent specificity for the pancreatic enzyme (as shown by tissue extracts) and its sensitivity (as shown by the limits of detectability), it is evidently a more reliable diagnostic indicator in less severe cases of pancreatitis.

There are two major differences between the two methods: pH and inclusion of bile salts. The pH optimum for serum lipase activity has generally been accepted as pH 7–8. However, as shown by Tietz and Fiereck (*3*), this optimum pH range is shown only by normal sera, whereas serum from patients with pancreatitis do not show this optimum and show virtually no change in activity between pH 7–9. Vogel and Zieve (*5*), however, have shown that at pH 9.1 in the presence of bile salts, very little activity can be measured in normal serum, but that this is the preferred pH for studying pancreatic lipase. Tietz and Repique (*8*), using an unbuffered system while maintaining pH with a pH-stat, have confirmed these findings, suggesting that pH 8.8 is the optimum for serum lipase estimations. The use of pH 9.1 at 25 °C in the diffusion plate will result in a working pH of 8.79 at 37 °C, owing to the large temperature coefficient of Tris buffers. Thus, although comparison statistics between the two methods of lipase estimation will give a numerical value, its validity is somewhat dubious, and is, hence, omitted.

However, this study has brought out several pertinent questions. Why do normal sera show no activity by diffusion analysis? Is the technique not sensitive enough to assay the low normal enzyme activity in serum? Our studies on the limits of detectability show the method to be sensitive to activities as low as 15 U/liter. Is the titrimetric assay nonspecific, measuring in addition to pancreatic lipase the activities of other enzymes such as lipoprotein lipase, nonspecific esterases, and perhaps even proteases? This has been suggested by Tietz and Repique (*8*). Within the wide range of lipase activities found in healthy individuals, it is possible for a patient with a basal lipase activity of 60 U/liter, assayed titrimetrically, to quadruple this value because of the appearance of pancreatic lipase and still remain within the expected limits for the population. Hence the assay of lipase of diffusion lends itself to an excellent screening procedure because of the positive/negative nature of the results.

Table 4. Measurement of Clearing Zone Diameters (mm) from Figure 1

Well No.	Activity U/liter	Outer diameter d_3	Inner diameter d_2	Well diameter d_1	$(d_3 - d_2) + d_1$
1	806	7.7	3.0	3.0	7.7
2	403	7.7	5.4	3.0	5.3
3	202	7.7	6.4	3.0	4.3
4	101	7.7	7.1	3.0	3.6

Another question posed by the diffusion analysis is the phenomenon of the double-ring ("bulls-eye") appearance of the plate for sera containing <500 U of lipase activity per liter. Why is there a zone of no activity around the sample well surrounded by a zone of clearing? In all other enzyme diffusion assays as exemplified by the amylase assay of Ceska (*9*) and the lysoplate method of Osserman and Lawlor (*10*) for lysozyme assay, the kinetics of the assay show a logarithmic proportionality between enzyme activity (A) and the diameter of the zone of activity (d)—i.e., log A = d. This relationship is also true for the lipase diffusion assay when saline is used as the diluent. However, the data shown in Table 4, taken from the plate in Figure 1, show no relationship for any diffusion assay published (*11*). Because all the outer diameters (d_3) are equal in this case and the diameter of the sample well is a constant (d_1), the only variable is the inner diameter of the zone of clearing (d_2). The only relationship that shows any linearity is the expression $(d_3 - d_2) + d_1 = \mathrm{A}$. One must therefore look at the parameters of diffusion in gels to understand what might cause this phenomenon. Experimentally (Goldberg, unpublished) the following relationships are observed for molecules diffusing from a 3-mm well into agarose gel (10 g/liter of water):

$$d = [(\sqrt{\mathrm{t}} \times \log \mathrm{T})/\log \mathrm{M_r}] \times k$$

where d = diameter of diffusion zone; t = time in minutes; T = temperature in °C; M_r = molecular weight of diffusible molecule; and k = a constant (parameters unknown, but empirically found to be 2.28 for diffusion in agarose). However, when one is considering diffusion of enzymes in substrate gels, several other factors must be taken into account, including the concentration of the substrate, the affinity of the enzyme for this substrate, and the sensitivity of the method used to detect the enzyme in the gel. Therefore, in a straightforward enzyme diffusion in a substrate gel, all factors are constant except the diameter of the zone of enzyme activity, which is dependent only on the detectability limit. Assuming constant sensitivity, detectability will therefore depend on the number of active enzyme molecules at any given point, which itself will depend on the initial concentration (hence activity) of enzyme in the fluid placed in the sample well, and the relationship d = log A holds true. How then can we explain why the outer diameters of the zones of activity are equal in this lipase diffusion plate? Do all samples contain equal amounts of enzyme? Obviously not. Therefore, we must postulate free diffusion of the enzyme in the gel until it can bind (and hence hydrolyze) its substrate. This, therefore, assumes some agent in serum, but not in urine or saline, which can prevent the binding of the enzyme to the substrate, and that this agent is in excess when the serum activity of lipase is <500 U/liter. According to the formula governing diffusion in gels, the lipase molecule must be of a much smaller molecular weight than this inhibiting agent to enable it to diffuse into a zone of enzyme excess where it can exhibit its activity, which accounts for the larger zone of inhibition as the enzyme concentration diminishes. The characterization of this inhibitor and its mode of action is still being studied, but preliminary data suggest a macromolecule that binds not to the enzyme, but to the substrate.

Studies on urinary lipase by enzyme diffusion suggest that lipase is not excreted via the kidneys, at least not in an active form. One urine that exhibited the highest amylase activity ever found in this laboratory (350 000 dye units/100 ml) did not show any lipase activity. The possibility of an inhibitor in urine was excluded by the observation that dilution of the Enzatrol standard with pooled urine gave results indistinguishable from those for dilutions made with saline.

There are several drawbacks to the use of enzyme diffusion as a routine method. The first is the standardization of the plate. Use of a secondary standard (or calibrator) is of course undesirable, because these calibrators are themselves standardized by what appears to be a less specific method. Nevertheless, as a pragmatic interim solution, these control sera do serve as workable standards to generate clinically useful data. The second major drawback is the measurement of small diameters. This problem is especially acute when the lipase activity is less than 100 U/liter. A pragmatic solution to this problem in our routine clinical laboratory is visual comparison of these low activity sera to standard sera. Again, this solution, although not ideal, gives clinically useful information, because the maximum error (50 U/liter) is of little clinical importance at this low level of lipase activity and the positive/negative nature of the test is sufficient.

In conclusion, it appears that estimation of serum lipase by radial enzyme diffusion, while clinically more useful than other methods because of its specificity for the pancreatic enzyme, has posed many new questions about this enzyme and we believe that all methods currently in use should be reassessed before any reference procedure is adopted.

This study was supported in part by NIH Research Training Grant in Clinical Chemistry, NI GMS/DADPA IT01 GM02122-01A1, under which Peter Pagast was a postdoctoral trainee, and by a grant from the Park Ridge Health Foundation, Park Ridge, Ill. Jack Goldberg acknowledges affiliation with Advanced Biomedical Methods, Inc.

References

1. Tietz, N. W., *Fundamentals of Clinical Chemistry,* Saunders, New York, N. Y., 1970, pp 419–420.

2. Cherry, J. S., and Crandall, L. A., Jr., The specificity of pancreatic lipase: Its appearance in the blood after pancreatic injury. *Am. J. Physiol.* **100,** 266 (1932).

3. Tietz, N. W., and Fiereck, E., Serum lipase. *Stand. Methods Clin. Chem.* **7,** 19 (1972).

4. Yang, J. S., and Biggs, H. G., A rapid and reliable method for the measurement of serum lipase activity. *Clin. Chem.* **17,** 512 (1971).

5. Vogel, W. C., and Zieve, L., A rapid and sensitive turbidimetric method for serum lipase based upon differences between the lipases of normal and pancreatitis serum. *Clin. Chem.* **9,** 168 (1963).

6. Burlind, G., and Galzigna, L., Turbidimetric procedure for the determination of lipase activity. *Clin. Chem.* **19,** 384 (1973).

7. Goldberg, J. M., Serum lipase method and medium. *U. S. Patent 3917515,* Nov. 4 (1975).

8. Tietz, N. W., and Repique, E. V., Proposed standard method for measuring lipase activity in serum by a continuous sampling technique. *Clin. Chem.* **19,** 1268 (1973).

9. Ceska, A., A new approach for quantitative and semiquantitative determinations of enzymic activities with simple laboratory equipment. Detection of amylase. *Clin. Chim. Acta* **33,** 135 (1973).

10. Osserman, E. F., and Lawlor, D. P., Serum and urinary lysozyme (muramidase) in monocytic and monomyelocytic leukemia. *J. Exp. Med.* **124,** 921 (1966).

11. Berne, B. H., Differing methodology and equations used in quantitating immunoglobulins by radial immunodiffusion—a comparative evaluation of reported and commercial techniques. *Clin. Chem.* **20,** 61 (1974).

CLIN. CHEM. 22/5, 638–642 (1976)

Diagnostic Use of Pancreatic Lipase Determination by Radial Enzyme Diffusion, and Design of a Routine Pancreatic Profile

Jack M. Goldberg

I show that detection of pancreatic lipase in serum by radial enzyme diffusion, when used in conjunction with amylase clearance/creatinine clearance ratio and alkaline phosphatase isoenzyme determination, provides a diagnostically meaningful representation of several forms of pancreatic disease.

Additional Keyphrases: *pancreatic disease, differential diagnosis • ratio of amylase clearance/creatinine clearance • liver disease*

The differential diagnosis of diseases of the pancreas remains an acute problem area in medicine today. It can be stated with some certainty that no single test has the capability of 100% accuracy in the diagnosis of pancreatic disease, much less in the determination of the etiology of the condition.

Basically, from the viewpoint of the clinical laboratory, inflammatory diseases of the pancreas can be placed in three broad categories: (*a*) acute, (*b*) chronic end stage, and (*c*) those cases that fall between *a* and *b*, including subacute pancreatitis, chronic relapsing pancreatitis, and space-occupying lesions of the pancreas. In addition, each group can be subdivided into obstructive and nonobstructive diseases and further subdivided into those with involvement of the common duct or simple pancreatic obstruction.

Various tests have been proposed to differentiate these conditions, but each measures a different metabolic aspect of the patient's physiology. Serum amylase activity is perhaps the most widely used and accepted index to pancreatic function. However, amylase is produced by several organs including pancreas, salivary glands, liver and kidney, and so an abnormally high value for serum amylase is only consistent with, but not diagnostic for, acute pancreatitis. An additional complication in the interpretation of serum amylase values is the kidney function of the patient. Amylase is excreted in the urine and, as such, the renal status of the patient can greatly influence its activity in serum and urine. Warshaw and Fuller (*1*) have proposed normalizing the amylase clearance rate to the creatinine clearance rate. Our experience with this clearance ratio will be discussed.

Departments of Biochemistry, Biophysics, and Pathology, Stritch School of Medicine, Loyola University of Chicago, Maywood, Ill. 60153; and Department of Pathology, Resurrection Hospital, Chicago, Ill. 60631.

Received Dec. 11, 1975; accepted Feb. 24, 1976.

Measurement of serum lipase activity is also commonly used as a pancreatic test. However, serum lipase estimations have not proven generally useful because of problems in quality control. Evidence for this statement is found in the Illinois regional quality-control program, in which CV's of 50 to 90% are not uncommon (although CV's this high admittedly usually are a reflection of poor technique rather than basically bad methodology). As pointed out by Tietz and Repique (*2*) and Goldberg and Pagast (*3*), this may be due in part to the nonspecificity of most titrimetric and turbidimetric methods in routine use. However, the specificity of lipase determination by radial enzyme diffusion for the pancreatic enzyme indicates that it can be a useful test of pancreatic status. Our experience with this test in routine clinical use is also discussed here.

Several enzymes have been proposed as useful tests for detecting obstructive diseases of the liver, among them γ-glutamyltransferase (EC 2.3.2.2) and 5′-nucleotidase (EC 3.1.3.5), but these are not specific enough to be diagnostic for hepatobiliary obstruction and their activities are often above normal in simple pancreatic disease. Rhone et al. (*6*) have shown that alkaline phosphatase isoenzymes, determined by electrophoresis, can be useful in establishing the diagnosis of hepatobiliary disease, owing to the presence of an alkaline phosphatase that is specific to the biliary tree. We have therefore incorporated alkaline phosphatase isoenzyme determination into our proposed pancreatic diagnostic profile.

The use of this profile and the clinical significance of the findings are the subject of this paper.

Methods and Materials

Amylase activity was measured in both serum and urine with the "Amylochrome" kit (Roche Diagnostics, Nutley, N.J. 07110). Creatinine was assayed with the Du Pont *aca* chemistry analyzer. Lipase was assayed with the "Diffuzyme Lipase" kit from Advanced Biomedical Methods, Inc., Niles, Ill. 60648. Alkaline phosphatase was assayed by the Calbiochem (La Jolla, Calif. 92037) "Stat Pack" procedure with the ABA-100 (Abbott Diagnostics, S. Pasadena, Calif. 91030) at 30 °C. All reagents for alkaline phosphatase isoenzyme determination were purchased from Sigma Chemical Co., St. Louis, Mo. 63178. "Noble Agar" (Difco Laboratories, Detroit, Mich. 48232) was used for the substrate support

Table 1. Screening Unselected Sera for Lipase Activity by Radial Enzyme Diffusion[a]

No. of positives	Other abnormalities
8	Elevated serum urea or creatinine.
7	Hyperglycemic fasting sera.
3	Bone fracture patients.
14	Pancreatitis (acute and chronic).

[a] n = 500; positives = 32; negatives = 468.

agar. The detailed method we used for alkaline phosphatase isoenzymes was as follows.

Sera for analysis were divided into two samples, one of which was heated at 56 °C for *exactly* 10 min, then cooled rapidly in running tap water. Sera that could not be analyzed within 4 h of blood drawing were frozen at −15 °C until analyzed.

Electrophoresis was performed with home-made equipment, essentially as described by Nerenberg et al. (7), with use of solid support for the cellulose acetate membrane. Two-microliter samples were applied to the membrane ("Sepraphore III"; Gelman Instrument Co., Ann Arbor, Mich. 48106) which had been soaked in tris(hydroxymethyl)aminomethane/barbital buffer (pH 8.8, 50 mmol of each per liter). The same buffer was used in the electrode chambers. Samples were applied to the membrane, heated and unheated samples adjacent to each other, together with a liver-extract control, a cord-blood (or bone) control and a commercial preparation of placental and intestinal enzymes (Dade, Miami, Fla. 33512). A sample of any available serum was applied at one side of the membrane as a further reference sample. Electrophoresis was at 200 V for 30 min. Cooling with an ice pack over the membrane did not improve the results and was not done routinely.

While electrophoresis was in progress, the substrate buffer was prepared as follows: 5 mg of α-naphthol AS-MX phosphate was dissolved in 5 ml of 2-amino-2-methyl-1-propanol buffer (625 mmol/liter, pH 10.2) and mixed with 5 ml of a 20 g/liter solution of melted agar that had been cooled to about 50 °C. The mixture was poured into a shallow plastic dish, large enough to hold the cellulose acetate membrane, and allowed to cool. (We used the plastic plates from the Hyland Agar Gel IEP system). After electrophoresis, the unselected reference serum (the serum on the side) was carefully cut from the membrane and stained for serum proteins with a solution containing 10 g of Ponceau S per liter of trichloroacetic acid (50 g/liter), then destained in dilute acetic acid (50 ml/liter). The rest of the cellulose acetate membrane was carefully placed over the substrate agar and incubated for 30 min at 37 °C. At this time the isoenzyme pattern was viewed and assessed under a long wavelength (365 nm) ultraviolet lamp. For a permanent record, the strip was covered with a 1 g/liter aqueous solution of Fast Blue RR salt (Sigma, Grade III) until all the isoenzyme bands were fully visible, then removed from the agar and rinsed in a bath of dilute acetic acid. Both sections of the cellulose acetate membrane were

Table 2. Selective Screening of Possible False Positives for Pancreatic Lipase Activity by Radial Enzyme Diffusion

Classification	No. sera	No. positive lipase results (range, U/liter)
Uremic patients (creatinine range 17–140 mg/liter)	30	30 (14–140)
Hyperglycemic patients (fasting serum glucose 1300–3200 mg/liter)	50	4 (28–280)
Bone-fracture patients	10	3 (28–56)

Table 3. Summary of Pancreatic Profiles on Selected High-Risk Patients

No. of patients	Final diagnosis	Lipase, U/liter	Clearance ratio, % ±2 SD, or range	Alkaline phosphatase, total (U/liter)	Isoenzymes
85	No proven pancreatic disease	0	1.4 ± 1.2	28–103	α_2
17	Biliary tree disease	0	1.5 ± 1.2	36–469	α_1 α_2
4	Edema of common duct	56–112	1.1–2.4	60–180	α_1 α_2
3	Acute pancreatitis	280–560	3.2–15.6	33–58	α_2
4	Chronic relapsing pancreatitis	56–112	1.6–2.4	49–74	α_2
11	Acute pancreatitis with common duct obstruction	120–1120	2.6–16.1	47–580	α_1 α_2

Table 4. Typical Biochemical Variables in Pancreatic Disease

Patient	Diagnosis	Lipase, U/liter	Amylase dye, U/liter		Creatinine, mg/liter		Amylase clearance / Creatinine clearance	Alkaline phosphatase	
			Serum	Urine	Serum	Urine		Total (U/liter)	Isoenzymes
	"Normal"	0	450–2000	660–5430	8–15	Variable	2.5%	19–64	α_2 liver
E.R.	Duodenal ulcer	0	770	2600	7	1270	1.9	88	α_2
R.M.	Gastritis	0	1650	6800	10	3120	1.3	59	α_2
B.S.	Chronic end stage pancreatitis	0	910	4200	12	1880	2.9	30	α_2
A.F.	Chronic end stage pancreatitis	0	1270	3200	11	950	2.9	53	α_2
V.T.	Common duct stone	280	1630	5460	9	810	3.7	220	α_1 α_2
J.W.	Cholecystitis with edema of common duct	27	1470	2105	9	5560	2.3	540	α_1 α_2
A.H.	Stone in ampulla of Vater	1120	7780	36000	22	1500	6.8	242	α_1 α_2
A.M.	Cancer of common duct	2780	40000	30000	—	—	—	520	α_1 α_2
F.W.	Cholangitis	0	860	1310	3	770	0.6	469	α_1 α_2
J.P.	Cholangitis	0	860	2220	5	1090	1.2	265	α_1 α_2
B.C.	Acute pancreatitis	560	2850	12000	8	1050	3.2	33	α_2
A.P.	Acute pancreatitis	280	3500	15300	9	950	4.1	58	α_2
A.A.	Acute pancreatitis	560	4750	36250	9	440	15.6	58	α_2
C.P.	Chronic relapsing pancreatitis	56	820	1660	9	790	2.3	74	α_2
	Chronic relapsing pancreatitis	56	1670	3870	9	990	2.1	59	α_2
B.S.	Chronic relapsing pancreatitis	84	1810	1620	7	400	1.6	49	α_2

adjoined by mounting on a plastic sheet ("Cronar," Du Pont) and dried. The alkaline phosphatase isoenzymes were then referenced to the serum protein mobility and the isoenzyme controls.

Diagnosis was based on evidence found at laparotomy, autopsy, radiography, endoscopy, and on clinical evaluation.

Results

Unselected sera from 500 admissions to the hospital were screened for the presence of pancreatic lipase by radial enzyme diffusion. Results are summarized in Table 1. Selective screening of uremic, hyperglycemic, and fracture patients are summarized in Table 2. A summary of 125 full pancreatic profiles is given in Table 3. Typical profile results are shown in Table 4.

Discussion

The diagnostic use of pancreatic lipase determination by radial enzyme diffusion depends on the specificity (true-negative rate) and sensitivity (true-positive rate) of the results (*8*).

Results of screening hospitalized patients yielded a prevalence of 6.4% of positive results regardless of the activity. Table 1 suggests a true-positive percentage of at least 2.8%, and probably closer to 4.2% if one includes those patients exhibiting hyperglycemia, a common finding in chronic pancreatitis. This leaves a false-positive rate of 2.2%, comprised entirely of uremic and fracture patients. Hence the specificity of the test appears to be 98%.

Sensitivity, on the other hand, is more difficult to assess. Only two false negatives have so far been proven.

Both were cases of end stage pancreatitis, which at autopsy showed little or no functional pancreas tissue left. However, assuming that the prevalence of false negatives is even higher, this would give a sensitivity (based on 240 cases of pancreatitis over an 18-month span) of about 96%.

Before one can judge the predictive value of a test or its efficiency, the prevalence of the disease must be known (*8*). Little is found in the literature on the prevalence of pancreatitis. (Prevalence is defined as the number of patients per 100 000 population who have the disease whether in active or healed form at the time of the study.) The only reliable information I have with regard to prevalence is data from autopsy cases. This is a highly select and biased group, but it does provide at least a model for the statistical tests of predictive value and efficiency. Reviewing 100 consecutive autopsy reports, 40 specifically mentioned abnormal findings on microscopic examination of the pancreas. These findings included acute hemorrhagic disease, chronic fibrosis with inflammatory response, cysts, abscesses, metastatic carcinoma, and pancreatic carcinoma. Thus a prevalence of 40 000 per 100 000 deaths was found, and a more conservative prevalence figure of 25 000 was used in the tables of Galen and Gambino (*8*). In summary, if one uses a sensitivity of 96% and a specificity of 98% with a prevalence of 25 000 per 100 000 population, the predictive value of a positive lipase is 91%, the predictive value of a negative result is 99%, and the overall efficiency of the test is 97%. However, this efficiency is for screening a population without regard to symptomatology, and hence the lipase test, when applied specifically to patients with symptoms consistent with pancreatitis, will have an even greater predictive value and efficiency.

The incidence of falsely positive results localized to uremic, hyperglycemic and fracture patients was of major significance with regard to the specificity of the lipase test. Systematic analysis of these patients (Table 2) shows that 100% of uremic patients evidently have a positive lipase serum. Is this due to pancreatitis associated with uremia or to a concentration effect of serum lipase due to diminished renal clearance of the enzyme? The more probable explanation is the latter. However, even in the most severe cases of uremia (serum urea nitrogen >750 mg/liter; creatinine >100 mg/liter) the highest activity of lipase observed was 140 U/liter. This observation suggests that pancreatic lipase is a natural constituent of serum, but that its activity is below the threshold of detection in healthy individuals (<14 U/liter). The only positive lipase data should then be from individuals with pancreatitis or uremia. If this is so, why should lipase activity be positive in sera from hyperglycemic patients? Systematic analysis of hyperglycemic patients' sera yielded a positive lipase rate of 8% (four patients of 50). The prevalence of hyperglycemia in this hospital is about 15 to 20% of all sera analyzed. If one assumes a 20% incidence, this would suggest that 100 of the 500 unselected sera screened for lipase (Table 1) would be hyperglycemic and that, of these, 8% (eight samples) would be positive for lipase. This compares well with the seven samples actually found. Further investigation of the four patients who were positive for lipase in the hyperglycemia survey showed three with diabetic-type oral glucose-tolerance curves and above-normal triglycerides, with lipoprotein fractionation resembling type IV lipoproteinemia (*9*). Two of these gave histories of abdominal pain. The fourth patient in this group had metastatic adenocarcinoma of the colon and diabetes mellitus. Hence, hyperglycemia and positive serum lipase was consistent with pancreatitis and the lipase results were considered true positives.

Bone-fracture patients were the only other group that gave positive serum lipase. The most likely explanation of this observation is the presence of a nonpancreatic lipase liberated into the plasma from fat cell necrosis, a common feature of fractures. In this case, the positive serum lipase activity would represent an actual false-positive. However, the presence of this enzyme should not interfere with the diagnosis of pancreatitis, with the possible exception of traumatic pancreatitis with multiple fractures, such as might occur in an automobile accident. Nevertheless, any case of fat necrosis should be classified as a false positive unless further evidence, such as serum amylase activities, confirms the suspicion of pancreatitis.

It is for this reason that, even though the diffusion lipase assay has excellent specificity and sensitivity, it must be used in conjunction with other tests for full diagnostic utility.

Several comments must be made on the use of the pancreatic profile as described above and typified in Table 4. After about 200 such profiles on patients with pain in the upper left quadrant, with full data on about 125 of these, I concluded that there is wide biological variability in the results, probably due in great part to the time relationship between profiling and time of onset of symptoms. However, general remarks can be made on the profile. The most consistent finding in cases of pancreatic inflammation is an increased serum lipase. Pancreatic lipase has been observed in all such patients with both acute and chronic relapsing pancreatitis unless, as in patients B.S. and A.F. (Table 4), there is little or no functional pancreas.

Urinary amylase is the most misleading of the tests because of the great variability in the degree of concentration of the urine specimens obtained, as shown by the variation in the urinary creatinine. Serum amylase activity did not show this wide variation, even though activity is certainly related to the renal status of the patient. Applying the formula of Warshaw and Fuller (*1*) to normalize the amylase clearance rate to the creatinine clearance rate has certainly been most effective in our hands in discriminating the unaffected patient from the patient with pancreatic disease. However, there is disagreement on the discriminatory cut-off level. Warshaw and Fuller suggest an upper limit of 5.3 for the clearance ratio, whereas the present study suggests 2.6 as the 95% confidence limit of the clearance

Table 5. Diagnostic Implications of Proposed Pancreatic Profile

Serum lipase activity	Amylase clearance / Creatinine clearance	Serum alkaline phosphatase: Total activity	Isoenzymes	Most likely diagnosis
Normal	Normal	Normal	α_2	Normal function or no pancreatic function.
Normal	Normal	Above normal	α_1 α_2	Hepatobiliary disease.
Above normal	Above normal	Above normal	α_1 α_2	Common-duct obstruction.
Above normal	Above normal	Normal	α_2	Acute pancreatitis.
Above normal	Normal	Normal	α_2 or bone or α_1 α_2	Minimal pancreatic inflammation. Rule out chronic relapsing pancreatitis, small space occupying lesion, or cholecystitis with edema of common duct.

ratio. (The clearance ratios among unaffected patients has a normal distribution.) Levine et al. (*10*) report a normal range of clearance ratios between 1.33 and 3.12. These widely differing ranges are probably due to differences in the methods used to estimate amylase activity. All cases in the present study for whom the clearance ratio was above normal were also positive for serum lipase. The wide range of values obtained reflected the time reference between onset of symptoms and profiling, because the highest results obtained were for patients in the acute phase of the disease and the lower figures were obtained for convalescent patients. It should be noted that the two cases of end-stage chronic pancreatitis both have elevated clearance ratios. A similar finding was reported by Levine et al. (*10*) for a patient with anaplastic, spindle-cell carcinoma replacement of pancreatic tissue.

Including the data on alkaline phosphatase isoenzymes was most helpful to the interpretation of the profile. In all cases of obstructive liver disease, including both those with and without pancreatitis, the presence of the α_1 biliary tree enzyme was established. This information can only be obtained by electrophoretic fractionation of the isoenzymes, because liver contains at least two isoenzymes with similar heat stabilities. The mere statement that the increase was of liver origin (information gained from heat and chemical fractionation studies) is insufficient to distinguish hepatobiliary disease from hepatocellular disease.

In conclusion, pancreatic lipase estimation by radial enzyme diffusion is a clinically useful tool in the diagnosis of pancreatic disease. When used in conjunction with the other tests in the proposed profile it is capable of detecting inflammatory pancreatic disease, even chronic pancreatitis. However, before chronic pancreatitis can be diagnosed, the presence of azotemia, bone fractures, and fat necrosis must be ruled out. The routine use of this profile over a limited series of cases has led to a more consistent and more frequently accurate diagnosis than any single test. The entire profile can be completed in less than 3 h. In emergency situations, an interim partial profile, consisting of the clearance ratio and total alkaline phosphatase activity, can be performed within 30 min with the completed profile results following later. Interpretation of the profile is summarized in Table 5. Although these results and conclusions are based on a relatively small series of cases, it does provide a working diagnostic tool subject to modification of content and interpretation.

Supported by a grant from the Park Ridge Health Foundation, Park Ridge, Illinois.

References

1. Warshaw, A. L., and Fuller, A. F., Jr., Increased renal clearance of amylase in diagnosis of acute pancreatitis. *New Engl. J. Med.* **292,** 325 (1975).

2. Tietz, N. W., and Repique, E. V., Proposed standard method for measuring lipase activity in serum by a continuous sampling technique. *Clin. Chem.* **19,** 1268 (1973).

3. Goldberg, J. M., and Pagast, P., Evaluation of lipase activity in serum by radial enzyme diffusion. *Clin. Chem.* **22,** 633 (1976).

4. Lum, G., and Gambino, R., Serum gamma-glutamyl transpeptidase activity as an indicator of diseases of liver, pancreas or bone. *Clin. Chem.* **18,** 358 (1972).

5. Bodansky, O., and Schwartz, M. K., 5′-Nucleotidase. *Adv. Clin. Chem.* **11,** 277 (1968).

6. Rohne, D. P., White, F. M., and Gidaspow, H., Isoenzymes of alkaline phosphatase in serum of patients with hepatobiliary disorders. *Clin. Chem.* **19,** 1142 (1973).

7. Nerenberg, S. T., DeMarco, L., and Ganger, C., Rapid large-scale screening of blood proteins by use of cellulose acetate on a solid support. *Clin. Chem.* **18,** 145 (1972).

8. Galen, R. S., and Gambino, S. R., *Beyond Normality: The Predictive Value and Efficiency of Medical Diagnoses.* Wiley, New York, N.Y., 1975.

9. Fredrickson, D. S., and Lees, R. S., System for phenotyping hyperlipoproteinemia. *Circulation* **31,** 321 (1965).

10. Levine, R. I., Glauser, F. L., and Berk, J. E., Increased amylase-creatinine clearance ratio in nonpancreatic disorders. *New Engl. J. Med.* **292,** 329 (1975).

CLIN. CHEM. 22/5, 643–646 (1976)

The Anion Gap: Its Use in Quality Control

David L. Witte, John L. Rodgers, and David A. Barrett II

Because the anion gap is useful in classifying acid–base disorders, quantitative information on this variable should be readily available. Three populations were studied and means and central 90% ranges were determined for the anion gap, calculated as sodium−(chloride + bicarbonate). In 1047 hospitalized patients the mean was 12 mEq/liter with a central 90% range of 6–20 mEq/liter, 86 fasted volunteers had a mean of 13 mEq/liter with a 90% range of 9–17 mEq/liter, and 203 plasmaphoresis donors had a mean of 11 mEq/liter with a 90% range of 7–16 mEq/liter. Most of this variability can be accounted for by analytical rather than physiological variation. This quantitation of the anion gap is useful for interchecking electrolyte values as an additional and inexpensive means of laboratory quality control. In 73 of 75 abnormal anion gaps, for which the data were verified to be correct, the clinical information provided a reasonable explanation for the abnormality.

Additional Keyphrases: *organic acidosis* • *multiple myeloma* • *normal values*

Since the introduction by Gamble (*1*) in 1950 of the "Gamblegram" as a method of expressing the interrelationship of anions and cations, most physicians have become familiar with the concept that there exists a balance between these ions. In the common methods for expressing this balance, a difference between the anions and cations is generally present and this has been referred to as the "anion gap" (*2*). This gap has been shown to have clinical and laboratory significance, but few data are available on the expected ranges in different population groups. In addition, various equations have been proposed to define the anion gap or delta (Δ); the common ones being sodium−(chloride + bicarbonate), which will be referred to as Δ_1, and (sodium + potassium) − (chloride + bicarbonate), which will be referred to as Δ_2. Another expression of the expected balance which has been proposed is sodium + potassium + 12 = chloride + bicarbonate + 24 (*3*).

Department of Pathology, College of Medicine, University of Iowa, Iowa City, Iowa 52242.
Received Oct. 13, 1975; accepted Feb. 25, 1976.

The anion gap (Δ_1 or Δ_2) is often referred to in the clinical literature on organic acidosis; most notably that of lactic acidosis and ketoacidosis (*4, 5*). Normal ranges for Δ_1 of 8–12 mEq/liter (*6*) or 5–12 mEq/liter (*7*) are quoted without supporting data. It is our contention that these ranges are too narrow and the entire concept of quantitative electrolyte balance is in need of further clarification. In addition, there have been several recent brief reports (*6, 8, 9*) regarding the clinical value of using the electrolyte balance or anion gap in patient diagnosis and management. These articles, in which Δ_2 was used, reported ranges as shown in Table 1. Here, we present quantitative data by utilizing the definition of the anion gap as given by Δ_1.

Methods

The values for Na^+, K^+, Cl^-, and CO_2 were measured with an unmodified continuous-flow analyzer (SMA 6/60; Technicon Instruments Corp., Tarrytown, N. Y. 10591). The anion gap was calculated as sodium −(chloride + bicarbonate) = Δ_1.

The data on anion gaps were gathered for hospitalized patients during three months from SMA 6/60 runs chosen without conscious bias. The plasmaphoresis samples were consecutive plasmaphoresis samples obtained by the blood donor center. The 86 "normal" samples were obtained from fasting workers at a local

Table 1. Previous Reports of Normal Anion Gaps

Population	No.	Normal anion gap (Δ_2) (range)	Reference
Hospital patients	3920	10–25	(*9*)
Blood donors	210	9–17	(*9*)
Volunteer staff	198	11–19	(*9*)
Hospital patients	1518	7–25	(*8*)
Hospital patients with normal values for electrolytes	466	10–20	(*9*)

Table 2. Precision of Electrolyte Measurements and Anion Gap

Variable	n	$\bar{x}$ (mEq/liter)	SD (mEq/liter)
Na	60	144	1.0
Cl	60	104	1.0
CO_2	60	21	1.0
Na − (Cl + CO_2)	111	18.8	1.9

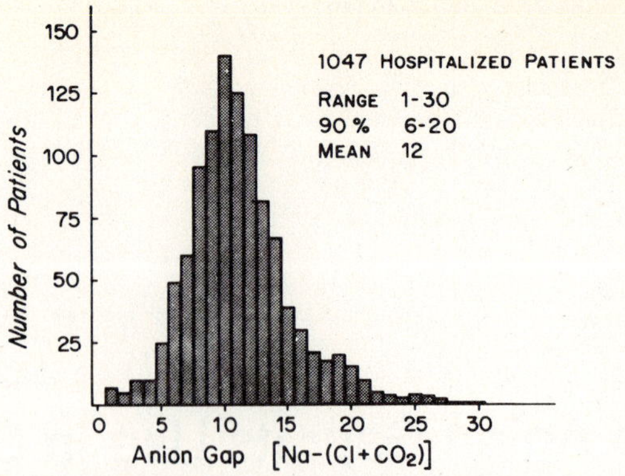

Fig. 1. Distribution of anion gaps [Na − (Cl + CO_2)] in 1047 hospitalized patients

production plant. The study group of patients were those found to have abnormal Δ values during a two-month period. Because this institution has an active hemodialysis and renal transplant program, many abnormal Δ_1's were found in this patient population. The cause of these abnormal anion gaps was easily explainable, so we did not include all of these patients in this study.

Because a recent study (*10*) reported lower anion gaps in patients with multiple myeloma, we also examined the charts with regard to electrolytes, blood urea nitrogen, and Δ_1 determinations of 46 patients with an immunolectrophoretic diagnosis of multiple myeloma.

Results

Precision data: The repetitive analysis of a frozen human serum pool yielded the results shown in Table 2.

Population data: The range of anion gaps observed in 1047 hospitalized patients was 1–27 mEq/liter (mean, 12 mEq/liter). A histogram of these results is shown in Figure 1 and the statistical parameters in Table 3. Nonparametric percentiles yielded a central 90% range of 6–20 mEq/liter. In 86 fasting volunteers the central 90% was 9–17 mEq/liter, and in 203 plasmaphoresis donors the central 90% was 7–16 mEq/liter (Figures 2 and 3, and Table 3).

The data on abnormal patients, collected during two months, are categorized in Table 4. The relative frequencies are not meaningful because we did not include all of the high anion gap results for patients with renal failure.

The range of anion gaps for the 46 patients with multiple myeloma was from 1–16 mEq/liter, with a mean of 8.7 mEq/liter. Of these 46 patients, 16 had a blood urea nitrogen exceeding 250 mg/liter. If this group with an abnormally high blood urea nitrogen is excluded, the anion gap range is from 1–15 mEq/liter (mean, 7.5 mEq/liter). The distribution is shown in Figure 4 and Table 3.

Discussion

Before discussing our results, let us consider the commonly proposed mechanisms leading to abnormal anion gaps. In our experience, most low anion gaps are not substantiated on repeated analysis, indicating previous laboratory error. In a three-month study of abnormal anion gaps, only four verified low gaps were found, two of which were explained by clinical information (Table 4). Murray et al. (*10*) have reported that multiple myeloma patients have low anion gaps because of the accumulation of cationic proteins. Our data likewise show a lower anion gap, with a mean of 8.7 mEq/liter. To separate the opposing effects of renal failure and myeloma on the anion gap we excluded patients with blood urea nitrogen exceeding 250 mg/liter. The remaining 30 patients had a mean anion gap of 7.5 mEq/liter, substantiating the presence of a low anion

Table 3. Observed Anion Gaps

Population	Range	$\bar{x}$	SD	Cumulative percentile 3%	5%	50%	95%	97%
1047 hospital patients	1–30	12	4.0	5	6	11	20	21
86 volunteers	8–18	13	2.4	9	9	13	17	17
203 plasma donors	4–20	11	2.8	6	7	11	16	18
46 multiple myeloma patients	1–16	8.7						
30 multiple myeloma patients with normal BUN	1–15	7.5						
16 multiple myeloma patients with BUN >25	3–16	11						

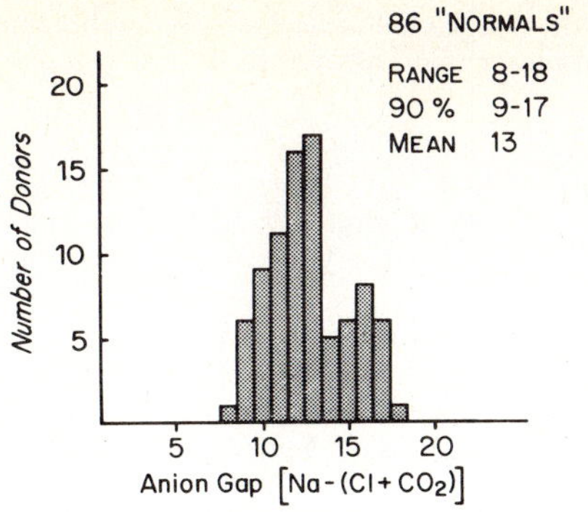

Fig. 2. Distribution of anion gaps [Na − (Cl + CO_2)] in 86 normal individuals

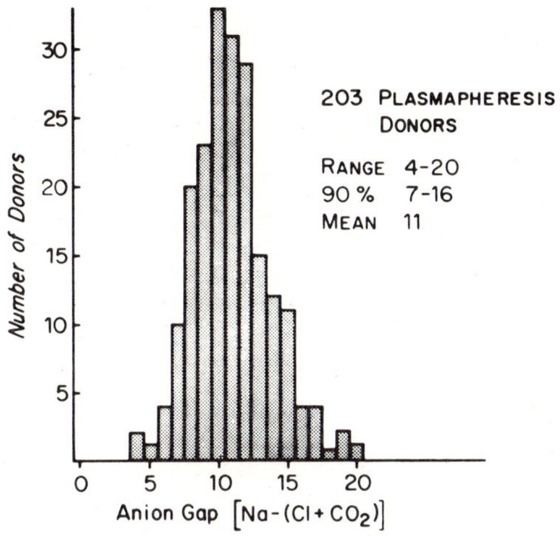

Fig. 3. Distribution of anion gaps [Na − (Cl + CO_2)] in 203 plasmaphoresis donors

gap in patients with multiple myeloma. The presence of bromide, which causes an overestimation of the chloride (*11, 12*), may also lead to an erroneously low gap.

In reviewing the case histories of patients with an elevated anion gap we found that 70 of the 71 gaps were explainable (Table 4). Because high values for anion gaps can arise from many causes, an increased gap is not a specific diagnostic datum. However, assessment of the anion gap may be useful in monitoring of patients. In cases of organic acid excess, the anion gap can provide an easily measured quantitative estimate of the degree of organic acid excess. As expected, the most frequent cause for a large anion gap was renal disease.

Any estimation of normal range includes the physiological variability and the analytical error. Martin et al. (*13*) analyzed this problem by using the mathematical tools of "convolution" and "de-convolution." The observed variance in the population is the sum of the true variance in the population plus the variance of the analytical method (equation 1) (*14*). In addition, the analytical variance of the anion gap is equal to the sum of the variances of the individual measurements (equation 2).

Table 4. Classification of Patients with Abnormal Anion Gaps

Group		No. patients
High anion gaps		
Renal failure		27
Patients with low chloride & CO_2		27
Dehydration	8	
Diuretic therapy	10	
Steroids + diuretic therapy	9	
Organic acid excess		10
Patients receiving Ringers–lactate		2
Androgenic disorder		1
Storage diseases		2
Hyperosmolar syndrome		1
Unclassifiable		1
		71
Low anion gaps		
Bromism		1
Chronic obstructive pulmonary disease		1
Unexplained		2
		4

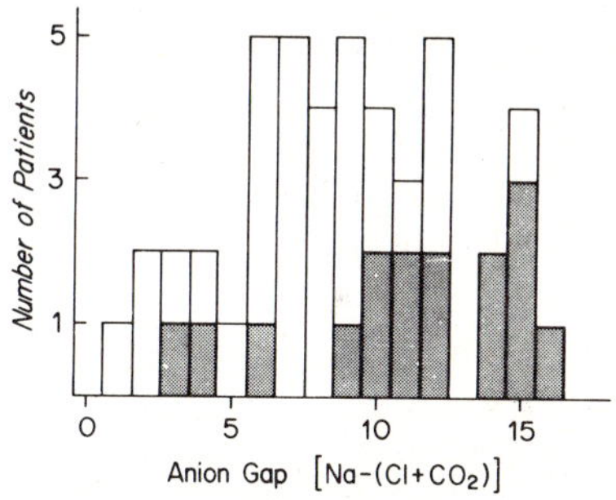

Fig. 4. Distribution of anion gaps [Na − (Cl + CO_2)] in 46 myeloma patients
Solid bars, patient's BUN greater than 250 mg/liter (n = 16); $\bar{X}$ = 11. Open bars, patient's BUN less than 250 mg/liter (n = 30); X = 7.5

$$SD^2_{observed} = SD^2_{population} + SD^2_{method} \quad (1)$$

$$SD^2_{gap} = SD^2\ Na + SD^2\ Cl + SD^2\ CO_2 \quad (2)$$

The analytical variances are given in Table 2 and the observed population variances in Table 3. By using equation 1 the calculated $SD_{population}$ for the hospitalized patients is 3.5 mEq/liter; for the normal fasting individual it is 1.4 mEq/liter; and for the plasmaphoresis donors it is 1.5 mEq/liter. As one would expect, the physiological variation in the anion gap in normal individuals is quite small and more than half the observed variation is due to analytical error. Also, not unexpectedly, the hospitalized patients show greater physiological variability. No attempts have been made to separate individual variation of anion gaps.

The use of the anion gap for quality control has been discussed by Buckley-Sharp and Miller (*8*). They believed that the gap was a poor substitute for quality control on the individual variables. However, the anion gap can be a useful and economical quality-control tool. Because much of the clinical chemistry data from a modern laboratory is generated on multiple-channel instruments, the concept of comparing the results of multiple determinations on a given patient can provide an additional means of quality control. Use of this concept to detect unsuspected random errors in electrolyte results in a single patient could be called "intercheck." Any electrolytes that give a calculated anion gap outside the usual range should be double checked, as well as any abnormally high or low value for Na^+, K^+, Cl^-, or bicarbonate. By doing this, errors are discovered that would have gone unnoticed if one relied completely on the individual results of control specimens included in the analytical run. In addition to this, it is useful to look at an analytical run of patient electrolytes for trends. If all the patients in a run have anion gaps that range from 7 to 10 mEq/liter, for example, one should suspect a systematic error that may not be detected from the quality-control data on individual channels. As more laboratories obtain computer systems, the flagging of abnormal anion gaps should be included. It should be evident that even though a patient's individual electrolytes are normal, an abnormal anion gap indicates further investigation of the patient.

We thank Mr. Douglas Schoemacher, Ms. Sandy Streeter, and Ms. Sandy Barker for technical assistance.

References

1. Gamble, J., *Chemical Anatomy, Physiology and Pathology of Extracellular Fluid.* Harvard University Press, Cambridge, Mass., 1950.

2. Davidson and Henry, *Clinical Diagnosis by Laboratory Methods,* Saunders, Philadelphia, Pa., 1974, p 781.

3. Brackett, N. C., Cohen, J. J., and Schwartz, W. B., Carbon dioxide titration curve of normal man. *New Engl. J. Med.* **272,** 6 (1965).

4. Lubowitz, H., Crespin, S., Wessler, S., and Avidi, L. V., Lactic acidosis. *Arch. Intern. Med.* **134,** 148 (1974).

5. Anon., Lactic acidosis. *Lancet* **ii,** 27 (1973). Editorial.

6. Kassirer, J. P., Serious acid-base disorders. *New Engl. J. Med.* **291,** 773 (1974).

7. Bear, R. A., and Gribik, M., Assessing acid base imbalances through laboratory parameters. *Hosp. Pract.* **9,** 157 (1974).

8. Buckley-Sharp, M. D., and Miller, A. L., The anion gap. *Lancet* **ii,** 206 (1973).

9. Thomas, D. W., Pain, R. W., and Duncan, B. M., The anion gap. *Lancet* **ii,** 848 (1973).

10. Murray, T., Long, W., and Narins, R. G., Multiple myeloma and the anion gap. *New Engl. J. Med.* **292,** 574 (1975).

11. Blume, R. S., MacLowry, J. D., and Wolff, S. M., Limitations of chloride determination in the diagnosis of bromism. *New Engl. J. Med.* **279,** 593 (1968).

12. Driscoll, J. L., and Martin, H. F., Detection of bromism by an automated chloride method. *Clin. Chem.* **12,** 314 (1966).

13. Martin, H. F., Gudzinowicz, B. J., and Fauger, H., *Normal Values in Clinical Chemistry,* Marcel Dekker, New York, N. Y., 1975.

14. Harris, E. K., Kanofsky, P., Skakarji, G., and Cotlove, E., Biological and analytical components of variation in long term studies of serum constituents in normal subjects. *Clin. Chem.* **16,** 1022 (1970).

Decreased Radioassay Values for Folate after Serum Extraction When Pteroylglutamic Acid Standards Are Used

Gary A. Mitchell, Sharon P. Pochron, Philip V. Smutny, and Rogelia Guity

Radioassay values for folate in protein-denatured (extracted) sera are compared with values obtained by individual serum blank correction. Lower folate values are reported for sera extracted at pH 1.3, 7.6, 10.5, and 12.4 when pteroylglutamic acid (PGA) calibration standards are used. The results are unchanged when ascorbate added to the sera is increased from 1 to 20 g/liter and when [^{3}H]PGA is substituted for ^{125}I-labeled PGA. However, a higher mean value for extracted serum is reported when *N*-5-methyltetrahydrofolic acid calibration standards are substituted for PGA. Because both patients' samples and assay calibrators were subjected to the same extraction methods, our results suggest that serum folate behaves differently from PGA during the extractions.

Abnormally high concentrations of folate-binding proteins are present in a significant number of patients' sera (*1–7*). A blank correction for the binding proteins is sometimes used in radioassays because interference from elevated binding proteins can result in inaccurately low values for folate in serum. Because the usefulness of serum blank corrections is debatable, some workers instead use extraction procedures to decrease serum protein interference (*2, 3, 5*). The effect of four different extraction methods on serum folate values determined by radioassay is presented and the results are compared with values obtained on using individual serum blank corrections.

Materials and Methods

The diluent in all assays was lysine buffer, 0.10 mol/liter, adjusted to pH 9.3 with NaOH and containing, per liter, 1.0 g of 100 Bloom type B, laboratory-grade gelatin (Fisher Scientific Co., Fair Lawn, N. J. 07410), 100 mg of thimerosal, and 100 mg of mercaptoethanol. Folate-binding protein was prepared from fresh whole milk by the general procedures of Ford et al. (*8*). The protein concentration of the preparation was estimated from the absorbance at 260 and 280 nm, calculated from the following formula: protein, g/liter = $1.45A_{280} - 0.74A_{260}$ (*9*). Aliquots of the protein solution, 16 g/liter, were stored at −20 °C. Crystalline folic acid (PGA), mol wt 441.4 (ICN Pharmaceuticals, Inc., Cleveland, Ohio 44128), was prepared in the lysine buffer and aliquots of a stock solution, 0.2 g/liter, were stored at −20 °C. The extinction coefficient of the PGA was determined in phosphate buffer (pH 7.0, 0.1 mol/liter) at 282 nm as $\epsilon = 26.7 \times 10^3$ liter mol^{-1} cm^{-1} and compares to the reported value of $\epsilon = 27 \times 10^3$ liter mol^{-1} cm^{-1} (*10*).

The diammonium salt of *N*-5-methyltetrahydrofolic acid (MTHF) from Terra-Marine Bioresearch, La Jolla, Calif. 92037, was also prepared in the lysine buffer at 0.2 g/liter and stored at −20 °C. ^{125}I-labeled folate, 0.24 mCi/liter was obtained from Diagnostic Biochemistry, Inc., San Diego, Calif. 92121, and [^{3}H]folate from Diagnostic Products Corp., Los Angeles, Calif. 90064. Both were used without additional purification or dilution. A suspension of Norit A charcoal, 10 g/liter, containing dextran of 60 000 to 90 000 mol wt, 1 g/liter, was used for separation of free folate from that bound to milk protein. The extraction reagents tested were:

1. HCl, 50 mmol/liter, pH 1.3
2. lysine, 25 mmol/liter, pH adjusted to 10.5 with NaOH (*2*)
3. NaOH, 0.38 mol/liter, containing 50 g/liter trichloroacetic acid, final pH 12.4 (*11*)
4. sodium phosphate, 50 mmol/liter, pH 7.6 (*5*)

Nonfasting serum from five men and five women was supplemented with 1 mg of ascorbate per milliliter of serum and stored in aliquots at −20 °C. The sera were assayed within two weeks from the date of collection.

Polypropylene tubes were used for assays requiring incubation in boiling water for protein denaturation; polystyrene tubes were used in the other assays. An "Iso-Lect" gamma counter (DADE) and a LS-100 Liquid Scintillation System (Beckman Instruments, Fullerton, Calif. 92634) were used for counting radioactivity.

Procedure

When patients' serum blanks were used, 1.0 ml of the lysine buffer was added to all tubes, with an additional 0.10 ml placed in the charcoal separation blank (or nonspecific binding) and patients' serum blank tubes. Ten microliters of standard or patient's serum was then added to appropriately labeled tubes followed by the addition of 0.10 ml (~10 μg) of milk protein to all tubes except for the blanks already mentioned. The tubes were vortex-mixed and then incubated in the dark at room temperature for 30 min. ^{125}I-labeled folate, 0.10 ml, was then added, the tubes vortex-mixed and again incubated in the dark at room temperature for 30 min. During this incubation period, a mean total cpm value

DADE Division, American Hospital Supply Corp., Miami, Fla. 33152.

Received Aug. 4, 1975; accepted Feb. 27, 1976.

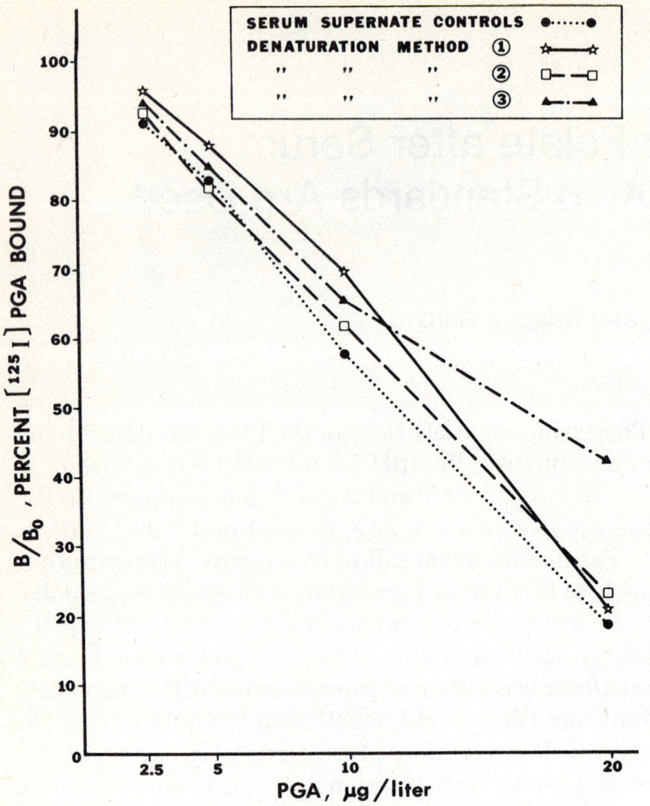

Fig. 1. PGA calibration curves for radioassays, with use of patient's serum blanks (●····●) and three methods of preliminary denaturation of patient serum (see Table 1)

was determined by counting the radioactivity in a representative number of tubes. The assay was terminated by adding 0.50 ml of the charcoal suspension to all tubes. The tubes were vortex-mixed, incubated at room temperature for 10 min and centrifuged to sediment the charcoal. The supernates were aspirated from the tubes and discarded. The ^{125}I-labeled folate in each charcoal pellet was determined by counting the radioactivity and was subtracted from the mean total cpm to give the supernate cpm. Standard folate results, including a "0" standard, were corrected by subtraction of the charcoal separation blank value; the patient samples were corrected with the corresponding serum blanks. A ratio of each supernate cpm to the cpm contained in the "0" standard supernate was then determined, B/B_0, which represents the percentage of the maximum amount of ^{125}I-labeled folate that could be bound by the binding protein (*12*). The B/B_0 values for the standards were plotted on linear paper vs. the standard concentrations in µg/liter (Figure 1). The concentration of folate in patients' sera was determined directly from the standard curve.

When the extraction methods (Table 1) were used, 0.20 ml of extraction reagent was added to all tubes including the blanks and standards (patient serum blanks not included in these assays). Ten microliters of standard or patient sample was then added to appropriately labeled tubes. When extraction methods 1, 2, or 4 were used, the tubes were boiled in a water bath for 10 min.

Table 1. Radioassay Values for Serum Folate, as Determined by Serum Blank Correction and after Three Methods of Preliminary Protein Denaturation (Sera from 10 Patients)

Serum blank correction	Extraction methods[a] (1) HCl, pH 1.3	(2) Lysine, pH 10.5	(3) NaOH-TCA, pH 12.4
	Folate, µg/liter		
5.2	4.6	3.7	3.5
4.1	3.2	2.5	2.6
8.0	6.1	4.2	4.5
12.0	11.3	8.4	6.9
9.3	4.9	6.0	5.3
19.2	18.2	16.8	15.5
6.1	5.0	3.7	4.6
8.9	7.6	6.6	5.6
8.7	6.8	5.4	6.2
6.0	3.9	2.8	2.8
Mean 8.8	7.2	6.1	5.8

[a] Reagents and methods are described in the text.

When method 3 was used, the assay tubes were incubated at room temperature for 10 min. Lysine buffer, 0.80 ml, was then added to all tubes to adjust the final pH to 9.3 and an extra 0.10 ml of buffer was added to the blank tubes. The remainder of the protocol was the same as previously described.

Results and Discussion

An initial set of experiments was performed, with use of pH 1.3, 10.5, or 12.4 for the serum extractions. After the extractions, lysine buffer was added to all tubes to adjust the pH to 9.3, because pteroylglutamate and *N*-5-methyltetrahydrofolate reportedly have equal affinities for the milk protein at that pH (*13*). ^{125}I-labeled folate and PGA calibration standards were used in these preliminary assays. The assay calibration curves are shown in Figure 1. Differences in these curves are probably related in part to the effects of the extraction reagents on the binding proteins as well as reagent effects on the folate calibrators. The maximum binding was about 60% for both the assay employing serum blanks and extraction method 2, while the maximum bindings were 68.5% and 46.5%, respectively, when extraction methods 1 and 3 were used. The blank values for unextracted patient sera were equivalent to the charcoal separation blank values of 3–5%, which may be attributed to the small amount of serum assayed, 10 µl. Mean values were determined from the results of each assay method (Table 1) and when compared show reductions in measured serum folate for the three extraction methods tested. Possible explanations for the smaller values observed for extracted serum would include: (*a*) ^{125}I-labeled folate was trapped in the supernates by denatured serum proteins, (*b*) the extractions

Table 2. Values for Folate in Unextracted and Extracted Serum on Using Different Tracers, Calibrators, Extraction Methods, and Quantities of Antioxidant

Tracer	Ascorbate in serum, mg/ml	Extraction method[a]	Calibrator	Serum sample 1	2	3
^{125}I	1	none	PGA	9.4	11.3	13.7
^{125}I	20	none	PGA	9.8	10.6	13.1
^{3}H	1	none	PGA	8.7	12.0	12.7
^{125}I	1	none	MTHF	9.1	11.8	12.5
^{125}I	1	phosphate buffer, pH 7.6	PGA	7.1	8.4	11.4
^{125}I	20	HCl, pH 1.3	PGA	4.9	6.9	9.3
^{3}H	1	HCl, pH 1.3	PGA	8.0	9.6	11.4
^{125}I	1	HCl, pH 1.3	MTHF	9.7	11.6	14.7

[a] Reagents and methods are described in the text.

were performed at the extremes of the pH range, (*c*) insufficient antioxidant was used, and (*d*) serum folate and PGA calibration standards did not behave identically during the extractions. To clarify these results, we made additional determinations on three different sera. After extraction at pH 1.3, serum supernate blank values were 1192, 1107, and 1251 cpm as compared to 1194 cpm for the assay separation blank. Unextracted serum supernate blank values were 1352, 1283, and 1206 cpm as compared to 1224 cpm for the assay separation blank. These results demonstrate that the lower folate values for extracted serum are not a result of tracer binding by extracted sera. The values for the same serum samples unextracted and extracted were then compared by using iodinated and tritiated folate tracers, different concentrations of antioxidant added to the sera, neutral and acidic pH extraction methods, and PGA and MTHF calibrators (Table 2).

In summary, substitution of [^{3}H]folate for ^{125}I-labeled folate did not eliminate the observed folate reductions. Using the pH 1.3 extraction method, we obtained smaller folate values, even when the antioxidant added to the sera was increased to 20 mg of ascorbate per milliliter. Smaller folate values were also observed after serum extractions performed at pH 1.3, 7.6, 10.5, and 12.4. Values for extracted serum were the same or increased only when MTHF was substituted for the PGA calibration standard. These results demonstrate that PGA and serum folate do not behave identically during extraction and suggest that there is destruction of endogenous serum folate by the extraction methods tested.

References

1. Archibald, E. L., Mincey, E. K., and Morrison, R. T., Estimation of serum folate levels by competitive protein binding assay. *Clin. Biochem.* **5,** 232 (1972).
2. Dunn, R. T., and Foster, L. B., Radioassay of serum folate. *Clin. Chem.* **19,** 1101 (1973).
3. Rothenberg, S. P., DaCosta, M., and Rosenberg, Z., A radioassay for serum folate: Use of a two-phase sequential incubation, ligand-binding system. *New Engl. J. Med.* **286,** 1335 (1972).
4. Waxman, S., and Schreiber, C., Measurement of serum folate levels and serum folic acid-binding protein by ^{3}H-PGA radioassay. *Blood* **42,** 281 (1973).
5. Kamen, B. A., and Caston, J. D., Direct radiochemical assay for serum folate: Competition between ^{3}H-folic acid and 5-methyl-tetrahydrofolic acid for a folate binder. *J. Lab. Clin. Med.* **83,** 164 (1974).
6. Eichner, E. R., Paine, C. J., Dickson, V. L., and Hargrove, M. D., Clinical and laboratory observations on serum folate-binding protein. *Blood* **46,** 599 (1975).
7. Zettner, A., and Duly, P. E., New evidence for a binding principle specific for folates as a normal constituent of human serum. *Clin. Chem.* **20,** 1313 (1974).
8. Ford, J. E., Salter, D. N., and Scott, K. J., The folate binding protein in milk. *J. Dairy Res.* **36,** 435 (1969).
9. Kalckar, H. M., Differential spectrophotometry of purine compounds by means of specific enzymes. *J. Biol. Chem.* **167,** 461 (1947).
10. Blair, J. A., and Saunders, K. J., A convenient method for the preparation of *dl*-5-methyltetrahydrofolic acid (*dl*-5-methyl-5,6,7,8-tetrahydropteroyl-L-monoglutamic acid). *Anal. Biochem.* **34,** 376 (1970).
11. Premachandra, B. N., and Ibrahim, I. I., A simple and rapid immunoassay for serum triiodothyronine. *Abstr., Fed. Am. Soc. Exp. Biol.* **34,** 313, Abstr. 531 (1975).
12. Rodbard, D., Rayford, P. L., and Ross, G. T., Statistical quality control of radioimmunoassays. In *Statistics in Endocrinology,* J. W. McArthur and T. Cotton, Eds. MIT Press, Cambridge, Mass., 1970, pp 411–429.
13. Givas, J. K., and Gutcho, S., pH dependence of the binding of folates to milk binder in radioassay of folates. *Clin. Chem.* **21,** 427 (1975).

CLIN. CHEM. 22/5, 650–656 (1976)

Creatine Kinase in Serum: 1. Determination of Optimum Reaction Conditions

Gabor Szasz,[1] Wolfgang Gruber,[2] and Erich Bernt[2]

To establish optimum conditions for creatine kinase (EC 2.7.3.2) activity measurement with the creatine phosphate → creatine reaction, we re-examined all kinetic factors relevant to an optimal and standardized enzyme assay at 30 and 25 °C. We determined the pH optimum in various buffers, considering the effect of the type and concentration of the buffer, as well as the influence of various buffer anions on the activity. The relation between activity and substrate concentration was shown and the apparent Michaelis constants of creatine kinase for creatine phosphate and ADP were evaluated. We tested the effect on creatine kinase measurement of the concentration of substrates (glucose and $NADP^+$) in the auxiliary and indicator reactions, especially the influence of the added auxiliary (hexokinase) and indicator (glucose-6-phosphate dehydrogenase) enzymes on the lag phase, at different temperatures. The $NADP^+$ concentration proved to be the factor limiting the duration of constant reaction rate. We studied the inhibition of creatine kinase and adenylate kinase by AMP and established a convenient AMP concentration. For reactivation of creatine kinase, *N*-acetyl cysteine as sulfhydryl compound was introduced. Finally, we examined the relationship between activity and temperature.

Creatine kinase (ATP:creatine *N*-phosphotransferase; EC 2.7.3.2) in serum is of outstanding clinical significance in the enzymology of heart and skeletal muscle because of its high sensitivity and relative specifity. According to recent investigations, only skeletal and heart muscle contain large amounts of creatine kinase (*1*). Thus, considerable increases in this activity in serum almost exclusively reflect diseases and damage of skeletal or heart muscle.

Creatine kinase catalyzes the reversible phosphorylation of creatine by ATP:

$$\text{creatine} + \text{ATP} \underset{\text{pH } 6.7}{\overset{\text{pH } 9.0}{\rightleftharpoons}} \text{phosphocreatine} + \text{ADP}$$

Because phosphocreatine (creatine phosphate) has a significantly higher energy than ATP, the equilibrium is largely shifted into the reverse direction. The equilibrium position depends also upon the pH. At pH optimum the reverse reaction proceeds four to six times faster than the forward reaction and should be preferred therefore in the development of an assay method. On the other hand, for the most desirable method only measurement techniques should be considered that follow the progress of the reaction directly and continuously (*2*). Such requirements are met only by the procedure in which the ATP formed is measured by means of an auxiliary and indicator enzyme:

$$\text{ATP} + \text{D-glucose} \overset{\text{hexokinase}}{\rightleftharpoons} \text{ADP} + \text{D-glucose-6-phosphate}$$

$$\text{D-Glucose-6-phosphate} + \text{NADP}^+ \underset{\text{dehydrogenase}}{\overset{\text{D-glucose-6-phosphate}}{\rightleftharpoons}} \text{D-glucono-}\delta\text{-lactone 6-phosphate} + \text{NADPH}$$

The course of the reaction can be monitored spectrophotometrically by measuring the conversion of $NADP^+$ to NADPH, which is done by following the increase in absorbance at 340 or 334 nm.

The method was described first by Oliver (*3*) and modified later by Rosalki (*4*) and Hess et al. (*5*) and others. We report here our re-examination of all kinetic factors relevant to the optimization and standardization of the creatine kinase assay at 30 °C (*2*) and 25 °C (*6*). A preliminary presentation[3] was given in 1974. In forthcoming papers we shall describe details of methodology, reference values, problems of inactivation and reactivation, the phenomenon of the "dilution effect," and the various interferences with the measurement that may be encountered.

Materials and Methods

Creatine phosphate, ADP, AMP, $NADP^+$, hexokinase (EC 2.7.1.1), and D-glucose-6-phosphate dehydrogenase (EC 1.1.1.49) (both enzymes from baker's

Presented at the Second International Symposium on Clinical Enzymology, Chicago, Ill., Oct. 27–29, 1975.

[1] Institute of Clinical Chemistry, University Medical School, Klinikstrasse 32b, 63 Giessen, Germany.

[2] Research Center, Boehringer Mannheim GmbH, 8132 Tutzing, Germany.

Received Dec. 29, 1975; accepted Mar. 1, 1976.

[3] Szasz, G., Bernt, E., Staehler, F: Proposal for a selected method for creatine kinase in serum. Sixth International Symposium on Clinical Enzymology, Venice, 1974.

Table 1. Assay Conditions for Creatine Kinase Activity Measurement in Human Serum[a]

	Author				
	This paper	Rosalki (*4*) 1967	Hess (*5*) 1968	German Standard Method (*16*) 1970	Warren (*7*) 1972
Buffer	100 (Imidazole)	50 (Tris)	50 (Triethanolamine)	100 (Triethanolamine)	70 (Imidazole)
pH	6.7	6.8	6.9	7.0	6.5
Creatine phosphate	30	10	20	35	15
ADP	2	1	1	1	3
Mg^{2+}	10	30	10	10	37.5
D-Glucose	20	20	20	20	10
$NADP^{+}$	2	0.8	0.8	0.6	2
Hexokinase	2500	600	1000	1200	4000
Glucose-6-phosphate dehydrogenase	1500	300	500	1200	2000
AMP	5	10	none	10	5
Thiol compound	20 (*N*-acetyl cysteine)	5 (Cysteine)	10 (Cysteine)	9 (Glutathione)	5 (DTT)

[a] The final reagent concentrations in the reaction mixture are given, in mmol/liter for the chemicals and in U/liter for the enzymes.

yeast) were from Bio-Dynamics/bmc, subsidiary of Boehringer Mannheim, Indianapolis, Ind. 46250. 2-(*N*-Morpholino)ethane sulfonic acid (MES), morpholinopropane sulfonic acid (MOPS), and 1,4-piperazinediethanesulfonic acid (PIPES) were from Calbiochem, San Diego, Calif. 92112. *N*-Acetyl cysteine was from Diamalt AG., Munich. All other compounds, in the purest quality available, were from E. Merck, Darmstadt. Fresh solutions of the reagents were prepared each working day.

Sera of patients with skeletal muscle lesions or myocardial infarction served as the source of creatine kinase.

Table 1 lists the final reagent concentrations in the reaction mixture. The serum sample comprised about 0.02 of this mixture by volume at the assay temperature of 30 °C and about 0.04 at 25 °C. After a 3- to 5-min pre-incubation the reaction was usually started with creatine phosphate. Taking into consideration the 2-min lag phase, we continuously monitored the increase in absorbance for several minutes at 334 nm. If the reaction was started with serum instead of creatine phosphate the time required for reactivation and lag phase amounted to 5 min. These "standard" conditions were used throughout except where specifically mentioned in the text or figure legends.

Results

Buffer and pH

In the optimum pH range for creatine kinase—between pH 6.5 and 7.0—only a few buffers are effective, especially PIPES (pK, 6.8), imidazole (pK, 7.1) and MOPS (pK, 7.2). In comparison, the pK values for triethanolamine (pK, 7.9) and Tris (pK, 8.2) are too high and that for MES (pK, 6.15) is too low. With imidazole acetate buffer, a broad pH optimum was observed between pH 6.5 and 7.0 (Figure 1). The evaluation of pH activity curves of 16 different sera showed the pH optimum to be at pH 6.7, but the difference in activity between pH 6.7 and 6.8 was only 2%. The pH–activity relationship seemed to be independent of the assay temperature (30 or 25 °C) and the type of the buffer used (imidazole or triethanolamine acetate).

Comparison among five different buffers (Table 2), all at 100 mmol/liter concentration and pH 6.7, showed almost identical creatine kinase activity in imidazole and triethanolamine, whereas in MOPS, MES, and PIPES buffers slightly to significantly lower activity was

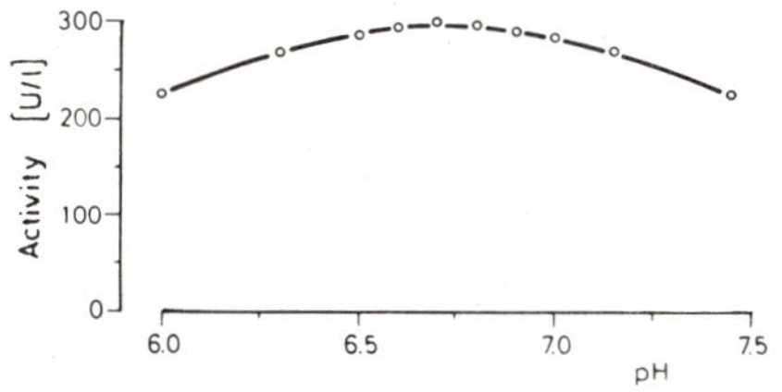

Fig. 1. Dependence of creatine kinase activity on pH (100 mmol/liter imidazole acetate buffer)

Table 2. Effect of Type of Buffer on Creatine Kinase Activity

	Imidazole acetate	Triethanolamine acetate	Sodium MOPS	Sodium MES	Sodium PIPES
U/liter[a]	166	165	163	159	150

[a] Mean activity of 12 sera, duplicate assays. Concentration of the buffers was 100 mmol/liter, the pH was 6.7.

Table 3. Effect on Creatine Kinase Activity of the Acid Used to Adjust the pH

Acid:	Formic	Hydro-chloric	Acetic	Nitric
U/liter[a]	137	135	134	133

[a] Mean activity of 12 sera, duplicate assays. Imidazole buffer, 100 mmol/liter, pH 6.7.

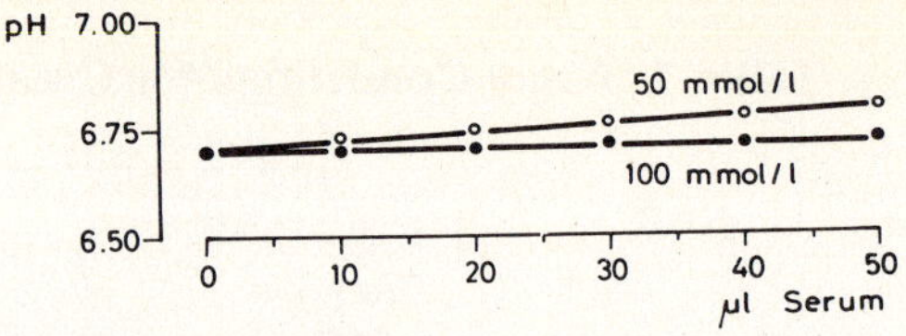

Fig. 4. Dependence of pH upon the volume fraction of the serum in the assay solution (0 to 0.9), in imidazole acetate buffer

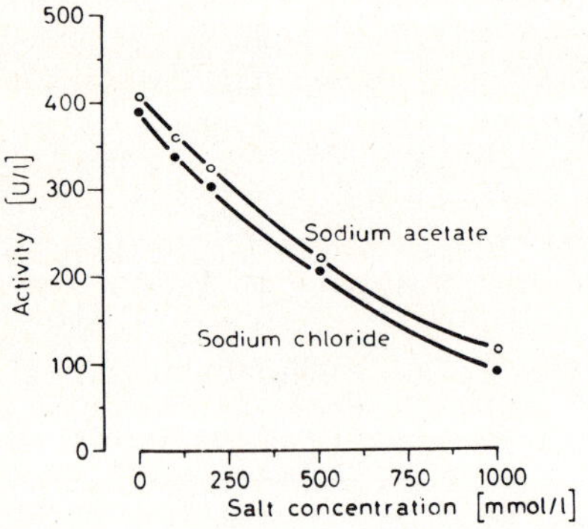

Fig. 2. Effect of some salts on creatine kinase activity

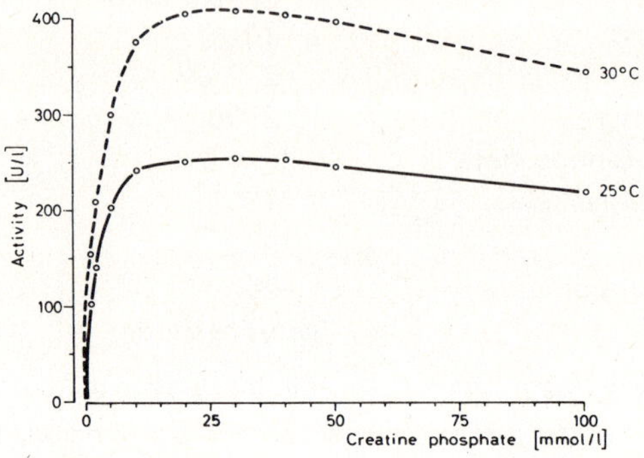

Fig. 5. Dependence of creatine kinase activity on creatine phosphate concentration

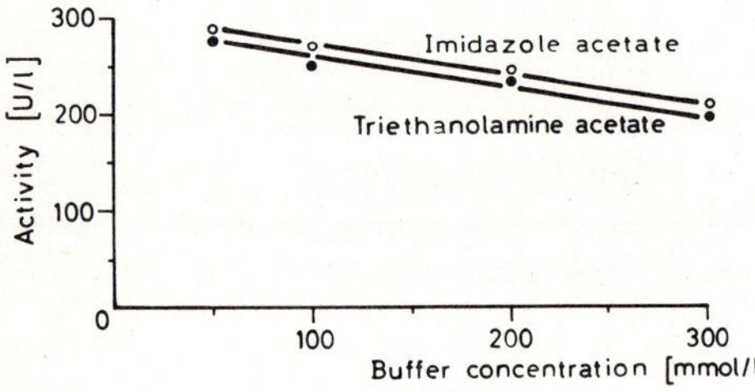

Fig. 3. Dependence of creatine kinase activity on buffer concentration

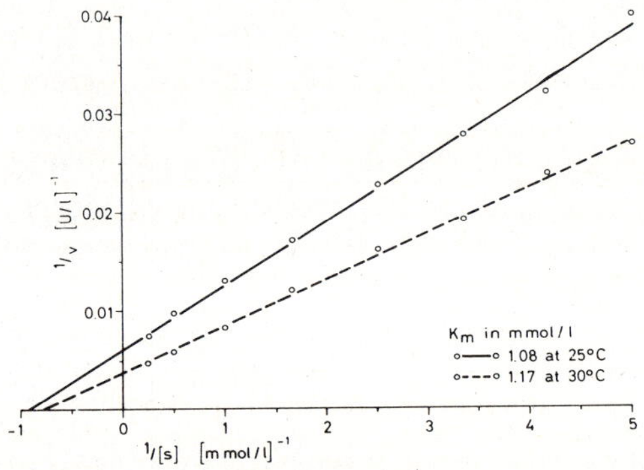

Fig. 6. Michaelis constants of creatine kinase for creatine phosphate—Lineweaver–Burk plot

measured. Thus the buffers of Good et al. (*8*) are not the best to use in measuring creatine kinase activity.

The type of acid used to adjust the pH only slightly affected the creatine kinase activity in imidazole buffer (Table 3). Acetic acid is the most practicable.

The effect of the buffer anions was additionally tested by adding increasing amounts of the corresponding sodium salt (Figure 2). Both sodium acetate and chloride inhibited creatine kinase markedly and to about the same extent.

Creatine kinase was inhibited by both imidazole and triethanolamine buffers (Figure 3). The activity without buffer, calculated by extrapolating the curves to 0 mmol/liter buffer concentration, is about 5% higher than at 50 mmol/liter, and an additional loss in activity of as much as 10% was observed on increasing the buffer concentration to 100 mmol/liter.

A larger proportion of serum in the assay mixture leads to an increase in pH (Figure 4). At 50 mmol/liter imidazole acetate buffer the increase in pH (ΔpH) per 10 μl of added serum to 500 μl reagent is 0.02, but only 0.005 at 100 mmol/liter. This is true also for freeze-dried sera with high pH values, up to pH 9.2. Moreover, the starting reagent, containing creatine phosphate in high concentration, may also cause a shift in pH. To maintain a constant pH in the reaction mixture, a buffer concentration of 100 mmol/liter is necessary.

Creatine Phosphate

Creatine kinase activity increases up to 30 mmol of creatine phosphate per liter; at greater concentrations we began to see inhibition (Figure 5). The relation between activity and creatine phosphate concentration is similar at both 25 and 30 °C.

The apparent Michaelis constants were calculated according to Lineweaver and Burk by means of regression analysis (Figure 6). For three different sera, the mean Michaelis constants of creatine kinase in human

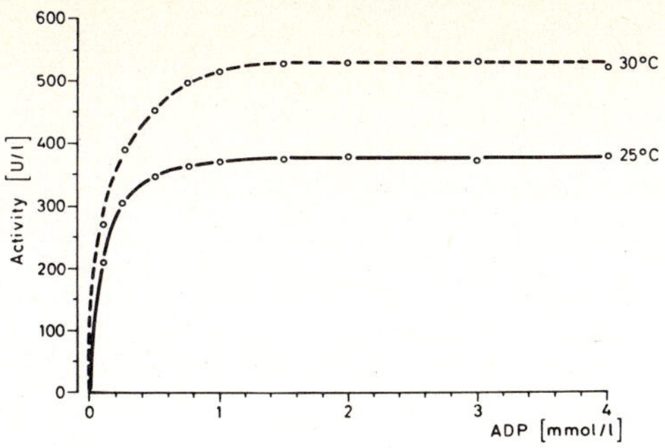

Fig. 7. Dependence of creatine kinase activity on ADP concentration

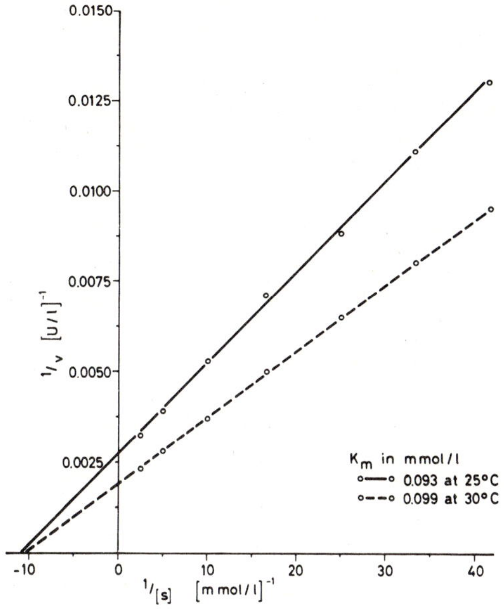

Fig. 8. Michaelis constants of creatine kinase for ADP—Lineweaver–Burk plot

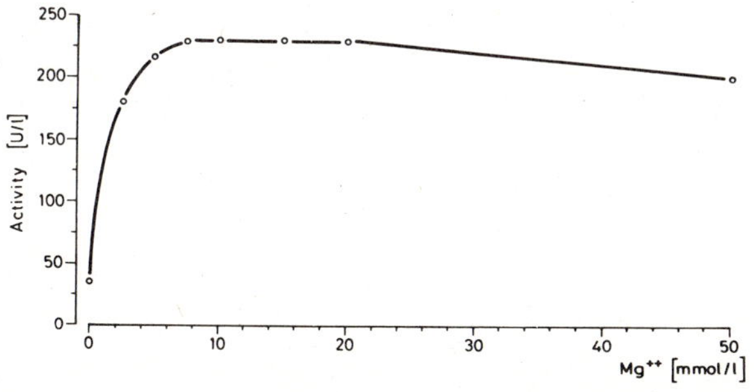

Fig. 9. Effect of magnesium ions on creatine kinase activity

serum for creatine phosphate were 1.08 mmol/liter at 25 °C and 1.17 mmol/liter at 30 °C.

Adenosine Diphosphate

For maximum creatine kinase activity, 2 mmol of ADP per liter was required (Figure 7). For ADP concentrations between 1 and 2 mmol/liter an increase was observed, especially at 30 °C, but there was no inhibition of activity with concentrations up to 4 mmol/liter.

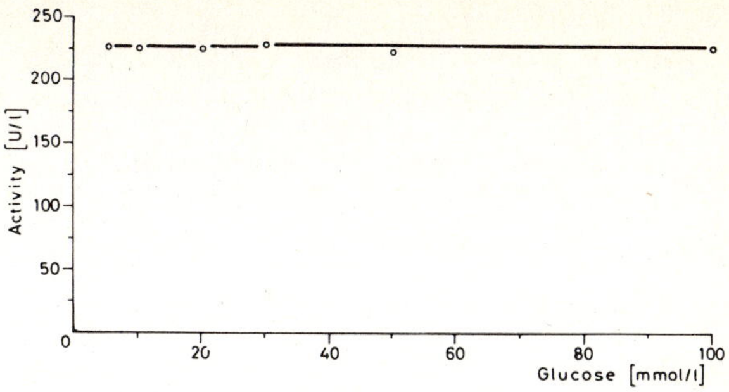

Fig. 10. Effect of glucose concentration on the value obtained for creatine kinase activity

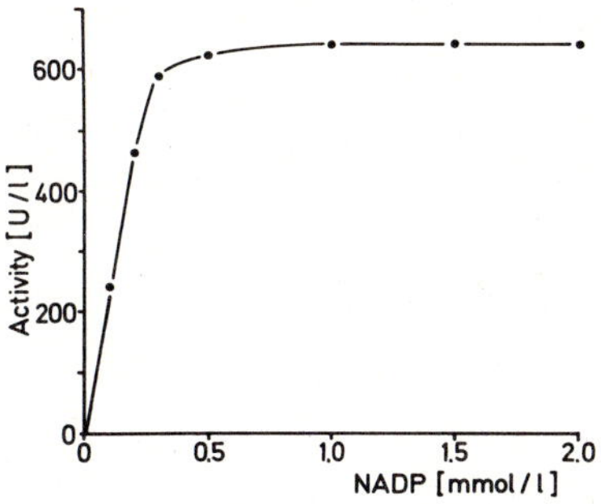

Fig. 11. Dependence of the value obtained for creatine kinase activity on the $NADP^+$ concentration at a volume fraction of sample of 0.02

The necessity to use 2 mmol of ADP per liter was corroborated by the K_m values. For ADP, the mean Michaelis constants for creatine kinase in three human sera were 93 μmol/liter at 25 °C and 99 μmol/liter at 30 °C (Figure 8). Thus the twentyfold K_m value is reached just at 2 mmol of ADP per liter.

Magnesium Salts

Magnesium ions are essential for creatine kinase activity. Without added magnesium salt only 10% of the maximum activity was observed (Figure 9). The highest activity will be obtained with concentrations of 10 to 20 mmol/liter. Magnesium acetate and chloride were equally effective.

Glucose

At glucose concentrations between 5 and 100 mmol/liter, creatine kinase activity was the same (Figure 10). Because the reading for the reagent blank—i.e., the assay solution without sample—was very small and independent of glucose concentration, we saw neither contaminant activity nor side activity of the auxiliary or indicator enzyme.

$NADP^+$

Creatine kinase activity is indicated by the production of NADPH from $NADP^+$. Between 1.0 and 2.0 mmol/liter, measurement of the creatine kinase activity, up to 600 U/liter, is independent of $NADP^+$ concentration for 10 min (Figure 11).

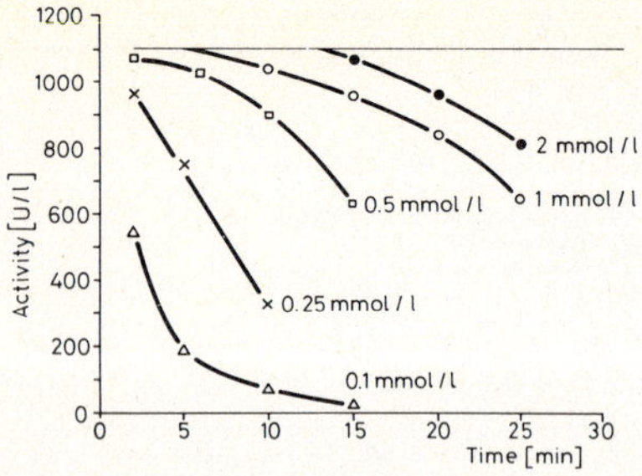

Fig. 12. Period of constant reaction rate at different $NADP^+$ concentrations
Volume fraction of sample: 0.02

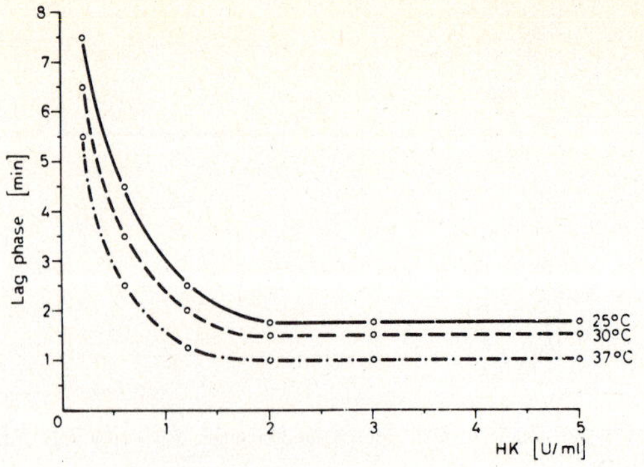

Fig. 14. Lag phase as a function of hexokinase activity (U/ml at 25 °C) in an assay mixture containing 2 U of glucose-6-phosphate dehydrogenase per milliliter

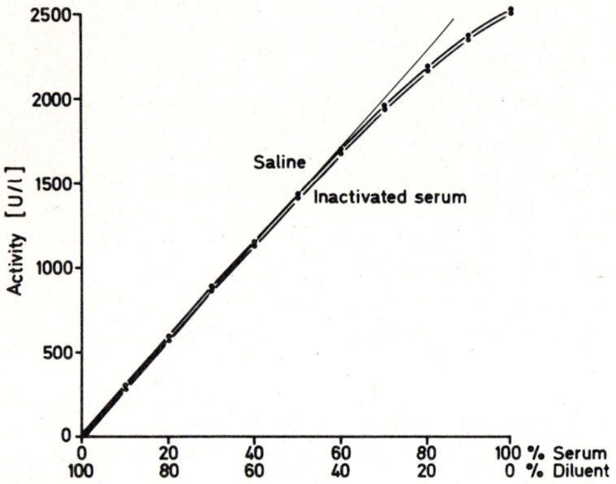

Fig. 13. Creatine kinase activity as a function of the amount of enzyme in the assay solution
Volume fraction of sample: 0.02

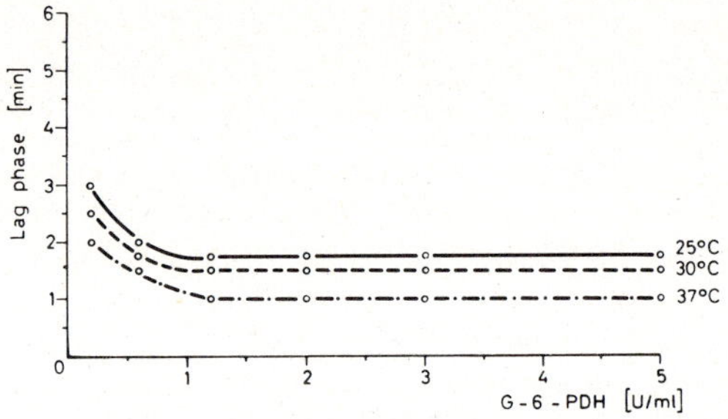

Fig. 15. Lag phase as a function of glucose-6-phosphate dehydrogenase activity (U/ml at 25 °C) in an assay mixture containing 2 U of hexokinase per milliliter

The duration of constant reaction rate, however, depends greatly on $NADP^+$ concentration (Figure 12). Including a lag phase of 2 min, the reaction rate decreases at 1.0 mmol of $NADP^+$ per liter in the presence of sera with activity of 1100 U/liter after 10 min total reaction time, although only a tenth of the $NADP^+$ in the assay solution has been reduced to NADPH. At 2.0 mmol of $NADP^+$ per liter the reaction rate remains constant for almost 15 min.

Enzyme Concentration

The relationship between enzyme concentration (i.e., the amount of serum in the assay solution) and enzyme activity remained linear up to 1500 U/liter whether physiological saline or inactivated serum was used as diluent (Figure 13). The data were obtained immediately after a lag phase of 2 min and at a volume fraction of sample of 0.02. At higher enzyme concentrations, the actually measured activities remain under the expected values, although—e.g., at 2000 U/liter—only a tenth of the $NADP^+$ that originally was present in the assay mixture is transformed within 5 min.

Hexokinase

The duration of the lag phase depends on the activity of the added auxiliary and indicator enzymes. The "true" lag phase—after 3 min of pre-incubation and starting the reaction with creatine phosphate—could be shortened by increasing the hexokinase activity to 2000 U/liter of reaction mixture. A greater hexokinase activity did not affect the duration of the lag phase (Figure 14).

As with every chemical reaction, the duration of the lag phase also depends on temperature. At 37 °C the lag phase is 1 min, at 25 °C it is 2 min, but it does not disappear at any temperature.

Glucose-6-phosphate Dehydrogenase

The lag phase is less influenced by glucose-6-phosphate dehydrogenase (Figure 15). Because the reagent blank increases gradually with added indicator enzyme, being 1.6, 4, and 8 U/liter at 1000, 2000, and 4000 U of glucose-6-phosphate dehydrogenase per liter, respectively, it is advisable to use a relatively low glucose-6-phosphate dehydrogenase activity.

In this study we used only baker's yeast glucose-6-phosphate dehydrogenase linked with $NADP^+$. The combination *Leuconostoc mesenteroides* enzyme and NAD^+ is now being studied.

N-Acetyl Cysteine

Creatine kinase in serum is rapidly inactivated (*9, 10*) but can be reactivated by adding sulfhydryl reagents (*4, 7, 11–14*). Such a sulfhydryl compound must quickly reactivate the enzyme without interfering with the measurement. Not only efficiency but also practicability

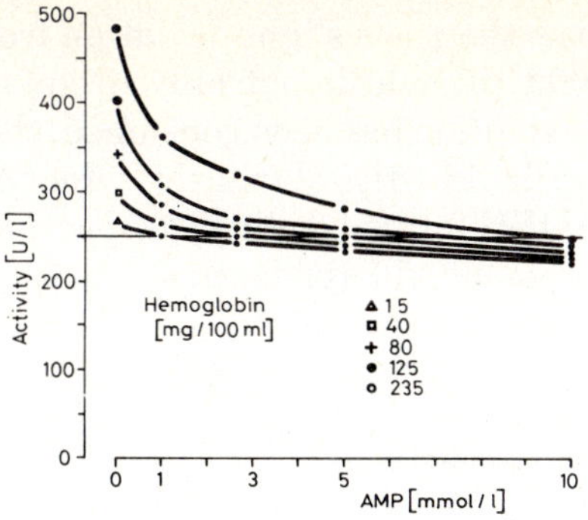

Fig. 16. Inhibition of adenylate kinase and creatine kinase by AMP

Apparent creatine kinase activity of human serum with added hemolysate, in the presence of 2 mmol of ADP per liter

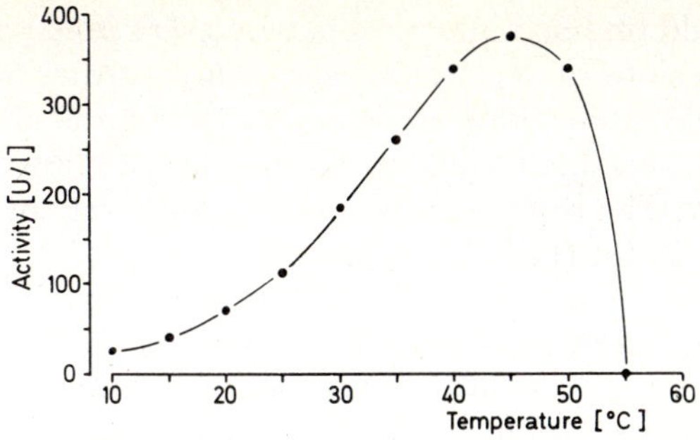

Fig. 17. Creatine kinase activity as a function of reaction temperature

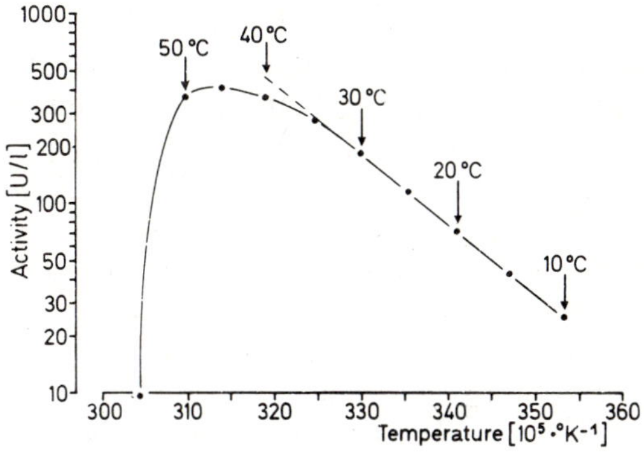

Fig. 18. Dependence of creatine kinase activity upon reaction temperature, plotted according to Arrhenius

should be considered: solubility, stability (even in solution), odor, and price.

By these criteria, of 27 thiol compounds tested, *N*-acetyl cysteine was the most suitable. At a concentration of 20 mmol of *N*-acetyl cysteine per liter, a constant creatine kinase activity was achieved within 3 min of pre-incubation and an additional 2 min for lag phase after starting the reaction with creatine phosphate. Prolonging the pre-incubation up to 6 h did not further increase the activity. If the reaction is started with serum, a total of 5 min is necessary. *N*-Acetyl cysteine was stable in the assay solution at pH 6.7 for at least 24 h at 25 °C and a week at 4 °C, as assessed both by determination of free sulfhydryl groups and by analytical recovery of creatine kinase activity.

We have reported on our investigations into the problem of inactivation and reactivation of creatine kinase in a preliminary paper,[4] and details will soon be published in this series.

AMP

ADP is also acted upon by adenylate kinase (EC 2.7.4.3), generating additional amounts of ATP. The normal range of adenylate kinase activity in human sera lies between 0–50 U/liter at 25 °C (unpublished observation), but is markedly greater in hemolytic specimens.

Figure 16 illustrates the extent of this interference. The apparent creatine kinase activity proportionately increased with the amount of hemolysate added to the serum. Such interference could be diminished by adding AMP. Because not only adenylate kinase but also creatine kinase will be inhibited by AMP, the AMP concentration must be a compromise. The inhibition is competitive and therefore depends on the ADP concentration. In the presence of 2 mmol of ADP per liter, 3 mmol of AMP per liter is sufficient in the case of sera with slight to moderate hemolysis. Markedly hemolyzed sera require 5 mmol of AMP per liter, but 10 mmol/liter is too much even for grossly hemolytic sera. Creatine kinase is inhibited by 5 to 10% by the presence of 5 mmol of AMP per liter.

[4] Bernt, E., Gruber, W., and Szasz, G., Vergleich von Reaktivatoren der Creatinkinase im Serum. *Z. Klin. Chem. Klin. Biochem.* **12**, 256 (1974) (Abstract).

Temperature

Creatine kinase activity increases with increasing reaction temperature up to 45 °C. At higher temperatures the activity rapidly decreases, and at 55 °C there is no detectable activity (Figure 17).

The activity–temperature relationship, plotted according to Arrhenius (Figure 18), was linear for temperatures between 10–35 °C; for higher temperatures the curve slopes downward. In an earlier study *(15)* in which a suboptimized method *(16)* was used, there was a deviation from linearity even at 30 °C. We used our "standard" conditions, except that the pH had to be adjusted because of the significant effect of temperature on the pH of the imidazole acetate buffer. If the pH is 6.7 at 25 °C, it will be, e.g., 7.2 at 10 °C or 6.4 at 55 °C.

Discussion

The total creatine kinase activity in serum can be a contribution from different isoenzymes. In cases of skeletal muscle damage the activity in serum is attributable almost exclusively to the presence of the MM isoenzyme, whereas in patients with myocardial infarction not only the MM, but also a variable MB isoenzyme activity (0–30%) is also present. The kinetic properties of the creatine kinase isoenzymes differ significantly *(17)*.

With respect to the affinity of the enzyme for its substrates or in the temperature activity relationship, we could find no differences between sera from patients with lesions of skeletal muscle or myocardial muscle. The MM isoenzyme obviously predominates in every serum, overshadowing the MB isoenzyme almost completely. The conditions we describe here are therefore optimum for the MM isoenzyme.

Table 1 compares the conditions described here and those formerly published by others (*4, 5, 7, 16*). It shows that almost all conditions we found to be optimal have already been used previously, although in none of the methods cited are all the conditions simultaneously optimal. Rosalki (*4*) recommends too-low concentrations of ADP, creatine phosphate, and $NADP^+$, and a too-low auxiliary and indicator enzyme activity. The Standard Method of the American Association for Clinical Chemistry by Swanson and Wilkinson (*18*) corresponds exactly to the method of Rosalki (*4*). The method of Hess et al. (*5*) is better, but still not optimal. Apart from the too-low ADP and (especially) $NADP^+$ concentrations, the main problem of the German Standard Method (*16*) arises from the use of reduced glutathione as reactivator. There may be an interference with creatine kinase activity measurement if the reagent contains considerable amounts of oxidized glutathione and the sample has a relatively high glutathione reductase (EC 1.6.4.2) activity. In this case NADPH, the product of the creatine kinase assay, will react with oxidized glutathione and the results for creatine kinase activity are incorrectly low.

Closest to the optimum are the conditions of Warren (*7*), but in that method the pH and the creatine phosphate concentration are too low and the magnesium ion concentration is too high.

The assay conditions we recommend are optimum at assay temperatures of either 30 °C (*3*) or 25 °C (*6*), probably even at 37 °C.[5] There are now only two possibilities for further enhancement of creatine kinase activity at a fixed temperature: to use a lower buffer and (or) AMP concentration. In fact, in almost all methods buffer concentrations lower than 100 mmol/liter are specified. A decrease to 50 mmol/liter would increase the activity by about 5%, but there would be problems in maintenance of a constant pH, especially when the reaction is started with creatine phosphate. A still-justifiable decrease of the AMP/ADP molar ratio from 2.5 to 1.5 would increase the creatine kinase activity by only 2–3%.

How long the reaction rate remains constant definitely depends on the $NADP^+$ concentration. With 2 mmol/liter, the linear range of activity could be extended to 1500 U/liter at a volume fraction of serum of 0.02. Because there is a slight deviation from linearity even at 2000 U/liter, although only 10% of the $NADP^+$ in the assay solution has been consumed, the deflection from zero-order kinetics obviously is due to the inhibition by NADPH formed during the reaction. Evidence for this statement will appear in a subsequent paper.

[5] W. Gerhardt, personal communication.

We thank Miss Elfriede Kinne for her conscientious technical assistance, and Mr. Harald Glaucke and Miss Eva-Beate Nittel for assistance with the manuscript. This work was supported by the Deutsche Forschungsgemeinschaft.

References

1. Smith, A. F., Separation of tissue and serum creatine kinase isoenzymes on polyacrylamide gel slabs. *Clin. Chim. Acta* **39**, 351 (1972).

2. Bowers, G. N., Bergmeyer, H. U., and Moss, D. W., Provisional Recommendation (1974) on IFCC methods for the measurement of catalytic concentration of enzymes. *Clin. Chim. Acta* **61**, F11 (1975). [*Clin. Chem.* **22**, 384 (1976)].

3. Oliver, I. T., A spectrophotometric method for the determination of creatine phosphokinase and myokinase. *Biochem. J.* **61**, 116 (1955).

4. Rosalki, S. B., An improved procedure for serum creatine phosphokinase determination. *J. Lab. Clin. Med.* **69**, 696 (1967).

5. Hess, J. W., Murdock, K. J., and Natho, G. J. W., Creatine kinase—A spectrophotometric method with improved sensitivity. *Am. J. Clin. Pathol.* **50**, 89 (1968).

6. Communication of the German Society for Clinical Chemistry. Recommendations for a uniform temperature for the estimation of enzyme activities in clinical chemistry. *Z. Klin. Chem. Klin. Biochem.* **9**, 464 (1971).

7. Warren, W. A., Activation of serum creatine kinase by dithiothreitol. *Clin. Chem.* **18**, 473 (1972).

8. Good, N. E., Winget, G. D., Winter, W., et al., Hydrogen ion buffers for biological research. *Biochemistry* **5**, 467 (1966).

9. Hughes, B. P., A method for the estimation of serum creatine kinase and its use in comparing creatine kinase to aldolase activity in normal and pathological sera. *Clin. Chim. Acta* **7**, 597 (1962).

10. Okinaka, S., Sugita, H., Momoi, H., et al., Cysteine stimulated serum creatine kinase in health and disease. *J. Lab. Clin. Med.* **64**, 299 (1964).

11. Kar, N. C., and Pearson, C. M., Activation of creatine phosphokinase by sulfhydryl compounds in normal and muscular dystrophy sera. *Proc. Soc. Exp. Biol. Med.* **118**, 662 (1965).

12. Bishop, C., Chu, T. M., and Shihabi, Z. K., Single stable reagent for creatine kinase. *Clin. Chem.* **17**, 548 (1971).

13. Dalal, F. R., Cilley, J., Jr., and Winsten, S., A study of the problems of inactivation of creatine kinase in serum. *Clin. Chem.* **18**, 330 (1972).

14. Miyada, D. S., Dinovo, E. C., and Nakamura, R. M., Creatine kinase reactivation by thiol compounds. *Clin. Chim. Acta* **58**, 97 (1975).

15. Szasz, G., The effect of temperature on enzyme activity and on the affinity of enzymes to their substrates. *Z. Klin. Chem. Klin. Biochem.* **12**, 166 (1974).

16. Recommendations of the German Society of Clinical Chemistry. Standardization of methods for the estimation of enzyme activities in biological fluids. *Z. Klin. Chem. Klin. Biochem.* **8**, 659 (1970).

17. Witteveen, S. A. G. J., Sobel, B. E., and DeLuca, M., Kinetic properties of the isoenzymes in human creatine phosphokinase. *Proc. Nat. Acad. Sci. USA* **71**, 1384 (1974).

18. Swanson, J. R., and Wilkinson, J. H., Measurement of creatine kinase activity in serum. *Stand. Methods Clin. Chem.* **7**, 33 (1972).

CLIN. CHEM. 22/5, 657-662 (1976)

Profile Analysis of Blood Proteins with a Centrifugal Analyzer

Mogens Blom and Niels Hjørne

We describe a procedure for routine analysis of a profile composed of eight blood proteins with a GEMSAEC centrifugal analyzer. The end-point technique is used and four standards are included in each run in the immunochemical analysis of the individual proteins. Additional computer programs fit the absorbance readings from the samples to the (nonlinear) standard curve and store the results in a patient's file for a final printout, which also presents the patient's data and reference values. The proteins are analyzed in a given order, which allows common blank runs to be used. Antisera are used in suitably high concentrations, so that the "antigen in excess" problem only appears for analysis of IgA and IgM when sera contain high amounts of the M-components of these two classes. The capacity, accuracy, and precision of the method are satisfactory.

Specific proteins were first immunochemically quantitated in liquid medium by Gitlin and Edelhoch (*1*), using a manual method. This principle has gained new interest after automation in continuous-flow systems with either turbidimetric or nephelometric recording of the antigen–antibody reactions (*2, 3*). Recently the technique has been transferred to centrifugal analyzers, which have a high precision in photometric measurements. Tiffany et al. (*4*) used a miniature centrifugal analyzer modified for nephelometry, and found a coefficient of variation (run-to-run precision) of 5.5% for equilibrium values and of 15.0% for rate measurements. Buffone et al. (*5*) also used two-point fixed-time kinetics on a laser-equipped system and demonstrated good precision in analysis for IgA, IgG, and IgM.

In our laboratory, quantitation of several proteins has been performed turbidimetrically with an unmodified GEMSAEC analyzer. The basic principles of the method have been published earlier, with albumin determination as a model (*6*). Because of the high initial velocity of the reactions (*7*) and the fact that the earliest possible reading on the standard model of the instrument is 30 s from the start, we have chosen the end-point technique and the use of a calibration curve in each run.

The following blood proteins have hitherto been determined with centrifugal analyzers: IgA, IgG, and IgM (*4, 5*); α_1-antitrypsin and C′3 complement (*4*); and albumin, orosomucoid, coeruloplasmin, haptoglobin, and transferrin (*8*).

The purpose of the present study has been to evaluate a procedure for routinely obtaining an analytical profile, mainly composed of those specific proteins that a panel of experts has considered most relevant as a supplement to the conventional electrophoretic separation of serum proteins (*9*). Furthermore, we have found it essential to complete the computerized data handling, so that the results for each patient are presented on an individual printout sheet.

Materials and Methods

Apparatus

The instrument we used was the GEMSAEC centrifugal analyzer (Electro-Nucleonics Inc., Caldwell, N. J. 07006; Model 400535-3) without any modification of the hardware.

An additional program to the original FOCAL programs has been published earlier (*6*). This program has been prepared in order to fit the absorbance readings from the individual samples to the nonlinear standard curve (precipitation curve) obtained from four standards included in each run. The program also calls attention to values outside the range of the standard curves and performs a check for unusual shapes of the curve (e.g., erroneous order of the four standard solutions in the transfer disc). A usual "GEMSAEC header" is used for each protein. In such a header, the concentration of the undiluted standard is indicated by the value of the "variable" SC. If a new concentration is brought into use, only this variable has to be changed when the values of the four working standards are calculated by the program.

Another special program,[1] to make maximum use of the capacity of the computer that is not being occupied by the original GEMSAEC procedures, has been devised to store the results of the individual sample in a patient

Department of Clinical Chemistry, Aalborg Hospital, P.O. Box 561, DK 9100 Aalborg, Denmark.

Received Feb. 2, 1976; accepted Mar. 5, 1976.

[1] Detailed information on the computer programs is available either from one of the authors (N.H.) or from Electro-Nucleonics Inc.

file on the magnetic tape deck. When all proteins comprised in the profile have been determined, a sheet for each patient is printed out that presents the patient's data, results, and the reference values.

Reagents

Antisera. Anti-human antisera against the proteins in question were obtained commercially (Technicon Instruments Corp., Tarrytown, N. Y. 10591; and Dakopatts A/S, Copenhagen, Denmark). These antisera were diluted 30- to 100-fold with a solution of sodium chloride (6 g/liter) and polyethylene glycol (60 g/liter) (polyethylene glycol, mol wt 4000, pure, cat. No. 4807 h; Koch-Light Laboratories Ltd., Colnbrook, England). Before use, solutions showing visible turbidity were clarified by passage through a 0.22-μm (av pore size) filter (Millipore Corp., Bedford, Mass. 01730.; cat. No. GSWP 02500). Clarification was necessary only for dilutions of antisera prepared as whole sera, but not for purified immunoglobulin fractions.

Blank reagent. The polyethylene glycol/saline solution was used without antibody for sample blank correction. This solution was not filtered.

Standards and human sera. A serum pool from persons negative for hepatitis B surface antigen served as a substandard. This pool was to some extent clarified by passage through a 1.2-μm (av pore size) filter (Milipore Corp.; cat. No. RAWP 04700) after storage at −20 °C for one month. The concentrations of the proteins concerned were determined by single radial immunodiffusion against "Standard Human Serum" (Behringwerke, Marburg, Germany; cat. No. ORDT 03) or, in the case of α_1-antitrypsin, against "Standard Human Plasma" (Behringwerke; cat. No. OTFI 03). The serum pool and sera from hospitalized patients were prediluted manually with saline (9 g/liter), which also was used for "flush" in the pipetting unit (Rotoloader). The predilution of the samples was 21-fold for determination of all the proteins except for albumin (251-fold).

Procedure

The transfer disc is loaded with the Rotoloader as follows: sample volume 7, 10, 15, or 40 μl. The sample is placed in well B and the antibody solution in well C. The 16 positions of the transfer disc are loaded according to the following arrangement of the sample cups: a water blank in position 1, standards of increasing concentrations in positions 2–5, samples in positions 6–15, and position 16 available for a control serum.

The following analyzer settings are used in the analysis:

Filter position	335–385 nm
Wavelength	340 nm
Reaction temp	37 °C
Reaction mode	End point
Running mode	Auto
Initial reading	(IR) 240 s
Reading interval	(RI) 60 s
No. readings	(NR) 01

The header information necessary for each protein is the following:

IR = 240
RI = 60
NR = 1
SC = standard concentration (different for each protein).
KT = 0 (not used)
TF = 0 (not used)
TC = specifies the values of the four standards for each protein.
AD = 4
HI = 0 (not used)
LO = 0 (not used)
SA = 0 (not used)
RM = 0 (not used)
XX = 0 (not used)
CD = 0, 1, or 2

The additional program used in handling the patients' data and the results of the analysis is self-explanatory, which means that storing and retrieval of data as well as all relevant information is obtained by following a series of simple instructions to the operator. The first step is to create a patient file containing names, dates of birth, and other information on the magnetic tape deck (DEC-tape). All results obtained during the runs of the individual protein analysis will be collected in this file and later printed out on a separate sheet for each patient on request from the operator. Blank readings are taken in a separate run 15 s after

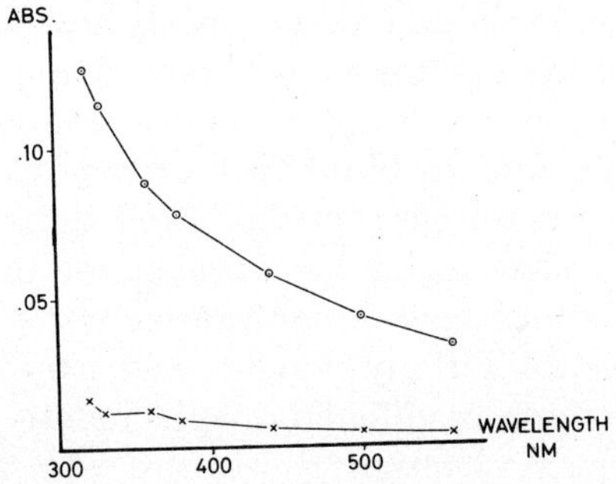

Fig. 1. Absorbances from reaction of a serum pool with blank reagents (*bottom curve*) and antihuman transferrin (*top curve*) at different wavelengths

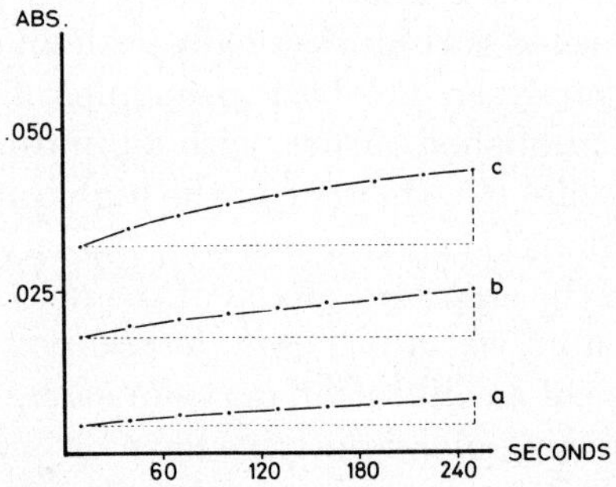

Fig. 2. Blank readings for a clear sample (*a*), a filtered serum pool (*b*), and a turbid nonfiltered pool (*c*) in the time interval 10–250 s after air-mixing in the cuvettes

Table 1. Essentials of Procedure for a Specific Protein Profile

Protein	Source of antiserum	Diln	Calibration pool diln		Sample prediln	Vol, μl	Range (calibrn. curve)	"Safe" concn	Blank run
Albumin	Dakopatts	1:100	1:701 1:241	1:351 1:181	1:251	10	15.2–58.9 g/l	101 g/l	—
Orosomucoid	Dakopatts	1:50	1:61 1:13	1:21 1:9	1:21	15	10–67 μm/l[a]	101 μmol/l	+
IgA	Technicon	1:50	1:61 1:13	1:21 1:9	1:21	15	69–450 int. units/ml[b]	1050 int. units/ml	+
Transferrin	Dakopatts	1:100	1:61 1:13	1:21 1:9	1:21	15	8–57 μm/l[c]	67 μmol/l	+
Haptoglobin	Technicon	1:50	1:176 1:13	1:31 1:9	1:21	15	0.3–6.5 g/l	11.8 g/l	+
α_1-Antitrypsin	Technicon	1:40	1:61 1:13	1:21 1:9	1:21	7	17–117 μm/l[d]	149 μmol/l	(+)
IgG	Dakopatts	1:50	1:61 1:13	1:21 1:9	1:21	7	56–411 int. units/ml[e]	959 int. units/ml	(+)
IgM	Dakopatts	1:30	1:41 1:13	1:21 1:9	1:21	40	72–327 int. units/ml[f]	980 int. units/ml	+, 240 s

[a] Mol. wt. = 44 100 [b] 1 mg = 59.5 U [c] Mol. wt. = 90 000 [d] Mol. wt. = 45 000 [e] 1 mg = 11.5 U [f] 1 mg = 115 U

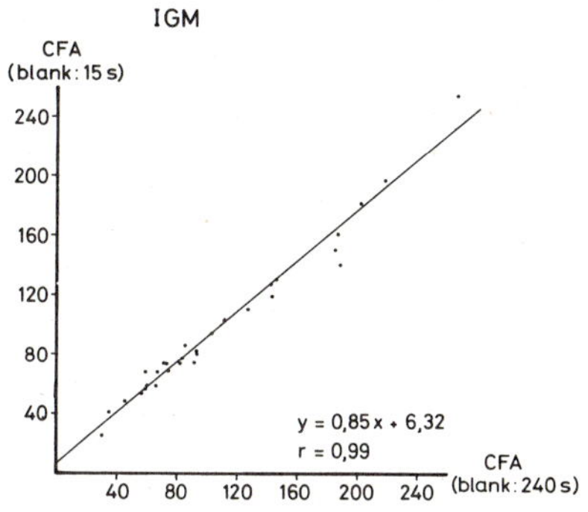

Fig. 3. Correlation between results from IgM analysis of 30 samples
Abscissa: blank readings after 240 s. *Ordinate:* blank readings after 15 s. Units as in Table 1

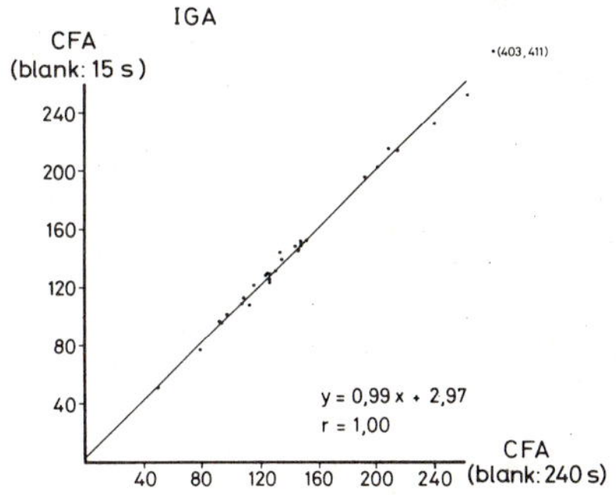

Fig. 4. Correlation between results from IgA analysis of 30 samples
Abscissa: blank readings after 240 s. *Ordinate:* blank readings after 15 s. Units as in Table 1

mixing. Blank values are subtracted automatically by use of the cuvette calibration procedure before the subsequent determination of the proteins. However, when IgM is being measured it is necessary to run a blank for fully 240 s.

Table 1 specifies a practical procedure for running a profile consisting of eight proteins. Dilutions of antisera, dilutions of the calibration pool, and sample volumes are given. Blank run is necessary when indicated by "+" in the last column; a "(+)" indicates that a blank run is of importance only if the disc contains visibly turbid samples. For albumin an ordinary cuvette calibration with water is sufficient because of the high final sample dilution (21 600-fold).

The eight proteins were analyzed in the order given in the table. Albumin requires separate sample dilution. For orosomucoid, IgA, and transferrin, a common blank run is made for each disc. Haptoglobin determination requires a separate blank run, because of the extended range of the calibration curve. α_1-Antitrypsin and IgG both require a sample volume of 7 μl, which makes possible a common blank run for these proteins. For IgM, a blank run of 240 s is required, because of the high volume (40 μl).

For comparison studies, electroimmunoassays were done according to Laurell (*10*) or with a turbidimetric continuous-flow system, which has undergone certain modifications since it was described (*11*).

Results

Wavelength: Figure 1 shows the absorbance values obtained for a serum pool, with blank reagent and with anti-human transferrin. Evidently, although the blank value is increasing with the decrease in wavelength, the net turbidity from the reaction is significantly higher in this part of the spectrum than at 440 nm, the traditionally preferred wavelength for turbidimetric measurements of antigen–antibody reactions. Because of

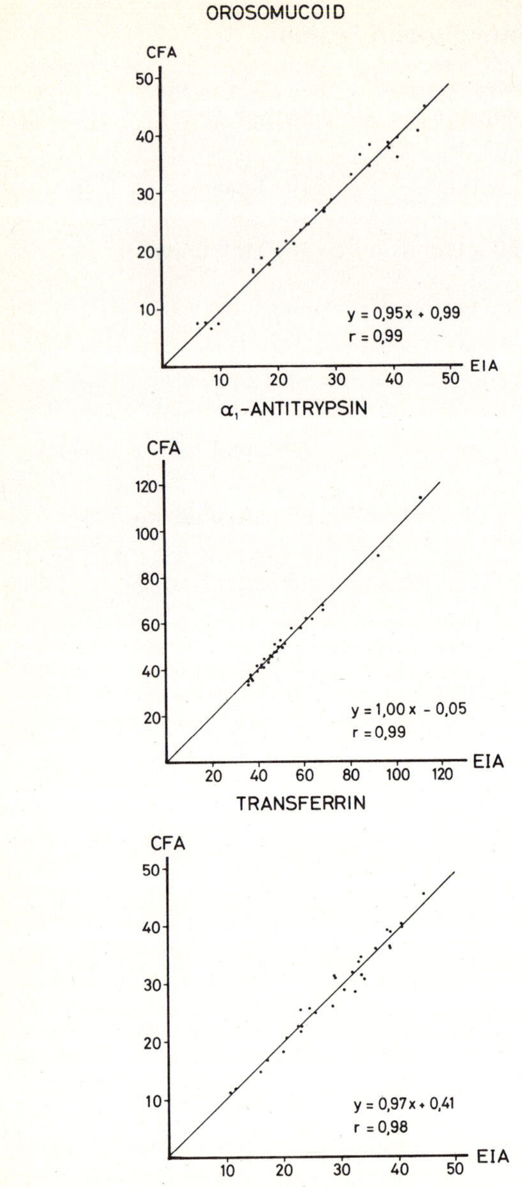

Fig. 5. Correlation between 30 orosomucoid, α_1-antitrypsin, and transferrin values given by electroimmunoassay (*EIA*) and by the present method (*CFA*)
Units as in Table 1

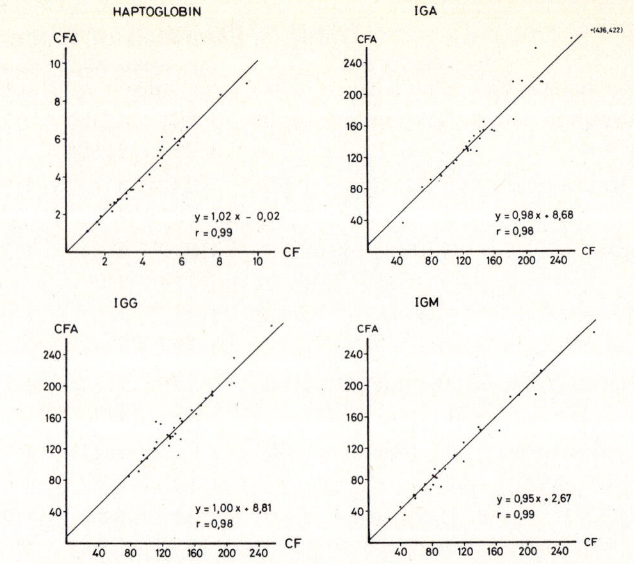

Fig. 6. Correlation between 30 haptoglobin, IgA, IgG, and IgM values given by the continuous-flow technique (*CF*) and the present method (*CFA*)
Units as in Table 1

suboptimal function of the instrument at 320 nm, we used 340 nm.

Time for blank reading: Figure 2 shows blank readings for a clear sample, a filtered serum pool, and a visibly turbid nonfiltered pool in the interval 10–250 s after the air-mixing step in the cuvettes. The sample volume was 40 μl.

It is seen that absorbance increases with time, the increase being about proportional to the value after 10 s. Thus a fundamental error is made when blank values read after 15 s are used. This is so because the nonspecific blank reaction adds a relatively greater amount of turbidity to the antigen–antibody reaction in the unclear standard than it does to the samples. Thus results for the samples will be too low, especially when they represent high concentrations of the protein in question. Samples with low concentrations are compared to relatively higher dilutions of the standard with more normal blanks. This means that low values are estimated more precisely.

To investigate the influence of this matter in practice, we compared results from IgM and IgA determinations from runs with blank correction after 15 s and after 240 s. Figure 3 demonstrates that blank runs of only 15 s could not be used in the measurement of IgM, where the final sample dilution was 300-fold. The same time (240 s) as used in reaction runs was necessary. In determination of IgA—and of the remaining proteins—15 s was found to be sufficient for practical purposes (Figure 4), because the final sample dilutions were at least 800-fold, which minimized the influence from the unspecific blank reaction.

Precision: Within-run precision was estimated by running three control sera with a concentration of the protein concerned within the low, medium, and high sections of the calibration curve 24 times each, equally distributed over eight discs. Day-to-day precision was assessed by measuring a control serum once daily for 18 days. The results are given in Table 2. Precision for albumin determination has been given earlier (*6*).

Method comparison: Sera from 30 hospitalized patients were analyzed for eight proteins (not including albumin) by the present method. For comparison, the sera were also analyzed for α_1-antitrypsin, orosomucoid, and transferrin by electroimmunoassays (Figure 5). Values for IgA, IgG, IgM, and haptoglobin were compared to values obtained by a continuous-flow technique (Figure 6). In the case of albumin, the method has earlier been compared to the Laurell technique (*6*). Figure 7 shows a printout of the albumin results for a single disc. These are kept in the laboratory, while the final printout sheets containing the values for the proteins for each patient (Figure 8) are forwarded to the clinician.

Table 2. Precision of Each Determination

Protein	Within-day: Low concn	CV, %	Within-day: Medium concn	CV, %	Within-day: High concn	CV, %	Day-to-day: Concn	CV, %
Orosomucoid, μmol/l	12	3.64	34	3.93	54	2.55	26	2.83
α_1-Antitrypsin, μmol/l	26	3.66	66	3.56	95	2.46	50	2.42
Haptoglobin, g/l	1.3	4.76	3.0	1.77	5.9	1.97	1.7	1.86
Transferrin, μmol/l	15	3.57	25	3.97	40	2.44	25	2.40
IgA, K U/l	83	3.41	153	2.68	250	1.54	131	3.29
IgG, K U/l	89	4.03	158	3.92	258	2.20	135	4.26
IgM, K U/l	88	6.22	210	4.15	273	2.41	130	6.36

```
*G

TYPE OF RUN?G

ROTOR:PROF-1

HOW MANY SAMPLES IN THIS DISC ARE PROFILE-ANALYSES ? 10

IR:    240    AD:      0     DET: ALBUMIN
RI:     60    CD:      0     DATE: 12.1.76.B6     RUN:     34
NR:      1    TC:   20.0     ROTOR: PROF-1

HI:   110.0000
LO:     0.0000
SA:     0.0000

10/40/500   340 NM

*G

 CUV     P-NR.      ABS.      GRAM/L

   2               0.0432     14.31   STAND.  1
   3               0.0809     28.56   STAND.  2
   4               0.1141     40.75   STAND.  3
   5               0.1499     57.00   STAND.  4
   6       1       0.1084     39
   7       2       0.0819     29
   8       3       0.0764     27
   9       4       0.1139     41
  10       5       0.0797     28
  11       6       0.0936     33
  12       7       0.0974     35
  13       8       0.0842     30
  14       9       0.0859     30
  15      10       0.0727     25
  16               0.1097     39

SET 'WRITE ENABLE' AND PRESS CR
```

Fig. 7. Printout of results for albumin from a single disc

```
AALBORG SYGEHUS NORD                                 DATO: 12-01-1976
CENTRALLABORATORIET
                                                      AFD: MED-1

PROTEIN-PROFILANALYSE                                REKV-NR: 3457

PATIENT(    2):  HANS ERIKSEN                        CPR-NR: 221238045

     ANALYSE                RESULTAT            REFERENCEOMRAADE

     ALBUMIN                32.0  GRAM/L        38.0 - 48.0  GRAM/L
     OROSOMUCOID            35.4  UMOL/L        11.1 - 28.4  UMOL/L
     ALFA-1-ANTITRYPSIN     72.0  UMOL/L        24.4 - 55.6  UMOL/L
     HAPTOGLOBIN            6.10  GRAM/L        0.40 - 3.50  GRAM/L
     TRANSFERRIN            22.1  UMOL/L        21.9 - 39.7  UMOL/L
     IMMUNOGLOBULIN-A        184  IU/ML           44 - 182  IU/ML
     IMMUNOGLOBULIN-G        220  IU/ML           83 - 173  IU/ML
     IMMUNOGLOBULIN-M        210  IU/ML           26 - 153  IU/ML
```

Fig. 8. Printout of the protein profile for a single patient

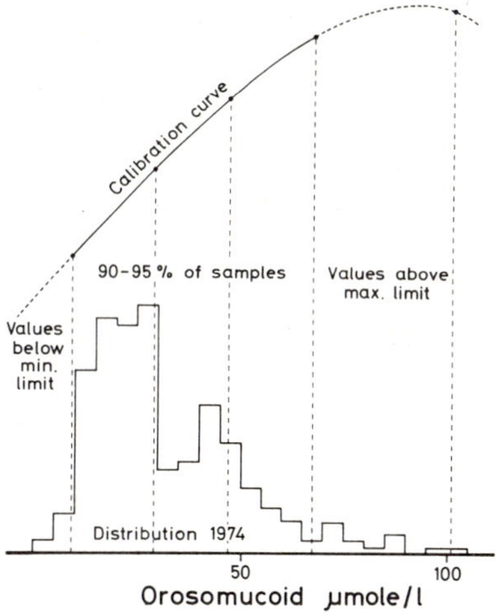

Fig. 9. The principle for choice of antiserum concentration

A concentration is chosen that allows 90–95% of the expected results to fall on the calibration curve and that ensures that the highest values will cause a turbidity greater than the absorbance for the most concentrated standards

Discussion

On the centrifugal analyzer one absorbance reading actually consists of the average of eight readings. This improves the signal-to-noise ratio to an extent that makes precise recordings of small absorbance differences possible, and is one of the main reasons why the protein determinations can be made with sufficiently high precision.

Results by the present method compared to those obtained by electroimmunoassays show good correlations for albumin, orosomucoid, α_1-antitrypsin, and transferrin. For the remaining proteins—haptoglobin and the immunoglobulins—which all are characterized by molecular heterogeneity in the individual samples, a good correlation between this method and continuous-flow technique can be demonstrated. However, in the case of IgM the comparison is characterized by a lower precision with both methods. As mentioned earlier, it is necessary in IgM determination to run the blank for 240 s because of the relatively low sample dilution, and the fact that an unspecific reaction with the blank reagent is taking place. In the two-point kinetic method described by Buffone et al. (*5*) the reactants are mixed again just before the readings, probably because a sedimentation of large antigen–antibody complexes is suspected. However we have never observed unstability or significant differences between readings taken before and after a second mix. Note that in our procedure the final concentration of both antigen and antiserum is lower than in the kinetic method.

In contrast to continuous-flow procedures, the present method does not allow detection of samples containing an excess of a specific protein in relation to the antiserum concentration used, as will appear from Figure 9. But for all the proteins except IgA and IgM it is possible to determine and use an antibody concentration that ensures that the highest expected value of a sample will give rise to a turbidity greater than the absorbance of the highest standards. In this case the printout of the results always will be: "Value above maximum limit," even though the sample could be situated beyond the point of equivalence. In Table 1 the "safe concentration," that with certainty will cause this warning flag, is given for each of the proteins (under the assumption that the antisera are diluted as recommended).

For this reason the antibody concentrations in this method will often be higher than in continuous-flow systems, but because of the wide ranges of the standard curves, which for the same reasons are made possible, only 5–10% of the samples have to be re-analyzed after another predilution. The number of samples that can be analyzed per milliliter of undiluted antiserum varies from 42 (for IgM) to 138 (for transferrin and albumin). In these calculations the consumption of antiserum by the four standards in each disc has been taken in consideration. In contrast to the continuous-flow systems, the GEMSAEC does not waste any reagent when being changed from one analysis to another.

As mentioned, "antigen in excess" will be a problem only in IgA and IgM determination, and only when an M component of one of these two classes is present. In case of IgG it is most unlikely that a concentration of 959 int. units/ml (Table 1), which corresponds to 83.2 g/liter, should be exceeded, even in sera from patients with severe myeloma. On the other hand, M-components belonging to the classes IgA and IgM may appear in concentrations higher than 1050 int. units/ml (17.6 g/liter) and 980 int. units/ml (8.5 g/liter), respectively. Thus the method is not applicable in screening for M components; it is generally accepted that such a screening should be done by electrophoretic separation of serum as well as of urine, Bence-Jones proteins otherwise would be missed.

The capacity of the method seems to be satisfactory compared to that of other procedures for measurement of specific proteins. Albumin, which does not need a separate blank run, can be measured at a rate of 100 samples per hour. If blank correction is necessary for a given protein, the rate will still be as high as 75 samples per hour. Only about 70 min is needed to complete a profile of all eight proteins in 11 sera. No manual calculations are necessary and only 5–10% of the samples have to be re-analyzed in another pre-dilution, which for routine purposes can be put off until the following day.

The method is based upon end-point measurements, but we agree with the point of view (*5*) that a kinetic method would be preferable even if it also requires four standards in each run. The advantages of a kinetic method are that separate blank runs could be avoided and the reaction time shortened. However, kinetic measurement has so far only been done on prototypes of centrifugal analyzers. We believe that a main advantage of the described method is the use of an unmodified instrument, which already is present in many laboratories and which can be used for other purposes in the daily routine.

References

1. Gitlin, D., and Edelhoch, H., A study of the reaction between human serum albumin and its homologous equine antibody through the medium of light scattering. *J. Immunol.* **66,** 67 (1951).

2. Kahan, J., and Sundblad, L., Automated immunochemical determination of β-lipoproteins. In *Automation in Analytical Chemistry, Technicon Symposia 1966;* **2,** E. Kawerau et al., Eds., Mediad, White Plains, N. Y., 1967, p 361.

3. Eckman, I., Robbin J. B., Van den Hamer, C. J. A., et al., Automation of a quantitative immunochemical microanalysis of human serum transferrin: A model system. *Clin. Chem.* **16,** 558 (1970).

4. Tiffany, T. O., Parella, J. M., Johnson, W. F., and Burtis, C. A., Specific protein analysis by light-scatter measurement with a miniature centrifugal fast analyzer. *Clin. Chem.* **20,** 1055 (1974).

5. Buffone, C. J., Savory, J., Cross, R. E., and Hammond, J. E., Evaluation of kinetic light scattering as an approach to the measurement of specific proteins with a centrifugal analyzer. 1. Methodology. *Clin. Chem.* **21,** 1731 (1975).

6. Blom, M., and Hjφrne, N., Immunochemical determination of serum albumin with a centrifugal analyzer. *Clin. Chem.* **21,** 195 (1975).

7. Savory, J., Buffone, G., and Reich, R., Kinetics of the IgG–anti-IgG reaction, an evaluation by conventional and stopped-flow nephelometry. *Clin. Chem.* **20,** 1070 (1974).

8. Blom, M., and Hjφrne, N., Immunochemical determination of blood proteins. In *Protides of the Biological Fluids,* 23rd Colloquium, H. Peeters, Ed., 1976, p 299.

9. Laurell, C.-B., Electrophoresis, specific protein assay, or both in measurement of plasma proteins? *Clin. Chem.* **19,** 99 (1973).

10. Laurell, C.-B., Quantitative estimation of protein by electrophoresis in agarose gel containing antibodies. *Anal. Biochem.* **15,** 45 (1966).

11. Blom, M., and Sorensen, D., A turbidimetric continous-flow system for immunochemical quantitation of blood proteins by use of a modified photometer. *Clin. Chem.* **19,** 1148 (1973).

CLIN. CHEM. 22/5, 663–666 (1976)

Technical Pitfalls in Measurement of Venous Plasma NH_3 Concentration

Glynda G. Gerron, Joseph D. Ansley, James W. Isaacs, Michael H. Kutner, and Daniel Rudman

Measurement of venous plasma NH_3 in normal subjects by the ion-exchange method of Forman [*Clin. Chem.* **10**, 497 (1964)] in a hospital clinical laboratory gave a mean value of 640 μg/liter (range, 300–1320 μg/liter; intra-assay, intra-individual, and inter-individual coefficients of variation, 8, 47, and 47%, respectively). The following conditions adversely affect the reproducibility of the test: pollution of laboratory atmosphere and glassware by NH_3-containing detergents; smoking by patient or analyst; delay, turbulence, or use of heparin lock in venipuncture; delay or warming of plasma above 0 °C before mixing it with resin; and delay in colorimetric analysis of resin eluate. When these sources of error were eliminated, the mean value for normals was reduced to 330 μg/liter, the range was narrowed to 220–470 μg/liter, and the above-mentioned CV's were 5, 16, and 17%, respectively. With the precautions cited, furthermore, the intra-assay and intra-individual CV's for fasting NH_3 concentration in cirrhotic patients were similarly reduced. An NH_3 tolerance test was done by administering a standard dose of NH_4Cl to patients and measuring venous plasma NH_3 at 0, 15, 30, 60, and 90 min; the NH_3 tolerance was quantified from the area under the curve relating concentration to time (μg · min/liter). As measured in the clinical laboratory, NH_3 tolerance of cirrhotic patients showed intra-assay and intra-individual CV's of 50 to 90%. When the tolerance tests were repeated in the same subjects with the laboratory precautions listed above, these CV's were reduced to 8–15%.

Additional Keyphrases: *NH_3 tolerance test • evaluating patency of portacaval shunts • diagnosis of hepatic encephalopathy • normal values • variation, source of • inter- and intra-individual variation • cirrhosis*

Measurement of venous plasma NH_3 concentration is useful in the differential diagnosis of hepatic encephalopathy (*1–3*). Furthermore, measurement of NH_3 concentration before and after ingestion of a standard dose of NH_4^+ salt ("NH_3 tolerance test") is useful in evaluating the patency of portacaval shunts (*4*).

Until 1961, measurement of plasma NH_3 was based on the microdiffusion method (*5–9*), which gave 600 to 1200 μg/liter as the normal range for fasting subjects. Since 1961, the ion-exchange method introduced by Hutchinson and Labby (*10*), and subsequently modified by Miller and Rice (*11*) and by Forman (*12*), has generally been used: plasma ammonium is adsorbed onto a cation-exchange resin, eluted with 4 mol/liter NaCl or 0.1 mol/liter NaOH, and measured colorimetrically. The normal range for fasting subjects with this method was reported to be 180 to 480 μg/liter by Miller and Rice (*11*), 230 to 700 μg/liter by Forman (*12*), and 240 to 750 μg/liter by Hutchinson and Labby (*10*). Neither the coefficient of variation (CV) of the measurement nor the variability in terms of intra-assay, intra-individual, and inter-individual components were reported by these investigators.

The intra-assay component represents the variability associated with replicate measurements, i.e., multiple determinations on a single blood sample. The intra-individual component represents the variability associated with replicate blood samples from the same subject. Finally the inter-individual component represents the variability associated with a single determination for each subject within a group of individuals.

We recently began to measure plasma NH_3 according to Forman (*12*), both in fasting patients and during NH_3 tolerance tests conducted according to Conn (*4*), to compare the effects of various types of shunt operation (*13*) on NH_3 metabolism. The range of plasma NH_3 in normal subjects reported by our hospital clinical laboratory was 300 to 1320 μg/liter; intra-assay CV [i.e., (SD/mean) × 100] was 8%, intra-individual CV 47%. Furthermore, the score for the standard NH_3 tolerance curve, calculated according to Conn (*4*), showed an inter-individual CV of 88%.

We investigated the sources of these unacceptably high CV's in the fasting plasma NH_3 and in the tolerance test, and identified five technical sources of error in the laboratory analysis. When these were corrected, the fasting normal range for NH_3 agreed closely with Miller and Rice (*11*)—viz., 180–480 μg/liter—and the intra-assay, intra-individual, and inter-individual variability in fasting plasma NH_3 for normal individuals was markedly decreased.

Departments of Medicine, Surgery and Biometry, Emory University School of Medicine and Clinical Research Facility, Emory University Hospital, Atlanta, Ga. 30322.

Received Jan. 30, 1976; accepted Mar. 3, 1976.

Methods

Subjects

Subjects were (*a*) 15 normal volunteers (11 men, four women), 18 to 30 years old, whose plasma NH_3 was measured on an outpatient basis and whose diet was not controlled; (*b*) 15 patients (eight men, seven women) 39 to 60 years old, with biopsy-documented alcoholic or post-necrotic cirrhosis, who had received a portacaval, mesocaval, mesorenal, or splenorenal shunt operation (*13*) three to 60 months previously because of portal hypertension and variceal hemorrhage. NH_3 studies were done within the hospital after three or more days during which the subject consumed 40 g of protein and 1800 to 2300 Cal daily.

We measured plasma NH_3 concentration in heparinized venous blood from the antecubital vein according to the method of Forman (*12*) either in the hospital's clinical laboratory or in the laboratory of the metabolic research unit, with various modifications as described under *Results*. The plasma NH_3 concentration was measured in two settings: (*a*) fasting NH_3 at 0800 hours, after a 14-h fast, and (*b*) after an overnight fast, the 0-h blood sample was drawn, the patient ingested the standard dose of NH_4Cl dissolved in 225 ml noncaloric lemonade,[1] and additional samples were taken at 15, 30, 60, and 90 min for NH_3 analysis. The standard dose[2] of NH_4Cl, in grams, was: (patient's ideal body weight)$^{0.75}$/(70 kg$^{0.75}$). Ideal body weight was estimated according to ref. *14*. Each NH_3 analysis was done in duplicate, to permit estimation of intra-assay variability. For each subject, fasting NH_3 was measured twice within one week, and the NH_3 tolerance test was also done twice within the same week, to permit estimation of the intra-individual variability for these two tests. As suggested by Conn (*4*), the NH_3 tolerance test was quantified in two ways: the 15-min plasma NH_3 concentration, and the area under the concentration-vs.-time curve during the period 0–90 min (Figure 1).

Results

Results from the clinical laboratory. Normal subjects' fasting plasma NH_3 averaged 640 μg/liter; the normal range was 300 to 1320 μg/liter (Table 1). CV's for fasting NH_3 within the normal group—intra-assay, intra-individual and inter-individual—were 8, 47, and 47, respectively. Neither k-factor normal nor nonparametric tolerance limits are reported, because skewness is apparent and our sample sizes are extremely small.

The NH_3 tolerance tests in normals, as reported by Conn (*4*), were flat (Figure 1). The average 15-min value was 930 μg/liter (range, 490 to 1700 μg/liter; intra-assay, intra-individual, and inter-individual CV's, 9, 25, and

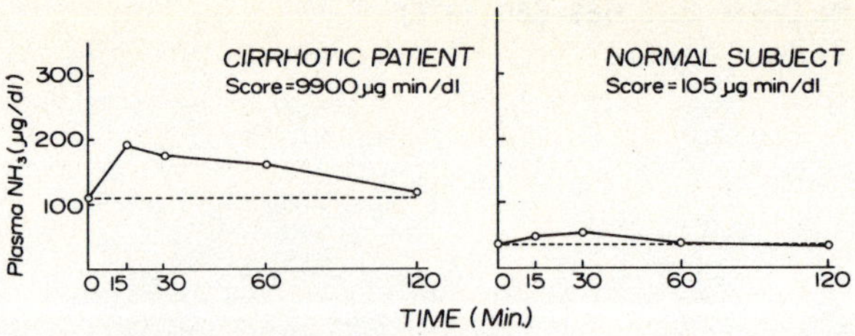

Fig. 1. Results of NH_3 tolerance test in a normal and in a cirrhotic subject

Score represents area between solid and dotted lines. Both results from the "special laboratory"

31%, respectively). When the NH_3 tolerance was scored by the area method, the range for normals was 0 to 2930 (mean 868; intra-assay, intra-individual and inter-individual CV's, 55, 82, and 88%). In cirrhotic patients, the average concentration of NH_3 in the plasma of fasting patients was 1180 μg/liter (range, 430–2630) with intra-assay and intra-individual CV's of 10 and 16%, respectively. In the NH_3 tolerance tests, 15-min values averaged 1840 μg/liter (intra-assay and intra-individual CV's of 6 and 23%), and scores averaged 79800 (intra-assay and intra-individual CV's were each 51%).

Identification of pitfalls. The high intra-assay and intra-individual CV's for fasting NH_3 in the normal group compared to other standard chemical analyses of plasma (*16*) suggested uncontrolled technical errors in the analysis. The high inter-individual CV in the normal individuals implied the same, although this finding in the cirrhotics could be explained by clinical heterogeneity in severity of the disease.

Accordingly, we now investigated the influence on the plasma NH_3 procedure of environmental, clinical, and analytical conditions prevailing in the clinical laboratory, and could identify five factors that adversely affect intra-assay and intra-individual CV of the test: (*a*) pollution of laboratory atmosphere or laboratory glassware by NH_3-containing detergents; (*b*) smoking by patient or staff; (*c*) delay, turbulence, or use of heparin lock in venipuncture; (*d*) delay or warming the plasma above 0 °C before mixing it with resin; and (*e*) delay in colorimetric analysis of the resin eluate.

Accordingly a "special NH_3 laboratory" was set up where blood NH_3 was measured under the following conditions:

- Patients do not smoke after midnight (one cigarette smoked 1-h before venipuncture was found to increase fasting blood NH_3 by 100–200 μg/liter).
- Technologists are nonsmokers.
- The "special laboratory" is used only for drawing blood for plasma NH_3 analysis and performing these analyses; it is closed and unoccupied at other times.
- This room is washed down (ceiling to floor) with a 52.5 g/liter sodium hypochlorite (Clorox) solution every other week.
- Traffic in and out of the special laboratory is restricted at all times, and prohibited when a test is in progress.

[1] Recipe: 225 ml of de-ionized water, 20 ml of lemon juice, 2 g of sugar substitute. Contains 3.3 g of carbohydrate, 0.1 g of protein, <0.1 g of fat, and Na, K, Cl, Ca, P, and Mg.

[2] Thus, the dose for a 70-kg subject was 1.0 g. Dose was adjusted to (body weight)$^{0.75}$ because of evidence (*15*) that this term more closely reflects metabolic mass of the body than does body weight or surface area.

Table 1. Summary of Values for Fasting Plasma NH_3 Concentration and NH_3 Tolerance, in Normal and Cirrhotic Subjects, as Measured in the Routine and Special Laboratories

	Clinical laboratory				Special laboratory			
n	Mean	Range	SD	CV, %	Mean	Range	SD	CV, %
			Fasting NH_3, µg/liter					
			50.39(A)[a]	8.4			10.53(A)[a]	4.7
15 N[b]	630.93	300–1320	290.40(B)[a]	46.7	320.80	220–470	50.24(B)[a]	16.0
			290.40(C)[a]	46.7			50.65(C)[a]	17.2
			120.18(A)[a]	10.4			20.74(A)[a]	2.9
15 C[b]	1170.57	430–2630	180.24(B)[a]	15.5	940.63	300–1850	200.76(B)[a]	21.9
			560.37(C)[a]	47.9			490.61(C)[a]	52.4
			NH_3 tolerance test: 15 min NH_3 concn, µg/liter					
			80.29(A)[a]	9.0			20.28(A)[a]	6.2
9 N[b]	920.58	490–1700	230.16(B)[a]	25.0	360.89	290–500	40.62(B)[a]	12.5
			290.10(C)[a]	31.4			50.36(C)[a]	14.5
			110.64(A)[a]	6.3			30.78(A)[a]	2.8
9 C[b]	1840.28	850–3800	410.99(B)[a]	22.8	1360.00	590–2440	200.41(B)[a]	15.0
			930.00(C)[a]	50.5			620.80(C)[a]	46.2
			NH_3 tolerance test: area under the curve, µg·min/liter					
			4730.70(A)[a]	54.6			840.50(A)[a]	7.8
9 N[b]	8680.36	0–29 300	7150.80(B)[a]	82.4	1080.50	20–4280	960.66(B)[a]	8.9
			7670.51(C)[a]	88.4			1080.07(C)[a]	10.0
			40 280.06(A)[a]	50.5			5360.63(A)[a]	9.7
9 C[b]	79 800.30	10 080–265 000	40 280.06(B)[a]	50.5	55 590.05	13 400–150 600	17 580.88(B)[a]	31.6
			76 350.97(C)[a]	95.7			47 840.09(C)[a]	86.1

[a] A, intra-assay; B, intra-individual; and C, inter-individual
[b] N, normal; C, cirrhotic

- The patient (if a heavy smoker) showers and puts on fresh pajamas before the test.
- Blood is drawn into an evacuated tube by a swift, accurate venipuncture, and the tube is filled completely. Each of the following factors increases the NH_3 value by 100–200 µg/liter: use of heparin lock; probing for a vein; drawing blood into a syringe and transferring it to an anticoagulated tube; partly filling the evacuated tube, with subsequent entry of air.
- The blood sample is placed on ice and centrifuged immediately at 0 °C in the filled, stoppered tube for 5 min.
- The plasma is placed on a column containing the resin within 8 min after venipuncture.
- Eluates from the resin are analyzed within 2 h (if eluates are stored overnight before analysis, NH_3 value is artifactually increased by 100–300 µg/liter).
- All glassware is chemically clean, soaked in a 52.5 g/liter solution of sodium hypochlorite ("Clorox"), and rinsed thoroughly in demineralized water the day before use.

Results from the "special laboratory". Within three months after the analysis in the clinical laboratory, each normal and cirrhotic subject was restudied in the "special laboratory." The results are shown in Table 1 and Figure 2. Data for the NH_3 tolerance tests could be obtained only from nine of the normals and nine of the cirrhotics. The average fasting values were now 20–50% less in both normals and cirrhotics, the ranges were 30–45% as wide, and the intra-assay and intra-individual CV's for normals were 38–66% less than had been determined in the regular clinical laboratory.

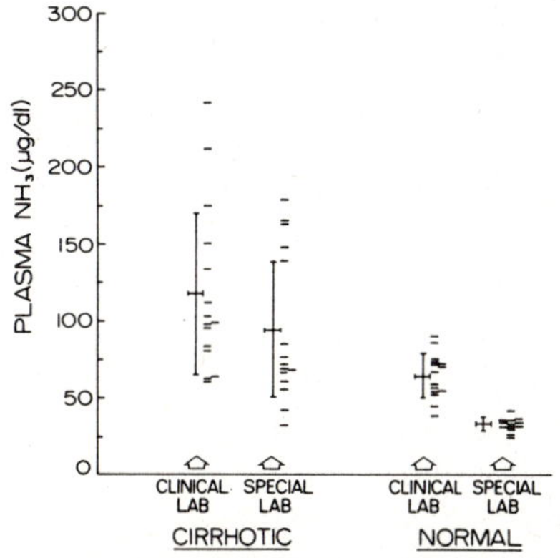

Fig. 2. Values for fasting plasma NH_3 concentration of nine to 15 normal or cirrhotic subjects in the two laboratories (regular and "special")
Mean ± SD is also shown for each set of values

The improvement in reproducibility was even more marked in the NH_3 tolerance tests (Table 1). For example, the intra-individual CV of NH_3 tolerance in normal subjects, calculated as the area under the curve, was 9% in the special laboratory compared to 82% in the clinical laboratory.

Discussion

Our initial experiences with fasting blood NH_3 values from the clinical laboratory showed a 2.1-fold higher normal mean than had been reported by the originators of the ion-exchange method of analysis, and our range was ±1020 μg/liter as compared with their range of about ±400. Consequently, the difference between normals and post-shunt cirrhotics (Table 1) was not statistically significant by the Wilcoxon rank sum test. Furthermore the venous NH_3 tolerance test described by Conn (*4*), when applied to the cirrhotics, was poorly reproducible in each individual (CV, 23–51%). In these respects our data resembled those of several clinical investigators (*17–21*) who reported wide day-to-day variations in degree of hyperammonemia of cirrhotic patients.

Most of the variation in our data clearly was not inherent in the NH_3 metabolism of the subjects; rather, it originated in the laboratory. Pollution of environment, glassware, staff, and patient with NH_3, and in vitro accumulation of plasma NH_3 because of suboptimal conditions of venipuncture technique, time, and temperature were the main causes. When these sources of error were removed, the normal range was lowered and narrowed, and the CV's for NH_3 in the plasma of fasting normal persons became comparable to those for K^+, glucose, cholesterol, and phosphate in plasma (*16*). The difference between normals and post-shunt cirrhotics (Table 1) was now statistically significant ($P < .005$) by the Wilcoxon rank sum test. Furthermore, the CV for the NH_3 tolerance test performed in the special laboratory was now comparable to that of the oral glucose tolerance test (*22*).

Studies of plasma NH_3 concentration in cirrhotic patients reported in the literature (*1–3, 17–21*) give conflicting views on the correlation between hyperammonemia and hepatic encephalopathy. Some of the disagreements in this field may well have originated in the laboratory errors identified in the present investigation. Re-examination of the relation of plasma NH_3 concentration and NH_3 tolerance to the natural history of liver disease, with attention to the technical pitfalls identified in this study, may be constructive.

Supported by USPHS Grants RR00039 and AM15736.

References

1. Stahl, J., Studies of the blood ammonia in liver disease. Its diagnostic, prognostic, and therapeutic significance. *Ann. Intern. Med.* **58,** 1 (1963).
2. Sherlock, S., Pathogenesis and management of hepatic coma. *Am. J. Med.* **24,** 805 (1958).
3. Reynolds, T. B., Redeker, A. G., and Davis, P., A controlled study of the effects of L-arginine on hepatic encephalopathy. *Am. J. Med.* **25,** 359 (1958).
4. Conn, H. O., Studies of the source and significance of blood ammonia IV. Early ammonia peaks after ingestion of ammonium salts. *Yale J. Biol. Med.* **45,** 543 (1972).
5. Conway, E. J., Apparatus for the microdetermination of certain volatile substances. IV. The blood ammonia, with observation on normal human blood. *Biochem. J.* **29,** 2755 (1935).
6. Seligson, D., and Seligson, H., A microdiffusion method for the determination of nitrogen liberated as ammonia. *J. Lab. Clin. Med.* **38,** 324 (1951).
7. Seligson, D., and Katsugi, H., The measurement of ammonia in whole blood, erythrocytes, and plasma. *J. Lab. Clin. Med.* **49,** 962 (1957).
8. Nathan, D. G., and Rodkey, F. L., Laboratory methods. A colorimetric procedure for the determination of blood ammonia. *J. Lab. Clin. Med.* **49,** 779 (1957).
9. Stone, W. E., A new colorimetric reagent for micro determination of ammonia. *Proc. Soc. Exp. Biol. Med.* **93,** 589 (1956).
10. Hutchinson, J. H., and Labby, D. H., New method for microdetermination of blood ammonia by use of cation exchange resin. *J. Lab. Clin. Med.* **60,** 170 (1962).
11. Miller, G. E., and Rice, J. D., Determination of the concentration of ammonia nitrogen in plasma by means of a simple ion exchange method. *Am. J. Clin. Pathol.* **39,** 97 (1963).
12. Forman, D. T., Rapid determination of plasma ammonia by an ion-exchange technic. *Clin. Chem.* **10,** 497 (1964).
13. Warren, W. D., Rudman, D., Millikan, W., et al., The metabolic basis of portasystemic encephalopathy and the effect of selective vs non-selective shunts. *Ann. Surg.* **180,** 573 (1974).
14. Metropolitan Life Insurance tables.
15. Kleiber, M., The fire of life. In *An Introduction to Animal Energetics,* John Wiley, New York, N.Y., 1961, p 177.
16. Cotlove, E., Harris, E. K., and Williams, G. Z., Biological and analytic components of variation in long-term studies of serum constituents in normal subjects. 3. Physiological and medical implications. *Clin. Chem.* **16,** 1028 (1970).
17. Dawson, A. M., and Sherlock, S., The effect of the amine oxidase inhibitor Marsilid on ammonium metabolism in liver disease. *Clin. Sci.* **17,** 587 (1958).
18. Zieve, L., Pathogenesis of hepatic coma. *Arch. Intern. Med.* **118,** 211 (1966).
19. Walker, C. O., and Schenker, S., Pathogenesis of hepatic encephalopathy with special reference to the role of ammonia. *Am. J. Clin. Nutr.* **23,** 619 (1970).
20. Warren, K. S., Iber, F. L., Doele, W., et al., Effect of alterations in blood pH on distribution of ammonia from blood to cerebrospinal fluid in patients in hepatic coma. *J. Lab. Clin. Med.* **56,** 687 (1960).
21. Summerskill, W. H. J., Wolfe, S. J., and Davidson, C. S., The metabolism of ammonia and alpha-keto-acids in liver disease and hepatic coma. *J. Clin. Invest.* **36,** 361 (1957).
22. Wilkerson, H. L., Hyman, H., Kaufman, M., et al., Diagnostic evaluation of oral glucose tolerance tests in nondiabetic subjects after various levels of carbohydrate intake. *New Engl. J. Med.* **262,** 1047 (1960).

CLIN. CHEM. 22/5, 667–672 (1976)

Method for Measuring the Concentration of Urinary Proteins According to Their Molecular Size Category

Amadeo J. Pesce, A. Hsu, C. Kornhauser,[1] K. Sethi, B. S. Ooi, and V. E. Pollak

We combined the use of a concentrating device (Minicon) and polyacrylamide gel electrophoresis in the presence of sodium dodecyl sulfate to semi-quantitate the concentration of (*a*) the collective low-molecular-weight proteins and (*b*) of albumin excreted in the urine of patients after renal transplantation. Analytical recovery of many serum proteins from samples concentrated 100-fold in the Minicon apparatus was about 70%. It was possible to examine many urine samples by polyacrylamide gel electrophoresis after concentration with this device. The reproducibility (CV) of the technique was on the order of 20% when albumin and low-molecular-weight protein were in about equal concentration. The method was adequate to differentiate glomerular and tubular proteinuria, because in glomerular proteinuria the ratio of albumin to low-molecular-weight proteins is about 20/1, whereas in tubular proteinuria the ratio is about 1/1.

Additional Keyphrases: *glomerular vs. tubular proteinuria • β_2-microglobulin • concentration technique • screening proteinurias*

In making diagnostic use of the urinary proteins in disease, it is important to differentiate these proteins on the basis of their molecular size (*1–5*). Most proteins excreted in the urine are from serum (*6*); albumin, transferrin, and γ-globulin predominate, but there are some serum proteins with molecular weight of less than 70 000 (*7, 8*). Proteinuria of glomerular origin can be distinguished from that associated with tubular disease by the molecular size of the proteins excreted in the urine (*1, 3*). Until recently, the most rigorous techniques for examining urinary proteins have been limited to Sephadex-gel column chromatography and radial immunodiffusion (*4, 8*); both of these are time consuming, and therefore few urines can be examined. Methods used for the biochemical assessment of tubular proteinuria for large numbers of samples include zone-electrophoretic methods on paper, starch gel, and polyacrylamide gel (*9*); in none of these is mobility of a protein proportional to its molecular size. Thus conflicting data can be obtained with similar patient populations (*10, 11*). A method is needed for study of many urine protein samples that is also suitable for examining a broad spectrum of proteins in terms of molecular size.

In this paper we describe a method for concentrating many samples of urinary protein by using the "Minicon" concentration device. We also report slight modifications of the method for the semi-quantitative measurement of urinary proteins based on moleular size, by using polyacrylamide gel electrophoresis in the presence of detergent (*12*).

Methods

Apparatus

Minicon concentrators. Type B-15 "Minicon" concentrators were obtained from the Amicon Corp., Lexington, Mass. 02173. These were all from lot No. C0028A.

Acrylamide gel system. We used the Model R-113 acrylamide gel system (Beckman Instruments, Inc., Fullerton, Calif. 92634).

Scanning densitometer. We used the "Quick Scan Electrophoresis Densitometer" (Helena Laboratories, Beaumont, Tex. 77704).

Reagents

Acrylamide and bisacrylamide were purchased from Eastman Organic Chemicals, Rochester, N. Y. 14650, and used without further purification; sodium dodecyl sulfate from Sigma Chemical Co., St. Louis, Mo. 63178; lysozyme from Worthington Biochemical Corp., Freehold, N. J. 07728; human albumin from the Research Division of Miles Laboratories, Kankakee, Ill. 60901; and Coomassie Brilliant Blue (sodium anazolene) from Schwarz/Mann Corp., Orangeburg, N. Y. 10962. All other chemicals were reagent grade.

Working Solutions

SDS/Tris/glycine pH 8.4 electrophoresis buffer.[2] Dissolve 21.8 g of ammonia-free glycine, 4.5 g of

Division of Nephrology, Department of Medicine, University of Cincinnati Medical Center, Cincinnati, Ohio 45267.

[1] Present address: Escuela de Medicina de León, 20 de Enero No. 915, León, Guanajuato, Mexico.

Received May 26, 1975; accepted Mar. 5, 1976.

[2] Nonstandard abbreviations used: SDS, sodium dodecyl sulfate; Tris, tris(hydroxymethyl)aminomethane [more properly, tris(hydroxymethyl)methylamine]; PAGE, polyacrylamide-gel electrophoresis; and ID, immunodiffusion.

tris(hydroxymethyl)aminomethane, and 1 g of sodium dodecyl sulfate in 80 ml of water and dilute to 1 liter.

Coomassie Blue staining solution. Add 1.25 g of Coomassie Blue to a mixture of 454 ml of methanol, 454 ml of water, and 46 ml of glacial acetic acid.

Destaining solution. Mix 650 ml of water, 250 ml of methanol, and 100 ml of glacial acetic acid.

Acetic acid solution. Add 20 ml of glacial acetic acid to 1 liter of water.

SDS solution. Dissolve 100 mg of sodium dodecyl sulfate in 10 ml of water.

Bovine serum albumin standards. Dissolve 300 mg of bovine plasma albumin (Armour Laboratories, Kankakee, Ill.) in 150 ml of water. Separate into 10 aliquots and freeze. For use, add 0.1, 0.2, 0.3, 0.5, 1.0, and 1.5 ml of this to a series of tubes and dilute to 5 ml with water.

Urine samples

Collect 24-h urine specimens with thymol preservative. Refrigerate, centrifuge, freeze, thaw, and re-centrifuge all urines to precipitate most of the phosphates and urates.

Procedures

Biuret test procedure. Add 5 ml of trichloroacetic acid solution (200 g/liter) to three 5-ml samples from each patient and to the standards. Mix and allow the solutions to stand for 20 min. Centrifuge for 15 min at 1800 × *g* in a clinical centrifuge. Decant the supernatant solutions. Dissolve the precipitate in 1 ml of 1 mol/liter NaOH. Add 2 ml of the usual biuret reagent to two of the three samples and 2 ml of NaOH to the third. Mix and allow the solutions to stand for 20 min. Read the absorbance at 540 nm. Subtract the absorbance of the sample redissolved in 1 mol/liter NaOH from those with biuret reagent. Read the value of the protein content from a curve of the absorbance of the albumin solutions vs. amount of albumin.

Protein Electrophoresis on Polyacrylamide Gel

The procedure used is similar to that described previously (*12*) but the staining procedure is changed as described below.

Sample preparation. Good results are obtained when the protein content of the samples is about 10 g/liter. The results of the biuret test on urine were used in calculating the sample concentration. All samples were concentrated by adding 10 ml to each well of the Minicon apparatus and allowing the sample to concentrate to the 25× mark (50-fold concentration). The protein concentration was adjusted to 10 g/liter by dilution with the Tris/glycine/detergent buffer. If the protein solution was so dilute that this concentration could not be attained, we made several applications of the sample from the Beckman dispenser.

Samples were prepared for application by mixing 50 μl of the concentrated urine protein, 5 μl of the SDS solution and one crystal of sucrose (to increase sample density). The samples were incubated for 15 min before being added to the gel. For comparison, a sample of normal serum and a mixture, standardized by weight, of 5 mg of lysozyme, 10 mg of human γ-globulin, and 8 mg of human albumin per milliliter were included in each gel.

Procedure. Dissolve 0.125 g of *N,N′*-methylenebisacrylamide and 2.375 g of acrylamide in 35 ml of the Tris/glycine buffer and then filter through Reeve Angel filter paper No. 802. To prepare the main bottom gel, dissolve 20 mg of ammonium persulfate in 22 ml of the filtered acrylamide solution. Add 33 μl of *N,N,N′,N′*-tetramethylethylenediamine, quickly mix thoroughly and pour into the mold, place the sample well mold into its proper place, and allow the gel to polymerize for 45 min. Prepare the top gel mixture by dissolving 10 mg of ammonium persulfate in 11 ml of the acrylamide filtrate, add 17 μl of the *N,N,N′,N′*-tetramethylenediamine mixture, and pour into a gel mold until full. Immediately apply the samples with the applicator into the preformed wells. Each delivery of the applications is about 5 μl. Up to five applications may be made without decreasing the resolution. After polymerizing for 45 min, start the cooling water, insert the wicks, and place the unit into the electrophoresis chamber. Apply a voltage of 400 V (about 40 mA) for 45 min. Remove the gel, place in the staining solution, and incubate for 45 min at 55 °C.

Rinse off the stain several times with destaining solution and place in the Beckman destaining apparatus for 12 min with the dilute acetic acid solution. Continue removing the excess dye by incubating the gel in the destaining solution at 55 °C for several hours and then soaking for several days at room temperature.

Dry the gels between two membranes under tension, as recommended by the manufacturer.

Scan the gels with the Helena Densitometer, using the wide slit opening and the long-scan and fast-speed settings. Adjust the albumin value for each sample to about 80 arbitrary intensity units. Reset this to a smaller value when the low-molecular-weight material has an intensity greater than 90 units. Obtain the amount of albumin, γ-globulin, and low-molecular-weight protein from the integration-pen markings.

Recovery of Proteins from the Minicon Concentrator

Preliminary studies were done in which normal human serum was diluted and concentrated with the Minicon Concentrator. Estimates of quantitative recovery were limited by the difficulties in establishing the amount of protein that had adsorbed to the apparatus or leaked into the absorbent pads. To overcome this problem, radiolabeled albumin was added to the diluted serum.

Rat serum albumin was labeled by the method of Gaizutis et al. (*13*), except that no carrier bovine serum albumin was added to the iodinated albumin before it was applied to the Sephadex G-25 column. One milliliter of human serum was diluted with 99 milliliters of phosphate-buffered saline, and 20 μl of labeled rat al-

Table 1. Recovery of ^{125}I-labeled Rat Serum Albumin Added to Serum Diluted 100-fold in Phosphate-Buffered Saline and Concentrated 100-fold with the Minicon B 15 Membrane[a]

				% Counts retained by the membrane					% Protein retained	
	(1)[b]	(2)[c]	(3)[d]	Adsorbed to membrane (4)	Extracted by washing (5)	Lost in pipet during transfer (6)	In concd solution (7)	Total (4+5+6+7) (8)	Readily Extract-able (7) ÷ (1) (9)	Total (8) ÷ (1) (10)
Actual measurements	94.3 ± 3.1	1.2 ± 0.2	12.1 ± 2.1	8.9 ± 2.6	4.4 ± 1.3	8.4 ± 2.8	59.5 ± 3.6	81.1		
Protein-bound, corrected for 4.71% free ^{125}I	94.3	1.2	7.7	9.3	4.6	8.8	62.4	85.2		
Corrected for 1.22% loss in initial transfer	94.3	. . .	7.8	9.4	4.7	8.9	63.2	86.2	67.1	91.4

[a] Results are expressed as the mean percentage recovery, ±SD, for eight experiments.
[b] % of total counts recovered from all sources.
[c] % counts lost in initial transfer into the apparatus.
[d] Counts lost by transfer through the membrane into the absorbent.

bumin was added. Ten milliliters of this mixture of diluted human serum and labeled rat albumin was added to each of the eight wells of the Minicon apparatus, and the solutions allowed to concentrate to the 50× mark on the apparatus. The net concentration was 100-fold. The concentrated sample was removed with a Pasteur pipet. Each sample well of the apparatus was then flushed with 2 milliliters of phosphate-buffered saline, labeled as the wash solution. The apparatus was then split with a hammer and screw driver, and the pad, sponge, and membrane for each section separated and placed into counting vials. A significant amount of radioactive material was also found on the transfer pipet; this value was recorded. There was a negligible amount of labeled material on the clear plastic. The amount of material found on the sponge was very small and, for purposes of reporting, was combined with that found in the absorbent pad.

Radial Immunodiffusion

Use the procedure of Mancini (*14*), with "Behring M Partigen Immunodiffusion" plates (Behring Diagnostics, Somerville, N. J. 08816). Add 5 μl of sample, allow the reaction to equilibrate for 48 h.

β_2 Microglobulin Assay

Use the "Phadebas β_2-microtest" (Pharmacia Diagnostics, Piscataway, N. J. 08854).

Results

Table 1 summarizes the results of experiments in which ^{125}I-labeled rat serum albumin was added to normal serum diluted 100-fold and concentrated 100-fold with the Minicon B-15 membrane. In all, 94.3% of the total counts added were accounted for from all sources. In the second and third lines of Table 1, corrections were made for the 4.7% free ^{125}I in the labeled rat serum albumin added, and for the 1.2% lost in the pipet during the initial transfer into the concentrating apparatus.

Table 2. Effect on Recovery of Nine Serum Proteins of Dilution and Subsequent Concentration of Four Sera Through the Minicon B-15 Concentrator[a]

Protein	Mean	±SD
^{125}I-labeled rat albumin	78.6	8.5
Albumin	74.8	6.1
Transferrin	70.5	3.7
IgG	73.8	2.7
Prealbumin	63.8	8.5
α_2 Gc-globulin	76.5	3.6
α_2 HS-glycoprotein	75.5	4.8
α_1-Antitrypsin	85.3	13.0
α_1-Acid glycoprotein	69.3	4.3
β_2-Glycoprotein	65.3	5.3

[a] As estimated from radial immunodiffusion results are expressed as (protein concentration in diluted and concentrated serum/protein concentration in native serum) × 100.

The amount of material recovered in the concentrated solution when the usual pipetting procedure was used was about 63%. An additional 9% was recovered from the pipet, and additional material was extracted by washing the apparatus with 2 milliliters of buffer. The total recovery by this procedure (Table 1, columns 5, 6, and 7) was about 77%. However, the amount readily obtained from the concentrating apparatus (columns 5 and 7) was only 67% of the starting material. Thus for normal operating procedures, about 33% of the starting material was lost, 9% because of adsorption to the

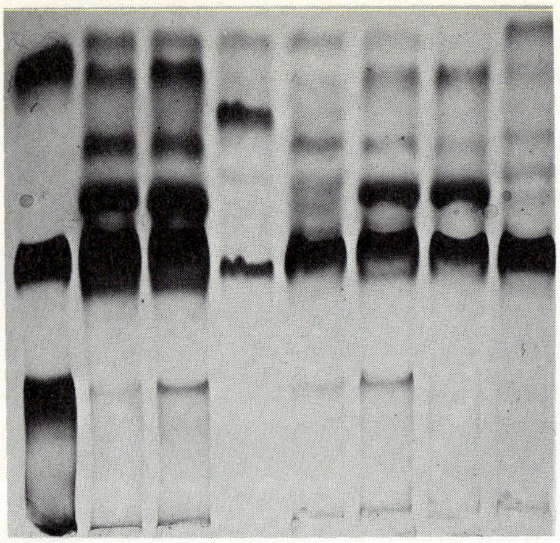

Fig. 1. Representative gel of a series of urines from patient F.L. (concentrated 50-fold)

Origin is at the bottom of the figure and proteins are represented as migrating to the top of the figure. *From left to right,* sample 1 is standard protein solution of albumin, γ-globulin, and lysozyme; samples 2–8 are from days 126–131 after transplantation

membrane or passage into the absorbent and the rest during transfer pipetting. The latter was not extractable without a wash solution. The data on line 1 of Table 1 indicate that the apparatus gave good reproducibility from sample to sample.

In a second experiment, four different samples of human serum from normal individuals were added to ^{125}I-labeled rat albumin; each sample was then diluted 50-fold in phosphate-buffered saline and concentrated in the Minicon B-15 concentrator. The amounts of nine human serum proteins were estimated by radial immunodiffusion in the native serum and in the diluted and concentrated samples (Table 2). Recovery of added ^{125}I-labeled rat albumin averaged 78.6%; that of the nine native serum proteins varied from 63.8 to 85.3%; thus there was no differential loss of any protein.

Reproducibility of the Polyacrylamide Gel Sodium Dodecyl Sulfate Technique on Urine Samples

A single urine sample was placed in the gel, as well as two- and fourfold dilutions of this sample. In all, eight replicates at three different concentrations each were quantitated on three different gels. Mean values for albumin and low-molecular-weight proteins were respectively 73 and 27%, i.e., an albumin/low-molecular-weight ratio of 2.7/1. The coefficient of variation for the estimate of albumin was 9%; that for low-molecular-weight protein was 26%.

The reproducibility was tested similarly on the urine of a single patient with glomerular disease. Mean values for albumin and low molecular-weight proteins were 92

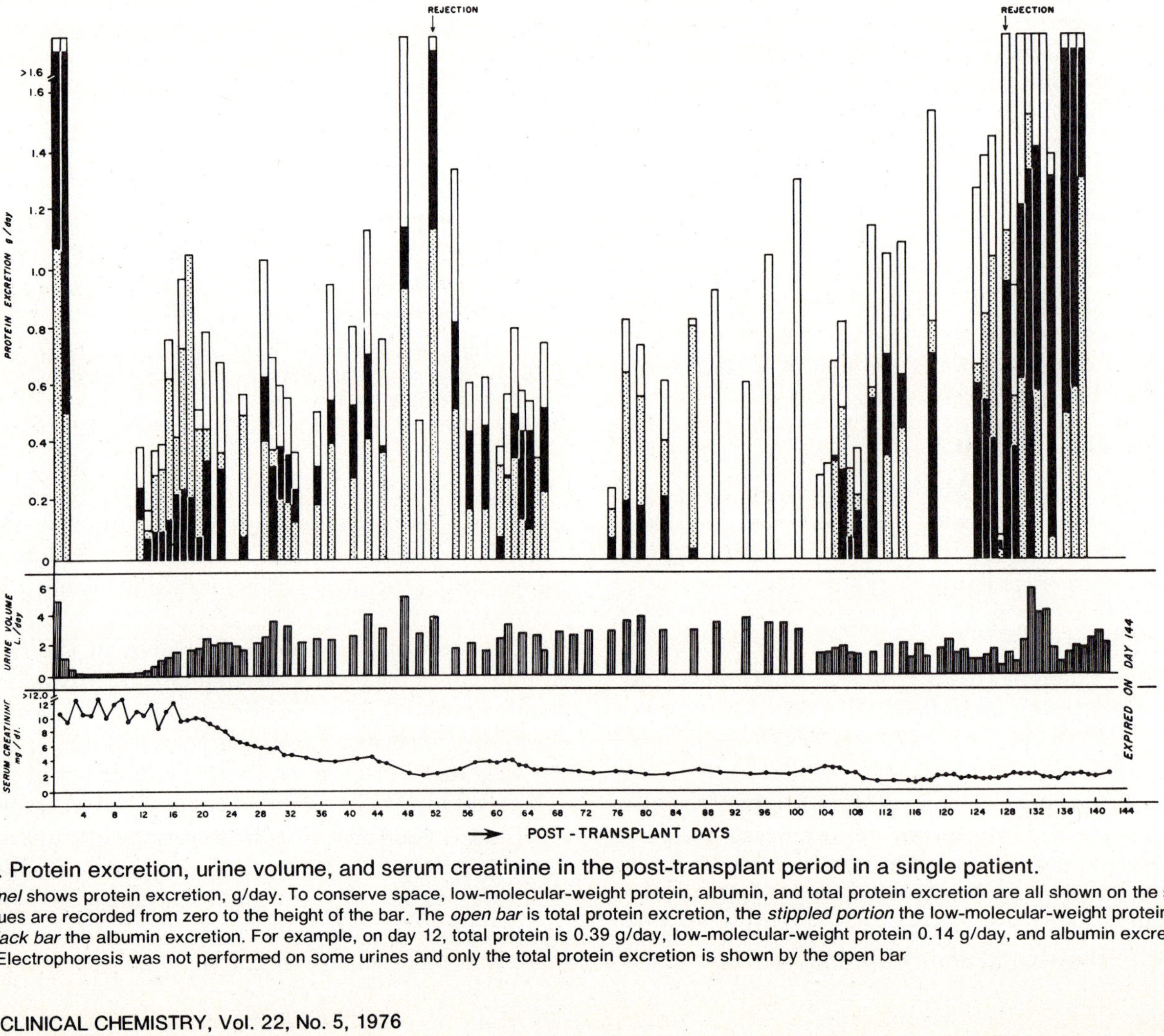

Fig. 2. Protein excretion, urine volume, and serum creatinine in the post-transplant period in a single patient.

Top panel shows protein excretion, g/day. To conserve space, low-molecular-weight protein, albumin, and total protein excretion are all shown on the same bar and values are recorded from zero to the height of the bar. The *open bar* is total protein excretion, the *stippled portion* the low-molecular-weight protein, and the *solid black bar* the albumin excretion. For example, on day 12, total protein is 0.39 g/day, low-molecular-weight protein 0.14 g/day, and albumin excretion 0.25 g/day. Electrophoresis was not performed on some urines and only the total protein excretion is shown by the open bar

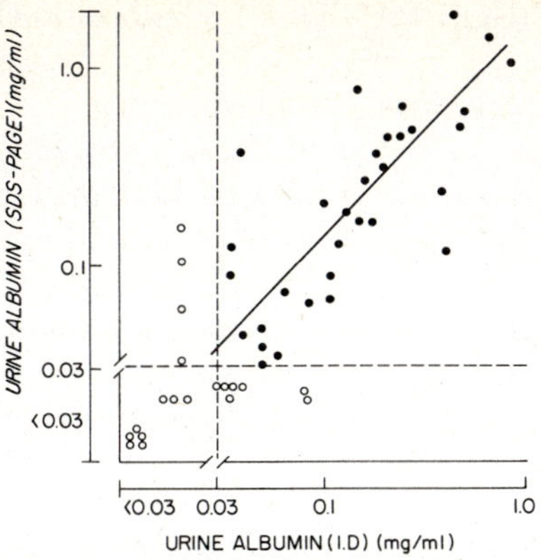

Fig. 3. Urine albumin concentration in 51 urine samples from patients with renal tubular disorders, as measured by immunodiffusion (*ID*) and by sodium dodecyl sulfate/polyacrylamide-gel electrophoresis (*SDS-PAGE*)

The *interrupted lines* denote the lower limits of accurate measurement by each technique, the *open circles* values below these limits. The *solid line* was calculated by regression analysis

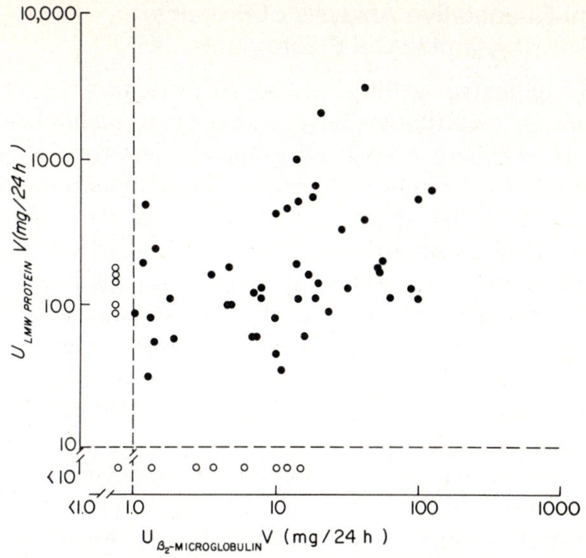

Fig. 4. Urinary excretion rates of β_2-microglobulin and low-molecular-weight protein compared

The 63 samples were from patients with renal tubular disorders. The *interrupted lines* denote the lower limits of accurate measurement by each technique, the *open circles* values below these limits

and 8%, respectively—i.e., a ratio of 11.5/1. The CV for the estimate of albumin was 4.6%; that for low-molecular-weight protein was 53%.

Serial Observations on Urine

Figure 1 shows a representative series of gels in which the proteinuria in a single patient after renal transplantation is assessed. In all urines, albumin and low-molecular-weight proteins predominated. Figure 2 shows the results of studies over a period of 134 days in this patient.

Measurement of Protein Concentration by SDS/Polyacrylamide-Gel Electrophoresis and by Quantitative Immunochemical Techniques

To evaluate the results obtained with the SDS/polyacrylamide gel electrophoretic method (SDS-PAGE) in urines from patients with tubular disorders, we also analyzed 51 urine samples studied by this method for albumin content, by radial immunodiffusion (ID). The results are shown in Figure 3. The equation describing this relationship was:

$$\text{Albumin (SDS-PAGE)} = 1.54 \text{ albumin (ID)} - 0.001$$

A similar relationship was observed whether the 19 paired specimens with the low values for albumin ($\leq$30 mg/liter) were included in or excluded from the regression analysis.

The β_2-microglobulin content of these 63 urine samples was measured by radioimmunoassay, and the results compared with the estimate of low-molecular-weight protein content measured by SDS/polyacrylamide gel electrophoresis (Figure 4). Overall, the correlation between $U_{\beta_2 \text{ microglobulin}}V$ and $U_{LMW}V$ was poor. Nevertheless, both methods predicted equally well the increased amount of low-molecular-weight protein in urine from patients with tubular disease. The normal and upper limit of normal of $U_{LMW}V$ is ≈6–10 mg/24 h (*8, 14*) and of $U_{\beta_2 \text{ microglobulin}}V$ is ≈82 and 370 µg/24 h (*15*). Using these criteria for the upper limit of normal, the relative diagnostic value is summarized in Table 3. Concordant results were obtained in 50 of the 63 specimens, and discordant results in 13. Of interest is the observation that six of the seven urines with high β_2-microglobulin excretion and normal low-molecular-weight protein excretion were from a single one of the eight patients studied; and that four of the six urines with normal β_2-microglobulin content and high low-molecular-weight protein content were from another patient.

Table 3. Relation between Excretion of Low-Molecular-Weight Protein ($U_{LMW}V$) and of β_2-Microglobulin (n = 63 Paired Urines)

	U_{β_2} microglobulin V	
$U_{LMW}V$	Normal	Increased
Normal	1	7
Increased	6	49

Discussion

Use of the Minicon Concentrator

Although some protein loss did occur, the Minicon Concentrator gave very reproducible results. Mechanical loss amounted to about 13%, and there definitely was some adsorption of protein to the membrane. Despite this loss, there was no selective loss of any serum protein measured. The convenience of the device and its reproducibility make it well suited for the study of a large number of samples.

Semi-Quantitative Analysis of Proteins by Polyacrylamide Gel Electrophoresis

We indicated earlier (*13*) that the procedure was not accurately quantitative; the destaining method has been improved. There is less background and less variability, so that the gel can be scanned by using a densitometer with minimal background interference. Because there are now no standards for the many low-molecular-weight proteins excreted in urine, absolute quantitation of all low-molecular-weight proteins by this or any other method is not possible. Nor is it practical to make use of any method such as Sephadex-gel chromatography or quantitative immunoassay of many serum proteins in urine.

For these reasons, the semiquantitative SDS/polyacrylamide gel electrophoretic method can only be evaluated against specific methods for certain selected proteins. Increased β_2-microglobulin excretion is considered to be an important marker for dysfunction of the renal tubules (*16*). The data in Table 3 indicate that, for the diagnostic purpose of detecting tubular dysfunction, the two methods did not differ. As there are many low-molecular-weight proteins in the urine, it is not surprising that some urines should show only a high β_2-microglobulin excretion whereas a few others with an increased amount of low-molecular-weight protein did not show a high excretion of β_2-microglobulin. The fact that most of these differences did not occur randomly but in urines from two particular patients suggests biological rather than technical factors.

Different results will be obtained when albumin is measured by different methods, particularly when one method is specific and the second measures albumin and other proteins within a certain range of molecular size. Qualitatively, analysis of tubular proteinuria by SDS/PAGE and column chromatography on Sephadex G-75 gave similar results (*12*). In the detailed analysis (at 280 nm) of the molecular size distribution of protein molecules in tubular proteinuria Dillard et al. reported (*8*): albumin, 30%; mol wt 60 000–40 000, 33%; mol wt ≤20 000, 27%; and mol wt >70 000, 9%. The Minicon B-15 concentrator, in contrast to the Amicon UM-10 membrane used in their study (*8*), has a nominal cut-off point of 15 000 mol wt and a significant proportion of proteins of mol wt <20 000 will have been excluded from analysis. As the albumin concentration using SDS/PAGE is estimated by the equation:

$$\text{Albumin (SDS/PAGE)} = \text{total protein} - \text{low-molecular-weight protein}$$

the exclusion of up to 27% of the total protein (molecules of <20 000 mol wt) leads to a corresponding overestimate of the albumin content. Also γ-globulin and proteins of high molecular weight bind the Coomassie Blue so poorly that the small amounts (9%) present in urine were not estimated and were therefore ignored. This also leads to an overestimate of the amount of albumin. Taking these factors into consideration the following relationship would be anticipated:

$$\text{Albumin (SDS/PAGE)} = 1.57 \text{ albumin (ID)}$$

This figure is very close to that observed.

The observations reported herein show clearly that the SDS/PAGE technique for analyzing urine proteins is a valid method for the study of proteinuria associated with renal tubular dysfunction. Although the technique is not strictly quantitative and does not measure individual serum proteins in urine with precision, it does measure proteins of the size of albumin and of smaller molecular size with reasonable accuracy. We think it is better than any other relatively simple technique for studying the ratio between these two categories of serum proteins in urine. Because most proteins with a molecular size less than that of albumin can be measured as a group, the method is superior to a method in which a single protein can be measured.

This work was supported in part by NIH Grants AM 17196 and AM 17330. We thank Drs. K. V. Rao and J. P. Fidler for their help in obtaining urines for these studies.

References

1. Schultze, H. E., and Heremans, J. F., *Molecular Biology of Human Proteins with Special Reference to Plasma Proteins,* **I**, Elsevier Pub. Co., Amsterdam, 1966.

2. Hardwicke, J., Cameron, J. S., Harrison, J. F., et al., Proteinuria, studied by clearances of individual macromolecules. In *Proteins in Normal and Pathological Urine.* Y. Manuel, J. P. Revillard, and H. Betuel, Eds. University Park Press, Baltimore, Md., 1970, pp 111–152.

3. Butler, E. A., and Flynn, F. V., The proteinuria of renal tubular disorders. *Lancet* **ii**, 978 (1958).

4. Harrison, J. F., and Northam, B. E., Low molecular weight urine proteins investigated by gel filtration. *Clin. Chim. Acta* **14**, 679 (1966).

5. Harrison, J. F., and Blainey, J. D., Low molecular weight proteinuria in chronic renal disease. *Clin. Sci.* **33**, 381 (1967).

6. Pesce, A. J., Gaizutis, M., and Pollak, V. E., Selectivity of proteinuria—an evaluation of the immunochemical and gel filtration techniques. *J. Lab. Clin. Med.* **75**, 586 (1970).

7. Bienenstock, J., and Poortmans, J., Renal clearance of 15 plasma proteins in renal disease. *J. Lab. Clin. Med.* **75**, 297 (1970).

8. Dillard, M. G., Pesce, A. J., Pollak, V. E., and Boreisha, I., Proteinuria and renal protein clearances in patients with renal tubular disorders. *J. Lab. Clin. Med.* **78**, 203 (1971).

9. Manuel, Y., and Laterre, B. C., Tubular proteinuria: Biochemical assay. In ref *2*, pp 172–187.

10. Laterre, E. C., van Ypersele de Strihou, C., and Alexandre, G. P. J., Proteinuria in human renal allograft with special reference to glomerular permeability in acute rejection crises. In ref. *2*, pp 300–308.

11. Revillard, J. P., Manuel, Y., Betuel, H., et al., Proteinuria in human renal allografts sequential studies. In ref. *2*, pp 309–318.

12. Pesce, A. J., Boreisha, I., and Pollak, V. E., Rapid differentiation of glomerular and tubular proteinuria by sodium dodecyl sulfate polyacrylamide gel electrophoresis. *Clin. Chim. Acta* **40**, 27 (1972).

13. Gaizutis, M., Pesce, A. J., and Lewy, J. E., Determination of nanogram amounts of albumin by radioimmunoassay. *Microchem. J.* **17**, 327 (1972).

14. Poortmans, J. R., and Jeanloz, R. W., Quantitative immunological determination of 12 plasma proteins excreted in human urine collected before and after exercise. *J. Clin. Invest.* **47**, 386 (1968).

15. Evrin, P. E., and Wibell, L., The serum levels and urinary excretion of β_2-microglobulin in apparently healthy subject. *Scand. J. Clin. Lab. Invest.* **29**, 69 (1972).

16. Peterson, P. A., Evrin, P. E., and Berggård, I., Differentiation of glomerular, tubular, and normal proteinuria: Determination of urinary excretion of β_2-macroglobulin, albumin, and total protein. *J. Clin. Invest.* **48**, 1189 (1969).

CLIN. CHEM. 22/5, 673–678 (1976)

Interference of Fatty Acids in the Competitive Protein-Binding Assay for Serum Thyroxine

William Shaw, Ivey Lois Hubert, and Francis W. Spierto

An increase in apparent thyroxine values obtained by competitive protein-binding assay on storage of sera is well documented. We find that the major source of this positive bias is probably the unsaturated nonesterified fatty acids. Nonesterified fatty acids cause a positive bias in the competitive protein-binding assay for serum thyroxine because they inhibit the binding of radioactive thyroxine by the serum-binding reagent (probably thyroxine-binding globulin). This inhibition by fatty acids may be due to the formation of a fatty acid/thyroxine complex. The degree of inhibition caused by the fatty acids depends on the length of the carbon chain of the fatty acid and the degree of saturation. Short-chain fatty acids are more potent inhibitors of thyroxine binding than those with a longer chain, and unsaturated fatty acids are more potent inhibitors of thyroxine binding than are saturated fatty acids. The polyunsaturated fatty acid, arachidonic acid, was the most potent inhibitor of all the fatty acids tested. Triglycerides (triacylglycerols) insignificantly inhibit thyroxine binding in this assay.

Additional Keyphrases: *structure as related to interference • variation, source of • thyroid status • radioassay*

Serum thyroxine (T_4) values obtained by competitive protein-binding assay (CPBA) reportedly increase with storage time (*1–4*); unpublished stability studies in our laboratory confirm these reports. Because serum T_4 values obtained with the T_4-by-column method (a colorimetric assay for iodide after chromatographic purification) are stable during storage (*2*), we considered the possibility that T_4 itself may be stable during storage but that some compounds or compounds formed during storage competitively inhibit binding of radioactive T_4 to the binding reagent in serum used as a source of thyroxine binding globulin in CPBA's for T_4. Because nonesterified fatty acids have been reported to cause an increase in values obtained in the free T_4 test (*5, 6*), we guessed that nonesterified fatty acids would similarly interfere in the CPBA for T_4.

Immunochemistry Section, Metabolic Biochemistry Branch, Clinical Chemistry Division, Bureau of Laboratories, Center for Disease Control, Department of HEW, Atlanta, Ga. 30333.

Received Jan. 5, 1976; accepted Mar. 2, 1976.

Materials and Methods

The CPBA we used for T_4 was the ethanol-extraction method modified (*8*) from that of Ekins et al. (*7*). Briefly, the method involves extraction of T_4 from serum with ethanol, evaporation of the extract, and a competitive protein binding step, with use of ^{125}I-labeled T_4 and thyroxine-binding globulin from diluted human serum as the binding reagent. This is an equilibrium-type assay; the binding reaction takes place with the mixture in an ice bath. Bound and free thyroxine are separated by adsorbing free thyroxine on an anion-exchange resin. Nonspecific binding controls from which the binder was omitted were routinely used; the percentage of radioactive T_4 bound in these tubes was less than 2% of the total radioactivity and was not affected by the concentrations of fatty acids we used in this study. In addition, we checked for adsorption of radioactive thyroxine to the glass test tubes used in our CPBA assay system by the use of controls containing all reagents except anion exchange resin. The contents of these control tubes were decanted following the binding reaction and residual radioactivity in the test tubes was determined. The amount of residual radioactivity in these tubes was less than 3% of the total radioactivity added and was not affected by the concentrations of fatty acids we used in this study.

Fatty acids were obtained from the following companies: lauric and palmitic from Eastman Organic Chemicals, Rochester, N.Y. 14650;[1] stearic and oleic from Fisher Scientific, Atlanta, Ga. 30324; myristic and linoleic from Chem Services, Inc., West Chester, Pa. 19380; and arachidonic, linolenic, arachidic, and palmitoleic from Sigma Chemical Co., St. Louis, Mo. 63178. Tripalmitin was obtained from Supelco, Inc., Bellefonte, Pa. 16823, and triolein from Analabs, North Haven, Conn. 06473.

The stated purity of the fatty acids was 99% for the products obtained from Chem Services, Sigma, Supelco, and Analabs. The oleic acid from Fisher was USP grade. Because lauric, stearic, and palmitic acids were not the highest grade available, the purity of these acids was checked by gas chromatography and found to be about 90%.

Fatty acids were dissolved at 25 °C in absolute ethanol. The triglycerides were less soluble in absolute ethanol at 25 °C than the fatty acids. Therefore, the triglycerides were dissolved in chloroform. In the method of Ekins et al. (*7*), serum samples are extracted with ethanol and the extracts evaporated. Thus, to simulate the conditions of this method, we evaporated aliquots of the fatty acid solutions (sufficient to give the amounts shown in Figure 1) in a manner identical to that used for the samples and then analyzed them as samples. In some experiments (Table 1) the aliquots of the fatty acids (sufficient to give the amounts shown in Table 1) were mixed with 0.2-ml aliquots of the serum extracts (equivalent to 67 μl of whole serum) and the mixed aliquots were then evaporated before analysis. This procedure was used to assess the influence of the serum extract itself on fatty acid inhibition of T_4 binding.

Recently, in some commercial kits for CPBA of T_4, the T_4 ethanol extraction methods have been shortened by assaying alcoholic extracts of serum without evaporating the alcohol. To simulate the conditions of these methods, we treated aliquots of fatty acid solutions in ethanol (sufficient to give the amounts shown in Table 2) as samples without prior evaporation of the ethanol. Because ethanol itself inhibits the binding of T_4 to the serum binding reagent, results were corrected for ethanol interference by use of blanks containing equivalent amounts of ethanol but no fatty acids.

The method used for the analysis of ethanol extracts of serum by gas chromatography of the trichloroethyl ester derivatives of the fatty acids was previously described (*9*). The identity of the major fatty acids in the ethanol extracts of serum was also confirmed as previously described (*10*) by combined gas chromatography–mass spectrometry of the methyl esters of the fatty acids with a Model 491-B gas chromatograph-mass spectrometer (Dupont Instruments, Monrovia, Calif. 91016). Thin-layer chromatography of both whole serum and serum extracts was performed on glass plates coated with Silica Gel G, as previously described (*11*).

[1] Use of trade names is for identification only and does not constitute endorsement by the Public Health Service or by the U.S. Department of HEW.

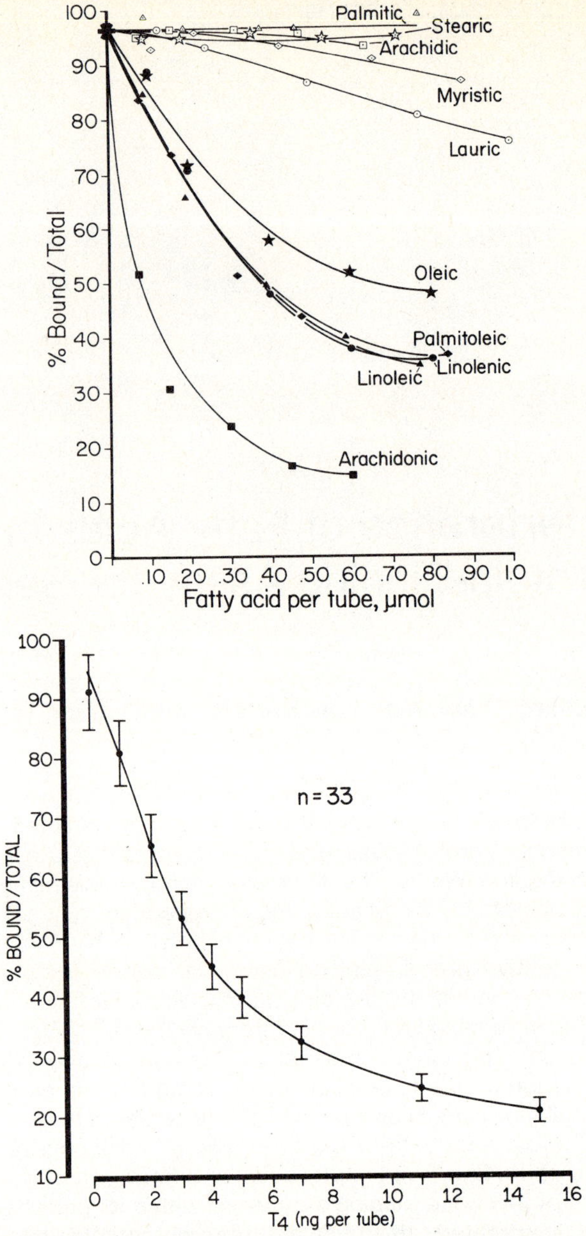

Fig. 1. (*Top*) Cross reactivity of nonesterified fatty acids in the CPB assay for T_4

The assay was conducted exactly like the routine CPB assay (see *bottom* figure) except that various fatty acids were added. Each assay tube contains the appropriate quantity of fatty acid, about 1 ng of ^{125}I-labeled T_4, and diluted serum used as the binding reagent, equivalent to 12 μl of whole human serum. Thus, each assay tube is equivalent to the zero concentration of thyroxine standard (*bottom* figure) except for the added fatty acids. *% Bound/Total* is the percentage of the total radioactive thyroxine bound by the serum binding reagent. Final molarity of the barbital buffer was 90 mmol/liter, pH 9.0. The reaction mixtures were incubated for 30 min at 0 °C, and the anion-exchange resin IRA-400 was used as the separating agent (*8*). Each point is the mean of duplicate determinations

(*Bottom*) T_4 Calibration curves obtained with the present CPBA

Each point is the average of duplicate determinations obtained on 33 separate runs. The distance between the vertical bars represents two standard deviations. *% Bound/Total* is the percentage of the total radioactive thyroxine bound by the serum used as binding reagent

Results and Discussion

Using thin-layer chromatography, we found that nonesterified fatty acids were increased and triglycerides were decreased in serum pools stored at room temperature for four weeks, as compared with aliquots

Table 1. Effect of Adding Various Fatty Acids to Ethanol Extracts of Serum on the Apparent T_4 Values Obtained by Competitive Protein-Binding Assay[a]

Fatty acid added	μmol added per 0.2 ml serum extract	Apparent serum T_4 value, μg/liter Pool 1	Pool 2	Pool 3
None	—	44	85	141
Arachidic ($C_{20:0}$)	0.32	50	90	144
Stearic ($C_{18:0}$)	0.36	50	88	142
Palmitic ($C_{16:0}$)	0.38	50	91	152
Myristic ($C_{14:0}$)	0.44	62	104	158
Lauric ($C_{12:0}$)	0.50	69	116	172
Oleic ($C_{18:1}$)	0.40	82	132	186
Palmitoleic ($C_{16:1}$)	0.32	119	171	242
Linoleic ($C_{18:2}$)	0.39	116	174	227
Linolenic ($C_{18:3}$)	0.40	102	160	211

[a] Solutions of the fatty acids in ethanol were mixed with the ethanol extracts of serum before the evaporation of the extracts; the assay was then conducted as usual. Values are the means of duplicate determinations.

Table 2. Comparison of the Interference of Fatty Acids in the CPBA for T_4, Analyzed with or without Prior Evaporation of the Ethanol

Palmitic: Fatty acid per tube, μmol	With[a] evapn	Without[b] evapn	Oleic: Fatty acid per tube, μmol	With[a] evapn	Without[b] evapn
	ng T_4 equivalent[c]			ng T_4 equivalent[c]	
0.78	0.2	0.3	0.80	3.7	6.5
	0.3	0.3		3.5	6.1
0.59	0.4	0.4	0.60	3.1	6.0
	0.5	0.9		3.7	6.4
0.39	0.05	1.1	0.40	3.0	4.5
	0.10	0.1		2.7	4.3
0.20	0.20	0.0	0.20	1.4	2.0
	0.05	0.1		1.4	2.0

[a] Assay was conducted exactly as in footnote b except that the ethanol in fatty acid solution was evaporated under nitrogen and 0.1 ml of distilled water was added to compensate for the volume of the evaporated ethanol.

[b] To each tube was added a 0.1-ml aliquot of an appropriate quantity of fatty acid dissolved in absolute ethanol, 0.5 ml of ^{125}I-labeled T_4 (approximately 1 ng) in 0.1 mol/liter barbital buffer, pH 9.0, and 0.4 ml of diluted serum binding reagent (equivalent to 12 μl whole human serum) in 0.1 mol/liter barbital buffer, pH 9.0. For blank tubes, 0.1 ml of absolute ethanol was substituted for the fatty acid. The reaction mixtures were incubated for 30 min at 0 °C, and then bound and free thyroxine was separated by adding 0.1 ml of a slurry of the anion-exchange resin IRA-400, as described more fully in reference *8*.

[c] Calibration curves for T_4 were performed at the same time as the fatty acid assays. The "ng T_4 equivalent" per tube represents the amount of T_4 standard per tube that would be needed to displace a quantity of radioactive T_4 equivalent to that displaced by the amounts of fatty acids given in Table 1. Results in assays without evaporation were corrected for ethanol interference by subtraction of the "ng T_4 equivalent" per tube for controls containing 0.1 ml ethanol. Results in assays with evaporation did not require correction since the amount of radioactive T_4 in controls in which ethanol was evaporated was equivalent to controls in which ethanol was not evaporated.

of the same serum pools stored at −20 °C. Exact quantitative data for nonesterified fatty acids in stored serum pools were not obtained. The apparent T_4 value obtained with CPBA of the sera stored at room temperature was 75–200% greater than that of the sera stored at −20 °C.

We analyzed ethanol extracts of pooled sera stored at −20 °C or at room temperature by gas chromatography and identified fatty acids with carbon-chain lengths between C_2 and C_{20} by comparing their retention times with those of pure standards. The major fatty acids in the ethanol extracts of serum stored for several weeks at room temperature or at −20 °C were tentatively identified as palmitic, oleic, stearic, and linoleic on the basis of retention time and the identity of these acids was confirmed with combined gas chromatography–mass spectrometry. We did not quantitate the concentration of each of the fatty acids in extracts of fresh or stored sera. However, we are now pursuing this quantitation.

Figure 1 demonstrates that fatty acids inhibit the binding of T_4 in the competitive protein-binding assay because it shows that the amount of ^{125}I-labeled T_4 bound to the binding protein in serum decreases with increasing concentrations of many of the fatty acids. It also shows that unsaturated fatty acids inhibit thyroxine binding much more than do saturated fatty acids. Chain length of saturated fatty acids and their inhibitor potency are related. For example, there is no significant inhibition of T_4 binding by fatty acids with a chain length exceeding 16 carbon atoms, but there is a significant inhibition by myristic acid ($C_{14:0}$) and an even greater inhibition by lauric acid ($C_{12:0}$).

For the unsaturated fatty acids there were insufficient data to establish a firm relationship between chain length and inhibition of T_4 binding, but the same inverse relationship between chain length and degree of inhibition appears to hold for them. For example, oleic acid ($C_{18:1}$) is a less potent inhibitor of T_4 binding than is palmitoleic acid ($C_{16:1}$). Evidently, the number of unsaturated bonds also significantly affects the potency of inhibition of thyroxine binding: stearic acid ($C_{18:0}$) has essentially no inhibitory effect on thyroxine binding, but oleic acid ($C_{18:1}$) has a marked effect, and linoleic acid ($C_{18:2}$) has an even greater effect. Linolenic acid ($C_{18:3}$), however, did not have an effect significantly different from that of linoleic acid. Arachidonic acid, with four unsaturated bonds ($C_{20:4}$) was the most potent inhibitor of thyroxine binding of all the fatty acids tested.

We obtained further information on fatty acid structure required for inhibition of T_4 binding by testing the effect of the triglycerides tripalmitin and triolein, in which the fatty acids are esterified with glycerol. Triolein and tripalmitin (the glycerol triesters of oleic and palmitic acids) did not inhibit T_4 binding at the highest concentrations used: 0.800 μmol of triolein and 0.380 μmol of tripalmitin per reaction tube, respectively. (Triglycerides are expressed here in terms of moles of fatty acids that would be obtained after hydrolysis.) The lack of inhibition by the triglycerides was not surprising because these compounds are relatively insoluble in aqueous solutions, but we did not take extraordinary measures to attempt to solubilize them, because our main purpose was to see whether the triglycerides in an ethanol extract of serum would interfere with the CPBA for T_4.

To determine if the serum extract itself might influence the inhibition of the fatty acids, we mixed ethanolic solutions of the fatty acids with ethanolic extracts of pooled serum containing three different concentrations of thyroxine (Table 1). The results were essentially the same as those presented in Figure 1, in which no serum extract was present. This experiment also demonstrates that chain length and degree of unsaturation greatly influence the extent of interference by the individual fatty acid.

These experiments establish that fatty acids can interfere in the serum T_4 assay and that the individual fatty acids differ markedly in their ability to inhibit T_4 binding. Because the solvents in the fatty acids and triglyceride solutions in the preceding experiments were evaporated before the other reagents were added, we could not be certain that the differences in inhibition with each of the fatty acids are not merely attributable to differences in the ability of the different acids to resolubilize in the incubation mixture after the solvent is evaporated. Therefore, aliquots of ethanol solutions of palmitic or oleic acids were analyzed as samples, both with and without prior evaporation of ethanol. Appropriate corrections for the interference of ethanol itself were made. As in the previous experiments, we found that oleic acid was a much more significant interference (Table 2) in the CPBA for T_4 than was palmitic acid, regardless of whether or not the ethanol was evaporated, although oleic acid interfered more strongly when it was added without prior evaporation. The reason for this difference is not completely clear but may be due to (*a*) a decreased stability of the unsaturated fatty acids during the evaporation step, or (*b*) increased solubility of the fatty acids when analyzed without prior evaporation. These results are also of interest because, in several commercial CPBA kit procedures for T_4 assay, T_4 is measured in the extract. It is apparent from these results that such methods may be especially liable to interference from nonesterified unsaturated fatty acids.

How significantly do fatty acids interfere in the competitive protein binding assay for thyroxine? Our results show that the extent of interference depends on the concentration of each individual fatty acid present. Unsaturated nonesterified fatty acids in serum extracts are a much greater source of error than are saturated fatty acids in the CPBA for T_4. The general range of concentrations of nonesterified fatty acids in serum is 0.2–1.5 mmol/liter whereas values as large as 4.0 mmol/liter may be found under certain experimental conditions (*5*). In our T_4 assay, an amount of extract equivalent to 67 μl of serum is used per reaction tube. If the free fatty acids are completely extracted, the amount of nonesterified fatty acid in the aliquot of serum extract used for analysis would be about 0.1 μmol for a sample at the upper limit of the normal range for nonesterified fatty acids. Figure 1 shows that, in the T_4 competitive protein-binding assay, all of the unsaturated fatty acids interfere substantially, and that arachidonic acid (0.1 μmol/tube) especially interferes. However, each serum sample may differ greatly with respect to the amounts of each of the nonesterified fatty acids (*12*), and we find no definitive study concerning the percentage of individual fatty acids in a wide variety of serum samples. In a study of the nonesterified fatty acids in the plasma of 11 persons who had fasted overnight, Chlouverakis and Harris (*12*) in 1960 found that the unsaturated fatty acids accounted on the average for about 70% of the major fatty acid peaks seen on gas–liquid chromatography. Oleic acid accounted for an average of 45% of the major fatty acid peaks and palmitic acid was the major unsaturated fatty acid, accounting for an average of about 24% of the major fatty acid peaks. Arachidonic acid, which would cause the most serious interference, is reported to be present at very low concentrations in plasma in comparison with the other nonesterified fatty acids (*13*). The exact quantitative interference in fresh serum samples cannot be assessed until the individual nonesterified fatty acids in serum have been quantitated in a large reference population.

However, our study indicates that the fatty acids probably interfere significantly in stored samples and serum calibrators if there is much conversion of various esters of fatty acids (phospholipids, triglycerides, and cholesterol esters) to their nonesterified form. Published data (*13*) on the lipid content of plasma or serum suggest that the concentration of esterified fatty acids at the upper limit of the normal range is about 21 mmol/liter of serum. Thus, even the hydrolysis of 10% of the esterified fatty acids could double the free fatty acid concentration (0.2–1.5 mmol/liter). An increase of 38–50% in the nonesterified fatty acid concentration in 24 h has been reported for sera stored at 25–30 °C and an increase of 12–25% in 24 h at −10 °C. Forbes and Camlin (*14*) reported increases in serum nonesterified fatty acids as great as 63% after storage of serum for 24 h at −15 °C. Such increases during storage are probably catalyzed by various serum enzymes. For example, lecithinase A (phosphatide 2-acyl-hydrolase, EC 3.1.1.4) in serum catalyzes the conversion of lecithin to lysolecithin (*13*) and a nonesterified fatty acid. "True" serum lipase (triacylglycerol acylhydrolase, EC 3.1.1.3) catalyzes the conversion of triglycerides to glycerol and nonesterified fatty acids (*15*). Carboxylic acid esterase (carboxylic-ester hydrolase, EC 3.1.1.1) and lipoprotein lipase (diacylglycerol acylhydrolase, EC 3.1.1.34) are also present in serum and catalyze the hydrolysis of esters to nonesterified fatty acids (*15*). Thus, the stability of serum fatty acid esters and, in turn, results for thyroxine by CPBA probably depend on the concentration of various lipids, lipolytic enzymes, their activators and inhibitors, and the storage conditions of the samples.

Seth (*1*) reported that storage of serum at room temperature for two days resulted in increases of 16% to 25% over the initial serum thyroxine value obtained by CPBA. Lee et al. (*2*) reported that storage of specimens for several days at room temperature or a week in the refrigerator results in spurious elevations in a CPBA. Results for protein-bound iodine or T_4-iodine were not affected. Frings and Hochholzer (*3*) reported that T_4 values for sera stored for four days at room temperature averaged 17% higher than those for fresh sera and cautioned against sending T_4 samples to distant laboratories by mail.

These findings seem to have a particular relevance to the widespread practice of using serum-based material for calibration of the CPBA and for proficiency-testing surveys. For example, the T_4 value of an unrefrigerated serum sample, mailed from Atlanta, Ga. to New Mexico and then returned, had doubled as compared to an aliquot of the sample stored frozen. The report that nonesterified fatty acids increase substantially at −15 °C indicates that a re-evaluation of the common practice of storing samples for several days or a week before analysis is in order. Many of these calibrators and proficiency-testing samples may be exposed to high temperatures during preparation and shipment, with resulting falsely elevated thyroxine values by CPBA. Indeed, the results of the Center for Disease Control's Proficiency Testing Program show that thyroxine values obtained by CPBA generally exceeded those obtained by the T_4-by-column colorimetric assay for iodide. Many different extraction techniques are now used in the CPBA for T_4; fatty acid interference may be obviated in some of these modifications because the thyroxine, but not the fatty acids, is extracted selectively from the serum. For example, Watson and Lees (*4*) reported that T_4 values obtained with CPBA did not change during storage of sera when thyroxine in serum was purified by Sephadex chromatography, but that T_4 values obtained with CPBA did change when T_4 was extracted from serum with ethanol.

The binding protein used as a binding reagent in the CPBA for T_4 is thyroxine-binding globulin (*7*). Thus, it is likely that fatty acid inhibition of T_4 binding in the CPBA is due to inhibition of T_4 binding by thyroxine-binding globulin. Tabachnik et al. (*16*), using a starch gel electrophoresis system, reported that oleic acid inhibits T_4 binding to highly purified thyroxine-binding globulin; they did not evaluate the effects of other fatty acids. Korcek and Tabachnik (*17*) have recently shown that a number of fatty acids are bound to thyroxine-binding globulin.

What is the mechanism for the fatty acid inhibition of T_4 binding to thyroxine-binding globulin? Two possibilities exist. The first possibility is that fatty acids interact directly with thyroxine-binding globulin. Preliminary evidence in our laboratory indicates that nonesterified unsaturated fatty acids increase the rate of dissociation of T_4 from thyroxine-binding globulin. However, the magnitude of this effect is not sufficient to account for the extent of a fatty acid inhibition of T_4 binding to thyroxine binding globulin. A second possibility is that the unsaturated fatty acids bind thyroxine directly. In 1965, Hoch et al. (*18*) reported that a low-molecular-weight substance extracted from a methanolic ammonia extract of a dialysate of human serum appeared to form a complex with T_4. This substance in an aqueous solution containing the major serum electrolytes decreased the rate coefficient of escape of T_4 through cellophane membranes. In a more recent study, Irvine (*19*) reported that a substance extracted with ethanol from human plasma bound T_4 and altered the distribution of T_4 in an equilibrium dialysis system in which an aqueous solvent was used but not in a system in which ethanol solutions were used. Based on the solubility of this substance in various solvents, Irvine concluded that this substance was a lipid, but did not further characterize this substance. At present, our data do not allow us to select either of the two possible mechanisms as the correct one. Nevertheless, the possibility that T_4 binds directly to unsaturated fatty acids is consistent with the previous studies of both Hoch and Irvine. Our finding that the amount of radioactive T_4 bound in the nonspecific binding controls was not increased by the concentrations of fatty acids employed was not unexpected and does not disprove the existence of a fatty acid/T_4 complex, because fatty acids are anions at the pH of the incubation mixture in our CPBA for T_4. The anion-exchange resin used as separating agent would be expected to bind fatty acids as well as the putative fatty acid/T_4 complex. Such a complex would be of considerable interest since, as Hoch suggested, it might play an important role in modifying the physiological effect of T_4 and might also be of significance in the investigation of both disorders of thyroid metabolism and other diseases.

Finally, the finding that fatty acids interfere with the CPBA for T_4 led us to consider whether the fatty acids would also interfere in the radioimmunoassay for T_4. A full evaluation of the possible effects of fatty acids on T_4 methods is now in progress. Preliminary data suggest that such interference in the radioimmunoassay for T_4 is essentially negligible.

Note added in proof: After this manuscript had been submitted we found that Rootwelt [*Scand. J. Clin Lab. Invest.* **35,** 649 (1975)] had reached similar conclusions concerning the interference of fatty acids in the CPBA for T_4.

We wish to acknowledge the assistance of Jackie Williams of the Lipid Section at the Center for Disease Control for the serum triglyceride analyses and for assisting us in setting up the thin-layer chromatography system in our laboratory. Dr. Claude Moss, Dr. John Brooks, and Ms. Cynthia Alley, of the Analytical Bacteriology Section, performed the gas chromatography and the combined GC-MS analyses.

References

1. Seth, J., Work simplification of a competitive protein binding analysis for serum thyroxine, and a study of some laboratory factors affecting assay results. *Clin. Chim. Acta* **46,** 431 (1973).

2. Lee, N. D., Catz, B., Margolese, M., and Pileggi, V. J., Comparison of laboratory test results for assessing thyroid function in normal subjects and treated and untreated hyper- and hypothyroid patients. *Clin. Chem.* **17,** 174 (1971).

3. Frings, C. S., and Hochholzer, J. M., Stability of serum thyroxine as measured by competitive protein binding methods. *Clin. Chem.* **19,** 680 (1973).

4. Watson, D., and Lees, S., Comparative study of thyroxine assays employing kit radio-ligand reagents. *Ann. Clin. Biochem.* **10,** 14 (1973).

5. Hollander, C. S., Free fatty acids: A possible regulator of free thyroid hormone levels in man. *J. Clin. Endocrinol. Metab.* **27,** 1219 (1967).

6. Braverman, L. E., Effect of physiological variations in free fatty acid concentration on the binding of thyroxine in the serum of euthyroid and thyrotoxic subjects. *J. Clin. Invest.* **48,** 878 (1969).

7. Ekins, R. P., Williams, E. S., and Ellis, S., The sensitive and precise measurement of serum thyroxine by saturation analysis. *Clin. Biochem.* **2,** 253 (1969).

8. Shaw, W., Hubert, I. L., and Spierto, F. W., Improvement of serum thyroxine competitive protein binding radioassay by kinetic analysis. CDC Proficiency Testing Publication. Available on request from: Immunochemistry Section, Clinical Chemistry Division, Center for Disease Control, 1600 Clifton Road, Atlanta, Ga. 30333.

9. Alley, C., Brooks, J., and Choudhary, G., Electron capture gas liquid chromatography of short chain acids as their 2,2,2-trichloroethyl esters. *Anal. Chem.* **48,** 387 (1976).

10. Moss, C., and Dees, S., Identification of microorganisms by gas chromatographic-mass spectrometric analysis of cellular fatty acids. *J. Chromatogr.* **112,** 595 (1975).

11. Mangold, H., Thin-layer chromatography of lipids. *J. Am. Oil Chem. Soc.* **38,** 708 (1961).

12. Chlouverakis, C., and Harris, P., Composition of the free fatty acid fraction in the plasma of human arterial blood. *Nature* **888,** 1111 (1969).

13. Wynbenga, D., and Inkpen, J., Lipids. In *Clinical Chemistry, Principles and Techniques,* R. Henry, D. Cannon, and J. Winkelman, Eds. Harper and Row, New York, N. Y., 1974.

14. Forbes, A., and Camlin, J., Effects of storage on serum nonesterified fatty acid concentrations. *Proc. Soc. Exp. Biol. Med.* **102,** 709 (1959).

15. Kachmar, J. F., Enzymes. In *Fundamentals of Clinical Chemistry,* N. Tietz, Ed., Saunders, Philadelphia, Pa., 1970, p 416.

16. Tabachnik, M., Hao, Y. L., and Korcek, L., Effect of oleate, diphenylhydantoin, and heparin on the binding of ^{125}I-thyroxine to purified thyroxine-binding globulin. *J. Clin. Endocrinol. Metab.* **36,** 392 (1973).

17. Korcek, M., and Tabachnik, M., Further characterization of human thyroxine binding globulin. *Biochim. Biophys. Acta* **371,** 323 (1974).

18. Hoch, H., Sinnett, S., Miller, P., and Mahady, I., Dialyzable thyroid hormone-binding material in human serum. *Biochemistry* **4,** 931 (1965).

19. Irvine, C., The effect of an ethanol-extractable thyroxine binding substance in plasma on the measurement of thyroxine by competitive binding. *J. Clin. Endocrinol. Metab.* **38,** 468 (1974).

CLIN. CHEM. 22/5, 679–680 (1976)

Chemistry of the Kober Reaction

Ronald W. A. Oliver, Søren B. Jensen,[1] and Gordon Crossley[2]

The main findings of a systematic study of the Kober reaction between pure estriol and aqueous sulfuric acid (with and without additives) are presented and discussed. We propose that the physico-chemical properties of the reaction products may only be understood if they are considered to be hydrophobic colloidal suspensions of differing particle size.

The female sex hormones, the estrogens, are currently being assayed by many clinical chemical laboratories because their excretion provides the best single biochemical monitor of fetal–placental function during pregnancy (*1*). In the most commonly used techniques the Kober reaction (*2*) produces a colored mixture, which is then measured by absorption (*3*) or fluorescence (*4*) procedures. Lately, these methods have been adapted to continuous-flow systems so as to increase the precision and analysis rate of the assays (*5*). In spite of the widespread interest in this assay, its chemistry has been relatively little studied (*6, 7*) and has remained obscure.

There are many modifications to the original Kober reaction, but essentially it consists of heating the estrogens with a strong aqueous sulfuric acid mixture containing an organic additive, usually quinol, followed by dilution with water to give a red mixture that is suitable for colorimetry. The Kober chromogen may be extracted into various organic solvents—e.g., chloroform—if other organic additives such as *p*-nitrophenol or trichloroacetic acid are present, to yield mixtures with enhanced color yield and strong fluorescence. The basic problem encountered in this assay method is the lack of reproducibility of the red color yield *between* batch, both for pure estrogens and biological fluids. We have therefore studied systematically the effect of various compositions of the aqueous sulfuric acid mixtures on the reaction and the effect of additives, light, and temperature on the red color yield obtained from chromatographically pure estriol. The latter was used because it forms the bulk of estrogen production during pregnancy (*1*). Its standard solutions were assayed in methanol, with use of the following spectral data (*8*); λ_{max} = 280 nm; ϵ_{max} = 1950 $mol^{-1} \cdot cm^{-1}$.

This is Paper No. 18 from the Biological Materials Analysis Unit, Dept. of Chemistry and Applied Chemistry, University of Salford, Peel Park, Salford 5, Lancs., U. K.

[1] Present address: Messrs J. Sturge and Co., Birmingham, U. K.

[2] Present address: Dept. of Clinical Chemistry, Bury General Hospital, Bury, Lancs., U. K.

Received Dec. 3, 1974; accepted Feb. 11, 1976.

Results

We found that pure estriol and aqueous sulfuric acid alone form three distinctly colored mixtures, yellow, red, and blue, by a single-stage heating process, and we designated these as Kober chromogens I, II, and III, respectively. Another distinct deep-blue mixture is produced by a two-stage heating-dilution-reheating process, and this is assigned to the formation of a Kober IV chromogen. A total of four other distinctly colored mixtures—orange, apple-green, green, and red-violet—can also be produced by two- or three-stage heating-dilution/concentration-reheating procedures. These colors are not, however, ascribable to additional Kober chromogens because they may be explained in terms of mixtures of the previous four chromogens. Full details for the optimal production of the assigned Kober chromogens, and their spectral properties, are summarized in Table 1.

The four chromogens defined in Table 1 may also be distinguished by their differing behavior upon subsequent adjustment of the acid concentration and reheating. Thus, the yellow Kober I species alone can only exist in sulfuric acid/water (75/25 by vol), even though it may be formed from mixtures containing Kober's II and III by increasing the acid concentration. The red Kober II species can exist in both the 75/25 and 28/72 acid/water mixtures in addition to the 55/45 mixture in which it is normally prepared. The Kober III chromogen can only be formed by heating estriol in 28/72 by vol acid/water, and its spectrum is unique in that it is temperature dependent: λ_{max} shifts to shorter wavelengths (550–560 nm) when the mixture is heated to 100 °C. Finally, the various deep-blue mixtures resulting from a number of interconversion experiments are all attributable to the formation of Kober IV chromogens. Thus the colors of certain acid mixtures of estriol depend upon their history and not entirely upon the final acid concentration.

When parallel experiments to those summarized in Table 1 were performed with various acid mixtures to which quinol had been added, only two colored mixtures, a yellow and a red, could be obtained by a single heating process. These colors may be assigned to an enhanced production of Kober I and II chromogens, respectively, on the basis of the spectral data. It was not possible to prepare the Kober III chromogen in the presence of quinol, and the deep-blue mixtures that could be prepared by various two-stage processes were assigned, by reference to Table 1, to Kober IV. Only two additional colored mixtures could be obtained in this series of experiments, orange and straw-yellow, and their spectra may be completely

Table 1. Optimal Spectral Properties of the Colored Mixtures Obtained by Heating Chromatographically Pure Estriol with Aqueous Sulfuric Acid Mixtures at 100 °C

Process[a]	Vol. % of aqueous H_2SO_4	Heating time, min	Visible color	λ_{max}, nm	a[b]	"Kober chromogen" no.
A	75	10	Yellow	456–460	1035	I
A	55	45	Red	508–512	485	II
A	28	60	Navy-blue	580–600	40	III
B(i)	98	1.5	Yellow		Not measured	
B(ii)	12.5	5.0	Deep-blue	650	275	IV

[a] A, single heating process; B(i), heating; B(ii), cooling-dilution-reheating process.
[b] a = absorptivity

interpreted in terms of mixtures of Kober chromogens I, II, and IV.

Because the Kober II chromogen corresponds to the analytical red mixture, this was next studied. We found that the color yield by the normal single-stage heating process was significantly affected by trace amounts of metal salts. Group IA metal ions and Group IIA metal ions decreased the color yield by 10% and 5%, respectively, but did not affect the rate of production of the chromogen. If the metal salts were added after the Kober II chromogen had been formed, they had no effect on color yield. On the other hand, the presence of trace amounts of iron, cobalt, nickel, or copper salts markedly affected the rate of production of the chromogen. Natural light ($\lambda > 360$ nm) affects the color yield because it alters the ferrous ion/ferric ion ratio of the iron impurities in the reagent-grade sulfuric acid (*9*). This finding probably explains some of the reported variations in color yield between batch, as also does our finding of the critical nature of the heating program and final heating temperature on the color yield of the Kober II chromogen.

In a final series of experiments, we found that the red mixtures of Kober II prepared by two different methods—(*a*) the reaction of H_2SO_4/water (55/45 by vol) with separate aliquots of a standard estriol solution, or (*b*) by dilution with H_2SO_4/water (55/45 by vol) of a strong Kober II mixture from a concentrated solution of estriol—both obeyed Beer's law over a limited range of concentration. However, there were large (80%) differences between the average absorptivities given by these mixtures of Kober II prepared by the two distinct methods, and although the mixtures both gave linear Lambert's law plots, these failed to pass through the origin and indicated higher absorbances than expected. On prolonged standing the absorption spectra of Kober II mixtures significantly changes; black precipitates were finally formed.

Discussion

We suggest that the only logical explanation for these unusual and diverse experimental findings is that the Kober reaction mixtures are lyophobic colloidal suspensions of differing particle size. It is not proposed at this time to speculate upon the chemical nature of the colloidal particles beyond pointing out that a red form of carbon has been reported (*10*) and that a suspension of colloidal graphite (Aquadag) in sulfuric acid/water (55/45 by vol) gave a very similar absorption spectrum to that for the Kober II mixture.

Once one realizes that the Kober reaction products are sols, the practical importance of strict controls over the purity of the reagents, reaction vessels, and temperature, and the need for knowledge of the history of the reaction mixtures may be understood from classical experiments in colloid chemistry (*11*). Further, the need to use organic additives when the Kober chromogens are extracted into organic solvents may also be understood in terms of the general requirement for protective agents when forming organosols from aquasols or vice versa. As a direct result of this interpretation of these experiments we have been able to *design* fast assay procedures for estriol, based upon the Kober reaction, which have high between-batch precision. We are now extending the colloidal hypothesis to guide us in our studies of other important analytical procedures involving strong sulfuric acid mixtures.

This work was supported in part from a grant from the National Society for Mentally Handicapped Children (Northwest Region) to S. B. J., and by grants from the Heinz and Anna Kroch Foundation and the Lawson Tate Medical Research Trust.

References

1. Wilde, C. E., and Oakey, R. E., Biochemical tests for the assessment of feto-placental function. *Ann. Clin. Biochem.* **12**, 83 (1975).

2. Kober, S., Eine kolorimetrische Bestimmung des Brusthormons. *Biochem. Z.* **239**, 209 (1931).

3. Oakey, R., Bradshaw, L., Eccles, S., et al., The rapid estimation of estrogens in pregnancy to monitor foetal risk. *Clin. Chim. Acta* **15**, 35 (1967).

4. Ittrich, G., Eine neue Methode zur chemischen Bestimmung der ostrogenen Hormone in Harn. *Hoppe-Seylers Z. Physiol Chem.* **312**, 1 (1958).

5. Hainsworth, I. R., and Hall, P. E., A simple automated method for the measurement of estrogens in the urine of pregnant women. *Clin. Chim. Acta* **35**, 201 (1971).

6. Jones, H. A., and Hahnel, R., Specificity and mechanism of the Kober reaction (for estrogen assay in biological fluids). *Steroids* **13**, 693 (1969).

7. Kimura, M., Kawata, M., Akiyama, K., et al., Chromogenic reactions of steroids with strong acids. IV. Specificity of the Kober reaction. *Chem. Pharm. Bull.* **21**, 1720 (1973).

8. Jensen, S. B., Some studies on the reaction between oestriol and aqueous sulphuric acid mixtures. Ph.D. thesis, University of Salford, Lancs., U. K., 1973.

9. Crossley, G., A low temperature assay for oestriol. M.Sc. Thesis, University of Salford, Lancs., U. K., 1975.

10. Schmidt, L., Boehm, H. P., and Hofmann, U., *Proc. 3rd Conference on Carbon.* Pergamon Press, 1957, p 235.

11. Hatschek, E., *The Foundations of Colloid Chemistry,* Ernest Benn Ltd., London, 1925.

CLIN. CHEM. 22/5, 681–682 (1976)

Specificity and Reproducibility of Acetone Precipitation in Identifying Surface-Active Phosphatidylcholine in Amniotic Fluid

L. L. Penney,[1] Dwain D. Hagerman, and Catherine A. Sei

We show the theoretical and actual variability in the amount of surface-active lecithin precipitated in the acetone-precipitation step of determining lecithin/sphingomyelin (L/S) ratios in the clinical laboratory. Lecithins precipitated may range from 60 to 90% of the total surface-active lecithins present. The range is sufficient to account for the occasional "immature" L/S ratios (less than 2/1) found in amniotic fluid from women bearing mature fetuses.

Additional Keyphrases: *fetal status • lipids • lecithin/sphingomyelin ratio • respiratory distress syndrome • lecithins*

Gluck et al. (*1*) reported that the RDS[2] in the newborn was predictable from measurements of the L/S ratio in the amniotic fluid. Many modifications of the method have been published since the original appeared (*2*). Depending on the technique used, fetal pulmonary maturity has been defined by densitometrically determined L/S ratios as low as 1.2/1 (*3*), although Gluck found 2/1 to be the value beyond which no fetus will be at risk for RDS (*4*). Some amniotic fluids with L/S ratios below the specified minimum will, however, be associated with no or very mild RDS.

The surface-active lecithins present in amniotic fluid are believed to reflect most accurately the status of the developing lung. Most naturally occurring lecithins are insoluble in cold acetone (*5, 6*), and in the lungs this fraction is also surface-active. Accordingly, cold-acetone precipitation is an integral step in determining the L/S ratio (*3, 4*). Longer-chain, fully-saturated acyl constituents would predictably be more abundant in the precipitable fraction (*6*). DPL is known to be surface-active (*3*) and has been demonstrated to be a major lecithin in the acetone-precipitable lecithins of human amniotic fluid and the alveolar wash and lung of various animals including the rabbit (*7*). The fact that cold-acetone precipitation is unlikely to be a quantitative procedure in the clinical laboratory, either with regard to a given molecular species of phosphatidylcholine or to surface-active molecules in general, led us to calculate the probabilities for the presence of selected molecular species in the acetone-insoluble and -soluble fractions and to test the theoretical prediction in a clinical laboratory setting.

Department of Obstetrics and Gynecology and Department of Biochemistry, University of Colorado School of Medicine, Denver, Colo. 80220.

[1] Present address: William Beaumont Army Medical Center, El Paso, Texas 79920. Address correspondence to D. D. H.

[2] Nonstandard abbreviations used: L/S, lecithin/sphingomyelin; RDS, respiratory distress syndrome; DPL, dipalmitoyl phosphatidylcholine; and DOL, dioleoyl phosphatidylcholine.

Received Dec. 15, 1975; accepted Feb. 15, 1976.

Materials and Methods

A portion of Gluck's data (*7*, p 356) was used to calculate the probable composition of the lecithin. Although it has not been shown in lung, and indeed is contrary to the usual teaching in so far as liver is concerned (*8*), we assumed that the probability of selection of a fatty acid for esterification in the β position in glycerol with a specified constituent in the α position was independent, and vice versa. Therefore, the probability P(x) for a fatty acid known to occur with $P(\alpha)$ at the α position simultaneously occupying a molecule with a fatty acid known to occur with $P(\beta)$ at the β position is $P(\alpha) \times P(\beta)$ (*9*).

Pure DPL and DOL and [*β-palmitoyl*-9,10-^{3}H]dipalmitoyl (^{3}H-DPL) phosphatidylcholine were purchased from Applied Science Laboratories, State College, Pa. 16801. The volume of amniotic fluid we use to determine the L/S ratio is customarily 3 ml, and according to Nelson (*10*) a "mature" fluid would contain at least 0.01 μmol/3 ml. Chloroform stock solutions containing, per 100 μl, 11.4 nmol of DPL and 9.1 nmol of DOL were distributed into 10 tubes so that each contained either 50, 100, or 200 μl of DPL stock solution plus 100 μl of DOL stock solution and 50 μl of ^{3}H-DPL (about 2220 dpm/μl). The contents of each of the 30 tubes were evaporated under a gentle stream of oxygen-free nitrogen and the residue was redissolved in about 30 μl of chloroform. Three milliliters of mature amniotic fluid from a single patient and 50 μl of ^{3}H-DPL were added to another 20 tubes and the contents mixed thoroughly. An experienced analyst was requested to analyze the amniotic fluid samples, identified only by a code number, by the Gluck extraction procedure, and by acetone precipitation at 0 °C as routinely done in our clinical laboratory. Both the acetone-precipitable and -soluble fractions were then dissolved in $CHCl_3$/methanol (2/1) and were transferred to counting vials with capillary pipets. A Packard Tri-Carb Model 3380 Liquid Scintillation Spectrometer was used to measure the radioactivity, counting long enough to decrease the counting error to a CV of less than 2%.

Table 1. Percentage of Total Lecithin That Theoretically is Acetone Precipitable in Rabbit Alveolar Wash and Residual Lung for Selected Molecular Species[a]

Molecular species	Alveolar wash	Residual lung
16:0, 16:0	70	73
16:0, 16:1	36	31
16:0, 18:1	24	39
16:0, 18:2	20	16

[a] From ref. *7*.

Table 2. Mean Values for Lecithin, Acetone-Precipitated and Soluble

Category	Mean (cpm)	SD (cpm)
Lecithin ppt., artificial samples	6496	1041
Lecithin ppt., amniotic fluid	8499	1292
Lecithin sol., artificial samples	3722	1534
Lecithin sol., amniotic fluid	2736	1042

Results

Table 1 shows selected examples of the most abundant molecular species, recalculated in terms of predicted percentage of each that is precipitable.

The mean radioactivity in both the precipitable and the soluble fractions was compared by Wilcoxon rank sum test. Within the artificial preparations the mean value at each concentration was the same but the means for both precipitable and soluble fractions were statistically different between amniotic fluid and the artificial preparations (Table 2). Using these four means and their standard deviations, we eliminated all values exceeding two standard deviations from the mean as "outliers." Table 3 shows the lecithin "precipitated" to lecithin "soluble" ratios as well as the range and mean of DPL precipitated. Based on standards of 50 μl ^{3}H-DPL counted with the same run, the total analytical recoveries were 63, 62, and 60, respectively, for the 50-μl, 100-μl, and 200-μl samples of DPL and 67% for the samples of amniotic fluid. These differences are not statistically significant by the rank sum test ($P < .01$).

Table 3. Lecithin Precipitable/Lecithin Soluble Ratios, by Category

	50 μl DPL, n = 8	100 μl DPL, n = 8	200 μl DPL, n = 9	Amniotic fluid, n = 9
	1.40	2.89	3.58	2.85
	2.49	1.59	4.36	2.80
	1.29	3.01	3.19	1.48
	1.52	1.12	1.19	2.61
	1.53	1.29	1.57	2.44
	3.33	2.60	2.12	3.33
	2.41	2.37	1.12	8.38
	1.70	1.49	1.84	2.23
			2.17	2.21
				3.00
				2.07
				2.22
				3.62
				9.18
				2.22
				3.46
				3.04
				7.36
				3.73
Range ppt'd.	58–77%	53–75%	53–81%	60–90%
Mean ppt'd.	66%	67%	70%	78%[a]

[a] Significantly different from other means ($P < .01$) by rank sum test.

Discussion

The proportion of DPL precipitated is about that predicted from theoretical considerations, but it appears to increase with the amount of extraneous lipid present and varies appreciably among analyses. As much as 10–40% of the desired lecithins may be lost into the acetone-soluble fraction. Measurement of total saturated lecithins, of a saturated/unsaturated lecithin ratio in amniotic fluid, or of DPL alone are measurements that conceivably could detect falsely low L/S ratios. We are currently evaluating these techniques.

These investigations were supported in part by HD-05085, NICHD.

References

1. Gluck, L., Kulovich, M. V., Borer, R. C., et al., Diagnosis of the respiratory distress syndrome by amniocentesis. *Am. J. Obstet. Gynecol.* **109,** 440 (1971).

2. Gluck, L., Kulovich, M. V., Borer, R. C., and Keidel, W. N., The interpretation and significance of the lecithin/sphingomyelin ratio in amniotic fluid. *Am. J. Obstet. Gynecol.* **120,** 142 (1974).

3. Gebhardt, D. O. E., Beintema, A., De Rooij, R. E., et al., A study of the lecithin/sphingomyelin ratio of amniotic fluid. *Clin. Chim. Acta* **64,** 133 (1975).

4. Gluck, L., and Kulovich, M. V., Lecithin/sphingomyelin ratios in amniotic fluid in normal and abnormal pregnancy. *Am. J. Obstet. Gynecol.* **115,** 539 (1973).

5. Artom, C., Labeled compounds and phospholipid metabolism. In *Methods in Enzymology* **IV,** S. P. Colowick and N. O. Kaplan, Eds. Academic Press, New York, N. Y., 1957, p 823.

6. Dervichian, D. G., The physical chemistry of phospholipids. *Prog. Biophys. Mol. Biol.* **14,** 26d (1964).

7. Gluck, L., Landowne, R. A., and Kulovich, M. V., Biochemical development of surface activity in mammalian lung. III. Structural changes in lung lecithin during development of the rabbit fetus and newborn. *Pediatr. Res.* **4,** 352 (1970).

8. White, A., Handler, P., and Smith, E. L. *Principles of Biochemistry,* McGraw Hill, New York, N. Y., 1973, p 581.

9. Remington, R. D., and Schork, M. A., *Statistics with Applications to the Biological and Health Sciences.* Prentice-Hall, Englewood Cliffs, N. J., 1970, p 75.

10. Nelson, G. H., Relationship between amniotic fluid lecithin concentration and respiratory distress syndrome. *Am. J. Obstet. Gynecol.* **112,** 827 (1972).

CLIN. CHEM. 22/5, 683–685 (1976)

Four Commercial Urease Reagents and a Laboratory-Prepared Reagent Compared for Analysis of Blood Urea Nitrogen with the Beckman Analyzer

Norbert S. Norkus, Norman P. Kubasik, and Harrison E. Sine, Jr.

Three laboratory-prepared urease reagents were compared with a commercial preparation supplied for routine use on the Beckman Blood Urea Nitrogen Analyzer. There were discrepancies in results for urea nitrogen among the four urease reagents when matching serum and the corresponding oxalate/fluoride treated plasma were compared as measured with the Beckman Analyzer and continuous-flow (AutoAnalyzer) method. All four urease preparations were affected by fluoride, but to different extents. We believe that an effective laboratory reagent can be prepared in the laboratory at significantly lower cost.

Additional Keyphrase: *effect of fluoride on urea nitrogen values (by urease)*

In the Beckman BUN Analyzer a conductivity rate method is used to determine urea nitrogen (*1*):

$$Urea + H_2O \xrightarrow{urease} 2NH_4^+ + HCO_3^-$$

The formation of ammonium and bicarbonate ions results in an increased conductivity of the reaction mixture, which is monitored by a conductivity electrode. The rate of ammonium bicarbonate formation is directly proportional to the urea concentration of the sample.

Use of commercially available reagents usually presents a significant savings relative to the preparation of such a reagent. This note describes our attempts to prepare a laboratory reagent that provides results equivalent to the commercial product, but at a smaller cost.

Materials and Methods

Urea nitrogen was assayed with a Beckman BUN Analyzer (Beckman Instruments, Inc., Fullerton, Calif. 92634) and the AutoAnalyzer II System (AA-II) for BUN and glucose (Technicon Instruments Corp., Tarrytown, N. Y. 10591). In the AA-II system a modification of the diacetylmonoxime method as described by Marsh et al. (*2*) is used.

The Clinical Laboratories, The Genesee Hospital, 224 Alexander St., Rochester, N. Y. 14607.
Received Oct. 6, 1975; accepted Mar. 3, 1976.

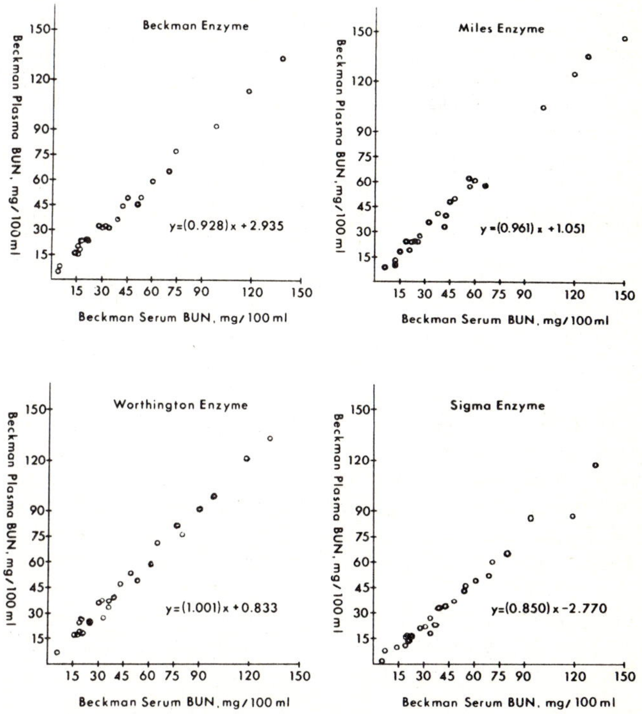

Fig. 1. Comparison of results for urea nitrogen in corresponding plasma and serum samples, as determined with the Beckman BUN Analyzer with use of four commercial urease preparations
n = 27 for all except Worthington, for which n = 26

A commercially available urease (EC 3.5.1.5) reagent, Beckman BUN Reagent Pack (Beckman Instruments) was compared to three laboratory-prepared reagents. The commercial reagent requires mixing two separately included reagents, urease and a tris(hydroxymethyl)aminomethane buffer, which results in a final urease activity of 35–45 kU/liter. The laboratory-prepared reagents were prepared from three different sources of jackbean-derived urease: (*a*) 3.4 kU/g (Sigma Chemical Co., St. Louis, Mo. 63178), (*b*) 120 kU/g

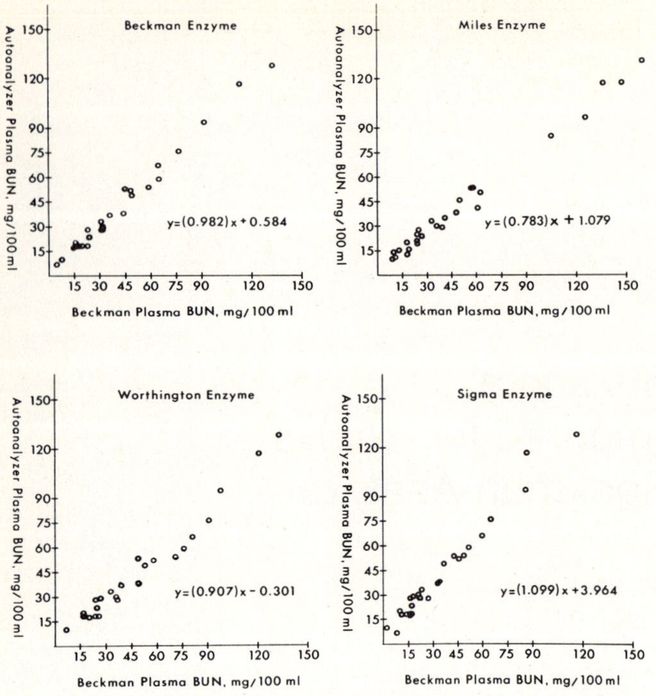

Fig. 2. Comparison of results for urea nitrogen in plasma as measured with the Beckman BUN Analyzer and an AutoAnalyzer method, with use of four commercial urease preparations
n = 27 for all except Worthington, for which n = 26

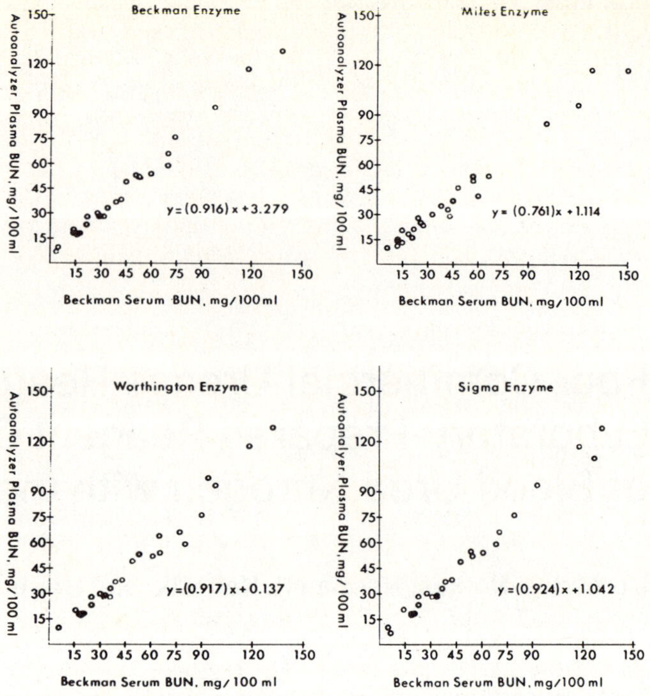

Fig. 3. Same as Figure 2, except the samples were serum

(Miles Labs., Elkhart, Ind. 46514), and (*c*) 120 kU/g (Worthington Biochemical Corp., Freehold, N. J. 07728). All were prepared by dissolving 100 mg of urease in 5 ml of 0.124 mol/liter tris(hydroxymethyl)aminomethane, pH 7.3 (preadjusted with glacial acetic acid/water, 30/70 by vol) and diluting this mixture to a final volume of 250 ml with a resulting urease activity of approximately 48 U/ml for the Miles and Worthington enzyme. However, attempts to increase the final urease activity of the Sigma product to more than 2 U/ml resulted in a reagent that was incompatible with the Beckman BUN Analyzer. This appeared to be related to the initial conductivity, which was several orders of magnitude greater than was so for the other urease preparations. A final Sigma urease activity of about 1.4 U/ml, consistent with the reagent preparation described above, was found to be compatible with the Beckman BUN Analyzer.

Blood samples were collected in red-stoppered Vacutainer tubes with no additive (cat. No. 4670-M3200), and gray-stoppered Vacutainer tubes containing 14 mg of potassium oxalate and 17.5 mg of sodium fluoride (cat. No. 4500-M3204PS), both from Becton, Dickinson and Co., Rutherford, N. J. 07070.

Results and Discussion

Figure 1 demonstrates the results observed when we compared matching plasma and serum samples from patients on the Beckman BUN Analyzer. Worthington urease demonstrated the best correlation, followed by Miles, Beckman, and Sigma, which all demonstrated higher values for serum urea nitrogen than for plasma urea nitrogen. With the Sigma urease, plasma values for urea nitrogen were only 85% of serum values.

Figure 2 compares plasma urea nitrogen as assayed with the Beckman BUN Analyzer and the AA-II system. Results with Miles urease correlated the poorest of the four tested, the

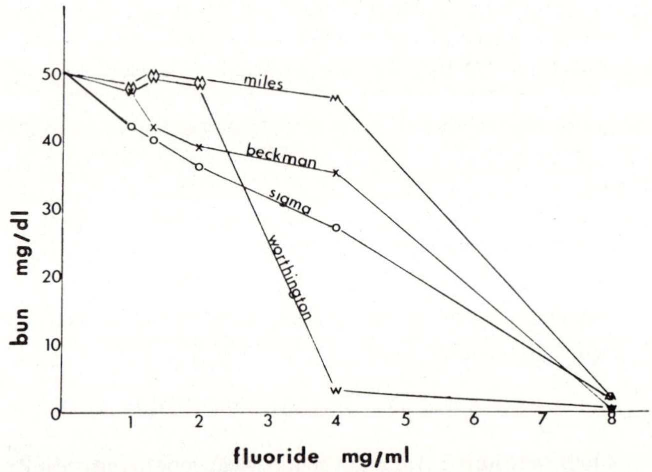

Fig. 4. Effect of fluoride on the assay of aqueous urea nitrogen with the Beckman BUN Analyzer, with use of four commercial urease preparations

Beckman BUN Analyzer results being about 22% higher than AA-II values. The Beckman reagent and Worthington urease correlated best.

Figure 3 demonstrates the similarly poor results for the Miles urease when serum urea nitrogen values (Beckman BUN Analyzer) were compared to plasma values (AA-II). Worthington, Sigma, and Beckman reagents showed about 8% higher values for serum.

All of the urease reagents were inhibited by fluoride (Figure 4), the Sigma enzyme being the most sensitive, which explains the lower values for plasma urea nitrogen (assayed on the Beckman BUN Analyzer) observed in Figures 1 and 2. The Miles enzyme showed the least effect of fluoride inhibition, but correlation was poor with the AA-II system (Figures 2 and 3). The Worthington enzyme and Beckman reagent exhibit a fluoride inhibition intermediate to the aforementioned enzymes.

We have found in practice that if an oxalate/fluoride Vacutainer tube is used for a urea nitrogen assay on the Beckman BUN Analyzer and contains between 4 and 8 ml of whole blood, only the Worthington preparation gives results comparable to those from the AA-II system.

A cost analysis of the Beckman-packaged reagent with the same reagent prepared in the laboratory (inclusive of reagents and labor) suggests a savings well in excess of $100.00 per liter of laboratory reagent.

We recommend that either the Beckman Reagent Pack or the laboratory-prepared reagent (with use of Worthington urease) be used with the Beckman BUN Analyzer.

References

1. Horak, E., and Sunderman, W., Jr., Measurements of serum urea by conductimetric urease assay. *Ann. Clin. Lab. Sci.* **2**, 425 (1972).

2. Marsh, W. H., Fingerhut, B., and Miller, H., Automated and manual direct methods for determination of blood urea. *Clin. Chem.* **11**, 624 (1965).

CLIN. CHEM. 22/5, 685–687 (1976)

Use of Blood Specimens Collected on Filter Paper in Screening for Abnormal Hemoglobins

Robert M. Schmidt,[1] Effie M. Brosious,[1] Solomon Holland,[1] Jane M. Wright,[1] and Graham R. Serjeant[2]

Both cellulose acetate electrophoresis and citrate agar electrophoresis were performed on 834 blood samples collected on filter paper in Jamaica and shipped for testing to the National Hemoglobinopathy Standardization Laboratory at the U.S. National Center for Disease Control. Additionally, 30 blood samples collected locally were stored on filter paper, in microhematocrit capillary tubes, and as whole blood specimens; at selected times the samples were tested for stability to determine the best sample-collection technique for hemoglobin electrophoresis. Results were most nearly accurate when both cellulose acetate electrophoresis and citrate agar testing were used. The methods are easy to perform, but results are unreliable if the blood samples on filter paper are stored at 4 °C for longer than two weeks before they are tested.

Additional Keyphrases: *hemoglobinopathies • sickle cell anemia • electrophoresis*

Several recent reports have suggested that blood specimens collected on filter paper for hemoglobinopathy testing are quite suitable for mass-screening programs (*1–3*). In addition, Garrick et al. (*4*) suggested that specimens collected on filter paper can be used to detect sickle cell anemia and to identify other hemoglobinopathies in newborns. Although the work of these investigators indicated that this is a reliable, efficient method of detecting abnormal hemoglobins, their results were not definitive because their 2435 cord-blood specimens included no FS phenotypes and only 14 FAS phenotypes. If blood samples collected on filter paper from a fingerprick can in fact be stored and shipped to a central laboratory, this method of collection would be particularly useful for hemoglobinopathy screening programs. Our study was designed to investigate whether accurate results can be obtained with such samples.

Materials and Methods

Cord-blood specimens from 834 consecutive deliveries at the Royal Victoria Jubilee Hospital in Kingston, Jamaica, were collected in heparinized tubes and on filter paper. Staff of the Medical Research Council Epidemiology Unit, University of the West Indies, screened the blood specimens collected in tubes for abnormal hemoglobins by the methods described by Serjeant et al. (*5*). The corresponding filter paper samples were stored at 4 °C for two weeks during the entire collection/screening procedure and then were air-mailed in refrigerated containers to the National Hemoglobinopathy Standardization Laboratory located at the Center for Disease Control.

When the specimens arrived at the Atlanta laboratory, 0.6-cm (diameter) discs of filter paper containing the blood spots were punched out and placed in labeled test tubes. About 0.2 ml of a tetrasodium ethylenediaminetetraacetate (EDTA) solution, 2.5 g/liter, was added to each tube to elute the hemoglobin from the paper discs. The tubes were left overnight at 4 °C. The next day, cellulose acetate electrophoresis of the eluted hemoglobin was performed as described previously (*6*). Subsequently, citrate agar electrophoresis was also done on the eluted hemoglobin samples by the method of Milner and Gooden (*7*). All specimens were tested in Atlanta no longer than four weeks after the initial testing in Jamaica.

[1] Hematology Division, Center for Disease Control, PHS, U. S. Dept. of HEW, Atlanta, Ga. 30333.

[2] Medical Research Council Epidemiology Unit, University of the West Indies, Kingston, Jamaica, West Indies.

The use of trade names is for identification only and does not constitute endorsement by the PHS or the U. S. Dept. of HEW.

Address reprint requests to Dr. Schmidt, Center for Disease Control, Atlanta, Ga. 30333.

Received Jan. 7, 1976; accepted Mar. 4, 1976.

Table 1. Phenotypes of 834 Cord Blood Samples as Determined by Three Methods

Electrophoretic method and sample	Total no. specs.	Phenotype: FA	FAS	FAC	FS	FA Bart's	FAS Bart's	Homozygous Hb A½	FS Bart's	F-Victoria Jubilee
Immediate screen (both cellulose acetate & citrate agar)	834	699	76	26	3	24	3	1	1	1
Cellulose acetate on mailed filter paper specimens	834	769	32	22	3	7	0	0	1	0
Cellulose acetate & citrate agar on mailed specimens	834	728	70[a]	25	3	7	0	0	1	0

[a] One sample here was a true FA or normal specimen, but was categorized as FAS because of the extreme electrophoretic smearing.

Table 2. Errors Made in Phenotyping 834 Cord Blood Samples Mailed on Filter Paper and Tested by Electrophoresis on Cellulose Acetate and Citrate Agar

	Phenotype: FAS	FAC	FA Bart's	FAS Bart's
No. false positives	1	0	0	0
No. false negatives	5	1	17	3

In addition, 10 normal and 20 abnormal specimens of whole blood were obtained from a local Atlanta hospital. Within 4 h of blood collection each of the 30 specimens was divided for storage into three aliquots. One portion was stored in an evacuated blood-collection tube containing Na_2EDTA, one was stored in a heparinized microhematocrit tube, and the third was spotted on filter paper. Half of each of the three aliquots was kept at room temperature for 30 days, the other half in the refrigerator for 30 days. On days 3, 7, 14, 20, and 30, cellulose acetate electrophoresis and solubility tests were run on one sample from each aliquot. The electrophoresis was graded as to the amount of smearing present and as to whether discernible bands could be seen in the areas where bands had been found in initial testing.

Results

Table 1 lists the phenotypes assessed in Atlanta with the cellulose acetate electrophoresis and citrate agar electrophoresis methods and the phenotypes assessed in Jamaica. Separations on cellulose acetate strips were generally poor, with much streaking and smearing of hemoglobin. Citrate agar patterns showed more definite bands, but substantial smearing between bands persisted. Over 57% of the sickle cell traits and 15% of the hemoglobin C traits were missed when cellulose acetate alone was used. Only 9.2% of the hemoglobin S traits and 4% of the hemoglobin C traits were missed when the combination of methods was used. The citrate agar procedure was needed to detect the hemoglobin S in almost half of the known FAS samples sent. The cellulose acetate procedure was virtually useless for detecting small amounts of hemoglobin. Hemoglobin Bart's, known to be relatively unstable, was not seen in most instances in the patterns obtained with the mailed filter-paper specimens. Table 2 summarizes these findings as the number of false-positive and false-negative results obtained. Results from part two of this study indicate that, if kept refrigerated, venous blood stored in evacuated blood-collection tubes can be tested satisfactorily after storage for longer than a month; in contrast, samples collected in heparinized microhematocrit tubes and on filter paper can be used satisfactorily for only two weeks. Because the problem of smearing increases with time, specimens stored on filter paper for longer than two weeks are not suitable for testing.

Discussion

The detection of abnormal hemoglobins at birth is important because it enables the physician to begin appropriate preventive-medicine procedures in babies with sickle cell disease, including hydration and early treatment of infections (*8*). Because hemoglobins S, C, D, and G and other β-chain variants are found only in small concentrations in the blood of newborns, it is generally believed that these variants cannot be detected until the concentration of fetal hemoglobin decreases. However, several investigators have independently reported success in detecting abnormal hemoglobins in cord blood (*5, 9–12*).

Blood samples collected on filter paper are now being obtained from newborns in 43 states for phenylketonuria screening (*13*), and this method also appears to be practical for obtaining samples for an abnormal hemoglobin screen. However, storage time and conditions must be considered if this technique is used. The current study indicates that storage of such samples for longer than two weeks results in smearing of hemoglobins, which produces major errors in interpretation of electrophoretic patterns.

References

1. Schneider, N. J., and Chan, M. S., Laboratory screening of hemoglobinopathies. *Health Lab. Sci.* **12,** 91 (1975).

2. Thambipillai, S., Senewiratne, B., and Chir, M., A simple finger-prick method of screening for abnormal hemoglobins. *Am. J. Clin. Pathol.* **63,** 836 (1975).

3. Hosty, T. S., Tomlin, G., and Atkins, R., Testing for hemoglobinopathies in a public health laboratory. *Public Health Lab.* **30,** 102 (1972).

4. Garrick, M. D., Dembue, P., and Guthrie, R., Sickle cell anemia and other hemoglobinopathies. Procedures and strategy for screening employing spots of blood on filter paper as specimens. *New Engl. J. Med.* **288,** 1265 (1973).

5. Serjeant, B. E., Forbes, M., Williams, L., and Serjeant, G. R., Screening cord bloods for the detection of sickle cell disease in Jamaica. *Clin. Chem.* **20,** 666 (1974).

6. Schmidt, R. M., Laboratory diagnosis of hemoglobinopathies. *J. Am. Med. Assoc.* **224,** 1276 (1973).

7. Milner, P. R., and Gooden, J., Rapid citrate-agar electrophoresis in routine screening for hemoglobinopathies using a simple hemolysate. *Am. J. Clin. Pathol.* **64,** 58 (1975).

8. Pearson, H. A., Progress in early diagnosis of sickle cell disease. *Children* **18,** 222 (1971).

9. Metters, J. S., and Yawson, G. I., The use of the cord blood sample for the detection of sickle cell anemia in the newborn. *J. Obstet. Gynaecol. Br. Commonw.* **77,** 935 (1970).

10. Pearson, H. A., O'Brien, R. T., McIntosh, S., et a al., Routine screening of umbilical cord blood for sickle cell diseases. *J. Am. Med. Assoc.* **227,** 420 (1974).

11. Schroeder, W. A., Jakway, J., and Powars, D., Detection of hemoglobins S and C at birth: A rapid screening procedure by column chromatography. *J. Lab. Clin. Med.* **82,** 303 (1973).

12. Schneider, R. G., Gustavson, Z. P., and Haggard, M. E., The incidence of genetically determined hemoglobin abnormalities in 11,247 cord blood samples. Hemoglobin F Dickenson, a new fetal variant. Abstracts of the Thirteenth International Congress of Haematology (1970).

13. Levy, H. L., Newborn metabolic screening: Past and prospect. *New Engl. J. Med.* **293,** 824 (1975).

Corrections

Volume 21

p 1668: In Figure 2, as shown, R_2 and C_2 are connected to the ac side of the bridge rectifier. The correct schematic would show the upper end of R_2 connected to the anode of the *SCR* and the lower end of C_2 to the cathode of the *SCR*.

p 1905: Figures corresponding to legends for Figures 3A and 3B are reversed, i.e., 3A is a negative sample, 3B a positive sample.

Volume 22

p 102: In both Tables 1 and 2, headings "630 nm" and "410 nm" should be reversed; caption under Fig. 1 should end ". . . solution No. 2."

p 156: Tenth line of last paragraph: change "100 ml" to "100 mol."

p 219, Table 1, fourth item in fourth column: "±68.8" should read "±8.8".

p 264, column 1: Source of *p*-HBAH is Aldrich Chemical Co., Milwaukee, Wis. 53233 (cat. No. H2,010-5).

p 273, under *Reagents:* "ferric nitrate (68.5 g/liter)" should read "mercuric nitrate (68.5 g/liter)"; "mercuric nitrate (202 g/liter)" should read "ferric nitrate (202 g/liter)." In Figure 1 (p 274), 620 μg, 530 μg, and 440 μg should be changed to 62 mg, 53 mg, and 44 mg.

p 344: under *Specificity,* "1.0 mg/liter" should read "100 mg/liter."

p 379: under *Procainamide assay,* sentence should be changed to read "Place the containers in an ice bath, add 2.0 ml of hydrochloric acid *and 1.0 ml of sodium nitrite,* mix the contents . . . ."

letters

Methaqualone Assay by Radioimmunoassay and Gas Chromatography

To the Editor:

Methods available for the analysis of samples for methaqualone or its metabolites (or both) include thin-layer chromatography (*1*), gas chromatography (*2*), and mass spectrometry (*3*). Although the last two techniques are quite sensitive, they require time-consuming chemical cleanup and, in some cases, may also require preparation of derivatives, procedures that consume additional time. Berman et al. (*4*) showed that radioimmunoassay is a sensitive method for assay of methaqualone in urine and that this method requires minimal preliminary sample handling. As a complement to their work on urine, we report here a radioimmunoassay of serum samples for methaqualone and its metabolites.

Using a commercially available radioimmunoassay kit and following its enclosed directions, we assayed drug-free sera to which were added, respectively, various amounts of methaqualone and each of its five metabolites: 4′-hydroxy-, 3′-hydroxy-, 6-hydroxy-, and 3′6-dihydroxymethaqualone, and 2-nitrobenzo-*o*-toluidide. Figure 1 illustrates the responses obtained for each of these compounds. We assayed each concentration of each solution in triplicate. The points plotted in Figure 1 represent the average percent of free drug for each sample; the range of values observed was within ±2% of the average for each sample. ("Percent free" was calculated by dividing the cpm for the supernate by the cpm for the amount of antigen used for each sample and multiplying by 100.) Methaqualone and its 3′- and 4′-hydroxy metabolites gave comparable responses over the concentration range studied. The 6-hydroxy metabolite gave a lesser response (~40% of that for methaqualone) and the 3′,6-dihydroxy metabolite gave a smaller (~25% of that for methaqualone) yet still observable response. Obviously, the radioimmunoassay is not specific for methaqualone and any radioimmunoassay response must be interpreted in terms of "methaqualone equivalents." The method is extremely sensitive, giving a response ≥ 30% of the blank for concentrations as low as 2 ng/ml (2 μg/liter).

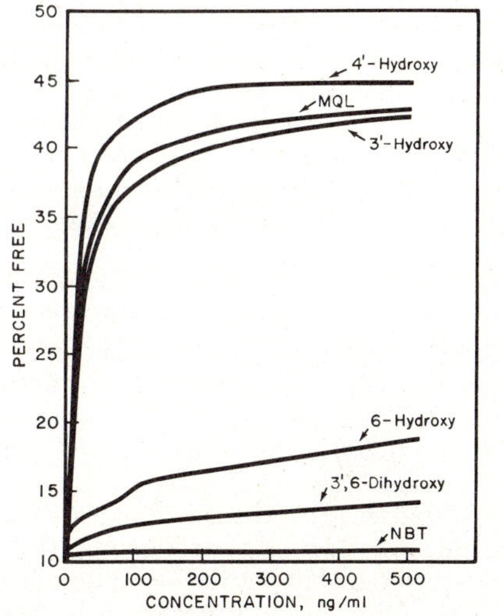

Fig. 1. Reactivities of methaqualone and of five unconjugated metabolites with RIA

"Percent Free" is defined in the text

In an effort to resolve the lack of specificity, we tried to resolve the parent drug and its metabolites by gas chromatography, but under the conditions used only the methaqualone gave a satisfactory response in the flame-ionization detector at the concentrations checked. We used a slight modification of the extraction procedure reported by Chin and Fastlich (*5*) and assayed the extracts on a Perkin-Elmer Model 3920 gas chromatograph. The column was coiled glass, 1.82 m × 2 mm i.d., packed with 3% OV-17 on 100/120 mesh Gas Chrom Q. Oven temperature was held at 230 °C.

Two explanations are possible for our not observing the metabolites chromatographically. First, as hydroxylated metabolites, they are phenols and thus not likely to extract from alkaline media into organic solvent. Changing the pH of the medium being extracted gave no different results. Secondly, as underivatized phenols, any amount that was extracted would not be eluted from the chromatographic column under our conditions, as we confirmed by preparing solutions of each metabolite in ethanol, injecting each of them under the above conditions, and not observing a response.

In order to compare both these methods, a series of solutions of methaqualone in serum were prepared, randomized, and assayed in a blind fashion by both methods (Table 1). Samples for radioimmunoassay analysis were appropriately diluted to bring them into the linear range before randomization. Radioimmunoassays were performed on triplicate aliquots of each sample. The tabulated results represent the average concentration determined and the range of values observed. For the gas-chromatographic analyses, standards were analyzed in the concentration range 0.2–50.0 mg/liter. Of this set, the lowest concentration for which an observable response was detected was 0.8 mg/liter. The calculated linear regression equation for these standards was $y = 0.144x(\text{mg/liter}) - 0.14$, with a correlation coefficient of 0.993. The "unknowns" were then assayed and the concentrations determined by comparison with the standard curve.

Table 1. Comparison of Results by GLC and RIA

Actual concn	Concn determined by GLC	Concn determined by RIA (range)
0.2	ND[a]	0.20 (.16–.23)
0.4	ND	0.42 (.32–.52)
0.8	0.79	0.78 (.73–.82)
1.0	1.01	0.88 (.81–.90)
2.0	2.04	1.61 (1.52–1.67)
4.0	3.89	4.28 (3.93–4.40)
8.0	7.93	8.18 (7.2–8.8)
10.0	9.59	8.20 (7.1–8.4)
20.0	19.82	17.57 (16.1–18.8)
30.0	28.10	28.30 (21.5–34.8)

[a] ND, not detected.

In conclusion, radioimmunoassay can be used as a screening procedure if a "yes or no" answer is satisfactory. If radioimmunoassay analysis of a specimen indicates the presence of methaqualone or one of its metabolites and if information regarding the concentration of the parent is required, then gas chromatography can be useful. However, neither assay technique will provide identity or concentration of any of the metabolites.

References

1. Sleeman, H. K., Cella, J. A., Harvey, J. L., and Beach, D. J., Thin-layer chromatographic detection and identification of methaqualone metabolites in urine. *Clin. Chem.* **21**, 76 (1975).

2. Mitchard, M., and Williams, M. E., An improved quantitative gas-liquid chromatographic assay for the estimation of methaqualone in biological fluids. *J. Chromatogr.* **72**, 29 (1972).

3. Bonnichsen, R., Marde, V., and Ryhage, R., Identification of free and conjugated metabolites of methaqualone by gas chromatography–mass spectrometry. *Clin. Chem.* **20**, 230 (1974).

4. Berman, A. R., McGrath, J. P., Permisohn, R. C., and Cella, J. A., Radioimmunoassay of methaqualone and its monohydroxy metabolites in urine. *Clin. Chem.* **21**, 1878 (1975).

5. Chin, D., and Fastlich, E., Improved extraction technique for gas-liquid chromatographic determination of methaqualone in serum. *Clin. Chem.* **20**, 1382 (1974).

R. O. Bost
C. A. Sutheimer
I. Sunshine

Cuyahoga County Coroner's Office and Institute of Pathology
Case Western Reserve University School of Medicine
Cleveland, Ohio 44106

Enzymatic Determination of Total Serum Cholesterol with the Vickers D-300 Analyzer

To the Editor:

We would like to contribute to the discussion (*1*) on the enzymatic determination of cholesterol. As soon as the methods of Richmond and Allain et al. appeared in *Clinical Chemistry* (*2, 3*), we tried to set up the totally enzymatic method on our mechanized analyzers (Vickers D-300 and CentrifiChem). As a first approach, we tested manually, with use of a Spectrophotometer Unicam SP 1700, and "Liponorm" (Nyegaard & Co. A/S, Oslo) test serum in different serum/reagent ratios, the kinetic development of the reaction, and we noticed that there is an induction step of about 2 min at 37 °C during which no color development is detected, and that an intense opalescence develops at concentrations of cholesterol exceeding 7.0 g/liter, which we obtained by adding a triple amount of test serum.

The reagents used in these preliminary studies were the same as Allain's et al. (*3*) with the following modifications: Carbowax-6000 (Fluka) 0.34 mmol/liter, cholesterol ester-hydrolase 28 U/liter, cholesterol oxidase 80 U/liter, peroxidase (500 kU/liter in $(NH_4)_2SO_4$, 3.2 mol/liter) 10 000 U/liter. The source of the above-mentioned enzymes is indicated below.

Table 1. Optimal Composition of Reagent Solutions

	per liter	
Solution No 1		
Sodium dihydrogen phosphate	100	mmol
Disodium hydrogen phosphate	100	mmol
4-Aminophenazone	1.64	mmol
Cholesterol ester hydrolase	28	U
Cholesterol oxidase	80	U
Peroxidase	10 000	U
Solution No 2		
Phenol	28	mmol
Triton X-100	40	ml

Reaction solution: equal volumes of solutions 1 and 2 ($pH_{25\,°C}$ = 6.6 ± 0.1).

Both of these unfavorable factors were easily overcome by simply adding to the test tube a few drops of Triton X-100 surfactant. With respect to the first point, it is known (*4*) that Triton X-100 is an activator for ester-hydrolases; with respect to the second, Triton X-100 evidently solubilizes both proteins and cholesterol. This hypothesis was confirmed in the course of the second approach we used, which will be described subsequently. In fact, on increasing the amount of enzymes added, there was an increasing opalescence as soon as temperatures higher than room temperature were reached.

Once we eliminated the above-mentioned troubles, we tried to reduce the cost of the test, which is quite high in this country owing to the high cost of the enzymes involved, particularly cholesterol oxidase. We purchased from Biochemia (Boehringer Mannheim) the following pure enzymes: cholesterol ester-hydrolase (EC 3.1.1.13) 10 U/mg, cholesterol oxidase (EC 1.1.3.6) 20 U/mg, and peroxidase (EC 1.11.1.7) grade II, 50 U/mg; all the listed activities are evaluated at 25 °C. We found that more Triton X-100 could replace both the sodium cholate that Allain et al. found to be "required for hydrolysis of cholesterol esters by cholesterol ester-hydrolase" and the Carbowax-6000 (polyethylene glicol, mol wt 6000–7000) "included in the formulation to aid in maintaining free cholesterol in solution" (*3*). Moreover, under these conditions, starting from a limit concentration of 0.25 ml of Triton X-100 per 100 ml, at which concentration the reagent solution (which is clear at room temperature) becomes opalescent as soon as the temperature of 33 °C is reached, there is a linear relationship between the limit at which opalescence is detectable and the cholesterol concentration. To be on the safe side, we used in our reagents a concentration of 20 ml of Triton X-100 per liter, with which no opalescence was produced up to 13.0 g of cholesterol per liter. The only negative effect of the addition of Triton X-100 was an increase in the blank absorbance with increasing concentrations of surfactant.

Table 2. Protocol for Vickers D-300

Syringe No.	Color code	Reagent	Station	Volume setting, ml
1 (outer)	brown	Solution No 1	57	1.50
7 (outer)	purple	Solution No 2	0	1.50
9 (outer)	white	Sample	0	0.03
Photometer pick-up station			10	
Rate of analysis			200 samples/h	
Rotor temperature			37 °C	
Sample blank			Not required	
Filter			505 nm	

The test was performed by incubating 30 µl of serum at 37 °C with 3.0 ml of the reagents shown in Table 1. Under these conditions we got a linear calibration in 10 min up to 3.0 g of cholesterol per liter; on prolonging the reaction time to 15 min we got a linear calibration curve up to 5.0 g of cholesterol per liter. On keeping, in the final reagent, the cholesterol ester-hydrolase concentration to 28 U/liter and the cholesterol oxidase concentration to 120 U/liter we got a linear calibration up to 6.0 g of cholesterol per liter in 10 min, and up to 10.0 g of cholesterol per liter in 15 min.

The control-of-procedure calibration was made both with solutions of recrystallized cholesterol in isopropanol and with serial dilutions or different serum/reagent ratios of Liponorm and Precilip (Biochemia, Boehringer Mannheim) in de-ionized water.

We correlated our results with results obtained by the enzymatic procedure of Röschlau et al. (*5, 6*), made available in kit form by Boehringer Mannheim Corp. This method was correlated by us with the Abell method (*7*) and gave the following correlation parameters: $y = -0.42 + 0.999x$ (y: Röschlau method, x: Abell method), $r = 0.99$, $s_{xy} = 4.09$,[1] n = 34. The comparison between our method and that of Röschlau et al. can be statistically summarized as follows: $y = 0.087 + 0.993x$ (where x is the method of Röschlau et al.), $r = 0.997$, $SD_d = 5.6$, n = 130. Their method was performed by us manually, while our method was performed on the Vickers D-300 according to the protocol illustrated in Table 2. We found the following statistical relationship between the method of Röschlau et al. and a manual Liebermann–Burchard (*8*) method, used routinely in our laboratory: $y = -21.61 +$

[1] s_{xy} is elsewhere (*9*) called SD_d.

$0.9829x$, $r = 0.9972$, $\bar{x} = 228.8$, $\bar{y} = 203.3$, $SD_d = 5.12$, $n = 56$. We think that very nearly the same statistical relationship must exist between our method and the above-mentioned comparison methods.

We hope we have given a useful indication to people interested in setting up economically an enzymatic method for determining total serum cholesterol.

We thank Dr. A. Peracino, Head, Servizio di Laboratorio per Ricerche Chimico-Cliniche e Microbiologiche, Ospedale Provinciale Consorziale di Treviglio e Caravaggio, for his invaluable help and suggestions at all stages of our study.

References

1. Tarbutton, P. N., and Gunter, C. R., Enzymatic determination of total cholesterol in serum. *Clin. Chem.* **20**, 724 (1974). Letter to the Editor.

2. Richmond, W., Preparation and properties of a cholesterol oxidase from *Nocardia* sp. and its application to the enzymatic assay of total cholesterol in serum. *Clin. Chem.* **19**, 1350 (1973).

3. Allain, C. C., Poon, L. S., Chan, C. S. G., et al., Enzymatic determination of total serum cholesterol. *Clin. Chem.* **20**, 470 (1974).

4. Allen, S. L., Allen, J. M., and Licht, B. M., Effect of Triton X-100 upon the activity of some electrophoretically separated acid phosphatases and esterases. *J. Histochem. Cytochem.* **13**, 434 (1965).

5. Röschlau, P., Bernt, E., and Gruber, W., Enzymatische Bestimmung des gesamt Cholesterin im Serum. *Z. Klin. Chem. Klin. Biochem.* **12**, 226 (1974).

6. Röschlau, P., Bernt, E., and Gruber, W., Enzymatic determination of total cholesterol in serum. Brochure edited by Boehringer Mannheim GmbH, Biochemica Werk Tutzing, 1974.

7. Abell, L. L., Levy, B. B., Brodie, B. B., and Kendall, F. E., Cholesterol in serum. *Stand. Methods Clin. Chem.* **2**, 26 (1958).

8. Spandrio, L., Analisi Biochimico-Cliniche, Piccin Editore, Padua, Italy, 1972, p 276; see also Huang, T. C., Chen, C. P., Wefler, V., and Raftery, A., A stable reagent for the Liebermann-Burchard reaction. Application to rapid serum cholesterol determination. *Anal. Chem.* **33**, 1405 (1961).

9. Westgard, J. O., and Hunt, M. R., Use and interpretation of common statistical tests in method-comparison studies. *Clin. Chem.* **19**, 49 (1973).

Francesco Zoppi
Domenico Fenili

Ospedale Provinciale Consorziale
24047 Treviglio, Italy

Collection of Blood Uncontaminated with Ca, Cu, Mg, or Zn, for Trace-Metal Analysis

To the Editor:

Contamination of blood samples that are to be assayed for trace-metals is a major problem unless stringent precautions are taken to eliminate it in equipment used to obtain and store blood specimens from the patient. For this reason, acid-washed glassware or plastic containers are usually used.

For mass screening of blood for trace-metals it would be convenient to collect blood in commercially available evacuated tubes, such as "Vacutainers" (Becton-Dickinson, Rutherford, N.J. 07070); however, these tubes contain significant amounts of zinc, predominantly in the rubber stopper (*1*), a finding we have confirmed and extended to include other brands of commercially available evacuated tubes.

We assayed three brands of tubes for calcium, copper, magnesium, and zinc by adding aliquots of a pool of human serum to 10 evacuated tubes from each of the commercial manufacturers, allowing it to remain in contact with the tubes for 45 min, and then assaying it for the metals of interest by atomic absorption spectroscopy. In every case, zinc contamination was detected in significant amounts. The results, including the associated standard deviations for the human serum pools, are shown in Table 1.

Table 1. Evaluation of Evacuated Blood-Collecting Tubes for Trace-Metal Contamination (Value: Mean of 10 Values)

	Brand		
	B-D[a]	Lab tube[b]	Venoject[c]
Ca, mg/dl[d]			
Before contact	9.7	9.7	9.7
After contact	9.6	9.7	9.8
Mg, mg/dl[d]			
Before contact	2.1	2.1	2.1
After contact	2.1	2.1	2.1
Cu, μg/dl[e]			
Before contact	105	105	133
After contact	105	104	135
Zn, μg/dl[f]			
Before contact	122	122	94
After contact	169	219	118

[a] Becton-Dickinson and Co., Rutherford, N.J. 07070
[b] Abbott Scientific Products Division, South Pasadena, Calif. 91030
[c] Kimble Glass Company, Toledo, Ohio 43601
[d] Method standard deviation = 0.1 mg/dl
[e] Method standard deviation = 3.2 μg/dl
[f] Method standard deviation = 3.5 μg/dl

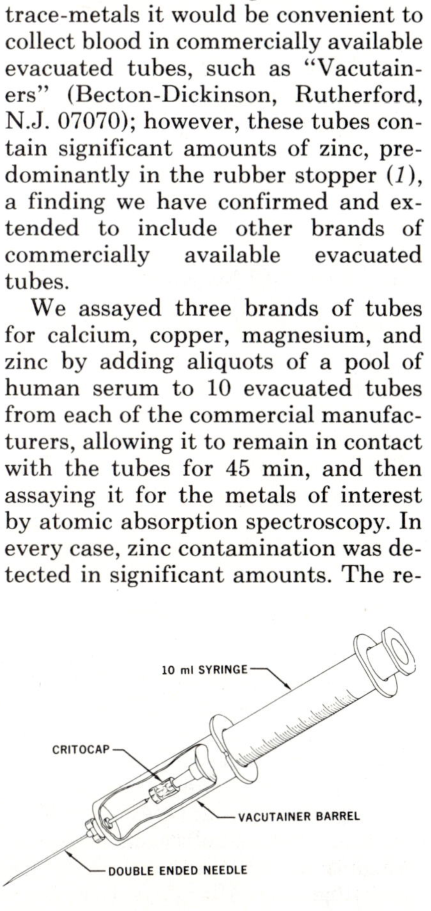

Fig. 1. 10-ml syringe with an attached "Critocap" inserted into a "Vacutainer" barrel

In our laboratory we must assay blood specimens for several metals, including zinc. However, the requirement for a large amount of blood to provide both serum and plasma for other tests precludes the use of zinc-free syringes for routine venipuncture.

Recently, a plastic tube closure, designed for use with glass capillary tubes, has become commercially available ("Critocap J"; Scientific Products, McGraw Park, Ill. 60085). This closure can be easily fitted on the nipple end of a 10-ml plastic syringe (Burron Medical Products, Inc., Bethlehem, Pa. 18018). The syringe can then be inserted into a Vacutainer barrel during the course of a multi-sample venipuncture. In this manner, blood can be drawn into the syringe and transferred to uncontaminated glass tubes (Figure 1).

We have determined that the Critocaps contain no calcium, copper, magnesium, or zinc. Ten of them were removed from five separate packages and attached to syringes. Aliquots of a human serum pool were drawn through Monoject 216 double-ended needles (Sherwood Medical Industries, Inc., Deland, Fla. 32720) into the syringes and transferred to glass tubes. These specimens were assayed for the metals by atomic absorption spectroscopy, and the results were compared to an aliquot of the pooled specimen that had not come into contact with the Critocaps. All other implements (needles, syringes, etc.), used in collecting and processing blood specimens for trace-metal analysis, were similarly examined, with negative results.

These tube closures can easily be used when multiphasic health screening is desired; we have used this method for six months, with no difficulties. The resulting data provide a more realistic normal range for trace-metals, particularly for serum zinc.

Reference

1. Helman, E. Z., Wallick, D. K., and Reingold, I. M., Vacutainer contamination in trace element studies. *Clin. Chem.* **17**, 61 (1971).

Robert O. Hughes
Dorothy F. Wease
Raymond G. Troxler

Clinical Pathology Branch/NGP
Clinical Sciences Division
USAF School of Aerospace Medicine
Brooks Air Force Base, Tex. 78235

Nonleakage of Radioiodide through Plastic

To the Editor:

In a recent Letter [*Clin. Chem.* **21**, 1691 (1975)] the implication was made that radioimmunoassays should not be run in polyethylene "Microfuge" tubes (Beckman 314326) because the tubes are permeable to free *iodine.* As described here, we have performed additional tests, which show that polyethylene tubes are permeable neither to iodine-labeled antigens nor to radiolabeled iodide ion, and that free $^{125}I_2$ is not produced in measurable quantities by radiolysis of ^{125}I-labeled antigens. We conclude that the problem cited in the earlier note is caused by the specific reagent systems used in that study and is not applicable to recommended radioimmunoassay practice, where free iodine is prudently avoided.

We tested three types of plastic tubes for permeability to radiolabeled antigens: the 400-μl polyethylene Microfuge tube (Beckman 314326), 1.5-ml polyethylene Microfuge B tube (Beckman 338802), and the 1.5-ml polypropylene Microfuge B tube (Sarstedt 39/10). To measure the migration of antigen through these tubes, we put 200 μl of radiolabeled antigen into the smaller tube and 1.0 ml of radiolabeled antigen into the two larger tubes. For each labeled antigen tested, the specified amount of material was added to each of five tubes. After capping, we suspended the tubes inside a 12 × 55 mm "Biovial" counting vial containing enough water to immerse the liquid portion of the inner vial. After 188 h at room temperature, the inner vials were removed and the radioactivity in the Biovials was counted for 10 min. With 10-min counts and five replicates for each antigen, we were able to detect as little as 5 counts per minute above background. In all cases this represented a limit of detectability of 0.01% to 0.02% of the added radioactivity.

The above experiment was performed on samples of freshly prepared ^{125}I-labeled T4, TSH, T3, and digoxin used routinely in Beckman radioimmunoassay test kits. To test the hypothesis that covalently bound iodine is converted to free iodine by radiolysis, we also tested samples of ^{125}I-labeled T4, TSH, and digoxin that were prepared 12 weeks before testing. For all seven antigen samples run in the three different plastic tubes at room temperature for 188 h, we were unable to detect *any* radioactive leakage through the tubes, within the limits of detectability (0.02%).

A similar experiment was run with a solution of carrier-free $Na^{125}I$ as the sample. Incubation time in this experiment was 48 h and counting time was 1 min. Under these conditions, 171 ± 70 counts above background of the original radioactivity migrated through the polyethylene Microfuge B tube (Beckman 31436), a migration of 0.17 ± 0.07% of the original sample. The other tubes showed no detectable migration of $Na^{125}I$ under the same test conditions.

It is not surprising to find that free iodine will permeate polyethylene. Iodine is a nonpolar molecule, relatively insoluble in water (0.34 g/liter), and very soluble in organic solvents (benzene, 100 g/liter; alcohol, 80 g/liter; carbon tetrachloride, 19 g/liter). On the basis of its solubility alone, one would suspect that iodine could migrate through hydrocarbon plastics such as polyethylene, polypropylene, and even polystyrene.

The migration observed by M. Kuhn and F. Naftolin with ^{125}I-labeled follitropin can be explained if one assumes the original sample contained some free $^{125}I_2$. This would not be surprising, because the Chloramine T iodination method used to synthesize the ^{125}I-labeled follitropin is known to result in the formation of free iodine under certain conditions, by oxidation of iodide with Chloramine T.

In summary, our experiments indicate that iodide ion and ^{125}I-labeled T4, T3, TSH, and digoxin do not permeate Microfuge or Microfuge B tubes. Further, there is no indication that significant quantities of free $^{125}I_2$ are formed by radiolysis of the labeled antigens tested. We have used these Microfuge and Microfuge B tubes in the development and evaluation of new radioimmunoassays as well as in routine testing with no difficulties of the nature described in the Letter. We conclude, therefore, that the Microfuge and Microfuge B tubes are indeed appropriate for micro- and semi-micro radioimmunoassays in which the volume requirements do not exceed 1.0 ml.

William W. Miller

Beckman Instruments, Inc.
Scientific Instruments Division
Irvine, Calif. 92664

Plasma Renin Activity and Radioimmunoassay of Angiotensin I (cont.)

To the Editor:

Following the publication of the "Selected Method" for plasma renin activity (PRA) (*1*), we submitted our comments to the senior author as well as to the Chairman of the AACC Committee on Selected Methods. Two comments (*2*, *3*) have appeared thus far in *Clinical Chemistry* as Letters to the Editor and we wish to comment now in a similar fashion.

The angiotensin I generation step in the assay of PRA has been the subject of intense controversy both at the academic and commercial levels and is clearly in need of standardization. Until such time, Schwarz/Mann will retain and recommend for its PRA protocol generation of angiotensin I at physiological pH. The user may, of course, disregard our recommendation and use the kit reagents solely for assaying angiotensin I.

The Schwarz/Mann protocol for the generation of angiotensin I by plasma renin calls for the addition of 0.1 ml of 4 mol/liter Tris chloride buffer to 1 ml of plasma containing EDTA, 8-hydroxyquinoline, and dimercaprol as inhibitors of angiotensinase. It has been shown that at pH 7.4, the pH of the buffered plasma, this choice of inhibitors will assure survival of angiotensin I during incubation at 37 °C (*4*). The small volume of buffer added to the plasma avoids a dilution effect upon the activity of the enzyme while its buffering capacity assures constancy of pH, a critical parameter disregarded in the Selected Method (*1*). Rate of generation varies with the pH of the plasma and buffering is essential. Some unbuffered plasmas may attain a pH of greater than 8 upon storage, with a resulting inactivation of renin (*5*). The incubation time in the Schwarz/Mann protocol is 3 h. Linearity of generation for as much as 5 h has been found for pools of plasma of both low and high PRA, buffered as described at pH 7.4.

On theoretical grounds, suboptimal generation of angiotensin I at pH 7.4 not only mimics in vivo conditions, but should also lessen substrate depletion in the substantial number of normal plasmas containing insufficient substrate for renin saturation. The rate constants for angiotensin I generation (K_m) under antibody capture conditions have indeed been shown to be less affected at pH 7.4 than at pH 5.5 (*5, 6*). Dramatic decreases in K_m as a function of decreasing substrate concentration were noted in both cases on prolonged (18-h) incubations.

The potential complications arising from the physiological variability of both substrate and renin levels concentrations, reviewed in the Letter of Heise (*2*), further underscore the need for standardization of generation conditions or development of the more significant PRC (direct-renin) assays.

Our PRA kit contains a highly purified monoiodinated angiotensin I prepared by a modification of the method of Nielsen et al. (*7*). However, we label to high specific activity and completely remove unlabeled, diiodinated, and damaged peptides. The Schwarz/Mann tracer is highly immunoreactive (typically, 90%) and has high specific activity (typically, 1000–1200 Ci/g). A new lot must meet radiochemical specifications for purity and limits of impurities (iodide and ^{125}I-labeled angiotensin II) as well as kit functionality tests comprising B_0, max. B_0, slope, and intercept. Each new tracer is also cross-checked against a previously accepted lot of tracer, with use of the same antiserum and standards. Stability tests are routinely conducted for the duration of the kit shelf life as part of our re-assay program. Storage of the radioactive angiotensin I in our laboratory for two half-lives (four months) has shown that the product can still be used in the radioimmunoassay of angiotensin I.

We feel that preparation of ^{125}I-labeled angiotensin I by individual users, as recommended by Latta (*3*), cannot be justified on economic or technical grounds. The user currently has a choice of at least three unit sizes costing $1.60 to $25 per μCi, depending on the quantity, and availability, from at least two reliable manufacturers. Potential personnel, equipment, and laboratory contamination must also be considered when handling millicurie quantities of $Na^{125}I$ in the Hunter–Greenwood iodination.

The angiotensin I used for the preparation of standards was synthesized in our laboratory by a solid-phase technique and characterized with respect to homogeneity, amino acid composition, and bioactivity. Solutions are calibrated spectrophotometrically and then diluted to prepare the kit standards. In our quality-control program, each new preparation of kit standard is cross-checked against a previously accepted lot of standard, using in each case the same preparations of antiserum and tracer. In order for a lot to be accepted for inclusion in a new kit, it must compare favorably with the previous lot and the assay data must meet all applicable specifications.

Early Schwarz/Mann preparations dating back to 1972 and 1973 were formulated with carrier proteins containing trace amounts of peptidase impurities, which selectively degraded angiotensin I and caused the reported variability in the standards (*8–10*) and in some tracer lots. The observed presence of peptidases even in some highly purified, crystalline carrier proteins necessitated implementation of strict quality-control tests for the selection of suitable lots (*11*). Our records show that our methods of standardization, interlot cross checks, and carrier selection have reduced interlot variation in our kit standards to insignificant levels. In addition, reassays of standards at one- and two-month intervals have shown no loss of potency for standards contained in our kits during the past two years.

We have surveyed the standards in a number of commercially available PRA kits and also have found variability of potency of the angiotensin I standards. In a comparison of these standards with angiotensin I (9 μg/ampoule) obtained from the National Institute of Biological Standards and Control, Mill Hill, England, we have found the following relationship:

Standard	Relative potency at 50% B_0: Schwarz/Mann data 8/73	Schwarz/Mann data 12/74	Hospital laboratory data 2/75
Mill Hill	100	100	100
Schwarz/Mann	79	82	89
Source A	—	38	29
Source B	55	—	58
Source C	67	—	—
Source D	46	—	—
Source E	10	—	—

Although the Mill Hill angiotensin I has not been established as a standard for radioimmunoassay it does serve as a point of reference in the preparation of kit standards.

High-affinity antisera are selected for our PRA kit. The current antiserum (K_a = 6.2 × 10^{10}; titer in assay, 1/60 000) has been used in our kits for more than two years and will detect 10 pg of angiotensin I at 90% B_0 while another antiserum (K_a = 5.6 × 10^{10}; titer in assay, 1/150 000) planned for future kits will detect 5 pg.

The sensitivity of these antisera permits efficient detection of the relatively lower PRA levels of angiotensin I generated at pH 7.4 and the accurate determination of low PRA values, approximately 0.035 ng/ml per hour. The antisera do not demand, for the RIA, generation of larger amounts of angiotensin I at an acidic pH in order to develop detectable levels of angiotensin. In addition, generation at pH 7.4, which is compatible with the quality of these antisera, avoids risks involved in adjusting of the pH of plasma to an acidic pH, such as dilution of the substrate and destruction of renin by careless acidifications.

The generation of PRA and the RIA of angiotensin require skill and care on the part of the analyst. Data obtained in our laboratory with our kits show that the standard curves, prepared as logit-log plots, are reproducible and that a wide range of plasma renin activities can be measured.

Proposals have been made to standardize conditions for the PRA and the RIA (*5*). Standardization may be forthcoming and this may demonstrate value for both manufacturers and users. We feel confident that Schwarz/Mann radioimmunoassay reagents can also meet the future requirements of a standardized RIA methodology for PRA.

References

1. Lash, B., and Fleischer, M., Radioimmunoassay of angiotensin I, for estimation of plasma renin activity. *Clin. Chem.* **20**, 620 (1974). Selected Method.

2. Heise, C. M., Measurement of plasma renin activity. *Clin. Chem.* **21**, 447 (1975). Letter to the Editor.

3. Latta, J., Improved measurement of plasma renin activity and concentration. *Clin. Chem.* **21**, 1344 (1975). Letter to the Editor.

4. Oparil, S., Koerner, T. J. and Haber, E., Effects of pH and enzyme inhibitors on apparent generation of angiotensin I in human plasma. *J. Clin. Endocrinol. Metab.* **39**, 965 (1974).

5. Poulsen, K., Important factors and pitfalls in radioimmunoassay for renin and angiotensin. Symposium: Measurement of angiotensin I and renin. Sponsored by SCOR (Hypertension), National Heart and Lung Institute, Cleveland, Oct. 9 and 10, 1974.

6. Poulsen, K., Kinetics of the renin system. The basis for determination of the different components of the system. *Scand. J. Clin. Lab. Invest.* **31**, *Suppl.* 132 (1973).

7. Nielsen, M. D., Jorgensen, M., and Giese, J., ^{125}I-Labeling of angiotensin I and II. *Acta Endocrinol.* (Copenhagen) **67**, 104 (1971).

8. Viol, G. W., Keane, P. M., Speed, J. F., and Smith, E. K. M., Assay of plasma renin activity using commercially available reagents. *Clin. Biochem.* **5**, 251 (1972).

9. Sealey, J. E., and Laragh, J. H., Searching out low renin patients: Limitations of some commonly used methods. *Am. J. Med.* **55**, 303 (1973).

10. Goldberg, S. D., and Spierto, F. W., Plasma renin activity: A method for rapid screening by radioimmunoassay and a comparison of two commercially available kits. *Clin. Chem.* **19**, 1396 (1973).

11. Rutner, H., Gutcho, S., Johnson, J., and Dodd, T., Peptidase activity of carrier proteins used in radioimmunoassays. *J. Nucl. Med.* **15**, 557 (1974).

Herman Rutner
Sidney Gutcho

Schwarz/Mann
Division of Becton, Dickinson and Co.
Orangeburg, N. Y. 10962

Ethchlorvynol Interference with Oxidimetric Determination of Ethanol in Urine

To the Editor:

Gas-chromatographic methods for ethanol quantitation provide greater specificity than traditional oxidimetric methods. The specificity of oxidimetric methods such as those of Kozelka–Hine (*1*) and Widmark (*2*) rely on the arguments that: (a) the sample came from a living person and (b) drugs or chemicals that would appreciably react with potassium dichromate could not be expected to be present in a living person, or that (c) interfering substances present are removed by chemical reaction (Kozelka–Hine) or constraints of the reaction conditions (Widmark).

Such reasoning has received the blessing of the California Administration Code in its regulations on Forensic Alcohol Analysis:

> §1220.1.4 The method shall be capable of the analysis of ethyl alcohol with a specificity which is adequate and appropriate for traffic law enforcement and
>
> §1220.1.4 Blood alcohol results on post mortem samples shall not be reported unless the oxidizable substance is identified as ethyl alcohol by qualitative test.

Our laboratory recently received an alcohol-free urine that gave an appreciable value for apparent ethanol by Kozelka–Hine oxidimetric analyses. The subject, a 28-year-old man, was arrested at 12:30 p.m. after leaving the scene of an accident in which he struck a legally parked vehicle. Blood and urine were obtained at 1:30 p.m.

The blood and the urine were both examined by an automated gas-chromatographic procedure (Hewlett-Packard) and found negative for alcohol. The urine was also analyzed in duplicate by the method of Kozelka–Hine and showed an apparent ethanol concentration of 600 and 700 mg/liter in the two analyses.

The urine was found negative for opiates and cocaine (Enzyme Multipled Immunoassay Technique). The blood was examined for common sedatives found in cases of impaired driving (*3*). Ethchlorvynol was identified by the Haux reaction (*4*) and by gas chromatography.

Ethchlorvynol in the blood was quantitated at about 10 mg/liter by a modification (ethyl acetate extraction) of the method of Haux.

The urine was examined and found to contain about 2000 mg of ethchlorvynol per liter. An aliquot of the sample was examined by another forensic laboratory by the method of Wallace et al. (*5*) and reported as 1750 mg/liter.

Standard ethchlorvynol solutions of these concentrations did not produce the oxidation reaction observed in the subject's urine, indicating that the observed interferences may, in part, be attributed to metabolites.

Although the interference encountered in this case produced a noticeable discoloration of the mercuric oxide "scrubber" tube in the Kozelka–Hine apparatus, which signaled to the analyst that some interference was probably present, this should be considered a potential source of error for similar methods of analysis for alcohol in urine.

References

1. Kozelka, F., and Hine, C., Method for determination of ethyl alcohol for medicolegal purposes. *Ind. Eng. Chem.* **13**, 905 (1941).

2. Smith, H., The specificity of the desiccation method for determining alcohol in biological fluids. *J. Lab. Clin. Med.* **38**, 762 (1951).

3. White, J., and Graves, M., The detection of sedative/hypnotic drugs in the impaired driver. *J. Chromatogr. Sci.* **12**, 219 (1974).

4. Haux, P., Ethchlorvynol (Placidyl) estimation in urine and serum. *Clin. Chim. Acta* **48**, 139 (1972).

5. Wallace, J., et al., A rapid and specific method for determining ethchlorvynol. *J. Forensic Sci.* **9**, 342 (1964).

James M. White

Orange County Sheriff–Coroner
Laboratory of Criminalistics
550 N. Flower St.
Santa Ana, Calif. 92702

Computer Program for Serum Protein Electrophoresis Calculations

To the Editor:

The Hewlett-Packard 65 Pocket Calculator has true programming capability in that it is able to store and automatically execute the steps required to solve a particular problem. These steps can be stored on a magnetic card that is loaded into the calculator, which then produces the program after the data have been keyed in.

A program of 79 steps has been prepared for doing all the calculations usually performed in serum electrophoresis. The input data consist of the integration counts from the densitometer for the five common protein bands—albumin, α_1, α_2, β, and γ-globulins—and the total serum protein concentration is determined chemically. The computer calculates the percent of total and the grams per deciliter for each protein constituent, and the albumin/globulin ratio.

I will be glad to send any one interested the program description and listing of the 79 steps, with user instructions, upon receipt of a stamped, self-addressed, number 10 envelope. The calculations can be done on the HP-65, for which the user can prepare his own magnetic card, and also on the HP-55 calculator, into which the programs can be keyed, but which does not permit the use of magnetic cards.

Arthur L. Levy

Chemistry Laboratory
St. Vincent's Hospital &
Medical Center of New York
153 W. 11th St.
New York, N.Y. 10011

Interference with Serotonin Determination

To the Editor:

Waalkes [*J. Lab. Clin. Med.* **53**, 824 (1957)] suggested the use of a "mixed-salt" of anhydrous sodium sulfate and trisodium phosphate for the recovery of serotonin from blood. We found that the combined salt reagent did indeed greatly improve our results in the estimation of serotonin in human platelets at the subnanogram level by fluorometry. Recently we have found that sodium sulfate purchased from J. T. Baker or Fisher Scientific contains a substance which gives a very high "blank" so that it is difficult to overcome its interference even at the nanogram level. We have found that Matheson Coleman & Bell's sodium sulfate is free of this contamination. We recommend the Waalkes "mixed-salt" for serotonin estimation in any body fluid or tissue, but suggest a check of the sodium sulfate be run through the procedure before use with biological materials.

Gregory S. Duboff

The Thomas Henry Simpson
Memorial Institute for
Medical Research
The University of Michigan
Ann Arbor, Mich. 48109

Table 1. Observed vs. Calculated Vitamin A Values[a]

Drug	No.	Observed av.	Calcd. av.	t	P
No drug	129	38.7	39.1	0.51	N.S.
Diphenylhydantoin	195	41.5	39.1	3.24	<0.01
Isosorbide dinitrate	4	62.4	42.5	3.78	<0.01
Phenobarbital	259	40.7	38.8	2.84	<0.01
Thioridazine	267	44.1	40.5	5.37	<0.001

[a] "Drug" is the medication received regardless of dose, schedule or other medication; "number" is the number of individuals receiving this medication; "observed" and "calculated" averages are explained in the text; t is the Student's t-value for matched pairs; and P is the probability. "N.S." is not significant.

Effects of Medication on Plasma Vitamin A Concentrations

To the Editor:

In the recent tabulation of effects of drugs on clinical laboratory tests by Young et al. (*1*), two drugs are shown to increase serum vitamin A concentrations and two to decrease them.

In 1974 we surveyed 1018 mentally retarded individuals for plasma vitamin A concentrations, by the method of Thompson et al. (*2*). As a part of this survey, we recorded the medication each patient was receiving at the time the blood was drawn. Because most of the patients were on long-term medication, it was impossible to establish premedication vitamin A values. Curtis and Swicord (*3*) have demonstrated that vitamin A concentrations in serum are a function of sex and age and that this relationship can be expressed mathematically to yield a calculated vitamin A value. We used their formula to calculate what the normal drug-free vitamin A value would be for each individual.

We divided the population by drug (regardless of amount, schedule, or any other medication) and compared the observed and calculated values for vitamin A for each individual by use of the paired t-test (*4*). As a control on our approach, we also compared those within the population who were drug free, using the same procedure. The observed and calculated values for the no-drug population of 129 were not significantly different and the average values differed by about 1% (Table 1).

As shown in Table 1, diphenylhydantoin, isosorbide dinitrate, phenobarbital, and thioridazine cause a highly significant increase in values for plasma vitamin A. (Thirty-six other medications had no apparent influence on vitamin A values).

This increase could either be the result of a measurement artifact caused by the presence of the medication or an in vivo increase in the homeostatic control level. We added 1 mg/100 ml of each of the drugs to drug-free plasma and again checked the apparent vitamin A. Only thioridazine caused an increased value. The apparent increased vitamin A concentrations in individuals taking the other drugs is probably a change in the homeostatic level.

Obviously this was purely a retrospective study. However, these data indicate that more investigations in the area of drug/vitamin A interaction are needed and indicate that four additional drugs influence actual or apparent plasma vitamin A values.

References

1. Young, D. S., Pestaner, L. C., and Gibberman, V., Effects of drugs on clinical laboratory tests. *Clin. Chem.* **21**, 387D (1975) (Special Issue).
2. Thompson, J. N., Erdody, R., and Maxwell, W. N., Simultaneous fluorometric determination of vitamin A and E in human serum and plasma. *Biochem. Med.* **8**, 403 (1973).
3. Curtis, J. L., and Swicord, W. F., Plasma vitamin A levels—a diagnostic indicator of hepatitis in an institutionalized mentally retarded population. *Am. J. Ment. Defic.*, in press.
4. Roscoe, J. T., *Fundamental Research Statistics for Behavioral Sciences.* Holt, Rinehart, & Winston, New York, N.Y., 1969.

Jerry L. Curtis
Wynette Swicord

Research Department
Regional Mental Health Center
Central State Hospital
Milledgeville, Ga. 31061

Enzymatic Determination of Cholesterol in High-Density Lipoprotein Fractions Prepared by Polyanion Precipitation

To the Editor:

The Note of Steele et al. (*1*) was of great interest to me because we have had the same problem for almost a year. When we started to assay the HDL-cholesterol of the local population by the enzymatic technique we quickly realized that the heparin–manganese procedure produced too high and irreproducible results. We are running our cholesterol and triglyceride determinations on a two-channel AutoAnalyzer (Technicon), using the enzyme solutions from Boehringer (Mannheim). Because control experiments demonstrated that heparin by itself had no influence on the assay, we circumvented the problem with Mn^{2+} salts, not by adding chelating agents (EDTA) to the solutions, but rather by searching for a substitute bivalent cation. After trial and error it was found that the method described below gave reliable and repducible results: 1 ml of serum (not plasma) was mixed with 50 μl of 2 mol/liter $MgCl_2$ and 50 μl of a 20 g/liter solution of dextran sulfate 500 (Pharmacia), allowed to stand for 5 min, and centrifuged. By immunochemical techniques we ascertained that this method precipitated quantitatively all the VLDL plus LDL up to a serum concentration of at least 20 g/liter. The excess of $MgCl_2$ had no influence on the enzymatic cholesterol assay and neither had the dextran sulfate. We isolated some HDL (*d* 1.065–1.121) by preparative ultracentrifugation (*2*) and assayed them with the AutoAnalyzer at various concentrations in the presence and absence of the precipitating agents. Absolutely no difference was found for results for cholesterol and triglycerides. The coefficient of variation of our enzymatic assay (day-to-day) is less than 3% for cholesterol, less than 4% for triglycerides. In addition it is possible to solubilize the precipitated VLDL + LDL in 0.1 mol/liter sodium citrate and assay them directly on the machine as a separate control. In all cases the sum of VLDL + LDL and HDL cholesterol was 97–103% of the value for the parent serum.

We therefore propose as an alternative to the procedure described by Steel et al. (*1*) to change the precipitating agents and use the enzyme solutions in the conventional way. An additional advantage of this procedure might be that no background staining at all is produced by dextran sulfate–$MgCl_2$; an apparent cholesterol of 10 ± 6 mg/liter in the HDL-reagent blank is reported from the heparin–Mn^{2+} procedure (*1*).

References

1. Steele, W. B., Koehler, D. F., Azar, M. M., et al., Enzymatic determinations of cholesterol in high-density-lipoprotein fractions prepared by a precipitation technique. *Clin. Chem.* **22**, 98 (1976).
2. Kostner, G., and Alaupovic, P., Studies of the composition and structure of plasma lipoproteins. Separation and quantification of lipoprotein families occurring in the high density lipoproteins of human plasma. *Biochemistry* **11**, 3419 (1972).

Gerhard M. Kostner

Institute of Medical Biochemistry
University of Graz
A-8010 Graz, Austria

Circle No. 389 on Reader's Service Card

book reviews

Urinalysis in Clinical Laboratory Practice. A. H. Free and H. M. Free. CRC Press, Inc., Cleveland, Ohio 44128, 1975, 284 pp. $47.50.

The authors' avowed purpose is to present information relating to the practical utility of urine study, and it would seem that this objective has been met. This volume is not a manual of laboratory procedures, but rather a compendium of information relative to the diagnostic potential of various urinary studies.

The book is organized into 50 separate sections, beginning with historical considerations of urinalysis and its implications and terminating in speculation on future potential of urine study. Included in the chapters are considerations of virtually all sorts of urinary study, ranging from urinary bacteriology and cytology through toxicology and hormone assays.

This book is probably of primary interest to those responsible for training of laboratory technicians who will be engaged in various analytic studies of urine. Indeed, one chapter deals with "Creative Approaches to Teaching Urinalysis", which will be of interest not only to the laboratory technician but to the instructor as well. The most significant criticism might be the price of this volume, which is only of average quality and lacks any color illustrations or other embellishments.

James F. Glenn

Division of Urologic Surgery
Duke University Medical Center
Durham, N. C. 27710

Normal Values in Clinical Chemistry. A Guide to Statistical Analysis of Laboratory Data. H. F. Martin, B. J. Gudzinowicz, and H. Fanger. Eds. Marcel Dekker, Inc., New York, N. Y. 10016. viii + 504 pp. $37.50.

The authors intend that this book has practical application in clinical laboratories and bring to it considerable statistical and clinical chemical experience. The subtitle of the book is a better indication of its content than its main title.

The book consists of only six chapters. The first is an interesting historical review of the concept of normal ranges. The second chapter is the only one in which the various factors that are known to influence laboratory data, other than a disease state, are mentioned. Yet these are mentioned in passing only, and adherents to the concept of reference values must feel that their viewpoint has been given short shrift. The third chapter includes simple rules to cope with both gaussian and nongaussian distribution of raw data. Methods for assuring quality assurance of analytical methods are also presented. The fourth chapter is a discussion of the influence of physiological variation and analytical error on normal ranges. The authors discuss several tests, each of which is affected by different physiological processes, e.g., BSP and creatinine clearances, and plasma cortisol. In the fifth chapter the authors develop "normal ranges" from typical hospital populations. In this chapter the authors discuss the Neumann, Bhattacharya, and Hoffman procedures for dissecting mixed populations. The authors also evaluate the Gram–Charlier series for isolating a "normal" population from a population containing both healthy and sick individuals. The final chapter is concerned with specificity and sensitivity of analytical methods in detecting disease with a discussion of the cause of false positive and negative indications. Each of the chapters is supported by a comprehensive bibliography and the book contains both detailed author and subject indices.

The book is simply written and is easy to follow. The content is presented in a logical sequence and the book provides all the information that a laboratory director need know to develop "normal ranges" from the mixed laboratory data that he is likely to produce in his laboratory. Whether these are the best data to use for the interpretation of patient values remains to be tested. This is a book that should be read by laboratory scientists. It should remove much of their doubts and suspicions of the statistical manipulation of laboratory data.

Donald S. Young

Clinical Chemistry Laboratory
NIH, Bethesda, Md. 20014

Books Received

Chemical Cycles and the Global Environment—Assessing Human Influences. R. M. Garrels, F. T. Mackenzie, C. Hunt. William Kaufmann, Inc., Los Altos, Calif. 94022. 222 pp. Paperback, $4.95. Pub. 1975.

Quantitative Analysis by Gas Chromatography, 5 (Chromatographic Science Series). J. Novák. Marcel Dekker, Inc., New York, N. Y. 10016. ix + 218 pp. $16.75. Pub. Sept. 1975. "This book is devoted primarily to the theoretical aspects of the problem; the main goal is to show that gas chromatography can be looked upon as a self-contained analytical discipline having its own consistent theory. Includes evaluation of result reliability."

Subunits in Biological Systems (Biological Macromolecules Series Volume 7—Part C). S. N. Timasheff and G. D. Fasman, Eds. Marcel Dekker, Inc., New York, N. Y. 10016. vii + 343 pp. $39.50. Pub. Nov. 1975.

the clinical chemist

Compiled by J. S. King, Executive Editor

AACC Award Winners, 1976

Norman G. Anderson will receive the 1976 *AACC Award for Outstanding Contributions to Clinical Chemistry,* sponsored by the Ames Co., at the 28th National Meeting of the AACC. This will be the 25th year that this award has been given.

Dr. Anderson is a native of Davenport, Washington, and obtained his B.A., M.A., and Ph.D. degrees from Duke University. His research interests are many, a basic one being the description of cell function and cell pathology at the molecular level. He has been concerned with the development of some of the instrumentation and separations systems required for this purpose, including the zonal ultracentrifuge (1955–1968), high-pressure chromatography for nucleic acid derivatives and urinary constituents, development of large-scale continuous-flow-with-banding ultracentrifuges for the large-scale purification of influenza and other viral vaccines (1964–68), development of the GeMSAEC computer-interfaced centrifugal analyzer (1968–71); development of methods for protein concentration dependent on the Mazur effect (1973–74); and development of cyclum systems for cyclic affinity chromatography (1972–74). The GeMSAEC has become a valuable and unique tool in the clinical laboratory. A miniaturized version, which occupies only one cubic foot, was developed for NASA's Skylab program.

Dr. Anderson has over 300 publications in cell physiology and fractionation, virus and vaccine purification, zonal and vaccine centrifuge development, high-pressure chromatography, centrifugal analyzer development, and fetal antigens in cancer and immunochemistry.

He has received many awards: the Van Slyke Award from the New York Section of the AACC, 1974; West Germany Academy of Sciences, 1973; Biomedical Engineering Society, 1973; John Scott Medal and Award, 1972, for the invention of the zonal ultracentrifuge (previous winners include Fleming, Land, J. J. Thompson, and Madame Curie); AEC Citation for contributions to the development of the influenza vaccine, 1972; award from the German Association for Clinical Chemistry for the GeMSAEC Analyzer as the most outstanding analytical advance worldwide in biochemical and clinical analysis during a two-year period, 1972; Eli Lilly Lectureship; Sigma Xi Award; IR100 Award; and a Special Citation by Edward Steichen for submarine photography.

In keeping with his many interests, Dr. Anderson belongs to a variety of societies: AACC, American Association for the Advancement of Science, American Institute of Biological Sciences, American Association for Cancer Research, American Physiological Society, Academy of Clinical Laboratory Physicians and Scientists, Biophysics Society, Biomedical Engineering Society, Society of Experimental Biology and Medicine, and the Society of General Physiologists.

Dr. Anderson was the Director of the Molecular Anatomy Program at Oak Ridge National Laboratory, 1968–1975, and a faculty member of the University of Tennessee–Oak Ridge Graduate School of Biomedical Sciences. His present position is Professor, Department of Surgery, Medical University of South Carolina, Charleston, South Carolina, and Associate Director for Basic Sciences, South Carolina Memorial Cancer Institute.

Robert S. Melville will receive the 1976 (eleventh) *AACC Award for Outstanding Contributions Through Service to Clinical Chemistry as a Profession,* sponsored by the Fisher Scientific Co.

Dr. Melville, originally from Worcester, Massachusetts, received his A.B. from Clark University and his Ph.D. degree from the State University of Iowa. Before joining the National Institute of General Medical Sciences in 1965, where he has served as Chief of the Automated Clinical Laboratory Section in the Biomedical Engineering Program since 1968, Dr. Melville progressed from research chemist at Massachusetts General Hospital to Chief Biochemist at St. Luke's Hospital, Chicago, via the Department of Biochemistry at the State University of Iowa, where he was a research assistant. He was also with the Veterans Administration for several years, where he served as chief bio-

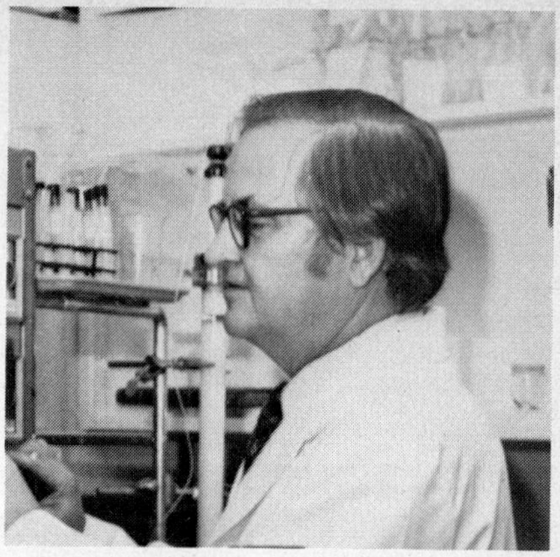

Norman G. Anderson

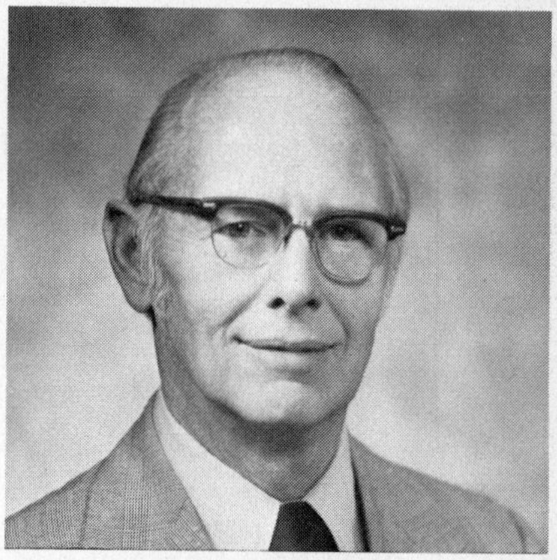

Robert S. Melville

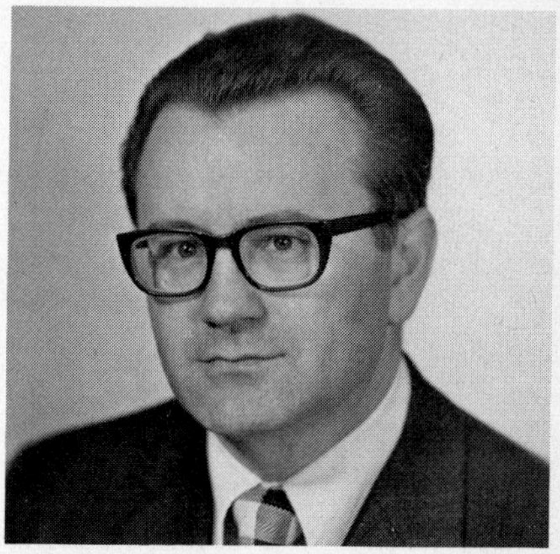

Norbert W. Tietz

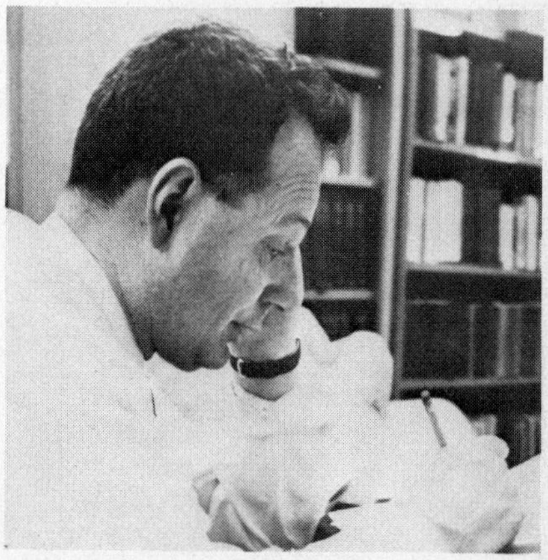

Nathan O. Kaplan

chemist at the VA Hospital in Iowa City and in the Central Office in Washington, D.C.

Dr. Melville has been active in the AACC for the past 25 years. He was its president in 1970–71, and has been a diplomate of the American Board of Clinical Chemists since 1952. He received the Joseph H. Roe Award in 1972 from the Capital Section, AACC. This award, sponsored by the American Instrument Co., is presented in recognition of contributions in the field of clinical chemistry.

Dr. Melville has a sustained record of unique contributions to the field of clinical chemistry, especially in recent years, which have by themselves greatly enhanced recognition of clinical chemistry and its standing as a separate discipline. Three of these many accomplishments deserve special mention. As Chief Biochemist of the Veterans Administration, Dr. Melville instituted policies and practices relating to clinical chemistry that endure to this day and that have done much to strengthen staffing and operational patterns in the clinical laboratory services of VA Hospitals all over the country.

Dr. Melville's outstanding contribution to the field of laboratory science is the major role he has played in the creation of a national program for the automation of clinical laboratories, in particular clinical chemistry laboratories. In 1968, he helped begin the national program on automated clinical laboratory sciences at the National Institute of General Medical Sciences of the NIH, and established the Automation in the Medical Laboratory Sciences Review Committee, which has reviewed and recommended funding of several of the most outstanding practical developments in the field. These include the Standard Reference Materials Program at the National Bureau of Standards, the development of the GeMSAEC centrifugal analyzer in collaboration with the Atomic Energy Commission at the Oak Ridge National Laboratory and (at an earlier time) the review of training and fellowship grants in clinical chemistry. The overall effect has been to interest many highly qualified young scientists in this important field. In addition, with Dr. Charles D. Scott of the Oak Ridge National Laboratory, Dr. Melville originated and has co-chaired the annual Oak Ridge *Symposia on Advanced Analytical Concepts for the Clinical Laboratory.* Now in their eighth year, these symposia provide a major forum for the interchange of ideas between basic and clinical laboratory scientists and members of the industrial sector.

Dr. Melville has been a highly effective and stabilizing influence in the provision of credentials for clinical chemists for some years. A founder of the National Registry in Clinical Chemistry and its immediate past-president, he has helped to develop and expand that program for more than 1000 persons working in clinical chemistry laboratories. As a director and current vice president of the American Board of Clinical Chemistry, he has also participated in the formulation of policies and practices that have greatly expanded and extended the peer system of providing credentials at the top of the profession through certification of ABCC diplomates.

In addition to his activities in clinical chemistry, Dr. Melville is a senior member of the Instrument Society of America, a member of the Association for Advancement of Medical Instrumentation, a fellow of the American Institute of Chemists, and the American Association for the Advancement of Science, and a member of the American Chemical Society, Sigma XI, Phi Lambda Upsilon, Gamma Alpha, and the American Society of Biomedical Engineering.

Norbert W. Tietz will receive the 1976 *AACC Award for Outstanding Efforts in Education and Training* sponsored by SmithKline Corp. This

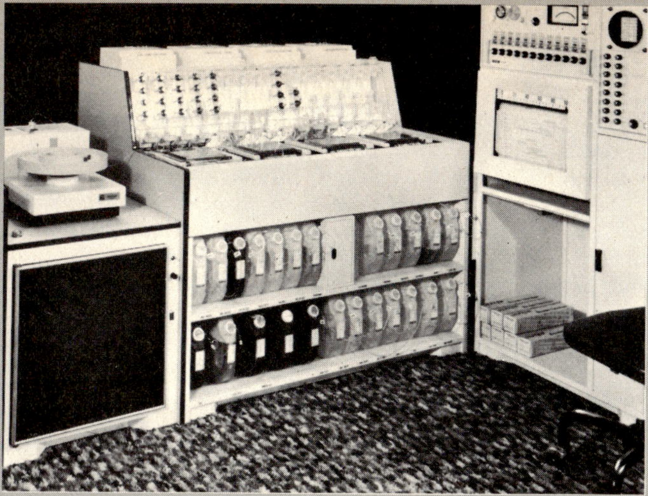

We sell very few "used" 12/60's.... most of them are fully reconditioned!

(and warranted)

Our used 12/60 systems are very low in price — our reconditioned systems are a little more. We put an exhaustive amount of work into our reconditioned systems so we can warrant them for 90 days and provide you with references of very satisfied customers. Our only business is support of Auto Analyzer* systems. We manufacture reagents and accessories, provide exchange modules, can even put Triglycerides on your 12/60.

EXCHANGE PUMP?

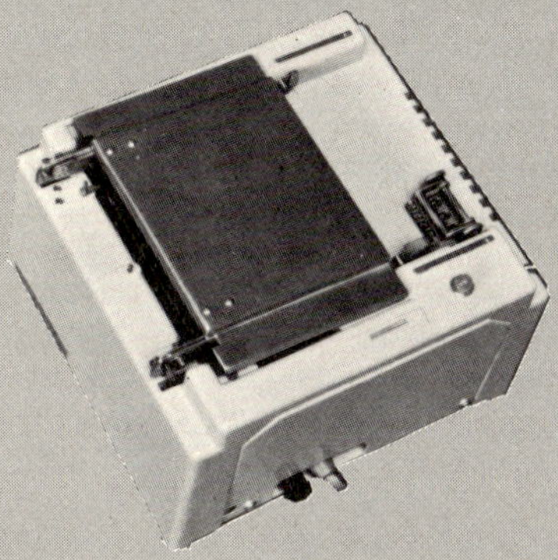

Is the pump III on your 12/60 or 6/60 getting tired? Is that wash valve sticky or leaking air? Why not exchange it for a fully reconditioned module that is warranted for 90 days? Call us toll free, we ship the unit to you and you return your old one in the same box. Simple as that. An example of a few exchange prices:

Pump III	**$500.00**
Sampler II or III	**$400.00**
Heating Bath, block type	**$150.00**
Wash valve	**$250.00**
Colorimeter 5a	**$600.00**

includes all new flowcells and phototubes

satisfaction fully guaranteed

Exchange Flowcells

1.5 and 2.0mm

FOR 12/60, 6/60 AND AAII

ALPKEM will send you a new flowcell exchange for $70.00 and your old broken flowcell and guarantee the quality of the new flowcell to be equal to that of a new one — any new one — or your money back —

available in any quantity!

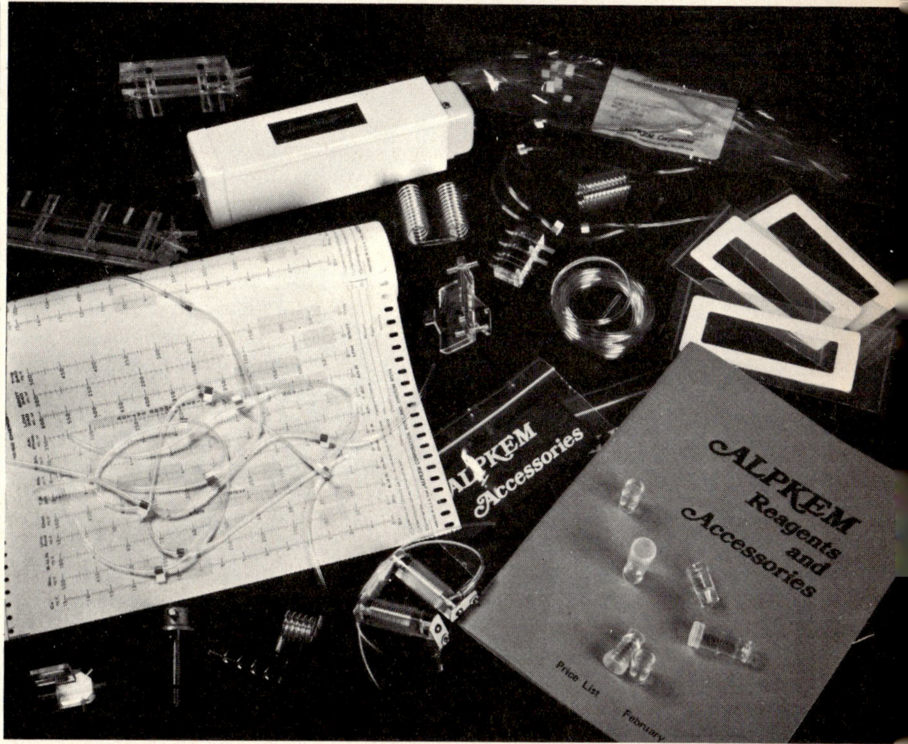

A complete supply of Auto Analyzer accessories is in stock for air shipment anywhere. Ask for our catalog.

*AUTO ANALYZER IS A TRADEMARK OF TECHNICON INSTRUMENTS CORP., TARRYTOWN, N.Y.

ALPKEM Corporation

1234 S.E. Union Avenue, Portland, Oregon 97214

Call us toll free — **800-547-5535***

*If busy or if calling from Oregon, dial **503-233-3626**

In CANADA contact *ALPKEM* CANADA, 403-243-6195

ALPKEM is a leading supplier of reconditioned 12/60, 6/60, AAII and basic AA systems. We maintain a substantial stock and can respond to your needs rapidly, be it a cartridge or an entire system. Let us send you more information. Thanks.

will be the sixth year that this award has been given.

Dr. Tietz was born and educated in Germany, and received a doctorate in Natural Sciences from the Technical University of Stuttgart. He came to the United States in 1954 as Research Fellow in the Department of Pathology, University of Chicago. Later Chairman of the Department of Chemistry, Reid Memorial Hospital, Richmond, Indiana, he went on to Mount Sinai Hospital Medical Center, Chicago, where he held a position as Director of Clinical Chemistry until early this year. He started as Associate in Pathology at the Chicago Medical School/University of Health Sciences and advanced to Professor of Clinical Chemistry in 1969 and Professor of Biochemistry in 1970. He was also Consultant to the State of Illinois, Department of Health.

During his years at the Chicago Medical School, Dr. Tietz has restructured the clinical chemistry portion of the course in clinical pathology for medical students. In the school of graduate and postdoctoral studies he established one of the first M.S. degree programs in clinical chemistry; this program has subsequently been expanded into a Ph.D. program. He was also involved in the organization of a degree program for medical technologists in the School of Related Health Sciences. He directed the teaching programs for residents in clinical pathology and the continuing-education programs in clinical chemistry for employees at the Mount Sinai Hospital Medical Center. Earlier this year, Dr. Tietz accepted a position as Director of Clinical Chemistry and Professor of Pathology, College of Medicine, University of Kentucky Medical Center, Lexington, Kentucky.

Dr. Tietz is editor of and contributor to the text *Fundamentals of Clinical Chemistry* (W. B. Saunders, 1970). A forthcoming second edition includes foreign as well as American authors.

He has coordinated and directed workshops: Electrolyte Institute and Workshop, Catholic Hospital Association of the USA, 1965; Gas Chromatography in Clinical Chemistry, Mount Sinai Hospital, Chicago, 1967; the International Seminar and Workshop in Enzymology, Mount Sinai Hospital Medical Center in 1972; and the Second International Symposium on Clinical Enzymology, Mount Sinai Hospital Medical Center, 1975. He has served on the faculty of many other national, regional, and local workshops.

Dr. Tietz has served as member of the AACC Committee on Education. He participated in the Conference of Program Directors in Columbus, Ohio, in 1972 and in Chicago in 1975, serving as Chairman of the M.S. Degree Study Group. He also served as a member of the AACC Committee on Standards, as chairman of the Sub-Committee on Enzymes, and as consultant to the Board of Editors of *Selected Methods of Clinical Chemistry*. Dr. Tietz is the 1976 President-Elect, AACC.

His research interests are in methodology related to clinical chemistry, and fat metabolism related to atherosclerosis.

He received the Clinical Chemist Award from the AACC Chicago Section in 1971 and was Chairman of the Chicago Section, 1965–7. He is a member of the American Institute of Chemists (Fellow), American Association for the Advancement of Science (Fellow), American Chemical Society, American Society of Clinical Pathologists (Associate), Sigma Xi, American Association of University Professors, and the Institute of Medicine of Chicago.

Nathan O. Kaplan will receive the fourth *AACC Award for Outstanding Contributions to Clinical Chemistry in a Selected Area,* sponsored by the Boehringer Mannheim Corporation.

Dr. Kaplan, a native New Yorker, received his A.B. from the University of California, Los Angeles, and his Ph.D. from the same university at Berkeley. He began his career as Assistant Biochemist, University of California, became a research chemist on the Manhattan Project, associate research biochemist at Massachusetts General Hospital, and Instructor, Harvard Medical School. He then went on to Assistant Professor, Associate Professor, and Professor of Biology, McCollum–Pratt Institute, The Johns Hopkins University. From 1957–68 he was Professor and Chairman of Biochemistry at Brandeis University. From 1968 to the present he has been Professor of Chemistry at the University of California at La Jolla.

Dr. Kaplan's main interest has been the study of enzymes from both a theoretical and applied point of view. On the practical level he has been involved in developing instrumentation for the automated determination of enzymes on a clinical level. From prototypes, these instruments have evolved into sophisticated instruments that are produced by a number of different manufacturers. He has made basic contributions in developing kinetic methods that can be used to distinguish isoenzymes. Analyzers based on this type of approach are appearing that determine isoenzymes by kinetic measurements, an example being the stopped-flow instruments for determining lactate dehydrogenase isoenzymes. A microcalorimeter developed by Dr. Kaplan has been used in the determination of the kinetics of uricase and lactate dehydrogenase of particular biochemical interest and is routinely used in clinical chemistry laboratories.

Analyse nanomoles of peptides and metabolites in 30 minutes...

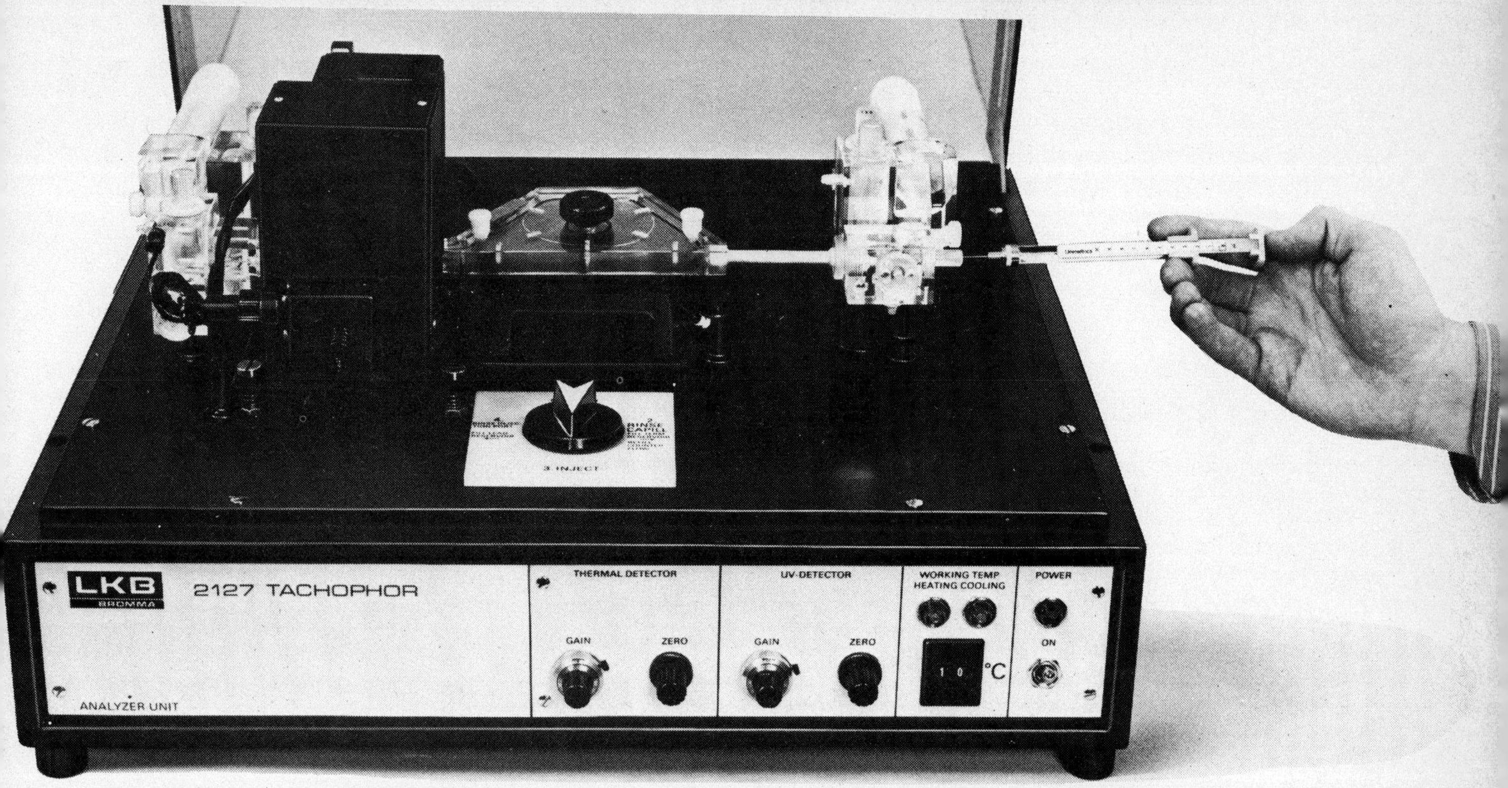

...with the LKB Tachophor

The LKB 2127 Tachophor utilizes the isotachophoresis principle for separating ions to give you results in 30 minutes or less. Ion species from metals to proteins can be separated easily and with high resolution. No pretreatment of the sample such as deproteinization or concentration is necessary. A typical separation of nucleotides or low molecular protolytes takes only 20 to 30 minutes.

The length of a zone is directly proportional to the amount of sample ions in the zone, so that quantitative determinations can simply be made by measuring the peak-width on the UV recording (as shown below).

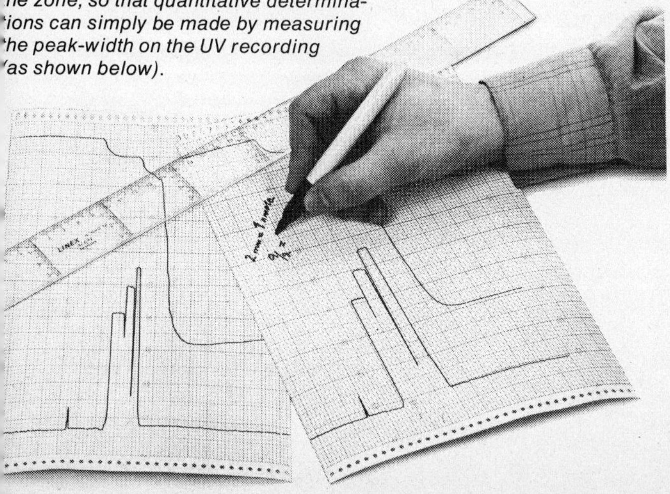

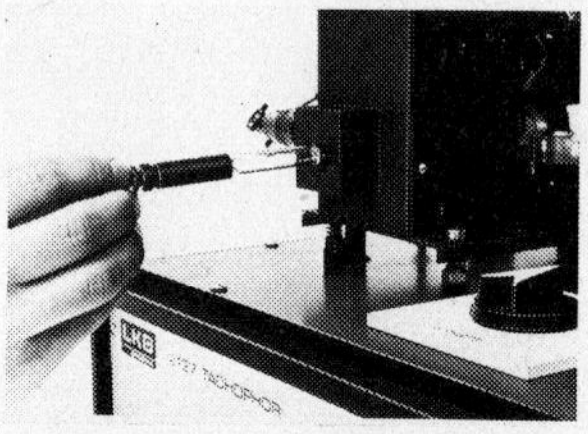

A twin-detector system, UV and thermal, gives you a complete picture of an analysed sample in the 0.1 to 50 μl range. The twin-buffer system using Ampholine® carrier ampholytes as 'spacers' gives you excellent separation and resolution of difficult peaks. And no stabilizing medium is required as in other electrophoresis methods. The UV lamp used in the LKB Tachophor detector system is a plug-in type that is very easy to change. The LKB Tachophor is easy to operate and maintain, with

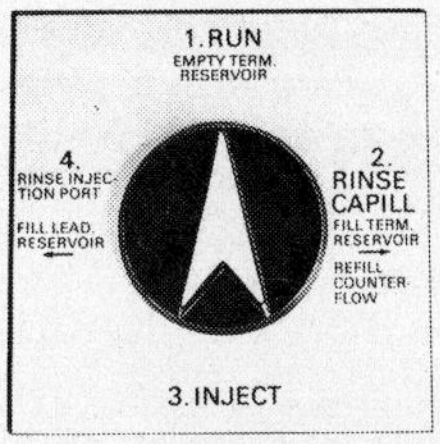

a 4-position control and simple sample injection, plus counter-flow capability for analysis of large volume dilute samples. For more information, contact your LKB representative or write to us at one of the adresses listed below.

LKB

LKB Instruments Inc.
12221 PARKLAWN DRIVE, ROCKVILLE MD. 20852
(301) 881-2510.
TELEX 89-682.

Circle No. 347 on Reader's Service Card

Dr. Kaplan is the author or co-author of about 350 publications, most of them dealing with enzymes. He is best known probably as co-editor (with S. P. Colowick) of *Methods in Enzymology* (Academic Press). His research interests have been in enzymology, immobilized enzymes, affinity chromatography, and cancer chemotherapy.

Dr. Kaplan is a member of the National Academy of Sciences and the American Academy of Arts and Sciences. His awards are: Honorary Fellow of the Harvey Society; Sigma Xi; Sugar Research Award; Nutritional Research Award; Eli Lilly Award in Biochemistry; Commonwealth Travel Fellowship; and John Simon Guggenheim Fellowship (1964–5 and 1975).

Ages of New AACC Members

An analysis was made of the ages of the persons accepted for membership in 1975. The results are shown in Figure 1, which represents 625 new members, including 67 student affiliates. The top of each bar represents the total number of each age and the distance between the x-axis and the lower end of the bar, the students of that age. The median age (left arrow) for all new members was 32 years, 33 years (middle arrow) when students were not included. The arrow

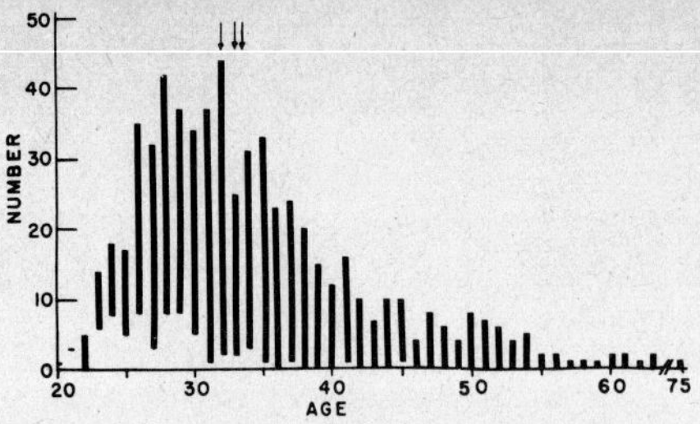

Fig. 1.

on the right is the calculated mean value. Most of the students were below 30, but two persons became student affiliates when over 40. Perhaps the youngest person ever to become a member of the Association is Lawrence L. Taylor, III, who became a student affiliate at the age of 20. The oldest person who was accepted as a member in 1975, perhaps the oldest ever accepted, was Dr. Elliott T. Adams of the Northeast Section. He became a Fellow at the age of 75, but would have been eligible earlier as he is a diplomate of the ABCC.

—**Albert A. Dietz**
Advisory Member
Committee on Membership

Publications

The *Proceedings of the Second National Conference on Proficiency Testing* for medical laboratories are now available; a copy was received in the Editorial Office on March 6.

The conference, sponsored by the National Council on Health Laboratory Services, which represents 17 member organizations active in conducting medical laboratories throughout the U.S., was held in Washington, D.C., on October 6 and 7, 1975. About 200 laboratorians, including several from England and the Netherlands, attended.

The first national conference on proficiency testing, held in Atlanta, Georgia, in 1971, was devoted primarily to discussions of the complexities of applying proficiency testing to laboratory medicine. The recent conference brought the previous discussions up to date and developed recommendations for the future. Separate study groups for nine areas of laboratory operation—bacteriology, blood banking, chemistry, hematology, histopathology and cytology, immunology, parasitology, radioimmunoassay, and toxicology—focused on questions and problems compiled in advance by the program committee. Their conclusions, along with recommendations to industry, government, and professional societies concerned with proficiency testing, are given in the *Proceedings.*

The 73-page publication also reprints 19 papers presented at the conference, with 14 summaries prepared by program and study-group chairmen.

Copies of the *Proceedings* may be ordered for $10 each from Information Services, 9650 Rockville Pike, Bethesda, Md. 20014. Checks should be made payable to the National Council on Health Laboratory Services.

RIA for Physicians, a clinically oriented newsletter; $30/yr ($35 to subscribers of *Radioassay News*). Write: Scientific Newsletters, Inc., 2421 W. Broadway, P. O. Box 4546, Anaheim, Calif. 92803.

Proceedings of the 1st Invitational Symposium on the Serodiagnosis of Cancer (AFRRI SP74-1, March, 1974) has been received (Mar. 12) from the Armed Forces Radiobiology Research Institute, Defense Nuclear Agency, Bethesda, Md. It reports proceedings of this meeting, held at the National Naval Medical Center, Bethesda, Md., Sept. 29, 1973.

Bicentennial Events at Brookhaven Lab

An Energy Fair, Open House, and Summer Saturdays are three events planned at ERDA's Brookhaven National Laboratory on Long Island for greeting the public in '76.

"The Laboratory, which has considerably broadened its initial mission of research on the peaceful aspects of the atom to helping ERDA develop all energy sources, will host the Energy Fair to provide visitors with a sampling of ex-

isting and planned energy technology," announced Dr. R. C. Anderson, Assistant Director. The 5-day exhibition, beginning on Wednesday, May 12, and ending on Sunday, May 16, will overlap with BNL's Open House on the weekend, May 15 and 16. Designed as a learning environment and as a stimulus for public response, interaction, and investigation of energy alternatives, the Fair will house dozens of exhibits from all over the country as well as from the Greater New York metropolitan area.

Movies and other audiovisuals will complement many exhibits.

Energy Fair and Open House visitors may also tour the building housing Brookhaven's historic Graphite Research Reactor and displays of the work of the Laboratory.

The new-style Open House on the weekend will highlight research in progress. The actual scientists and technicians involved will explain and demonstrate research methods and tools as well as answer questions about their work. "It's a 'hands on' approach that proved extremely popular during last year's Open House," Dr. Anderson said.

The public is invited to visit 14 separate research areas including laboratories in the Medical, Biology, Chemistry, Physics, Accelerator, Applied Mathematics, and Applied Science Departments. To be viewed, in addition, are BNL's large research machines: the Alternating Gradient Synchrotron, one of the world's largest proton accelerators; two Tandem Van de Graaff electrostatic accelerators, the largest tandem accelerator facility used to accelerate nuclei of atoms to velocities one-tenth the speed of light; and the High Flux Beam Reactor, one of the most advanced research reactors providing neutrons for research in medical and energy fields.

A series of Saturday bus tours of the Lab site will run all summer (except July 3). Featured will be a long stop at BNL's Exhibition Hall. More details on the Summer Saturdays will be released at a later date.

"Because of the number of areas that can be toured during Open House and the broad scope of the Energy Fair exhibits and seminars, visitors may wish to set aside two days for attending these special free events," suggested Dr. Anderson. "Hours are 10:00 a.m. to 4:00 p.m. daily, food is available, and no reservations are required. School groups or other large touring groups may, however, wish to contact the Public Relations Office at (516) 345-2345 for further information. Announcements regarding seminar scheduling will be made shortly."

The entrance to Brookhaven National Laboratory is on the William Floyd Parkway, approximately one mile north of Exit 68 of the Long Island Expressway.

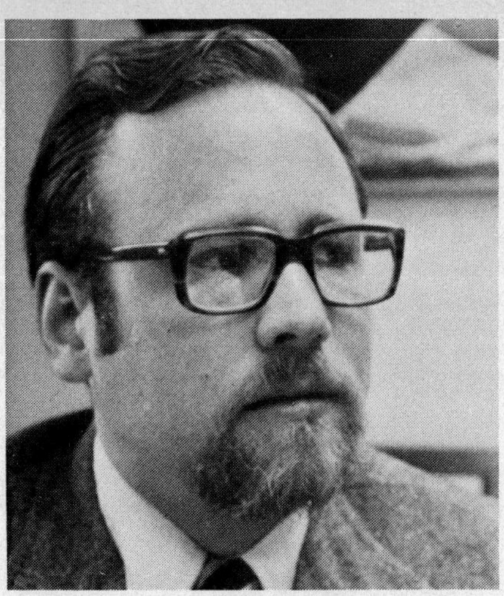

C. S. Frings

Awards

At the 27th Pittsburgh Conference on Analytical Chemistry and Applied Spectroscopy, Cleveland, Ohio, on March 3, 1976, Dr. C. S. Frings received the first Pittsburgh Applied Analytical Chemistry Award. This award is presented by the Society of Analytical Chemists of Pittsburgh, "to the author of a paper published within the preceding five years which has been especially useful in solving real problems in analytical chemistry". The award paper was entitled, "Drug Screening" and appeared in CRC Critical Reviews in Clinical Laboratory Sciences, CRC Press Inc., Vol 4, No. 4, pages 357–382, 1973. The award is a plaque and $1000.00.

Prix André Lichtwitz. This prize (8800 francs) for 1976 is awarded by the Institut National de la Santé et de la Recherche Médicale to a French or foreign research worker, or team, for outstanding work on calcium or phosphorus metabolism during the previous year. Ten copies of fully documented applications should reach the Director of the INSERM, c/o le Docteur Bonnot, 101, rue de Tolbiac, 75645 Paris Cedex 13, by June 29.

Meetings and Continuing Education

Northeast Section: This section announces two meetings: May 12, E. J. Ariëns, AACC National Tour Speaker, at Carney Hospital, Dorchester, Mass.; and June 16, H. E. Spiegel speaks on federal legislation in the clin. lab. area, at Old Sturbridge Village, Sturbridge, Mass. Write: H. C. Clemson, Lynn Hosp., Lynn, Mass. 01904.

Interpretative Enzymology, June 29–July 2, 1976, Univ. Calif., San Diego School of Med. Particulars from: David Allan, M.D., Associate Dean for Continuing Education, UCSD School of Medicine (M-002), La Jolla, Calif. 92093. (Tel. 714/452-3707).

Seventh International Congress on Automation (Technicon). This will be held Dec. 13–15, 1976, at the New York Hilton, New York City. Theme: "Tomorrow's Technology Today." Particulars from Michele Barth, Technicon Corp., Tarrytown, N.Y. 10591 (Tel. 914/631-8000).

Squibb National Nuclear Medicine Seminar, a four-day program (ASMT-approved) will be conducted without charge in 14 U.S. cities during 1976. Write: Daniel J. Murphy, E. R. Squibb & Sons, Inc., P. O. Box 4000, Princeton, N.J. 08540.

Expo-Medical 76—Symposium, Exhibition Gardens, Tel Aviv, Israel, Sept. 15–20, 1976. Features symposia on Emerging Diagnostic Systems in Medicine, Inborn Metabolic Errors, Nutritional Status. Write: Organizing Committee and Secretariat, P. O. Box 16271, Tel Aviv.

In Vitro Nuclear Medicine, Oct. 11–13, 1976. A three-day course of lectures for persons interested in the in vitro application of radioactive tracers. Procedures such as radioimmunoassay, competitive protein-binding assay, immunoradiometric assay, enzymatic assay, and other radiometric techniques will be presented. The theoretic basis, practical aspects of the procedures, and clinical application will be discussed. The course will stress the recent progress and clinical aspects of the field. Cost: $200. Write: Office of Continuing Medical Education, The Johns Hopkins Medical Institutions, Turner Building, Room 17, 720 Rutland Ave., Baltimore, Md. 21205.

Fed Up?

There is a feeling in the country that we might be able somehow to get along as well if some large part of the bureaus and agencies of the federal government were to magically vanish and government were to confine itself to the business of governing. Some recent quotes:

> Another question asked [of 2074 persons] was, 'In which of the areas listed would you most like (and least like) to have your taxes spent for science and technology?' The replies, in 1972 and 1974 indicate a great incongruity between what the people say they want and what the government actually does in this matter. Topping the list in both 1972 and 1974, with 65 and 69 percent was "improving health care." Next came "reducing and controlling pollution," with 60 and 50 percent.
>
> —Daniel S. Greenberg, *The New England Journal of Medicine,* March 25, 1976, discussing the NSB report, *Science Indicators—1974.*

> Second, we need to put our health care delivery system in perspective. We cannot expect our health care institutions to cure all our illnesses, nor solve all of our health problems. With this perspective, we might be better able to curb the rising costs of health

You talk English. It talks FORTRAN.

The Unique ROTOCHEM® IIa Centrifugal Fast Analyzer

It's fast. It's accurate. It will print test results for lab or ward use. And it's simple to operate.

What makes it all possible is computer technology coupled with a proven analytical technique — to make testing easier and faster. The ROTOCHEM IIa Analyzer, directed by a computer that utilizes FORTRAN language programs, provides a flexibility of operation and output which will resist obsolescence for years to come — as new methods are developed, you can develop new programs to operate your ROTOCHEM unit. The output is fantastic — batch testing, stat tests, test status reports, and patient test result printouts are all part of the norm. Computer technology in the modern clinical lab.

Want to computerize your lab? Start with a ROTOCHEM Analyzer. You talk English. It talks FORTRAN. It's an easy first step.

Today's Technology for Today AND Tomorrow.

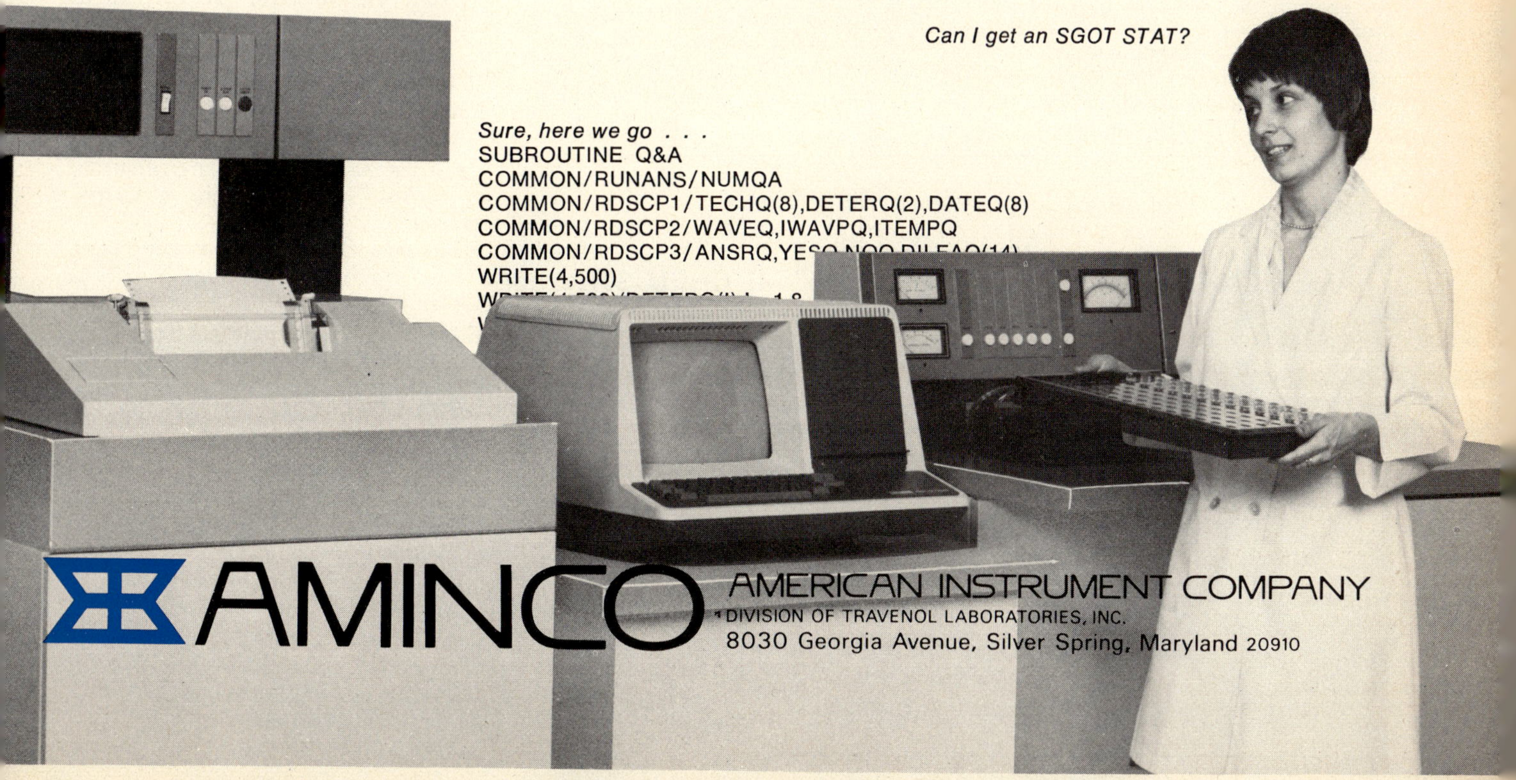

Circle No. 329 on Reader's Service Card

care. I think the American public has expected too much from the delivery system. If those of us who serve the system every day help the public understand the limitations of the delivery system, we just might help curb both its rising costs *and growing regulation by government.* (italics ours).

—Remarks by Karl D. Bays, Chairman and Chief Executive Office, American Hospital Supply Corp., before the Scientific Apparatus Makers Association, Phoenix, Ariz., November 10, 1975.

The past decade has seen a runaway growth of bureaucracy, restrictive legislation, and squandering of taxpayers' money on such high-sounding but ill-planned undertakings as regional medical programs and comprehensive medical care—all this with the seeming approval, and urging, of many of the faculty of our medical schools. . . .

—Irvine H. Page, M.D., Editorial in *Modern Medicine,* Feb. 15, 1976

Has the rising cost of government involvement in health care been worth the price?

The Commerce Department forecasts that total US health care spending will rise another 10% this year to $135 billion—up from $40 billion 10 years ago. During the same span, Washington upped its share of the health care tab from 19 to nearly 40%, largely through such massive programs as Medicare. But look at Medicare itself. Before it began, the over-65 population paid about 70% of its medical bills out of pocket. Today, although senior citizens pay only 40% themselves, rising costs have forced them to pay almost as many actual dollars for medical care as they did in 1965.

"Washington Report," in *Modern Medicine* Feb. 15, 1976, p 20

A tide is turning and the public is becoming fed up with the extent that government over-involves itself in the lives of the citizens, their activities and their businesses. People have witnessed the promises of successive administrations and congressional laws, only to note that they fall far short in delivery, that they cost unbelievably more than projected, and that with them comes an overlay of suffocating regulations.

—Warren L. Bostick, M.D., President, ASCP, in *Laboratory Medicine* **7,** No. 3, March 1976, p 2

As a result of the debate on forthcoming legislative proposals, it is hoped that the vital need for prompt clinical feedback in drug discovery will be increasingly realized and, above all, that regulations will be avoided that impose cumbersome and often redundant constraints on clinical studies.

It is certainly appropriate that government should regulate clinical experimentation, but it is vitally important that all parties constantly seek means that allow this vital process to proceed as efficiently and expeditiously as possible. The view that the sole function of drug regulation is the protection of the public from harm should be replaced by a new and broadened conception of the regulators' mission. The public interest would be best served if the Congress broadened the mandate of FDA to include a positive responsibility to encourage drug innovation and to expedite the development and availability of new drugs.

—from *Annual Report 1975,* Pfizer

—J.S.K.

A Footnote on Nomenclature

Readers may have noticed the use of the title 'Chairholder' in the preceding reports. This results from a letter from Professor D. N. Baron of the Royal Free Hospital in London, England who wrote to the Editor:

"Sir, I am sorry that you are using the grotesque word 'Chairperson' on page 1 of the December 1975 issue. If you have to degenderise the Chairman, then 'Chairholder' is much better English and has the same meaning (compare 'Office-holder').

Yours faithfully, D. N. Baron"

Perhaps this suggestion of Professor Baron's should be taken up by all those responsible for organising congresses, symposia, and meetings!

—from *IFCC Newsletter* No. 13 March 1976, p 7

Some Forthcoming Papers (Special Issue)

Analysis of Results of Toxicological Examinations Performed by Coroners' or Medical Examiners' Laboratories in 2000 Drug-Involved Deaths in Nine Major U.S. Cities
Eugene C. Dinovo, Louis A. Gottschalk, Frederick L. McGuire, Herman Birch, and Jon F. Heiser

Results of a Nine-Laboratory Survey of Forensic Toxicology Proficiency
Eugene C. Dinovo and Louis A. Gottschalk

Automated Enzymic Determination of Ethanol in Blood, Serum and Urine with a Miniature Centrifugal Analyzer
T. P. Hadjiioannou, S. I. Hadjiioannou, J. Avery, and H. V. Malmstadt

Improved Micro-Radioimmunoassay of Digoxin in Serum, with use of ^{125}I-Labeled Digoxin
Benjamin Calesnick and Annette Dinan

Analytical Toxicology: Applications of Element-Selective Electrolytic Conductivity Detection for Gas Chromatography
Brian E. Pape

Enzymatic Assay for Methotrexate in Serum and Cerebrospinal Fluid
Larry C. Falk and Dennis R. Clark

Relative Merits of Some Methods for Amphetamine Assay in Biological Fluids
Robert O. Bost, Craig A. Sutheimer, and Irving Sunshine

Serum Quinidine Concentrations: Comparison of Fluorescence, Gas-Chromatographic, and Gas-Chromatographic–Mass-Spectrometric Methods
David H. Huffman and Charles E. Hignite

Gas-Chromatographic Quantitation of Theophylline in Small Volumes of Plasma
Donald Perrier and Evangeline Lear

Gas-Chromatographic Determination of an Antifibrinolytic Drug, δ-Aminocaproic Acid
Thomas R. Keucher, Elizabeth B. Solow, John Metaxas, and Robert L. Campbell

Gas-Chromatographic Micro-Scale Procedure for Theophylline, with use of a Nitrogen-Sensitive Detector
Charles J. Least, Jr., George F. Johnson, and Harvey M. Solomon

Monitoring Drug Concentrations in a Case of Combined Overdosage with Primidone and Methsuximide.
George F. Johnson, Charles J. Least, Jr., James W. Serum, Elizabeth B. Solow, and Harvey M. Solomon

Gas-Chromatographic Analysis for Therapeutic Concentrations of Amitriptyline and Nortriptyline in Plasma, with Use of a Nitrogen Detector
David N. Bailey and Peter I. Jatlow

editorial

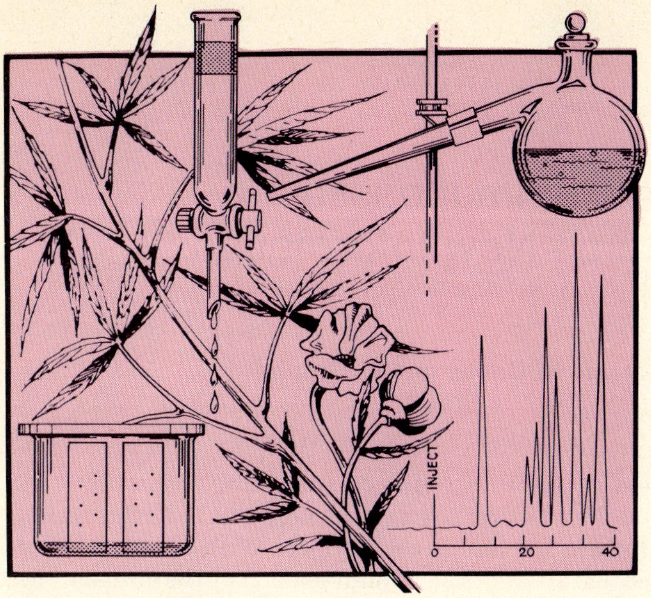

A New Role for the Clinical Chemist

If you will peruse the contents of this journal 15 or even 10 years ago, you will see why a special issue such as this one could hardly have appeared then. Measurement of the vanishingly small concentrations of drugs in the blood or urine was beyond the limits of the methods then in general use in clinical chemistry laboratories: colorimetric, ultraviolet spectrophotometric, or fluorometric. All of them left much to be desired in specificity or sensitivity, and most were deficient in both. The specificity problem was often further complicated by the presence of active and (or) inactive metabolites and conjugates.

Because of improvements in existing instrumentation and the newer techniques, exemplified by those described and applied in this issue, clinical chemists have recently assumed a new and extremely important responsibility. It is important, in some cases critically so, to be able to follow the patient's compliance with the prescribed medication, to know what concentrations of drugs are reaching the intended site(s) and how long a given dosage or dosage form maintains this concentration—in sum, to know the optimum regimen for a specific patient (including such special problems as the infant, the pregnant woman, the aged, and the patient with liver disease or renal disease). Now, in an ever-increasing number of instances, it is practicable to do so. This is an enormous stride toward more rational and effective therapy, as has been discussed before in this journal [*Clin. Chem.* **21,** 1368 (1975)].

The clinical chemist has an accordingly greater role in treatment as well as in diagnosis, a role that first came to the fore when screening for and monitoring drug abuse became so widely necessary.

Such procedures are also useful in detecting, assessing, and monitoring the treatment of the patient who has taken a suicidal or unintentional overdose (as is illustrated by the Case Report in this issue), as well as in helping some of the estimated 300 000 people who are hospitalized annually in the U. S. because of a drug reaction, of whom about a tenth die as a consequence.

Some day we shall be able routinely to measure drugs in their target organ or tissue. For the moment, we must generally be content with measuring them in serum or, on occasion, in cerebrospinal fluid or urine. Fortunately, monitoring is necessary or useful for only a minority of the 1200 different drugs currently on the market.

The Editors directed that this issue be in essence a sequel to our issue on "Toxicology and Drug Assay" [*Clin. Chem.* **20**/2 (1974)], which was well received. As the issue came together, the distinction between the *results* of actual monitoring of drug concentrations and the *techniques* for doing so became rather blurred.

Not incidentally, at about the time copy for this issue started on its way to the printer the second AACC-sponsored Pine Mountain Conference [*cf. Clin. Chem.* **21,** 1696 (1975)] was in progress, this one on "Basic Principles of Therapeutic Drug Monitoring," and our Canadian counterparts will also hold a symposium on this theme at their July annual meeting. Perhaps other such meetings were and are being held elsewhere, I cannot say. In any event, this illustrates the topicality of this issue.

We hope that not only clinical chemists, but also clinicians, forensic chemists, toxicologists, pharmacologists, et al. will find this issue useful.

Again we thank our contributors and express our appreciation both for their heart-warming enthusiasm for this issue and their patience in allowing a rather longer than usual delay in the publication of their work in some cases.

References[1]

1. Wilder, J., and Perchalski, R. J., How assay methods can guide drug therapy for epileptic patients. *Mod. Med.* **43,** 68 (July 1, 1975).

2. Lamy, P. P., and Vestal, R. E., Drug prescribing for the elderly. *Hosp. Pract.* **11**/1, 111 (January 1976).

3. Sheiner, L. B., Melmon, K. L., and Rosenberg, B., Instructional goals for physicians in the use of blood level data—and the contribution of computers. *Clin. Pharmacol. Ther.* **16,** 260 (1974).

4. La Du, B. N., Jr., The genetics of drug reactions. *Hosp. Pract.* **6**/6, 97 (June 1971).

5. Koch-Weser, J., and Sellers, E. M., Binding of drugs to serum albumin. *New Engl. J. Med.* **294,** 311, 326 (1976).

J.S.K.

Art courtesy of Waters Associates

[1] The references are "selected" only on the basis of having come to my attention and having unusual relevance to the problems mentioned above.

review

CLIN. CHEM. 22/6, 712–725 (1976)

Detection of Drugs of Abuse by Radioimmunoassay: A Summary of Published Data and Some New Information

R. Cleeland, J. Christenson, M. Usategui-Gomez, J. Heveran, R. Davis, and E. Grunberg

We review the status of radioimmunoassays for detection of abused drugs. Individual assays with use of ^{125}I-labeled antigens are all performed in an identical manner and can be completed in 30 min to 1 h. Combined assays for simultaneous detection of two or more such drugs or assays in which a tritium-labeled antigen is used require 1–2 h for completion. All tests can be performed with 0.1 ml or less of specimen. The assays involving ^{125}I reliably detect urinary concentrations of, per liter, 40–100 μg of morphine, 100 μg of barbiturates, methadone, methaqualone, or benzoylecgonine, and 1000 μg of amphetamine. The assay for morphine involving ^{3}H detects 60 μg/liter. Each assay is capable of providing a qualitative and quantitative estimate of the drugs sought. The ^{125}I-labeled antigens have a usable shelf life of at least two to four months after the antigen is iodinated; the tritium assay is stable for six months. The assays can be performed with use of paper discs that have been suspended in urine and then dried, in place of the liquid specimen. The assays appear to be equally applicable to detection of drugs in urine, blood, saliva, and tissues. All of them are done at ambient temperature and can be used equally well for emergency (stat) tests or mass screening. Except for the benzoylecgonine assay, the clinical reliability of these tests has been demonstrated.

Additional Keyphrases: *"cutoff" values • assay of drugs in blood, urine, saliva • assay of samples on paper discs • technical considerations • blank values • disappearance rates from blood • screening*

The use of radioimmunoassays (RIA) for detection of drugs of abuse has been documented (*1–8*). Comparative studies on drug detection by physical and immunological means, including RIA, have also appeared (*9–14*). In most instances, radioimmunoassays have been used for screening urine specimens, although detection by RIA of barbiturates or morphine and its analogs in blood (*1, 3*) and of morphine and its analogs or methadone in autopsy tissues has also been reported (*15, 16*).

Development of these radioimmunoassays was based on the original work of Spector and Parker (*17*), who first successfully obtained antibodies to morphine by coupling 3-*O*-carboxymethylmorphine to bovine serum albumin for use as the antigen. With a derivative of secobarbital for the hapten portion of the antigen, the feasibility of a radioimmunoassay for detection of barbiturates was later demonstrated (*18, 19*). These experimental studies were done with ^{3}H- or ^{14}C-labeled antigens.

During our initial development of RIA's for use to detect abused drugs, it became apparent that ^{125}I-labeled antigens would be preferable to tritiated or ^{14}C-labeled antigens for widespread application as a rapid, less-expensive assay. Therefore, our efforts were primarily directed toward development of assays utilizing derivatives of the appropriate antigen that could be readily iodinated. However, an assay with use of tritiated dihydromorphine is also currently available.

To date, radioimmunoassays have been developed in our laboratories for detection of morphine, barbiturates, amphetamine, methadone, methaqualone, and benzoylecgonine, as well as combination assays to test for two or more of these drugs simultaneously. To facilitate multiple testing for several drugs of abuse, the various individual radioimmunoassays have been designed to be performed in an identical manner. The combined assays are done like the individual assays, except that two or more iodinated antigens and specific antibodies are combined, stored, and used in this premixed form.

Here, we review the status of these assays as to their applicability to rapid drug screening, quantitation of drugs in biological specimens, limits of sensitivity, specificity, and stability in terms of usable shelf life of the reagents. In addition, general problems related to development of all assays such as preparation of antibody pools with consistent specificity and binding characteristics will be discussed.

Methodology

Table 1 lists the reagents for the individual and combined RIA's utilizing ^{125}I-labeled antigens, while Table 2 contains a general outline of the assay procedures.

Research Division, Hoffmann-La Roche, Nutley, N. J. 07110.
Received Feb. 4, 1976; accepted Mar. 4, 1976.

Table 1. Reagents Utilized in Radioimmunoassays for Drugs of Abuse

Separate reagents	
Antigen reagent,	^{125}I-labeled morphine,[a] secobarbital, amphetamine, methaqualone, methadone, and benzoylecgonine derivatives. All labeled antigens were diluted in 0.01 mol/liter phosphate-buffered saline (PBS, pH 7.2) to give radioactive concentrations ranging from 5 to 70 Ci/g.
Antibody reagent,	Antiserum prepared against specific haptens by procedures similar to those described by Spector and Parker (*17*). Antisera were diluted in serum from unimmunized animals, then further diluted with an equal volume of PBS.
Saturated ammonium sulfate solution,	Prepared in de-ionized water and used without neutralization.
Standards,	All standards prepared from pools of urine tested and found by RIA not to give appreciable differences in counts per minute from expected background. Standards were prepared as concentrated solutions in appropriate solvents and then diluted in pooled urine to give the desired concentration.
Combined reagents	
Antigen–antibody,	^{125}I-labeled morphine and ^{125}I-labeled secobarbital derivative combined (dual assay) or containing an additional ^{125}I-labeled amphetamine derivative (triple assay). The combined labeled antigens were diluted in PBS, pH 7.2, to appropriate radioactive concentrations. Goat antiserum to each of the antigens was diluted in normal goat serum to appropriate concentrations and mixed with an equal volume of PBS. The diluted antibody reagent was added to an equal volume of combined antigen reagent and allowed to equilibrate for at least 24 h at 4 °C.

[a] An assay in which [^{3}H]7,8-dihydromorphine is used as a label is available, and reagents utilized in this test have been described previously (*1*).

Temperature requirements. The temperature used with any of these RIA's is not critical; all steps may be done at ambient temperature. Because temperature is not a critical factor, automation of these assays has been facilitated.

Qualitative estimation. For screening urine, positive urine controls supplied with each set of reagents are tested in duplicate or triplicate. Unknowns are then tested singly or in duplicate and the average counts per minute (cpm) of the positive controls are compared with the cpm of the unknowns. Only those unknowns with cpm values equal to or greater than the average cpm value of the positive control are considered positive.

Table 2. Radioimmunoassay Protocol for Drugs of Abuse (^{125}I-Labeled Antigens)[a]

Separate reagents

Into 10 × 75 or 12 × 75 mm glass tubes:

1. Add 0.1 ml of standards and unknowns to separate tubes.
2. Add 0.2 ml of antigen reagent to each tube, mix well.
3. Add 0.2 ml of antibody reagent to each tube, mix well.
4. Incubate for at least 10 min at ambient temperature.
5. Add 0.5 ml of saturated ammonium sulfate solution, mix well.
6. Incubate for 5–10 min at ambient temperature.
7. Centrifuge in swinging bucket rotor for 10 min at 1250–2500 × *g*. Withdraw 0.5 ml of supernate from each tube and transfer it to appropriate tube for counting in a gamma scintillation counter.

Combined reagents

Into 10 × 75 or 12 × 75 mm glass tubes:

1. Add 0.1 ml of standards and unknowns to separate tubes.
2. Add 0.4 ml of combined reagents to each tube, mix well.
3. Incubate for at least 1 h at ambient temperature.
4. Continue as above from step 5.

[a] Assay procedure with use of tritiated morphine has been described previously (*1*).

Quantitation. For quantitation of each assay, a calibration curve is prepared by assaying, in duplicate or triplicate, several standard solutions containing different concentrations of each drug in urine (or other biological fluids) that has been tested and found to give an acceptable background count. The average cpm of each drug concentration is plotted on the y-axis and the concentration of drug on the x-axis. Calibration curves usually have, at lower drug concentrations, a relatively linear portion with a relatively steep slope, which gradually decreases at higher concentrations. Best quantitative results are obtained by using the more linear portion of the curve. The cpm for each unknown sample is then converted to nanogram equivalents per milliliter by use of the calibration curve. Each unknown is quantitated in one of two ways. (*a*) If the cpm value of the unknown falls outside the linear portion of the calibration curve, the unknown is diluted serially 10-fold in diluent that has previously been found to give an acceptable background count. The diluted unknown is assayed and that dilution which gives a value within the linear portion of the curve is used to estimate the concentration of the unknown present. (*b*) Alternatively, smaller volumes (e.g., 20 μl) of the undiluted or diluted unknown can be assayed. The standards are tested by using 0.1-ml amounts. The result obtained with the volume(s) of unknown that falls within the linear portion of the standard curve is used for quantitation.

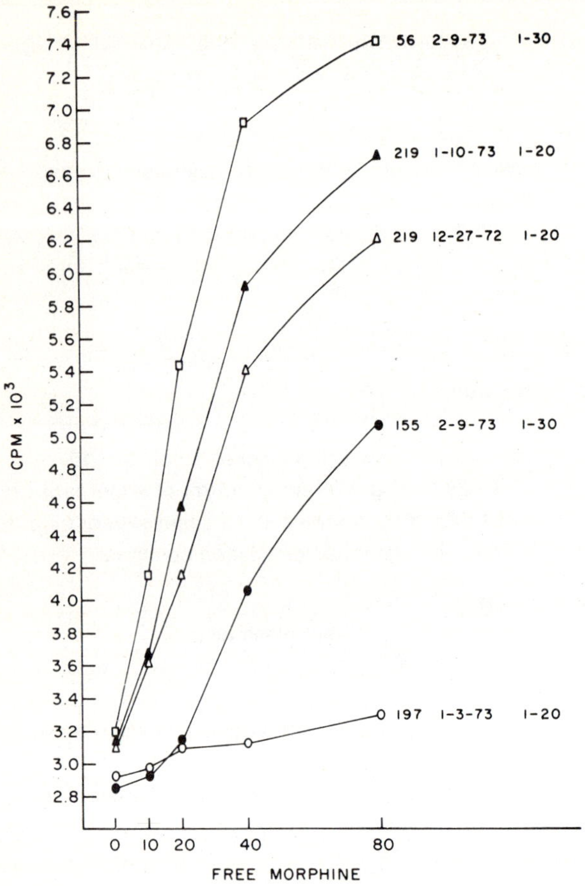

Fig. 1. Response curves for individual bleedings from goats immunized with the morphine immunogen
Abscissa, µg/liter

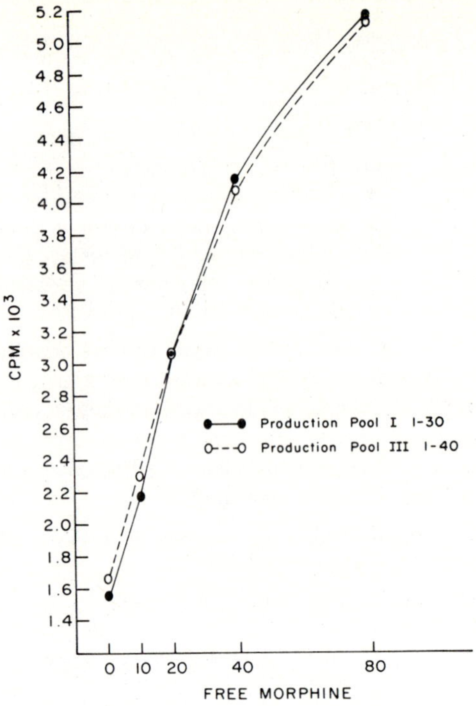

Fig. 2. Response curves for two individual pools of morphine goat antiserum
Abscissa, µg/liter

The linear range of an assay may be expanded by increasing the amounts of reagents used. Manning et al. (*16*), using 2.5-fold the recommended amounts of methadone reagents, expanded the linear range of the methadone standard curve from 50–150 µg/liter to 50–600 µg/liter and thus decreased the number of dilutions required for quantitation.

General Characteristics of the RIA's

Antibody avidity and specificity. Any immunoassay is only as specific as the antibody used and, as with immunoassays in general and RIA's in particular, only highly reproducible if the avidity of the antibody is maintained from lot to lot.

The procedure for obtaining desired antibody has been to immunize between 30 and 70 goats or rabbits per immunogen and to test individual bleedings from each animal for binding capacity. Once binding has been established, the avidity of the antibody, as measured by displacement of labeled antigen by unlabeled antigen, is determined. To illustrate this procedure, Figure 1 shows the reactivity of several individual goat bleedings to the same ^{125}I-morphine antigen in terms of the ability of unlabeled morphine to displace labeled antigen from antibody. For a bleeding to be acceptable, it must have displacing activity equivalent to or greater than a standard reference serum (here equivalent to a difference of at least 3000 cpm between the negative urine control and the 80 µg/liter morphine standard). The bleedings from goats 56 and 219 would be acceptable for use in the antibody pool while the bleedings from goats 155 and 197 would be rejected. Each of the acceptable bleedings is then tested for ability to detect low concentrations of morphine added to "normal" urines, lack of cross-reactivity to methadone and dextromethorphan, and sensitivity for morphine glucuronide comparable to that for morphine.

Acceptable bleedings are pooled and filtered and the new pool matched to a reference pool, to ensure that each lot of reagents prepared, regardless of the pool of antiserum used, will give a similar response curve as shown in Figure 2.

From the data presented in Figure 2 one can see that a 30-fold dilution of Pool 1 gives a standard curve very similar to that seen with a 40-fold dilution of Pool 3. Pool 1 is the reference antiserum pool for both avidity and cross-reactivity.

Similar procedures are followed for obtaining proper antibody pools for the other RIA's. For example, as has been observed by others (*2, 5, 14*), certain aromatic amines other than amphetamines are reactive in immunoassays for amphetamine detection. We have found phenylpropanolamine and phentermine to be particularly reactive. Consequently, all bleedings from goats immunized with the amphetamine immunogen are tested against 10 000 µg/liter solutions of potentially cross-reacting compounds in "normal" human urine. The results of tests for cross reactivity and avidity of each bleeding are analyzed by using a computer program based on orthogonal polynomials and the method

Table 3. Compounds Routinely Evaluated for Cross-Reactivity in Amphetamine Radioimmunoassay

Compound (10 000 μg/liter)	Range of reactivity[a] (amphetamine equivalents, μg/liter)
Phenmetrazine HCl	0–400
Dextromethorphan HCl[b]	0–250
Phenylpropanolamine HCl	1–2000
Propylhexedrine	1–750
Phentermine	8–1600
L-Ephedrine[b]	0–200
Isoproterenol HCl[b]	0–68
Tyramine HCl	47–520
Norepinephrine bitartrate[b]	0–10
Dopamine HCl	0–100
Methamphetamine	1–520

[a] A typical range of reactivity for multiple bleedings from a random group of 20 animals is given for the 10 000 μg/liter solutions.

[b] After a pattern of low reactivity had been set over a period of several months, these compounds were no longer routinely tested.

Table 4. Cross-Reactivity of a Typical Pooled Amphetamine Antiserum

Compound (10 000 μg/liter)	Cross-reactivity (amphetamine equivalents, in μg/liter)
Phenmetrazine HCl	5
Phenylpropanolamine HCl	260
Propylhexedrine	14
Phentermine	170
Tyramine HCl	150
Methamphetamine	28

of least squares. The program uses calculated cpm values to determine whether the tested serum sample meets the required specifications. Because the determination of acceptable avidity depends on differences in cpm between individual points, the use of calculated cpm values minimizes the effect of random error. Using the equation for the fitted line and cpm values associated with the cross-reactants, amphetamine equivalents for each cross-reactant are calculated. Only those sera that are acceptable under criteria for both avidity and cross-reaction are pooled for use in the assay. Table 3 shows the compounds tested, with ranges of cross-reactivity encountered, while Table 4 shows cross-reactivity data for a typical acceptable amphetamine antiserum pool. It is clear that a relatively specific antiserum reagent can be obtained by this procedure.

Sensitivity limits. Each radioimmunoassay developed for drug detection can detect the corresponding drug in concentrations ranging from the high picogram range (250–999 ng/liter) to the low nanogram range (1–50 μg/liter), depending on the concentration of antibody used. However, for use in screening of urine specimens, two factors dictate practical limitations on sensitivity. The first factor is the normal background variation of urine not containing the drug sought, but containing all of the products found in urines from people consuming other drugs, including ethanol, caffeine, and nicotine. Table 5 shows results of tests of urines from 100 people known not to be taking morphine or related analogs and assaying with either ^{125}I-labeled or ^{3}H-labeled morphine. It is evident that any assay set to detect less than 30 μg of morphine equivalents per liter with use of the ^{125}I label and less than 50 μg of morphine equivalents per liter with use of the ^{3}H label would result in unacceptable numbers of falsely positive results. The actual detection limits, because of expected urine interference, have therefore been set at 40 μg/liter for assays with ^{125}I-labeled morphine and 60 μg/liter with [^{3}H]morphine. Whenever tritiated labels (e.g., [^{3}H]morphine, [^{3}H]phenobarbital) are used, we have noted that values for normal urines tend to be higher than when the corresponding ^{125}I-labeled antigen was used, which may be attributed to chemiluminescence of the urine in the scintillation fluid.

Table 5. Apparent Concentration of Morphine in Urines of 100 Normal Individuals

μg ME/liter[a]	^{125}I assay %	^{3}H assay %
0–9	90	70
10–19	8	17
20–29	2	6
30–39	0	5
40–49	0	2

[a] Results expressed as morphine equivalents (ME).

The second limitation on sensitivity of these assays is an even more practical one: the need to confirm positive RIA tests by a nonimmunologic assay. Use of concentration steps and gas–liquid chromatography allows reliable detection of many agents at concentrations as low as 100 μg/liter, while only by use of gas chromatography/mass spectrometry can lower values be detected (*12*).

A cutoff value of 100 μg/liter is used for all assays except the amphetamine RIA, for which it is 1000 μg/liter. In addition, a 40 μg/liter cutoff for the ^{125}I-labeled morphine and 60 μg/liter cutoff for the [^{3}H]morphine assay are available. These lower cutoff values allow for a longer detection time after drug intake, but can present problems in confirmation of positives. The reagents for the amphetamine radioimmunoassay have been so formulated as to provide a reliable cutoff value of 1000 μg/liter. This higher cutoff value in relation to the other assays is intended to minimize problems of cross reactivity of closely related substances (see Table 3).

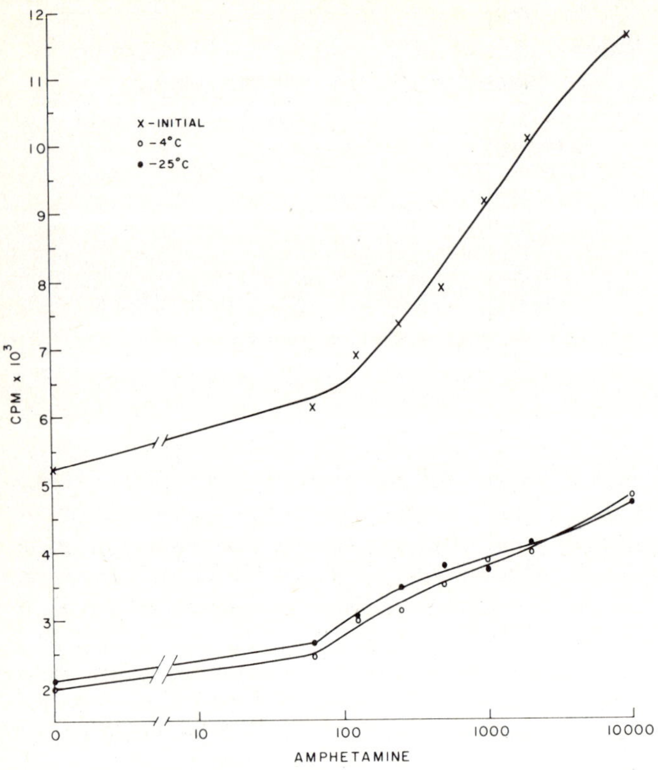

Fig. 3. Radioactivity (cpm) vs. amphetamine concentration after three months at 4 and 25 °C
Abscissa, μg/liter

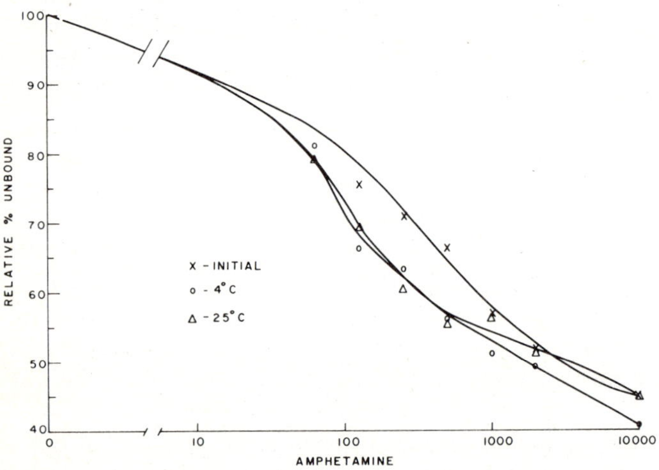

Fig. 4. Relative percent unbound ^{125}I-labeled antigen vs. amphetamine concentration after three months at 4 and 25 °C
Abscissa, μg/liter

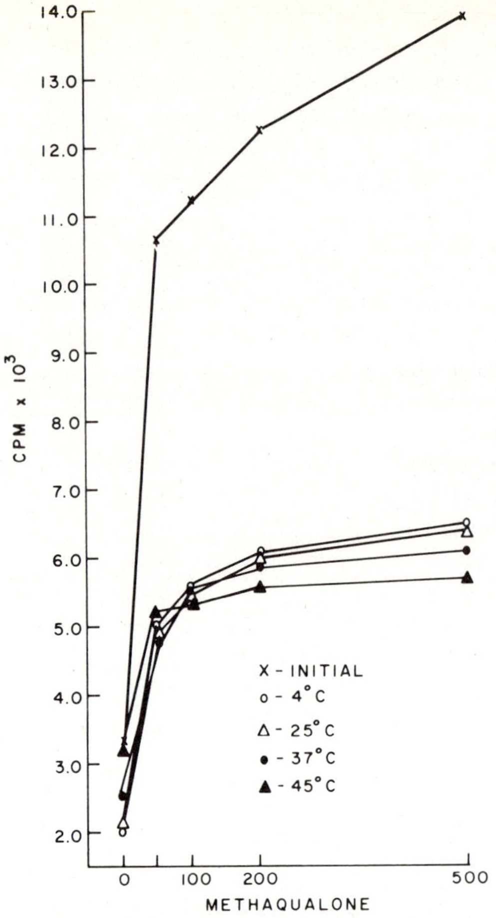

Fig. 5. Radioactivity (cpm) vs. methaqualone concentration after three months at 4, 25, 37, and 45 °C
Abscissa, μg/liter

Reagent stability. For practical use, it is essential that RIA reagents have a reasonable shelf life. Therefore, each assay has been evaluated for stability of the test components in the following manner. The reagents are tested soon after iodination of the antigen and then stored at 4, 25, 37, and 45 °C. The stored reagents are tested at one week, two weeks, and then at monthly intervals from the time at which the ^{125}I-labeled antigen was prepared. The criteria used to assess the stability of the reagents are: acceptability of the standard curve as a function of time and temperature, and determination of relative percent binding. The latter differentiates radioactive decay from antigen/antibody degradation.

We have previously reported that the stability of the morphine assay at 4 °C was directly related to radioactive decay while at higher temperatures (i.e., 37 °C and above) antigen degradation appeared to be the major factor (*7*). However, even after four months at 4 °C, satisfactory response curves could be obtained and the assay used without difficulty.

We have also shown that the barbiturate assay was relatively unaffected at 4 °C or ambient temperature after three months of storage, while at 37 °C the percent-binding curve for the reagent was somewhat flattened compared to that observed when the reagents were held at the lower temperatures (*3*). At 45 °C, this trend was accelerated and the reagents after two months at this temperature were not usable (*3*).

Amphetamine stability data for reagents held at 4 and 25 °C for three months are summarized in Figures 3 (response curve) and 4 (relative percent binding). It is evident that a satisfactory response performance is obtained at 4 and 25 °C for at least three months (Figure 3) with little antigen or antibody degradation observed (Figure 4). After storage at 37 °C and above, satisfactory performance was observed for two months (37 °C) and one month (45 °C).

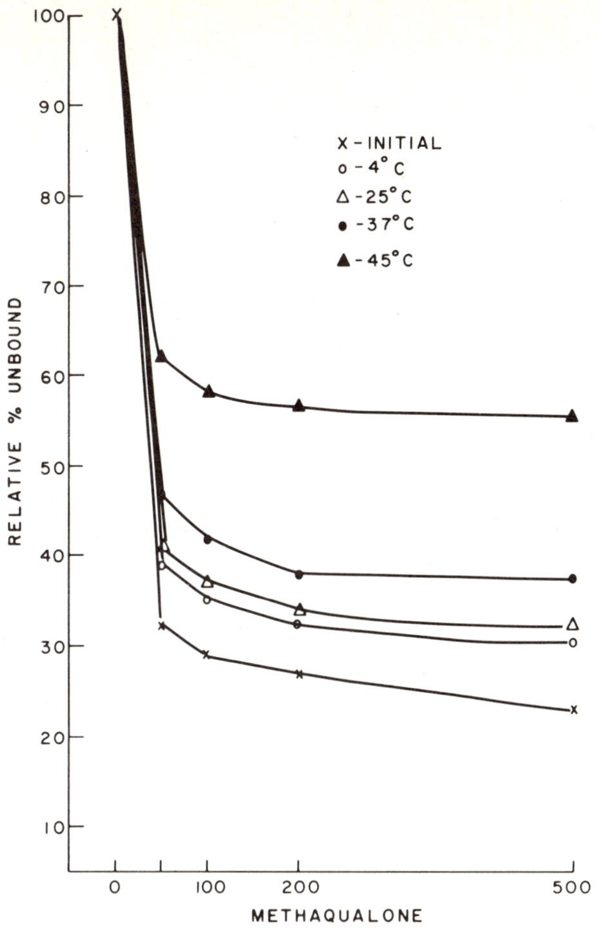

Fig. 6. Relative percent unbound ^{125}I-labeled antigen vs. methaqualone concentration after three months at 4, 25, 37, and 45 °C

Abscissa, μg/liter

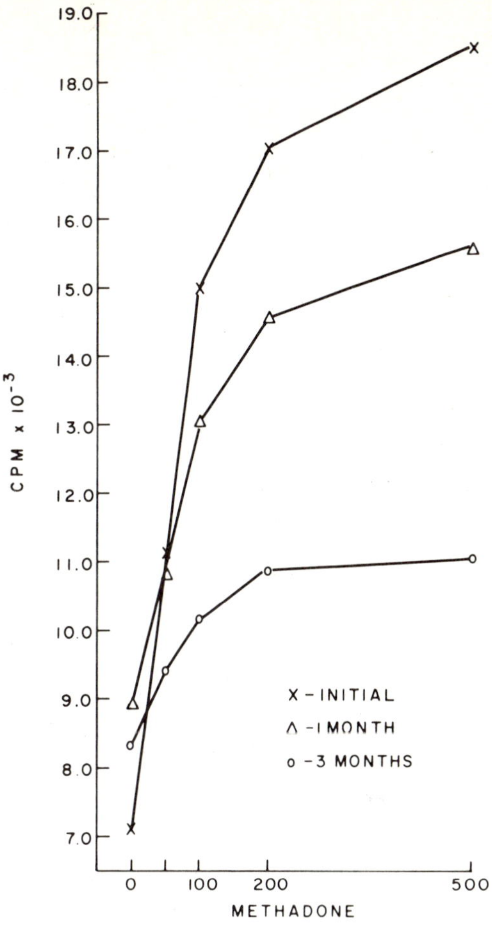

Fig. 7. Radioactivity (cpm) vs. methadone concentration after storage at 4 °C

Abscissa, μg/liter

Representative data for stability of the methaqualone reagents held for three months are shown in Figures 5 (response curve) and 6 (relative percent binding). Satisfactory performance was obtained for at least three months at 4, 25, and 37 °C but not at 45 °C.

For the methadone reagents, performance in terms of response (Figure 7) was satisfactory for at least three months at 4 °C. However, the relative percent binding curves (Figure 8) show a marked trend toward reduced binding, indicating degradation of antigen or antibody. This degradation was greatly accelerated when the reagents were held at elevated temperatures. At 25 °C the reagents were stable for two weeks; at 37 and 45 °C, for only one week.

The stability profile for the combined barbiturate/morphine assay has been previously reported (*6*). We observed that the relative percent of unbound antigens were essentially unchanged at 4 and 25 °C after storage for three months. During the same time the actual radioactivity (cpm) decreased as expected while the curves remained paired (*6*).

The stability profile of a triple reagent (barbiturates/morphine/amphetamine) as a function of time and temperature was studied to determine if degradation of any one component would have a deleterious effect

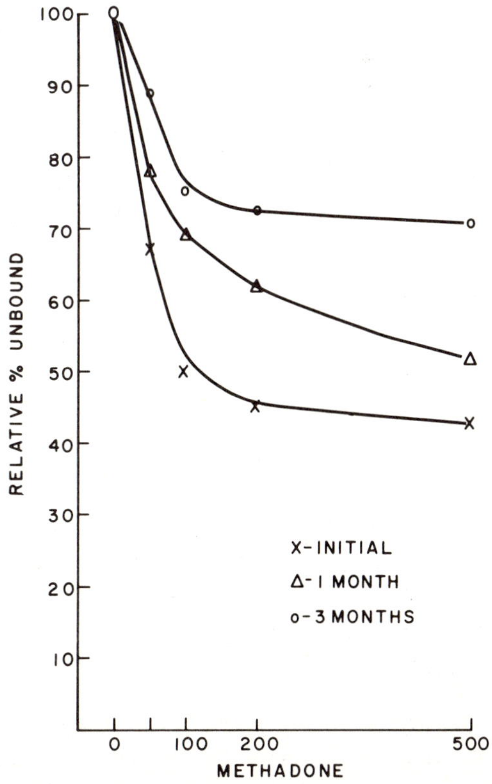

Fig. 8. Relative percent unbound ^{125}I-labeled antigen vs. methadone concentration at 4 °C

Abscissa, μg/liter

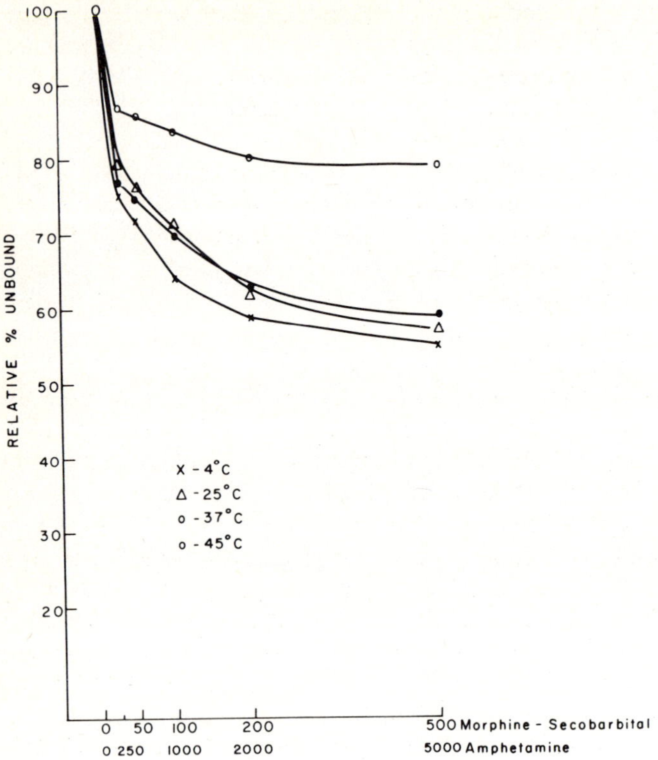

Fig. 9. Relative percent unbound ^{125}I-labeled antigens vs. concentration after three months at 4, 25, 37, and 45 °C
Abscissa, µg/liter

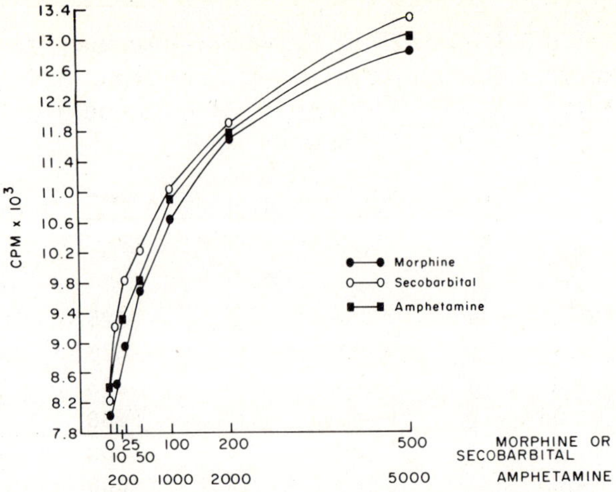

Fig. 10. Radioactivity (cpm) vs. concentration at time of preparation
Abscissa, µg/liter

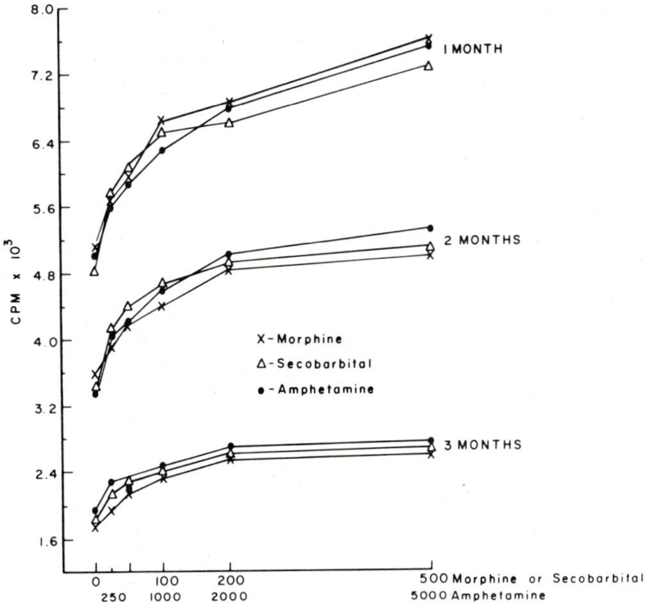

Fig. 11. Radioactivity (cpm) vs. concentration after 1, 2, and 3 months at 4 °C
Abscissa, µg/liter

on the matched response of the individual drugs. The performance of the triple reagent was determined initially and at monthly intervals for six months after storage at 4, 25, 37, and 45 °C. The data (Figure 9) indicated that the relative percentages of unbound ^{125}I-labeled antigens were essentially unchanged at 4, 25, and 37 °C after storage for three months. At 45 °C, a decreased response was evident. In terms of response curve, the reagent was stable at 4 °C during the three month period. The counts per minute at each drug concentration decreased owing to radioactive decay, but the individual curves remained well matched (See Figures 10 and 11).

Our preliminary data suggest to us that the reagents for the benzoylecgonine assay are stable for about three months at 4 and 25 °C.

Clinical and Experimental Results

Morphine

Because the morphine RIA is available with either ^{3}H- or ^{125}I-labeled antigen, it was important to demonstrate that the reagents prepared with either label would quantitatively detect morphine or its metabolite, morphine glucuronide, with comparable sensitivity. Therefore, a volunteer was given 10 mg of morphine per 70 kg body weight, intravenously, and urine samples were collected over a 72-h period and the amount of drug, in terms of morphine equivalents, determined both by the tritium and the iodine assay (Table 6). Evidently both assays detect the morphine or morphine glucuronide in this individual's urine to about the same extent.

The specificity of the morphine RIA for morphine and related analogs (i.e., codeine, heroin, and levorotatory morphinans) has been previously described (*1, 5, 13*). The sensitivity of this RIA for detection of morphine in the urine of addicts or volunteers for periods of at least 72 h after heroin or morphine administration has also been demonstrated (*1, 9, 10;* see Tables 6, 12, and 14 herein).

Barbiturates

In the barbiturate assay, secobarbital derivatives were used to prepare both antigen and antibody. When other barbiturates were used as the unlabeled standards the sensitivity of the assay could be increased (Table 7) without significantly increasing the prevalence of false-positive reactions (*3*). Thus, for example, with

Table 6. Detection by Radioimmunoassay of Morphine and Morphine Analogs in Urine, with ^{3}H-Labeled or ^{125}I-Labeled Morphine as the Antigen

	Morphine equivalents, µg/liter [a]	
Time, h	^{3}H	^{125}I
0	5 [b]	1 [b]
0–8	3166	2525
8–16	2616	2475
16–24	1300	883
24–36	292	238
36–48	295	308
48–60	258	205
60–72	140	178

[a] Single dose of morphine administered intravenously, 10 mg/70 kg body weight, to a volunteer, urine collected at the time intervals shown.
[b] Each value in this column is average of three separate determinations.

Table 7. Relative Activity of Five Barbiturates (100 µg/liter Secobarbital Standard)

Secobarbital	100 [a]
Pentobarbital	45
Butabarbital	45
Amobarbital	35
Phenobarbital	25
Barbital	10

[a] Secobarbital equivalents, µg/liter of urine.

Table 8. Apparent Concentration of Methadone in Urines from 118 Individuals Attending a Methadone Clinic

Methadone equivalents, µg/liter	No. individuals
≥500	46
200–500	58
100–200	11
50–100	1
<50	2

barbital as the unlabeled standard, the sensitivity could be increased 10-fold over that seen when secobarbital was the unlabeled standard. The ability of this RIA to detect barbiturates after administration of clinically acceptable doses of different barbiturates has been previously shown for urine (*3, 5*) and plasma (*3*). Cross-reactivity does not appear to be a problem (*3, 5*).

Methadone

Methadone is metabolized by successive *N*-demethylation and intramolecular condensations to 2-ethylidene-1,5-dimethyl-3,3-diphenyl-1-pyrrolidine (MM1) and 2-ethyl-5-methyl-3,3-diphenyl-1-pyrroline (MM2). Furthermore, it is known that MM1 is excreted in man in larger quantities than methadone itself, while MM2 is excreted only in trace amounts.

We have attempted to determine the distribution of amounts of methadone one could encounter in the urines from individuals who had been attending a methadone clinic. Table 8 shows our results. With 100 µg of methadone per liter as the cutoff point, 97% of the urines tested were positive, with 88% containing more than 200 µg/liter.

Manning et al. (*16*) tested the ^{125}I-labeled methadone RIA for cross reactivity against the 29 most commonly encountered drugs and the two major metabolites MM1 and MM2. They found none with any of these drugs in concentrations of 2500 µg/liter, as compared to a 100 µg/liter standard. The methadone antibody, therefore, seems to be highly specific. They further confirmed the ability of the RIA to detect methadone by assaying urines from 100 individuals in methadone maintenance programs and 100 urines from people not receiving methadone. By thin-layer chromatography and gas chromatography the 200 samples were shown to be positive or negative for methadone. The RIA detected 99 of the positive and all 100 of the negative urines correctly.

In a "blind" study (*16*) these authors tested 292 samples by RIA, including 88 proficiency samples from the N. Y. State Department of Health and the United States Communicable Disease Center. The samples were then submitted for thin-layer and gas-chromatographic confirmation. All methadone positive and negative proficiency samples were correctly identified and of 68 specimens identified as positive by RIA, 58 were identified as positive by the confirmation methods. Four of the nonconfirmed, RIA-positive urines were from people on a methadone maintenance program.

Amphetamine

Amphetamine is not notably metabolized in humans, so the greater portion of an administered dose appears as amphetamine in the urine. Thus, the amphetamine RIA was designed to detect amphetamine itself.

A clinical study that we did with human volunteers showed that the assay can detect the use of moderate doses of amphetamine with a high degree of reliability. Four subjects received oral doses of either 15 or 30 mg of *d*-amphetamine sulfate (three doses of either 5 or 10 mg over a period of about 12 h). The total urine volume excreted during fixed time intervals up to five days after the first dose was collected and assayed. Table 9 shows that there was individual variation in the pattern of amphetamine excretion. Three of the four subjects had high urinary amphetamine concentrations within 1 h of the first dose (i.e., >1000 µg/liter). High concentrations were detected in the urines of all four subjects for as long as two days after the first dose, and one of the four had a high value for three days after the first dose.

In a similar study, 18 volunteer subjects received single oral doses of drugs other than amphetamine

Table 9. Testing of Urines from Four Volunteers Who Ingested *d*-Amphetamine Sulfate

Dose, mg	Amphetamine equivalents (μg/liter) in urine collected during specified time interval (h) 0	0–1	1–4	4–8	8–12	12–24	24–48	48–72	72–96	96–120
15	23	3300	~10 000	2000	1100	6500	3200	450	110	26
15	0	0	140	900	500	2300	2700	260	170	46
30	8	1700	3600	5400	8400	7800	3800	440	220	17
30	2	6400	4400	4100	6500	4600	4400	4900	600	370

Table 10. Drugs Administered to Human Subjects for Cross-Reactivity Study with the Amphetamine Radioimmunoassay

Drug	Dose, mg
Phentermine (resin form)	15 or 30
Chlorophentermine HCl	65 (free base)
Phenmetrazine HCl	25
Chlorpheniramine maleate	4
Promethazine HCl	25
Isoproterenol HCl	10
Diethylpropion HCl	25
Pargyline HCl	25

Two subjects received the indicated dose of each of the drugs listed (two subjects received 15 mg each of phentermine resin and two received 30 mg each).

(Table 10) and their urines were monitored for five days thereafter. Of the 162 specimens, 160 had amphetamine-equivalent values below 100 μg/liter. One specimen gave a value of 400 μg/liter 12 to 24 h after the ingestion of 15 mg of phentermine (in resin form) and one specimen a value of 110 μg/liter 72 to 96 h after the ingestion of 65 mg (free base) of chlorphentermine HCl.

As is clear from Table 4, the assay is relatively insensitive to methamphetamine. However, because amphetamine is a metabolite of methamphetamine, it is possible that the use of methamphetamine can also be detected. To test this, four human volunteers were given 30 mg (three doses of 5 mg per day for two days) of methamphetamine hydrochloride orally and urine specimens collected at 6-h intervals up to 144 h after the initial doses were assayed. Urines from all four subjects showed high values for amphetamine equivalents, the highest values ranging from 450 to 1500 μg/liter. However, only one of the four subjects had urine levels above 1000 μg/liter, and then, only at 42 and 48 h after the initial dose. Thus, the assay is not a reliable test for the use of methamphetamine, although amphetamine equivalents may be detected in some cases.

Mulé et al. (*5*) compared a variety of methods for detection of amphetamine in urine in a drug-abuse screening laboratory. The methods used, in addition to radioimmunoassay, were enzyme multiplied immunoassay technique ("EMIT"), "routine" thin-layer chromatography (*20, 21*), and differential elution thin-layer chromatography (*22*). The differential elution procedure was used to confirm results by the other methods. Of the 130 specimens tested, 15.4% were positive (>0.25–0.5 μg/ml) by radioimmunoassay, 4.6% (>1.5 μg/ml) by enzyme multiplied immunoassay technique ("EMIT"), 11.5% (>2–3 μg/ml) by routine thin-layer chromatography, and 8.5% (1.5 μg/ml) by differential elution thin-layer chromatography. Of the 20 specimens that were positive by radioimmunoassay, nine were confirmed. However, an additional eight of the 20 samples contained less than 0.5 μg/ml by radioimmunoassay, which is well below the limit of sensitivity of the differential elution method. All but one of the 110 specimens that were negative by radioimmunoassay was confirmed.

Methaqualone

Methaqualone is extensively metabolized in humans, so that very little of an administered dose of the drug appears as such in the urine. The metabolites are mainly glucuronides of monohydroxylated derivatives (*23*). Because of quantitative and qualitative variations among individuals in the excretion of these metabolites, the assay is standardized with methaqualone. The antiserum reacts equally well with the unconjugated forms of two of the major metabolites (3′- and 4′-monohydroxy) as it does with methaqualone, and the conjugated forms react less strongly (*4*).

The reagents for the assay have been so formulated as to provide a cutoff value of 100 μg/liter. Tests of urines from normal populations have yielded results as high as 39 μg of methaqualone equivalents per liter. However, in a typical random sample of 100 normal urines, 90 tested at less than 20 μg/liter of methaqualone equivalents. Thus, the cutoff value of 100 μg/liter provides a generous margin against false positives.

This cutoff is sufficiently sensitive to detect methaqualone and (or) metabolites in the urine for at least five days. Four human volunteers were administered oral doses of either 150 or 300 mg of methaqualone. The total urine excreted within fixed time intervals up to 120 h following ingestion of the drug was collected and tested by radioimmunoassay. In all four subjects, the first specimen (0–1 h) gave a value exceeding 500 μg/liter (the most concentrated standard used) and remained so for the duration of the study. After appropriate dilutions of these specimens in normal human urine, drug concentrations in the specimens were found to range from 1550 μg/liter (at 96–120 h) to about 55 000 μg/liter (at 1–4 h) in terms of methaqualone equivalents.

Table 11. Drugs Administered to Human Subjects for Cross-Reactivity Study with the Methaqualone Radioimmunoassay

Drug	Dose, mg
Methyprylon	300
Aprobarbital	40
Phenobarbital sodium	64
Secobarbital sodium	100
Glutethimide	500
Diphenylhydantoin sodium	100
Primadone	250
Diazepam	10
Oxtriphylline	200
Caffeine, citrated	250
Thioridazine hydrochloride	25
Quinine sulfate	325
Imipramine hydrochloride	25
Phenylbutazone	100
Flurazepam hydrochloride	30

For each drug, two subjects received the indicated dose.

In another experiment, human volunteers were administered standard doses of the drugs listed in Table 11 and the total urine excreted within fixed time intervals up to 120 h was collected and assayed. The highest value for methaqualone equivalents encountered was 32 μg/liter, which is within the normal range. Of the 267 specimens assayed, 260 (97%) tested at 20 μg/liter or less.

Berman et al. (*4*) reported no cross-reactions with normal urines that had been supplemented with high concentrations of drugs of abuse other than methaqualone.

Benzoylecgonine

O-Benzoylecgonine is the major urinary metabolite of cocaine. A radioimmunoassay with a ^{125}I-labeled antigen to detect this metabolite has been developed and tested, but is still in an experimental stage. The following summary is based on the data available.

A random sample of 100 "normal" urines was tested, to determine the range of apparent benzoylecgonine concentrations to be expected in a normal population. The results ranged from 0 to 11 μg/liter. Thus, a cutoff value of 100 μg/liter for the qualitative assay appears to be well above the normal range.

The test appears to be quite specific for benzoylecgonine. Some potentially cross-reacting compounds were dissolved in normal human urine and tested. Cocaine at 10 000 μg/liter was equivalent to 590 μg of benzoylecgonine per liter (5.9% as reactive as benzoylecgonine). However, the response to cocaine in terms of benzoylecgonine equivalents was not proportional to the concentration of cocaine. For example, 1000 μg of cocaine per liter was equivalent to 330 μg of benzoylecgonine per liter (33% as reactive as benzoylecgonine). Ecgonine, 10 000 μg/liter, produced a response equivalent to only 53 μg/liter of benzoylecgonine. Atropine and (−)scopolamine hydrobromide, both of which are also tropine derivatives, gave negligible responses. Procaine hydrochloride, 10 000 μg/liter, produced a response equivalent to only 5 μg/liter of benzoylecgonine.

Combined Radioimmunoassays

Because of the independent, flexible nature of RIA's, two single assays can be combined to give a dual assay by carefully manipulating the concentrations of antigens and antibodies. A positive result in such a test indicates the presence of either or both drugs, which can then be identified by using the individual RIA's. The feasibility of simultaneously testing for two classes of drugs of abuse while maintaining stability, specificity, and sensitivity equivalent to the individual assays has been demonstrated with morphine and barbiturate (*5*, *6*).

The possibility of developing a radioimmunoassay for three drugs—namely, morphine, barbiturates, and amphetamine—was investigated. The triple-assay reagent was prepared as a mixture of labeled antigens and corresponding antibodies. Figure 10 shows that the individual response curves for morphine, barbiturate, and amphetamine can be closely superimposed.

Our data make it apparent that a combined RIA for detection of the presence of one or more of three drugs can be developed. Clinical evaluation of the assay for three drugs has not been done.

Use of Discs Impregnated with Urine

In any large-scale drug testing program involving urine specimens, the problems of transportation, storage, and identification can be significant. We therefore investigated the feasibility of using paper discs impregnated with test urines, to eliminate the need for liquid urine samples for testing.

Standard 6.35-mm Schleicher and Schuell (S&S) discs No. 740-E were soaked for 30 min in urine of individuals receiving known drugs; the discs were then dried at 37 °C for 2 h on plastic sheets and stored at room temperature until used about one week later. These discs, when saturated, absorb 50 μl of fluid and can be assayed directly by folding them in half and dropping them into 12 × 75 mm tubes to which the RIA reagents are then added. After incubation at ambient temperature for 1 h, the procedure outlined in Table 2 (precipitation with saturated ammonium sulfate solution, centrifugation, and removal of 0.5 ml of supernate for counting) is done without removing the disc from the tube.

For the morphine assay, two calibration curves were prepared. One with use of urines containing 0, 20, 40, 80, and 160 μg of morphine per liter. In the other we used discs that were soaked in the same urine standards, dried, and used without further treatment. Similar calibration curves were prepared for the barbiturate assays, with 0, 50, 100, 200, 400, 800, and 1600 μg/liter secobarbital standards. The calibration curves, after

Table 12. Determination of Morphine Equivalents in Urines from Volunteers Receiving 10 mg i.v. Morphine per 70 kg Subject[a]

	Counts/min		ME, μg/liter[b]	
Time, h	Disc	Liquid	Disc	Liquid
Subject 1				
0	2245	2073	0	0
0–8	18310	17624	>80	>80
8–16	16727	16191	>80	>80
16–24	17382	17068	>80	>80
24–36	14949	16566	>80	>80
36–48	12763	13928	>80	>80
40–60	9380	11945	64	>80
60–72	10265	12758	72	>80
72–84	7845	10123	38	63
Subject 2				
0	2167	2393	1	1
0–8	18818	18594	>80	>80
8–16	18230	18508	>80	>80
16–24	17180	17131	>80	>80
24–36	14889	17958	>80	>80
36–48	14494	16502	>80	>80
48–60	13153	16239	>80	>80
60–72	10845	12349	80	>80
72–84	7403	9088	42	52
Subject 3				
0	2207	2152	1	0
0–8	18402	19149	>80	>80
8–16	18090	18783	>80	>80
16–24	15460	17437	>80	>80
24–36	14700	17208	>80	>80
36–48	14018	16010	>80	>80
40–60	13688	15737	>80	>80
60–72	9083	12720	60	>80
72–84	8219	9931	50	60

[a] Comparison of values obtained by using liquid urine specimens or standard paper discs soaked in each urine specimen.

[b] ME, μg/liter = micrograms morphine equivalents per liter, determined by reading the corresponding cpm value for discs from a reference curve obtained for discs soaked in urines containing the morphine standards and the corresponding cpm value for liquid from a reference curve with use of the morphine urine standards.

correction for the difference in volume between disc (0.05 ml) and liquid standards (0.1 ml), were superimposable on each other for both morphine and secobarbital.

Table 12 shows results of assays with urines from three individuals receiving morphine and Table 13 shows those for urines from three individuals receiving secobarbital, butabarbital, and glutethimide, respectively. In both tables, the raw cpm counts for discs and liquid specimens as well as μg/liter equivalents after interpolation from the disc and liquid reference curves are presented. At the 72–84 h test period for subject 1 (Table 12), the μg/liter morphine equivalents were above the 40 μg/liter cutoff for liquid samples and borderline for the discs. Otherwise all samples (Tables 12 and 13) that were positive for liquid specimens were also positive for the discs and those negative for liquid specimens were also negative for the discs. Evidently paper discs can be substituted for liquid samples. These discs would offer several advantages: (*a*) after saturation in urine and drying they can be stored at ambient temperature; (*b*) they eliminate the problems associated with storage and transportation of bulk urine; (*c*) they can be used directly in the assay and will not interfere in the separation step; (*d*) either disc or liquid standards can be used; and (*e*) the discs are easily handled with tweezers.

One disadvantage is in quantitation of a drug. If for example, the amount of drug on the disc lies outside the linear portion of the calibration curve, accurate values require careful elution and subsequent dilution. Quantitation of samples containing high drug concentrations by this method is more difficult than using urine specimens directly. In addition, at least two discs per specimen must be submitted for quantitation and the ability to confirm by standard methodology (e.g., thin-layer chromatography) when discs are used is problematical.

Table 13. Determination of Secobarbital Equivalents in Urines from Volunteers Receiving Single Oral Doses of Barbiturates or Glutethimide[a]

	Counts/min		SE, µg/liter[b]	
Time, h	Disc	Liquid	Disc	Liquid
Subject 1				
Secobarbital 100 mg				
0	1820	2872	0	0
0–1	16679	21511	>800	>800
1–4	17212	22449	>800	>800
4–8	17440	20845	>800	>800
8–12	18660	19691	>800	>800
12–24	18960	21696	>800	>800
24–48	19045	19904	>800	>800
48–72	17011	18402	>800	>800
Subject 2				
Butabarbital 100 mg				
0	4357	6723	0	15
0–1	12293	13878	265(280)[c]	200
1–4	12960	14360	325(320)	240
4–8	13585	13924	385(270)	200
8–12	12370	13820	265(280)	200
12–24	11955	12960	225(250)	165
24–48	12696	14811	300(310)	290
48–72	13310	12014	360(350)	130
Subject 3				
Glutethimide 500 mg				
0	3684	4946	0	5
1	4468	5035	5	5
4	4674	4610	5	3
8	6003	6932	15	20
16	5394	6599	10	15

[a] Comparison of values obtained by using liquid urine specimens or standard paper discs soaked in each urine specimen.

[b] SE, µg/liter = micrograms secobarbital equivalents per liter, determined by reading the corresponding cpm value for discs from a reference curve obtained by using discs soaked in urines containing the secobarbital standards and the corresponding cpm value for liquid from a reference curve obtained with the secobarbital urine standards.

[c] Numbers in parentheses refers to SE µg/liter calculated by reading µg/liter for disc cpm off reference curve for liquid standards and multiplying by two, because the liquid reference curve was calculated with 0.1 ml samples while the discs took up about 0.05 ml.

Other Biological Fluids and Tissues

While the radioimmunoassays described have been used mainly for urine screening, their sensitivity and reliability also make them potentially very valuable for qualitatively or quantitatively determining abused drugs in other tissues or fluids. Coumbis and Kaul (*15*) showed, using the ^{3}H-labeled morphine assay, that morphine and analogs could easily by detected in urine, vitreous fluid, whole blood, and bile obtained after autopsy. In addition, using simple physiological saline extraction of organ homogenates, they could also readily detect morphine and analogs in liver, kidney, and brain, as well as in lung, heart, spleen, and skin. Only in the case of highly viscous materials (some bile specimens), highly hemolyzed bloods, and biological fluids with acid reactions was interference observed with the assay. This could be easily corrected by preparing standards in the appropriate biological materials known to be devoid of the drug sought. Manning et al. (*16*) have shown that methadone can easily be detected in blood, brain, urine, or bile as well as in kidney and liver homogenates by the methadone RIA. For all fluids or tissues except kidney and liver, standards prepared in water gave a satisfactory calibration curve. For kidney and liver, standards prepared in homogenates of negative tissues appear to give more nearly accurate calibration curves.

Using a ^{3}H-labeled morphine assay, we attempted to correlate the morphine in urine, serum, and saliva from individuals receiving a known dose of morphine. Calibration curves were prepared with standards prepared in urine, serum, and saliva that were negative for morphine. Table 14 summarizes our results. The levels of morphine and metabolites were higher in urine than in the serum and could be detected for a considerably longer period of time (i.e., 72 vs. 6–8 h), confirming our earlier observations (*1*). It is also apparent that the concentrations of morphine in saliva are in most instances lower than those in serum and can be detected reliably only for 2–6 h.

We also examined how well RIA can detect barbiturates in plasma and saliva as compared to urine. Tri-

Table 14. Morphine Concentration, by ^{3}H-Radioimmunoassay, in Urine, Serum, and Saliva of Individuals Receiving 10 mg Morphine (i.v.) per 70-kg Subject

Urine:

Time, h	Subject 1	2	3	4	5	6
			μg morphine/liter			
0	7	0–2	—	0–9	0	0–5
0–8	>12 000	>1200	7900	>12 000	>1200	4700
8–16	2900	>1200	1275	1080	920	5200
16–24	>1200	>1200	930	3400	970	1590
24–36	725	910	690	825	1300	565
36–48	300	590	550	490	740	720
48–60	191	229	100	158	144	340
60–72	60	90	73	180	44	310

Serum-saliva:

	Subject 1		2		3		4		5		6	
Time, h	Serum	Saliva	Serum	Saliva	Serum	Saliva	Serum	Saliva	Serum	Saliva	Serum	Saliva
0	0	0	0	0	0	0	0	6	0	0	0	0
2	92	74	117	18	127	32	107	>160	126	67	105	44
4	72	0	65	65	85	0	83	12	81	0	73	20
6	36	0	40	0	63	0	43	12	20	0	51	0
8	16	0	10	0	28	0	11	0	13	0	21	0
15	0	0	0	0	0	0	0	0	0	0	1	0
24	0	0	0	0	0	0	0	0	0	0	0	0
36	0	0	0	0	0	0	0	3	0	0	0	3
48	0	0	0	0	0	0	0	0	0	2	0	0
60	0	0	0	0	0	0	0	0	0	0	0	0
72	0	0	0	0	0	0	0	0	0	1	0	0

tium-labeled phenobarbital (New England Nuclear) served as the label and phenobarbital standards were prepared in urine, serum, and saliva from an individual known to be free of barbiturates and other drugs. The assay and test procedure was similar to that used for the morphine RIA. Three individuals were given orally 30 mg phenobarbital, 100 mg pentobarbital, and 100 mg secobarbital, respectively, and urines were collected at 0, 4–8, 24–48, and 48–72 h after drug administration. Plasma and saliva specimens were collected at 0, 4, 24, 48, and 72 h after drug administration. The barbiturate (in micrograms of phenobarbital equivalents per liter) was determined by interpolation from calibration curves prepared with phenobarbital diluted in the appropriate negative biological fluids. Barbiturates were readily detected for 72 h in all urine, serum and saliva specimens (Table 15). Although values were generally higher in urine than in serum or saliva, both serum and saliva values exceeded 100 μg/liter even after 72 h. These results suggest that for detection of barbiturates, serum and saliva would both be acceptable test specimens.

The ability to detect methaqualone and benzoylecgonine by RIA in various biological fluids other than urine is now being investigated.

Discussion

It is apparent that these radioimmunoassays are sensitive and specific for detecting abused drugs, not only in urine, but in various other biological fluids and tissues.

The advantage of using this type of assay is two-fold:

1. A negative result is strong evidence that clinically significant amounts of the drug in question are not present and therefore more laborious analytical procedures are not necessary.

2. Because of the sensitivity, it is usually possible to detect the agent sought for a longer time after drug administration than is possible with other methods.

The assays are so formulated that they are simple to do and can be quickly completed. Thus they lend themselves very well to emergency tests and screening.

Moreover, use of combined RIA's can further increase the efficiency of screening, because the need to test for two or more agents is reduced to retesting only the positive specimens. As with any immunoassay, these RIA's lack absolute specificity. When positive results are obtained, it is necessary to use a nonimmunologic confirmatory test to establish the presence of a drug with certainty.

Table 15. Barbiturate Concentration, by ^{3}H-Radioimmunoassay, in Urine, Plasma, and Saliva of Individuals Receiving Known Oral Doses of Barbiturates

	Type of barbiturate and dose		
Urine Time, h	Phenobarbital, 30 mg	Pentobarbital, 100 mg	Secobarbital, 100 mg
0	0	26[a]	0
4–8	710	5900	2200
24–48	590	6700	3600
48–72	440	7300	2200

Plasma, Saliva Time, h	Plasma	Saliva	Plasma	Saliva	Plasma	Saliva
0	0	64	26	15	0	2
8	590	300	1250	510	500	450
24	660	200	1000	550	740	220
48	550	180	550	410	670	345
72	490	160	420	240	310	105

[a] Micrograms phenobarbital equivalents per liter.

We gratefully acknowledge the cooperation of Drs. Robert Pocelinko and Mia Parsonnet in the clinical studies involving the amphetamine and methaqualone RIA's and of Dr. Eliot Vesell in the clinical studies with the morphine RIA.

References

1. Catlin, D. H., Cleeland, R., and Grunberg, E., A sensitive, rapid radioimmunoassay for morphine and immunologically related substances in urine and serum. *Clin. Chem.* **19,** 216 (1973).

2. Cheng, L. T., Kim, S. Y., Chung, A., and Castro, A., Amphetamines: New radioimmunoassay. *FEBS Lett.* **36,** 339 (1973).

3. Cleeland, R., Davis, R., Heveran, J., and Grunberg, E., A simple rapid ^{125}I radioimmunoassay for the detection of barbiturates in biological fluids. *J. Forensic Sci.* **20,** 45 (1975).

4. Berman, A. R., McGrath, J. P., Permisohn, R. C., and Cella, J. A., Radioimmunoassay of methaqualone and its monohydroxy metabolites in urine. *Clin. Chem.* **21,** 1878 (1975).

5. Mulé, S. J., Whitlock, E., and Jukofsky, D., Radioimmunoassay of drugs subject to abuse: Critical evaluation of urinary morphine-barbiturate, morphine, barbiturate, and amphetamine assays. *Clin. Chem.* **21,** 81 (1975).

6. Usategui-Gomez, M., Heveran, J. E., Cleeland, R., et al., Simultaneous detection of morphine and barbiturates in urine by radioimmunoassay. *Clin. Chem.* **21,** 1378 (1975).

7. Davis, R., Feldhaus, J., Heveran, J., et al., Iodination of morphine and dihydromorphine as related to radioimmunoassay. *Clin. Chem.* **21,** 1498 (1975).

8. Harwood, C. T., Radioimmunoassay: Its application to drugs of abuse. *Pharmacology* **11,** 52 (1974).

9. Catlin, D. H., Urine testing: A comparison of five current methods for detecting morphine. *Am. J. Clin. Pathol.* **60,** 719 (1973).

10. Gorodetzky, C. W., Angel, C. R., Beach, D. J., et al., Validity of screening methods for drugs of abuse in biological fluids. Heroin in urine. *Clin. Pharmacol. Ther.* **15,** 461 (1973).

11. Bidanset, J. H., Drug analysis by immunoassays. *J. Chromatogr. Sci.* **15,** 293 (1974).

12. Mulé, S. J., Methods for the analysis of morphine and related surrogates: Current status. *J. Chromatogr. Sci.* **12,** 245 (1974).

13. Mulé, S. J., Bastos, M. L., and Jukofsky, D., Evaluation of immunoassay methods for detection in urine of drugs subject to abuse. *Clin. Chem.* **20,** 243 (1974).

14. Mulé, S. J., and Bastos, M. L., In *Immunoassays for Drugs Subject to Abuse.* S. J. Mulé, I. Sunshine, M. Braude, and R. E. Willette, Eds., CRC Press, Cleveland, Ohio, 1974, pp 99–106.

15. Coumbis, R. J., and Kaul, B., Distribution of morphine and related compounds in human tissues and biological fluids using radioimmunoassay techniques. *J. Forensic Sci.* **19,** 307 (1974).

16. Manning, T., Bidanset, J. H., Cohen, S., and Lukash, L., Evaluation of the Abuscreen for methadone. *J. Forensic Sci.* **21,** 112 (1976).

17. Spector, S., and Parker, C. W., Morphine: Radioimmunoassay. *Science* **168,** 1347 (1970).

18. Spector, S., and Flynn, E. J., Barbiturates: Radioimmunoassay. *Science* **174,** 1036 (1971).

19. Flynn, E. J., and Spector, S., Determination of barbiturate derivatives by radioimmunoassay. *J. Pharm. Exp. Ther.* **181,** 547 (1972).

20. Mulé, S. J., Bastos, M. L., Jukofsky, D., and Saffer, E., Routine identification of drugs of abuse in human urine: II. Development and application of the XAD-2 resin column method. *J. Chromatogr.* **63,** 289 (1971).

21. Bastos, M. L., Jukofsky, D., Saffer, E., et al., Modifications of the XAD-2 resin column method for the extraction of drugs of abuse from human urine. *J. Chromatogr.* **71,** 549 (1972).

22. Bastos, M. L., Jukofsky, D., and Mulé, S. J., Routine identification of drugs of abuse in human urine. III. Differential elution of the XAD-2 resin. *J. Chromatogr.* **81,** 93 (1973).

23. Bonnichsen, R., Fri, C. G., Negoita, C., and Ryhage, R., Identification of methaqualone metabolites from urine extract by gas chromatography–mass spectrometry. *Clin. Chim. Acta* **40,** 309 (1972).

review

CLIN. CHEM. 22/6, 726–732 (1976)

Radioimmunoassay of Antibiotics and Chemotherapeutic Agents

Alan Broughton and James E. Strong

Therapeutic monitoring of drugs has become of major importance, and has stimulated development of new assay systems. Chemotherapeutic agents, many of which are toxic, have until recently been assayed by microbiological systems or other complex techniques that are impractical for a clinical laboratory. Radioimmunoassays have now been developed for some of these agents. We review the techniques for producing hapten protein conjugates and radiolabeling at specific sites on the drug molecule, and the use of these assays in clinical medicine and pharmacology.

The assay of drugs in biological fluids has attracted much attention in recent years, primarily for two reasons: first, for investigations into their absorption, distribution, metabolism, and excretion (pharmacokinetics) and second, for monitoring therapy (*1*). The therapeutic monitoring of drugs is justified by the finding that response to therapy is often better correlated with the concentration of the drug in the blood than with prescribed dosage (*2*). An additional indication for routine clinical assay for many toxic therapeutic agents is that as much as 8% of hospitalizations may be because of drug-induced illness (*3*). Werner et al. (*4*) have described concepts for the rational selection of drugs suitable for assay on a routine clinical basis. These included drugs that displayed the following characteristics: dangerously toxic, with poorly defined clinical end points; narrow therapeutic range; used in life-threatening disease; used chronically, widely used; and, finally, a technologically and pharmacologically valid assay must be available.

Many antibiotics fulfill the above criteria but are not measured routinely in the clinical laboratory. Interestingly, a microbiological assay for a chemotherapeutic agent was outlined in Fleming's original paper on penicillin (*5*). This assay was later described by Florey and his colleagues (*6*) as being laborious and not having much clinical application. In the same paper, they also described what today is the standard microbiological assay system: radial diffusion, producing zones of inhibition. This method remains essentially unchanged, having the same disadvantages—i.e., imprecision, and lack of sensitivity and specificity—as described in the original paper. In a subsequent paper, Heatley (7) described in detail the microbiological assay of penicillin by this technique. The earliest chemical method for determination of a chemotherapeutic agent appeared in 1937 when Marshall et al. reported an assay for *p*-aminobenzenesulfonamide, based on a diazotization technique (*8*). This was later improved to become the basis of the present technique for determination of the sulfonamide drugs (*9*). Few antibiotics can be chemically assayed directly, most conventional methods requiring time-consuming solvent extraction procedures followed by spectrophotometry, or chromatography. Gas–liquid chromatography, which has sufficient sensitivity and specificity to monitor chemotherapy, is a heavy consumer of human and instrumental time and is not readily amenable to automation (*1*).

Radioimmunoassay techniques, originally used in drug assays for the detection of cardiac glycosides (*11*) but later extended to other drugs, offer an alternative approach for the assay of antibiotics. The procedure is suitable for semi-automation or full automation in clinical laboratories and can potentially be used for almost any antibiotic. Moreover, the assay is usually so specific that other naturally occurring compounds or drugs do not interfere. The theoretical sensitivity of radioimmunoassay is also equivalent to or greater than any conventional technique. However, development of a radioimmunoassay requires the production of a specific antibody and the development of a suitable radioactively labeled drug.

Antibody Production

Most chemotherapeutic agents have a molecular weight of less than 1000 and are therefore not immunogenic by themselves. Landsteiner (*12*) showed that small molecules could be coupled to a carrier protein as

Department of Pathology, University of Texas Medical School, P.O. Box 20708, 6400 W. Cullen St., Houston, Tex. 77025.
Received Feb. 9, 1976; accepted Mar. 8, 1976.

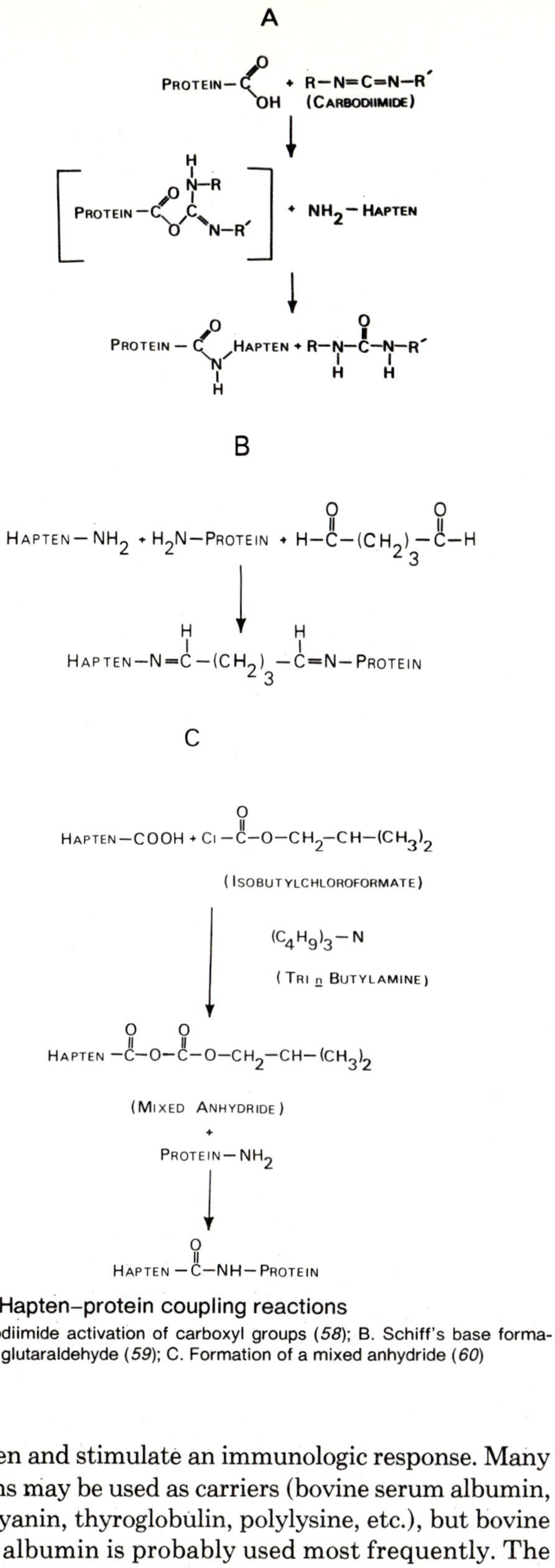

Fig. 1. Hapten–protein coupling reactions

A. Carbodiimide activation of carboxyl groups (*58*); B. Schiff's base formation with glutaraldehyde (*59*); C. Formation of a mixed anhydride (*60*)

a hapten and stimulate an immunologic response. Many proteins may be used as carriers (bovine serum albumin, hemocyanin, thyroglobulin, polylysine, etc.), but bovine serum albumin is probably used most frequently. The chemotherapeutic agents can be conjugated to a protein by coupling amine or carboxyl functional groups on the antibiotic molecule with either carboxyl or amine groups on the carrier protein (Figure 1). Antibiotics lacking the necessary functional groups for direct conjugation can be modified as shown in Figure 2 to form the appropriate derivatives. The resulting conjugate is purified by dialysis and chromatography and the molar ratio of drug to carrier protein determined spectrophotometrically or by incorporation of a radioactive tracer.

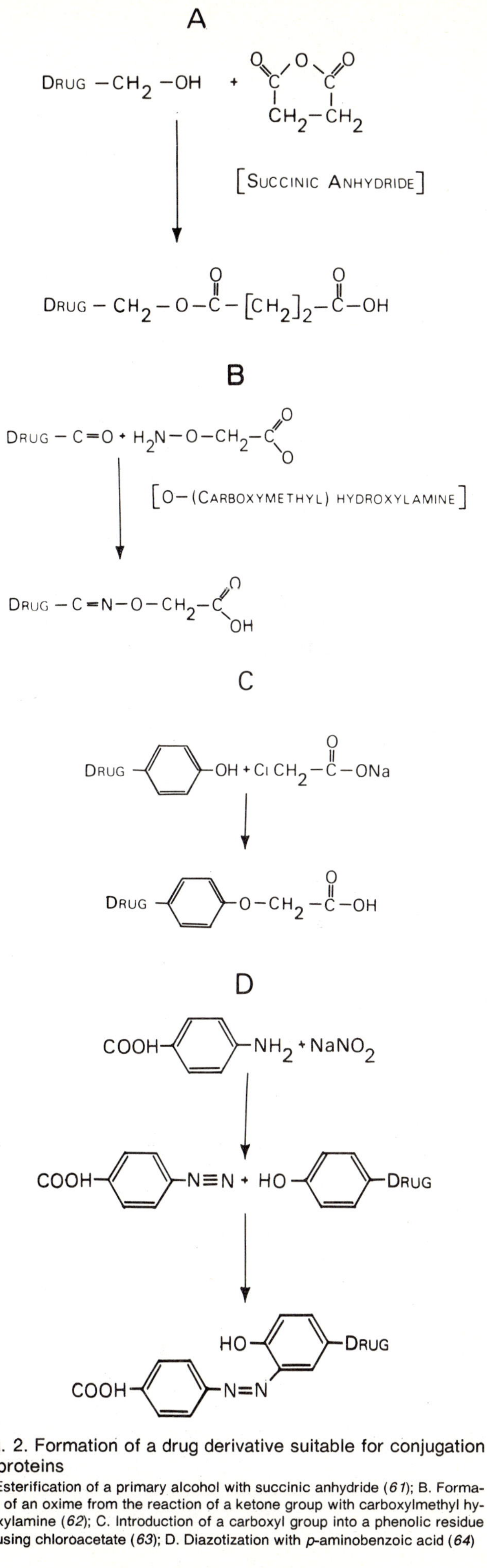

Fig. 2. Formation of a drug derivative suitable for conjugation to proteins

A. Esterification of a primary alcohol with succinic anhydride (*61*); B. Formation of an oxime from the reaction of a ketone group with carboxylmethyl hydroxylamine (*62*); C. Introduction of a carboxyl group into a phenolic residue by using chloroacetate (*63*); D. Diazotization with *p*-aminobenzoic acid (*64*)

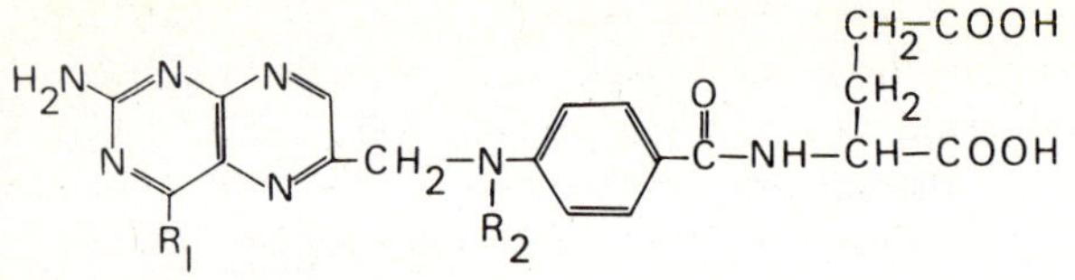

Fig. 3. Folic acid analogs
Folic acid: R_1 = OH; R_2 = H
Methotrexate: R_1 = NH_2; R_2 = CH_3
Aminopterin: R_1 = NH_2; R_2 = H

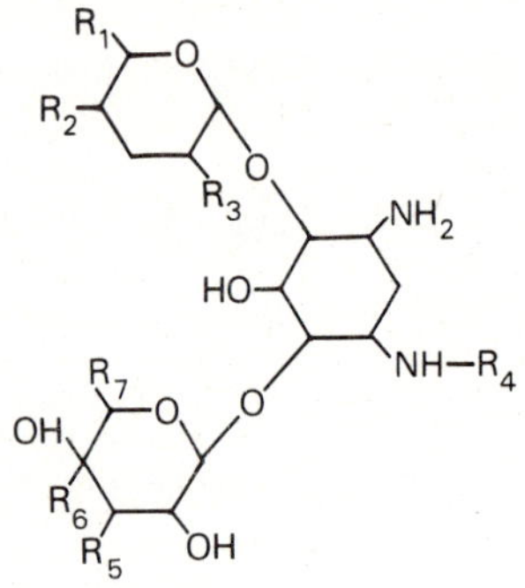

Fig. 4. Structure of the aminoglycoside antibiotics
Gentamicin C_1: R_1 = $CH(CH_3)NHCH_3$, R_2 = H, R_3 = NH_2, R_4 = H, R_5 = $NHCH_3$, R_6 = CH_3, R_7 = H
Sisomicin*: R_1 = CH_2NH_2, R_2 = H, R_3 = NH_2, R_4 = H, R_5 = $NHCH_3$, R_6 = CH_3, R_7 = H
Tobramycin: R_1 = CH_2NH_2, R_2 = OH, R_3 = NH_2, R_4 = NH_2, R_5 = NH_2, R_6 = H, R_7 = CH_2OH
Kanamycin A: R_1 = CH_2NH_2, R_2 = OH, R_3 = OH, R_4 = NH_2, R_5 = NH_2, R_6 = H, R_7 = CH_2OH
Amikacin: R_1 = CH_2NH_2, R_2 = OH, R_3 = OH, R_4 = $NHCOCOHCH_2CH_2NH_2$, R_5 = NH_2, R_6 = H, R_7 = CH_2OH

* Sisomicin also contains a double bond in the pyranose ring between the carbon atoms adjacent to R_1 and R_2.

There have been numerous regimens proposed for the production of antisera, and the subject has been extensively reviewed (*13, 14*). Although no method has been clearly established as superior, we have had success with the method of Hurn and Landon (*15*), with use of New Zealand white rabbits and monthly intramuscular injections of conjugate emulsified in Freund adjuvant. After several booster injections, the resulting antiserum is evaluated for specificity and avidity.

The antibody recognition site (determinate group) on the hapten is generally the group most removed from the region of conjugation to the carrier protein. Therefore, the specificity of the immunoassay depends upon the site of drug–protein conjugation (*16*). Thus the biologically active region of the drug or the moieties of the drug that differ from metabolic products should not be used for conjugation to the carrier protein. Radioimmunoassays that can differentiate between the cancer-treatment drug, methotrexate, and folic acid have been produced by conjugation through the carboxyl groups of the glutamic acid residue on the molecule (Figure 3), thus leaving the amine-substituted pteroic acid portion exposed for antibody recognition (*17*). Radioimmunoassays for aminoglycoside antibiotics also demonstrate the specificity of antisera produced by using drug–protein conjugates. Antibodies produced

Table 1. The Specificity of Antisera Produced Against Gentamicin or Tobramicin Bovine Serum Albumin Conjugates

	% Cross reaction	
Drug	**Anti-gentamicin/BSA**	**Anti-tobramicin/BSA**
Gentamicin	100	< 1
Sisomicin	65	< 1
Tobramycin	< 1	100
Kanamycin	< 1	12.2
Amikacin	< 1	< 1

against gentamicin–bovine serum albumin conjugates do not cross react significantly with kanamycin, differing in the substitution of four functional groups, but cross react 65% with sisomicin, which differs only in the substitution of one functional group (Figure 4). An antibody produced against a tobramycin–bovine serum albumin conjugate cross reacts 12.2% with kanamycin but is relatively nonreactive with gentamicin or sisomicin (Table 1). In addition to specificity, the sensitivity of an immunoassay is determined by the avidity of the antisera.

The affinity constant of an antisera can be calculated by using a Scatchard plot (*18*) or by an equilibrium technique (*19*). Affinity constants so determined for an antisera produced with gentamicin–bovine serum albumin conjugates were 8×10^9 and 10.5×10^9 liter/mol, respectively (*20*), values that compare favorably with affinity constants reported for polypeptide hormones (*14, 21*). Zettner (*22*) has proposed formulas, based on the affinity constant, for determining the optimum concentrations of antibody and labeled antigen to produce maximum sensitivity.

Production of Radiolabeled Antibiotics

Because most drugs lack suitable residues for direct iodination, tritium or carbon-14 labeled antibiotics are used in many radioimmunoassays. The inherent technical difficulties involved with beta-emitting isotopes make gamma emittors, such as iodine-125, desirable for any radioimmunoassay (*23*). Chemical manipulations similar to those used in the conjugation of antibiotics to carrier proteins may also be used to form iodinatable derivatives. Hunter (*24*) has demonstrated this technique using ^{125}I-labeled tyramine, tyrosine methyl ester, and histamine. Edwards et al. (*25*) found that ^{125}I-labeled histamine conjugated compounds in steroid immunoassays showed superior performance because of their increased affinity for antibodies when compared with ^{3}H-labeled steroids. Bolton and Hunter (*26*) used a preiodinated hydroxyphenylsuccinimide ester to label human growth hormone; the resulting compound had a high specific activity with minimal iodination damage. We have modified this procedure to label gentamicin (*20*), sisomicin (*27*), and tobramycin (manuscript in preparation). This technique (Figure 5) has many advantages, which include not exposing the drug to oxidizing agents used in standard iodination techniques

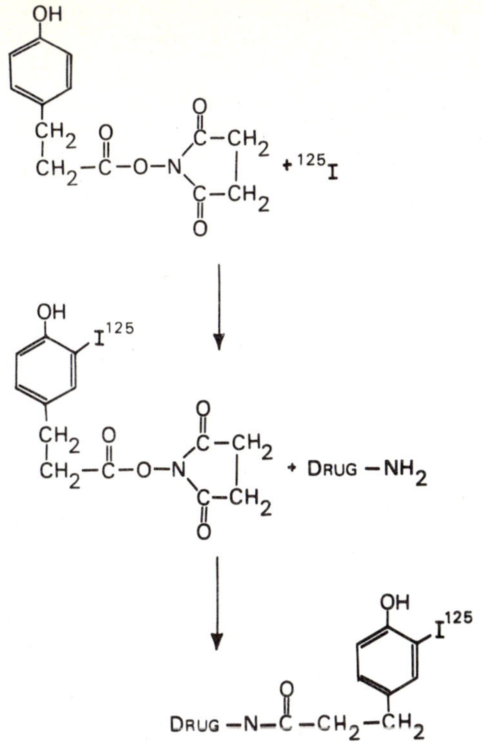

Fig. 5. The reaction of 3-(*p*-hydroxyphenyl)propionic acid *N*-hydroxysuccinimide ester with amine groups to produce an iodine-labeled drug derivative

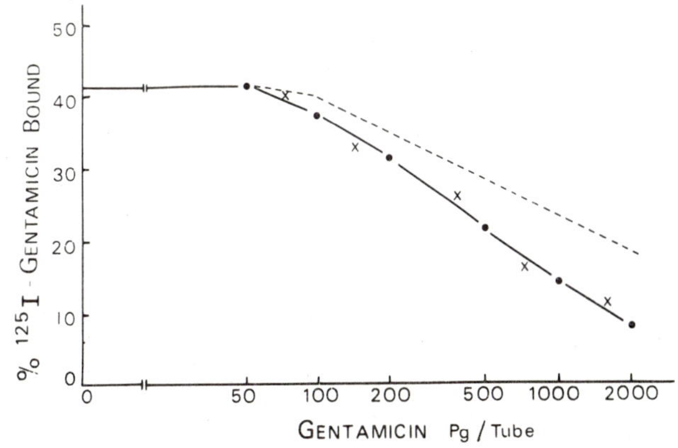

Fig. 6. Assessment of the immunoreactivity of ^{125}I-labeled gentamicin

●, Unlabeled gentamicin; x, ^{125}I-labeled gentamicin; - - - -, form of a curve expected if the ^{125}I-labeled gentamicin is damaged during preparation

(*26*) and attaching the preiodinated hydroxyphenyl succinimide ester to the same site used in drug-carrier protein conjugation. Thus, the iodinated derivative does not interfere with antibody binding of gentamicin (Figure 6).

Occasionally, antibiotics contain moieties that can be directly iodinated. Bleomycin, an antitumor antibiotic, contains an imidazole group as well as primary amine groups. These amine groups were unreactive with the conjugation procedure in which Bolton and Hunter's acylating ester was used. Therefore, an alternative method was selected. The imidazole group was iodinated using the Chloramine-T technique (*28*) at an alkaline pH (*29*). The resulting labeled compound, although of low specific activity, was suitable for developing a radioimmunoassay (*30*). Meyers et al. (*31*), recently reported the production in high yield of an iodinated bleomycin of high specific activity, by the iodine monochloride technique. Although their compound was produced for use in in vivo scanning techniques, it should also be appropriate for use in radioimmunoassay.

Specific Assays

Penicillin. Dismukes et al. (*32*) described the specificity of antibodies raised against benzyl penicillin, oxacillin, and 6-amino-penicillinic acid conjugated with bovine gamma globulin. The beta lactam ring in these penicillins spontaneously cleaves to produce penicilloyl derivatives, which then covalently bind to epsilon amino groups of lysine. The antibodies so produced were specific for the penicilloyl derivatives of the native penicillin, but their activity against the native penicillins was greatly reduced. These results indicated that the method of conjugating haptens to protein carriers must be one that least disturbs the native configuration if radioimmunoassays are to be specific for an antibiotic and not its degradation products. Wal and Bories (*33*) produced an assay for the penicilloyl derivatives in biological fluids by using preiodinated bovine serum albumin conjugated to penicillin groups. There was no cross reaction between the penicilloyl groups and penicillin G in the radioimmunoassay. This assay was designed to detect penicilloyl groups in dairy products and other biological fluids where they may be present in trace amounts. Such biologically inactive penicilloyl derivatives can be formed in man or animals treated with penicillin and allergies have been reported following consumption of products from animals thus treated (*34*).

Isoniazid. Schwenk et al. (*35*) recently reported an assay for this anti-tuberculosis agent. Antibodies were raised against an isoniazid–bovine serum albumin conjugate, and the drug was radioactively labeled with tritium. The sensitivity of this assay was 50 μg/liter and cross reactivity was 2% with acetylisoniazid, 1% for isonicotinic acid, 48% with isonicotinamide, and less than 1% with *p*-aminosalicylic acid. Isoniazid is metabolized by acetylation, and patients can be divided into two genetically distinct groups based on their metabolic rates (*36*). The authors recommended that the radioimmunoassay for isoniazid be used to detect fast and slow metabolizers of the drug and thus enable optimization of chemotherapy.

Aminoglycoside antibiotics. The aminoglycoside antibiotics are active against infections with Gram negative bacilli but are potentially ototoxic and nephrotoxic (*37*). Thus, it is important to monitor aminoglycoside chemotherapy, particularly in patients with impaired renal or cardiac function. The first aminoglycoside radioimmunoassay was developed by Lewis et al. (*38*) for gentamicin. They prepared antibodies by using a carbodiimide activated conjugation of gentamicin to a variety of carrier proteins. A sensitivity of 2 ng was achieved in the radioimmunoassay with a tritium-labeled antibiotic. There was little or no cross reactivity with other aminoglycoside antibiotics: neomycin, kanomycin, and streptomycin. Mahon et al. (*39*) improved the sensitivity of this assay by chromatographic purification of the tritium-labeled drug. An iodinated gentamicin radioimmunoassay was developed in our laboratory (*20*) by use of the pre-iodinated hydroxyphenyl succinimide ester technique, which further improved the assay sensitivity to 80 pg. Comparison of results for this assay with those for a microbiological assay gave a correlation coefficient of 0.87. The antisera did not cross react with kanomycin, tobramycin, or streptomycin, but displayed 65% cross reactivity with sisomicin. This cross reactivity facilitated the development of a sisomicin radioimmunoassay (*27*) with a sensitivity of 140 pg. Comparison of the sisomicin radioimmunoassay with a microbial assay yielded a correlation coefficient of 0.85. Radioimmunoassays for other aminoglycosides have been reported: Lewis et al. (*40*) produced an assay for amikacin with a sensitivity of 5 ng; our laboratory has also developed one for tobramycin with a sensitivity of 280 pg (manuscript in preparation).

In addition to microbiological and radioimmunoassays, there are also radioenzymatic assays for aminoglycosides (*41, 42*). These assays are based on the following principle: An enzyme mediated by *Escherichia coli* "R" factor adenylates aminoglycosides, utilizing ATP in the reaction. The ATP in the assay is labeled with ^{14}C and serves as the source of the adenyl group. Quantitation is achieved by measuring the amount of ^{14}C incorporated onto the aminoglycoside. A comparison of the radioimmunoassay of ^{3}H-labeled gentamicin with the radioenzymatic assay by Minshew et al. (*43*) resulted in a correlation coefficient of 0.9 and a linear-regression line with a slope of 0.99. This indicated that both methods yield comparable results, which are not statistically significantly different.

Cancer chemotherapeutic agents. These drugs are highly toxic by virtue of their pharmacological action. Radioimmunoassays have been developed for a few of the agents and used to investigate their pharmacokinetics and metabolism in patients. The capacity to monitor chemotherapeutic drugs routinely may provide a basis for monitoring therapy and avoiding or minimizing toxicity.

Methotrexate. Methotrexate, a folate antagonist that binds to folate reductase (EC 1.5.1.3), was first assayed by radioimmunoassay with use of an antibody raised in rabbits immunized with a carbodiimide activated methotrexate/methylated bovine serum albumin conjugate and a tritium-labeled drug (*17*). The antibody prepared in this manner cross reacted less than 0.1% with folate. Levine and Powers (*44*) also reported a radioimmunoassay for methotrexate in which hemocyanin was used as the carrier protein for antibody production. This assay could detect 80 pg of the drug and was applicable for determining methotrexate concentrations in patients receiving folinic acid "rescue" therapy (*45*). The antisera used in this radioimmunoassay cross

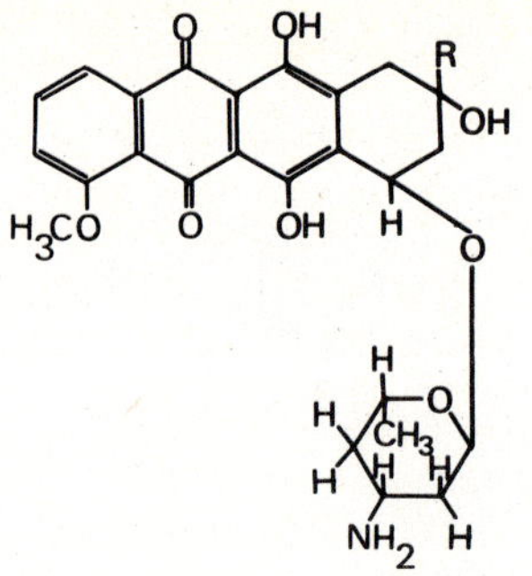

Fig. 7. Structure of adriamycin (R = $COCH_2OH$) and daunomycin (R = $COCH_3$)

reacted five orders of magnitude less with folate, tetrahydrofolate, or folinic acid, which lack either the 4-amino or 10-methyl group of methotrexate (Figure 3). The authors suggested this indicated an immunodominance of either one or both of these groups (*44*). Raso and Schrieber (*46*) also developed a radioimmunoassay for methotrexate and investigated the characteristics of their antisera (similarly developed using methotrexate/methylated bovine serum albumin conjugates). They found that compounds resembling methotrexate lacking the 10-methyl substitution but having the 4-amino substitution (aminopterin) showed 10% cross-reactivity whereas compounds lacking the 4-amino substitution displayed less than 0.01% cross reactivity. These data suggested that the 4-amino substitution in methotrexate was immunodominate (*46*). Arons et al. (*47*) used the binding of methotrexate to dihydrofolate reductase (EC 1.5.1.4) instead of an antibody as the basis of a radioassay for methotrexate. Their sensitivity was 500 pg, and they reported no interference in the assay by physiological concentrations of folate and other analogs.

Adriamycin. This anthracycline antibiotic, isolated from *Streptomyces pencilius* is used in treating several different types of neoplastic disorders (*48, 49*). At therapeutic concentrations, this drug can sometimes produce toxic side effects, of which cardiotoxicity is the most serious (*57*). Van Vunakis et al. (*51*) described a radioimmunoassay for adriamycin and the related compound, daunomycin (Figure 7), with a sensitivity of about 1 μg/liter of serum. Antisera were produced by using carbodiimide- or glutaraldehyde-activated conjugates of adriamycin to human serum albumin or hemocyanin. These conjugates were injected into rabbits, monkeys, and a goat. The goat immunized with a glutaraldehyde-activated conjugate of adriamycin to human serum albumin produced an antibody that gave the most sensitive assay. The other antibodies that were produced varied in specificity with the species of animal and type of conjugate. The radioactively labeled drug used in this assay was prepared by carbodiimide conjugation of *p*-hydroxyphenylacetic acid to adriamycin. The resultant adriamycin derivative was iodinated by the lactoperoxidase method. This conjugation technique produced an amide derivative at the same site on the adriamycin molecule as used in carbodiimide conjugation of the drug with the carrier protein. The goat antisera recognized this bond with the carrier protein, as indicated by its increased affinity for *N*-acetyladriamycin compared with adriamycin.

Langone et al. (*52*) used a combination of radioimmunoassay and high-pressure liquid chromatography to identify and measure adriamycin and its metabolites in biological fluids. This procedure demonstrated the advantage of combining the sensitivity of radioimmunoassay with the separation achieved by liquid chromatography for identifying variations in drug metabolism among individual patients.

Bleomycin. This antineoplastic antibiotic, isolated from a mutant strain of *Streptomyces verticillus,* has been effective against a variety of neoplasms, including squamous cell carcinoma, lymphoma, and testicular carcinoma (*53*). The most common toxic effect of the drug is a minor cutaneous reaction. However, pulmonary toxicity occurs in about 10% of the patients, resulting in pulmonary fibrosis in about 1% (*54*).

Investigations into the toxicity and pharmacokinetics of this drug have been hampered by lack of a precise and sensitive assay (*55*). The published microbiological assays (*56, 57*) lack accuracy and sensitivity at bleomycin concentrations below 1 mg/liter of serum. We have developed a radioimmunoassay for this antibiotic with antisera produced in rabbits by using carbodiimide-activated conjugation of bleomycin to bovine serum albumin, and iodinated bleomycin prepared as described above (*30*). The assay was sensitive to 250 pg (2.5 μg/liter) and did not cross react with other antineoplastic agents. Comparison with a microbial assay for bleomycin gave a correlation coefficient of 0.978. Studies on patients receiving bleomycin by continuous infusion indicate that the assay can be used to monitor steady-state concentrations and estimate pharmacokinetic variables in patients receiving multiple drug therapy (Broughton, Strong, and Holoye; manuscript in preparation).

Therapeutic monitoring of drug concentrations in blood will be requested more frequently by physicians to optimize therapy and avoid toxicity (*2*). The clinical laboratory is the logical department to perform these assays, using methods that are rapid, precise, sensitive, specific and suitable for automation. Previously, assays for antibiotics have involved microbiological techniques or complicated procedures requiring highly sophisticated instrumentation and personnel. Radioimmunoassays, however, are eminently suitable for routine use. Therefore, the continued development of reliable radioimmunoassays for antibiotics and other chemotherapeutic agents will allow clinical laboratory medicine more fully to participate in the delivery of health care by providing a quantitative basis for rational modification of chemotherapy.

We appreciate the supply of bleomycin from Bristol Laboratories, Syracuse, New York, and the aminoglycosides from Dr. Gerald P. Bodey, Sr., M. D. Anderson Mospital, Houston, Texas. Dr. Bodey also performed the microbiological assays of these drugs. Dr. S. T. Crooke of Bristol Laboratories performed the microbiological assays of bleomycin.

References

1. Marks, V., Lindup, W. E., and Baylis, E. M., Measurement of therapeutic agents in blood. *Adv. Clin. Chem.* **16,** 47 (1973).

2. Vesell, E. S., and Passonanti, Q. T., Utility of clinical chemical determinations of drug concentrations in biologic fluids. *Clin. Chem.* **17,** 851 (1971).

3. Werner, M., and Sutherland, E. W., The contribution of laboratory medicine to clinical pharmacology. *Hum. Pathol.* **6,** 135 (1975).

4. Werner, M., Sutherland, E. W., and Abramson, F. P., Concepts for the rational selection of assays to be used in monitoring therapeutic drugs. *Clin. Chem.* **21,** 1368 (1975).

5. Fleming, A., On the antibacterial action of cultures of a penicillium with special reference to their use in the isolation of *B. influenzae. Br. J. Exp. Pathol.* **10,** 226 (1929).

6. Abraham, E. P., Chain, E., Fletcher, C. M., et al., Further observations on penicillin. *Lancet* **ii,** 177 (1941).

7. Heatley, N. G., A method for the assay of penicillin. *Biochem. J.* **38,** 61 (1944).

8. Marshall, E. K., Emerson, K., and Cutting, W. C., Para-aminobenzenesulfonamide absorption and excretion: Method of determination in urine and blood. *J. Am. Med. Assoc.* **108,** 953 (1938).

9. Bauer, J. D., Ackermann, P. G., and Toro, G., *Clinical Laboratory Methods,* C. V. Mosby, St. Louis, Mo., 1974, p 800.

10. Castro, A., Clinical applications of radioimmunoassays of drugs in humans. *Medikon* **4,** 17 (1975).

11. Oliver, G. C., Parker, B. M., Brasfield, D. L., and Parker, C. W., The measurement of digitoxin in human serum by radioimmunoassay. *J. Clin. Invest.* **47,** 1035 (1968).

12. Landsteiner, K., *The Specificity of Serological Reactions,* Harvard University Press, Cambridge, Mass., 1946.

13. Lader, S., Hurn, B. A. L., and Court, G., A comparative assessment of immunization procedures for radioimmunoassay. In *Radioimmunoassay and Related Procedures in Medicine.* International Atomic Energy Agency, Vienna, 1974, pp 31–44.

14. Odell, W. D., Abraham, G. A., Skowsky, W. R., et al., In *Principles of Competitive Protein Binding Analysis,* Chap. III, W. D. Odell and W. H. Daughaday, Eds., J. B. Lippincott Co., Philadelphia, Pa., 1971, pp 57–88.

15. Hurn, B. A. L., and Landon, J., Antisera for radioimmunoassay. In *Radioimmunoassay Methods,* K. E. Kirkham, and W. M. Hunter, Eds., Churchill Livingstone, London, 1973, pp 121–142.

16. Linder, H. R., Perel, E., Friedlander, A., and Zeitlin, A., Specificity of antibodies to ovarian hormones in relation to the site of attachment of the steroid hapten to the peptide carrier. *Steroids* **19,** 357 (1972).

17. Bohoun, C., Duprey, F., and Boudene, C., Radioimmunoassay of methotrexate in biological fluids. *Clin. Chim. Acta* **57,** 263 (1974).

18. Scatchard, G., The attractions of proteins for small molecules and ions. *Ann. N.Y. Acad. Sci.* **51,** 660 (1949).

19. Odell, W. D., Abraham, G., Raud, H. R., et al., Influence of immunization procedures on the titer, affinity, and specificity of antisera to glycopeptides. *Acta Endocrinol.* (Copenhagen) **142** (*Suppl*), 54 (1969).

20. Broughton, A., and Strong, J. E., Radioimmunoassay of iodinated gentamicin. *Clin. Chim. Acta* **66,** 125 (1976).

21. Keane, P. M., Walker, W. H. C., Gauldie, J., and Abraham, G. E., Thermodynamic aspects of some radioimmunoassays. *Clin. Chem.* **22,** 70 (1976).

22. Zettner, A., Principles of competitive binding assays (saturation analysis). 1. equilibrium techniques. *Clin. Chem.* **19,** 699 (1973).

23. Parker, C. W., Radioimmunoassays. In *Progress in Clinical Pathology.* M. Steffanini, Ed., Grune and Stratton, New York, N. Y., 1972, pp 103–141.

24. Hunter, W. M., Preparation and assessment of radioactive tracers. *Br. Med. Bull.* **30,** 18 (1974).

25. Edwards, R., Gilby, E. D., and Jeffcoate, S. L., Iodine-125 tracers in steroid radioimmunoassay. In *Radioimmunoassay and Related Procedures in Medicine.* International Atomic Energy Agency, Vienna, 1974, pp 31–44.

26. Bolton, A. E., and Hunter, W. M., The labelling of proteins to high specific activity by conjugation to a ^{125}I-containing acylating agent. *Biochem. J.* **133,** 529 (1973).

27. Broughton, A., Strong, J. E., and Bodey, G. P., Radioimmunoassay of sisomicin. *Antimicrob. Agents Chemother.* **9,** 247 (1976).

28. Hunter, W. M., and Greenwood, F. C., Preparation of ^{131}I-labeled human growth hormone of high specific activity. *Nature* **194,** 495 (1962).

29. Schutle, L., and Havinga, E., Base catalysts in aromatic iodination, kinetics and mechanism of the iodination of *p*-cresol, 2,6-dimethylphenol, imidazole and dimethylaminobenzenesulfonic acid. *Tetrahedron* **26,** 2297 (1970).

30. Broughton, A., and Strong, J. E., Radioimmunoassay of bleomycin. *Cancer Res.* **36,** 1418 (1976).

31. Meyers, J., Krohn, K., and De Nardo, G., Preparation and chemical characterization of radioiodinated bleomycin. *J. Nucl. Med.* **16,** 835 (1975).

32. Dismukes, W. E., de Riel, K., and Hyslop, N. E., Jr., Specificity of antipenicilloyl antibodies: Utility in radioimmunoassays of penicillins. *Clin. Res.* **21,** 1059 (1975).

33. Wal, J. M., and Bories, G., Radioimmunoassay of penicilloyl groups in biological fluids. *FEBS Lett.* **57,** 9 (1975).

34. Gounell, H., and Szakvary, A., Antibiotiques et aliments. I-les accidents allergiques lies aux residus. *Bull. Acad. Med.* **150,** 76 (1966).

35. Schwenk, R., Kelly, K., Tse, S. K., and Sehon, A. H., A radioimmunoassay for isoniazid. *Clin. Chem.* **21,** 1059 (1975).

36. Radhakrishna, S., Fox, W., Mitchison, D. A., and Menon, N. K., A controlled comparison of a twice weekly and three once weekly regimens in the initial treatment of pulmonary tuberculosis. *Bull. WHO* **43,** 143 (1970).

37. Jackson, G. G., and Riff, J. J., Pseudomonas bacteria: Pharmacologic and other basis for failure of treatment with gentamicin. *J. Infect. Dis. (Suppl.)* **124,** 185 (1971).

38. Lewis, J. E., Nelson, J. C., and Elder, H. A., Radioimmunoassay of an antibiotic: Gentamicin. *Nature, New. Biol.* **239,** 214 (1972).

39. Mahon, W. A., Ezer, J., and Wilson, T. N., Radioimmunoassay for measurement of gentamicin in blood. *Antimicrob. Agents Chemother.* **3,** 585 (1973).

40. Lewis, J. E., Nelson, J. C., and Elder, H. A., Amikacin: A rapid and sensitive radioimmunoassay. *Antimicrob. Agents Chemother.* **7,** 142 (1975).

41. Smith, D. H., Otto, B. Van., and Smith, A., A rapid chemical assay for gentamicin. *New Engl. J. Med.* **286,** 583 (1972).

42. Stevens, P., Young, L. S., and Hewett, W. L., Improved acetylating radioenzymatic assay of amikacin, tobramycin and sisomicin in serum. *Antimicrob. Agents Chemother.* **7,** 374 (1975).

43. Minshew, B. H., Holmes, R. K., and Baxter, C. R., Comparison of a radioimmunoassay with an enzymatic assay for gentamicin. *Antimicrob. Agents Chemother.* **7,** 107 (1975).

44. Levine, L., and Powers, E., Radioimmunoassay for methotrexate. *Res. Commun. Chem. Pathol. Pharmacol.* **9,** 543 (1974).

45. Mitchell, M. S., Wawro, N. W., De Conti, R. C., et al., Effectiveness of high dose infusions of methotrexate followed by leneovorin in carcinoma of head and neck. *Cancer Res.* **28,** 1088 (1968).

46. Raso, V., and Schreiber, R., A rapid and specific radioimmunoassay for methotrexate. *Cancer Res.* **35,** 1407 (1975).

47. Arons, E., Rothenberg, S. P., da Costa, M., et al., A direct ligand-binding radioassay for the measurement of methotrexate in tissues and biological fluids. *Cancer Res.* **35,** 2033 (1975).

48. Bachur, N. R., Interdisciplinary session report. Current status of studies with adriamycin (NSC 123127). *Cancer Chemother. Rep.* **4,** 47 (1973).

49. Carter, S. K., Di Marco, A., Ghione, M., et al., Eds., *International Symposium on Adriamycin.* Springer Verlag, Berlin, 1972.

50. Reinchart, J. J., Lewis, R. P., and Balcerzak, S. P., Adriamycin cardiotoxicity in man. *Ann. Intern. Med.* **81,** 475 (1974).

51. Van Vunakis, H., Langone, J. J., Riceberg, L. J., and Levine, L., Radioimmunoassays for adriamycin and daunomycin. *Cancer Res.* **34,** 2546 (1974).

52. Langone, J. J., Van Vunakis, H., and Bachur, N. R., Adriamycin and metabolites: Separation by high pressure liquid chromatography and quantitation by radioimmunoassay. *Biochem. Med.* **12,** 283 (1975).

53. Blum, R. H., Carter, S. K., and Agre, K., A clinical review of bleomycin—a new antineoplastic agent. *Cancer* **31,** 903 (1973).

54. Carter, S. K., and Blum, R. H., The current status of bleomycin and adriamycin. *Cancer* **24,** 322 (1974).

55. Chabner, B. A., Myers, C. E., Coleman, C. N., and Johns, D. G., The clinical pharmacology of antineoplastic agents. *New Engl. J. Med.* **292,** 1159 (1975).

56. Umezawa, H., Suhara, Y., Takita, T., and Maeda, K., Purification of bleomycins. *J. Antibiot.* **19,** 210 (1966).

57. Ohnuma, T., Holland, J. F., Masuda, H., et al., Microbiological assay of bleomycin: Inactivation tissue distribution and clearance. *Cancer* **33,** 1230 (1974).

58. Goodfriend, G. L., Levine, L., and Fasman, G. D., Antibodies to bradykinin and angiotensin: A use of carbodiimides in immunology. *Science* **144,** 1344 (1964).

59. Avrameas, S., and Ternynck, T., The cross linking of proteins with glutaraldehyde and its use for the preparation of immunoadsorbents. *Immunochemistry* **6,** 53 (1969).

60. Erlanger, B. F., Beiser, S. M., Borek, F., et al., In *Methods in Immunology and Immunochemistry.* C. A. Williams and M. W. Chase, Eds., Academic Press, New York, N.Y., 1967, p 149.

61. Abraham, G. E., and Grover, P. K., Covalent linkage of steroid hormones to protein carriers for use in radioimmunoassay. In *Principles of Competitive Protein-Binding Assays.* W. D. Odell, and W. H. Daughaday, Eds., J.B. Lippincott Co., Philadelphia, Pa., 1971, pp 140–157.

62. Erlanger, B. F., Borek, F., Beiser, S. M., and Lieberman, S., Preparation and characterization of conjugates of bovine serum albumin with progesterone, deoxycorticosterone, and estrone. *J. Biol. Chem.* **234,** 1090 (1959).

63. Spector, S., and Parker, C. W., Morphine radioimmunoassay. *Science* **168,** 1347 (1970).

64. Fabachnick, M., and Sobotka, H., A spectrophotometric study of the coupling of diazotized arsanilic acid with proteins. *J. Biol. Chem.* **235,** 1051 (1960).

CLIN. CHEM. 22/6, 733–738 (1976)

review

Quantitative Enzyme Immunoassay: Current Status

Simon L. Scharpé, Walter M. Cooreman, Walter J. Blomme, and Gert M. Laekeman

The current status of this group of techniques for assay of endogenous and exogenous compounds in biological fluids is briefly reviewed.

Additional Keyphrases: *enzyme-linked immunoabsorbent assay • homogeneous enzyme immunoassay (EMIT) • drug screening in urine • toxicology • radioassay • monitoring of therapy*

Since the development of the competitive binding assay based on the use of radiolabeled ligands as published in 1959 by Yalow and Berson (*1*), this technique has found widespread and diversified application in the biochemical field. The enthusiastic acceptance of this methodological principle appears to be related to the inherent specificity of this technique. The sensitivity of radioimmunoassay in the 10^{-11} to 10^{-17} mole range allows accurate quantitative estimations of a great variety of biologically active compounds encountered in nanogram to picogram amounts in biological systems. However, compounds labeled with gamma-emitting isotopes have a relatively short shelf-life, and health hazards are involved in their preparation. Radiation damage may also affect the immunochemical reactivity of the labeled substance. Application of beta-emitting isotopes necessitates the use of expensive liquid scintillants and may consume prolonged counting times owing to low specific activity of the labeled product. Therefore, it is not surprising that alternative analytical procedures are being developed that take full advantage of the specificity and sensitivity that result from the application of antibodies but avoid the use of radionuclides.

Spin labeling (*2–4*) also has an intrinsic sensitivity that is within the same range as radioimmunoassay, but requires very expensive equipment. In these assays, known amounts of antibodies to the drug to be detected are mixed with an analog of the drug that has been labeled with a nitroxide radical (spin label). The specimen of biological fluid to be assayed is then added to this mixture. As a result of competition between the spin-labeled drug and the free drug for the limited number of antibody binding sites, some of the spin-labeled drug becomes detached from the antibody. The presence of free spin-labeled drug is signaled by the appearance of a sharp three-line electron spin resonance spectrum superimposed on the broad spectrum produced by the bound label. The signal intensity is a direct measure of the drug concentration in the unknown sample.

Faculty of Medicine, Clinical Biochemistry Unit, University of Antwerp, Universiteitsplein 1, Wilrijk 2610, Belgium.

Received Nov. 18, 1975; accepted Mar. 29, 1976.

Conjugates between enzyme and antibody and between enzyme and antigen have been used in histochemistry and immunochemistry to detect antigens and antibodies (*5*). Such conjugates can also be used instead of radiolabeled antibodies and antigens in radioimmunoassay. The use of an enzyme label in immunoassay was introduced in 1971 (*6–8*). This approach has several interesting features: (*a*) stability of the label for months, possibly for years, (*b*) detection of enzymatic activity requires only photometric equipment, (*c*) sensitivity is a function of the marker, and (*d*) the need for a separation step may be obviated.

Assays in which a bacteriophage label is used have a sensitivity in the same range as radio- or enzyme-immunoassay, also because of its amplifying effect (*9, 10*), but the determination of free phage requires time. The technique consists of chemically attaching haptens and antigens to a bacteriophage in such a way that the resulting conjugated phage is still viable but now possesses new antigenic determinants. The chemically modified bacteriophage may be inactivated with antibodies directed toward the substances attached to the phage, and this inactivation may be selectively inhibited by the free hapten or antigen.

General features of quantitative radio- or enzyme-immunoassay. The reaction between a test substance (P), the same substance labeled with an enzyme or radioisotope (P^*), and a specific binding agent (Q), that can bind both P and P^* can be written as (*11*):

$$\{P + P^*\} + \{Q\} \underset{k_2}{\overset{k_1}{\rightleftarrows}} \{PQ + P^*Q\}$$

$$k_1 \gg k_2 \text{ (* denotes labeling)}$$

In the case of competitive protein binding, Q is the naturally occurring receptor or transport molecule for P. In the case of immunoassay, Q is the antibody for P.

Because the only variable in this test system is P, the test substance, the quantity of P^*Q will be inversely proportional to the initial molar concentration of P.

Usually PQ and P^*Q differ so much chemically or physically from P and P^*, that $PQ + P^*Q$ can be easily separated from P and P^*. On measuring the amount of marker in $PQ + P^*Q$, or in $P + P^*$, or in both fractions, for various initial concentrations of P, a dose–response curve is obtained that can be used as a reference curve. The theoretical and practical aspects of the most widely used methods for separating bound ($PQ + P^*Q$) and free ($P + P^*$) fractions in the equilibrium mixture of radioimmunoassay, such as adsorption on coated charcoal of the free fraction and fractional precipitation of the bound fraction by organic solvents or neutral salts, are reviewed elsewhere (*12*).

However, an enzyme label differs from isotope labels by its molecular dimensions. The small difference between the bound and free fractions with regard to molecular weight and charge prohibits the use of many of the conventional separation methods used in radioimmunoassay. Two separation techniques are applied in enzyme immunoassay: precipitation of the bound fraction by addition of an excess of a second antibody directed against IgG of the species used to raise antibodies for the actual assay (*13–16*), and solid-phase systems in which the antibody is linked to an insoluble matrix. The latter includes the adsorption of antibody to the wall of the assay tube (*17–24*) and its covalent linking to activated cellulose (*8, 25*), Biogel (*26*), Sephadex (*27*), or Sepharose 4B (*28*). A combination of the two, a second antibody covalently coupled to cellulose (double-antibody solid phase, abbreviated DASP), is also used successfully (*8, 25, 29, 30*).

Enzyme-linked immunosorbent assay. In the immunoradiometric assay and in the enzyme-linked immunosorbent assay (sometimes abbreviated ELISA), labeled antibodies and antigen are used that have been made insoluble by virtue of attachment to a solid carrier (tubes, insoluble polymer):

$$\vdash P + P + Q^* \rightleftarrows \vdash PQ^* + PQ^*$$

where $\vdash$ denotes the carrier, and * denotes the radioisotope in the immunoradiometric assay or the labeled enzyme in the enzyme-linked immunosorbent assay. In this case, the amount of P is reflected in the distribution of Q^* between $\vdash PQ^*$ and PQ^*.

This procedure has been applied in the assay of many protein and peptide hormones (Table 1).

Table 1. Applications of Enzyme Immunoassay in Diagnosis

Substance to be measured	Label	Separation technique	References
Anti-adenosine antibody	β-galactosidase		(*49*)
Anti-DNA antibody	peroxidase	solid phase (coated tube)	(*17*)
Antibodies to *Salmonella* O antigens	alkaline phosphatase	solid phase (coated tube)	(*18*)
Estrogens (total)	peroxidase	double-antibody solid phase	(*29*)
α-Fetoprotein (rat)	alkaline phosphatase	solid phase (coated tube)	(*19*)
α-Fetoprotein (human)	peroxidase	double antibody	(*13, 14, 40*)
	glucose oxidase	solid phase	(*50*)
	alkaline phosphatase	double antibody	(*15*)
Haptoglobin	alkaline phosphatase	solid phase (coated tube)	(*20*)
HCG	peroxidase	solid phase (cellulose)	(*8, 25*)
	peroxidase	double-antibody solid phase	(*8, 25*)
α_2H-globulin	peroxidase	double antibody	(*16*)
HPL	peroxidase	double-antibody solid phase	(*29*)
IgE	alkaline phosphatase	solid phase (coated tube)	(*21*)
IgG	alkaline phosphatase	solid phase (coated tube)	(*22, 23*)
	peroxidase	solid phase (Biogel)	(*26*)
	glucose oxidase	solid phase (Sepharose 4 B)	(*28*)
Insulin	glucose oxidase	solid phase (Sephadex)	(*27*)
	peroxidase	solid phase (coated tube)	(*61*)
Estradiol, estriol	peroxidase	double-antibody solid phase	(*30*)
Pregnancy-associated α-macroglobulin	peroxidase	solid phase (coated tube)	(*24*)
Thyroxine	malate dehydrogenase		(*51*)

Wide (*31*) introduced in 1971 the "sandwich" technique, in which:

$$\vdash Q + P \rightleftarrows \vdash QP + Q^* \rightleftarrows \vdash QPQ^*$$

If $\vdash Q$ and Q^* are present in excess, the amount of $\vdash QPQ^*$ is proportional to the initial amount of P. Obviously, this technique will only work for multivalent P molecules.

Homogeneous enzyme immunoassay (*32*) uses antibodies (Q) that attach themselves to a specific drug molecule (P) (or another small antigen) that has been covalently linked to an enzyme (*). The enzyme in the P^*Q complex is thus deactivated until the antibody "releases" it upon coming into contact with a free drug molecule, allowing the enzyme to react with its substrate:

$$\text{(Enzyme–drug):antibody + drug} \rightleftarrows \text{(enzyme–drug) + antibody:drug}$$

$$P^*{:}Q + P \rightleftarrows P^* + Q{:}P$$

$$\text{Substrate} \xrightarrow{P^*} \text{product}$$

The inhibition of enzyme activity by antibody is probably caused either by conformational changes induced by antibody binding to an "active" group of the enzyme or by prevention of conformational changes necessary for catalytic activity (*33*).

Because there is no need for a separation step, this type of assay is called homogeneous enzyme immunoassay. Homogeneous enzyme immunoassay or enzyme-multiplied immunoassay (abbreviated EMIT) is now perhaps the most widely used enzyme immunoassay methodology, particularly for drug monitoring. The *choice of the enzyme label* to be used in enzyme immunoassay depends on several criteria: (*a*) it should possess a high specific activity at a pH value that does not impair antigen-antibody binding; (*b*) it should be simply and very sensitively detectable; (*c*) it should be readily available in a highly purified, soluble, and stable form at reasonable cost; (*d*) it should possess reactive groups through which it can be linked to other molecules without significantly impairing either the enzyme activity or antigen–antibody binding; and (*e*) it should not be inhibited by substances present in biological fluids and also not occur in significant concentrations in biological fluids. Table 2 lists the enzymes now being used for labeling. Experience has shown that lysozyme (EC 3.2.1.17), glucose-6-phosphate dehydrogenase (EC 1.1.1.49) and malate dehydrogenase (EC 1.1.1.37) are well suited to use in homogeneous enzyme immunoassay.

Homogeneous enzyme immunoassay can be used in *drug screening of urine* (*3, 35–37*) (Table 3). The urine test result can be available 5 to 10 min after the urine is received, because the actual test only requires about 1 min each for controls and samples. Because the system depends on the activity of lysozyme, for which the pH optimum is 6 to 7, it may be necessary to buffer urine samples that are alkaline as a result of prolonged storage to pH 6 to 7 before assay. False positives caused by endogenous lysozyme in urine may be eliminated by the use of proper controls. The EMIT method is more sensitive for detection of psychoactive drugs than are the thin-layer chromatographic techniques, but less sensitive than radioimmunoassay. A limitation of immunoassays is that specificity for a drug is not absolute and drugs of similar chemical structure may cross-react, as indicated in Table 3. The EMIT opiate assay is designed to detect morphine and morphine glucuronide, the major metabolites of heroin. However, the assay will also detect other opiates, including heroin, codeine, the analgesic meperidine, and somewhat higher concentrations of the narcotic antagonist nalorphine. High or abuse concentrations of such nonopiate substances as chlorpromazine and dextromethorphan may also cross-react. Mulé et al. (*38, 39*) compared EMIT results with those of thin-layer chromatography. Using thin-layer chromatography as the comparison method, they found 2.6%, 5.6%, 12.5%, 5.1%, and 10.0% "false" positives for methadone, opiates, amphetamines, barbiturates, and cocaine, respectively, for the EMIT method. The "false" negatives they reported were 2.3%, 0.1%, 0.7%, 0.2%, and 1.9%, respectively. These low percentages of false negatives encourage the judicious use of these tests to rule out toxic concentrations in cases of suspected drug overdose. However, after a positive re-

Table 2. Enzymes Now Being Used for Labeling

Enzyme	EC no.	Source	M_r	Used to detect
Malate dehydrogenase	1.1.1.37	pig-heart mitochondria	70 000	NADH
Glucose-6-phosphate dehydrogenase	1.1.1.49	*Leuconostoc mesenteroides*	102 000	NADPH
Peroxidase	1.11.1.7	horse-radish root	40 000	H_2O_2/chromogen
Alkaline phosphatase	3.1.3.1.	calf intestine	100 000	*p*-nitrophenol
Exo-1,4-α-glucosidase	3.2.1.3.	*Rhizopus niveus*		glucose > NADPH
Lysozyme	3.2.1.17.	chicken egg-white	14 000	cell wall fragments of *Micrococcus luteus*
β-Galactosidase	3.2.1.23.	*Escherichia coli*	518 000	*o*-nitrophenol

Table 3. Applications of Homogeneous Enzyme Immunoassay in Monitoring Drugs in Urine and Plasma

Drugs to be measured	Sensitivity, mg/liter	Some drugs known to cross-react	References
In urine[a]			
Amphetamines	2	ephedrine	(*3, 37, 39*)
		phenmetrazine	
Barbiturates	2	glutethimide	(*3, 34, 37, 39*)
Benzodiazepine			b
Benzoyl ecgonine	1.6		(*3, 37, 39*)
Methadone	0.5	chlorpromazine	(*3, 37, 39, 43*)
		dextromethorphan	
		promethazine	
Opiates	0.5	chlorpromazine	(*32, 44–46*)
		dextromethorphan	(*3, 37, 39*)
	0.001		(*33*)
Propoxyphene			b
In plasma[c]			
Carbamazepine	1		b
Digoxin	0.001		(*47*)
Diphenylhydantoin	2.5		(*41, 42, 48*)
Ethosuximide	10		b
Phenobarbital	5		(*41, 42, 48*)
Primidone	2.5		(*41*)

[a] Label is lysozyme in each case, except for second listing under "Opiates," for which the label is malate dehydrogenase.
[b] Syva Corp., 3181 Porter Drive, Palo Alto, Calif. 94304.
[c] Label is glucose-6-phosphate dehydrogenase in each case.

sult, additional analysis by a nonimmunological procedure must be performed for confirmation.

Applications of enzyme immunoassay for the determination of various biochemical entities are listed in Table 1. At the moment only a few definitive data about their evaluation and correlation with conventional techniques are available (*40*). The introduction of enzyme immunoassays for *monitoring concentrations of drugs in plasma* (Table 3) will soon allow routine drug monitoring during treatment of epilepsy, dosage adjustment programs during therapy with digoxin, or monitoring of gentamicin therapy in renal failure. Legaz and Raisys (*41*) evaluated the EMIT antiepileptic drug assay and compared results for it with those by a gas–liquid chromatographic procedure. They obtained a correlation coefficient of 0.97 for diphenylhydantoin, phenobarbital, and primidone. Booker and Darcey (*42*) report similar results. Experience with the antiepileptic drug diphenylhydantoin has shown that with commonly used doses (300–400 mg daily in adults), this drug decreases or abolishes seizures in most patients. However, a few develop symptoms of toxicity on this dosage and some others appear to derive no benefit. Diphenylhydantoin is metabolized, predominantly in the liver, to *p*-hydroxyphenytoin and there are large interindividual differences in the steady-state concentrations of the drug. Therapeutic concentrations in serum at steady state (*52*) fall between 10–20 mg/liter (mean, 12 mg/liter) for diphenylhydantoin, 5–11 mg/liter (mean, 8 mg/liter) for primidone, and 40–60 mg/liter (mean, 45 mg/ml) for ethosuximide. Only the unbound fraction of these drugs in plasma is available for penetration into the central nervous system. Diphenylhydantoin, for example, is about 90% bound to plasma proteins at therapeutic concentrations (*53*). The decreased binding of diphenylhydantoin by plasma proteins in hyperbilirubinemic infants (*54*) and uremic patients (*55*) explains why this drug controls seizures in these two situations at very low concentrations in plasma, concentrations usually considered to be ineffective in adult epileptics with normal liver and kidney function. From the practical point of view, indications for determining these antiepileptic drugs in serum may be: (*a*) to ascertain whether the drug is biologically available in cases where the therapeutic dose has been prescribed and seizure control is incomplete; (*b*) when there is need for concomitant administration of drugs that are enzyme inducers, or when a patient is receiving multiple antiepileptic drugs and is experiencing toxicity or uncontrolled seizures; and (*c*) when an epileptic patient presents symptoms of intoxication, because it is difficult to distinguish the clinical signs of neurologic dysfunction from the toxic effects of antiepileptic drugs. The antiepileptic effect of phenobarbital is correlated with plasma concentrations of 20–40 mg/liter (mean, 25 mg/liter). However, concentrations of this drug in plasma vary only slightly among individual patients who are on the same dose. Several investigators have shown a well-established relationship between the concentration of digoxin in plasma and its therapeutic and toxic effects (*56*). Different methods are currently available: the ^{86}Rb uptake inhibition assay, ATPase inhibition, and competitive protein binding assays of either the radioimmunoassay or the enzymatic displacement type. They have been reviewed recently (*57*). The availability of a homogeneous enzyme immunoassay for digoxin (*47*) will add new possibilities for the estimation of plasma concentrations under clinical conditions. Assaying plasma digoxin provides the clinician with information of considerable value because the therapeutic concentrations of digoxin required by individual patient are not readily predictable from consideration of dose of digoxin, body weight, serum creatinine concentration, urinary excretion rate of creatinine, age, and height (*58*). Frequently toxicity occurs in an important number of patients treated, and moreover this diagnosis is frequently very difficult to make on clinical grounds because increasing heart failure and a wide variety of arrhythmias may be attributable either to overdigitalization or to the underlying condition for which the drug was being administered. The value of the quantitation of concentrations of plasma digitalis glycosides in therapy has been discussed by several authors recently (*56, 58*). As exemplified throughout this short review, the capability of enzyme immunoassay to make quantitative measurements of an increasing number of biochemical variables and drug concentrations with a high degree of sensitivity and specificity will be of value to different areas of clinical chemistry.

Adaptation of homogeneous enzyme immunoassay to centrifugal analysis (*59, 60*) will reduce time and reagent cost and allow the processing of large numbers of specimens. Continued research is needed on selection of more suitable enzymes for labeling, together with more detailed studies on the mechanism of antibody inhibition of enzyme activity.

References

1. Yalow, R., and Berson, S., Assay of plasma insulin in human subjects by immunological methods. *Nature* **184,** 1648 (1959).

2. Leute, R., Ullman, E., Goldstein, A., and Herzenberg, L., Spin immunoassay technique for determination of morphine. *Nature, New Biol.* **236,** 93 (1972).

3. Schneider, R., Bastiani, R., Leute, R., et al., Use of enzyme and spin labeling in homogeneous immunochemical detection methods. In *Immunoassay for Drugs Subject to Abuse,* S. Mulé, I. Sunshine, M. Braude, and R. Willette, Eds., CRC Press, Cleveland, Ohio, 1974, p 45.

4. Montgomery, M., Holtzman, J., Leute, R., et al., Determination of diphenylhydantoin in human serum by spin immunoassay. *Clin. Chem.* **21,** 221 (1975).

5. Sternberger, L., *Immunocytochemistry,* Prentice-Hall, Englewood Cliffs, N. J., 1974.

6. Avrameas, S., and Guilbert, B., Dosage enzymo-immunologique de protéines à l'aide d'immunosorbants et d'antigènes marqués aux enzymes. *C.R. Acad. Sci., Ser. D,* **273,** 2705 (1971).

7. Engvall, E., and Perlmann, P., Enzyme-linked immunosorbent assay (ELISA). Quantitative assay of immunoglobulin G. *Immunochemistry* **8,** 871 (1971).

8. Van Weemen, B., and Schuurs, A., Immunoassay using antigen-enzyme conjugates. *FEBS Lett.* **15,** 232 (1971).

9. Sela, M., Highly sensitive immunoassay of proteins and other compounds with bacteriophage. *Triangle (Engl. Ed.)* **11,** 61 (1972).

10. Andrieu, J., Mamas, S., and Dray, F., Viroimmunoassay of steroids: Method and principles. In *Steroid Immunoassay,* E. Cameron, S. Hillier, and K. Griffiths, Eds., Alpha Omega Pub. Co., Cardiff, Wales, U.K., 1975, p 189.

11. Zettner, A., Principles of competitive binding assays (saturation analyses). I. Equilibrium techniques. *Clin. Chem.* **19,** 699 (1973).

12. Ratcliffe, J., Separation techniques in saturation analysis. *Br. Med. Bull.* **30,** 32 (1974).

13. Alpert, E., Coston, R., and Perroto, J., Immunoenzymatic assay for alpha-fetoprotein. *Lancet* **i,** 626 (1974).

14. Alpert, E., Immunoenzymatic assay for alpha-fetoprotein. *Lancet* **i,** 807 (1975).

15. Belanger, L., Hamel, D., Dufour, D., and Pouliot, M., Double-antibody enzyme immunoassay applied to human α_1-fetoprotein. *Clin. Chem.* **22,** 198 (1976).

16. Fuccaro-Decaens, C., Meriadec, B., Buffe, D., and Burtin, P., Étude comparative de deux techniques sensibles de dosage immunologique: Le dosage radioimmunologique et le dosage enzymoimmunologique, appliqués à la détection de l'α_2H-globuline sérique. *Ann. Immunol.* **125** C, 747 (1974).

17. Pesce, A., Mendoza, N., Boreisha, I., et al. Use of enzyme-linked antibodies to measure serum anti-DNA antibody in systemic lupus erythematosus. *Clin. Chem.* **20,** 353 (1974).

18. Carlsson, H., Lindberg, A., and Hammarström, S., Titration of antibodies to Salmonella O antigens by enzyme-linked immunosorbent assay. *Infect. Immun.* **6,** 703 (1972).

19. Belanger, L., Sylvestre, C., and Dufour, D., Enzyme-linked immunoassay for alpha-fetoprotein by competitive and sandwich procedures. *Clin. Chim. Acta* **48,** 15 (1973).

20. Miedema, K., Boelhouwer, J., and Otten, J., Determinations of proteins and hormones in serum by an immunoassay using antigen-enzyme conjugates. *Clin. Chim. Acta* **40,** 187 (1972).

21. Hoffman, D., Estimation of serum IgE by an enzyme-linked immunosorbent assay (ELISA). *J. Allergy Clin. Immunol.* **51,** 303 (1973).

22. Engvall, E., Jonsson, K., and Perlmann, P., Enzyme-linked immunosorbent assay. II. Quantitative assay of protein antigen, immunoglobulin G, by means of enzyme-labelled antigen and antibody-coated tubes. *Biochim. Biophys. Acta* **251,** 427 (1971).

23. Engvall, E., and Perlmann, P., Enzyme-linked immunosorbent assay, ELISA. III. Quantitation of specific antibodies by enzyme-labeled anti-immunoglobulin in antigen-coated tubes. *J. Immunol.* **109,** 129 (1972).

24. Stimson, W., and Sinclair, J., An immunoassay for pregnancy-associated α-macroglobulin using antibody–enzyme conjugates. *FEBS Lett.* **47,** 190 (1974).

25. Van Weemen, B., and Schuurs, A., Immunoassay using antibody–enzyme conjugates. *FEBS Lett.* **43,** 215 (1974).

26. Avrameas, S., and Guilbert, B., Enzyme-immunoassay for the measurement of antigens using peroxidase conjugates. *Biochimie* **54,** 837 (1972).

27. Ishikawa, E., Enzyme immunoassay of insulin by fluorimetry of the insulin-glucoamylase complex. *J. Biochem.* **73,** 1319 (1973).

28. Masseyeff, R., Maiolini, R., and Bouron, Y., A method of enzyme immunoassay. *Biomedecine* **19,** 314 (1973).

29. Bosch, A., van Heli, H., Brands, J., et al., Methods for the determination of total estrogens (TE) and human placental lactogen (HPL) in plasma of pregnant women by enzyme-immunoassay (EIA). *Clin. Chem.* **21,** 1009 (1975). Abstract.

30. Van Weemen, B., and Schuurs, A., Immunoassay using hapten-enzyme conjugates. *FEBS Lett.* **24,** 77 (1972).

31. Wide, L., Solid phase antigen-antibody systems. In *Radioimmunoassay Methods,* K. Kirkham and W. Hunter, Eds., Livingstone, Edinburgh, 1971, p 405.

32. Rubenstein, K., Schneider, R., and Ullman, E., "Homogeneous" enzyme immunoassay, a new immunochemical technique. *Biochem. Biophys. Res. Commun.* **47,** 846 (1972).

33. Rowley, G., Rubenstein, K., Huisjen, J., and Ullman, E., Mechanism by which antibodies inhibit hapten-malate dehydrogenase conjugates. *J. Biol. Chem.* **250,** 3759 (1975).

34. Walberg, C., Correlation of the "EMIT" urine barbiturate assay with a spectrophotometric serum barbiturate assay in suspected overdose. *Clin. Chem.* **20,** 305 (1974).

35. Brattin, W., and Sunshine, I., Immunological assays for drugs in biological samples. *Am. J. Med. Technol.* **39,** 223 (1973).

36. Bastiani, R., Phillips, R., Schneider, R., and Ullman, E., Homogeneous immunochemical drug assays. *Am. J. Med. Technol.* **39,** 211 (1973).

37. Brattin, W., and Sunshine, I., A comparison of available immunoassays for drugs of abuse in urine. In ref. *3*, p 107.

38. Mulé, S., Bastos, M., and Jukofsky, D., Evaluation of immunoassay methods for detection, in urine, of drugs subject to abuse. *Clin. Chem.* **20,** 243 (1974).

39. Mulé, S., and Bastos, M., A comparison of immunoassay methods for the detection of drugs subject to abuse. In ref *3*, p 99.

40. Alpert, E., and Coston, R. L., Serum alpha-fetoprotein (AFP) in benign and malignant gastrointestinal diseases: Evaluation of an immunoenzymatic assay. *Clin. Chim. Acta* **58,** 77 (1975).

41. Legaz, M., and Raisys, V., Correlation of the "Emit" antiepileptic drug assay with a gas liquid chromatographic method. *Clin. Biochem.* **9,** 35 (1976).

42. Booker, H., and Darcey, B., Enzymatic immunoassay vs. gas/liquid chromatography for determination of phenobarbital and diphenylhydantoin in serum. *Clin. Chem.* **21,** 1766 (1975).

43. McIntyre, J., Armandi, A., Risen, L., et al., Thin-layer chromatography and enzyme immunoassay of L-alpha-acetyl methadol and methadone metabolites in urine. *Clin. Chem.* **21,** 109 (1975).

44. Mulé, S., Methods for the analysis of morphine and related surrogates: Current status. *J. Chromatogr. Sci.* **12,** 245 (1974).

45. Schneider, R., Lindquist, P., Tong-in Wong, E., et al., Homogeneous enzyme immunoassay for opiates in urine. *Clin. Chem.* **19,** 821 (1973).

46. Gorodetzky, C., and Kullberg, M., Validity of screening methods for drugs of abuse in biological fluids. II. Heroin in plasma and saliva. *Clin. Pharmacol. Ther.* **15,** 579 (1974).

47. Chang, J., Crowl, C., and Schneider, R., Homogeneous enzyme immunoassay for digoxin. *Clin. Chem.* **21,** 967 (1975).

48. Spiehler, V., Sun, L., Miyada, D., and Jessen, B., Evaluation of radioimmunoassay (RIA), enzyme immunoassay (EMIT) and spectrophotometry for clinical determination of the anticonvulsant drugs: Phenobarbital and diphenylhydantoin. *Clin. Chem.* **21,** 946 (1975). Abstract.

49. Lauer, R., and Erlanger, B., An enzyme-immunoassay of antibody specific for adenosine using β-galactosidase. *Immunochemistry* **11,** 533 (1974).

50. Maiolini, R., Ferrua, B., and Masseyeff, R., Enzymoimmunoassay of human alpha-fetoprotein. *J. Immunol. Methods* **6,** 355 (1975).

51. Ullman, E., Blakemore, J., Leute, R., et al., Homogeneous enzyme immunoassay for thyroxine. *Clin. Chem.* **21,** 1011 (1975). Abstract.

52. Penry, J., Usefulness of serum antiepileptic drug levels in the treatment of epilepsy. In *Drug Interactions,* P. Morselli, S. Cohen, and S. Garattini, Eds. Raven Press, New York, N. Y., 1974, p 299.

53. Lunde, P., Rane, A., Yaffe, S., et al., Plasma protein binding of diphenylhydantoin in man: Interaction with other drugs and the effect of temperature and plasma dilution. *Clin. Pharmacol. Ther.* **11,** 846 (1970).

54. Rane, A., Lunde, P., Jalling, B., et al., Plasma protein binding of diphenylhydantoin in normal and hyperbilirubinemic infants. *J. Pediatr.* **78,** 877 (1971).

55. Reidenberg, M. M., Odar-Cederloff, I., von Bahr, C., et al., Protein binding of diphenylhydantoin and desmethylimipramine in plasma from patients with poor renal function. *New Engl. J. Med.* **285,** 264 (1971).

56. Smith, T., and Haber, E., Clinical value of the radio-immunoassay of the digitalis glycosides. *Pharmacol. Rev.* **25,** 219 (1973).

57. Smith, T., and Haber, E., The current status of cardiac glycoside assay techniques. *Prog. Cardiol.* **2,** 49 (1973).

58. Wagner, J., Yates, J., Willis, III, P., et al., Correlation of plasma levels of digoxin in cardiac patients with dose and measures of renal function. *Clin. Pharmacol. Ther.* **15,** 291 (1974).

59. Strasser, B., and Zinterhofer, L., Rapid enzyme immunoassay of phenobarbital and dilantin on a centrifugal fast analyzer. *Clin. Chem.* **21,** 946 (1975). Abstract.

60. Broughton, A., and Ross, D., Drug screening by enzymatic immunoassay with the centrifugal analyzer. *Clin. Chem.* **21,** 187 (1975).

61. Kleinhammer, G., Lenz, H., Linke, R., and Gruber, W., Bestimmung von Serum-Insulin im solid phase Enzymimmunoassay unter verwendung antikörper-beschichteter Polystyrolgläschen. *Z. Anal. Chem.* in press.

CLIN. CHEM. 22/6, 739–748 (1976)

Analytical Toxicology: Applications of Element-Selective Electrolytic Conductivity Detection for Gas Chromatography

Brian E. Pape

We applied a commercially available microelectrolytic conductivity detector to toxicological problems of qualitative and quantitative analysis by gas chromatography. The detector can be used for the sensitive and selective detection of halogen-, nitrogen-, and sulfur-containing compounds. Relative response in different element-selective detector variables such as reaction gas, reaction catalyst, and furnace temperature can be used to further improve qualitative identification by gas chromatography.

Additional Keyphrases: *drug assay • flame ionization detector • electron capture analysis • detection of N-, S-, and halogen-containing compounds in blood*

Gas–liquid chromatography (GLC)[1] is a fundamental analytical tool in most clinical and forensic toxicology laboratories. Most such instrumentation in these laboratories makes use of flame ionization detection (FID) because of its good general response, adequate sensitivity for most common analysis, excellent linear range and detector stability, and few problems with the instrumental interface and operational variables such as combustion gases, ion collection, and signal amplification. Analytical requirements, however, continually arise for which greater detector sensitivity and selectivity is needed than FID can supply. Some examples are halogen-containing volatiles in complex mixture, specificity for sulfur-containing phenothiazines and phenothiazine metabolites, and selectivity for nitrogen-containing organic compounds as compared with hydrocarbon co-extractables. Improved detector sensitivity is most often required in analyses for basic drugs in blood and tissues.

A summary of some common types of detectors (thermal conductivity, gas density balance, electron capture, alkali flame, helium ionization, and cross section) by McNair and Bonelli (*1*) illustrates the compromises that must often be made in increasing detector sensitivity and (or) selectivity for an element or functional group while retaining the required flexibility in GLC instrumentation. Other detector systems used in GLC include the thermistor, argon, microwave emission, photoionization, nonradioactive helium ionization, radiofrequency, ultrasonic, microcoulometric, reaction coulometric, electrolytic conductivity, infrared spectrometer, photometric, mass spectrometer, far ultraviolet, and spectrofluorometric systems. The performance characteristics of these have been reviewed by Hartman (*2*). The flame photometric detector and electron capture detector have been used to detect sulfur- and halogen-containing drugs, respectively. Photometric systems are adequately sensitive and quite selective, but their response is nonlinear and their application limited. Most applications of electron capture detection involve the formation of halogenated derivatives, requiring additional analytical preparation. Functional-group chemistry of some major drug classes is not favorable to such derivitization reactions (e.g., unsubstituted nitrogen heterocyclics and tertiary amines). As a result of these limitations, other element-selective detector systems are receiving increased attention. For example, Toseland et al. (*3*) have applied to thermionic nitrogen-selective detector to the GLC determination of anticonvulsants and barbiturates in plasma and tissues.

The electrolytic conductivity detector represents another element-selective system that as yet has been investigated only casually. The application of electrolytic conductivity detection (ElCD) to gas chromatography was first reported by Piringer and Pascalau (*4*). Coulson (*5*) later developed a modified ElCD system that allowed the selective and sensitive detection of organic halogen-, sulfur-, and nitrogen-containing compounds. Jones and Nickless (*6*) constructed a modified Coulson detector with a slightly greater sensitivity for halogenated compounds. The commercially available Coulson ElCD system, while quite sensitive, suffered from its large size, its required interfacing, and its lower sensitivity as compared to electron capture detection of halogenated pesticides. The instrumental evolution and applications of ElCD have been reviewed by Selucky (*7*). Hall (*8, 9*) subsequently reported the enhancement of the sensitivity and selectivity of the Coulson detector and constructed an improved mi-

Department of Pathology—Toxicology Laboratory, School of Medicine, University of Missouri-Columbia, Columbia, Mo. 65201.

[1] Nonstandard abbreviations used: GLC, gas–liquid chromatography (-ic); FID, flame ionization detector; and ElCD, electrolytic conductivity detection (-or).

Received Sept. 4, 1975; accepted Feb. 26, 1976.

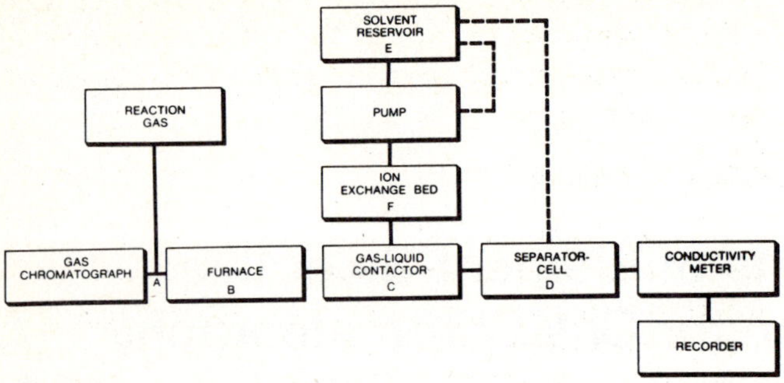

Fig. 1. Block diagram of the ElCD system

croelectrolytic conductivity detector, which is now commercially available (*10*).

The principle of ElCD operation. Effluent from a gas chromatograph undergoes thermal decomposition under predetermined conditions of furnace temperature, reaction gas, reaction catalyst, and abstractors, and is then combined with a stream of de-ionized liquid in a simple gas–liquid contractor. The electrical conductivity of the liquid is continuously measured with an a.c. bridge circuit and auxiliary recorder. Only those components are detected in the gas chromatographic effluent that are decomposed to yield products that are both readily soluble and ionized in the conductivity liquid. Figure 1 shows the relationship of the principal components in the ElCD system, all of which are contained in a single unit.

The pyrolyzer section (*A* and *B*) contains the detector furnace, the quartz or nickle reaction tube, and the reaction gas inlet. The cell assembly (*C* and *D*) consists of an integrated one-piece Teflon gas–liquid contractor and micro-conductivity cell made of stainless steel and Teflon. The liquid circulation system (*E* and *F*) consists of a glass liquid reservoir, liquid pump, needle valve for flow regulation, and an ion-exchange bed. Components of the conductivity bridge include a fixed-voltage a.c. power supply, current-suppression bridge, and signal attenuator. Conductivity-bridge and electrometer-output controls consist of an attenuator, which selects one of eight binary levels of output signal attenuation; a conductivity range switch, which selects one of seven ranges of conductivity measurement representing full-scale pen deflection, from 1–1000 $\mu\Omega^{-1}$; a coarse and fine zero control, which balances the a.c. bridge to allow positioning of recorder pen; and a display meter selectable for furnace temperature or cell conductivity. Additional components of the detector system include a furnace temperature controller, and furnace power and detector power monitors.

An appreciation of detector variables is critical to an understanding of ElCD element-selectivity. Thermal decomposition of the GLC effluent is based on the reduction (H_2 reaction gas), oxidation (O_2 or air reaction gas), or pyrolysis (no reaction gas) of the organic species at high temperature (usually 800 to 900 °C). Decomposition may involve either catalytic (quartz reaction tube and nickle wire, or nickel reaction tube) or non-catalytic (quartz reaction tube) conditions. The particular mode of decomposition may be referred to as the "furnace chemistry." The reaction products obtained depend on the molecular structure, furnace chemistry, and the use of post-furnace abstractors that trap acidic or basic products. Solubilization and ionization of the reaction product(s) (NH_3, HCl, Cl_2, S_xO_x, etc.) at the gas–liquid contactor may be referred to as "cell chemistry." Cell chemistry is based on effective gas–liquid contact and separation, on ionization processes, and the use of reactive solutes in the liquid phase. Changes in conductivity attributable to specific conductance, liquid flow rate, and electrometer settings are often termed "conductance variables."

Selectivity and sensitivity are determined by a particular combination of furnace chemistry, cell chemistry, and conductance variables (*8*). In the reduction mode, H_2S, HCl, NH_3, and CH_4 are the major reaction products obtained from organic compounds containing sulfur, chlorine, or nitrogen. H_2S has a low ionization constant and gives no appreciable response, HCl can be removed by a scrubber such as $Sr(OH)_2$ or $AgNO_3$, and the formation of NH_3 often requires the use of nickle catalyst. In the oxidative mode, SO_2 and SO_3, HCl, CO_2, H_2O, and N_2 are produced from the thermal decomposition of sulfur-, chlorine-, and nitrogen-containing organics. The response produced by CO_2 is low, owing to poor solubilization (short gas–liquid contact time) or the use of an organic conductivity solvent (usually alcohols); water and N_2 give little or no response; sulfur oxides can be removed from the furnace reaction products by using a CaO scrubber; and HCl can also be removed with an acid scrubber ($AgNO_3$). Consequently, a proper choice of reaction conditions—abstractors—and of conductivity liquid allows the highly selective detection of either sulfur-, halogen-, or nitrogen-containing compounds.

Further selectivity among organochlorine compounds (example: aliphatic as compared with aromatic chlorine) may be realized by choice of furnace temperature (*8*). The highly sensitive detection of organic nitrogen with use of an HCl/ethanol conductivity solvent has also been recommended by Hall (*9*). The neutralization reaction ($NH_3 + H_3O^+ \rightarrow NH_4^+ + H_2O$) is believed to produce a greater change in conductance as compared to solubilization and partial ionization ($NH_3 + H_2O \rightarrow NH_4^+ + OH^-$; $pK_b = 4.76$) (*6*). Moreover, dilute HCl conductivity solutions may be used to differentiate chlorine- and nitrogen-containing organics (reductive mode, nickle catalyst) without the use of selective abstractors (*6*). Differentiation is based on the decrease in conductivity caused by NH_3 neutralization reactions, as opposed to the increase caused by HCl. By analogy, the selective enhancement of ElCD response to sulfur (as H_2S) in the reductive mode may be realized by using a reactive conductivity solvent (*6*). Increased sensitivity is based on the rapid oxidation of H_2S in dilute acid solution containing iodine ($H_2S + I_2 \rightleftharpoons 2H^+ + 2I^- + S$).

We have used the commercial Hall ElCD system (*10*) in routine and special toxicological analysis for some nine months and believe it offers significant advantages in element-selective GLC screening procedures and in quantitation of nanogram amounts of sample.

Selected ElCD applications to analytical toxicology and a discussion of general detector principles are the subject of this report.

Materials

Gas Chromatograph and Detectors

GLC analyses were done with a four-column Model MT 222 gas chromatograph equipped with ElCD, FID, and flame photometric detector systems (TRACOR Inc., Austin, Tex. 78721). The conventional ElCD reaction-gas inlet was modified with two nupro metering valves and a bypass valve to a soap-bubble flowmeter, allowing convenient switching between H_2 and O_2 reaction-gas sources and measurement of reaction-gas flow. Helium carrier gas (25 ml/min) was used because of the slight reduction of N_2 to NH_3 when N_2 carrier gas is used in conjunction with the ElCD in the reductive mode. The 1-mm and 4-mm (i.d.) furnace reaction tubes were made of quartz, and were obtained from TRACOR Inc. When using the 1 mm reaction tubes, and H_2 and O_2 reaction-gas flow rate was 20 ml/ min in the reductive and oxidative mode, respectively. With the 4 mm reaction tubes, reaction-gas flow rate was increased to 75 ml/min to avoid peak broadening owing to increased residence time in the reaction tube. The 4-mm reaction tubes were only used for the analysis of 1,4-benzodiazepines and 1,4-benzodiazepin-2-ones, tricyclic antidepressants, and phenothiazines (*discussed below*). When nonhydrocarbon solvents were injected and 4-mm reaction tubes were used, the solvent front was vented ahead of the ElCD furnace, to avoid carbonization of the reaction tube. The ElCD reaction catalyst, when used, consisted of fine nickle wire, tightly coiled and positioned in the center of the furnace heating zone (quartz reaction-tube). The ElCD conductivity solvent used for all analyses except 1,4-benzodiazepines and 1,4-benzodiazepin-2-ones, tricyclic antidepressants, and phenothiazines was isopropanol/distilled water (5/95 by vol) at a flow rate of 0.5–1.0 ml/min cell flow, and was maintained at pH 6.5–7.0 by a mixed bed ion-exchange resin (Amberlite IRN-150; Rohm and Haas, Philadelphia, Pa. 19105; or from TRACOR Inc.). The other analyses (*noted above*) were done by using a conductivity solvent of isopropanol/distilled water (15/85 by vol), maintained at an alkaline pH with a coventional stacked ion-exchange resin tube containing 70% Soxhlet-extracted IRN-78 on the pump side and 30% Soxhlet-extracted IRN-150 on the cell side (IRN-78 from Rohm and Haas or TRACOR Inc.).

GLC Columns and Column Packings

GLC packings are denoted as follows. The "3% OV-17" packing was 30 g of OV-17 per kilogram of the support, 100/120 mesh Chrom Q (Applied Science Laboratories, Inc., State College, Pa. 16801). The "4% OV-17" packing was 40 g of OV-17 per kilogram of the support, Chromsorb G AW DMCS 80/100 mesh HP (Analabs, New Haven, Conn. 06510). Poropak Q-S, 100/120 mesh, was obtained from Waters Associates, Milford, Mass. 01757. All GLC columns were glass, 180 cm × 2 mm i.d.

Other Chemicals

All chemicals were AR grade. Drugs for use as standards were obtained from pharmaceutical manufacturers. Tolylbarbital (5-ethyl-5-*p*-tolylbarbituric acid) was obtained from Aldrich Chemical Co., Inc., Milwaukee, Wis. 53233.

Methods

Extraction and GLC quantitation of ethchlorvynol in plasma. Five milliliter aliquots of plasma containing 20 mg ethchlorvynol per liter were extracted at pH 7 with differing volumes of *n*-hexane, in Teflon-lined, screw-capped extraction tubes. The extract was directly analyzed by GLC (2-μl injection) or, alternatively, was first dehydrated with anhydrous sodium sulfate and then analyzed by GLC without concentration of the hexane. GLC was done on a column containing 3% OV-17, at an injector and oven temperature of 125 °C isothermal (ethchlorvynol retention time, 2.5 min). The ElCD was operated in the reductive mode, with use of Ni catalyst and a furnace temperature of 820 °C. The conductivity electrometer (range, attenuation) was 100 $\mu\Omega^{-1} \times 2$ (100 μmho × 2).

Extraction and GLC quantitation of methaqualone in plasma. One milliliter of a saturated solution of sodium monobasic phosphate added to 1 ml of plasma containing 18 mg of methaqualone per liter was extracted with 0.5 ml of *n*-hexane, and the extract was processed as discussed above. GLC was on a 4% OV-17 column with an injection temperature of 300 °C and column temperature of 275 °C isothermal. Methaqualone retention time was 8.0 min. The ElCD was operated in the reductive mode (H_2 + Ni catalyst) at 830 °C.

Plasma drug screening. Two milliliters of plasma containing 15 mg each of methyprylon, amobarbital, meprobamate, glutethimide, phenobarbital, and methaqualone per liter was extracted with 25 ml of chloroform at pH 7. The chloroform phase was isolated, dehydrated with anhydrous sodium sulfate, decanted, and evaporated. The residue was redissolved in 50-μl of methanol and analyzed by GLC on 3% OV-17 (injector temperature 250 °C, oven temperature programmed from 125 to 300 °C at 8 °C/min). The ElCD was operated in the reductive mode without catalyst, at a furnace temperature of 820 °C. Comparative chromatograms were obtained with use of 3% OV-17 column interfaced to an FID system.

Effect of ElCD furnace variables. The effects of furnace temperature and reaction gas on ElCD response were studied under defined conditions. The GLC standard consisted of a solution of 1 mg/ml each of methyprylon, amobarbital, pentobarbital, secobarbital, meprobamate, glutethimide, phenobarbital, tolylbarbital, methaqualone, and diphenylhydantoin in methanol. A volume of 1 μl was routinely used. GLC was done on a 4% OV-17 column with an injector temperature of 250 °C and with column temperature programmed from 125 to 300 °C at 8 °C/min. A quartz reaction tube (no catalyst) was used to study the effect of furnace temperature (650 to 850 °C) and reaction-gas conditions (per minute, 10 and 20 ml H_2, 20 ml O_2, pyrolytic) on ElCD response.

Extraction and GLC quantitation of meprobamate. One milliliter of chloroform, containing 200 μg of *p*-dimethylaminobenzaldehyde, was added to 5-ml plasma aliquots containing meprobamate at 40, 30, 20, 10, and 0 mg/liter. Ten milliliters of chloroform was added and the mixtures were extracted in Teflon-lined, screw-capped culture tubes. After the phases were separated by centrifugation, the aqueous phase was aspirated, and the chloroform phase was dehydrated with anhydrous sodium sulfate, decanted, and evaporated. The residue was redissolved in 100-μl of methanol, and 2-μl was analyzed by GLC on 3% OV-17, with an injector temperature of 225 °C and column temperature programmed from 175 to 250°C at 8 °C/min. The ElCD was operated in the reductive mode with Ni catalyst, a furnace temperature of 820 °C, and electrometer setting of 300 $\mu\Omega^{-1} \times 1$.

GLC of volatile chlorinated hydrocarbons. Two-microliter aliquots of an aqueous solution of dichloromethane, chloroform, and 1,2-dichloroethane (100 mg of each per liter) were analyzed on a Poropak Q-S column with injector and column temperatures of 190 and 175 °C, respectively, and ElCD electrometer set at 30 $\mu\Omega^{-1} \times 2$. Comparative chromatograms were obtained with use of a Poropak Q-S column interfaced to an FID system.

GLC of phenalkylamines. An injection of 100 ng each of amphetamine and metamphetamine in 2-μl of *n*-hexane was analyzed by GLC on a 4% OV-17 column. The temperature of both the GLC injector and the column was 125 °C. The ElCD was operated in the reductive mode with use of a nickle catalyst, a furnace temperature 825 °C, and a conductivity electrometer setting of 100 $\mu\Omega \times 1$.

Extraction and GLC analysis of barbiturates in plasma. Plasma, 5 ml, containing about 15 mg each of amobarbital, secobarbital, pentobarbital, and phenobarbital per liter was extracted with 1 ml of isopropyl ether in a Teflon-lined, screw-capped culture tube, and the tube centrifuged to separate the phases; 2 μl of the isopropyl ether phase was analyzed by GLC on 4% OV-17 (injector temperature 250 °C, oven temperature programmed from 175 to 300 °C at 8 °C/min). The ElCD was operated in the reductive mode without catalyst, furnace temperature 820 °C, and an electrometer setting of 3 $\mu\Omega^{-1} \times 1$.

Analysis of 1,4-benzodiazepines and 1,4-benzodiazepin-2-ones. The 1,4-benzodiazepines (medazepam and *N*-desmethyl medazepam) and 1,4-benzodiazepin-2-ones (diazepam, *N*-desmethyl diazepam, oxazepam, nitrazepam, flurazepam, *N*-1-hydroxyethyl flurazepam, and *N*-1-desalkyl flurazepam) were analyzed by GLC on a column containing 3% OV-17 with an injector and column temperature of 235 °C isothermal. The ElCD was operated in the reductive mode (H_2 + Ni catalyst) at 850 °C for qualitative analyses. A 4-mm i.d. quartz reaction tube and $Sr(OH)_2$ scrubber were used in all analyses. The GLC/ElCD quantitative analysis of medazepam and diazepam and their major metabolites in plasma was done by a modified procedure of de Silva and Puglisi (*11*). The procedure involves the extraction of 4-ml plasma standards (see *Results and Discussion*) buffered to pH 9.0 into diethyl ether; the back extraction of drugs into 2 mol/liter HCl; and final alkalinization of the acidic back extract followed by partitioning of drug into diethyl ether. The modification consisted of the re-extraction of the alkalinized HCl back-extract phase into chloroform rather than diethyl ether to avoid the requirement for the 30 min drying under reduced pressure to eliminate residual water.

Tricyclic antidepressants. Imipramine, desipramine, amitriptyline, nortriptyline, protriptyline, and doxepen were analyzed by GLC on a column containing 3% OV-17, with isothermal injector and column temperature of 245 and 225 °C respectively. The ElCD was operated in the reductive mode with Ni catalyst, 4-mm quartz reaction tube, $Sr(OH)_2$ scrubber, and IRN-78/IRN-150 stacked ion-exchange tube. The injection solvent was routinely vented prior to ElCD furnace. The extraction of the tricyclic drugs from 4-ml plasma standards was according to a modified procedure of Ervik and Ehrsson (*12*). Plasma standards of individual tricyclic drugs at a concentration of 100–500 μg/liter were prepared with the respective HCl salts; 500 ng of promazine HCl internal standard was added to 5 ml of each plasma standard; and these were made alkaline with 0.5 ml of 1 mol/liter NaOH and extracted into 5 ml of benzene. The extraction tube was centrifuged, the benzene removed for evaporation, and the final residue redissolved in 25 μl of benzene/methanol (19/1 by vol) for analysis of 2 μl by GLC/ElCD. Drug and internal standard were chromatographically resolved on OV-17, and the drug was quantitated with the internal standard technique (see *Results and Discussion*).

Phenothiazines. Phenothiazine and the hydrochloride salts of promazine, chlorpromazine, and trifluoperazine were analyzed by GLC/ElCD on a column containing 3% OV-17 (injector and column temperature 245 and 230 °C, respectively). Nitrogen-selective detection was achieved with H_2 reaction-gas + Ni catalyst, and a $Sr(OH)_2$ scrubber to remove acids such as HCl and HF. Furnace temperature was 850 °C.

Results and Discussion

Ethchlorvynol. Ethchlorvynol was quantitated by direct extraction of plasma and GLC, with use of the Hall ElCD in the reductive mode with nickle catalyst, and demonstrated selectivity and sensitivity at the nanogram level when hydrocarbon solvents are used (Figure 2). Additionally, GLC/ElCD analysis without further cleanup or concentration of the organic extract saves time and avoids analytical error arising from

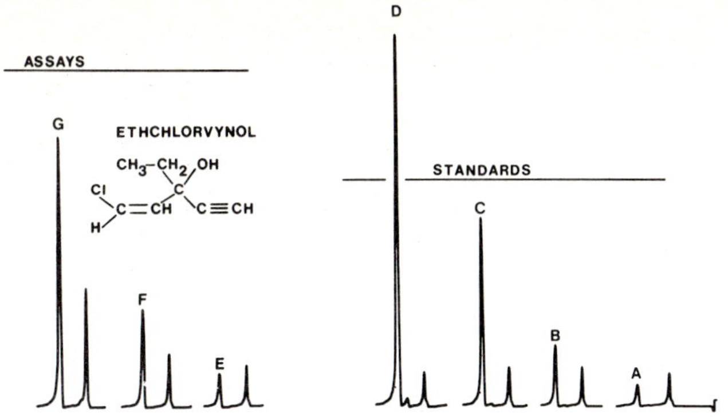

Fig. 2. GLC-ElCD chromatograms of ethchlorvynol standards and plasma extractions

Chromatograms *A, B, C,* and *D* are for 10, 20, 100, and 200 ng of ethchlorvynol in 2-μl of hexane. Chromatograms *E, F,* and *G* are for direct GLC analyses of hexane extracts (10, 5, 1 ml of extract) of 100 ng of ethchlorvynol in 5 ml of plasma

possible volatilization of ethchlorvynol during solvent evaporation. The analytical sensitivity necessary for micro-scale analysis can be achieved by a combination of electrometer attenuation (200-fold increase available), optimization of furnace-chemistry variables such as H_2/He carrier gas ratio and decrease in conductivity cell liquid-flow rate, to which detector response is inversely proportional. Factors limiting cell flow-rate to not less than 0.1 ml/min include peak broading (solute diffusion) and the operation of the gas–liquid contactor and separator.

Methaqualone. Nitrogen-selective ElCD response to methaqualone was linear over the range of 10–1000 ng studied. The sensitivity and element-selectivity of the detector are reflected in lower detection limits, greatly enhanced drug-to-solvent peak response, and absence of plasma interference peaks produced by plasma co-extractables. The extraction with buffered hexane permits the use of smaller solvent volumes (less emulsion) and direct GLC analysis because the relative detector response to hydrocarbons in the reductive mode is very low.

A slight negative pen deflection seen immediately preceding the leading edge of the methaqualone peak suggests a solvent-mediated neutralization reaction ($NH_3 + H_3O^+ \rightarrow NH_4^+ + H_2O$). Such a neutralization phenomenon (conductivity solvent too acidic) will be the factor limiting detectability unless a basic exchange-resin bed mixture is used to maintain the pH of the conductivity solvent at greater than 7.

Meprobamate. Quantitation of meprobamate in plasma by GLC/ElCD by use of *p*-dimethylaminobenzaldehyde as the internal standard, required the use of H_2 reaction gas and nickle catalyst. Chromatograms demonstrated a linear ElCD response, the elimination of significant interference from co-extractables, and more definitive qualitative identification (i.e., based on both retention time and element-selectivity) as compared to FID analysis. Additionally, change in relative detector response (meprobamate vs. internal standard) with different furnace chemistries can be used to confirm qualitative identification. For example, without nickle catalyst, the primary amino groups of meprobamate are still detected as NH_3 via a reductive decomposition mechanism at 820 °C furnace temperature, while the tertiary amine of the internal standard produces no ElCD response unless nickle catalyst is used. Thus, GLC retention time, ElCD element-selectivity, and relative ElCD response together with the use of appropriate furnace chemistries provide a set of complementary analytical data that allow more nearly certain qualitative identification and quantitation. However, GLC/FID analysis produces questionable data when nonselective extraction and cleanup procedures are used.

The choice of ElCD furnace chemistry or internal standard for drug quantitations requires considerable care until more is known about the principles of detector response. In addition to the choice of an internal standard based on mutual co-extraction with the drug of interest and their adequate resolution and detection by chromatographic instrumentation, principles of ElCD response and detector variability should be considered. Variations in ElCD that may cause nonlinearity in detector response ratio with differing concentration ratios of drug and internal standard include: (*a*) specific requirement for furnace chemistry mode, which may affect the working linear range of drug or internal standard detection; (*b*) gaseous or solution-phase reactivity of furnace products (e.g., NH_3 + HCl or S_xO_x); (*c*) differential effects of post-furnace abstractors; and (*d*) fluctuations in pH of conductivity solvent that differently affect dissociation constants of furnace reaction products from drug and internal standard. These detector variables must be considered rather distinctly

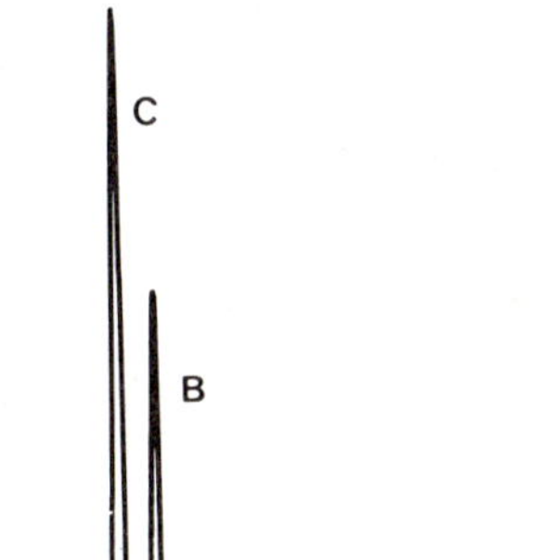

Fig. 3. GLC/ElCD chromatogram of 100 ng of amphetamine (*B*) and methamphetamine (*C*) in 2 μl of hexane (*A*)

Furnace chemistry: reductive mode, with catalyst

from those traditionally encountered in GLC/FID analysis—i.e., different relative extraction efficiencies at different drug/internal standard concentration and differential thermal or chromatographic decomposition. Criteria for choosing an internal standard to be used in GLC/ElCD analysis include: (*a*) compounds containing only the one reactive element (N, halogen, S) present in the drug to be quantitated; (*b*) compounds with functional group chemistry as similar to that of the drug of interest as possible; and (*c*) compounds with an optimum furnace chemistry similar to that of the drug being measured. The quantitation of drugs with two or more reactive elements (e.g., phenothiazines) or the need to use reaction gas abstractors may present additional analytical problems, and these problems are being actively considered in this laboratory.

Phenalkylamines. ElCD sensitivity and selectivity (relative to hydrocarbons) for nitrogen-containing phenalkylamine congeners was demonstrated by the analysis of 100 ng each of amphetamine and methamphetamine in a 2-μl hexane injection (Figure 3). Hall (*13*) has successfully detected 5 ng of amphetamine in combination with 10 ng of methamphetamine on a column containing alkaline Carbowax, with a good signal/noise ratio. He used the ElCD reductive mode with nickle catalyst, but substituted electrolytic-grade hydrogen for helium as the carrier gas.

With GLC/ElCD, sensitivity is a function of chromatographic phenomena (decomposition, sorption processes, peak shape, etc.), detector variables, cell chemistry, and residual detector noise. The choice of ElCD furnace-chemistry variables such as reaction tube, reaction catalyst, reaction gas, furnace temperature, and reaction product abstractors is critical to maximizing detector sensitivity. These variables affect conversion (reaction products of the drug) and throughput (the proportion of the reaction products that is delivered to the conductivity cell for a particular furnace chemistry mode and compound). Conversion rate is not only determined by the decomposition mechanisms operative with a particular furnace chemistry, but also by the residence time of the GLC effluent in the reaction tube. Sorption–desorption processes involving reaction tube and nickle catalyst surface phenomena may also play a minor role in affecting conversion-and-throughput and peak shape, as do the physical configuration and chemistry of acidic or basic abstractors in the post-furnace reaction tube. Contamination from solvent or drug carbonization processes or GLC "bleed" in the reaction tube or post-furnace transfer line will increase detector background and may trap furnace reaction products. A consideration of cell chemistry must include the processes of effective gas–liquid mixing—solubilization—and ionization, which may limit trace analysis. Mixing and solubilization may be improved by using low flow rates for the conductivity solvent (0.1–0.5 ml/min) to both increase contact time and increase effective conductance. Optimum solvent pH is important to prevent neutralization reactions, while solvent impurity and contamination from the ion-exchange bed will affect background conductivity. A quantitative discussion of some detector variables and residual detector noise has been presented by Hall (*8, 9*).

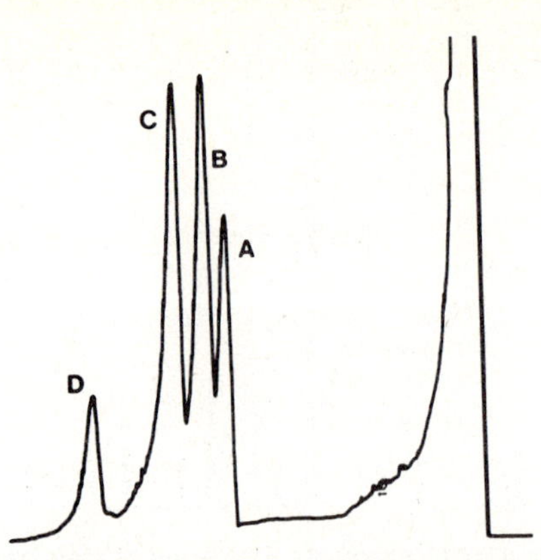

Fig. 4. GLC/ElCD chromatogram of isopropyl ether extract of amobarbital (*A*), pentobarbital (*B*), secobarbital (*C*), and phenobarbital (*D*) in plasma, 15 mg of each per liter

Barbiturates. Figure 4 shows the GLC/ElCD chromatogram for a 2-μl injection of the isopropyl ether extract from a sample of plasma containing 15 mg of the indicated barbiturates per liter. If one assumes 100% extraction, each peak represents less than 75 ng of drug. Differences among these compounds in the percentage content of nitrogen or their relative extractability do not explain the dramatic differences in detector response, which more probably are attributable to the furnace chemistry of the individual drugs.

To study furnace chemistry and detector response, we varied ElCD reaction gas conditions while holding constant the conductivity solvent flow-rate, solvent pH, and furnace temperature. Use of the reductive mode greatly improved peak resolution. With decreased H_2 reaction gas glow rate, detector response became increasingly similar to that obtained under pyrolytic conditions. Under reductive conditions, methaqualone was not detected without the use of a nickle catalyst. The inability to detect diphenylhydantoin under the conditions noted was due to short reaction-tube residence time; this may be corrected by using a larger (4 mm i.d.) reaction tube.

The effect of ElCD furnace temperature on detector response and peak resolution was studied under reductive conditions (H_2, no catalyst). Peak shape and peak height were optimum with an 800–850 °C furnace temperature. At present, the recommended furnace chemistry for barbiturate screening is 20 ml of H_2 reaction gas per minute, no catalyst (barbiturates poison nickle catalyst), and furnace temperature of 820 °C. Figure 5 shows a chromatogram obtained from a 1-μl injection of a 1 mg/ml methanolic drug mixture with ElCD, at the recommended furnace and detector settings.

Plasma drug screening. Figure 6 demonstrates the comparative advantage of ElCD over FID in the GLC screening of serum or plasma for weakly acidic and neutral drugs. Chromatogram *A* illustrates reduced ElCD response to co-extractable interferences and the

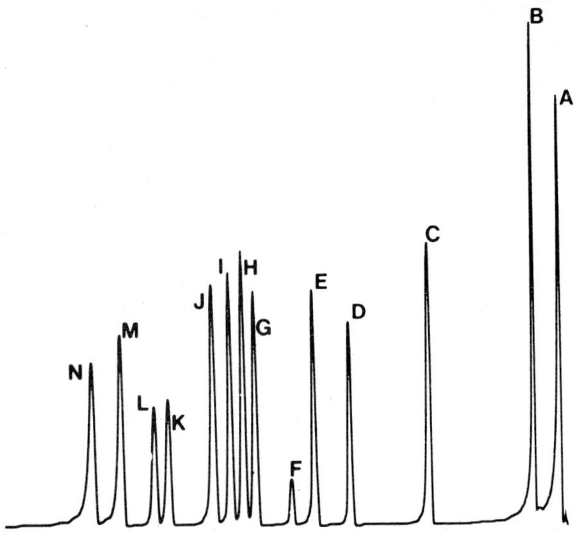

Fig. 5. GLC/EICD chromatogram (reductive mode, no catalyst) of acidic-neutral drug mixture

Methanol solvent front (*A*), ethchlorvynol (*B*), ethosuximide (*C*), metharbital (*D*), barbital (*E*), methyprylon (*F*), butabarbital (*G*), amobarbital (*H*), pentobarbital (*I*), secobarbital (*J*), glutethimide (*K*), mephobarbital (*L*), phenobarbital (*M*), and tolylbarbital (*N*)

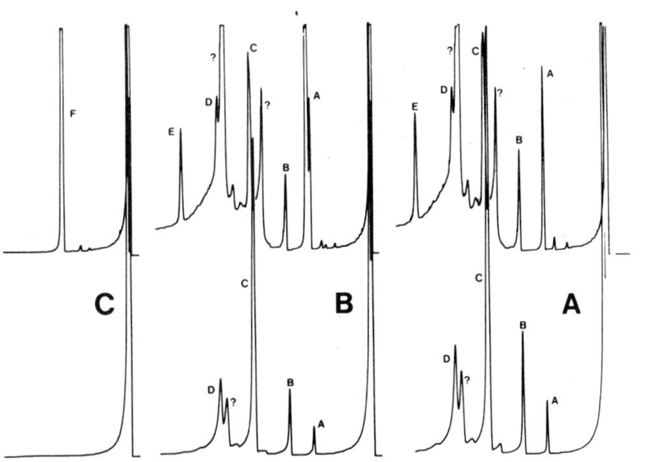

Fig. 6. Comparative GLC/FID (*upper*) and GLC/EICD (*lower*) chromatograms of plasma extracts containing methyprylon (*A*), amobarbital (*B*), meprobamate and glutethimide (*C*), phenobarbital (*D*), methaqualone (*E*), phthalate ester (*F*), and unidentified plasma co-extractable (?)

Analyses include: chromatogram *A*, routine plasma extraction; chromatogram *B*, plasma in contact with "serum skimmer"; chromatogram *C*, extraction of "serum skimmer"

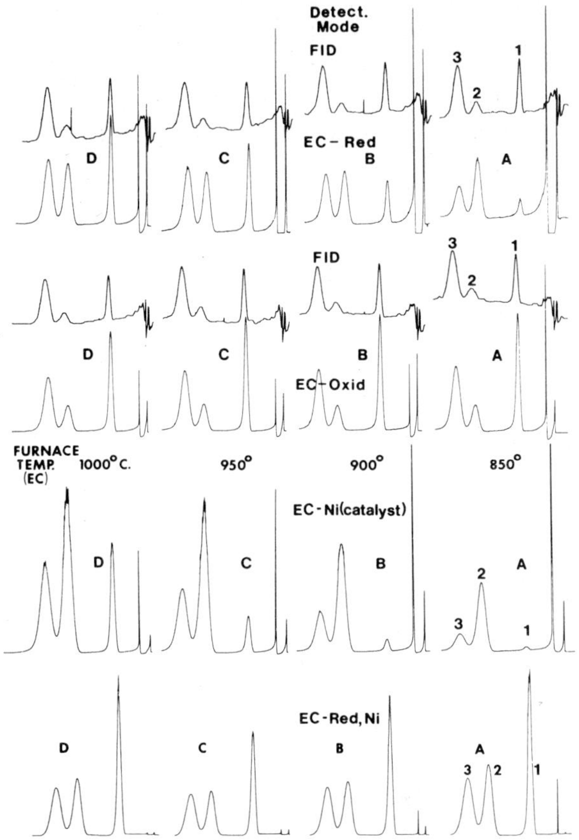

Fig. 7. Comparative GLC chromatograms of dichloromethane (*1*), chloroform (*2*), and dichloroethane (*3*) by electrolytic conductivity (*EC*) and FID

ElCD furnace modes included: reductive without catalyst (*EC-Red*); oxidative without catalyst (*EC-Oxid*); pyrolytic with catalyst (*EC-Ni*); and reductive with catalyst (*EC-Red, Ni*). ElCD furnace temperatures were 850 (*A*), 900 (*B*), 950 (*C*), and 1000 °C (*D*)

capability of obtaining a more nearly accurate quantitative analysis. Additionally, there are fewer misinterpretations of "serum peaks" as unidentified drug constituents. The FID response in chromatogram *B* demonstrates an additional interference from a phthalate ester (identified by mass spectrometry), caused by contact of the plasma with a commercial "serum skimmer" for 20 min before the extraction. This contaminant would make quantitation of methyprylon by FID more difficult. Chromatogram *C*, another dual FID/ElCD tracing obtained from a chloroform extract of the "serum skimmer", shows no ElCD response to the carbon-, hydrogen-, oxygen-containing phthalate ester.

Volatile chlorinated hydrocarbons. Volatile chlorinated hydrocarbon chromatograms obtained from matched Poropak Q-S columns are summarized in Figure 7. Variations in ElCD furnace chemistry are reflected in changes in relative detector response between dichloromethane:chloroform:dichloroethane and total "chlorine response":water peak as a function of reaction-gas composition, catalyst, and furnace temperature. In addition to the improved sensitivity and selectivity of ElCD for halogenated volatiles compared to FID, GLC/ElCD improves the certainty of correct qualitative identification by allowing the use of a type of "pattern recognition." This "pattern recognition" refers to the comparative change in detector response for the unidentified peak as compared to that for a cholorinated internal standard with change in furnace chemistry. Although Dolan and Hall (*8*) have commented on dechlorination mechanisms for polychlorinated systems, the elucidation of the competitive decomposition mechanisms involved in these chlorinated aliphatic systems is incomplete.

Figure 8 demonstrates a potential application of ElCD vs. FID with regard to the relative selectivity in the analysis for chlorinated volatiles. Chromatograms *A* are matched FID and ElCD detector response to a 2-μl injection of a 100 mg/liter solution of chlorinated

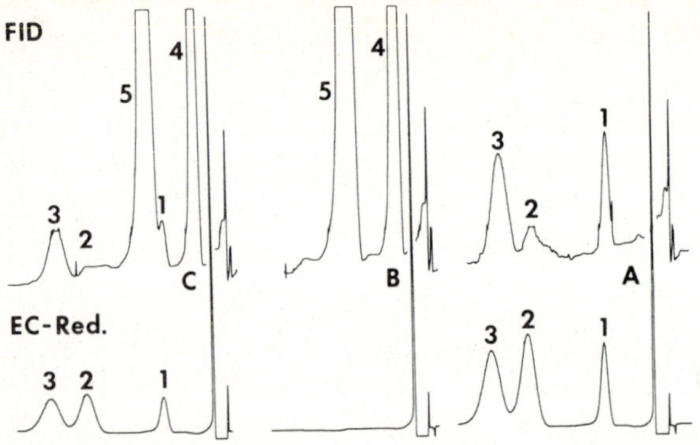

Fig. 8. GLC/ElCD and GLC/FID chromatograms of dichloromethane (*1*), chloroform (*2*), and dichloroethane (*3*)

Chromatogram *A*, 2 μl of *1, 2,* and *3* (100 mg/liter). Chromatogram B, 2 μl of ethanol (*4*) and *n*-propanol (*5*) (800 mg/liter). Chromatogram C, 2 μl of *1, 2,* and *3* (50 mg/liter) in solution with 400 mg of *4* and *5* per liter

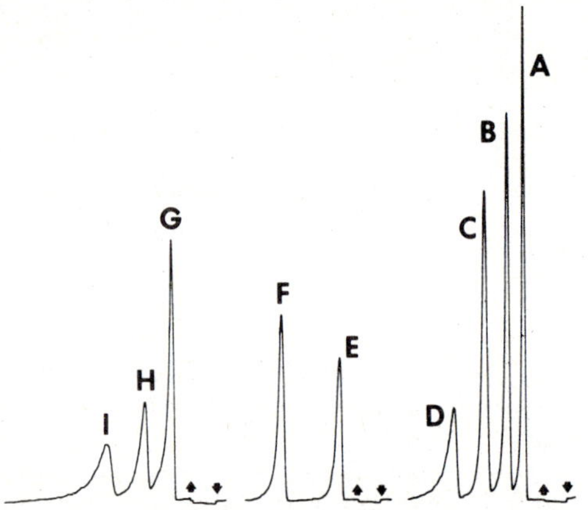

Fig. 9. GLC/ElCD chromatograms of 50 ng of medazepam (*A*), *N*-desmethyl medazepam (*B*), diazepam (*C*), *N*-desmethyl diazepam (*D*), oxazepam (*E*), flurazepam (*F*), *N*-1-desalkyl flurazepam (*G*), *N*-1-hydroxyethyl flurazepam (*H*), and nitrazepam (*I*)

Furnace chemistry: reductive mode, with catalyst and $Sr(OH)_2$ scrubber. Arrows indicate the venting of injection solvent

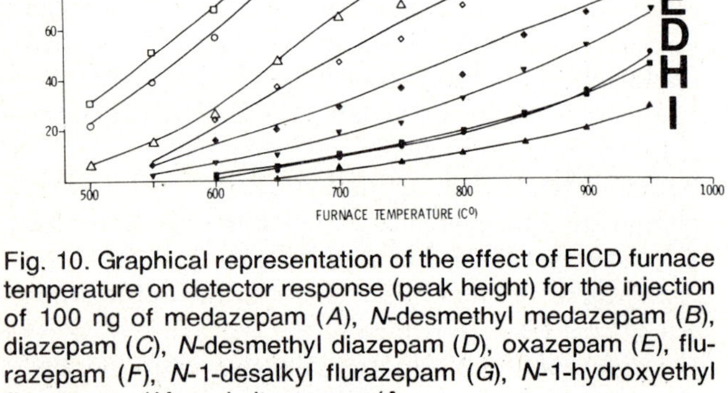

Fig. 10. Graphical representation of the effect of ElCD furnace temperature on detector response (peak height) for the injection of 100 ng of medazepam (*A*), *N*-desmethyl medazepam (*B*), diazepam (*C*), *N*-desmethyl diazepam (*D*), oxazepam (*E*), flurazepam (*F*), *N*-1-desalkyl flurazepam (*G*), *N*-1-hydroxyethyl flurazepam (*H*), and nitrazepam (*I*)

Furnace chemistry: reductive mode, with catalyst and $Sr(OH)_2$ scrubber

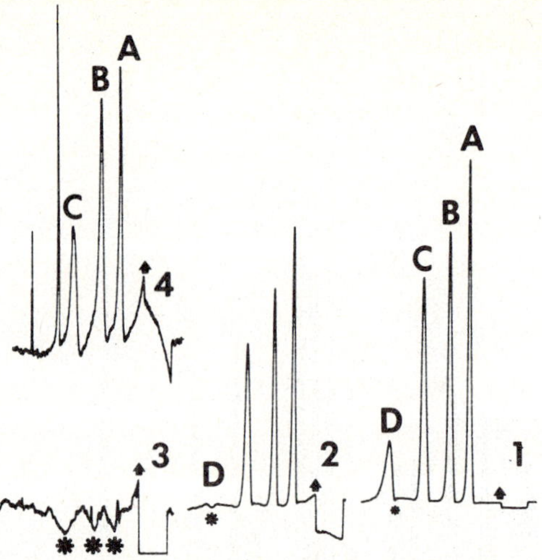

Fig. 11. GLC/ElCD chromatograms of medazepam (*A*), *N*-desmethyl medazepam (*B*), diazepam (*C*), and *N*-desmethyl diazepam (*D*), demonstrating the effect of neutralization reactions and $Sr(OH)_2$ scrubber

Furnace chemistry: reductive mode, with catalyst and $Sr(OH)_2$ scrubber. Chromatogram *1*, 100 ng *A–D*, electrometer 100 $\mu\Omega^{-1} \times 2$ attenuation, and 10 mg of scrubber. Chromatogram *2*, 20 ng *A–D*, electrometer 30 $\mu\Omega^{-1} \times 1$ attenuation, and 10 mg of scrubber. Chromatogram *3*, 2 ng *A–D*, electrometer 3 $\mu\Omega^{-1} \times 1$ attenuation, and 10 mg of scrubber. Chromatogram *4*, 2 ng *A–D*, electrometer 3 $\mu\Omega^{-1} \times 1$, and 20 mg of scrubber. Arrow indicates venting of injection solvent. (*) indicates neutralization reaction causing negative peak

volatiles in water. Chromatograms *B* demonstrate the selectivity of ElCD (reductive mode, no catalyst) against aliphatic alcohols (ethanol and *n*-propanol, 800 mg/liter, 2-μl injection). Matched FID and ElCD chromatograms *C* of a 2-μl injection of 400 mg/liter each of ethanol and *n*-propanol in solution with 50 mg/liter chlorinated hydrocarbons illustrates that ElCD affords a more nearly certain qualitative identification and quantitation.

1,4-Benzodiazepines and 1,4-benzodiazepin-2-ones. The sensitive nitrogen-selective analysis of these halogen- and nitrogen-containing congeners required the use of a 4-mm i.d. reaction tube to allow longer reaction-tube residence time and the use of a $Sr(OH)_2$ scrubber to remove HCl and HF reaction products that would otherwise result in peak tailing and neutralization reactions (e.g., gas-phase: $NH_3 + HX \rightarrow NH_4X$; solution-phase: $NH_4^+ + OH^- + HX \rightarrow NH_4^+ + X^- + H_2O$). Under the prescribed ElCD furnace and GLC conditions (see *Methods*), a cell flow-rate of 0.5 ml/min, and electrometer setting of 100 $\mu\Omega^{-1} \times 1$, the on-column injection of 50 ng of drug is easily detected (Figure 9). With these GLC and cell flow-rate conditions, the minimum detectable quantity with a signal/noise ratio of 2/1 was 500 pg of medazepam (*A*), 500 pg of *N*-desmethyl medazepam (*B*), 1 ng of diazepam (*C*), 20 ng of *N*-desmethyl diazepam (*D*), 2 ng of oxazepam (*E*), 2 ng of flurazepam (*F*), 2 ng of *N*-1-desalkyl flurazepam (*G*), 15 ng of *N*-1-hydroxyethyl flurazepam (*H*), and 20 ng of nitrazepam (*I*).

A lower minimum detectable quantity may be achieved by decreasing cell flow-rate, optimizing the H_2 reaction-gas flow-rate, and increasing furnace temperature (see Figure 10 for temperature effect). A lower

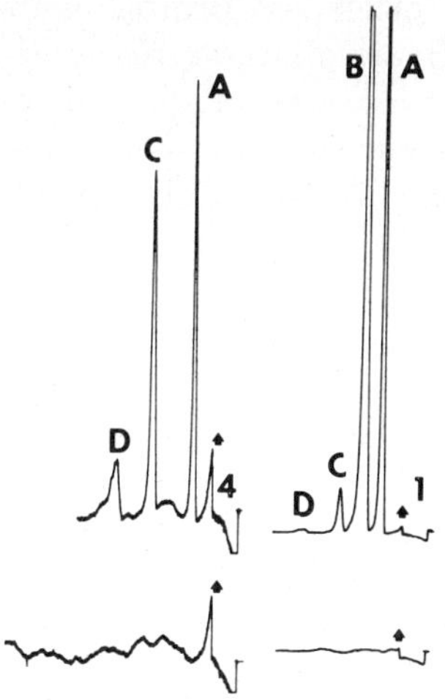

Fig. 12. GLC/ElCD chromatograms of extracts of medazepam, diazepam, and metabolites in plasma

Furnace chemistry: reductive mode, with catalyst and $Sr(OH)_2$ scrubber. Chromatogram *1*, analysis of 4 ml of plasma containing 200 μg medazepam (*A*), 300 μg of *N*-desmethyl medazepam (*B*), 40 μg of diazepam (*C*), and 80 μg of *N*-desmethyl diazepam (*D*) per liter; electrometer 30 $\mu\Omega^{-1} \times 1$ attenuation. Chromatogram *4*, analysis of 4 ml of plasma containing 40 μg of internal standard *A*, 40 μg of *C*, and 80 μg of *D* per liter; electrometer 3 $\mu\Omega^{-1} \times 1$ attenuation. Arrow indicates venting of injection solvent. Lower chromatograms represent the analysis of blank plasma

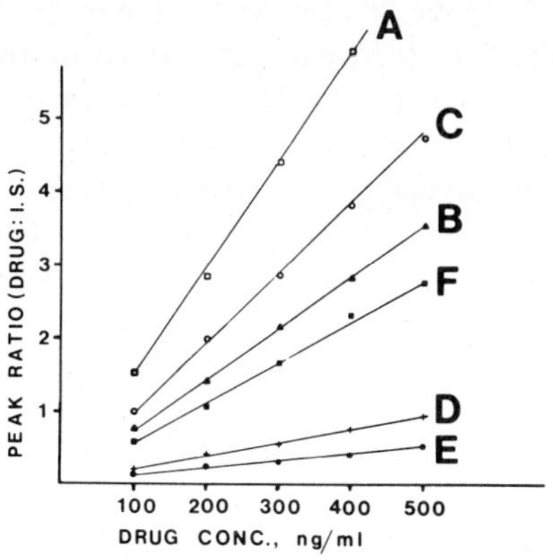

Fig. 13. Standard curves of the GLC/ElCD response to the analysis of extracts of plasma containing various concentrations of imipramine (*A*), desipramine (*B*), amitriptyline (*C*), nortriptyline (*D*), protriptyline (*E*), and doxepen (*F*), with 500 ng of promazine HCl as internal standard per 4 ml of plasma analyzed

Furnace chemistry: reductive mode, with nickle catalyst and $Sr(OH)_2$ scrubber

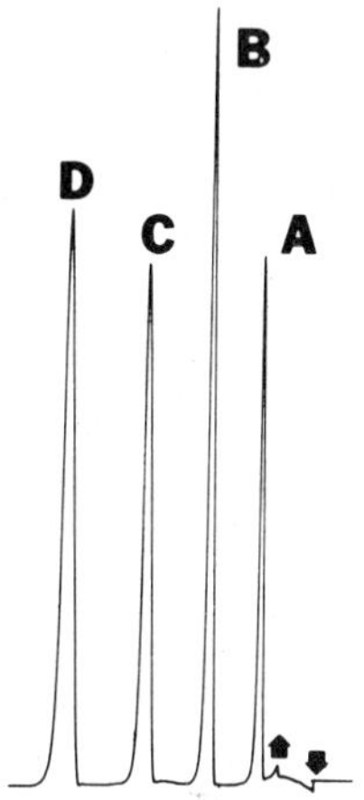

Fig. 14. GLC/ElCD chromatograms of 20 ng of phenothiazine (*A*), 32 ng of promazine HCl (*B*), 35 ng of chlorpromazine HCl (*D*), and 48 ng of trifluoperazine 2HCl (*D*)

Furnace chemistry: reductive mode, with catalyst and $Sr(OH)_2$ scrubber; electrometer 10 $\mu\Omega^{-1} \times 2$ attenuation. These quantities of *A–D* represent 1.4, 2.8, 2.8, and 4.2 ng of nitrogen, respectively

minimum detectable quantity for congeners such as *B, D, E, G, H,* and *I* might also be realized by derivatization to improve GLC volatility and peak shape, and to reduce adsorption losses (*14*). The quantity of $Sr(OH)_2$ scrubber used also affects the minimum detectable quantity (Figure 11). The "operative" phenomena in determining the *detector's* minimum detectable quantity include the relative production of HCl or HF vs. NH_3 under a specific set of reaction conditions, the trapping efficiency of $Sr(OH)_2$ for HX, and the throughput of NH_3 and HX to the conductivity cell. For example, chromatograms 3 and 4 in Figure 11 demonstrate the importance of the scrubber in trapping HCl and preventing neutralization reactions.

The quantitative analysis of medazepam and diazepam, and their major biotransformation products present in plasma, was done by the modified extraction method of de Silva and Puglisi (see *Methods*) and GLC/ElCD (Figure 12). Chromatogram 1 is the GLC/ElCD analysis of a 4-ml plasma extract containing 200 μg of *A*, 300 μg of *B*, 40 μg of *C*, and 80 μg of *D* per liter. Based upon reported recovery efficiencies (*11*), the chromatogram represents the on-column injection of approximately 60 ng of *A*, 90 ng of *B*, 12 ng of *D*, and 24 ng of *D*. The quantitative analysis, as judged by GLC/ElCD, was linear over at least a 10-fold increase in drug concentrations. Chromatogram 4 illustrates the analysis of 4 ml of plasma containing 40 μg of *C* and 80 μg of *D* per liter. The analysis of plasma resulted in no significant interference peaks. The quantitation of medazepam, diazepam, and metabolites in plasma according to the more straightforward protein precipitation/extraction/direct GLC analysis of de Silva et al. (*14*) using ElCD also resulted in chromatograms free of interference peaks and allowed the quantitation of therapeutic drug concentrations.

A comparison between nitrogen- and chlorine-selective ElCD and electron capture analysis for these drugs and drug metabolites is presently underway in this laboratory.

Tricyclic antidepressants. The quantitative analysis of tricyclic drugs in plasma was linear over the 100–500 μg/liter concentration range (Figure 13). Differences in the individual calibration curves representing ElCD response to drug vs. internal standard are due to the weight-percent of nitrogen in the individual compounds, the furnace chemistry mechanisms resulting in NH_3 production, and relative efficiencies of extraction and GLC. Although of about the same molecular weight, imipramine (*A*) and desipramine (*B*) contain a nitrogen in the ring structure not present in *C–F.* A ranking of ElCD response ($A > B > C \sim F \dot{>} D > E$) to equimolar injections of these tricyclic compounds at optimized furnace conditions demonstrated that ElCD response to *N,N*-dimethyl analogs was greater that the response to their respective N-methyl congeners (e.g. $A > B$ and $C > D$). ElCD response to protriptyline was the lowest because of both its weight-percent nitrogen and the furnace chemistry associated with its secondary alkylamino substituent. Further differences in the quantitative analytical response (Figure 13) to equivalent drug concentrations of A and C compared to their N-methyl analogs B and D is most probably due to the greater adsorptive loss of B and D during extraction and GLC.

Drug and drug metabolite combinations such as A–B and C–D are not resolved by GLC on a column containing OV-17. However, derivatization with acetic anhydride will allow separation by GLC (retention order: N,N-dimethyl analog, promazine, N-methyl acetamide derivative) and accurate quantitation at drug concentrations of greater than 75 μg/liter of plasma. Nonlinearity at low drug concentrations is due to loss in extraction, GLC, and ElCD reaction-product throughput to the conductivity cell. These phenomena are being investigated in an attempt to develop a reliable quantitative analysis in the 5–40 μg/liter concentration range encountered in the therapeutic monitoring of tricyclic antidepressant drug concentrations.

Phenothiazines. Phenothiazines analyzed by GLC/ElCD were detected in the nitrogen-selective mode (Figure 14). Detector response was quantitatively related to the nitrogen content and did not show the variations caused by side chain chemistry that were noted for the tricyclics. The minimum detectable quantity of phenothiazine was less than 100 pg.

A quantitative comparison of the element-selectivity of the ElCD in the nitrogen-, halogen-, and sulfur-selective modes vs. flame photometric and electron capture detectors is being undertaken by this laboratory.

I conclude that the Hall ElCD is a more sensitive and element-selective detector than FID, and permits GLC analysis with less sample clean-up, direct injection of sample extracts without concentration of the organic solvent, and a more certain qualitative identification. Various ElCD furnace chemistry modes permit the detection of organic nitrogen, halogen, sulfur, or carbon, as contrasted to other less flexible element-selective detectors (e.g., flame photometric—sulfur and phosphorus, thermionic or alkali flame—nitrogen or phosphorous, and electron capture—halogens). The current cost of the ElCD ($2995) is not prohibitive, and is available as part of a complete GLC/ElCD instrument (TRACOR Inc.) or it may be interfaced with most commercial gas chromatographs.

I thank Ken Mahler, of TRACOR Inc., for support of this study, and Timothy Flynn for technical assistance.

References

1. McNair, H. M., and Bonelli, E. J., *Basic Gas Chromatography,* 5th ed., Varian Aerograph, Walnut Creek, Calif., 1969, pp 118–119.

2. Hartman, C. H., Gas chromatograph detectors. *Anal. Chem.* **43,** 124A (1972).

3. Toseland, P. A., Albani, M., and Gauchel, F. D., Organic nitrogen-selective detector used in gas-chromatographic determination of some anticonvulsant and barbiturate drugs in plasma and tissues. *Clin. Chem.* **21,** 98 (1975).

4. Piringer, O., and Pascalau, M. J., Ein neuer Detektor fur die Gaschromatographie. *J. Chromatogr.* **8,** 410 (1962).

5. Coulson, D. M., Electrolytic conductivity detector for gas chromatography. *J. Gas Chromatogr.* **3,** 134 (1965).

6. Jones, P., and Nickless, G., Versatile electrolytic conductivity detector for gas chromatography. *J. Chromatogr.* **73,** 19 (1972).

7. Selucky, M. L., Specific gas chromatography detectors. Part II: Electrolytic conductivity detector. *Chromatographia* **5,** 359 (1972).

8. Dolan, J. W., and Hall, R. C., Enhancement of the sensitivity and selectivity of the Coulson electrolytic detector to chlorinated hydrocarbon pesticides. *Anal. Chem.* **45,** 2198 (1973).

9. Hall, R. C., A highly sensitive and selective microelectrolytic conductivity detector for gas chromatography. *J. Chromatogr. Sci.* **12,** 152 (1974).

10. Product description: Model 310 Hall electrolytic conductivity detector (TRACOR Inc., Austin, Tex. 78721).

11. de Silva, J. A. F., and Puglisi, C. V., Determination of medazepam (Nobrium), diazepam (Valium) and their major biotransformation products in blood and urine by electron capture gas-liquid chromatography. *Anal. Chem.* **42,** 1725 (1970).

12. Ervik, M., Walle, T., and Ehrsson, H., Quantitative gas chromatographic determination of nanogram levels of desipramine in serum. *Acta Pharm. Suec.* **7,** 625 (1970).

13. Hall, R. C., *Retention Times* (TRACOR Bulletin), TRACOR Inc., Austin, Tex. 78721 (1974).

14. de Silva, J. A. F., Bekersky, I., Puglisi, C. V., et al., Determination of 1,4-benzodiazepines and -diazepin-2-ones in blood by electron-capture gas-liquid chromatography. *Anal. Chem.* **48,** 10 (1976).

CLIN. CHEM. 22/6, 749–753 (1976)

Radioimmunoassay, Enzyme Immunoassay, Spectrophotometry, and Gas–Liquid Chromatography Compared for Determination of Phenobarbital and Diphenylhydantoin

Vina Spiehler,[1] Lilla Sun,[1] Don S. Miyada,[2] Steve G. Sarandis,[2] E. Richard Walwick,[3] Marston W. Klein,[3] Dennis B. Jordan,[3] and Barbara Jessen[4]

Sera from epileptic patients were assayed for phenobarbital and diphenylhydantoin by four different analytical procedures. Quantitative results obtained by radioimmunoassay (**I**) and enzyme immunoassay (**II**) were compared to each other and to the results obtained on aliquots of the same sample by gas–liquid chromatography (**III**) and ultraviolet spectrophotometry (**IV**). For phenobarbital the correlation coefficients were **I** vs. **II**, 0.909; **I** vs. **III**, 0.947; **II** vs. **III**, 0.917; **I** vs. **IV**, 0.950; **II** vs. **IV**, 0.953. For diphenylhydantoin the correlation coefficients were **I** vs. **II**, 0.953; **I** vs. **III**, 0.951; **II** vs. **III**, 0.957; **I** vs. **IV**, 0.862; **II** vs. **IV**, 0.898. The immunoassays can be substituted for liquid chromatography or ultraviolet spectrophotometry without changing the resulting clinical interpretations.

Diphenylhydantoin (Dilantin, Parke-Davis), phenobarbital, and primidone (Mysoline, Ayerst), are the drugs most commonly used in the treatment of grand mal, psychomotor epilepsy, and other forms of focal epilepsy. Because the clinical symptoms of epilepsy are not conveniently monitored, clinicians have turned to the measurement of these antiepileptic drugs in the blood to determine the adequacy of dosage and the possibility of toxicity. Concentrations of the drug in serum and therapeutic or toxic effects have been correlated (*1*). Such monitoring allows the physician (*a*) to detect non-compliance; (*b*) to evaluate the patient with inadequate seizure control, or a change in degree of seizure control caused by poor absorption or rapid metabolism of the drug; and (*c*) to establish baseline concentrations and to confirm suspected intoxication. Moreover, in the case of a patient with symptoms of drug intoxication, who is receiving several drugs, the offending drug may be precisely identified and the dose corrected.

Because of the importance of monitoring antiepileptic drug blood concentrations, new or improved methods have been continually introduced. Our objective was to compare the quantitative results obtained for phenobarbital and diphenylhydantoin by radioimmunoassay (RIA) and enzyme-mediated immunoassay (EMIT) (*2–6*) with results from spectrophotometric (*7–10*) and gas–liquid chromatographic (GLC) (*11–14*) procedures.[5]

Materials and Methods

Samples

We assayed sera from 90 epileptic patients referred by physicians for antiepileptic drug screen and from 50 patients admitted to a hospital emergency room for suspected drug overdose. Samples were assayed by the two immunoassay methods and by either spectrophotometry or chromatography.

Methods

Phenobarbital

EMIT

The reagents for the enzyme immunoassay of phenobarbital were obtained from Syva Corp., Palo Alto, Calif. 94304, and used according to the manufacturer's

[1] Beckman Instruments, Inc., Irvine, Calif. 92664. Address correspondence to Lilla Sun.
[2] Orange County Medical Center, Orange, Calif. 92668.
[3] Hospital-Pathologist Central Laboratory of Orange County, Garden Grove, Calif. 92640.
[4] Hoag Memorial Hospital, Newport Beach, Calif. 92660.
Received Oct. 16, 1975; accepted Dec. 30, 1975.

[5] Nonstandard abbreviations used: RIA, radioimmunoassay; EMIT, enzyme-mediated immunoassay; and GLC, gas-liquid chromatography.

instructions. Absorbance was measured at 340 nm on a Model 24/25 double-beam spectrophotometer with a heated sipper cell and a Model 701 Printer/Calculator (all from Beckman Instruments, Inc., Irvine, Calif. 92664).

The antibody to phenobarbital, obtained from Syva Corp., showed the following cross reactivity: phenobarbital 100.0%, mephobarbital 20.0%, secobarbital 1.0%, amobarbital 0.7%, pentobarbital 0.5%, diphenylhydantoin 0.5%, and primidone 0.5%.

RIA

The reagents for radioimmunoassay of barbiturates were obtained from Roche Diagnostics, Hoffmann-La Roche, Inc., Nutley, N.J. 07110 and used according to the manufacturer's protocol for quantitative assay. Phenobarbital solutions of 1000, 500, 250, 125, 63, 32 and 16 μg/liter were used in constructing the standard curve. The supernate was counted on a "Biogamma" gamma counter (Beckman Instruments).

The antibody to barbiturates, obtained from Roche Diagnostics, showed the following cross reactivity: secobarbital 100.0%, pentobarbital 45.0%, butabarbital 45.0%, amobarbital 35.0%, phenobarbital 25.0%, and barbital 10.0%. The manufacturer has found no significant cross reactivity with diphenylhydantoin.

GLC

The gas–liquid chromatographic analysis was performed according to the method of Perchalski et al. (*14*). Methylene chloride was substituted for ethyl ether as the extraction solvent. "Concentratubes" (Laboratory Research, Los Angeles, Calif. 90036) were used for the final extraction. Trimethylanilinium hydroxide in methanol, 25 ml/100 ml, from Southwest Analytical Chemicals, Austin, Tex., was used to methylate the drugs on the column as described elsewhere (*10, 12–14*). 5-Methyl-phenylhydantoin (Aldrich Chemical Co., Milwaukee, Wis. 53233) was used as an internal standard. A Model 5710A gas chromatograph was used for this assay with 3% OV-17 on Gas Chrom Q in a 1.82 m × 2 mm (i. d.) column (Hewlett-Packard, Avondale, Pa. 19311).

Spectrophotometry

Spectrophotometry was performed according to the method of Goldbaum (*7*) as modified by Bogan and Smith (*8*). Absorbance of the unknown at 260 nm was compared with that of a butabarbital standard.

Diphenylhydantoin

EMIT

The reagents for the enzyme mediated immunoassay of diphenylhydantoin (Syva Corp.) were used according to the manufacturer's instructions. Absorbance was read as described previously.

The antibody to diphenylhydantoin obtained from Syva Corp. showed the following cross reactivities: diphenylhydantoin 100.0%, 5-hydroxyphenyl-5-phenylhydantoin 0.5%, phenobarbital 0.5%, primidone 0.5%, methsuximide 0.5%, ethosuximide 0.5%, and mephobarbital 0.5%.

RIA

The reagents for radioimmunoassay of diphenylhydantoin (Wien Laboratories, Inc., Succasunna, N. J. 07876) were used according to the manufacturer's instructions. The supernate was counted on a Model 350 liquid scintillation counter (Beckman Instruments).

The antibody to diphenylhydantoin, obtained from Wien Laboratories, showed the following cross reactivities: diphenylhydantoin 100.0%, 5-hydroxy-phenyl-5-phenylhydantoin 76.5%, 5-ethyl-5-phenylhydantoin 1.0%, phenobarbital 0.1%, mephobarbital 0.1%, and primidone 0.1%.

GLC

The method of Perchalski et al. (*14*), modified as described in the above GLC section, was used for the gas–liquid chromatographic analysis.

Spectrophotometry

The procedure of Wallace (*9*) as modified by Dill et al. (*10*) was used for the ultraviolet spectrophotometric analysis of diphenylhydantoin. The absorption of the oxidation product, benzophenone, in isooctane was measured at 247 nm vs. a reagent blank.

Table 1. Statistical Comparison of Immunoassay, Spectrophotometry and Gas-Chromatography for Determining Phenobarbital and Diphenylhydantoin

	m	b	S_{xy}	r	n	t
		mg/liter				
Phenobarbital						
a. RIA vs. EMIT	.867	1.19	5.15	.909	59	15.17
b. RIA vs. GLC	.795	1.45	3.84	.947	47	19.62
c. EMIT vs. GLC	.901	.797	4.65	.917	32	12.58
d. RIA vs. spectr.	.995	−2.36	3.57	.950	15	15.25
e. EMIT vs. spectr.	.898	−1.47	3.03	.953	18	12.63
Diphenylhydantoin						
f. RIA vs. EMIT	1.11	−.12	2.78	.953	59	23.76
g. RIA vs. GLC	.661	1.61	2.19	.951	47	21.16
h. EMIT vs. GLC	.786	.976	2.04	.957	60	26.47
i. RIA vs. spectr.	.718	1.78	1.93	.862	33	14.52
j. EMIT vs. spectr.	.711	1.98	1.63	.898	36	11.89

m = slope of the least-squares regression line
b = intercept of the least-squares regression line
S_{xy} = standard error of the estimate
r = correlation coefficient
n = number of cases
t = *t*-statistics testing linear regression

Statistical Analysis

Concentrations of phenobarbital found by radioimmunoassay and enzyme immunoassay were compared to each other and to concentrations of phenobarbital found by gas–liquid chromatography or ultraviolet spectrophotometry on aliquots of the same sample. Errors were estimated from the least-squares parameters (slope of the least-squares line, y intercept, standard error of estimates S_{xy}) as recommended by Westgard and Hunt (*15*).

Systematic errors may be constant (a systematic error in concentration units) or proportional (a systematic error in percentage units). Using a simulated test set of data, Westgard and Hunt (*15*) demonstrated that constant error is reflected exactly in the intercept of the least-squares line, as well as in the bias. The slope, standard error, correlation coefficient, and standard deviation are not sensitive to constant error. The exact magnitude of proportional error is quantitated by changes in the slope, m.

Westgard and Hunt (*15*) pointed out that both the standard error and the standard deviation reflect the magnitude of the random error. The correlation coefficient decreases as random error increases, but the changes are small.

Cases showing large discrepancies (±3 SD) were not included in the linear regression and statistical calculations (*16*).

Results

Phenobarbital (Table 1)

Radioimmunoassay vs. enzyme immunoassay (Table 1, line *a*). The slope of the line is 0.867, which indicates a proportional error of 13.3%. Constant error is estimated at 1.19 mg/liter from the intercept. The random error is estimated at 5.15 mg/liter from the standard error of the estimate, S_{xy}. The correlation coefficient is 0.909. For example, a radioimmunoassay value of 30 mg of phenobarbital per liter would correspond to an average value of 27.4 mg/liter ±5.2 (SD) by enzyme immunoassay.

Immunoassays vs. gas chromatography (Table 1, lines *b* and *c*). The slope is 0.795 for radioimmunoassay and 0.901 for enzyme immunoassay, which indicates a proportional error of 20% and 10%, respectively. Constant error is estimated as 1.45 mg/liter (RIA) and 0.79 mg/liter (EMIT). Random error estimated from the standard error is 3.84 mg/liter (RIA) and 4.65 mg/liter (EMIT). The correlation coefficients were 0.947 and 0.917, respectively. For example, a phenobarbital value of 30 mg/liter by gas–liquid chromatography would correspond to an average value by RIA of 34.9 ± 3.84 mg/liter and an average value by EMIT of 32.4 ± 4.65 mg/liter.

Immunoassays vs. spectrophotometry (Table 1, lines *d* and *e*). From the least-squares parameters, proportional error between the immunoassays and Goldbaum's method (*7*) was much less than that found when comparing immunoassays to gas–liquid chromatography. Proportional error was estimated at 0.5% (RIA) and 10.0% (EMIT), constant error as −2.36 mg/liter (RIA) and −1.47 mg/liter (EMIT), and random error as 3.5 mg/liter (RIA) and 3.0 mg/liter (EMIT). The correlation coefficients were 0.950 and 0.953, respectively. For example, a phenobarbital value of 30 mg/liter obtained by spectrophotometry would correspond to an average value by radioimmunoassay of 32.5 ± 3.5 mg/liter and an average value by enzyme immunoassay of 35.0 ± 3.0 mg/liter.

Diphenylhydantoin (Table 1)

Concentrations of diphenylhydantoin found by radioimmunoassay and enzyme immunoassay were compared to each other and to concentrations of diphenylhydantoin found by gas–liquid chromatography and by spectrophotometry according to Wallace (*9*) as modified by Dill et al. (*10*).

Radioimmunoassay vs. enzyme immunoassay (Table 1, line *f*). Error estimates based on the least-squares parameters as described by Westgard and Hunt (*15*) indicate a proportional error of 10% and a constant error of 0.12 mg/liter. Random error is estimated as 2.78 mg/liter. The correlation coefficient is 0.953. A diphenylhydantoin concentration of 10 mg/liter by radioimmunoassay would correspond to an average value of 9.14 ± 2.78 mg/liter by enzyme immunoassay.

Immunoassay vs. gas–liquid chromatography (Table 1, lines *g* and *h*). The slopes were 0.661 and 0.786, which suggest 34% and 22% proportional error for RIA and EMIT when gas chromatography is taken as the reference method. The constant error is small, 1.61 mg/liter and 0.976 mg/liter, and the random error was 2.19 and 2.04 mg/liter, respectively. The correlation coefficients were 0.951 and 0.957.

A diphenylhydantoin value of 10 mg/liter by gas chromatography would correspond to an average value

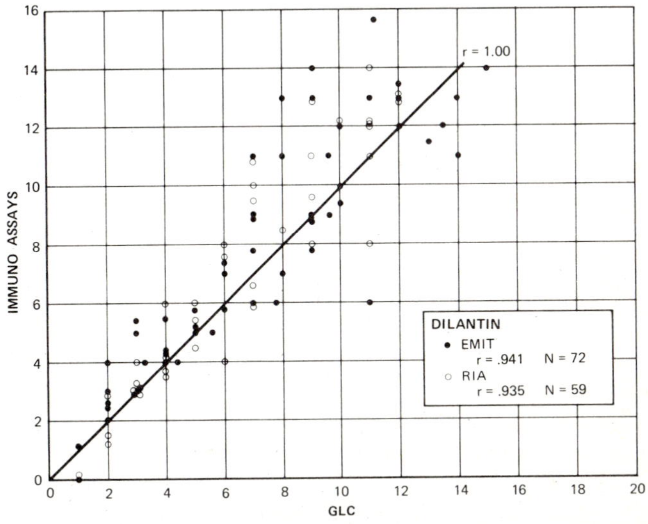

Fig. 1. Immunoassay vs. gas–liquid chromatography compared for diphenylhydantoin determination

of 12.7 ± 2.2 mg/liter (RIA) or 11.5 ± 1.0 mg/liter (EMIT).

Immunoassays vs. spectrophotometry (Table 1, lines *j* and *i*). Estimated from the linear regression parameters, the proportional error was about 30%, the constant error was 1.8 mg/liter, and the random error range was 1.6 to 1.9 mg/liter for both immunoassays. The correlation coefficients were 0.862 and 0.898, respectively.

In our hands, concentration of 10 mg/liter as determined by the method of Wallace (*9*) as modified by Dill et al. (*10*) would correspond to an average value of 11.4 ± 1.9 mg/liter (RIA) or 11.3 ± 1.6 mg/liter (EMIT).

Interferences

A scattergram of the immunoassay results for diphenylhydantoin plotted against the results obtained by gas–liquid chromatography is shown in Figure 1. When the case histories were investigated some of the outlying points seen on this scattergram (and on the corresponding graphs for the other comparisons) could be explained in some cases by the different cross reactivities of the immunoassays and by interference from other drugs taken by the patient.

Patients receiving mephobarbital gave different apparent phenobarbital concentrations by the different methods. For example, in one of the cases in which the patient received both mephobarbital and phenobarbital, the apparent phenobarbital concentrations (mg/liter) were: 54 (GLC), 50 (EMIT), 42 (RIA), and 32 (spectrophotometric).

The gas–liquid chromatographic method involving methylation does not distinguish between phenobarbital and mephobarbital (*12*). The two drugs cannot be separately measured by this procedure. The extraction efficiency for mephobarbital by this method is not known. However, since the apparent phenobarbital concentrations by GLC in these cases were the highest values, it may be that GLC results represent the sum of the two drugs present.

According to the manufacturer (Syva Corp.), the enzyme immunoassay for phenobarbital cross reacts 20% with mephobarbital. For a mixture of equal amounts of mephobarbital and phenobarbital the phenobarbital result by EMIT would be 20% too high. This appeared to be true in several cases encountered in this study.

In our study, the radioimmunoassay results were slightly less than those obtained by enzyme immunoassay.

The spectrophotometric procedure of Goldbaum gives the sum of 5,5-substituted barbiturates. However, the 1,5,5-substituted barbiturates (hexobarbital, mephobarbital, metharbital, etc.) have characteristically different absorption spectra and do not show a shift in absorption between pH 14.0 and 9.0 (*17*). For this reason the spectrophotometric method probably suffered the least interference and gave the most nearly accurate value for phenobarbital in these cases.

No other systematic interference from other drugs given concurrently was noted in the phenobarbital or diphenylhydantoin assay. The drugs prescribed concurrently included amitriptyline, primidone (Mysoline, Ayerst), ethosuximide (Zarontin, Parke-Davis) and thioridazine (Mellaril, Sandoz).

Discussion

The immunoassays fill the requirements for an acceptable assay method for antiepileptic drugs. They require very little sample; the Wien radioimmunoassay for diphenylhydantoin requires only 10 µl of serum, the EMIT procedures require 50 µl, and the Roche Diagnostics procedure, 100 µl. The immunoassays can be performed more quickly than the methods now in use, because no extraction or concentration is involved. The fastest procedure is EMIT, which requires less than 2 min per tube; thus, it allows a standard curve and several samples to be run in less than 15 min from receipt of serum. The radioimmunoassays each require 1 h to obtain quantitative results. Because the immunoassays are sensitive in the nanogram range, it was necessary to dilute patients' serum.

By contrast, gas–liquid chromatography permits simultaneous analysis for several drugs (primidone, phenobarbital, and diphenylhydantoin) which, with batching of specimens, lends itself well to nonemergency analysis. We found the method we used (*14*) to be convenient and reliable for routine laboratory use.

The immunoassay results for phenobarbital correlate well with each other and with the values found by gas chromatography and spectrophotometry. Plaa and Hine (*18*) reported that the average phenobarbital concentration in the blood of 30 adult subjects receiving 200 mg of phenobarbital per day for control of seizures was 32 ± 18 mg/liter (range, 7 to 56 mg/liter). As calculated from the least-squares regression parameters, the immunoassays would give average values of 34.9 mg/liter (RIA) and 32.4 mg/liter (EMIT) for a gas-chromatographic value of 30 mg/liter or 32.5 mg/liter (RIA) and 35.0 mg/liter (EMIT) for a spectrophotometric value of 30 mg/liter. Therefore, if the faster, more convenient immunoassays were used in place of the other methods, this substitution would have little effect on the clinical interpretation of blood drug concentrations.

The immunoassay results for diphenylhydantoin correlate well with each other and with the gas–liquid chromatographic method, and somewhat less well with the spectrophotometric procedure of Dill et al. (*10*). Kutt et al. (*19*) showed that symptoms of intoxication (nystagmus) caused by diphenylhydantoin begin to appear when its concentration in the blood approaches 20 mg/liter (range 15–25 mg/liter). As calculated from the least-squares regression parameters described above, use of the immunoassays for diphenylhydantoin determination would give average values of 27.8 mg/liter (RIA) and 24.2 mg/liter (EMIT) for a gas chromatographic value of 20 mg/liter and (or) average values of 25.2 mg/liter (RIA) and 25.4 mg/liter (EMIT) for a spectrophotometric value of 20 mg/liter. Therefore, here again, the use of the immunoassay results would not change the clinical interpretation.

References

1. Kutt, H., Pharmacodynamic and pharmacokinetic measurements of antiepileptic drugs. *Clin. Pharmacol. Ther.* **16,** 243 (1974).

2. Cleeland, R., Davis, R., Heveran, J., and Grunberg, E., A simple ^{125}I-radioimmunoassay for the detection of barbiturates in biological fluids. *J. Forensic Sci.* **20,** 45 (1975).

3. Spector, S., and Flynn, E. J., Barbiturates—radioimmunoassay. *Science* **174,** 1036 (1971).

4. Flynn, E. J., and Spector, S., Determination of barbiturate derivatives by radioimmunoassay. *J. Pharmacol. Exp. Ther.* **181,** 547 (1972).

5. EMIT Antiepileptic Drug Asays, Package Insert, Syva Corp., Palo Alto, Calif. 94304, 1975.

6. Tigelaar, R.E., A radioimmunoassay for diphenylhydantoin. *Clin. Chim. Acta* **45,** 231 (1973).

7. Goldbaum, L. R., Determination of barbiturates. *Anal. Chem.* **24,** 1604 (1952).

8. Bogan, J., and Smith, H., Analytical investigations of barbiturate poisoning—description of methods and a summary of results. *J. Forensic Sci. Soc.* **7,** 37 (1967).

9. Wallace, E., Microdetermination of diphenylhydantoin in biological specimens by ultraviolet spectrophotometry. *Anal. Chem.* **40,** 978 (1968).

10. Dill, W. A., Chucot, L., Chang, T., and Glazko, A. J., Simplified benzophenone procedure for determination of diphenylhydantoin in plasma. *Clin. Chem.* **17,** 1200 (1971).

11. Brockmann-Hansen, E., and Oki, O. T., Gas chromatography of barbiturates, phenolic alkaloids and xanthine bases: Flash heater methylation by means of trimethylanilinium hydroxide. *J. Pharm. Sci.* **58,** 370 (1969).

12. Kupferburg, H. J., Quantitative estimation of diphenylhydantoin, primidone and phenobarbital in plasma by gas-liquid chromatography. *Clin. Chim. Acta* **29,** 283 (1970).

13. Kananen, G., Osiewicz, R., and Sunshine, I., Barbiturate analysis—a current assessment. *J. Chromatogr. Sci.* **10,** 283 (1972).

14. Perchalski, R. J., Scott, K. N., Wilder, B. J., and Hammer, R. H., Rapid, simultaneous GLC determination of phenobarbital, primidone and diphenylhydantoin. *J. Pharm. Sci.* **62,** 1735 (1973).

15. Westgard, J. O., and Hunt, M. R., Use and interpretation of common statistical tests in method-comparison studies. *Clin. Chem.* **19,** 49 (1973).

16. Barnett, R. N., A scheme for the comparison of quantitative methods. *Am. J. Clin. Pathol.* **43,** 562 (1965).

17. Sunshine, I., and Gerber, S. R., *Spectrophotometric Analysis of Drugs.* Charles C Thomas, Springfield, Ill., 1963.

18. Plaa, G. L., and Hine, C. H., Hydantoin and barbiturate levels observed in epileptics. *Arch. Int. Pharmacodyn. Ther.* **128,** 375 (1960).

19. Knutt, H., Winters, W., Kokenge, R., and McDonell, F., Diphenylhydantoin metabolism, blood levels and toxicity. *Arch. Neurol.* (Chicago) **11,** 642 (1964).

CLIN. CHEM. 22/6, 754–760 (1976)

Efficacy of Activated Charcoal Hemoperfusion in Removing Lethal Doses of Barbiturates and Salicylate from the Blood of Rats and Dogs

John B. Hill, Frank L. Palaia,[1] J. Lawrence McAdams, Phyllis J. Palmer, and S. Melissa Maret

Rats were injected intraperitoneally with lethal doses of sodium pentobarbital (115 mg/kg) or a lethal mixture of sodium salicylate (500 mg/kg) and sodium acetazolamide (25 mg/kg). Within about 20 min, part of each group was connected to an extracorporeal circuit containing uncoated activated charcoal and part to an empty control circuit. After a 90-min hemoperfusion, the treated groups showed a significantly decreased mortality (58% to 14% for pentobarbital; 100% to 0% for salicylate). Dogs were injected intravenously with lethal doses of sodium phenobarbital (175 mg/kg). One group was treated by hemoperfusion through an empty device in a control extracorporeal circuit, a second group was treated with loose-bed activated charcoal devices, and a third group with fixed-bed activated charcoal devices. For both the fixed and loose-bed devices, a 5-h hemoperfusion markedly decreased mortality (100% to ≤15%). The lethal combination of salicylate and closed-circuit methoxyflurane anesthesia was also successfully treated in dogs. This study clearly demonstrates the lifesaving potential of uncoated activated charcoal hemoperfusion.

Additional Keyphrases: *toxicology • hypotension and extracorporeal perfusion of blood • rats, dogs • emergency procedure • salicylate and methoxyflurane anesthesia*

Removal of poisonous substances from the body by flowing the blood through an activated charcoal[2] bed in an extracorporeal circuit was first described by Hippocrates Yatzidis in 1964 (*1*). Since then, several investigators have used hemoperfusion through activated charcoal and have shown the removal of a number of drugs and toxins (*1–18*); however, the design of these experiments does not allow the lifesaving potential of this technique to be evaluated. Because charcoal hemoperfusion is being used more frequently in the clinic (*14–16, 18*), we thought that its lifesaving efficacy should be more clearly demonstrated and evaluated.

In our experiments, no active form of therapy other than charcoal hemoperfusion was used to save the experimental animals. The substances chosen for study were administered in such a way that we had adequate time to establish the extracorporeal flow of blood through the activated charcoal (or a control device lacking activated charcoal) before the animal died. These conditions are not those likely to be found in an actual poisoning situation, but were used because they enabled us to treat the animals by hemoperfusion without other supportive therapy. This approach allows comparisons of efficacy under well-defined conditions by eliminating the variability associated with oral administration, respiratory support, and cardiovascular support. Under these experimental conditions, we obtained clear evidence of efficacy in rats with the use of loose-bed uncoated activated charcoal devices and in dogs with the use of loose and fixed-bed uncoated activated charcoal devices.

Becton, Dickinson and Company Research Center, P. O. Box 12016, Research Triangle Park, N. C. 27709.

[1] Present address: Hospital Products Division, Research & Development, Building 4, Department No. 973, Abbott Laboratories, North Chicago, Ill. 60064.

Received Jan. 22, 1976; accepted Feb. 13, 1976.

[2] The terms "activated charcoal," "charcoal," and "activated carbon" have been used interchangeably in the literature. Engineers, as represented by the American Society for Testing and Materials, and some manufacturers of "activated carbon" use that term. The *United States Pharmacopeia* and most of the medical community and other manufacturers of charcoal use the term "activated charcoal." Because charcoal contains carbon and other substances as well, "activated impure carbon" would seem more precise than "activated carbon." Publications in the hemoperfusion literature show a preference of 5 to 1 for "charcoal" over "carbon." We prefer to use the term "activated charcoal." "Activated" refers to the treatment of charcoal with a mild oxidizing process to rid the charcoal of organic matter and thus increase the adsorptive properties. All charcoals used for hemoperfusion are activated. Much work in the charcoal hemoperfusion field has been done with activated charcoal with a polymer membrane on its surface. We use the terms "uncoated activated charcoal" and "coated activated charcoal" to distinguish between charcoal with a polymer-free surface and that with a polymer-coated surface. In this publication, the term "activated charcoal" and "charcoal" are used interchangeably and refer to uncoated activated charcoal. The terms "loose-bed" and "fixed-bed" refer to loose granular charcoal and immobilized granular charcoal, as described in the text.

Materials and Methods

Studies on Rats

In experiments designed to demonstrate a decrease in mortality associated with an overdose of sodium pentobarbital, an intraperitoneal dose of 115 mg/kg body wt was administered and served as the anesthetic as well as the poison. Sprague–Dawley strain male albino rats weighing 275–410 g were used. In the experiments designed to demonstrate a decrease in salicylate toxicity, an intraperitoneal injection of 500 mg of sodium salicylate per kilogram body weight plus 25 mg of sodium acetazolamide per kilogram body weight was given to Wistar male albino rats weighing 300–360 g. These rats were anesthetized with ether. The use of two strains of rats has no significance other than availability at the time of the experiment. Polyethylene cannulas (Intramedic No. PE50; Clay Adams, Parsippany, N. J. 07054) were tied into the surgically exposed femoral vein and artery, and the other end was connected to larger tubing (No. PE90) with appropriate size Tygon sleeving cut from AutoAnalyzer (Technicon Corp., Tarrytown, N. Y. 10591) pump tubing. The activated charcoal granules were held in 2.5- or 20-ml "Plastipak" syringes (Becton-Dickinson, Rutherford, N. J. 07070) as pictured in Figure 1. Rubber washers, cut from the syringe rubber plunger tips, were used to hold the polyester monofilament screen filters (DAFAB D-120, 43-μm square openings; Wire Cloth Enterprises, Inc., Pittsburgh, Pa. 15238) in place. In this study on rats, we used activated charcoal made from coconut shell (North American Carbon, Inc., Columbus, Ohio 43219), screened through U. S. sieve series No. 30 and collected on No. 50 screens, yielding particles about 0.3–0.6 mm in diameter. The activated charcoal was washed in a loose-bed column with upward-flowing tap water until the effluent was free of visible particulate matter. Unless otherwise noted in the text, the extracorporeal system was primed with heparinized donor rat blood from etherized rats. Within about 20 min, blood was pumped from the artery with an AutoAnalyzer Pump I (Technicon) or a micro-infusion roller pump (Model RL175; The Holter Co., Extracorporeal Medical Specialties, Inc., Bridgeport, Pa. 19405) through the activated charcoal granule bed and back into the femoral vein at a rate of about 3 ml/min. Control circuits of comparable volume contained the tubing and priming solution, but no charcoal. All circuits were cleaned but were not sterilized. Rats were injected with a single intravenous dose of sodium heparin (5 mg/kg body wt) at the start of the perfusion and were given 3 mg of protamine sulfate per kilogram body weight, intravenously, after being disconnected from the circuit. Two control and three treated rats that showed respiratory or blood-flow problems in less than 10 min of extracorporeal circulation were discarded from the pentobarbital series. The drugs to be removed were administered before the surgical procedures necessary for establishing the extracorporeal circuit. These procedures were completed in about 15–20 min. No artificial respiration or other supportive therapy was allowed.

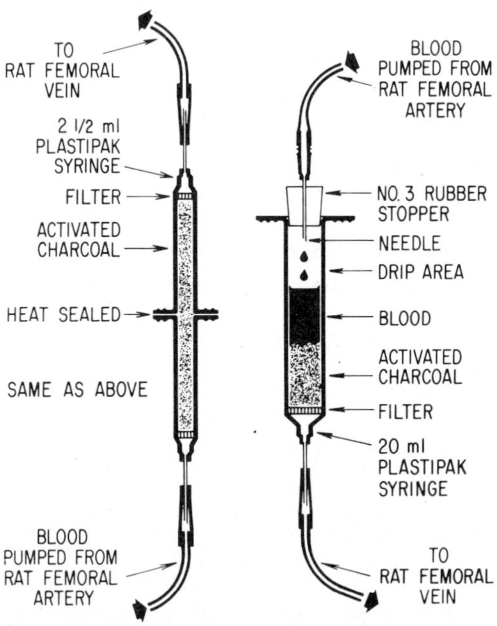

Fig. 1. Two types of loose-bed activated charcoal devices used in rat experiments

Studies on Dogs

The charcoal-containing devices used in the dog studies were of two types, loose and fixed-bed. The loose-bed devices were similar in design to the column (left half of Figure 1) just described for the rat studies, except they were larger, containing from 80 to 200 g of activated charcoal granules, and were made from polycarbonate. Polyester monofilament screen filters (DAFAB D-120) kept the granules within the device. For the most part, they were used without sterilization but were autoclaved before use in a few experiments. No effects of this difference were seen.

The dog studies were conducted with coconut-shell charcoal obtained from two sources. One source was the same as that used in the rat studies just described. The second source was type PCB (Pittsburgh Activated Carbon Co., Pittsburgh, Pa. 15230) and was screened through U. S. sieve series No. 20 and collected on No. 50 screens, yielding particles about 0.3–0.8 mm in diameter. These two types of activated charcoal were compared in dog experiments for solute removal and were not found to differ significantly. Three of 15 loose-bed devices and 21 of 27 fixed-bed devices used in the dog experiments were made with type PCB activated charcoal.

We developed the fixed-bed devices to minimize fragmentation and decrease the infusion of particulates into the body. These devices (B-D Hemodetoxifier; B-D Life Support Systems, Sharon, Mass. 02067) decrease particulate production by at least two orders of magnitude (*13*). The device (Figure 2) was made of uncoated activated charcoal granules deposited on a sheet of polyester film that had been coated with a thin layer of

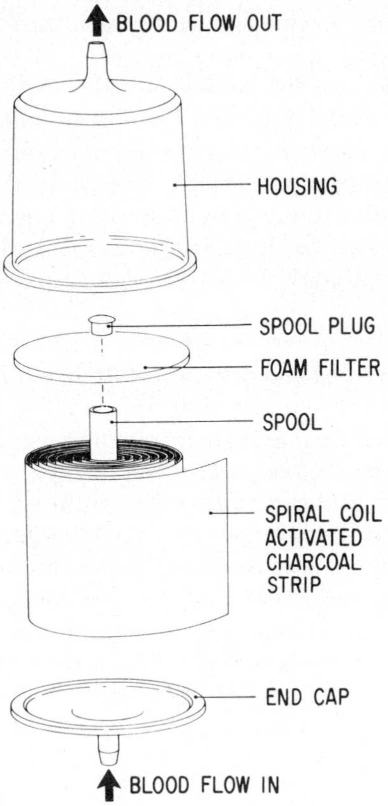

Fig. 2. Components of fixed-bed activated charcoal device used in dog experiments

chlorosulfonated polyethylene, a synthetic rubber with demonstrated blood compatibility (*19*). The charcoal adhered to the tacky coating and thus to the 8 cm × 6 m polyester film. Excess charcoal was removed and the polyester strip was rolled on a polycarbonate spool. A polyurethane foam filter was attached to one end of the coil. The completed coil was inserted into a rigid polycarbonate housing and was held in place with an epoxy resin in such a manner as to ensure blood flow through the spaces between the turns of the coil. The devices were washed free of loose particulates, filled with physiological saline, and were sterilized with 2.5 Mrad (1 rad = 0.01 J/kg) of gamma radiation from a ^{60}Co source. The devices contain about 100 g of charcoal, and a volume of about 170 ml is required to prime them.

Male purebred beagles were used in these studies after the preliminary experiments. Initially, however, male mongrels supplied by local dealers were used. Four of the control dogs (no charcoal) and 11 of the test dogs (loose-bed charcoal) were mongrels. All the rest were beagles.

On the morning of a typical experiment, the dog was weighed and a lethal dose of sodium phenobarbital (175 mg/kg) administered intravenously: 0.50 to 0.66 of the dose was given initially; the rest 10–15 min later. This technique was used because we wanted to avoid an immediate death caused simply by too-rapid infusion of this drug. In experiments in which phenobarbital was not given, we used an intravenous dose of short-acting barbiturate (pentobarbital, 30 mg/kg) and administered a mixture of 100% oxygen and methoxyflurane inhalation anesthesia to maintain anesthesia by means of a veterinary anesthesia machine (Pitman-Moore, Inc., Fort Washington, Pa. 19304). All dogs had cuffed endotracheal tubes, but ventilation was not supported.

When the animal was anesthetized, the femoral artery and vein were exposed and cannulas (Clay Adams tubing No. PE240-280, 1.5–2.0 i.d., or equivalent) were threaded into them and secured with ties. Heparin, 5 mg/kg, was administered to ensure anticoagulation.

After waiting an additional 15–30 min for the administered drug to equilibrate, we pumped blood from the artery and through the circuit shown in Figure 3. The device in the circuit had been rinsed previously with sterile saline and the circuit primed with 500 ml of dextran (mol wt 80 000), 60 g/liter, in physiological saline. The dextran solution from the circuit was allowed to flow into the femoral vein. An infusion of glucose, 50 g/liter, was pumped into the venous line at a rate of about 100 ml/h for 4 h of the perfusion with the microinfusion roller pump.

When animals given phenobarbital began to require anesthesia as the phenobarbital effects lessened (about 1 h after the start of hemoperfusion), methoxyflurane inhalation or electroanesthesia (Stoelting Co., Chicago, Ill. 60623) was begun and continued until the extracorporeal flow was terminated and the circuit removed from the dog. Extracorporeal treatment time was 5 h. When completed, the vessels were ligated and the wounds stitched closed. Penicillin, 300 000 arb. units, and streptomycin, 37 mg, were given intramuscularly to prevent postoperative infection.

A roller pump (Drake-Willock, Portland, Ore. 97222) was used in the occlusive position to pump blood at 150 ml/min through the circuit composed of appropriate modifications of existing hemodialysis tubing sets (see Figure 3). Blood pressure and circuit pressure were monitored continuously with pressure transducers (Hewlett-Packard, Palo Alto, Calif. 94304).

Phenobarbital concentrations in plasma were determined by the method of Butler et al. (*20*). Whole-blood salicylate concentrations were determined by an automated fluorometric procedure (*21*). Blood pH was determined with a temperature-controlled microelectrode unit and a Radiometer Model 4 pH meter (The London Co., Cleveland, Ohio 44145). Statistical probabilities in the mortality experiments were taken from 2 × 2 contingency tables as described by Finney (*22*).

Results

Studies on Rats

Table 1 summarizes the results for the series of rats to which 115 mg of pentobarbital was administered intraperitoneally per kilogram body weight. With no treatment, 88% of the rats succumbed to this dose. With activated charcoal treatment, only 14% of the rats succumbed (P = 0.001). The empty-column control perfusion resulted in 58% mortality, not a statistically significant difference from the 88% mortality, but sig-

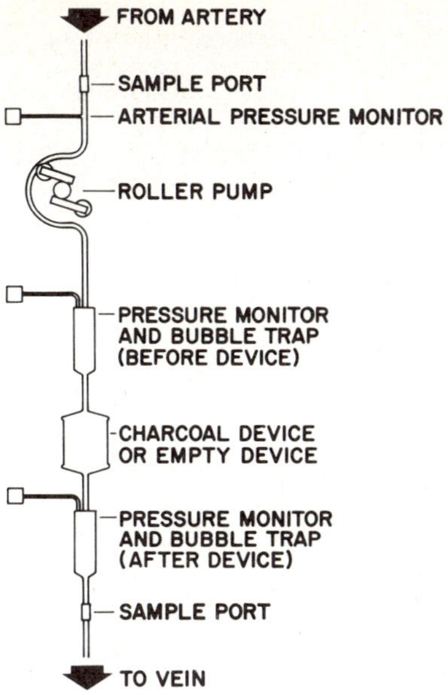

Fig. 3. Extracorporeal circuit used in dog experiments

Table 1. Rat Mortality after Intraperitoneal Sodium Pentobarbital (115 mg/kg)

No treatment	Empty circuit	Activated charcoal circuit
7/8	7/12	2/14
		1/9[a]

[a] These columns were primed with saline rather than donor blood.

nificantly ($P = 0.03$) different from the mortality for the test animals. Dilution of the rat's blood with drug-free blood plus the addition of plasma proteins, which bind the pentobarbital and help to keep it out of the tissue, might be expected to lessen mortality.

In another experiment of this sort, instead of priming the activated charcoal column with donor rat blood, we used physiological saline. These animals, too, showed a low mortality (11%) as compared to the control rats.

Salicylate, 1500 mg/kg, given intraperitoneally, kills rats within 10 min. The observation that acetazolamide increased the toxicity of salicylate and that rats so treated survived a little longer suggested a means of producing salicylate poisoning with time for the extracorporeal circuit to be established. Acetazolamide increases salicylate mortality by decreasing the blood pH, thus allowing the salicylate easier access to the brain and other tissues (*23*). This combination (500 mg sodium salicylate plus 25 mg sodium acetazolamide per kilogram), given intraperitoneally, killed all of seven untreated rats. As seen in Table 2, statistically significant results favoring the activated charcoal-treated animals were obtained. After the hemoperfusion, concentrations of salicylate in blood are lower in the treated animals. The activated charcoal column decreased the effect of acetazolamide on pH, either by removing acetazolamide

Table 2. Data on Rats Injected Intraperitoneally with, per Kilogram Body Weight, 500 mg of Sodium Salicylate Plus 25 mg of Sodium Acetazolamide

Treatment	Empty circuit	Activated charcoal
No. rats	3	3
Blood salicylate, mg/liter, before treatment	544–680	500–684
Blood salicylate, mg/liter, after 86–90 min on circuit or at death	684–820	236–292
Blood pH after treatment	7.10–7.14	7.20–7.28
Results ($P = 0.05$)	All dead in 45–93 min	All alive and well

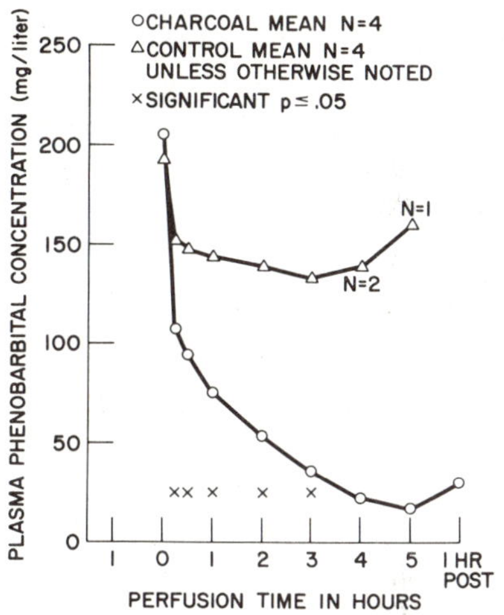

Fig. 4. Plasma phenobarbital concentrations in dogs given a 175 mg/kg intravenous dose of sodium phenobarbital followed by treatment with a fixed-bed activated charcoal device or a charcoal-free control circuit

X's refer to the times at which the two groups differed significantly

or by increasing the blood pH in some other manner. Both the pH-elevating effect and the salicylate-lowering effect of the charcoal may have contributed to the elimination of mortality.

Studies on Dogs

In one series of experiments, eight beagle dogs were given an intravenous 175 mg/kg dose of sodium phenobarbital. Four, chosen without conscious bias, were treated by use of fixed-bed activated charcoal devices and four had their blood perfused through an empty chamber with a 170-ml void volume. Perfusions were continued for 5 h unless death intervened. Three of the four control dogs died before the end of the extracorporeal treatment and one died 16 h after hemoperfusion; none regained consciousness. All four of the dogs treated with activated charcoal were fully conscious within 1 h after perfusion. Figure 4 compares the phenobarbital

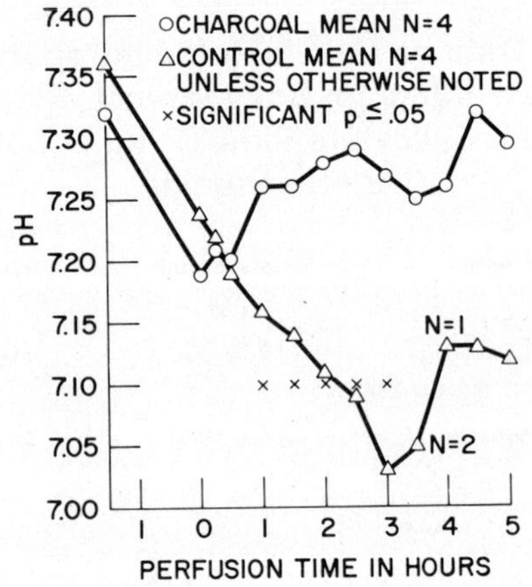

Fig. 5. Blood pH in dogs given a 175 mg/kg intravenous dose of sodium phenobarbital followed by treatment with a fixed-bed activated charcoal device or a charcoal-free control circuit
X's refer to the times at which data for the two groups differed significantly

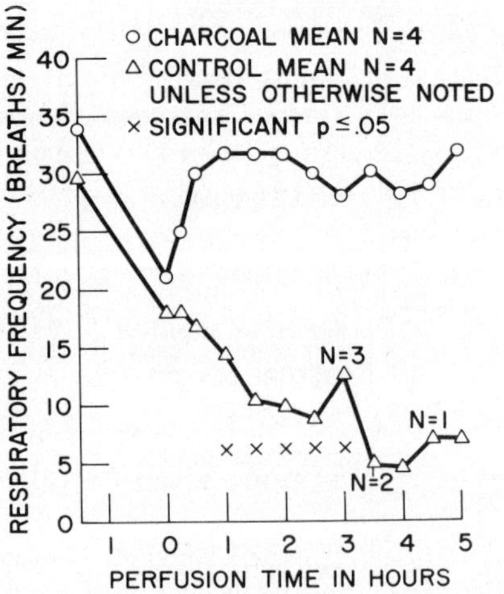

Fig. 6. Respiratory rate in dogs given a 175 mg/kg intravenous dose of sodium phenobarbital followed by treatment with a fixed-bed activated charcoal device or a charcoal-free control circuit
X's refer to the times at which data for the two groups differed significantly

concentrations in the plasma of the two groups of dogs. Both show an immediate decrease of about 20%, owing to dilution of the blood with the drug-free dextran priming solution in the circuit. The treated animals' plasma phenobarbital concentrations continued to decline during the perfusion but a slight rebound was seen in the 1-h postperfusion sample. In the control group, the values declined slowly after the initial dilution, reflecting the slow elimination of that drug. The plotted mean values increase as the dogs with the lower plasma-drug concentrations die and are not included in the average. This apparent contradiction (that the animals with lower values died sooner) is easily explained by the data in Figure 5, which show the blood pH changes for the two groups. The blood pH declined after administration of the drug. It continued to decrease in the control animals while increasing toward pre-drug values in the animals treated with activated charcoal. It also appears to increase in the control group as those animals with the lower blood pH values die. This is in keeping with the studies of Waddell and Butler (*24*), who found a concurrent increase in tissue phenobarbital and a decrease in plasma phenobarbital concentrations as blood pH decreased. Figure 6, showing respiratory rates for the two groups of animals, is strikingly similar to the blood-pH curves and suggests that one reason for the blood-pH differences may well be depressed respiration and the accumulation of carbon dioxide.

Table 3 contains the mortality figures for all dogs on the "no supportive therapy" protocol given 175 mg of sodium phenobarbital per kilogram intravenously and treated with an arterio-venous extracorporeal circuit and with use of either an empty column, a loose-bed or a fixed-bed device. One dog treated by use of a loose-bed device, which survived the perfusion but died from an excessive dose of polybrene (given to antagonize the heparin) after the perfusion, was excluded from this tabulation. The data in Table 3 include the eight-dog series previously described. This larger series differs in that it includes experiments in which "tracer" doses of creatinine or salicylate were administered to the animals treated with activated charcoal as a second check on successful functioning of the adsorbent.

Table 3. Summary of Experiments on Lethal Doses of Phenobarbital (175 mg/kg)

Device used	No. dogs	No. surviving	Mortality, %	*P* value (vs. control)
Empty column (control)	10	0	100	—
Loose-bed activated charcoal	15	13	13	<0.001
Fixed-bed activated charcoal	27	23	15	<0.004

A strikingly decreased mortality may be seen in the activated charcoal-treated animals. Of the two dogs dying in the loose-bed group, one was found to have a postperfusion arterial glucose value of 100 mg/liter, and probably died of hypoglycemia. Once this possibility was recognized, routine glucose infusions were used in all experiments. As much as 9 g of glucose could be removed per 100 g of charcoal. The four dogs in the fixed-bed device group that died all did so within 7 min of starting the perfusion. All were hypotensive before perfusion was begun. With this protocol, no attempt could be made to correct this hypotension, but these four deaths provided evidence that hypotension must be corrected before any extracorporeal therapy is begun. Recently, some phenobarbital-treated dogs, not included in this strict protocol, that were hypotensive before extracorporeal therapy were treated with a norepinephrine infusion or elevation of the foot of the operating table, to correct the hypotension. These animals survived.

A 232 mg/kg dose of sodium salicylate may be given to a normal conscious dog intravenously without producing symptoms or toxicity. This dose was used, therefore, as a "tracer" in certain experiments to ascertain whether the devices were adsorbing properly. In the anesthetized dog breathing a methoxyflurane/oxygen mixture administered through a tracheal tube by a closed-circuit anesthesia device, this dose of salicylate is highly toxic; indeed, in our experience, it is uniformly fatal. This combination produces a marked hyperthermia and an increased respiratory rate. Other investigators have made similar observations on salicylate and halothane anesthesia (J. D. Andrade and A. Temple, personal communication). In the series of dogs treated with methoxyflurane anesthesia and 232 mg of sodium salicylate per kilogram body weight, three had their blood perfused through empty devices and all died with hyperthermia while 12 dogs whose blood was perfused through fixed-bed activated charcoal devices all lived. Figure 7 shows blood salicylate concentrations in these two groups of animals. Clearly, this laboratory-produced salicylate toxicity may be reversed by fixed-bed activated-charcoal hemoperfusion. Inasmuch as this condition has occurred in one dog with salicylate and pentobarbital anesthesia and a cuffed endotracheal tube alone, it is probably the result of interference with heat loss during concomitant increased heat production. The metabolic stimulatory action of salicylates in excess is well known.

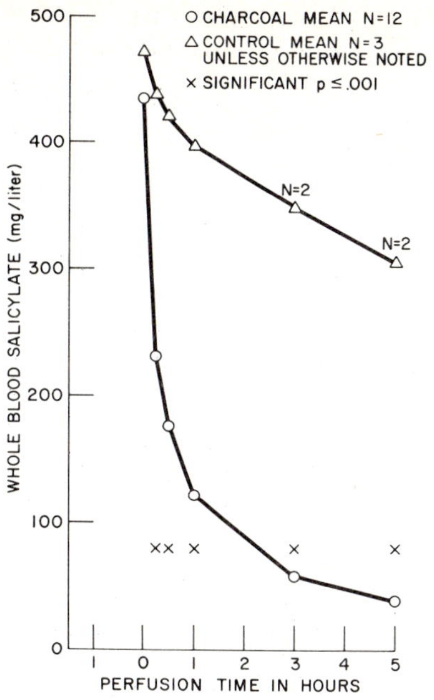

Fig. 7. Salicylate concentrations in whole blood of dogs given a 232 mg/kg intravenous dose of sodium salicylate followed by treatment with a fixed-bed activated charcoal device or a charcoal-free control circuit

X's refer to the times at which data for the two groups differed significantly

Discussion

These experiments show that under the described conditions lethal doses and mixtures of certain drugs may become nonlethal through the intervention of uncoated activated charcoal hemoadsorption alone.

Other investigators have studied poison removal in animal experiments not designed to show the lifesaving potential of charcoal hemoperfusion (*1–8*). Hagstam et al. (*9*) administered 130 mg of phenobarbital per kilogram to 13 rabbits by deep intramuscular injection. All were treated with activated charcoal hemoperfusion and lived. Although another rabbit was left untreated, the fate of that rabbit is unclear. These authors compare their results with the control group of other authors (*25*) who, administering the same dose, killed six of 18 rabbits. Varying conditions from laboratory to laboratory make such comparisons extremely hazardous. DeMyttenaere et al. (*10*) used activated charcoal hemoperfusion to treat glutethimide poisoning in dogs. They administered 400 mg/kg by mouth to six dogs. The four treated survived; the two controls died. These experiments, which are suggestive, fall short of statistical significance. Our own experience in administering a 400 mg/kg oral dose of glutethimide bears this out in that our control dog, left untreated, survived. Maini and Winchester (*11*) studied the removal of paraquat, a herbicide that produces pulmonary fibrosis, from the blood of dogs with activated charcoal or a cation-exchange resin hemoperfusion. They showed a statistically significant decrease in the concentrations of the herbicide in blood when both adsorbent-treated groups were compared with the controls. No other information on the effects of the paraquat on the dogs was given.

The degree of difficulty in showing clear evidence of efficacy in the clinical use of charcoal hemoperfusion for poison removal will depend on the criterion to be met. If a decrease in mortality is required, it may well be impossible. Reported mortality figures, for example, are already low for the management of acute barbiturate poisoning (*26*). Assessing the role played in any given case by the other forms of therapy and supportive measures, which ethically could not be withheld, would be extremely difficult. If efficacy can be equated with a decrease in morbidity as compared with existing treatments, such evidence may be forthcoming. The role played by adjunct therapies such as gastric lavage, orally administered activated charcoal, emetics, purges, diuresis, and supportive nursing techniques—plus the variation in substances and amounts taken by patients coupled with the unreliability of the histories obtained—makes the matching of case histories with and without charcoal hemoperfusion a hazardous exercise. It might be wise to accept evidence of toxic substance removal by the device used as the clinical criterion for efficacy. Then, safety becomes the deciding issue in whether or not to use the technique.

Detailed evidence for the safety of charcoal hemoperfusion is not a part of this communication. However, experience with single activated charcoal hemoperfusion in over 200 dogs, some of which have been kept as long as five years after treatment, has as yet failed to reveal any untoward effects. An important clinical consideration that this report does not encompass is the risk to acutely poisoned patients from the establishment of extracorporeal circuits.

Coated activated charcoal has been used by several investigators (*3, 4, 6–8, 15–18*), but none of these showed clear efficacy of coated charcoal in removing poisonous substances from animals. Weston et al. (*17*) did show a statistically significant increase in the mean survival time in dogs with a surgically induced ischemic hepatic failure. No extracorporeal circulation, however, was described for the control group. Inasmuch as the molecular size of the toxic substances accumulating in liver failure is unknown and the findings of Denti et al. (*27*) have shown that coating can markedly interfere with the adsorption of larger molecules, the results of Weston et al. (*17*) may have been more impressive had uncoated charcoal been used. In any case, the results of the present study in rats and dogs with uncoated charcoal should not be extrapolated to coated charcoal.

We gratefully acknowledge the support and encouragement of K. Abel, G. B. Phillips, T. J. Bauer, and W. J. Howe throughout this study, and the roles played by J. Critcher, R. K. Hanson, J. K. Walrath, and C. R. Horres in the preparation of this manuscript.

References

1. Yatzidis, H., A convenient haemoperfusion micro-apparatus over charcoal for the treatment of endogenous and exogenous intoxications. Its use as an effective artificial kidney. *Proc. Eur. Dial. Transplant Assoc.* **1,** 83 (1964).

2. Rosenbaum, J. L., Ronquillo, E., and Argyres, S. N., Column hemoperfusion and hemodialysis techniques to treat barbiturate intoxication in dogs. *J. Albert Einstein Med. Cent.* **16,** 67 (1968).

3. Andrade, J. D., Kunitomo, K., Van Wagenen, R., et al., Coated adsorbents for direct blood perfusion: HEMA/activated carbon. *Trans. Am. Soc. Artif. Intern. Organs* **17,** 222 (1971).

4. Chang, T. M. S., *Artificial Cells.* Charles C Thomas, Springfield, Ill., 1972, p 137.

5. Barakat, T., and MacPhee, I. W., Experiments with an extracorporeal carbon column as a simplified artificial kidney. *Br. J. Surg.* **57,** 580 (1970).

6. Willson, R. A., Thompson, R. P. H., Winch, J., and Williams, R., Rapid removal of paracetamol by haemoperfusion through coated charcoal. *Lancet* **i,** 77 (1973).

7. Widdop, B., Medd, R. K., Braithwaite, R. A., et al., Experimental drug intoxication: Treatment with charcoal haemoperfusion. *Arch. Toxicol.* **34,** 27 (1975).

8. Winchester, J. F., Edwards, R. O., Tilstone, W. J., and Woodcock, B. G., Activated charcoal hemoperfusion and experimental acetaminophen poisoning. *Toxicol. Appl. Pharmacol.* **31,** 120 (1975).

9. Hagstam, K. E., Larsson, L. E., and Thysell, H., Experimental studies on charcoal haemoperfusion in phenobarbital intoxication and uraemia, including histopathologic findings. *Acta Med. Scand.* **180,** 593 (1966).

10. DeMyttenaere, M. H., Maher, J. F., and Schreiner, G. E., Hemoperfusion through a charcoal column for glutethimide poisoning. *Trans. Am. Soc. Artif. Intern. Organs* **13,** 190 (1967).

11. Maini, R., and Winchester, J. F., Removal of paraquat from blood by haemoperfusion over sorbent materials. *Br. Med. J.* **iii,** 281 (1975).

12. Dunea, G., and Kolff, W. J., Clinical experience with the Yatzidis charcoal artificial kidney. *Trans. Am. Soc. Artif. Intern. Organs* **11,** 178 (1965).

13. Hill, J. B., Palaia, F. L., McAdams, J. L., et al., The rationale for fixed-bed charcoal in hemoperfusion. *Kidney Int.* In press.

14. Barbour, B. H., LaSette, A. M., and Koffler, A., Fixed-bed charcoal hemoperfusion for the treatment of drug overdose. *Kidney Int.* In press.

15. Vale, J. A., Rees, A. J., Widdop, B., and Goulding, R., Use of charcoal haemoperfusion in the management of severely poisoned patients. *Br. Med. J.* **i,** 5 (1975).

16. Martin, A. M., Mitchell, D. C., Gibbons, J. K., et al., Charcoal haemoperfusion in the management of severe poisoning. *Br. Med. J.* **i,** 392 (1975).

17. Weston, M. J., Gazzard, B. G., Buxton, B. H., et al., Effects of haemoperfusion through charcoal or XAD-2 resin on an animal model of fulminant liver failure. *Gut* **15,** 482 (1974).

18. Amdahl, T., and Peterson, J., Treatment of chronic uremia with albumin/collodion-coated activated charcoal—a preliminary report. *Lakartidningen* **72,** 587 (1975).

19. Wright, J. S., Johnston, J. B., and Luber, L. J., Thrombus resistance of intravascular implants of chlorosulphonated polyethylene. *J. Thorac. Cardiovasc. Surg.* **52,** 740 (1966).

20. Butler, T. C., Mahaffee, C., Waddell, W. J., Phenobarbital: Studies of elimination, accumulation, tolerance and dosage schedules. *J. Pharmacol. Exp. Ther.* **111,** 425 (1954).

21. Hill, J. B., and Smith, R. M., An automated microfluorimetric determination for salicylate in body fluids and tissue extracts. *Biochem. Med.* **4,** 24 (1970).

22. Finney, D. J., The Fisher-Yates test of significance in 2 × 2 contingency tables. *Biometrika* **35,** 145 (1948).

23. Hill, J. B., Experimental salicylate poisoning: Observations on the effects of altering blood pH on tissue and plasma salicylate concentrations. *Pediatrics* **47,** 658 (1971).

24. Waddell, W. J., and Butler, T. C., The distribution and excretion of phenobarbital. *J. Clin. Invest.* **36,** 1217 (1957).

25. Alwall, N., Lindgren, P., and Lunderquist, A., On the artificial kidney. XX. Treatment of severe phenobarbital poisoning in rabbits, by means of forced polyuria, exchange ultrafiltration and dialysis and a preliminary report on dialytic treatment of barbiturate poisoning in patients. *Acta Med. Scand.* **143,** 299 (1952).

26. Matthew, H., and Lawson, A. A. H., Acute barbiturate poisoning—a review of two years experience. *Q. J. Med.* **35,** 539 (1966).

27. Denti, E., Luboz, M. P., and Tessore, V., Adsorption characteristics of cellulose acetate coated charcoals. *J. Biomed. Mater. Res.* **9,** 143 (1975).

CLIN. CHEM. 22/6, 761–764 (1976)

Rapid Radioisotopic Procedure for Determination of Nortriptyline in Plasma

K. P. Maguire,[1] G. D. Burrows,[1] J. P. Coghlan,[2] and B. A. Scoggins[2]

With the widespread use of tricyclic antidepressant drugs, the relationship between the concentration of the drug in the plasma and the therapeutic response is of considerable interest. We describe a double-isotope derivative dilution procedure for measuring plasma nortriptyline. In the method, [^{14}C]nortriptyline is used for estimating procedural losses and [^{3}H]acetic anhydride for derivative formation. The assay is rapid and adequately specific, sensitive, precise, and reproducible for routine clinical use. We used it to investigate the variation in steady-state drug concentrations in plasma of persons who were on a 150 mg/day dose of nortriptyline. Intra-individual variation from day to day was 10–14%. This variation was not significantly affected by the dosage schedule, the time of sampling after an oral dose, or the storage of the plasma samples. For 19 patients on 150 mg of nortriptyline per day, the mean concentration in plasma was 181 ± 22 (SE) μg/liter, a value that compares well with our previous findings and those of other groups.

We report a rapid double-isotope derivative dilution assay for measuring nortriptyline, based on a modification (*1*) of an isotope-derivative dilution assay (*2*). In the method [^{14}C]nortriptyline is used to correct for procedural losses and [^{3}H]acetic anhydride for derivative formation. Chromatography of the radiolabeled derivative has been included to improve specificity.

The double-isotope derivative dilution assay has advantages over the isotope-derivative assay. Because each sample has its own recovery indicator, a standard curve for each assay is unnecessary, as is also the duplicate analysis of samples. Moreover, the method has advantages over other currently available procedures such as gas–liquid chromatography (*3–5*) and mass-fragmentography (*6, 7*), both of which are more time-consuming and require expensive, sophisticated equipment. Suitable radioimmunoassay procedures have yet to be described.

Measurement of plasma nortriptyline is important in monitoring an individual patient's therapeutic response because there can be large inter-individual differences for patients who are on the same dosage regimen.

[1] Department of Psychiatry, University of Melbourne, Parkville, Victoria, Australia.

[2] Howard Florey Institute of Experimental Physiology and Medicine, Parkville, Victoria, Australia.

Received Dec. 14, 1975; accepted Jan. 26, 1976.

Materials and Methods

Purification of [^{14}C]Nortriptyline

[^{14}C]Nortriptyline (18 mCi/g) was purified every 14 days by thin-layer chromatography in the system benzene/dioxane/ethanol/diethylamine, 50/40/5/5 by volume (*8*). Purified material was stored in ethanolic solution in the dark at 4 °C.

Extraction of Plasma Samples

Plasma samples (acidified with ⅕-volume of 0.1 mol/liter HCl) were stored at −20 °C until assay. Siliconized 7-ml glass-stoppered tubes were used in all steps.

After addition of [^{14}C]nortriptyline (1.8×10^{-4} μCi), 1-ml plasma samples were alkalinized with 0.4 ml of 1 mol/liter NaOH. Treated samples were gently extracted with 3 ml of *n*-heptane by rotation for 15 min. Any emulsions were broken by freezing the samples in liquid nitrogen and allowing them to thaw. A 2-ml aliquot of each heptane extract was transferred to clean tubes for acetylation.

Derivative Formation

Anhydrous pyridine, 100 μl, and 50 μl of 0.02% vacuum-distilled [^{3}H]acetic anhydride (330 Ci/mol) (The Radiochemical Centre, Amersham, U. K.) in anhydrous benzene were added to each sample. The method of purification and determination of specific activity of the [^{3}H]acetic anhydride has been described previously (*9*). After thorough mixing of their contents, the stoppered tubes were placed in a water bath at 60 °C for 1 h.

Purification of the Derivative

Hydrolysis and re-extraction. The solvent was evaporated in an air stream and 2 ml of 0.1 mol/liter NaOH was added per sample. The stoppered tubes were returned to the 60 °C water bath for 15 min, then cooled to room temperature. *n*-Heptane, 2 ml, was added to each tube and the acetylated derivative extracted by rotation for 10 min. After phase separation (about 10 min), the aqueous phase was aspirated. A further 2 ml of 0.1 mol/liter NaOH was added and the samples were rotated again for 10 min. After phase separation, 1-ml aliquots of the heptane phase were transferred to clean tubes.

Thin-layer chromatography. After addition of 10 μg of nortriptyline acetate (prepared by reacting nortriptyline with unlabeled acetic anhydride in a similar manner to that described above) as ultraviolet marker, we evaporated the solvent. The samples were applied to aluminum sheets precoated with silica-gel (20 cm × 20 cm × 0.25 mm, Silica-Gel GF254/5554; Merck) in three successive 0.2-ml portions of methanol in methylene chloride (40/60 by vol). Twelve samples were applied per sheet. The sheets were developed at room temperature in the ascending system benzene/acetone 1/1 by vol (*2*). The samples were located by the absorption of the added marker at 254 nm, and the appropriate area of the silica gel was scraped with the help of vacuum into glass "transpettes" (Clay-Adams) plugged with glass wool. Samples were eluted into glass vials by passing 10 ml of the methanol/methylene chloride mixture through the pipettes. The solvent was evaporated and 10 ml of a phosphor solution was added (4 g PPO and 40 mg dimethyl POPOP/liter of toluene, Packard Instrument Co.). (The thin-layer chromatography step can be omitted, in which case, after hydrolysis and reextraction, the 1-ml aliquots of the solvent phase are transferred to glass vials, the solvent is evaporated, and phosphor solution added.)

Determination of Mass

The radioactivity of samples was counted for 20 min in a liquid scintillation spectrometer (Packard). Standard vials for the determination of machine background, ^{3}H and ^{14}C counting efficiencies, specific activity of the [^{3}H]acetic anhydride, recovery of [^{14}C]nortriptyline indicator, and leakage between channels were counted with each assay.

Equations for the estimation of the mass of double-labeled samples by use of isotope derivative dilution techniques have been described previously (*10, 11*). We followed the latter method (*11*) in estimating nortriptyline.

Results

Analytical Variables

Precision. Plasma pools of known nortriptyline concentration, 100 and 200 μg/liter, were used to evaluate the precision of the assay. In most patients treated clinically, concentrations of the drug in plasma lie between these values. The precision (CV) of the assay at the two concentrations was ±7%. Analysis of a quality-control sample (about 100 ng of nortriptyline per milliliter of water) in each assay gave a result of 90.4 ± 7.0 μg/liter (mean ± SD; n = 34) and a CV of 8%. Reproducibility was further demonstrated by re-assay of 19 samples. Results for first assay were 158 ± 65 μg/liter (mean ± SD) and on second assay after 120 days, 159 ± 70 μg/liter.

Analytical recovery. Accuracy was reflected by a linear recovery of nortriptyline over the range 25–200 μg/liter. Recovery of the [^{14}C]indicator through the method was 23.9 ± 3.5% (mean ± SD; n = 43). Losses during the early extraction steps predominantly accounted for the low recovery. The chromatography step accounted for 7% of losses, because the recovery without chromatography was 31.3 ± 3.0% (mean ± SD; n = 43).

Interferences. Inclusion of the chromatography step eliminated interference by the major metabolite of nortriptyline, 10-hydroxy-nortriptyline. R_F values for the acetylated derivatives were 0.32 (metabolite) and 0.37 (nortriptyline).

Salicylic aldehyde was used by Gram and Fredricson-Overo (*12*) to block primary amines; hence desmethylnortriptyline could not interfere in the acetylation reaction. Assay of samples by this method and by the present double-isotope procedure lead to no significant difference in the plasma levels obtained ($P > 0.9$, Student's *t*-test).

Nonspecific interference was also decreased significantly ($P < 0.05$) by inclusion of the chromatography step. The nonspecific blank of the assay was 14.6 ± 10.9 μg/liter (mean ± SD) without, and 2.7 ± 2.9 μg/liter with chromatography (n = 42).

Comparison with Other Methods

Close correlation was obtained between the isotope-derivative assay used previously (*1*) and the new assay. Samples analyzed by both methods resulted in a mean of 158 ± 17 (old assay, ±SE) and 181 ± 22 (new assay) μg/liter. These were not significantly different (n = 19, $P > 0.05$).

Our results for persons on a daily dose of 150 mg compare favorably with other published data (*1, 14–16*). In our most recent study by use of our method, we found a mean drug concentration in plasma of 181 ± 15 μg/liter (±SE) for 22 patients [2 men, 20 women; mean age, 41.6 ± 9.7 y (±SD)] (*13*). This compares with mean values of 171 ± 19 (±SE; n = 32) and 171 ± 13 (n = 65) mg/liter obtained in two previous studies (*1, 14*).

Results reported by other groups also compare well. Lyle et al. (*15*) found a mean plasma nortriptyline concentration of 170 ± 24 μg/liter (±SE, n = 14, on 150 mg/day) and Braithwaite (*16*) found a mean of 166 μg/liter (n = 10, 80–200 mg/day); both used the gas-chromatographic method of Braithwaite and Widdop (*3*).

Variation

Within-individual. In a study of two individuals, plasma nortriptyline was measured daily for 10 days. Variations of ±10% and ±12% were observed in their steady-state values (Table 1). Patient *a* was studied for a further 30 days and a variation of ±14% was observed for 23 samples taken during the total period.

Variation in steady-state concentrations in plasma. Some factors that could contribute to the variation observed in steady-state plasma values were examined. As shown in Figure 1, the time of sampling after the last oral dose did not appear to contribute importantly, because no significant change occurred during an 8-h period.

When persons were on different dosage schedules, all

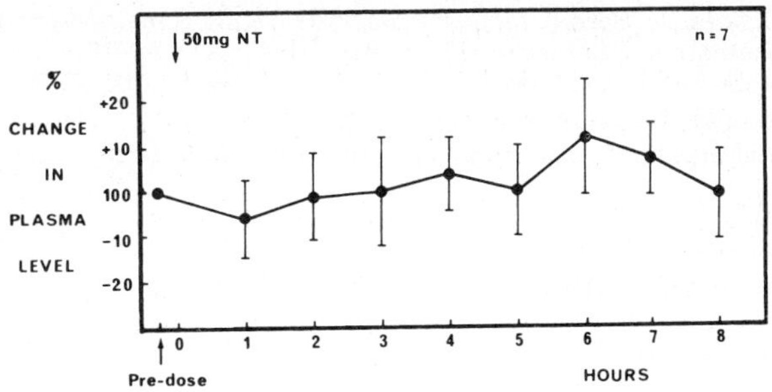

Fig. 1. Percentage change in plasma concentrations (mean ± SD; n = 7) during 8 h after last 50-mg dose of nortriptyline; the pre-dose value is taken as 100%

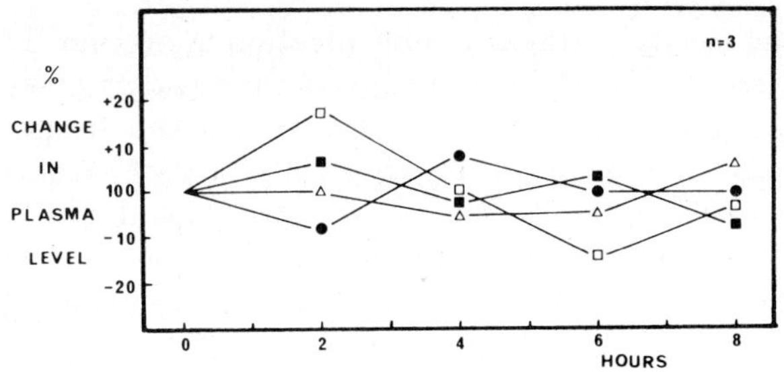

Fig. 2. Percentage change in plasma-drug concentrations (mean, n = 3) during 8 h (from 0800 h) is shown for four dosage schedules

150 mg of nortriptyline per day was given as follows: ■ 50 mg 0800, 1400, 2200 h; □ 150 mg 2200; △ 100 mg 0800, 50 mg 2200; ● 50 mg 0800, 100 mg 2200. In the absence of samples at 0 time, an average of the values at 2, 4, 6, and 8 h was taken as 100%. SD's are omitted, for clarity, but were similar to those in Figure 1

Table 1. Between-day Variation in Steady-state Concentrations of Nortriptyline in Plasma of Two Patients

	Drug concn, µg/liter	
Day	*a*	*b*
1	251	70
2	269	60
3	263	78
4	311	67
5	235	52
6	274	63
7	246	74
8	237	78
9	225	72
10	—	74
Mean ± SD	257 ± 26	69 ± 8
CV	10.2%	12.2%

Both patients were treated with 150 mg/day for 21 days before and during this study. Patient *b* was also receiving 0.25 mg of digoxin, 0.5 mg of navidrex, 1 tab. of slow-release K, 5–10 mg of nitrazepam, and 1 tab. Glyceryl trinitrate when necessary.

Table 2. Effect of Plasma Storage Conditions on Apparent Nortriptyline Value

	Nortriptyline, µg/liter	
Day of assay	−4 °C	22 °C
0	236	233
2	218	216
7	234	234
13	249	200
27	225	164

Nortriptyline (about 200 µg/liter) was added to drug-free human plasma. Half was stored frozen, half stored at room temperature. 1-ml aliquots analyzed on the days shown.

totalling 150 mg of nortriptyline per day, little difference was found in plasma concentrations, and they varied similarly for the four such schedules (Figure 2). This has important clinical implications, because a once-nightly dose minimizes side-effects and takes full advantage of the sedative effects of the drug.

Effects of storage. The method of storage of the plasma samples may be important. It appears that after separation of the plasma, the nortriptyline is stable for several days at room temperature (Table 2). If kept frozen, no measurable change occurs during 120 days.

Discussion

For routine clinical use, an assay must be specific, sensitive, precise, and reproducible. If possible, it should be simple, quick, and inexpensive. The described double-isotope derivative dilution assay fulfills most of these requirements.

Specificity was achieved by inclusion of a chromatography step, which adequately separates nortriptyline from its major plasma metabolites, 10-hydroxy-nortriptyline and desmethylnortriptyline (*17*). We found a close correlation between results obtained by this new assay and the isotope-derivative assay (*1*), further indicating the specificity of both techniques.

The lower limit of sensitivity of the assay is 5 µg/liter, as determined primarily by the low specific activity of the [^{14}C]nortriptyline. If this could be brought closer to the theoretical (65 Ci/mol) then the sensitivity would be greatly improved. Reduction in the nonspecific blank value by further chromatography would also improve sensitivity. However, the sensitivity obtained with this assay is more than adequate for routine clinical use.

Our results obtained with this assay compare favorably with those from our earlier studies and those from the workers who used gas-chromatography. The one exception is the Scandinavian group, who observe lower values for plasma in their studies by gas-chromatography–mass-spectrometry (*18–20*). The reasons for the differences between these studies and others have been discussed (*21*).

A double-isotope derivative dilution method for measuring concentrations in plasma of a similar antidepressant, maprotiline ("Ludiomil"; Ciba-Geigy) has been published (*22*), but the author did not take full advantage of the principle of double-isotope dilution because standards were used in calculating the mass of the drug in unknown plasma samples.

Once the assay is established, two important considerations when measuring plasma nortriptyline are the between-day variations within individuals on a fixed dose and the within-day within-individual variations in the steady-state drug concentration in plasma. The latter is largely (83%) genetically determined as a result of genetic control over the metabolism of the drug (*23, 24*). Alexanderson (*24*) also found that only 17% of the variation in nortriptyline plasma levels was due to between-day (13%) and within-day (4%) fluctuations. The oral dose is obviously an important factor (*13*) as also may be other drugs administered at the same time (*12, 25, 26*). The time of sampling after an oral dose, the dosage schedule on a fixed regimen, and the method of handling plasma do not appear to contribute significantly to the variations observed in steady-state values for plasma drug concentration.

A between-day, within-individual variation of 10–14% has been found, which is close to the results of Alexanderson (*24*). Because the amount of variation likely to occur in steady-state values has been established, daily measurement of plasma nortriptyline is probably unnecessary. Weekly or twice-weekly samples would be quite satisfactory. Frequent sampling is necessary when studying pharmacokinetics or drug interactions.

For routine clinical use, the double-isotope assay without the chromatography step is satisfactory. Although some sensitivity and precision is lost, less time is required to complete each assay and more samples can be analyzed per assay.

We thank H. Lundbeck & Co., Denmark, for the supply of [^{14}C]-nortriptyline, Drs. R. Mulhearn and W. Zylstra of Roche Products for financial support, and Ms. B. Maddison for technical assistance.

References

1. Burrows, G. D., Davies, B., and Scoggins, B. A., Plasma concentration of nortriptyline and clinical response. *Lancet* **ii,** 619 (1972).

2. Hammer, W. H., and Brodie, B. B., Application of isotope derivative technique to assay of secondary amines: Estimation of desipramine by acetylation with H^3-acetic anhydride. *J. Pharmacol. Exp. Ther.* **157,** 503 (1967).

3. Braithwaite, R. A., and Widdop, B., A specific gas-chromatographic method for the measurement of "steady-state" plasma levels of amitriptyline and nortriptyline in patients. *Clin. Chim. Acta* **35,** 461 (1971).

4. Hucker, H. B., and Stauffer, S. C., G.L.C. method for quantitative determination of amitriptyline in human plasma. *J. Pharm. Sci.* **63,** 296 (1974).

5. Gifford, L. A., Turner, P., and Pare, C. M. B., Sensitive method for the routine determination of tricyclic antidepressants in plasma using a specific nitrogen detector. *J. Chromatogr.* **105,** 107 (1975).

6. Borga, O., Palmer, L., Linnarson, A., and Holmstedt, B., Quantitative determination of nortriptyline and desmethylnortriptyline in human plasma by combined gas-chromatography–mass spectrometry. *Anal. Lett.* **4,** 837 (1971).

7. Frigerio, A., Belvedere, G., Nadai, F de., et al., A method for the determination of imipramine in human urine by gas-liquid chromatography–mass fragmentography. *J. Chromatogr.* **74,** 201 (1972).

8. Garriott, J. F., and Stohlman, A., Detection of some psychotherapeutic drugs and their metabolites in urine. *Clin. Toxicol.* **4,** 225 (1971).

9. Coghlan, J. P., Wintour, M., and Scoggins, B. A., The measurement of corticosteroids in adrenal vein blood of sheep. *Aust. J. Exp. Biol. Med. Sci.* **44,** 639 (1966).

10. Okita, G. T., Kabara, J. J., Richardson, F., and LeRoy, G. V., Assaying compounds containing H^3 and C^{14}. *Nucleonics* **15,** 111 (1957).

11. Coghlan, J. P., and Scoggins, B. A., Measurement of aldosterone in peripheral blood of man and sheep. *J. Clin. Endocrinol. Metab.* **27,** 1470 (1967).

12. Gram, L. F., and Fredricson-Overo, K., Drug interaction: Inhibitory effect of neuroleptics on metabolism of tricyclic antidepressants in man. *Br. Med. J.* **i,** 463 (1972).

13. Burrows, G. D., Scoggins, B. A., Stevenson, J., et al., Plasma nortriptyline and clinical response—A study using changing plasma levels. *Psychol. Med.*, in press.

14. Burrows, G. D., Scoggins, B. A., Turecek, L. R., and Davies, B., Plasma nortriptyline and clinical response. *Clin. Pharmacol. Ther.* **16,** 639 (1974).

15. Lyle, W. H., Brooks, P. W., Early, D. F., et al., Plasma concentration of nortriptyline as a guide to treatment. *Postgrad. Med. J.* **50,** 282 (1974).

16. Braithwaite, R. A., Interindividual differences in steady-state plasma nortriptyline in patients. *Br. J. Clin. Pharmacol.* (1976). In press.

17. Borga, O., and Garle, M., A gas-chromatographic method for the determination of nortriptyline and some of its metabolites in human plasma and urine. *J. Chromatogr.* **68,** 77 (1972).

18. Kragh-Sorensen, P., Asberg, M., and Eggert-Hansen, C., Plasma-nortriptyline levels in endogenous depression. *Lancet* **i,** 7795 (1973).

19. Kragh-Sorensen, P., Eggert-Hansen, C., Larsen, N. E., et al., Long-term treatment of endogenous depression with nortriptyline with control of plasma levels. *Psychol. Med.* **4,** 174 (1974).

20. Kragh-Sorensen, P., Eggert-Hansen, C., Baastrup, P. C., and Hvidberg, E. F., Self-inhibiting action of nortriptyline's antidepressive effect at high plasma levels. *Psychopharmacologia* (1976). In press.

21. Scoggins, B. A., Coghlan, J. P., Maguire, K. P., et al., The measurement of plasma levels of tricyclic antidepressant drugs. *Aust. N.Z. J. Psychiatry* (1976). In press.

22. Riess, W., The double radio-isotope derivative technique for the assay of drugs in biological material. Part I. The determination of maprotiline. *Anal. Chim. Acta* **68,** 363 (1974).

23. Hammer, W. H., and Sjoqvist, F., Plasma levels of monomethylated tricyclic antidepressants during treatment with imipramine-like compounds. *Life Sci.* **6,** 1895 (1964).

24. Alexanderson, B., Pharmacokinetics of nortriptyline in man after single and multiple oral doses: The predictability of steady-state plasma concentrations from single dose plasma level data. *Eur. J. Clin. Pharmacol.* **4,** 82 (1972).

25. Alexanderson, B., Price-Evans, D. A., and Sjoqvist, F., Steady-state plasma levels of nortriptyline in twins: Influence of genetic factors and drug therapy. *Br. Med. J.* **iv,** 764 (1969).

26. Burrows, G. D., and Davies, B., Antidepressants and barbiturates. *Br. Med. J.* **iv,** 113 (1971).

CLIN. CHEM. 22/6, 765–768 (1976)

Gas-Chromatographic Micro-Scale Procedure for Theophylline, with Use of a Nitrogen-Sensitive Detector

Charles J. Least, Jr., George F. Johnson, and Harvey M. Solomon

We report a micro-scale procedure for determination of theophylline by use of gas chromatography with nitrogen-sensitive detection. The procedure requires only 20 µl of serum, plasma, or saliva. This sample size makes the determination especially appropriate for monitoring in a pediatric population. With the sample volume used, background interference is equivalent to about 0.1 mg/liter and 0.5 mg of theophylline per liter can easily be measured. The new method correlates well with our earlier flame ionization gas-chromatographic procedure that required 1 ml of sample [*Clin. Chem.* **21,** 1038 (1975)]. The selectivity of the nitrogen detector allows a simplified extraction procedure. Between-run precision (CV) is 2.8% at a theophylline concentration of 14.8 mg/liter.

Additional Keyphrases: *theophylline in saliva, serum, plasma* • *pediatric chemistry* • *therapy for asthma and for apnea, bradycardia in the newborn* • *nitrogen/phosphorus detector* • *interference from evacuated blood-collection tubes*

During the past year, several new methods have appeared for determining theophylline in biological fluids by gas chromatography or high-pressure liquid chromatography (*1–4*). The usefulness of monitoring serum theophylline concentration in the management of patients with asthma has been well established. More recently, it has been demonstrated that theophylline is effective in the treatment of apnea and bradycardia of the low-birth-weight infant (*5*). Safe and effective use of theophylline in this context also depends on information obtained from measuring the concentrations of this drug in the serum. We describe a new gas-chromatographic procedure for theophylline, with use of a nitrogen/phosphorus detector. The sensitivity of this detector allows the assay to be performed on sample volumes of 20 µl; its selectivity allows simplified sample preparation.

Materials and Methods

Chemicals

Theophylline, theobromine, phenobarbital, caffeine, and hypoxanthine were from Sigma Chemical Co., St. Louis, Mo. 63178. Xanthine, 3-methylxanthine, 3-isobutyl-1-methylxanthine, and *N,N*-dimethyl-acetamide were from Aldrich Chemical Co., Milwaukee, Wis. 53233. Uric acid was from the National Bureau of Standards, Washington, D. C. Iodopentane was from Eastman Kodak Co., Rochester, N. Y. 14650. Tetramethylammonium hydroxide (TMH) 24 g/100 ml methanol was from Matheson, Coleman, and Bell, East Rutherford, N. J. 07073. Chloroform and hexane ("Nanograde") were from Mallinckrodt Chemical Works, St. Louis, Mo. 63147. Isopropanol was from J. T. Baker Chemical Co., Phillipsburg, N. J. 08865.

Therapeutic Drug Monitoring Laboratory, Department of Laboratory Medicine, The Johns Hopkins Hospital, Baltimore, Md. 21205.
Received Nov. 20, 1975; accepted Feb. 8, 1976.

Reagents

Tetramethylammonium hydroxide (24 g/liter of methanol): Stock TMH, 24 g/100 ml of methanol, was diluted 1:10 with methanol and stored at 4 °C.

N,N-*Dimethylacetamide/TMH mixture:* Eight volumes of *N,N*-dimethylacetamide was combined with one volume of TMH (24 g/liter of methanol).

3-Isobutyl-1-methylxanthine stock solution (100 mg/liter): 3-Isobutyl-1-methylxanthine, 10 mg, was dissolved in 100 ml of ethanol. To prepare the internal standard solution (0.1 µg of 3-isobutyl-1-methylxanthine per milliliter) 1 ml of this solution was evaporated under nitrogen in a water bath, and the residue was dissolved in 1 liter of chloroform/isopropanol (20/1 by vol).

Procedure

Add 20 µl of serum, plasma, or saliva (with an Eppendorf pipet) to 100 µl of 1 mol/liter HCl in a 16 × 100 mm test tube with Teflon-lined screw cap. Add 3 ml of the internal standard solution and extract for 5 min (we used an Eberbach shaker at 250 oscillations/min). Centrifuge (2000 rpm, 5 min) and remove the aqueous phase by aspiration. Decant the remaining organic phase into "Concentratubes" (Laboratory Research Co., Los Angeles, Calif. 90036) and evaporate under nitrogen in a water bath at 50 °C. To the residue, add 100 µl of the *N,N*-dimethylacetamide/TMH mixture and vortex mix for 10 s. Add 50 µl of iodopentane, vortex mix for 10 s, and allow the tube to stand for 10 min at room temperature. Centrifuge for 5 min at 2500 rpm to sediment the precipitate formed, and with a Pasteur pipet transfer the supernate to a 1-ml "Reacti-Vial" (Pierce Chemical Co., Rockford, Ill. 61105) and evaporate it under nitrogen in a 50 °C water bath. Add 20 µl of hexane to the residue and vortex mix for 10 s. Prepare standards of 5, 10, 15, and 20 mg of theophylline per liter by evaporating 50, 100, 150, and 200 µl of a solution of theophylline in ethanol (100 mg/liter) and adding 1 ml of drug-free plasma to each residue. Extract and analyze 20 μl of these standards. Construct a standard curve by plotting the ratio of the peak height of theophylline to that of the internal standard as a function of the concentration of theophylline.

Instrument and Instrumental Conditions

We used a Model 3920 gas chromatograph (Perkin-Elmer Corp., Norwalk, Conn. 60856) equipped with dual nitrogen/phosphorus detectors and an all-glass receiver system. The recorder (Hitachi–Perkin-Elmer, Model 165) was operated at 1 mV full scale and chart speed of 10 mm/min. The glass columns were 91 cm × 2 mm (i.d.), configured for the all-glass version utilizing heated on-column injectors. Column packing was 3% OV-17 on 100/120 Gas Chrom Q (Applied Science Labs, State College, Pa. 16801). Injector temperature was 250 °C, detector temperature 280 °C, and oven temperature was programmed from 180–260 °C at 8 °C/min. The carrier gas (nitrogen) flow rate was 35 ml/min; air, 100 ml/min; and hydrogen, 4 ml/min. The detector was operated in the nitrogen/phosphorus mode with the jet-potential control in position 3. After flow rates of the support gases were set, the potentiometer controlling the bead temperature was increased from zero until the recorder deflection caused by background was 15% of full-scale with the electrometer attenuation set at ×10. This procedure ensured reproducible detector sensitivity from day to day, and resulted in similar potentiometer settings if the same rubidium silicate bead was used.

A Model 3370B integrator (Hewlett-Packard, Avondale, Pa. 19311) was used to measure peak areas (in microvolt seconds) for sensitivity calculations.

Results and Discussion

At first, we used the micro-alkylation procedure of Greeley (*6*) to prepare volatile derivatives of xanthines suitable for gas chromatography (*1*). The pentyl derivatives were chosen to optimize the separation of theophylline, theobromine, phenobarbital, and the internal standard on OV-17 (*2*). When we extended this procedure to the nitrogen/phosphorus detector, the nitrogen-containing solvent *N,N*-dimethylacetamide used in the alkylation procedure was removed by evaporation and the residue re-dissolved in hexane before chromatography. If this step was omitted—i.e., if the nitrogen-containing solvent was not removed—the resulting large solvent peak obscured the derivative peaks.

Figure 1 shows representative chromatograms of a reagent blank and of biological specimens extracted and derivatized according to our procedure. Chromatogram *A* (reagent blank) was obtained by extracting 20 μl of a sodium chloride solution (155 mmol/liter). Chromatograms *B* and *C*, in which the internal standard was omitted, were obtained for saliva and plasma of individuals not receiving theophylline or phenobarbital. Background peaks from extracted biological specimens (saliva or serum) contributed a response equivalent to

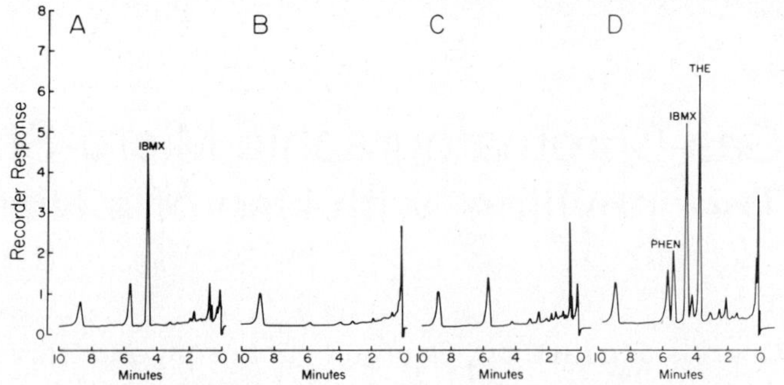

Fig. 1. Chromatograms of a reagent blank and biological specimens

Temperature was programmed from 180 to 260 °C, at 8°/min. Column packing: 3% OV-17 on 100/120 Gas Chrom Q. *A*. Reagent blank, 20 μl of 155 mmol/liter sodium chloride substituted for sample; internal standard included. *B*. Saliva blank, 20 μl of drug-free saliva; internal standard omitted. *C*. Serum blank, 20 μl of drug-free serum; internal standard omitted. *D*. Serum standard, 20 μl of serum to which theophylline and phenobarbital (15 mg/liter) were added; internal standard included. Chromatographic peaks represent 24 ng of each compound injected on the column; electrometer attenuation was ×100

<0.10 mg of theophylline per liter when a 20-μl sample was used. Chromatogram *D* was obtained with plasma from a normal individual, to which theophylline and phenobarbital (15 mg of each per liter) were added. This chromatogram represents 24 ng of each compound injected onto the chromatographic column. The pentyl derivatives of theophylline and phenobarbital are well separated from each other and from 3-isobutyl-1-methylxanthine, the internal standard. Caffeine and theobromine are also extracted in our procedure; however, their retention times (2.1 and 4.2 min, respectively) are such that they do not interfere with the compounds of interest. The relative retention times for caffeine, theophylline, theobromine, and phenobarbital—calculated relative to 3-isobutyl-1-methylxanthine—are 0.48, 0.81, 0.92, and 1.26, respectively.

Other xanthines investigated for possible interference with our assay included hypoxanthine, 3-methylxanthine, xanthine, and uric acid. These compounds, added to serum at concentrations of 25 mg/liter, produced no peaks with retention times equivalent to those of the derivatives of interest or of the internal standard, 3-isobutyl-1-methylxanthine.

Figure 2 illustrates chromatograms obtained by analysis of concurrently collected specimens of saliva and serum from a patient receiving theophylline. The saliva was collected in a 50-ml screw-cap plastic tube (Falcon Plastics, Oxnard, Calif. 93030), and blood was collected without an anticoagulant in a micro-hematocrit capillary tube (No. 1021; Clay Adams, Parsippany, N. J. 07054) and a "Vacutainer" tube (No. 3202; Becton-Dickinson, Rutherford, N. J. 07070). In contrast to chromatograms *A* and *B*, chromatogram *C*, the serum sample collected in the Vacutainer, showed not only the peaks observed for theophylline and 3-isobutyl-1-methylxanthine, but also a large peak with a retention of 5.8 min. Analysis of additional patients' samples collected in Vacutainers (No. 3206PS and No. 3202 for plasma and serum, respectively) also showed this prominent peak. The contaminating peak is not completely resolved from the pentyl derivative of pheno-

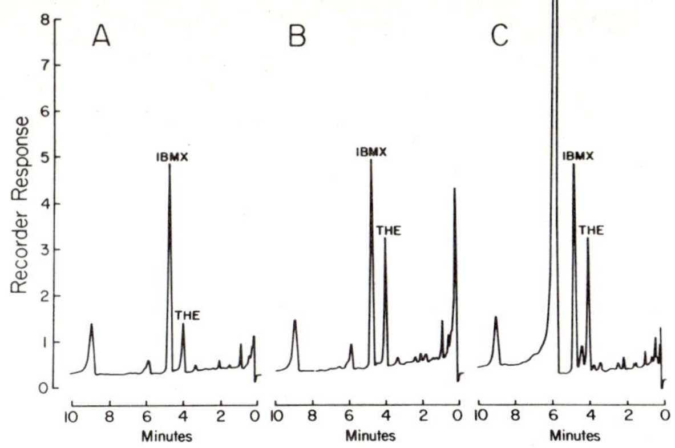

Fig. 2. Chromatograms obtained by analysis of 20 µl of saliva and serum specimens

Samples collected concurrently from a patient receiving theophylline. *A.* Saliva specimen, collected in screw-cap plastic tube. *B.* Serum specimen, collected in a micro-hematocrit capillary tube. *C.* Serum specimen, collected in a red-stoppered B-D Vacutainer tube (No. 3202)

barbital, which has a retention time of 5.4 min. When an aqueous solution of sodium chloride (155 mmol/liter) was added to Vacutainers, and the contents mixed thoroughly and then analyzed with our procedure for theophylline, the same chromatographic peak was observed as with serum and plasma specimens collected in these Vacutainers. Another commercially available evacuated blood-collection tube ("J-Vac"; Jelco Laboratory, Raritan, N. J. 08869) showed no evidence of this contaminant when saline was similarly used. Other experiments with Vacutainers showed that the contaminating peak was not dependent on alkylation with pentyl iodide.

To further characterize this interfering peak, 2 ml of the sodium chloride solution was added to a Vacutainer, mixed well, and 20 µl removed. This sample was extracted with chloroform/isopropanol, according to our procedure. The extract was evaporated and the residue was dissolved in 20 µl of hexane. The solution was analyzed further by gas-chromatography with the Perkin-Elmer nitrogen/phosphorus detector in the phosphorus mode and by gas chromatography/mass spectrometry.[1] The chemical ionization mass spectral data obtained from this sample showed ions at 399, 355, 299, and 199. These data are consistent with the mass spectral results of Finkle et al. (7), who identified this compound as tri-2-butoxyethyl phosphate, a plasticizer from Vacutainers.

Analytical recovery of theophylline in our procedure was established as follows. We added 0.3 µg of theophylline to 20 µl of drug-free plasma and extracted, with use of the internal standard solution, as described in the *Methods* section. A second standard was prepared by extracting 20 µl of drug-free plasma, and before derivatization, adding 0.3 µg of theophylline. We compared the peak height ratio of the extracted standard to the ratio obtained from the standard to which theophylline was added after extraction. The recovery so measured was 82%.

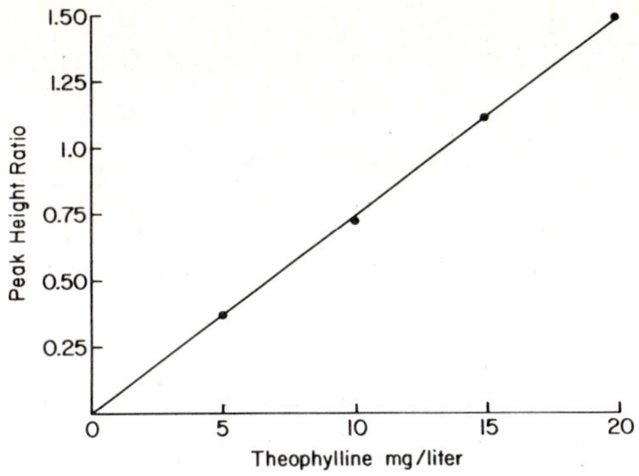

Fig. 3. Standard curve for theophylline

Figure 3 illustrates a typical standard curve obtained by our procedure. The ratio of the peak height of theophylline to the peak height of the internal standard was linearly related to concentration up to 20 mg/liter in serum. If recovery was 100% at all steps in our procedure, the 20 mg/liter standard would correspond to the on-column injection of 40 ng of theophylline.

The within-run coefficient of variation (CV) of the assay at 14.8 mg of theophylline per liter was 2.1% ($n = 10$), and 4.4% at 0.5 mg/liter ($n = 12$). Assessed during three months, between-run precision at 14.8 mg/liter was 2.8% ($n = 20$). Although a complete standard curve was included with each analytical run from which our overall precision data was derived, we found that the absolute variation in relative peak-height ratios of the 10 mg/liter standard and the above control plasma were only 2.3% and 2.9%, respectively. These data demonstrate excellent detector stability and indicate that especially urgent determinations may be made without preparing a standard curve if proper reagent and instrumental control are maintained.

Extracted plasma standards were used to determine both salivary and plasma theophylline concentrations, because equivalent amounts of theophylline added to and extracted from both saliva and plasma gave the same relative peak-height ratios.

Twenty-six specimens of serum and 25 specimens of saliva obtained from patients attending the Pediatric Allergy Clinic were analyzed for theophylline by our previously described gas-chromatographic macro-scale method (2), which requires 1 ml of sample and a double-extraction procedure before derivatization, and by the micro-scale procedure for theophylline we describe here. Concentrations of theophylline in the sera ranged from 1.0 to 46.6 mg/liter. The mean value observed with the macro-scale procedure was 15.8 mg/liter and with microscale procedure 16.0 mg/liter. When values for this micro-scale procedure were regressed against values for the macro-scale method, the slope of the unweighted linear least-squares regression line was 1.01, the intercept was 0.07 mg/liter, and the coefficient of correlation was 0.993. Concentrations of theophylline in saliva ranged from 0.5 to 19.6 mg/liter; the mean value observed with our former procedure was 8.4 mg/liter, with

[1] We thank Frank Vandemark and Reginald F. Adams, Laboratory Medicine Department, Perkin-Elmer Corp., Norwalk, Conn. 60856 for the gas-chromatographic and mass spectral analysis of this sample.

Table 1. Sensitivity of the Nitrogen/Phosphorus Detector to Selected Nitrogen-Containing Compounds

	Detector sensitivity[a]	
	Coulombs/g of compounds[b]	Coulombs/g of nitrogen[b]
Caffeine[c]	0.103	0.33
Theophylline	0.095	0.31
Theobromine	0.088	0.30
3-Isobutyl-1-methylxanthine	0.082	0.32
Phenobarbital	0.031	0.27

[a] Instrumental conditions as outlined in the methods section.

[b] Electrometer sensitivity (A/mV) × attenuation × peak area (μV-s)/quantity of compound (gram) ×1000 = coulomb/gram.

[c] All compounds except caffeine were chromatographed as their pentyl derivatives.

our micro-scale procedure it was 8.3 mg/liter. When values for the micro-scale procedure were regressed against values for the macro-scale method, the slope of the unweighted linear least-squares line was 0.93, with an intercept of 0.5 mg/liter and a correlation coefficient of 0.990.

Detector sensitivity is presented in Table 1 as both coulombs per gram of compound and coulombs per gram of nitrogen, under the instrumental conditions outlined in the methods section. The manufacturer states that a sensitivity of at least 0.5 C/g of nitrogen is attainable with the nitrogen/phosphorus detector. The instrumental conditions we used for the analysis of theophylline according to the method described in this paper resulted in a detector sensitivity of 0.33 C/g of nitrogen for caffeine. We found that a response of 6.0 C/g of nitrogen for caffeine could be attained when the temperature of the bead was increased. At such high levels of sensitivity, however, analysis with the nitrogen/phosphorus detector is limited by the presence of impurities in the solvents used. A peak height contribution equivalent to 1 mg of theophylline per liter was observed when a 2-μl sample of plasma was analyzed. This background peak, however, is equivalent to only 0.1 mg of theophylline per liter when the sample volume is 20 μl.

It can be seen from Table 1 that the pentyl derivative of theophylline exhibits about a threefold greater sensitivity than the pentyl derivative of phenobarbital when results are expressed as coulombs per gram of compound injected. However, when results are expressed as coulombs per gram of nitrogen, these compounds show equal sensitivity. Studies of a series of alkylated derivatives of theophylline, with alkyl chain length varying from three to seven carbon atoms, demonstrated that detector sensitivity is independent of chain length when sensitivity is expressed as coulombs per gram of nitrogen. The data presented on sensitivity of xanthine derivatives are consistent with the mechanism suggested by Kolb and Bishoff (*8*) for the response of the nitrogen/phosphorus detector to compounds containing nitrogen. They postulate that the sensitivity exhibited by nitrogen-containing compounds results from their ability to produce cyan radicals when burned in the detector.

The major advantage of our procedure for theophylline is that it requires a smaller sample. Our previous flame ionization gas-chromatographic procedure (*2*) for this drug required a 1-ml sample of serum or saliva; the present procedure requires only 20 μl, a sample size that is particularly appropriate for monitoring serum concentrations of theophylline in (e.g.) management of apnea in premature infants (*5*). Because there is marked variation between premature infants in their rates of metabolism of theophylline, concentrations in serum should be measured repetitively to ensure safe and effective use of the drug. Until now, the smallest sample volume reported in the literature for monitoring theophylline concentrations has been 0.1 ml (*3, 4*).

Because of the selectivity of the nitrogen/phosphorus detector for nitrogen-containing compounds, we could use a simplified extraction procedure for this drug. With this procedure a single determination can be performed in about 45 min.

References

1. Johnson, G. F., Dechtiaruk, W. A., and Solomon, H. M., Gas-chromatographic determination of theophylline in human serum and saliva. *Clin. Chem.* **21**, 144 (1975).

2. Dechtiaruk, W., Johnson, G. F., and Solomon, H. M., Faster gas-chromatographic procedure for theophylline. *Clin. Chem.* **21**, 1038 (1975).

3. Weinberger, M., and Chidsey, C., Rapid analysis for theophylline in serum by use of high-pressure cation-exchange chromatography. *Clin. Chem.* **21**, 834 (1975).

4. Arbin, A., and Edland, P., Determination of theophylline in biological material by means of electron capture gas chromatography. *Acta Pharm. Suec.* **12**, 119 (1975).

5. Shannon, D. C., Gotay, F., Stein, I. M., et al., Prevention of apnea and bradycardia in low-birthweight infants. *Pediatrics* **55**, 589 (1975).

6. Greeley, R. H., New approach to derivatization and gas-chromatographic analysis of barbiturates. *Clin. Chem.* **20**, 192 (1974).

7. Finkle, B. S., Foltz, R. L., and Taylor, D. M., A comprehensive GC-MS reference data system for toxicological and biomedical purposes. *J. Chromatogr. Sci.* **12**, 304 (1974).

8. Kolb, B., and Bischoff, J., A new design of a thermionic nitrogen and phosphorus detector for GC. *J. Chromatogr. Sci.* **12**, 625 (1974).

CLIN. CHEM. 22/6, 769–771 (1976)

Simultaneous Gas-Chromatographic Analysis for Phenobarbital, Diphenylhydantoin, Carbamazepine, and Primidone in Serum

Chempithera V. Abraham and Harry D. Joslin

We describe a simple, sensitive determination of phenobarbital, diphenylhydantoin, carbamazepine, and primidone in serum, by use of gas–liquid chromatography with temperature programming. The methylated derivatives of these anticonvulsants are well resolved, as was 5-(*p*-methylphenyl)-5-phenylhydantoin, the internal standard. The proposed procedure requires only 0.20 ml of serum and can be done in less than 30 min. The lower limit of detection for each of the drugs is 0.5 mg/liter. Analytical recoveries of drug from serum were excellent and peak height and concentration were linearly related up to twice the toxic concentration for serum.

Gas–liquid chromatography is widely used for determining antiepileptic drugs (*1–3*). Its sensitivity and specificity allows simultaneous measurement of anticonvulsant drugs. Here, we describe a simple method for simultaneously determining phenobarbital, diphenylhydantoin, primidone, and carbamazepine in 1 ml of plasma or serum in less than 30 min.

Materials and Methods

Reagents and standards

Drugs used as standards were diphenylhydantoin (Dilantin; Parke-Davis & Co., Detroit, Mich. 48232), carbamazepine (Tegretol; CIBA Pharmaceutical Co., Summit, N. J. 07901), phenobarbital (Eli Lilly and Co., Indianapolis, Ind. 46206), primidone (Ayerst Laboratory Inc., New York, N. Y. 10017) and 5-(*p*-methylphenyl)-5-phenylhydantoin (Aldrich Chemical Co., Milwaukee, Wis. 53200).

Trimethylphenylammonium hydroxide, 0.2 mol/liter. This was prepared from trimethylphenylammonium iodide (Fisher Scientific Co., Silver Spring, Md. 20910) that had been recrystallized three times from absolute ethanol as follows. Into a 250-ml glass-stoppered Erlenmeyer flask with a Teflon stirrer, add 6.94 g of silver oxide, 10.52 g of trimethylphenylammonium iodide, and 200 ml of absolute methanol. Stir (magnetic stirrer) for 2.5 h and store at 4 °C. The supernatant solution is stable for at least a month. Filter appropriate amounts of it through Whatman No. 1 filter paper immediately before use.

Lynchburg Training School and Hospital, P.O. Box 1098, Lynchburg, Va. 24505.
Received Nov. 21, 1975; accepted Feb. 2, 1976.

Standards

Internal standard. Dissolve 18 μg of 5-(*p*-methylphenyl)-5-phenylhydantoin per milliliter of chloroform, and use 5 ml of this solution for the extraction.

Drug standards. The stock drug standards were prepared in the following concentrations: phenobarbital, 2 g/liter; carbamazepine, 0.5 g/liter; primidone, 1 g/liter; and diphenylhydantoin, 2 g/liter. The stock drug standards were added to a drug-free pool of serum to obtain five standards with the concentrations listed in Table 1. All four drugs were added to the same serum. These standards were kept frozen in screw-cap, Teflon-coated tubes until use.

Standard curve. Standard curves were prepared for each drug. Each serum standard was extracted and chromatographed in duplicate as if it were a patient sample. The mean value of the relative peak height ratios from the duplicate analyses of each standard were plotted against the concentration of the respective standard (Figure 1).

Instrumentation

We used a Model 2400 gas chromatograph (Fisher Scientific Co., Pittsburgh, Pa. 15219) with dual hydrogen flame-ionization detectors and borosilicate glass columns (200 cm × 2 mm i.d.) packed with 3% SP 2250 on 100/120 mesh "Supelcoport," type 50-50 Me-Ph (Supelco, Inc., Bellefonte, Pa. 16823). Before use, the columns were heat conditioned at 310 °C for 24 h with a carrier gas (nitrogen) flow rate of 50 ml/min.

Table 1. Concentration of Working Standards in Serum

Standard	Phenobarbital	Diphenylhydantoin	Primidone	Carbamazepine
		mg/liter		
1	5	2.5	2.5	1
2	10	5	5	2.5
3	20	10	10	5
4	40	20	15	7.5
5	80	40	20	10

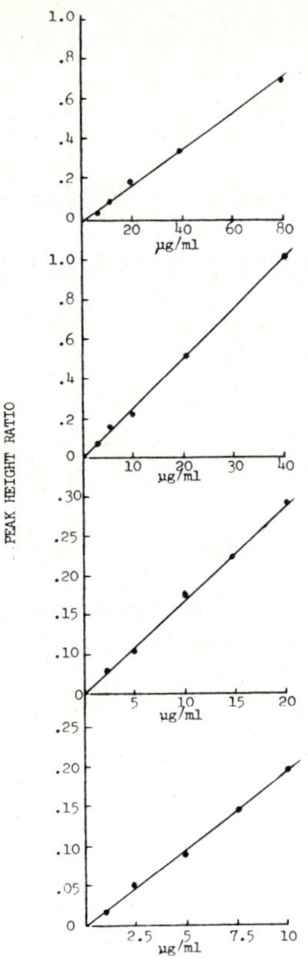

Fig. 1. Standard curve for (*top to bottom*) phenobarbital, diphenylhydantoin, primidone, and carbamazepine
Each point is mean value for two runs

Oven temperature was maintained at 190 °C during periods of inactivity, with a carrier-gas flow rate of 50 ml/min. The injection ports were sealed with 10-mm septums (Supelco). Detectors and injection ports were heated to 310 and 250 °C, respectively. Electrometer output was monitored with a Fisher Model 5000 series dual-pen recorder, at a chart speed of 25 mm/min. The electrometer was operated at a range of 10^{-11} A/mV and the amplifier output was attenuated at 128.

Chromatographic conditions. Oven temperature was programmed from 190 to 300 °C at a rate of 15 °C/min, the program being started immediately after the sample extract was injected. Gas-flow rates were: nitrogen, 160 ml/min; hydrogen, 30 ml/min; and air, 300 ml/min.

Extraction Procedure

One milliliter of serum or plasma was combined with 0.5 ml of 0.25 mol/liter hydrochloric acid in a 13 × 150 mm test tube (Teflon-lined screw cap). Five milliliter of chloroform containing 90 μg of the internal standard was added to the screw-cap tube, which was then shaken for 1 min on a vortex-type mixer. The aqueous (upper) phase was aspirated and the organic phase filtered through a Whatman No. 1 filter paper (the filter paper was rinsed before use with few milliliters of chloroform) into a conical centrifuge tube and evaporated in a warm water bath (40 °C) under a stream of nitrogen. The tubes were closed tightly with a cork until the residues were to be injected into the gas chromatograph.

Table 2. Between-day Analytical Recoveries (n = 31)

Drug added to serum	Mean concn: Added	Found	SD	Recovery, %
		mg/liter		
Phenobarbital	20	19.8	1.1	99
Diphenyl-hydantoin	10	9.9	0.4	99
Primidone	15	15.1	1.0	101
Carbamazepine	10	10.4	0.6	104

Chromatography

The residue in the centrifuge tube was reconstituted with 100 μl of the trimethylphenylammonium hydroxide solution. One to two microliters of this extract was chromatographed at a programmed temperature on the SP 2250 column. Peaks were identified by comparing their retention times relative to the retention time for the internal reference peak to such data for known standards. Drug concentrations were calculated from the standard curve.

The precision of the proposed method was checked by using aliquots of drug-supplemented serum pools, which were stored frozen. The serum pool contained all four drugs.

Results

Figure 1 shows standard curves for primidone, diphenylhydantoin, carbamazepine, and phenobarbital, prepared by the peak-height ratio technique. All four curves are linear to approximately twice the toxic concentration. Analytical recovery of the drugs from the serum was measured by adding known amounts of these four drugs to the same sample and analyzing it for 31 consecutive days. Recovery ranged from 99 to 104% (Table 2).

Chromatograms of serum specimens extracted and methylated according to our procedure are presented in Figure 2. Chromatogram *A*, with the internal standard, is a typical pattern for serum from a normal individual not receiving anticonvulsants. The three predominant peaks marked *S* are attributable to normal serum constituents. Chromatogram *B* is from a patient who was receiving all four of the antiepileptic drugs. The concentrations calculated from this serum sample were: primidone, 4 mg/liter; phenobarbital, 20 mg/liter; carbamazepine, 3 mg/liter; and diphenylhydantoin, 10 mg/liter. Chromatogram *C* is our standard 4 (Table 1), prepared by adding the drugs to pooled serum. All four drug peaks were well separated and there were no interfering peaks.

Precision

The between-day precision of the proposed method was evaluated (Table 2). The standard deviation varied from 0.4 to 1.1 mg/liter. Analytical recoveries varied from 99 to 104%.

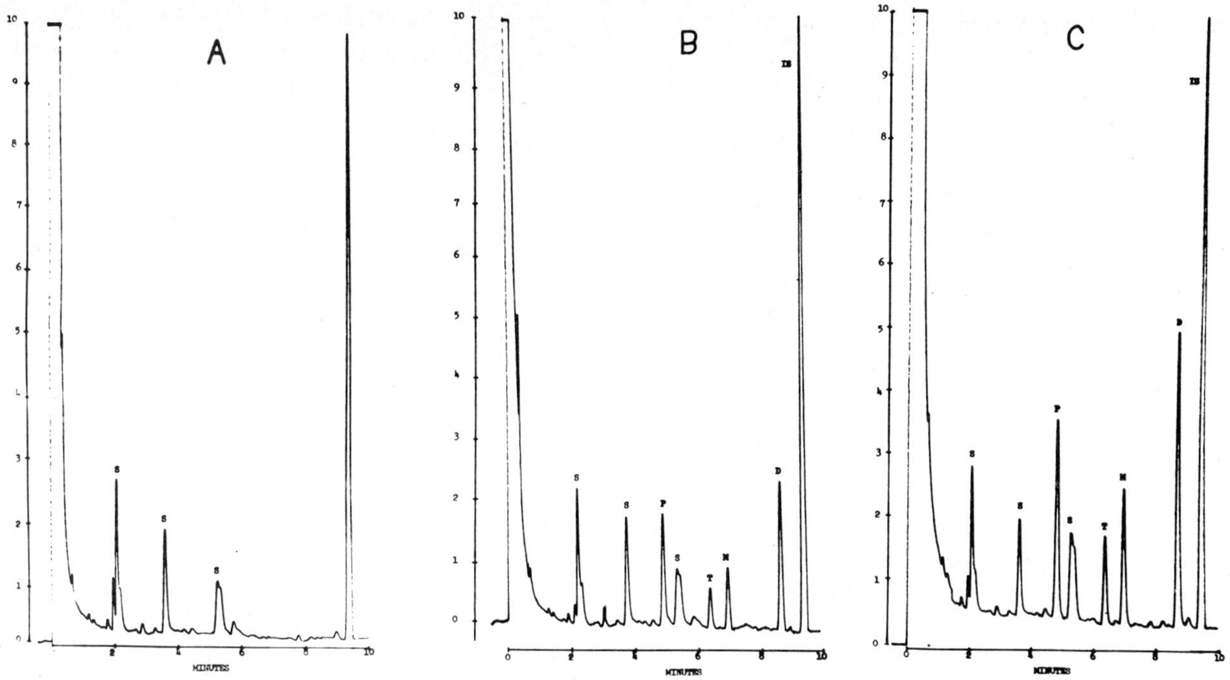

Fig. 2. Chromatograph obtained by methylation of serum extract

Temperature programmed from 190 to 300 °C at 15 °C/min. Column packing 3% SP 2250 on 100/200 mesh Supelcoport-type 50–50 Me-Ph. *P*, phenobarbital; *T*, carbamazepine; *M*, primidone; and *D*, diphenylhydantoin; *I.S.*, internal standard, 5-(*p*-methylphenyl)-5-phenylhydantoin; *S*, peak due to serum constituents. *A*, drug-free serum (1.0 ml) with internal standard. *B*, serum (1.0 ml) from patient receiving phenobarbital, diphenylhydantoin, carbamazepine, and primidone. *C*, serum (1.0 ml) to which these four drugs have been added

The usual sample volume used was 1 ml of serum or plasma. In pediatric cases, similar results can be obtained by decreasing the amounts of serum, chloroform, and reagent proportionately. In some instances we successfully used as little as 0.2 ml of serum.

Drug concentrations as low as 0.5 mg/liter were easily measured by adjusting the sensitivity of the analysis, e.g., injecting a more concentrated extract, increasing the volume of injection, or increasing the electrometer output.

Discussion

Rose et al. (*4*) emphasize that determinations of antiepileptic drugs are not readily available to most physicians who prescribe these medications. Laboratories are reluctant to establish anticonvulsant assays because of the considerable capital investment and commitment of experienced technical personnel. However, such monitoring is important to better treatment.

Our method is simple and well-suited for the clinical laboratory. A single extraction and chromatographic system is used to analyze for all four of the anticonvulsant drugs. Use of a single internal standard and one temperature programming reduces the technical difficulties and standardization procedure, and gives well-separated peaks for all of the four drugs. The on-column methylation, and the use of glass column and SP 2250 gives good peak characteristics and a linear standard curve.

The five standards that contain all the four drugs were prepared on the basis of a report on observed concentrations in serum (*5*). In our proposed method the concentration in standard 5 is about twice the toxic concentration, standard 1 is less than a third the therapeutic concentration.

With this procedure one can determine the most commonly used antiepileptic drugs in a single operation within 30 min.

References

1. Baumel, I. P., Gallagher, B. B., and Mattson, R. H., Phenylethylmalonamide (PEMA), an important metabolite of primidone. *Arch. Neurol.* (Chicago) **27**, 34 (1972).

2. Kananen, G., Osiewicz, R., and Sunshine, I., Barbiturate analysis—a current assessment. *J. Chromatogr. Sci.* **10**, 283 (1972).

3. Friel, P., and Green, J. R., Quantitative assay for carbamazepine serum levels by gas-liquid chromatography. *Clin. Chim. Acta* **43**, 69 (1973).

4. Rose, S. W., Smith, L. D., and Penry, J. K., Blood level determinations of antiepileptic drugs: Clinical value and methods. U. S. Dept. HEW, Bethesda, Md., 1971.

5. Kutt, H., and Penry, J. K., Usefulness of blood levels of antiepileptic drugs. *Arch. Neurol.* (Chicago) **31**, 283 (1974).

CLIN. CHEM. 22/6, 772–776 (1976)

Gas-Chromatographic Determination of 5-Fluorocytosine in Human Serum

Sally A. Harding, George F. Johnson, and Harvey M. Solomon

We describe a sensitive and precise gas-chromatographic method, in which cytosine is used as the internal standard, for determination of an antifungal agent, 5-fluorocytosine, in serum. The trimethylsilyl derivative of this drug is well separated from the internal standard and from normal serum constituents. Amphotericin B does not interfere with the determination of 5-fluorocytosine. The lower limit of detection for 5-fluorocytosine is 1 mg/liter when 200 μl of serum is analyzed. Within-run precision (CV), established by analysis of 10 replicates, was 4.5% at a concentration of 19.9 mg/liter. Twenty-five serum samples were analyzed for 5-fluorocytosine by a microbiological assay and by the gas-chromatographic method. Mean value observed with the bioassay was 78.5 mg/liter and with our procedure was 69.4 mg/liter. When values for our assay were regressed against values for the bioassay, slope of the least-squares line was 0.85, intercept was 2.7 mg/liter, and *r* was 0.93.

Many clinical microbiologists still use biological assays to estimate various antibiotics in physiological fluids, even though such procedures are inherently less precise, more difficult to control, and subject to greater interferences than are modern chemical assays. The first chemical method for quantitative determination of sulfonamides was introduced in 1939 by Bratton and Marshall (*1*) and this colorimetric procedure is still widely used to measure these compounds. Moreover, when an initial hydrolysis step is included, the biologically inactive *N*-acetyl metabolite of various sulfonamides can also be determined; hence, it is possible to determine whether patients acetylate these drugs slowly or rapidly (*2*). Although chemical and immunochemical methods for the determination of antibiotics have improved greatly in accuracy, precision, sensitivity, and specificity (*3, 4*) since the introduction of the Bratton–Marshall technique for sulfonamides, some clinical microbiologists (*5*) still claim that chemical assay methods for antibiotics are nonspecific, detecting (e.g.) metabolites of these drugs that possess little if any biological activity.

Patients with serious bacterial and fungal infections are frequently treated concurrently with several chemotherapeutic agents. When the antibiotics involved in such therapy cannot be separated by relatively simple physical techniques and when assay organisms possessing selective sensitivity to individual drugs in such therapeutic regimens are not available, it is difficult if not impossible to determine drug concentrations meaningfully by biological assay.

5-Fluorocytosine is an antifungal agent frequently utilized in combination with amphotericin B for treatment of deep-seated mycotic infections (*6, 7*). Monitoring of serum concentrations of 5-fluorocytosine has been recommended to provide optimum therapeutic benefit and avoid toxicity (*8*). To our knowledge, such determinations have been performed only by bioassay. The yeasts utilized in these bioassays for 5-fluorocytosine are, however, also inhibited by amphotericin B, and various techniques—including ultra-filtration (*8*) and differential diffusion through yeast nitrogen base agar from filter paper disks—have been used to separate these drugs (*9*).

5-Fluorocytosine, which has a relatively simple chemical structure, is readily converted to a volatile trimethylsilyl derivative. We describe an accurate and precise gas-chromatographic method that is specific for 5-fluorocytosine and is suitable for the routine determination of this drug in serum.

Therapeutic Drug Monitoring Laboratory, Department of Laboratory Medicine, The Johns Hopkins Hospital, Baltimore, Md. 21205.

Received September 4, 1975; accepted Sept. 22, 1975. (At the authors' request, this paper was held so that it could appear in this special issue.)

Materials and Methods

Reagents

5-Fluorocytosine was kindly provided by Hoffmann-La Roche, Inc., Nutley, N. J. 07110; cytosine was purchased from Aldrich Chemical Co., Milwaukee, Wis. 53233. We prepared stock solutions (100 mg/liter) of each of these compounds by dissolving 10 mg in 100 ml of ethanol. A working solution of 5-fluorocytosine (10 mg/liter) was prepared by diluting the stock solution 10-fold with ethanol.

Amphotericin B was purchased from E. R. Squibb and Sons, Inc., Princeton, N. J. 08540. A stock solution (100 mg/liter) was prepared by suspending 50 mg of the drug in 10 ml of distilled water and then diluting this solution 50-fold with distilled water.

n-Butanol and ethanol were purchased from Fisher Scientific Co., Fair Lawn, N. J. 07410. Regis silylation mix was obtained from Regis Chemical Co., Morton Grove, Ill. 60053.

Procedure for Extraction and Silylation

Serum (200 μl) was combined in a 16 × 125 mm test tube (with a Teflon-lined screw cap) with 800 μl distilled water, 30 μl HCl (2 mol/liter) and 1 ml of phosphate buffer (0.1 mol/liter, pH 3.0) containing 10 mg/liter of the internal standard, cytosine. The buffer solution was stored at 4 °C and was dispensed from an automatic pipet (Repipet; LabIndustries, Berkeley, Calif. 94710). The contents of the tubes were mixed on a vortex-type mixer for 30 s and 5 ml of butanol was then added to each tube with a Repipet. The tubes were shaken for 10 min in an Eberbach shaker at 250 oscillations per minute and centrifuged at 2000 rpm for 10 min. The butanol layers were aspirated and discarded. One milliliter of phosphate buffer (1 mol/liter, pH 7.9) was added to the aqueous phase to adjust the pH to 7.4, 5 ml of butanol was added with the Repipet, and the contents of the tubes were mixed and extracted as just described. The phases were separated by centrifugation as described above. The butanol layers were transferred to 7-ml screw-capped silylation vials and evaporated under nitrogen in a water bath at 55 °C. Regis Silylation mix, 50 μl, was added to each vial and the contents of the vials were mixed thoroughly on a vortex-type mixer. Two-microliter samples were injected into the gas chromatograph.

Standard curves were prepared from pooled normal human serum that contained known amounts of 5-fluorocytosine. These serum standards (10, 25, 50, 75, and 100 mg/liter) were prepared by evaporating appropriate amounts of the working solution of 5-fluorocytosine under nitrogen and adding 200 μl of drug-free serum to the residue.

Gas Chromatography

A Model 5711A dual-column gas chromatograph equipped with flame-ionization detectors (Hewlett-Packard, Avondale, Pa. 14311) was used. The glass columns (122 cm × 2 mm i.d.) were packed with 3% OV-17 on 100/120 Gas Chrom Q (Applied Science Labs., Inc., State College, Pa. 16801). Injector port temperature was 250 °C, detector temperature was 300 °C, and oven temperature was programmed from 100 to 240 °C at 16 °C/min. The nitrogen flow rate was 50 ml/min.

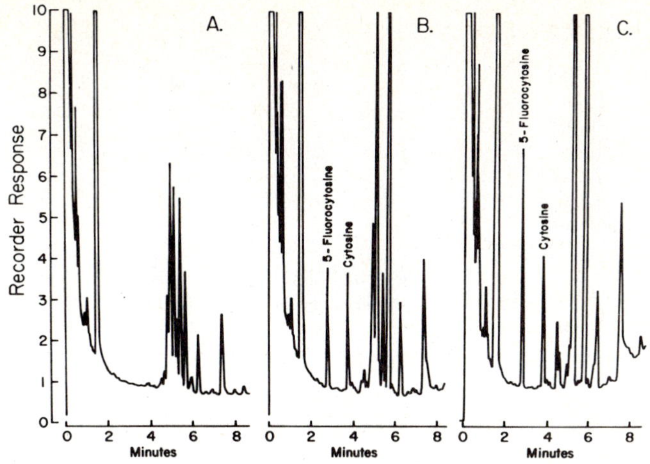

Fig. 1. Chromatograms obtained by silylation of serum extracts
A, drug-free serum (200 μl); internal standard not included; *B*, serum (200 μl) to which 25 mg/liter cytosine and 25 mg/liter 5-fluorocytosine were added; *C*, serum (200 μl) from a patient receiving amphotericin B and 5-fluorocytosine. 5-Fluorocytosine concentration in this sample was 48.4 mg/liter

Microbiological Assay for 5-Fluorocytosine

Specimens were analyzed for 5-fluorocytosine according to a modification of the bioassay procedure of Block and Bennett (*8*). In the original procedure standard solutions of the drug, prepared in pooled, normal human serum, were not ultrafiltered through collodion membranes while serum samples obtained from patients treated concurrently with 5-fluorocytosine and amphotericin B were ultrafiltered. In the modified procedure both standard solutions and patient samples were ultrafiltered. All bioassays for 5-fluorocytosine were performed in the laboratory of Dr. John E. Bennett, Clinical Mycology Section, Laboratory of Clinical Investigation, National Institute of Allergy and Infectious Diseases, Bethesda, Md. 20014.

Results

When sera from normal individuals were extracted and derivatized according to the procedure we have described, several chromatographic peaks were observed; however, none interfered with either 5-fluorocytosine or cytosine (Figure 1*A*). Normal sera and sera from patients treated with 5-fluorocytosine did not contain endogenous cytosine. The chromatogram presented in Figure 1*B* was obtained from a normal serum to which 5-fluorocytosine and cytosine were added. A single chromatographic peak was observed for each compound, with a retention time of 2.65 min for 5-fluorocytosine and 3.62 min for cytosine. No interference from amphotericin B was noted with specimens obtained from any of the patients on combined drug therapy or with normal serum samples to which were

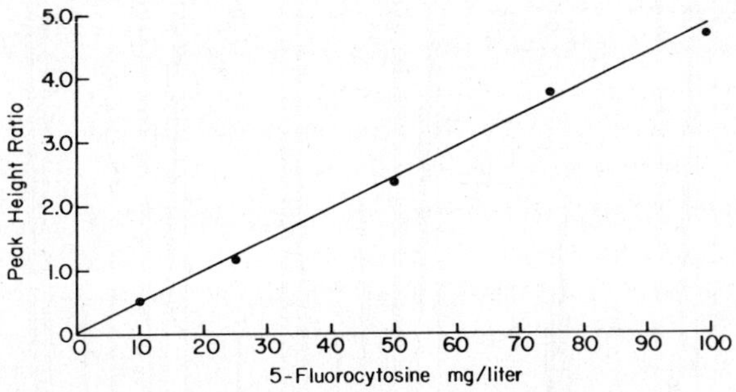

Fig. 2. Standard curve for 5-fluorocytosine in serum

added amphotericin B in final concentrations of 12.5, 25.0, or 50.0 mg/liter and 5-fluorocytosine in final concentrations ranging from 20 to 100 mg/liter. Figure 1*C* shows a chromatogram obtained with serum from a patient on combined therapy with 5-fluorocytosine and amphotericin B. The concentration of 5-fluorocytosine in this clinical specimen was 48.4 mg/liter.

A typical standard curve obtained with our procedure is shown in Figure 2. Linearity was observed over the range of 0–200 mg of 5-fluorocytosine per liter. The lower limit of detection for 5-fluorocytosine, based on twice the standard deviation of baseline noise, was 1 mg/liter when the sample volume was 200 μl.

Recovery of 5-fluorocytosine from serum was measured in the following way: a solution of 30 μg of the compound in methanol was evaporated and to the residue was added 1 ml of drug-free serum. This sample was extracted as described in the *Methods* section; however, volume transfers were quantitated. A second (non-extracted) standard was prepared concurrently by evaporating 30 μg of the same compound to dryness, and both sample and standard were derivatized by addition of 50 μl of silylating reagent. Two microliters of each sample were chromatographed. The peak height of the serum sample was corrected for solvent transfers. Absolute recovery of the drug from serum was calculated by comparing the ratio of corrected peak height of the extracted serum sample to that of the non-extracted standard. The absolute recoveries of 5-fluorocytosine and cytosine determined by this procedure were 30.3% and 30.9%, respectively. When concentrations of 5-fluorocytosine ranging from 25–150 mg/liter were prepared in pooled normal sera and assayed according to our procedure, the mean recovery of this drug relative to the internal standard was 95.9% (n = 12).

Within-run reproducibility (CV) for our assay was 4.5% at a concentration of 19.9 mg/liter (n = 10). Between-run reproducibility was 7.5% as determined by the use of paired duplicates according to the following formula: $SD = \sqrt{\Sigma d^2/2n}$, where d = difference between duplicate pairs. The mean value for this group of samples was 48.1 mg/liter, with a range of 4.1 to 187.8 mg/liter (n = 23).

Twenty-five serum samples were analyzed for 5-fluorocytosine by the microbiological assay and with the gas chromatographic method we have described (Figure 3). Seventeen of these samples were prepared by adding various amounts of 5-fluorocytosine to pooled normal sera and eight were obtained from patients receiving both amphotericin B and 5-fluorocytosine. The mean value for the bioassay was 78.5 mg/liter (range, 5.0 to 194.0 mg/liter). The mean value by the gas chromatographic procedure was 69.4 mg/liter (range, 4.5 to 156.0 mg/liter). When values obtained by the gas-chromatographic assay were regressed against those obtained with the bioassay, the slope of the linear least-squares line was 0.85, the intercept was 2.7 mg/liter, and the coefficient of correlation was 0.93.

Discussion

The incidence of systemic fungal infections has risen progressively with increased use of such drugs as steroids, antibiotics, and immunosuppressants, and as a result of larger numbers of renal-transplant recipients and more prolonged survival of patients with neoplastic diseases (*10, 13*). Systemic yeast infections are the most frequently encountered of these opportunistic mycoses and the prognosis in such systemic infections is poor, the overall mortality being 75% (*14*).

In vitro and clinical studies indicate that 5-fluorocytosine is effective in treating infections from sensitive strains of *Candida, Torulopsis*, and *Cryptococcus* (*15, 17*).

In man, about 90% of the administered dose of 5-fluorocytosine is excreted unchanged in the urine and the remainder appears in the feces (*18*). Concentrations of this drug in serum are greater in patients with impaired renal function and clearance is prolonged compared to that observed in patients with normal renal function (*8, 15, 19*). Toxic effects of 5-fluorocytosine on the bone marrow and liver have been observed more commonly in patients with renal insufficiency treated with usual therapeutic doses of 5-fluorocytosine (*19, 20*), which suggests that rational dosage regimens in such patients should be based on measurements of serum concentrations. Block and Bennett (*8*) indicate that peak serum concentrations of 5-fluorocytosine as great as 120 mg/liter can be attained without risk of drug-induced toxicity. Concentrations of at least 25 mg/liter

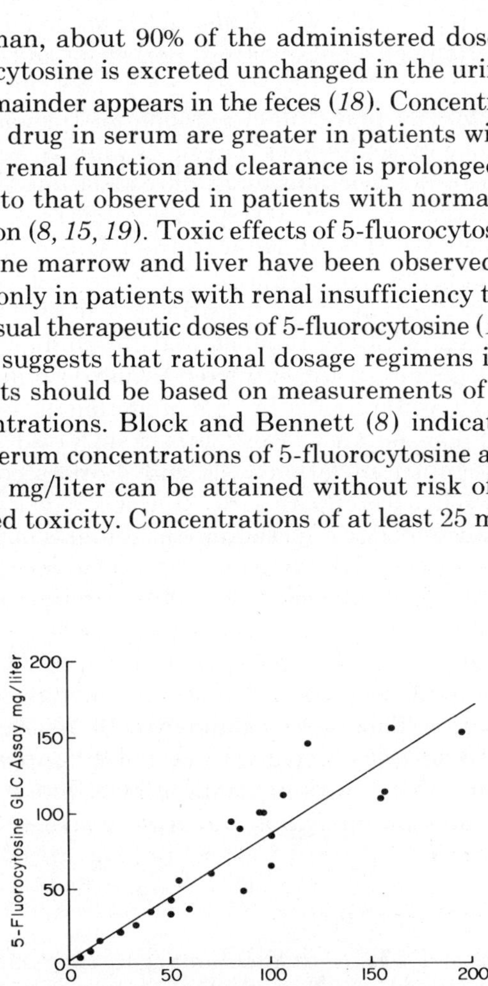

Fig. 3. Comparison of a microbiological assay and gas chromatographic assay for 5-fluorocytosine in serum

of serum should be attained during therapy, because many resistant mutants emerge at lower concentrations (*21*).

Treatment of a number of fungal diseases is frequently undertaken with 5-fluorocytosine and amphotericin B, because this combination is synergistic and reduces the development of resistance to 5-fluorocytosine by the infecting organism (*6, 7*). The usual therapeutic doses of amphotericin B often produce nephrotoxicity; hence serum concentrations of 5-fluorocytosine should also be monitored in this population to provide safe and effective therapy with the drug.

Although several bioassay procedures for estimating 5-fluorocytosine in serum have been reported, it is difficult to determine their precision because no meaningful information has been published concerning within- or between-run reproducibility (*8, 9*). It is likely, however, that the precision of these assays is rather limited, because one procedure involves processing all specimens in triplicate and the other in quadruplicate. The within-run coefficient of variation of our assay for 5-fluorocytosine was 4.5% at a concentration of 19.9 mg/liter and the between-run precision (CV) was 7.5 percent. These data suggest that our gas-chromatographic assay has adequate precision to permit determinations on single samples rather than on replicates as required by the bioassays. The relatively good reproducibility of this procedure is due primarily to use of cytosine, a closely related compound, as the internal standard in the assay. When normal human serum was extracted and derivatized according to our procedure without addition of this internal standard, a chromatographic peak with the retention time of the trimethylsilyl derivative of cytosine was not observed. This is consistent with the observations of Bishop et al. (*22*), who did not detect free purines or pyrimidines in normal human blood. Our procedure is not interfered with by normal constituents in serum or by amphotericin B, which suggests that it also has requisite specificity for 5-fluorocytosine.

Although chemical methods for analysis of 5-fluorocytosine in biological fluids have not been previously described, several procedures have been reported for the quantitative determination of 5-fluorouracil, an antimetabolite used in cancer chemotheraphy (*23, 25*). This drug, a weak acid ($pK_a = 8.0$), can be separated from plasma by various techniques, including dialysis, anion-exchange chromatography, and extraction with a mixture of *n*-propanol in ether. The trimethylsilyl derivative of 5-fluorouracil has good chromatographic characteristics on OV-1 and SE-30 and the drug can also be derivatized by on-column alkylation with trimethylanilinium hydroxide. Recently Pantarotto et al. (*26*) determined by gas chromatography–mass spectrometry that the product of this alkylation is *N,N*-dimethyl-5-fluorouracil.

The double-extraction procedure we use involves an initial extraction with butanol at pH 3.0 to remove interfering neutral and acidic compounds. 5-Fluorocytosine is not extracted into butanol at this pH. The pH is then adjusted to 7.4 and the drug and internal standard are extracted into butanol. The extraction efficiency of 5-fluorocytosine is only 30.3% and that of the internal standard is 30.9%, which indicates that these compounds have similar partition characteristics. The trimethylsilyl derivatives of 5-fluorocytosine and cytosine prepared in our assay have excellent chromatographic characteristics and are stable for as long as 24 h if they are protected from moisture. We have also established that 5-fluorocytosine can be alkylated with trimethylanilinium hydroxide; however, this derivative is absorbed to the column and is therefore not suitable for the quantitative determination of the drug.

Because of the variation inherent in the bioassay it is difficult to know whether the slope (0.85) that we found for the regression line is statistically different from unity.

Safe and effective treatment with many potent drugs having narrow margins of safety depends in part on measurements of their concentrations in serum (*27*). Therapeutic monitoring of antiarrhythmic drugs, anticonvulsants, cardiac glycosides, and the bronchodialator theophylline are increasingly utilized to ensure optimum therapeutic benefit and to avoid drug toxicity. Rapid, specific, accurate, and precise chemical methods are available for these compounds, and it is mandatory that similar techniques be developed for the quantitative determination of antibiotics.

We thank John E. Bennett, M.D., Head, Clinical Mycology Section, LCI, National Institute of Allergy and Infectious Diseases, National Institutes of Health, Bethesda, Md. 20014, for providing the microbiological assay for 5-fluorocytosine used in this study.

References

1. Bratton, A.C. and Marshall, E. K., Jr., A new coupling component for sulfanilamide determination. *J. Biol. Chem.* **128,** 537 (1939).

2. White, T. A., and Evans, D. A. P., The acetylation of sulfamethazine and sulfamethoxypyridazine by human subjects. *Clin. Pharmacol. Ther.* **9,** 89 (1968).

3. Resnick, G. L., Corbin, D., and Sandberg, D. H., Determination of serum chloramphenicol utilizing gas-liquid chromatography and electron capture spectrometry. *Anal. Chem.* **28,** 582 (1966).

4. Minshen, B. H., Holmes, R. K., and Baxter, C. R., Comparison of radioimmunoassay with an enzymatic assay for gentamicin. *Antimicrob. Agents Chemother.* **7,** 107 (1975).

5. Washington, J. A., II, *Laboratory Procedures in Clinical Microbiology,* Little, Brown and Co., Boston, Mass., 1975, p 309.

6. Modoff, G., Comfort, M., and Kobayashi, G. S., Synergistic action of amphotericin B and 5-fluorocytosine against yeast-like organism. *Proc. Soc. Exp. Biol. Med.* **138,** 571 (1971).

7. Rabinovich, S., Shaw, B. D., Bryant, T., and Danta, S. T., Effect of 5-fluorocytosine and amphotericin B on *Candida albicans* infection in mice. *J. Infect. Dis.* **130,** 28 (1974).

8. Block, E. R., and Bennett, J. E., Pharmacological studies with 5-fluorocytosine. *Antimicrob. Agents Chemother.* **1,** 476 (1972).

9. Kaspar, R. L., and Drutz, D. J., Rapid, simple bioassay for 5-fluorocytosine in the presence of amphotericin B. *Antimicrob. Agents Chemother.* **7,** 462 (1975).

10. Bodey, G. P., Fungal infections complicating acute leukemia. *J. Chronic Dis.* **19,** 668 (1966).

11. Hart, P. D., Russell, E., and Remington, J. S., The compromised host and infection. II. Deep fungal infection. *J. Infect. Dis.* **120,** 172 (1969).

12. Hutter, R. V. S., and Collins, H. S., The occurrence of opportunistic fungus infections in a cancer hospital. *Lab. Invest.* **11,** 1036 (1962).

13. Rifkind, D., Marchioro, T. L., Schneck, S. A., and Hill, R. B., Systemic fungal infections complicating renal transplantation and immunosuppressive therapy. *Am. J. Med.* **43,** 29 (1967).

14. Taschdjian, C. L., Seelig, M. S., and Kozinn, P. J., Serological diagnosis of candidal infections. *CRC Crit. Rev. Clin. Lab. Sci.* **4,** 19 (1973).

15. Steer, P. L., Marks, M. I., Klite, P. D., and Eickhoff, T. C., 5-Fluorocytosine: An oral antifungal compound. *Ann. Intern. Med.* **72,** 15 (1972).

16. Vandevelde, A. G., Mauceri, A. A., and Johnson, J. E., III, 5-Fluorocytosine in the treatment of mycotic infections. *Ann. Intern. Med.* **77,** 43 (1972).

17. Fass, R. J., and Perkins, R. L., 5-Fluorocytosine in the treatment of cryptococcal and candida mycoses. *Ann. Intern. Med.* **74,** 535 (1971).

18. Koechlin, B. A., Rubio, F., and Palmer, S., The metabolism of 5-fluorocytosine-$2^{14}C$ and cytosine-^{14}C in the rat and the disposition of 5-fluorocytosine-$2^{14}C$ in man. *Biochem. Pharmacol.* **15,** 435 (1966).

19. Record, C. O., Skinner, J. M., Sleight, P., and Speller, D. C. E., Candida endocarditis treated with 5-fluorocytosine. *Br. Med. J.* **i,** 262 (1972).

20. Davies, R. R., and Reeves, D. S., 5-Fluorocytosine and candidiasis. *Br. Med. J.* **i,** 577 (1971).

21. Normark, S., and Schonebeck, J., In vitro studies of 5-fluorocytosine resistance in *Candida albicans* and *Torulopsis glabrata. Antimicrob. Agents Chemother.* **2,** 114 (1972).

22. Bishop, C., Rankine, D. M., and Talbott, J. H., The nucleotides in normal human blood. *J. Biol. Chem.* **234,** 1233 (1959).

23. Windeheuser, J. J., Sutter, J. L., and Aven, E., 5-Fluorouracil and derivatives in cancer chemotherapy: Determination of 5-fluorouracil in blood. *J. Pharm. Sci.* **51,** 301 (1972).

24. Cohen, J. L., and Brennan, P. B., GLC assay for 5-fluorouracil in biological fluids. *J. Pharm. Sci.* **62,** 572 (1973).

25. Rao, K. V., Killion, K., and Tanrkiut, Y., GLC determination of fluorouracil. *J. Pharm. Sci.* **63,** 1328 (1974).

26. Pantarotto, C., Martini, A., Blevedere, G. et al., Application of gas chromatography chemical ionization mass fragmentography in the evaluation of bases and nucleoside analogues used in cancer chemotherapy. *J. Chromatogr.* **99,** 519 (1974).

27. Koch-Weser, J., Serum drug concentrations as therapeutic guides. *New Engl. J. Med.* **287,** 227 (1972).

CLIN. CHEM. 22/6, 777-781 (1976)

Gas-Chromatographic Analysis for Therapeutic Concentrations of Amitriptyline and Nortriptyline in Plasma, with Use of a Nitrogen Detector

David N. Bailey and Peter I. Jatlow

We describe a gas-chromatographic procedure for the simultaneous determination of amitriptyline and its active metabolite, nortriptyline, in therapeutic concentrations in human plasma, with use of a nitrogen detector. Both drugs are extracted at pH 10.5 into hexane/isoamyl alcohol, back-extracted into dilute HCl, and re-extracted into hexane/isoamyl alcohol after alkalinization of the HCl. The solvent is evaporated and the residue gas-chromatographed. Protriptyline is used as the internal standard. As little as 5 μg of amitriptyline or nortriptyline can be detected per liter of plasma. The coefficients of variation, for a concentration of 200 μg/liter, are 4.6% and 4.3% within-day and 8.6% and 3.4% day-to-day for amitriptyline and nortriptyline, respectively. The procedure was applied to patients receiving therapeutic doses of both drugs and also to patients who had taken overdoses of amitriptyline.

Additional Keyphrases: *values after overdose* • *toxicology*

Amitriptyline ("Elavil," Merck Sharp & Dohme) and its active *N*-desmethyl metabolite, nortriptyline, also a commercially available therapeutic agent ("Aventyl," Eli Lilly and Co.), are among the most widely administered tricyclic antidepressants (Figure 1). There have been reports of large individual differences in steady-state concentrations in the plasma of patients receiving the same therapeutic doses of these tricyclics, and monitoring these compounds in plasma has become of interest in the treatment of depression (*1–4*). Concentrations of amitriptyline and nortriptyline in plasma after therapeutic doses range from 20 to 300 μg/liter (*5*), and, for nortriptyline, intermediate concentrations (50–140 μg/liter) may provide better clinical response than either lower or higher concentrations (*6*).

While mass fragmentography, with its superior sensitivity and specificity, is ideally suited for the determination of these drugs at such low concentrations (*7*), it is not widely available. Gas–liquid chromatography has been used to measure amitriptyline and nortriptyline (*5, 8–11*); however, in most of these procedures conventional flame-ionization gas chromatography is used, and the lower limit of detection has been at best 20 μg/liter, and involves a rather laborious extraction and derivatization (*5*). Borga and Garle (*8*) reported an electron-capture gas-chromatographic procedure that is sensitive to 10 μg/liter, but it was described only for nortriptyline and also requires an involved extraction and derivatization with heptafluorobutyric anhydride. Wallace et al. (*11*) recently reported another electron-capture gas-chromatographic assay sensitive to 5 μg/liter, but their method requires prior oxidation of both amitriptyline and nortriptyline to the same compound (anthraquinone), so that only a value for total tricyclics is obtained.

Here, we report a relatively simple gas-chromatographic procedure for the simultaneous, direct determination of underivatized amitriptyline and nortriptyline in human plasma at concentrations as low as 5 μg/liter, with use of a selective nitrogen ("alkali flame") detector. Karmen and Guiffrida (*12*) originally described this type of detector.

Materials and Methods

Apparatus

We used a Model 3920 gas–liquid chromatograph equipped with a nitrogen/phosphorus detector (Perkin-Elmer Corp., Norwalk, Conn. 06852). The column was coiled glass (2 mm i.d., 1.8 m long) containing 3% OV-17 on Gas-Chrom Q, 100/120 mesh (Applied Science Laboratories, Inc., State College, Pa. 16801). Relative retention times and peak areas were determined with a PEP-1 data processor (Perkin-Elmer Corp.)

Reagents

All reagents were analytical (AR) grade.

Hexane. This was redistilled and then passed through a 4 cm by 26 cm column of alumina A-540, 80/200 mesh (Fisher Scientific Co., Pittsburgh, Pa. 15219).

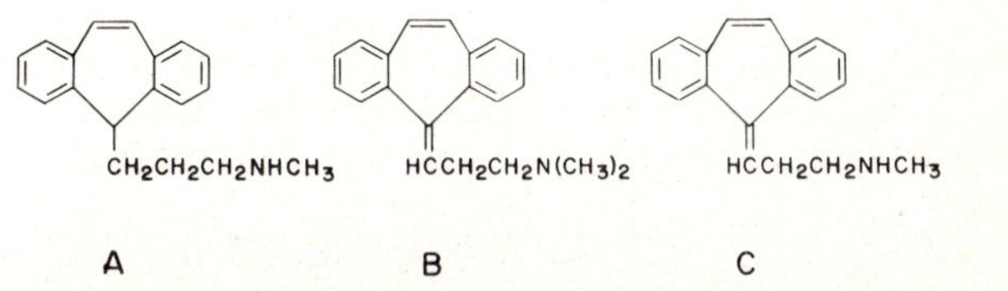

Fig. 1. Structures of (*A*) protriptyline, (*B*) amitriptyline, and (*C*) nortriptyline

Department of Laboratory Medicine, Yale University School of Medicine, New Haven, Conn. 06510.
D.N.B. is an NIH postdoctoral fellow.
Received Oct. 16, 1975; accepted Dec. 10, 1975.

Isoamyl alcohol. This was redistilled.

Methanol. This was redistilled.

Hexane/isoamyl alcohol, 98/2 by vol.

Na_2CO_3, anhydrous.

Saturated Na_2CO_3. This reagent was washed with hexane/isoamyl alcohol before use.

HCl, 0.1 mol/liter. The distilled water used to prepare this solution was first washed with hexane/isoamyl alcohol.

Na_2SO_4, anhydrous.

Standards in Methanol

Store all standards in the freezer (−15 °C). The first three listed should be re-prepared at least once a month.

Protriptyline hydrochloride (internal standard), 1.00 g/liter. Dissolve 10 mg of protriptyline hydrochloride (Merck Sharp & Dohme, Rahway, N. J. 07066) in 10 ml of methanol.

Amitriptyline base, 1.00 g/liter. Dissolve 11.32 mg of amitriptyline hydrochloride (Merck Sharp & Dohme), equivalent to 10 mg of amitriptyline base, in 10 ml of methanol.

Nortriptyline base, 1.00 g/liter. Dissolve 11.38 mg of nortriptyline hydrochloride (Eli Lilly and Co., Indianapolis, Ind. 46206), equivalent to 10 mg of nortriptyline base, in 10 ml of methanol.

Mixed amitriptyline and nortriptyline standard, 100 mg/liter. Dilute 100 μl of each of the 1.00 g/liter solutions of amitriptyline and nortriptyline with 0.8 ml of methanol. Prepare this standard just before each run.

Dilute internal standard in hexane/isoamyl alcohol, 100 μg/liter. Add 10 μl of the 1.00 g/liter protriptyline hydrochloride solution to each 100 ml of the hexane/isoamyl alcohol prepared for the initial extraction. This provides 333 ng of internal standard per milliliter of plasma extracted. Prepare with each run.

Standards in Plasma

Concentrated standard in plasma, 500 μg/liter. Dissolve 100 μl of the mixed standard in 20 ml of drug-free plasma. We prepared the concentrated standard with each run, but it is stable for at least one month if frozen.

Working standards in plasma. For each run, appropriately dilute the concentrated standard with drug-free plasma to achieve the desired concentrations (usually 10–300 μg/liter).

Procedure

All glassware was washed with HCl (1 mol/liter) and rinsed with hexane/isoamyl alcohol before use. Blood from patients receiving therapeutic doses of amitriptyline or nortriptyline was sampled into heparinized glass syringes. Blood from patients who had taken overdoses of amitriptyline was collected into evacuated glass tubes containing no anticoagulant (Vacutainers; Becton-Dickinson, Division of Becton, Dickinson and Co., Rutherford, N. J. 07070). If they were not to be analyzed promptly, the samples were centrifuged and the plasma (or serum) frozen (−15 °C).

Place 3 ml of plasma (samples, drug-free plasma, and plasma standards) into 15-ml glass tubes equipped with Teflon-lined screw caps. Adjust the pH to 10.5 by adding 0.5 ml of saturated Na_2CO_3. Add 10 ml of hexane/isoamyl alcohol *containing the internal standard* and extract for 3 min. Centrifuge at 3000 rpm for 3 min and transfer the upper solvent layer to a clean 15-ml screw-capped tube. Add 1 ml of HCl (0.1 mol/liter), extract for 3 min, and, after centrifugation, aspirate and discard the upper solvent phase. Wash the acid for 1 min with 2 ml of hexane/isoamyl alcohol (*without internal standard*), centrifuge, and discard the upper solvent layer. Add 1 scoopful (about 500 mg) of anhydrous Na_2CO_3 to saturate the aqueous phase, mix well, and extract for 3 min with 2 ml of hexane/isoamyl alcohol (*without internal standard*). After centrifugation, dehydrate the upper solvent layer over anhydrous Na_2SO_4 in a 10-ml test tube. Transfer the solvent to a 5-ml glass centrifuge tube and evaporate it in a stream of nitrogen at room temperature.

Dissolve the residue in 20 μl of methanol and chromatograph 4 μl under the following conditions: column temperature, 235 °C (isothermal); injector temperature, 255 °C; nitrogen detector temperature, 300 °C (detector current setting of 5.9–6.9, corresponding to rubidium glass bead temperatures of about 350–400 °C); carrier gas (helium) flow rate, 20 ml/min; air flow, 400 ml/min; hydrogen, 1 ml/min; and amplifier setting, ×1. Calculate the peak-area ratio (amitriptyline or nortriptyline/protriptyline internal standard) for each sample and determine the plasma concentration by comparison to the peak-area ratios of the extracted standards.

Results

We analyzed 24 different drug-free plasmas, and 16 gave slight responses corresponding in retention time to amitriptyline and nortriptyline, equivalent to 3 μg/liter or less of both. The detection limit for each drug was thus considered to be about 5 μg/liter for the proposed method. The relationship between relative peak area and plasma concentration of amitriptyline and nortriptyline was linear over the range 5 to 300 μg/liter ($r = 0.99$). Nonlinearity was observed at concentrations exceeding 300 μg/liter, and samples were diluted and re-analyzed if above this concentration.

For precision studies, drug-free plasma was supplemented to a concentration of 200 μg each of amitriptyline and nortriptyline per liter. Twelve aliquots of this plasma were analyzed in one day to determine within-day precision and the remaining plasma was frozen (−15 °C). One aliquot of the frozen supplemented plasma was thawed and analyzed on 11 different days during 30 days, to determine day-to-day precision and sample stability. The coefficients of variation were 4.6% and 4.3% within-day and 8.6% and 3.4% day-to-day for amitriptyline and nortriptyline, respectively.

The analytical recovery was 45–50% for both amitriptyline and nortriptyline, determined by comparison of relative peak areas of extracted supplemented plasmas with those of nonextracted methanolic standards.

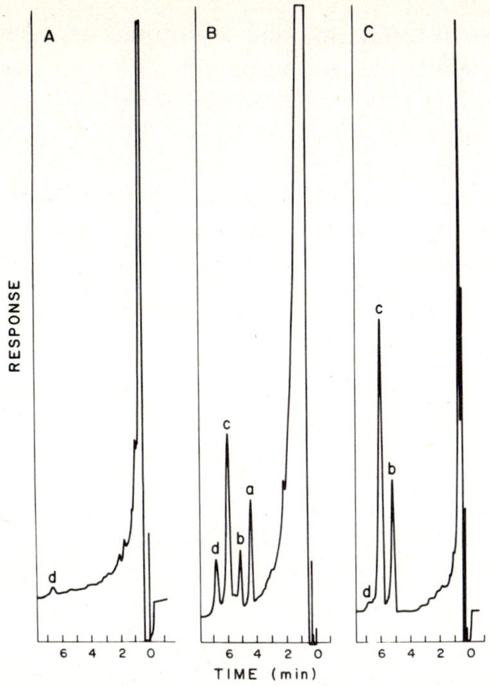

Fig. 2. Chromatograms of plasma extracts of (*A*) a normal volunteer on no medication, no internal standard added; (*B*) a patient on 250 mg of amitriptyline daily (plasma amitriptyline = 133 μg/liter, plasma nortriptyline = 110 μg/liter); and (*C*) a patient on 150 mg of nortriptyline daily (plasma amitriptyline = 0, plasma nortriptyline = 130 μg/liter)

Attenuation, ×128. (*a*, amitriptyline, RRT 0.74; *b*, nortriptyline, RRT 0.86; *c*, protriptyline internal standard, RRT 1.00; *d*, noninterfering contaminant peak, RRT 1.14). RRT: retention time relative to that of the internal standard, protriptyline

This incomplete recovery is corrected for by the use of extracted plasma standards in the proposed procedure.

The stability of the drugs in plasma was established to be at least one month when frozen at −15 °C. The extract residues were stable at least overnight when stored at 4 °C in a desiccator.

When plasma was collected in heparinized glass syringes, essentially "clean" chromatograms were obtained, the background response being equivalent to 3 μg/liter or less for amitriptyline and nortriptyline. In addition, a small noninterfering peak at retention time 1.14 relative to the internal standard was usually seen (peak *d*, Figure 2). This peak was much more pronounced in specimens that had been collected in Vacutainers.

Forty-seven commonly used basic drugs (Table 1) were screened for interference in the assay by comparing the relative retention time of their nonextracted methanolic solutions with those of amitriptyline (0.74) and nortriptyline (0.86) under the chromatographic conditions of the assay. (Acidic drugs, such as barbiturates, would not be recovered under the alkaline extraction conditions of the assay.) Doxepin ("Sinequan," Pfizer) had a relative retention time identical to that of nortriptyline, and, when drug-free plasma was supplemented with doxepin, it extracted and chromatographed as nortriptyline. Desipramine, the active *N*-desmethyl metabolite of imipramine ("Tofranil," Geigy), and itself a commercially available antidepressant ("Pertofrane," USV Pharmaceutical; "Norpramin," Lakeside), was extracted and chromatographed; its retention time corresponded to that of the internal standard, protriptyline. Thus, plasma from patients receiving doxepin would give falsely positive results for nortriptyline, and patients receiving either imipramine or desipramine in addition to amitriptyline or nortriptyline (an unlikely occurrence) would have falsely depressed values for the last two drugs because the response of the internal standard would be enhanced by desipramine. No other interfering drugs were found, although three of the drugs indicated in Table 1 had retention times near those of amitriptyline or nortriptyline, or both.

Table 1. Forty-Seven Common Basic Drugs Screened for Interference

atropine[a]	ethosuximide	perphenazine
benztropine	fluorazepam	phenacetin
caffeine	fluphenazine	phenylpropanol-amine
chlorazepate	haloperidol	prochlorperazine
chlordiazepoxide	hydrochlorothiazide	propoxyphene
chlorothiazide	imipramine[a]	quinine
chlorpheniramine	meperidine	scopolamine[a]
chlorpromazine	methadone	sulfamethoxazole
chlorzoxazone	methamphetamine	tetracycline
cocaine	methapyrilene	thioridazine
codeine	methaqualone	thiothixene
desipramine[b]	methyl phenidate	trihexyphenidyl
dextroamphetamine	morphine	tripelennamine
diazepam	neostigmine	tranylcypromine
diphenhydramine	nicotine	trifluoperazine
doxepin[c]	oxazepam	

[a] Retention time within 0.5 min of that of amitriptyline or nortriptyline.
[b] Extracts and chromatographs like protriptyline (internal standard).
[c] Extracts and chromatographs like nortriptyline.

Plasmas from patients receiving therapeutic doses of the following medications (often administered concomitantly with the tricyclics) were analyzed, to see whether their metabolites interfered: perphenazine, chlorpromazine, thioridazine, and benztropine. None did.

We analyzed 12 plasmas from nine patients in whom therapeutic doses of amitriptyline and (or) nortriptyline had been stabilized (Table 2). In addition, we analyzed 25 samples from 17 patients, each of whom had ingested a nonfatal overdose of medications including amitriptyline. Plasma drug values in overdose ranged up to 1080 μg/liter for amitriptyline, up to 337 μg/liter for nortriptyline, and up to 1260 μg/liter for total tricyclics (sum of both). Data on three overdoses involving amitriptyline alone without other drugs are also shown in Table 2.

To validate the procedure further, we determined four consecutive values for amitriptyline and nortriptyline in one patient who had taken an overdose of amitriptyline, and drew decay curves for amitriptyline,

Table 2. Plasma Concentrations of Amitriptyline and Nortriptyline in Patients

Patient no.	Daily dose	Other medication	Plasma concn, μg/liter: Amitriptyline	Nortriptyline
		Patients on therapeutic doses of nortriptyline:		
1	50 mg	none	0	31
	150 mg	none	0	185
2	50 mg	none	0	50
	200 mg	none	0	208
3	150 mg	none	0	130
	200 mg	none	0	261
4	150 mg	none	0	215
5	200 mg	none	0	278
		Patients on therapeutic doses of amitriptyline:		
6	50 mg	[a]	18	52
7	150 mg	[b]	64	73
8	200 mg	none	28	75
9	250 mg	none	133	110
		Patients who had overdosed with amitriptyline alone:		
10	0.50–0.75 g	none	456	77
11	1.20 g	none	333	204
12	1.25–250 g	none	740	210

[a] Chlorpromazine, 125–150 mg daily.
[b] Thioridazine, 200 mg daily; trihexyphenidyl, 4 mg daily; diphenylhydantoin, 300 mg daily.

nortriptyline, and total tricyclics (the sum of both). All three semilog curves were linear (Figure 3).

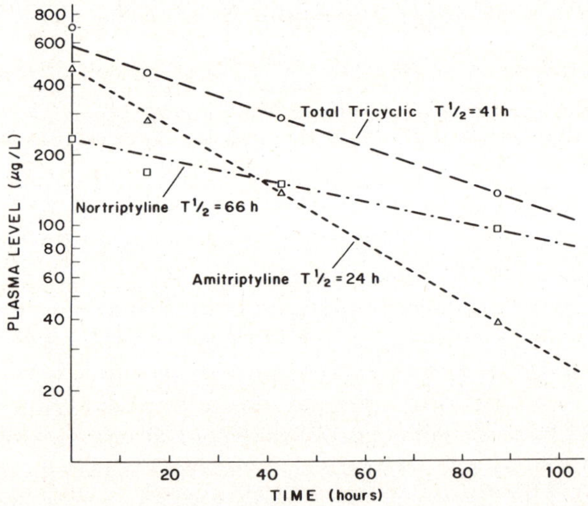

Fig. 3. Semilogarithmic decay curves for plasma amitriptyline, nortriptyline, and total tricyclics (sum of amitriptyline and nortriptyline) in a patient who had taken an overdose of amitriptyline

Discussion

The interest in optimizing drug therapy by monitoring concentrations in blood is increasing, and this is true for the tricyclic antidepressants as well. Values for our series of patients, stabilized on therapeutic doses (Table 2), were similar to those obtained by others (*1–3, 5, 6, 9, 13, 14*), and they displayed moderate individual variation, as has also been previously reported (*1–4*). As expected, both amitriptyline and its desmethyl metabolite nortriptyline were found in the plasmas of patients receiving amitriptyline, but only nortriptyline in patients receiving nortriptyline. Some of our patients were on lower initial doses (50 mg) than in the other reported studies (*1–3, 6, 9, 13, 14*) so that initial values were occasionally lower in our series. As doses were increased, the concentrations in plasma also increased.

Values for amitriptyline after acute amitriptyline overdose were usually greater than those for nortriptyline, probably reflecting insufficient time for mono-*N*-demethylation of the parent drug. Except for three patients, all of our overdose cases had consumed other drugs in addition to amitriptyline, and so we do not now have sufficient data to make adequate clinical correlations. Fatalities have been frequent in other reports of amitriptyline overdose (*10, 15–18*); all our patients survived.

Because concentrations of amitriptyline and nortriptyline in plasma after therapeutic doses are low, conventional flame-ionization gas chromatography at best affords marginal sensitivity, and derivatization is required to enhance the response. These low values, however, are well within the range of measurement achieved by gas chromatography with a selective nitrogen detector, and derivatization is not required.

Because protriptyline is both an isomer of nortriptyline and a structural homolog of amitriptyline (Figure 1), has about the same solubility properties that they have, and is itself only a rarely administered tricyclic antidepressant, we selected it as the internal standard for the assay. It has been used as an internal standard by others in the assay of amitriptyline and nortriptyline (*9, 16*).

Back-extraction of amitriptyline and nortriptyline into dilute HCl provides sufficiently "clean" extracts, free from neutral lipids, and has been used by others (*9*). Our day-to-day use of the nitrogen detector has been described previously (*19*).

We did not study the more polar 10-hydroxyamitriptyline and 10-hydroxynortriptyline metabolites. However, it is unlikely that they would be extracted under the conditions of the proposed method.

Of 47 common basic drugs, only doxepin and desipramine interfered. Doxepin and desipramine, however, themselves tricyclic compounds, would not be administered with amitriptyline or nortriptyline, although hypothetically they could be combined in an overdose situation.

We specifically analyzed plasma from patients receiving therapeutic doses of chlorpromazine, perphenazine, thioridazine, and benztropine (all included in Table 1), to exclude their metabolites as potential interferences, because these drugs are often given in combination with amitriptyline or nortriptyline and one (perphenazine) is combined with amitriptyline in two commercial preparations ("Triavil," Merck Sharp & Dohme; "Etrafon," Schering). No interferences were found. The noninterfering contaminant peak at relative retention time 1.14 (peak *d*, Figure 2) was considerably enhanced in specimens drawn into Vacutainers. It may represent tri(2-butoxyethyl)phosphate, which has been identified by others (*20*). When blood was collected into heparinized glass syringes, as was the case for all our patients on therapeutic doses of the tricyclics, this peak was small.

This work was supported in part by Training Grant 2-T01-GM00696-13 from the NIH and Research Grant DA 01294-06 from the National Institute on Drug Abuse.

We thank Drs. Craig Van Dyke, Donald Sweeney, and Craig Nelson for providing clinical specimens.

Amitriptyline hydrochloride and protriptyline hydrochloride were gifts from Merck Sharp & Dohme, Rahway, N. J. Nortriptyline hydrochloride was a gift from Eli Lilly and Co., Indianapolis, Ind.

References

1. Braithwaite, R. A., Goulding, R., Theano, G., et al., Plasma concentration of amitriptyline and clinical response. *Lancet* **i,** 1297 (1972).

2. Hammer, W., Martens, S., and Sjoqvist, F., A comparative study of the metabolism of desmethylimipramine, nortriptyline, and oxyphenylbutazone in man. *Clin. Pharmacol. Ther.* **10,** 44 (1969).

3. Asberg, M., Cronholm, B., Sjoqvist, F., and Tuck, D., Correlation of subjective side effects with plasma concentrations of nortriptyline. *Br. Med. J.* **iv,** 18 (1970).

4. Glassman, A. H., and Perel, J. M., Plasma levels and tricyclic antidepressants. *Clin. Pharmacol. Ther.* **16,** 198 (1974).

5. Braithwaite, R. A., and Widdop, B., A specific gas-chromatographic method for the measurement of "steady-state" plasma levels of amitriptyline and nortriptyline in patients. *Clin. Chim. Acta* **35,** 461 (1971).

6. Asberg, M., Cronholm, B., Sjoqvist, F., and Tuck, D., Relationship between plasma level and therapeutic effect of nortriptyline. *Br. Med. J.* **iii,** 331 (1971).

7. Borga, O., Palmer, L., Linnarsson, A., and Holmstedt, B., Quantitative determination of nortriptyline and desmethylnortriptyline in human plasma by combined gas chromatography-mass spectrometry. *Anal. Lett.* **4,** 837 (1971).

8. Borga, O., and Garle, M., A gas chromatographic method for the quantitative determination of nortriptyline and some of its metabolites in human plasma and urine. *J. Chromatogr.* **68,** 77 (1972).

9. Hucker, H. B., and Stauffer, S. C., GLC method for quantitative determination of amitriptyline in human plasma. *J. Pharm. Sci.* **63,** 296 (1974).

10. Norheim, G., The simultaneous determination of amitriptyline and nortriptyline in post mortem blood and urine using gas-liquid chromatography. *J. Chromatogr.* **88,** 403, (1974).

11. Wallace, J. E., Hamilton, H. E., Goggin, L. K., and Blum, K., Determination of amitriptyline at nanogram levels in serum by electron capture gas-liquid chromatography. *Anal. Chem.* **47,** 1516 (1975).

12. Karmen, A., and Guiffrida, L., Enhancement of the response of the hydrogen flame ionization detector to compounds containing halogen and phosphorous. *Nature* **201,** 1204 (1964).

13. Sjoqvist, F., A pharmacokinetic approach to the treatment of depression. *Int. Pharmacopsychiatry* **6,** 147 (1971).

14. Asberg, M., Individualization of treatment with tricyclic compounds. *Med. Clin. North Am.* **58,** 1083 (1974).

15. Spiker, D. G., Weiss, A. N., Chang, S. S., et al., Tricyclic antidepressant overdose: Clinical presentation and plasma levels. *Clin. Pharmacol. Ther.* **18,** 539 (1975).

16. Gard, H., Knapp, D., Walle, T., and Gaffney, T., Qualitative and quantitative studies on the disposition of amitriptyline and other tricyclic antidepressant drugs in man as it relates to the management of the overdosed patient. *Clin. Toxicol.* **6,** 571 (1973).

17. Norheim, G., Distribution of amitriptyline and nortriptyline in fatal amitriptyline intoxications with different survival times. *Forensic Sci.* **4,** 187 (1974).

18. Glogner, P., Heni, N., Herkel, L., and Hoefer, G., Toedliche Limbratril-F-Intoxikation. *Dtsch. Med. Wochenschr.* **98,** 2472 (1973).

19. Jatlow, P. I., and Bailey, D. N., Gas-chromatographic analysis for cocaine in human plasma with use of a nitrogen detector. *Clin. Chem.* **21,** 1918 (1975).

20. Costello, C. E., Hertz, H. S., Sakai, T., and Biemann, K., Routine use of a flexible gas chromatograph-mass spectrometer computer system to identify drugs and their metabolites in body fluids of overdose victims. *Clin. Chem.* **20,** 255 (1974).

Liquid Chromatographic Method for Monitoring Therapeutic Concentrations of L-Dopa and Dopamine in Serum

Ralph M. Riggin, Richard L. Alcorn, and Peter T. Kissinger[1]

We describe a new method for the simultaneous assay of 3,4-dihydroxyphenylalanine (L-dopa) and dopamine in serum. Both compounds have been determined quantitatively at concentrations as low as 10 μg/liter with a coefficient of variation of less than 4%. Peak heights were linearly related to concentration up to 10 mg/liter for each compound. Assay of human sera gave within-run and day-to-day coefficients of variation of 2.8% and 3.1% for L-dopa, and 2.9% and 3.7% for dopamine. The linear relationship between readings (nA, y-axis) and concentration (μg/liter) is described by the following equations: $y = (21.0 \pm 0.082)x + (0.46 \pm 0.31$ SD) for L-dopa and $y = (17.0 \pm 0.10)x + (0.08 \pm 0.04$ SD) for dopamine. The procedure combines liquid/solid extraction, liquid chromatography, and controlled-potential electrochemistry. The simplicity, sensitivity, and accuracy of this method make it suitable for routine clinical analysis of serum samples to optimize bioavailability for individual patients. After the extraction procedure is completed, samples can be analyzed at the rate of 10/h.

Additional Keyphrases: *monitoring efficacy of dopa decarboxylase inhibitors • electrochemical detection of eluate • dopamine sulfate esters*

The importance of L-dopa (3,4-dihydroxyphenylalanine) in the treatment of Parkinson's disease is well established (*1*). Therapy with L-dopa consists of gradually increasing the daily dosage until the optimum response is reached, usually within two to three weeks (*2*). The amount of drug required can be reduced significantly by concomitant dosing with extracerebral dopa decarboxylase (EC 4.1.1.28) inhibitors such as carbidopa (*3*). The ratio of dopamine to L-dopa in the serum indicates the effectiveness of the dopa decarboxylase inhibitor. The bioavailability of the unaltered drug and the effectiveness of the inhibitor are not routinely evaluated for individual patients because of the lack of a satisfactory assay. There is a definite need for a clinically feasible simultaneous method for L-dopa and dopamine in serum.

The most widely used methods of analysis for catecholamines have been variations of the classical fluorometric approach (*4–7*). These procedures involve conversion of the previously isolated and separated catecholamines to fluorescent derivatives. Simultaneous assay of the individual catecholamines by these methods is difficult and not well suited to routine clinical application. Most commonly, "total catecholamines" are measured, referring only to norepinephrine and epinephrine, but not L-dopa and dopamine. Recently, other techniques for catecholamine analysis have been introduced. Various groups have advocated gas chromatography with flame ionization (*8*), electron capture (*9*), or mass spectrometric detection (*9, 10*).

Because of the similarity of the molecules, many of the classical methods for L-dopa analysis will work equally well for the hypotensive drug α-methyl dopa. The fluorescent and colorimetric methods are not highly selective, and therefore any L-dopa present, if not first separated, may interfere with the α-methyl dopa analysis. Gas chromatographic (*11*) and electrochemical methods (*12*) are superior in this regard.

This paper describes an assay for L-dopa and dopamine (3,4-dihydroxyphenethylamine) in serum by high-performance liquid chromatography with electrochemical detection (*13*). Our approach consists of isolating and preconcentrating the catechols by liquid/solid extraction, then separating them on a high-performance strong cation-exchange resin (*14*). L-Dopa and dopamine are determined in a single chromatogram in 6 min. The dopa decarboxylase inhibitor, carbidopa, does not interfere in the analysis.

Materials and Methods

Reagents

Hydrochloric acid, 6 mol/liter, and 370 ml/liter.

Disodium ethylenediaminetetraacetate, 100 g/liter.

Sodium metabisulfite, 50 g/liter. Store refrigerated and prepare freshly every two weeks.

Phosphate buffer, pH 7.4. Dissolve 1.18 g of potassium monobasic phosphate and 8.16 g of sodium dibasic phosphate heptahydrate in 1 liter of distilled water.

Sodium hydroxide, 500 g/liter, 3 mol/liter, and 1 mol/liter.

Acetic acid, 1 mol/liter.

Mobile phase, 10 mmol/liter H_2SO_4 and 40 mmol/liter Na_2SO_4.

Alumina. Acid wash Woelm W200 neutral alumina, according to the method of Anton and Sayre (*15*).

Aqueous standards. Dissolve 61.6 mg of dopamine hydrochloride and 50.0 mg of L-dopa in individual

Department of Chemistry, Purdue University, West Lafayette, Ind. 47907.

[1] Address correspondence to this author.

Received Sept. 9, 1975; accepted Jan. 6, 1976.

500-ml volumetric flasks. Dilute to the mark with 0.1 mol/liter $HClO_4$. These solutions are stored refrigerated. No degradation was detected after 10 weeks.

Serum pool. Collect about 100 ml of blood from healthy humans. Store aliquots of the serum in 5-ml vials at −35 °C so that only the required amount of serum need be thawed for each analysis. Working standards are prepared daily by adding 10-μl aliquots of the aqueous standards of dopamine and L-dopa (100 mg/liter, in 0.1 mol/liter $HClO_4$) to 1 ml of the serum pool. The working standard will then contain 1 mg of each compound per liter.

Apparatus

The liquid chromatographic system was identical to that previously described (*13*), with the addition of a 2-cm precolumn (*15*) and a pneumatically actuated 20-μl slider valve for sample injection (Laboratory Data Control, Riviera Beach, Fla.; Model CSVA-20). We used a commercial electrochemical detector based on our earlier work (Bioanalytical Systems Inc., P.O. Box 2206, West Lafayette, Ind. 47906; Model LC-2). The strong cation-exchange resin was dry packed in a 50 cm × 2 mm i.d. glass column (Altex Scientific, 1450 Sixth St., Berkeley, Calif. 94710; Model 251-02). The pellicular resin used was a Vydac bonded-phase cation-exchange resin (The Separations Group, 8738 Oakwood Ave., Hesperia, Calif. 92345; Model 232CX). Water was circulated through a jacket (Altex, Model 251-10) surrounding the column to maintain a temperature of 28 °C. The mobile phase was pumped at a rate of 0.40 ml/min. The detector potential was set at +0.72 V vs. an Ag/AgCl reference electrode.

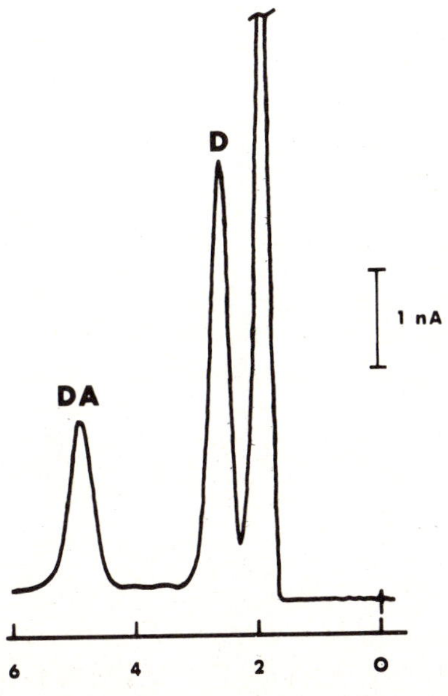

Fig. 1. Recorder tracing of results of liquid-chromatographic assay of L-dopa and dopamine isolated from serum

D (L-dopa): 1.1 ng injected; 140 μg/liter of serum; *DA* (dopamine): 0.35 ng injected; 44 μg/liter of serum

Procedure

Place 1 ml of blood serum, 3.5 ml of saturated sodium chloride solution, and 100 μl of concentrated hydrochloric acid in a 15-ml polypropylene centrifuge tube. Shake well and centrifuge for 15 min at 15 000 × *g* to precipitate the protein. Pour the supernate into a 12-ml glass centrifuge tube. Hydrolyze sulfate conjugates by heating in a 90 °C water bath for 20 min. Cool the tubes and then add 0.5 g of ammonium sulfate. Extract twice with ethyl acetate and once with hexane (5-ml portions of each). Centrifuge briefly, aspirate, and discard the nonaqueous layers.

Place the aqueous layer in a 10-ml beaker with a magnetic stirrer. Add 100 μl of both the ethylenediaminetetraacetate and the sodium metabisulfite solutions. While stirring the mixture, adjust the pH to 8.5 ± 0.1 by rapid addition of 3 mol/liter sodium hydroxide and then 1 mol/liter sodium hydroxide. Shake with 60 mg of acid-washed alumina in a 5-ml conical screw-cap vial (Pierce Chemical Co., Box 117, Rockford, Ill. 61105; Reacti-Vials) for 12 min. Allow the alumina to settle and then aspirate and discard the serum solution. Wash the alumina once with the phosphate buffer and twice with distilled water. Dry the alumina in a vacuum oven for 10 min at 40 °C.

Elute the L-dopa and dopamine from the alumina with 300 μl of 1 mol/liter acetic acid. Gently shake the vials for 10 min on a mechanical shaker. Transfer about 200 μl of the eluent to a second vial. Inject 20 μl of this solution onto the chromatographic column. Measure the peak heights and calculate the concentrations by comparison with the peak heights obtained for the working standard containing a known concentration (1 mg/liter) of L-dopa and dopamine.

Results and Discussion

Figure 1 depicts a chromatogram for a sample isolated from the serum of a patient undergoing L-dopa therapy. This example was chosen because the concentration of L-dopa (140 μg/liter) is lower than is normally expected for a therapeutic dose and because most previous methods have a detection limit of about 1 mg/liter. Because the amount of L-dopa present in the blood of Parkinson's disease patients on L-dopa therapy is frequently about 1 mg/liter (*2*), it is desirable to be able to measure lower concentrations, particularly for pharmacokinetic studies. The present method permits measurements down to 10 μg/liter with a precision of better than ±4%. In addition, dopamine can be quantitated simultaneously down to the same limit, which makes the method well suited to following the efficacy of decarboxylase inhibitors. This latter capability is unique to the present assay. The two dopamine sulfate esters cannot yet be monitored directly and thus a hydrolysis procedure is necessary, to establish the total dopamine present. These esters are known to constitute a major part of the serum dopamine (*17*).

We know of no probable endogenous interferences with this assay, because of the highly specific combination of liquid chromatography and electrochemistry.

Table 1. Precision Data for the Chromatographic Assay

	L-Dopa (n = 8)	Dopamine (n = 8)
Within-run, CV, %	2.8	2.9
Day-to-day, CV, %	3.1	3.7
Analytical recovery, %	95.1	98.8
Analytical recovery, CV, %	3.0	3.7

We are now using the method routinely for clinical samples. Very similar procedures have been devised for monitoring other catechol-based drugs in serum (e.g., α-methyl dopa and carbidopa). We believe that the approach described here has general applicability to compounds of this type, although slight modifications in conditions may be necessary to optimize the assay for a particular drug. Other commercial column packings (e.g., Du Pont "Zipax SCX") than that used here will improve the resolution in certain situations. For example, when both carbidopa and L-dopa are administered together, they are better resolved with Zipax SCX as the stationary phase.

Table 1 summarizes precision and recovery data for the assay. The linear relation between readings and concentration was tested by adding standard amounts of each compound to the serum pool over a range from 50 μg/liter to 10 mg/liter and analyzing. The linear response in nanoamperes (y) vs. μg/liter (x) is described by the following equations:

$$y = (21.0 \pm 0.082)x + (0.46 \pm 0.31 \text{ SD}) \text{ for L-dopa}$$

and

$$y = (17.0 \pm 0.10)x + (0.08 \pm 0.04 \text{ SD}) \text{ for dopamine.}$$

After the extraction procedure is completed, samples can be analyzed at the rate of 10 per hour.

This investigation was supported by grants from the NIGMS, NIH (grants GM21580-01 and GM22713-01), the National Science Foundation (grant GP-42452X), and the Showalter Trust Fund. We thank Dr. David C. Wenke (Erie County Laboratory, Buffalo, N. Y.) for helpful discussion and exchange of samples.

References

1. Marka, J., *The Treatment of Parkinsonism with L-Dopa,* American Elsevier, New York, N. Y., 1974.

2. Hare, T. A., Beaseley, B. L., Chambers, R. A., et al., Dopa and amino acid levels in plasma and cerebrospinal fluid of patients with Parkinson's disease before and during treatment with L-dopa. *Clin. Chim. Acta* **45,** 273 (1973).

3. Vickers, S., Stuart, E. K., Hucker, H. B., and VandenHeuvel, W. J. A., Further studies on the metabolism of carbidopa, (−)-L-α-hydrazino-3,4-dihydroxy-α-methylbenzenepropanoic acid monohydrate, in the human, rhesus monkey, dog and rat. *J. Med. Chem.* **18,** 134 (1974).

4. Hare, T. A., and Vogel, W. H., Rapid estimation of DOPA in physiological fluids using the amino acid analyzer. *Biochem. Med.* **4,** 277 (1970).

5. Johnson, J. C., Gold, G. J., and Clouet, D. H., An improved method for the assay of dopa. *Anal. Biochem.* **54,** 129 (1973).

6. Atack, C. V., The determination of dopamine by a modification of the dihydroxyindole fluorimetric assay. *Br. J. Pharmacol.* **48,** 699 (1973).

7. Spiegel, H. E., and Tonchen, A. E., Semiautomated method for measurement of dopa in plasma. *Clin. Chem.* **16,** 763 (1970).

8. Watson, J. R., Determination of levodopa and levodopa products by GLC. *J. Pharm. Sci.* **63,** 96 (1974).

9. Lhuguenot, J-C., and Maume, B. F., Improvements in quantitative gas phase analysis of catecholamines in the picomole range by electron-capture detection and mass fragmentography of their pentafluorobenzylamine–trimethyl derivatives. *J. Chromatogr. Sci.* **12,** 411 (1974).

10. Curtius, H. Ch., Wolfensberger, M., Steinmann, B., et al., Mass fragmentography of dopamine and 6-hydroxydopamine. *J. Chromatogr.* **99,** 529 (1974).

11. Watson, J. R., and Lawrence, R. C., Specific quantitative gas-liquid chromatography of methyl dopa and some foreign related amino acids in raw material and commercial tablets. *J. Chromatogr.* **103,** 63 (1975).

12. Riggin, R. M., Rau, L-D., Alcorn, R. L., and Kissinger, P. T., Determination of phenolic sympathetic stimulants in pharmaceuticals by liquid chromatography with electrochemical detection. *Anal. Lett.* **7,** 791 (1974).

13. Kissinger, P. T., Felice, L. J., Riggin, R. M., et al., Electrochemical detection of selected organic components in the eluate from high performance liquid chromatography. *Clin. Chem.* **20,** 992 (1974).

14. Kissinger, P. T., Riggin, R. M., Alcorn, R. L., and Rau, L-D., Estimation of catecholamines in urine by high performance liquid chromatography with electrochemical detection. *Biochem. Med.* **13,** 299 (1975).

15. Pachla, L. A., and Kissinger, P. T., Precolumn for high performance liquid chromatography. *Anal. Chem.* **48,** 237 (1976).

16. Anton, A. H., and Sayre, D. F., A study of the aluminum oxide trihydroxyindole procedure for the analysis of catecholamines. *J. Pharmacol. Exp. Ther.* **138,** 360 (1962).

17. Tyce, G. M., Sharpless, N. S., and Meunter, M. D., Free and conjugated dopamine in plasma during levodopa therapy. *Clin. Pharmacol. Ther.* **16,** 782 (1974).

CLIN. CHEM. 22/6, 785–788 (1976)

Enzymatic Assay for Methotrexate in Serum and Cerebrospinal Fluid

Larry C. Falk,[1] Dennis R. Clark,[2] Sumner M. Kalman,[2] and Thomas F. Long[3]

We describe an assay for methotrexate in biological fluids. The assay is based on inhibition by methotrexate of dihydrofolate reductase from *Lactobacillus casei*. The lower limit of sensitivity in serum is 2×10^{-8} mol (about 10 μg) of methotrexate per liter. Within-run precision is ±5% (coefficient of variation) and day-to-day variation is 18%. Advantages of the assay are ease of manipulation, high sensitivity, and specificity.

Additional Keyphrases: *cancer treatment • psoriasis treatment • drug assay*

Methotrexate (MTX) is a folic acid antagonist widely used in cancer chemotherapy (*1–4*) and sometimes in severe psoriasis (*5*). In recent years high doses of MTX followed by citrovorum factor "rescue" have been used in treating certain tumors (*6*). The citrovorum factor restores the body pools of tetrahydrofolate cofactors, which are depleted in the presence of MTX. MTX blocks the reduction of folic acid and dihydrofolic acid to tetrahydrofolic acid by inhibiting the enzyme tetrahydrofolate dehydrogenase (EC 1.5.1.3). Although it is thought that MTX damages sensitive tumors more than other rapidly proliferating tissues (*1*), such selectivity is not complete, and serious toxicity—including skin rash, myelosuppression, mucosal ulceration, and renal damage—can result. Monitoring serum methotrexate to predict toxicity after high-dose MTX therapy is reported (*7–9*). In addition, a correlation has been demonstrated between cerebrospinal fluid MTX concentrations and neurotoxicity after intrathecal administration of MTX (*10*). Use of serum MTX values to adjust the citrovorum factor dose and avert impending toxicity has also been reported (*7*). Such monitoring is likely to assume a greater role in the treatment of cancer and psoriasis with MTX in the future.

[1] Department of Pharmacology, Stanford University, [2] Drug Assay Laboratory, Stanford University Hospital, and [3] Children's Hospital, Stanford, Calif. 94305.

Received Nov. 3, 1975; accepted Feb. 25, 1976.

The enzyme-inhibition assay for MTX has been available for over a decade (*11, 12*) and has been used in studies of the pharmacology of MTX (*1, 8, 9, 13*). Unfortunately, descriptions of this assay have not been sufficiently detailed to enable clinical laboratories without expertise in enzyme kinetics to adopt the method. In addition, handling and storage of dihydrofolate, the substrate for the method, has required special care. The commercial availability of the enzyme and of dihydrofolic acid has prompted us to develop a simple procedure for measuring MTX. The method is accurate, fast, sensitive, and precise, and can be used with any recording spectrophotometer capable of monitoring absorbance at 340 nm, although the instrument described below has proved particularly efficient. We have been using this assay to monitor high-dose therapy with MTX in children since September 1974 in a drug-assay laboratory staffed by medical technologists.

Materials and Methods

Instrumentation

Spectrophotometer. Absorbances were measured with a Model 300N Microsample Spectrophotometer with a 3017-T aspirating thermocuvette (Gilford Instrument Laboratories, Inc., Oberlin, Ohio 44074). The wavelength was 340 nm; the cuvette was maintained at 30 °C, and was set to aspirate 0.9 ml.

Data presentation. Changes in absorbance (ΔA) were measured and recorded by a Timer/Printer (Syva Corp., Palo Alto, Calif. 94304). The program was set on "ΔA", the delay time at 20 s, and the read time at 120 s. We found this Timer/Printer ideally suited to this task, although the assay can be performed by any instrument, including a strip-chart recorder, capable of accurately recording ΔA.

Dihydrofolate dispenser. A PB 600-1 Repeating Dispenser (Hamilton Co., Reno, Nev. 89502) was used, fitted with a 1.0-ml Hamilton gas-tight syringe, so that it dispensed precise 20-μl aliquots.

Reagents

Reaction buffer. A mixture of 0.7 ml of β-mercaptoethanol (Eastman Organic Chemicals, Rochester, N.Y. 14650), 50 ml of tris(hydroxymethyl)aminomethane buffer (1 mol/liter, pH 7.5) and 20 ml of ethylenediaminetetraacetic acid (50 mmol/liter) was diluted to 1 liter. The reaction buffer is stable for at least two months when stored at 4 °C.

Methotrexate calibrators. Sodium methotrexate (supplied by the National Cancer Institute, NIH, Bethesda, Md. 20014) was diluted with water to obtain five concentrations between 2.0×10^{-8} and 3.0×10^{-7} mol/liter (calculated as the free acid). Stored frozen in 1-ml aliquots, these calibrators were stable for at least seven weeks.

Dihydrofolate buffer. A mixture of 25 ml of tris(hydroxymethyl)aminomethane buffer (1.0 mol/liter, pH 7.5) and 5.3 ml of β-mercaptoethanol was diluted to 250 ml with distilled water. This buffer is stable at least two months at 4 °C.

Dihydrofolic acid. This was purchased from Sigma Chemical Co., St. Louis, Mo. 63178, in 25-mg ampules. The contents of an ampule were washed into a beaker with 10.0 ml of a mixture of 5 mmol/liter HCl and 14 mmol/liter β-mercaptoethanol. The resulting suspension was stirred while 0.3 ml was withdrawn and dissolved in 2.7 ml of the dihydrofolate buffer. When 20 μl of this solution was added to 1.0 ml of reaction buffer, the absorbance in the 1-cm pathlength cell of the spectrophotometer was 0.075 ± 5 *A*. (If necessary, the concentration of the suspension was adjusted to bring the absorbance into the proper range.) The suspension was stored in 0.3-ml aliquots in plastic culture tubes. Stored capped and frozen at −20 °C in the dark, this preparation is stable for at least two months.

Dihydrofolate solution. An aliquot of dihydrofolic acid for the assay was prepared each day by thawing a tube of the suspension and diluting it with 2.7 ml of the dihydrofolate buffer. The resulting solution was then loaded into the 1.0-ml Hamilton Dispenser. Both the filled dispenser and the tube containing the unused dihydrofolic acid solution were stored in crushed ice. The dispenser was refilled from the tube as needed, and the unused portion was discarded at the end of the day.

Dihydrofolate reductase (EC 1.5.1.3). We used an enzyme preparation from *Lactobacillus casei.* (This enzyme is now available from the New England Enzyme Center, Boston, Mass. 02111.) The specific activity was 90 μmol/h per milligram of protein. The enzyme is stored in a desiccator at −20 °C. Individual tubes containing 0.25-mg samples of the enzyme for use in the assay were prepared by dissolving 25 mg of the powder in 10 ml of distilled water, and dividing the solution into 100-μl aliquots in 12 × 75 mm disposable plastic culture tubes. Stored capped and frozen, this preparation is stable for at least two months.

NADPH was purchased from Sigma Chemical Co. in vials containing 1.0 mg each.

Reaction mixture. This was prepared freshly each day. Seventy milliliters of reaction buffer was measured into a graduated cylinder. The contents of one 1-mg vial of NADPH and one tube of enzyme were rinsed into a 100-ml amber-colored bottle with the buffer. The bottle was capped and inverted gently several times to mix the contents. This mixture was kept in crushed ice and any unused portion was discarded at the end of the day.

Patient samples. Serum, cerebrospinal fluid, and plasma (containing heparin, fluoride, oxalate, or EDTA anticoagulants) were used. Serum specimens were stable for at least six months when stored frozen at −20 °C, but only for three days at room temperature.

Procedure

A set of calibrators and a methotrexate control sample were thawed in a beaker of water at room temperature. The reaction mixture and dihydrofolate solution were prepared as above. Twenty microliters of a calibrator was pipetted with an Eppendorf pipet or a suitable dilutor into a 12 × 75 mm disposable glass culture tube. One milliliter of the reaction mixture was then added. The spectrophotometer cuvet was rinsed with distilled water, then purged with air for 5 s. Dihydrofolate solution, 20 μl, was dispensed into the reaction tube from the Hamilton Dispenser. The tube was then vortex-mixed briefly (1–2 s) and the entire solution was aspirated into the cuvet of the spectrophotometer. This aspiration automatically started the timer and, after a delay of 20 s, the initial absorbance was printed. The change in absorbance (Δ*A*) was printed 120 s later. The five calibrators were each assayed once, and a "zero calibrator" of distilled water was included. The values of Δ*A* were plotted vs. the methotrexate concentration (Figure 1) to obtain a calibration curve. Patients' samples (serum or cerebrospinal fluid), and the methotrexate control were assayed in the same way. Serial tenfold dilutions with water were made to obtain a Δ*A* value which fell within the range of the calibrators.

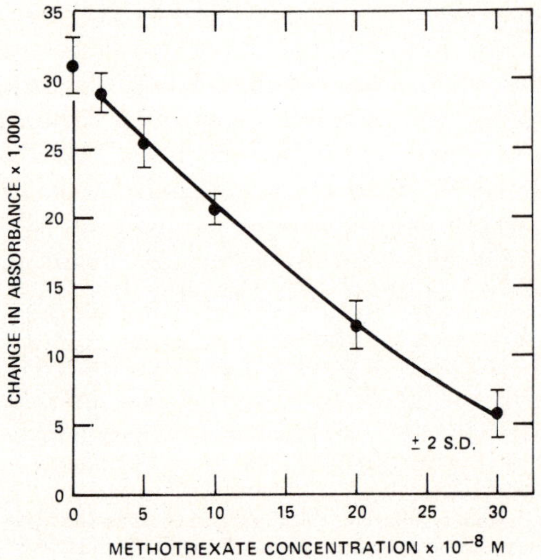

Fig. 1. Calibration curve for MTX assay

Results for patient samples were checked by making a further dilution with water to obtain another value of ΔA for each sample that fell within the range of the calibrators. A separate calibration curve was run with each batch of reaction mixture and dihydrofolic acid. A control containing 5.0×10^{-7} mol of MTX per liter of plasma was diluted 10-fold and assayed daily.

A calibration curve was stable for 12 h. Individual patient's samples could be analyzed in about 5 min, once the calibration curve was established.

Results

The assay measures MTX in concentrations of 2.0×10^{-8} to 3.0×10^{-7} mol/liter. Samples were diluted in 10-fold steps with water to obtain a concentration in this range. Serum samples were obtained from 50 hospitalized patients receiving various drugs other than MTX. Included were icteric, lipemic, and hemolyzed specimens. Each sample gave the expected result when analyzed as a blank (no MTX) and with MTX added to a concentration of 1.0×10^{-7} mol/liter.

Within-run precision was measured by 20 replicate assays of a plasma standard that contained 8.0×10^{-6} mol/liter MTX. The range of values obtained was 6.8×10^{-6} to 8.0×10^{-6} mol/liter (corresponding to $\pm 0.001A$) with an average of 7.5×10^{-6} mol/liter and a standard deviation (SD) of 0.43×10^{-6} mol/liter. Day-to-day precision was monitored by running a plasma control standard containing 5.0×10^{-7} mol/liter. These were run daily under routine assay conditions by six different technologists during 29 days. The mean of the 29 determinations was $6.3 \pm 1.2 \times 10^{-7}$ mol/liter.

Samples were sent to two other laboratories for comparison analysis. The results are indicated in Table 1. The range of MTX concentrations encountered in monitoring high-dose MTX therapy of osteosarcoma in children is from approximately 10^{-3} mol/liter to less than 10^{-8} mol/liter, depending on the dose and time of sampling (*7–9*).

Table 1. Concentration of Methotrexate in 18 Sera, as Measured in Three Laboratories

Our lab.	Lab. 1[a]	Lab. 2[b]
	mol/liter	
8.5×10^{-6}	7.73×10^{-6}	
6.5×10^{-6}	4.49×10^{-6}	
4.4×10^{-6}	2.58×10^{-6}	
2.4×10^{-3}	2.49×10^{-3}	
7.0×10^{-7}	3.47×10^{-7}	
1.4×10^{-3}	1.24×10^{-3}	
9.7×10^{-6}	8.4×10^{-6}	
3.6×10^{-7}	3.86×10^{-7}	
1.7×10^{-3}	1.32×10^{-3}	
6.4×10^{-6}	3.73×10^{-6}	
1.7×10^{-6}	1.28×10^{-6}	
4.7×10^{-6}	3.86×10^{-6}	
1.5×10^{-3}		1.98×10^{-3}
1.5×10^{-3}		1.32×10^{-3}
3.0×10^{-4}		5.51×10^{-4}
4.0×10^{-4}		6.61×10^{-4}
5.9×10^{-6}		1.1×10^{-5}
4.8×10^{-5}		4.3×10^{-5}

[a] Similar enzymatic methods: Linear-regression analysis of the logs of the results yields $y = 0.974x - 0.0316$; $r = 0.998$

[b] Fluorometric method (*16*): Linear-regression analysis of the logs of the results yields $y = 0.990x - 0.026$; $r = 0.990$

Discussion

Methotrexate has found increasing application in cancer chemotherapy and continues to be used in the treatment of severe psoriasis. Laboratory evidence indicates that serum methotrexate concentrations in mice can be correlated with inhibition of DNA synthesis in tissues (*13*). Clinical studies indicate that serum methotrexate determinations can help predict toxicity and guide supportive therapy during methotrexate treatment (*7–10*). These studies and the expanding use of this drug underscore the need for a simple assay suitable for routine use by clinical laboratories.

At least five assays are currently available for MTX quantification: fluorometric (*16*), bacteriological (*15*), radioimmunological (*17*), direct ligand binding (*18*), and enzyme inhibition (*11, 12, 19*). Fluorometric methods require difficult manipulations and are at least an order of magnitude less sensitive than enzyme inhibition techniques. The microbiological assay, although sensitive, requires a 36-h incubation period and suffers from a large variability that limits its clinical usefulness. The relatively new radioimmunoassay of MTX has good inherent sensitivity for aqueous solutions, however, interference from serum constituents currently limits its usefulness. The direct ligand binding assay, while sensitive, requires time-consuming manipulation, complicated calculations, and expensive equipment. In existing enzymatic methods, the stability and availability of reagents has been a serious problem. These difficulties have precluded its use as a routine, fast, analytical method.

The method described in this paper suffers from none of the above limitations. It is sensitive, precise, accurate, and specific. It uses a common clinical laboratory instrument and commercially available reagents. Details are given for the manipulation and storage of reagents. We believe that this method can be adopted by most clinical chemistry laboratories and that it is a vital adjunct to MTX therapy.

The cooperation and advice of Dr. Roy Kisliuk of Tufts University, who also supplied the enzyme we used in this method, is gratefully acknowledged. We also thank Mr. Jerry Derr (National Cancer Institute) for his cooperation and helpful discussions, Dr. Marian Freeman-Narrod (Albert Einstein Medical Center, Northern Division, Philadelphia, Pa.) and Dr. Terry Schultz (Mountain States Tumor Institute, Boise, Idaho) for analysis of comparison samples. This work was supported in part by USPHS-NIH Training Grant GM-0322-15.

References

1. Frei, E., III, Jaffe, N., Tattersall, M. H. N., et al., New approaches to cancer chemotherapy with methotrexate. *New Engl. J. Med.* **292,** 846 (1975).

2. Hertz, R., Lewis, J., Jr., and Lipsett, M. B., Five years' experience with the chemotherapy of metastatic choriocarcinoma and related trophoblastic tumors in women. *Am. J. Obstet. Gynecol.* **82,** 631 (1961).

3. Capizzi, R. L., DeConti, R. C., Marsh, J. C., and Bertino, J. R., Methotrexate therapy of head and neck cancer; improvement in therapeutic index by the use of leucovorin "rescue." *Cancer Res.* **30,** 1782 (1970).

4. Djerassi, I., Rominger, C. J., Kim, J. S., et al., Phase I study of high doses of methotrexate with citrovorum factor in patients with lung cancer. *Cancer* (Philadelphia) **30,** 22 (1972).

5. Weinstein, G. D., Methotrexate for psoriasis. *J. Am. Med. Assoc.* **225,** 412 (1973).

6. Djerassi, I., High-dose methotrexate (NSC-740) and citrovorum factor (NSC-3590) rescue: Background and rationale. *Cancer Chemother. Rep.* **6,** Part 3, pp 3–6 (1975).

7. Falk, L. C., Long, T. F., and Kalman, S. M., The use of serum methotrexate levels to reduce toxicity during high dose methotrexate leucovorin rescue therapy for osteogenic sarcoma in children. *Pharmacologist* **17,** 201 (1975).

8. Tattersall, M. H. N., Parker, L. M., Pitman, S. W., and Frei, E. III, Clinical pharmacology of high-dose methotrexate (NSC-740). *Cancer Chemother. Rep.* **6,** Part 3, p 25 (1975).

9. Stoller, R. G., Jacobs, S. A., Drake, J. C., et al., Pharmacokinetics of high-dose methotrexate (NSC-740). *Cancer Chemother. Rep.* **6,** Part 3, p 19 (1975).

10. Bleyer, W. A., Drake, J. C., and Chabner, B. A., Neurotoxicity and elevated cerebrospinal fluid MTX concentration in meningeal leukemia. *New Engl. J. Med.* **289,** 770 (1973).

11. Bertino, J. R., and Fischer, G. A., VI Techniques for study of resistance to folic acid antagonists. *Methods Med. Res.* **10,** 297 (1964).

12. Werkheiser, W. C., Zakrzewski, S. F., and Nichol, C. A., Assay for 4-amino folic acid analogues by inhibition of folic acid reductases. *J. Pharmacol. Exp. Ther.* **137,** 162 (1962).

13. Chabner, B. A., and Young, R. C., Threshold MTX concentration for *in vivo* inhibition of DNA synthesis in normal and tumorous target tissues. *J. Clin. Invest.* **52,** 1804 (1973).

14. Pratt, C. B., Roberts, D., Shanks, E., and Warmath, E. L., Response toxicity and pharmacokinetics of high-dose methotrexate (NSC 740) with citrovorum factor (NSC 3590) rescue for children with osteosarcoma and other malignant tumors. *Cancer Chemother. Rep.* **6,** Part 3, p 13 (1975).

15. Noble, W. C., White, P. M., and Baker, H., Assay of therapeutic doses of MTX in body fluids of patients with psoriasis. *J. Invest. Dermatol.* **64,** 69 (1975).

16. Freeman, M. V., A fluorometric method for the measurement of a 4-amino-10-methyl pteroylglutamic acid (amethopterin) in plasma. *J. Pharmacol. Exp. Ther.* **120,** 1 (1957).

17. Raso, V., and Schreiber, R., A rapid and specific radioimmunoassay for methotrexate. *Cancer Res.* **35,** 1407 (1975).

18. Arons, E., Rothenberg, S. P., da Costa, M., et al., A direct ligand-binding radioassay for the measurement of methotrexate in tissues and biological fluids. *Cancer Res.* **35,** 2033 (1975).

19. Overdijk, B., Van der Kroef, W. M. J., Visser, A. A. M., and Hooghwinkel, G. J. M., The determination of methotrexate in serum and urine. *Clin. Chim. Acta* **59,** 177 (1975).

CLIN. CHEM. 22/6, 789–801 (1976)

Relative Merits of Some Methods for Amphetamine Assay in Biological Fluids

Robert O. Bost, Craig A. Sutheimer, and Irving Sunshine

We describe principles and details that we use for amphetamine determination in blood and urine by photometric, thin-layer chromatographic, gas-chromatographic, and immunologic (EMIT and radioimmunoassay) procedures. Results, interferences, stabilities, and economic considerations are intercompared and recommendations are made.

Additional Keyphrases: *inter-method comparison • drug assay • economics of laboratory operation • screening*

Selecting the most suitable method for determining amphetamine from among the many (*1*) is difficult. The laboratory director usually has little or no time to evaluate alternatives.

This paper is intended to provide objective data on various features of some methods for amphetamine—precision, accuracy, sensitivity, range, interfering substances, personnel and equipment demands, and costs for reagents and personnel.

Many different methods were examined, and those which seemed to us to be the most useful were subjected to detailed evaluation.

Principles

There are two fundamental steps in most of the procedures described below: (*a*) separation of amphetamine from the biological matrix and (*b*) identification and quantitation of the material so isolated. Although many separation techniques have been described and used successfully, the separation method we chose for these experiments was solvent extraction from basic solutions. Methods for identification and quantitation are detailed. They include: (*a*) formation of an ion pair by reaction of methyl orange with amphetamine, which is measured photometrically (*2*); (*b*) development of fluorophores in the thin-layer chromatographic procedures (*3–6*); (*c*) formation of the acetamide by reaction with acetic anhydride in one of the flame-ionization procedures (*7*); (*d*) formation of the isothiocyanate by reaction with carbon disulfide in a second flame-ionization procedure (*8*); (*e*) formation of the trichloroacetamide by reaction with trichloroacetyl chloride in the electron-capture detector procedure (*9*); and (*f*) determination of free amphetamine by use of a nitrogen/phosphorus-sensitive detector (*10*).

Cuyahoga County Coroner's Office; and The Institute of Pathology, School of Medicine, Case Western Reserve University, Cleveland, Ohio 44106.

Received Jan. 15, 1976; accepted Feb. 25, 1976.

Some immunoassays (*11–13*) for amphetamine were also studied, and we present the principles of their use subsequently in the text.

Sample Handling

All chemicals used were analytical-reagent grade unless otherwise noted. All drugs were of "reference standard" quality. All reagents were stored in glass containers at 4 °C. All samples were also stored at 4 °C if not analyzed as soon as received or processed for analysis. Samples were usually analyzed within 24 h and never more than a week after receipt. No preservative was added to urine samples; a solid anticoagulant, sodium oxalate or sodium fluoride, was added to blood samples.

Photometric Methods

Methyl orange. A procedure that was frequently used at a time when more elegant techniques were not available, this procedure was evaluated according to the method described by Frings et al. (*2*). We obtained the data recorded in Table 2. These indicate the limited specificity and sensitivity of this method, hence we give no further details.

(4-Chloro-7-nitrobenzo-2-oxa-1,3-diazole) chloride. This procedure was developed in our laboratory (*3*), and so we have not rigorously re-evaluated it.

Thin-Layer Chromatographic Methods

Reagents

Amphetamine sulfate stock solution, 100 mg/liter, 3.70 × 10^{-4} mol/liter (Smith, Kline and French, Philadelphia, Pa 19101): Dissolve 13.6 mg of amphetamine sulfate in water and dilute to 100 ml with water.

Control solutions, 1.0 and 5.0 mg/liter: Dilute 5.0 ml of the amphetamine stock solution to 50.0 ml with drug-free urine; the resulting solution has a concentration of 10 μg/ml. Into two 10.0-ml volumetric flasks, place 1.0 and 5.0 ml of this solution, respectively, and dilute to 10.0 ml with drug-free urine.

Interfering-substance solutions, 100 mg/liter: Dissolve an appropriate amount of the drugs suspected of being present in the specimen(s) (see list in Table 1) in water and dilute to 100 ml.

Ammonium chloride buffer, pH 9.2: Add 1 liter of water to 450 g (8.4 mol; an excess to ensure saturation) of ammonium chloride, mix well, and let the mixture stand overnight. Adjust the pH of this saturated ammonium chloride solution to 9.2 by adding concentrated ammonium hydroxide.

Chloroform/isopropanol: Combine 100 ml of isopropanol and 900 ml of chloroform, and mix well.

Ethanolic sulfuric acid: Place 5 ml of 95% ethanol in a 10.0-ml flask. Cautiously add 2.0 ml of concentrated (18 mol/liter) sulfuric acid, cool to room temperature, and fill to the mark with 95% ethanol.

Potassium hydroxide, 2.0 mol/liter: Dissolve 112 g of potassium hydroxide in water and dilute to 1 liter with water.

Potassium phosphate buffer, 0.26 mol/liter, pH 10: Dissolve 4.56 g of dibasic potassium phosphate in about 90 ml of water. Adjust the pH to 10.0 with the aqueous potassium hydroxide (2.0 mol/liter). Dilute to 100 ml with water.

Developing solvent: Ethyl acetate/methanol/ammonium hydroxide, 85/10/5 by vol. Prepare this solvent just before use.

Ninhydrin spray reagent: Dissolve 400 mg of ninhydrin in acetone and dilute to 100 ml with acetone. This reagent must be freshly prepared.

Ninhydrin spray reagent, pH 10: Dissolve 400 mg of ninhydrin in 100 ml of pH 10 potassium phosphate buffer. Readjust the pH to 10.0 with potassium hydroxide (2.0 mol/liter). This solution is stable for several days.

Phenylacetaldehyde spray reagent: Dissolve 0.50 ml of phenylacetaldehyde in 95% ethanol and dilute to 100 ml with 95% ethanol. This reagent is stable for three months at 4 °C.

4-Phenylspiro(furan-2[3H]-1′-phthalan)-3,3′dione (fluorescamine or "Fluram") spray reagent (Roche Diagnostics, Nutley, N. J. 07110): Dissolve 5.0 mg of Fluram in acetone and dilute to 25.0 ml with acetone. (*Note:* The manufacturer claims this reagent to be stable for as long as three months, but we find that for optimum sensitivity it should be freshly prepared every two to three days.)

Triethylamine spray reagent: Dissolve 10 ml of triethylamine in acetone and dilute to 100 ml with acetone.

4-Chloro-7-nitrobenzo-2-oxa-1,3-diazole reagent: Dissolve 25 mg of this compound (Eastman Organic Chemicals, Rochester, N. Y. 14650) in chloroform and dilute to 25 ml with chloroform. This reagent must be prepared freshly each working day.

Equipment

Thin-layer chromatographic plates: "Silica Gel G" plates 20 × 20 cm (Analtech, Newark, Del. 19711).

Water bath, approximately 45 °C. A beaker of water on a hot plate will serve.

Thin-layer chromatographic developing tanks: Any standard unit will suffice.

Culture tubes, 25 × 150 mm, 50 ml, fitted with Teflon-lined screw caps (Kimble, Toledo, Ohio 41901).

Culture tubes, 25 × 100 mm, 30 ml, fitted with Teflon-lined screw caps (Kimble).

Rotator. ("Rugged Rotator", Model RD-250; Kraft Apparatus Co., S. Richmond Hill, N. Y. 11419).

Ultraviolet light source, providing both 254-nm and 313-nm radiation. ("Chromato-Vue", Model C5; Ultra-Violet Products, Inc., San Gabriel, Calif. 91778).

Oven, for drying plates.

Procedure

Place the developing solvent in the tank to allow equilibration. Seal the tank and proceed to the next step.

Place 5.0 ml of each sample (sample urines and both control solutions) in separate 30-ml screw-capped culture tubes. Add 2.0 ml of the ammonium chloride buffer and 20.0 ml of the chloroform/isopropanol mixture.

Extract by rotating for 20 min at 5–10 rpm.

Centrifuge the tubes at 2500 rpm for 5 min.

Aspirate and discard each aqueous upper layer.

Filter each lower layer through Whatman No. 1 paper into clean 30-ml screw-capped culture tubes. (*Note:* When using 4-chloro-7-nitrobenzo-2-oxa-1,3-diazole as the detection reagent, add 1.0 ml of the reagent solution to the filtrate before beginning the evaporation and delete the addition of the ethanolic sulfuric acid. The rest of the procedure is unchanged.)

Evaporate nearly to dryness in a 45 °C water bath under a gentle stream of air. When the volume has been reduced to about half, add 2 drops of the ethanolic sulfuric acid to avoid loss of the volatile amphetamine. Continue to concentrate the extract to a final volume of 5–10 μl.

Dissolve the cooled residue in 20 μl of methanol and spot the solution on a thin-layer chromatographic plate, 1.5 cm above the lower edge of the plate.

Place the plate in the equilibrated developing tank and develop the plate until the solvent front is 15 cm above the origin.

Remove the plate from the tank, dry it in an oven at 60 °C for 10 min, remove it from the oven, and allow it to cool.

Apply the detection system of choice.

Detection Systems

Ninhydrin

a. Spray the cooled plate lightly with the ninhydrin-in-acetone spray reagent.

b. Expose the plate to 254-nm radiation for 5 min. (Support the plate 10–15 cm from the light source.)

c. Heat the plate at 100 °C for 4 min.

d. Repeat steps b and c.

e. Look for pink-grey spots. If necessary, repeat the entire sequence.

Ninhydrin/phenylacetaldehyde

a. Spray the cooled plate lightly with the pH 10 ninhydrin spray reagent.

b. Immediately over-spray the plate more heavily with phenylacetaldehyde spray reagent.

c. Let the plate stand at room temperature for 10–15 min.

d. View the plate under 313-nm radiation. Look for bright-green fluorescence.

Fluram

a. Spray the cooled plate with triethylamine spray reagent.

b. Over-spray the plate with the Fluram spray reagent.

c. Over-spray the plate with triethylamine spray reagent.

d. Let the plate stand at room temperature for 10–15 min.

e. View the plate under 313-nm radiation. Look for blue fluorescence.

4-Chloro-7-nitrobenzo-2-oxa-1,3-diazole

a. Observe the plate under 313-nm radiation. Look for yellow spots. Highly concentrated samples may yield spots that are observable under visible light.

Gas-Chromatographic Methods

Reagents

Amphetamine sulfate stock solution, 100 mg/liter, 3.70 × 10^{-4} mol/liter (Smith, Kline and French, Philadelphia, Pa. 19101): Dissolve 13.6 mg of amphetamine sulfate in water and dilute to 100 ml with water.

Reference amphetamine solutions, 0.1, 0.5, 1.0, 2.5, 5.0, 7.5, and 10.0 mg/liter: Dilute 5.0 ml of the amphetamine stock solution to 50.0 ml with drug-free urine or blood; the resulting solution has a concentration of 10 μg/ml. In each of several 10.0 ml volumetric flasks, respectively, place 0.1, 0.5, 1.0, 2.5, 5.0, and 7.5 ml of the 10 μg/ml amphetamine solution and dilute each to 10.0 ml with drug-free urine or blood.

Interfering substance solutions, 100 mg/liter: Dissolve an appropriate amount of the drugs under suspicion (see list in Table 1) in a small amount of water and dilute to 100 ml with water.

Tranylcypromine sulfate (internal standard, 1, 25 mg/liter, 1.88 × 10^{-4} mol/liter; Smith, Kline and French): Dissolve 17.0 mg of tranylcypromine sulfate in water and dilute to 500 ml with water.

Methoxyphenamine hydrochloride (internal standard 2, 6.5 mg/liter, 3.62 × 10^{-4} mol/liter: Upjohn, Kalamazoo, Mich. 49001): Dissolve 15.6 mg of methoxyphenamine hydrochloride in water and dilute to 200 ml with water. Dilute 10.0 ml of this stock to 100.0 ml to obtain the desired 6.5 μg/ml.

Methoxyphenamine hydrochloride (internal standard 3, 1.6 mg/liter, 9.05 × 10^{-5} mol/liter): Dissolve 9.50 mg of methoxyphenamine hydrochloride in water and dilute to 500 ml with water. Dilute 10.0 ml of this stock to 100 ml to obtain the desired 1.6 μg/ml.

Sodium hydroxide, 6.0 mol/liter: Dissolve 240 g of sodium hydroxide in water and dilute to 1 liter with water.

Sodium hydroxide, 2.5 mol/liter: Dissolve 100 g of sodium hydroxide in water and dilute to 1 liter with water.

Lead acetate, 1.4 mol/liter: Add 54 g (an excess) of lead acetate trihydrate to water and dilute to 100 ml with water. Stir the mixture at about 35 °C for 2 h and then allow it to cool to room temperature (this produces a saturated solution of lead acetate).

Ammonium hydroxide, 15 mol/liter (concentrated).

Ammonium chloride buffer, pH 9.2: Add 1000 ml of water to 450 g of ammonium chloride, mix well, and let the mixture stand overnight. Adjust the pH of this saturated ammonium chloride solution to 9.2 by adding concentrated ammonium hydroxide.

Diethyl ether/ethyl acetate: In a liter flask combine 500 ml of diethyl ether and 500 ml of ethyl acetate. Mix well.

Ethanolic hydrochloric acid: Place 5 ml of 95% ethanol in a 10.0-ml flask. Cautiously add 0.5 ml of concentrated (12 mol/liter) hydrochloric acid. Cool to room temperature and fill to the mark with 95% ethanol.

Toluene ("Nanograde"; Mallinckrodt Chemical Works, St. Louis, Mo. 63160).

Chloroform ("Spectrograde"; Matheson, Coleman and Bell, Norwood, Ohio 45212).

Carbon disulfide.

Trichloroacetyl chloride (Eastman Kodak Co., Rochester, N. Y. 14650). Redistill and use the 114 °C fraction.

Acetic anhydride.

Equipment

Gas chromatograph A: A gas chromatograph (Perkin-Elmer 3920) equipped with a flame ionization detector, or a nitrogen/phosphorus detector as the experiment requires, a coiled glass column, 1.82 m × 2 mm i.d., packed with 3% OV-17 on 100/120 mesh Gas-Chrom Q and a 1 mV strip-chart recorder such as the Coleman 165 (Perkin-Elmer Corp., Norwalk, Conn. 06856).

Gas chromatograph B: A gas chromatograph (Hewlett-Packard 5713A) equipped with a linear ^{63}Ni electron-capture detector, a coiled glass column, 0.91 m × 4 mm i.d., packed with 5% OV-7 on 80/100 mesh high-performance Chromosorb W, and a 1 mV strip-chart recorder, Model 7143A (Hewlett-Packard, Avondale, Pa. 19311).

Rotator. ("Rugged Rotator", Kraft).

"Concentratubes", 18 × 114 mm. (Laboratory Research Co., P.O. Box 36509, Los Angeles, Calif. 90036).

Culture tubes, 16 × 125 mm, 15 ml, with Teflon-lined screw caps (Kimble, Toledo, Ohio 41901).

Glass syringes, 10.0 μl (Hamilton Co., P.O. Box 10030, Reno, Nev. 89510).

Water bath, controllable at 35 °C.

Procedures

(a) Isothiocyanate derivative by flame ionization detection:

To each of a series of Concentratubes add 2.0 ml of each sample (urine samples and each reference solution 0.5 mg/liter and greater). Add 0.5 ml of the tranylcypromine solution (internal standard 1).

Vibrate the contents of tubes on a vortex-type mixer to ensure that the solutions are well mixed.

Add 0.1–0.15 ml of the lead acetate solution and 0.5 ml of ammonium hydroxide and vortex-mix again for 5–10 s.

Add 0.25 ml of carbon disulfide and vortex-mix for

30 s. (This simultaneously extracts and converts the drugs to their dithiocarbamates.)

Centrifuge (2500 rpm, 5 min) to separate the phases. (If emulsions form, the mixtures should be stirred with a glass rod and the tubes recentrifuged.)

Aspirate and discard the aqueous phases (this is only for convenience).

Withdraw a 5-μl aliquot of the carbon disulfide phase into a 10-μl syringe and inject *slowly* into the injection port of gas chromatograph A, using the flame ionization detector. (This slow injection improves reproducibility and converts the dithiocarbamate derivatives of primary amines to their isothiocyanates (8).) *Note:* Rinse the syringe thoroughly with a solvent such as chloroform to prevent its becoming clogged.

For each analysis, obtain the peak area ratio by dividing the peak area for the amphetamine derivative by that of the derivative of the internal standard.

(For interference study only.) To determine the extent to which other substances interfere with this determination, assay aliquots of all of the test solutions for interfering substances by the procedure described above.

Gas-chromatographic conditions.

Temperatures, °C	Injection port—250	
	Detector—300	
	Column—hold at 160 °C for 1 min, program at 4 °C per min from 160 to 190 °C	
Gas flows, ml/min:	N_2	40
	H_2	38
	Air	320

Under these conditions, the amphetamine derivative emerges from the column at 3.9 min, the tranylcypromine derivative at 5.8 min.

If the objective is to screen large numbers of samples for absence or presence of amphetamine rather than to obtain quantitative data, the column temperature can be held at 210 °C. The amphetamine derivative will emerge from the column in about 1.3 min and the tranylcypromine derivative in about 1.8 min. The time interval between injections is shortened to 2.5–3 min. When combined with the technique of injecting a pooled mixture of 3-μl aliquots from each of two extracts, the isothermal conditions can increase sample assay rate from four per hour with the quantitative procedure to 40 per hour for the screening procedure. (Pooled samples can be justified if the number of samples to be analyzed is large and the proportion of positive results is expected to be relatively low, as is the usual situation in most laboratories concerned with screening procedures for drugs subject to abuse. Of course, any positive result requires that each of the component samples in the pool be re-analyzed.)

(*b*) *Acetamide derivative by flame ionization detection:*

To each of a series of Concentratubes, add 6.0 ml of each sample (urine samples and all reference solutions 0.5 mg/liter and greater), 0.25 ml of methoxyphenamine hydrochloride (internal standard 2), and 0.3 ml of the 6.0 mol/liter sodium hydroxide solution, in that order.

While vigorously vortex-mixing the contents of each tube, add 0.25 ml of chloroform and continue mixing for 30 s.

Centrifuge the tubes (2500 rpm, 5–10 min).

Aspirate and discard the aqueous phases (this is only for convenience).

Aspirate 3 μl of the chloroform layer into a 10-μl Hamilton syringe, followed by 1.5 μl of acetic anhydride.

Slowly inject this mixture into the injection port of chromatograph A, and use the flame ionization detector. (A slow injection improves the on-column derivatization and reproducibility.)

For each analysis, obtain the peak-area ratio by dividing the peak area of the amphetamine derivative peak by that of the peak for the internal-standard derivative.

(For interfering substances study only.) To determine the extent to which other substances interfere with this determination, analyze aliquots of the interfering substance test solutions by the procedure described above.

Gas-chromatograph conditions:

Temperature, °C	Injector—250	
	Detector—300	
	Column—140 for 1 min program at 16 °C per min from 140 °C to 240 °C and then hold at 240 °C for at 4 min	
Gas flows, ml/min:	N_2	40
	H_2	38
	Air	320

Under these conditions, the amphetamine derivative has a retention time of 4.9 min, the methoxyphenamine derivative a retention time of 7.2 min.

If the objective is simply to screen many samples for presence or absence of amphetamine, the column temperature can be held at 190 °C. The amphetamine derivative will emerge in about 2.5 min and the methoxyphenamine derivative in about 3.5 min. The time interval between injections is shortened to 4.5–5 min. When combined with the technique of injecting a pooled mixture, 2-μl aliquots from each of two extracts plus 2 μl of acetic anhydride, the isothermal conditions can increase sample throughput from five per hour with the quantitative procedure to 25 per hour for the screening procedure. (See the above note on pooled samples.)

(*c*) *Trichloroacetamide derivative by electron-capture detection:*

To a series of the 15-ml culture tubes add, in the order mentioned, 1.0 ml of each sample (urine samples and all their reference solutions or blood samples and all their reference solutions), 0.5 ml of the 2.5 mol/liter NaOH, 0.5 ml of the methoxyphenamine hydrochloride solution (internal standard 3), and 2.0 ml of "Nanograde" toluene.

Place the tubes in a rotator and extract the samples for 30 min at 8 rpm.

Transfer each upper layer to a clean 15-ml tube. Try not to aspirate any aqueous phase. Add 25 μl of trichloroacetyl chloride to each tube.

Vortex-mix the mixtures vigorously for 30 s and incubate them at room temperature for 30 min. (Any trace of water carried over in the previous step will cause turbidity, but this can be tolerated.)

Add 2.0 ml of the 6.0 mol/liter NaOH to the mixtures and vigorously vortex-mix for 30 s (any turbidity will now clear).

Centrifuge the tubes (2500 rpm, 5 min).

Withdraw 2.0 μl of the organic phase into a 10.0-μl syringe and inject on gas chromatograph B.

For each analysis, obtain the peak-area ratio by dividing the peak area of the amphetamine derivative by that of the internal-standard derivative.

(For interfering substances study only.) To determine the extent to which other substances interfere with this determination, analyze aliquots of the reference interfering substance test solutions by the procedure described above.

Gas-chromatographic conditions:

Temperatures, °C	Injection port—200 Detector—300 Column—Start at 180 °C for 2 min, then program at 16 °C per min to 260 °C, then hold at 260 °C for 2 min
Gas flow, ml/min	Argon/methane (95/5 by vol) 60

Under these conditions, the amphetamine derivative emerges from the column at 3.3 min, the methoxyphenamine derivative at 5.4 min.

If the objective is simply to screen large numbers of samples for the presence or absence of amphetamine, pooled samples may be assayed and chromatographed isothermally. At 275 °C the amphetamine derivative appears in 0.5 min, the methoxyphenamine derivative in 0.8 min. The time interval between injections is shortened to 1 min. Thus, analysis rate can be increased from five samples per hour to nearly 180 per hour by pooling three 2-μl extracts. (See previous note on pooled samples.)

(*d*) *Free amphetamine by nitrogen/phosphorus detection:*

To a series of the 15-ml culture tubes add, in the order mentioned, 5.0 ml of each sample (urine samples and all their reference solutions or blood samples and all their reference solutions), 0.25 ml of the 2.5 mol/liter NaOH, 1.0 ml of the methoxyphenamine hydrochloride solution (internal standard 2), and 5.0 ml of the diethyl ether/ethyl acetate solution.

Place the tubes in a rotator and extract the samples for 30 min at 8 rpm.

Centrifuge the resulting mixture to separate the phases. (Emulsions may be broken with a stirring rod.)

Transfer each upper layer to clean Concentratubes, add 3 drops of ethanolic hydrochloric acid, and slowly evaporate the solution to about 100 μl in a 35 °C water bath, under a gentle stream of dried air.

To the concentrated extracts add 1 drop of pH 9.2 ammonium chloride buffer and vortex-mix.

Centrifuge the resulting mixtures.

Aspirate 5 μl of the organic (upper) phase into a 10.0-μl syringe and inject onto gas chromatograph A, and use the nitrogen/phosphorus detector.

For each analysis, obtain the peak-area ratio by dividing the peak area of the amphetamine by that of the internal standard.

(For interfering substances study only.) To determine the extent to which other substances interfere with this determination, we analyzed aliquots of the reference interfering substance test solutions by the procedure described above.

Gas-chromatographic conditions:

Temperatures, °C	Injection port—250 Detector—300 Column—Start at 110 °C for 1 min, then program at 8 °C per min to 170 °C, then hold at 170 °C for 4 min.	
Gas flow, ml/min	He	35
	H_2	3
	Air	100

Using these conditions, the amphetamine emerges from the column at 3.0 min, the methoxyphenamine at 7.0 min.

Because of this technique's nonspecific extraction procedure and the detector's extreme sensitivity, isothermal determinations of pooled samples is not advised for fear of overloading the detector with nitrogenous organic compounds and thus slowing down total output rather than speeding it. We suggest that after about every 5 to 10 sample runs the column be baked at 250 °C for 5 min, to eliminate eventual "organic-nitrogen poisoning."

Standardization and calculation: The output of the detector is recorded by any conventional means that permits determination of retention times and peak areas. The retention times are used to characterize the compounds; peak areas are used for quantitation.

Peak-area ratios obtained for the reference solutions are plotted vs. their respective amphetamine concentrations to provide a standard curve. The concentration of any test sample is then determined by interpolation of its peak-area ratio from the standard curve.

Use of a data processor simplifies calculations. We used the Perkin-Elmer PEP-1 data processor.

Principles of Immunoassays

Immunoassay of drugs is based on classical immunochemical procedures; antigen/antibody reaction is used as an analytical tool. All immunoassays are based on a similar principle—the competitive displacement of the labeled drug from the antigen/antibody complex by unlabeled drug in the sample. The concentration of the drug in the sample can then be determined by measuring the amount of the displaced radiolabeled drug or alternatively, by measuring the amount of radiolabeled drug still bound to the antibody. In some immunoassays this involves separating the free and bound drug forms, usually easily done by established techniques. In homogeneous immunoassay procedures this separations step is not required, and so fewer manipulations are required.

Immunological Methods

Principle of Enzyme Multiplied Immunoassay Technique (EMIT)

The Enzyme Multiplied Immunoassay Technique (EMIT) for amphetamine is based on use of an enzyme, lysozyme (EC 3.2.1.17), which is linked to the drug in question in the antigen reagent. This enzyme catalyzes hydrolysis of the mucopolysaccharide component of the cell walls of certain bacteria—specifically, 1,4-β-linkages between *N*-acetylmuramic acid and 2-acetamido-2-deoxy-*D*-glucose residues in a mucopolysaccharide or mucopeptide. The antibody binds the drug and its attached enzyme, rendering the enzyme inactive. In the assay, any drug present in the sample competes with the enzyme/drug complex (antigen reagent) for binding to the antibody; any unbound enzyme is free to hydrolyze the cell walls of the bacteria used in the assay (*Micrococcus lysodeikticus*). There is no need to separate components of the reaction, because in a negative sample there is no competition for the antibody sites, the enzyme is completely bound, and no activity ensues. If the drug in question is present in the sample, the enzyme-labeled drug is unbound and its activity—and hence the drug concentration—can be determined by measuring the rate of clearing of the suspension of the cell walls (the decrease in absorbance) as the enzyme hydrolyzes them into small, soluble fragments.

Reagents

All reagents except the interfering substance solutions were obtained in kit form from Syva Corp., Palo Alto, Calif. 94304:

Antibody solution (Reagent A).

Antigen/lysozyme solution (Reagent B).

Tris(hydroxymethyl)aminomethane/maleate buffer, pH 6.0, 0.25 mol/liter. Pour the entire contents of the EMIT Buffer Concentrate into the plastic bottle labeled "EMIT Buffer Solution" and add distilled water to the inscribed fill-line on the bottle.

Bacterial cell-wall suspension, 75 mg of *Micrococcus lysodeikticus* in 100 ml of the buffer.

Urine controls (containing 1.0, 5.0, and 50.0 mg of amphetamine per liter).

"Normal" urine, or pooled urine from "normal" drug-free individuals.

Interfering substance solutions, 100 mg/liter: Dissolve an appropriate amount of the drugs under suspicion (see list in Table 1) in a small amount of water and dilute to 100 ml with water.

Equipment

Disposable continuous-flow analyzer sample cups, conical, 2-ml (Fisher Scientific Co., Pittsburgh, Pa. 15219).

Spectrophotometer with flow-through cuvette and constant temperature control (Model 300N; Gilford Instrument Laboratories, Inc., Oberlin, Ohio 44074) with a timer/printer/calculator (Seiko S-100; Cavro Scientific Instruments, Los Altos, Calif. 94022).

Micro sampler/dilutor (Model 1500; Cavro).

Procedure

Into the 2-ml conical sample cups dispense 0.5 ml of the bacterial cell-wall suspension. (Be sure to resuspend the bacteria before each use.)

Using the automatic sampler/dilutor, add to the suspension in the sample cup, in the order listed: (*a*) 50 μl of the urine sample or standard plus 0.25 ml of the buffer; (*b*) 50 μl of the antibody solution (Reagent A) plus 0.25 ml of the buffer; and (*c*) 50 μl of the antigen/lysozyme solution (Reagent B) plus 0.25 ml of the buffer.

Immediately aspirate the reaction mixture into the temperature-controlled (37 $\pm$ 0.5 °C) flow-through cuvette of a spectrophotometer set at 436 nm. Set the timer/printer/calculator to record the absorbance after 10 s, to allow for temperature equilibration, and again at 50 s, after the cuvette is filled. Calculate the decrease in absorbance over this 40s span.

Determine the concentration of the drug in the a standard curve. Even a negative sample will give some decrease in absorbance; therefore, a positive sample must have a greater decrease than that of the lowest detectable concentration of the drug to which the antibody is specific. All positive samples should be tested for exogenous lysozyme (which is a naturally occurring body constituent) to eliminate possible false positives. To check for this, re-analyze the positive samples just as described above in the procedure, substituting 50 μl of the buffer for both the antibody and antigen/lysozyme solutions (Reagents A and B). Subtract this decrease from the original decrease, and if this difference is still greater than that of the lowest detectable concentration, the sample is indeed positive.

(For interfering substances study only.) To determine the extent to which other substances interfere with this determination, assay aliquots of the various interfering substance solutions by the procedure described above.

Principle of Radioimmunoassay (RIA)

Another immunoassay that has become very popular and has been applied to many different substances (rather than only drugs of abuse) is radioimmunoassay (RIA). In this technique the antigen is labeled with a suitable radioactive isotope, usually either ^{125}I, ^{3}H, or ^{14}C. The usual antigen/antibody reaction is performed, and either the bound or (usually) the displaced radioactive drug in the resulting mixture is separated and measured. The measuring device used depends on the label. ^{125}I-labeled products are measured in a gamma counter; ^{3}H-labeled compounds require a scintillation counter.

Reagents

All reagents except for the interfering substance solutions were obtained in kit form (Roche Diagnostics, Nutley, N. J. 07110):

Antibody reagent.

Radiolabeled antigen reagent.

Positive urine control (1.0 mg/liter).

"Normal" urine control: Use "normal" urine or a pooled urine from "normal" drug-free individuals.

Ammonium sulfate, saturated solution.

Interfering substance solutions, 100 mg/liter: Dissolve an appropriate amount of the drugs listed in Table 1 in a small amount of water and dilute to 100 ml with water.

Equipment

Disposable culture tubes, 10 × 75 mm.

Semiautomatic pipets (Eppendorf pipets or Schwarz/Mann "Biopipettes") or glass transfer pipets (Lang/Levy). (Because this procedure involves both low concentrations and small volumes, carry-over, accuracy, and reproducibility of measurements are critical factors which must be in rigid control.)

Gamma scintillation counter (for ^{125}I).

Procedure

In a 10 × 75 mm culture tube, mix 0.1 ml of urine sample or standard and 0.4 ml of the combined antibody reagent and radio-labeled antigen reagent. *Note:* Alternatively, 0.2 ml of each reagent may be added separately, without pre-mixing. (Always analyze a positive and "normal" urine control in duplicate with each set of samples.) Allow 1 h for equilibrium to be approximated.

Add 0.5 ml of the saturated ammonium sulfate solution, to precipitate the antibody and antibody/antigen complex. Mix, and wait 5 to 10 min to ensure that precipitation is complete. Centrifuge (10 to 20 min, 1000 to 1500 × *g*).

Place 0.5 ml of the clear supernate into a counting vial for the gamma scintillation counter. *Note:* Be extremely cautious to avoid aspirating any precipitate into the supernate. Measure the radioactivity by the appropriate method.

Table 1. Interfering Substances[a]

	Methyl[b] orange	TLC[c,e]	CS_2[c,e]	Ac_2O[c,e]	ECD[c,e]	EMIT[d,e]	RIA[d,e]
Amitriptylene	No	No	N.P.	No	N.C.	No	No
Benzoic acid	No	No	N.P.	No	No	No	No
Benzphetamine	No	No	N.P.	No	N.C.	24 mg/liter	No
Brompheniramine	No	No	N.P.	N.P.	No	N.C.	N.C.
Chlorpheniramine	No	No	N.P.	N.P.	No	No	No
Cyclopentamine	No	Yes	No	>10 mg/liter	>5 mg/liter	N.C.	N.C.
Diethylpropion	No	No	Yes	>10 mg/liter	N.C.	No	No
Ephedrine	21 mg/liter	Pos/Neg	N.P.	No	N.C.	20 mg/liter	No
p-Hydroxyamphetamine	No	Pos/Neg	N.P.	No	1.1 mg/liter	No	>10 mg/liter
Imipramine	No	No	N.P.	No	No	No	No
Indomethacin	No	No	N.C.	N.C.	N.C.	1.2 mg/liter	No
Isoproterenol	No	No	No	N.P.	No	N.C.	N.C.
Isoxsuprine	No	Pos/Neg	N.P.	N.P.	No	N.C.	N.C.
Mephentermine	No	No	No	Pos/Neg	No	N.C.	N.C.
Meprobamate	No	No	N.P.	No	No	No	No
Methadone	No	No	N.P.	Pos/Neg	N.P.	No	No
Methamphetamine	45 mg/liter	Yes	N.P.	Pos/Neg	No	>50 mg/liter	Pos/Neg
Methoxamine	16 mg/liter	Yes	N.P.	No	No	No	No
Methoxyphenamine	N.C.	Yes	N.P.	No	No	N.C.	N.C.
Methylphenidate	N.C.	No	No	No	No	N.C.	N.C.
Norepinephrine	No	No	N.P.	Yes	No	No	No
Nylidrin	N.C.	Yes	N.P.	No	No	N.C.	N.C.
Phenformin	N.C.	No	N.P.	N.P.	No	N.C.	N.C.
Pheniramine	N.C.	No	N.P.	No	No	N.C.	N.C.
Phenmetrazine	37 mg/liter	Yes	Yes	No	No	40 mg/liter	No
Phentermine	N.C.	N.C.	N.P.	N.C.	N.C.	N.C.	N.C.
Phenylephrine	No	No	N.P.	Pos/Neg	No	No	No
Phenylpropanolamine	13 mg/liter	No	N.P.	No	N.P.	9 mg/liter	1.3 mg/liter
Propylhexadrine	N.C.	Yes	N.P.	Pos/Neg	No	N.C.	N.C.
Tranylcypromine	5 mg/liter	No	N.P.	No	No	14 mg/liter	1.6 mg/liter
Tuaminoheptane	46 mg/liter	Pos/Neg	N.P.	No	N.P.	20 mg/liter	>10 mg/liter

[a] Entries in the table are explained as follows: NC, not analyzed; NP, no peak, i.e., compound was assayed but did not produce a gas-chromatographic peak on the gas chromatograph; No, compound was assayed but did not interfere; Yes, interferes. Numbers indicate the amphetamine concentration that would give a response equivalent to the 100 mg/liter test solution.

[b] A compound was considered to interfere if it displayed an absorbance at 515 nm.

[c] A compound was considered to interfere if its R_F or R_t was within 10% of the value for amphetamine.

[d] A compound was considered to interfere if it produced counts (RIA) or if it resulted in an absorbance decrease (EMIT) greater than that of the low cut-off standard.

[e] TLC, thin-layer chromatography; CS_2, carbon disulfide; Ac_2O, acetic/anhydride; ECD, electron-capture detector; EMIT, Enzyme Multiplied Immunoassay Technique; RIA, radioimmunoassay.

Determine the amount of drug present by use of a standard curve. If the drug concentration in a sample is found to exceed that in the positive urine control and if quantitative results are desired, the sample should be diluted (to yield a final concentration lower than that of the positive control, but discernible from the "normal" control urine) and re-analyzed.

(For interfering substances study only.) To determine the extent to which other substances interfere with this determination, assay aliquots of the various interfering substance solutions by the procedure described above.

Results

Interfering Substances

We determined whether the compounds listed in Table 1 might interfere with the determination of amphetamine. Aqueous solutions (100 μg/ml) of these compounds were prepared. Aliquots of each of these solutions were assayed according to the described procedures. Table 1 shows the results.

Comparison Studies—Urine

To compare the various methods, we assayed urine samples by several of the described methods (Table 2). All samples were not analyzed by all methods. Quantitative results were given for all tests except thin-layer chromatography, for which results were reported as either positive or negative.

Table 2 indicates that half of the results of the methyl orange procedure were falsely positive; this is attributable to the method's lack of specificity and sensitivity. Statistical calculations were performed on those nonzero samples listed in Table 2 that the ECD method indicated were positive, comparing each of the immunoassays with the electron capture results. Regression lines were calculated, with the following results:

$$\text{RIA } y = 1.11\,x + .062; \quad r = 0.96$$

$$\text{EMIT } y = 0.31\,x + 0.78; \quad r = 0.21$$

The slopes and correlation coefficients both reveal that the RIA technique is in better agreement with ECD than is the EMIT procedure. However, it should be remembered that EMIT is intended to be, at best, semiquantitative and thus good quantitative correlation should not be expected.

The manufacturers of both immunoassay systems set a cut-off value of 1.0 μg/ml, below which all results are to be called negative. Accepting the ECD results as the reference values, the RIA results include one false positive, whereas the EMIT results include one false negative and three false positives. EMIT is known to detect both methamphetamine and amphetamine, whereas RIA and the ECD procedure monitor only amphetamine. The uncertain history of the samples analyzed suggests that the presence of methamphetamine in some samples would have passed unnoticed by RIA and the ECD and may account for the false positives reported for the EMIT results.

The gas-chromatographic data (Table 2) indicate that below a concentration of 0.4 mg/liter the standard curves for the isothiocyanate and acetamide methods become nonlinear and the signal-to-noise ratio diminishes, so that determinations below this value should not be considered valid without confirmation by an alternative method.

Comparison Studies—Blood

Amphetamine was added to blood known to be drug-free, and these samples were analyzed (as "blind" samples) by gas chromatography with use of both electron-capture and nitrogen detectors (Table 3).

The isothiocyanate and acetamide methods were not used. Analytical recovery of amphetamine from blood by these two methods was so poor that even the sought-for highest concentration could not be detected. Their poor extractability caused too many interfering artifacts, so that we found it impossible to identify and quantitate amphetamine accurately.

Extraction Efficiency

To ascertain the efficiency of extraction for each of the previously described procedures, we extracted aliquots of reference solutions containing tritiated as well as unlabeled amphetamine and analyzed aliquots of the original sample and final extract for radiolabeled amphetamine. Extraction efficiencies were calculated, correcting for the aliquoting steps (Table 4).

Stability Study

Samples of urine from persons known to have ingested amphetamine were collected in glass containers, and portions were assayed several times during the following four weeks, to determine whether or not storage conditions affected the amphetamine concentration. The samples were stored at 4 °C and aliquots were analyzed one and four days after collection. On the eighth day, the samples were subdivided; one portion was stored in a glass container, one was adjusted to pH 2 and stored in a glass container, one was stored in a plastic container, and one was adjusted to pH 2 and stored in a plastic container. Storage for all was at 4 °C. Each of these portions was assayed on the tenth day and again on the twenty-ninth day. Analyses were performed according to the trichloroacetamide/electron-capture detector method. Peak-area ratios (peak area for the amphetamine derivative divided by that of the internal standard derivative) were calculated for each sample. We saw no significant change in peak-area ratio or detectable change in pH, regardless of length of time or mode of storage.

Discussion

Photometric Methods

We do not recommend use of the methyl orange method because (*a*) its precision and accuracy are unacceptable, (*b*) its sensitivity limit is considerably above the required 1 mg/liter, and (*c*) many false-positives were obtained (see Table 2).

The fluorometric procedure, with use of 4-chloro-

Table 2. Comparison of the Results (mg/l) of Several Techniques for Urine Analyses for Amphetamine[a]

Methyl orange	TLC[c]	RIA[c]	EMIT[c]	ECD[c]
		Drug, mg/liter		
1.0	Pos	0.74	3.30	0.68
1.5	Pos	1.45	1.48	1.09
2.3	Pos	1.75	1.75	1.21
1.0	Pos	0.50	0.81	0.43
6.8	Pos	0.37	0.32	0.25
1.0	Pos	0.64	0.42	0.28
2.6	Pos	0.18	0.72	0.20
3.0	Pos	0.40	1.10	0.27
1.0	Pos	0.54	0.26	0.53
1.0	Pos	0.58	0.34	0.64
2.3	Pos	2.10	0.50	1.73
2.3	Pos	1.48	1.18	1.55
2.6	Pos	1.75	1.18	1.54
1.0	Pos	1.05	1.05	0.97
2.8	Neg	0.0	0.0	0.0
1.4	Neg	0.0	0.0	0.0
3.5	Neg	0.0	0.0	0.0
6.5	Pos/Neg	0.0	0.0	0.0
2.6	Neg	0.13	0.0	0.0
5.5	Neg	0.0	0.30	0.0
1.8	Neg	0.0	0.30	0.0
7.8	Pos/Neg	0.0	0.18	0.0
1.0	Neg	0.0	0.0	0.0
1.0	Neg	0.0	0.0	0.0
7.4	Neg	0.0	0.68	0.0
2.3	Neg	0.0	0.0	0.0
8.4	Neg	0.0	0.0	0.0
1.8	Neg	0.0	0.0	0.0
1.0	Neg	0.0	0.32	0.0
3.5	Neg	0.0	0.0	0.0
1.0	Neg	0.16	0.0	0.0
1.0	Neg	0.0	0.0	0.0
1.0	Neg	0.0	0.0	0.0
2.6	Neg	0.0	0.0	0.0
1.0	Neg	0.0	0.0	0.0
8.1	Neg	0.15	0.0	0.0
9.0	Neg	0.21	0.58	0.0
1.0	Neg	0.0	0.0	0.0

CS_2[c]	Ac_2O[c]	ECD[b,c]
0.0	0.33	0.0
0.18	0.26	0.26
1.83	2.07	2.02
1.51	1.56	1.13
1.16	1.15	0.83
1.67	2.06	1.96
0.55	0.46	0.59
0.0	0.0	0.0
0.0	0.0	0.0
0.57	0.44	0.45
3.39	QNS	3.68
1.54	1.51	1.67
0.79	1.28	0.86
1.00	0.96	1.03
0.0	0.0	0.0
0.0	0.0	0.0
0.18	0.03	0.29
0.20	0.03	0.30
0.32	0.03	0.37
1.16	0.01	1.06
1.16	1.17	1.16
3.64	6.80	3.81
0.0	0.34	0.62
4.08	7.98	4.04
1.23	1.37	1.31
1.56	1.80	1.57
1.30	1.60	1.46
0.0	0.0	0.0
0.0	QNS	0.0
0.0	0.0	0.0
2.82	1.82	2.46

ECD[c]	NPD[b,c]
1.55	1.64
2.18	1.96
1.06	0.86
1.04	0.86
0.69	0.63
0.01	0.03
0.79	0.69
2.01	1.90
1.75	1.66
1.16	1.31
2.37	2.46
1.98	1.90
0.04	0.06
2.09	2.10
0.60	0.73
0.53	0.30
QNS	QNS
0.11	0.11
0.80	0.70
0.06	QNS
0.80	0.90
1.29	1.10
0.10	0.10
0.10	0.30
1.08	1.20
0.49	0.40
0.61	0.61
0.01	QNS

[a] All results were obtained by using the procedures described in the text. The TLC detection system was 4-phenylspiro(furan-2[3H]-1-phthalan)-3,3′-dione.

[b] Analysis performed and data supplied by Dr. R. F. Adams, Perkin-Elmer, Norwalk, Conn.

[c] TLC, thin-layer chromatography; RIA, radioimmunoassay; EMIT, Enzyme Multiplied Immunoassay Technique; CS_2, carbon disulfide; Ac_2O, acetic anhydride; ECD, electron-capture detector; NPD, nitrogen/phosphorus detector.

Table 3. Comparison of the Results (mg/l) of ECD[a] and NPD[a] Analyses of Blood for Amphetamine

Aqueous			Serum		
Drug added (mg/l)	ECD[a]	NPD[a]	Drug added (mg/l)	ECD[a]	NPD[a]
0.10	0.11	0.05	0.0	0.0	0.0
2.50	2.57	2.46	2.50	2.44	2.70
2.50	2.65	2.45	5.00	5.05	5.65
1.00	2.09	0.89	1.00	0.88	0.96
7.50	7.45	7.81	10.00	10.10	10.06
10.00	10.07	10.06	0.10	0.11	0.0
0.0	0.0	0.0	0.50	0.54	0.37
10.00	10.08	9.85	0.0	0.0	0.0
1.00	1.01	0.85	7.50	7.49	7.36
5.00	5.07	4.75	0.50	0.54	0.37
0.10	0.10	0.07	2.50	2.54	2.50
0.0	0.0	0.0	7.50	7.44	6.63
0.50	0.46	0.50	0.10	0.12	0.14
0.50	0.57	0.66	10.00	10.02	9.81

Statistical Evaluation

ECD:		NPD:	
A: Accuracy 5%	S: Accuracy 1%	A: Accuracy 7%	S: Accuracy 1%
Precision ±.07 mg/liter	Precision ±.05 mg/liter	Precision ±.13 mg/liter	Precision ±.09 mg/liter
$r = .994$	$r = 1.005$	$r = .994$	$r = .996$

Regression line (x) abscissa: true value
($y = mx + b$) (y) ordinate: experimental value

ECD:		NPD:	
$y = .976x + .25$ mg/liter	$y = 1.01x - .037$ mg/liter	$y = .092x + .747$ mg/liter	$y = .977x - .08$ mg/liter

[a] ECD, electron-capture detector; NPD, nitrogen/phosphorus detector.

7-nitrobenzo-2-oxa-1,3-diazole, can meet the sensitivity requirement at nominal reagent cost. However, analysis rate is low and specificity is not good—other primary amines as well as methamphetamine will interfere. Some degree of differentiation is possible by running excitation spectra (*3*), but still no definitive identification is obtainable.

Thin-Layer Chromatographic Methods

This technique can be used to test large numbers of samples for the presence or absence of amphetamine with more than satisfactory sensitivity to meet screening requirements. The high cost of an assay is primarily a function of the cost of the chromatographic plates, but this is offset by the minimal initial investment for capital equipment. Also, less technical expertise is required of the laboratory personnel. Several steps in the procedure (extraction, development) do not require continuous attention, thus setting the analyst free for other activities. Interference from other drugs is not a major problem, except for methamphetamine, for which amphetamine is a metabolite. If these two compounds have to be resolved, then confirmation by alternative procedures is necessary.

Of the 38 samples we assayed in the comparison study (Table 2), only two were listed as "pos/neg" (i.e., results not clear). The rest were consistent with the results of other methods, indicating that the thin-layer chromatographic procedure gives accurate results.

All four of the detection procedures attain the required sensitivity at approximately equivalent reagent cost, but because the Fluram spray is the most sensitive, we recommend it for assays requiring detection of concentrations far lower than 1 mg/liter.

Gas-Chromatographic Methods

These methods can be effectively used either to screen large numbers of samples qualitatively or to assay fewer samples quantitatively. All four methods will easily detect 1 mg/liter. In addition, methods involving use of the electron-capture detector and the nitrogen/phosphorus detector are potentially useful for pharmacokinetic studies or for therapeutic monitoring, because very low concentrations can be detected with either, as may be required in monitoring amphetamine in blood after its therapeutic use. Per-assay costs for reagents and expendables are low, but the initial capital investment is fairly large. Analyst time per assay is comparable to the other methods. About 5 to 7 h is required to process 20 samples quantitatively, but there are time intervals when the analyst would be free for other activities. Of the samples analyzed (Table 2), very few false results were obtained, the acetamide/flame ionization detector method being the least reliable (one

Table 4. Comparison of Analytical Parameters of the Indicated Methods for the Analysis for Amphetamine

	Photometric			TLC[i]		
	Colorimetric	Fluorometric	Ninhydrin	Ninhydrin/phenyl-acetaldehyde	Fluram®	NPD[i]
Volume (ml)	5.0	2.0	5.0	5.0	5.0	10.0
Minimal detectable concentration (mg/liter)[a]	5.0	1.0	0.5	0.1	0.05	0.1
Percent extraction[b]	7	60	60	60	60	60
Absolute sensitivity (ng)[c]	1750	1200	2000	400	200	400
Linearity						
Range (mg/liter)	5.0–100.0	1.0–10.0	—	—	—	—
Regression coefficients[d] (m)	+0.05					
(y = m (mg/liter) + b) (b)	+0.03	—	—	—	—	—
Correlation coefficient (r)	.848	—	—	—	—	—
P values for regression and r[e]	> 0.05	—	—	—	—	—
Accuracy & Precision						
Accuracy (%)[f]	20%	8%	—	—	—	—
Standard deviation (mg/liter)	± 0.60	± 0.10	—	—	—	—
Cost analysis						
Time/assay for 1 assay (h)	1	2	3	3	3	2.75
Time/assay for 20 assays (h)	0.3	0.3	0.3	0.3	0.3	0.3
Reagent cost/assay (1 assay) (cents)[g,h]	4	3	62	62	63	60
Reagent cost/assay (20 assays) (cents)[g,h]	3	3	8	8	8	8
Sample load/technician 8-h day	25	30	50	50	50	50

	Immunoassay		GLC[i]			
	EMIT[i]	RIA[i]	FID-CS_2[i]	FID-Ac_2O[i]	ECD[i]	NPD[i]
Volume (ml)	0.05	0.10	2.0	6.0	1.0	5.0
Minimal detectable concentration (mg/liter)[a]	1.0	1.0	0.4	0.4	0.05	0.01
Percent extraction[b]	80	85	20	30	85	80
Absolute sensitivity (ng)[c]	40	85	3	9	0.04	1.7
Linearity						
Range (mg/liter)	1.0–10.0	0.5–10.0	0.5–10.0	0.5–10.0	0.5–10.0	0.5–10.0
Regression coefficients[d] (m)	—	—	+0.25	+0.48	+2.13	+0.97
(y = m (mg/liter) + b) (b)			−0.06	−0.07	−0.04	−0.10
Correlation coefficient (r)	—	—	.987	.995	.993	.992
P values for regression and r[e]			< 0.01	< 0.01	< 0.01	< 0.01
Accuracy & Precision						
Accuracy (%)[f]	8%	3%	8%	2%	3%	6%
Standard deviation (mg/liter)	±0.02	±0.04	±0.14	±0.16	±0.03	±0.08
Cost analysis						
Time/assay for 1 assay (h)	0.02	1	1	1	1	1.5
Time/assay for 20 assays (h)	0.03	0.1	0.4	0.4	0.3	0.2
Reagent cost/assay (1 assay) (cents)[g,h]	90	100	0.1	0.05	1	1
Reagent cost/assay (20 assays) (cents)[g,h]	90	100	0.1	0.05	1	1
Sample load/technician 8-h day	200	200	25	25	25	30

[a] "Minimal detectable concentration" is the lowest amphetamine concentration required to elicit a response from the detection system that is obviously greater than the response from a drug-free sample.

[b] "Percent extraction" is the percentage of added amphetamine that reaches the detector system. These data were obtained by using radiolabeled amphetamine.

[c] "Absolute sensitivity" is the smallest amount that the detection system can recognize as amphetamine.

[d] Regression coefficients: In all cases a ratio response or absolute response was plotted vs. concentration to determine the linearity of the response. The slope (m), and the intercept (b) were calculated from these plots.

[e] The statistical significance of the regression and correlation coefficients were obtained from a table (*14*), after calculating a t-statistic for the values.

[f] "Accuracy percent" is expressed by the equation A% = $[(\bar{X}_i - \hat{X})/\hat{X}] \times 100$, where $\bar{X}_i$ is the experimental values' mean and $\hat{X}$ is the true value. This was calculated from the daily standard curves.

[g] Immunoassay costs can be significantly decreased if reagents are purchased in bulk amounts.

[h] These costs do not reflect the cost of running standards or controls with the samples of interest.

[i] TLC, thin-layer chromatography; NDD, 7-chloro-4-nitrobenzo-2-oxa-1,3-diazole; EMIT, Enzyme Multiplied Immunoassay Technique; RIA, radioimmunoassay; FID, flame ionization detector; CS_2, carbon disulfide; Ac_2O, acetic anhydride; ECD, electron-capture detector; NPD, nitrogen/phosphorus detector.

false positive and four false negatives in 30 samples analyzed). Several of the drugs tested for interference (Table 1) had a retention time similar to that of amphetamine by at least one gas-chromatographic method. However, only four (methadone, methamphetamine, *p*-hydroxyamphetamine, and phenylephrine) are likely to appear in screening samples. The first two are commonly abused drugs, the third is a metabolite of amphetamine, and the last is a nasal decongestant. If the user must resolve these drugs, then another analysis by an alternative gas-chromatographic procedure is required to provide this answer.

The data obtained with the electron-capture detector and the nitrogen/phosphorus detector were analyzed statistically. The calculated *t*-value was 0.11 with 54 degrees of freedom $[(n_1 - 1) + (n_2 - 1)]$, consistent with a 93% probability that the concentrations obtained by the two methods were identical (*14*).

Immunological Methods

Immunotechniques are sensitive and relatively specific, can be performed easily and rapidly by personnel with modest scientific training, and most of them provide objective results. These attributes are designed to suit those laboratories that must continually analyze many samples for a given substance, particularly in screening many specimens that are expected to be predominantly negative. Many other elegant procedures satisfy similar needs for one or more of the attributes listed, but few combine them all, as do the immunoassays.

The inherent advantage of the RIA technique is that because the radiolabeled drug has a high specific radioactivity, its concentration can be sensitively and precisely determined. Standard curves are obtained by plotting counts per minute vs. concentration. Usually, these have a limited linear portion, and above these concentrations, unless the sample is diluted, all one can determine is that the sample is positive for the specific drug. One attribute of RIA over most of the EMIT assays is that it can be applied to serum, something that until now is not the case for EMIT.

The general objections to all immunoassays also prevail for this RIA procedure, plus some additional ones. Because radioactive substances are involved, additional precautions and safety measures are required—all reasonable and easily met. Shelf life may be a problem also, particularly for I^{125}-labeled compounds. The time for a single determination is relatively long (40 min), but when many are done concomitantly, as they can be, the time per sample decreases significantly.

The EMIT determination requires only 1 min to complete and is simple to perform. Its primary advantages are its speed and its relatively moderate instrument cost, currently about $6000 to $8000. Of course, the cost of the antiserum is high—currently $0.50 to $0.60 a test for amphetamine—but when prompt results are required, this system is the one that can provide the necessary results.

One difficulty with the EMIT system is that lysozyme is naturally present in some samples and may be a source of falsely positive results. Of course, one can easily check for this sort of interference by adding the urine sample to the bacterial suspension and noting if any clearing results. This check is inexpensive, because no antibody is required. Another problem is that in rather alkaline urines the activity of the lysozyme released from the antigen/lysozyme solution is almost eliminated, leading to many falsely negative results.

The greatest defect of immunoassays is their lack of specificity. Very few antisera exist that are specific for a single compound, although some have been prepared with very high specificity when cost was no object. Hence, one should confirm all positive results by some other procedure if specificity is important. Clearly, it is essential to know precisely what specific substance is present in certain forensic medicine problems, because (e.g.) a job may be in jeopardy or a potential parole violator incarcerated.

Summary

In all of these procedures the analyst must recognize that an absolute physical property is not being measured. A positive result is a necessary but is not a sufficient proof of identity. Additional tests may be required, depending on the specificity required. Our purpose was objectively to determine the various analytical factors of importance in several different methods now available for analysis for amphetamine. These data are recorded in Table 4 and complement those on specificity (Table 1). Included in Table 4 are sensitivity or detection limits; experimental linear range (for quantitative assays) or minimum observable concentration (in the case of thin-layer chromatography); statistics to indicate reproducibility and accuracy; time required; and reagent-cost, tabulated two ways; for running only one sample and on a per-assay basis when 20 samples are analyzed concomitantly.

The amphetamine method best suited to a given laboratory depends on that laboratory's needs. Factors to be considered include (*a*) number of samples to be processed, (*b*) type of equipment available, (*c*) personnel available and their background, (*d*) acceptable turnaround time, (*e*) the ultimate use of the results, and (*f*) funds available.

For pharmacokinetic studies or for monitoring therapeutic concentrations in blood, the most sensitive method must be selected, i.e., gas chromatography—assaying either the trichloroacetamide derivative with an electron-capture detector or free amphetamine directly with the nitrogen detector. Radioimmunoassay has the necessary sensitivity, but quantitative analyses require serial dilutions of the sample, which increases the cost of the analysis dramatically.

In most clinical/toxicology laboratories, many amphetamine analyses are requested of samples from individuals involved in drug-abuse programs. In these samples, qualitative answers are sufficient, a positive result being defined as a concentration of 1 mg/liter or more. Thin-layer chromatographic procedures are well suited for this purpose. The initial expense for equipment is minimal, reagent costs are low, and modest technical expertise is required of the laboratory personnel. In those laboratories that already have a gas chromatograph and qualified personnel, one of the gas-chromatographic methods would be very adequate. These methods can be adjusted to provide either qualitative or quantitative data, as the need requires. Either of the immunological methods would be a suitable choice for those laboratories that have the equipment and personnel available.

We gratefully acknowledge our debt to Roche Diagnostics and Syva Corp. for their contribution of many reagents (RIA, FLURAM, EMIT) used in this study, which was supported in part by grant DA-00687-01 from the Center for Study of Narcotics and Drug Abuse of the NIMH, NIH, USPHS.

References

1. Bastos, M. L., and Hoffman, D. B., Comparison of methods for detection of amphetamines, cocaine, and metabolites. *J. Chromatogr. Sci.* **12,** 269 (1974).

2. Frings, C. S., Queen, C., and Foster, L. B., Improved colorimetric method for assay of amphetamines in urine. *Clin. Chem.* **17,** 1016 (1971).

3. Monforte, J., Bath, R. J., and Sunshine, I., Fluorometric determination of primary and secondary amines in blood and urine after thin-layer chromatography. *Clin. Chem.* **18,** 1329 (1972).

4. (*a*) Klein, B., Sheehan, J. E., and Grunberg, B., Use of fluorescamine ("Fluram") to detect amphetamine in urine by thin-layer chromatography. *Clin. Chem.* **20,** 272 (1974). (*b*) Meola, J. M., and Brown, H. H., Fluorescamine as a fluorogenic reagent for *d*-amphetamine identification by TLC. *Clin. Chem.* **20,** 88 (1974). Letter to the Editor.

5. Samjima, K., Dairman, W., and Udenfriend, S., Condensation of ninhydrin with aldehydes and primary amines to yield highly fluorescent ternary products. 1. Studies on the mechanism of the reaction and some characteristics of the condensation product. *Anal. Biochem.* **42,** 222 (1971).

6. Mulé, S. J., Routine identification of drugs of abuse in human urine. I. Application of fluorometry, thin-layer and gas-liquid chromatography. *J. Chromatogr.* **55,** 255 (1971).

7. Toseland, P. A., and Scott, P. H., Determination of amphetamine as its *N*-acetyl derivative by gas-liquid chromatography. *Clin. Chim. Acta* **25,** 75 (1969).

8. Beckett, A. H., Tucker, G. T., and Moffatt, A. C., Routine detection and identification in urine of stimulants and other drugs, some of which may be used to modify performance in sport. *J. Pharm. Pharmacol.* **19,** 273 (1967).

9. Änggård, E., and Hankey, A., Derivatives of sympathomimetic amines for gas chromatography with electron capture detection and mass spectrometry. *Acta Chem. Scand.* **23,** 3110 (1969).

10. Kolb, B., Linder, M., and Kempken, B., Der thermionische Phosphor-Stickstoff-Detektor (PND). *Angew. Chromatogr.* **21,** 1 (1974).

11. Sunshine, I., Immunoassays. In *Methodology for Analytical Toxicology,* I. Sunshine, Ed., CRC Press, Cleveland, Ohio, 1975, pp 399–400.

12. Lorenzo, B., Enzyme Multiplied Immunoassay Technique (EMIT). In *Methodology for Analytical Toxicology,* I. Sunshine, Ed. CRC Press, Cleveland, Ohio, 1975, pp 401–403.

13. Lorenzo, B., Radioimmunoassay (RIA). In *Methodology for Analytical Toxicology,* I. Sunshine, Ed., CRC Press, Cleveland, Ohio, 1975, pp 403–406.

14. Beyer, W., *Handbook of Tables for Probability and Statistics,* W. Beyer, Ed., CRC Press, Cleveland, Ohio, 1966, pp 225–232.

Automated Enzymic Determination of Ethanol in Blood, Serum, and Urine with a Miniature Centrifugal Analyzer

T. P. Hadjiioannou,[1] S. I. Hadjiioannou, J. Avery, and H. V. Malmstadt[2]

We describe an automated spectrophotometric reaction-rate method for determination of ethanol in serum and urine with a miniature centrifugal analyzer. The ethanol is selectively oxidized in the presence of alcohol dehydrogenase and NAD^+ to form NADH, which is measured by the rate of change of its absorbance. Reaction rates are determined automatically, and unknown concentrations are calculated from a computer-generated working curve based on aqueous ethanol standards. Blood, serum, or urine specimens need not be deproteinized. The method permits duplicate analysis of at least 30 samples per hour. Coefficients of variation and relative errors are about 2–3% for ethanol concentrations of 0.3–3.0 μg per 2 μl of sample. Analytical recovery of ethanol added to serum is 92–103% (average, 98.5%). Comparisons with distillation-oxidation, gas-chromatographic, and conventional enzymic procedures give satisfactory agreement.

Ethanol determinations are the most frequent analyses required in the forensic and clinical toxicology laboratory (*1*). The increased demand for ethanol determinations, largely in response to traffic safety legislation, has resulted in the development of a variety of analytical methods. Gas-chromatographic methods, by virtue of their ability to separate and quantitate sample components, have been widely used (*2, 3*).

During the past 20 years, enzymic methods (*4–13*) have been increasingly favored over the chemical oxidation methods, because of their high specificity, great sensitivity, and simplicity. The basis of the enzymic methods is the reaction:

$$CH_3CH_2OH + NAD^+ \overset{ADH}{\rightleftarrows} CH_3CHO + NADH + H^+ \quad (1)$$

where ADH is alcohol dehydrogenase (EC 1.1.1.1), which catalyzes the reaction, and NAD^+ and NADH are the oxidized and reduced forms of the coenzyme. Automated versions of both the chemical oxidation and enzymic methods exist, mainly for use on continuous-flow analyzers (*8*). An automatic reaction-rate method has also been used in which the time required for a small, fixed amount of NADH to form is related directly to the ethanol concentration (*9*).

Modifying the enzymic reaction rate method (*9*) for use on an automated miniature centrifugal analyzer makes it possible to increase sample analysis rate substantially while greatly decreasing sample size. Amounts of ethanol in the range 0.3–3.0 μg per 2 μl of body fluid (blood, blood serum, or urine) are determined with relative errors and coefficients of variation of about 2 to 3%. The method permits duplicate analysis of at least 30 samples per hour.

Materials and Methods

Apparatus

Hardware. The instrumental system is based upon the original ORNL design (*14–18*), but it incorporates extensive modifications as previously described (*19*). Further improvements have been made for the present work.

The centrifugal analyzer disc in this study contains 16 separate 100-μl measurement cuvettes. Radially connected with each measurement cuvette are a sample and a reagent fill well, each of which can hold 50 μl of solution. Distilled water is loaded into the fill wells for cuvette No. 1, which is designated the reference cuvette (100% transmittance). The position corresponding to cuvette No. 2 is blocked with opaque material. The signal measured at cuvette position 2 provides the "background" or zero transmittance output. The remaining 14 cuvettes are used for samples or standards. Measurements are made on each rotation of the disc at each cuvette position. Values from each cuvette are

School of Chemical Sciences, University of Illinois, Urbana, Ill. 61801.

[1] Visiting Professor of Analytical Chemistry from the Laboratory of Analytical Chemistry, University of Athens, Athens, Greece.

[2] Send reprint requests to this author.

Received July 21, 1975; accepted Mar. 1, 1976.

summed, and an average for each cuvette is calculated 20 times during the measurement interval. The transmittance for any cuvette is calculated from the ratio of the background-corrected sample average to the background-corrected reference average.

Samples and reagents are loaded into the fill wells with a Pipetman P-200 adjustable pipet (Cole Scientific, Canoga Park, Calif. 91303) and an Eppendorf 50-μl pipet (Brinkman Instruments, Westbury, N.Y. 11590).

Accurate temperature control is not required because standards are run together with samples on each disc, under the same conditions.

Software. A reaction-rate computer program written for the present work is available from us (write to H. V. M.) Twenty absorbance values are calculated for each sample and standard cuvette as the reaction proceeds. The reaction rate, expressed in change-in-absorbance per second, is calculated for each cuvette by fitting a least-squares line through the data points. Calibration curves that relate the reaction rate to the concentration of the standards are determined by least-squares fit. The software provides for the absorbance vs. time curves for any cuvette or the calibration curve to be displayed on either an oscilloscope or a high-speed line printer. Display of the absorbance vs. time curves allows the user to choose the optimum concentrations and measurement time during the development of the method. The effects of different concentrations of reagent and standards on the slope and linearity of the calibration curve can be observed by simply running the various mixtures in parallel on a single disc and comparing results based on the calibration curve for each mixture. Once optimum concentrations are determined, the appropriate number of standards necessary for a calibration curve can be determined. Examples of such an approach in the development of the procedure for ethanol are discussed.

Reagents

Pyrophosphate buffer, 75 mmol/liter, pH 8.7. Dissolve 33.4 g of $Na_4P_2O_7 \cdot 10H_2O$, 8.4 g of semicarbazide hydrochloride (AR, alcohol-free), and 1.6 g of glycine in about 800 ml of distilled water, adjust to pH 8.7 with about 66 ml of 1 mol/liter NaOH, and dilute to 1 liter with distilled water. Refrigerate when not in use.

NAD^+, 3.6 mmol/liter. Dissolve 2.5 mg of NAD^+ (Sigma; β-NAD, Grade III) per milliliter of the above buffer solution. Refrigerate when not in use.

Phosphate buffer, 100 mmol/liter, pH 7.5. Dissolve 1.86 g of $NaH_2PO_4 \cdot H_2O$ and 12.26 g of Na_2HPO_4 in distilled water and dilute to 1 liter. To prepare the working solution (1 mmol/liter), dilute the stock solution 100-fold with distilled water.

Alcohol dehydrogenase (ADH; EC 1.1.1.1), from Sigma Chemical Co. Dissolve 1.6 mg of ADH in 10.0 ml of the working phosphate buffer solution and refrigerate when not in use. Dilute this solution 10-fold with working phosphate buffer solution just before use to give the working ADH solution. This solution must be kept refrigerated, except during loading of the disc.

Ethanol standards. Absolute ethanol (U.S. Industrial Chemicals, New York, N.Y. 10016) was used to prepare standard solutions. Dilute 1.90 ml of absolute ethanol to 100 ml with distilled water. Then dilute a 10.0-ml aliquot of this solution to 100 ml to give a solution containing 1.50 mg of ethanol per milliliter. Prepare working standards containing 0.75, 3.0, and 7.5 mg of ethanol per 100 ml from this solution by dilution. These standards are stable for several weeks. Before use, dilute the working standards fivefold with NAD^+ solution. The resulting composite standards are labeled $St_{0.75}$, St_3, and $St_{7.5}$.

Procedure

Dilute the sample 20-fold with water to prepare dilute sample solution S. For an analysis in duplicate, only 80 μl of solution S are needed, equivalent to 4 μl of sample; however, larger quantities are usually prepared to minimize the effect of pipetting error. Dilute solution S fivefold with the NAD^+ solution to prepare composite sample solution S_c. Pipet 50 μl of water into both fill wells of the first (reference) cuvette, and 50 μl of working ADH solution into all 14 remaining outer (reagent) fill wells of the disc. The second cuvette is not used for samples since it is used for a background reading. Pipet 50 μl of composite ethanol standards $St_{0.75}$, St_3, and $St_{7.5}$ each in duplicate, into six of the inner cavities of the sample cuvettes and 50 μl each of the composite sample solutions S_c in duplicate into the remaining inner cuvettes. Use the teletypewriter to set the following operating variables: a premeasurement delay time of 12 s, which includes a mixing time of 11.3 s during which four rapid acceleration and braking operations take place, and a measurement time of 20 s, during which 20 absorbance readings are taken for each cuvette. Place the loaded disc on the rotor. The analysis is started and run under computer control. At the end of the analytical run, remove the disc, empty it by aspiration, wash thoroughly with distilled water, and allow it to air dry.

If the original sample contains more than 160 mg of ethanol per 100 ml, the dilution factor should be such that dilute solutions S does not contain more than 8 mg of ethanol per 100 ml.

Data reduction. The maximum reaction rates in each cuvette are automatically determined by a special least-squares program. The slope and y-intercept of the calibration curve are calculated by fitting concentrations of the standards and rates measured for the ethanol standards to a straight line. These values are used to calculate the concentrations of unknown samples from their reaction rates.

Results and Discussion

Basic considerations concerning ethanol-free reagents, their stability, contamination, and interfering substances are similar to those previously reported (*9*). Delay and measurement times were properly adjusted to ensure that mixing is thorough and that absorbance data are collected during the period of maximum reaction rate.

Application of the miniature centrifugal analyzer provides a convenient way to study the linear range, precision, and accuracy of the ethanol assay. Various initial NAD^+ concentrations and ADH activities can be used. By running the various mixtures in parallel on a single disc and using arbitrary subsets of the standards in the construction of the calibration curve, the effects of different concentrations of reagents and standards on the linearity and slope of the calibration curve can be observed and the optimal concentrations chosen. Several combinations of NAD^+ and ADH were tried, in the ranges 3.6×10^{-3} to 3.6×10^{-2} mol of NAD^+ per liter and activities of about 1.6 to 13 U/ml of working ADH solution, equivalent to final concentrations after the mixing of 3.6×10^{-4} to 3.6×10^{-3} mol of NAD^+ per liter and activities of 0.8 to 6.5 U/ml. The most accurate results for the range 0.75–8 mg of ethanol per 100 ml of standard solution, equivalent to 15 to 160 mg of ethanol per 100 ml of body fluid before the 20-fold dilution, were obtained with the combination 3.6×10^{-3} mol of NAD^+ per liter and 2.5 to 3 U of working ADH solution per milliliter. These reagent concentrations were chosen as optimum for the determination of ethanol in body fluids. Under the selected conditions there is a linear relationship between reaction rate and ethanol concentrations in the range 0.75–8 mg of ethanol per 100 ml. The ethanol concentrations of the samples should be brought into this range by appropriate dilution because the slopes of the working curves decrease at higher concentrations.

A delay time of 12 s and a measurement time of 20 s were chosen, so that at least 10 of the 20 absorbance measurements are taken when the rate is at the maximum.

In this work the only temperature control is room temperature to ±1 °C, but accurate results are obtained because calibration materials are included among the samples in each disc. Because legal protocol may require standards to be run concurrently with samples, the lack of temperature control is not a problem. With accurate temperature control to within 0.1 °C, however, it should be feasible to run only one control standard on each disc. This is indicated by results obtained during six runs completed over a 90-min period. The CV for the slopes of the calibration curves was 3.7%, and the average error increased by only 1% when each calibration curve was used for all discs.

The accuracy of the proposed method was estimated by recovery experiments done by adding various amounts of ethanol to pooled ethanol-free sera to produce concentrations of 15–150 mg of ethanol per 100 ml. The results are shown in Table 1. Analytical recovery ranged from 92 to 103%, with an average of 98.5% for the entire series.

To check the precision, we did a series of determinations on several of the aforementioned pooled sera containing known amounts of added ethanol, as well as on blood samples. The proposed method shows a high degree of reproducibility, with coefficients of variation ranging from 0.5 to 2.9% ($n = 5$–8), which includes errors arising from pathlength variation, pipetting, and other instrumental factors.

Table 1. Recovery of Ethanol Added to Human Serum

Ethanol concn, g/liter		Recovery, %
Added	Found	
0.150	0.138	92.0
0.300	0.308	102.7
0.600	0.618	103.0
1.200	1.136	94.7
1.500	1.498	99.9

Table 2. Results of Ethanol Analysis in Aqueous Solutions, Urine, and Blood

		Ethanol concn, g/liter	
No.[a]	Medium	ATEP[b]	Present method[c,d]
54	aqueous	1.14	1.12
55	aqueous	1.99	1.95
61	aqueous	2.96	3.33
62	aqueous	1.60	1.79
57	urine	2.44	2.43
58	urine	3.18	3.39
63	urine	0.90	1.01
64	urine	2.03	2.18
59	blood	0.82	0.94
60	blood	2.91	2.77
65	blood	2.55	2.62
66	blood	3.24	3.16

[a] Refers to specimen numbering at ATEP.
[b] Alcohol Testing Evaluation Program, Madison, Wis. Samples analyzed by 28 laboratories by distillation-oxidation, gas-chromatographic, and enzymic procedures. Mean value.
[c] Average of two values.
[d] Samples analyzed without deproteinization.

We tested the proposed method by analyzing several aqueous samples and specimens of pooled blood and urine, which were analyzed by distillation-oxidation, gas-chromatographic, and enzymic procedures at the Alcohol Testing Evaluation Program (ATEP), Madison, Wis., by 28 laboratories participating in the program (*20*). The results are shown in Table 2. The correlation coefficient for 12 samples was 0.986. The good correlation demonstrates the accuracy of the present method.

The chief advantages of the present work are sensitivity and speed with very small sample volumes, and also that no sample pretreatment, such as distillation or deproteinization, is necessary. The miniature centrifugal analyzer method for the determination of ethanol in body fluids performs well, as demonstrated by good precision, nearly 100% recovery, and agreement of results with those obtained by conventional methods.

This research was supported in part by NIH Grant HEW PHS GM21984-01. J.P.A. received an industrial fellowship supported by Rohm and Haas.

References

1. Sunshine, I., Alcohol in biological material. *Stand. Methods Clin. Chem.*, **3**, 1 (1961).

2. Laessig, R. H., Submicro sampling and solvent extraction system for rapid gas chromatographic determination of blood alcohol. *Anal. Chem.* **40**, 2205 (1968).

3. Battista, H. J., Computerized blood alcohol analysis. *Chromatographia* **5**, 206 (1972).

4. Bonnichsen, R., and Theorell, H., An enzymatic method for the microdetermination of ethanol. *Scand. J. Clin. Lab. Invest.* **3**, 58 (1951).

5. Bücher, T., and Redetzki, H., Eine spezifische photometrische Bestimmung von Äthylalcohol auf fermentative Wege. *Klin. Wochenschr.* **29**, 615 (1951).

6. Brink, N. G., Bonnichsen, R., and Theorell, H., A modified method for the enzymatic microdetermination of ethanol. *Acta Pharmacol. Toxicol.* **10**, 223 (1954).

7. Bonnishsen, R., and Lundgren, G., Comparison of the ADH and the Widmark procedures in forensic chemistry for determining alcohol. *Acta Pharmacol. Toxicol.* **13**, 256 (1957).

8. Goldberg, L., and Rydberg, U., Automated enzymatic microdetermination of ethanol in blood and urine. In *Automation in Analytical Chemistry. Technicon Symposia 1965,* L. T. Skeggs, Jr., et al., Eds., Mediad, New York, N.Y., 1966, p 595.

9. Malmstadt, H. V., and Hadjiioannou, T. P., Specific enzymatic determination of alcohol in blood by an automatic spectrophotometric reaction rate method. *Anal. Chem.* **34**, 455 (1962).

10. Laessig, R. H., A convenient submicro sampling and enzymatic analysis technique for the determination of blood alcohol. *Microchem. J.* **13**, 561 (1968).

11. Ellis, F. W., and Hill, J. B., An automated fluorometric procedure for the enzymatic determination of ethanol in fingertip blood. *Clin. Chem.* **15**, 91 (1969).

12. Jones, D., Gerber, L. P., and Drell, W., A rapid enzymatic method for estimating ethanol in body fluids. *Clin. Chem.* **16**, 402 (1970).

13. Rosalki, S. B., A new colorimetric procedure for blood alcohol determination. *Anal. Lett.* **4**, 819 (1971).

14. Anderson, N. G., Basic principles of fast analyzers. *Am. J. Clin. Pathol.* **53**, 778 (1970).

15. Anderson, N. G., Burtis, C. A., Mailen, J. C., et al., Feasibility of miniaturization of a fast analyzer. *Anal. Lett.* **5**, 153 (1972).

16. Burtis, C. A., Mailen, J. C., Johnson, W. F., et al., Development of miniature fast analyzer. *Clin. Chem.* **18**, 753 (1972).

17. Scott, C. D., and Burtis, C. A., Miniature fast analyzer systems. *Anal. Chem.* **45**, 327 (1973).

18. Burtis, C. A., Johnson, W. F., Mailen, J. C., et al., Development of an analytical system based around a miniature fast analyzer. *Clin. Chem.* **19**, 895 (1973).

19. Avery, J., Gregory, R. P., IV, Renoe, B. W., et al., A centrifugal analyzer with a new all-digital measurement system. *Clin. Chem.* **20**, 942 (1974).

20. Laessig, R. H., Becker, R. V., Basteyns, B. J., and Field, P. H., Performance evaluation of Wisconsin laboratories performing implied-consent alcohol determinations. *Health Lab. Sci.* **12**, 82 (1975).

CLIN. CHEM. 22/6, 806–809 (1976)

Gas-Chromatographic Determination of an Antifibrinolytic Drug, ϵ-Aminocaproic Acid

Thomas R. Keucher, Elizabeth B. Solow,[1] John Metaxas, and Robert L. Campbell

We describe a modified method for assay of ϵ-aminocaproic acid. Serum or cerebrospinal fluid is deproteinized, followed by cation-exchange column-chromatography, and *N*-trifluoroacetyl-*n*-butyl derivatives of amino acids are formed and separated by gas chromatography. Tranexamic acid, a nonprotein amino acid, was used as an internal standard. The assay is sensitive and precise, and results correlate adequately with those obtained with an automated amino acid analyzer (ion-exchange chromatography).

Additional Keyphrases: *analysis for the drug in serum, plasma, cerebrospinal fluid, urine • results by ion-exchange chromatography compared • assay for tranexamic acid*

ϵ-Aminocaproic acid is used in therapy for hemorrhage (*1*), angioneurotic edema (*2*), intracranial aneurysms (*3*), and other diseases (*1*) ("AMICAR"; Lederle Laboratories, Div. of American Cyanamid Co.). It is an antifibrinolytic agent, inhibiting conversion of plasminogen into plasmin (*4, 5*). Hitherto, its concentrations in plasma and biological fluids have been evaluated by electrophoresis (*6*), paper chromatography (*7–9*), cation-exchange column chromatography (*10*), coagulation analysis (*9*), clot lysis time (*11, 12*), or by gas-chromatographic separation of a dinitrophenyl derivative (*13*). Disadvantages of the previous techniques—high analytical error, insensitivity, inprecision at low concentrations, and the relatively large volumes of specimen required—led us to investigate gas–liquid chromatographic methods for this assay.

Ikekawa et al. (*13*) reported that a dinitrophenyl derivative of this drug could be used as an internal standard for derivatives of free amino acids in serum for their gas–liquid chromatographic method. Raulin et al. (*14*) noted the elution position of ϵ-aminocaproic acid, a nonprotein amino acid, relative to those of the common amino acids. They showed that the compound was not separated from aspartic acid under their chromatographic conditions.

This paper describes a gas-chromatographic method for separating ϵ-aminocaproic acid from the amino acids normally present in biological fluids, with emphasis on the determination of the drug in serum. We adapted the gas–liquid chromatographic method of Gehrke et al. (*15–17*) for determining amino acids as their *N*-trifluoro-acetyl-*n*-butyl esters. Tranexamic acid [4-(aminomethyl)-cyclohexanecarboxylic acid] is not a normal component of biological fluids, and so it is useful as an internal standard. Moreover, it not only possesses the functional groups for monitoring the reaction, but also can be advantageously used to assess the performance of the ion-exchange column procedure, thereby increasing the reliability of the quantitative analysis in this complex mixture of amino acids (*17*).

Materials and Methods

Reagents

Tranexamic acid and ϵ-aminocaproic acid were supplied by Lederle Laboratories, Div. of American Cyanamid Co., Pearl River, N. Y. 10965.

HCl in methanol (1.25 mol/liter), HCl in butanol (3 mol/liter), and trifluoroacetic acid anhydride were obtained from Regis Chemical Co., Chicago, Ill. 60610.

The cation-exchange resin (Amberlite CG-120, 110-120 mesh) was purchased from Mallinckrodt Chemical Works, St. Louis, Mo. 63160.

Special Equipment

Disposable columns (0.1 × 4 cm) were from Bio-Rad Laboratories, Richmond, Calif. 98494 (cat. no. 7311110).

We used an infrared lamp (Model HS 250-3; Instrumentation for Research and Industry, Cheltenham, Pa. 19012) to dry the eluates.

Instrumentation

Our gas chromatograph, Series 7300, equipped with flame-ionization detector, was from Packard Instruments Co., Downers Grove, Ill. 60015.

Division of Neurological Surgery, Department of Surgery, Indiana University School of Medicine, 1100 W. Michigan St., Indianapolis, Ind. 46202.

[1] Address communications to this author.
Received Jan. 23, 1975; accepted Feb. 9, 1976.

For the column packing, we used ethylene glycol adipate, 0.65% on Chromosorb W, 80/100 mesh, which was prepared for us (Analytical Biochemistry Laboratory, Inc., Columbia, Mo. 65201). The glass column was in a glass U-shaped configuration, 180 cm × 4 mm i.d.

The following temperatures were used: inlet port 200 °C; flame-ionization detector, 260 °C; and oven temperatures programmed from 100 °C with an increase of 3 °C/min to a final temperature of 200 °C.

The flow rate of the carrier gas, nitrogen, was adjusted to achieve good resolution.

The "VIDAR" digital integrator, Model No. 6300, was from Autolab, Mountain View, Calif. 94049.

Procedure

Prepare the cation-exchange resin as described by Gehrke et al. (*15*), and then store it in an equal volume of distilled water, under refrigeration. Add 2 ml of the resin suspension to the disposable column, allow it to settle well, and then wash the resin with distilled water.

Add 2.5 ml of picric acid solution (10 g/liter) to 0.5 ml of serum, to remove proteins, and 0.5 ml of tranexamic acid solution (100 mg/liter of distilled water) as the internal standard. Mix well, and centrifuge. Decant the supernatant fluid to the resin column and remove excess picric acid by washing with distilled water.

Elute the amino acids with two 1-ml volumes of 7 mol/liter ammonium hydroxide. Pool the eluates directly into a 20-ml vial with a flat bottom and a screw cap, and evaporate the fluid under an infrared lamp with the maximum heat adjusted so that it is 100 °C at the level of the bottom of the vial.

Add 200 µl of HCl in methanol (1.25 mol/liter) to the dried sample, cap the vial tightly, and mix well with a vortex-type mixer. Allow esterification (methyl ester) to proceed at room temperature for 30 min, transfer the liquid to a micro-reaction vial, and evaporate the solvent on a sandbath at 100 °C with the aid of a stream of nitrogen. To transesterify the amino acids, forming the more soluble butyl ester of ε-aminocaproic acid, add 200 µl of HCl in butanol (3 mol/liter) to the dried sample, cap the vial tightly, and mix well. Return the vial to the sandbath (100 °C) for 5 min. Again evaporate the excess solvents with the aid of a stream of nitrogen in order that no residual butanol remains in the vial or in its screw-cap. Add 100 µl of dichloromethane and evaporate the solvent. Repeat with a second aliquot of dichloromethane and again evaporate the solvent completely. This is done to assure the complete azeotropic removal of water. Cool the capped vial before the final derivatization step.

To acylate the amino acids, add 100 µl of dichloromethane and 50 µl of trifluoroacetic acid anhydride to the reaction vial. Immediately cap the vial tightly, mix well, and allow the *N*-trifluoroacetyl acylation reaction to progress for 5 min in another sandbath, preadjusted to 150 °C. Cool the vial before removing the screw-cap, and then evaporate the excess reagents in the 100 °C sandbath. Reconstitute the derivatized amino acid residue in 50 µl of dichloromethane.

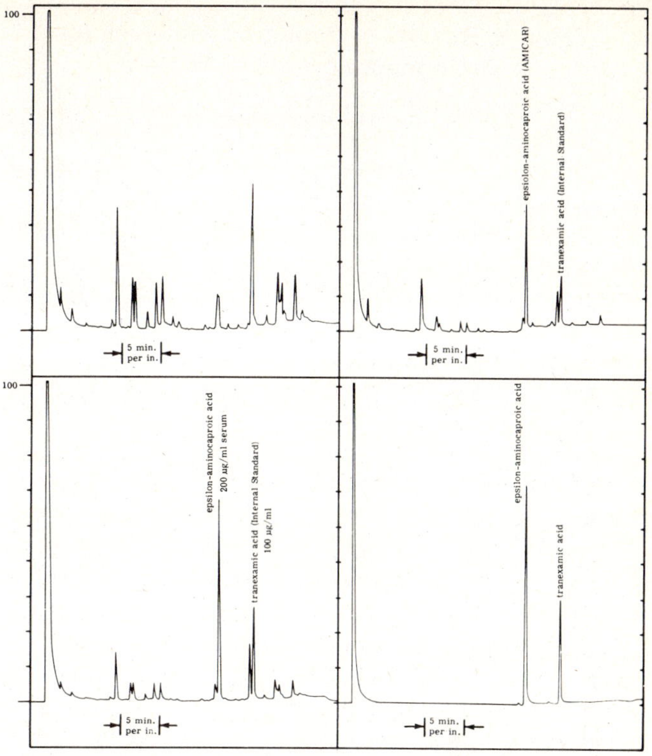

Fig. 1. Gas–liquid chromatograms of N-trifluoroacetyl-*n*-butyl amino acids, illustrating positions of ε-aminocaproic acid and tranexamic acid

Upper left: blood-bank plasma, unsupplemented. *Upper right:* serum from a patient receiving therapy with ε-aminocaproic acid. *Lower left:* blood-bank plasma plus drug and internal standard (200 and 100 mg/liter, respectively). *Lower right:* aqueous solution of drug and internal standard

Inject 1 or 2 µl into the chromatograph.

To prepare cerebrospinal fluid specimens, combine 0.5 ml of the fluid with 0.5 ml of the tranexamic acid solution (20 mg/liter of distilled water) as the internal standard, and continue with the procedures as described above for serum assay.

Urine samples may be similarly assayed, but because the concentration of ε-aminocaproic acid in the urine is expected to be high, dilute the sample 100-fold with distilled water.

Quantitation

Routinely use two standards in serum or plasma to prepare a calibration curve. Supplement the two sera with ε-aminocaproic acid to contain 100 and 300 mg/liter, then follow the complete procedure as described above for unknown samples.

Calculate the integration ratio of ε-aminocaproic acid to tranexamic acid for both standards. For each standard, graph the integration ratio on the ordinate vs. drug concentration (mg/liter) on the abscissa, and draw an appropriate line through zero.

Results

Figure 1 shows some typical chromatograms of *N*-trifluoroacetyl-*n*-butyl derivatives of free amino acids. The ε-aminocaproic acid was resolved from aspartic acid

Table 1. Results of Duplicate Analyses for ϵ-Aminocaproic Acid in 16 Sera

Drug concn, mg/liter				
		Mean	SD	CV, %
33	27	30	4.24	14.1
92	97	94	3.54	3.7
126	120	123	4.24	3.4
159	148	154	7.79	5.1
158	158	158	0	0
166	162	164	2.83	1.7
161	188	174	22.90	13.2
182	179	180	2.12	1.2
181	200	190	13.40	7.1
251	211	231	28.30	12.3
271	274	272	2.12	0.8
285	264	274	14.80	5.4
288	275	282	9.19	3.3
320	282	301	26.90	8.9
326	362	344	25.50	7.4
420	392	406	19.80	4.9
				Av 5.8

and phenylalanine, and appears between these two peaks. The peak corresponding to the tranexamic acid derivative appeared after glutamic acid.

To verify the linearity of our method, ratios as described above were determined for known concentrations of ϵ-aminocaproic acid from zero to 500 mg/liter. The relationship was linear; the curve passed through the origin with a slope of 0.0103 and a variance of 2 SD = 0.0004.

Reproducibility of the standardization method was evaluated by examining 50 consecutive daily calibration ratios during three months. The average slope of these lines was 0.0104 (SD ±0.0009). The individual ratios were then combined to provide a common line, which passed through the origin with a slope of 0.0104 ± 0.0002. The agreement of these slopes is indicative of consistent standardization from day to day.

A series of 16 serum samples was analyzed in duplicate (Table 1). The coefficient of variation for paired duplicates averaged 5.8% (range, 0–14%).

Results from the gas-chromatographic procedure were compared to results from an amino acid ion-exchange analyzer (Table 2). The serum and cerebrospinal fluid determinations were done by the present method without knowledge of results from the amino acid analyzer.[2] Between 10–150 mg/liter, values for the drug as obtained with the amino acid analyzer were somewhat lower than those obtained by the present method; for drug concentrations exceeding 150 mg/liter the reverse was true.

[2] This group of specimens was received from D. W. Nibbelink, M.D., Department of Neurology, and Louis Stegink, Ph.D., Department of Biochemistry and Pediatrics, University Hospital, University of Iowa, Iowa City, Iowa 52240. The amino acid analyzer (Technicon) results are their data.

Table 2. Results for ϵ-Aminocaproic Acid in Samples of Serum and Cerebrospinal Fluid by Our Method (GLC) and as Measured with an Amino Acid Analyzer (AA)

Concn in serum		Concn in cerebrospinal fluid	
mg/liter			
by GLC	by AA	by GLC	by AA
115	80	7.0	6.6
147	118	13.5	9.0
99	80	14.0	9.0
158	132	8.0	7.0
264	330	48.0	14.0
156	132	107.0	95.0
179	262	11.0	12.2
360	420	12.0	12.2
		8.0	13.9
		Trace	8.0
		none evident	0.7

Although not in complete agreement, the two chromatographic methods do provide similar results over a wide range in drug concentrations.

Discussion

The swift renal clearance of ϵ-aminocaproic acid (*8*) necessitates large and frequent doses of the drug (about 15 mg/kg body weight every 1 to 2 h) to maintain therapeutic serum concentrations in the range of 100–400 mg/liter. With this dosage, cerebrospinal fluid drug concentrations are usually 10–20% of those for serum. Also because of its rapid clearance, serum concentrations of the drug can fluctuate widely with relatively slight changes in the dosage schedule. Therapy with this drug must, therefore, be monitored more closely than would be the case for a drug that is excreted more slowly. Assay, preferably daily, of the concentration of the drug in serum assures maintenance of a therapeutic concentration. Toxic accumulation of this nonprotein amino acid should be avoided.

In earlier methods for measuring ϵ-aminocaproic acid the degree of fibrinolytic inhibition was measured (*9, 11, 12*); such semiquantitative assay suffered from the biological variability of the fibrinolytic systems among patients (*18*). Paper chromatography (*7–9*) is not adequately sensitive. McNichol et al. (*8*) found that for concentrations <50 mg/liter the error exceeded 25%. They considered this technique to be unreliable for concentrations <20 mg/liter, but even for concentrations greater than 100 mg/liter the mean error was 20%. Markwardt et al. (*9*) state that with thin-layer chromatography of a dinitrophenyl derivative they could detect ϵ-aminocaproic acid at concentrations of 10 mg/liter, although no information regarding precision of this technique was given; furthermore, much time was required for each determination. Takada et al. (*10*) reported a column-chromatographic technique that could be used to detect ε-aminocaproic acid in concentrations as low as 13 mg/liter without concentrating the specimen to increase sensitivity. A distinct disadvantage of this method was the large ("several-milliliter") sample volume required. Moreover, they could not resolve tranexamic acid and ε-aminocaproic acid, and no other internal standard was used.

Finally, although tranexamic acid has not yet been approved for general clinical trial in the United States, it is also an antifibrinolytic drug, and is perhaps more extensively used worldwide than is ε-aminocaproic acid. By exchanging the drug and internal standard ratio in this procedure, an equally sensitive and reliable method for the determination of tranexamic acid is available. This is of great importance, because tranexamic acid is 7- to 10-fold more potent than ε-aminocaproic acid (*19*). The therapeutic serum concentration for tranexamic acid is considered to be 10–50 mg/liter.

We thank Kathy Redelman, R.N., for her assistance in collecting the samples and coördinating medication schedules.

References

1. Nilsson, I. M., Andersson, L., and Bjorkman, S. E., Epsilonaminocaproic acid (E-ACA) as a therapeutic agent based on 5 year's clinical experience. *Acta Med. Scand.* (*Suppl.*) **448,** 5 (1966).

2. Frank, M. M., Sergent, J. S., Kane, M. A., and Alling, D. W., Epsilon aminocaproic acid therapy of hereditary angioneurotic edema. *New Engl. J. Med.* **286,** 808 (1972).

3. Mullan, S., and Dawley, J., Antifibrinolytic therapy for intracranial aneurysms. *J. Neurosurg.* **28,** 21 (1968).

4. Ablondi, F. B., Hagan, J. J., Philips, M., and DeRenzo, E. C., Inhibition of plasmin, trypsin and the streptokinase-activated fibrinolytic system by ε-aminocaproic acid. *Arch. Biochem.* **82,** 153 (1959).

5. Alkjaersig, N., Fletcher, A. P., and Sherry, S., ε-Aminocaproic acid: An inhibitor of plasminogen activation. *J. Biol. Chem.* **234,** 832 (1959).

6. Sjoerdsma, A., and Hanson, E. A., Determination of ε-aminocaproic acid in urine by means of high-voltage paper electrophoresis. *Acta Chem. Scand.* **13,** 2150 (1959).

7. McNichol, G. P., Fletcher, A. P., Alkaersig, N., and Sherry, S., Plasma amino acid chromatography with ion-exchange resin loaded paper: Assay of ε-aminocaproic acid. *J. Clin. Lab. Med.* **59,** 7 (1962).

8. McNichol, G. P., Fletcher, A. P., Alkjaersig, N., and Sherry, S., The absorption, distribution and excretion of ε-aminocaproic acid (ε-ACA) following its oral or intravenous administration to man. *J. Clin. Lab. Med.* **59,** 15 (1962).

9. Markwardt, F., Klöcking, H. P., and Richter, M., Die Bestimmung synthetischer Antifibrinolytica in Korperflussingkeiten und Organen. *Pharmazie* **22,** 83 (1967).

10. Takada, Y., Takada, A., and Okamoto, U., A new method of determination of epsilon-aminocaproic acid and aminomethyl cyclohexanecarboxylic acid. *Keio J. Med.* **13,** 115 (1964).

11. Wolosowicz, N., Niewiarowski, S., and Czerepko, K., Method of determining ε-aminocaproic acid (EACA) in blood plasma, based on the antifibrinolytic properties of this compound. *Thromb. Diath. Haemorrh.* **10,** 309 (1964).

12. Wolosowicz, N., and Niewiarowski, S., A simple method for determining ε-aminocaproic acid (EACA) in urine. *Clin. Chim. Acta* **12,** 555 (1965).

13. Ikekawa, N. Hoshino, O., Watanuki, R., et al., Chromatographic separation of DNP amino acids and its application to the analysis of serum amino acids. *Anal. Biochem.* **17,** 16 (1966).

14. Raulin, F., Shapshak, P., and Khare, B. N., Quantitative gas–liquid chromatography of non-protein amino acids in the presence of twenty protein amino acids. *J. Chromatogr.* **73,** 35 (1972).

15. Gehrke, C. W., Roach, D., Zumwalt, R. W., et al., Quantitative gas–liquid chromatography of amino acids in proteins and biological substances. Publication of Analytical Biochemistry Laboratories, Inc., Columbia, Mo. 65201, 1968.

16. Zumwalt, R. W., Kuo, K. C., and Gehrke, C. W., Application of a gas–liquid chromatographic method for amino acid analysis: A system for analysis of nanogram amounts. *J. Chromatogr.* **55,** 267 (1971).

17. Gehrke, C. W., Kuo, K., and Zumwalt, R. W., The complete gas–liquid chromatographic separation of twenty protein amino acids. *J. Chromatogr.* **57,** 209 (1971).

18. Mikata, I., Hasegawa, M., Igarashi, T., and Matsuki, Y., Studies on plasmin and fibrinogen by new method with ε-aminocaproic acid. *Keio J. Med.* **11,** 185 (1962).

19. Okamoto, S., Sato, S., Takada, Y., and Okamoto, U., An active stereo-isomer (*trans*-form) of AMCHA and its antifibrinolytic (anti-plasminic) action in vitro and in vivo. *Keio J. Med.* **13,** 177 (1964).

CLIN. CHEM. 22/6, 810-812 (1976)

Serum Quinidine Concentrations: Comparison of Fluorescence, Gas-Chromatographic, and Gas-Chromatographic/Mass-Spectrometric Methods

David H. Huffman and Charles E. Hignite

Serum quinidine concentrations were determined in patients on chronic therapeutic doses. Although results were higher by a protein precipitate–fluorescence method as compared to a specific extraction fluorescence method, there was substantial correlation between results by the two methods ($r = 0.945$, $P < 0.001$). We established the specificity of the extraction method by a methylation gas-chromatographic method and by a gas-chromatographic/mass spectrometric method in which the base peak in the mass spectra of the methylated products of both quinidine and cinchonidine, the internal standard, was monitored. We conclude that the protein precipitate method should be discarded.

Additional Keyphrase: *cardiac arrythmias*

Knowledge of serum quinidine concentrations assists the physician in the management of patients who are receiving quinidine (*1–4*). Until recently, quinidine concentrations have been determined by a protein precipitate–fluorescence method (*5*). For this method, a therapeutic range of 3–6 mg/liter has been suggested (*6*). Hartel and Korhonen (*7*) identified several polar metabolites of quinidine and dihydroquinidine by thin-layer chromatography, and modified an extraction method (*8*) to measure quinidine concentrations, in which benzene is used as the organic solvent. In a further modification of this method, Kessler et al. (*9*) studied the pharmacokinetics of quinidine in patients with renal failure and congestive heart failure, and recommended that the protein-precipitate method be abandoned in favor of the more specific extraction method.

We have determined quinidine concentrations in the sera of 27 patients who were receiving quinidine sulfate as therapy for cardiac arrhythmias. This report compares the quinidine concentrations determined by the two fluorescence methods with those by a specific gas-chromatographic method (*10*), the validity of which we have confirmed by gas chromatography/mass spectrometry (GC/MS).

Medical and Research Services (KCVAH Project 3794-05), Veterans Administration Hospital; and the Departments of Medicine and Pharmacology, University of Kansas School of Medicine.

Address correspondence to D.H.H. at the Research Service (151), VA Hospital, 4801 Linwood Boulevard, Kansas City, Mo. 64128.

Received Jan. 30, 1976; accepted Feb. 25, 1976.

Materials and Methods

Patients

All patients were hospitalized on a general medical service and had been receiving quinidine sulfate for at least three days. Blood for quinidine concentration was obtained by venipuncture 4–6 h after the last oral dose of quinidine sulfate. The blood was centrifuged, and the serum was either promptly assayed or frozen at −20 °C until assay. Creatinine clearances for the patients were either measured or were estimated with use of a nomogram involving the patient's serum creatinine value, age, sex, and weight (*11*).

Fluorescence Assays

Fluorescence method I was the protein precipitate method described by Brodie and Udenfriend (*5*). Fluorescence method II was the extraction method of Hartel and Kohronen (*7*) as modified by Kessler et al. (*9*).

For both methods fluorescence was measured in a Farrand spectrophotofluorometer (activation wavelength, 350 nm; fluorescence wavelength, 445 nm) and compared with quinidine standards that had been carried through the entire procedure. All quinidine concentrations are given in micrograms of quinidine base per milliliter of serum.

Gas Chromatography

We used a modification of the flash methylation procedure of Midha and Charette (*10*). To duplicate 1-ml serum samples, 1 ml of water containing the internal standard, cinchonidine (2 μg/ml), 0.5 ml of NaOH (1 mol/liter), and 5 ml of benzene were added. The mixture was shaken for 10 min, centrifuged, and the benzene layer transferred to a conical tube and evaporated at 70 °C under air. The residue was reconstituted

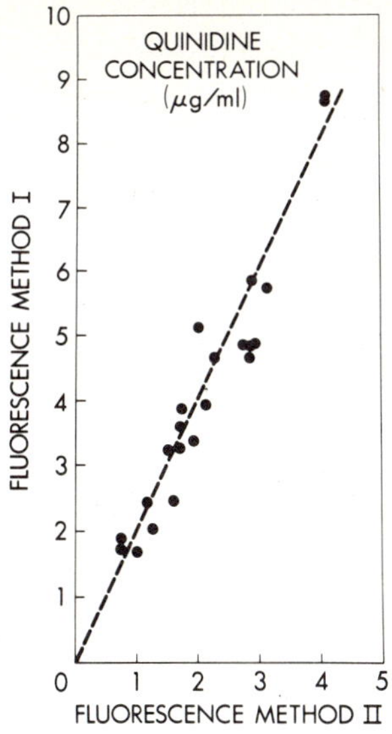

Fig. 1. Relationship between serum quinidine concentrations as determined by two fluorescence methods

See text for details

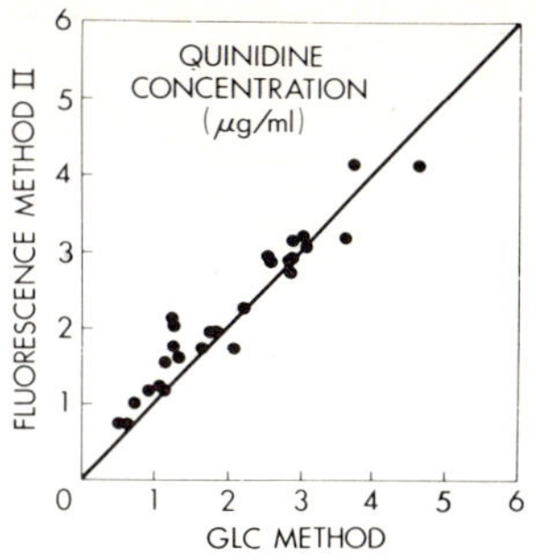

Fig. 2. Relationship between serum quinidine concentrations as determined by the extraction-fluorescence method (II) and by a gas-chromatographic method that involves flash methylation of quinidine and the internal standard

Each point is the mean of duplicate samples from the same patient. See text for details

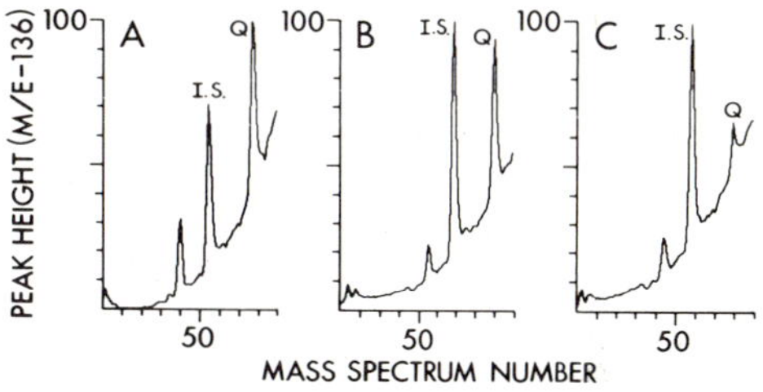

Fig. 3. Mass chromatograms for *m/e* 136, the base peak in the mass spectra of the methylated products of both quinidine (*Q*) and cinchonidine (*IS*) for a 5 μg/ml quinidine standard (panel A), and two patients (panels B and C)

Column conditions identical to the GC analyses except that helium was the carrier gas (30 ml/min) and the column temperature was programmed from 220 to 320 °C at 10 °C/min

in 25 μl of trimethylanilinium hydroxide (0.2 mol/liter in methanol; "Methelute"; Pierce Chemical Co., Rockford, Ill. 61105). Two microliters of the Methelute solution were injected into a Varian Aerograph, Model 2400, equipped with a hydrogen flame detector. Nitrogen was the carrier gas, with a flow rate of 30 ml/min. The column was a 180-cm glass column packed with 3% OV-17 on Gas Chrom Q, 80–100 mesh. The temperatures of the injection port, column, and detector were 320, 245, and 285 °C, respectively. Under these conditions the retention times for methylated cinchonidine and quinidine were 4.25 and 7.2 min, respectively. There were no interfering peaks in blank plasma carried through the entire procedure, but two later-eluting peaks were present in the blank plasma. The sensitivity limit for serum quinidine concentration was 50 ng/ml. Quinidine concentrations were determined by the peak-height ratio for quinidine and the internal standard. Four quinidine standards (1, 3, 5, and 7 μg/ml) were prepared in blank plasma and assayed together with the patient's sera. Because quinidine sulfate was used to prepare the standards, it was necessary to multiply the determined quinidine concentrations by 0.82, to obtain the quinidine concentrations as micrograms of quinidine base per milliliter of serum. The coefficient of variation for 10 determinations on the same day was 4.7%.

Gas Chromatography/Mass Spectrometry

To substantiate the results determined by GC analysis, portions of selected samples were also analyzed by GC/MS. The GC/MS computer system was the Finnigan 3300, operated on line with a Finnigan 6000 data system. The electron impact mass spectra were continuously monitored throughout the complete temperature-programmed gas chromatographic analysis, 5–10 mass spectra being recorded for each effluent component. The mass chromatogram for *m/e* 136, the base peak in the mass spectra of the methylated products of both quinidine and cinchonidine (*10*) was used to determine the concentration of quinidine in each sample. The computer system was used to determine the areas of the peaks in the mass chromatogram for both quinidine and internal standard. The ratio of the areas of the two peaks in the unknown sample was then compared to the area ratio for a standard sample containing known amounts of quinidine and internal standard, carried through the same procedure.

Results and Discussion

In agreement with earlier reports (*1, 7–9*), quinidine concentrations as determined by the protein precipitate method (fluorescence method I) are higher than those determined by the extraction method. Despite these differences there was a substantial correlation (Figure 1) between results by the two methods ($r = 0.945$, $P < 0.001$). To determine which method was the more nearly accurate, the same serum samples were assayed by the GC method. As demonstrated in Figure 2, there was an excellent correlation between results by gas chromatography and by fluorescence method II ($r = 0.959$, $P < 0.001$), which indicated that the extraction method was more specific than the protein precipitate method.

To further substantiate the accuracy and specificity of the second fluorescence method, we used the GC/MS system. Methylated quinidine and cinchonidine both have base peaks at *m/e* 136, and so we could use a single mass chromatogram for quantitation. The correct peaks for each compound in the mass chromatogram were chosen on the basis of both retention times and examination of the complete mass spectra. Figure 3 shows three such mass chromatograms. The areas of the peaks corresponding to quinidine and the internal standard were determined with the aid of the computer. Panel *A* was the mass chromatogram of *m/e* 136 for a 5 μg/ml quinidine standard. Panels *B* and *C* were mass chromatograms of *m/e* 136 for sera from two of the patients. Quinidine concentrations for these patients were 2.57 and 0.63 mg/liter. This related well to concentrations of 2.75 and 0.60 mg/liter, as determined by the extraction fluorescence method. A similar close comparison was obtained for a third patient (2.63 vs. 2.75 for the GC/MS and fluorescent method II, respectively).

From these data, we conclude that the extraction fluorescence method (II) is both accurate and specific and should therefore be used when the pharmacokinetics of quinidine are to be studied. However, under certain circumstances, the protein precipitate method may be preferred for monitoring clinical response to quinidine in patients: it is easier than the extraction method and, after the initial protein precipitation step, could be done by an automated procedure. However, if the protein precipitate method is used, the resulting quinidine concentrations should be divided by two to obtain an estimate of the actual quinidine concentration.

An objection to using the protein precipitation method was raised by Kessler et al. (*9*). They determined the ratio of quinidine concentrations determined by the two methods (I/II), related this ratio to the renal function of that patient, and found a significant inverse correlation between these variables. That is, as creatinine clearance decreased, the ratio (I/II) increased. They interpreted this to indicate a greater retention of the water-soluble metabolites of quinidine and dihydroquinidine relative to quinidine in renal failure. The varying amounts of these metabolites changed the ratio of the quinidine concentrations determined by the two methods, and this was the basis of their recommendation that the protein precipitate method be discarded.

In our experience, however, this relationship was not as evident. The mean (±SD) ratio for quinidine concentration determined by the two methods (I/II) was 2.0 ± 0.29 (range, 1.55 to 2.54). The endogenous creatinine clearances of these patients varied from 15 to 85 ml/min, and there was no correlation between the ratio and creatinine clearance. It is possible, however, that an increased ratio (I/II) might occur in patients with more severe renal-function impairment. Because results of the fluorescence method II agree well with those of GC and GC/MS methods, and because fluorescence method I gives quinidine concentrations that average twice those obtained by fluorescence method II, then fluorescence method I, the protein precipitate method, gives erroneous results and should be discarded.

Supported in part by USPHS Grant No. 15956.

References

1. Resnekov, L., Gibson, D., Waich, S., et al., Sustained-release quinidine (Kinidin Durules) in maintaining sinus rhythm after electroversion of atrial dysrhythmias. *Br. Heart J.* **33,** 220 (1971).

2. Edwards, I. R., Hancock, B. W., and Saynor, R., Correlation between plasma quinidine and cardiac effect. *Br. J. Clin. Pharmacol.* **1,** 455 (1974).

3. Sokolow, M., and Edgar, A. L., Blood quinidine concentrations as guide in the treatment of cardiac arrhythmias. *Circulation* **1,** 576 (1950).

4. Ditlefsen, E. M. L., and Knudson, B., Quinidine treatment in chronic auricular fibrillation. 1. Conversion to sinus rhythm related to quinidine serum concentration. *Acta Med. Scand.* **156,** 1 (1956).

5. Brodie, B. B., and Udenfriend, S., The estimation of quinine in human plasma, with a note on the estimation of quinidine. *J. Pharmacol. Exp. Ther.* **78,** 154 (1943).

6. Koch-Weser, J., Serum drug concentrations as therapeutic guides. *New Engl. J. Med.* **287,** 227 (1972).

7. Hartel, G., and Korhonen, A., Thin layer chromatography for the quantitative separation of quinidine and quinidine metabolites from biological fluids and tissues. *J. Chromatogr.* **37,** 70 (1968).

8. Cramér, G., and Isaksson, B., Quantitative determination of quinidine in plasma. *Scand. J. Clin. Lab. Invest.* **15,** 553 (1963).

9. Kessler, K. M., Lowenthal, D. J., Warner, H., et al., Quinidine elimination in patients with congestive heart failure or poor renal function. *New Engl. J. Med.* **290,** 706 (1974).

10. Midha, K. K., and Charette, C., GLC determination of quinidine from plasma and whole blood. *J. Pharm. Sci.* **63,** 1244 (1974).

11. Siersback-Nielsen, K. K., Moholm-Hanson, J., Kampman, J., and Kristenson, M., Rapid evaluation of creatinine clearance. *Lancet* **i,** 1133 (1971).

CLIN. CHEM. 22/6, 813–816 (1976)

Rapid Radioimmunoassay for Methotrexate in Biological Fluids

Jørn Hendel, Lydia J. Sarek, and Eigill F. Hvidberg

We report a radioimmunoassay for the cytostatic folic acid antagonist methotrexate. Antiserum was raised in rabbits immunized with a conjugate of methotrexate and methylated bovine serum albumin. The calibration curve of the assay is linear from 1 to 100 ng methotrexate per 100-μl sample, 0.1 ng methotrexate still inhibiting the binding of the tracer by 20%. The coefficient of variation ranged from 4.04% to 11.58%. The reaction of the antiserum proved to be specific for methotrexate, as only insignificant interference could be demonstrated with folic acid, folinic acid (leucovorin), or tetrahydrofolic acid. With the method, results are available about 20 h after blood sampling at a daily capacity of at least 48 samples (i.e., about 15 determinations), depending on the equipment. Concentrations of methotrexate in plasma and erythrocytes were determined in five patients who were on continuous treatment with the drug. In one patient the concentration/time curves were followed in plasma and erythrocytes by frequent determinations for 24 h after a parenteral dose. The results indicate that the procedure is well suited for clinical investigations.

Additional Keyphrases: *cancer* • *pharmacokinetics* • *monitoring drugs* • *erythrocytes*

The folic acid antagonist methotrexate (Mtx) was introduced almost three decades ago (*1*). Since then, this cytostatic drug has proved to be of considerable value in the treatment of several malignant diseases (*2–4*). During recent years it has also been demonstrated to be effective against some non-neoplastic disorders (*5–8*). However, its clinical use is limited by its toxicity, of which bone marrow depression (*9*), hepatotoxicity (*10*), nephrotoxicity (*11*), and pulmonary complications (*12*) are the most serious consequences. If given appropriately, folinic acid (leucovorin) acts as an antidote by preventing the depletion of hydrogenated folates that is caused by Mtx (*13*), but the optimal timing and the dose required are poorly defined. With the possible exception of hepatotoxicity, the above-mentioned toxic effects seem to be dose related, and it is therefore quite possible that they could be prevented or decreased if concentrations of Mtx in plasma are monitored in the patients. This is further emphasized by the present knowledge of the fate of Mtx in the body. It is predominantly excreted unchanged by the kidneys, the rate being highly dependent on the glomerular filtration rate (*14, 15*). A better understanding of the pharmacokinetics of Mtx in man is therefore of importance if therapeutic monitoring by means of determinations in plasma is to be a reality. This, in turn, will depend on reliable methods. Most kinetic studies have been done with radiolabeled Mtx (*16, 17*), but several analytical procedures have also been published. However, their practical value seems to have been limited.

The aim of the present study was, therefore, to develop an assay for Mtx in plasma and in other biological materials such as erythrocytes, which could be used for more extensive kinetic studies in man and also for assisting in clinical use of this drug.

Materials and Methods

Preparative Measures

Synthesis of immunogen: Three different immunogens were synthesized and tested in different immunization schedules (to be published elsewhere). The immunogen and the immunization procedure described were those found to be the most efficient and reproducible.

To ensure proper coupling between Mtx-COOH groups and the free-NH_2 groups of the protein, all accessible carboxylic groups in the bovine serum albumin molecule were methylated as follows: 2.0 g bovine serum albumin was dissolved in 500 ml of dehydrated methanol. Dry HCl gas was passed through the chilled solution, with stirring, for 3 h. After the mixture was kept for 24 h at 4 °C in the dark, the precipitate was washed several times with cold diethyl ether, separated from the liquid by centrifugation, and dried in a desiccator.

Five hundred milligrams of Mtx, 900 mg of methylated bovine serum albumin, 196 mg of 1-ethyl-3-(3′-dimethylaminopropyl)-carbodiimide hydrochloride were mixed in a stoppered vial and shaken for 24 h. Methylene chloride was removed from the mixture by evaporation under reduced pressure, 50 ml of water was added, and the vial was shaken for a further 24 h. The clear-yellow solution was transferred to a dialysis sack and dialyzed vs. 0.01 mol/liter NaOH until no Mtx could be detected in the dialysate. After lyophilization, the dialyzed protein was a bright-yellow powder.

Immunization procedure: Four male New Zealand white rabbits, six months old and weighing about 2 kg, were treated with 10 to 15 intradermal injections of a mixture of Freund complete adjuvant (2 parts) and a solution of the immunogen in isotonic saline (1 part). The emulsion contained 3 mg of the conjugate per milliliter, and a total of 2 ml of the emulsion was injected

Clinical Pharmacology Research Unit, Department of Pharmacology and Rigshospitalet, University of Copenhagen, Denmark.

Address correspondence to: Jørn Hendel, M.D., whose present address is: Department of Clinical Chemistry, Finsen Institute, 49, Strandboulevarden, DK-2100 Copenhagen O, Denmark.

Received Mar. 1, 1976; accepted Mar. 23, 1976.

into each rabbit. The procedure was repeated every 4 to 5 weeks. After three to six months all the rabbits showed specific antibodies against Mtx in appropriate titers.

Assay Description

Reagents and apparatus: Rabbit antiserum against Mtx.

Tracer: [^{3}H]3′,5′,9(*N*)-methyltrexate, sodium salt (Radiochemical Centre, Amersham).

Standard Mtx, 94% purity (American Cyanamide Company, Pearl River, N.Y.).

Blind plasma: ultracentrifuged, granulocyte-free human plasma.

Polyethylene glycol, "Carbowax 6000," Merck, for synthesis.

Diluent buffer: 0.1 mol/liter Na_2HPO_4, adjusted to pH 7.4.

Solubilizer: "Soluen-350" (Packard Instrument Company).

Liquid scintillator: "Insta-Gel" (Packard Instrument Co.).

All samples were counted in a liquid scintillation spectrometer (Packard Tri-Carb, Model 8 2450).

Procedure: We tested several methods for separating free and antibody-bound fractions (to be published elsewhere). The method described here was found to be the most suitable. The radioimmunoassay procedure was done as follows: In 4-ml polypropylene tubes were mixed: 500 μl of rabbit antiserum, diluted 1000-fold; 100 μl of patient's sample or standard of Mtx; and 100 μl of tracer, i.e., 9 ng of [^{3}H]-Mtx.

As controls, 14 vials containing known Mtx standard concentrations were run in parallel with the patients' samples. Two blanks were run for every series as controls for nonspecific binding. The samples were mounted on an agitator and incubated overnight at 21 °C. Polyethylene glycol solution, 0.7 ml, was added to each tube, mixed on a vortex-type mixer and centrifuged in a refrigerated centrifuge (3200 × *g*) at 4 °C for 45 min. The supernatant fluid was decanted and any

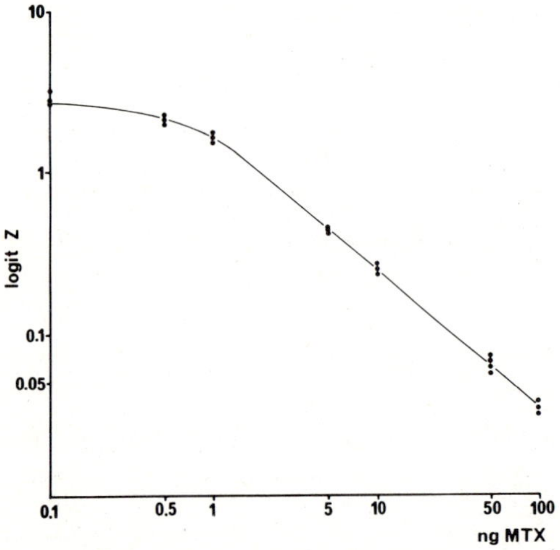

Fig. 1. Standard curve (logit Z/log concn) for displacement of ^{3}H-labeled Mtx from antibody binding sites by Mtx

supernate remaining on the tube walls was removed. The precipitate was dissolved in 1.0 ml of Soluen-350 at 60 °C, cooled, and transferred to 20-ml counting vials. The vials were shaken vigorously and the radioactivity was counted. Quench correction was estimated by automatic external standard ratio. To simulate quenching, we used plasma or erythrocyte lysate.

All samples were run in duplicate and the results were calculated separately for each tube.

Standard curve: The amount of Mtx in an unknown sample was determined by the degree to which it displaced the binding of the ^{3}H-labeled Mtx to the antibodies. Standard curve was obtained by plotting logit Z vs. unlabeled Mtx present, on a log scale. The response metameter Z is defined by

$$Z = \frac{b/f}{b_0/f_0}, \text{ logit } Z = \frac{Z}{1 - Z}$$

b_0 = cpm of antibody-bound tracer in control without unlabeled Mtx; b = cpm of antibody-bound tracer in the assay system; f_0 = cpm of unbound tracer in supernatant without unlabeled Mtx; and f = cpm of unbound tracer in supernatant in assay system.

Patients and Blood Sampling

Five patients were examined, to check the applicability of the method (Table 2). All patients were on continuous treatment with Mtx. One patient (the second listed) was also investigated by assaying a series of blood samples after a parenteral dose. Blood samples were drawn into heparinized tubes and centrifuged. Erythrocytes were washed twice with saline (9 g/liter) and lysed by freezing at −20 °C. All samples were stored at −20 °C until analyzed.

Results

The standard curve (Figure 1) for the Mtx-radioimmunoassay utilizes the logit Z–log dose relationship introduced by Rodbard and Lewald (*18*). Transformed in this way, the assay data yield a rectilinear response curve over a wide range.

The significance of the antiserum dilution for the shape of response curve is demonstrated in Figure 2.

Precision and reproducibility: For 20 tubes assayed the coefficient of variation was less than 1%. A similar analysis was performed to test the interassay precision by performing repeated measurements of five calibration curves in several ranges. The results are presented in Table 1.

Sensitivity: The calibration curve is linear from 1 to 100 ng per 100-μl sample. Even 0.1 ng of Mtx inhibits binding of the tracer by 20%. With the method one can easily detect a concentration of 2 ng of Mtx per milliliter of plasma. By decreasing the amount of the tracer added, sensitivity can be increased, but the linear range of the assay is also reduced considerably (Figure 2).

Specificity: Folic acid, folinic acid (leucovorin), and tetrahydrofolic acid were tested for possible interference in the present assay. Each of these compounds showed a considerable weaker affinity toward the antibody than Mtx (Figure 3).

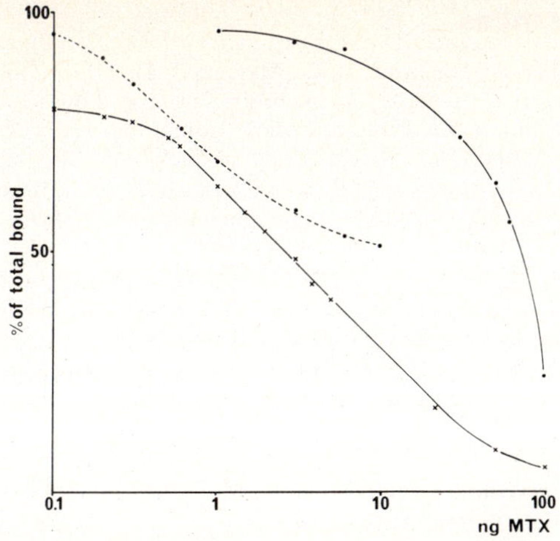

Fig. 2. Variations in the inhibition curves obtained when variously diluted antiserum or various amounts of tracer added
X—X—X, antiserum dilution, 1000-fold, tracer 9 ng. ●—●—●, antiserum dilution, 100-fold, tracer 9 ng. ● - - - - ● - - - - ●, antiserum dilution, 1000-fold, tracer 4.5 ng

Table 1. Interassay Variation of Mtx in Plasma in Different Concentration Ranges

Mtx in the assay, ng	CV, %
0.1	8.43
0.5	7.58
1.0	6.11
5.0	4.04
10.0	6.82
50.0	10.46
100.0	11.58

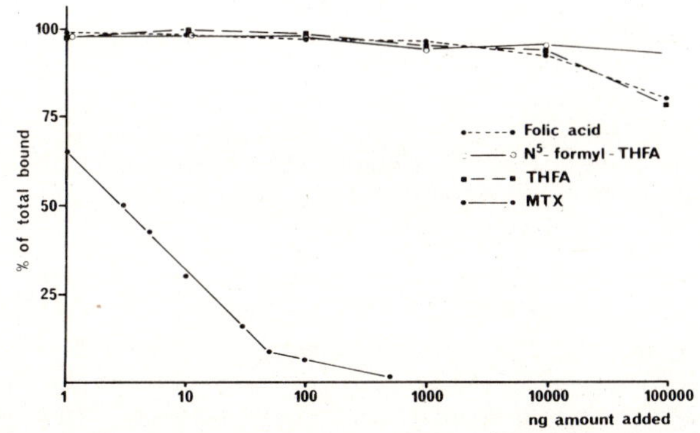

Fig. 3. Serologic specificity of the utilized antiserum tested for cross reactions with folic acid, tetrahydrofolic acid (*THFA*) and N^5-formyltetrahydrofolic acid (N^5-formyl-*THFA*, leucovorin)

Nonspecific binding of the total amount of the tracer in any sample never exceeded 2%.

Applicability to blood samples from patients: Table 2 gives results of Mtx determinations in five patients immediately before they received their next dose in a continuous treatment. In most patients, measurable concentrations are found in both plasma and erythrocytes one week after the last dose. The concentration/time curve after a single injection of 20 mg intrathecally plus 40 mg intramuscularly to one of the patients is shown in Figure 4. In plasma, the peak concentration is reached quickly and is very high, but then declines sharply (Figure 4*a*). Much lower concentrations are present in the erythrocytes, the peak value being less distinct and obtained much later (Figure 4*b*).

Capacity and speed of the procedure: The number of samples that can be assayed per day mainly depends on the size of the refrigerated centrifuge, but in our hands 48 samples—representing, e.g., 15 different

Table 2. Mtx Concentrations Measured Immediately before Next Dose in Five Outpatients on Long-term Treatment

Sex	Age (y)	Dosage schedule	Duration (weeks)	Mtx, ng/ml: Plasma	Mtx, ng/ml: Erythrocytes
M	33	60 mg i.m. weekly	6	28	12
M	38	alternating weekly between 60 mg i.m. and 20 mg intrathecally + 40 mg i.m.	5	16	10
F	48	60 mg i.m. weekly	8	5	21
M	65	60 mg i.m. weekly	10	3	18
M	47	60 mg i.m. weekly	7	<1	3

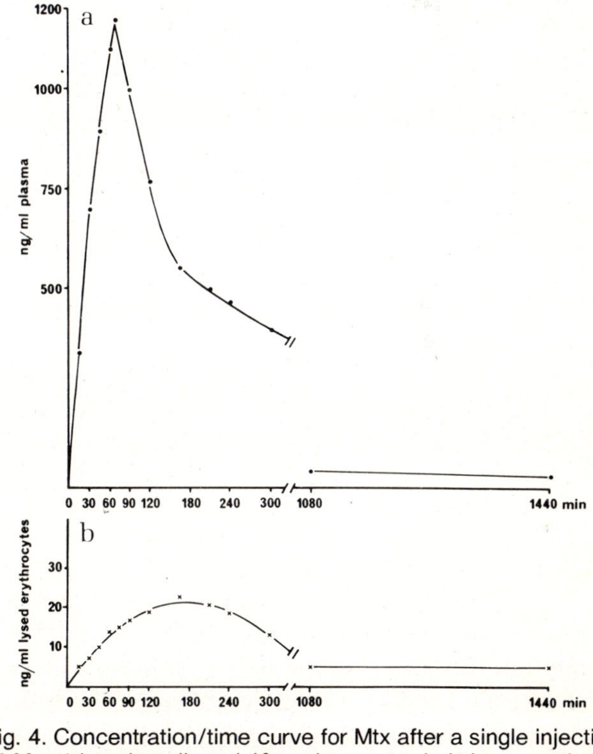

Fig. 4. Concentration/time curve for Mtx after a single injection of 20 mg intrathecally and 40 mg intramuscularly in one patient's plasma (*a*) and in erythrocytes (*b*)

plasma determinations—were processed by one laboratory assistant in a day. Because antibody coupling is allowed to react to equilibrium overnight, it is possible to split up a larger series after incubation if the precipitation with polyethylene glycol is done immediately before the centrifugation. In this way the capacity can be increased. The results of about 15 different Mtx determinations can be available about 20 h after the blood sampling, if this is done before noon.

Discussion

Several methods have been published for determining Mtx in biological fluids. Freeman (*19*) used the fact that the difference between the fluorescence before and after oxidation of the drug is proportional to its concentration. The sensitivity of the fluorometric methods is about 50 ng/ml plasma and all pteridines are co-determined. An enzymatic method (*20*) and a radio-enzymatic modification (*21*) measure Mtx by its inhibiting effect on dihydrofolate dehydrogenase (EC 1.5.1.4). The assay is quite sensitive (10 ng/ml plasma), but tedious and time consuming. Furthermore, it cannot be used in patients treated with leucovorin. A microbiological method for folic acid antagonists was described (*22*) and modified (*23*). The sensitivity of these assays is also about 10 ng/ml, but the specificity is poor, because both folic acid and certain antibiotics interfere.

Recently two radioimmunoassays were described (*24, 25*) for Mtx determination in biological material. Both methods make use of the double-antibody technique. The antisera are highly specific serologically, but the double-antibody technique is quite time consuming. Our assay overcomes this problem by separating antibody-bound Mtx with polyethylene glycol, thereby saving the lengthy second incubation and improving the sensitivity (*26*).

The method seems to be highly specific and may be used in patients treated simultaneously with leucovorin. The usefulness of the method in clinical practice should be examined closely, but our results for a few patients show that the procedure is well suited for routine purposes, if a sufficiently good quality and amount of antiserum has been produced.

Measurement of Mtx in erythrocytes is of particular interest, not only from a clinical point of view. The lipophilic erythrocyte membrane could explain the delayed entry of Mtx into erythrocytes. Inside them, the drug is very strongly bound to the dihydrofolate dehydrogenase, and this could account for the slow release of Mtx from these cells (*cf.* Figure 4*b*). In the case of folate, the concentrations in erythrocytes serve as an indirect index of the concentrations in liver cells (*27*). Our preliminary observations may suggest that similar conditions could exist for Mtx. The erythrocyte kinetics of this drug should therefore be explored in more detail.

Medical Department A, Rigshospitalet, is thanked for providing blood samples from patients. Pure standard Mtx was kindly supplied by Lederle, American Cyanamide Co.

This study was supported by grants from The Danish State Medical Research Council.

References

1. Farber, S., Diamont, L. K., Mercer, R. D., et al., Temporary remissions in acute leukemia in children produced by folic acid antagonist, 4-aminopteroylglutamic acid, (Aminopterin) *New Engl. J. Med.* **238,** 787 (1948).

2. Haghbin, M., Tan, C. C., and Clarkson, B. D., Intensive chemotherapy in children with acute lymphoblastic leukemia (L-2 protocol). *Cancer* (Philadelphia) **33,** 1491 (1974).

3. Li, H. C., Hertz, R., and Bergenstal, D. M., Therapy of choriocarcinoma and relayed trophoblastic tumors with folic acid and purine antagonists. *New Engl. J. Med.* **259,** 66 (1958).

4. Hertz, R., Lewis, J., Jr., and Lipsett, M. B., Five years experience with the chemotherapy of metastatic choriocarcinoma and related trophoblastic tumors in women. *Am. J. Obstet. Gynecol.* **82,** 631 (1961).

5. Weinstein, G. D., and Frost, P., Methotrexate for psoriasis. *Arch. Dermatol.* **103,** 33 (1971).

6. Van Leden, H., and Schiff, M., Antimetabolite therapy in midline lethal granulomas. *Arch. Ophthalmol.* **80,** 460 (1964).

7. Capizzi, R. L., and Bertino, J. R., Methotrexate therapy of Wegeners granulomatosis. *Ann. Intern. Med.* **74,** 74 (1971).

8. Lacher, M. J., Spontaneous remission or response to methotrexate in sarcoidosis. *Ann. Intern. Med.* **69,** 1247 (1968).

9. Philips, F. S., Tiersch, J. B., and Ferguson, F. C., Studies on the action of 4-aminopteroylglutamic acid and its congeners in mammals. *Ann. N. Y. Acad. Sci.* **52,** 1349 (1950).

10. Dahl, M. G., Gregory, M. M., and Scherer, P. J., Methotrexate hepatotoxicity in psoriasis-comparison of different dose regimens. *Br. Med. J.* **1,** 654 (1972).

11. Condit, P. T., Chanes, R. E., and Joel, W., Renal toxicity of methotrexate. *Cancer* (Philadelphia) **23,** 126 (1969).

12. Everts, C. S., Westcott, J. L., and Brag, D. G., Methotrexate therapy and pulmonary disease. *Radiology* **107,** 539 (1973).

13. Levitt, M., Mosher, M., DeConti, R. C., et al., Improved therapeutic index of methotrexate with "leucovorin rescue". *Cancer Res.* **33,** 1729 (1973).

14. Kristensen, L. O., Wiesmann, K., and Hutters, L., Renal function and the rate of disappearance of methotrexate from serum. *Eur. J. Clin. Pharmacol.* **8,** 439 (1975).

15. Huffman, D. H., Wan, S. H., Azarnoff, D. L., and Hoogstraten, B., Pharmacokinetics of methotrexate. *Clin. Pharmacol. Ther.* **14,** 572 (1973).

16. Dedrick, R. L., Zaharko, D. S., and Lutz, J., Transport and binding of methotrexate in vivo. *J. Pharm. Sci.* **62,** 882 (1973).

17. Anderson, L. L., Collins, G. J., Ojima, Y., and Sullivan, R. D., A study of the distribution of methotrexate in human tissues and tumors. *Cancer Res.* **30,** 1344 (1970).

18. Rodbard, D., and Lewald, J. E., Computer analysis of radioligant assay and radioimmunoassay. *Acta Endocrinol.* **147,** 79 (1970).

19. Freeman, M. V., A fluorometric method for the measurement of 4-amino-10-methyl-pteroylglutamic acid (aminopterin) in plasma. *J. Pharmacol. Exp. Ther.* **120,** 1 (1957).

20. Werkheiser, W. C., Zakrzewski, S. F., and Nichol, C. A., Assay for 4-amino folic acid analogues by inhibition of folic acid reductase. *J. Pharmacol. Exp. Ther.* **137,** 162 (1962).

21. Rothenberg, S. P. A., A radioenzymatic assay for folic acid antagonist in biological fluids. *J. Lab. Med.* **66,** 294 (1965).

22. Burchenal, J. H., Waring, G. B., Ellison, R. R., and Reilly, H. C., A simple method for determination of levels of amethopterin in blood and urine. *Proc. Soc. Biol. Med.* **78,** 603 (1951).

23. Shapiro, W. R., Dean, D. M., Young, F., and Metha, B. M., Methotrexate: Distribution in cerebrospinal fluids after intravenous ventricular and lumbar injections. *New Engl. J. Med.* **24,** 161 (1975).

24. Bohuon, C., Dubrey, F., and Boudene, C., Radioimmunoassay of methotrexate in biological fluids. *Clin. Chim. Acta* **57,** 263 (1974).

25. Levine, L., and Powers, E., Radioimmunoassay for methotrexate. *Res. Commun. Chem. Pathol. Pharmacol.* **9,** 543 (1974).

26. Desbuquois, B., and Aurbach, G. D., Use of polyethylene glycol to separate free and antibody-bound peptide hormones in radioimmunoassays. *J. Clin. Endocrinol.* **33,** 732 (1971).

27. Hoffbrand, A. V., Newcombe, B. F. A., and Mollin, D. L., Method of assay of red cell folate activity and the value of the assay as a test for folate deficiency. *J. Clin. Pathol.* **19,** 17 (1966).

CLIN. CHEM. 22/6, 817–823 (1976)

Determination of Clomipramine and Desmethyl-Clomipramine in Plasma or Urine by the Double-Radioisotope Derivative Technique

G. Carnis, J. Godbillon,[1] and J. P. Metayer

A double radioisotope derivative method was developed for the determination of clomipramine and desmethyl-clomipramine in plasma or urine. After addition of ^{14}C-labeled clomipramine and desmethyl-clomipramine as internal standards and extractive isolation of both compounds, desmethyl-clomipramine is acetylated with [^3H]acetic anhydride. The [^3H]acetamide is separated from clomipramine by thin-layer chromatography and its radioactivity is measured. Clomipramine, extracted from the silica gel, is reacted with trichloroethyl chloroformate. The urethane is saponified and decarboxylated. The resulting desmethyl-clomipramine is acetylated with [^3H]-acetic anhydride. The [^3H]acetamide is purified by thin-layer chromatography and its radioactivity is measured. The sensitivity of the method is 15 μg/liter for clomipramine and 2 μg/liter for desmethyl-clomipramine. Its specificity was made sure by a cross-check with a gas chromatography–mass spectrometry technique.

Additional Keyphrases: *gas chromatography/mass spectrometry • determination of tertiary-amine drugs*

Very few analytical methods have been reported for the determination of clomipramine (Anafranil®, Geigy) in biological materials.

Colorimetric (*1, 2*) or fluorometric (*3*) methods lack specificity and sensitivity. These drawbacks were partly overcome by gas chromatography (*4–8*).

Gas chromatography–mass spectrometry with deuterated internal standards appears to be the most satisfactory method: clomipramine can be determined at concentrations as low as 1 ng/ml.[2]

However, since gas chromatography–mass spectrometry equipment is costly, there is still a demand for more chemically oriented methods with comparable sensitivity and precision.

The double-radioisotope derivative technique reported in detail for the determination of maprotiline (Ludiomil®, Geigy) (*9*) seemed to fulfill such requirements.

The present paper describes a double-radioisotope derivative technique for the assay of clomipramine (**I**) and its main metabolite (*10*), desmethyl-clomipramine (**II**). It is based on the tertiary amine degradation by trichloroethyl chloroformate and subsequent acetylation. Variabilities of the yields of derivatization and losses are corrected by using two ^{14}C-labeled internal standards—^{14}C-**I** and ^{14}C-**II**—introduced into the sample at the beginning of the assay.

Material and Methods

Apparatus

Shaker, model TRI; Infors AG, 4149 Hofstetten bei Basel, Switzerland.

Liquid scintillation spectrometer: Tri-Carb Model 3385 (Packard Instrument Co. Inc., Downers Grove, Ill. 60515).

Thin-layer chromatography plates: 20 × 20 cm silica gel (Merck F_{254}; E. Merck A. G., D-61 Darmstadt, Germany).

Reagents

All reagents and solvents were analytical grade.

Dioxane: distilled under nitrogen over $LiAlH_4$ and stored at +4 °C in fused glass ampoules under nitrogen.

The unlabeled *N*-acetyl derivative of desmethyl-clomipramine (**III**), used as carrier, was prepared in our laboratory.

Labeled compounds: ^{14}C-labeled-clomipramine (64.9 μCi/mg), desmethyl-clomipramine (66.8 μCi/mg), and [^3H]maprotiline (65 μCi/mg) were synthesized in our radioisotope laboratory.

[^3H]acetic anhydride solution: [^3H]acetic anhydride (100 Ci/mol; Radiochemical Centre, Amersham, Buckinghamshire, England HP7 9LL) was diluted with unlabeled acetic anhydride in dried heptane to yield 2 ml/liter solution with 50 Ci/mol specific activity. This solution was stored at +4 °C, in portions of 1 ml, in fused glass ampoules.

Standard solutions: Losses were observed when handling solutions of both compounds in distilled water at low concentrations. When using acidic solutions (10 mmol/liter HCl) of **I** and **II**, the adsorption on glass or plastic surfaces was minimized.

Scintillation mixture: Scintillator "Butyl-PBD" (Ciba-Geigy) at a concentration of 8 g/liter in toluene (scintillation grade Merck).

Procedure

Figure 1 summarizes the procedure. The principle of reaction is as follows:

Ciba-Geigy Biopharmaceutical Research Center, B. P. 130, 92505 Rueil-Malmaison, France.

[1] Address correspondence to this author, including reprint requests.

[2] J. P. Dubois, this issue, p 892.

Received Feb. 16, 1976; accepted March 23, 1976.

$$\mathrm{I} \xrightarrow[\text{DIPEA}]{\mathrm{ClCOOCH_2CCl_3}} \mathrm{IV} \xrightarrow{\mathrm{OH^-}} \mathrm{II} \xrightarrow{\mathrm{^3H\text{-}Ac_2O}} \mathrm{^3H\text{-}III}$$

DIPEA = diisopropylethylamine

R_1	R_2	Compound
CH_3	CH_3	Clomipramine (I)
CH_3	H	Desmethyl-clomipramine (II)
CH_3	$COCH_3$	Acetyl-desmethyl-clomipramine (III)
CH_3	$COOCH_2CCl_3$	Clomipramine carbamate (IV)
H	H	Bis-desmethyl-clomipramine (V)

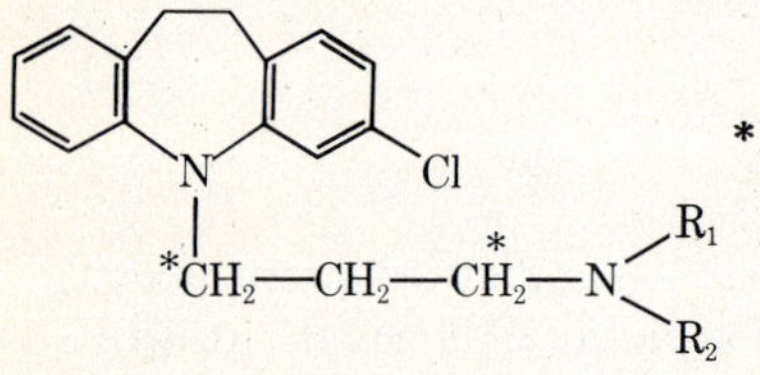

*Position of the ^{14}C in the internal standards ^{14}C-I and ^{14}C-II.

Extraction. Introduce into a plastic centrifuge tube 2 ml of plasma or urine, 40 ng of ^{14}C-**I**, 10 ng of ^{14}C-**II**, 2 ml of pH 10 buffer, and 10 ml of heptane containing isoamyl alcohol (1/100 by vol). Shake for 15 min at 400 rpm and centrifuge for 5 min at 3000 rpm. Transfer the organic phase into a 10-ml glass ampoule, shake with 1 ml of 0.05 mol/liter sulfuric acid, and centrifuge. Discard the organic phase. Add 0.5 ml of 1 mol/liter sodium hydroxide and 5 ml of heptane to the aqueous phase. After shaking, collect the heptane, and evaporate it under nitrogen. Store the residue in a vacuum desiccator for 1 h.

Acetylation (in a glove box). Add 50 μl of [^{3}H]acetic anhydride solution (added amount: 1 μmol, 50 μCi) and 100 μl of dioxane to the evaporation residue. Heat at 60 °C for 15 min. Evaporate the excess [^{3}H]acetic anhydride and dioxane by heating at 60 °C for 5 min while aspirating off the vapors through two wash bottles containing 5 mol/liter sodium hydroxide. Add 2 ml of heptane and 0.5 ml of 10 mmol/liter sodium hydroxide. After shaking, collect the heptane and evaporate under nitrogen.

Thin-layer chromatographic purification. Add 50 μl of a chloroform solution of unlabeled **III** (about 10 μg) to the evaporation residue. Spot this solution and a chloroform solution of **I** (about 5 μg), respectively, on positions *a* and *b* as indicated on Figure 2. Develop in the first dimension with benzene/ethyl acetate (5/5) then in the second dimension with benzene/ethyl acetate/triethylamine (7/2/1). Dry the chromatograms at room temperature and observe the spots under ultraviolet light. The two reference spots of **I** permit one to locate clomipramine from the sample. Scrape the zone corresponding to **I** (dotted rectangle on Figure 2) into a 10-ml glass ampoule with a funnel-shaped neck.

*Radiometry—determination of **II**.* Scrape the spot corresponding to ^{3}H-**III** into a plastic counting vial. Add 0.2 ml of methanol and 20 ml of scintillation mixture. Together with four blank counting samples to correct all other samples for background activity, count four radiometric ^{3}H-standard samples (methanolic solution of [^{3}H]maprotiline) to measure the channel ratio, and four radiometric ^{14}C-standard samples with the same amount of ^{14}C-**II** used as internal standard. ^{3}H and ^{14}C activities are measured by the discriminator ratio method (*11*).

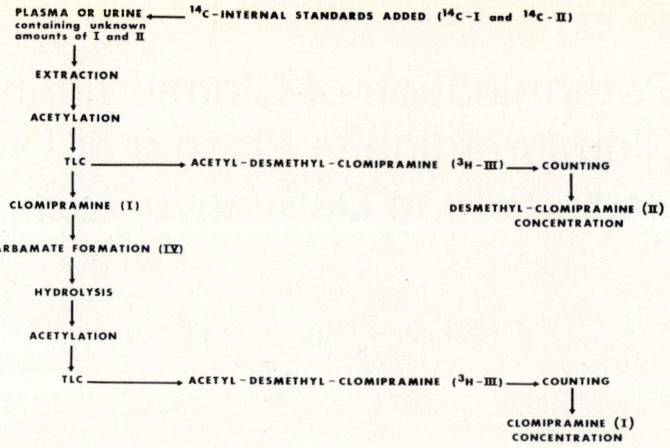

Fig. 1. Procedure scheme

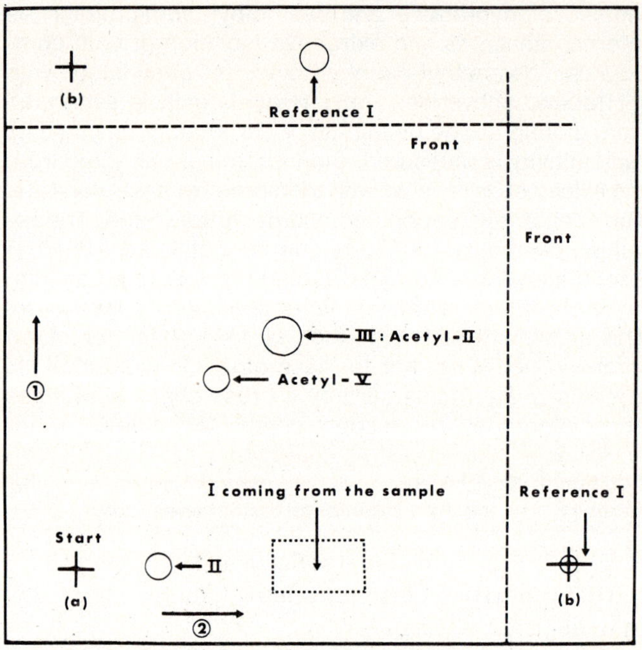

Fig. 2. Thin-layer chromatographic separation of **I**, **II**, **III**, and acetyl-**V**
① Benzene/ethyl-acetate (5/5); ② Benzene/ethyl-acetate/triethylamine (7/2/1)

*Extraction of **I** from silica gel.* Extract **I** from the silica gel with 1 ml of pH 10 buffer and 4 ml of heptane. After shaking, collect the heptane and evaporate it under nitrogen.

Formation of the carbamate. To the evaporation residue add successively 1 ml of benzene, 10 μl of trichloroethyl chloroformate, and 20 μl of diisopropylethylamine. Keep the ampoule at room temperature for 10 min. Evaporate the solvent and reagents under nitrogen. Add 1 ml of 0.05 mol/liter sulfuric acid and 3 ml of heptane. After shaking, collect the heptane and evaporate it under nitrogen.

Hydrolysis of the carbamate. Add 300 μl of diethylene glycol monoethyl ether/aqueous 8 mol/liter sodium hydroxide (4/1) to the evaporation residue. Heat the ampoule at 180 °C for 5 min. Add 1 ml of 0.5 mol/liter sulfuric acid and 3 ml of heptane. Shake and discard the organic phase. Add 0.5 ml of 2 mol/liter sodium hy-

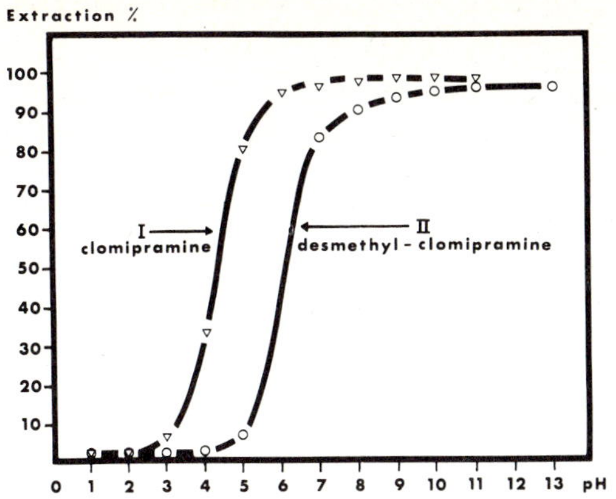

Fig. 3. Distribution of clomipramine (**I**) and desmethyl-clomipramine (**II**) between aqueous phase and heptane +1% isoamyl alcohol as a function of pH

Table 1. Recovery of Clomipramine (I) and Desmethyl-clomipramine (II) from Human Plasma or Urine

	Human plasma		Urine	
Compound	Concn, ng/ml	Recovery, %	Concn, ng/ml	Recovery, %
	47	95.4	47	93.7
I	92	100.0	235	100.0
	185	92.1	470	96.1
	47	95.6	49	90.4
II	94	96.6	244	92.3
	188	98.9	488	87.1

droxide and 3 ml of heptane. After shaking, collect the heptane and evaporate it under nitrogen at room temperature.

Acetylation. Use the conditions described above.

Thin-layer chromatographic purification. Add the chloroform solution of the carrier **III** to the evaporation residue and spot it on the plate. Develop in the first dimension with chloroform/acetone (9/1) then in the second dimension with benzene/ethyl acetate (5/5). Mark the carrier spot that is seen under ultraviolet light.

*Radiometric determination of **I**.* Operate as described for determination of **II.** The ^{14}C-**II** is replaced by ^{14}C-**I** in radiometric samples.

Data processing. ^{14}C-radiometric standards allow calculation of the overall yield of ^{14}C-internal standard in each sample. This yield permits one to correct the recovered ^{3}H activity to a theoretical 100% yield. The resulting ^{3}H activity value is converted to concentration units from a calibration curve, established at each run, giving the ^{3}H response (cpm/ml) vs. the concentration (ng/ml) of references samples.

Further details for the calculation appear elsewhere (*9*).

Results and Discussion

Elaboration of Optimal Conditions

Extraction. **I** and **II** are extracted from aqueous solutions by heptane above pH 9 (Figure 3). They can be

Table 2. Correlation of Clomipramine and Desmethyl-clomipramine Concentrations in Plasma and ^{3}H-Activity of the *N*-Acetyl Derivative[a]

Concn, ng/ml	Overall yield of ^{14}C-internal standard, %	^{3}H-activities 100% yield, mean ± 2 SD (cpm/ml)
Desmethyl-clomipramine[b]		
0	45.7	327 ± 71
42	45.5	3225 ± 225
85	42.4	6300 ± 229
127	48.7	9131 ± 303
Slope, cpm/ng = 69.5		
Intercept, cpm/ml = 330		
Correl. coeff. = 0.9994 (*14*)		
Clomipramine[c]		
0	4.1	1199 ± 32
46	3.7	4268 ± 60
92	6.2	7326 ± 416
138	6.3	10529 ± 562
Slope, cpm/ng = 67.5		
Intercept, cpm/ml = 1174		
Correl. coeff. = 0.9991 (*10*)		

[a] Sample volume, 2 ml. Specific activity of ^{3}H-acetic anhydride, 50 Ci/mol.
[b] Four values per concentration.
[c] Three values per concentration.

re-extracted from the organic phase into aqueous phase at pH 1 and extracted again with heptane in basic medium, so that only endogenous lipophilic bases can be extracted together with **I** and **II.**

Table 1 indicates that good extraction yields are obtained from human plasma and urine at various concentrations.

Acetylation. The acetylation is completed in 15 min at 60 °C with dioxane as solvent and 1 μmol of acetic anhydride (2 ml/liter solution in heptane).

Formation of the carbamate. **I** reacts quantitatively with 2,2,2-trichloroethyl chloroformate in benzene solution in the presence of diisopropylethylamine to yield the carbamate, **IV.** The carbamate is extracted as a neutral compound and thus separated from unreacted base.

Hydrolysis of the carbamate. The basic hydrolysis (*12, 6*) of **IV** proceeds only at high temperature. At 180 °C for 5 min, saponification and decarboxylation of **IV** give **II** with 87% yield. At this temperature, reaction times longer than 5 min decrease the yield of **II**. Generally, the cleavage of carbamates such as **IV** is easily performed by reduction with zinc dust in acetic acid or methanol (*13, 14*). Using such conditions, yields of **II** were lower than with the proposed basic hydrolysis.

Thin-layer chromatographic purification. The first thin-layer chromatography system was introduced to separate ^{3}H-**III** from the acetyl-derivatives of extractable biogenic amines and unreacted **II** from **I**. If the acetylation is not quantitative, the remaining **II** will react with the chloroformate to yield the same carbamate as **I**. That system was also chosen to separate **III** from the acetyl-derivative of **V** (see Figure 2).

Amounts of internal standards. The amounts of internal standards to be used in the procedure depend on the overall yields of the assay. They must be chosen so as to get good counting precision. Using ^{14}C-labeled compounds with about a 6 μCi/mg specific activity, 200 ng of ^{14}C-**I** and 100 ng of ^{14}C-**II** must be used. The same accuracy and precision are obtained when compounds with a 10-fold higher specific activity are used: only 10 ng of ^{14}C-**II** and 40 ng of ^{14}C-**I** need be used; in such conditions, the sensitivity of the determination of **II** is improved.

Correlation of the Concentrations of I and II in Plasma or Urine with ^{3}H-Activity of the *N*-Acetyl Derivative

Determinations were performed from several solutions of **I** and **II** in human plasma or urine (concentrations between 0 and 130 ng/ml). Forty nanograms of ^{14}C-**I** and 10 ng of ^{14}C-**II** were used as internal standard. The ^{3}H activity was corrected to 100% by means of the percentage of ^{14}C activity accounted for. The numerical data for several independent determinations per concentration are given in Table 2. For **I** and **II**, a linear relationship between ^{3}H activity of the *N*-acetyl derivative and concentration was obtained in the range 0–130 ng/ml.

For routine analysis, a calibration curve is established with each analytical run. It is sufficient to determine the intercept of the regression line with the ordinate (^{3}H activity corresponding to plasma blank samples containing only the ^{14}C-labeled internal standard) and to measure the ^{3}H response of three reference samples containing known amounts of each compound.

Assay specificity. Bis-desmethyl-clomipramine (**V**), a metabolite of I with a primary amino group, is quantitatively extracted together with **I** and **II**.

The specificity of the method was checked by determining **I** and **II** in the presence of **V**. We prepared four plasma samples, each containing 25.9 and 77.4 ng of **I** and **II** per milliliter, respectively. In two of these samples, 500 ng/ml of **V** was added and the whole analytical procedure applied.

As indicated in Table 3, there is no interference of **V** on the determination of **I** and **II**.

The specificity of the assay was made sure by a cross-check with a gas chromatography–mass spectrometry technique.[2] Plasma concentrations of clomipramine were measured by both techniques in patients after repeated administration of Anafranil®, 50-mg capsules. As indicated in Table 4, the results are in agreement with a mean difference of 6.1%.

Although gas chromatography–mass spectrometry appears to give slightly lower figures, the proposed technique can be considered as specific for **I** and **II** determination.

Table 3. Determination of I and II in Presence or Absence of Bis-desmethyl-clomipramine (V)[a]

Amount of V	Clomipramine (I) found	Desmethyl-clomipramine (II) found
	ng/ml	
0	23.8	62.7
	22.6	69.7
500	25.5	69.1
	25.9	68.6

[a] Clomipramine (I) concentration, 25.9 ng/ml; desmethyl-clomipramine (II) concentration, 77.4 ng/ml.

Table 4. Assay Specificity[a]

Concn found, ng/ml		Difference	
DRID	GC-MS	ng	%
40	37	3	7.5
39	35	4	10.3
54	47	7	13.0
77	69	8	10.4
103	98	5	4.8
56	56	—	—
64	62	2	3.1
66	64	2	3.0
314	288	26	8.3
303	283	20	6.6
361	375	14	3.9
537	507	30	5.6
562	530	32	5.7
592	556	36	6.1
161	155	6	3.7
198	210	12	6.1

[a] Clomipramine concentrations in plasma after repeated administration of Anafranil®, 50-mg capsules. Comparison of results obtained by double-radioisotope derivative technique (*DRID*) and gas chromatography–mass spectrometry (*GC-MS*).

Assay Precision, Accuracy, and Sensitivity

Precision, reproducibility. Various concentrations of **I** and **II** were determined several times. The data summarized in Tables 5 and 6 indicate good precision and reproducibility at concentrations greater than 15 ng/ml and 2 ng/ml for **I** and **II**, respectively.

Table 7 summarizes results of replicate analyses of three reference samples that were introduced in every series of determinations over a seven-month period.

Accuracy. To simulate a real assay, solutions of **I** and **II** in plasma or urine were prepared at various concentrations and analyzed in duplicate. The results (Table

Table 5. Clomipramine Assay, Precision and Reproducibility

Introduced, ng/ml	7.6	10.4	15	41.1	82.2	123.3	201
	4.4	5.6	14.4	39.4	79.3	128.0	198.4
Found	7.5	10.5	18.2	38.7	81.9	121.7	204.5
	6.8	7.3	14.8	37.6	82.4	123.5	205.4
	7.2	7.6	15.3	39.8	89.4	119.6	198.8
Mean	6.5	7.75	15.7	38.9	83.2	123.2	201.8
Confidence limits (P = 0.95), and range	4.2–8.7	4.5–11.0	12.9–18.4	37.3–40.4	76.4–90.1	117.5–128.9	195.9–207.6

Table 6. Desmethyl-clomipramine Assay: Precision and Reproducibility

Introduced, ng/ml	1	2	5	10	30.3	217.4
	0.9	2.9	5.0	8.8	30.7	229.3
	0.9	2.9	4.9	10.2	31.1	214.8
Found	0.9	2.4	5.2	11.0	31.0	217.6
	1.1	2.9	4.4	9.7	32.8	227.7
	0.6	2.1	6.0	9.1		
Mean	0.9	2.6	5.10	9.8	31.4	222.3
Confidence limits (P = 0.95), and range	0.65–1.1	2.2–3.1	4.4–5.8	8.7–10.8	29.9–32.9	210.9–233.8

Table 7. Assay Precision: Replicate Analyses of Identical Reference Samples during Seven Months

Compound	Concn, ng/ml	Mean	SD	CV, %
Clomipramine (I)	57.6	55.6 (n = 22)	4.3	7.7
	115.3	117.8 (n = 12)	11.8	10.0
	230.7	231.9 (n = 22)	12.2	5.3
Desmethyl-clomipramine (II)	53.0	51.7 (n = 22)	3.9	7.5
	106.0	108.5 (n = 12)	7.5	6.9
	212.1	212.1 (n = 22)	8.1	3.8

Table 8. Test Analysis of Clomipramine and Desmethyl-clomipramine: Assay Accuracy

Clomipramine				Desmethyl-clomipramine			
ng/ml			Deviation from theory, %	ng/ml			Deviation from theory, %
Introduced	Found	m		Introduced	Found	m	
4.5	3.1 7.0	5.0	+11.1	1.0	0.9 1.0	1.0	—
9.0	10.6 11.4	11.0	+22.2	2.5	2.5 1.7	2.1	−16.0
13.6	15.3 14.4	14.8	+ 8.8	4.9	5.6 5.0	5.3	+8.2
20.8	18.3 19.0	18.7	−10.0	9.9	8.9 9.5	9.2	−7.1
33.3	29.3 32.9	31.1	− 6.6	14.8	14.6 15.3	14.9	+0.7
51.4	56.5 53.2	54.8	+ 6.5	54.3	53.7 54.4	54.0	−0.6
310.0	309.4 327.1	318.2	+ 2.2	321.0	330.6 335.8	333.2	+3.8

Table 9. Influence of the Specific Activity of the ^{14}C-labeled Internal Standard on the Sensitivity of the Technique[a]

Compound	^{14}C-labeled internal standard: Spec. act., μCi/mg	Used amount, ng	Sensitivity, ng/ml
Clomipramine	6.0	200	20
	64.9	40	10–15
Desmethyl-clomipramine	6.5	100	15
	66.8	10	2

[a] [^{3}H] acetic anhydride: 50 Ci/mol

Table 10. Clomipramine (I) and Desmethyl-clomipramine (II) in Plasma (ng/ml) after a Single Oral Dose of 50 mg or 100 mg of Clomipramine

Time, h	Subject 01, Dose, 50 mg: I	II	Subject 02, Dose, 100 mg: I	II
0	0	0	0	0
1	0	0	0	<S.L.[a]
3	22	4	46	9
6	21	6	39	12
24	<S.L.[a]	<S.L.[a]	<S.L.[a]	10

[a] Sensitivity limit: 15 ng/ml for **I**, 2 ng/ml for **II**

8) indicate good agreement between found and introduced amounts that exceeded the sensitivity limits.

Sensitivity. The sensitivity of the assay—defined as the lowest amount of drug that can be assayed with acceptable reproducibility (±10% error)—depends on the specific activities of the ^{14}C-labeled internal standards and the ^{3}H-labeled reagent.

^{14}C-labeled internal standards with two different specific activities were used. It appeared that use of small amounts of internal standards with high specific activity greatly improved the sensitivity in the determination of **II** (see Table 9). The assay procedure of **I** is much more complicated than for **II** (three derivatization steps after chromatographic separation). This probably is the reason why only a slight improvement could be achieved for **I.**

^{3}H-labeled acetic anhydride was used at two specific activities: 50 and 250 Ci/mol. No further improvement was achieved when using 250 Ci/mol acetic anhydride because the ^{3}H response of impurities originating from the plasma is increased and the chromatographic separation does not entirely remove this contamination.

Using ^{3}H-labeled acetic anhydride with 50 Ci/mol specific activity and 40 ng of ^{14}C-**I** as internal standard, we found that the method enables **I** to be determined in plasma or urine at concentrations down to 10–15 ng/ml in 2-ml samples; lower amounts are detectable. **II** can be assayed at concentrations down to 2 ng/ml with use of the same reagent and 10 ng of ^{14}C-**II** as internal standard.

Plasma Concentrations of Clomipramine and Desmethyl-Clomipramine in Man

Single dose administration. Plasma concentrations of **I,** measured in two volunteers after administration of a single oral dose of Anafranil® tablets, are given in Table 10.

Steady-state plasma concentrations. Concentrations of **I** and **II** in plasma were measured in patients on different days during chronic administration of Anafranil®,

Table 11. Clomipramine (I) and Desmethyl-clomipramine (II) in Plasma after Repeat Doses of Anafranil® Capsules

Subjects	Daily dose, mg during plasma collection period	Concn, ng/ml: 1st sampling day[a] I	II	2nd sampling day[a] I	II	3rd sampling day[a] I	II
		20.1	65.8	16.8	70.0	42.4	65.2
1	100[b]	40.2	74.3	39.2	66.3	54.0	76.1
		49.4	84.7	52.6	72.8	57.0	81.5
		77.3	112.5	56.5	96.8	51.5	89.1
2	150[c]	76.1	104.1	64.5	97.8	65.9	98.3
		103.2	115.9	66.6	96.0	62.6	94.5
		108.0	175.4	135.5	187.2	135.9	199.8
3	200[d]	133.3	197.0	168.9	221.3	155.4	218.5
		167.2	243.3	162.3	228.2	153.4	210.8

[a] Sampling on days 1, 8, and 15 for subjects 1 and 2, on days 1, 3, and 6 for subject 3.
[b] One 50-mg capsule each in the morning and at bedtime.
[c] One 50-mg capsule each in the morning, afternoon, and at bedtime.
[d] One 50-mg capsule each in the morning and afternoon, two capsules at bedtime.

50-mg capsules (daily dose, between 100 and 200 mg). The data given in Table 11 reveal considerable variability.

Concentrations of desmethyl-clomipramine tended to exceed the corresponding clomipramine concentrations and showed less variability.

We conclude that the technique described in this paper permits one to determine clomipramine and its major metabolite in plasma or urine, and to monitor concentrations in plasma or urine in clinical pharmacology experiments or during the course of a therapeutic treatment. The sensitivity of the assay might be insufficient to accurately determine the low concentrations achieved in single dose studies when low dosages are given.

Should ^{14}C-labeled bis-desmethyl-clomipramine be available, this metabolite could be assayed without any additional step together with clomipramine and desmethyl-clomipramine.

This double-radioisotope derivative technique, based on desmethylation by ethyl chloroformate, could be extended to the determination of other tertiary amine drugs for which only few sensitive and specific analytical methods are available; imipramine (Tofranil®, Geigy) and desipramine (Pertofran®, Geigy) have been assayed in plasma or urine down to 20 ng/ml and 5 ng/ml, respectively (J. Godbillon and W. Riess, unpublished results.)

The sensitivity obtained for desmethyl-clomipramine when using small amounts of internal standards with high specific activity indicates that nanogram amounts can be determined by the double-radioisotope derivative technique if the derivatization reaction is simple.

We thank W. Küng (Radioisotope Laboratory, Ciba-Geigy, Basle) for providing ^{14}C-labeled clomipramine and desmethyl-clomipramine and [^{3}H]maprotiline; W. Theobald (Medical Department, Ciba-Geigy, Basle) for the clinical experiment with a single oral dose; B. C. Schiele (Saint Paul Ramsey Hospital, Saint Paul, Minn.) and I. Wilson (Dorothea Dix Hospital, Raleigh, N.C.) for the clinical experiment with repeated doses; and E. Renk and W. Riess (Ciba-Geigy, Basle) for valuable suggestions.

References

1. Viala, A., Gouezo, F., and Gola, C., Séparation et identification par chromatographie sur couche mince de cinq antidépresseurs thymoanaleptiques dérivés de la benzodiazépine. *J. Chromatogr.* **45,** 94 (1969).

2. Lemontey, Y., Meunier, J., and Lafargue, P., Recherche, identification et dosage en toxicologie d'urgence des 5-*H*-dibenzo-(*b, f*)-azépines dans les milieux biologiques. *Clin. Chim. Acta* **30,** 713 (1970).

3. Moody, J. P., The biological availability of clomipramine (Anafranil). *J. Int. Med. Res.* **1,** 325 (1973).

4. Viala, A., Cano, J. P., Gola, C., and Gouezo, F., Identification des antidépresseurs tricycliques dérivés de l'imipramine par chromatographie en phase gazeuse. *J. Chromatogr.* **59,** 297 (1971).

5. Viala, A., Gola, C., Cano, J. P., and Gouezo, F., Méthode de recherche des antidépresseurs imipraminiques dans l'urine par chromatographie en phase gazeuse et par chromatographie sur couche mince. *Ann. Pharm. Fr.* **30,** 445 (1972).

6. Hartvig, P., and Vessman, J., Electron capture gas-chromatography of tertiary amines after a demethylation reaction to secondary amines. *Acta Pharm. Suec.* **11,** 115 (1974).

7. Riedman, M., Specific gas chromatography determination of phenothiazines and barbiturate tranquillizers with the nitrogen flame ionization detector. *J. Chromatogr.* **92,** 55 (1974).

8. Gifford, L. A., Turner, P., and Pare, C. M. B., Sensitive method for the routine determination of tricyclic antidepressants in plasma using a specific nitrogen detector. *J. Chromatogr.* **105,** 107 (1975).

9. Riess, W., The double radioisotope derivative technique for the assay of drugs in biological samples. Part I. The determination of maprotiline. *Anal. Chim. Acta* **68,** 363 (1974).

10. Faigle, J. W., and Dieterle, W., The metabolism and pharmacokinetics of clomipramine (Anafranil). *J. Int. Med. Res.* **1,** 281 (1973).

11. Okita, G. T., Kabara, J. J., Richardson, F., and Leroy, G. V., Assaying compounds containing ^{3}H and ^{14}C. *Nucleonics* **15,** 111 (1957).

12. Seidlova, V., and Protiva, M., Neurotrope und psychotrope Substanzen XIII. Beiträge zur Synthese von Amitriptylin, Nortriptylin und ähnlichen Substanzen. *Coll. Czech. Chem. Commun.* **32,** 2826 (1967).

13. Windholz, T. B., and Johnston, D. B. R., Trichloroethoxy carbonyl: A generally applicable protecting group. *Tetrahedron Lett.* **27,** 2555 (1967).

14. Montzka, T. A., Matiskella, J. D., and Partyka, R. A., 2,2,2-Trichloroethyl chloroformate: A general reagent for demethylation of tertiary methylamines. *Tetrahedron Lett.* **14,** 1325 (1974).

Simultaneous Measurement of Phenobarbital, Diphenylhydantoin, and Primidone in Blood by High-Pressure Liquid Chromatography

Pokar M. Kabra,[1] George Gotelli, Robert Stanfill, and Laurence J. Marton[2,3]

We describe a sensitive, precise high-pressure liquid chromatographic method in which 5-(*p*-methylphenyl)-5-phenylhydantoin is used as the internal standard for simultaneous determination of diphenylhydantoin, phenobarbital, and primidone in whole blood and plasma. These anticonvulsant drugs are well separated from each other and from normal blood constituents in less than 10 min. The lower limit of detection for each drug is 100 ng for primidone, 200 ng for dilantin, and 300 ng for phenobarbital. The eluted drugs were detected by their absorption at 254 nm, and evaluated from their peak heights as compared to internal standard. The method was successfully adapted for pediatric samples (100 to 500 μl of whole blood or plasma). Fifty specimens were analyzed for phenobarbital and diphenylhydantoin and 25 specimens for primidone by a standard gas-chromatographic method and by our liquid-chromatographic method; the resulting correlation coefficient was >0.98.

Additional Keyphrases: *pediatric chemistry • relation between concn in whole blood and plasma • single-step extraction • gas chromatography compared*

Diphenylhydantoin (DPH) and phenobarbital are the two drugs most often used for the control of epileptic seizures. Primidone, a drug widely used in the management of seizures, is partly metabolized to phenobarbital and phenethylmalonamide. Because both primidone and its metabolite, phenobarbital, possess anticonvulsant activity (*1*), it is advisable to monitor the concentration of both compounds in serum or whole blood after therapy with primidone. The value of information on concentrations in blood for therapeutic monitoring of these drugs has been the subject of recent reviews (*2, 3*). These determinations are most often made by spectrophotometric (*4*) or gas–liquid chromatographic methods (*5–7*). Recently, Evans (*8*) reported a method for simultaneous determination of diphenylhydantoin and phenobarbital in serum by high-pressure liquid chromatography. However, the method required a multi-step sample preparation procedure with critical pH adjustments, and no provision was made for use of an internal standard. While our studies were in progress, two additional methods were reported for the analysis of anticonvulsants by high-pressure liquid chromatography (*9, 10*). The first method (*9*) measures the concentration of phenobarbital and diphenylhydantoin in serum, but no provision was made to determine primidone concentration. The second method (*10*) measures the concentration of several anticonvulsants in serum. However, the authors reported recovery rates for the drugs of only 40–73% from serum, with use of the charcoal-adsorption technique. Their detection of column effluent at 195 nm is fairly nonspecific, and the method is not adaptable with instruments equipped with a fixed-wavelength ultraviolet detector. Their use of phenacetin, a commonly used analgesic drug, as an internal standard is a potential source of error in the quantitation of these drugs. In contrast to the above methods, our method offers: (*a*) rapid, sensitive, and simultaneous assay of diphenylhydantoin, phenobarbital, and primidone in small volumes of whole blood or plasma; (*b*) rapid, quantitative, single-step solvent extraction of these drugs from whole blood and plasma; and (*c*) easy adaptation of the method to determination of these drugs in pediatric samples (100–500 μl of blood or plasma). Values for

Division of Clinical Chemistry, Department of Laboratory Medicine, School of Medicine, University of California, San Francisco, San Francisco, Calif. 94143.

[1] Advanced Fellow in Clinical Chemistry (NIH Grant, GM 0193).

[2] L. J. M. is the recipient of NCI Research Career Development Award No. CA-00112.

[3] Also Department of Neurosurgery.

Received Dec. 15, 1975; accepted Mar. 2, 1976.

whole blood or plasma from the same subject on anticonvulsant therapy did not differ significantly; hence the method could be used interchangeably for either. Total chromatographic time is less than 10 min.

Materials and Methods

Chromatography

We used a Model 601 (Perkin-Elmer Corp., Norwalk, Conn. 06856) high-pressure liquid chromatograph equipped with a variable-wavelength ultraviolet detector (Perkin-Elmer LC 55), a 1-mV Honeywell Electronic 194 recorder, and a 30 cm × 4.0 mm (i.d.) silicic acid ("m-Poracil"; Waters Associates Inc., Milford, Mass. 01757). The column effluent was monitored at 254 nm. The column was eluted with a chloroform/methanol/28% ammonium hydroxide mixture (95/4.5/0.5, by vol), at the rate of 1 ml/min.

Reagents and Reference Materials

Chloroform and methanol, AR grade (J. T. Baker Chemical Co., Phillipsburg, N. J. 08865).

Ammonium hydroxide, 28% (Mallinckrodt Chemical Works, St. Louis, Mo. 63160).

Diphenylhydantoin (Eastman Organic Chemicals, Rochester, N. Y. 14650).

Primidone was supplied as a gift from Ayerst Laboratories Inc., New York, N. Y. 10017.

Phenobarbital (Mallinckrodt).

5-(p-*Methylphenyl*)-*5-phenylhydantoin,* our internal standard, was purchased from Aldrich Chemical Co., Milwaukee, Wis. 53233.

A stock internal standard, 250 mg/liter, was prepared in methanol, and was stable for at least a month at 4 °C. A working internal standard (25 mg/liter) was prepared by diluting the stock solution 10-fold in water. This solution was stable for at least two days at 4 °C.

Drug reference standard. A standard solution of diphenylhydantoin, phenobarbital, primidone, and the internal standard was prepared by dissolving 25 mg of each in 100 ml of ethanol. This solution was stable for at least a month at 4 °C.

Procedure

Whole blood or plasma, 2 ml, was combined with 2 ml of the diluted internal standard. Glacial acetic acid, 75 μl, was added with immediate vortex-mixing for 20 s. Ten milliliters of chloroform were added and the mixture was mechanically shaken for 5 min, followed by centrifugation for 5 min at 210 × *g* (2000 rpm). The blood coagulum ring or plasma layer was aspirated off and the chloroform poured into a conical centrifuge tube and evaporated at 70 °C with a vacuum evaporator. The residue was redissolved in 50 μl of ethanol, and 2 to 5 μl was injected into the high-pressure liquid chromatograph. A control was run daily, prepared by adding sufficient diphenylhydantoin, primidone, and phenobarbital to pooled whole blood. For pediatric samples, the blood or plasma (100 to 500 μl) was mixed with an equal volume of internal standard and similarly processed, except that the residue was redissolved in 15 μl of ethanol, and 10 μl of the specimen was injected into the high-pressure liquid chromatograph. Washing the column with 150 ml of tetrahydrofuran once weekly significantly increased the usable lifespan of our column.

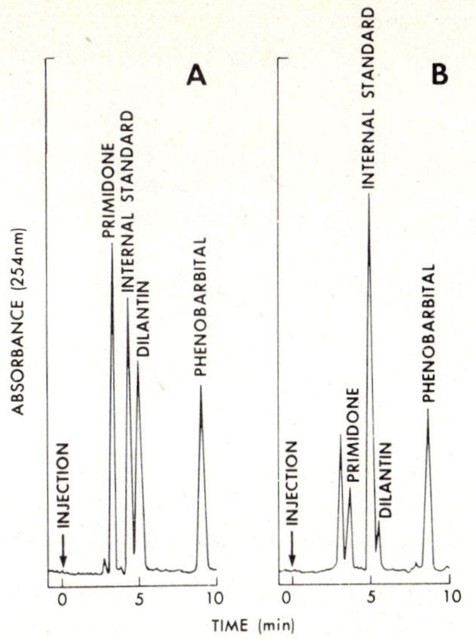

Fig. 1. High-pressure liquid chromatogram of primidone, diphenylhydantoin, and phenobarbital

Trace *A* shows a typical chromatogram for the drug reference standard, trace *B* the chromatogram from whole blood of a patient receiving all three of these drugs

Results

Figure 1 shows representative chromatograms of the drug reference standard and whole blood extracted specimens. Figure 1*A* shows a typical chromatogram for the drug reference standard, Figure 1*B* a chromatogram from whole blood of a patient receiving all three of these drugs. Primidone, diphenylhydantoin, and phenobarbital could each be quantitated at a concentration of 1 mg/liter—far below the therapeutic range.

Linearity: Whole blood and plasma standards were prepared containing various known amounts of each drug, equivalent to 2 to 100 mg/liter. A constant amount of internal standard was added to each sample. Concentration and reading were linearly related from 2 mg/liter to at least 50 mg/liter for primidone and diphenylhydantoin, and from 2 mg to at least 100 mg/liter for phenobarbital.

Recovery: When known amounts of drug were added to whole blood and plasma, analytical recovery rates for each drug were between 95–110% for the entire linear range. This agrees well with Evenson et al. (*11*) and Pippenger et al. (*12*), who reported 90–100% recovery with similar chloroform-extraction techniques.

Precision. Table 1 presents precision data for the drugs analyzed by our procedure. Within-run precision was estimated by 10 analyses of the same samples, in duplicate.

Comparison between Whole Blood and Plasma

Whole blood and plasma specimens from patients on anticonvulsant therapy were processed and drug con-

Table 1. Precision of Assays for Anticonvulsants in Whole Blood

Drug	Within-run (n = 10) Range, mg/liter (±SD)	Within-run CV, %	Day-to-day (n = 22) Range, mg/liter (±SD)	Day-to-day CV, %
Primidone	10.7 ± 1.6	7.4	17.0 ± 2.0	6
Diphenylhydantoin	10.6 ± 1.8	5.7	24.0 ± 2.8	5.9
Phenobarbital	10.7 ± 1.6	7.4	18.0 ± 2.4	6.8

Table 2. Comparison between Concentrations of Diphenylhydantoin, Primidone and Phenobarbital in Whole Blood and Plasma

Drug	n	Range, mg/liter	Slope	Intercept	Correl. coeff.
Phenobarbital	26	2–86	1.011	0.070	0.993
Diphenylhydantoin	30	2–39	1.008	0.398	0.987
Primidone	10	2–16	0.97	0.538	0.94

Table 3. Comparison between Micro-Scale and Regular Specimens

Drug	n	Range, mg/liter	Slope	Intercept	Corr. coeff.
Diphenylhydantoin	27	2–27	0.925	0.78	0.970
Phenobarbital	22	2–63	1.057	−0.494	0.994
Primidone	10	3–12	0.700	2.15	0.957

centrations determined by high-pressure liquid chromatography. Concentrations of phenobarbital, diphenylhydantoin, and primidone determined from whole blood and plasma were compared. Table 2 shows the results.

Comparison between Micro-Scale and Regular Samples

Micro-scale samples (100 to 500 μl) of whole blood or plasma from patients on these drugs were assayed and compared with regular (2 ml) samples (Table 3). We could easily detect 2 mg/liter of these drugs when only 100 μl of sample was used.

Quantitation and Identification of the Drugs

Quantitation was done by measuring the peak heights of the drugs relative to the internal standard. The drugs were identified by retention time. Effluent corresponding to several of the resulting peaks for each drug was collected and subjected to chemical ionization mass-spectroscopy. The mass spectrum of each was identical with that of the authentic drug.

Table 4. Retention Times of Some Other Drugs

Drug	Retention time, min[a]
Ethosuximide	4.5
Carbamazepine	3.5
Mesentoin	3
Chlorodiazepoxide	3
Primidone	4
Mephobarbital	7
5-(p-Methylphenyl)-5-phenylhydantoin	5
Diphenylhydantoin	5.5
Phenobarbital	8
5-(p-Hydroxyphenyl)-5-phenylhydantoin	25

[a] From time of injection onto column

Table 5. Gas- and Liquid-Chromatographic Measurement of Diphenylhydantoin, Primidone, and Phenobarbital in Whole Blood Compared

Drug	n	Range, mg/liter	Slope	Intercept	Corr. coeff.
Phenobarbital	50	1.0–40.0	0.963	0.411	0.987
Diphenylhydantoin	50	1.0–25.0	0.936	0.931	0.982
Primidone	25	2.0–16.0	1.020	0.208	0.988

Interference from Other Drugs

To determine the potential usefulness of the procedure, we checked for possible interference from several other drugs by chromatographing pure standards and physiological samples. Table 4 shows the retention times for the drugs tested.

Comparison with Gas Chromatography

Table 5 presents the comparison data for the assay of these three drugs by our procedure and by a gas chromatographic method.

Discussion

High-pressure liquid chromatography of phenobarbital, primidone, and diphenylhydantoin is more rapid and specific than are spectrophotometric and gas-chromatographic techniques, and does not necessitate derivatization of these compounds in order to achieve sufficient sensitivity and resolution as do most gas-chromatographic methods. High-pressure liquid chromatographic columns allow for the injection of significantly larger amounts of sample than is true for gas-chromatographic columns; thus the total volume of an extract of whole blood or plasma may be used for the analysis. We successfully applied our procedure to pediatric samples, volumes that were previously too small for accurate measurement. Results obtained by high-pressure liquid chromatography and gas-chromatography on the same sample correlated well for these drugs.

References

1. Baumel, I. P., Gallagher, B. B., and Mattson, R. H., Phenyl ethyl malonamide (PEMA), an important metabolite of primidone. *Arch. Neurol.* (Chicago) **27,** 34 (1972).

2. Rose, S. W., Smith, L. D., and Penry, J. K., Blood level determinations of antiepileptic drugs. Clinical value and methods. Obtainable from the National Institute of Neurological Diseases and Stroke, NIH, Bethesda, Md. 20014, 1971.

3. Buchtal, F., and Lennox-Buchtal, M. A., Relation of anticonvulsant effect to concentration in serum. In *Antiepileptic Drugs,* D. M. Woodbury, J. K. Penry, and R. P. Schmidt, Eds. Raven Press, New York, N. Y., p 193.

4. Plaa, G. L., and Hine, C. H., A method for the simultaneous determination of phenobarbital and diphenylhydantoin in blood. *J. Lab. Clin. Med.* **47,** 649 (1956).

5. Least, C. J., Johnson, G. F., and Solomon, H. M., Therapeutic monitoring of anticonvulsant drugs: Gas-chromatographic simultaneous determination of primidone, phenylethyl malonamide, carbamazepine, and diphenylhydantoin. *Clin. Chem.* **21,** 1658 (1975).

6. Toseland, P. A., Grove, J., and Berry, D. J., An isothermal GLC determination of the plasma levels of carbamazepine, diphenylhydantoin, phenobarbitone, and primidone. *Clin. Chim. Acta* **38,** 321 (1972).

7. Davis, H. L., Falk, K. J., and Bailey, D. G., Improved method for the simultaneous determination of phenobarbital, primidone, and diphenylhydantoin in patients serum by gas-liquid chromatography. *J. Chromatogr.* **107,** 61 (1975).

8. Evans, J. E., Simultaneous measurement of diphenylhydantoin and phenobarbital in serum by high performance liquid chromatography. *Anal. Chem.* **45,** 2428 (1973).

9. Atwell, S., Green, V., and Haney, W., Development and evaluation of method for simultaneous determination of phenobarbital and diphenylhydantoin in plasma by high pressure liquid chromatography. *J. Pharm. Sci.* **64,** 806 (1975).

10. Adams, R. F., and Vandemark, F. L., Simultaneous high pressure liquid chromatographic determination of some anticonvulsants in serum. *Clin. Chem.* **22,** 25 (1976).

11. Evenson, M. A., Jones, P., and Darcey, B., Simultaneous measurement of diphenylhydantoin and primidone in serum by gas-liquid chromatography. *Clin. Chem.* **16,** 107 (1970).

12. Pippenger, C. E., and Gillen, H. W., Gas chromatographic analysis for anticonvulsant drugs in biological fluids. *Clin. Chem.* **15,** 582 (1969).

CLIN. CHEM. 22/6, 828–831 (1976)

Radioimmunoassay for Clindamycin

Terry J. Gilbertson and R. P. Stryd

We describe a radioimmunoassay for measuring clindamycin in serum extracts that is more accurate than the microbiological assay because of the minimal response of the metabolite, *N*-demethylclindamycin. The assay is not affected by the presence of other antiobiotics. As described it is as sensitive as the microbiological assay, but can be made more sensitive.

Additional Keyphrases: *antibiotics in serum and urine* • *comparison with microbiological assay* • *drug assay*

Clindamycin is a semisynthetic antibiotic in which a 7(S)-chloro group is substituted for the 7(R)-hydroxyl group on the parent compound, lincomycin (*1*). We needed to measure more accurately the concentrations of clindamycin in serum, both alone and in the presence of other antibiotics. Accordingly, we developed the radioimmunoassay reported here.

Materials and Methods

Preparative Methods

[N-methyl-^{3}H]*clindamycin·HCl·CH_3CH_2OH.* *N*-Demethylclindamycin·HCl, 100 mg (0.22 mmol), was dissolved in 5 ml of water. The solution was cooled to 5 °C in an ice bath. Formaldehyde (370 g/liter, in water) 40 µl (0.53 mmol) was added. After 15 min, most of the *N*-demethylclindamycin was converted to the reactive intermediate, as shown by thin-layer chromatography (TLC) on silica gel with ethylacetate, acetone, and water (8/5/1 by vol) as developing solvent. Sodium borohydride, 10 mg (0.26 mmol), equivalent to 1.04 mmol of H, was added. Hydrogen evolution began immediately, and the product began to separate as an oil. After 75 min, the reaction was complete as shown by the previously used TLC system. The basic reaction mixture was extracted with $CHCl_3$ (5 × 10 ml). The $CHCl_3$ solution was dehydrated with Na_2SO_4 and evaporated to about 3 ml. The $CHCl_3$ solution was applied to a 20-mm (i.d.) column of dry-packed silica gel, 50 g, which had been stirred with a 10/1 by volume mixture of $CHCl_3$/methanol, 80 g being added per kilogram of gel. The column was eluted with the same solvent and 10-ml fractions were collected. The product was located, by TLC of effluent fractions, in tubes 9 and 10.

Clinical Research Laboratories, The Upjohn Company, Kalamazoo, Mich. 49001.

Received Jan. 26, 1976; accepted Mar. 3, 1976.

The contents of tubes 9 and 10 were combined and the solvent was evaporated. The residue was dissolved in 0.5 ml absolute ethanol, and three drops of ethanolic HCl were added. Crystallization occurred on cooling. The product was filtered and washed with ethylacetate/ethanol, 10/1 by volume. The yield was 61.9 mg, 57.3%, mp 156–160 °C (dec.). The infrared spectra was identical with that from an authentic sample. The final labeling was done by Mallinckrodt/Nuclear, St. Louis, Mo. 63160, using this procedure. Figure 1 shows the reaction.

Clindamycin-2-hemisuccinate. Clindamycin-2-hemisuccinate was synthesized by the method of Sinkula et al. (*2*). The workup after the acid hydrolysis is a modification of that supplied by W. Morozowich (*3*). 3,4-*O*-*p*-Anisylideneclindamycin·HCl, 5.0 g (8.6 mmol), and succinic anhydride, 5.0 g (50 mmol), were added to 50 ml of pyridine in a 500-ml flask fitted with a condenser and drying tube. The mixture was heated for 2.5 h at about 90 °C. After cooling, diethyl ether (500 ml) was added to precipitate the product as a gum. The precipitate was dissolved in 75 ml of glacial acetic acid. Water, 10 ml, was added and the mixture was heated for

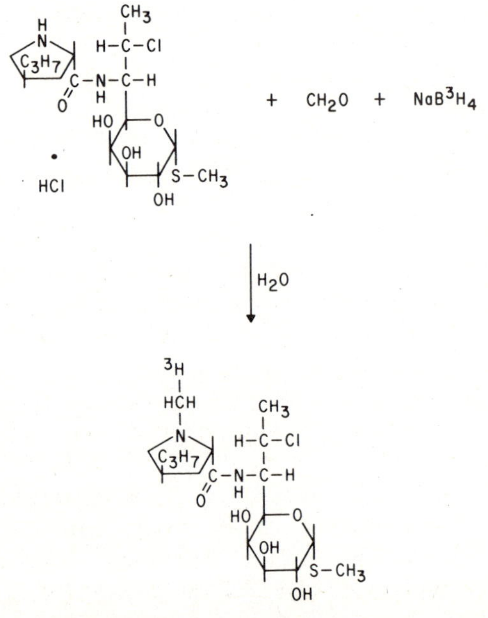

Fig. 1. Synthesis of [*N-methyl*-^{3}H]clindamycin

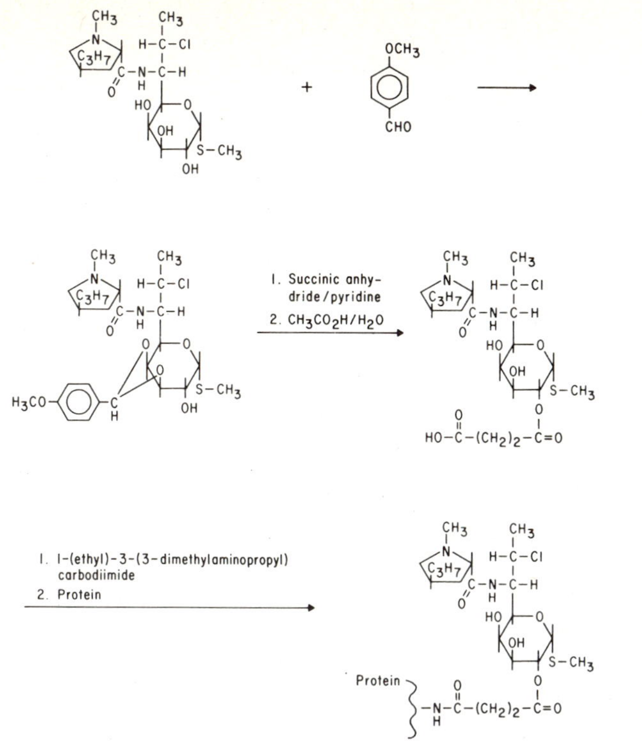

Fig. 2. Synthesis of the protein conjugate of clindamycin

45 min at about 90 °C. The solvent was evaporated and the residue dissolved in 25 ml of $CHCl_3$, and the solution seeded with succinic acid. The succinic acid was filtered off and washed with cold $CHCl_3$. Ether was added to the combined $CHCl_3$ extracts to precipitate the product, which was then dissolved in water and the pH adjusted to 6.0 with NH_4OH. The product crystallized from this mixture. It was recrystallized by dissolving in the minimum amount of $CHCl_3$ followed by the addition of hexane until crystals appeared (yield: 1.02 g, 22%; mp 169–172 °C). The infrared and nuclear magnetic resonance spectra were identical to those for an authentic sample obtained from W. Morozowich.

Clindamycin-2-hemisuccinyl/bovine serum albumin. Bovine serum albumin, 100 mg, was dissolved in 4 ml of water. The pH was adjusted to 5. Clindamycin-2-hemisuccinate, 100 mg, was added to 4 ml of water and 1-ethyl-3-(3-dimethylaminopropyl) carbodiimide·HCl, 100 mg, was added. The clindamycin-2-hemisuccinate mixture was added to the bovine serum albumin solution, the pH adjusted to 5, and the mixture allowed to remain at room temperature overnight. The mixture was dialyzed against distilled water and freeze dried. The yield was 116 mg. This conjugation procedure is shown in Figure 2.

The number of derivatized lysines attached to each bovine serum albumin molecule as determined by the trinitrobenzene sulfonic acid method (*4*) was 30.

Induction of antiserum. Two rabbits were injected intradermally with 10.0 mg of conjugate in an equivolume 50/50 mixture of saline (9 g of NaCl per liter) and Freund complete adjuvant (Difco Laboratories, Detroit, Mich. 48232). This was followed by 0.5 ml of pertussis vaccine (Eli Lilly & Co., Indianapolis, Ind. 46206). The rabbits then received monthly injections of 100 μg of conjugate in the saline/incomplete adjuvant mixture. After seven months, titers of 1/150 or greater were induced in both rabbits.

Sample preparation. Add 0.5 ml of serum to 2.5 ml of $CHCl_3$ and mix for 30 s. Centrifuge at 2000 rpm for 5 min, and aspirate the serum layer. Transfer an 0.1-ml aliquot of the $CHCl_3$ extract to a 1.5 × 5-cm polyethylene vial and evaporate under nitrogen. The sample is now ready for assay.

This extraction recovered an average of 90.4% of [^{3}H]clindamycin added with the same amounts of unlabeled clindamycin as reported in the recovery and precision studies.

Standards. Dissolve clindamycin·HCl·H_2O in distilled water. The range is 1 to 250 ng/0.1 ml (10 to 2500 μg/liter).

Assay Procedure

Add 0.5 ml of phosphate buffer (50 mmol/liter phosphate, 9 g/liter NaCl, and 0.1 g/liter NaN_3; pH 8) to the residue in the sample vials to dissolve the antibiotic. Add an identical volume to the total-bound count vials. Only 0.4 ml of buffer is added to the standard vials, followed by 0.1 ml of standard solution. Add 0.1 ml of [^{3}H]clindamycin (~1800 cpm) to all vials. To the mixture of labeled and nonlabeled antibiotic in all vials add 0.2 ml of first antiserum diluted to bind 65–70% of label. Mix contents of all vials and allow to stand at room temperature for 2 h. After this initial incubation, add 0.2 ml of second antiserum diluted to bind all of first antibody. Mix and allow to stand overnight at 4 °C. After the second incubation, add 2.5 ml of buffer to each vial and centrifuge at 3000 rpm for 20 min. Decant the vials and allow to drain for 1 min. To each vial add 6 ml of scintillation cocktail containing 7570 ml of toluene, 250 ml of "Bio-Solv BBS-3" (Beckman Instruments, Fullerton, Calif. 92634) and 318 ml of "Liquifluor" (New England Nuclear, Boston, Mass. 02118). Mix to disperse the precipitated antibody–antibiotic complex. Count in a liquid scintillation counter until 500 counts have accumulated for the highest standard. If the samples contain concentrations of antibiotic greater than those in the highest standard, they can be assayed by taking a smaller aliquot of $CHCl_3$ extract or by diluting the serum before extraction. Repeated checking by means of the automatic, external-standard-channels ratio method showed little variation in quench when extracts were used as samples. The tritium counting efficiency was about 45%. Figure 3 shows an example of a standard curve in the log-logit transform.

Results

Analytical Variables

Cross-reactivity. The antiserum had a large cross-reactivity with clindamycin-2-phosphate (171%) and low cross-reactivity with clindamycin-2-palmitate (2.4%). This was the reverse of what was expected on the basis of structural similarity to clindamycin-2-hemi-

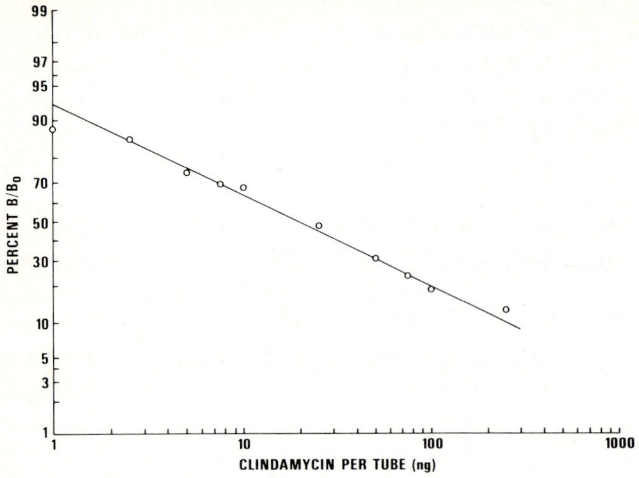

Fig. 3. Standard curve for clindamycin radioimmunoassay

succinate. A possible explanation is that the long palmitate side-chain hydrophobically bonds to another portion of the clindamycin molecule, making it unrecognizable by the antibodies. This is not possible for the smaller, charged phosphate molecule. The phosphate group must satisfactorily mimic the carbonyl group of the hemisuccinate to render it more tightly bound than clindamycin.

The metabolite, clindamycin sulfoxide, cross-reacts 41.8%. This cross-reactivity is not desirable because this compound is a major urinary metabolite and a minor serum metabolite. A new conjugate has been prepared with freshly recrystallized hemisuccinate in an attempt to induce antiserum without this problem.

Only lincomycin, of the other antibiotics tested, cross-reacted to a measurable degree (2.4%).

None of the components of the antibiotic or the common sugars cross-reacted. The results are shown in Table 1.

Recovery and precision studies. Recovery studies were on sera supplemented with five different concentrations of drug, from 5.00 to 0.100 mg/liter. Each value was measured four times in a single day for each of five days. The percent deviation and day-to-day CV are shown in Table 2. The average within-day CV for 20 determinations on two serum samples, containing ~1 and ~2 mg/liter, was 8.9%.

Sensitivity. The sensitivity of this procedure for clindamycin in serum is about 0.1 mg/liter, about the same as for the microbiological assay. However, the sensitivity of this assay depends primarily on the specific activity of the [^{3}H]clindamycin, so this could be readily increased. Sodium [^{3}H]borohydride is now available with specific activities of 15–20 kCi/mol. Synthesis with this borohydride could change the sensitivity to 5.0 μg/liter.

Comparison with Microbiological Assay (*5*)

Our assay generally produces values that are lower than those found with the microbiological assay. The difference tends to increase as the time after adminis-

Table 1. Cross-Reactivities[a]

Clindamycin derivatives	
Clindamycin-2-phosphate	171.0%
Clindamycin-2-palmitate	2.4%
N-(β-Hydroxyethyl)clindamycin	8.1%
Clindamycin metabolites	
N-Demethylclindamycin	4.8%
Clindamycin sulfoxide	41.4%
Other antibiotics	
Lincomycin	2.4%
Penicillin G	0
Penicillin O	0
Gentamycin	0
Erythromycin	0
Spectinomycin	0
Other compounds	
D-Glucose	0
D-Galactose	0
Epi-7-chloro-methylthiolincosaminide	0
Propylhygric acid	0

[a] Defined as:

$$\frac{\text{Mass of unlabeled clindamycin at midpoint of standard curve} \times 100}{\text{Mass of test compound at midpoint}}$$

Table 2. Recovery and Precision

Found[a]	Added	Deviation, %	CV, %
mg/liter			
4.90 ± 0.23	5.00	− 2.0	4.69
2.00 ± 0.15	2.00	0.0	7.50
1.03 ± 0.13	1.00	+ 3.0	12.6
0.48 ± 0.068	0.50	− 4.0	14.2
0.11 ± 0.017	0.10	+10.0	15.4

[a] Mean of 20 determinations (±SD)

Table 3. Comparison of Results of Present Method with Those of Microbiological Assay, in Two Patients

	Patient 3		Patient 6	
Time, h[a]	Microbiol.	RIA	Microbiol.	RIA
	mg/liter			
0	1.08	0.778	2.44	1.22
0.5	1.07	0.884	2.13	1.16
1.0	2.80	2.49	3.52	1.86
1.5	2.90	2.77	3.90	2.61
2.0	2.24	2.63	3.84	2.31
4.0	1.82	1.35	2.42	1.41
6.0	0.95	0.70	1.56	0.60
12.0	0.82	0.47	1.39	0.59
18.0	0.90	0.64	1.31	0.54

[a] After a 150-mg oral dose

tration of the drug increases. The difference can be attributed to two factors. The microbiological assay is more sensitive to *N*-demethylclindamycin than to clindamycin (*6*). Brodasky et al. (*7*) have shown that when both *N*-demethylclindamycin and clindamycin are measured in serum at 1 and 8 h, the amount of *N*-demethyl averages 2.7% and 21% of the total, respectively. Therefore, *N*-demethyl makes a larger contribution to the microbiological assay as time after administration of drug increases. Except in patients who produce high concentrations of sulfoxide in the serum, this should be a more accurate assay than the microbiological one. In urine, with the high concentrations of sulfoxide, the microbiological assay would be more accurate.

Results for serum, as measured by both methods for two subjects after receiving a 150-mg oral dose of clindamycin·HCl, are shown in Table 3.

Discussion

Clindamycin is indicated in serious infections caused by susceptible aerobic Gram-positive cocci and anaerobic bacteria for which less toxic alternatives are not indicated. The minimum inhibitory concentration range for Gram-positive cocci is ≤1.0 mg/liter (*8*). The minimum inhibitory concentration range for anaerobic bacteria is 1.6–6.2 mg/liter; however, *Clostridia* are more resistant than are most anaerobes (*9*).

Clindamycin and other antibiotics produce colitis in sensitive individuals (*10*). Present data suggest that the concentrations in blood or stool are not related to this effect.

One case of hepatotoxicity has been reported (*11*). This was associated with high (25.6 mg/liter) concentrations in serum. Monitoring of serum concentrations in patients with markedly reduced renal or hepatic function may be indicated during high-dose therapy.

Measurement of clindamycin in serum is helpful in diseases such as osteomyelitis (*12*), when the patient is switched to oral clindamycin after initial intravenous administration. This assay measures only clindamycin and not *N*-demethylclindamycin, which is also microbiologically active. Therefore, to assess serum antimicrobial concentrations realistically, blood must be drawn between 1 and 2 h after an oral dose, when the parent compound represents 90% or more of the pharmacologically active drug (*7*). Methylation to convert all of the microbiologically active drug back to the parent drug may provide information on total pharmacologically active drug concentrations at other times. This suggestion (by a reviewer) is being investigated.

We thank the microbiological section of The Upjohn Clinical Research Laboratories, especially W. L. Lummis and M. A. Burnett, for supplying information about the microbiological assay and the results of that assay.

References

1. Magerlein, B. J., Birkenmeyer, R. D., and Kagan, F., Chemical modification of lincomycin. *Antimicrob. Agents Chemother.* **1966,** 727 (1967).

2. Sinkula, A. A., Morozowich, W., and Rowe, E. L., Chemical modification of clindamycin: Synthesis and evaluation of selected esters. *J. Pharm. Sci.* **62,** 1106 (1973).

3. Morozowich, W., Personal communication.

4. Habeeb, A. F. S. A., Determination of free amino groups in proteins by trinitrobenzene sulfonic acid. *Anal. Biochem.* **14,** 328 (1966).

5. Wagner, J. G., Novak, E., Patel, N. C., et al., Absorption, excretion and half life of clindamycin in normal adult males. *Am. J. Med. Sci.* **256,** 25 (1968).

6. Argondelis, A. D., Coats, J. H., Mason, D. J., and Sebek, O. K., Microbial transformation of antibiotics III: Conversion of clindamycin to 1′-demethylclindamycin and clindamycin sulfoxide by streptomyces species. *J. Antibiot.* **22,** 309 (1969).

7. Brodasky, T. F., Argondelis, A. D., and Eble, T. E., The characterization and thin layer chromatographic quantitation of the human metabolite of clindamycin. *J. Antibiot.* **21,** 327 (1968).

8. "Performance Standards for Antimicrobial Disc Susceptibility Tests," National Committee for Clinical Laboratory Standards, 1975, Villanova, Pa.

9. Staneck, J. L., and Washington, J. A., Antimicrobial susceptibilities of anerobic bacteria: Recent clinical isolates. *Antimicrob. Agents Chemother.* **6,** 311 (1974).

10. Keeffe, E. B., Katon, R. M., Chan, T. T., et al., Pseudomembranous enterocolitis: Resurgence related to newer antibiotic therapy. *West. J. Med.* **121,** 462 (1974).

11. Elmore, M., Rissing, J. P., Rink, L., and Brooks, G. F., Clindamycin-associated hepatotoxicity. *Am. J. Med.* **57,** 627 (1974).

12. Feigin, R. D., Pickering, L. K., Anderson, D., et al., Clindamycin treatment of osteomyelitis and septic arthritis in children. *Pediatrics* **55,** 213 (1975).

CLIN. CHEM. 22/6, 832–836 (1976)

Tabulation of Therapeutic, Toxic, and Lethal Concentrations of Drugs and Chemicals in Blood

Charles L. Winek

These data represent information from the literature and personal experience.

References to the data may be found in previous articles (*1–7*). Other authors have also presented such data (*8–11*).

Special attention must be paid to the utilization of these data. Interpretation of test results based on the data presented must be with the usual consideration of factors affecting the pharmacological response of a drug as well as other factors. Table 1 lists general factors that must be considered in interpreting the data. The factors listed cover most aspects for which blood-concentration data may be used: therapeutic monitoring, generic equivalency, efficacy of treatment in poisonings, cause of death, etc.

The intended effect and corresponding dose of a drug will certainly affect the therapeutic blood concentration. For example, a person receiving 25 mg of chlorpromazine rectally will have a lower blood drug concentration than a person receiving 300 mg of chlorpromazine orally, the former dose being used as an antinauseant and the latter as an antipsychotic. The therapeutic concentration is, of course, the most important value, as this serves as a guide to what might be expected vis-à-vis toxic or lethal situations.

Data of this sort are useful for several medical and legal purposes. One of these is monitoring drugs used in the treatment of chronic disorders. Several classes of drugs used for chronic disorders include the digitalis group, the anticonvulsant group, the antipsychotic group, and the antibiotic group. Drug-concentration data for antibiotics are not included in the table.[1]

Because the method of analysis can affect the information on concentrations in blood, information in Table 2 will change as data are generated from newer and better analytical methods.

Many industrial chemicals have not yet been monitored in humans and therefore data on expected concentrations consistent with "safe" occupational exposure are lacking. Several values are contained in Table 2 that indicate exposure to a toxic substance. Monitoring substances such as lead, mercury, cadmium, etc. is routine in some industries. Legislation affecting toxic substances in the industrial environment will require monitoring of other chemicals and this will result in establishing "safe" blood concentrations for many materials.

The general concept of assessing concentrations of chemicals in blood is relatively new, and I have prepared this Table to provide a concise, single source of data to be used as a guide. I reemphasize that the values should

Table 1. Factors Affecting Concentrations in Blood

Drug and Chemical Factors
- Dosage form
- Use and dose
- Route of administration
- Concentration of toxicant
- Duration of exposure

Human Factors
- Age
- Weight
- Time of sampling
- Method of analysis and presence of metabolites
- Treatment given, if any
- Time interval between sampling and analysis
- Storage of specimen

Pathological Factors
- Disease state (esp. renal and hepatic)
- Body water (normal or dehydration)
- Menstruation
- Anatomical abnormalities (congenital or surgically and (or) traumatically caused)
- Genetic disorders (pharmacogenetics)

Pharmacological/Biochemical Factors
- Gastrointestional absorption
- Tissue binding at active and inactive sites
- Rate of elimination (excretion)
- Storage (bone, hair, nails, fat)
- Induction or inhibition of microsomal enzymes
- Synergistic or antagonistic action of other drugs
- Tolerance (from prolonged use or use of drugs with cross tolerance)
- Rate of detoxication (metabolism or biotransformation)
- Additive drug effects

Toxicology Departments, Allegheny County Coroner's Office and Duquesne University, Pittsburgh, Pa. 15219.

[1] But a list of peak antibiotic concentrations in serum can be found in Appendix II to a chapter by A. L. Barry and L. D. Sabath, p 431, 2nd ed. of *Manual of Clinical Microbiology* (Amer. Soc. of Microbiology, Washington, D.C., 1974), E. H. Lennette et al., Eds.

Received and accepted Mar. 5, 1976.

Table 2. Drug and Chemical Blood Concentrations[a]

Compound	Therapeutic or "normal" concn	Toxic concn	Lethal concn
Acetaminophen (Tylenol)	10–20 mg/liter	400 mg/liter	1500 mg/liter
Acetazolamide (Diamox)	10–15 mg/liter		—
Acetohexamide (Dymelor)	21–56 mg/liter		—
Acetone		200–300 mg/liter	550 mg/liter
Aluminum	0.13 mg/liter	—	—
Ammonia	500–1700 mg/liter		—
Aminophylline (Theophylline)	20–100 mg/liter		—
Amitriptyline (Elavil)	50–200 μg/liter	400 μg/liter	10–20 mg/liter
Amphetamine	20–30 μg/liter	—	2 mg/liter
Arsenic	0.0–20 μg/liter	1.0 mg/liter	15 mg/liter
Barbiturates			
Short-acting	1 mg/liter	7 mg/liter	10 mg/liter
Intermediate-acting	1–5 mg/liter	10–30 mg/liter	30 mg/liter
Phenobarbital	~10 mg/liter	40–60 mg/liter	80–150 mg/liter
Barbital	~ 10 mg/liter	60–80 mg/liter	100 mg/liter
Benzene	—	any measurable	0.94 mg/liter
Beryllium	Tissue levels generally used (lung & lymph)	—	—
Boron (boric acid)	0.8 mg/liter	40 mg/liter	50 mg/liter
Bromide	50 mg/liter	0.5–1.5 g/liter	2 g/liter
Brompheniramine (Dimetane)	8–15 μg/liter		
Cadmium	0.1–0.2 μg/liter	50 μg/liter	—
Caffeine	—	—	>100 mg/liter
Carbamazepine (Tegretol)	2 mg/liter	8–10 mg/liter	—
Carbon monoxide	1% saturation of Hb	15–35% saturation of Hb	50% saturation of Hb
Carbon tetrachloride	—	20–50 mg/liter	—
Carisoprodol (Rela, Soma)	10–40 mg/liter	—	—
Chloral hydrate (Noctec)	10 mg/liter	100 mg/liter	250 mg/liter
Chloroform	—	70–250 mg/liter	390 mg/liter
Chlordiazepoxide (Librium)	1.0–3.0 mg/liter	5.5 mg/liter	20 mg/liter
Chlorpheniramine	—	20–30 mg/liter	—
Chlorpromazine (Thorazine)	0.5 mg/liter	1–2 mg/liter	3–12 mg/liter
Chlorpropamide (Diabinese)	30–140 mg/liter	—	—
Chlorprothixine (Taractan)	0.04–0.3 mg/liter	—	—
Codeine	25 μg/liter	—	—
Copper	1–1.5 mg/liter	5.4 mg/liter	—
Cyanide	0.15 mg/liter	—	>5 mg/liter

(continued)

Table 2. Continued

Compound	Therapeutic or "normal" concn	Toxic concn	Lethal concn
DDT	13 μg/liter	—	—
Desipramine (Norpramin)	0.59–1.4 mg/liter	—	10–20 mg/liter
Dextropropoxyphene (Darvon)	50–200 μg/liter	5–10 mg/liter	57 mg/liter[b]
Diazepam (Valium)	0.5–2.5 mg/liter	5–20 mg/liter	>50 mg/liter
Dieldren	1.5 μg/liter	—	—
Digitoxin	1.7–2.1 μg/liter	—	320 μg/liter
Digoxin	0.6–1.3 μg/liter	2–9 μg/liter	—
Dinitro-*o*-cresol	—	30–40 μg/liter	75 mg/liter
Diphenhydramine (Benadryl)	5 mg/liter	10 mg/liter	—
Ethinamate (Valmid)	5–10 mg/liter	—	—
Diphenylhydantoin (Dilantin)	5–22 mg/liter	50 mg/liter	100 mg/liter
Divinyl oxide	—	—	700 mg/liter
Doxepin (Sinequan)	—	—	>10 mg/liter
Ethanol	—	1.5 g/liter	>3.5 g/liter
Ethchlorvynol (Placidyl)	5 mg/liter	20 mg/liter	150 mg/liter
Ethosuximide (Zarontin)	25–75 mg/liter	—	—
Ethyl chloride	—	—	400 mg/liter
Ethyl ether	0.9–1.0 g/liter	—	1.4–1.89 g/liter
Ethylene glycol	—	1.5 g/liter	2–4 g/liter
Fluoride	0.5 mg/liter	—	2 mg/liter
Gold (sodium aurothiomalate)	3–6 mg/liter	—	—
Glutethimide (Doriden)	0.2 mg/liter	10–80 mg/liter	30–100 mg/liter
Halothane (Fluothane)	—	—	200 mg/liter
Hydrogen sulfide	—	—	0.92 mg/liter
Hydromorphone (Dilaudid)	—	—	0.1–0.3 mg/liter
Imipramine (Tofranil)	0.05–0.16 mg/liter	0.7 mg/liter	2 mg/liter
Isopropanol	—	3.4 g/liter	—
Iron	500 mg/liter (erythrocytes)	6 mg/liter (serum)	—
Lead	0.05–1.3 mg/liter	0.7 mg/liter	—
LSD (lysergic acid diethylamide)	—	1–4 μg/liter	—
Lidocaine	2 mg/liter	6 mg/liter	—
Lithium	4.2–8.3 mg/liter	13.9 mg/liter	13.9–34.7 mg/liter
Magnesium	0.8–1.3 mmol/liter	—	0.5 mmol/liter
Manganese	0.15 mg/liter	4.6 mg/liter	—
Mercury	60–120 μg/liter	—	—
Meperidine (Demerol)	600–650 μg/liter	5 mg/liter	30 mg/liter

Table 2. Continued

Compound	Therapeutic or "normal" concn	Toxic concn	Lethal concn
Meprobamate	10 mg/liter	100 mg/liter	200 mg/liter
Methadone	480–860 μg/liter	2 mg/liter	>4 mg/liter
Methamphetamine	—	5 mg/liter	40 mg/liter
Methanol	—	200 mg/liter	>890 mg/liter
Methapyrilene	2 μg/liter	30–50 mg/liter	>50 mg/liter
Methaqualone (Quaalude)	5 mg/liter	10–30 mg/liter	>30 mg/liter
Methsuximide (Celontin)	2.5–7.5 mg/liter	—	—
Methylene chloride	—	—	>280 mg/liter
Methylenedioxyamphetamine (MDA)	—	—	4–10 mg/liter
Methyprylon (Noludar)	10 mg/liter	30–60 mg/liter	100 mg/liter
Morphine	0.1 mg/liter	—	0.05–4 mg/liter
Nickel	0.41 mg/liter	—	—
Nicotine	—	10 mg/liter	5–52 mg/liter
Nitrofurantoin (Furadantin)	1.8 mg/liter	—	—
Nortriptyline (Aventyl)	1.2–1.6 μg/liter	5 mg/liter	13 mg/liter
Orphenadrine	—	2 mg/liter	4–8 mg/liter
Oxalate	2 mg/liter	—	10 mg/liter
Papaverine	1 mg/liter	—	—
Paramethoxyamphetamine (PMA)	—	—	2–4 mg/liter
Paraldehyde	50 mg/liter	200–400 mg/liter	500 mg/liter
Pentazocine (Talwin)	0.14–0.16 mg/liter	2–5 mg/liter	10–20 mg/liter
Perphenazine (Trilafon)	—	1 mg/liter	—
Phencyclidine	—	<.5 mg/liter	1.0 mg/liter
Phenmetrazine	—	—	4 mg/liter
Phensuximide (Milontin)	10–19 mg/liter	—	—
Phenylbutazone (Butazolidin)	100 mg/liter	—	—
Phosphorus	concn in tissues usually used		
Primidone (Mysoline)	10 mg/liter	50–80 mg/liter	100 mg/liter
Probenecid (Benemid)	100–200 mg/liter	—	—
Procaine amide	6 mg/liter	10 mg/liter	—
Prochlorperazine (Compazine)	—	1 mg/liter	—
Promazine (Sparine)	—	1 mg/liter	—
Propoxyphene	50–200 μg/liter	5–20 mg/liter	57 mg/liter[b]
Propranolol (Inderal)	0.025–0.2 mg/liter		8–12 mg/liter

(continued)

Table 2. Continued

Compound	Therapeutic or "normal" concn	Toxic concn	Lethal concn
Propylhexedrine (Benzedrex)	—	—	2–3 mg/liter
Quinidine	3–6 mg/liter	10 mg/liter	30–50 mg/liter
Quinine	—	—	12 mg/liter
Salicylate (acetylsalicylic acid)	20–100 mg/liter	150–300 mg/liter	500 mg/liter
Sulfadiazine	80–150 mg/liter	—	—
Sulfadimethoxine (Madribon)	80–100 mg/liter	—	—
Sulfaguanidine	30–50 mg/liter	—	—
Sulfanilamide	100–150 mg/liter	—	—
Sulfisoxazole (Gantrisin)	90–100 mg/liter	—	—
Strychnine	—	2 mg/liter	9–12 mg/liter
Theophylline	20–100 mg/liter	—	—
Thioridazine (Mellaril)	1–1.5 mg/liter	10 mg/liter	20–80 mg/liter
Tin	0.12 mg/liter	—	—
Tolbutamide (Orinase)	53–96 mg/liter	—	—
Toluene	—	—	10 mg/liter
Tribromoethanol	—	—	90 mg/liter
Trichloroethane	—	—	0.01–1 g/liter
Trimethobenzamide (Tigan)	1.0–2.0 mg/liter	—	—
Warfarin	1.0–10 mg/liter	—	—
Zinc	0.68–1.36 mg/liter	—	—
Zoxazolamine (Flexin)	3–13 mg/liter	—	—

[a] Some common brand names that may be more familiar than the generic name, alternative forms (e.g., aminophylline/theophylline), and the like are given parenthetically.

[b] McBay reports much lower values.

not be considered absolute in light of the factors that can affect blood concentrations. The values represented are for adult man generally and via the oral route of administration, with obvious exceptions (e.g., chemicals that are inhaled).

It is my intent to periodically update the data as new information becomes available. Information, comments, and criticisms are welcome.

References

1. Winek, C. L., Drug and chemical blood levels. In *Wecht's Legal Medicine Annual.* Appleton, New York, N.Y., 1970, chap. 5.
2. Winek, C. L., Laboratory criteria for the adequacy of treatment and significance of blood levels. *Clin. Toxicol.* **3,** 541 (1970).
3. Winek, C. L., A role for the hospital pharmacist in toxicology and drug blood level information. *Am. J. Hosp. Pharm.* **28,** 351 (1971).
4. Winek, C. L., *Narcotics and Narcotic Addiction,* 4th ed. D. W. Maurer and V. H. Vogel, Eds., C. C Thomas, Springfield, Ill., 1973.
5. Winek, C. L., Drug and chemical blood levels—Update, In *Wecht's Legal Medicine Annual.* Appleton, New York, N.Y., 1973, chap. 5.
6. Winek, C. L., Forensic toxicology. In *Methods in Radioimmunoassay, Toxicology, and Related Areas.* I. L. Simmons and G. W. Ewing, Eds. Plenum, New York, N.Y., 1975.
7. Winek, C. L., Drug and chemical blood levels. In *Toxicology Annual 1974,* C. L. Winek, Ed., Marcel Dekker, New York, N.Y., 1975.
8. Niyogi, S. K., Drug levels in cases of poisoning. *Forensic Sci.* **2,** 67 (1973).
9. McBay, A. J., Toxicological findings in fatal poisonings. *Clin. Chem.* **19,** 361 (1973).
10. McBay, A. J., Chemical findings in poisonings. *New Engl. J. Med.* **274,** 1257 (1966).
11. Curry, A. S., *Poison Detection in Human Organs,* 3rd ed. Charles C Thomas, Springfield, Ill., 1975.

CLIN. CHEM. 22/6, 837–842 (1976)

Assessment of Interference by Aspirin with Some Assays Commonly Done in the Clinical Laboratory

Joseph I. Routh and William D. Paul

We have assessed the interference of acetylsalicylic acid (aspirin) with some common clinical laboratory assays, because of its widespread use and reported interference. The therapeutic regimens involved ingestion of 10 325-mg tablets daily for three days or eight tablets for five days or two weeks. Twenty-one commonly done determinations were run on control sera, and sera were collected during and after drug therapy. Significant changes in *t*-test values, indicating the significance of the standard deviation of the difference between controls and specimens drawn after drug therapy, were observed for chloride (increased), and for total protein, calcium, cholesterol, uric acid, bilirubin, and thyroxine (decreased). Aspirin therapy depressed the apparent concentrations of these constituents progressively in the three-day regimen and initially in the long-term regimens, followed by recovery toward zero *t*-values at the end of the longer regimens.

Additional Keyphrases: *variation, source of • salicylate in blood after aspirin ingestion • analytical error*

There have been many reports in the literature of drug interference with laboratory assays. In 1962, Caraway (*1*) stimulated interest in drug interference with a comprehensive discussion of problems in the laboratory. Several authors have compiled such data into tables of drugs that interfere with individual determinations in whole blood, serum, spinal fluid, and urine. This series was initiated by Wirth and Thompson in 1965 (*2*), followed by Elking and Kabat in 1968 (*3*) and by Constantino and Kabat in 1973 (*4*), but the most ambitious undertaking to date is the computer-assisted listing of drug interference in 1972 (*5*) updated and much expanded in 1975 (*6*) by Young et al. The common theme in these tabulations has been the expression of the effect of the drug as an increase or decrease in the value obtained for the constituent being analyzed. The compilations by Young et al. also attempt to differentiate between an in vivo physiological effect and a direct chemical methodological interference.

Departments of Biochemistry and Orthopedic Surgery, The University of Iowa, Iowa City, Iowa 52242.
Received Feb. 9, 1976; accepted Mar. 8, 1976.

There have been few attempts to quantitate the effect of a drug on clinical chemistry determinations. There are obviously many problems involved in such a study, but we have started to explore this field. The drug chosen for study was acetylsalicylic acid (aspirin) for three major reasons: (*a*) aspirin ingestion reportedly affects a number of laboratory determinations; (*b*) our laboratory has more than 30 years of research experience with the chemistry, methodology, and metabolism of the drug; and (*c*) people often ingest aspirin without being aware that it is a drug, and so may neglect to mention it when asked about drugs taken. It is difficult to estimate the number of apparently normal patients whose blood specimens contain salicylates when drawn for laboratory profiles. The large number of over-the-counter medications that contain aspirin and are used for self-medication compounds this problem. Two major factors must be taken into account in exploratory studies: the therapeutic regimen and the salicylate concentrations in the blood.

In the present study we used apparently normal subjects (laboratory and hospital personnel), who followed four different regimens of aspirin ingestion. Serum was sampled at the beginning and during each regimen and analyzed for total salicylates and for 13 to 20 biochemical constituents.

Methods

Serum samples were analyzed for total protein, albumin, calcium, phosphate, cholesterol, glucose, urea nitrogen, uric acid, alkaline phosphatase (EC 3.1.3.1), lactate dehydrogenase (EC 1.1.1.27), aspartate aminotransferase (EC 2.6.1.1; AST), total bilirubin, Na, K, Cl, CO_2, and creatinine on the SMA 12/60 and SMA 6/60 continuous-flow analyzers (Technicon). Amylase was determined by the Amylochrome method of Klein et al. (*7*), triiodothyronine (T-3) uptake by the method of Sterling and Tabachnick (*8*) (Abbott), thyroxine (T-4) by the method of Murphy and Jachan (*9*) (Dade), and total salicylates by a modification of the Brodie method developed in our laboratory (*10*). To improve repro-

Table 1. Significance of the Effect of Aspirin Ingestion on Common Laboratory Determinations as Indicated by *t*-Test Values[a]

		First day		Second day		Third day	
Determination	**Control Mean ± SD**	**Mean ± SD**	t^b	**Mean ± SD**	t^b	**Mean ± SD**	t^b
Salicylates	2.8 ± 1.06	131.0 ± 24.2	—	165.4 ± 12.4	—	177.2 ± 14.0	—
Total protein	7.6 ± 0.36	7.5 ± 0.40	−1.19	7.5 ± 0.35	*−2.30*	7.4 ± 0.39	*−4.06*
Albumin	4.9 ± 0.28	4.7 ± 0.25	*−4.61*	4.5 ± 0.23	*−7.81*	4.4 ± 0.19	*−10.12*
Calcium	10.1 ± 0.47	10.0 ± 0.40	−1.14	10.0 ± 0.95	−2.00	9.9 ± 0.28	*−2.63*
Inorg. phos.	3.8 ± 0.41	3.8 ± 0.44	0.14	3.7 ± 0.56	−0.33	3.8 ± 0.49	0.07
Cholesterol	185 ± 34.7	180 ± 35.8	*−2.28*	179 ± 33.2	*−2.79*	177 ± 30.3	*−3.19*
Glucose	91 ± 13.9	84 ± 12.0	*−4.59*	82 ± 12.5	*−5.24*	84 ± 10.4	*−3.82*
Urea N	15 ± 3.9	16 ± 4.3	1.90	16 ± 3.2	1.77	16 ± 3.5	1.03
Uric acid	5.0 ± 1.3	4.3 ± 1.7	*−3.83*	3.4 ± 1.8	*−6.09*	2.9 ± 1.6	*−9.12*
Alk. phos.	52 ± 17.8	53 ± 16.0	0.49	52 ± 14.6	−0.15	52 ± 14.7	−0.53
LDH	123 ± 20.9	125 ± 23.1	0.49	128 ± 16.7	1.14	135 ± 19.9	*2.94*
Tot. bilirubin	0.5 ± 0.14	0.4 ± 0.11	*−5.41*	0.3 ± 0.11	*−5.85*	0.3 ± 0.08	*−6.07*
AST	24 ± 7.9	24 ± 13.3	0.26	22 ± 5.8	−1.33	21 ± 4.8	−1.61
Sodium	144 ± 1.8	144 ± 2.2	0.94	144 ± 2.5	1.65	145 ± 2.0	*2.49*
Potassium	4.3 ± 0.28	4.4 ± 0.32	1.53	4.4 ± 0.29	0.43	4.4 ± 0.30	0.68
Chloride	105 ± 3.1	106 ± 2.9	0.91	107 ± 3.3	*2.64*	107 ± 3.3	*2.83*
CO_2	26 ± 3.0	26 ± 3.1	−0.32	26 ± 2.8	−0.30	26 ± 3.7	−0.90
Creatinine	1.0 ± 0.20	1.0 ± 0.19	−0.56	0.9 ± 0.19	−0.65	1.0 ± 0.16	0.41
Amylase	93 ± 18.5	93 ± 17.7	0.26	88 ± 13.3	−1.79	89 ± 15.3	−1.09
T-3	26 ± 3.6	27 ± 3.6	1.44	27 ± 3.5	*2.21*	27 ± 3.8	1.95
T-4	8.5 ± 1.52	7.6 ± 1.87	*−3.58*	7.5 ± 1.66	*−4.39*	7.0 ± 1.53	*−8.98*

[a] All values are expressed in mg/dl except salicylate is in µg/ml, T-4 in µg/100 ml, T-3 in % uptake, amylase in Somogyi units/100 ml, and alk. phos., LDH, and AST in U/liter.

[b] $t = 2.08$ at 95% level.

Table 2. Significance of the Effect of Aspirin Ingestion on Common Laboratory Determinations as Indicated by *t*-Test Values[a]

Determination	**Control 1, Mean ± SD**	**5 days, Mean ± SD**	t^b	**Control 2, Mean ± SD**	**5 Days, Mean ± SD**	t^b	t^b **(Controls)**
Salicylates	0.3 ± 0.44	95.3 ± 44.9	—	4.9 ± 2.4	59.5 ± 44.1	—	—
Total protein	7.4 ± 0.39	7.2 ± 0.30	*−2.85*	7.4 ± 0.36	7.2 ± 0.30	*−2.39*	−0.30
Albumin	4.6 ± 0.29	4.5 ± 0.18	−1.46	4.6 ± 0.32	4.5 ± 0.26	−1.62	0.88
Calcium	9.9 ± 0.27	9.9 ± 0.30	0.30	9.9 ± 0.38	9.7 ± 0.35	*−2.76*	0.01
Inorg. phos.	3.5 ± 0.35	3.5 ± 0.43	−0.39	3.4 ± 0.35	3.2 ± 0.43	−1.42	−0.80
Cholesterol	199 ± 32.8	186 ± 29.6	*−3.25*	191 ± 33.6	190 ± 34.6	−0.15	*−2.38*
Glucose	83 ± 14.4	82 ± 15.6	−0.14	73 ± 7.6	86 ± 13.8	*4.21*	−2.07
Urea N	15 ± 4.1	16 ± 4.1	1.21	15 ± 4.4	16 ± 4.6	0.95	−0.30
Uric acid	5.2 ± 0.98	4.0 ± 2.4	*−4.33*	5.2 ± 0.94	4.4 ± 1.8	*−2.83*	0.06
Alk. phos.	55 ± 17.3	55 ± 16.6	−0.05	55 ± 18.2	52 ± 15.5	−1.60	−0.46
LDH	163 ± 30.8	161 ± 23.6	−0.58	167 ± 29.9	164 ± 26.0	−0.70	0.59
Tot. bilirubin	0.5 ± 0.16	0.4 ± 0.13	*−2.77*	0.4 ± 0.15	0.4 ± 0.15	0.05	*−3.32*
AST	27 ± 5.8	18 ± 8.5	*−5.98*	23 ± 7.0	23 ± 6.8	0.18	*−4.18*
Na	144 ± 2.7	142 ± 1.7	*−4.27*	144 ± 1.9	144 ± 2.0	−0.69	0.84
K	4.4 ± 0.31	4.8 ± 0.30	*4.99*	4.5 ± 0.29	4.4 ± 0.34	−0.13	0.01
Cl	105 ± 3.0	104 ± 1.8	−1.03	104 ± 2.4	106 ± 2.6	*3.96*	−1.67
CO_2	22 ± 1.5	24 ± 2.9	*2.97*	25 ± 2.3	23 ± 2.5	*−4.49*	*5.48*
Creatinine	1.0 ± 0.17	1.0 ± 0.17	*3.24*	1.0 ± 0.17	1.0 ± 0.15	−0.21	1.28
Amylase	160 ± 32.8	140 ± 22.9	*−4.60*	123 ± 22.1	125 ± 26.0	0.51	*−7.57*
T-4	9.3 ± 1.51	7.9 ± 1.81	*−5.08*	8.1 ± 1.57	7.8 ± 1.48	−1.14	*−3.25*

[a] All values are expressed in md/dl except salicylate is in µg/ml, T-4 in µg/dl, amylase in Somogyi units/100 ml, and alk. phos., LDH, and AST in U/liter.

[b] $t = 2.09$ at the 95% level.

Table 3. Significance of the Effect of Aspirin Ingestion on Common Laboratory Determinations as Indicated by *t*-Test Values[a]

Determination	Control, Mean ± SD	First week Mean ± SD	First week t^b	Second week Mean ± SD	Second week t^b	Control, Mean ± SD	Third week Mean ± SD	Third week t^b	Fourth week Mean ± SD	Fourth week t^b
Salicylates	0.6 ± 1.0	62.1 ± 40.9	—	55.5 ± 30.0	—	2.5 ± 1.0	53.5 ± 15.4	—	39.8 ± 16.9	—
Total protein	7.6 ± 0.42	7.4 ± 0.35	*−6.09*	7.5 ± 0.35	*−3.04*	7.6 ± 0.35	7.3 ± 0.44	*−3.29*	7.5 ± 0.36	−1.52
Albumin	4.6 ± 0.32	4.6 ± 0.27	−1.17	4.7 ± 0.27	0.35	4.7 ± 0.34	4.6 ± 0.35	*−2.84*	4.7 ± 0.28	−0.64
Calcium	10.1 ± 0.66	9.8 ± 0.53	*−5.05*	9.9 ± 0.81	*−2.36*	10.1 ± 0.56	9.4 ± 0.39	*−5.55*	9.8 ± 0.51	*−2.75*
Inorg. phos.	3.5 ± 0.51	3.5 ± 0.58	0.05	3.2 ± 0.53	−2.13	3.9 ± 0.61	3.7 ± 0.41	*−2.65*	3.7 ± 0.36	−1.82
Cholesterol	230 ± 39.1	216 ± 39.6	*−4.05*	216 ± 38.8	−1.91	217 ± 36.6	215 ± 34.4	−0.36	214 ± 31.6	−0.67
Glucose	81 ± 10.3	79 ± 6.4	−0.39	72 ± 8.4	*−4.47*	79 ± 9.4	78 ± 5.1	−0.39	86 ± 8.6	*5.75*
Urea N	16 ± 3.7	17 ± 5.1	1.68	16 ± 3.2	0.73	17 ± 5.0	16 ± 5.7	−0.47	17 ± 4.1	0.38
Uric acid	4.9 ± 1.01	3.9 ± 1.63	*−3.97*	4.0 ± 1.67	*−2.61*	5.3 ± 1.08	4.3 ± 1.92	*−3.13*	4.5 ± 1.75	*−2.98*
Alk. phos.	50 ± 12.4	47 ± 11.1	*−3.38*	45 ± 7.9	*−2.34*	44 ± 7.9	42 ± 8.9	−1.86	42 ± 8.1	−1.92
LDH	130 ± 10.8	130 ± 16.3	0.17	128 ± 7.2	−0.66	127 ± 13.4	122 ± 14.3	−1.25	127 ± 10.5	0.04
Tot. bilirubin	0.5 ± 0.17	0.5 ± 0.15	−1.73	0.5 ± 0.13	−1.78	0.5 ± 0.09	0.4 ± 0.10	*−3.98*	0.4 ± 0.08	*−2.71*
AST	26 ± 7.8	24 ± 7.8	−1.24	24 ± 9.3	−0.84	27 ± 8.8	25 ± 7.8	−0.99	26 ± 6.7	−0.86
Na	146 ± 2.3	146 ± 2.1	0.86	147 ± 3.0	1.83	147 ± 1.7	144 ± 2.9	*−2.92*	146 ± 2.1	−0.64
K	4.4 ± 0.26	4.4 ± 0.19	0.20	4.4 ± 0.32	−0.19	4.8 ± 0.56	4.2 ± 0.22	*−11.10*	4.5 ± 0.26	*−3.71*
Cl	105 ± 3.4	107 ± 3.8	*2.71*	107 ± 2.9	*3.94*	107 ± 2.0	106 ± 2.0	−2.00	107 ± 2.1	−0.66
CO_2	25 ± 2.5	24 ± 3.1	−1.62	24 ± 2.8	−1.64	25 ± 2.5	25 ± 2.4	−0.49	26 ± 3.2	2.06
Creatinine	0.9 ± 0.18	0.9 ± 0.22	2.17	1.0 ± 0.19	*2.91*	1.0 ± 0.15	1.0 ± 0.16	1.03	1.0 ± 0.16	0.17
Amylase	145 ± 30.6	151 ± 33.0	0.13	150 ± 29.6	1.00	163 ± 31.9	172 ± 22.0	1.31	167 ± 36.1	0.60
T-3	25 ± 4.3	25 ± 4.5	−0.30	24 ± 3.2	−0.39	26 ± 3.2	27 ± 2.0	0.62	25 ± 3.3	−1.10
T-4	8.5 ± 1.62	7.4 ± 1.67	*−2.67*	7.6 ± 1.58	−2.07	7.5 ± 2.08	6.4 ± 2.06	*−2.31*	7.0 ± 1.44	−0.62

[a] All values are expressed in mg/dl except salicylate in μg/ml, T-4 in μg/100 ml, T-3 in % uptake, amylase in Somogyi units/100 ml, and alk. phos., LDH, and AST in U/liter.

[b] t = 2.31 at the 95% level (third and fourth weeks).

ducibility of the results all serum specimens from the control period or experimental period in each regimen were frozen and analyzed in a single run on the SMA 12/60 and SMA 6/60 and in the amylase, triiodothyronine uptake and thyroxine determinations. It had previously been determined that frozen samples gave essentially the same values as did fresh serum.

Regimens and Results

Because research reports (*11, 12*) suggest that the ingestion of one or two 325-mg (5-grain) aspirin tablets may affect clotting factors and platelet aggregation, the first therapeutic regimen involved the administration of only 650 mg of aspirin to 20 fasting subjects, to test for biochemical changes. A blood sample was drawn, the subject ingested two 325-mg aspirin tablets with 200 ml of water, and another blood sample was drawn 60 min later. Because we recognized that in these studies inter- and intra-individual variations in values for the constituents would occur (*13*), each subject served as his own control. The statistical operation that seemed most pertinent for a comparison of control values and those obtained after drug therapy was the paired *t*-test, which gives an indication of the significance of the standard deviation of the difference (d) between the control specimens and those drawn after drug therapy regimens. The formulas used for the calculation of the *t*-values are as follows:

$$t = \frac{\bar{d}}{S_d}\sqrt{n} \text{ where } S_d = \sqrt{\frac{\Sigma d^2 - \frac{(\Sigma d)^2}{n}}{n-1}} \text{ and } \bar{d} = \frac{\Sigma d}{n}$$

When we calculated the mean values ±SD for total salicylates and 13 serum constituents,[1,2] three significant differences were observed, but we concluded that ingestion of two aspirin tablets causes no marked changes in values obtained for these chemical constituents of serum.

The second regimen was a short-term, intensive dosage to simulate that practiced by many people as therapy for influenza or coryza: two 325-mg aspirin tablets were ingested every 4 h (0800, 1200, 1600, 2000, and 2400 hours) for three days by 22 subjects. A control specimen and specimens at 0800 hours on the following three days (before aspirin ingestion) were drawn before the first meal of the day. Table 1 summarizes the results for total salicylate and 20 chemical constituents. Of the 60 *t*-test values, 26 were significant, with 23 showing a decrease and three an increase. During all three days of aspirin ingestion there were significant decreases in apparent values for albumin, cholesterol, glucose, uric acid, bilirubin, and thyroxine.

To assess the effect of the chemical presence of the drug in vitro and on the various reagents in the individual determinations, we added sodium salicylate, in an amount equal to the concentration of total salicylate on the third day, directly to the control sera of 15 of the 22 subjects. The only values significantly affected by direct addition of salicylate to the serum control were those for albumin, a result of interference by salicylate with the binding of "HABA" dye by the albumin.[2] (A method using bromcresol green was used throughout the remaining studies.)

The third regimen involved 20 subjects, who ingested eight 325-mg aspirin tablets daily (two at 0800, 1200, 1600, and 2000 hours) for five days, followed by eight days during which no aspirin was ingested and then another five-day period similar to the first. Blood samples were drawn for each control period and at the end of each five-day period. Table 2 shows the results of the analysis for total salicylate and 19 other constituents. Of the 38 *t*-test values, 17 were significant, with 12 showing a decrease and five an increase. Total protein and uric acid exhibited significant decreases during both five-day periods, while values for cholesterol, bilirubin, aspartate aminotransferase, Na, amylase, and thyroxine decreased significantly in the first but not in the last five-day period.

A smaller group (13 subjects) was used to study effects of long-term aspirin therapy similar to that followed by patients with arthritis. They ingested two 325-mg aspirin tablets four times a day (at 0800, 1200, 1600, and 2000 hours) for two weeks, ingested no aspirin for one week, and then repeated the two-week regimen. Blood was sampled at the beginning of each period and at the end of the first, second, third, and fourth weeks on aspirin therapy. Table 3 shows our results. Of the 80 *t*-test values 28 were significant, 24 showing a decrease and four an increase. Values for calcium and uric acid decreased during all four weeks, total protein during the

Table 4. Mean Serum Salicylate Values (±SD) in Different Regimens

Regimen	Control	End of period
	mg/liter	
60-min	1.1 ± 0.84	55.6 ± 9.79
Three-day		
First day	2.8 ± 1.06	131.0 ± 24.2
Second day	2.8 ± 1.06	165.4 ± 12.4
Third day	2.8 ± 1.06	177.2 ± 14.0
Five-day		
First 5 days	0.3 ± 0.44	95.3 ± 44.9
Second 5 days	4.9 ± 2.4	59.5 ± 44.1
Two-week		
First week	0.6 ± 1.0	62.1 ± 40.9
Second week	0.6 ± 1.0	55.5 ± 30.0
Third week	2.5 ± 1.0	53.5 ± 15.4
Fourth week	2.5 ± 1.0	39.8 ± 16.9

[1] Calcium increased, urea nitrogen and aspartate aminotransferase decreased; *t* values 2.24, −2.33, and −2.27, respectively ($t = 2.09$ at 95% level).

[2] Detailed data will be made available to interested individuals who direct their request to one of the authors (J.I.R.) or to the Editorial Office.

first three, alkaline phosphatase in the first two weeks, bilirubin and potassium during the third and fourth weeks, thyroxine during the first and third, and cholesterol in the first week. Chloride showed a significant increase over the control period in the first and second weeks.

The salicylate concentrations in the serum specimens for each subject in the four regimens were measured, and the data are available.[2] Mean serum salicylate values for the different regimens are summarized in Table 4. Because specimens for analysis were drawn before 0800 hours on each control or sample day or week, the salicylate values are low, and in the case of the last three regimens represent concentrations in serum about 8 to 12 h after aspirin ingestion.

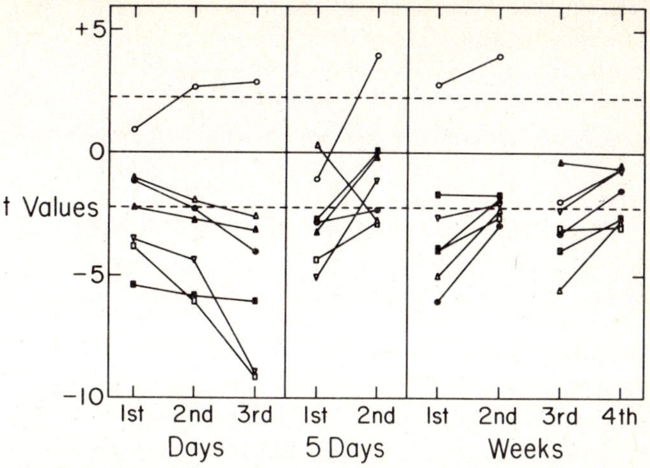

Fig. 1. Changes in *t*-values of constituents most affected by aspirin therapy. All *t*-values above or below the dotted lines are significant at the 95% level
○—○, chloride; ●—●, total protein; △—△, calcium; ▲—▲, cholesterol; □—□, uric acid; ■—■, bilirubin; and ▽—▽, T-4

Discussion

To facilitate comparison of the last three therapeutic regimens, Table 5 lists the *t*-values for the 3-day, 5-day, and 2-week periods. The changes in the six constituents, which demonstrate five or more significant differences in a negative direction (total protein, calcium, cholesterol, uric acid, bilirubin, and thyroxine) and in chloride, which shows five differences in a positive direction, are expressed graphically in Figure 1.

The three-day short-term intensive regimen was characterized by a progressive decrease in the *t*-values for the six constituents listed above. This was in contrast to the five-day or two-week aspirin therapy regimens, in which the major changes were a decline in the *t*-values at the end of the first five days or first week of the periods, followed by a recovery or increase in them. Except for chloride values, only two other *t*-values of those depicted in Figure 1 were above zero: a calcium of 0.30 and a bilirubin of 0.05.

The results reported in Table 5 indicate that the presence of the salicylate ion in the serum, as would occur after aspirin ingestion, does not interfere with the reagents used in any of the 20 methods used in this study except for the HABA dye method for albumin.

Table 5. Compilation of *t*-Values Obtained in Three Different Regimens[a]

	Days			5 Days		Weeks			
Determination	1st	2nd	3rd	1st	2nd	1st	2nd	3rd	4th
Total protein	−1.19	*−2.30*	*−4.06*	*−2.85*	*−2.39*	*−6.09*	*−3.04*	*−3.29*	−1.52
Albumin	*−4.61*	*−7.81*	*−10.12*	−1.46	−1.62	−1.17	0.35	*−2..84*	−0.64
Calcium	−1.14	−2.00	*−2.63*	0.30	*−2.76*	*−5.05*	*−2.36*	*−5.55*	*−2.75*
Inorg. phos.	0.14	−0.33	0.07	−0.39	−1.42	0.05	−2.13	*−2.65*	−1.82
Cholesterol	*−2.28*	*−2.79*	*−3.19*	*−3.25*	−0.15	*−4.05*	−1.91	−0.36	−0.67
Glucose	*−4.59*	*−5.24*	*−3.82*	−0.14	*4.21*	−0.39	*−4.47*	−0.39	*5.75*
Urea N	1.90	1.77	1.03	1.21	0.95	1.68	0.73	−0.47	0.38
Uric acid	*−3.83*	*−6.09*	*−9.12*	*−4.33*	*−2.83*	*−3.97*	*−2.61*	*−3.13*	*−2.98*
Alk. Phos.	0.49	−0.15	−0.53	−0.05	−1.60	*−3.38*	*−2.34*	−1.86	−1.92
LDH	0.49	1.14	*2.94*	−0.58	−0.70	0.17	−0.66	−1.25	0.04
Tot. bilirubin	*−5.41*	*−5.85*	*−6.07*	*−2.77*	0.05	−1.73	−1.78	*−3.98*	*−2.71*
AST	0.26	−1.33	−1.61	*−5.98*	0.18	−1.24	−0.84	−0.99	−0.86
Sodium	0.94	1.65	*2.49*	*−4.27*	−0.69	0.86	1.83	−2.92	−0.64
Potassium	1.53	0.43	0.68	*4.99*	−0.13	0.20	−0.19	*−11.10*	*−3.71*
Chloride	0.91	*2.64*	*2.83*	−1.03	*3.96*	*2.71*	*3.94*	−2.00	−0.66
CO_2	−0.32	−0.30	−0.90	*2.97*	*−4.49*	−1.62	−1.64	−0.49	2.06
Creatinine	−0.56	−0.65	0.41	*3.24*	−0.21	2.17	*2.91*	1.03	0.71
Amylase	0.26	−1.79	−1.09	*−4.60*	0.51	0.13	1.00	1.31	0.60
T-3 uptake	1.44	2.21	1.95			−0.30	−0.39	0.62	−1.10
T-4	*−3.58*	*−4.39*	*−8.98*	*−5.08*	−1.14	*−2.67*	−2.07	*−2.31*	−0.62

[a] Italicized values are significant at the 95% level.

(This method was changed after the second regimen.) The recent tabulation of drug effects (*6*) lists only one methodological interference applicable to the seven constituents in Figure 1: a decrease in calcium caused by a depression of the fluorescence of calcein. Such an interference was not uniform in the present study, especially in the short-term regimens (Tables 1 and 2).

The changes summarized in Table 5 therefore all appear to be the result of a physiological action of aspirin or the resulting salicylate ion. The competition for binding of salicylate and normal serum constituents to albumin has often been quoted as the cause of aspirin interference in the determination of calcium, bilirubin, and uric acid. A search of the report of Young et al. (*6*) fails to substantiate this supposition. No such effects are reported for calcium or uric acid, and one study reports an increase in apparent bilirubin owing to the competition for albumin binding. A decrease in thyroxine after aspirin ingestion has been attributed to a displacement of thyroxine from the binding sites of thyroxine-binding pre-albumin (*11*). The concentration of thyroxine-binding prealbumin versus that of thyroxine-binding globulin in the serum would suggest a much smaller decrease in thyroxine than reported in the present study. The interference of aspirin ingestion with results for total protein, thyroxine, and cholesterol in serum is more difficult to explain and represents an effect of the drug that has not commonly been recognized.

Evidently aspirin therapy depresses the values for the six constituents progressively in the three-day regimen and initially in the first five days or first week of the two-week regimens. This is followed by a recovery toward zero t-values at the end of 10 days or the second week of each two-week period. Because the t-values are the lowest after three days, five days, or one week, it must take the physiological mechanisms of the body a reasonably long time to adjust to aspirin therapy.

References

1. Caraway, W. T., Chemical and diagnostic specificity of laboratory tests. *Am. J. Clin. Pathol.* **37,** 445 (1962).

2. Wirth, W. A., and Thompson, R. L., The effect of various conditions and substances on the results of laboratory procedures. *Am. J. Clin. Pathol.* **43,** 579 (1965).

3. Elking, M. P., and Kabat, H. F., Drug-induced modifications of laboratory test values. *Am. J. Hosp. Pharm.* **25,** 485 (1968).

4. Constantino, N. V., and Kabat, H. F., Drug-induced modifications of laboratory test values—revised, 1973. *Am. J. Hosp. Pharm.* **30,** 24 (1973).

5. Young, D. S., Thomas, D. W., Friedman, R. B., and Pestaner, L. C., Effects of drugs on clinical laboratory tests. *Clin. Chem.* **18,** 1041 (1972).

6. Young, D. S., Pestaner, L. C., and Gibberman, V., Effects of drugs on clinical laboratory tests. *Clin. Chem.* **21,** No. 5, (1975). Special (April) issue.

7. Klein, B., Foreman, J. A., and Searcy, R. L., New chromogenic substrate for determination of serum amylase activity. *Clin. Chem.* **16,** 32 (1970).

8. Sterling, K., and Tabachnick, M., Resin uptake of ^{131}I-triiodothyronine as a test of thyroid function. *J. Clin. Endocrinol.* **21,** 456 (1961).

9. Murphy, B. E. P., and Jachan, C., The determinations of thyroxine by competitive protein-binding analysis employing an anion-exchange resin and radiothyroxine. *J. Lab. Clin. Med.* **66,** 161 (1965).

10. Routh, J. I., Paul, W. D., Arredondo, E., and Dryer, R. L., Semimicro method for the determination of salicylate levels in blood. *Clin. Chem.* **2,** 432 (1956).

11. Sunderman, F. W., Jr., Effect of drugs on hematological tests. *Ann. Clin. Lab. Sci.* **2,** 1 (1972).

12. Rossi, E. C., and Levin, N. W., Inhibition of primary ADP-induced platelet aggregation in normal subjects after administration of nitrofurantoin. *J. Clin. Invest.* **52,** 2457 (1973).

13. Harris, E. K., Kanofsky, P., Shakarji, G., and Cotlove, E., Biological and analytic components of variation in long-term studies of serum constituents in normal subjects. II. Estimating biological components of variation. *Clin. Chem.* **16,** 1022 (1970).

CLIN. CHEM. 22/6, 843–846 (1976)

Results of a Nine-Laboratory Survey of Forensic Toxicology Proficiency

Eugene C. Dinovo[1] and Louis A. Gottschalk

Toxicological determinations are crucial to coroners' or medical examiners' judgments that drugs are significantly involved in a death. However, differences in laboratory procedures, thoroughness of screening, and limits of detection may result in artifactual differences in the toxicological results and the subsequent interpretations of them. To test this possibility, we conducted a toxicology proficiency-testing survey of nine collaborating laboratories. The results for the proficiency samples point out startling interlaboratory differences in accuracy and precision of detection of drugs. These observed variations in toxicological proficiency may introduce a significant source of error in drug-death statistics and in epidemiological deductions based on these statistics.

A brief proficiency-testing program was performed, to assist the National Institute on Drug Abuse in its efforts to improve the investigating and reporting of drug-related deaths in nine major U. S. cities (Chicago, Cleveland, Dallas, Los Angeles, Miami, New York, Philadelphia, San Francisco, and Washington, D. C.). The program covered a time period from February to August 1974.

Drug-death determination depends in part on test results obtained in toxicology laboratories. The toxicological results are often crucial to coroners' or medical examiners' judgments that drugs are significantly involved in a death. However, interlaboratory differences in procedures, thoroughness of screening, or limits of detection may result in artifactual differences in mortality statistics from various reporting areas. Therefore, in conjunction with a research project collecting detailed information on 2000 drug-related deaths (*1, 2*) in these nine cities, a brief proficiency survey was also conducted to assess the differences and variations in the extent and quality of toxicological examinations performed by the laboratories of the participating coroners and medical examiners.

Methods

Five standard drug samples were used in the study. Three samples consisted of drugs added to drug-free urine and two of drugs added to a 30 g/liter solution of human albumin. Some drugs were at the same concentration in different samples. Each of the five specimens contained 6.5 mg of secobarbital per liter, in order to measure the variations in the secobarbital assay for a given laboratory over a period of time.

The concentrations chosen were those associated with low toxicity (*3, 4*) to provide a moderate challenge to the toxicological methodologies. The 25-ml urine samples and the 10-ml albumin samples were lyophilized and capped under reduced pressure. For each sample, either one urine vial or two albumin vials were sent out to the cities; if requested, more of the sample was sent.

Reference assays were performed by three laboratories.[2] We identified the drugs present and asked the laboratories to perform quantitative assays. Reference assays were not performed to find the correct experimental value but to check the preparation and manufacture of the drug specimens. The results of the reference assays demonstrated that all the drugs were present in the manufactured standards and that no gross errors in preparation had occurred.

Some samples were sent as complete unknowns; for some, partial information was supplied such as "drugs in this vial are neutrals and volatiles," or "this vial contains barbiturates"; and some samples were sent with their drug content qualitatively identified. This was done to simulate the situation in coroners' and medical examiners' offices, where different amounts of information are presented with each case.

It was understood by the medical examiners and coroners that our specimens were artifactual ones, that several drugs but no metabolites were present, and that routine assays were to be performed. The results were to be returned to us and the laboratory's identity was to be kept confidential by us. We emphasize that the term "false negative," as used in this paper, means a drug was present in the sample and not found by the laboratory, whether or not the laboratory screened or tested for that drug.

Some laboratories raised questions as to the concentrations used and the sample size; they pointed out that urine and albumin solutions are not representative of the actual postmortem specimens presented to them, and that a specimen history was needed to outline the toxicological examination. We believed, however, that it was practically impossible to simulate actual post-

Department of Psychiatry and Human Behavior, California College of Medicine, University of California, Irvine, Calif. 92717.

[1] Present address: Department of Pathology, VA Hospital, Sepulveda, Calif. 91343.

Received Dec. 8, 1975; accepted Feb. 9, 1976.

[2] Reference assays were performed by our laboratory, by the Orange County Sheriff-Coroner's Office laboratory, and by Reference Laboratory of North Hollywood, Calif. However, all drugs were not assayed by each laboratory.

Table 1

Results for Albumin Sample I, Sent As a General Unknown

	Secobarbital	Pentobarbital	Salicylic acid
Drugs present, mg/liter	6.5	6	400
Results reported by participating laboratories, mg/liter			
	4	3	340
	6	6	360
	5	3.8	-
	7.17	5.41	402
	——— 11.1 ——— [a]		567
	7.5	7.1	390
	+	+	+
	6	6	380
	——— 9.5 ——— [a]		360
Mean	5.7	5.2	400
STANDARD DEVIATION	1.2	1.3	76
Reference assays			
	6.2	4.9	410

[a]: Secobarbital and pentobarbital were reported together by this laboratory.

+: Drug found but not quantitated.

-: Drug was not found.

Table 2

Results for Urine Sample II, Sent As a General Unknown

	Secobarbital	Methadone	Morphine	Methaqualone	Flurazepam	Ethanol	False positives
Drugs present, mg/liter	6.5	2.5	3.5	20	30	0.15%	
Results reported by participating laboratories, mg/liter							
	7.0	2.8	4.1	27.4	36	0.12	
	4	10	3	-	-	0.12	
	3.8	-	-	1.8	-	-	
	7.0	-	+	+	+	0.12	
	6	3	3	28, 25	42, 38	0.10	
	5.2	-	+	5.1	-	-	
	+	+	+	+	-	-	Salicylic acid
	5	-	-	-	-	0.12	
	+	+	+	+	-	-	
Mean	5.4	5.3	3.4	17.5	38.7	0.12	
SD	1.3	4.1	0.6	12.9	3.0	0.01	
Reference assays							
	4.6	2.2	3.6	16	+	N/R	

+: Drug was found but not quantitated.

-: Drug was not found.

N/R: No response.

Table 3

An Association of Toxicologists;

Results for Urine Sample II

	Secobarbital	Methadone	Morphine	Methaqualone	Flurazepam	False positives
Drugs present, mg/liter	6.5	2.5	3. 5	20	30	
Results reported by members, mg/liter						
	6.5	-	+	21.7	-	
	9.0	+	+	+	-	
	5.0	17.0	+	24.0	-	
	5.0	-	5.0	-	-	Darvon, 20
	11.0	6.0	+	-	+	Cocaine, 37
	-	-	+	-	-	
	5.0	0.8	3.1	18.0	13.0	
	5.6	-	+	21.0	23.0	
	7.0	+	+	16.6	+	
	+	+	+	-	-	
	4.0	+	+	30.0	-	Meperidine +
	2.0	-	4.0	20.0	-	
	7.0	+	5.0	-	-	Propoxyphene +
	+	-	+	-	-	
	+	+	+	-	-	
	2.0	+	+	20.0	25.0	
	3.5, 5.6	2.1, 2.2	3.4,2.7,4.6	15.0, 16.7	+	
	-	4.45	-	-	-	
	7.1	-	+	21.0	-	Pentobarbital +
Mean	5.35	5.4	3.97	20.3	---	
SD	0.815	1.75	0.40	1.4	---	

+: Drug found but not quantitated.

-: Drug not found.

mortem specimens; that a fictional history might lead as well as mislead; that clearly specified information was better than a history; and that manufactured specimens should render the assays less difficult because no metabolites or other interfering substances were present.

Results

Table 1 shows the results for Sample I, the albumin solution with added secobarbital, pentobarbital, and salicylic acid at a calculated concentration of 6.5, 6.0, and 400 mg/liter, respectively. Sample I was sent out as a general unknown. The results of the assays were generally quite good for these three drugs. Only one false negative was reported. Most of the laboratories assayed the barbiturates by gas-liquid chromatography, using a chloroform extraction at acidic or neutral pH values ranging from pH 3 to 7.5. Salicylate was assayed by ultraviolet spectrophotometry after chloroform extraction of the specimen at acidic pH values ranging from pH 1 to 6. The extraction pH within the range given did not seem to influence the quantitative results for either barbiturate or salicylate.

In contrast to the one false negative reported for Sample I, reports on Sample II (urine), also sent out as a general unknown, showed 18 (33%) false negatives out of a possible 54 findings (Table 2). Only two laboratories identified and quantitated all of the drugs. One false positive was reported, salicylic acid. All nine laboratories found secobarbital. Seven laboratories quantitated it with a mean of 5.4 mg/liter, about equal to that of Sample I, 5.7 mg/liter. Of the other drugs, ethanol was quantitated by five laboratories, methaqualone was found by seven laboratories and quantitated by four, morphine was found by seven and quantitated by three, and methadone was found by five and quantitated by three. Of these drugs, only for ethanol and morphine do the reported values agree reasonably with the actual concentration. One of the three values for methadone and two of the five values for methaqualone are grossly inconsistent with the calculated value, the reference assay, and the mean for the nine laboratories.

It is of interest to compare the results reported by coroners' or medical examiners' laboratories with those obtained with the same sample by members of an association of toxicologists, a mixed group of forensic, commercial, and clinical laboratories. Table 3 shows that 31 false negatives were reported out of a possible total of 95 findings, or 33% false negatives, exactly equal to the false negative percentage of the coroners' and medical examiners' laboratories in the nine target cities. The situation is evidently the same, regardless of lab-

Table 4

Results for Albumin Sample III[a]

	Drugs present, mg/liter						
	Seco-barbital	Meprobamate	Chlorodia-zepoxide	Diazepam	Acetone	Ethanol	False positives
	6.5	25	20	25	0.05%	0.15%	
	Results reported by participating laboratories, mg/liter						
	3.3, 2.6	11	13	12	0.036	0.076	
	3.8	-	10	20	0.043	0.088	
	4.3	13.2	+	+	0.03	0.08	
	-	34	-	-	0.048	0.085	
	-	10, 10	-	-	0.031	0.075	Tyrosine +
	1.8	-	-	24.1	-	-	
	-	-	-	3.6	0.034	0.029	Isopropanol, 0.01%
Mean	3.1	15.6	11.5	14.9	0.037	0.07	
SD	1.0	10.3	2.1	9.0	0.003	0.02	
	Reference assays						
	5.8	30	10	18.6	0.04	0.09	

[a]: Drugs in this sample were identified as neutrals and volatiles.

+: Drugs found but not quantitated.

-: Drugs not found.

Table 5

Results for Urine Sample IV[a]

	Drugs present, mg/liter							
	Seco-barbital	Methaqua-lone	Diazepam	Amphet-amine	Morphine	Methadone	Codeine	False positives
	6.5	20	25	3.5	3.5	2.5	3.0	
	Results reported by participating laboratories, mg/liter							
	2.5	10	4	0.8	3, 4	1.6	1.6	
	5.8	18.3	22.2	3.5	3.2	2.4	2.9	
	5.4	11.9	19.2	3.7	+	2.4	3.2	
	5.2	33	+	+	5.5	8.3	-	Cocaine +
	5.3	15.7	24.2	4.1	5.8	0.7	3.7	
	3.2	-	3.9	-	-	6.8	5.2	
	6.7	17.7	2	3.8	1.3	7	2.1	
	8	12	20	3	7.5	3	2.5	
	4.9	27.0	37.0	5.0	11.0	2.5	8.0	
Mean	5.2	18.2	16.6	3.4	5.2	3.9	3.6	
SD	1.6	8.0	12.3	1.3	3.0	2.7	2.1	
	Reference assays							
	6.2	15	30	1.5	1.9	1.7	2.3	

[a]: This sample was sent out with all drugs present specified.

+: Drugs found but not quantitated.

-: Drugs not found.

Table 6

Results for Urine Sample V[a]

	Drug present, 6.5 mg/liter	
	Secobarbital	False positives
	Results reported by participating laboratories, mg/liter	
	9.5	
	4	
	6	
	4.4	Phenobarbital +
	8.5, 6.4	
	5.8	
	5	
	384[b]	Doriden, 3.6
Mean	6.2	
SD	1.9	
Reference assay	5.4	

[a]: Drug class was identified for this sample.

[b]: Not used in statistics.

+: Drug found but not quantitated.

-: Drug not found.

Table 7

Time Study of Secobarbital (6.5 mg/liter) Measurements, by City

Sample	City 1	City 2	City 3	City 4	City 5	City 6	City 7	City 8	City 9
	Secobarbital found, mg/liter								
Serum I (February)	5.55[a]	4	4.75[a]	7.5	7.17	5.0	+	6.0	6.0
Urine IV (March)	+	4	5.2	7.0	3.8	5	+	6	7
Serum III (May)	-	N/R	-	3.3	-	4.3	1.8	N/R	3.8
Urine II (June)	5.2	8	4.9	5.8	6.7	5.3	3.2	2.5	5.4
Urine V (August)	384[b]	5	4.4	8.5, 6.4	6.0	4	9.5	-	5.8
Mean	5.4	5.3	4.8	6.4	5.9	4.7	4.8	4.8	5.6
SD	0.25	1.9	0.33	1.8	1.5	0.5	4.1	2.0	1.2

[a]: One-half of barbiturate (secobarbital and pentobarbital) concentration.

[b]: Not included in statistics.

N/R: No response.

+: Drug found but not quantitated.

-: Drug not found.

oratory affiliation. The major difference seems to lie in the rate of false positives: five false positives for the association of toxicologists (19 laboratories) vs. one false positive for the nine forensic laboratories.

Every drug was assayed by a variety of methods and with use of various extraction pH's. Traditional methodologies such as ultraviolet spectrophotometry, gas-chromatography, and thin-layer chromatography predominated. None of the new methods such as radioimmunoassay, enzyme-multiplied immunoassay, or free-radical assay were being used by the coroners' and medical examiners' laboratories. Most of the quantitations were done by ultraviolet spectrophotometry and gas chromatography, except for morphine, which was chiefly quantitated by fluorometry.

Table 4 shows the results for Sample III (albumin). The drugs in this sample were identified in a covering letter as being neutrals and volatiles. Seven of the nine laboratories responded to this sample. Six of the seven quantitated the volatiles (acetone and ethanol). Secobarbital and meprobamate were found and quantitated by four of the seven laboratories; chlordiazepoxide was identified by three laboratories and quantitated by two; and diazepam was found and quantitated by four. The mean for secobarbital in this sample (3.1 mg/liter) was much lower than for the previous two samples (5.7 and 5.4 mg/liter).

Fourteen (33%) false negatives were reported out of 42 possible findings; there were two false positives (tyrosine and isopropanol). Only one laboratory identified and quantitated all the drugs in the sample.

Sample IV (urine) was sent out with all the drugs in the mixture specified, to check the quantitative procedures by bypassing the screening procedures. Four (6%) false negative findings out of 63 possible findings were reported—a significant improvement over the previous three samples for which false negatives averaged 29%. One false positive was reported (cocaine). Table 5 shows these results.

A preponderance of the gas-chromatographic method is again apparent for all classes of drugs in this sample. Theoretically, because all drugs were identified, there should have been no false negatives for Sample IV, but one laboratory either did not assay for these drugs or looked for them and could not find them. The other false negative is probably a clerical error, the typing of "cocaine" for "codeine."

The last sample sent out, Sample V (urine), contained only secobarbital, 6.5 mg/liter. The drug(s) in the vial were identified as barbiturates in the covering letter. No false negatives were reported, but two false positives were found (phenobarbital and glutethimide). The one result reported as 384 mg/liter is, we hope, a transcriptional error in its omission of the decimal point (Table 6). Both false positives were found by gas chromatography, with use of a chloroform extraction at acidic pH, conditions similar to those used for the true positives.

Table 7 shows the results, by city, for secobarbital measurement in each of the samples, assayed at different times. Secobarbital was present at the same concentration in all five samples. Only three of the nine laboratories consistently found secobarbital, and, of these three, only one laboratory had a coefficient of variation of 10% or less. The results presented in Table 7 clearly demonstrate significant intra-laboratory variations as well as large interlaboratory differences for a rather well-established and supposedly routine assay. Most laboratories used a chloroform extraction at pH values ranging from 3 to 7.5. Even so, the reports contained four false negatives, three unquantitated results, and one probable clerical error.

The forensic pathologists and toxicologists from these nine cities commented concerning their impressions of the usefulness of this kind of quality-control analysis of their toxicological examinations. They all believed that seeing the results of their analyses compared to those of other laboratories, in a confidential manner, helped spur them on toward further self-examination and improvement of their detection and assay procedures.

Discussion

The major finding of this proficiency study was that the toxicological laboratories with which the nine medical examiners and coroners were associated varied considerably in the precision and accuracy with which they performed drug assays. Another important finding was that accuracy and precision of the quantitation increased greatly with the amount of information supplied to the analyst with each sample. Examination of Tables 2 and 3, tabulating the results of a urine sample sent as an unknown, and Table 5, tabulating the results of a urine sample sent with all the drugs present identified, is sufficient to indicate the improvement. Tables 2 and 3 contain a large proportion of negative and unquantitated results (33% false negatives and 26% unquantitated findings), while Table 5 contains 6% false negatives and 5% unquantitated findings, clearly a great improvement. In the case of the unknown sample (Table 2), four laboratories failed to identify, and two others failed to quantitate, methadone; in the case of the known sample (Table 5), all nine laboratories quantitated methadone. Evidently all these laboratories have adequate instrumentation and methodologies to quantitate these drugs when they are known to be in the sample. This problem seems to lie more in screening for drugs and not in quantitating them. If one can improve the screening accuracy, perhaps the whole toxicological examination will improve.

We must conclude at this point that, since there exists a wide interlaboratory variance in the detection, accuracy, and precision of toxicological analysis, this wide variance is probably reflected in the drug-death statistics and drug-death certification in these and other cities in the United States. Epidemiological considerations based on these drug-death statistics will need to be re-evaluated in this light.

Finally, the collective evaluations of this toxicological quality-control survey by the toxicologists and forensic pathologists most directly involved in death investigation and certification definitely supported the continuation of some similar program of proficiency testing by a neutral organization or agency. All individuals concerned believed that improvement in the accuracy of mortality statistics for drug-related deaths would result.

The research upon which this paper is based was funded by the National Institute on Drug Abuse, Department of Health, Education, and Welfare, under Contract No. 271-75-3004. We thank our collaborators: F. L. McGuire, J. F. Heiser, H. Birch, and B. R. Nandi. Thanks are due to Dr. Larry Tolle, Manager of Research Administration, and Anthony Fontana, Associate Clinical Chemist, of Hyland Laboratories, Costa Mesa, Calif., for assistance in the preparation and lyophilization of the drug specimens, and to Robert H. Cravey, Chief Toxicologist of the Orange County Sheriff-Coroner's Office, for collaborating with us in performing reference assays.

References

1. Gottschalk, L. A., McGuire, F. L., Heiser, J. F., and Alexander, P. B., *The Development of a Uniform System for Reporting and Recording Drug-Related Deaths,* vols. I and II. U. S. Dept. of HEW, National Institute of Mental Health. Report on NIMH Contract No. HSM-42-72-139 for the period June 26, 1972–June 25, 1973.

2. Gottschalk, L. A., McGuire, F. L., Dinovo, E. C., et al., *The Investigation and Reporting of Drug-Involved Deaths.* U. S. Dept. of HEW, Alcohol, Drug Abuse, and Mental Health Administration, National Institute on Drug Abuse. Report on NIDA Contract No. HSM-42-72-139 for the period June 26, 1973–June 25, 1975.

3. Niyogi, S. K., Drug levels in cases of poisoning. *Forensic Sci.* **2,** 67 (1973).

4. Baselt, R. C., Wright, J. A., and Cravey, R. H., Therapeutic and toxic concentrations of more than 100 toxicologically significant drugs in blood, plasma, or serum: A tabulation. *Clin. Chem.* **21,** 44 (1975).

CLIN. CHEM. 22/6, 847-850 (1976)

Analysis of Results of Toxicological Examinations Performed by Coroners' or Medical Examiners' Laboratories in 2000 Drug-Involved Deaths in Nine Major U. S. Cities

Eugene C. Dinovo,[1] Louis A. Gottschalk, Frederick L. McGuire, Herman Birch, and Jon F. Heiser

Data were collected on 2000 deaths in which psychoactive drugs were involved. The data were submitted by medical examiners or coroners in nine U. S. cities from their case files. The 2000 cases comprise a representative sample from each of these cities of deaths from psychoactive drugs between 1972 through 1974. This report details inter-city differences in methods and practices of the toxicological examination as well as in the type and numbers of drugs reported. Even when the same analytical method was used in various cities, there were differences in extraction solvent and extraction pH. Of the 3909 drugs detected, 2945 were quantitated; the number of drugs quantitatively measured per case studied ranged from a low of 0.82 for New York to a high of 2.20 for Washington, D. C. The number of different drugs quantitatively measured varied from 16 for New York to 30 for San Francisco; however, New York qualitatively assayed for the presence of a total of 25 drugs. The number and type of drugs found per case varied. Methadone, for example, was found in 60% of the cases reported by New York and in 49% of the cases from Washington, D. C., but in only about 10% of cases reported by Philadelphia, Dallas, Miami, and San Francisco, and in less than 1% of Los Angeles and Cleveland cases; it was not reported by Chicago. Phenmetrazine-caused deaths were reported only by Dallas (one case) and Washington, D. C. (29 cases). From the data as a whole, information is presented for 33 drugs as to the concentration in physiological tissues and fluids. Analysis of single psychoactive drug cases and single-drug-plus-ethanol cases shows that, in the presence of ethanol, the toxic blood concentration of imipramine, amytriptyline, meprobamate, thioridazine, morphine, propoxyphene, methaqualone, and all barbiturates was decreased by an average of 50%.

Our research group, under the auspices of the National Institute on Drug Abuse, has collected extensive data on 2000 psychoactive drug-involved deaths from nine major United States cities. The U.C.I. Reporting Form for Drug-Involved Deaths, developed by this group (*1*), was used to obtain the data (*2*). It consists of about 135 items of inquiry in such areas as biographic, demographic, on-site investigation, toxicological examination, postmortem examination, treatment before death, and suicide.

This paper deals solely with the toxicological examinations as reported by the cities on the U.C.I. Reporting Form for Drug-Involved Deaths. Analysis of these data clearly demonstrates large variations among cities in procedures, methods, test results, and drugs tested for.

Methods of Data Collection

A collaborative working relationship was first established with the medical examiner or coroner in each of the nine cities and with his associated toxicological laboratory. "Psychoactive drug-involved death" was defined as any death referred to a medical examiner or coroner in which psychoactive pharmacological agents were considered to be related to or involved in the fatal event. Instances in which ethanol was the sole chemical agent involved in the death were not acceptable for this study, but instances in which ethanol in combination with other psychoactive chemical substances was involved with the death were acceptable.

The National Institute on Drug Abuse limited this study to the collection of psychosocial and biomedical data on 2000 cases from nine cities (one laboratory per city), which included such large cities as New York, Chicago, Los Angeles, and Philadelphia, a well as the smaller cities of Cleveland, Dallas, Miami, San Francisco, and Washington, D. C.

Based on 1970 census figures, quotas were set for each urban jurisdiction on the basis of the ratio between its population and that of the others. Thus, if City A had twice the population of City B, City A would be expected to contribute about twice as many cases. Smaller cities were assigned smaller quotas, but slightly more than their share so that there would be enough data for valid statistical analysis. In the opinion of each medical examiner or coroner, the cases reported are representative of all such cases occurring in each city during 1972–1974. We assumed that, when cases were gathered at different time intervals from different cities within the total time-frame, month-to-month biases arising from seasonal influences were negligible or nonexistent. This assumption was considered warranted by all participating data-collection centers.

All cases selected for this series had to be, in the opinion of the referring medical examiner or coroner,

Department of Psychiatry and Human Behavior, California College of Medicine, University of California, Irvine, Calif. 92717.

[1] Current address: Department of Pathology, Veterans Administration Hospital, Sepulveda, Calif. 91343. Address reprint requests to this author at Department of Psychiatry and Human Behavior, College of Medicine, University of California, Irvine, Calif. 92717.

Received Dec. 8, 1975; accepted Feb. 16, 1976.

Table 1. Results of Assays, by City

RESULTS REPORTED	Chicago	Cleveland	Dallas	Los Angeles	Miami	New York	Philadelphia	San Francisco	Washington D.C.	Total
Zero or traces										
No.	8	13	5	5	12	66	49	1	0	159
Column %	1.7	4.2	2.2	0.9	4.4	6.7	14.2	0.2	0	4.1
Qualitative presence										
No.	0	81	5	1	47	587	84	0	0	805
Column %	0	26	2.2	0.2	17	59.5	24.4	0	0	20.6
Quantitated										
No.	465	216	214	527	216	334	211	432	330	2945
Column %	98.3	69.7	95.6	98.8	78.5	33.8	61.3	98.8	100.0	75.3
Drugs quantitated per case										
	1.58	1.44	2.14	1.76	1.43	0.82	1.06	1.72	2.20	1.47
Total drugs										
	473	310	224	533	275	987	344	433	330	3909
Total drugs per case										
	1.60	2.07	2.24	1.78	1.82	2.44	1.73	1.73	2.20	1.95

Table 2. Number of Quantitative Assays for Alcohol, Diazepam, Morphine, Barbiturates and Propoxyphene (i.e., ADMBP) and Total Number of Drug Quantitated, by City

	No. of Quantitative Assays for ADMBP [a]	Total No. of Quantitative Assays	ADMBP [a] % of Total	No. of Drugs Quantitated
Chicago	358	465	77.0	21
Cleveland	141	216	65.3	25
Dallas	133	214	62.1	29
Los Angeles	449	527	85.2	25
Miami	103	216	47.7	25
New York	222	334	66.5	16
Philadelphia	141	211	66.8	21
San Francisco	322	432	74.5	30
Washington, D.C.	126	330	38.2	25

[a] ADMBP is an acronym for the following drugs: alcohol (ethanol), diazepam, morphine, barbiturates (phenobarbital, amobarbital, pentobarbital and secobarbital), and propoxyphene.

Table 3. Examples of Differences in Drug Assay Patterns, by City

		Chicago	Cleveland	Dallas	Los Angeles	Miami	New York	Philadelphia	San Francisco	Washington D.C.
METHADONE Quantitative and Qualitative	N	0	1	6	2	7	242	21	6	73
% of total drugs tested			0.3	2.7	0.4	2.5	24.5	6.1	1.4	22.1
% of cases			0.7	6	0.7	4.6	59.8	10.6	2.4	48.6
MORPHINE Quan/Qual	N	127	30	14	145	10	93	49	78	45
% of total drugs tested		26.8	9.6	6.3	27.2	3.6	9.4	14.2	18	13.6
% of cases		43.1	20	14	48.3	6.6	23.0	24.6	31.2	30.0
QUININE Quan/Qual	N	0	1	0	0	2	122	54	0	45
% of total drugs tested			0.3			0.7	12.4	15.7		13.6
% of cases			0.7			1.3	30.1	28.6		30.0
PHENMETRAZINE Quan/Qual	N	0	0	1	0	0	0	0	0	29
% of total drugs tested				0.4						8.8
% of cases				1						19.3
METHAMPHETAMINE and AMPHETAMINE Quan/Qual	N	0	1	1	0	3	1	27	12	·25
% of cases			0.3	0.4		1.1	0.1	7.8	2.8	7.6
% of cases			0.7	1		2.0	0.2	13.6	4.8	16.7

a psychoactive drug-involved death in which the drug—alone, in combination with another psychoactive drug or alcohol, or in combination with a pre-existing medical disease or an external circumstance (auto accident or gunshot)—led to a fatality. Each data-collection center was also advised to select consecutive cases on which all data necessary to complete the forms were available.

These data on 2000 psychoactive drug-related deaths are most likely not representative of the entire United States during 1972–1974, but probably give a fair picture of urban America, and certainly allow a meaningful and accurate analysis of regional variations in characteristics of the toxicological examination.

Results

The toxicological laboratories of these cities tested for a total of 3909 drugs (1.95 per case). Of these, 2945 were quantitated, traces or no drugs were found in 159, and 805 drugs were simply reported as being present. Table 1 lists the type of result reported by the laboratory of each city. Definite patterns of toxicological examination clearly emerge. Washington, D. C., quantitated all of the drugs detected. In contrast, New York quantitated 33.8%, reported a qualitative "present" for 59.5%, and found a trace or no drug for 6.7% of the drugs that were tested for. The other cities lay somewhere between these two extremes. Qualitative presence was reported by Miami for 17%, by Philadelphia for 24.4%, and by Cleveland for 26% of their tested drugs. Chicago, Dallas, Los Angeles, and Washington reported a qualitative presence for less than 2% of their drugs. The same four cities reporting high percentages of drugs as qualitatively present also reported higher percentages of zero or traces found, as follows: Miami, 4.2%; Cleveland, 4.4%; New York, 6.7%; and Philadelphia, 14.2%. The other five cities reported less than 2% zero or traces.

Another way to view these differences is to look at the number of quantitated drugs per case studied. By this analysis, New York and Philadelphia were clearly different from the other seven laboratories in the number of drugs quantitated per case: 0.82 and 1.06, respectively. A middle group of cities reported quantitation of drugs per case as follows: Miami, 1.43; Cleveland, 1.44; Chicago, 1.58; San Francisco, 1.72; and Los Angeles, 1.76 drugs per case, while Dallas and Washington quantitated 2.14 and 2.20 drugs per case, respectively.

Chicago, Los Angeles, San Francisco, Dallas, and Washington quantitated in their toxicological laboratories practically all the drugs found, and the number of drugs reported per case nearly equals the number of drugs quantitated per case. On the other hand, more drugs were reported per case than were quantitated by Cleveland (1.14-fold), Miami (1.27-fold), and Philadelphia (1.63-fold). New York reported per case three times as many drugs as they quantitated.

Alcohol (ethanol), diazepam, morphine, barbiturates (phenobarbital, amobarbital, pentobarbital, and secobarbital), and propoxyphene comprised 68% of the total drugs quantitated by the nine cities, as shown in Table 2. The percentages of the total comprised by these drugs ranged from a low of 38.2% for Washington, D. C., to a high of 85.2% for Los Angeles. These same drugs accounted for 89% of the qualitative assays performed by New York. Miami's low percentage for these drugs (47.7%) was due to a relatively large number of glutethimide, ethchlorvynol, and methaqualone assays. New York showed an overwhelming proportion of methadone assays, more than three times the proportion of the other cities combined. Philadelphia showed a relatively high number of amphetamine, methamphetamine, and methadone assays, and Washington a large number of methadone, methamphetamine, qui-

Table 4. Drugs Quantitated in Physiological Fluids and Tissues

Location:	Blood	Urine	Bile	Liver	Lung	Kidney	Stomach	Other
PART A								
Drugs reported								
N	3216	1928	1517	1234	185	258	1629	291
% of total	31.4	18.8	14.8	12.0	1.8	2.5	15.9	2.8
PART B								
Drug reported	Ethanol	Morphine	Morphine	Methadone	Methadone	Methadone	Methadone	Methadone
N	639	476	695	328	65	71	326	73
% of total	19.8	24.7	45.8	26.6	35.1	27.5	20.0	25.0
Drug reported	Morphine	Methadone	Methadone	Quinine	Quinine	Quinine	Quinine	Quinine
N	450	363	318	167	27	29	142	46
% of total	14.0	18.8	21.0	13.5	14.6	11.2	8.7	15.9
Drug reported	Methadone	Quinine	Quinine	Propoxyphene	Phenmetrazine	Phenmetrazine	Morphine	Ethanol
N	372	194	192	79	24	25	134	29
% of total	11.6	10.1	12.7	6.4	13.0	9.7	8.2	10.0
Drug reported	Secobarbital	Ethanol	Propoxyphene	Secobarbital	Propoxyphene	Propoxyphene	Propoxyphene	Phenmetrazine
N	238	121	68	72	15	19	113	23
% of total	7.4	6.3	4.5	5.8	8.1	7.4	6.9	7.9
Drug reported	Pentobarbital	Propoxyphene	Amitriptyline	Pentobarb.	Methamphet.	Methamphet.	Secobarbital	Secobarbital
N	180	98	43	68	14	17	112	16
% of total	5.6	5.1	2.8	5.5	7.5	6.6	6.9	5.5

Table 5. Quantitative Assays of Drugs

	SINGLE DRUG & POLYDRUG CASES			SINGLE DRUG CASES			SINGLE DRUG-ETHANOL CASES		
GENERIC NAME OF DRUG	Number and Location	Mean Concentration mg/liter	SD	Number in Blood	Mean Concentration mg/liter	SD	Number in Blood	Mean Concentration mg/liter	SD
Meprobamate	17 blood	64	77	3	105.3	46.9	3	89.3	52.2
Thioridazine	11 blood	4.8	2.6	5	5.0	2.1	1	3	—
Diazepam	67 blood	18	80	3	4.8	2.7	5	5.2	6.6
Imipramine	16 blood	7.8	8.8	6	10.7	13.2	1	2	—
Amitriptyline	18 liver	52	72	7	17.5	10.0	2	11.5	2.12
Amobarbital	95 blood	35	133	6	16.5	27.7	—	—	—
Pentobarbital	151 blood	20	19	56	25.2	19.7	29	19.3	18.8
Secobarbital	202 blood	18	50	57	20.2	17.0	30	13.6	10.7
Phenobarbital	130 blood	36	96	34	88.6	176.9	20	11.3	13.0
Methadone	99 blood	34	155	33	2.6	5.9	11	55.5	180
Salicylate	39 blood	525	1170	9	607	282	—	—	—
Propoxyphene	93 blood	20	94	16	18.3	27.7	15	9.7	11.4
Pentazocine	7 blood	14	13	3	15.7	15.1	—	—	—
Glutethimide	34 blood	70	177	14	42.1	33.2	3	62.1	18.1
Methaqualone	39 blood	14	18	3	112.7	136	3	57	60.3
Chloral hydrate	13 blood	47	47						
Meperidine	9 blood	8.0	13						
Morphine	371 bile	54	256						
Methamphetamine	40 urine	43	106						
Cocaine	2 blood	399	555						
Quinine	16 bile	2.0	1.0						
Ethanol	583 blood	1375	1042						
Codeine	16 bile	11	—						
Ethchlorvynol	37 blood	47	49						
Barbiturate sedative	47 blood	33	76						
Chlorpromazine	7 liver	50	64						
Lidocaine	10 blood	254	527						
Phenothiazine	2 urine	52	39						
Chlordiazepoxide	21 blood	6.9	9.7						
Flurazepam	8 blood	13	30						
Phenmetrazine	22 urine	24	44						
Piphenylhydantoin	9 blood	45	43						

nine, and phenmetrazine assays. Among all the cities, only Washington (29 cases) and Dallas (one case) reported phenmetrazine cases.

The number of different drugs quantitated by the cities varied as well, from a low of 16 drugs for New York to a high of 30 for San Francisco. New York, however, qualitatively assayed for 25 drugs.

Table 3 summarizes the laboratory results for five drugs, listing in each cell the number of tests performed quantitatively or qualitatively, the percentage of the total drugs reported, and percentage of cases positive for the drug for each city. There were large differences among cities. In New York and Washington, methadone represented 24.5% and 22.1%, respectively, of all drugs tested for and was found in 60% of the cases for New York and 49% of the cases for Washington—very high percentages indeed. In contrast, methadone was found in much smaller proportions in Philadelphia, Dallas, Miami, and San Francisco, in less than 1% of cases reported by Los Angeles and Cleveland, and was not reported at all by Chicago.

Morphine was found in significant numbers by all cities, ranging from a low of 3.6% of total drugs (reported by Miami) to a high of 27.2% of total drugs (reported by Los Angeles). Morphine was found in 48.3% and 43.1% of the cases reported by Los Angeles and Chicago, respectively, and in only 6.6% of Miami cases. Quinine was not reported in four cities, including both Chicago and Los Angeles, the leaders in percentage of cases containing morphine. It was reported found in about 30% of the cases in New York, Washington, and Philadelphia. These northeastern seaboard cities seemed to observe a very high incidence of methadone- and morphine-related cases, much more so than the rest of the participating cities. In contrast, Washington alone among the nine cities found a substantial number of cases of phenmetrazine-involved death, 20% of their cases. Washington and Philadelphia showed the greatest proportion of amphetamine-involved deaths. About 15% of the cases reported by these cities were found to involve amphetamine, whereas the average for the other cities was 1.2%.

One possible source of the differences would seem to be the drug-analysis methodology used by each city. If, for example, Los Angeles had used a more specific and accurate method for measuring morphine, and the other cities had used other, less-specific or less-reliable methods, this might explain the large representation of morphine-involved deaths in Los Angeles. Unfortunately, the methodologies used by the various cities for morphine assays were quite similar: gas–liquid chromatography predominated, followed by spectrofluorometry, immunoassays, fluorescent assays, and color tests. Perhaps the chief difference was not in the final assay method, but in earlier steps of the assays—in the extraction procedure, the extraction solvent, or the pH used in the extraction. One can use gas–liquid chromatography to measure a drug after it has been concentrated from the specimen by a wide variety of extraction methods and solvents. Therefore, though the final assay methods were similar, the earlier steps might have been different. The answer to this question must await further data collection and analysis. The other clear possibility is that these are genuine epidemiological differences.

Table 4 lists in Part A the total number of drugs detected in various body tissues and fluids and the percent of the grand total for all sites. Of this total, 93% was on the blood, urine, bile, liver, or stomach contents. The frequency of tests on other body fluids or tissues depends largely on the city and on the drug in question. Phenothiazines, amphetamine, metamphetamine, and quinine are preferentially assayed in urine; bile is the preferred specimen for morphine assays.

Part B of Table 4 lists the five major drugs tested for in each tissue or physiological fluid and the percent of the total per site. Morphine was the most commonly tested-for drug in the blood, urine, and bile, closely followed by methadone in these same three fluids. Methadone, however, was the most commonly assayed-for drug in all tissues and fluids, possibly representing the large number of methadone treatment programs in the northeastern seaboard cities, New York, Philadelphia, and Washington, D. C. These three cities represented 45% of all drugs reported, and from Table 3 it can be seen that they showed much larger percentages of morphine and methadone than did the other cities combined. The data on phenmetrazine in Table 4 were primarily due to reports by Washington. Part B of Table 4 would hardly be different if only New York, Philadelphia, and Washington were considered.

Table 5 lists the drugs most commonly found, representing more than 90% of the drugs reported. Some drugs were detected by the laboratory more often then they were listed as being involved in the death in another part of the form, indicating that in some instances the presence of a drug in body fluid or tissues was judged not to be a factor in the death.

The first three columns of Table 5 list the number of cases, the type of specimen studied, the mean concentration found, and the standard deviation of the concentration reported for these drugs. The large number of cases and the standard deviations presented in Table 5 add immeasurably to the usefulness of the data, giving a range—for some drugs a rather wide range—of toxic concentrations. This table complements other tabulations of toxic concentrations (*3, 4*).

The remainder of Table 5 gives data on the concentration of only those drugs that were found alone and the concentration of those drugs found in combination with alcohol. With the possible exception of diazepam, methadone, and glutethimide, all the other drugs when present alone show a higher toxic blood concentration than when they are present in combination with ethanol. Such synergism not only involves barbiturates, but also includes a great variety of drugs such as imipramine, amytriptyline, meprobamate, thioridazine, morphine (in blood and bile), propoxyphene, and methaqualone. The decrease in toxic concentration when the drug was present in combination with ethanol was usually considerable; only about half as great a concentration was toxic.

The exceptions noted above, upon further investigation and collection of data, may not really disagree with the trend. Diazepam, for example, appeared in these data in concentrations only slightly greater when in combination with alcohol than when alone, diazepam in combination with alcohol was reported in only five cases, and glutethimide in combination with alcohol in only three. Data on more cases may easily alter the pattern for these two drugs. Methadone is a different story: its concentration in blood when present in combination with ethanol was more than 20-fold that when it was present alone. The standard deviation for this combination is more than three times the mean, indicating a very wide range of results (Table 5). On further inspection of these data, one finds that New York represents 70% of the cases of blood methadone reported, whether alone or in combination. New York, however, did not report assays for methadone in urine. The results for methadone in urine, alone and in combination with alcohol, contrast sharply with the results for blood. For all cities, the mean concentration of methadone in urine when present alone was 10.3 mg/liter (n = 27; SD = 11.9 mg/liter), but when methadone was present in combination with alcohol, the mean was 4.5 mg/liter (n = 13; SD = 2.7 mg/liter). These results for urine imply that ethanol is toxicologically synergistic with methadone and that New York's large influence on the blood data obscures possible synergism in blood. In contrast to the pattern in drug combinations with alcohol, the concentration of a drug in blood when it is present alone or when in combination (Table 5, first six columns) does not seem to follow any clear pattern.

A toxicology proficiency survey was done concurrently with the data collection (*5*). The analysis of the toxicological examinations performed on 2000 drug-involved deaths by the nine participating cities demonstrated a wide interlaboratory variance in the quality of the toxicological examinations from these cities.

In summary, it is clear that definite and potentially significant differences exist in the toxicological examinations performed by the various laboratories to give rise to the disparities noted. Regional psychosocial and biomedical differences have also been found (*6*). A question that must be asked about the interlaboratory toxicological differences in psychoactive drug-involved deaths presented to medicolegal offices is: to what extent are these true differences, representing regional epidemiological differences, and to what extent do these differences represent toxicological, instrumental, and methodological availability or sophistication, personal or forensic laboratory departmental emphasis, personnel training, case load, resource limitations, or other factors? This is a critical question and needs to be considered in interpreting drug-death statistics and related toxicological findings.

Supported in part by a research contract (No. 271-75-3004) from the National Institute on Drug Abuse, ADAMHA, Department of HEW.

References

1. Gottschalk, L. A., McGuire, F. L., Heiser, J. F., and Alexander, P. B., *The Development of a Uniform System for Reporting and Recording Drug-Related Deaths*, vols. I and II. U. S. Dept. of HEW, National Institute of Mental Health. Report on NIMH Contract No. HSM-42-72-139 for the period June 26, 1972–June 25, 1973.

2. Gottschalk, L. A., McGuire, F. L., Dinovo, E. C., et al., *The Investigation and Reporting of Drug-Involved Deaths.* U. S. Dept. of HEW, Alcohol, Drug Abuse, and Mental Health Administration, National Institute on Drug Abuse. Report on NIDA Contract No. HSM-42-72-139 for the period June 26, 1973–June 25, 1975.

3. Niyogi, S. K., Drug levels in cases of poisoning. *Forensic Sci.* **2**, 67 (1973).

4. Baselt, R. C., Wright, J. A., and Cravey, R. H., Therapeutic and toxic concentrations of more than 100 toxicologically significant drugs in blood, plasma, or serum: A tabulation. *Clin. Chem.* **21**, 44 (1975).

5. Dinovo, E. C., and Gottschalk, L. A., Results of a nine-laboratory survey of forensic toxicology proficiency. *Clin. Chem.* **22**, 843 (1976).

6. Gottschalk, L. A., McGuire, F. L., Heiser, J. F., et al., Regional psychosocial and biomedical differences in psychoactive drug-involved deaths in the United States. In preparation, 1976.

CLIN. CHEM. 22/6, 851–855 (1976)

Serum Theophylline Analysis by High-Pressure Liquid Chromatography

Merle A. Evenson and Brenda L. Warren

We have developed and evaluated a rapid, high-pressure liquid-chromatographic method for theophylline in serum. Only 0.2 ml of serum is required for each determination, and the sensitivity of this method is 0.5 mg/liter. This method, involving liquid extraction and silica adsorption chromatography, provides adequate selectivity, accuracy, and precision for routine or research applications. Little sample preparation is required before chromatography. We found no endogenous or exogenous interferences. Use of β-hydroxypropyl theophylline as the internal standard provides reproducible results for this micro-scale method.

Additional Keyphrases: *pediatric chemistry* • *adsorption* • *liquid extraction* • *internal standard* • *drug assay*

Theophylline, a stimulant and an alkaloid naturally occurring in tea leaves, is a drug which produces several pharmacological actions of therapeutic interest. A methylated xanthine (1,3-dimethylxanthine), it stimulates the central nervous system, acts on the kidney to produce diuresis, stimulates cardiac muscle, and relaxes smooth muscles. A most important use is to relax the smooth muscles of the bronchi in the bronchial constriction which occurs in asthma. Treatment with theophylline definitely increases vital capacity of the bronchi (*1–6*).

Slow intravenous injection and a quantitative analytical method for measuring drug concentrations in serum are highly desired to alleviate or minimize the adverse side-effects when theophylline is given intravenously (*1, 7–9*).

As shown by Jenne et al. (*3*), the metabolism of theophylline varies widely in rate, and a therapeutic dose for one patient may be toxic for another.

Therapeutic concentrations in plasma are about 10 mg/liter; concentrations in excess of 20 mg/liter may cause nausea, headache, palpitation, a decrease in blood pressure, and occasionally death (*1, 10, 11*).

Methods described in the literature for measuring theophylline in serum are by ultraviolet spectrophotometry, gas chromatography, and high-pressure liquid chromatography (HPLC). Schack and Waxler (*12*) describe an ultraviolet absorption method in which theophylline was extracted with chloroform and isopropanol, back-extracted with sodium hydroxide, and absorbance measured at 277 nm and 310 nm. The differential readings compensate for the blank. Gupta and Lundberg (*13*) developed a differential spectrophotometric method at 285 nm in which the same extract at two different pH's is used for the sample and reference solutions.

Johnson et al. (*14*) reported a gas-chromatographic procedure in which volatile butyl derivatives of theophylline are prepared and injected into the column. This method separated theophylline from theobromine and phenobarbital, two major interfering substances in classical methods. (*Ed. note:* see also Perrier and Lear, this issue.)

Thompson et al. (*15*) developed an HPLC method for determining theophylline in serum and urine. The procedure involves preliminary separation of the xanthines on Aminex A-5, a cation-exchange resin column. Weinberger and Chidsey (*16*) adapted this method for use with pediatric samples.

Although the above HPLC methods are selective for theophylline, at least 27 min of instrument time is required for each injection.

Sitar et al. (*17*) present an HPLC method for theophylline in plasma, in which a column packed with silica is used. Their method requires 0.5 ml of plasma and at least 35 min of processing time before the evaporation step. Their method requires less than 10 min for chromatography and no interferences were observed. Manion et al. (*18*) describe a HPLC method for 1.0 ml of plasma, with organic phase extraction and chromatography on silica.

We have developed a HPLC method for the analysis of theophylline which requires only 8 min after injection onto the column. A liquid inlet pressure of 17.25 MPa (2500 pounds per square inch) and a flow rate of 0.4 ml/min are used with the column at ambient temperature. We also have eliminated the need for a pre-column by making a chloroform/isopropanol extract of 200 μl of serum (7–8 min processing time before evaporation) and injecting a 5-μl sample of the reconstituted extract. The mobile phase is 6% by vol absolute ethanol and 94% by vol chloroform/heptane/acetic acid mixture, the latter prepared by mixing 300 ml of water-saturated chloroform, 200 ml of heptane, and 400 μl of glacial acetic acid.

Materials and Methods

Equipment and Reagents

All HPLC analyses were performed with a Du Pont

Department of Medicine and the Clinical Toxicology Laboratories, University of Wisconsin Hospitals, Madison, Wis. 53706.
Received Feb. 5, 1976; accepted Mar. 17, 1976.

830 Liquid Chromatograph (Du Pont Instruments, Wilmington, Del. 19898) with a 254-nm ultraviolet detector.

Comparison data were obtained by a modified Schack and Waxler method developed by and used in our service toxicology laboratory, with use of a 402 UV-Visible Spectrophotometer (Perkin-Elmer Corp., Norwalk, Conn. 06856).

A 10-μl syringe (cat. No. 701; Hamilton Co., Reno, Nev. 89504) was used to make injections directly into the column without interruption of flow.

For extractions, we used 15-ml centrifuge tubes with ground glass stoppers. A 200-μl adjustable "Pipetman" pipet (Rainin Instrument Co., Inc., Boston, Mass. 02215) was used for delivery of samples, standards, and controls. Ten-milliliter dispensers (Glenco Scientific, Inc., Houston, Tex. 77007) were used to deliver 8 ml of chloroform/isopropanol (see below) and 1 ml of acetate buffer (5 mol/liter, pH 6.5).

All reagents used were AR grade unless otherwise noted.

A "ZORBAX" SIL 25 cm × 2.1 mm (i.d.) column (Du Pont Instruments) pre-packed with 6–8 μm spherical silica particles was purchased.

Water-saturated chloroform ("Nanograde") was prepared by adding 3.0 ml of distilled water per liter of chloroform and mixing with a magnetic stirrer for 2–3 h. Any undissolved water was aspirated from the top of the chloroform. The water-saturated chloroform was used in preparation of the mobile phase as well as in reconditioning the column.

Methanol and acetone for column reconditioning were prepared by adding 1.0 ml of distilled water per liter with thorough mixing.

Isopropanol, absolute ethanol, and heptane are used without prior treatment or special precautions.

The chloroform/isopropanol used for the extractions is a combination of 20 parts of non-water-saturated chloroform plus 1 part of isopropanol.

The 5 mol/liter acetate buffer was prepared from AR grade anhydrous sodium acetate. The pH was adjusted to 6.5 with 5 mol/liter acetic acid.

"Acetic methanol" (acetic acid/methanol, 5/95 by vol) was used for reconditioning the column.

"Basic methanol" was methanol adjusted to pH 8.0 with sodium hydroxide; it was used for reconditioning the column. (*Care:* a higher pH will cause rapid deterioration of the column packing.)

Standards and Controls

We used crystalline theophylline (cat. No. T1633; Sigma Chemical Co., St. Louis, Mo. 63178), theobromine (No. T-4500, Sigma), caffeine (Sandoz Pharmaceuticals, Hanover, N. J. 07936), and β-hydroxypropyl theophylline (β-HPT; C. H. Boehringer Sohn, Ingelheim im Rhein, West Germany; distributed in the U. S. by Henley and Co., New York, N. Y. 10004).

Stock 200 mg/liter standards of theophylline and β-HPT were prepared in distilled water.

Working standards of theophylline—5, 10, 20, 30, and 40 mg/liter—were prepared from the stock solution by dilution with distilled water.

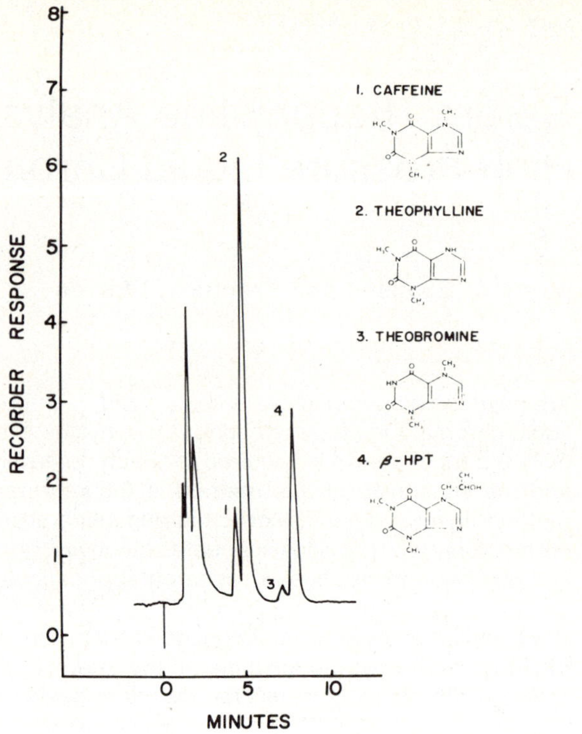

Fig. 1. Extraction of human serum sample containing caffeine (*1*), theophylline (*2*), theobromine (*3*), and β-HPT (*4*)
Full-scale recorder response represents a scale expansion of 8×10^{-2} *A*. The theophylline (peak *2*) represents a 40 mg/liter concentration in serum. Chart speed, 0.2 inches/min

A 30 mg/liter working standard of β-HPT was prepared from the stock solution and diluted with distilled water. Used as an internal standard, this is taken through the extraction procedure during sample preparation.

Extraction and Procedure

The sample is prepared as follows: Extract 200 μl of human serum samples, standards, or controls in the presence of the acetate buffer into chloroform/isopropanol. Evaporate 5 ml of the chloroform/isopropanol extract, redissolve in 50 μl of chloroform, and inject 5 μl onto the column. From the recorder chart, obtain peak-height measurements for theophylline and β-HPT and calculate the ratio of theophylline to β-HPT. Plot ratios for the standards and calculate sample values from the working curve (Figure 1).

The extraction is done as follows: Deliver 1.0 ml of acetate buffer at pH 6.5 into each 15-ml centrifuge tube. With the Pipetman pipet, deliver 0.2 ml of the 30 mg/liter β-HPT internal standard into each tube, followed by 0.2 ml of drug-free plasma pool. Pipet 0.2 ml of each standard solution into separate tubes and add the internal standard and the drug-free plasma pool. Deliver 0.2 ml of control pool, serum samples, and internal standard into the respective control and sample tubes. Vortex-mix each tube 2–3 s to thoroughly mix the buffered aqueous phases. Deliver 8.0 ml of chloroform/isopropanol into each tube and insert the ground-glass stopper. Vortex-mix each tube for 20 s,

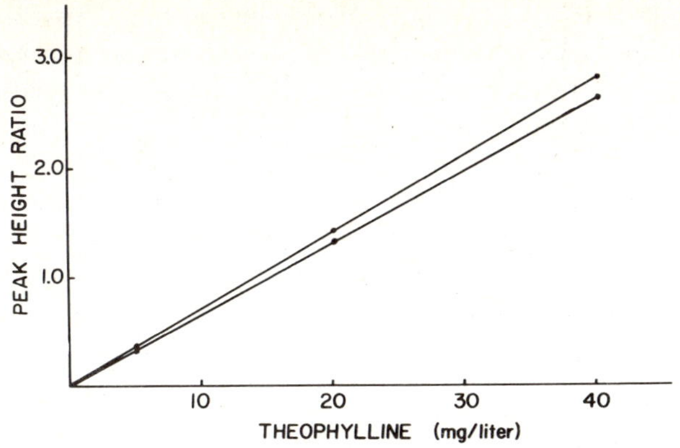

Fig. 2. Theophylline standard curves obtained for the present method on different days, showing the change in sensitivity

then centrifuge for 5 min. Aspirate and discard the aqueous (top) layer from each tube, transfer 5.0 ml of the organic extract into thin-walled tubes, and evaporate it in a 60 °C water bath with dry air turbulence. Stopper the tubes until ready to inject the samples. Immediately before injection, pipet 50 μl of chloroform into the residue in the tube, stopper, and vortex-mix to reconstitute. With the Hamilton syringe, remove 5 μl of the reconstituted extract and inject it onto the column.

Buffers of pH 4.0, 6.5, and 8.0 were examined; the pH 6.5 buffer extracted the most theophylline: about 5% more than at pH 4.0 and about 20% more than at pH 8.0. The extraction coefficient doubled when isopropanol was added to the chloroform as compared to extracting with chloroform alone. We used the proportions of 20:1 for chloroform and isopropanol; proportions of 2:1 and 50:1 gave insignificant differences. About 90% of the theophylline is extracted by our protocol from either serum or aqueous standards.

Vortex-mixing times of 20 s, and 1, 2, and 4 min were evaluated; extraction was as complete in 20 s as in 4 min.

Results

Precision and Accuracy

A standard curve (theophylline, 5, 20, 40 mg/liter) was prepared with each set of extractions. The maximum variation in sensitivity observed is shown with the standard working curves in Figure 2. These curves were obtained on different days and represent the extremes in sensitivity changes. As a column ages, sensitivity decreases and the retention time increases. The intercept of the standard working curve will move up the y axis.

Within-run precision (Table 1) was determined on 10 separate extractions of 5 and 20 mg of theophylline per liter of serum. A non-serum-based standard in chloroform was also analyzed for within-run precision. The within-run coefficient of variation (CV) is 2.82% for 5 mg/liter and 1.04% for 20 mg/liter in serum. The CV for the 30 mg/liter theophylline in chloroform standard is 1.07%.

Between-run precision was established on two drug-free plasma pools. Theophylline had been added to concentrations of 10 and 20 mg/liter, respectively. Five-milliliter aliquots were frozen and a new tube of pool was used for each set of extractions. Between-run precision was also established for a 10 mg/liter standard.

A typical set of extractions includes the three standards, the two pooled plasma samples, and the human serum samples.

Table 1. Precision of HPLC

Within-run	5 mg/liter serum	20 mg/liter serum	30 mg/liter $CHCl_3$
n	10	10	10
$\bar{X}$	5.2	20.1	30.5
1 SD	0.14	0.21	0.32
CV	2.82%	1.04%	1.07%
Between-run	**Pool A (10 mg/liter)**	**Pool B (20 mg/liter)**	**10 mg/liter aqueous**
n	26	26	10
$\bar{X}$	9.17	18.18	9.76
1 SD	0.49	0.64	0.29
CV	5.34%	3.52%	2.97%

Table 2. Analytical Recovery of Theophylline in Sera

Already in serum, mg/liter	Plus theophylline 10 mg/liter		20 mg/liter	
8.6 ± 0.5	18.2 ± 0.6	96%	30 ± 1	107%
8.8 ± 0.5	18.6 ± 0.6	98%	29 ± 1	101%
13.6 ± 0.7	23.8 ± 0.8	102%	33 ± 1	97%
6.6 ± 0.4	16.6 ± 0.6	100%	26.4 ± 0.9	99%
12.2 ± 0.7	21.8 ± 0.8	96%	32 ± 1	99%
11.0 ± 0.6	20.8 ± 0.7	98%	31 ± 1	100%
$\bar{X}$ =		98.3%		100.5%
	5 mg/liter		**10 mg/liter**	
17.0 ± 0.6	21.8 ± 0.8	96%	26.8 ± 0.9	98%
17.4 ± 0.6	22.6 ± 0.8	104%	28 ± 1	106%
23.0 ± 0.8	28 ± 1	100%	33 ± 1	100%
20.0 ± 0.7	24.6 ± 0.9	92%	30 ± 1	100%
18.8 ± 0.6	23.6 ± 0.8	96%	28 ± 1	92%
19.4 ± 0.7	24.2 ± 0.9	96%	29 ± 1	96%
$\bar{X}$ =		97.3%		98.7%

Interferences

A known negative serum blank shows peaks of less than 1% of full scale in the theophylline and β-HPT areas. Occasionally serum blanks with peaks with a re-

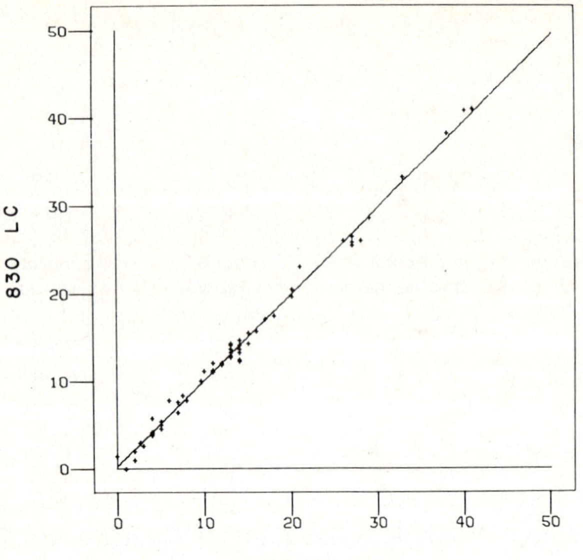

Fig. 3. Theophylline as measured by the present method vs. the spectrophotometric method
Units are mg/liter

tention time like that of theobromine of up to 5% full scale will be observed, but this is of no consequence for this method.

The following drugs produce no peaks in the time interval from the caffeine peak (3.00 min) to the β-HPT peak (9.25 min): phenobarbital, diazepam, chlorpromazine, acetazolamide, furosemide, chlordiazepoxide, uric acid, 8-chlorotheophylline and dihydroxytheophylline. A peak for chloramphenicol has a retention time of 6.25 min, between theophylline (5.50 min) and theobromine (8.50 min), but does not interfere with either. Serum samples were analyzed before and after hemolysis and before and after addition of bilirubin; in neither case was the value obtained statistically different.

To evaluate the accuracy of the method we performed a series of standard addition (analytical recovery) studies. Two groups of serum samples were obtained, one with values near 10 mg/liter and another with values near 20 mg/liter. Each sample was individually analyzed with and without theophylline added. The sera with values near 10 mg/liter had added 10 and 20 mg/liter; the 20 mg/liter group had added 5 and 10 mg of theophylline per liter. Table 2 gives the recovery data. For the first group the recovery of added theophylline was 98.3% for the 10 mg/liter addition and 100.5% for the 20 mg/liter addition. For the second group the recovery was 97.3% for 5 mg/liter addition, 98.7% for the 10 mg/liter addition. Theophylline in the serum is evidently analytically indistinguishable from added theophylline.

We compared results for theophylline in human sera as measured by the HPLC and the spectrophotometric method. The data were obtained during seven months, with no more than 5 samples being analyzed each day. Duplicate extractions were conducted for the HPLC method, single analyses were done by the other method.

The spectrophotometric method is in routine use and is adequate for samples without interferences. These interferences are usually apparent from the spectra obtained. There are interferences with many samples, and this prompted us to develop the more specific present method.

The following statistical summary of the 56 comparisons and Figure 3 illustrate the comparison data for the individual samples. The values ranged from 0.0 to 41 mg/liter and the samples included specimens that were icteric, hemolyzed, or lipemic. The slope is 0.983, the y-intercept 0.278, Student's t-test value is 0.413, the bias is 0.049, and the correlation coefficient is 0.995.

Discussion

Our method is accurate, precise, and rapid. It has several advantages over other HPLC methods: only 0.2 ml of serum is needed, sample-processing time is shorter, water-based rather than serum-based standards are used along with an internal standard, and we have found no interferences after seven months during which we analyzed more than 50 sera from a hospital population. Recovery studies indicate that the HPLC method is accurate. Moreover, in separate experiments, we determined that the signal obtained when the complete sample preparation protocol is followed is about 90% of that obtained with a direct injection of a standard solution. Precision is excellent, as shown by the within-run and between-run precision data.

Concentration and peak height are linearly related between 5 to 40 mg/liter, which amply covers the range of values found in hospital populations, but drops off rapidly between 40 and 50 mg/liter. Although sensitivity changes slightly from day to day, this is unimportant because a standard curve with an internal standard is established with each group of extractions.

Because of interferences commonly occurring with our present spectrophotometric method for theophylline, the comparisons were performed on sera samples which gave no obvious interferences by that method. Such screening will bias the comparison data. Evaluation of the comparison data shows that the two methods correlate quite well. The Student's t-test value at the 95% confidence level when n is 25 is 2.06. For our method, 56 values were compared and gave a t-test value of 0.413. Thus there are considerably fewer than 5 chances in 100 that the difference between the values obtained by the two methods is statistically significant. The correlation coefficient gives an estimate of the reliability with which results of the two methods may be compared. In each instance when the spectrophotometric method gave higher results than the HPLC method, extraneous peaks occurred. These extra peaks were resolved and did not interfere with quantitation but did interfere with the spectrophotometric method.

A disadvantage of this HPLC method is the useful lifetime and the rate of deterioration of the column. This usefulness was extended by injecting acid methanol onto the column at the beginning of each day, or, with much use, every 4 h or after every 20 to 25 injections. Therefore, from our experience it is best to prepare not more than 25 extractions at one time.

Periodic reconditioning of the column was necessary after about every 200 to 250 injections. Reconditioning consisted of about 30 min pumping time for each of the following, in the sequence presented: water-saturated chloroform, acetone, methanol, water, methanol, acetone, and water-saturated chloroform. Following this sequence the mobile phase is pumped through the column for about 4 h or overnight. Indications that reconditioning is necessary are shown by increased peak widths, decreased sensitivity, and a non-zero intercept on the standard curve. We have been able to recondition the column twice after the initial conditioning but a third conditioning has not been successful.

Proportions of the mobile phase are critical to the separation, sensitivity, and retention time of the peaks. Ethanol has the most pronounced effect on the characteristics of the peaks. It is stored in the secondary reservoir under nitrogen. The primary reservoir contains the chloroform, heptane, and acetic acid mixture. By changing the proportioning potentiometer, the percentage of ethanol in the mobile phase can be altered. Increasing the percentage of ethanol will increase the sensitivity, shorten the retention time, and decrease the resolution. Increasing the concentration of heptane substantially above that suggested will decrease resolution. On the other hand, with no heptane, theophylline and theobromine peaks have nearly the same retention times. The acetic acid is added to increase sensitivity. However, too much acetic acid will result in an unstable baseline. The optimum proportions of the primary reservoir solutions are water-saturated chloroform, 300 ml; heptane, 200 ml; and acetic acid, 400 μl. The optimum mobile phase contains 6% of the secondary reservoir (ethanol) and 94% of the primary reservoir (chloroform/heptane/acetic acid).

For reproducible activity of the silica surface, it is necessary to use a water-containing mobile phase. Snyder and Kirkland (*19*) describe a convenient and reproducible method for adjusting the water content of nonpolar solvents. They recommend use of about 50% water-saturated mobile phase. By diluting the water-saturated chloroform with 200 ml heptane, we have attained a 60% water-saturated solution.

The available scale expansion is 80-fold that we are using. Thus the detection limit when the noise is low is a function of the scale expansion and the volumes of sample and organic phases used. We therefore believe that, realistically, the lower limit of detection for the scale expansion used here and the method discussed is 0.50 mg/liter.

In summary, this HPLC method for theophylline, like others in which organic phase extractions and adsorption chromatography on silica are used (*17, 19*), shows no endogenous or exogenous interfering substances. Further, this method has adequate linearity, precision, and accuracy in serum for the concentration range from 5 to 40 mg/liter. The high sensitivity allows the method to be useful for micro-scale samples usually obtained from pediatric patients.

We thank Gary Lensmeyer, Michael Poquette, and Sherry Burney for the theophylline comparison data for the spectrophotometric method; Henley and Co. for supplying the β-hydroxypropyl theophylline, 8-chlorotheophylline, and dihydroxytheophylline used in this method development; and the Clinical Chemistry Laboratory for supplying the statistical analysis of the comparison data. Loan of the Du Pont Model 830 high-pressure liquid chromatograph from the Instrument Products Division, E. I. du Pont de Nemours and Co. (Inc.), Wilmington, Del. 19898, is gratefully acknowledged.

References

1. Goodman, L. S., and Gilman, A., *The Pharmacological Basis of Therapeutics*. 4th ed., Macmillan Co., New York, N. Y., 1970.

2. Cornish, H. H., and Christman, A. A., A study of the metabolism of theobromine, theophylline and caffeine in men. *J. Biol. Chem.* **288,** 315 (1959).

3. Jenne, J. W., Wyze, E., Rood, F. S., and MacDonald, F. M., Pharmacokinetics of theophylline. *Clin. Pharmacol. Ther.* **13,** 349 (1972).

4. Kern, H., Schilling, P., and Muller, S. H., *Gas Chromatographic Analysis of Pharmaceuticals and Drugs.* Varian Instrument Division, Park Ridge, Ill., 1968.

5. Dorfman, L. J., and Jarvik, M. E., Comparative stimulant and diuretic actions of caffeine and theobromine in man. *Clin. Pharmacol. Ther.* **11,** 869 (1970).

6. Ehret, C. F., Potter, V. R., and Dobra, K. W., Chronotypic action of theophylline and of pentobarbital as circadian zeitgebers in the rat. *Science* **188,** 1212 (1975).

7. Mitenko, P. A., and Ogilvie, R. I., Rapidly achieved plasma concentration plateaus, with observations on theophylline kinetics. *Clin. Pharmacol. Ther.* **13,** 329 (1971).

8. Intravenous aminophylline. *Lancet* **ii,** 950 (1973). Editorial.

9. Zwillich, C. W., Sutton, F. D., Neff, T. A., *et al.,* Theophylline induced seizures in adults. *Ann. Intern. Med.* **82,** 784 (1975).

10. Levy, G., Ellis, E. F., and Koysooko, R., Indirect plasma theophylline monitoring in asthmatic children by determination of theophylline concentration in saliva. *Pediatrics* **53,** 873 (1974).

11. Clarke, E. G., *Isolation and Identification of Drugs.* The Pharmaceutical Press, London, England, 1969.

12. Schack, J. A., and Waxler, S. H., An ultraviolet spectrophotometric method for the determination of theophylline and theobromine in blood and tissues. *J. Pharmacol. Exp. Ther.* **97,** 283 (1949).

13. Gupta, R. C., and Lundberg, G. D., Quantitative determination of theophylline in blood by differential spectrophotometry. *Anal. Chem.* **45,** 2403 (1973).

14. Johnson, G. F., Dechtiaruk, W. A., and Solomon, H. M., Gas chromatographic determination of theophylline in human serum and saliva. *Clin. Chem.* **21,** 144 (1974).

15. Thompson, R. D., Nagasawa, H. T., and Jenne, J. W., Determination of theophylline and its metabolites in human urine and serum by high-pressure liquid chromatography. *J. Lab. Clin. Med.* **84,** 584 (1974).

16. Weinberger, M., and Chidsey, C., Rapid analysis for theophylline in serum by use of high-pressure cation-exchange chromatography. *Clin. Chem.* **21,** 834 (1975).

17. Sitar, D. S., Piafsky, K. M., Rangno, R. E., and Ogilvie, R. I., Plasma theophylline concentrations measured by high-pressure liquid chromatography. *Clin. Chem.* **21,** 1774 (1975).

18. Manion, C. V., Shoeman, D. W., and Azarnoff, D. L., High pressure liquid chromatographic assay of theophylline in biological fluids. *J. Chromatogr.* **101,** 169 (1974).

19. Snyder, L. R., and Kirkland, J. J., *Modern Liquid Chromatography.* Wiley-Interscience, New York, N. Y., 1974.

CLIN. CHEM. 22/6, 856–859 (1976)

Rapid Micromethod for Measuring Anticonvulsant Drugs in Serum by High-Performance Liquid Chromatography

S. J. Soldin and J. Gilbert Hill

We describe an assay system for measuring phenobarbital, diphenylhydantoin, primidone, ethosuximide, and carbamazepine in 25 μl of serum. The procedure involves precipitation of proteins with an acetonitrile solution containing cyheptamide as an internal standard, and reverse-phase chromatography on a 4 mm × 30 cm column containing "μBondapak C18." The anticonvulsants are eluted with an equivolume mixture of potassium phosphate buffer (10 mmol/liter, pH 8.0) and acetonitrile at a flow rate of 0.8 ml/min, detected by their absorbance at 200 nm, and quantitated by measuring peak areas. When measurement of primidone is not required, a 254-nm detector may be used. Each analysis requires 10 min. Optimum column temperature has been found to decrease with use. Analytical recoveries for the five drugs varied from 92% to 102% with good precision (coefficients of variation between 2.8% and 8.2% for therapeutic and toxic concentrations). The results obtained with this method compare favorably with results obtained by gas–liquid chromatography (correlation coefficients between 0.77 and 0.98). In over 1300 patients' samples analyzed to date, the only drugs known to have interfered with the assay are gentamicin, diazoxide, and mephobarbital.

Additional Keyphrases: *reverse-phase chromatography • fast, small-sample simultaneous analysis • pediatric chemistry*

The ideal procedure for assay of anticonvulsant drugs will be one that provides for the reliable, rapid, economical quantitation, in a micro-scale sample, of all of the commonly used anticonvulsant drugs. The frequency with which new methods for these assays are published indicates the high degree of interest in achieving this goal, but it has not yet been reached.

Gas–liquid chromatographic analysis (GLC) of anticonvulsant drugs requires a relatively large sample (frequently as much as 1 ml) and a significant amount of time on sample clean-up and derivatization. In addition, no single set of analytical conditions has as yet been described that is suitable for more than four of the common anticonvulsant drugs.

Enzyme immunoassays are rapid and are applicable to micro-scale samples, but have the disadvantage of relatively high cost, and the limitation of requiring separate assay systems for each drug.

Service Division, Department of Biochemistry, The Hospital For Sick Children, and Department of Clinical Biochemistry, University of Toronto, Toronto, Canada.

Received Mar. 1, 1976; accepted Mar. 17, 1976.

The use of high-performance liquid chromatography (HPLC) for the analysis of anticonvulsant drugs has been reported in a number of recent publications. However, the method for phenobarbital and diphenylhydantoin described by Atwell et al. (*1*) and Evans (*2*) require extensive sample preparation before chromatography, and the method described by Gauchel et al. (*3*) has been applied only to the assay of carbamazepine. More recently, Adams and Vandemark (*4*) described the use of reverse-phase HPLC for measurement of anticonvulsant drugs in 0.5 ml of serum. With their method, six different drugs can be measured simultaneously, but sample preparation involves many time-consuming steps that apparently contribute to poor recoveries.

In contrast, the HPLC method we describe can be performed on 25 μl of plasma, requires minimal sample work-up, provides almost complete analytical recovery of phenobarbital, primidone, ethosuximide, diphenylhydantoin, and carbamazepine, and requires only 10 min for completion.

Materials and Methods

Apparatus. Throughout these studies we used a high-performance liquid chromatograph, Model ALC/GPC-204/6000 A, with a Model U6P injection system, and a 4 mm × 30 cm "μBondapak C-18" column mounted in a temperature control block (cat. No. 27486), all from Waters Associates, Inc., Milford, Mass. 07157. The detector was a Waters Model 440 with 254-nm wavelength kit, or the Model LC55 variable-wavelength spectrophotometer (Perkin-Elmer Corp., Norwalk, Conn. 06856). The recorder was a Honeywell Electronic Model 196 (Honeywell Inc., Fort Washington, Pa. 19034) equipped with an Autolab Minigrator (Spectra-Physics, Santa Clara, Calif. 95051).

Reagents. We obtained acetonitrile, methanol, and dimethyl sulfoxide from Burdick and Jackson, and standards from Applied Science Laboratories (phenobarbital), Parke–Davis (diphenylhydantoin and ethosuximide), Ayerst Laboratories (primidone and cyheptamide), and Geigy (carbamazepine).

Procedures

Procedure 200 (applicable to all five drugs, uses 200-nm detector). Add 25 μl of acetonitrile containing 0.3 μg of cyheptamide (as an internal standard) to 25 μl of serum or plasma in a 6 × 50 mm glass test tube.

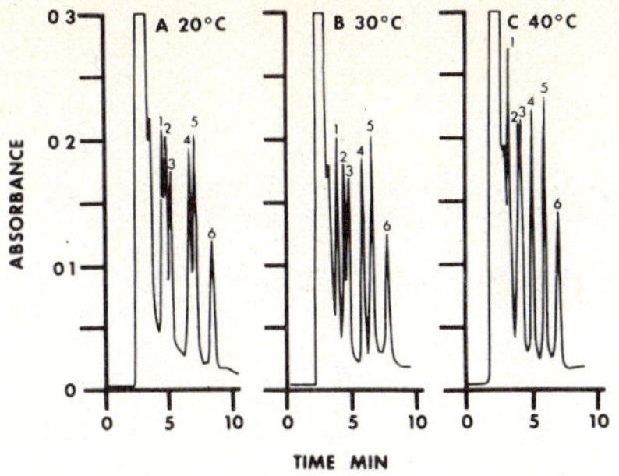

Fig. 1. Effect of temperature on the resolution of anticonvulsant drugs by procedure 200

The plasma specimen analyzed contained, per liter, 21.6 mg of phenobarbital (*1*), 32.9 mg of primidone (*2*), 32.7 mg of ethosuximide (*3*), 19.8 mg of diphenylhydantoin (*4*), and 39.1 mg of carbamazepine (*5*). Peak *6* represents the internal standard

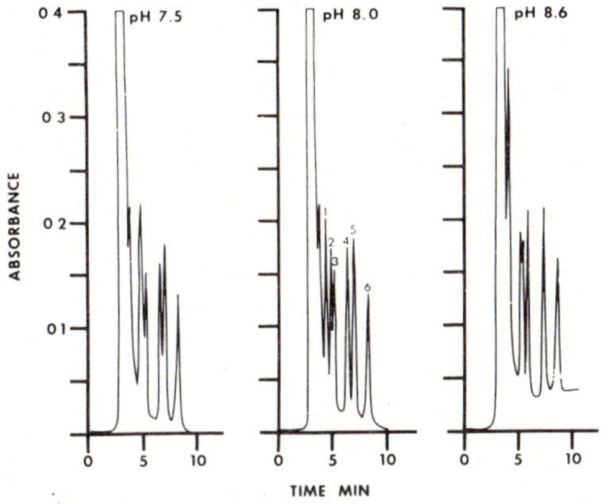

Fig. 2. Effect of pH on the resolution of anticonvulsant drugs for procedure 200

The plasma specimen analyzed contained, per liter, 21.6 mg of phenobarbital (*1*), 32.9 mg of primidone (*2*), 32.7 mg of ethosuximide (*3*), 19.8 mg of diphenylhydantoin (*4*), and 39.1 mg of carbamazepine (*5*). Peak *6* represents the internal standard

Vortex-mix the mixture for 30 s, then centrifuge for 1 min. Inject about 3 μl of the supernate directly into the chromatograph and elute with an equal-volume mixture of potassium phosphate buffer (10 mmol/liter, pH 8.0) and acetonitrile, at a flow rate of 0.8 ml/min. Detector sensitivity setting should be 0.05 *A* full scale.

Procedure 254 (applicable if measurement of primidone is not required). Procedure 254 is identical to procedure 200, except that the amount of internal standard in the original acetonitrile is 4.1 μg in 25 μl, and a 254-nm detector is used. The detector sensitivity setting should be 0.01 *A* full scale.

Peaks on the chromatogram are identified on the basis of their retention times relative to the internal standard. Drug concentrations are calculated from the peak areas according to the formula:

$$\text{Concentration of drug} = (\text{peak area for drug}/\text{peak area for internal standard}) \times (1/\text{R.R}) \times \text{concentration of internal standard}$$

where R.R. equals relative response (in terms of peak area) of drug compared to an equal amount of internal standard.

Table 1. Relative Response of Drugs Compared with Internal Standard

	Detector wavelength	
Drug	254 nm	200 nm
Phenobarbital	8.86	0.57
Primidone	0.42	0.34
Ethosuximide	0.47	0.39
Diphenylhydantoin	2.48	0.86
Carbamazepine	20.48	0.51
Cyheptamide	1.00	1.00

Table 2. Precision and Relative Recovery Studies for Measurement of Anticonvulsant Drugs in Plasma

Within-day precision by replicate analysis			Between-day precision and relative recoveries by replicate analysis			
n	Concn, mg/liter	CV, %	n	Concn, mg/liter	CV, %	Mean rel. recov., %
			Phenobarbital			
10	9.3	8.2	10	10.8	8.6	92
10	18.7	4.7	10	21.6	11.1	95
10	66.2	2.8	10	64.9	6.4	100
			Primidone			
10	14.1	6.3	10	16.4	8.8	99
10	28.7	5.2				
			Ethosuximide			
10	32.1	5.4	10	32.7	12.2	97
10	104.5	3.5	10	98.1	12.8	97
			Dilantin			
10	9.1	5.6	10	9.9	8.1	96
10	18.9	5.1	10	19.8	7.9	102
10	63.3	3.1	10	59.4	8.3	96
			Carbamazepine			
10	22.5	7.0	10	19.6	9.0	98

Table 3. Analytical Recovery of Drugs Added to Plasma

Drug	Concn, mg/liter	Mean recovery, % (n = 5)
Phenobarbital	15.8	84
Primidone	14.2	80
Ethosuximide	31.2	83
Diphenylhydantoin	10.9	93
Carbamazepine	10.9	88
Cyheptamide	11.2	94

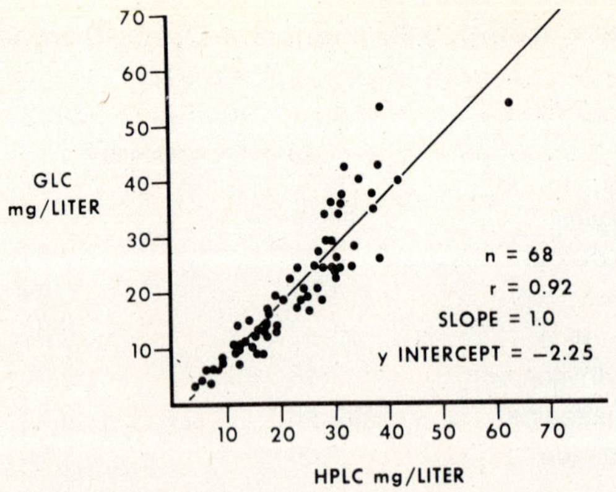

Fig. 3. Comparison of the HPLC method with the GLC method for phenobarbital

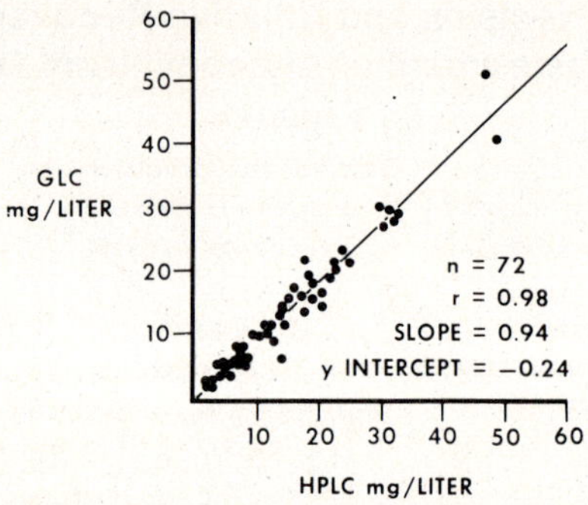

Fig. 4. Comparison of the HPLC method with the GLC method for diphenylhydantoin

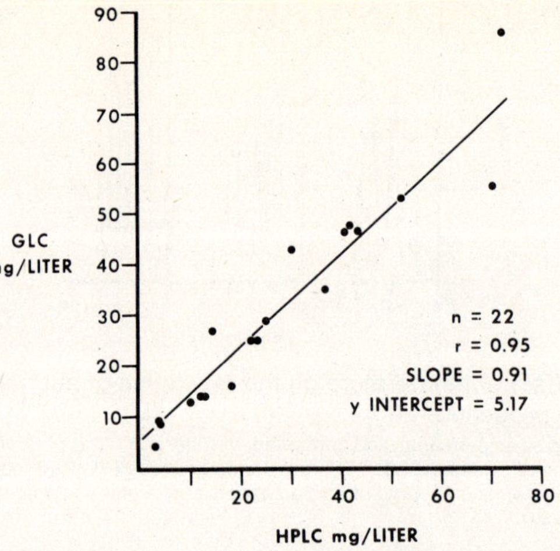

Fig. 5. Comparison of the HPLC method with the GLC method for ethosuximide

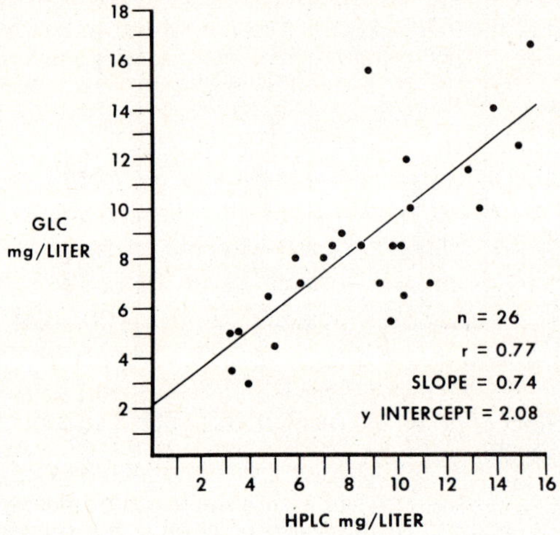

Fig. 6. Comparison of the HPLC method with the GLC method for primidone

The μBondapak columns are washed daily with methanol, and weekly with acetonitrile and dimethylsulfoxide. Under the conditions described, a column may be used for about 1200 analyses before requiring replacement.

Results and Discussion

Analytical Variables

Detector wavelength. Solutions of primidone and ethosuximide absorb well at 200 nm, but poorly at 254 nm, so that maximum sensitivity for the analysis of these two drugs is provided by the use of a 200-nm detector. In practice, however, the concentration of ethosuximide is usually high enough to permit its measurement at either 200 nm or 254 nm. Phenobarbital, diphenylhydantoin, and carbamazepine absorb well at both of these wavelengths, so that either detector may be used for their measurement.

Column temperature. With a new column, optimum separation of these drugs was observed at 30 °C (Figure 1). Decreasing the temperature improves the primidone–ethosuximide separation, but worsens the phenobarbital–primidone separation, whereas increasing the temperature has the opposite effect. With use and loss of resolving power a lower column temperature is required to provide adequate separation of the primidone–ethosuximide pair.

Composition of eluent. Satisfactory separation of the five anticonvulsant drugs was obtained only when the phosphate buffer component of the eluent had a pH of between 7.8 and 8.1, and the ratio of buffer to acetonitrile was one (Figure 2).

Method of Calculation

By taking known amounts of the five drugs and the internal standard through the procedure we demonstrated a linear relationship between peak area and drug concentration over a concentration range far in excess of that required for clinical purposes. In addition, by dividing the peak area for a known amount of each drug by the peak area for an equal amount of the internal standard, we established the relative response factors used in final calculations (Table 1).

Precision

We assessed the precision of the method by repeated analyses (procedure 200) of plasma specimens containing therapeutic and toxic concentrations of the drugs being investigated. As shown in Table 2, within-

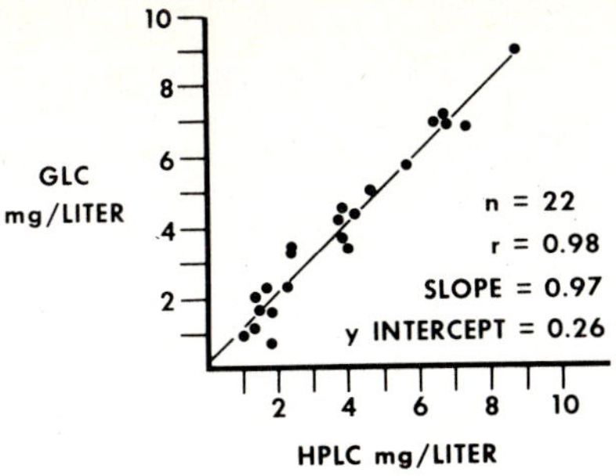

Fig. 7. Comparison of the HPLC method with the GLC method for carbamazepine

day precision varied between 2.8% and 8.2%, between-day precision between 6.4% and 12.8%. The same experiment, repeated with procedure 254, gave very similar results. These values are acceptable for most clinical purposes, and compare well with previously reported values obtained with GLC (*5–7*) and HPLC (*4*).

Accuracy

We measured the absolute recovery from plasma of the five drugs and the internal standard in the following way. The six compounds were added to drug-free plasma to achieve the concentrations shown in Table 3. This plasma was then analyzed by procedure 200, except that the acetonitrile used to precipitate protein did not contain cyheptamide. Carefully measured aliquots of the supernate were then chromatographed and the peak areas determined. Percentage recovery was calculated by comparing these peak areas with the peak areas obtained by the direct injection of the pure compounds. As shown in Table 3, absolute analytical recoveries of the drugs ranged from 80% for primidone to 93% for diphenylhydantoin. The absolute recovery of cyheptamide was 94%. The same experiment with procedure 254 yielded similar results. In Table 2 we have shown that the relative recoveries of the five drugs at therapeutic and toxic concentrations vary between 92% and 102%. These results confirm that cyheptamide is a suitable internal standard in this assay system.

Accuracy was further evaluated by analyzing a series of patients' specimens by GLC (*8–10*) and the proposed HPLC system, and comparing results. For these comparisons, procedure 200 was used for specimens containing primidone, and procedure 254 was used for all others. As may be seen in Figures 3–7, the correlation coefficients varied between 0.77 and 0.98. The relatively poor correlation between GLC and HPLC for primidone is not yet explained, but in view of the precision and recovery data shown in Tables 2 and 3, we speculate that the differences may be attributable to deficiencies in the GLC method rather than the HPLC method.

Drug Interference

Although no systematic analysis of drugs that might interfere with the procedure has been undertaken, we have processed over 1300 patients' specimens and the only interfering drugs found to date are gentamicin, diazoxide, and mephobarbital. In uremic patients the diphenylhydantoin metabolite 5-(*p*-hydroxyphenyl)-5-phenylhydantoin will interfere with the analysis of primidone and ethosuximide, causing falsely high values.

GLC/HPLC comparison studies were made possible through the kind cooperation of Dr. A. L. Sherwin of the Montreal Neurological Institute, Montreal (for carbamazepine), and Dr. J. A. Lowden, Research Institute, The Hospital For Sick Children, Toronto (for diphenylhydantoin, phenobarbital, primidone and ethosuximide). The skilled technical assistance of Mrs. T. Gero is gratefully acknowledged.

References

1. Atwell, S. H., Green, V. A., and Haney, W. G., Development and evaluation of method for simultaneous determination of phenobarbital and diphenylhydantoin in plasma by high-pressure liquid chromatography. *J. Pharm. Sci.* **64,** 806 (1975).

2. Evans, J. E., Simultaneous measurement of diphenylhydantoin and phenobarbital in serum by high performance liquid chromatography. *Anal. Chem.* **45,** 2428 (1973).

3. Gauchel, G., Gauchel, F. D., and Birkofer, L., A. micromethod for the determination of carbamazepine in blood by high speed liquid chromatography. *Z. Klin. Chem. Klin. Biochem.* **11,** 459 (1973).

4. Adams, R. F., and Vandemark, F. L., Simultaneous high-pressure liquid-chromatographic determination of some anticonvulsants in serum. *Clin. Chem.* **22,** 25 (1976).

5. Least, C. J., Jr., Johnson, G. F., and Solomon, H. M., Therapeutic monitoring of anticonvulsant drugs: Gas-chromatographic simultaneous determination of primidone, phenylethylmalonamide, carbamazepine and diphenylhydantoin. *Clin. Chem.* **21,** 1658 (1975).

6. Booker, H. E., and Darcey, B. A., Enzymatic immunoassay vs. gas/liquid chromatography for determination of phenobarbital and diphenylhydantoin in serum. *Clin. Chem.* **21,** 1766 (1975).

7. Ritz, D. P., and Warren, C. G., Single extraction GLC analysis of six commonly prescribed antiepileptic drugs. *Clin. Toxicol.* **8,** 311 (1975).

8. MacGee, J., Rapid identification and quantitative determination of barbiturates and glutethimide in blood by gas-liquid chromatography. *Clin. Chem.* **17,** 587 (1971).

9. Sherwin, A. L., Eisen, A. A., and Sokolowski, C. D., Anticonvulsant drugs in human epileptogenic brain. *Arch. Neurol.* (Chicago) **29,** 73 (1973).

10. Wilensky, A. J., and Lowden, J. A., Inadequate serum levels after intramuscular administration of diphenylhydantoin. *Neurology* **23,** 318 (1973).

CLIN. CHEM. 22/6, 860-862 (1976)

Rapid Gas-Chromatographic Measurement of Anticonvulsant Drugs in Serum

Floyd Dorrity, Jr.[1,3] and Markku Linnoila[2]

We describe a rapid method for precisely measuring concentrations of anticonvulsant drugs in serum. The simple procedure, adaptable to the clinical laboratory, can be used for the routine simultaneous measurement in sera of phenobarbital, primidone, dephenylhydantoin, and (or) ethosuximide. The extraction procedure requires no solvent evaporation and gives a good yield for primidone and quantitative extraction for the other drugs. The relatively small amount of "early phenobarbital" formed during on-column methylation permits a precise analysis of phenobarbital based on a single peak. Results can be made available directly, without manual measurements or calculations.

Methods in which concentrated trimethylanilinium hydroxide or tetramethylammonium hydroxide are used to extract anticonvulsant drugs, as proposed by MacGee for diphenylhydantoin (*1*), eliminate the need for solvent evaporation and offer a rapid and simple analysis, but usually lack sensitivity or precision for phenobarbital and primidone. Recently, Joern (*2*) reported that extraction with an equivolume mixture of diethyl ether and toluene results in an improved recovery of primidone from serum.

We have used a similar solvent mixture, ether/toluene (3/7 by vol), to determine values for more than 5000 patients' sera since January 1974. Our experience indicates that the use of this mixed solvent improves the extraction efficiency for ethosuximide, phenobarbital, and primidone over that obtained with toluene alone. There is no difference between the extraction efficiencies obtained with 3/7 (by vol) and 1/1 (by vol) ether/toluene mixtures.

[1] Laboratory Service, Veterans Administration Hospital, Durham, N. C. 27710.

[2] Department of Psychiatry, Duke University Medical Center, Durham, N. C. 27710.

[3] Mr. Dorrity's current address is: Department of Psychiatry and Clinical Chemistry Laboratory, Duke University Medical Center, Durham, N. C. 27710.

Received Dec. 23, 1975; accepted Mar. 21, 1976.

Our extraction procedure differs from that reported by Joern in the ionic strength of the NaH_2PO_4 used to buffer the serum. We achieve a 57% extraction of primidone with 3 mol/liter buffer, but only 43% extraction with 1 mol/liter buffer. The larger peak area obtained by using the more concentrated buffer permits more precise quantitation of primidone.

We markedly improved the precision of phenobarbital analysis by minimizing the degradation of phenobarbital during flash-heater methylation. A single large *N,N*-dimethylphenobarbital peak permits quantitation that is simpler and more precise than by other methods.

Materials and Methods

Extraction Procedure

One milliliter of serum, 1 ml of 3 mol/liter NaH_2PO_4 dissolved in methanol/water (1/9 by vol), and 10 ml of ether/toluene (3/7 by vol) containing 2.50 μg of 5-(4-methylphenyl)-5-phenylhydantoin per milliliter as an internal standard are placed in a 15-ml, glass-stoppered, round-bottom tube. The mixture is shaken vigorously by hand for 30 s, then centrifuged (1000 × *g*, 2 min).

After centrifugation, about 9 ml of the organic (upper) phase is decanted into a 12-ml, glass-stoppered, conical tube. Fifty microliters of 2 mol/liter tetramethylammonium hydroxide in methanol (Southwestern Analytical Chemicals, Inc., Austin, Tex.) is added and the tube is shaken and centrifuged as described above.

After centrifugation, the ether/toluene (upper) layer is aspirated. The last traces of the solvent are carefully aspirated from the interface. Fifty microliters of methanol is added to the remaining tetramethylammonium hydroxide (approximately 20 μl) and the tube is agitated briefly by hand. Most of the diluted tetramethylammonium hydroxide is transferred to a micro sample vial (Wheaton Scientific, Millville, N. J. 08332) with a Pasteur pipet, and 1 μl is injected into the chromatograph.

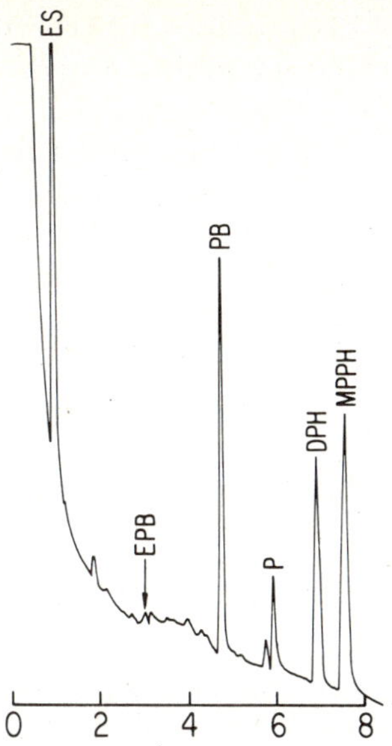

Fig. 1. Gas chromatogram from sample of pooled sera containing: ethosuximide (*ES*) 41 μg/ml, phenobarbital (*PB*) 23 μg/ml, primidone (*P*) 9 μg/ml, and diphenylhydantoin (*DPH*) 13 μg/ml. 25 μg of 5-(4-methylphenyl)-5-phenylhydantoin (*MPPH*) added per milliliter of serum as an internal standard. Attenuation = 2^8. *EPB*, "early phenobarbital"

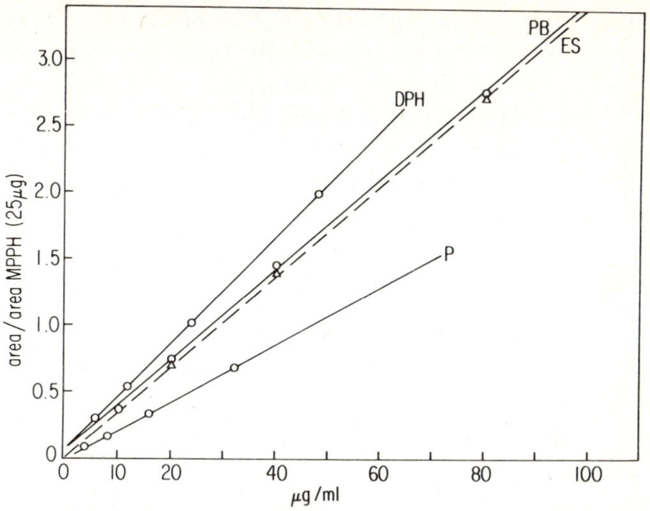

Fig. 2. Peak area ratio of anticonvulsant drugs extracted from sera, as a function of drug concentration

Each point represents the mean of six determinations. The best straight line for each set of data was determined by the method of least squares. The point representing an ethosuximide concentration of 160 μg/ml and a peak area ratio of 5.53 is not shown

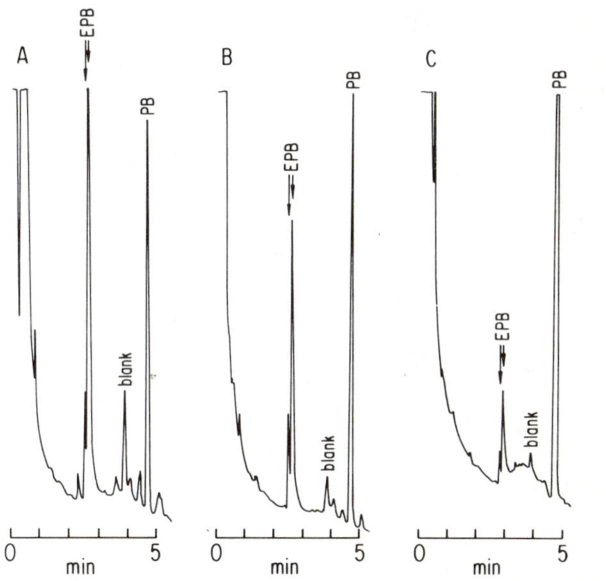

Fig. 3. Gas chromatogram of 100 μg of phenobarbital per milliliter, added to drug-free serum

Attenuation = 2^9. *N,N*-Dimethylphenobarbital, *PB*. "Early phenobarbital," *EPB*. (*A*) trimethylanilinium hydroxide extract injected into a 2-mm injection port liner. PB/Σ EPB, PB = .35, CV = 6.1 (n = 10); (B) tetramethylammonium hydroxide extract injected into a 2 mm injection port liner. PB/Σ EPB, PB = .58, CV = 2.6 (n = 6); (C) tetramethylammonium hydroxide extract injected into a 1 mm injection port liner. PB/Σ EPB, PB = .80, CV = 1.6 (n = 7)

The blank found for drug-free sera is diminished by conditions that diminish EPB

Gas Chromatography

The flame-ionization detector is operated in a single mode because, under the conditions of analysis, there is no appreciable column bleed. The column is 180 cm × 2 mm (i.d.) "Chromatoglass," continuous from septum to detector (Apollo Associates, Ardsley, N. Y. 10502) packed with 3% OV 17 on Chromosorb WHP 80/100 mesh (Supelco, Inc., Bellefonte, Pa. 16823).

The column is conditioned before use for 1.5 h at 310 °C without carrier-gas flow and overnight at 280 °C with a nitrogen flow of 40 ml/min. Injector temperature is 350 °C, detector temperature 300 °C. Carrier gas is nitrogen at a flow rate of 40 ml/min. The automatic sampler (Hewlett-Packard, Avondale, Pa. 19311) is equipped with a 1-μl syringe (Hamilton Co., Reno, Nev. 89502)

Temperature programming permits the simultaneous determination of four drugs relative to a single internal standard (Figure 1). Column temperature is held at 150 °C for 1 min, programmed from 150 to 260 °C at 20 °C/min, and held at 260 °C for 2 min.

We have recently adapted the method to an automatic data-reduction system (Hewlett-Packard Model 5830).

Results

Calibration. Calibration standards are prepared by dissolving pure drugs (obtained from the respective manufacturers) in methanol. To facilitate calibration, mixtures of all four drugs are prepared at four concentrations. One milliliter of drug-free serum, 100 μl of calibration standard, and 0.9 ml of 3.3 mol/liter NaH_2PO_4 are combined and the extraction is done as described earlier. The resulting calibration curves are linear over the range of concentrations normally found in sera of patients undergoing anticonvulsant drug therapy (Figure 2).

Stability. Several authors have commented on the instability of phenobarbital in concentrated trimethylanilinium hydroxide (*3–5*), an important consideration if automated sampling of preloaded samples is used. To determine the stability of the four drugs in tetramethylammonium hydroxide, we ran a single extract from serum to which a mixture of the four drugs had been added at 4-h intervals for 16 h (i.e., five runs). The resulting CVs were: 1.6% for 43.3 μg/ml ethosuximide, 1.1% for 23.0 μg/ml phenobarbital, 1.2% for 9.6 μg/ml primidone, and 1.4% for 13.4 μg/ml diphenylhydantoin. In samples held for 24 h there is a significant decrease in the response for primidone.

Precision. The inclusion of multiple internal standards for specific anticonvulsants has been suggested as a means of enhancing the repeatability of drug-concentration measurements (*6*). For results to be reported directly as concentrations in serum with the data-reduction system, each drug must be quantitated on the basis of a comparison with the area of a single internal-standard peak. We obtain excellent precision by this method and eliminate manual calculations. We determined the overall precision of the method during one month by daily extraction of a serum pool to which a mixture of the four drugs had been added. The CVs were 3.0% for 42.0 μg/ml ethosuximide, 2.2% for 22.7 μg/ml phenobarbital, 2.4% for 9.5 μg/ml primidone, and 2.8% for 13.7 μg/ml diphenylhydantoin ($n = 22$).

Carry-over. Carry-over, expressed as a percentage of the previously injected sample, varied from 4% for diphenylhydantoin to 1% for phenobarbital. This is of little importance, because a clinically significant increase in apparent concentrations owing to carry-over requires a previous injection representing extremely toxic concentrations. The sample following such a sample should be repeated.

Degradation. Degradation of phenobarbital during flash heater methylation has been examined by several authors (*3–5*). In our experience, samples extracted into tetramethylammonium hydroxide give a larger proportion of *N,N*-dimethylphenobarbital than those extracted into trimethylanilinium hydroxide (Figure 3, *A* and *B*). The proportion of dimethyl derivative formed is increased if the inner diameter of the portion of the glass column into which the sample is injected is decreased (Figure 3, *B* and *C*). This effect may be due to the increased linear flow rate through the smaller volume of the narrow injection port liner. Reduction of the early phenobarbital peak permits a more precise calculation of phenobarbital concentration based on a substantially larger *N,N*-dimethylphenobarbital peak. Use of a single peak to quantitate phenobarbital permits automatic data reduction, so that concentrations in serum are directly calculated.

We thank Mrs Helen Farrell for her assistance in the preparation of the manuscript, and Dr. Robert L. Habig for his critical review of the manuscript.

References

1. MacGee, J., Rapid determination of diphenylhydantoin in blood plasma by gas–liquid chromatography. *Anal. Chem.* **42,** 421 (1970).

2. Joern, W. A., Gas chromatography of anticonvulsant drugs, with no solvent evaporation. *Clin. Chem.* **21,** 1548 (1975).

3. Perchalski, R. J., Scott, K. N., Wilder, B. J., and Hammer, R. H., Rapid, simultaneous GLC determination of phenobarbital, primidone, and diphenylhydantoin. *J. Pharm. Sci.* **62,** 1735 (1973).

4. VanMeter, J. C., and Gillen, H. W., A source of variation in the gas chromatographic assay of phenobarbital treated with trimethylanilinium hydroxide. *Clin. Chem.* **19,** 359 (1973).

5. Osiewicz, R., Aggarwal, V., Young, R. M., and Sunshine, I., The quantitative analysis of phenobarbital with trimethylanilinum hydroxide. *J. Chromatogr.* **88,** 157 (1974).

6. Solow, E. B., Metaxas, J. M., and Summers, T. R., Antiepileptic drugs: A current assessment of simultaneous determination of multiple drug therapy by gas–liquid chromatography–on column methylation. *J. Chromatogr. Sci.* **12,** 256 (1974).

CLIN. CHEM. 22/6, 863–867 (1976)

Method for Alcohol Determination in Biological Liquids by Sensing with a Solid-State Detector

Kurt M. Dubowski

I describe a new method for quantitative alcohol determination in equilibrated headspace gas of biological liquids by means of a solid-state metal-oxide semiconductor (MOS) detector. After equilibration of the NaCl-saturated specimen at 40 °C or other convenient temperature in a closed vessel, a Taguchi MOS sensor is momentarily exposed to the headspace vapor. The resulting dc voltage change from the baseline conditions accurately reflects the alcohol concentration of the liquid specimen, and can be read in direct alcohol-concentration units. Calibration is linear to 3.00 g/liter (300 mg/dl). Values for analytical recovery ranged from 98 to 102%. Correlation of results for blood alcohol concentration by this method (y_i) and an automated gas-chromatographic reference method (x_i) was y, g/liter = $0.991x + 0.014$, with $r = 0.997$ for 103 blood specimens having concentrations ranging from 0 to 2.89 g/liter (0–289 mg/dl), with a mean difference ($x_i - y_i$) = −6 mg/liter (0.6 mg/dl). The method is sensitive to 0.01 g/liter (1 mg/dl) and can be readily automated. An internal standard is not required.

Additional Keyphrases: *screening • toxicology • solid-state metal-oxide semiconductor detector • vapor analysis • gas-chromatography compared*

Ambient sensing of alcohol[1] in breath by physical-chemical means with use of solid-state devices has been recently introduced for breath-alcohol screening tests (*1, 2*). Thus, the A.L.E.R.T.™ portable electronic breath-alcohol tester (*3, 4*) detects alcohol with an *n*-type MOS[2] device, the Taguchi Gas Sensor (*5*). This consists of a small (4.4 × 1.7 × 1.2 mm) porous stannic oxide semiconductor element, the electrical conductance of which increases in proportion to the alcohol concentration of vapor specimens to which it is exposed, through reversible surface adsorption of the gaseous molecules (*6*). Integral noble-metal electrodes and heating elements are contained in the MOS sensor element, and suitable electronic circuitry is used to "condition" the detector and reproducibly to convert the conductance changes to dc voltages that actuate lamp signals indicative of the breath-alcohol concentration (*7*).

This breath-alcohol screening test procedure is inherently simple, rapid, sensitive, and reagentless. These characteristics are also desirable in a method for alcohol determination in blood and other biological liquids for clinical purposes. We therefore combined this solid-state alcohol sensing scheme with the well-established principle of equilibrium partition of volatiles between liquids and "headspace" gas in a closed system at controlled temperature (*8*) to develop a new *quantitative* method for alcohol analysis in biological liquids. The resulting method is conceptually analogous to gas-chromatographic determination of alcohol in biological liquids by headspace analysis (*9–11*). However, the instrumentation is simpler and less expensive, it can be used intermittently without lengthy or complicated preparation, and it yields a final result (e.g., blood-alcohol concentration) without computations—i.e., by direct digital readout.

Materials and Methods

Apparatus

For solid-state alcohol sensing. This consisted of a constant-temperature water bath (Model K-4 Lauda Water Bath; Brinkmann Instruments, Inc., Westbury, N. Y. 11590) maintained at 40 ± 0.02 °C; a Taguchi Gas

Departments of Medicine, Biochemistry & Molecular Biology, and Pathology; and Toxicology Laboratories, University of Oklahoma Health Sciences Center, Oklahoma City, Okla. 73190.

Presented in part at the 8th Annual Symposium on Advanced Analytical Concepts for the Clinical Laboratory, Oak Ridge National Laboratory, Oak Ridge, Tenn., March 26, 1976.

[1] The unmodified word *alcohol* in this article refers to ethanol.

[2] Nonstandard abbreviations used: MOS, metal-oxide semiconductor; BAC, blood alcohol concentration.

Received Feb. 23, 1976; accepted Mar. 8, 1976.

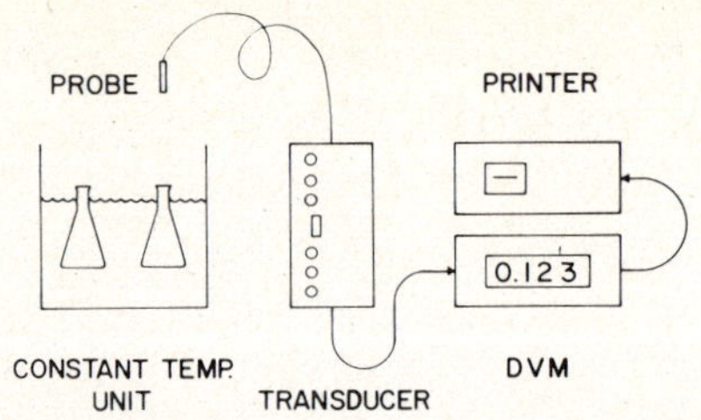

Fig. 1. Block diagram of the apparatus for solid-state sensing of alcohol in headspace gases

Sensor (No. 109; Figaro Engineering, Inc., Osaka 560, Japan) mounted at the inlet of a 2-ml Cornwall-type glass hypodermic syringe; an A.L.E.R.T.™ breath-alcohol test device (Borg-Warner Corp., Des Plaines, Ill. 60018) modified to serve as the signal conditioner; a digital voltmeter (Model 351 Multimeter; Data Technology Corp., Santa Ana, Calif. 92704); and, optionally, an electronic digital printer (Model 2000; Electro-Numerics Corp., Santa Clara, Calif. 95051). A variable resistance (150 kΩ maximum) potentiometer was connected in series between the signal conditioner and the digital voltmeter. Screw-capped Erlenmeyer flasks with Teflon-coated elastomer septa (Products No. 13320 and 13310, 25- and 10-ml "Reacti-Flasks"; Pierce Chemical Co., Rockford, Ill. 61105) or standard 24-ml Machata cylindrical glass headspace vials were used to equilibrate the liquid specimens with headspace gas. Figure 1 schematically shows the apparatus arrangement.

For gas-chromatographic analyses. Gas chromatography, as a comparison procedure, was done with an automated gas-chromatographic headspace analyzer (Model F-40 Multifract; Perkin-Elmer Corp., Norwalk, Conn. 06856). The flame ionization detector response was recorded with a 250 mm potentiometric strip-chart recorder (Model 194; Honeywell, Inc., Ft. Washington, Pa. 19034).

Reagents

The only reagents required are crystalline sodium chloride (AR) and aqueous ethanol reference solutions containing 1.00 and 2.00 g/liter (100 and 200 mg/dl).[3] These dilute ethanol solutions are stable for at least one year, when stored in borosilicate glass containers at 4 °C.

Procedures

Detector-sensing. One milliliter of well-mixed whole blood was placed in a 25-ml Erlenmeyer septum flask containing 1 g of sodium chloride, mixed by swirling, and the flask was immersed to the screw-cap level in a water bath at 40 °C for at least 30 min. An ethanol reference solution, usually 1.00 g/liter (100 mg/dl), was identically prepared and incubated. After equilibration at 40 °C for 30 min or longer, a fixed volume (about 2 ml) of headspace gas was withdrawn from the reference flask and immediately directed past the previously purged Taguchi Gas Sensor. The resulting peak digital voltmeter reading was adjusted to the nominal volume of the ethanol reference sample (e.g., 100 for a 1.00 g/liter sample), and the purge-headspace withdrawal-sensing result-reading process then repeated for each biological specimen. Purging of the detector between samples involved a 25-s heating cycle, during which room air was repeatedly aspirated into the Cornwall syringe and directed past the Sensor. In serial analyses, standardization was checked after every tenth specimen. A micro-modification of this procedure consisted of placing 100 μl of well-mixed whole blood into a 10-ml Erlenmeyer septum flask containing 0.1 g of sodium chloride and proceeding as above.

Gas-chromatography. These analyses on aqueous and biological specimens were done by the automated gas-chromatographic headspace method of Machata (*12, 13*), modified by Dubowski (*14*). Aqueous reference specimens were used in this modification, and all samples were saturated with sodium chloride (1 g of sodium chloride + 1 ml of liquid sample) before equilibration at 40 °C and subsequent gas-chromatographic analysis. The detector responses were recorded on a 250-mm wide chart, and the concentrations of test samples were calculated by comparison with the reference samples by using either electronic integration of the curves or peak-height measurements. Both quantitation procedures yielded the same results in our hands. A 1.8 meter × 3.2 mm (o.d.) stainless-steel column packed with 0.4% "Carbowax 1500" on 60/80 mesh "Carbopack A" (Supelco, Inc., Bellefonte, Pa. 16823) was used. Typical operating conditions for the gas-chromatograph were: nitrogen (carrier gas) flow, 35 ml/min at 117.7 kPa; hydrogen flow, 35 ml/min at 107.9 kPa; air flow, 300 ml/min at 117.7 kPa; column temperature, 80 °C; dosing line temperature, 178 °C; and detector temperature, 150 °C. The instrument was programmed as follows: pressurization 60 s, injection 3 s, analysis 240 s, dosing line

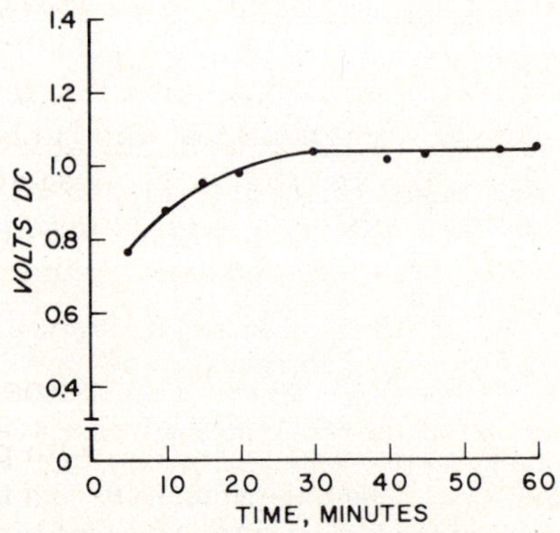

Fig. 2. Time course of dc voltage output of Taguchi Gas Sensor, showing time required for equilibration of headspace gas at 40 °C

[3] Alcohol concentrations are expressed herein in g/liter or mg/liter. In deference to established medicolegal usage and the universally accepted interpretation of blood-alcohol concentrations, the corresponding concentrations in mg/dl are also stated. 1.00 g/liter = 100 mg/dl = 21.71 mmol ethanol/liter.

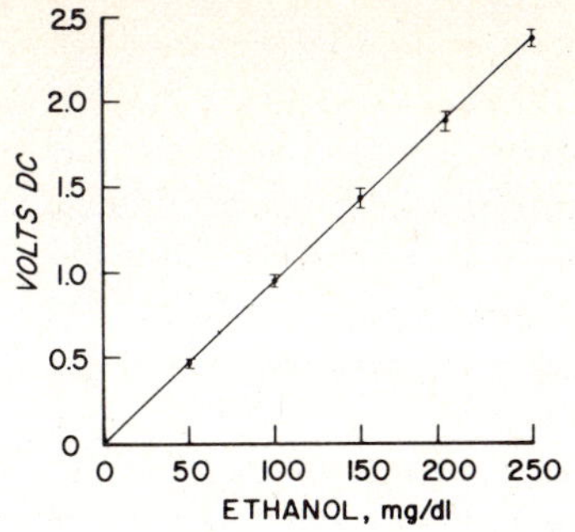

Fig. 3. Calibration curve for alcohol determination by solid-state detector sensing at 40 °C

Points = mean of six determinations, 2 SD in brackets. The curve corresponds to $x = 105.6y + 0.14$ ($r = 0.997$)

purge 12 s, stabilization 12 s, one analysis per sample vial. Duplicate injections of the sample headspace vapor were made, from separate vials, for each specimen, and reference ethanol samples, 1.00 and 2.00 g/liter (100 and 200 mg/dl), were included at the beginning, in the middle, and at the end of each turntable run of 30 samples.

Results

Standardization and Linearity

The time required for complete equilibration between the liquid and vapor phases varied with the incubation temperature and other factors such as shape and volume of the equilibration vessel. Figure 2 shows the relation between elapsed time and Taguchi Gas Sensor output voltage for equilibration at 40 °C, for sodium chloride-saturated liquids. At higher temperatures, equilibration is more rapid. Figure 3 shows the basic calibration curve for this system for equilibration at 40 °C, illustrating linearity to 2.50 g of ethanol per liter (250 mg/dl) and the greater relative precision of the measurement at higher concentrations. (In other experiments, linearity of calibration to 3.00 g/liter (300 mg/dl) at 40 °C was demonstrated.) At 40 °C, the calibration curve corresponded to the least-squares linear regression equation $x = 105.6y + 0.14$ ($r = 0.997$), where x = blood alcohol concentration, mg/dl and y = Taguchi Gas Sensor output, in volts dc, without attenuation for direct-reading results. The corresponding calibration equation is $x = 1.056y + 0.0014$, where x = blood alcohol concentration, g/liter. Increased equilibration temperatures yielded higher dc voltage outputs and hence increased sensitivity; e.g., the instrument response at 65 °C was approximately fivefold that at 35 °C for equal alcohol concentrations in the liquid phase, in the presence of salt.

Precision, Accuracy, Sensitivity, and Specificity

Precision. Within-run and between-run precision of the procedure for a control specimen with a target value of 1.00 g/liter (100 mg/dl) are given in Table 1; the latter represents data for runs on successive days. Recovery experiments with 0.50, 1.00, 1.50, and 2.00 g of added ethanol per liter of specimen (50, 100, 150, 200 mg/dl) yielded the following results (mean ± SD): 0.509 ± 0.03, 1.005 ± 0.06, 1.477 ± 0.06, and 1.990 ± 0.05 g/liter, for corresponding mean recoveries of 102, 101, 98, and 100%.

Table 1. Precision of TGS-Headspace Procedure for Ethanol Determination

Test	Ethanol, g/liter: Within-run	Between-run
1	1.05	0.97
2	1.01	1.01
3	0.98	1.02
4	1.04	1.04
5	1.03	1.05
6	1.01	0.96
7	0.98	0.98
8	1.00	0.96
9	0.98	1.01
10	1.03	0.94
11	0.97	1.03
12	0.96	0.97
13	0.96	1.01
14	1.02	0.98
15	0.98	0.98
16	0.99	1.03
17	1.02	1.01
18	1.02	0.96
19	0.99	1.02
20	1.00	1.00
21	1.00	1.03
22	1.00	
23	1.00	
24	1.01	
25	0.97	
Mean	1.000	0.998
SD	±0.024	±0.031
CV	2.43%	3.11%

Inter-method comparison. Figure 4 compares results of this new method of analysis for alcohol in 103 random blood specimens submitted for routine forensic alcohol determination with those of our automated gas-chromatographic headspace reference method, for analyses done independently in the same laboratory. Least-squares linear regression analysis of these data yielded y, g/liter = $0.991x + 0.014$, with $r = 0.997$, $\bar{x} = 1.233$ g/liter, and $\bar{y} = 1.236$ g/liter (123 mg/dl) where x_i and y_i are the blood alcohol concentrations determined by the reference method and the new procedure, respectively. The mean difference in results for blood alcohol concentration obtained by the two procedures ($x_i - y_i$) was −6 mg/liter (−0.6 mg/dl) for the 103 blood specimen pairs; 53 of the ($x_i - y_i$) differences were positive, 50 negative. For another 16 blood specimens, varying in blood alcohol concentration from 1.30 to 3.10 g/liter (130

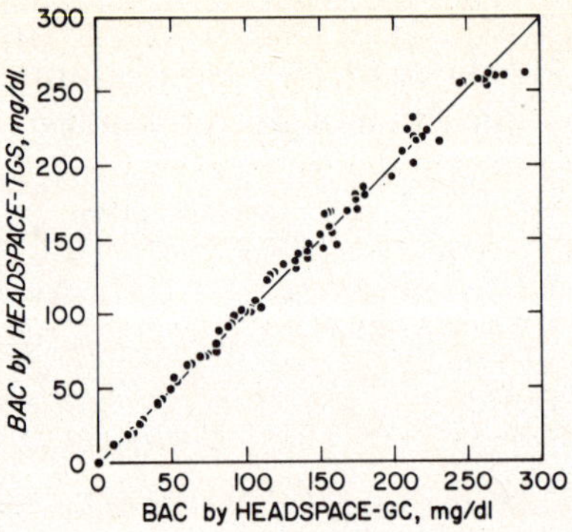

Fig. 4. Correlation of the results of 103 blood alcohol determinations by the reference "headspace-GC" method and the present method

The least-squares linear regression equation for the correlation is $y_i = 0.991x_i + 1.38$ ($r = 0.997$), and the mean difference ($x_i - y_i$) = −0.6 mg/dl (6.0 mg/liter). The perfect correlation line is shown, for comparison

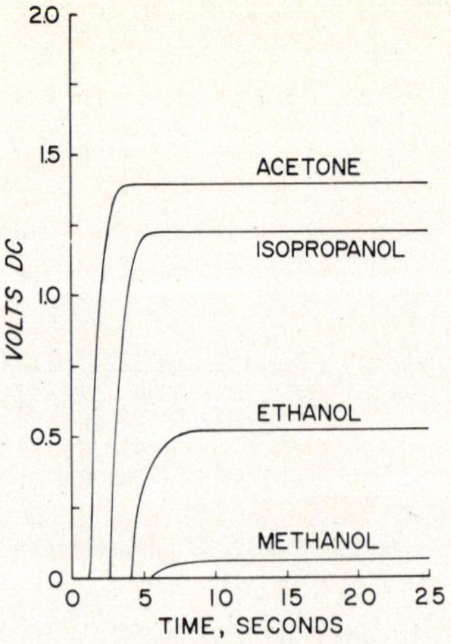

Fig. 5. Time course of dc voltage output of the solid-state detector for analysis of headspace gas at 40 °C above equimolar (12 mmol/liter) solutions of acetone, ethanol, isopropanol, and methanol in the presence of sodium chloride

Detector output was attenuated in order to keep all values on the recorder chart, and the recorder tracings shifted horizontally for clarity

to 310 mg/dl), independently analyzed in double-blind fashion in two different laboratories, by the new method (y_i) and by the automated gas-chromatographic headspace analysis method (x_i), the least-squares linear regression equation was y, g/liter = $0.929x + 0.151$, with $r = 0.988$, $\bar{x} = 2.131$ g/liter, $\bar{y} = 2.131$ g/liter (213 mg/dl), and a mean difference ($x_i - y_i$) of 0. For paired results on the 103 blood specimens, paired-t calculations yielded $t_{calc} = |0.473|$ (n = 103, DF = 102) with a table value $t_{0.995} = 2.617$.

Differences of 0.01 g of alcohol per liter of specimen (1 mg/dl) were readily detectable by this procedure. Analysis of blood from abstaining subjects consistently yielded results for apparent blood alcohol concentration of less than 0.02 g/liter (2 mg/dl), with a mean = 0.006 ± 0.0062 g/liter (0.6 ± 0.62 mg/dl) for n = 18. The time course of the dc voltage output of the Taguchi Gas Sensor, attenuated to keep all values on the recorder chart, is shown in Figure 5 for equimolar (12 mmol/liter) aqueous solutions of acetone, ethanol, isopropanol, and methanol in the presence of sodium chloride at 40 °C.

Discussion

The novelty of this method lies in the application of a solid-state detector to fully *quantitative* determination of ethanol in the equilibrated headspace above liquid specimens. Because the sensor output is an electrical signal, direct readout in desired concentration terms is readily obtainable. The inherent sensitivity of the procedure allows analysis of microliter specimens without additional manipulations, and permits unknown and reference samples to be equilibrated at room temperature. Increases in sensitivity are achievable with higher equilibration temperatures, which also reduce the time required for equilibration. Separation of the alcohol from biological liquids by passive isothermal diffusion provides a "headspace" vapor sample of convenient volume to which the Taguchi Gas Sensor can be momentarily exposed. Because the sensor reproducibly responds to the ambience and the response does not critically depend on a known sample volume or mass, an internal standard is not needed. The sensing period and turnaround time between samples are short (6 s and 40 s, respectively) and the method is, therefore, practical for mass alcohol "screening" applications in medical examiner toxicology laboratories or in intake centers for alcoholic subjects. Simplicity of the required manipulations and absence of elaborate preparations make the method practical for intermittent use on brief notice.

Standardization is done in parallel with the analysis of unknown specimens and aqueous reference samples are used. When a liquid sample is saturated with an inorganic salt such as sodium sulfate or sodium chloride before equilibration, its original solid content becomes immaterial, as demonstrated by Bassette et al. (*15*) and widely relied upon in the analysis of volatiles in blood and other biological specimens (*9–11, 14*). The linearity of the procedure allows use of a single reference-sample concentration.

The precision of this method compares favorably with that of leading manual procedures for blood-alcohol analysis. Its accuracy, as reflected in the analytical recovery of added ethanol and the comparison with a highly accurate and precise automated reference method (*14, 16*), is very satisfactory. The bias of the new method is negligible, as shown by regression analysis, the sign test at the 99% confidence level, and the paired-t computation of the paired results at the 99% confidence level, which justify acceptance of the null hypothesis that there is no statistically significant difference between results obtained by the two methods on identical specimens.

The Taguchi Gas Sensor responds to various combustible gases or vapors (*6*) and is therefore not a specific ethanol detection device. However, as illustrated in Figure 5, the initial slope of the voltage-vs.-time response differs appreciably in this system for different volatile organic substances in equimolar concentrations. This suggests that suitable selectivity for ethanol (or other desired volatile substance) might be attained by electronic "gating" of the acceptable voltage vs. time course. Simple chemical manipulation can also be used, such as trapping of acetone by passing the headspace vapor through a short sodium bisulfite column before sensing.

The feasibility of alcohol detection and determination in biological specimens by means of a solid-state detector device has been demonstrated in a manual method. The method could be automated by relatively simple means, such as use of a controlled-temperature turntable and timed, mechanical penetration of equilibration vials for headspace aspiration, with intervening detector-purge phases.

This work was supported in part by the Insurance Institute for Highway Safety. Grateful acknowledgment is also made to Alcohol Countermeasure Systems, Borg-Warner Corp., Des Plaines, Ill., for providing the modified A.L.E.R.T.™ unit used as the signal conditioner.

References

1. Dubowski, K. M., Recent developments in breath-alcohol analysis. In *Alcohol, Drugs and Traffic Safety (Proceedings of the Sixth International Conference on Alcohol, Drugs, and Traffic Safety, Toronto, Sept. 1974)*, S. Israelstam and S. Lambert, Eds., Addiction Research Foundation of Ontario, Toronto, 1975, pp 483–494.

2. Mason, M. F., and Dubowski, K. M., Breath-alcohol analysis: Uses, methods, and some forensic problems-review and opinion. *J. Forensic Sci.* **21**, 9 (1976).

3. A.L.E.R.T.™ Brochure ABW-2-411. Alcohol Countermeasure Systems, Borg-Warner Corp., Des Plaines, Ill. 60018, 1974.

4. Dubowski, K. M., Evaluation of the Borg-Warner breath-alcohol screening device. *Ann. Clin. Lab. Sci.* **3**, 308 (1973).

5. Taguchi, N., Semiconductor Gas Detecting Device. U. S. Patent 3,732,519 (May 8, 1973).

6. *TGS Gas-Sensing Semi-Conductor.* Figaro Engineering, Inc., Osaka, Japan, Feb. 1974.

7. Dubowski, K. M., The analysis of breath alcohol by means of an instrumental screening device. In *Manual of Procedures for the Applied Seminar on the Clinical Pathology of Respiratory Diseases,* Institute for Clinical Science, Philadelphia, Pa., 1972, pp 189–199.

8. Harger, R. N., Raney, B. B., Bridwell, E. G., and Kitchel, M. F., The partition ratio of alcohol between air and water, urine, and blood. *J. Biol. Chem.* **183**, 197 (1950).

9. Wallace, J. E., and Dahl, E. V., Rapid vapor phase method for determining ethanol in blood and urine by gas chromatography. *Am. J. Clin. Pathol.* **46**, 152 (1966).

10. Dubowski, K. M., Ethanol-type C procedure. In *Methodology for Analytical Toxicology,* I. Sunshine, Ed., CRC Press, Inc., Cleveland, Ohio, 1975, pp 149–154.

11. Dubowski, K. M., Organic volatile substances. *Ibid.*, pp 407–411.

12. Machata, G., Über die gaschromatographische Blutalkoholbestimmung. *Blutalkohol* **4**, 252 (1967).

13. Machata, G., Determination of alcohol in blood by gas chromatographic headspace analysis. *Clin. Chem. Newsletter* (pub. by Perkin-Elmer Corp., Norwalk, Conn.) **4**, 29–32 (1972).

14. Dubowski, K. M., *A Study of Characteristics of a Reliable and Practical Breath Alcohol Screening Test: Part B-Manual for Analysis of Ethanol in Biological Specimens.* Contract No. DOT-TSC-472, U. S. Department of Transportation, Washington, D. C., 1976.

15. Bassette, R., Ozeris, S., and Whitnah, C. H., Gas chromatographic analysis of head space gas of dilute aqueous solutions. *Anal. Chem.* **34**, 1540 (1962).

16. Dubowski, K. M., Biological aspects of breath-alcohol analysis. *Clin. Chem.* **20**, 294 (1974).

review

CLIN. CHEM. 22/6, 868-878 (1976)

Pharmacokinetic Interpretation of Data Gathered during Therapeutic Drug Monitoring

Barry H. Dvorchik and Elliot S. Vesell

We review some pharmacokinetic principles that can facilitate interpretation of data obtained during therapeutic drug monitoring: the one- and two-compartment models, volume of drug distribution, drug clearance, organ clearance, bioavailability, first-pass effect, chronic or repetitive dosing, and use of urine and saliva to measure drug clearance and drug binding to plasma proteins, respectively. We also describe use of saliva to estimate rapidly, conveniently, and noninvasively the concentration of the free, pharmacologically active form of the drug as well as the fraction of drug bound to plasma protein.

Additional Keyphrases: *"biologic half-life" of a drug • drug distribution and clearance • drug binding to plasma proteins • urine or saliva as the sample in drug monitoring • dosage/concentration relations*

Clinical chemists are frequently requested to identify and quantitate a wide variety of drugs in the blood and urine of acutely poisoned patients. To this extent, responsibility for verification and treatment of drug toxicity rests with clinical chemists, because they furnish the information that forms the basis for therapy.

Recent developments in pharmacology and medicine indicate that under some circumstances measurement of drug concentration in blood is the best available guide to ascertain each patient's particular dose requirements (*1, 2*). Such circumstances include: (*a*) high incidence of toxicity resulting from certain drugs used alone or in combination; (*b*) failure to attain adequate pharmacologic responses after administration of potent drugs with low therapeutic indices given in the usual doses; (*c*) interactions of concomitantly administered drugs to change the peak effects and durations of action expected when each drug is used alone, which alterations can involve drug absorption from sites of drug administration, distribution of drugs among various compartments of the body, biotransformation, excretion, or a combination of these processes; (*d*) assessment of patient compliance, especially when the desired therapeutic effects are not obtained; (*e*) exposure to compounds abundantly distributed in our environment—such as caffeine, nicotine, ethanol, benzpyrene and DDT—that may change the capacity of an individual to eliminate therapeutic agents; (*f*) demonstration that individuals can differ greatly in their inherent capacity to absorb, distribute, metabolize, and excrete drugs. (large interindividual differences in these processes, but especially in rates of hepatic drug metabolism, render fallacious the tacit assumption that administration of a given drug solely by weight or by surface area to all patients with adequate cardiovascular, hepatic, and renal function results in closely similar drug concentrations in blood and other tissues); (*g*) the increasing number of pharmacogenetic conditions in which specific point mutations inherited in classical mendelian fashion affect the enzymes that metabolize drugs, thereby altering their safety, peak effects, and duration of action; and (*h*) development of new, convenient, accurate, inexpensive, and rapid methods for assay of many drugs in biological fluids, thereby permitting the physician to adjust the dosage of many drugs more precisely according to their concentrations in biological fluids (*1, 2*).

The physician and clinical chemist should discriminate between those drugs that can practically and usefully be measured in blood or some other biological fluid and those that cannot (*3*). Some drugs cannot be satis-

Departments of Pharmacology and Obstetrics and Gynecology, The Pennsylvania State University College of Medicine, Hershey, Pa. 17033.

Received Feb. 2, 1976; accepted Mar. 26, 1976.

factorily assayed in biological fluids because convenient methods are not yet available for their determination. Although for many drugs a close correlation exists between blood drug concentrations and pharmacological or therapeutic effects, this relationship does not apply for all drugs (*2*). Some drugs are bound so avidly by certain tissues that they may be virtually undetectable in biological fluids or present in such low concentrations that their true concentrations in other organs are concealed. Drugs of this type, as well as drugs that form irreversible covalent bonds with certain macromolecules, may continue to exert their effects long after they vanish from all other sites in the body.

The therapeutic and toxic properties of most pharmacological agents are determined in vivo by the absorption characteristics of the drug and the combined, simultaneously occurring processes of distribution, metabolism, and excretion. The intensity of these pharmacological effects depends on the amount of pharmacologically active substance that gets to the site of drug action (receptor site).

Pharmacokinetics is the study of the time course of absorption, distribution, metabolism, and excretion of drugs and their metabolites in the intact organism. The amounts of drug and metabolite(s) in readily available biological fluids are measured as functions of time and dosage. Mathematical models are then established to predict quantitatively these dynamic processes. Thus, knowledge of a drug's pharmacokinetic profile within any individual should allow the clinician to choose an adequate dosage schedule that will rapidly and safely produce and maintain a desired pharmacological effect. Obviously, for any pharmacokinetic analysis to be useful the assays on which the analysis is based must separate the parent drug from any metabolites. Most of the currently used analytical methods meet this requirement.

Most pharmacokinetic principles have been obtained by investigating the concentration of a drug in blood or plasma as a function of time (*4–7*). This paper does not review the enormous body of pharmacokinetic literature; instead, the interested reader is referred elsewhere (*5–11*). After a discussion of some basic pharmacokinetic principles, we intend to describe the applicability of using biological fluids other than blood, either alone or in combination with blood, to monitor therapeutic drug concentrations and to gain information about drug disposition that cannot be gained conveniently from blood alone.

Pharmacokinetic Models

Numerous observations performed in vivo on drug distribution, absorption, and excretion led to the concept that a biological system can be treated as if there were boundaries separating the system into parts ("compartments") and that a drug is transferred from one compartment to another in conformance with first-order kinetics. Although the assumption of first-order kinetics and rate coefficients that are constants is a gross approximation of a complex biological phenomenon, this approach, when utilized with discretion and understanding, has often proved rewarding; these kinetic assumptions have been validated by drug studies performed in vivo.

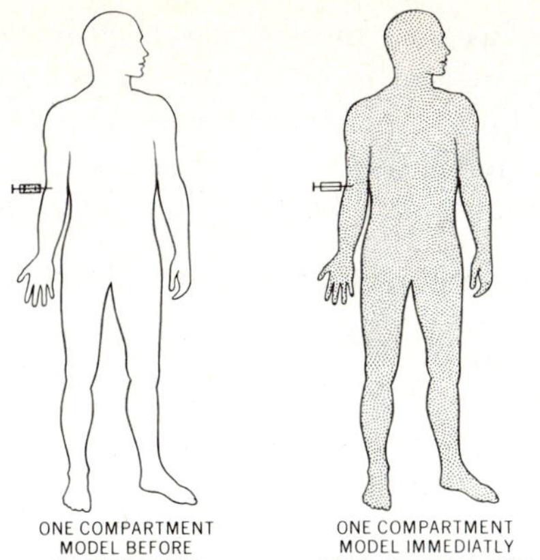

Fig. 1. The one-compartment model

The One-Compartment Pharmacokinetic Model

The simplest pharmacokinetic model, the "one-compartment model," assumes that after administration (and absorption for those drugs administered by routes other than intravenous injection) drugs are instantaneously and homogeneously distributed throughout the fluids and tissues of the body (Figure 1). This assumption does not necessarily mean that the concentration of drug in plasma and other body fluids and tissues is the same at the same time. What the one-compartment model does assume, however, is that changes in plasma drug concentration quantitatively reflect changes occurring in drug concentrations of other body fluids and tissues.

For drugs whose distribution in the body follows one-compartment pharmacokinetics, a plot of the logarithm of the plasma drug concentration against time will be a straight line. The equation describing the plasma decay curve is

$$C = Ae^{-(k_e)t} \tag{1}$$

where k_e is the first-order rate constant for the overall elimination of drug from the body, C is the concentration of drug at time t, and A is the concentration of drug at time 0, when all of the drug administered has been absorbed but none has been removed through metabolism or excretion. The apparent first-order rate constant, k_e, is usually the sum of the rate constants of a number of individual processes such as renal excretion, biliary excretion, and metabolism. The apparent first-order rate constant for elimination of drug from the body is related to the "biologic half-life" of the drug by the equation

$$t½ = \frac{0.693}{k_e} \tag{2}$$

Unfortunately, this simple model does not account accurately for the observed time course of most drugs in the body, because most drugs occupy two or three compartments, rather than one. Serious errors may be introduced into a pharmacokinetic analysis by the assumption that a drug distributes according to a one-compartment model if this assumption is false (*12, 13*).

The Two-Compartment Pharmacokinetic Model

For most pharmacokinetic purposes, the mammalian body may be considered a multicompartment system, with all compartments directly or indirectly in contact with blood. The rate at which exchange of drug between blood and tissues takes place depends on the blood flow through the tissues, the volume of the tissues, and the partition of drug between blood and tissues. On the basis of similarities in blood flow and partition coefficients between blood and tissues, various tissues may be grouped together so that the body may be regarded as a two- or three-compartment model (*12*). Owing to differences in vascularization among tissues, drug may rapidly exchange between blood and some tissues. Together with blood these tissues may be considered one compartment, commonly called the "central" compartment. It should be obvious that this central compartment has, in general, no real physiological meaning but varies in extent with the particular drug under study. The other tissues may be considered as a "peripheral" compartment, the number of peripheral compartments depending also on the properties of the drug. At some time a state of "distribution equilibrium" between the central and peripheral compartments is reached, whereupon loss of drug from plasma is described by a monoexponential process indicative of kinetic homogeneity with respect to drug concentrations in all fluids and tissues of the body. The central compartment and one peripheral compartment suffice to describe the pharmacokinetic properties of most drugs (Figure 2).

When, for purposes of pharmacokinetic analysis, the body has to be subdivided into a central compartment and one or more peripheral compartments, the semilogarithmic plot of blood concentration vs. time is not linear, but biphasic or triphasic (*14–17*). In the case of the two-compartment model represented schematically in Figure 3, where elimination occurs from the central compartment, a semilogarithmic plot of concentration of drug in the blood against time (Figure 4) can be separated into two distinct linear segments, described by the following equation:

$$C = Ae^{-\alpha t} + Be^{-\beta t} \quad (3)$$

The initial rapid decrease in drug concentration with time is due to the simultaneously occurring processes of drug distribution and drug elimination. The slope of the distributional phase, α, is obtained by subtracting the extrapolated portion of the β phase from the experimental data (Figure 4, also ref. *7, 8*). The half-life for the distributive process is determined from eq. 2, where α replaces k_e.

The terminal linear phase, or "beta" phase, describes irreversible loss of drug from the body, usually as a result of metabolism and renal excretion, although enterohepatic recirculation occurs with certain drugs. The first-order half-life of this terminal linear phase, commonly called the "biologic half-life" of drug in the body, can be calculated from eq. 2, where β replaces k_e. The slope, β, of the terminal linear portion of the curve relating log drug concentration to time does not equal the first-order elimination rate constant, k_e, from equations 1 and 2, but rather is a function of k_e, k_1, and k_2 (*7, 9*) where

$$\beta = k_e \bigg/ \left(1 + \frac{k_1}{k_2}\right) \quad (4)$$

See Figure 3 for definition of k_1 and k_2.

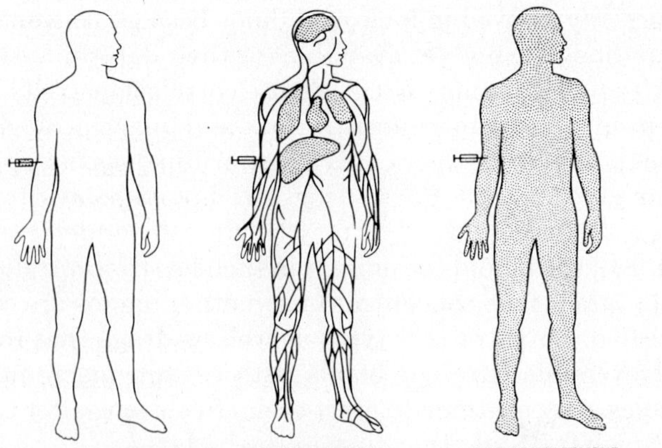

Fig. 2. The two-compartment model

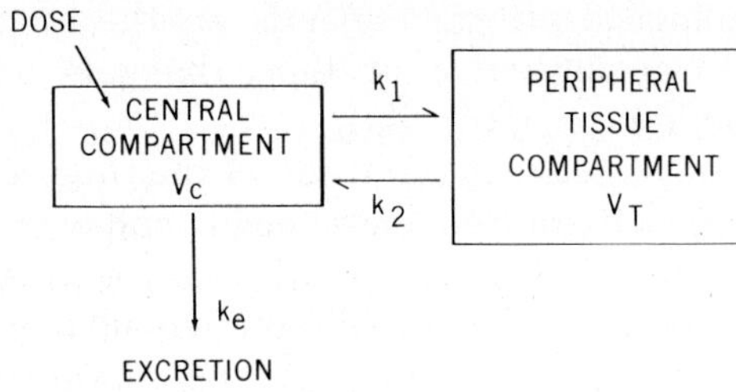

Fig. 3. Two-compartment model with elimination occurring from the central compartment

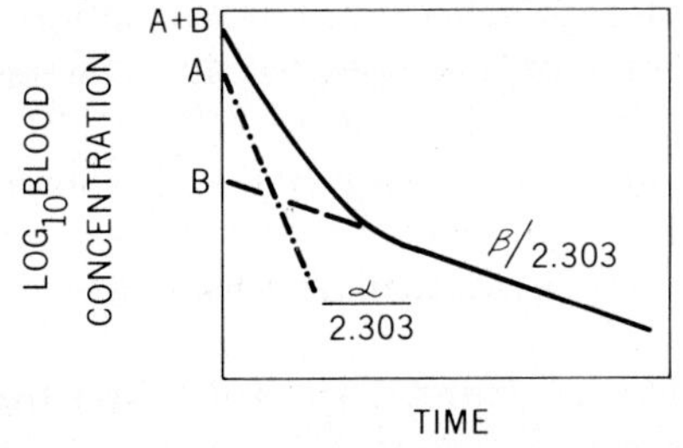

Fig. 4. The logarithm of the drug concentration in blood plotted against time (*solid line*) after intravenous administration of a drug whose disposition can be described by a two-compartment model

The dashed line (- -) represents extrapolation of the terminal (β) phase. The other line (- • • -) was obtained by the method of residuals (*7, 8*)

The coefficients A and B in eq. 3 are obtained from the intercepts of the α and β phase, respectively. The sum of A and B is taken as the drug concentration at $t = 0$, on the assumption that the drug is completely absorbed from its site of administration. Once the four terms in eq. 1 are determined, individual rate constants may be calculated. Equations used to calculate the individual pharmacokinetic parameters (i.e., k_1, k_2, k_e) are published elsewhere (*6–8*).

The apparent volume of the central compartment (V_c) expressed in liters or liters per kilogram of body weight can be determined from the following:

$$V_c = \text{dose administered}/(A + B) \tag{5}$$

Calculation of the apparent volume of the tissue compartment, V_T, requires knowledge of the "total apparent volume of distribution," V_d, since

$$V_d = V_c + V_T \tag{6}$$

V_d may be calculated by at least two methods (*7, 8, 18–23*). The first, in which the area under the blood-concentration–time curve (AUC) is used, provides the most useful estimate of V_d after single doses of drugs. AUC is one of the most useful parameters in pharmacokinetics because it is directly proportional to the total amount of drug that reaches the central compartment. The apparent volume of distribution determined by this method relates the amount of drug in the body to its concentration at all times during the beta phase of the curve (*7, 8, 20–23*)

$$(V_d)_\beta = \text{dose}/(\beta \times AUC) = \text{dose}\Big/\left(\frac{A}{\alpha} + \frac{B}{\beta}\right)\beta \tag{7}$$

Another method of calculating V_d is shown in eq. 8:

$$(V_d)_{ss} = V_c\left(1 + \frac{k_1}{k_2}\right) \tag{8}$$

$(V_d)_{ss}$ refers to the volume of distribution at steady state. This method is useful when dealing with constant drug concentrations in blood, attained after multiple dosing or constant intravenous infusion (*7, 8, 18, 19, 23*). This latter method is not recommended for calculating V_d after a single dose of a drug, because the condition under which it was derived applies only for that time at which the net transfer of drug between compartments is zero (*19, 20, 22*).

Clearance

Total Body Clearance

As stated above, for most drugs the biologic half-life, $(t½)_\beta$, is a complex function encompassing several discrete pharmacologic processes: drug distribution, biotransformation, and urinary elimination. Clearance, on the other hand, permits expression of rates of drug removal from the body in a way that is independent of these processes (*18, 24–26*). The total body clearance of a drug, that resulting from all processes of elimination, may be determined from the expression

$$\text{Clearance} = (V_c)(k_e) = \beta(V_d)_\beta = \text{dose}/AUC \tag{9}$$

Perrier and Gibaldi (*25*) demonstrated that clearance, and not β, is a direct measure of the intrinsic metabolic activity of the liver, if the liver is an integral part of the central compartment. For drugs subject to first-pass metabolism, where the liver is considered to be a compartment peripheral to the central compartment, the use of clearance as an index of hepatic metabolism is limited. Thus, for drugs whose disposition can be described by a two-compartment model (with elimination occurring from the central compartment), clearance is a more meaningful measurement of drug elimination than the disposition rate constant, β.

Organ Clearance

The concept of clearance may also be used to determine the efficiency of any organ in removing a drug irreversibly from the perfusing blood (first-pass effect). The question that arises is whether plasma or blood clearance is the parameter for physiological interpretation of clearance (*27–29*). For a further discussion of this aspect of pharmacokinetics, see references *24, 27–29.*

The rate at which a drug is delivered to the clearing organ(s) is also involved in clearance, because clearance reflects both removal of drug, expressed by the term extraction ratio, and blood flow to the organ(s). In pharmacokinetics, when relating drug clearance to blood flow, one should utilize blood drug clearances and blood flows (*27*).

Rowland et al. (*24*) and Perrier and Gibaldi (*26*), using different models, showed that the above interrelationships can be described by the equation

$$\text{Organ clearance} = Q\left[\frac{\text{Cl}_{\text{intrinsic}}}{Q + \text{Cl}_{\text{intrinsic}}}\right] \tag{10}$$

Q is the blood flow to the organ and $\text{Cl}_{\text{intrinsic}}$ is the maximal capacity of the organ to remove drug by all pathways in the absence of any flow limitations (i.e., intrinsic organ clearance). The fractional term in eq. 10 is equivalent to the extraction ratio. Figure 5 shows the relationship between liver blood flow and hepatic drug extraction for drugs with various extraction ratios. Figure 6 shows the relationship between liver blood flow and total hepatic clearance for drugs with various extraction ratios.

The pharmacokinetic behavior of a particular drug depends on the relative values of $\text{Cl}_{\text{intrinsic}}$ and Q. When $\text{Cl}_{\text{intrinsic}} >> Q$ (extraction ratio > 0.8), clearance becomes dependent upon blood flow to the eliminating organ. When $Q >> \text{Cl}_{\text{intrinsic}}$ (extraction ratio < 0.2), clearance becomes independent of organ blood flow and is approximately equal to $\text{Cl}_{\text{intrinsic}}$. For intermediate conditions (0.2 < extraction ratio < 0.8) clearance is partly flow-dependent (*24, 27–29*).

One cannot conveniently directly determine in vivo the organ clearance of a drug. However, the total body clearance (TBC) of a drug can be determined from eq. 9. If the drug is eliminated both by metabolism and excretion of the unchanged drug and if the fraction of drug excreted unchanged (f_e) is known, renal clearance

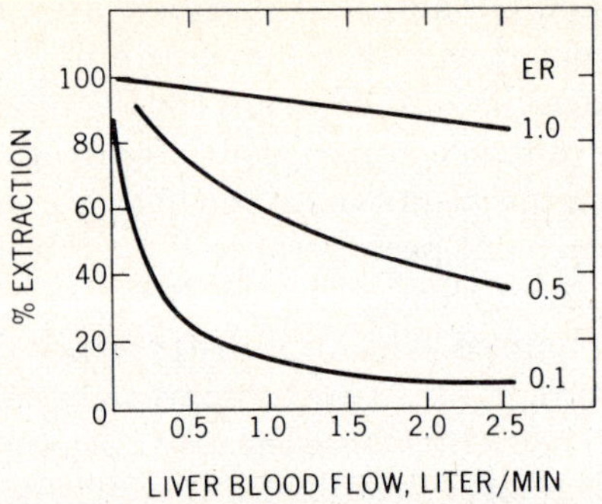

Fig. 5. Relationship between hepatic blood flow and hepatic extraction for drugs with various extraction ratios (*ER*)
Revised from Wilkinson and Shand (*29*)

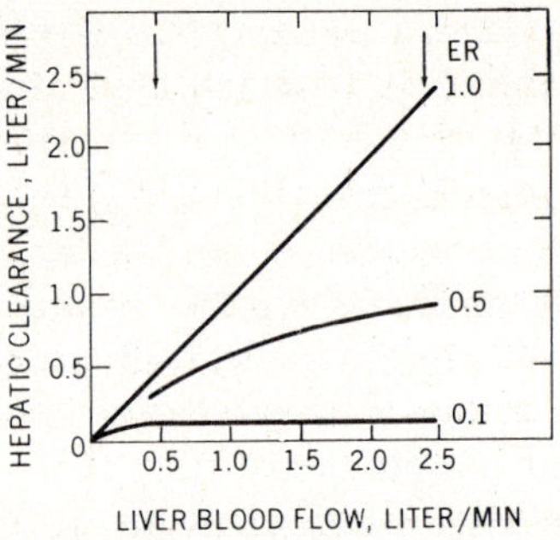

Fig. 6. Relationship between hepatic blood flow and total hepatic clearance for drugs with various extraction ratios (*ER*)
Arrows indicate normal physiological range of liver blood flow and the extraction values refer to a normal flow of 1.5 l/min. Revised from Wilkinson and Shand (*29*)

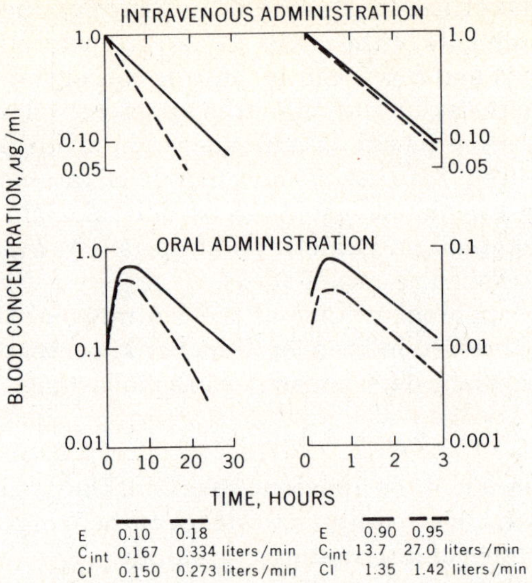

Fig. 7. Effect of increasing hepatic total intrinsic clearance ($Cl_{intrinsic}$) on the curves for total drug concentration in blood vs. time, after intravenous and oral administration of equal doses of two totally metabolized drugs
The *left panels* refer to a drug with an initial $Cl_{intrinsic}$ equivalent to an extraction ratio of 0.1 at a blood flow of 1.5 l/min. The *right panels* refer to a drug with an initial extraction ratio of 0.9. The *AUC*'s after oral administration are inversely proportional to $Cl_{intrinsic}$. From Wilkinson and Shand (*29*); reprinted with permission of the publisher

of the drug [$Cl_{renal} = (f_e)(TBC)$] can be calculated. The difference [$TBC - Cl_{renal}$] equals the metabolic clearance of the drug. If the liver is the only organ involved in metabolism of the drug, then this value equals the hepatic clearance of the drug.

Several physiological or pathological conditions that alter cardiac output, blood distribution, or both can change hepatic blood flow (*cf. 28*). One drug may also exert an effect on the elimination of another drug through a hemodynamic interaction or by altering intrinsic clearance (e.g., enzyme induction). Alterations in acid–base balance can also affect pharmacokinetic parameters (*7, 8, 10, 11*). When pharmacokinetic principles are used to describe the disposition of any drug in an individual patient one should also be aware of the possibility that supervention of these conditions can cause significant changes in pharmacokinetic parameters for certain drugs and hence in the dosage requirements for these drugs. Figures 7 and 8 show how changes in $Cl_{intrinsic}$ and hepatic blood flow, respectively, can alter the curves relating drug concentrations in the blood to time after intravenous or oral administration of totally metabolized compounds.

The pharmacokinetic parameters described above can be obtained for any drug by measuring in an individual the concentration of drug in plasma or blood as a function of time. One should be aware, however, that the parameters obtained always refer to the particular fluid used to measure the drug concentration. Thus, for example, if blood is used, the pharmacokinetic parameters refer to whole blood. Because only nonprotein-bound drug is pharmacologically active, it would appear to be beneficial to be able to refer all pharmacokinetic parameters, regardless of whether obtained from whole blood or plasma, to this fraction of the totally determined drug concentration. [Note that clearance may be an exception (*27–29*).] If the drug concentration is determined from whole blood, one needs to determine the plasma/erythrocyte partition coefficient and the fraction of the drug bound to plasma proteins. If plasma drug concentrations are measured, only the fraction of drug bound to plasma protein need be determined. Knowledge of these factors will permit any pharmacokinetic parameter to be obtained in terms of the nonprotein-bound drug concentration, total concentration in plasma, or total concentration in blood (*30*).

The clinical chemist rarely receives a sufficient number of samples from a given individual to perform a complete pharmacokinetic analysis. Nevertheless, the clinical chemist should be aware of these pharmacokinetic principles, to ensure that his half-life determinations of a drug are based solely on samples obtained during the beta phase.

Thus far, the pharmacokinetics of drugs administered only by a single intravenous injection have been discussed. However, most drugs are administered by other routes on an acute and chronic basis. The sections below describe certain aspects of pharmacokinetics after administration of drugs by routes other than single in-

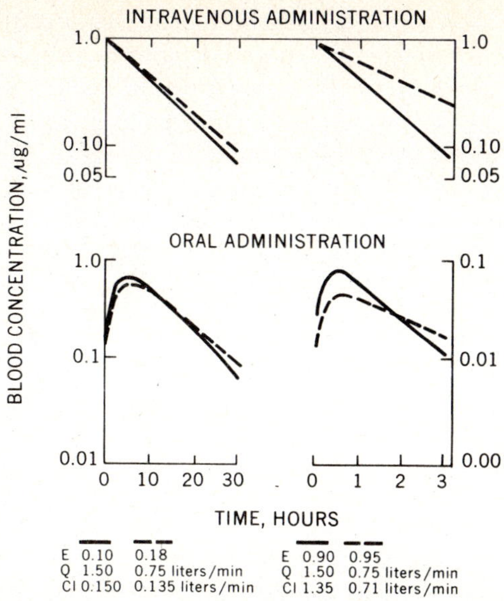

Fig. 8. Effects of decreasing hepatic blood flow on the total blood concentration–time curves after intravenous and oral administration of equal doses of two totally metabolized drugs

The *left panels* refer to a drug with a total intrinsic clearance equivalent to an extraction ratio of 0.1 when blood flow equals 1.5 l/min. The *right panels* refer to a drug with an intrinsic clearance equivalent to an extraction ratio of 0.9. From Wilkinson and Shand (*29*); reprinted with permission of the publisher

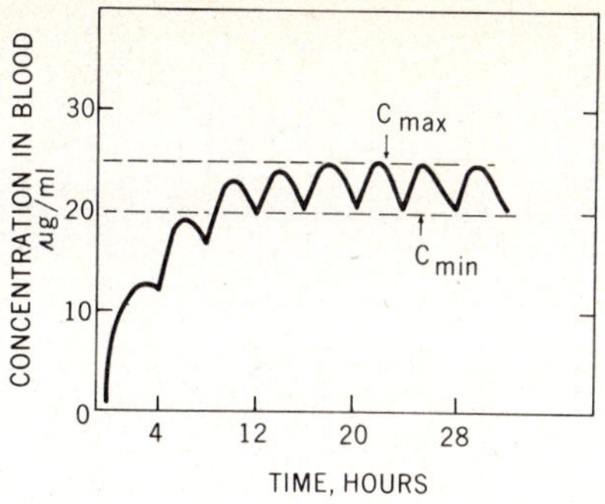

Fig. 9. Typical plot of the concentration of a drug in blood after repetitive oral administration of equal doses at equal time intervals

travenous injection. For more comprehensive discussions, the reader is referred to references *6–10, 27, 31–35*.

Bioavailability

The most popular mode of drug administration is the oral route. After administration of a drug by this route, the area under the blood drug concentration-time curve (AUC) reflects the amount of drug that reaches the systemic sampling site. The ratio of $AUC_{oral}/AUC_{i.v.}$ has been taken to be a measure of the bioavailability of the drug after oral administration.

All drugs, when administered orally, must pass through the gut wall and, when absorbed via the hepatic portal system, must traverse the liver before reaching the systemic sampling site. On the assumption of complete gastrointestinal absorption of drugs, it is possible that for a certain compound a fraction of the dose absorbed may not reach the sampling site because of metabolism within gut or liver. This "first-pass" effect, especially with respect to the liver, has received increasing recognition (*27–29, 31–40*). Thus far only a few drugs have been shown to exhibit this "first-pass" effect, most notably imipramine, lidocaine, meperidine, nortriptyline, phenacetin, and propranolol.

A hospitalized patient might initially receive drugs intravenously, rather than orally. As mentioned above, changes in the patient's physiological and pathological state may be reflected in altered body clearance of these drugs, thereby altering their therapeutic impact or effect. Pharmacokinetic considerations reveal that even if no discernible changes occur in the curve relating drug concentration to time (and thus total body drug clearance) when the patient is on intravenous therapy, a switch in the route of administration from intravenous to oral, which commonly occurs when a patient is discharged, can alter the pharmacokinetic profile and dosage requirements (Figures 7 and 8, bottom).

For example, consider a drug that stimulates the hepatic enzymes that metabolize drugs. If the hepatic clearance of this drug, or of a simultaneously administered drug, approaches hepatic blood flow (i.e., extraction ratio, ER, $\geq$ 0.9), then even though the hepatic enzymes are stimulated, changes in the clearance of the drug may not be observable while the drugs are given intravenously. If the drugs are administered orally, a decrease in bioavailability (as judged by AUC) will be evident (Figure 7, bottom right). Thus, while the body clearance of drug remains unchanged, the patient could be receiving as little as 50% of the intended dose.

Chronic or Repetitive Dosing

While some drugs, particularly analgesics, hypnotics, bronchodilators, antihistamines, and neuromuscular blocking agents, may be used effectively in a single dose, numerous therapeutic agents are given chronically. In many instances chronically administered drugs are taken sufficiently frequently that measurable and often pharmacologically significant concentrations of drug persist in the body at the time that a subsequent dose is received. Thus, the drug tends to accumulate at a decreasing rate with increasing number of doses until a steady-state plasma level of drug is achieved (Figure 9). For drugs whose disposition follows first-order kinetics, the average steady-state blood concentration is a function of the dose (D), fraction of dose absorbed (f), dosing interval (τ), biologic half-life ($t\frac{1}{2} = 0.693/\beta$), and apparent volume of distribution (V_d) (*41*). The relationship between the average steady-state blood concentration ($\bar{C}$) and the above factors is given by the equation (*42*)

$$\bar{C} = 1.44\,(t\tfrac{1}{2}) \cdot (fD)/V_d \cdot \tau \tag{11}$$

and

$$\text{Clearance} = (f)(D)/\bar{C}_{ss}(\tau) \tag{12}$$

In some cases the terminal exponential elimination phase is difficult if not impossible to observe, because it occurs only after drug concentrations have decreased

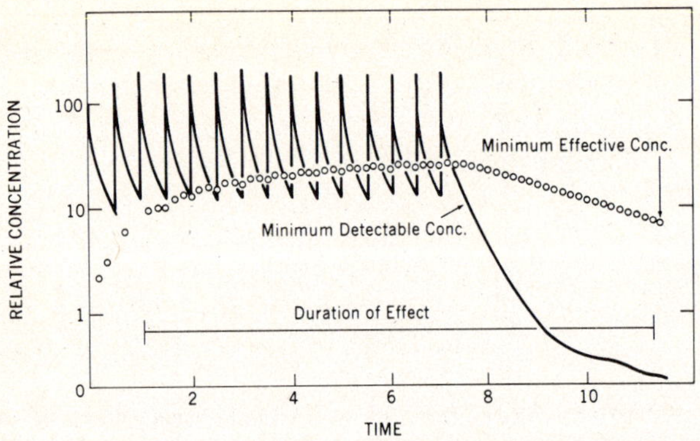

Fig. 10. Relative concentrations of a drug in the central and "deep" peripheral compartments of a three-compartment system during repetitive administration of equal doses at equal time intervals. The *curve* and the *circles* represent the central and the deep peripheral compartments, respectively
From Gibaldi et al. (*4*); reprinted with permission of the publisher

by two or more orders of magnitude from those occurring immediately after administration of a single dose. In this case, it is possible to reach an apparent steady-state concentration in plasma while the drug concentration in an organ or tissue that acts as a "deep" compartment continues to rise. If the site of drug action is in this "deep" compartment, then this discrepancy in pharmacokinetic behavior between plasma and deep compartment can account for (*a*) delayed onset of therapeutic activity, (*b*) increases in pharmacological effects at times when plasma drug concentrations appear to be at steady-state, and (*c*) occurrence of pharmacological effects despite negligible drug concentrations in the plasma (Figure 10).

Use of Urine or Saliva for Obtaining Pharmacokinetic Parameters

The pharmacokinetic data discussed above are usually obtained by following the concentration of drug or metabolites in blood as a function of time (*4–7*). The necessary blood samples must be drawn by skilled personnel in the clinic or hospital, and problems may occur with old or young patients or when serial samples are needed.

Use of more accessible body fluids, such as urine or saliva, simplifies sample collection for several reasons. Urine and saliva are more convenient and less discomforting or risky to obtain than blood. Furthermore, these noninvasive methods can offer information on drug disposition that may be either unavailable or difficult to acquire from blood.

Drug Kinetics from Urinary Excretion Data

Many potent therapeutic agents, especially those with large volumes of distribution, present problems for pharmacokinetic analysis, because even at their peak pharmacological effect the drug concentrations in blood are very low. Thus, depending on the selectivity and sensitivity of the analytical procedure, determination of the drug concentration in the blood may be insufficiently accurate (*3*).

Because a substantial fraction of the administered dose, either as the unchanged drug or metabolite(s), is usually excreted in the urine, it would be very useful if the urinary excretion data could be used to obtain an estimate of certain pharmacokinetic parameters. For drugs whose disposition can be described by a one compartment model and whose metabolites are rapidly excreted (*5*)

$$\log\begin{pmatrix}\text{rate of excretion of}\\ \text{drug or metabolites}\end{pmatrix} = \log(\text{constant}) - \left(\frac{k_e}{2.303}\right)t \quad (13)$$

This same relationship holds for drugs whose disposition conforms to a two-compartment model and whose metabolites are rapidly excreted, except that β replaces k_e (*43*). Thus, measurement of the rate of elimination of a drug or any of its metabolites permits estimation of the drug's biologic half-life.

In practice, the logarithm of the amount of drug excreted in a series of equal intervals is plotted vs. the mid-point of each time interval. This method requires no knowledge of the total amount of drug or metabolite excreted at infinity, so loss of a urine specimen does not invalidate the experiment. Furthermore, collection of urine can be discontinuous; it can be abandoned overnight and started again the following day. Thus, this method is particularly applicable to investigation of progressive changes in the rate of drug elimination that may occur during a course of drug therapy. This method has been successfully used to analyze data on urinary salicylamide excretion in adults (*44*) and diphenylhydantoin elimination in overdosed children (*45*). One problem with this method is that fluctuations in the rate of drug elimination cause appreciable departures from linearity (*43, 46*).

Another method that can be utilized is termed the "Sigma-minus" method (*43, 46, 47*). Derived from classical chemical kinetics, this method discloses the amount of drug in the body from knowledge of the amount of drug or metabolite excreted at any time (U) and the total amount excreted (U_∞). When elimination is first order

$$\log(U_\infty - U) = \log U_\infty - \left(\frac{\beta}{2.303}\right)t \quad (14)$$

Furthermore,

$$U_\infty = \frac{k_i A_0}{\beta} \quad (15)$$

where k_i is the first-order rate constant for either (*a*) elimination of metabolite (when elimination is slower than formation), (*b*) production of metabolite (when production is slower than elimination), or (*c*) elimination of unchanged drug (*43*). A_0 represents that fraction of the administered dose reaching the central compartment. When absorption is complete, A_0 is equal to the administered dose.

The "Sigma-minus" method requires knowledge of

U_∞ and so in theory requires total collection of urine until such time as drug excretion is essentially complete. It has been suggested (*48*) that urine be collected for a time period equal to 10 times the drug's half-life. This requirement applies to the laboratory concerned with defining the complete pharmacokinetic profile of a drug; the clinical chemist need only carry urine collections through three to five drug half-lives, because 87 to 96%, respectively, of a drug is eliminated from the body during this period.

The fraction of the dose of a drug excreted in the urine depends on the ratio of renal clearance to total body clearance. Thus, any factor affecting total body clearance can affect the ultimate fraction of the dose eliminated in urine. Furthermore, renal clearance is a complex function of glomerular filtration, tubular secretion, and tubular reabsorption (*49*), the precise combination varying from drug to drug. Any factor affecting one or more of the components of renal clearance will also affect the pharmacokinetic parameters (*50*). Alterations in protein binding and urinary pH can affect the urinary excretion and metabolism of certain drugs (*7, 8, 10, 50, 51*).

In summary, urinary excretion data permit determination of (*a*) the overall disposition constant, β, for loss of drug from the body; and (*b*) the rate constants for urinary elimination of unchanged drug, for production or elimination of metabolites, or for both. A further discussion of these methods is given in references *5–9, 11, 43, 46–48*. The use of urine for pharmacokinetic analysis is particularly promising in pediatric and geriatric patients.

Drug Kinetics from Salivary Excretion Data

Identification in saliva of most therapeutic agents after their oral or parenteral administration is well documented (*52–65*). For most drugs thus far examined, transfer from plasma to saliva appears to be passive, pH dependent, and proportional to the concentration of the compound in plasma (*43, 52, 60, 62–65*). Lithium is an exception in that transport from blood to saliva appears to be active, thereby accounting for higher lithium concentrations in saliva than plasma (*61*). The observation that salivary drug concentration is often proportional to plasma drug concentration led to use of saliva as a noninvasive technique for monitoring most drug concentrations in plasma and for obtaining various pharmacokinetic data (*43, 57–65*).

Measurement of drug concentrations in saliva offers several advantages over similar measurements performed in plasma. In the first place, many specimens can be obtained noninvasively, without loss of blood or exposure of pediatric and geriatric patients to discomfort and potential skin irritation and infection. More importantly, however, drug concentrations in saliva represent the free fraction of the drug, whereas data on concentrations in plasma represent both the free and protein-bound forms of the drug (*43, 52, 53, 57, 60, 62–65*). In plasma, the ratio of free to protein-bound drug varies with age and disease state and may also change appreciably in the same patient, owing to factors such as altered albumin concentrations and the presence of other compounds that can displace the drug from its binding site on albumin. Moreover, the clinical chemist cannot conveniently, inexpensively, and routinely separate the free drug from the bound drug in plasma. Only the free form of the drug is available to produce pharmacological effects, and so measurements of drug concentrations in saliva are more therapeutically meaningful because they represent the concentration of the free fraction of the drug.

Salivary drug concentration is proportional to plasma drug concentration. Thus, the same pharmacokinetic principles discussed above for blood and plasma can also be used when salivary drug concentrations are measured.

Drug transfer from blood to saliva is pH dependent (*52–65*); thus, the concentration of total drug in plasma can be calculated from salivary drug concentration by

Table 1. Fraction of Drug Bound to Plasma Proteins as Determined by (*a*) Equilibrium Dialysis and (*b*) Relationship between Drug Concentration in Saliva and Plasma[a,b]

	Calculated from		
Drug	Equilib. dial (ref. no)	Concns. in saliva and plasma[a,b] (ref. no)	Difference, %
Aminopyrine	0.15 (*71*)	0.20 (*43*)	33
Amobarbital	0.41 (*67*), 0.58 (*64*)	0.60 (*64*)	3.4
Antipyrine	<0.1 (*72*)	0.03 (*43*)	—
Digoxin	0.23 (*68*)	0.22 (*63*)	4.3
Diphenyl-hydantoin	0.86 (*67*), 0.90 (*69*)	0.90 (*65*)	0
Phenacetin	0.30 (*70*)	0.40 (*43*)	33
Phenobarbital	0.32 (*67*)	0.36 (*70*)	19
Salicylic acid	0.45–0.80 (*67*)	0.69–0.77 (*58*)	—
Theophylline	0.59 (*60*)	0.52 (*60*)	12
Tolbutamide	0.91 (*62*)	0.98 (*62*)	8

[a] Fraction of acidic drug bound to plasma proteins

$$= 1 - \left\{\frac{[S]}{[P]}\left(\frac{1 + 10^{(pH_p - pK_a)}}{1 + 10^{(pH_s - pK_a)}}\right)\right\}$$

and

Fraction of basic drug bound to plasma proteins

$$= 1 - \left\{\frac{[S]}{[P]}\left(\frac{1 + 10^{-(pH_p - pK_a)}}{1 + 10^{-(pH_s - pK_a)}}\right)\right\}$$

These equations are rearrangements of equations described by Matin et al. (*62*).

[b] Plasma pH = (pH_p) = 7.4 and salivary pH = (pH_s) = 6.5 for the equations above.

Table 2. *K* Factors for Determination of Plasma Protein Binding of a Drug from the Drug Concentration in Saliva and Plasma According to Equation 17

	K factor[a]			
	Plasma pH 7.4, saliva pH 6.5		Plasma pH 7.4, saliva pH 7.0	
Drug pK_a	Acids	Bases	Acids	Bases
<4	7.94	0.999	2.51	0.999
4.5	7.87	0.991	2.50	0.998
5.0	7.73	0.973	2.49	0.994
5.5	7.31	0.921	2.42	0.983
6.0	6.28	0.780	2.36	0.945
6.5	3.97	0.563	2.15	0.856
6.8	3.32	0.418	1.93	0.767
7.0	2.66	0.336	1.76	0.699
7.2	2.15	0.272	1.58	0.632
7.4	1.77	0.250	1.43	0.570
7.6	1.44	0.178	1.30	0.518
7.8	1.33	0.167	1.21	0.424
8.0	1.23	0.153	1.14	0.453
8.5	1.07	0.135	1.05	0.417
9.0	1.02	0.129	1.02	0.404
9.5	1.01	0.127	1.01	0.400
>10.0	1.00	0.126	1.00	0.399

[a] The *K* factor is derived as follows:

for acids, $K = 1 + 10^{(pH_p - pK_a)}/1 + 10^{(pH_s - pK_a)}$.

for bases, $K = 1 + 10^{-(pH_p - pK_a)}/1 + 10^{-(pH_s - pK_a)}$.

These equations are from Matin et al. (*62*).

use of a modification of the equations of Jacobs (*66*) as described by Matin et al. (*62*). To test the validity of these equations in estimating the fraction of drug bound to plasma proteins, we compared the fraction of drug bound to plasma proteins, as determined by equilibrium dialysis, with that obtained by use of the equations described by Matin et al. (*62*). Analysis of the data in Table 1 indicates that the values for the fraction of drug bound to plasma proteins derived from these equations agree closely with those obtained from equilibrium dialysis.

For most drugs measurement of the concentration in saliva provides a good estimate of the concentration of the free form of the drug in plasma *without correction for pH* (*43*). This generalization applies to acidic drugs whose pK_a is greater than 8.5 and basic drugs whose pK_a is 5.5 or less. Measurement of drug concentrations in simultaneously obtained samples of saliva and plasma permits accurate estimation of the percent binding of a drug to plasma proteins *without knowledge of plasma* or *salivary pH*. The following equation permits determination of the fraction of drug bound to plasma proteins (F_B) from the salivary and plasma drug decay curves (*43*):

$$F_B = 1 - K\left[\frac{(V_d)_p}{(V_d)_s}\right] \qquad (16)$$

which can be equated to the following simplified version of the formulas described by Matin et al. (*62*):

$$F_B = 1 - K\frac{[S]}{[P]} \qquad (17)$$

where K is a proportionality factor that takes into account plasma and salivary pH as well as the pK_a of the drug. For drugs whose pK_a lies within the ranges given above, $K = 1$ and thus plasma and salivary pH need not be determined. However, for drugs whose pK_a is outside this range, the effect of pH on the distribution of drug between these two biological fluids must be taken into account. Table 2 provides the value of K in equation 17 for various pK_a's at salivary pH's of 6.5 and 7.0. In normal individuals salivary pH appears to be generally between 6.5 and 7.2 (*62, 63*).

Finally, two methodological considerations arise in connection with the use of saliva to monitor drug concentrations. Precaution should be exercised to avoid having remnants of orally administered drug in the mouth when salivary specimens are collected. Chiou et al. (*73*) reported this source for several aberrantly high salicylate concentrations measured in saliva. This problem occurs mainly when specimens are collected shortly after drug administration. Washing the mouth before obtaining the specimen of saliva can eliminate this problem, if it should appear. In our experience, this difficulty never arose during measurement of drug concentrations in saliva; our salivary drug-decay curves have been as smooth and consistent with first-order kinetics as the plasma drug-decay curves (*43*). Saliva collected with or without salivary gland stimulation through the chewing of parafilm yielded similar drug concentrations; therefore, chewing parafilm did not alter the salivary concentrations of the drugs that we investigated (*43*).

In summary, measurement of drug in saliva as a function of time permits determination of pharmacokinetic data usually obtained from plasma. In addition, for most drugs saliva discloses the concentration of the free, pharmacologically active form of the drug, whereas plasma concentrations represent the total drug concentration (free plus protein-bound). If plasma and saliva samples are obtained simultaneously, measurement of their respective drug concentrations permits one to estimate the fraction of drug bound to the plasma proteins. Because binding of drug to plasma proteins can fluctuate widely both between and within patients, measurement of drug concentrations in plasma alone are of limited value, whereas salivary drug concentrations are of more value therapeutically.

This work was supported in part by grants 1-R01-DA 01180-01 and 1-R01-CA16536-01 from the NIH.

References

1. Vesell, E. S., and Passananti, G. T., Utility of clinical chemical determinations of drug concentrations in biological fluids. *Clin. Chem.* **17,** 851 (1971).

2. Vesell, E. S., Relationship between drug distribution and therapeutic effects in man. *Annu. Rev. Pharmacol.* **14,** 249 (1974).

3. Werner, M., Sutherland, E. W., III, and Abramson, F. P., Concepts for the rational selection of assays to be used in monitoring therapeutic drugs. *Clin. Chem.* **21,** 1368 (1975).

4. Gibaldi, M., Levy, G., and Weintraub, H., Drug distribution and pharmacological effects. *Clin. Pharmacol. Ther.* **12,** 734 (1971).

5. Nelson, E., Kinetics of drug absorption, distribution, metabolism and excretion. *J. Pharm. Sci.* **50,** 181 (1961).

6. Wagner, J. G., *Biopharmaceutics and Relevant Pharmacokinetics,* The Hamilton Press, Hamilton, Ill., 1971.

7. Notari, R. E., *Biopharmaceutics and Pharmacokinetics,* 2nd ed., Marcel Dekker, New York, N. Y., 1975.

8. Gibaldi, M., and Perrier, D., *Pharmacokinetics,* Marcel Dekker, New York, N. Y., 1975.

9. Garrett, E. R., Theoretical pharmacokinetics. In *Klinische Pharmakologie und Pharmakotherapie,* H. P. Kuemmerle, E. R. Garrett and K. M. Spitzy, Eds., Urban and Schwarzenberg, Munich, 1971.

10. van Rossum, J. M., Significance of pharmacokinetics for drug design and the planning of dosage regimens. In *Drug Design,* Volume **11, I,** E. J. Ariens, Ed., Academic Press, New York, N. Y., 1971.

11. O'Reilly, W. J., Pharmacokinetics in drug metabolism and toxicology. *Can. J. Pharm. Sci.* **7,** 66 (1972).

12. Riegelman, S., Loo, J. C. K., and Rowland, M., Shortcomings in pharmacokinetic analysis by conceiving the body to exhibit properties of a single compartment. *J. Pharm. Sci.* **57,** 117 (1968).

13. Sedman, A. J., and Wagner, J. G., Importance of the use of the appropriate pharmacokinetic model to analyze *in vivo* enzyme constants. *J. Pharmacokinet. Biopharm.* **2,** 161 (1974).

14. Balasubramaniam, K., Lucas, S. B., Mawer, G. E., and Simons, P. J., The kinetics of amylobarbitone metabolism in healthy men and women. *Br. J. Pharmacol.* **39,** 564 (1970).

15. Kaplan, S. A., Weinfeld, R. E., Abruzzo, C. W., and Lewis, M., Pharmacokinetic profile of sulfisoxazole following intravenous, intramuscular, and oral administration in man. *J. Pharm. Sci.* **61,** 773 (1972).

16. Gibaldi, M., Levy, G., and Hayton, W., Kinetics of the elimination and neuromuscular blocking effect of *d*-tubocurarine in man. *Anesthesiology* **36,** 213 (1972).

17. Shen, D., Gibaldi, M., Throne, M., et al., Pharmacokinetics of bethanidine in hypertensive patients. *Clin. Pharmacol. Ther.* **17,** 363, 1975.

18. Riggs, D. S., *The Mathematical Approach to Physiological Problems,* Williams and Wilkins, Baltimore, Md., 1963.

19. Riegelman, S., Loo, J., and Rowland, M., Concept of a volume of distribution and possible errors in evaluation of this parameter. *J. Pharm. Sci.* **57,** 128 (1968).

20. Benet, L. Z., and Ronfeld, R. A., Volume terms in pharmacokinetics. *J. Pharm. Sci.* **58,** 639 (1969).

21. Gibaldi, M., Effect of mode of administration on drug distribution in a two-compartment open system. *J. Pharm. Sci.* **58,** 327 (1969).

22. Gibaldi, M., Nagashima, R., and Levy, G., Relationship between drug concentration in plasma or serum and amount of drug in the body. *J. Pharm. Sci.* **58,** 193 (1969).

23. Perrier, D., and Gibaldi, M., Relationship between plasma or serum drug concentration and amount of drug in the body at steady state upon multiple dosing. *J. Pharmacokinet. Biopharm.* **1,** 17 (1973).

24. Rowland, M., Benet, L. Z., and Graham, G. G., Clearance concepts in pharmacokinetics. *J. Pharmacokinet. Biopharm.* **1,** 123 (1973).

25. Perrier, D., and Gibaldi, M., Clearance and biologic half-life as indices of intrinsic hepatic metabolism. *J. Pharmacol. Exp. Ther.* **191,** 17 (1974).

26. Perrier, D., and Gibaldi, M., Drug clearance in multicompartment systems. *Can. J. Pharm. Sci.* **9,** 11 (1974).

27. Rowland, M., Influence of route of administration on drug availability. *J. Pharm. Sci.* **61,** 70 (1972).

28. Wilkinson, G. R., Pharmacokinetics of drug disposition: Hemodynamic considerations. *Annu. Rev. Pharmacol.* **15,** 11 (1975).

29. Wilkinson, G. R., and Shand, D. G., A physiological approach to hepatic drug clearance. *Clin. Pharmacol. Ther.* **18,** 377 (1975).

30. Garrett, E. R., and Lambert, H. J., Pharmacokinetics of trichloroethanol and metabolites and interconversions among variously referenced pharmacokinetic parameters. *J. Pharm. Sci.* **62,** 550 (1973).

31. Harris, P. A., and Riegelman, S., Influence of the route of administration on the area under the plasma concentration-time curve. *J. Pharm. Sci.* **58,** 71 (1969).

32. Gibaldi, M., and Feldman, S., Pharmacokinetic basis for the influence of route of administration on the area under the plasma concentration-time curve. *J. Pharm. Sci.* **58,** 1477 (1969).

33. Gibaldi, M., and Feldman, S., Route of administration and drug metabolism. *Eur. J. Pharmacol.* **19,** 323 (1972).

34. Gibaldi, M., and Perrier, D., Route of administration and drug disposition. *Drug Metab. Rev.* **3,** 185 (1974).

35. Gibaldi, M., Boyes, R. N., and Feldman, S., Influence of first-pass effect on availability of drugs on oral administration. *J. Pharm. Sci.* **60,** 1338 (1971).

36. Perrier, D., and Gibaldi, M., Influence of first-pass effect on the systemic availability of propoxyphene. *J. Clin. Pharmacol.* **12,** 449 (1972).

37. Cleaveland, C. R., and Shand, D. G., Effect of route of administration on the relationship between β-adrenergic blockade and plasma propranolol level. *Clin. Pharmacol. Ther.* **13,** 181 (1972).

38. Saidman, L. J., and Eger, E. I., II, Uptake and distribution of thiopental after oral, rectal, and intramuscular administration: Effect of hepatic metabolism and injection site blood flow. *Clin. Pharmacol. Ther.* **14,** 12 (1973).

39. Gram, L. F., and Christiansen, J., First-pass metabolism of imipramine in man. *Clin. Pharmacol. Ther.* **17,** 555 (1975).

40. Gram, L. F., and Overo, K. F., First-pass metabolism of nortriptyline in man. *Clin. Pharmacol. Ther.* **18,** 305 (1975).

41. Levy, G., Pharmacokinetic control and clinical interpretation of steady-state blood levels of drugs. *Clin. Pharmacol. Ther.* **16,** 130 (1974).

42. van Rossum, J. M., and Tomey, A. H. M., Rate of accumulation and plateau plasma concentration of drugs after chronic medication. *J. Pharm. Pharmacol.* **20,** 390 (1968).

43. Vesell, E. S., Passananti, G. T., Glenwright, P. A., and Dvorchik, B. H., Studies on the disposition of antipyrine, aminopyrine, and phenacetin using plasma, saliva, and urine. *Clin. Pharmacol. Ther.* **18,** 259 (1975).

44. Levy, G., and Matsuzawa, T., Pharmacokinetics of salicylamide elimination in man. *J. Pharmacol. Exp. Ther.* **156,** 285 (1967).

45. Garrettson, L. K., and Jusko, W. J., Diphenylhydantoin elimination kinetics in overdosed children. *Clin. Pharmacol. Ther.* **17,** 481 (1975).

46. Martin, B. K., Drug urinary excretion data—some aspects concerning the interpretation. *Br. J. Pharmacol. Chemother.* **29,** 181 (1967).

47. Cummings, A. J., Martin, B. K., and Park, G. S., Kinetic considerations relating to the accrual and elimination of drug metabolites. *Br. J. Pharmacol. Chemother.* **29,** 136 (1967).

48. Wagner, J. G., Some possible errors in the plotting and interpretation of semilogarithmic plots of blood level and urinary excretion data. *J. Pharm. Sci.* **52,** 1097 (1963).

49. Pitts, R. F., *Physiology of the Kidney and Body Fluids,* 2nd ed., Year Book Med. Pub., Inc., Chicago, Ill., 1968.

50. Wagner, J. G., Equations for excretion rate and renal clearances of exogenous substances not actively reabsorbed. *J. Clin. Pharmacol.* **7,** 89 (1967).

51. Wagner, J. G., Pharmacokinetics. *Annu. Rev. Pharmacol.* **8,** 67 (1968).

52. Killmann, S. A., and Thaysen, J. H., The permeability of the human parotid gland to a series of sulfonamide compounds, *para*aminohippurate and inulin. *Scand. J. Clin. Lab. Invest.* **7,** 86 (1955).

53. Rasmussen, F., Salivary excretion of sulphonamides and barbiturates by cows and goats. *Acta Pharmacol. Toxicol.* **21,** 11 (1964).

54. Borzelleca, J. F., and Cherrick, H. M., The excretion of drugs in saliva. Antibiotics. *J. Oral Ther. Pharmacol.* **2,** 180 (1965).

55. Borzelleca, J. F., and Doyle, C. H., Excretion of drugs in saliva. Salicylate, barbiturate, sulfanilamide. *J. Oral Ther. Pharmacol.* **3,** 104 (1966).

56. Joselow, M. M., Ruiz, R., and Goldwater, L. J., The use of salivary (parotid) fluid in biochemical monitoring. *Am. Ind. Hyg. Assoc., J.* **30,** 77 (1969).

57. Borzelleca, J. F., and Putney, J. W., Jr., A model for the movement of salicylate across the parotid epithelium. *J. Pharmacol. Exp. Ther.* **174,** 527 (1970).

58. Graham, G., and Rowland, M., Application of salivary salicylate data to biopharmaceutical studies of salicylates. *J. Pharm. Sci.* **61,** 1219 (1972).

59. Glynn, J. P., and Bastain, W., Salivary excretion of paracetamol in man. *J. Pharm. Pharmacol.* **25,** 420 (1973).

60. Koysooko, R., Ellis, E. F., and Levy, G., Relationship between theophylline concentration in plasma and saliva of man. *Clin. Pharmacol. Ther.* **15,** 454 (1974).

61. Groth, U., Prellwitz, W., and Jähnchen, E., Estimation of pharmacokinetic parameters of lithium from saliva and urine. *Clin. Pharmacol. Ther.* **16,** 490 (1974).

62. Matin, S. B., Wan, S. H., and Karam, J. H., Pharmacokinetics of tolbutamide: Prediction by concentration in saliva. *Clin. Pharmacol. Ther.* **16,** 1052 (1974).

63. Huffman, D. H., Relationship between digoxin concentrations in serum and saliva. *Clin. Pharmacol. Ther.* **17,** 310 (1975).

64. Inaba, T., and Kalow, W., Salivary excretion of amobarbital in man. *Clin. Pharmacol. Ther.* **18,** 558 (1975).

65. Cook, C. E., Amerson, E., Poole, W. K., et al., Phenytoin and phenobarbital concentrations in saliva and plasma measured by radioimmunoassay. *Clin. Pharmacol. Ther.* **18,** 742 (1975).

66. Jacobs, M. H., Some aspects of cell permeability to weak electrolytes. *Cold Spring Harbor Symp. Quant. Biol.* **8,** 30 (1970).

67. Kudla, R. M., El-Bassionni, A., and Mattocks, A. M., Accelerated peritoneal dialysis of barbiturates, diphenylhydantoin and salicylate. *J. Pharm. Sci.* **60,** 1065 (1971).

68. Lukas, D. S., and DeMartino, A. G., Binding of digitoxin and some related cardenolides to human plasma proteins. *J. Clin. Invest.* **48,** 1041 (1969).

69. Lunde, P. K. M., Rane, A., Yaffe, S. J., et al., Plasma protein binding of diphenylhydantoin in man. *Clin. Pharmacol. Ther.* **11,** 846 (1970).

70. Brodie, B. B., and Axelrod, J., The fate of acetophenetidin (phenacetin) in man and methods for the estimation of acetophenitidin and its metabolites in biological material. *J. Pharmacol. Exp. Ther.* **97,** 58 (1949).

71. Brodie, B. B., and Axelrod, J., The fate of aminopyrine (Pyramidon) in man and methods for the estimation of aminopyrine and its metabolites in biological material. *J. Pharmacol. Exp. Ther.* **99,** 171 (1950).

72. Soberman, R., Brodie, B. B., Levy, B. B., et al., The use of antipyrine in the measurement of total body water in man. *J. Biol. Chem.* **179,** 31 (1949).

73. Chiou, W. L., Chang, K., and Peng, G. W., Precaution in the monitoring of drug levels in saliva: Abnormal salicylate levels after oral dosing. *J. Clin. Pharmacol.* **16,** 158 (1976).

CLIN. CHEM. 22/6, 879–883 (1976)

Gas-Chromatographic Method for Acetaminophen (*N*-Acetyl-*p*-Aminophenol) Based on Sequential Alkylation

Walter A. Dechtiaruk, George F. Johnson, and Harvey M. Solomon

A gas-chromatographic procedure for acetaminophen is described in which the drug is chromatographed as the *O*-heptyl-*N*-methyl derivative. This derivative is prepared by a sequential alkylation procedure in which the phenolic hydroxyl group of the parent compound is alkylated off-column with heptyl iodide and the amide group is derivatized on-column by reaction with trimethylanilinium hydroxide. The internal standard, *N*-propionyl-*p*-aminophenol, is subjected to the same derivatization procedure. This gas-chromatographic procedure correlates well with conventional colorimetric and spectrophotometric procedures for acetaminophen and is more sensitive. Within-run precision (CV) was 2.0% at a serum concentration of 10.0 mg/liter (n = 10) and between-run precision was 4.0% over a period of eight months. This method is particularly applicable to studies of the pharmacokinetics of acetaminophen.

Additional Keyphrases: *pharmacokinetics* • *saliva, serum*

In man, large doses of acetaminophen (*N*-acetyl-*p*-aminophenol) can produce severe liver necrosis and occasionally cause fatal hepatic coma. Prescott et al. reported that intravenous cysteamine protected patients against hepatic necrosis following massive overdosage with acetaminophen (*1*). The decision whether to administer cysteamine to patients who ingested large doses of acetaminophen was based on the concentration of this drug in the plasma. Thus measurements of acetaminophen in plasma are critical in selecting patients at risk of potentially serious liver injury and also in determining those for whom treatment with cysteamine is unnecessary.

Numerous methods for the determination of acetaminophen in various biological fluids have been reported, including a colorimetric procedure (*2*); differential ultraviolet spectrophotometry (*3*); and gas-chromatography of the free drug (*4*), the mono- and di-trimethylsilyl derivatives (*5*), the acetylated derivative (*6*), and the *O*-benzoyl, *N*-trimethylsilyl derivative (*7*). Recently a high-resolution liquid-chromatographic method has been described that permits determination of free acetaminophen as well as seven of its metabolites (*8*). However, this method was used for studies of the metabolism of acetaminophen and was not proposed for routine use in diagnosis and management of intoxication.

Of the various procedures described, the differential ultraviolet spectrophotometric method of Routh et al. (*3*) and the colorimetric procedure of Glynn and Kendal (*2*) are probably most applicable to the laboratory diagnosis of massive overdosage with acetaminophen, as they are relatively easy to perform and can be provided without delay. In contrast, the published gas-chromatographic procedures are more complex and take considerably longer to perform. Moreover, underivatized acetaminophen is strongly adsorbed to most chromatographic columns, the trimethylsilyl derivatives are unstable, and the extent of formation of the benzoyl *N*-trimethylsilyl derivative of acetaminophen is incomplete (*7*).

The gas-chromatographic method we described for acetaminophen is based on the formation of the stable *O*-heptyl-*N*-methyl derivative of the drug, which shows a symmetrical chromatographic peak without evidence of adsorption on the column. This procedure was used in our laboratory to validate both the differential spectrophotometric and the colorimetric method for the emergency determination of acetaminophen. Our gas-chromatographic procedure is sensitive and specific and is particularly suited to pharmacokinetic studies of acetaminophen.

Materials and Methods

Reagents and Comparison Materials

Acetaminophen, N,N-*dimethylacetamide, iodobutane, iodoheptane, and propionic anhydride* were obtained from Aldrich Chemical Co., Milwaukee, Wis. 53233. A stock solution of acetaminophen (100 mg/liter) was prepared by dissolving 10 mg in 100 ml of ethanol.

Therapeutic Drug Monitoring Laboratory, Department of Laboratory Medicine, The Johns Hopkins Hospital, Baltimore, Md. 21205.
Received Feb. 24, 1976; accepted Mar. 26, 1976.

4-Aminophenol was purchased from the Gallard-Schlesinger Chemical Mfg. Corp., Carle Place, N. Y. 11514. *N*-Propionyl-*p*-aminophenol, the internal standard, was prepared by reacting 4-aminophenol with propionic anhydride in ethyl ether at 25 °C for 1 h, similar to the procedure of Stewart and Willis for synthesis of *N*-butyryl-*p*-aminophenol (*9*). The product was recrystallized three times from ethanol by gradual addition of water until crystallization commenced. A stock solution of the internal standard (100 mg/liter) was prepared by dissolving 10 mg in 100 ml of ethanol. A working solution of the internal standard (1 mg/liter) was prepared by evaporating 10 ml of the stock solution to dryness under nitrogen in a water bath at 40 °C and then dissolving the residue in 1 liter of ether/toluene (40/60 by vol).

Trimethylanilinium hydroxide (TMAH), 25 g/liter, in methanol. This reagent was prepared by reacting trimethylanilinium iodide (Eastman Organic Chemicals, Rochester, N. Y. 14650) with silver oxide (Matheson, Coleman and Bell, East Rutherford, N. J. 07073) according to the method of Osiewicz et al. (*10*).

Methanol and toluene ("ChromatoQuality") and tetramethylammonium hydroxide (TMH) 240 g/liter, in methanol were purchased from Matheson, Coleman and Bell. The TMH was diluted 10-fold with methanol and stored at 4 °C.

Pentyl iodide and hexyl iodide were obtained from Eastman Organic Chemicals.

Procedure for Extraction and Alkylation before Gas Chromatography

Serum (1 ml) or saliva (1 ml) was combined in a 16 × 125 mm test tube (Teflon-lined screw cap) with 1 ml of distilled water, 1 g of NaCl, and 10 ml of ethyl ether/toluene (40/60 by vol) containing 10 μg of the internal standard, *N*-propionyl-*p*-aminophenol. The mixture was shaken for 15 min in an Eberbach shaker at 250 oscillations/min and centrifuged at 2500 rpm for 10 min. The organic (top) phase was transferred to 16 × 125 mm test tubes (Teflon-lined screw cap) containing 2 ml of 0.1 mol/liter NaOH. The tubes were shaken for 10 min and centrifuged for 5 min. The organic phase was aspirated and discarded. One-half milliliter of phosphate buffer (1 mol/liter, pH 6.8), 1 g of NaCl, and 10 ml of ether were added to the aqueous solution. The mixture was shaken for 10 min and centrifuged for 5 min. The ether was transferred to tubes with constricted tips ("Concentratubes"; Laboratory Research Co., Los Angeles, Calif. 90036) and evaporated under nitrogen in a water bath at 40 °C. Eighty microliters of *N,N*-dimethylacetamide, and 20 μl of dilute tetramethylammonium hydroxide (TMH in methanol 24 g/liter) was added to the residues. The tubes were mixed on a vortex-type mixer for 5 s after each addition. Iodoheptane, 20 μl, was added and the tubes were again mixed on a vortex-type mixer for 5 s and allowed to stand at room temperature for 10 min. Then the tubes were centrifuged for 1 min at 2000 rpm to sediment the tetramethylammonium iodide. The clear supernate was transferred to 1.0 ml "Reacti-Vials" (Pierce Chemical Co., Rockford, Ill. 61105) and evaporated under nitrogen in a water bath at 40 °C. Twenty-five microliters of dilute trimethylanilinium hydroxide (25 g/liter of methanol) was added to the residues and the contents of the tubes were mixed on a vortex-type mixer for 10 s. Of this solution, 1 μl was injected into the gas chromatograph.

Serum-based standards (5, 10, 15, and 20 mg/liter) were prepared by evaporating to dryness under nitrogen 50, 100, 150, and 200 μl of a solution of acetaminophen in ethanol (100 μg/ml) and adding 1 ml of serum. Similar standards were prepared with saliva.

Gas Chromatography

A Model 5710A (Hewlett Packard, Avondale, Pa. 19311) dual-column gas chromatograph equipped with flame ionization detectors was used. The glass columns (122 cm × 6 mm, 2 mm i.d.) were packed with 3% OV-17 on 100/120 mesh Gas Chrom Q (Applied Science Labs., Inc., State College, Pa. 16801). The injector temperature was 250 °C; the detector 300 °C; and the oven temperature was programmed at a rate of 16 °C/min from 150 to 260 °C. The flow rate of nitrogen was 40 ml/min.

Differential Spectrophotometric Method for Acetaminophen

The differential spectrophotometric absorbance method of Routh et al. (*3*) was used for the determination of acetaminophen in serum and saliva. One milliliter of serum or saliva was extracted with 10 ml of diethyl ether, and 8 ml of the organic phase was removed and extracted with 2.5 ml of $NaHCO_3$ (4 g/liter). One milliliter of the aqueous layer and 1 ml of water were pipetted into a silica cuvette (reference cell), 1 ml of the aqueous layer and 1 ml of 0.25 mol/liter NaOH into the other cuvette (sample cell). Absorbance was measured

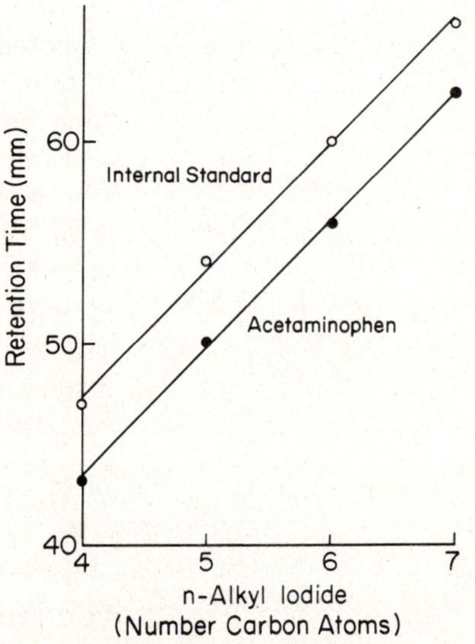

Fig. 1. Relationship between retention times of the *O*-alkyl-*N*-methyl derivatives of acetaminophen and the internal standard (*N*-propionyl-*p*-aminophenol) and chain length of the alkyl iodide used in derivatization

at 266 nm with a Beckman DB-GT spectrophotometer (Beckman Instruments, Inc., Fullerton, Calif. 92634).

Colorimetric Method for Acetaminophen

Acetaminophen in serum was determined by a modification of the method of Glynn and Kendal (*2*) based on the reaction of this drug with nitrous acid to yield the chromophore, 2-nitro-4-acetamidophenol (*10*).

To a 16 × 100 mm glass screw-cap culture tube, add 1 ml of serum and 2 ml of trichloroacetic acid (100 g/liter). Mix on a vortex-type mixer for 30 s and then centrifuge at 2000 rpm for 2 min. Decant the supernatant fluid into a 50-ml culture tube containing 1 ml of hydrochloric acid (6 mol/liter) and 2 ml of freshly prepared sodium nitrite (100 g/liter). Allow the tubes to stand for 2 min at room temperature. Then add 2 ml of ammonium sulfamate (150 g/liter) followed by 5 ml of NaOH (100 g/liter); mix thoroughly. Using a Beckman DB-GT Spectrophotometer, measure the absorbance at 430 nm of the solution against a blank, prepared with 1 ml of drug-free serum.

Results and Discussion

In preliminary experiments, we synthesized the *O*-methyl derivative of acetaminophen according to the classical method of Claisen (*11*), which is known to alkylate phenolic hydroxyl groups (*12*). The retention time of this compound on OV-17 was the same as that observed when acetaminophen was reacted with methyl iodide according to our modification of the method of Greeley (*13*). However, when acetaminophen was methylated on-column with trimethylanilinium hydroxide, a new chromatographic peak was observed with a different retention time than *O*-methyl acetaminophen, which suggests that under these conditions the amide nitrogen as well as the phenolic hydroxyl group of this drug might be alkylated. This alkylation would be analogous to that observed by Tanaka and Wien (*14*) in which on-column alkylation of substituted phenyl ureas with trimethylanilinium hydroxide yielded the 3-*N*-methyl analogs. When we subjected *O*-methyl acetaminophen to on-column methylation, we observed a single chromatographic peak, which had the same retention time as that noted when acetaminophen was methylated on-column. Subsequently, we studied the effect of on-column *N*-methylation on the gas-chromatograph characteristics of a series of *O*-alkyl derivatives of acetaminophen prepared with the corresponding alkyl iodide according to our modification of the method of Greeley (*13*). Retention times for the *O*-alkyl derivatives of acetaminophen and *N*-propionyl-*p*-aminophenol (the internal standard) were linearly related to the number of carbon atoms in the alkyl iodide used for derivatization (Figure 1). The difference between the retention times of the derivatives of acetaminophen and the internal standard remained constant as the alkyl chain length increased.

While the preparation of mixed derivatives for gas-chromatography is well known, the principle of sequential alkylation has to our knowledge not been applied previously to derivatization of drugs. Our studies with acetaminophen indicate the potential versatility provided by sequential alkylation when the compound has multi-functional groups, some of which cannot be alkylated by the mild procedure of Greeley but can be derivatized by on-column alkylation. By varying the chain length of the alkyl iodide used in the initial alkylation, it was possible to vary the retention time of the final product in order to minimize interference from background peaks. Although we used trimethylanilinium hydroxide for the on-column alkylation step in our procedure, it is apparent that other quaternary alkylating agents such as triethylphenylammonium hydroxide and tetrabutylammonium hydroxide could be used to further increase the versatility of sequential alkylation.

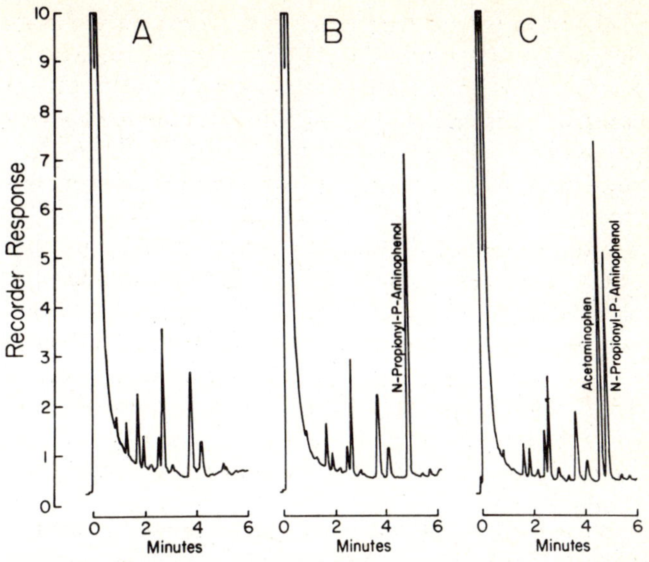

Fig. 2. Chromatograms of serum extracts derivatized according to our procedure

Temperature was programmed from 150 to 260 °C at 16 °C/min. Column packing was 3% OV-17 on 100/120 Gas Chrom Q. *A*, Drug-free serum (1.0 ml); internal standard not included. *B*, Serum (1.0 ml) to which 10 µg of internal standard *N*-propionyl-*p*-aminophenol, was added. *C*, Serum (1.0 ml) from healthy volunteer 0.5 hour after oral dose of 900 mg acetaminophen. The serum concentration of acetaminophen in this specimen was 26.0 mg/liter

Chromatograms of serum specimens extracted and derivatized according to our procedure are presented in Figure 2. Chromatogram *A*, with internal standard omitted, was obtained from serum not containing acetaminophen. Chromatogram *B*, with the internal standard included, represents serum from an individual prior to receiving acetaminophen. Chromatogram *C* was obtained from the same individual 0.5 hour after an oral dose of 900 mg. The serum concentration of acetaminophen in this sample was 26.0 mg/liter.

Figure 3 represents chromatograms of salivary specimens extracted and derivatized according to our procedure. Chromatogram *A*, with internal standard omitted, was obtained from saliva that did not contain acetaminophen. Chromatogram *B*, with the internal standard included, represents saliva from an individual prior to dosing with acetaminophen. Chromatogram *C* was obtained from the same individual 1 h after a oral

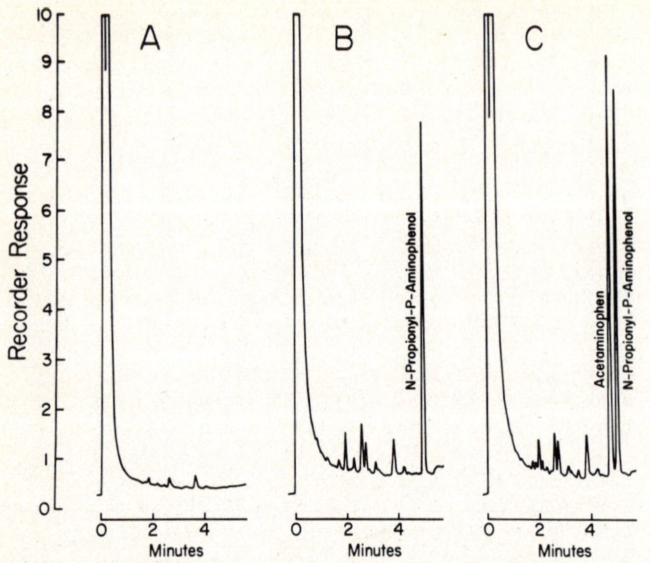

Fig. 3. Chromatograms of salivary extracts derivatized according to our procedure

A, Drug-free saliva (1.0 ml); internal standard not included. *B*, Saliva (1.0 ml) to which 10 μg of internal standard *N*-propionyl-*p*-aminophenol, was added. *C*, Saliva (1.0 ml) obtained from this subject 1.0 h after an oral dose of 900 mg acetaminophen. The saliva concentration of acetaminophen in this specimen was 16.4 mg/liter

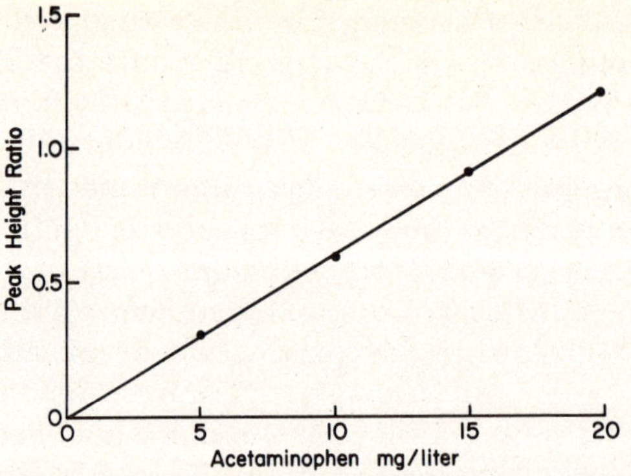

Fig. 4. Standard curve for acetaminophen from serum

Table 1. Concentrations of Acetaminophen in Serum and Saliva after an Oral Dose of 900 mg

	Concn in		
	Serum (A)	Saliva (B)	
Time, h	mg/liter		Ratio A/B
0	0.0	0.0	—
0.5	25.7	27.5	0.93
1.0	20.7	20.8	0.99
2.0	15.3	15.4	0.99
3.0	11.1	10.7	1.04
4.0	8.3	8.4	0.99
6.0	4.6	5.3	0.87

dose of 900 mg. The concentration of acetaminophen in the specimen of saliva was 16.4 mg/liter.

Figure 4 represents a typical standard curve obtained with our procedure for acetaminophen. There was a linear relation between the ratio of peak height of drug to internal standard and the concentration of drug in serum over the range of 0–20 mg/liter. Identical curves were obtained with standards prepared in serum and saliva. The lower limit of detection for acetaminophen based on twice the standard deviation of baseline noise, was 0.5 mg/liter when the sample volume was 1 ml.

Within-run reproducibility for our assay was 2.0% at a serum concentration of 10.0 mg/liter (n = 10) and 3.0% at this concentration in saliva (n = 10). Between-run reproducibility during eight months was 4.0% for serum and 3.4% for saliva.

Other drugs, including sodium salicylate, *p*-aminophenol, *p*-acetophenetidine, phenobarbital, primidone, and diphenylhydantoin, that may be present in serum or saliva were investigated for possible interference with our procedure for acetaminophen. None of these interfered except primidone, which had the same retention time as acetaminophen.

It is known from the work of Mrochek et al. (*8*) that large amounts of the glucuronide of acetaminophen and smaller quantities of acetaminophen sulfate are present in the serum of subjects receiving this drug. Our assay is designed to measure unconjugated acetaminophen. The stability of ether glucuronides and sulfate esters is well known (*15*). Because hot concentrated acid is required to hydrolyze an ether glucuronide, the mild conditions of our assay (pH 6.8) are unlikely to produce detectable hydrolysis of this metabolite. Moreover the polar nature of the conjugates would not lead to their extraction during our procedure.

Fifty-nine serum specimens were analyzed for acetaminophen by the differential spectrophotometric method and by our procedure. Concentrations of the drug ranged from 0.0 to 31.7 mg/liter. The mean value observed for the spectrophotometric method was 10.5 mg/liter and with our procedure was 10.6 mg/liter. When values for the gas-chromatographic procedure were regressed against values for the differential spectrophotometric method, the slope of the non-weighted linear least-squares regression line was 1.03; the intercept was −0.26 mg/liter, and the coefficient of correlation was 0.99.

Similar comparative studies were conducted with 52 specimens of saliva containing acetaminophen in concentrations ranging from 1.4 to 27.5 mg/liter. The mean value observed for the differential spectrophotometric method was 8.8 mg/liter and with our procedure was 10.1 mg/liter. The slope of the non-weighted linear least-squares regression line was 1.00; the intercept was 1.17 mg/liter, and the coefficient of correlation was 0.99.

Five clinical specimens were analyzed for acetaminophen by our gas-chromatographic procedure and by the colorimetric method of Glynn and Kendal (*2*). The mean value as determined by the gas-chromatographic assay was 24.3 mg/liter and by the colorimetric assay was 27.2 mg/liter. The maximum difference observed between the two methods was 6.6 mg/liter. The colorimetric procedure was less sensitive than either the gas-chromatographic method or the differential spectrophotometric procedure but is adequate for analysis of the toxic concentrations of acetaminophen.

The application of our gas-chromatographic procedure to pharmacokinetic studies with acetaminophen is demonstrated in Table 1. In this study, a healthy volunteer received 900 mg of acetaminophen orally after an overnight fast and serum and saliva were collected during the following six hours. Within 0.5 h of administration of the dose, the serum and salivary concentrations of acetaminophen were 25.7 and 27.5 mg/liter, respectively. Thereafter concentrations in serum and saliva declined exponentially with a half-life of 2.3 h, which is similar to that reported in normal subjects (*16, 17*). At the pH values normally observed for human serum and saliva, 7.4 and 6.8 to 7.2, respectively, acetaminophen ($pK_a = 9.51$) is uncharged, hence its distribution ratio between these fluids should reflect only the extent to which it binds to serum proteins. The observed equivalence of serum and salivary concentrations of acetaminophen in this subject indicates no significant binding of this drug.

References

1. Prescott, L. F., Swainson, C. P., Forrest, A. R. W., et al., Successful treatment of severe paracetamol overdosage with cysteamine. *Lancet* **i**, 588 (1974).

2. Glynn, J. P., and Kendal, S. E., Paracetamol measurement. *Lancet* **i**, 1147 (1975).

3. Routh, J. I., Shane, N. A., Arrendondo, E. G., and Paul, W. D., Determination of N-acetyl-*p*-aminophenol in plasma. *Clin. Chem.* **14**, 9 (1968).

4. Grove, J., Gas-liquid chromatography of *N*-acetyl-*p*-aminophenol (paracetamol) in plasma and urine. *J. Chromatogr.* **59**, 289 (1971).

5. Prescott, L. F., The gas-liquid chromatographic estimation of phenacetin and paracetamol in plasma and urine. *J. Pharm. Pharmacol.* **23**, 111 (1971).

6. Prescott, L. F., Gas-liquid chromatographic estimation of paracetamol. *J. Pharm. Pharmacol.* **23**, 807 (1971).

7. Street, H. V., Estimation and identification in blood plasma of paracetamol (*N*-acetyl-*p*-aminophenol) in the presence of barbiturates. *J. Chromatogr.* **109**, 29 (1975).

8. Mrochek, J. E., Katz, S., Christie, W. H., and Dinsmore, S. R., Acetaminophen metabolism in man, as determined by high-resolution liquid chromatography. *Clin. Chem.* **20**, 1086 (1974).

9. Stewart, M. J., and Willis, R. G., Simplified gas chromatographic assay for paracetamol. *Ann. Clin. Biochem.* **12**, 4 (1975).

10. Osiewicz, R., Aggarwal, V., Yong, R. M., and Sunshine, I., The quantitative analysis of phenobarbital with trimethylanilinium hydroxide. *J. Chromatogr.* **88**, 157 (1974).

11. Claisen, L., Über die Umlagenrung von Phenolallyl Äthern in die isomeren Allylphenole I. Mono-, Di-und Triallylierung des gewohnlichen Phenols. *Justus Liebigs Ann. Chem.* **69**, 418 (1919).

12. Kawahara, F. K., Microdetermination of derivatives of phenols and mercaptans by means of electron capture gas chromatography. *Anal. Chem.* **40**, 1009 (1968).

13. Greeley, R. H., New approach to derivatization and gas chromatographic analysis of barbiturates. *Clin. Chem.* **20**, 192 (1974).

14. Tanaka, F. S., and Wien, R. G., Gas chromatography of substituted phenylureas by flash-heater methylation with trimethylanilinium hydroxide. *J. Chromatogr.* **87**, 85 (1973).

15. Clarke, E. G. C., *Isolation and Identification of Drugs,* William Clowes & Sons, Ltd., London, Great Britain, 1971, pp 144–145.

16. Prescott, L. F., Roscie, P., Wright, N., and Brown, S. S., Plasma-paracetamol half-life and hepatic necrosis in patients with paracetamol overdosage. *Lancet* **i**, 519 (1971).

17. Levy, G., Khana, N. N., Soda, D. M., Tsuzuki, O., and Stern, L., Pharmacokinetics of acetaminophen in the human neonate: Formation of acetaminophen glucuronide and sulfate in relation to plasma bilirubin concentration and D-glucaric acid excretion. *Pediatrics* **55**, 818 (1975).

CLIN. CHEM. 22/6, 884-888 (1976)

Quantitative Gas-Chromatographic Flame-Ionization Method for *p*-Chlorophenoxyisobutyric Acid in Human Serum and Saliva

John N. Connor, George F. Johnson, and Harvey M. Solomon

We describe a gas-chromatographic method for *p*-chlorophenoxyisobutyric acid (**I**) the active metabolite of clofibrate. The drug and internal standards are separated from either serum or saliva by a double extraction procedure and converted to the corresponding butyl esters by reaction with iodobutane in a mixture of methanol and *N,N*-dimethylacetamide containing tetramethylammonium hydroxide. Within-run CV of this assay at a serum **I** concentration of 79.2 mg/liter was 2.3% and at a salivary **I** concentration of 2.5 mg/liter was 2.1%. Precision during four months of the serum and salivary assays at these concentrations was 4.1% and 6.2%, respectively. The mean serum concentration of **I** (12 h after dose) in patients receiving the drug at an average dose of 28.0 mg/kg per day was 109.6 mg/liter. Serum and salivary concentrations of **I** as determined by our procedure were used to calculate the unbound fraction of drug in human serum. Such measurements can be used to monitor therapy in patients with renal disease, where drug toxicity may arise from high concentrations of unbound **I**.

Additional Keyphrases: *clofibrate* • *therapy for hyperlipidemia* • *monitoring of drugs*

Clofibrate, the ethyl ester of *p*-chlorophenoxyisobutyric acid, is widely used in the treatment of hyperlipidemia. This ester is rapidly hydrolized to *p*-chlorophenoxyisobutyric acid (CPIB)[1] by serum and tissue esterases (*1*); the acid is cleared from the body almost entirely by renal secretion (*2*). It has been recommended that serum concentrations of CPIB be monitored in patients with chronic renal failure to reduce the risks of toxicity (*3*).

A spectrophotometric method for CPIB, based on hydrolysis of this compound to *p*-chlorophenol, was developed by Barrett and Thorp (*4*); however, it has limited application to clinical specimens because other acidic drugs in serum may interfere with the ultraviolet absorption of the derived *p*-chlorophenol. Several gas-chromatographic methods for CPIB have also been described (*5–8*). However, one of these procedures (*5*) requires a preliminary thin-layer chromatographic separation of CPIB from fatty acids in plasma, and in all the others diazomethane is used to prepare the methylated derivative (*6–8*). Because of these limitations, we did not consider these procedures appropriate for routine use in our Therapeutic Drug Monitoring Laboratory. The gas-chromatographic method of Gugler et al. (*9*) avoids the potential hazards of diazomethane by esterifying CPIB with dimethylsulfate in alcoholic potassium carbonate. These workers utilized clofibrate as their internal standard, and we were concerned that some individuals might, because of disease or the presence of other drugs, have significant amounts of the parent compound in their serum. Recently Karmen and Haut (*10*) described a method for CPIB in which they used a gas chromatograph equipped with flame-ionization detector selectively sensitive to halogen. When serum samples, extracted and derivatized according to their procedure, were analyzed with a conventional hydrogen flame ionization detector they observed large quantities of the methyl esters of other fatty acids, which far exceeded the amounts of CPIB present and made quantitation difficult. Bruderlein et al. (*11*) reported a gas-chromatographic procedure for CPIB based on flame-ionization detection of the methyl ester of this drug, which was prepared by reaction with methanolic HCl at room temperature. This method was precise and results correlated well with those from the ultraviolet spectrophotometric procedure when the latter results were corrected for the nonspecific background absorbance of control sera.

Therapeutic Drug Monitoring Laboratory, Dept. of Laboratory Medicine, The Johns Hopkins Hospital, Baltimore, Md. 21205.

[1] Nonstandard abbreviations used: CPIB, *p*-chlorophenoxyisobutyric acid; CPPA, 3-(*p*-chlorophenoxy)propionic acid; and CPAA, *p*-chlorophenoxyacetic acid.

Received Mar. 15, 1976; accepted Mar. 31, 1976.

Greeley described a procedure for the alkylation of organic acids in which the tetramethylammonium salt of the acid reacts with an excess of primary alkyl iodide in methanolic *N,N*-dimethylacetamide (*13*). This reaction is mild, rapid, and complete and has been used in our laboratory for the alkylation of theophylline (*13*), ethosuximide (*14*), and acetaminophen (*15*). We have investigated its application to the alkylation of CPIB and describe here a quantitative gas-chromatographic procedure involving flame-ionization detection of the *n*-butyl ester of the drug; the procedure is suitable for determination of CPIB in serum and saliva. This method has been used in our Therapeutic Drug Monitoring Laboratory on a routine basis for over one year, to assist physicians in evaluating patient compliance, in the design of appropriate therapeutic regimens, and for pharmacokinetic studies in patients with renal disease.

Materials and Methods

Chemicals and Comparison Materials

Ammonium hydroxide (14.8 mol/liter), ethyl ether (anhydrous), and phosphorus pentoxide were obtained from Fisher Scientific Co., Fair Lawn, N.J. 07410.

p-*Chlorophenoxyacetic acid and 1-iodobutane* (99% pure) were obtained from the Eastman Kodak Co., Rochester, N.Y. 14650.

*3-(*p*-Chlorophenoxy)propionic acid* was obtained from Pfaltz and Bauer, Inc., Flushing, N.Y. 11368.

p-*Chlorophenoxyisobutyric acid* (sodium salt) was obtained from Ayerst Laboratories, Montreal 101, P.Q. Canada.

N,N-*Dimethylacetamide* (spectrophotometric grade) was obtained from Aldrich Chemical Co., Milwaukee, Wis. 53233.

Methanol ("chromatoquality"), tetramethylammonium hydroxide (240 g/liter of methanol), and toluene ("chromatoquality") were obtained from Matheson, Coleman and Bell, East Rutherford, N.J. 07073.

Reagents

Prepare stock solutions (1 mg/ml) of CPIB, *p*-chlorophenoxyacetic acid (CPAA), and 3-(*p*-chlorophenoxy)propionic acid (CPPA) by dissolving 111 mg of the sodium salt of *p*-chlorophenoxyisobutyric acid and 100 mg of each of the other compounds in 100 ml of methanol. Prepare a working solution of CPIB (100 μg/ml) by diluting 10 ml of the stock solution to 100 ml with methanol and prepare a working solution containing both internal standards, CPAA (150 μg/ml) and CPPA (150 μg/ml), by combining 15 ml of each stock solution and diluting to 100 ml with methanol. Prepare 7.4 mol/liter NH_4OH in methanol freshly for each run by diluting concentrated NH_4OH with an equal volume of methanol.

Standards

Prepare serum standards (0, 40, 80, 120, 160 mg/liter) and saliva standards (0, 2, 4, 6, 8 mg/liter) by adding appropriate amounts of CPIB working solutions (0, 10, 20, 30, 40 μl) to 16 × 100 mm screw-cap culture tubes and evaporating the solutions under nitrogen at room temperature. Add 1 ml of 1 mol/liter HCl to each tube. For serum determinations, combine 25 μl of drug-free serum with the HCl; for saliva determinations combine 500 μl of drug-free saliva with the HCl.

Sample Preparation and Extraction

Combine serum (25 μl) or saliva (500 μl) with 1 ml of 1 mol/liter HCl in 16 × 100 mm culture tubes (Teflon-lined screw cap). To standards and patients' samples, add 25 μl of working internal standard solution, vortex mix, and add 8.0 ml of anhydrous ether with a "Repipet" (Lab Industries, Berkeley, Calif. 94710). Extract all samples for 15 min in an Eberbach shaker at 250 oscillations per minute and centrifuge at 2000 rpm for 15 min. Transfer (Pasteur pipette) the ether layer to 18 × 114 mm "Concentratubes" (Laboratory Research Co., Los Angeles, Calif. 95035) and evaporate under a gentle stream of nitrogen at room temperature.

Wash the walls of the tubes with 100 μl of the 7.4 mol/liter NH_4OH in methanol and vortex mix the contents of each tube. Add 5 ml of toluene with a Repipet, mix, and centrifuge as described above. Aspirate the toluene layer and evaporate the aqueous layer in a desiccator containing P_2O_5.

Add 40 μl of *N,N*-dimethylacetamide, 10 μl of tetramethylammonium hydroxide (24 g/liter of methanol), and 10 μl of iodobutane to each tube. After each addition vortex mix the samples. Let the tubes stand for 10 min, then centrifuge at 2000 rpm for 2 min. With a 10-μl syringe (Glenco Scientific, Inc., Houston, Texas, 77006), inject 2.5 μl of the supernatant fluid into the gas–liquid chromatograph.

Gas-Liquid Chromatography

We used a Model 5711A dual-column gas chromatograph equipped with flame ionization detectors (Hewlett-Packard, Avondale, Pa. 14311). The glass columns (120 cm × 2 mm i.d.), configuration 5 for on-column injection, were packed with 3% OV-17 on 100/120 Gas Chrom Q (Applied Science Laboratories, Inc., State College, Pa. 16801). Septa were type HT-9 (Applied Science Laboratories), high temperature, low bleed.

The injection-port temperature was 250 °C, detector temperature 300 °C; the oven temperature was programmed from 130 °C to 240 °C at a rate of 16 °C/min. The flow rate for the carrier gas, N_2, was set at 50 ml/min; the air flow rate was 250 ml/min; the H_2 flow rate was 40 ml/min; and the chart speed was 13 mm/min.

Results and Discussion

In preliminary studies, we prepared a series of *N*-alkyl esters of CPIB according to the procedure of Greeley (12). Of the compounds studied, the *N*-butyl ester exhibited a chromatographic peak that was not subject to interference by substances normally encountered in human serum or saliva. Accordingly, we selected this derivative for use in our routine procedure for CPIB.

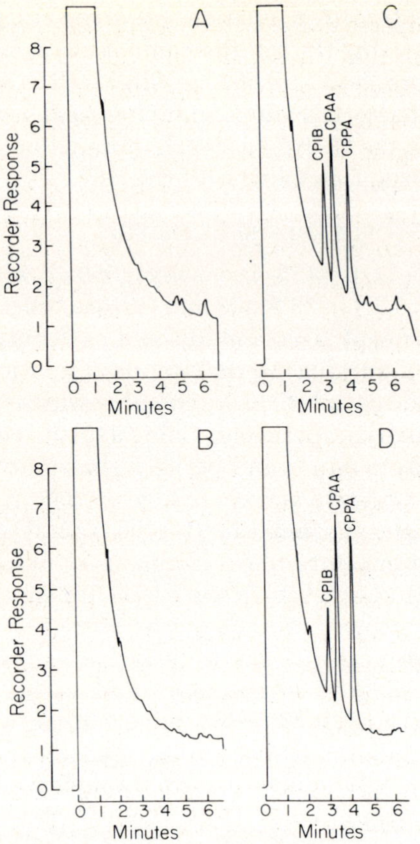

Fig. 1. Chromatograms obtained on analysis of normal serum and saliva, with and without added CPIB

Temperature was programmed from 130 to 240 °C, at 16 °C/min. Column packing was 3% OV-17 on 100/120 Gas Chrom Q. *A*, Normal serum, 25 μl of drug-free serum; internal standards omitted. *B*, Normal saliva, 500 μl of drug-free saliva; internal standards omitted. *C*, Serum standard, 25 μl of serum to which CPIB (80 mg/liter) was added; internal standards included. *D*, Saliva standard, 500 μl of saliva to which CPIB (2.5 mg/liter) was added; internal standards included

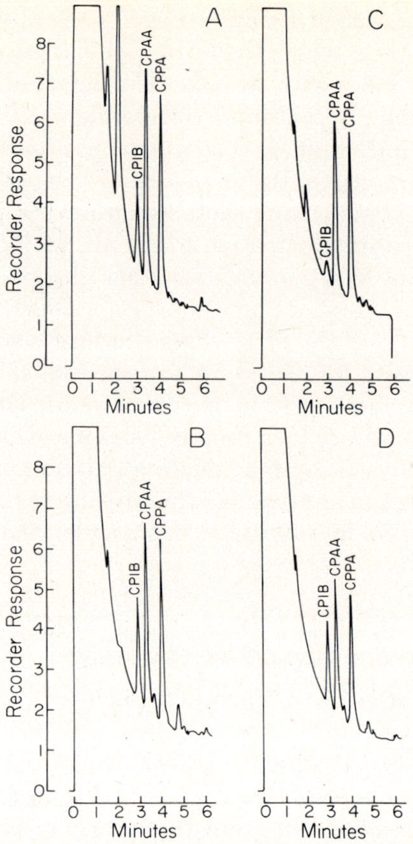

Fig. 2. Chromatograms of (*A*) saliva (500 μl) containing 2 mg of CPIB per liter, and (*B*) serum (25 μl) containing 56.0 mg of CPIB per liter, collected concurrently from a patient with markedly impaired renal function 48 h after a 0.5-g oral dose of ethyl chlorophenoxyisobutyrate. (*C*) saliva (500 μl) containing 0.5 mg of CPIB per liter, and (*D*) serum (25 μl) containing 62.6 mg of CPIB per liter, collected concurrently from a normal individual 10 h after an oral dose of 0.5 g of clofibrate

Representative chromatograms of serum and saliva extracted and derivatized according to our procedure are presented in Figure 1. Chromatograms *A* and *B*, with the internal standards omitted, were obtained from the serum and saliva of a normal individual not receiving CPIB. Chromatograms *C* and *D* were obtained from the serum and saliva of a normal individual, to which CPIB (80 and 2.5 mg/liter, respectively) was added. The butyl derivatives of the drug and internal standards were well separated from each other; the retention times of CPIB relative to CPAA and CPPA were 0.37 and 1.08, respectively.

CPAA and CPPA were used as internal standards because of their chemical similarity to CPIB. These compounds are all highly volatile and care must be exercised during the evaporation steps in our procedure, because it has been demonstrated by Karmen and Haut that they are not always lost in equal proportions (*10*). Although either CPAA and CPPA can be used for quantitative purposes, a consistently lower coefficient of variation was obtained with CPAA as the internal standard. However, CPPA was routinely included to call attention to interfering substances having the same retention time as CPAA and to the possibility of unequal loss of compounds during evaporation.

Figure 2 illustrates chromatograms obtained from saliva (*A*) and serum (*B*) collected concurrently from a patient with markedly impaired renal function, 48 h after a 0.5-g oral dose of ethyl chlorophenoxyisobutyrate (clofibrate). The concentration of CPIB in saliva was 2.0 mg/liter, in serum 56.0 mg/liter. Chromatograms *C* and *D* were obtained from saliva and serum collected concurrently from a normal individual 10 h after an oral dose of 0.5 g of ethyl chlorophenoxyisobutyrate. The salivary and serum concentrations of CPIB in this volunteer were 0.5 and 62.6 mg/liter, respectively.

Figure 3 (*A*) illustrates typical standard curves obtained by our procedure with serum. Linear relationships were observed between the ratios of the peak height of CPIB to CPAA and to CPPA over a concentration range of 0 to 160 mg/liter CPIB. Salivary standard curves prepared with use of these two internal standards also showed linear relationships between their ratios and the concentrations of CPIB.

Other compounds investigated for possible interferences included: caffeine, theophylline, diphenylhydantoin, phenobarbital, primidone, salicylic acid, acetyl salicylic acid, and acetaminophen. When these compounds were added to serum and saliva at a concentration of 50 mg/liter, no interfering peaks with reten-

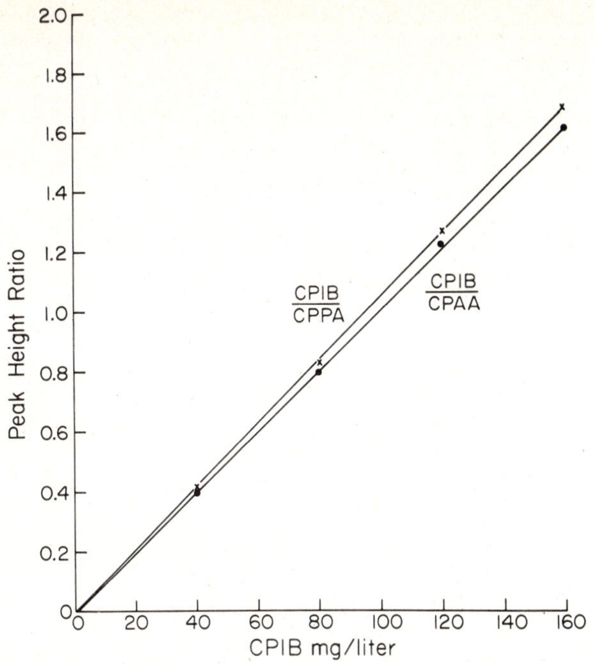

Fig. 3. Standard curves for CPIB in serum

tion times equivalent to CPIB, CPAA, or CPPA were observed.

Recovery of CPIB and of the two internal standards from serum and saliva was determined in the following manner: 25 μl of drug-free serum and 500 μl of drug-free saliva were added to separate tubes containing 80 μg of CPIB, CPAA, and CPPA. These samples were extracted as described above; however, all volume transfers were quantitated. A second, nonextracted standard containing 80 μg of each compound was prepared. All samples were derivatized as described in the *Methods* section and exactly 2.5 μl of each sample was chromatographed. The peak heights of the extracted samples were then corrected for solvent transfers. Absolute recoveries of the compounds were calculated by comparison of the ratio of the corrected peak height of the extracted samples to that of the nonextracted standard. The absolute recoveries of CPIB, CPAA, and CPPA from serum were 89.1%, 95.9%, and 99.8%, respectively, and from saliva were 91.5%, 90.9%, and 95.3%, respectively.

The within-run coefficient of variation (CV) of our assay at a serum CPIB concentration of 79.2 mg/liter was 2.3% (n = 10); at a saliva CPIB concentration of 2.46 mg/liter it was 2.1% (n = 10). During four months, the between-run precision of this assay at these concentrations was 4.1% for serum (n = 20) and 6.2% for saliva (n = 20).

Although separate standard curves for serum and saliva were included with each analytical run from which our precision data were derived, we subsequently determined that the relative peak-height ratios of the salivary standards did not differ significantly from those of the serum standards. Therefore, for routine determinations serum-based standards were used for the analysis of CPIB in both serum and saliva.

We compared our gas-chromatographic procedure for CPIB with that developed by Bruderlein et al. (*11*), which is based on gas chromatography of the methyl ester of the drug. Fifteen serum specimens were supplied, ranging in concentration from 0 to 140 mg of CPIB per liter, with a mean value of 74.1 mg/liter. The mean value observed with our procedure was 75.7 mg/liter (range, 0–136 mg/liter). When values obtained with our procedure were regressed against those obtained from Dr. Bruderlein, the slope of the nonweighted linear least-squares regression line was 1.02, the intercept was −0.21 mg/liter, and the coefficient of correlation was 0.99.

We measured concentrations of CPIB in the serum of 30 patients attending the Lipid Clinic of The Johns Hopkins Hospital, to evaluate their compliance with medication orders. These subjects received the drug at a dose of 28.0 ± 6.4 mg/kg body wt. per day (mean ± SD) and blood samples were obtained 12 h after the last dose. The mean serum concentration of CPIB was 109.6 mg/liter (SD, 28.2 mg/liter). Although there was considerable variability in the serum concentration of this drug among individuals, we failed to detect it in the serum of only two of the 30 patients, one of whom reported that he had exhausted his supply of drug during the week before his clinic visit. The striking degree of compliance in this patient population is in sharp contrast to that observed previously in outpatients with seizure disorders who were treated chronically with anticonvulsants (*16*) or in asthmatics on long-term therapy with theophylline (*13*).

Recent studies with salicylic acid (*17*), acetaminophen (*18*), tolbutamide (*19*), amobarbital (*20*), and several anticonvulsants, including diphenylhydantoin and phenobarbital (*21*), indicate that the unbound drug is in equilibrium between serum and saliva. Only the un-ionized form of a drug can diffuse across the epithelium of the salivary gland and the equilibrium distribution of any drug between serum and saliva will be influenced by the pK_a of the compound, the pH of saliva, and the pH of serum. Inaba and Kalow (*20*) measured amobarbital concentrations in serum and saliva of adult volunteers and used the following formula to estimate the unbound fraction in serum:

Percent unbound drug =

$$\frac{[\text{saliva}]}{[\text{serum}]} \times \frac{1 + 10^{7.4-pK_a}}{1 + 10^{pH\ \text{saliva}-pK_a}} \times 100$$

They also measured amobarbital binding to plasma proteins in these subjects directly by equilibrium dialysis and compared these results to values estimated with this formula. The calculated and observed values for the unbound fraction of amobarbital were in excellent agreement.

CPIB is an acid (pK_a = 3.1) and is extensively bound to human albumin. At usual therapeutic concentrations in individuals with normal renal function, the extent of binding of CPIB, as determined by equilibrium dialysis, was about 95–97% (*2, 9*). In contrast, 80 to 93% of the drug was bound to albumin in patients with the nephrotic syndrome (*2, 9*). It has been claimed that the higher concentrations of unbound CPIB in these patients are responsible for its toxic effects, which include muscle pain, stiffness, weakness, and general malaise (*3*). We used our gas-chromatographic method to indirectly estimate the extent of binding of CPIB to serum albumin. Serum and salivary concentrations of the drug were determined and the unbound fraction was calculated. In an individual with normal renal function, the bound fraction of CPIB was estimated to be 96.4%. In an individual with severe renal insufficiency (creatinine clearance less than 5 ml/min) the bound fraction was 88.8%. These values are in excellent agreement with those reported in the literature. The simultaneous determination of serum and salivary CPIB with our gas-chromatographic method can therefore be used to ascertain and avoid toxicity caused by high concentrations of unbound drug.

We thank Dr. H. Bruderlein of Ayerst Research Laboratories, Montreal, Quebec, for providing us with clinical samples for our comparative study.

References

1. Thorp, J. M., Experimental evaluation of an orally active combination of androsterone with ethyl chlorophenoxyisobutyrate. *Lancet* **i**, 1323 (1962).

2. Bridgman, J. F., Rosen, S. M., and Thorp, J. M., Complications during clofibrate treatment of nephrotic-syndrome hyperlipoproteinaemia. *Lancet* **ii**, 506 (1972).

3. Pierides, A. M., Alvarex-Ude, F., Kerr, D. N. S., and Skillen, A. W., Clofibrate-induced muscle damage in patients with chronic renal failure. *Lancet* **ii**, 1279 (1975).

4. Barrett, A. M., and Thorp, J. M., Studies on the mode of action of clofibrate: Effect on hormone-induced changes in plasma-free fatty acids, cholesterol, phospholipids, and total esterified fatty acids in rats and dogs. *Br. J. Pharmacol.* **133**, 381 (1968).

5. Sedaghat, A., Nakamura, H., and Ahrens, Jr., E. H., Determination of clofibrate in biological fluids by thin-layer and gas–liquid chromatography. *J. Lipid. Res.* **15**, 352 (1974).

6. Berlin, A., Quantitative gas chromatographic determination of clofibrinic acid in plasma. *J. Pharm. Pharmacol.* **27**, 54 (1975).

7. Cuong, T. C., and Tuong, A., Quantitative determination of *p*-chlorophenoxyisobutyric acid in blood plasma by gas–liquid chromatography. *J. Chromatogr.* **106**, 97 (1975).

8. Houin, G., Thebault, J. J., d'Athis, Ph., et al., A GLC method for estimation of chlorophenoxyisobutyric acid in plasma. Pharmacokinetics of a single oral dose of clofibrate in man. *Eur. J. Clin. Pharmacol.* **8**, 433 (1975).

9. Gugler, R., Shoeman, D. W., Hoffman, D. H., et al., Pharmacokinetics of drugs in patients with the nephrotic syndrome. *J. Clin. Invest.* **55**, 1182 (1975).

10. Karmen, A., and Haut, H., Assay of clofibrate in human serum by gas chromatography. *Biochem. Med.* **12**, 154 (1975).

11. Bruderlein, H., Robinson, W. T., Kraml, M., and Dvornik, D., A gas–liquid chromatographic determination of *p*-chlorophenoxyisobutyric acid and its comparison to an ultra violet method. *Clin. Biochem.* **8**, 261 (1975).

12. Greeley, R. H., Rapid esterification for gas chromatography. *J. Chromatogr.* **88**, 229 (1974).

13. Johnson, G. F., Dechtiaruk, W. A., and Solomon, H. M., Gas-chromatographic determination of theophylline in human serum and saliva. *Clin. Chem.* **21**, 144 (1975).

14. Least, C. J., Jr., Johnson, G. F., and Solomon, H. M., A quantitative gas chromatographic determination of ethosuximide based on *N*-butylation. *Clin. Chim. Acta* **60**, 285 (1975).

15. Dechtiaruk, W. A., Johnson, G. F., and Solomon, H. M., Gas-chromatographic method for acetaminophen (*N*-acetyl-*p*-aminophenol) based on sequential alkylation. *Clin. Chem.* **22**, 879 (1976).

16. Dawson, K. P., and Jamieson, A., Value for blood phenytoin estimation in management of childhood epilepsy. *Arch. Dis. Child.* **46**, 386 (1971).

17. Graham, G., and Rowland, M., Application of salivary salicylate data to biopharmaceutical studies of salicylates. *J. Pharm. Sci.* **61**, 1219 (1972).

18. Glynn, J. P., and Bastain, W., Salivary excretion of paracetamol in man. *J. Pharm. Pharmacol.* **25**, 420 (1973).

19. Matin, S. B., Wan, S. H., and Karam, J. H., Pharmacokinetics of tolbutamide: Prediction by concentration in saliva. *Clin. Pharmacol. Ther.* **16**, 1052 (1974).

20. Inaba, T., and Kalow, W., Salivary excretion of amobarbital in man. *Clin. Pharmacol. Ther.* **18**, 558 (1975).

CLIN. CHEM. 22/6, 889–891 (1976)

Diazepam Abuse: Incidence, Rapid Screening, and Confirming Methods

Thomas A. Rejent and Kenneth C. Wahl

We studied 2500 patients suspected to be drug-overdose victims. Blood samples were quantitatively screened for the most commonly abused drugs, including diazepam. Of these, 61% had positive findings, including diazepam in about one of every four. A new rapid, simple, and quantitative gas-chromatographic method for simultaneous analysis of diazepam and sedatives (in two instruments) is described. A single extraction at low pH is used, preserving the balance of the sample to be used for confirming methods via ultraviolet spectrophotometry and thin-layer chromatography. Prevalence of other positive findings is also listed, and findings for diazepam are categorized by age.

Additional Keyphrases: *gas chromatography • ultraviolet spectrophotometry • thin-layer chromatography • drug abuse • toxicology • screening*

Abuse of psychotropic drugs continues to increase steadily in the United States. Whereas 15 to 20 years ago, sedative intoxications predominated, many different compounds are reported now as causative factors in instances of drug-induced stupor and coma.

One of these, diazepam, reportedly is the drug most often prescribed to treat anxiety and thus becomes accessible to potential abusers. Its popularity is further attributed to the fact that it is readily available illicitly. A significant problem also arises because of its widespread use together with other drugs (*1, 2*).

The prevalence of diazepam was investigated in patients (brought to area hospitals' emergency rooms) who presented in drug-induced lethargy, stupor, or coma. Our facility exclusively serves about 40 area hospitals on an around-the-clock basis in all phases of clinical and forensic toxicology. We studied a total of 2500 cases during the last six months of 1975. The frequency with which diazepam was detected surprised us; its prevalence in certain age groups is likewise revealing.

Erie County Laboratories, Division of Toxicology, E. J. Meyer Memorial Hospital, Buffalo, N. Y. 14215.

Received Jan. 30, 1976; accepted April 1, 1976.

Diazepam (7-chloro-1,3-dihydro-1-methyl-5-phenyl-2*H*-1,4-benzodiazepin-2-one) can be extracted with organic solvents from biological fluids at various pHs with varying degrees of efficiency. This method improves upon previous reports by using a single acidic extraction for diazepam and sedatives. The subsequent gas chromatogram of diazepam is much cleaner than is the case after basic or neutral extraction. To expedite the analysis, the acid extract was injected into two gas chromatographs to detect soporifics and diazepam.

Alcohol was also determined for all samples. Diazepam was quantitatively reported if detected by this method and its presence subsequently was confirmed by ultraviolet spectrophotometry and thin-layer chromatography.

Materials

Diazepam stock solution, 1.00 g/liter in absolute ethanol.

Diazepam working standards. For spectrophotometry: 1, 3, 5, 7, and 10 mg/liter, aqueous. For chromatography: 10, 30, 50, 70, and 100 mg/liter, in ethyl acetate.

TLC plates: Silica Gel GF, 20 × 20 cm (Analtech, Inc., Newark, Del. 19711).

Instrumentation

Gas chromatography

Volatiles: Perkin-Elmer F-11. Detector: FID. Recorder: Honeywell Electronik 194, chart speed 2.54 cm/min. Column: 0.4% Carbowax 1500 on Carbopak A, 180.0 × 0.3 cm. Temperatures: oven, 85 °C; detector, 190 °C; injector, 190 °C. Carrier gas: helium. Flow rate: 45 ml/min.

Sedatives: F&M Model 400. Detector: FID. Recorder: Varian A25, chart speed, 2.1 cm/min. Column: 3.8% SE-30 on 80/100 Chromosorb W (AW-DMCS) 180.0 cm × 4 mm (i.d.). Temperatures: oven, 180 °C; detector, 205 °C; injector, 230 °C. Carrier gas: helium. Flow rate: 45 ml/min.

Diazepam

Gas chromatography: Perkin-Elmer Model 990. Detector: dual FID. Recorder: Linear Instruments, Model 252A, chart speed 1 cm/min. Column: 3.8% SE-30 on 80/100 Chromosorb W (AW-DMCS), 90.0 cm × 4 mm (i.d.). Temperature: oven, 240 °C; detector 290 °C; injector, 290 °C. Carrier gas: helium. Flow rate: 50 ml/min.

Ultraviolet spectrophotometry: Beckman Model ACTA-M-VI spectrophotometer. Scanning range, 340–220 nm, 1 nm/s. Silica cuvettes, 12 × 12 × 45 mm. Lightpath, 10 mm.

Thin-layer chromatography: Developing solvent: chloroform/acetone, 1/1 by vol. Visualization: ultraviolet (254 nm) light; and Dragendorff's reagent.

Methods

Gas chromatography. Alcohols (volatiles) were determined by a direct injection method, with 2-propanol as an internal standard (*3*); blood was diluted fourfold with 2-propanol, 500 mg/liter.

In assay for sedatives and diazepam, serum was analyzed essentially according to the method of Sine et al. (*4*). A 2-ml sample was acidified with 0.1 ml of HCl (6 mol/liter). An internal standard (aminopyrine, 300 mg/liter) was contained in the reconstituting solvent. Into each of the two chromatographs, set up as described above, we injected 2-μl aliquots. Diazepam concentration values are based solely on peak-height comparison with standards similarly run. The aminopyrine added as an internal standard is taken up in the solvent front at the 240 °C temperature required for diazepam. Diazepam standards (in ethyl acetate) are injected directly without extraction (See *Discussion*).

Ultraviolet spectrophotometry. A modified procedure (*5*) was used, wherein 6 ml of serum or standards was extracted with diethyl ether at pH 6.7. Acidic impurities were removed with 5 ml of NaOH (0.45 mol/liter); chlordiazepoxide and fluorazepam were extracted into 2 ml of H_2SO_4 (0.25 mol/liter), and diazepam was then extracted into 2 ml of HCl (2 mol/liter). Diazepam exhibits maxima at 241 and 284 nm, and was quantitated at the former by comparison to the standards. As little as 0.5 mg/liter can be so detected.

Table 1. Prevalence of Drugs in Positive Cases (Ethanol Not Included)

Drug	No. patients
Diazepam	369
Barbiturates	351
Salicylic acid	197
Methyprylon	36
Glutethimide	35
Meprobamate	16
Chlordiazepoxide	13
Amitriptyline	10
Acetaminophen	8
Phenothiazines	7
Ethchlorvynol	6
Fluorazepam	6
Isopropanol	6
Propoxyphene	6
Methapyrilene	3
Paraldehyde	2
Pentazocine	2
Carisoprodol	1
Methaqualone	1
Theophylline	1
Total	1076

Thin-layer chromatography. Each of the acid extracts previously scanned was diluted to 8 ml with water, saturated with solid sodium bicarbonate, and the supernate extracted with 20 ml of chloroform, which was filtered and then evaporated in a stream of warm air. The residues, reconstituted in a minimum amount of ethyl acetate, were spotted, developed (*6*) to 16 cm, and visualized first under ultraviolet light (254 nm) and then by spraying with Dragendorff's reagent. Diazepam is seen at an R_F of about 0.80.

Results and Discussion

Of the 2500 samples, 1521 gave positive results. Excluding ethanol, diazepam was the most frequently detected drug. Because therapeutic concentrations of diazepam are below the range of sensitivity of the gas-

Table 2. Diazepam and Other Drugs Detected, by Age Groups (2500 Cases)

Age group	Diazepam	Diazepam + ETOH[a]	Diazepam + other drugs	Diazepam, other drugs + ETOH	Total diazepam	Other drugs	ETOH	ETOH + other drugs	Total	Percent
0–9	2	—	—	—	2	5	6	—	13	0.9
10–19	39	29	11	6	85	109	165	28	387	25.4
20–29	44	42	30	14	130	126	189	39	484	31.8
30–39	30	33	10	5	78	84	104	19	285	18.7
40–49	10	23	8	4	45	42	82	12	181	11.9
50–59	11	9	—	—	20	34	45	13	112	7.4
60+	4	5	—	—	9	22	22	6	59	3.9
Totals	140	141	59	29	369	422	613	117	1521	100.0%

[a] ETOH, ethanol

chromatographic procedure, positive findings necessarily indicate overuse of the compound. When screening procedures gave negative results, different procedures were used to detect other compounds, especially in the case of a known ingestion.

Table 1 lists all drugs found, either singly or in combination, or with ethyl alcohol. Phenacetin and caffeine findings were not recorded. Ethyl alcohol was detected most frequently: 900 cases.

Table 2 shows the incidence of detection of diazepam, other drugs, and alcohol by age groups; the 20–29 year age group predominated (32%) in all categories.

The first 150 samples in which diazepam was detected by gas chromatography were re-quantitated by ultraviolet spectrophotometry and its identity confirmed by thin-layer chromatography. Some quantitative discrepancy was noted; ultraviolet spectrophotometry showed higher concentrations of diazepam in some cases, a difference attributable to the additional measurement of the *N*-desmethylmetabolite in the spectrophotometric method. The ratio of diazepam to metabolite depends on dose, time of ingestion, and duration of use (*7*). In a clinical emergency this information is not considered as significant as it is to establish the presence of the compound. No false positives were encountered.

None of the drugs in Table 1 interfere in the gas-chromatographic analysis of diazepam. It is important to optimize chromatographic conditions for separation of diphenylhydantoin, methaqualone, and diazepam. The other commonly used benzodiazepines—chlordiazepoxide, oxazepam, and fluorazepam—are poorly extracted at low pH and do not interfere.

Analytical recovery was studied by gas chromatographing ethanolic diazepam diluted with drug-free serum in the most common overdose range of 1 to 10 mg/liter, in increments of 1 mg/liter, and 10 to 100 mg/liter, in increments of 10 mg/liter. Peak height was compared to the peak height produced by direct injection of diazepam in ethyl acetate. For all concentrations, recovery was 91% or better, indicating ample recovery at low pH.

Significantly, 77% of all our values for diazepam in positive cases were 3 mg/liter or less. The large number of samples encountered indicates that values exceeding 1 mg/liter are consistent with acute ingestion of more than the normal therapeutic amount of the drug, in agreement with previous reports (*8–11*).

The abuse of drugs continues unabated in the United States. Awareness of "hard drug" use predominates in the news media and funded programs (*11*), but the facts concerning other drug misuse are generally hidden. Diazepam (and probably others) are heavily misused, but are not the subjects of critical editorialization.

Highly prescribed psychotropic drugs can easily end up in the hands of many others. Therefore, the clinical analyst should be aware of drug popularity, which in our present society leads to overuse, abuse, and often requires medical intervention in a clinical emergency.

References

1. Valium overuse cited in National Council report. In *Narcotics Control Digest,* 5 143, 5 (1975).

2. Firm disputes Valium abuse reported by Drug Council. *Ibid.,* No. 44, p 2.

3. *Chromatography-Lipid Newsletter,* 8/1, (1974). Supelco, Inc.

4. Sine, H. E., McKenna, M. J., Rejent, T. A., and Murray, M. H., Emergency gas liquid chromatographic determination of barbiturates and glutethimide in serum. *Clin. Chem.* **16,** 587 (1970).

5. Walberg, C. B., The determination of diazepam, type C procedure. In *Manual of Analytical Toxicology,* I. Sunshine, Ed. CRC Press, Cleveland, Ohio, 1971, pp 123–126.

6. Berry, D. J., and Grove, J., Emergency toxicological screening for drugs commonly taken in overdose. *J. Chromatogr.* **80,** 205 (1973).

7. de Silva, J. A. F., Koechlin, B. A., and Bader, G., Blood level distribution patterns of diazepam and its major metabolite in man. *J. Pharm. Sci.* **55,** 7 (1966).

8. de Silva, J. A. F., Schwartz, M. A., Stefanovic, V., et al., Detrrmination of diazepam in blood by gas liquid chromatography. *Anal. Chem.* **36,** 11 (1964).

9. Arnold, E. A., A simple method for determining diazepam and its major metabolites in biological fluids: Application in bioavailability studies. *Acta. Pharmacol. Toxicol.* **36,** 335 (1975).

10. Kanto, J., Kangas, L., and Surtola, T., Cerebro-spinal fluid concentrations of diazepam and its metabolites in man. *Ibid.,* p 328.

11. Viala, A., Cano, J. P., Dravet, C., et al., Blood levels of diazepam (valium) and N-desmethyldiazepam in the epileptic child. *Psychiatr., Neurol., Neurochir.* **74,** 153 (1971).

12. Holden, C., Drug abuse 1975: The "war" is past, the problem is as big as ever. *Science* **190,** 638 (1975).

CLIN. CHEM. 22/6, 892–897 (1976)

Measurement of Clomipramine, *N*-Desmethylclomipramine, Imipramine, and Dehydroimipramine in Biological Fluids by Selective Ion Monitoring, and Pharmacokinetics of Clomipramine

Jean-Pierre Dubois, Werner Küng, Walter Theobald, and Bernard Wirz

To quantitatively determine tricyclic antidepressant agents, we used a combined gas chromatograph/mass spectrometer system, and deuterium-labeled internal standards. Recovery exceeds 95% and the coefficient of variation is less than 4% for human whole-blood samples supplemented with 5 to 15 ng of clomipramine hydrochloride or 20 to 60 ng of dehydroimipramine hydrogen fumarate per milliliter. For both amines, the detection limit is 0.3 μg/liter. Six healthy volunteers who received a single oral dose of 50 mg of clomipramine hydrochloride showed peak drug concentrations in the blood 3 to 5 h after administration, ranging between 14.4 and 30.1 μg/liter. Plasma/whole blood concentration ratios varied from 0.70 to 1.20, and the cumulative renal elimination from 0 to 72 h is less than 0.2% of the dose. This method is suitable for in vivo bioavailability studies of unchanged clomipramine, dehydroimipramine, and imipramine after a single oral dose of as little as 25 mg.

Additional Keyphrases: *whole blood • urine • gas chromatography/mass spectrometry • monitoring tricyclic antidepressants*

Clomipramine, 3-chloro-5-[3-(dimethylamino)-propyl]-10,11-dihydro-5*H*-dibenz[*b,f*]azepine-hydrochloride, the active ingredient in "Anafranil" (Geigy, Switzerland), and imipramine, 5-[3-(dimethylamino) - propyl] - 10,11 - dihydro - 5*H* - dibenz[*b,f*]azepin-hydrochloride, the active ingredient in "Tofranil" (Geigy, Switzerland), are well-known antidepressant agents.

Different methods for measuring clomipramine and imipramine in biological fluids have been reported: fluorescence (*1, 2*), thin-layer chromatography/densitometry (*3–5*), radioimmunoassay (*6*), gas chromatography (*7, 8*), and gas chromatography/mass spectrometry (*9–11*), but only the last one of these methods is sensitive and specific enough for monitoring concentrations of the unchanged active compound in whole blood after a single oral dose of 50 or even 25 mg of a tricyclic antidepressant agent.

We describe here a gas chromatographic/mass spectrometric method for quantitatively determining clomipramine, desmethylclomipramine, imipramine, or dehydroimipramine in 1 ml of human whole blood, down to a concentration of 0.3 μg/liter. Deuterium-labeled internal standards are added to the biological sample before the extraction process. Urine samples have been analyzed in the same way.

Materials and Methods

Instrument

Analyses were done with a Model 9000 combined gas chromatograph/mass spectrometer system (LKB Producter AB, S-161 25 Stockholm-Bromma 1, Sweden) equipped with a mass marker and an accelerating voltage alternator from LKB, and a Speedomax G Model S millivolt high-speed recorder (Leeds & Northrup, North Wales, Pa. 19454). The chromatograph was fitted with 2.1-m glass columns, 3 mm i.d., packed with 3% OV-101 on 80–100 mesh Gas Chrom Q for clomipramine and desmethylclomipramine determinations, and 3% OV-17 on 80–100 mesh Supelcoport from Supelco, Bellefonte, Pa., for imipramine and dehydroimipramine determinations. Helium flow was 30 ml/min. Operating temperatures were: flash heater, 270 °C; column, 270 °C; molecular separator, 285 °C; ion source, 310 °C. The trap current was 60 μA, and the electron energy 30 eV. Entrance slit width was 0.4 mm, collector slit width, 0.6 mm. The accelerating voltage alternator was adjusted to monitor the intensities of two molecular ions: clomipramine (m/e = 314) and D_4-clomipramine containing one ^{37}Cl atom (m/e = 320); the pentafluoropropyl derivatives of desmethylclomipramine (m/e = 446) and D_5-desmethylclomipramine containing one ^{37}Cl atom (m/e = 453); imipramine (m/e

Research Department and Medical Department, Pharmaceuticals Division, Ciba-Geigy Limited, Basel, Switzerland.

Address correspondence to J.P.D., c/o Ciba-Geigy Limited, R-1055.6.23, CH-4002 Basel, Switzerland.

Received Feb. 2, 1976; accepted April 7, 1976.

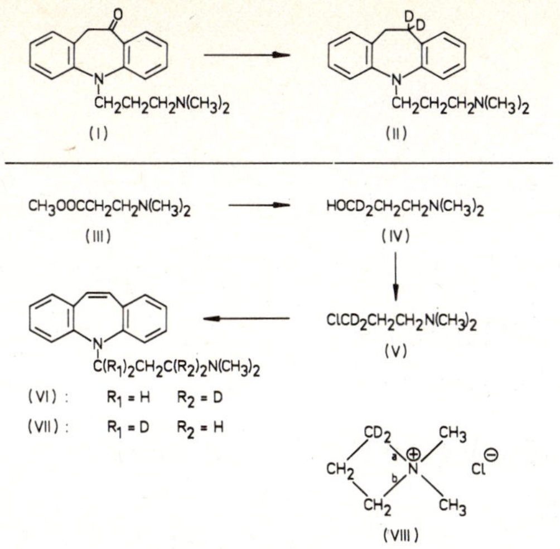

Fig. 1. Synthesis of D_2-imipramine (**II**) and D_2-dehydroimipramine (mixture of isomers **VI** and **VII**)

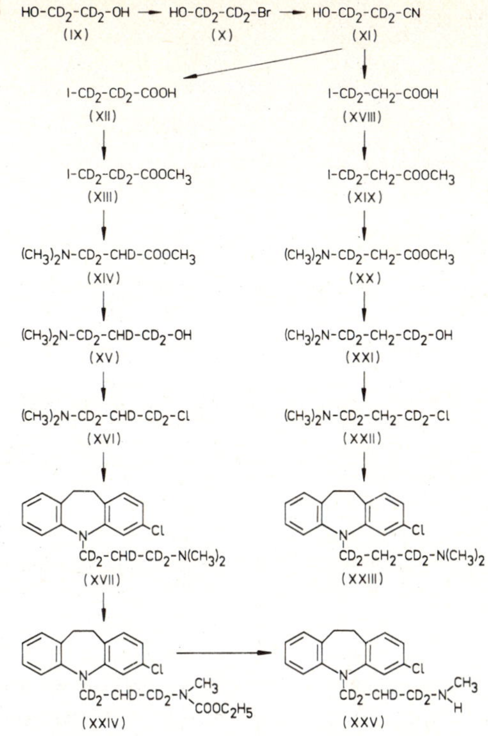

Fig. 2. Synthesis of D_4-clomipramine (**XXIII**) and D_5-desmethylclomipramine (**XXV**)

= 280) and D_2-imipramine (m/e = 282); dehydroimipramine (m/e = 278) and D_2-dehydroimipramine (m/e = 280). The third channel of the accelerating voltage alternator was used to control the stability of the magnetic field strength.

Reagents

All chemicals were of analytical grade and were specially tested for purity with blank runs.

Synthesis of the Deuterium-Labeled Internal Standards

The reaction pathway for the preparation of the deuterium-labeled internal standards is outlined in Figures 1 and 2.

D_2-Imipramine (**II**) carrying the deuterium atoms at one benzyl position of the azepine ring, was obtained by reduction of 5-[3-(dimethylamino)-propyl]-10,11-dihydro-5*H*-dibenz[*b,f*]azepin-10-one (I) with lithium aluminum deuteride.

D_2-Dehydroimipramine, D_4-clomipramine, and D_5-desmethylclomipramine were labeled with the deuterium atoms attached to the amino-propyl side chain.

D_2-Dehydroimipramine (mixture of isomers **VI** and **VII**) was obtained by reduction of 3-dimethylamino-propanoic acid methyl ester **III** with lithium aluminum deuteride, conversion of the resulting 3-dimethyl-amino-propanol **IV** to the chloride **V,** which was used as alkylating reagent in the *N*-alkylation of 5*H*-dibenz[*b,f*]azepine. The deuterium label of the resulting product is distributed in equal amounts to the 1- and 3-position of the propyl side chain, as shown by nuclear magnetic resonance and mass spectrometry. Confirmation of the specific deuterium labeling in the intermediate chloride **V** has also been established by nuclear magnetic resonance and mass spectrometry. The rearrangement of the deuterium atoms can be rationalized assuming the formation of an azetidinium intermediate **VIII,** followed by displacement on either bond "a" or bond "b" of **VIII** during the alkylation reaction (*12*), yielding the two isomers **VI** and **VII.** Solomon et al. (*13*) have reported the preparation of deuterated promazine, specifically labeled in either the 1-, 2-, or 3-position of the propyl side chain, by condensation of the corresponding 3-dimethylamino-propyl-4-toluenesulfonates with phenothiazine. No evidence is given, however, for the specific labeling of the resulting products.

D_4- and D_5-Clomipramine (**XXIII** and **XVII**). Dideutero- and tetradeutero-3-iodopropanoic acid **XVIII** and **XII** were prepared by reaction of D_4-ethylene glycol **IX** to ethylene bromohydrin **X** and hydracrylonitrile **XI,** and hydrolysis of the latter with hydroiodic acid or deuteroiodic acid, respectively. After methylation of the two 3-iodopropanoic acids and reaction of the esters **XIX** and **XIII** with dimethylamine, the same reaction pathway was followed as described above for dehydroimipramine. During substitution of tetradeutero-3-iodopropanoic acid methyl ester **XIII** with nondeuterated dimethylamine, one deuterium atom was lost, because of the elimination–addition mechanism of this substitution (*14*).

D_5-Desmethylclomipramine (**XXV**) was obtained after reaction of D_5-clomipramine **XVII** with ethyl chloroformate and hydrolysis of the carbamic acid ester **XXIV.**

Extraction Procedure

At pH values exceeding 10, the amines are extracted in high yield with *n*-heptane/isoamyl alcohol (99/1 by vol); at pH values below 2, the amines can be re-extracted from the solvent.

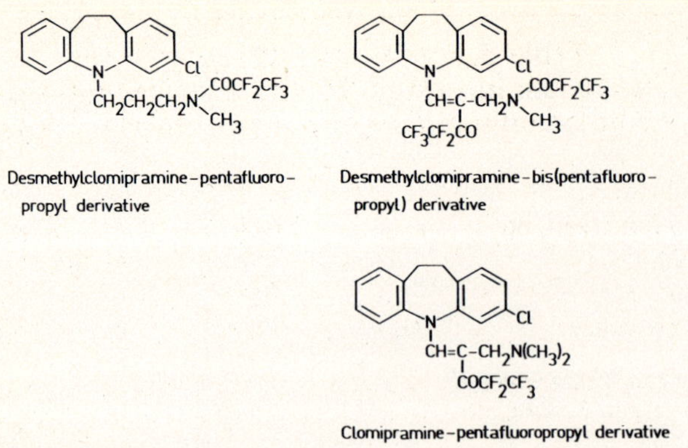

Fig. 3. Principle reaction products of desmethyl-clomipramine and clomipramine with pentafluoropropionic anhydride at different temperatures

Extraction scheme: Mix 0.5 ml of a 200 μg/liter solution of the internal standard in 10 mmol/liter HCl with 1 ml of the biological fluid. Add 1 ml of 2 mol/liter Na_2CO_3 and 4.5 ml of *n*-heptane/isoamyl alcohol (99/1 by vol). Agitate for 15 min and centrifuge for 10 min at 1100 × *g*. Remove the *n*-heptane phase and extract into 0.5 ml of 50 mmol/liter H_2SO_4. Discard the organic phase and add 0.3 ml of 1 mol/liter NaOH and 1.6 ml of *n*-heptane. Remove the *n*-heptane phase and evaporate under nitrogen. Redissolve the residue in 6 to 10 μl of pyridine. The sample is now ready for analysis.

If the concentration of the sample lies outside of the calibration range, as for urine samples, better results are obtained by adding more internal standard to 1 ml of the liquid and diluting this mixture to a concentration that is within the calibration range than by adding the usual amount of internal standard solution to a diluted biological sample.

Derivatization of Desmethylclomipramine

Desmethylclomipramine reacts with pentafluoropropionic anhydride at 30 °C to give the monopentafluoropropyl derivative. At 40 °C, the principal reaction product is a β,γ-unsaturated bis(pentafluoropropyl) derivative, which corresponds to the bis(trifluoroacetyl) derivative of desipramine described by Walle et al. (*15*). At 60 °C even clomipramine reacts with pentafluoropropionic anhydride to form a β,γ-unsaturated monopentafluoropropyl derivative (Figure 3).

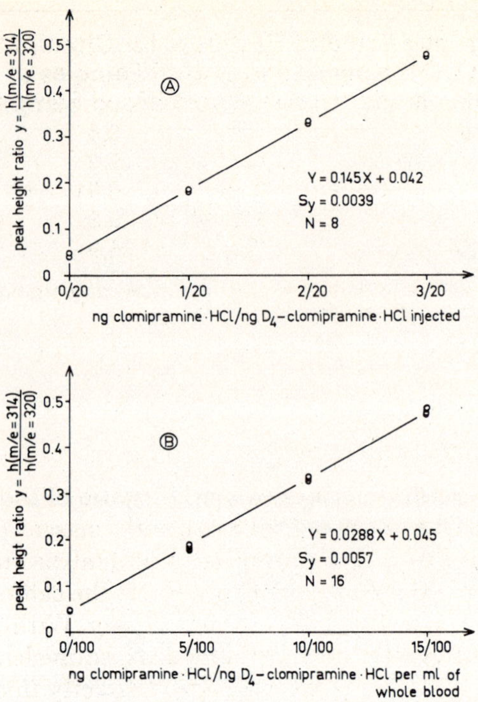

Fig. 4. Calibration curves for clomipramine hydrochloride with D_4-clomipramine hydrochloride as internal standard

A, Direct injection of salt-mixtures in pyridine. *B*, Injection of about 0.2 of the extract of 1 ml of drug-supplemented human whole blood

Desmethylclomipramine can also be derivatized in the *n*-heptane phase (concentration about 100 ng in 1.6 ml of *n*-heptane) by adding 20 μl of dimethylformamide, 20 μl of pyridine, and 100 μl of pentafluoropropionic anhydride to the *n*-heptane phase and heating at 60 °C for 1 h. The *n*-heptane phase is then washed with 1.5 ml of a water/methanol mixture (2/1 by vol) and evaporated. This method has been reported for the formation of the heptafluorobutyl derivative of desmethylnortriptyline by Borgå et al. (*16*).

Table 1. Calibration Curves for Dehydroimipramine·$C_4H_4O_4$, Imipramine·HCl, and Desmethylclomipramine·HCl (Pentafluoropropyl Derivative)[a]

Substance and internal standard	Calibration points	N	Least-squares line Y = mX + b	S_y
Dehydroimipramine·$C_4H_4O_4$ and	A) 0/20; 5/20; 10/20; 15/20	8	Y = 0.0454X + 0.023	0.0070
D_2-Dehydroimipramine·$C_4H_4O_4$	B) 0/100; 20/100; 40/100; 60/100	14	Y = 0.00906X + 0.028	0.0060
	Scaling factor 5			
Imipramine·HCl and	A) 0/12; 1/12; 2/12; 4/12; 6/12	10	Y = 0.0824X + 0.028	0.0035
D_2Imipramine·HCl	B) 0/120; 20/120; 40/120; 60/120	14	Y = 0.00841X + 0.024	0.0035
	Scaling factor 10			
Desmethylclomipramine·HCl and	A) 0/20; 0.5/20; 1/20; 1.5/20; 2/20	10	Y = 0.138X + 0.053	0.0051
D_5-Desmethylclomipramine·HCl	B) 0/100; 5/100; 10/100	6	Y = 0.0270X + 0.046	0.0051
(pentafluoropropyl derivative)	Scaling factor 5			

[a] A) Direct injection of salt-mixtures in pyridine (a/b means: a ng substance + b ng internal standard injected). B) Injection of about 1/5 of the extract of 1 ml of drug-supplemented human whole blood (a/b means: a ng substance + b ng internal standard in 1 ml of human whole blood).

Table 2. Precision and Recovery for Clomipramine·HCl Determinations in 1-ml Samples of Supplemented Human Whole Blood Samples[a]

Added, ng	4.8	9.6	14.4
Found mean, ng	4.6	9.3	14.2
SD, ng	0.16	0.31	0.48
CV, %	3.5	3.3	3.4
% recovery	95.8	96.9	98.6

[a] Single determinations of each of the three concentrations done on twelve different days (n = 12).

Table 3. Precision and Recovery for Dehydroimiproamine·$C_4H_4O_4$ Determinations in 1-ml Sample of Supplemented Human Whole Blood[a]

Added, ng	2.0	20.0	40.0	60.0
Found mean, ng	2.0	19.9	39.8	60.2
SD, ng	0.16	0.47	1.56[b]	0.93
CV, %	8.0	2.4	3.9	1.5
% recovery	100.0	99.5	99.5	100.3

[a] Single determinations of each of the three concentrations, 20.0, 40.0, and 60.0 ng, done on 12 different days (n = 12). For 2.0 ng, n = 10.

[b] SD = 0.82 ng, if two extreme values (42.7 and 36.3 ng) are eliminated.

Quantitative Evaluation

For quantitation, the peak-height ratio of the mass spectrometer response at the specific masses of the molecular ions of the substance to be analyzed and of the internal standard is compared with the calibration curve, which is prepared with each assay. With use of deuterium-labeled internal standards, equivalent calibration curves can be obtained by directly injecting mixtures of the salts of the substance to be analyzed and of the internal standard, or by injecting a portion of the extract of 1 ml of drug-supplemented samples of human whole blood.

The solutions containing 1 mg of labeled or nonlabeled clomipramine hydrochloride, imipramine hydrochloride, or dehydroimipramine hydrogen fumarate in 10 ml of pyridine are stable for a year at 4 °C. Therefore, we directly injected mixtures of these solutions for calibration and used the supplemented human whole blood samples, which were also run with each assay, for precision and accuracy documentation.

Results

Method

Figure 4 shows the calibration curves for clomipramine hydrochloride by direct injection of salt mixtures in pyridine (*A*) and by injection of a portion of the extract from 1 ml of drug-supplemented samples of human whole blood (*B*). Each least-squares line is characterized by three parameters: the slope *m*,[1] which is influenced by a proportional error, the *y*-intercept *b*, which is influenced by a constant error, and the standard error of estimate S_y, which quantitates the random error (*17, 18*).

The parameters *m*, *b*, and S_y of the calibration curves of dehydroimipramine hydrogen fumarate, imipramine hydrochloride, and the pentafluoropropyl derivatives of desmethylclomipramine are listed in Table 1. Day-to-day precision and recovery for clomipramine hydrochloride and dehydroimipramine hydrogen fumarate obtained from repeated analyses of 1 ml of drug-supplemented human whole blood are given in Tables 2 and 3. For both amines, the detection limit, equal to twice the standard deviation of the day-to-day precision of the samples supplemented with the lowest amount of drug, is 0.3 μg/liter.

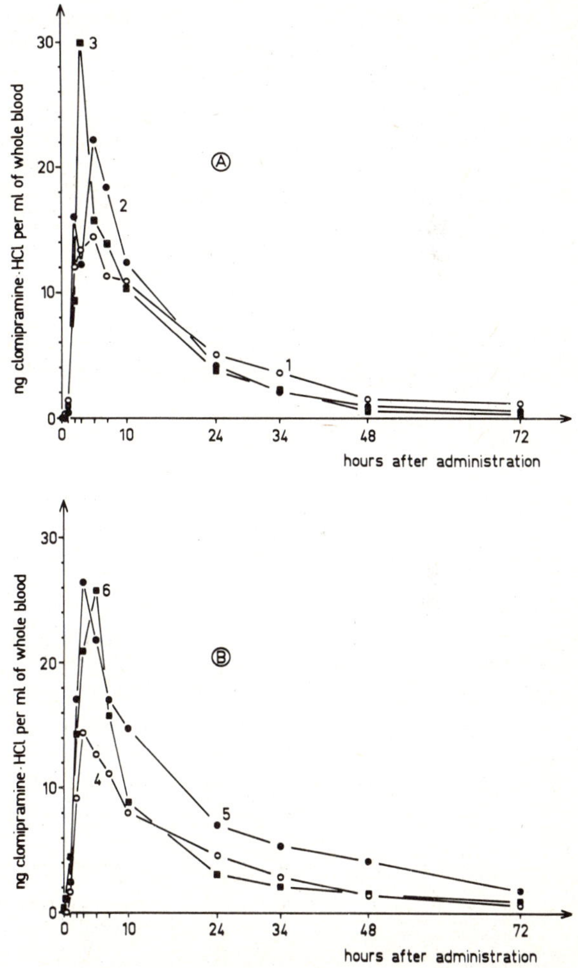

Fig. 5. *A* and *B*: Concentrations of unchanged clomipramine hydrochloride (ng/ml) in whole blood after a single oral dose of 50 mg of clomipramine hydrochloride (two 25-mg "Anafranil" sugar-coated tablets) to six healthy volunteers

[1] Nonstandard abbreviations used: $\bar{x}$ = arithmetic mean; SD = standard deviation; CV = coefficient of variation, CV = (SD:$\bar{x}$)·100; Σ = sum; n = number of calibration points; *m* = slope of the least-squares line; *b* = *y*-intercept of the least-squares line; S_y = standard error of estimate in the *y*-direction of the least-squares line,

$$S_y = \sqrt{\frac{\Sigma (y - Y)^2}{n - 2}}$$

Y = *Y*-value calculated from the least-squares equation $Y = mX + b$.

Pharmacokinetic Study with Clomipramine in Man

In a clinical study, six healthy volunteers received a single oral dose of 50 mg of clomipramine hydrochloride in the form of two 25-mg "Anafranil" commercial sugar-coated tablets. Whole-blood samples were drawn just before and 0.5, 1, 2, 3, 5, 7, 10, 24, 34, 48, and 72 h after administration, and urine was collected before and during the time intervals 0 to 24, 24 to 48, and 48 to 72 h. All these samples were kept frozen at −20 °C and analyzed within four weeks.

Figure 5 shows the whole blood concentrations of unchanged clomipramine hydrochloride, Table 4 contains the areas under the whole blood concentration curves from 0 to 72 h and the plasma/whole blood concentration ratios, and Figure 6 shows the cumulative renal elimination from 0 to 72 h for each of the six healthy volunteers.

Table 4. Area under the Concentration Curve for Whole Blood after a Single Oral Dose of 50 mg of Clomipramine·HCl Given to Six Healthy Volunteers, and Plasma/Whole Blood Concentration Ratio

Volunteer	Body weight [kg]	Area under concn curve from 0 to 72 h [ng/ml * hours]	$c_{Plasma}/c_{Whole\ blood}$ Mean value (N = 4)[a]	SD
1	70	330.7	1.00	0.14
2	77	330.7	1.14	0.06
3	76	295.9	0.70	0.08
4	70	276.9	0.83	0.10
5	79	521.3	1.20	0.13
6	64	316.8	1.04	0.12

[a] Measured 2, 5, 7, and 24 h after administration.

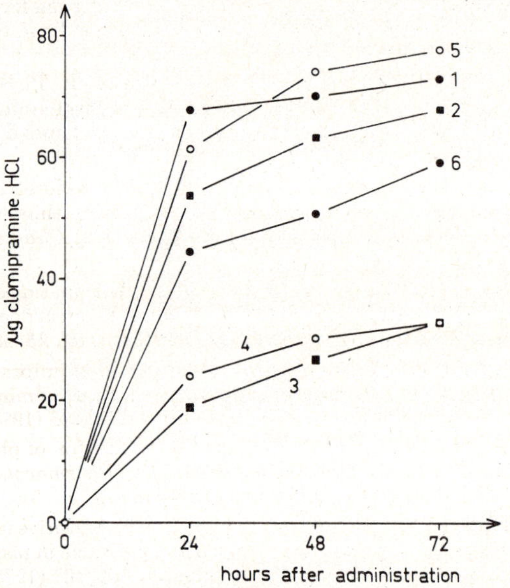

Fig. 6. Cumulative renal elimination of unchanged clomipramine hydrochloride (μg) after a single oral dose of 50 mg clomipramine hydrochloride given to six healthy volunteers

Discussion

Gas Chromatograph/Mass Spectrometer System

Excellent day-to-day precision of the gas chromatograph/mass spectrometer system has been found by directly injecting salt-mixtures of the substance and the internal standard in pyridine. The coefficient of variation of the slope *m* of these calibration curves was less than 1%.

For imipramine and dehydroimipramine, where internal standards labeled with two deuterium atoms were used, the calibration range for a given quantity of internal standard is limited because of the natural ^{13}C content of the nonlabeled material (*19*). To avoid a significant contribution of the substance to the signal on the specific mass of the internal standard, an excess of internal standard must be added to the biological sample. The excess of deuterium-labeled internal standard serves also as a carrier to minimize losses during the extraction procedure.

Drug-Supplemented Samples of Human Whole Blood

Comparison of the calibration curves obtained by injecting the extracts of drug-supplemented samples or by directly injecting salt-mixtures in pyridine permits adequate differentiation between random, constant, and proportional errors.

Random error. Equal values for the standard error of estimate S_y have been found for both types of calibration curves.

Constant error. Impurities contained in the solvent used before the evaporation may cause a constant error, indicated by a parallel shift of the least-squares line. Such constant errors can be eliminated by running blanks and zero values with each assay.

Proportional errors, indicated by a different slope of the least-squares line, have frequently been observed during the elaboration of this method; they are due to problems in preparation of solutions of the tricyclic antidepressant agents. Up to 20% of the substance have been lost when we prepared solutions containing 200 μg of substance per liter of water, ethanol, or *n*-heptane; for solutions in 10 mmol/liter HCl, these losses were less than 5%. The best results, however, were obtained by directly dissolving the substance in human whole blood. One-milliliter portions stored at −20 °C showed an analytical recovery of about 96% after two months and of about 90% after four months.

Pharmacokinetic Study with Clomipramine in Man

The rapid passage of the clomipramine to the body tissues and metabolism of the major part of the drug are the reasons for the low concentrations of unchanged clomipramine hydrochloride found in biological fluids (*20*). Nevertheless, the whole blood concentrations observed from 0 to 48 h after administration of a single oral dose of 50 mg of clomipramine hydrochloride to six healthy volunteers are two- to a 100-fold the detection limit of the method, and the six areas under the whole blood concentration curves differ by a factor of less than two.

The peak blood concentrations of unchanged clomipramine hydrochloride range between 14.4 and 30.1 μg/liter and the cumulative renal elimination from 0 to 72 h varies between 33.0 and 77.8 μg, corresponding to 0.07% and 0.16% of the dose. These results accord with previously reported studies on the pharmacokinetics of clomipramine (*20, 21*) and demonstrate the possibility to study in vivo the bioavailability of unchanged clomipramine hydrochloride in human whole blood after a single oral dose of 50 or even 25 mg with the gas chromatography/mass spectrometry method when a deuterium-labeled internal standard is used.

We thank Mr. R. Ackermann for skillful technical assistance.

References

1. Moody, J. P., Tait, A. C., and Todrick, A., Plasma levels of imipramine and desmethylimipramine during therapy. *Br. J. Psychiatry* **113**, 183 (1967).

2. Olivier-Martin, R., Marzin, D., Buschsenschutz, E., Pichot, P., and Boissier, J., Concentrations plasmatiques de l'imipramine et de la desmethylimipramine et effet anti-dépresseur au cours d'un traitement contrôlé. *Psychopharmacologia* **41**, 187 (1975).

3. Breyer, U., Petruch, F., and Villumsen, K., Plasme levels of tricyclic psychoactive drugs and metabolites in patients: A thin layer chromatographic assay. *Naunyn-Schmiedeberg's Arch. Pharmakol.* **287** *Suppl.*, R 91 (1975).

4. Nagy, A., and Treiber, L., Quantitative determination of imipramine and desipramine in human blood plasma by direct densitometry of thin-layer chromatograms. *J. Pharm. Pharmacol.* **25**, 599 (1973).

5. Nagy, A., and Johansson, R., Plasma levels of imipramine and desipramine in man after different routes of administration. *Naunyn-Schmiedeberg's Arch. Pharmakol.* **290**, 145 (1975).

6. Sathanathan, G. L., and Gershon, S., Correlation of plasma and cerebrospinal fluid levels of imipramine. *Clin. Pharmacol. Ther.* **15**, 218 (1974).

7. Gifford, L. A., Turner, P., and Pare, C. M. B., Sensitive method for the routine determination of tricyclic antidepressants in plasma using a specific nitrogen detector. *J. Chromatogr.* **105**, 107 (1975).

8. Reite, S. F., A gas chromatographic method for the simultaneous determination of imipramine and desipramine in human serum using nitrogen detection. *Medd. Nor. Farm. Selsk.* **37**, 76 (1975).

9. Frigerio, A., Belvedere, G., De Nadai, F., et al., A method for the determination of imipramine in human plasma by gas-liquid chromatography-mass fragmentography. *J. Chromatogr.* **74**, 201 (1972).

10. Belvedere, G., Burti, L., Frigerio, A., and Pantarotto, C., Gas chromatographic-mass fragmentographic determination of "steady state" plasma levels of imipramine and desipramine in chronically treated patients. *J. Chromatogr.* **111**, 313 (1975).

11. Taylor, P. A., and Egan, L. P., Mass fragmentography of imipramine extracted from serum. *Finnigan Spectra* **4**, December (1974).

12. Elderfield, R. C., and Ressler, C., Further study of the rearrangement occurring during the alkylation of 6-methoxy-8-aminoquinoline with 1-diethylamino-3-chloropentane. *J. Am. Chem. Soc.* **72**, 4059 (1950).

13. Solomon, M. D., Summons, R., Pereira, W., and Duffield, A. M., A study of the electron impact promoted fragmentation of promazine sulphoxide and promazine using specifically deuterated analogues. *Aust. J. Chem.* **26**, 325 (1973).

14. *Methoden der Organischen Chemie* (*Houben-Weyl*), Band V/4: Halogenverbindungen. Georg Thieme Verlag, Stuttgart, 1960, pp 701–702.

15. Walle, T., Ehrsson, H., and Bogentoft, C., Synthesis and structure of an enaminic bis(trifluoroacetyl) derivative of desipramine. *Acta Pharm. Suec.* **9**, 509 (1972).

16. Borgå, O., Palmér, L., Linnarsson, A., and Holmstedt, B., Quantitative determination of nortriptyline and desmethylnortriptyline in human plasma by combined gas chromatography-mass spectrometry. *Anal. Lett.* **4**, 837 (1971).

17. Westgard, J. O., and Hunt, M. R., Use and interpretation of common statistical tests in method-comparison studies. *Clin. Chem.* **19**, 49 (1973).

18. Sachs, L., *Angewandte Statistik: Planung und Auswertung, Methoden und Modelle*, Springer, Berlin und Heidelberg, 4. Ausgabe 1974, pp 316–321.

19. Holland, J. F., Teets, R. E., Bieber, M. A., and Sweeley, C. C., A proposed standardization of the mathematical methods used in the calculations and presentation of data from isotope dilution experiments. 21st Annual Conf. on Mass Spect. and Allied Topics. San Francisco, Calif., 20–25 May 1973, American Soc. for Mass Spectrom., N. C-4 pp 55–59.

20. Faigle, J. W., and Dieterle, W., The metabolism and pharmacokinetics of clomipramine (Anafranil). *J. Int. Med. Res.* **1**, 281 (1973).

21. Moody, J. P., The biological availability of clomipramine-(Anafranil). *J. Int. Med. Res.* **1**, 325 (1973).

scientific notes

CLIN. CHEM. 22/6, 898–900 (1976)

Gas-Chromatographic Quantitation of Theophylline in Small Volumes of Plasma

Donald Perrier and Evangeline Lear

We describe a rapid procedure for quantitating theophylline in 100-μl plasma samples by use of a gas–liquid chromatograph equipped with a flame ionization detector. This method is especially useful for monitoring theophylline concentrations in serum or plasma of infants, because sufficiently large blood samples can be readily obtained from a heel prick. The method is specific for theophylline in the presence of caffeine, theobromine and phenobarbital. For plasma concentrations equal to or greater than 5 mg/liter the average daily coefficient of variation was less than 7% while the coefficient of variation from day to day was less than 11%. The same approach can also be used to measure concentrations of phenobarbital in small volumes of plasma or serum, and is readily adapted to determination of theophylline and phenobarbital in larger samples.

Additional Keyphrases: *pediatric chemistry* • *drug assay*

Although the use of theophylline in the treatment of various respiratory disorders is well established, its use as a treatment for apnea in premature infants is recent (*1–4*). The pronounced intersubject differences in the biological half-life of theophylline in adults (*5, 6*) and children (*7*) are also apparent in infants. Shannon et al. (*2*) observed considerable variability in serum theophylline concentrations in infants receiving the same dose on a body-weight basis. This large variability in serum theophylline is of concern because of the rather narrow therapeutic range for theophylline (*2, 8*). Maximum therapeutic activity is observed to occur within the 10 to 20 mg/liter range (*5, 8*), while toxicity is more likely to be observed when concentrations exceed 20 mg/liter (*9*). Hence, administration of theophylline should be individualized based on plasma or serum theophylline concentrations and clinical assessment of the apnea.

School of Pharmacy, University of Kentucky, Lexington, Ky. 40506.
Received Nov. 6, 1975; accepted Feb. 17, 1976.

Theophylline has been quantitated in serum or plasma by titrimetry (*10*), spectrophotometry (*11–13*), high-pressure liquid chromatography (*14–16*), and gas–liquid chromatography (*17–24*). The shortcomings of the titration and spectrophotometric procedures, with respect to specificity and sample volume required have been discussed (*19–22*). Although the high-pressure chromatographic and most of the gas-chromatographic procedures reported for theophylline are specific, 1 to 3 ml of serum or plasma is generally required. For an analytical method to be suitable for routine use in the quantitation of blood drug concentrations in infants, the capability of using small volumes of plasma or serum is highly desirable. Arbin and Edlund (*24*) described a procedure for measuring theophylline in 100 μl of plasma by use of a gas-chromatograph equipped with an electron capture detector, but the procedure is too complex for routine use. A high-pressure liquid chromatographic procedure has been recently reported for the determination of theophylline in 0.1-ml serum samples (*16*).

We report here a rapid, specific gas-chromatographic method for measuring theophylline in volumes of plasma that can readily be obtained from infants via a heel prick. Assay time has been decreased relative to previous methods without sacrificing precision and accuracy.

Materials and Methods

Reagents

Monobasic sodium phosphate, isopropanol, chloroform, and toluene were obtained from Fisher Scientific Co, Cincinnati, Ohio 45242. Tetrabutylammonium hydroxide in methanol (25/75 by vol) was purchased from J. T. Baker Chemical Co., Phillipsburg, N. J. 08865. The theophylline was obtained from Matheson, Coleman and Bell, Norwood, Ohio 45212.

Procedures

To 100 μl of plasma in a centrifuge tube was added 100 μl of phosphate buffer (0.3 mol/liter, pH 5) plus 1 ml of isopropanol in chloroform (5/95 by vol) containing amobarbital USP

(3 mg/liter) as the internal standard. This tube was mixed for 15 s with a vortex-type mixer, then centrifuged for 5 min. The aqueous (upper) phase was aspirated and discarded. The organic phase was transferred to a 3-ml Pyrex ground-glass-stoppered conical centrifuge tube that had previously been modified by heating and drawing the conical end to a finer point. The isopropanol/chloroform was evaporated under nitrogen in a 60 °C water bath, 1 ml of toluene was added, and the contents of the tube were mixed with a vortex-type mixer. Ten microliters of a solution of tetrabutylammonium hydroxide (25 ml per deciliter of methanol/water, 1/1 by vol) was added to the 3-ml centrifuge tube containing the toluene. After mixing with a vortex-type mixer for 15 s and centrifuging for 1 min, 2.5 μl of the aqueous methanol phase was withdrawn and injected into the gas-chromatograph. This sample was obtained by passing the gas-chromatograph syringe needle through the toluene layer into the aqueous methanol (lower) phase. Dilution of the tetrabutylammonium hydroxide/methanol with water was necessary because the tetrabutylammonium hydroxide/methanol is miscible with the toluene. Standard curves were prepared by adding known amounts of theophylline to blank plasma and subjecting these samples to the above procedure.

We used a gas chromatograph (Model 1700, Varian Aerograph, Walnut Creek, Calif. 94598) equipped with a flame ionization detector. The Pyrex glass column (1.8 m × 2 mm i.d.) was packed with 3% OV-17 on Chromosorb G 100/120 mesh (Applied Sciences Labs Inc, State College, Pa. 16801) and conditioned overnight at 300 °C with a nitrogen flow of 10 ml/min. The operating conditions were as follows: injection port temperature, 350 °C; oven temperature, 250 °C; detector temperature, 300 °C; carrier gas (nitrogen) flow rate, 50 ml/min; hydrogen flow rate, 40 ml/min; and air flow rate, 300 ml/min.

Results and Discussion

Since MacGee (*25*) and Kupferberg (*26*) reported on-column methylation to be a convenient method for the gas–liquid chromatographic determination of various anticonvulsants in plasma, on-column alkylation has been used to quantitate several xanthines and barbiturates (*18–23, 27, 28*). Although on-column methylation has been used for the determination of theophylline (*21, 22*), this method is not suitable for the separation of xanthines (*28*). Theophylline (1,3-dimethylxanthine) and theobromine (3,7-dimethylxanthine) are both converted to caffeine (1,3,7-trimethylxanthine) and hence cannot be distinguished. However, on-column preparation of the propyl (*20*), butyl (*22, 28*), and pentyl (*23*) derivatives, in conjunction with (*22, 23*) or without (*20, 28*) temperature programming, has enabled the successful resolution of the xanthines theophylline, theobromine, and caffeine. Butylation of theophylline by reaction with tetrabutylammonium hydroxide was initially reported by Kowblansky et al. (*28*) and later utilized by Johnson et al. (*22*) for the measurement of theophylline in human serum and saliva. Although Johnson et al. (*22*) used temperature programming, theophylline was adequately separated from the other xanthines theobromine and caffeine, as well as from phenobarbital (a constituent of some theophylline dosage forms) under the present isothermal conditions. The retention times for caffeine, theophylline, theobromine, and phenobarbital were 1.8, 6.6, 7.5, and 8.4 min, respectively.

Figure 1 shows representative chromatograms of a blank plasma extract, a blank plasma extract with the internal standard amobarbital (retention time, 2.9 min) in the extracting solvent, and an extract of plasma to which theophylline has been added with amobarbital in the extracting solvent. As is evident, no peaks are present that interfere with the measurement of theophylline or amobarbital. Because amobarbital is used clinically, there is the possibility that a patient may be taking both theophylline and amobarbital. In such a case another internal standard would be required. The butyl derivatives of aprobarbital, alphenal, and 1-methylxanthine have retention times close to that for theophylline (*22, 28*) and hence would be suitable alternatives to amobarbital as internal standards.

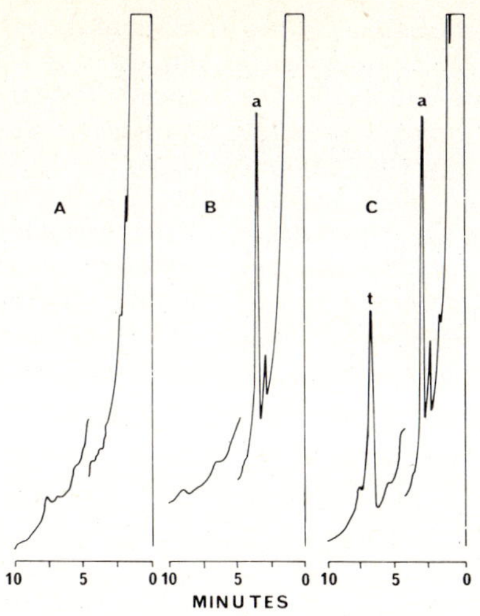

Fig. 1. Chromatograms obtained from an extract of blank plasma (*A*), an extract of blank plasma with amobarbital (*a*) in the extracting solvent (*B*), and an extract of plasma to which theophylline (*t*) has been added with amobarbital in the extracting solvent (*C*)

The attenuation was changed from 256×10^{-12} to 128×10^{-12} at five minutes

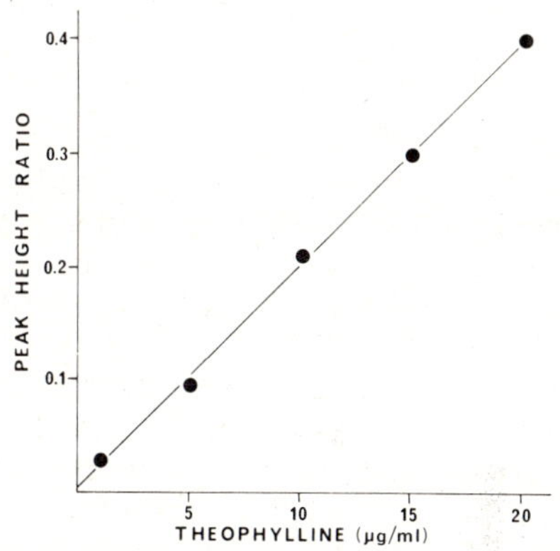

Fig. 2. Typical standard curve obtained for supplemented plasma samples

A typical standard curve is shown in Figure 2. The average coefficients of variation (*29*) for four runs, each run performed in triplicate on different days, at concentrations of 1, 5, 10, and 20 mg/liter were 10.3, 5.1, 6.8, and 2.4%, respectively. The respective coefficients of variation among runs were 18.5, 10.7, 3.4, and 7.9%. Thirteen plasma samples from patients on theophylline therapy were assayed in duplicate over a period of one week. The standard deviation of duplicate means (*30*) for the thirteen samples was 0.5 mg/liter. Theophylline concentrations in these plasma samples ranged from 1.4 to 15 mg/liter, with a mean concentration of 7.0 mg/liter.

Because only 10 μl of an aqueous methanolic solution of tetrabutylammonium hydroxide can extract the theophylline and amobarbital from the toluene, and bring about their butylation by direct injection of an aliquot of this extract into a gas-chromatograph, the quantitation of theophylline concentrations in 100-μl plasma samples is possible with a flame-ionization detector. This convenient approach for extraction and preparation of alkyl derivatives was first demonstrated by MacGee (*25*) for the methylation of hydantoins. The use of the internal standard in the first extraction step not only increases the precision of the method but requires only two accurate volumetric measurements: the plasma sample and the isopropanol/chloroform/internal standard solution. Furthermore, assay time is shortened by the decrease in the number of steps and in the time required for the evaporation, mixing, and centrifugation steps.

This method has also been successfully used to quantitate phenobarbital in small volumes of plasma, and is readily adapted to the quantitation of phenobarbital and theophylline in larger volumes. If only phenobarbital is being measured, it can be directly extracted from plasma with toluene that contains the internal standard.

Supported in part by a Merck Grant for Faculty Development.

References

1. Kuzemko, J. A., and Paala, J., Apnoeic attacks in the new born treated with aminophylline. *Arch. Dis. Child.* **48,** 404 (1973).
2. Shannon, D. C., Gotay, F., Stein, I. M., et al., Prevention of apnea and bradycardia in low-birthweight infants. *Pediatrics* **55,** 589 (1975).
3. Uauy, R., Shapiro, D. L., Smith, B., and Warshaw, J. B., Treatment of severe apnea in prematures with orally administered theophylline. *Pediatrics* **55,** 595 (1975).
4. Lucey, J. F., The xanthine treatment of apnea of prematurity. *Pediatrics* **55,** 584 (1975).
5. Jenne, J. W., Wyze, E., Rood, F. S., and MacDonald, F. M., Pharmacokinetics of theophylline. *Clin. Pharmacol. Ther.* **13,** 349 (1972).
6. Mitenko, P. A., and Ogilvie, R. I., Pharmacokinetics of intravenous theophylline. *Clin. Pharmacol. Ther.* **14,** 509 (1973).
7. Levy, G., Pharmacokinetic control of theophylline therapy. In *Clinical Pharmacokinetics, A Symposium,* G. Levy, Ed., APhA Academy of Pharmaceutical Sciences, Washington, D. C., 1974, pp 103–110.
8. Mitenko, P. A., and Ogilvie, R. I., Rational intravenous doses of theophylline. *New Engl. J. Med.* **289,** 600 (1973).
9. Piafsky, K. M., and Ogilvie, R. I., Dosage of theophylline in bronchial asthma. *New Engl. J. Med.* **292,** 1218 (1975).
10. Plummer, A. J., A method for the quantitative estimation of theophylline in blood and urine. *J. Pharmacol. Exp. Ther.* **93,** 142 (1948).
11. Truitt, E. B., Jr., Carr, C. J., Bubert, H. M., and Krantz, J. C., Jr., The quantitative estimation of theophylline in blood. *J. Pharmacol. Exp. Ther.* **91,** 185 (1947).
12. Schack, J. A., and Waxler, S. H., An ultraviolet spectrophotometric method for the determination ot theophylline and theobromine in blood and tissues. *J. Pharmacol. Exp. Ther.* **97,** 283 (1949).
13. Gupta, R. C., and Lundberg, G. D., Quantitative determination of theophylline in blood by differential spectrophotometry. *Anal. Chem.* **45,** 2403 (1973).
14. Thompson, R. D., Nagasawa, H. T., and Jenne, J. W., Determination of theophylline and its metabolites in human urine and serum by high-pressure liquid chromatography. *J. Lab. Clin. Med.* **84,** 584 (1974).
15. Manion, C. V., Shoeman, D. W., and Azarnoff, D. L., High-pressure liquid chromatographic assay of theophylline in biological fluids. *J. Chromatogr.* **101,** 169 (1974).
16. Weinberger, M., and Chidsey, C., Rapid analysis for theophylline in serum by use of high-pressure cation exchange chromatography. *Clin. Chem.* **21,** 834 (1975).
17. Chrzanowski, F. A., Niebergall, P. J., Nikelly, J. G., et al., Gas chromatographic analysis of theophylline in human serum. *Biochem. Med.* **11,** 26 (1974).
18. Arbin A., and Edlund, P. O., Determination of theophylline and probenecid in biological material. *Acta Pharm. Suec.* **11,** 249 (1974).
19. Wesley-Hadzija, B., A simple method for the estimation of theophylline in plasma by gas liquid chromatography. *Br. J. Clin. Pharmacol.* **1,** 515 (1974).
20. Shah, V. P., and Riegelman, S., GLC determination of theophylline in biological fluids. *J. Pharm. Sci.* **63,** 1283 (1974).
21. Dusci, L. J., Hackett, L. P., and McDonald, I. A., Gas-liquid chromatographic determination of theophylline in human plasma. *J. Chromatogr.* **104,** 147 (1975).
22. Johnson, G. F., Dechtiaruk, W. A., and Solomon, H. M., Gas-chromatographic determination of theophylline in human serum and saliva. *Clin. Chem.* **21,** 144 (1975).
23. Dechtiaruk, W., Johnson, G. F., and Solomon, H. M., Faster gas-chromatographic procedure for theophylline. *Clin. Chem.* **21,** 1038 (1975).
24. Arbin, A., and Edlund, P. O., Determination of theophylline in biological material by means of electron capture gas chromatography. *Acta Pharm. Suec.* **12,** 119 (1975).
25. MacGee, J., Rapid determination of diphenylhydantoin in blood plasma by gas-liquid chromatography. *Anal. Chem.* **42,** 421 (1970).
26. Kupferberg, H. J., Quantitative estimation of diphenylhydantoin, primidone and phenobarbital in plasma by gas-liquid chromatography. *Clin. Chim. Acta* **29,** 283 (1970).
27. MacGee, J., Rapid identification and quantitative determination of barbiturates and glutethimide in blood by gas-liquid chromatography. *Clin. Chem.* **17,** 587 (1971).
28. Kowblansky, M., Scheinthal, B. M., Cravello, G. D., and Chafetz, L., Specific gas chromatographic determination of xanthines and barbiturates by flash-heater N-butylation. *J. Chromatogr.* **76,** 467 (1973).
29. Sokal, R. R., and Rohlf, J., *Biometry.* W. H. Freeman and Co., San Francisco, Calif., 1969, pp 176–181.
30. Kimball, A. W., Queries. *Biometrics* **8,** 85 (1952).

CLIN. CHEM. 22/6, 901-902 (1976)

Primidone Analyses: Correlation of Gas-Chromatographic Assay with Enzyme Immunoassay

Lilla Sun[1] and E. Richard Walwick[2]

Serum specimens from patients on primidone therapy were assayed by two currently available procedures: a commercially available enzyme immunoassay (EMIT) and a published gas-chromatographic procedure. Both procedures were done with commercially available materials and equipment. Results by the two procedures agreed well, which suggests that the two methods could be used interchangeably. For the 94 specimens studied, the correlation coefficient was 0.98, and the least-squares values of slope and intercept were, respectively, 0.97 and 0.51 mg/liter.

Use of primidone (primaclone; 5-ethyl-dihydro-5-phenyl-4,6(1H,5H)-pyrimidinedione) is well established in therapy to control seizures, especially where patients do not respond well to the common barbiturate or hydantoin therapy (*1*). Interpatient variation in metabolism of primidone has not been extensively documented (*2*), but is of interest in monitoring therapy with primidone in specific patients.

A test system for the enzyme immunoassay of primidone has recently become available from Syva Co., Palo Alto, Calif. 94304, as one of their EMIT-AED tests. It offers a rapid means of drug assay appropriate to the emergency treatment situation. Primidone is assayed by gas chromatography in many laboratories. Comparison of results by these two procedures is therefore considered important, especially to laboratories intending to institute either or both of these methods. This work also supplements comparison studies reported for other analysis procedures for anticonvulsant drugs (*3, 4*).

An often-encountered limitation of the gas-chromatographic procedure results from the insolubility of primidone. The extraction/purification procedure we selected for this study gives reproducible analytical recovery of primidone, and the chromatographic pattern has a low background, relatively free of spurious peaks.

Materials and Methods

The samples we used were 94 serum samples from patients, submitted for assay of primidone during a three-month period.

The immunoassay procedure we used to measure primidone was that presented in the package insert supplied with the EMIT primidone assay system (Syva Co.) as described for the Model 24/25 spectrophotometer with sipper system (Beckman Instruments, Inc.). The Model 24/25 was used with the Model 701 printer/calculator (Beckman Instruments, Inc.). Samples were dispensed and diluted with a Model 1800 pipettor/diluter (Cavro Scientific Instruments, Los Altos, Calif. 94022). All components for analysis, including standards and controls,

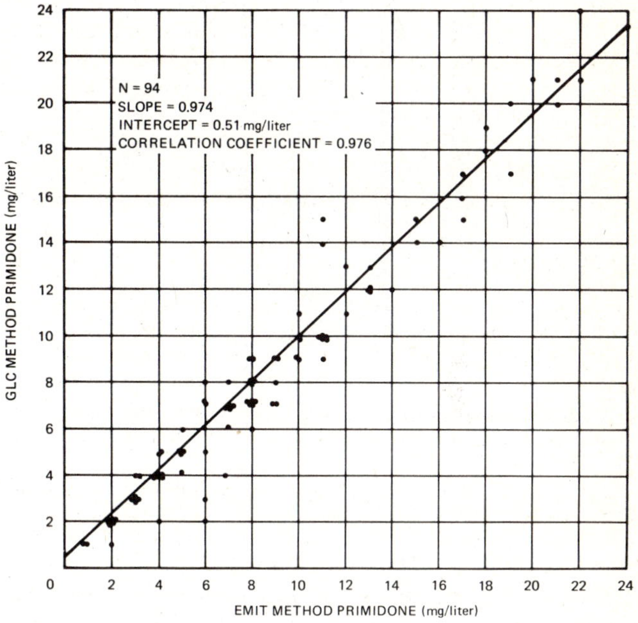

Fig. 1. Comparison of GLC to EMIT

were part of the assay system supplied by Syva Co., for evaluation of the procedure for primidone analysis. The antibody to primidone that they supplied was described as showing a cross reactivity, relative to primidone as 100%, of 1.25% for phenobarbital, 0.25% for mephobarbital, 0.28% for secobarbital, 1.25% for diphenylhydantoin, 0.25% for methsuximide, 0.25% for ethosuximide, and 1.25% for carbamazepine.

The gas-chromatographic analysis was done as described by Perchalski et al. (*5*), with only minor changes. Trimethylanilinium hydroxide in methanol 25/75 by vol. (Southwestern Analytical Chemicals, Inc., Austin, Tex. 87867) was used for methylation. Primidone for preparation of standards and serum pools was obtained from Ayerst Laboratories (685 3rd Ave., New York, N.Y. 10017). Methylene chloride "spectrograde" (J. T. Baker Chemical Co., Hayward, Calif. 94544) was substituted for ethyl ether as the extraction solvent. 5-Methyl-5-phenylhydantoin (Aldrich Chemical Co., Inc., Milwaukee, Wis. 53233) was used as internal standard, and micro nipple-tipped centrifuge tubes "Concentratubes" (Laboratory Research Company, Los Angeles, Calif. 90036) were used for final extraction. Control samples were prepared by pooling drug-free serum and introducing ethanolic primidone standard in the pool to a concentration of 20 mg/liter. The pooled serum control was stored at −40 °C in 1-ml volume until used. A Hewlett-Packard Model 5710A gas-liquid chromatograph (Avondale, Pa. 19311) was used for this assay with 3% OV17 on 100–120 mesh Gas Chrom Q (Applied Science Labs., Inc., State College, Pa. 16801) as the column packing in a 1.82 m × 2 mm (i.d.) column.

[1] Beckman Instruments, Inc., Irvine, Calif. 92713.
[2] Hospital-Pathologist Central Laboratory of Orange County, Inc., Garden Grove, Calif. 92640.
Received Nov. 29, 1975; accepted Dec. 22, 1975.

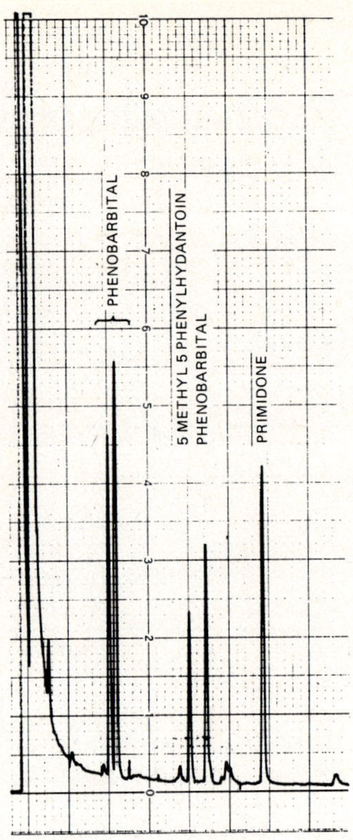

Fig. 2. Gas-liquid chromatography elution pattern of specimen from patient on primidone therapy

Results and Discussion

Figure 1 compares results by the two methods. They agree well. Least-squares regression analysis of the 94 specimens showed the slope of the line to be .974, which indicates a proportional error of 2.6%. From the value of the intercept, constant error is estimated at 0.5 mg/liter. Random error is estimated at 1.2 mg/liter from the standard error. The correlation coefficient is 0.976. Thus, for a chromatographic value of 10 mg/liter, the EMIT procedure would give an average value of 10.3 ± 1.2 mg/liter.

Figure 2 shows a gas-chromatographic elution pattern of a patient specimen. As suggested by the pattern, the phenobarbital in the specimen (summation of the three peaks representing phenobarbital) considerably exceeds the primidone concentration. Clinical data are not available to substantiate that all of the phenobarbital is derived from primidone, but this is the sort of pattern usually seen with serum from a patient being treated with primidone.

We find this chromatographic procedure to be highly reliable. It avoids problems encountered with other procedures relative to interfering plasma constituents and solubility of primidone (especially re-solution of the residue after evaporating the initial organic extract). Because both primidone and phenobarbital are quantitated simultaneously, the physician can see the relative amounts of primidone and phenobarbital in the specimen. Day-to-day reproducibility of the chromatographic procedure was determined by 25 replicate analyses of a serum containing primidone, 20 mg/liter. The average concentration was 21.0 mg/liter with a SD of 1.60 and a CV of 7.6%.

Because no concentration or extraction is required, the enzyme immunoassay can be done in 15 min from receipt of the specimen. In fact, the great sensitivity of the system requires that the specimen be diluted as part of the procedure. Day-to-day reproducibility of the EMIT system was determined by 20 replicate analyses of a serum containing primidone, 12 mg/liter. The average concentration was 12.2 mg/liter with a SD of 1.06 and a CV of 8.1%.

References

1. AMA Drug Evaluations, *AMA Department of Drugs,* 2nd ed., Publishing Sciences Group, Inc., Acton, Mass., 1973.

2. Woodbury, D. M., Penry, J. K., and Schmidt, R. P., *Antiepileptic Drugs,* Raven Press, New York, N. Y., 1972.

3. Brooker, H. E., and Darcey, B. A., Enzymatic immunoassay vs. gas/liquid chromatography for determination of phenobarbital and diphenylhydantoin in serum. *Clin. Chem.* **21,** 1766 (1975).

4. Spiehler, V., Sun, L., Miyada, D., et al., Radioimmunoassay, enzyme immunoassay, spectrophotometry, and gas-liquid chromatography compared for determination of phenobarbital and diphenylhydantoin. *Clin. Chem.* **22,** 749 (1976).

5. Perchalski, R. J., Scott, K. N., Wilder, B. J., and Hammer, R. H., Rapid simultaneous GLC determination of phenobarbital, primidone and diphenylhydantoin. *J. Pharm. Sci.* **62,** 1735 (1973).

CLIN. CHEM. 22/6, 903–905 (1976)

Improved Micro-Radioimmunoassay of Digoxin in Serum, with Use of ^{125}I-Labeled Digoxin

Benjamin Calesnick and Annette Dinan

A micro-radioimmunoassay of ^{125}I-labeled digoxin is described in which 10-μl rather than 50-μl aliquots of sera are required. The method is a modification of a simplified, rapid, and accurate procedure, which is commercially available as a kit. There is excellent correlation between results by these two methods, in which lyophilized digoxin standards and insoluble antibody polymer are used. The digoxin concentration in capillary sera was not significantly different from that in the corresponding venous blood. It is clinically useful to monitor digoxin therapy in capillary sera, particularly in patients in whom blood sampling by venipuncture is inconvenient or difficult.

Additional Keyphrases: *"kit" methods* • *pediatric chemistry*

Knowledge of concentrations of drugs in the blood is important to forensic scientists, toxicologists, medical investigators, and clinicians. However, the significance of these data depends on the accuracy of the methods used for their determinations. Numerous reports (*1–4*) indicate that the technical problems in radioimmunoassay have resulted in erroneous results and lack of reproducibility. We, too, have encountered such problems when using commercial kits with either ^{3}H- or ^{131}I-labeled digoxin. Thus we decided to evaluate a method that involves use of ^{125}I-labeled digoxin, lyophilized digoxin standards, and insoluble digoxin-antibody polymer. The labeled derivative is [^{125}I]-succinyl digoxin tyrosine, which has a high solubility and specific activity, prolonged stability, and is in a lyophilized form.

Materials and Methods

Our purpose was to (*a*) substantiate accuracy and reproducibility of the kit procedure (Curtis Nuclear Corp., Los Angeles, Calif. 90058), (*b*) validate reproducibility of a modification of this procedure involving a microtechnique, and (*c*) compare digoxin concentration in capillary and venous blood samples.

We used Curtis Digoxin RIA kits from nine different production lots in this study.

Blood samples for digoxin determinations were obtained from a total of 40 hospitalized patients, 45 to 83 years of age and weighing between 46 and 105 kg (104 to 233 pounds) who were under treatment for congestive heart failure. They were all maintained with single daily doses of either 0.125 mg (14 patients) or 0.25 mg (26 patients) of digoxin. All blood samples were collected at 1430–1530 hours, 6 h after ingestion of the medication, both by venipuncture of the antecubital vein and by finger prick.

Linear regression analysis was performed to test the precision of the original methodology and paired *t*-tests were used to determine differences between groups (*6*).

Procedure

The accuracy of these kits was first tested by determining the recovery of digoxin (USP grade) added to digoxin-free sera. These were primary standards and corresponded to 0, 1.2, 2.4, 4.0, and 4.8 μg of digoxin per liter. Assays were conducted according to the procedure prescribed for these kits, which contain secondary standards.

In this study we analyzed 50-μl aliquots of venous sera according to the method included with these kits and 10-μl aliquots of the same samples according to our modification of this method. We also analyzed samples of both capillary and venous sera from the same patients, collected within 1 min of one another and the sera frozen if not immediately assayed. All analyses were done in duplicate. We used a Gamma Scintillation Spectrometer, Model 5375 (Packard Instrument Co., Inc., Downers Grove, Ill. 60515), with 10-min counting times. The analytical procedure was:

All reagents and sera were brought to room temperature (15–30 °C) before use.

Each polymer tablet (from the kit) was dissolved in 0.5 ml of sodium chloride solution (9 g/liter). After the tablets were dissolved, forming the polymer tablet slurry, 100-μl aliquots were pipetted into test tubes, the solution being shaken before each aliquot to assure complete dissolution of polymer tablets. Then the samples were mixed gently by hand and left at room temperature for 10 min.

Aliquots, 10 μl, of standards and patients' sera were pipetted (Eppendorf Microliter pipets) directly into the antibody polymer slurry, mixed, and left at room temperature for 10 min.

Ten microliters of ^{125}I-labeled digoxin tracer (no less than 1 mCi/liter can be used in this method) were pipetted directly into the tubes, mixed, and left at room temperature for 30 min.

After 30 min, 1.0 ml of the saline was pipetted into each test tube, mixed with a vortex-type mixer until the precipitate was suspended, and centrifuged (3000 rpm, 5 min) at room temperature. The saline wash was carefully decanted, and dis-

Division of Human Pharmacology, The Hahnemann Medical College & Hospital of Philadelphia, 230 N. Broad St., Philadelphia, Pa. 19102.

Received May 9, 1975; accepted Feb. 27, 1976.

Table 1. Values Obtained with Six Lots of Curtis Nuclear Kit for Four Concentrations of USP Digoxin Added to Serum

		Lot no.								
n	USP digoxin stds	1100 06F4	1100 05F4	1100 04F4	1100 03F4	1100 02F4	1100 01F4	$\bar{X}$	SD	CV, %
		μg/liter								
		1.00	0.94	0.92	0.95	1.21	0.98			
18	1.2	1.00	0.99	0.88	1.00	1.26	0.99	1.01	0.108	10.68
		0.99	0.98	1.10	0.95	1.20	0.90			
		2.35	2.25	2.40	2.42	2.35	2.70			
18	2.4	2.42	2.20	2.50	2.50	2.45	2.60	2.43	0.139	5.73
		2.35	2.26	2.40	2.40	2.52	2.70			
		4.10	3.70	3.90	4.15	3.88	3.95			
18	4.0	4.20	3.78	3.80	3.98	3.75	4.15	3.95	0.162	4.10
		4.08	3.82	4.00	3.90	3.75	4.15			
		4.82	4.40	4.95	4.68	4.48	4.78			
17	4.8	4.89	4.52	5.20	4.92	4.48	4.46	4.75	0.256	5.38
		4.80	4.77	5.20	Broken tube	4.48	5.00			

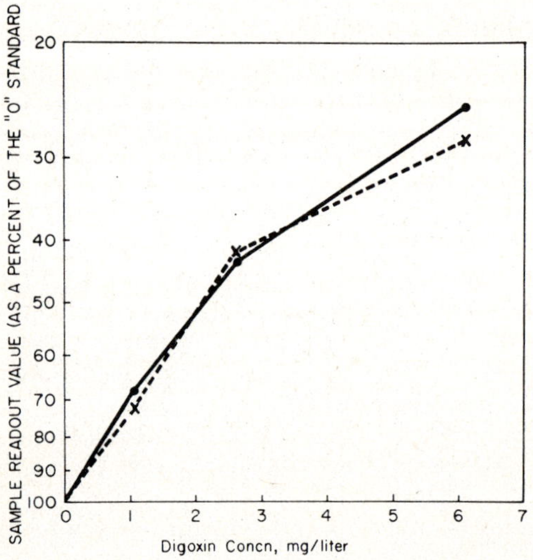

Fig. 1. Standard curves prepared with 10-μl (X) and 50-μl (●) samples

carded. The small packed precipitate button must not be disturbed. This step is repeated.

After the final washing, the test tubes were inverted, to drain. Each test tube was then washed thoroughly on the outside, rinsed with distilled water, dried, and the radioactivity of its contents counted.

Results

A line of regression was plotted from the data (Table 1) to determine the accuracy of the commercially available Curtis RIA kits. The slope was 1.1005 ± 0.0031, with an intercept of −0.49 + 0.09. The *t*-test for the slope was 350.6 and for the intercept −45.7. The correlation coefficient was 0.9997 and significant correlation was obtained between primary and secondary digoxin standards. The method is linear and satisfactorily accurate.

Standard curves were constructed for each assay (Figure 1). During the course of this study, four curves were obtained for each kit, and excellent reproducibility was obtained between them. The same control serum was used as an unknown in each assay.

Serum digoxin concentrations of our patients ranged between 0.23 to 2.90 μg/liter. Statistical analysis of data comparing paired samples of digoxin concentrations in 10-μl and 50-μl samples of venous sera obtained in this group of patients indicated an average difference ($\bar{X}$) = 0.022 ± 0.3052 (SD) (t = 0.456, and $P > 0.60 < 0.70$).

Digoxin concentrations were compared in capillary and venous blood of 20 patients. We compared results for 10- and 50-μl samples of venous blood and 10-μl samples of capillary and venous blood. Statistical analysis indicated that for the 10- vs. 50-μl samples, $\bar{X}$ = 0.110 ± 0.261 (SD), t = 1.89 and P >0.05 < 0.10; for the 10-μl capillary vs. venous samples, $\bar{X}$ = 0.0435 ± 0.1975 (SD), t = 0.986, and P >0.20 < 0.40.

Discussion

Our data confirm that the original radioimmunoassay kit for digoxin gives rapid, accurate results and is suitable for routine clinical use. Because special equipment and preparation of solutions required by other methods is obviated, there are fewer possible sources of laboratory error and less time is required to perform these assays. The simplification of radioimmunoassay of digoxin when ^{125}I-labeled digoxin is used has been confirmed by others (*6, 7*).

Our micro-radioimmunoassay for digoxin depends on the specific activity of ^{125}I-labeled digoxin supplied by the manufacturer being about 1 mCi/liter or greater, so that the 10-μl volumes we used in this method can be easily detected with a gamma counter. Our micro-method was compared to the manufacturer's prescribed method.

There was no significant difference between capillary and venous blood concentration of digoxin.

Therefore, from the practical clinical aspect, our procedure, which requires 10 μl rather than 50 μl aliquots of sera, can be used when venipuncture is difficult or undesirable, as in cases of extreme obesity, venous thrombosis, or peripheral vascular disease, or for infants and children.

We wish to acknowledge the support and assistance of Robert Rousseau, Ph.D., and Curtis Nuclear Corp.

References

1. Fogelman, A. M., LaMont, J. T., Finklestein, S., et al., Fallibility of plasma digoxin in differentiating toxic from nontoxic patients. *Lancet* **ii,** 727 (1971).

2. Anggard, E. E., Chew, L. F., and Kalman, S. M., A source of error in digoxin radioimmunoassay. *New Engl. J. Med.* **287,** 935 (1972).

3. Burnett, G. H., Conklin, R. L., Wasson, G. W., and MacKinney, A. A., Variability of standard curves in radioimmunoassay of plasma digoxin. *Clin. Chem.* **19,** 725 (1973).

4. Holtzman, J. L., Shafer, R. B., and Erickson, R. R., Methodological causes of discrepancies in radioimmunoassay for digoxin in human serum. *Clin. Chem.* **20,** 1194 (1974).

5. Holtzman, J. L., and Shafer, R. B., Discrepancies in the radioimmunoassay for digoxin. *J. Am. Med. Assoc.* **233,** 817 (1975).

6. Snedecor, G. W., and Cochran, W. G., *Statistical Methods,* 6th ed., Iowa University Press, Ames, Iowa, 1967.

7. Horgan, E. D., and Riley, W. J., Radioimmunoassay of plasma digoxin, with use of idodinated tracer. *Clin. Chem.* **19,** 187 (1973).

8. Drewes, P. A., and Pileggi, V. J., Faster and easier radioimmunoassay of digoxin. *Clin. Chem.* **20,** 343 (1974).

CLIN. CHEM. 22/6, 905–907 (1976)

Adaptation of "EMIT" Technique for Serum Phenobarbital and Diphenylhydantoin Assays to the Miniature Centrifugal Analyzer

Sheldon D. Brunk, Themis P. Hadjiioannou,[1] Semi I. Hadjiioannou, and Howard V. Malmstadt[2]

We used a miniature centrifugal analyzer in a spectrophotometric rate-measurement mode to determine the anticonvulsant drugs phenobarbital and diphenylhydantoin in serum, by use of a modified enzyme immunoassay ("EMIT", Syva Corp.) We decreased reagent cost per determination by at least sixfold by means of microscale techniques. Also, the analysis rate is increased by measuring multiple samples simultaneously. Our method requires only 3 μl of serum for duplicate determinations. Replicate analyses of sera containing phenobarbital and diphenylhydantoin gave reaction rates with a CV of 1.5%. Run-to-run CV was 15%. Analytical recovery for drug-supplemented serum samples was 98%, and results for a series of samples compared well with results obtained by gas chromatography (for phenobarbital, $r = 0.95$; for diphenylhydantoin, $r = 0.91$).

Routine monitoring of phenobarbital and diphenylhydantoin is a valuable aid in the management of patients with generalized epileptic seizures (*1*). Gas–liquid chromatography is the most widely used method for measuring anticonvulsants (*2*). This technique is reasonably sensitive, accurate, and reliable, but has several inherent disadvantages. It is relatively time-consuming. Usually, several milliliters of serum are required, which may not be in the best interest of the patient if day-to-day monitoring is desired. At least one sample pretreatment step must be performed, and the quality of results often strongly depends on the skill of the laboratory personnel. Finally, the overall cost of the determination is frequently high.

The recently introduced Enzyme Multiplied Immunoassay Technique ("EMIT", Syva Corp., Palo Alto, Calif. 94303) provides an alternative to conventional methods (*3*–*8*). EMIT assays are based on a binding process between antibody and antigen (drug). Initially, an enzyme-labeled drug is bound to binding sites on the antibody, and the activity of free enzyme is low. Free drug present in the sample competes with an enzyme-labeled drug for antibody binding sites, enzyme is correspondingly released, and enzymic activity of the sample increases. In the present analysis, free enzyme then catalyzes the conversion of the substrate, NAD^+, to NADH, which is reflected in an increased absorbance at 340 nm. The rate of increase is related to the concentration of free drug in the sample.

The technique is rapid, specific, reliable, and sensitive, and no sample pretreatment is required. The principal disadvantage, the high cost of reagents, can be offset by use of microscale techniques made possible by the miniature centrifugal analyzer. Here, we show that good quantitative results can be obtained at lower cost, at a higher rate, and with a smaller sample than with the usual EMIT procedure.

Materials and Methods

Apparatus

Hardware. The instrumental system, based on the original ORNL design (*9*), but incorporating extensive modifications, is described elsewhere (*10*). An automatic pipette (Model

School of Chemical Sciences, University of Illinois at Urbana-Champaign, Urbana, Ill. 61801.

[1] Visiting professor of chemistry. Permanent address: Laboratory of Analytical Chemistry, University of Athens, Greece.

[2] Address requests for reprints to this author.

Received July 21, 1975; accepted Mar. 1, 1976.

25000; Micromedic Systems, Inc., Philadelphia, Pa. 19105) was used for reagent handling. "Pipetman" adjustable pipettes (Models P-20 and P-200; Cole Scientific, Canoga Park, Calif. 91303) were used for sample handling. The centrifugal analyzer disc used in this study contains 16 measurement cuvettes. Associated with each are a sample and a reagent well, each of 50-μl capacity. Measurement cuvette No. 1 is used to set 100% transmittance. The optical path for cuvette No. 2 is blocked, so that this cuvette is used for background measurements. The remaining 14 cuvettes are used for samples or standards. We did not control temperature because standards were run on each disc.

Software. We did not use the Syva timer-printer or the EMIT AED graph paper. Instead we used a reaction-rate computer program and a log-log curve-fitting routine.[3] Twenty absorbance values were calculated per measurement cuvette during the measurement interval. A measurement was taken from each cuvette for every rotation of the disc. Since the rotation speed was 2000 rpm and the measurement time was 80 s, each of the twenty values represented the average absorbance during 133 rotations, or 4 s. An absorbance change of about 0.01 *A* usually took place during 4 s, a change that is at least 100-fold the instrumental drift. The reaction rate per cuvette, in absorbance change per second, was calculated by fitting a least-squares line through the data points. Calibration curves (log reaction rate vs. log concentration) were determined by least-squares fit.

Reagents. We obtained two EMIT serum assay kits, specifically for phenobarbital and diphenyhydantoin, respectively. Each kit contains an antibody/substrate reagent (reagent A) and a drug/enzyme reagent (reagent B). These reagents were reconstituted by adding 5.5 ml of distilled water to each vial. A buffer concentrate and a set of drug calibrators (common to both determinations) were also obtained from Syva. The buffer solution [tris(hydroxymethyl)aminomethane hydrochloride, 55 mmol/liter, pH 7.9] was reconstituted with 140 ml of distilled water. The lyophilized, serum-base drug calibrators were prepared by adding 3.0 ml of distilled water to each vial. Reagents A and B are stable for 12 weeks. The calibrators are stable for at least two months.

Procedure

We modified the method described in the Syva package inserts. With the centrifugal analyzer disc, a single reagent must be used along with a single sample solution. Thus either reagent A or reagent B must be mixed with the sample before the analysis. First, we mixed the sample with reagent A and loaded these solutions into the sample wells on the disc. When we reversed the procedure by mixing the sample with reagent B, we observed no significant difference in the results. The procedure we used in this study was the reversed mixing sequence.

With the automatic pipette, aliquot 139 μl of reagent B and deliver it with 1.09 ml of buffer into a disposable beaker. Allow this solution to stand for at least 1 min before adding the serum. Meanwhile, deliver 139 μl of reagent A and 1.11 ml of buffer into a second beaker. With a manual pipette, deliver 139 μl of diluted reagent B into each of seven sample cups. Three cups are used for standards, four for samples. Then add 3 μl of each serum standard or sample to its respective cup. After a 1-min wait, load 50 μl of each of the various serum solutions, in duplicate, into the sample wells on the disc. Then load 50 μl of diluted reagent A into each reagent well. This procedure provides a sufficient amount of reagent to load one disc, with a minimum of waste. These diluted reagent solutions should be used within 30 min. Place the loaded disc in the centrifugal analyzer, set for a delay time of 15 s, measurement time of 80 s, and a wavelength of 340 nm.

[3] Information available from the authors.

Table 1. Within-Run Precision of Reaction Rates

	A[a]			B[b]		
	Reaction rate[c]	SD	CV, %	Reaction rate[c]	SD	CV, %
Phenobarbital, mg/liter						
5	2.166	0.055	2.6	1.959	0.020	1.0
20	2.408	0.026	1.1	2.314	0.030	1.3
80	2.685	0.027	1.0	2.619	0.042	1.6
Diphenylhydantoin, mg/liter						
2.5	2.160	0.012	0.6	1.284	0.025	1.9
10	2.304	0.044	1.9	1.331	0.028	2.1
30	2.453	0.021	0.9	1.413	0.008	0.6

[a] Mixing sequence: usual EMIT procedure.
[b] Mixing sequence: reversed procedure.
[c] Rates expressed in change in milliabsorbance units per second.

Table 2. Results of Determinations in Calibration Sera

Present	Found, mg/liter	SD	CV, %
Phenobarbital			
5	5.5	1.03	19
10	8.9	1.14	13
20	20.3	3.25	16
40	40.4	4.45	11
80	75.2	11.05	15
Diphenylhydantoin			
2.5	2.45	0.44	18
10	10.4	2.57	25
30	30.4	3.16	10

Results

Table 1 shows the within-run precision (n = 14) of the reaction rates for the normal reagent mixing sequence and for the reversed sequence. The CV for both mixing sequences was very similar. Day-to-day variation in results obtained from the reversed mixing sequence (Table 2) was determined by analyzing various calibrators during two weeks (n = 8). Concentrations found differed from concentrations present by only ±1 mg/liter. Run-to-run CV was about 15%, not significantly different than the CV for the usual mixing sequence.

We compared the results of the EMIT procedure with those of a gas-chromatographic procedure, for 20 samples containing phenobarbital and 22 samples containing diphenylhydantoin. (Figures 1 and 2). For phenobarbital, r = 0.95, intercept = +0.68, and slope = 0.72. For diphenylhydantoin, r = 0.91, intercept = +0.14, and slope = 0.78.

We prepared three artificial standards by adding phenobarbital to the negative serum calibrator. Analytical recovery for such standards is given in Table 3.

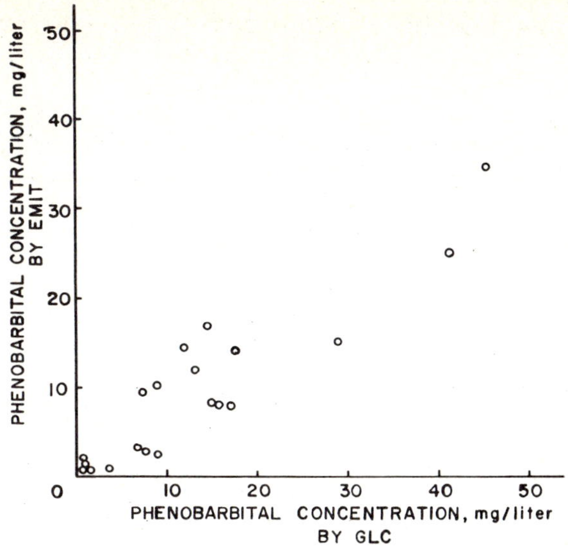

Fig. 1. Serum phenobarbital concentrations as measured by two methods

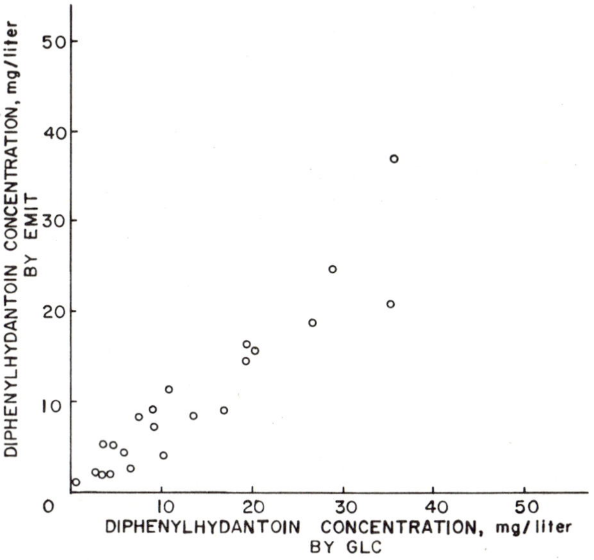

Fig. 2. Serum diphenylhydantoin concentrations as measured by two methods

Discussion

The recently introduced EMIT procedure for anticonvulsants offers several advantages when compared to gas chromatography. Sample size is substantially reduced, sample pretreatment is eliminated, and analysis time is greatly decreased. However, the EMIT procedure is expensive when conventional instrumentation is used. The miniature centrifugal analyzer offers a solution to this problem. Reagent cost can be reduced by at least sixfold through use of smaller volumes in the analysis. Two determinations can be performed on only 3 μl of serum; the usual procedure requires 10 μl per determination. Because the analysis and data reduction are done under computer control, calibration curves need not be plotted manually—an additional time saving.

Table 3. Analytical Recovery of Phenobarbital

Present	Found	
mg/liter		Recovery, %
5.0	4.6	92
20.0	20.4	102
80.0	78.8	98.5

Although the CV for the reaction rates was small (1.5%), the CV for the drug concentrations was quite large (15%), a difference attributable to pipetting errors, the high blank reading, and the small slope of the log-log working curves. No significant difference in results was seen when the usual mixing sequence was compared to the reversed mixing sequence.

The correlation between results by EMIT and gas chromatography was satisfactory ($r = 0.95$ for phenobarbital, 0.91 for diphenylhydantoin). The accuracy of the method was indicated by the 98% of drug accounted for in supplemented serum samples.

A 3-μl sample volume was chosen so that prepared reagents could be efficiently used within 30 min. Because 4 to 5 min is required to load the disc after reagent dilution, an additional lag phase is introduced. We observed a slow decrease in values after 30 min. The same may be expected with the usual EMIT procedure (*3*). A completely automated sample-handling system would help alleviate this problem and improve the precision.

This research was supported in part by NIH Grant HEW PHS GM21984-01.

References

1. Kutt, H., and Penry, J., Usefulness of blood levels of antiepileptic drugs. *Arch. Neurol.* (Chicago) **31,** 283 (1974).

2. Kupferberg, H., Quantitative estimation of dephenylhydantoin, primidone and phenobarbital in plasma by gas liquid chromatography. *Clin. Chim. Acta* **29,** 283 (1970).

3. Syva Corporation, Palo Alto, Calif., Package insert for the EMIT phenobarbital assay kit, April 1975.

4. Rubenstein, K. E., Schneider, R. S., and Ullman, E. F., "Homogeneous" enzyme immunoassay, a new immunochemical technique. *Biochem. Biophys. Res. Commun.* **47,** 846 (1972).

5. Schneider, R., Lindquist, P., Tong-in-Wong, E., et al., Homogeneous enzyme immunoassay for opiates in urine. *Clin. Chem.* **19,** 821 (1973).

6. Brattin, W. J., and Sunshine, I., Immunological assays for drugs in biological samples. *Am. J. Med. Technol.* **39,** 223 (1973).

7. Mulé, S. J., Bastos, M. L., and Jukofsky, D., Evaluation of immunoassay methods for detection, in urine, of drugs subject to abuse. *Clin. Chem.* **20,** 243 (1974).

8. Broughton, A., and Ross, D. L., Drug screening by enzymatic immunoassay with the centrifugal analyzer. *Clin. Chem.* **21,** 186 (1975).

9. Burtis, C., Mailen, J., Johnson, W., et al., Development of a miniature fast analyzer. *Clin. Chem.* **18,** 753 (1972).

10. Avery, J., Gregory, R., Renoe, B., et al., A centrifugal analyzer with a new all-digital measurement system. *Clin. Chem.* **20,** 942 (1974).

11. *Chemical and Biological Aspects of Drug Dependence,* Chemical Rubber Co., Cleveland, Ohio 44128, 1972, p 283.

12. Booker, H. E., and Darcy, B. A., Enzymatic immunoassay vs. gas chromatography for the determination of phenobarbital and diphenylhydantoin in serum. *Clin. Chem.* **21,** 1766 (1975).

CLIN. CHEM. 22/6, 908–911 (1976)

Simplified Fluorometric Assay for Diphenylhydantoin in Plasma

Wesley A. Dill, Amy Leung, Arlyn W. Kinkel, and Anthony J. Glazko

The fluorometric benzophenone procedure for diphenylhydantoin has been simplified by eliminating the need for preliminary extraction of plasma with an organic solvent. Assays are done directly on 0.2 ml of plasma by treating it with alkaline permanganate to form benzophenone, extracting the benzophenone with heptane, and then shaking the heptane layer with sulfuric acid and measuring the fluorescence of the acid layer. The assay is highly reproducible, and adequately sensitive to detect 1 μg of the drug per milliliter of plasma. Fluorometric and gas–liquid chromatographic assays of 154 plasmas gave results that were not significantly different, even in the presence of phenobarbital, other barbiturates and anticonvulsant drugs, or of various tranquilizers and other commonly used drugs. The assay is rapid, the unit cost per assay low.

Additional Keyphrases: *gas-chromatography compared* • *benzophenone*

Data on plasma concentrations of 5,5-diphenylhydantoin (phenytoin, "Dilantin", DPH) are particularly useful in adjusting dose schedules to suit the requirements of the individual patient (*1, 2*). The early colorimetric (*3*) and spectrophotometric (*4*) assay procedures were time consuming and subject to interference from phenobarbital and other drugs. Gas–liquid chromatographic (GLC) procedures (*5, 6*), introduced later, are highly specific, but generally require more than 1 ml of plasma and about 20 min per sample. Radioimmunoassays (*7*) appear to be highly specific and sensitive, but the prepared reagents are expensive.

The oxidation of DPH by heating with alkaline permanganate to yield benzophenone, first described by Wallace et al. (*8*), increases the specificity, because phenobarbital does not interfere with this assay. However, the method in its original form was unwieldy, requiring reflux operations during the oxidation step, and it lacked sensitivity. Numerous modifications in the extraction and oxidation step (*9, 10*) and development of a fluorometric assay procedure for benzophenone (*11, 12*) resulted in a highly sensitive assay procedure that is suitable for clinical use.

The present report describes a further simplified assay of this sort, in which the initial solvent extraction step is eliminated entirely, permitting direct oxidation of small volumes of plasma and subsequent fluorometric assay of the benzophenone. We assayed 154 clinical plasma samples by the modified fluorometric procedure and compared the results with GLC assays of the same specimens. Results by the two procedures agreed well, even in the presence of a wide variety of other drugs.

Research and Medical Affairs Division, Parke-Davis & Co., Ann Arbor, Mich. 48106.

Received Mar. 26, 1975; accepted Mar. 5, 1976.

Materials and Methods

Gas–liquid chromatography: Assays of 0.5-ml plasma samples were done in duplicate and the results averaged. The procedure included the use of 5-(*p*-methylphenyl)-5-phenylhydantoin as an internal standard (*5*), precipitation of cholesterol as the digitonide, extraction of DPH with diethyl ether (*13*), and GLC by on-column methylation with use of trimethylanilinium hydroxide reagent (*14*). The chromatograph was a Model 402 (Hewlett-Packard, Avondale, Pa. 19311), with use of a 180-cm column of 10% OV-17 on Gas Chrom Q and hydrogen-flame detection. Temperatures used were: flash heater, 300 °C; column, 235 °C; and detector, 265 °C.

Fluorometric procedure: The procedure is similar to that described earlier (*11*), except that the initial solvent-extraction step has been eliminated. Disposable glass tubes (Kimball Products, Owens-Illinois, Toledo, Ohio 43666; cat. No. 73000) were used throughout, to minimize glassware cleaning problems. Details of the procedure are as follows.

Using 18 × 150 mm disposable test-tubes, dilute 0.2 ml of plasma or serum with 2 ml of water and mix. Add about 0.5 g of crystalline potassium permanganate (reagent-grade; J. T. Baker Chemical Co., Phillipsburg, N.J. 08865) and 0.5 ml of a 500 g/liter sodium hydroxide solution (Mallinckrodt Chemical Works, St. Louis, Mo. 63147). Each tube is capped with a glass marble and the contents are mixed by using a vortex-type mixer. The tubes are then placed in a rack with the bottoms of the tubes in direct contact with a hot plate[1] at 200 °C, and heated for 10 min. Each tube is removed two or three times during the heating period and shaken by hand to mix the contents. They are then cooled to room temperature by immersion in a water bath, and 3 ml of acid-washed hep-

[1] The hot plate (Lindberg Type H-2, Chicago, Ill. 60612) was covered with a sheet of asbestos with round holes (18 mm diameter) cut out to correspond with the position of the test tubes. The bottom section of a test-tube rack was removed to permit direct contact of the tube bottoms with the hot plate.

Table 1. Summary of 20 Replicate Fluorometric Assays of a Series of Diphenylhydantoin Standards in Plasma, with Use of Two Different Photofluorometers

Instrument	DPH concn, $\mu g/ml$	Mean[a]	SD	SE	CV	Corrected mean per μg DPH[b]
Aminco-Bowman						
Spectrophoto-	0	5.65	0.72	0.16	0.127	0
fluorometer	5	37.76	1.63	0.37	0.043	6.42
(355/485 nm)	10	66.96	1.61	0.36	0.024	6.12
	15	92.90	1.72	0.38	0.018	5.82
Turner	0	7.97	1.28	0.29	0.160	0
Model 111	5	34.73	2.44	0.55	0.070	5.35
	10	60.11	1.34	0.30	0.022	5.21
	15	83.31	1.75	0.39	0.021	5.02

[a] Readings uncorrected for reagent blanks, which were nearly the same as those for normal plasma.
[b] Values corrected for plasma blank and divided by mg/liter concentration of DPH.

tane[2] is added to each tube and mixed for 30 s (vortex-type mixer) to extract the benzophenone.[3] All tubes are then centrifuged, and 2 ml of the heptane extract is pipetted into 13 × 100 mm disposable test-tubes. With an all-Pyrex glass dispenser (Labindustries, Berkeley, Calif. 94710), 1.2 ml of concentrated sulfuric acid[4] (AR grade, Mallinckrodt) is measured into each tube, the contents are vortex-mixed for 20 s and centrifuged. The tubes are then placed in a special holder[5] designed to be used in the fluorometer (*11*), and readings of the acid layer, activated at 355 nm, are made at 485 nm.[6] A series of 10 standards and blanks made up in bovine plasma are run with each set of unknowns, and the results are expressed as micrograms of DPH-acid equivalents per milliliter of plasma.

Assays were run in duplicate on the clinical specimens in this study, and the mean values reported. For replicate assays, DPH standards were made up in bovine plasma in final concentrations of 0, 5, 10, and 15 $\mu g/ml$, and assayed by the procedure described above.

Clinical procedures: Blood samples were drawn from 154 patients at the Sunland Training Center, Ft. Myers, Fla., who had been receiving daily doses of diphenylhydantoin along with other drugs. The heparinized blood was centrifuged, and the separated plasma was frozen and shipped to our laboratories. Upon arrival, the samples were divided for GLC and fluorometric assays in two separate laboratories (see acknowledgments).

Statistical methods: Means, standard deviations, standard errors, and coefficients of variation were calculated with a computer program for small numbers of samples (n-1). The *t*-test for the difference between the means of paired observations and correlation coefficients were calculated. Lines of regression were calculated by the method of least squares.

Results

Reproducibility and Sensitivity

Diphenylhydantoin standards made up in bovine plasma to contain 0, 5, 10, and 15 mg/liter were each assayed 20 times by the fluorometric assay procedure described under *Methods*. Each sample was read first in the Aminco-Bowman Spectrophotofluorometer, and then (in different cuvettes), in the Turner instrument. Table 1 gives the mean values for the readings, uncorrected for normal plasma blanks, together with the calculated standard deviations, standard errors, and coefficients of variation. The actual readings obtained with the two instruments were not directly comparable, because the sensitivity settings were different, the wavelengths used for measurement were different (diffraction grating vs. filters), and the test-tube cuvettes were different. However, for both instruments, the standard curves showed a very similar pattern: readings were directly proportional to DPH concentrations in the lower range, but there was a slight downward inflection in the curves at higher concentrations. For this reason, a series of standards made up in bovine plasma were included with each set of assays, and the concentrations of DPH were read directly from the standard curve. This also corrected for slight differences between the fluorescence generated for DPH assays in water or in plasma, the latter generally being slightly higher.

"Within-day" precision for 20 replicate assays of each of four standard solutions by one analyst can be evaluated from the coefficients of variation shown in Table 1. These were about 2% at high drug concentrations (10–15 mg/liter), about 4% at lower ones (5 mg/liter), and 13–16% for drug-free plasma. "Day-to-day" precision was estimated from results for six

[2] Heptane (glass-distilled, Burdick and Jackson Labs., Inc., Muskegon, Mich. 49442) was washed by shaking with sulfuric acid as previously described (*11*). On the day of assay, it is washed twice with one-quarter volumes of sulfuric acid to ensure the absence of interfering substances.

[3] The extraction step is time consuming and can be shortened by using two vortex-type mixers, holding one test tube in each hand.

[4] The selection of the sulfuric acid and its subsequent handling has been described previously (*11*). Fluorometer readings should be made within 30 min after the acid is added.

[5] The adapter for the 13 × 100 mm tubes consisted of a piece of brass tubing (15 mm o.d. × 10 mm) placed at the bottom of the Aminco-Bowman 12-mm square cuvette holder to elevate the tube and to keep it centered. The upper part of the tube passed through a round hole in a rubber gasket near the top of the holder, also designed to keep the tube centered. The adapter for the 12 × 75 mm disposable test-tubes used with the Turner Model 111 consisted of a brass tube with windows cut out to permit the passage of light. The test-tube was retained at the proper height by means of a plug at the base of the metal holder.

[6] The Aminco-Bowman Spectrophotofluorometer (Amer. Instr. Co., Silver Spring, Md. 20910) was used for most of the work reported here. However, the Turner Model 111 (G. K. Turner Assoc., Palo Alto, Calif. 94303), a filter-type instrument, proved to be equally effective. Readings were made with filters 7-60 (activation) and 65A (emission).

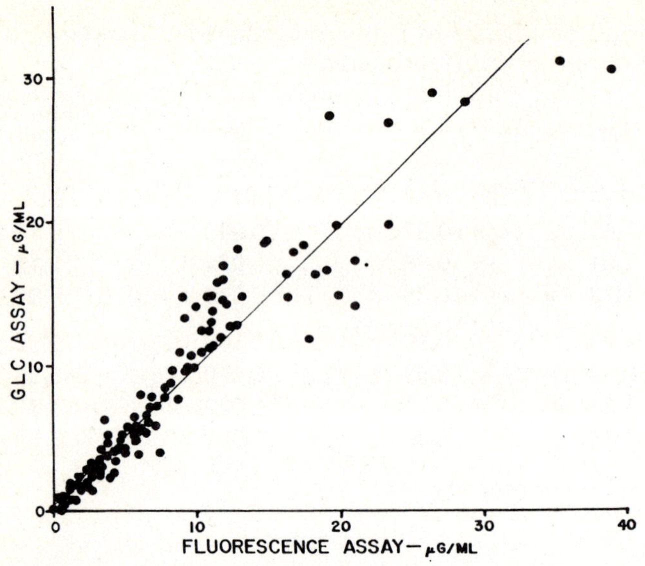

Fig. 1. Comparison of DPH assays on 154 plasma specimens by fluorometric and GLC assay procedures

Line of regression calculated by method of least squares. Mean ± SD for *y*-axis intercept = 0.26 ± 0.23; slope = 0.98 ± 0.02; correlation coefficient = 0.96

Table 2. Results for Diphenylhydantoin in Clinical Specimens, by Dosage Groups

Dosage groups	Mean dosage	No. subjects	Mean age, y	Mean body wt, kg	Mean, fluoro. assay	Mean, GLC assay	*t*-score[a]
mg/kg					mg/liter		
0–1	0.83	3	30.7	79.2	—	—	—
1–2	1.44	23	27.2	56.3	1.2	1.1	0.76
2–3	2.56	25	24.8	59.0	5.0	5.1	0.56
3–4	3.46	24	27.2	57.0	7.7	7.4	0.96
4–5	4.40	35	23.7	55.2	8.5	8.6	0.86
5–6	5.43	22	21.0	49.6	9.2	9.5	0.58
6–7	6.52	13	19.7	44.6	10.7	11.8	1.45
>7	8.41	8	15.3	35.0	14.3	13.7	0.68
All	3.97	153	23.9	54.0	7.1	7.2	0.86

[a] *t*-score calculated for the difference between the means of paired observations ($t > 2$ needed to indicate a significant difference between the fluorometric and GLC assays).

assays of 10 drug-supplemented plasma specimens and controls, obtained by two analysts on three consecutive days. The coefficient of variation averaged 7.3% (range, 4.6–8.8%) for DPH concentrations ranging from 2.5–20 mg/liter; but increased to 87% for the drug-free plasma specimens (mean "blank," 0.1 mg/liter; range, 0.0–0.4 mg/liter). For a series of DPH standards made up in bovine plasma (5, 10, and 20 mg/liter) and assayed 20 times during six weeks by two different analysts, the ratio of fluorometer readings at 20/10 mg/liter averaged 1.82 ± 0.12 (SD) with a coefficient of variation of 6.0%; the ratio of readings for 10 and 5 mg/liter concentrations averaged 1.94 ± 0.12 (SD), with a coefficient of variation of 6.7%. The sensitivity of this procedure was about 0.2 μg of DPH for the 0.2 ml volume of plasma used for the assay; i.e., about 1 mg of DPH per liter of plasma.

Assay of Clinical Specimens

The assay data are shown in Figure 1, in which the results of the fluorometric assays are plotted vs. those by GLC assay. (Individual assay values will be supplied to interested readers upon request.) The mean for all fluorometric assays was 7.09 ± 0.55 (SE) in comparison with the mean GLC assays of 7.23 ± 0.57 (SE), with a correlation coefficient of 0.96. Student's *t*-test for the difference between the means of paired observations gave a *t*-score of 0.89 ($P > 0.05$). The data indicate no significant differences between the fluorometric and GLC assays.

Table 2 summarizes assay values obtained by the GLC and fluorometric techniques, grouped by daily dosage of DPH. About 83% of the subjects received phenobarbital or primidone in addition to DPH; nearly half of the patients received phenothiazines or tricyclic antidepressants; about 15% of the patients were given barbiturates and other anticonvulsant drugs; and a number of other drugs were used.[7] No interference was encountered in this assay procedure with phenobarbital, primidone, ethosuximide, or diazepam, or with the DPH metabolites 5-(*m*-hydroxyphenyl)-5-phenylhydantoin and 5-(*p*-hydroxyphenyl)-5-phenylhydantoin. Some interference may be expected from drugs that form benzophenone upon oxidation with permanganate, such as diphenhydramine (*15*) and methadone (*16*). However, the usual concentrations of these drugs in plasma are too low to interfere significantly with DPH assays.

We thank William B. Barrow, M.D., and the patients at Sunland Training Center for their cooperation in the collection of blood specimens; Harold E. Machamer, Ph.D., and Frank B. Brandon, Ph.D., for organizing the trial; Robert A. Buchanan, M.D., Jan Turner, R.N., and Meiggs Haggerty for supporting the clinical portion of the work; Anne Horaczek for handling the plasma shipments and summarizing clinical information; and Barbara S. Eng for assistance with the GLC assays.

GLC assays were done under the direction of Dr. A. W. Kinkel in the Biopharmaceutics Section, Department of Pharmaceutical Research and Development, Parke-Davis & Co., Detroit, Mich.

Fluorometric assays were done in the Chemical Pharmacology Section, Pharmacology Department, Parke-Davis & Co., Ann Arbor, Mich.

References

1. Buchthal, F., and Lennox-Buchtal, M. A., Diphenylhydantoin: Relation of anticonvulsant effect to concentration in serum. In *Antiepileptic Drugs,* D. M. Woodbury, J. K. Penry, and R. P. Schmidt, Eds., Raven Press, N.Y., 1972, pp 193–209.

2. Lund, L., Anticonvulsant effect of diphenylhydantoin relative to plasma levels. *Arch. Neurol.* (Chicago) **31,** 289 (1974).

3. Dill, W. A., Kazenko, A., Wolf, L. M., and Glazko, A. J., Studies of 5,5-diphenylhydantoin (Dilantin) in animals and man. *J. Pharmacol. Exp. Ther.* **118,** 270 (1956).

4. Svensmark, O., and Kristensen, P., Determination of diphenylhydantoin and phenobarbital in small amounts of serum. *J. Lab. Clin. Med.* **61,** 501 (1963).

5. Chang, T., and Glazko, A. J., Quantitative assay of 5,5-diphenylhydantoin (Dilantin) and 5-(*p*-hydroxyphenyl)-5-phenylhydantoin by gas–liquid chromatography. *J. Lab. Clin. Med.* **75,** 145 (1970).

6. MacGee, J., Rapid determination of diphenylhydantoin in blood plasma by gas–liquid chromatography. *Anal. Chem.* **42,** 421 (1970).

[7] In addition to DPH and phenobarbital, drugs received by the patients (and the numbers of subjects who were receiving each drug) were as follows: Mysoline (34), Mellaril (33), Thorazine (22), Serentil (13), Dulcolax (11), Stelazine (9), Artane (9), Mebara (9), Valium (6), Zarontin (5), vitamins (5), Quide (3), Tridione (3), milk of magnesia (3), Metamucil (2), and 1 each of Haldol, Elavil, Prolixin, Mesantoin, Tegretol, Gemonil, Amesec, Cogentin, griseofulvin, Orinase, and Diamox.

7. Booker, H. E., and Darcey, B. A., Enzymatic immunoassay vs. gas–liquid chromatography for determination of phenobarbital and diphenylhydantoin in serum. *Clin. Chem.* **21**, 1766 (1975).

8. Wallace, J., Biggs, J., and Dahl, E. V., Determination of diphenylhydantoin by ultraviolet spectrophotometry. *Anal. Chem.* **37**, 410 (1965).

9. Dill, W. A., Chucot, L., Chang, T., and Glazko, A. J., Simplified benzophenone procedure for determination of diphenylhydantoin in plasma. *Clin. Chem.* **17**, 1200 (1971).

10. Dill, W. A., and Glazko, A. J., Comments on the determination of diphenylhydantoin (cont.). *Clin. Chem.* **20**, 915 (1974). Letter to the Editor.

11. Dill, W. A., and Glazko, A. J., Fluorometric assay of diphenylhydantoin in plasma or whole blood. *Clin. Chem.* **18**, 675 (1972).

12. Dill, W. A., Fluorometric assay of phenytoin. In *Methods of Analysis of Anti-Epileptic Drugs*. J. W. A. Meijer, H. Meinardi, C. Gardner-Thorp, and E. van der Kleijn, Eds., Excerpta Medica, Amsterdam; American Elsevier Co., Inc., New York, N.Y., 1973.

13. Driessen, O., and Emonds, A., Simultaneous determination of antiepileptic drugs in small samples of blood plasma by gas chromatography. Column technology and extraction procedure. *Proc. K. Ned. Akad. Wet.* **77**, 171 (1974).

14. Kupferberg, H. J., Quantitative estimation of diphenylhydantoin, primidone and phenobarbital in plasma by gas-liquid chromatography. *Clin. Chim. Acta* **29**, 283 (1970).

15. Glazko, A. J., Dill, W. A., Young, R. M., Smith, T. C., and Ogilvie, R. I., Metabolic disposition of diphenhydramine. *Clin. Pharmacol. Ther.* **16**, 1066 (1974).

16. Wallace, J. E., Hamilton, H. E., Payte, J. T., and Blum, K., Sensitive spectrophotometric method for determining methadone in biological specimens. *J. Pharm. Sci.* **61**, 1397 (1972).

CLIN. CHEM. 22/6, 911–914 (1976)

Assay of Phenytoin: Adaptation of "EMIT" to the Centrifugal Analyzer

Paul R. Finley, R. Jane Williams, and James M. Byers III

We describe adaptation to the centrifugal analyzer of the homogeneous enzyme immunoassay ("EMIT") for phenytoin (diphenylhydantoin). The assay was modified to give greater range and sensitivity, and less reagent is needed. Precision and accuracy are excellent, and results correlate well with those by gas–liquid chromatography; the slight systematic bias is of no clinical significance.

Measurement of phenytoin (diphenylhydantoin) in serum is used as an aid in managing treatment of patients who are subject to generalized epileptic seizures (*1*), to increase the efficacy and safety of therapy. Such monitoring facilitates individualization of dosage regimens, reveals irregular drug intake, and identifies the responsible agent in drug-intoxicated patients who are being administered several drugs simultaneously (*2*).

Frequent monitoring of the concentration of the drug in serum is necessary to achieve satisfactory seizure control in ambulant patients with grand mal epilepsy. Therapeutic concentrations may vary among individuals, and it is therefore important to measure them in each individual patient over periods of time. The estimation of phenytoin has been done for the most part by using gas–liquid chromatography or ultraviolet spectrophotometry. Rubenstein et al. (*3*) introduced the "enzyme multiplied immunoassay technique" (EMIT). The Syva Research Institute, Palo Alto, Calif. 94304, has developed this particular assay so that at the present time one can use the system for the measurement, in urine, of opiates as a class, amphetamine and methamphetamine, and barbiturates as a class including pentobarbital, phenobarbital, butabarbital, secobarbital, and amobarbital. Methods have also been developed for the measurement in urine of cocaine and cocaine metabolites as well as methadone. Broughton and Ross (*4*) have recently adapted the EMIT to the centrifugal analyzer in the measurement of the above classes of drugs in the urine.

It is now possible to use this system to measure phenytoin and phenobarbital in serum. Other antibodies are being prepared to measure other anti-epileptic drugs, including ethosuximide, primidone, and carbamazepine.

In EMIT assays, enzyme labels are used instead of radioactive labels. An antibody specific to phenytoin is used. An enzyme (from *Leuconostoc mesenteroides*), glucose-6-phosphate dehydrogenase (EC 1.1.1.49), which is not present in human serum, is attached to the phenytoin molecule in such a way that the enzyme cannot act on its substrate, glucose 6-phosphate, when the molecule is captured by the antibody. When the sample material, which in this case is serum, is mixed with the antibody and enzyme-labeled molecule, any free molecules of the compound of interest in the sample will compete with the enzyme-labeled molecules for the limited number of antibody binding sites. The more free molecules available in the sample, the more enzyme will remain unbound and therefore active in the mixture. NAD^+ is also added to the substrate mixture. The enzyme converts NAD^+ to NADH, resulting in an absorbance change that is measured at 340 nm. The assay, therefore, is essentially a competitive binding type of assay. Schneider et al. (*5*) have given a detailed discussion of the homogeneous enzyme immunoassay.

Department of Pathology, Arizona Medical Center, Tucson, Ariz. 85724.

Received Feb. 23, 1976; accepted April 1, 1976.

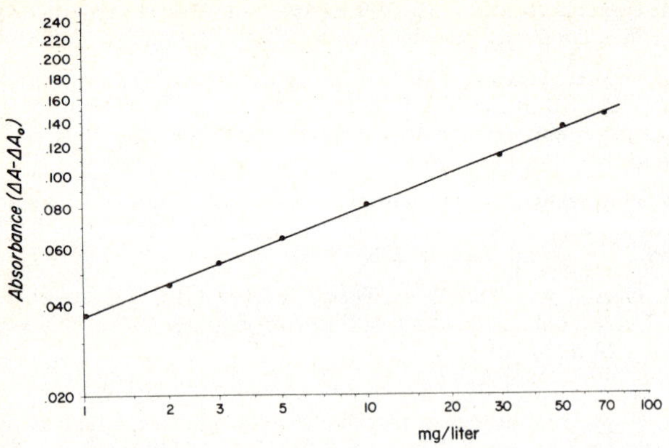

Fig. 1. Standard curve for phenytoin

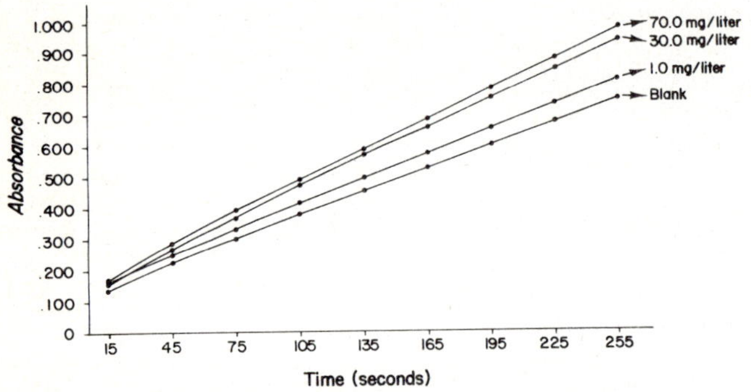

Fig. 2. Relation between absorbance and time, for a blank and 1-, 30-, and 70-mg/liter concentrations of phenytoin

The manufacturer recommends that the EMIT system be run with very careful automatic timing. The instrument suggested for use in analysis of urine and serum samples is the Model 300N spectrophotometer (Gilford Instrument Co., Oberlin, Ohio 44074). A timer-printer and a small automatic diluter (Syva Corp.) for the purpose of semi-automating the system is mandatory. Certain predilution steps are required, and assay time is exactly 80 s. The immunoassay of phenytoin has been shown to give a very close correlation with gas–liquid chromatography (*6, 7*).

A recent report (*8*) discusses measurement of phenytoin with a centrifugal analyzer and reports the adaptation of the EMIT system to the centrifugal analyzer. The reagents were prediluted; pipetting into the transfer discs was manual. The reported coefficient of variation was between 5 and 10%, depending on thermal conditions. A pre-incubation time of 3 min was used. There was no mention of correlation with results by ultraviolet or gas/liquid chromatographic methods, nor was the sensitivity of the assay mentioned.

We wished to adapt the EMIT assay of phenytoin to a centrifugal analyzer and to avoid the use of manual pipetting into the transfer discs. We also wished to expand the range of the assay substantially more than the present 2.5 to 30 mg/liter, because we not only must measure phenytoin as a drug of abuse in patients, but also must measure phenytoin half-lives.

Materials and Methods

Apparatus

We performed the immunoassays with an "Aminco Roto-Chem II" centrifugal analyzer (American Instrument Co., Silver Spring, Md. 20920).

Table 1. Phenytoin—Precision of GLC

	Within-day			Between-day		
	Mean	SD		Mean	SD	
Concn	mg/liter		CV, %	mg/liter		CV, %
Low	4.3	0.22	5.1	4.4	0.31	7.0
Therapeutic	13.2	0.71	5.4	13.4	0.91	6.8
High	52.6	3.11	5.9	54.2	4.12	7.6

Table 2. Phenytoin—Precision of EMIT

	Within-day			Between-day		
	Mean	SD		Mean	SD	
Concn	mg/liter		CV, %	mg/liter		CV, %
Low	4.6	0.25	5.4	4.8	0.34	7.2
Therapeutic	13.3	0.80	6.0	13.5	1.05	7.8
High	55.5	2.91	5.2	54.3	4.5	8.3

Reagents

All reagents used for the immunoassay procedure were those commercially available from the Syva Corp. Reagents A and B are provided as a matched set for each of the assays to be performed and are specific for phenytoin. The buffer solution and the calibrators are also supplied with the kit. Reagent A is the antibody/substrate reagent; it contains NAD^+, the specific antibody to phenytoin, and the substrate, glucose-6-phosphate. Reagent B is the drug/enzyme complex, phenytoin coupled to glucose-6-phosphate dehydrogenase. The two reagents are in lyophilized form. Reconstituted with distilled water, they are stable for four weeks if kept refrigerated.

Buffer solution. Tris(hydroxymethyl)aminomethane hydrochloride buffer (55 mmol/liter, pH 7.9) with added surfactant is prepared from a buffer concentrate supplied with each reagent kit; the solution is stable at room temperature.

Calibrators. A series of serum standards containing phenytoin in concentrations ranging from 0–30 mg/liter are provided as a lyophilized serum-based preparation.

We prepared another set of standards from our own stock diphenylhydantoin solution. The standards were made up using a stock solution added into a commercial control serum ("Chemvarion"; Clinton Laboratories, Santa Monica, Calif. 90404).

The gas–liquid chromatography method of Barrett (*9*) was used, with methylation and programmed temperature.

Procedure

Standard EMIT procedure. The procedure recommended by the manufacturer is as follows: Place 50 μl of standard or unknown serum plus 250 μl of buffer in a 1-ml disposable beaker. This step and the succeeding dilution steps may be done with a pipettor–dilutor. Before proceeding, at least 1 min should elapse. Deliver 50 μl of diluted serum from the first beaker plus 250 μl of buffer into a second beaker. Then dispense into the second beaker 50 μl of reagent A plus 250 μl of buffer. Next add 50 μl of reagent B plus 250 μl of buffer to the second beaker. Immediately upon addition of Reagent B, aspirate the contents of the second beaker into the spectrophotometer (Model 300N, Gilford Instrument Co.) flow cell. This automatically activates the printer/calculator to time and

Table 3. Phenytoin—Analytical Recovery Studies (EMIT) (n = 20)

Added concentration, mg/liter	4.0	15.0
Assayed mean, mg/liter	4.23	15.36
SD, mg/liter	0.36	1.16
CV, %	8.5	7.5

Table 4. Phenytoin—EMIT Linearity[a]

Dilution	Expected (mg/liter)	Found (mg/liter)	Difference (mg/liter)	Difference %
none	68	68	—	—
1:2	34	35	+ 1.0	2.9
1:4	17	17.5	+ 0.5	2.9
1:6	11.3	12.5	+ 1.2	10.6
1:10	6.8	7.1	+ 0.3	4.4
1:20	3.4	3.6	+ 0.2	5.8

[a] Actual patient sample (dilutions in "Chemvarion")

Table 5. Phenytoin—Regression Statistics

EMIT vs. GLC (105 patient samples)

r_2 (correlation)	.99625	
r	.99252	
SE of estimate	1.03259	
Intercept (A)	- .11573	
Significance of (A)	.21971	
SE of (A)	.14910	(t = −.771)
Slope (B)	1.04393	
Significance of (B)	.00001	
SE of (B)	.00893	(t = 4.919)
EMIT mean	12.7295	
GLC mean	12.3048	
Difference of means	.4248	
SD of difference	1.142	
SE of difference	.111	
Correlation	.996	
t-value	3.81	

record the measurement. Make two absorbance readings at 340 nm, the first at 15 s, the second at 95 s. The difference (ΔA) over the 80-s measurement period is used to calculate the results. Prepare a standard curve by plotting $\Delta A - \Delta A_0$ (ΔA_0 is the absorbance of the zero standard at 80 s) for each standard on EMIT graph paper (a modified logit function paper). A linear relation should be obtained.

Modification for centrifugal analyzer. We modified the EMIT procedure as follows:

1. The buffer is diluted twofold with water.
2. Reagent A is diluted 10-fold (rather than fivefold) with buffer.
3. Reagent B is diluted 10-fold (rather than fivefold) with buffer.
4. After dilution of Reagent A and Reagent B, these are allowed to set at room temperature for at least 1 h. The dilutions may be used for as long as five days if stored at 4 °C.
5. Load the sample cups as follows: cup 1, negative serum blank; cups 2–14, standards and sera. Set the Rotofil Automatic Samplet/Dilutor (American Instrument Co.) as follows: Serum/standard pump, 8 μl; buffer pump, 200 μl; Reagent A, 200 μl; Reagent B, 200 μl. Deliver sample, buffer and Reagent A to the inner well, and Reagent B to the middle well. Then place the transfer disc on the centrifugal analyzer. The assay may be begun immediately. The analyzer is controlled with Kinetic Rate III tape, a program supplied by the American Instrument Co. It allows the user to take initial and final absorbance readings at any time chosen. Analyses are run at 30 °C. Readings are taken at 45 and 225 s. This allows an elapsed reading time of exactly 3 min. The absorbance differences ($\Delta A - \Delta A_0$) are plotted on special EMIT graph paper.

Results

Standard curve. Figure 1 is a plot of the standard curve obtained with use of the centrifugal analyzer. The range has been extended so that the standard curve encompasses values from 1 mg/liter to 70 mg/liter. Figure 2 shows the relationship between absorbance change and time of reading, for a series of concentrations. These data were obtained by use of Kinetic Rate I tape, supplied by the American Instrument Co., which allows the user to take nine absorbance readings at equal intervals chosen by the operator. There is a slight nonlinearity between 15 and 45 s; the curve then becomes linear. The 3-min reading time ensured an adequate absorption change, for reasonable sensitivity.

Precision. Within-day and day-to-day precision for phenytoin measured on both the gas–liquid chromatograph (Table 1) and the Aminco Roto-Chem II (Table 2) are shown; the patients' samples include concentrations below, within, and above the therapeutic range. The within-day samples were analyzed 20 times on the same day by both procedures; the between-day analyses were done on 25 successive days. The precision of the EMIT system compares favorably with that of the comparison method.

Accuracy. The analytical recovery for the method is shown in Table 3. Two experiments were done. Phenytoin was added to the negative control serum (Chemvarion) to give concentrations of 4.0 and 15.0 mg/liter, respectively. The samples were analyzed on each of 20 separate days. The resulting coefficient of variation was satisfactory and the analytical recovery adequate.

Table 4 shows a linearity study of a serum with a high phenytoin concentration, diluted with the negative control serum (Chemvarion). Linearity is evidently satisfactory down to low concentration of the drug.

Thirty-two sera that contained both phenobarbital and phenytoin were obtained from patients undergoing maintenance therapy for convulsive disorders. Results for these particular samples compared well with measurements by gas–liquid chromatography; phenobarbital does not interfere in the EMIT method. (These sera are included in the comparison study between the EMIT system and gas/liquid chromatography.)

A linear regression analysis of the comparison study is shown in Table 5. The coefficient of correlation is acceptable. The standard error of the estimate shows very modest scatter about the line. The intercept is close to 0, and the standard error of the intercept has a t-score of −.771, essentially no significant difference from an 0 intercept. The slope, however, shows a t-score of 4.919, which is slightly significant. EMIT values evidently have a tendency to be slightly higher than the values obtained by gas/liquid chromatographic analysis. These data are very similar to the study of Booker and Darcey (7), in which the authors discuss the correlation between the enzymatic immunoassay as done by the recommended technique on the Gilford instrumentation vs. gas/liquid chromatography done in a standard manner. The *t*-value of 3.81 shows a definite but small difference in the two means.

Interferences. Bilirubin concentrations up to 150 mg/liter did not affect results of the assay. Extremely lipemic sera also had no effect. There was, however, a significant suppression of absorbance by hemoglobin. The following interferences were noted: at a hemoglobin concentration of 5000 mg/liter, 70%; at 2500 mg/liter, 55%; at 1250 mg/liter, 10%; and at 1000 mg/liter or less, no interference.

Discussion

The measurement of phenytoin is of great value clinically. Measurement by gas/liquid chromatography is slow and may be difficult technically. It also requires at least 1.0 ml of serum, whereas the modification of the EMIT system proposed uses only 8 microliters in the assay. The EMIT technique is simple, rapid, and many samples may be processed at one time. The accuracy is quite satisfactory. Our reproducibility is somewhat better than that reported by Booker and Darcey (7).

Our modification increases the detectable range over previous immunoassay techniques and is reliable from 1–70 mg/liter. There is a slight systematic proportional bias when comparing EMIT assay to gas/liquid chromatographic assay. The slight bias is not significant clinically. The greater dilution of the reagents than recommended by the Syva Corp. diminishes the expense of the test. The use of Chemvarion has proved very effective as the base serum for our own standards. The standards prepared in our laboratory compare extremely well with those supplied by the company. Up to 10 sera may be analyzed in 5 min; reagent cost per sample is about 40¢, as compared to $1 for the standard EMIT procedure.

When we performed the assay in a kinetic mode, we observed nonlinearity for the first 45 s. To ensure complete linearity, we therefore read the absorbance change from 45 to 225 s, a total elapsed time of 3 min.

The specificity of the antibody has been shown in this assay. This is particularly important because patients taking phenytoin are often taking other drugs as well. The only interference we have observed is that of hemolysis, and this appears to be a very substantial problem.

References

1. Lund, L., Anticonvulsant effect of diphenylhydantoin relative to plasma levels. *Arch. Neurol.* (Chicago) **31,** 289 (1974).

2. Kutt, H., and Penry, J. K., Usefulness of blood levels of antiepileptic drugs. *Arch. Neurol.* (Chicago) **31,** 283 (1974).

3. Rubenstein, K. E., Schneider, R. S., and Ullman, E. F., "Homogeneous" enzyme immunoassay. A new immunochemical technique. *Biochem. Biophys. Res. Commun.* **47,** 846 (1972).

4. Broughton, A., and Ross, D. L., Drug screening by enzymatic immunoassay with the centrifugal analyzer. *Clin. Chem.* **21,** 186 (1975).

5. Schneider, R. S., Lindquist, P., Wong, E. T., et al., Homogeneous enzyme immunoassay for opiates in urine. *Clin. Chem.* **19,** 821 (1973).

6. Pippenger, C. E., Sickler, D. L., and Lichtblau, L., Preliminary clinical evaluation of an experimental enzyme immunoassay system for diphenylhydantoin and phenobarbital in serum. *Clin. Chem.* **20,** 869 (1974). Abstract.

7. Booker, H. E., and Darcey, B. A., Enzymatic immunoassay vs. gas–liquid chromatography for determination of phenobarbital and diphenylhydantoin in serum. *Clin. Chem.* **21,** 1766 (1975).

8. Strasser, B., and Zinterhoffer, L., Rapid enzyme immunoassay of phenobarbital and Dilantin on a centrifugal fast analyzer. *Clin. Chem.* **21,** 946 (1975) Abstract.

9. Barrett, M. J., Determination of serum levels of diphenylhydantoin by gas/liquid chromatography. *Clin. Chem. Newsl.* **3,** 16 (1971).

Monitoring Drug Concentrations in a Case of Combined Overdosage with Primidone and Methsuximide

George F. Johnson, Ph.D., Charles J. Least, Jr., M.S.,[1] James W. Serum, Ph.D.,[2] Elizabeth B. Solow, M.S.,[3] and Harvey M. Solomon, M.D.

We describe a case of fatal overdosage with primidone and methsuximide. During the early phase of the patient's hospital course we found concentrations of methsuximide, *N*-desmethylmethsuximide, and primidone in serum that far exceeded the usual therapeutic concentrations, as determined by gas–liquid chromatography. Determination of *N*-desmethylmethsuximide in peritoneal fluid demonstrated concentrations comparable to those in serum. This led to the therapeutic decision to manage the patient by dialysis. Subsequently, serum samples collected during the course of hospitalization were analyzed quantitatively by gas–liquid chromatography for methsuximide, *N*-desmethylmethsuximide, primidone, phenobarbital, and diphenylhydantoin. Selected serum specimens were also analyzed by gas chromatography–mass spectrometry, and *N*-methyl-2-hydroxymethyl-2-phenylsuccinimide, a metabolite of methsuximide not previously described in human serum, was identified by analysis of its mass spectrum.

Additional Keyphrases: *gas chromatography • mass spectrometry • new metabolite, N-methyl-2-hydroxymethyl-2-phenylsuccimide • single-ion chromatography • toxicology*

Monitoring of therapeutic agents in serum is widely utilized by neurologists to ensure safe and effective treatment with various anticonvulsant drugs (*1, 2*). Several of these drugs are metabolized to compounds that also possess anticonvulsant activity or produce symptoms of central nervous system toxicity. In such circumstances, both the parent drug and its pharmacologically active metabolite(s) should be quantitated. Primidone and methsuximide, commonly used to manage various types of seizures, are converted to active metabolites in vivo. Recent studies in man indicate that methsuximide is demethylated to *N*-desmethylmethsuximide, and the plasma concentration of this metabolite greatly exceeds that of the parent compound in patients treated chronically with methsuximide (*3*). Primidone is converted in part to phenobarbital, which possesses profound pharmacologic activity, and to phenylethylmalonamide, for which the pharmacologic activity in man is not yet established (*4*).

Cases of acute overdosage with primidone (*5, 6*) and with methsuximide (*7*) have been reported and each drug, under this circumstance, produces profound central nervous system depression. Combined massive, fatal overdosage with these two drugs, such as occurred in the patient reported here, has not been described previously. We measured serum concentrations of these drugs and metabolites during the course of her hospitalization, which included management with both peritoneal and hemodialysis. In addition, the availability of sequential specimens from this unique case provided us with an opportunity to investigate further the metabolism of methsuximide and primidone, which we did by gas chromatography–mass spectrometry.

Case History

A 29-year-old unconscious white woman was admitted to the Emergency Room of The Johns Hopkins Hospital on March 28, 1975. She had a 10-year history of seizures and during the eight years before admission had been treated with diphenylhydantoin, phenobarbital, and primidone. In August 1973, her neurological status was re-evaluated because of occasional absence seizures, and methsuximide was added to the therapeutic regimen. She was also noted to have an abnormal glucose-tolerance test and was treated by dietary restriction in addition to tolbutamide.

During the month before admission, the patient became progressively more depressed and required

[1] Therapeutic Drug Monitoring Laboratory, Department of Laboratory Medicine, The Johns Hopkins Hospital, Baltimore, Md. 21205.

[2] Hewlett-Packard Co., Avondale, Pa. 19311.

[3] Division of Neurosurgery and the Department of Neurology, Indiana University School of Medicine, Indianapolis, Ind. 46202.

Received Jan. 23, 1976; accepted Feb. 2, 1976.

treatment with amitriptyline. She remained depressed, however, and was seen regularly by a psychiatrist. On the evening prior to admission the patient complained of general malaise and had a syncopal episode. Although she awoke later in the evening, she had difficulty walking and acted as if she were intoxicated; she then returned to bed and became unresponsive. Twelve hours later she could not be aroused and was brought to the Emergency Room.

Vital signs on admission included blood pressure, 95/72 mmHg; pulse, 90/min; respiration, 20/min; and temperature, 37.2 °C. The physical examination was unremarkable except for the neurological evaluation, which disclosed an unconscious patient with pupil diameter 7 mm, equal and nonreactive to light; corneal reflexes absent; no sensory response to deep pain; flaccid extremities; and no deep-tendon reflexes.

Laboratory studies demonstrated extremely high serum concentrations of methsuximide (98.5 mg/liter) and primidone (62 mg/liter), and she was admitted to the Medical Intensive-Care Unit.

The patient's hospital course was characterized by an initial respiratory arrest with ventricular tachycardia and cyanosis, but she was quickly resuscitated. Subsequently, she developed hypotension with urine output decreased to 3 ml/h and a systolic blood pressure of 50–60 mmHg. She was first treated with norepinephrine and thereafter she was maintained on dopamine. Because of her hypotension, peritoneal dialysis was begun; however, when her blood pressure stabilized, a shunt was created between her right femoral artery and saphenous vein, and she subsequently underwent two periods of hemodialysis. Her course was characterized by persistent bleeding from the shunt, which necessitated massive transfusion therapy. On the third hospital day, her pupils reacted to light for the first time, and a slight cold caloric reflex was noted. The next day neurological examination showed spontaneous extra-ocular movements and positive corneal reflexes; however, the patient remained flaccid without spontaneous movements. Her level of consciousness did not improve and on the fifth hospital day she had two cardiac arrests and marked hypotension recurred that required pressor therapy. Thereafter her course was further complicated by Gram-negative sepsis and disseminated intravascular coagulation, and she expired on the eleventh hospital day.

Materials and Methods

Comparison Materials

Diphenylhydantoin and phenobarbital (Sigma Chemical Co., St. Louis, Mo. 63178).

Primidone and phenylethylmalonamide (Ayerst Laboratories, Montreal 101, P.Q. Canada).

Tolbutamide (The UpJohn Co., Kalamazoo, Mich. 49001).

p-*Toluenesulfonamide* (Aldrich Chem. Co., Milwaukee, Wis. 53233)

N,*2-Dimethyl-2-(4-hydroxyphenyl) succinimide*, referred to hereafter as *p*-hydroxyphenylmethsuximide, and *2-methyl-2-(4-hydroxyphenyl)-succinimide* were kindly provided by Kenneth H. Dudley, Ph.D., of the Center for Research in Pharmacology and Toxicology, School of Medicine, University of North Carolina, Chapel Hill, N. C. 27514.

Methsuximide and N-*desmethylmethsuximide* were obtained from Parke-Davis & Co., Ann Arbor, Mich. 48106). Standard solutions (100 mg/liter) of each of these compounds were prepared by dissolving 10 mg in 100 ml of methanol.

An *internal standard solution* containing ethotoin (Abbott Laboratories, N. Chicago, Ill. 60064) and phensuximide (Parke-Davis & Co.) was prepared by dissolving 7.5 mg of each of these compounds in 1 liter of ethyl acetate.

Extraction Procedure

Serum (200 μl) was combined in a 16 × 100 mm culture tube (Teflon-lined screw cap) with 50 μl of 2 mol/liter HCl and 5 ml of the internal standard solution. The tubes were extracted for 10 min in an Eberbach shaker at 250 oscillations/min and centrifuged at 2000 rpm for 5 min. The organic phase was transferred to "Concentratubes" (Laboratory Research Co., Los Angeles, Calif. 90036) and concentrated under nitrogen in a water bath at 40 °C. When 5–10 μl of solvent remained in the Concentratube tip the tubes were removed from the evaporator and 50 μl of ethyl acetate was added to each. The tubes were vortex mixed, and 1 μl was injected into the gas chromatograph.

Standard curves were prepared by analyzing samples of normal human serum containing known amounts of methsuximide and *N*-desmethylmethsuximide. These serum standards were prepared by evaporating to dry-

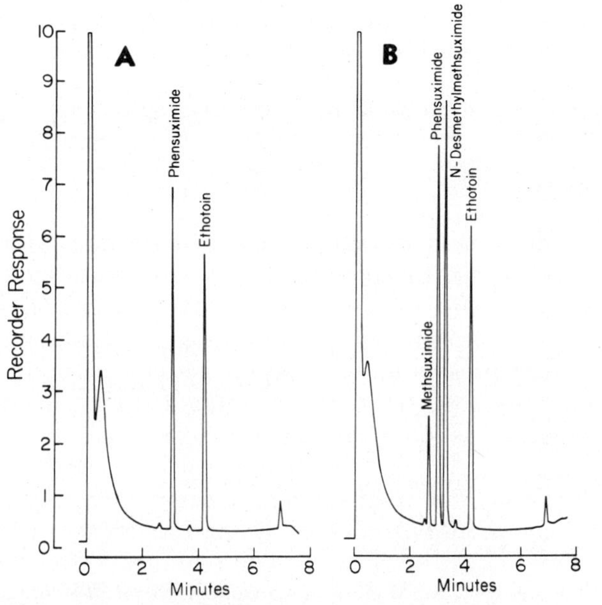

Fig. 1. Chromatograms obtained by extraction and chromatography according to our procedure

Oven temperature programmed from 150 to 270 °C at 16 °C/min. Column packing: 3% OV-17 on 100/120 Gas Chrom Q. *A*, drug-free serum (200 μl); internal standards included. *B*, serum (200 μl) to which 10 μg of methsuximide and 40 μg of *N*-desmethylmethsuximide were added; internal standards included

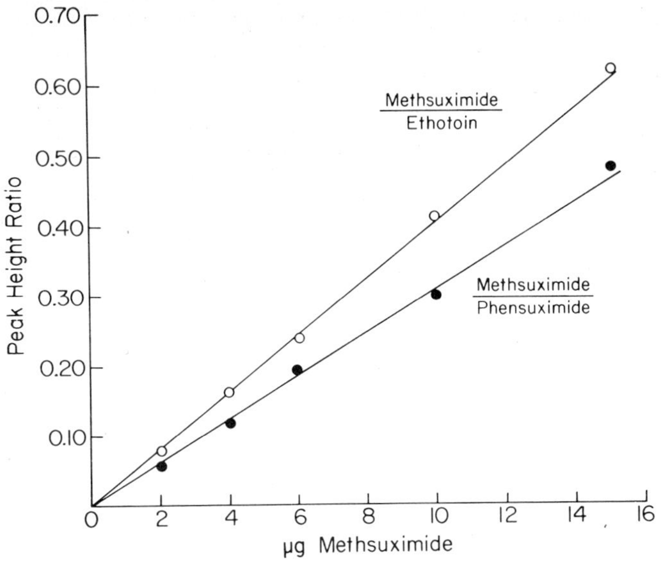

Fig. 2. Standard curves for methsuximide, with use of both ethotoin and phensuximide as internal standards

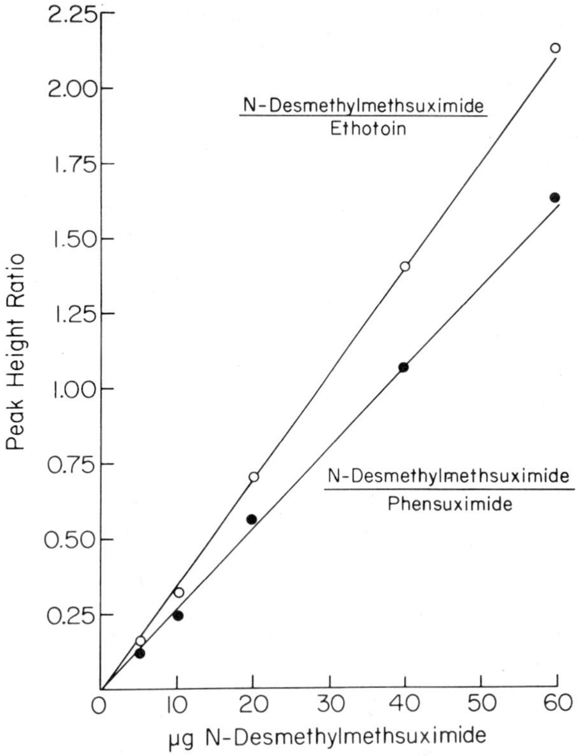

Fig. 3. Standard curves for *N*-desmethylmethsuximide, with use of both ethotoin and phensuximide as internal standards

ness under nitrogen appropriate amounts of the methanolic solutions of each compound and adding 200 μl of drug-free serum. Although phensuximide and ethotoin were equally suitable as internal standards, we used phensuximide to establish peak-height ratios for quantitation of methsuximide and *N*-desmethylmethsuximide.

Instrument and Instrumental Conditions for Gas Chromatography

We used a Model 5711A gas chromatograph equipped with dual flame-ionization detectors and a Model 7123A 1 mV recorder (both from Hewlett-Packard, Avondale, Pa. 19311). Columns were 122-cm glass, 2 mm i.d., configuration 5 for on-column injection (Hewlett-Packard), packed with 3% OV-17 on 100/120 Gas Chrom Q (Applied Science Labs., Inc., State College, Pa. 16801). The injector temperature was 250 °C, the detector was 300 °C and the oven temperature was programmed 150–270 °C at 16 °C/min.

Gas-Chromatographic Method for Other Anticonvulsant Determinations

Analyses of diphenylhydantoin, phenobarbital and primidone were performed by on-column methylation according to the method of Kananen et al. (*8*).

Gas Chromatography–Mass Spectrometric–Computer Analysis

For electron ionization mass spectra, we used a Model 5784A gas chromatograph equipped with a heated on-column injection port, interfaced through a membrane separator to a Model 5982A GC/MS system with a dodecapole analyzer, and coupled to a 5933A data system (all from Hewlett-Packard). The gas-chromatographic column was glass, 360 cm × 2 mm i.d., packed with 0.25% neopentyl glycol succinate plus 0.025% phosphoric acid on Chromosorb G-HP, 100/120 mesh (Johns-Manville, Denver, Colo. 80217) (*9*). The injector temperature was 250 °C; the oven temperature was held at 140 °C for 4 min and then programmed at 8 °C/min to 230 °C and held; and the transfer-line temperature was 250 °C. Mass spectra were recorded at 70 eV ionizing voltage, 200 μA emission current, and at an ion-source temperature of 190 °C. Chemical ionization spectra were obtained by using the same instrument in the chemical ionization mode with the following conditions: no separator was used, methane was used as both carrier and ionizing reagent gas, and spectra were recorded at an ionizing voltage of 300 eV and an emission current of 200 μA.

Results and Discussion

Controls and standards. Figure 1 depicts representative chromatograms of serum specimens extracted according to our procedure. Chromatogram *A*, with the internal standards phensuximide and ethotoin included, was obtained from serum of a normal individual not receiving anticonvulsants. Chromatogram *B* was obtained from serum of a normal individual, to which was added 10 μg of methsuximide and 40 μg of *N*-desmethylmethsuximide per 200 μl. The compounds of interest and the internal standards are well separated from each other and no significant interferences have been observed in serum from patients not on anticonvulsant therapy.

Figure 2 illustrates typical standard curves for methsuximide prepared by the peak-height ratio technique, with phensuximide and ethotoin as internal standards. Linearity was observed between the ratio of

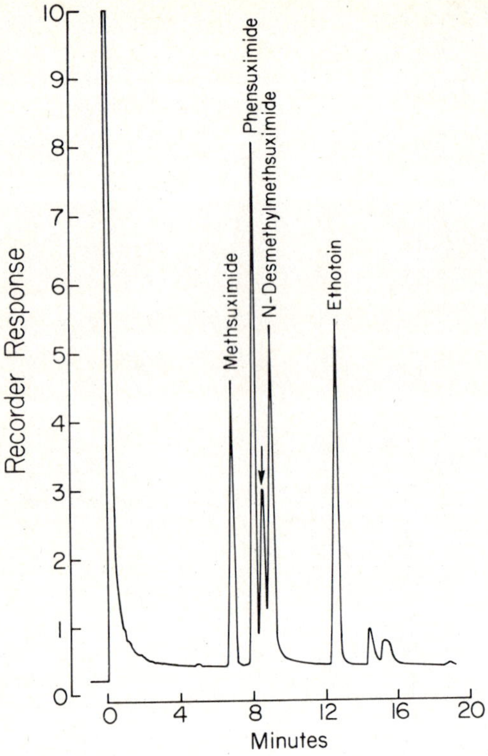

Fig. 4. Chromatogram obtained from the serum of the patient at time of admission
Methsuximide and *N*-desmethylmethsuximide concentrations in this sample are 98.5 and 125 mg/liter, respectively. Oven temperature programmed from 120 to 200 °C at 4 °C/min

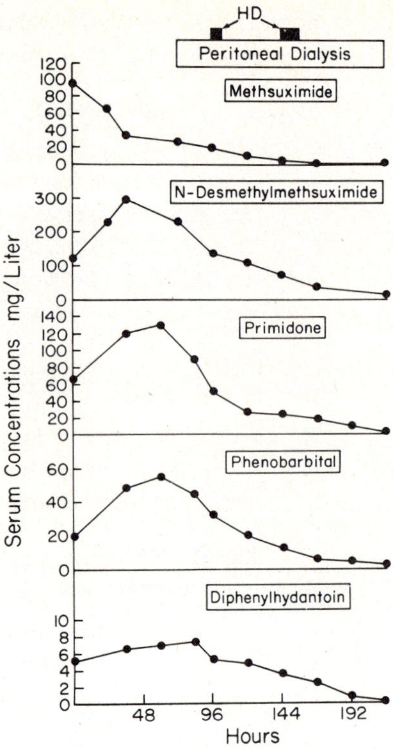

Fig. 5. Serum concentrations of (*top to bottom*) methsuximide, *N*-desmethylmethsuximide, primidone, phenobarbital, and diphenylhydantoin, as monitored throughout the course of the patient's hospitalization
The *solid blocks* marked *HD* correspond to periods of hemodialysis

peak height of drug to each internal standard and the amount of drug extracted from serum over the range of 0–15 μg methsuximide.

Figure 3 illustrates typical standard curves for *N*-desmethylmethsuximide prepared by the peak-height ratio technique, with phensuximide and ethotoin as internal standards. A linear relation was observed between the ratio of peak height of *N*-desmethylmethsuximide to each internal standard and the amount of *N*-desmethylmethsuximide extracted from serum over the range of 0–60 μg of this metabolite of methsuximide.

Data for the patient. A representative chromatogram of serum from the patient, obtained at the time of admission, is presented in Figure 4. The concentrations of methsuximide and *N*-desmethylmethsuximide in this specimen were 98.5 and 125 mg/liter, respectively. An unidentified peak was observed midway between the chromatographic peaks of phensuximide and *N*-desmethylmethsuximide. This peak was present in all of the patient's serum samples, and decreased with time, which suggests that it was also related to the drugs that she ingested.

Serum concentrations of methsuximide, *N*-desmethylmethsuximide, primidone, phenobarbital, and diphenylhydantoin were monitored throughout the course of hospitalization (Figure 5). At the time of admission, the serum concentrations of methsuximide and *N*-desmethylmethsuximide were 98.5 and 125 mg/liter, respectively. Thereafter, the serum concentrations of methsuximide declined progressively with time. In contrast, the concentration of *N*-desmethylmethsuximide in serum increased during the first 36 h of observation to a maximum of almost 300 mg/liter and then declined gradually. The serum concentration of primidone increased from 62 mg/liter at the time of admission to a maximum concentration of 130 mg/liter at 60 h and then decreased with time. The initial concentration of phenobarbital in the patient's serum was 20 mg/liter and the peak concentration (55 mg/liter), like that of primidone, was observed at 60 h. The concentration of diphenylhydantoin in serum increased from 5.2 mg/liter at the time of admission to a peak of 7.5 mg/liter at 84 h, then decreased progressively.

The initial pattern of high concurrent serum concentrations of methsuximide and its metabolite, *N*-desmethylmethsuximide seen in Figure 5 has been observed previously only in another case of massive overdosage with methsuximide (*7*). In contrast, patients treated chronically with therapeutic doses of this drug had plasma concentrations of the *N*-desmethylmetabolite 700-fold that of the parent compound (*3*). Strong et al. (*3*) have suggested a tentative therapeutic range for *N*-desmethylmethsuximide of 10 to 40 mg/liter, and observed ataxia and lethargy at concentrations exceeding 40 mg/liter. Possible explanations for the high initial serum concentrations of both methsuximide and *N*-desmethylmethsuximide observed in our patient as well as in the patient reported by Karch (*7*) included saturation of the enzyme responsible for demethylation of the parent compound or inhibition of this enzyme by the demethylated product.

At the time of admission, the patient's serum concentration of primidone was 62 mg/liter, six-fold the upper limit of the therapeutic range for this drug (2). Thereafter the primidone concentration increased to a maximum of 130 mg/liter at 60 h. This time course is most compatible with continued absorption of the drug from the gut. The presence of phenobarbital in our patient's serum could be due either to formation of this compound in vivo from primidone, or to ingestion of the barbiturate directly. The time course of appearance of phenobarbital in her serum (Figure 5) is compatible with continued absorption of its metabolic precursor, primidone, as well as with sustained absorption of the barbiturate itself.

Because of the high plasma concentrations of methsuximide, primidone, and their active metabolites, it was not possible to determine the contribution of the individual compounds to the profound coma seen in this patient.

After acute overdosage with the drugs this patient took, they would be cleared from the body only by metabolism. Under such conditions in the patient reported by Brillman et al. (5), the plasma half-life of phenobarbital observed in primidone overdosage was 4.5 days, as compared to 15 h for the parent compound. In our patient the concentrations of phenobarbital and primidone declined to about half their peak values by 60 h and 30 h, respectively. We have not calculated half-lives for the clearance of these drugs from serum because of concurrent removal of the compounds by peritoneal and hemodialysis (Figure 5). Peritoneal fluid obtained before the 60-h peritoneal dialysis was begun contained 225 mg of *N*-desmethylmethsuximide per liter, while serum obtained concurrently contained 278 mg of this drug per liter, which indicates that *N*-desmethylmethsuximide can cross the peritoneal membrane. This observation prompted the clinical staff to institute and sustain peritoneal dialysis. During the first 2 h of peritoneal dialysis, 280 mg of *N*-desmethylmethsuximide was removed. When the patient's blood pressure stabilized, she was also treated by hemodialysis. During a 2.5-h period of the first hemodialysis, approximately 1 g of *N*-desmethylmethsuximide accumulated in the dialyzer bath. As shown in Figure 5, after 216 h of treatment all drugs in her serum had decreased to either subtherapeutic or nonmeasurable concentrations.

Further information on some components. We thought that the unidentified peak observed in the routine gas-chromatographic analysis of the serum sample (Figure 4) might be another metabolite of methsuximide and therefore we conducted a more detailed investigation by use of combined gas chromatography–mass spectrometry (GC/MS). Three samples of serum were chosen for analysis by GC/MS: one obtained at the time of admission, a second 24 h after admission, and the third at 36 h. Ethyl acetate extracts of these sera were injected on column without derivatization. During the elution of the components from the column, the mass spectrometer was scanned approximately every 2 s through a 40–400 range of *m/e* and the data were stored on the computer for subsequent analysis. The mass intensities were summed for each spectrum and then normalized to produce a reconstructed chromatogram (Figure 6) analogous to the response from a flame-ionization detector on a gas chromatograph.

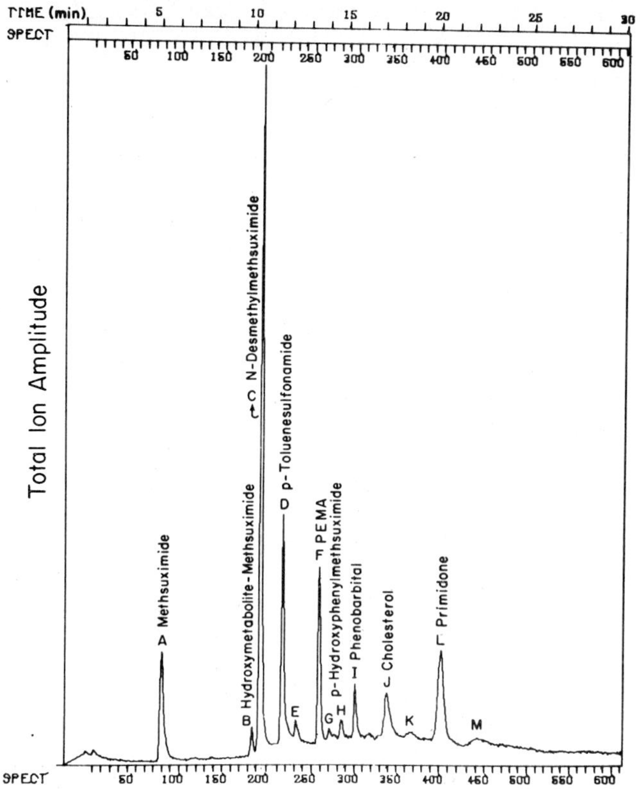

Fig. 6. Total-abundance chromatogram obtained by GC/MS analysis of serum collected 36 h after admission

The three extracted serum samples analyzed in this manner showed similar peaks in their total-abundance chromatograms; however, the peak heights differed considerably because they represented metabolites of the ingested drugs.

The presence of metabolites of methsuximide other than *N*-desmethylmethsuximide was investigated in the 36-h sample. Of the 14 peaks present in the chromatogram of this sample (Figure 6), peaks *A* and *C* were identified as methsuximide and *N*-desmethylmethsuximide, respectively, by plotting single-ion chromatograms of the two molecular ions, *m/e* 203 and 189. The corresponding mass spectra were consistent with literature spectra (*3, 10*) and spectra of the authentic compounds.

The technique of single-ion chromatography (*11*) was used to search the GC/MS data for the reported hydroxymethsuximide metabolites (*12, 13*). Underivatized monohydroxymetabolites of methsuximide exhibit a prominent molecular ion at *m/e* 219. Figure 7 shows the peaks (*B* and *H*) that represent ions of *m/e* 219. Ex-

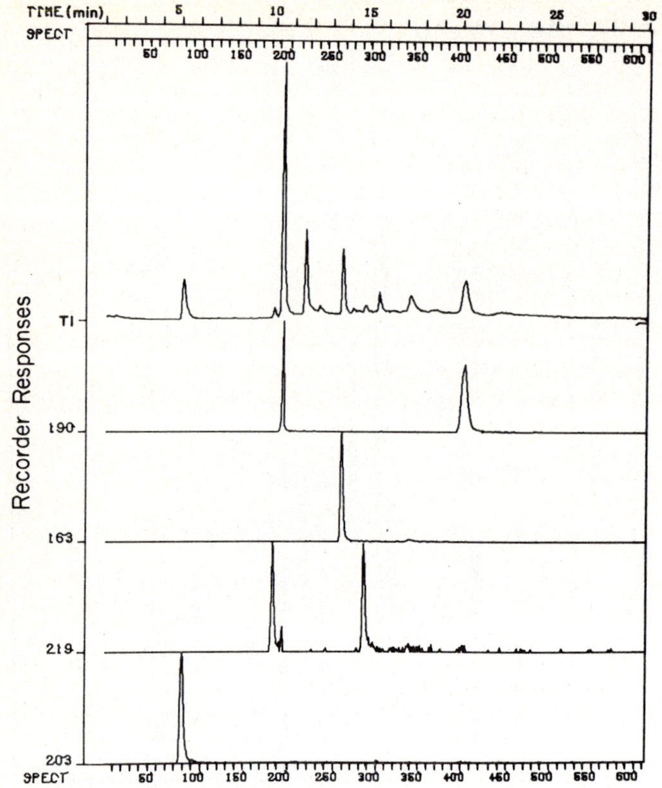

Fig. 7. Computer-reconstructed single-ion chromatograms of serum collected 36 h after admission

Total ion current is plotted as a function of spectrum number. Molecular ions of methsuximide (203) and hydroxy metabolites and methsuximide (219); the base peak of phenylethylmalonamide (163); and ions of *m/e* 190 prominent in the spectrum of primidone and the ^{13}C isotope of the molecular ion of *N*-desmethylmethsuximide are presented

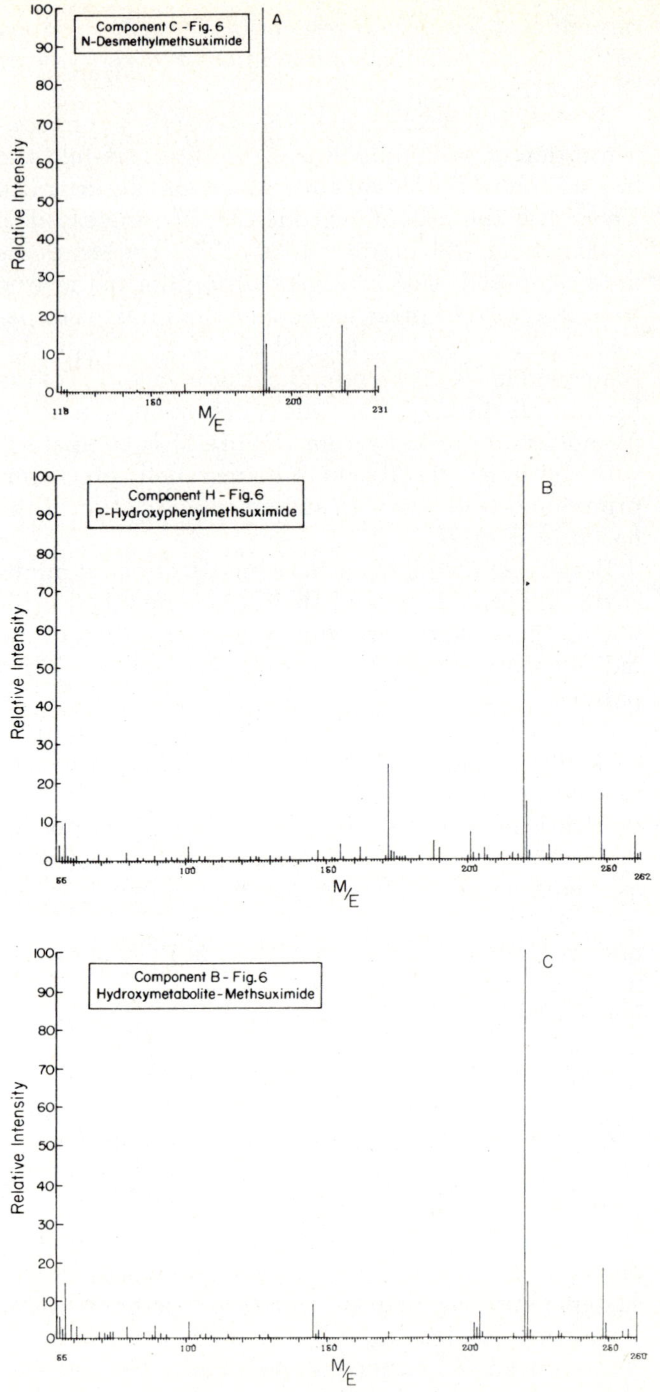

Fig. 8. Chemical-ionization mass spectra of compounds represented by gas-chromatographic peaks from patient's serum, obtained with methane as reagent gas

A, *N*-desmethylmethsuximide (MH^+ 190); B, *p*-hydroxyphenylmethsuximide (MH^+ 220); C, hydroxymetabolite of methsuximide, *N*-methyl-2-hydroxymethyl-2-phenylsuccinimide (MH^+ 220)

amination of the total mass spectra of these peaks indicate that both compounds have a molecular weight of 219.

An ethyl acetate solution of *p*-hydroxyphenylmethsuximide, one of the known methsuximide metabolites, was injected into the GC/MS and its retention time and mass spectrum were compared to those for components *B* and *H*. Component *H* was thus determined to be *p*-hydroxyphenylmethsuximide. If component *B* was also a metabolite of methsuximide, one of three structures was probable: *N*-methyl-2-hydroxymethyl-2-phenylsuccinimide, *N*,2-dimethyl-2-phenyl-3-hydroxysuccinimide, or *N*-hydroxymethyl-2-methyl-2-phenylsuccinimide. The first two of these compounds have previously been reported as urinary metabolites of methsuximide in the rat, guinea pig, and human (*13*). The *N*-hydroxymethyl compound was ruled out by the intense *m/e* 134, which is attributable to loss of the -$CONCH_3CO$- moiety similar to methsuximide itself. A tentative identification of component *B* as *N*-methyl-2-hydroxymethyl-2-phenylsuccinimide is based on the intense *m/e* 132 ion, which corresponds to the molecular ion of 2-phenyl propenal formed by the loss of hydrogen from the 134 ion.

Because of the large amount of *N*-desmethylmethsuximide present in the patient's serum, we also searched for its corresponding *p*-hydroxymetabolite. However, there was no peak present that had a retention time or mass spectrum corresponding to that of authentic 2-methyl-2-(4-hydroxyphenyl)-succinimide.

Several components could not be readily identified because their electron ionization spectra did not exhibit molecular ions. For this reason, we obtained a chemical-ionization (methane) GC/MS analysis from the 36-h sample. The chemical ionization spectra of components

L and *F* clearly showed their molecular weights to be consistent with those of primidone and phenylethylmalonamide, respectively. Chemical ionization spectra of *N*-desmethylmethsuximide, *p*-hydroxymethylmethsuximide, and the hydroxylated metabolite of the drug tentatively identified as *N*-methyl-2-hydroxymethyl-2-phenyl-succinimide, are shown in Figure 8. Because the process of chemical ionization involves a low energy transfer of a proton, the mass spectra show very little fragmentation, with the largest peak usually being the protonated molecular ion (MH^+), peaks appearing at M+29 ($M+C_2H_5$) and M+41 ($M+C_3H_5$) are also common when methane is used as the reagent gas (*14*).

Component *D* (Figure 6) was compared to authentic tolbutamide and to *p*-toluenesulfonamide, the thermal decomposition product of tolbutamide. The retention time and mass spectra of component *D* were identical to those of authentic *p*-toluenesulfonamide. Moreover, the chemical ionization mass spectrum of component *D* showed its major peak at *m/e* 172 consistent with the protonated molecular ion of *p*-toluenesulfonamide. Matin and Knight (*15*) reported that *N*-1-methyl tolbutamide, a closely related compound, decomposed in part to *N*-1-methyl-*p*-toluenesulfonamide both in the injector port and ion source of their GC/MS system.

Component *E* was identified as tri-2-butoxyethylphosphate, a plasticizer, from B-D Vacutainer stoppers, by comparison of its electron ionization mass spectrum to the published spectrum of this contaminant (*16*).

Component *J* was identified, from its mass spectrum, as cholesterol. Component *G* appears to have a molecular weight of 228. The base peak of its electron ionization spectrum is 130; however, this material has not been identified. The very minor components *K* and *M* appear to be steroidal type compounds. Diphenylhydantoin was detected in trace amounts by plotting the single-ion chromatogram of the molecular ion.

We thank the house staff of The Johns Hopkins Hospital for their diligence in collecting and identifying the large number of clinical samples obtained from this patient during her hospitalization and for providing us with a summary of her clinical course.

References

1. Solow, E. B., and Green, J. B., The simultaneous determination of multiple anticonvulsant drug levels by gas-liquid chromatography. *Neurology* **22,** 540 (1972).

2. Kutt, H., and Penry, J. K., Usefulness of blood levels of anti-epileptic drugs. *Arch. Neurol.* (Chicago) **31,** 382 (1974).

3. Strong, J. M., Abe, T., Gibbs, E. L., and Atkinson, A. J., Jr., Plasma levels of methsuximide and *N*-desmethylmethsuximide during methsuximide therapy. *Neurology* **24,** 250 (1974).

4. Baumel, I. P., Gallagher, B. B., DiMicco, J., and Goico, H., Metabolism and anticonvulsant properties of primidone in the rat. *J. Pharmacol. Exp. Ther.* **186,** 305 (1973).

5. Brillman, J., Gallagher, B. B., and Mattson, R. H., Acute primidone intoxication. *Arch. Neurol.* (Chicago) **30,** 255 (1974).

6. Bailey, D. N., and Jatlow, P. I., Chemical analysis of massive crystalluria following primidone overdose. *Am. J. Clin. Pathol.* **58,** 583 (1972).

7. Karch, S. B., Methsuximide overdose—delayed onset of profound coma. *J. Am. Med. Assoc.* **223,** 1463 (1973).

8. Kananen, G., Osiewicz, R., and Sunshine, I., Barbiturate analysis—a current assessment. *J. Chromatogr. Sci.* **10,** 283 (1972).

9. Bente, H. B., and Wisniewski, J. V., A new GC column for the analysis of phenobarbital, primidone and diphenylhydantoin. Application Note ANGC 6-75, Hewlett-Packard, Avondale, Pa. 19311.

10. Finkle, B. S., Foltz, R. L., and Taylor, D. M., A comprehensive GC-MS reference data system for toxicological and biomedical purposes. *J. Chromatogr. Sci.* **12,** 304 (1974).

11. McFadden, W. H., Ed., *Techniques of Combined Gas Chromatography/Mass Spectrometry: Applications in Organic Analysis.* John Wiley and Sons, Inc., New York, N. Y., 1973, pp 252–255.

12. Dudley, K. H., Bius, D. L., and Waldrop, C. D., Urinary metabolites of *N*-methyl-α-methyl-α-phenylsuccinimide (methsuximide) in the dog. *Drug Metab. Dispos.* **2,** 113 (1974).

13. Horning, M. G., Butler, C., Harvey, D. J., et al., Metabolism of *N*,2-dimethyl-2-phenylsuccinimide (methsuximide) by the epoxide-diol pathway in rat, guinea pig and human. *Res. Commun. Chem. Pathol. Pharmacol.* **6,** 565 (1975).

14. Munson, M. S. B., and Field, F. H., Chemical ionization mass spectrometry. I. General introduction. *J. Am. Chem. Soc.* **88,** 2621 (1966).

15. Matin, S. B., and Knight, J. B., The use of solid probe chemical ionization mass spectrometry and gas chromatography–chemical ionization mass spectrometry in quantitation of drugs in biological fluids. Determination of tolbutamide and its metabolites in human plasma. *Biomed. Mass Spectrom.* **1,** 323 (1974).

16. Costello, C. E., Sakai, T., and Biemann, K., Identification of drugs in body fluids particularly in emergency cases of acute poisioning. In ref. *11,* pp 377–384.

case report

Beta-Carotene Content of Certain Organs from Two Patients Receiving High Doses of Beta-Carotene

Micheline M. Mathews-Roth, M.D., [1] **Andreas A. Abraham, M.D.,** [2] **and Thomas G. Gabuzda, M.D.**[2]

We measured carotene in the livers of two patients receiving beta-carotene therapy for photosensitivity. In both patients, the amount of carotene was within reported ranges for patients on normal diets; no abnormal amounts of beta-carotene had accumulated in the livers after oral administration of large amounts of beta-carotene. Light-microscopic examination of the liver (specimen obtained at cholecystectomy) of one patient with erythropoietic protoporphyria and cholesterosis showed findings characteristic of these conditions. Electron-microscopically, semicrystalline inclusions were seen in the mitochondria of the hepatocytes; such inclusions have been reported in several conditions, including erythropoietic protoporphyria and porphyria cutanea tarda, and in control subjects. Microscopic examination of the liver of the other patient, who had Rothmund–Thomson syndrome and died of acute bacterial meningitis, revealed no abnormalities. The cerebrum of the latter patient contained 13 μg of carotene per kilogram (wet weight) of brain. No previous report of analysis of human brain for carotenoids could be found.

Additional Keyphrases: *brain, liver • erythropoietic protoporphyria • therapy for photosensitivity • Rothmund–Thomson syndrome • vitamin A • semicrystalline inclusions in hepatocytic mitochondria*

Treatment with high doses of crystalline beta-carotene is currently being used for amelioration of photosensitivity in erythropoietic protoporphyria and certain photosensitivity disorders (*1, 2*). To date, no reports have appeared of toxicity attributable to beta-carotene in the treated patients, nor has a search of the literature revealed any reports of toxicity from crystalline carotene. It is nevertheless necessary to continue to observe patients receiving high doses of beta-carotene for possible toxicity. It is also relevant to examine for carotene content the organs of any such patients who may come to autopsy or operation. Opportunities arose to study the carotenoid content of the liver of two patients taking beta-carotene, and also to study the brain of one of these.

[1] Channing Laboratory and Department of Medicine, Harvard Medical School, and Department of Medical Microbiology, Boston City Hospital, Boston, Mass. 02118.

[2] Division of Research, Lankenau Hospital, Philadelphia, Pa. 19151.

Received Mar. 25, 1976; accepted Mar. 29, 1976.

Materials and Methods

Patients. Patient A, a 4-year-old girl with Rothmund–Thomson syndrome, had been taking beta-carotene (30 mg/day) to alleviate the photosensitivity characteristic of this disease. This patient died suddenly of acute bacterial meningitis. At postmortem examination, the findings in the brain and meninges were consistent with meningitis. Also present was minimal evidence of a coagulopathy similar to that seen in fulminant meningitis, i.e., focal unilateral adrenal hemorrhage, and pulmonary capillary thrombosis. Gross and microscopic examination of the liver revealed no significant pathological changes. The last blood carotenoid value was 2.5 mg/liter.

Patient B, a 22-year-old female with erythropoietic protoporphyria (free erythrocyte protoporphyrin, 17 mg/liter), had been taking beta-carotene (180 mg/day) for about a year to alleviate the photosensitivity associated with the disease. Because of a history of several attacks of right upper quadrant and mid-epigastric pain after fatty meals, she underwent a cholecystectomy. Specimens of liver and gall bladder, and of gall-bladder contents, were obtained and analyzed for carotene content. At operation the liver was found to be grossly normal; the gall bladder contained rather thick, viscid bile, but no stones. The lining of the gall bladder was characteristic of cholesterosis on gross examination, and this was confirmed on microscopic examination. The patient's blood carotene concentration on the day before surgery was 8.64 mg/liter.

The patient reported that she had received steroids (cortisone) for the treatment of severe photosensitivity reactions, most recently in 1974, before starting beta-carotene therapy. She also stated that she had never taken any oral contraceptives.

Electron microscopic studies were done on the liver biopsy specimen of patient B. After fixation in glutaraldehyde (50 ml/liter, pH 7.4) for 60 min, the specimen was postfixed with 10 g/liter osmium tetroxide and then dehydrated and embedded in EPON 812. After toluidine blue staining, 1-μm sections were studies by light microscopy and ultrathin sections were stained with uranyl acetate and lead citrate and examined with a Philips 300 electron microscope.

Table 1. Carotene and Vitamin A in the Liver

Source (ref.)	Carotene, mg/kg wet wt Mean	Carotene, mg/kg wet wt Range	Vitamin A, int. kilounits/kg wet wt Mean	Vitamin A, int. kilounits/kg wet wt Range
Ralli et al. (*4*)				
diabetic patients	26.30	1.20–96.80	364.56	19.05–613.80
nondiabetic patients	10.08	1.50–37.50	305.90	88.00–1126.40
Dzialoszynski and Tomaszewski (*5*)	5.40	0–14.00	504.00	0–2500.00
Jensen and With (*6*)	20.42	1.12–42.59	201.42	20.16–483.20
Ralli et al. (*7*)	14.40	3.30–39.00	1210.00	34.00–6390.00
Blankenhorn (*8*)	7.64	2.31–27.30		
Hoppner et al. (*9*)				
males	8.40	0–35.50	341.28	0–2222.35
females	11.20	0–43.40	321.22	0–3852.32
Present report				
Patient A	21.88		57.57	
Patient B	11.92		96.29	
Patient with ASHD	3.06		22.10	

Results and Discussion

Table 1 gives the amount of carotene and vitamin A found in the livers of the two patients under study, and in the liver of an elderly patient who died of arteriosclerotic heart disease. Also listed are the liver carotenoid and vitamin A concentrations reported by several investigators (*4–9*). This includes a study done on diabetics (*4*), whose carotenoid values are often increased because of their increased intake of carotenoid-containing vegetables and fruits. There was no abnormally high accumulation of beta-carotene in the livers of the two patients taking carotene. Although the values are higher than those of the patient not taking carotene, the values fall within the ranges reported by other workers (Table 1). The lack of abnormal accumulation of beta-carotene in the liver has been seen in animal studies (*10*). The vitamin A concentrations of the patients taking carotene, although higher than those of the patient dying of arteriosclerosis, were still within the ranges reported by others for hepatic vitamin A content (Table 1).

Two reports were found of necropsies with microscopic examination of the liver (*11, 12*) and a third report of a liver biopsy (*13*) from patients with diabetes and carotenemia owing to overingestion of vegetables. Two of the reports noted the presence of yellow granules in some hepatic cells. None of the cases reported had any alteration in the normal anatomy of the liver, although in one case the presence of fat vacuoles in some cells was noted (*12*). In the third case no remarkable amount of pigment was seen, but fat globules were said to be present in about 80% of the cells (*13*).

Routine light-microscopic findings in patient B demonstrated normal overall hepatic architecture with intrahepatic and canalicular cholestasis. Red fluorescent deposits were seen by fluorescence microscopy. The Kupffer cells contained strongly periodic acid-Schiff positive cytoplasm resistant to diastase treatment. Doubly refractile material was present in occasional Kupffer cells. These findings have been previously reported in patients with erythropoietic protoporphyria (*14, 15*). Routine microscopic studies of patient A revealed no abnormality. In neither patient did we see the fatty changes and the marked pigmentation reported in the diabetic patients.

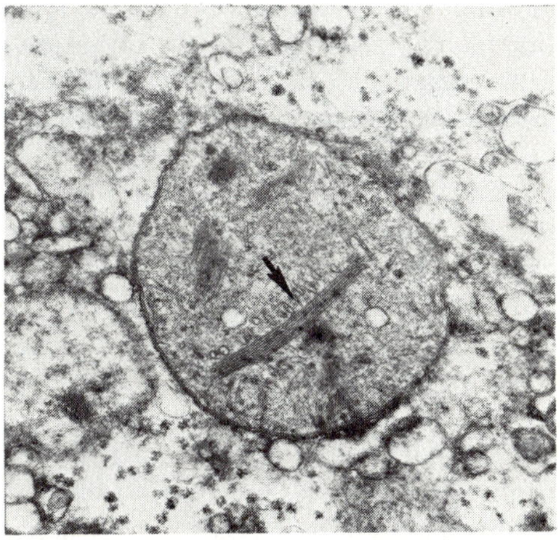

Fig. 1. Electron micrograph, showing semicrystalline structures within mitochondrion of an hepatocyte of patient B
Magnification, 62 000

Electron microscopic observations on the liver of patient B revealed the presence of semicrystalline inclusions of stacked laminar character in most of the mitochondria (exemplified in Figure 1). These were often multiple and were found in all of 55 hepatocytes examined. Crystalline inclusions have previously been seen in the hepatocyte cytoplasm of patients with erythropoietic protoporphyria (*14, 15*). Recently, Wolff et al. (*16*) have reported crystalline inclusions in the mitochondria of the hepatocytes of one of two patients with this disorder whom they studied. Hepatocyte mitochondrial crystalline inclusions have been reported in other conditions, including porphyria cutanea tarda, patients taking steroids, and control subjects (*17–19*). The significance of these inclusions remains unknown.

We found no detectable carotenoids in the gall-bladder wall or in the gall-bladder contents removed at operation. Only traces of carotenoids were found in the biliary drainage (180 μg/liter) and duodenal drainage (80 μg/liter) taken the day before operation.

We found no report of the quantitative determination of carotenoid pigments in human brain in the literature. Analysis for carotene content of the cerebral tissue of patient A revealed a content of 13 μg/kg wet weight of brain. The cerebrum of the patient who died of arteriosclerosis contained 27 μg of carotene/kg wet weight of brain. The greater content of carotenoids in the brain of the older patient seems to be consistent with the observations of Karnaukhov et al. (*20*) of higher carotenoid content in the brains of older animals as compared to younger ones, but this is, of course, only a single observation.

Our data suggest that, as in animal studies, abnormal amounts of beta-carotene and vitamin A do not accumulate in the liver as a result of the ingestion of crystalline beta-carotene. This may also be true for brain, although more studies are needed before this conclusion is certain.

Although two patients is a small number to study, such patients with photosensitivity do not come to operation or autopsy with great frequency. For this reason we wish to report the data we have obtained to date, and to urge other investigators to analyze for carotenoid content the organs of those patients receiving carotenoid therapy who may come to operation or autopsy. This is of special interest in patients with erythropoietic protoporphyria, as there are reports that suggest an increased incidence of gall bladder and hepatic dysfunction in occasional patients with this disease [for review, see (*21*)].

This work was supported by grant AM 14545-06 from the NIAMDD, NIH. We thank Dr. Ambrose Keeley for examining the liver sections, and Dr. Richard J. Sampson for providing the specimens.

References

1. Mathews-Roth, M. M., Pathak, M. A., Fitzpatrick, T. B., et al. Beta-carotene as an oral photoprotective agent in erythropoietic protoporphyria. *J. Am. Med. Assoc.* **228,** 1004 (1974).

2. Jansen, C. T., Beta-carotene treatment of polymorphous light eruption. *Dermatologica* **149,** 363 (1974).

3. Mathews-Roth, M. M., Presence of carotenoids in thé erythrocyte membranes of carotenemic and noncarotenemic individuals. *Clin. Chem.* **21,** 258 (1975).

4. Ralli, E. P., Brandaleone, H. P., and Mandelbaum, T., Studies on the effect of the administration of carotene and vitamin A in patients with diabetes mellitus. *J. Lab. Clin. Med.* **20,** 1266 (1934–1935).

5. Dzialoszynski, L., and Tomaszewski, W., Vitamin A content in human liver. *Edinburgh Med. J., New Ser.* **54,** 252 (1947).

6. Jensen, H. B., and With, T. K., Vitamin A and carotenoids in the liver of mammals, birds, reptiles and man, with particular regard to the intensity of the ultraviolet absorption and the Carr-Price reaction of vitamin A. *Biochem. J.* **33,** 1771 (1939).

7. Ralli, E. P., Papper, E., Paley, K., and Bauman, E., Vitamin A and carotene content of human liver in normal and in diseased subjects. *Arch. Intern. Med.* **68,** 102 (1941).

8. Blankenhorn, D. H., Carotenoids in man IV Carotenoid stores in normal adults. *J. Biol. Chem.* **229,** 809 (1957).

9. Hoppner, K., Phillips, W. E. J., Erdody, P., et al., Vitamin A reserves of Canadians. *Can. Med. Assoc. J.* **101,** 736 (1969).

10. Bagdon, R. E., Zbinden, G., and Studer, A., Chronic toxicity studies of beta-carotene. *Toxicol. Appl. Pharmacol.* **2,** 225 (1960).

11. Gordon, A. H., Connor, C. H., and Rabinowitch, I. M., An unusual case of diabetes mellitus: Death after thirteen years' observation: Necropsy. *Am. J. Med. Sci.* (*New Ser.*) **175,** 22 (1928).

12. Pariente, A. C., Present, C. H., and Ralli, E. P., A case of carotenemia and diabetes mellitus with necropsy report and analyses of liver for carotene, vitamin A, total fat and cholesterol. *Am. J. Med. Sci.* **192,** 365 (1936).

13. Lascano-Gonzalez, J. C., Dameno, E., and Traina, M. H., Carotinemia—A proposito de un caso estudiado desde el punto de vista clinico y humoral, y anatomopatologico por puncion-biopsia hepatica. *Prensa Med. Argent.* **41,** 3431 (1954).

14. Matilla, A., and Molland, E. A., A light and electromicroscopic study of the liver in case of erythrohepatic protoporphyria and in griseofulvin-induced porphyria in mice. *J. Clin. Pathol.* **27,** 698 (1974).

15. Bloomer, J. R., Phillips, M. J., Davidson, D. L., and Klatskin, G., Hepatic disease in erythropoietic protoporphyria. *Am. J. Med.* **58,** 869 (1975).

16. Wolff, K., Wolff-Schreiner, E., and Gschnait, F., Liver inclusions in erythropoietic protoporphyria. *Eur. J. Clin. Invest.* **5,** 21 (1975).

17. Waldo, E. D., and Tobias, H., Needle-like cytoplasmic inclusions in the liver in porphyria cutanea tarda. *Arch. Pathol.* **96,** 368 (1973).

18. Sternlieb, I., and Berger, J. E., Optical diffraction studies of crystalline structures in electron micrographs. II. Crystalline inclusions in mitochondria of human hepatocytes. *J. Cell Biol.* **43,** 448 (1969).

19. Martinez-Manautou, J., Aznar-Ramos, R., Bautista-O'Farrill, J., and Gonzalez-Angulo, A., The ultrastructure of liver cells in women under steroid therapy. II. Contraceptive therapy. *Acta Endocrinol.* (Copenhagen) **65,** 207 (1970).

20. Karnaukhov, V. N., Tataunas, T. B., and Petrunyaka, V. V., Accumulation of carotenoids in brain and heart of animals on aging; the role of carotenoids in lipofuschin formation. *Mech. Ageing Dev.* **2,** 201 (1972).

21. DeLeo, V., Poh-Fitzpatrick, M. B., Mathews-Roth, M. M., and Harber, L. C. Erythropoietic protoporphyria—10 years' experience. *Am. J. Med.* **60,** 8 (1976).

letters

N-Acetylglucosaminidase and γ-Glutamyltransferase in Urine of Patients with Renal Transplants: Not an Early Indicator of Rejection

To the Editor:

Renal transplant rejection, which can be difficult to diagnose clinically at an early stage, is often reversible by prompt treatment. Treatment might be more effective if there were advance warning of impending rejection, and with this in view a variety of tests have been proposed, including a number involving urinary enzyme measurements (*1–5*). Determination of urinary β-*N*-acetylglucosaminidase (EC 3.2.1.30; NAG) and γ-glutamyltransferase (EC 2.3.2.2; γ-GT) seemed promising, both because kidney tissue is rich in these enzymes and because increases in urinary NAG excretion reportedly (*4*) precede by up to three weeks the detection of acute rejection by established methods.

We studied urinary enzyme excretion in 76 renal transplant patients. Whenever possible we obtained 24-h urine specimens from the time of transplantation until discharge from the hospital, and further specimens when patients attended the clinic for followup. In most cases activities of both NAG and γ-GT were estimated, NAG by the method described by Barratt (*6*), with 4-methylumbelliferyl-2-acetamido-2-deoxy-β-D-glucopyranoside as substrate at 37 °C and measuring the liberated 4-methyl-umbelliferone fluorometrically at 450 nm, and γ-GT by the method of Szasz (*7*), with γ-glutamyl-*p*-nitranilide and glycylglycine, at 24–25 °C. No specimens that had been frozen were tested, because Stokke (*8*) has shown that freezing sometimes causes loss of γ-GT activity. Although Szasz (*9*) has reported the presence of dialyzable inhibitors of γ-GT in urine, Stokke (*8*) could not confirm this and concluded that dialysis of urine for determination of γ-GT activity should be unnecessary if the concentration of the urine in the incubation mixture is kept low. In a few experiments we assessed the effect of dialysis and found that it was associated with a slight loss of activity, so we did not adopt it routinely; the general similarity in the excretion patterns of NAG and γ-GT in our patients suggests that no great error was introduced by this omission. Routine biochemical tests such as the estimation of blood urea, serum creatinine, creatinine clearance, urinary electrolytes, urea, and protein, and measurement of the urinary volume, were also performed on all patients.

Altogether some 600 NAG and 700 γ-GT estimations were made. Results were expressed as international (IUB) units of enzyme excreted per 24 hours. (Similar results were obtained when excretion was expressed as units of activity per milligram of creatinine.)

An average baseline of enzyme excretion, excluding the initial period of high excretion immediately following the grafting operation, was calculated for each patient. In the absence of rejection or infection, the 24-h urinary excretion of NAG and γ-GT did not exceed twice this baseline, except in one patient after biopsy (see below). Each graft appeared to establish its own baseline of enzyme excretion (*cf. 10*), and for this reason we made no attempt to calculate a "normal" baseline for each enzyme that would apply to all patients. Also, in agreement with Sandman et al. (*10*), we could find no correlation between this baseline value for enzyme excretion and the course of recovery.

NAG. In a total of eight episodes of rejection NAG excretion was increased on every occasion, by as much as three- to 50-fold the individual patient's baseline value.

γ-GT. The γ-GT estimation had been in use for some time before we began to estimate NAG. In a total of 11 episodes of rejection, γ-GT excretion was likewise increased on every occasion, by as much as three- to 10-fold the individual patient's baseline.

Neither urinary NAG nor γ-GT estimations provided an early warning of rejection; we could find no evidence that elevation in the excretion of these enzymes preceded other indications of rejection. It is interesting to note that Sandman et al. (*10*), who studied the excretion of a number of enzymes (including NAG) after renal transplantation, made no claim that NAG estimation gave any earlier warning than did the other tests that they used in monitoring renal transplant rejection.

Increases in enzyme excretion in the absence of rejection occurred on 10 occasions with NAG and nine occasions with γ-GT. (These formed two series with only three patients in common.) Such "false-positive" increases, which ranged from about 2.5 to seven- or eight-fold the patient's baseline, could in most cases be correlated with the presence of a renal tract infection; in four patients the blood pressure was above normal and they were receiving treatment with methyldopa—though whether this is of significance is not clear. The possibility that this or other drugs may have influenced the results cannot be excluded. In one patient an increase to nearly threefold the baseline excretion of γ-GT was noted after biopsy of the grafted kidney.

We conclude that measurement of urinary NAG and γ-GT excretion may be useful in confirming evidence of rejection, but it appears to be of no value as an early indicator of a rejection episode. In view of the frequency of increases in enzyme excretion in the absence of rejection, and the fact that treatment with immunosuppressive agents is not without risk, we wish to caution against reliance on these enzyme measurements as evidence of rejection on their own. As was emphasized by Wellwood et al. (*4*), other causes of renal cell damage may be expected to increase the urinary excretion of enzymes and should be excluded.

We thank the technical staff of the laboratory for their help with many of the γ-GT estimations. Mr. Keith Allen, a student of the University of Surrey, helped with many of the preliminary experiments involved in setting up the γ-GT method, during a period of training in our laboratory.

References

1. Prout, G. R., Macalalag, E. V., Jr., and Hume, D. M., Serum and urinary lactic dehydrogenase in patients with renal homotransplants. *Surgery* **56,** 283 (1964).

2. Ballantyne, B., Wood, W. G., and Meffan, P. M., Sequential analysis of urinary enzymes in early diagnosis of parenchymal damage after renal homotransplantation. *Br. Med. J.* **ii,** 667 (1968).

3. Bergström, K., Blomstrand, R., Magnusson, G., and Werner, B., Some laboratory data, including enzymatic observations, in human renal homotransplantation. *Acta Chir. Scand.* **134,** 467 (1968).

4. Wellwood, J. M., Ellis, B. G., Hall, J. H., et al., Early warning of rejection? *Br. Med. J.* **i,** 261 (1973).

5. Dance, N., Price, R. G., Cattell, W. R., et al., The excretion of *N*-acetyl-β-glucosaminidase and β-galactosidase by patients with renal disease. *Clin. Chim. Acta* **27,** 87 (1970).

6. Barratt, A. J., In *Lysosomes: A Laboratory Handbook,* J. T. Dingle, Ed., North Holland, Amsterdam and London, 1972, p 116.

7. Szasz, G., A kinetic photometric method for serum γ-glutamyl transpeptidase. *Clin. Chem.* **15,** 124 (1969).

8. Stokke, O., Preservation of γ-glutamyl transpeptidase activity in human urine. *Clin. Chim. Acta* **57,** 143 (1974).

9. Szasz, G., γ-Glutamyltranspeptidase-Aktivität im Urin. *Z. Klin. Chem. Klin. Biochem.* **8,** 1 (1970).

10. Sandman, R., Margules, R. M., and Kountz, S. L., Urinary lysosomal glycosidases after renal allotransplantation: Correlation of enzyme excretion with allograft rejection and ischemia. *Clin. Chim. Acta* **45,** 349 (1973).

J. W. Keyser
G. Ll. Watkins
J. R. Salaman

Departments of Medical Biochemistry and Surgery
The Welsh National School of Medicine
Royal Infirmary
Cardiff, Wales

Calibration of Glucose Methods with Lyophilized Materials: A Caution

To the Editor:

Although it is generally agreed that calibration of analytical instruments is ideally achieved by use of aqueous solutions of pure reference material, many systems require the use of a protein-based calibrator. Accordingly, materials intended for calibration purposes are available that have a protein base and either (*a*) contain a "weighed in" quantity of reference material or (*b*) have been assayed for the desired analyte by a "reference" method. In general, the final product is supplied in lyophilized form.

Recent experience in our laboratory with two such products has convinced us that the report of Sternberg (*1*) concerning the use of such materials for calibration of some glucose methodologies may be largely unheeded. His report indicated that the process of lyophilization may cause bonding between glucose and protein, the result of which is that some analytical procedures do not recover the amount of glucose either weighed in or as determined by the "reference" method. In general, a glucose procedure with a strong acid (such as an *o*-toluidine method) will recover all of the glucose present in a lyophilized protein-based material whereas an enzymatic method will not. Thus, the values for glucose concentration supplied by a manufacturer may not be valid for all procedures even though all the methods purport to measure "true" glucose. Because the use of protein-based materials to calibrate glucose measuring systems is widespread, the point made by Sternberg deserves re-emphasis.

Our recent observations with "Standardize" (American Monitor Corp., Indianapolis, Ind. 46268), intended as a calibration material for the American Monitor Programachem 1040, and with "Auto Ref" (DADE Div. Amer. Hosp. Supply Corp., Miami, Fla. 33152), intended for calibration of automated analytical instruments, illustrate this problem. Standardize contains a protein base into which reference materials are weighed; Auto Ref is assayed by "reference" methods, the one for glucose being an *o*-toluidine procedure (*2*). We reconstituted each product as directed and assayed them in triplicate by each of the following glucose methods.

(i) Oxygen rate (OR) method as performed by the Beckman Glucose Analyzer (Beckman Instruments, Inc., Fullerton, Calif. 92634).

(ii) Glucose oxidase (GO) based procedure developed by American Monitor Corp. and performed on the Programachem 1040.

(iii) Hexokinase procedure (HK) performed on the Abbott ABA-100 with the use of Abbott "A-Gent" reagent (Abbott Laboratories, So. Pasadena, Calif. 91030).

(iv) *o*-Toluidine (OT) method (*2*).

Table 1. Method Dependence of Glucose Recovery

Method	"Auto Ref" Control Mean	SD	"Standardize" Control Mean	SD
	mg/liter			
OR	1850	6	1420	6
GO	1850	30	1380	32
HK	1810	0	1390	6
OT	1960	21	1490	13
Insert	2020	25	1570	—

We calibrated the OR, HK, and OT methods with a commercially prepared aqueous glucose standard containing 1500 mg of glucose per liter. For the GO method, the Programachem 1040 was calibrated with Dade "Lab-trol" (a control material supplied in liquid form) after the manufacturer's value for glucose was verified by the HK procedure. The glucose recovered by each procedure is given in Table 1, along with the value supplied by the manufacturer ("insert"). These results indicate that enzymatic methods (OR, GO, HK) will recover less glucose from a lyophilized protein-based material than will the OT method. Therefore, if a lyophilized material is analyzed for glucose by the OT method, the value derived cannot be used for calibration purposes with other glucose methods even though they all theoretically measure "true" glucose. In like manner, even if pure glucose is weighed into a protein-based solution, subsequent lyophilization will result in part of this compound becoming unrecoverable by enzymatic methods. Caution is therefore required when using the manufacturer-supplied glucose values accompanying lyophilized calibration materials. Where the use of lyophilized protein-based products is required, it may be necessary to determine the glucose concentration of such materials by using a procedure such as the OR or HK method and an aqueous glucose standard for instrument calibration.

References

1. Sternberg, J. C., Factors influencing precision and accuracy of glucose values obtained on control sera by the *o*-toluidine and oxygen rate glucose oxidase methods. *Clin. Chem.* **18,** 694 (1972). Abstract.

2. Feteris, W. A., A serum glucose method without protein precipitation. *Am. J. Med. Technol.* **31,** 17 (1965).

R. R. Swain
R. M. Carpenter
S. L. Briggs

Lilly Lab. for Clinical Research
Wishard Memorial Hospital
Indianapolis, Ind. 46202

Decomposition of 1,3-Dimethylphenobarbital in Trimethylanilinium Hydroxide

To the Editor:

Phenobarbital is frequently determined by a procedure that involves injecting a mixture of the drug and trimethylanilinium hydroxide (TMAH) into a gas chromatograph (*1*). This technique results in the formation of 1,3-dimethylphenobarbital, which is the peak quantitated on the gas chromatogram (*2*). There has been much discussion of the appearance of one or more peaks on the chromatogram for which the retention time is much shorter than that of 1,3-dimethylphenobarbital, and one of these in particular has been designated the "early peak" (*3–7*). This early peak has been identified as *N*-methyl-α-phenylbutyramide (*5, 7*). The presence of *N,N*-dimethyl-α-phenylbutyramide has also been demonstrated (*7*).

Because of the interest in the methylation of phenobarbital, we wish to report some observations we have made on the instability of 2,3-dimethylphenobarbital under conditions used in the gas-chromatographic procedure. Injection of 1,3-dimethylphenobarbital in methanol yielded a single peak at 6.7 min (Hewlett-Packard 5830A, 3% OV1 on 80–100 W.H.P., 180 cm × 4 mm (i.d.) column, nitrogen flow rate 30 ml min^{-1}, injection port temperature 250 °C, and column temperature 160 °C). However, injection of this compound with TMAH (0.2 mol/liter) yielded peaks at 1.8, 6.7, 7.0, and 8.2 min with integrated areas of 275 000, 38 940, 102 300, and 1581 (arbitrary units), respectively. The peak at 1.8 min was obtained when phenobarbital was injected with TMAH (0.2 mol/liter) and corresponds to the previously mentioned "early peak." The peak at 6.7 min is unchanged 1.3-dimethylphenobarbital, whereas the peaks at 7.0 and 8.2 min arise from the decomposition of this compound, because appropriate control experiments showed they did not originate from TMAH itself.

We established that 2,3-dimethylphenobarbital is relatively stable in TMAH at room temperature, and that the decomposition occurred after injection, by chromatographing a solution of the 1,3-dimethylphenobarbital in TMAH (0.2 mol/liter) that had been standing at room temperature for 10 days but was neutralized with dilute hydrochloric acid before injection. The chromatogram obtained showed a single peak at 6.7 min, the retention time for pure 1,3-dimethylphenobarbital.

A more detailed examination of the products of the reaction of 1,3-dimethylphenobarbital with TMAH by gas chromatography/mass spectrometry revealed a number of additional products and from our experiments we have concluded that the 1,3-dimethylphenobarbital is degraded to trimethyl- and tetramethyl-phenylethylmalonamides, *N*-methyl- and *N,N'*-dimethyl-α-phenylbutyramides, and methyl α-phenylbutyrate. The detailed chemistry of the decomposition will be presented later, but in view of our findings the results of any method for phenobarbital determinations based on quantitation of reaction products should be treated with caution.

References

1. Kupferberg, H. J., Quantitative estimation of diphenylhydantoin, primidone, and phenobarbital in plasma by gas-liquid chromatography. *Clin. Chim. Acta* **29**, 283 (1970).

2. Brochmann-Hansen, E., and Oke, T. O., Gas chromatography of barbiturates, phenolic alkaloids, and xanthine bases: Flash-heater methylation by means of trimethylanilium hydroxide. *J. Pharm. Sci.* **58**, 370 (1969).

3. Stevenson, G. W., On-column methylation of barbituric acids. *Anal. Chem.* **38**, 1949 (1966).

4. Van Meter, J. C., and Gillen, H. W., A source of variation in the gas-chromatographic assay of phenobarbital treated with trimethylanilium hydroxide. *Clin. Chem.* **19**, 359 (1973). Letter to the Editor.

5. Wu, A., Concerning on-column methylation of phenobarbital. *Clin. Chem.* **20**, 630 (1974), Letter to the Editor.

6. Perchalski, R. J., Scott, K. N., Wilder, B. J., and Hammer, R. H., Rapid simultaneous GLC determination of phenobarbital, primidone, and diphenylhydantoin. *J. Pharm. Sci.* **62**, 1735 (1973).

7. Osiewicz, R., Aggarwal, V., Young, R. M., and Sunshine, I., The quantitative analysis of phenobarbital with trimethylanilium hydroxide. *J. Chromatogr.* **88**, 157 (1974).

Patrick S. Callery
James Leslie

School of Pharmacy
University of Maryland
Baltimore, Md. 21201

Procedures Compared for Extracting Benzodiazepines from Blood

To the Editor:

Adsorption methods have recently been described, which include the use of activated charcoal (*1–3*), Amberlite XAD-2 ion-exchange resin (*4*), and Celite (*5*), to extract drugs from blood or serum. I wish to report a comparison of these extraction methods (suitably modified) for the analytical recovery from blood of therapeutic concentrations of some representative benzodiazepines, namely nitrazepam, diazepam, and its metabolite *N*-desmethyl diazepam.

For Celite extractions I modified the procedure of Ehrsson and Knapp (*5*) to the use of redistilled chloroform instead of water-saturated ethyl acetate. Use of the former solvent gave cleaner extracts and much better recoveries of therapeutic concentrations of benzodiazepines than did the water-saturated ethyl acetate. A small layer (about 5 mm) of Celite packed into each column below the Celite/blood mixture prevented the elution of pigments. In these extractions, optimum recoveries were achieved only when the columns were firmly packed.

To allow a direct comparison of the extraction procedures, the Amberlite XAD-2 method of Missen and Lewin (*4*) was adapted to the extraction of a 0.4 ml blood sample, using 1 ml of resin. When different solvents were compared for the elution of diazepam adsorbed onto XAD-2 resin (from aqueous solution), the order of recovery was: chloroform (96–97%) > diethyl ether (86–89%) > acetone (71–83%) > methanol (47–66%). Chloroform gave the most consistent and efficient recovery of diazepam and 2 × 10 ml was therefore used after 10 ml acetone (which removed residual water) to further elute drugs from XAD-2 resin. The eluates were combined and concentrated.

Charcoal extractions were also performed on a 0.4-ml blood sample following the procedure of Adams (*2*), but with the difference that I again eluted benzodiazepines with acetone followed by chloroform, to give optimum recoveries of these drugs. Use of chloroform alone gave poor recoveries of diazepam from charcoal, presumably because this solvent did not sufficiently penetrate the wet powder.

The extracts obtained in each case were analyzed by electron capture/gas chromatography under conditions similar to those published for quantitation of diazepam (*6*), and nitrazepam (*7, 8*).

The extraction methods outlined were applied to drug-supplemented blood samples, and also to samples taken postmortem and samples taken from intoxicated drivers. I found that for blood supplemented with diazepam (0.15 μg/ml) four replicate extractions with use of Celite, XAD-2, and charcoal gave mean recoveries of 91%, 73%, and 75%, respectively. For blood supplemented with nitrazepam (0.31 μg/ml), four replicate Celite, XAD-2, and charcoal extractions gave mean recoveries of 59%, 56%, and 47%, respectively. Individual recoveries lay within ±4% of the mean. The lower recovery of nitrazepam from the supplemented blood was only partly attributable to limitations in the analytical method followed, because when nitrazepam standards were hydrolyzed to 2-amino-5-chlorobenzophenone (*7, 8*), this compound was recovered in yields ranging from 82–92%.

When nitrazepam, diazepam, and *N*-desmethyl diazepam were extracted from authentic blood samples the Celite method gave only marginally higher recoveries of these drugs than did the XAD-2 procedure. The charcoal procedure gave reasonable recoveries of diazepam and its metabolite, but it gave poor recoveries of nitrazepam. It was noticeable that the results for authentic blood samples (analyzed by each of the three procedures) did not always correlate with corresponding recoveries from the supplemented bloods, indicating a danger in attaching too much significance to recoveries from drug-supplemented bloods.

In my hands, the Celite extraction was rapid and I could perform an extraction in about 10 min. By contrast, an Amberlite XAD-2 extraction took about 17 min plus 1 h on a rolling mill. However, the Celite method extracted large amounts (100–400 μg) of cholesterol from blood samples, whereas the other procedures extracted much less (about 10% of the amounts extracted by the Celite extracts).

At present we are using the Celite extraction method to rapidly screen drivers' blood samples for benzodiazepines. If we wish to screen for low concentrations of other drugs, we extract a larger volume of blood (2–10 ml) with Amberlite XAD-2. This combination of the two methods thus affords versatility in the efficient extraction of blood samples for drugs.

References

1. Meola, J., and Vanko, M., The use of charcoal in the qualitative and quantitative analysis of drugs. *Clin. Chem.* **18,** 713 (1972). Abstract.

2. Adams, R. F., Drug analysis by simultaneous dual-column GLC. Part I: Very rapid clinical screening for restricted drugs in serum. *Clin. Chem. Newsl.* (published by Perkin-Elmer Corp., Norwalk, Conn. 06856) **4,** 15 (1972).

3. Butler, T. J., Charcoal extraction of drugs from serum/plasma. *Clin. Chem.* **20,** 868 (1974). Abstract.

4. Missen, A. W., and Lewin, J. F., A nonionic resin extraction of drugs in blood. *Clin. Chim. Acta* **53,** 389 (1974).

5. Ehrsson, H., and Knapp, D., Rapid, efficient procedure for extraction of drugs for toxicological analysis. *Clin. Chem.* **20,** 1366 (1974).

6. Howard, A. G., Nickless, G., and Hailey, D. M., A rapid gas chromatographic method for the determination of diazepam and metabolites in body fluids. *J. Chromatogr.* **90,** 325 (1974).

7. Beharrell, G. P., Hailey, D. M., and McLaurin, M. K., Determination of nitrazepam (Mogadon) in plasma by electron capture gas-liquid chromatography. *J. Chromatogr.* **70,** 45 (1972).

8. Masuda, Y., Determination of nitrazepam in blood and urine by gas liquid chromatography. *Jpn. J. Legal Med.* **25,** 445 (1971).

Alan W. Missen

Chemistry Division
Department Scientific & Industrial Research
Private Bag
Petone, New Zealand

Quench-Correction Techniques in Liquid Scintillation

To the Editor:

The paper by Helman et al. (*1*) is long overdue in warning of potential problems caused by improper liquid scintillation quench-correction techniques in the clinical laboratory. The authors' point was well made; the *usual* sample channels ratio and external standard channels ratio methods do not correct for color quenching (the absorption of photons from the scintillator by chemical impurities in the sample).

In their interesting report on the solution to the problem, they proposed two methods of quench approximation: preparation of colored radioactive standards and chemical decolorization of samples.

The preparation of radioactive standards, let alone colored radioactive standards, is an exacting art, which can be performed accurately in perhaps a half-dozen laboratories in the world. Therefore, one would be hard pressed to recomend this technique for routine use in the clinical laboratory.

There are other problems. Standards cannot be sealed adequately in screw-cap vials, so flame-sealed ampoules should be used. Colored samples are bleached quite easily by ordinary sunlight and they become useless in a matter of hours. Radiolysis in solution produces peroxides, which quickly begin to decolorize the standard. The rate of decolorization is directly proportional to the total activity within the sample, and high-activity samples decolorize more rapidly than low-activity samples.

More importantly, there are a number of chromophores and combinations of chromophores of which bilirubin and hemoglobin are only two. Attempts to quantify color quenching by mimicking the sample absorbance spectrum work correctly only if the standard absorbance spectrum precisely matches the sample absorbance spectrum in the sensitive wavelength band of the photomultiplier tube. This would suggest the impractical alternative of preparing a quenched standard set for every sample, by using different amounts of the same serum.

There are, I believe, more realistic alternatives. The safest and most accurate means of color quench correction is internal standardization. Although two counts are required, internal standardization can be made far simpler than decolorization of samples and the preparation of colored standards, by adding standard with a Hamilton manual Repeating Dispenser (PB600-1).

Automated combustion methods that convert biological material to carbon dioxide and water (thus eliminating color quenching) are becoming routine for methods involving tritium. Lesser pulse height analysis, a newer instrumental technique recently described by Ediss et al. (*2*), appears very promising.

Proper quench-correction techniques *must* be used in liquid scintillation counting of colored samples in critical radioimmunoassays to ensure against misdiagnoses. Perhaps the emerging trend toward "gamma" labeled haptens will render further discussions on the point moot.

References

1. Helman, E. Z., Spiehler, V., and Holland, S., Elimination of error caused by hemolysis and bilirubin-induced color quenching in clinical radioimmunoassays. *Clin. Chem.* **20,** 1187 (1974).

2. Ediss, C., Noujaim, A. A., and Wiebe, L. Lesser pulse height analysis in liquid scintillation counting. In *Liquid Scintillation Counting: Recent Developments,* P. E. Stanley and B. A. Scoggins, Eds., Academic Press, New York, N. Y., 1974, pp 91–101.

Kent Painter

Dept. of Radiology and Radiation Biology
Colorado State University and Micromedic Diagnostics, Inc.
Fort Collins, Colo. 80523

The first author of the paper in question responds as follows:

To the Editor:

Data given in our paper (ref. *1* above) showed excellent recoveries of digoxin and T-3 uptake values when hemolyzed or jaundiced samples were corrected for quench by External Standard Channels Ratio *or* decolorization methods as described.

Radiolysis was not found to be a problem at the activity levels used.

Data in the papers supported the use of only one chromophore (hemoglobin) to make a general daily quench series for quench correction. It is not necessary that the spectra of the sample and quench standards be the same. The absolute concentrations of the bilirubin and hemoglobin in the quench standards do not have to be constant, just so the desired curve range of ESCR numbers is obtained and, of course, the standards must be run along with each batch of patients' samples.

Neither internal standardization nor combustion methods are practical for the clinical laboratory. While we did not make this comparison, it might be valuable to study results obtained when aliquots of patients' samples are corrected for quench as we described and as proposed by Dr. Painter.

Edith Zak Helman
Executive Editor
Radioassay News

P. O. Box 4546
Anaheim, Calif. 92803

Use of an Inhibitor in Kinetic Determination of Glucose with a Centrifugal Analyzer by the Glucose Dehydrogenase Reaction

To the Editor:

We recently (*1*) proposed a method for the kinetic determination of glucose with a centrifugal analyzer. Using the same enzyme preparation, Müller-Matthesius (*2*) proposed the addition of competitive inhibitors to increase the sensitivity of the reaction. We therefore investigated whether this could improve our reaction conditions. The influence of adding 410 mmol of potassium thiocyanate was studied. A Lineweaver–Burk plot indicated competitive inhibition and the Michaelis constant increased about 1.5-fold. With this inhibitor concentration, 3 mmol of NAD^+, and 500 mg (~ 900 U) of glucose-dehydrogenase per liter of Tris buffer (200 mmol, pH 7.8), the linearity of the reaction improved considerably. The deviation from linearity at 5 g of glucose per liter was now only 3.2% and the factor KT used previously by us (*1*) to correct for nonlinearity was reduced from 326 to 86. The method can now be used without this correction up to quite high glucose concentrations. Even with the correction for nonlinearity this modification has the advantage over the previously described method that the variation at higher substrate concentrations is slightly smaller because the error in measuring the standard absorption is less magnified by the quadratic term of the equation for linearity correction. This is clearly demonstrated in Figure 1, where the same analytical results were used for the calculation of the coefficient of variation with and without linearity corrections. The disadvantage, however, is that the shelf-life of the reagent is reduced. Potassium thiocyanate may be added to the buffer without any noticeable effect on stability for weeks, but the glucose dehydrogenase and the NAD^+ should be added immediately before use. This modification therefore seems to have its place where no correction for nonlinearity is or can be performed.

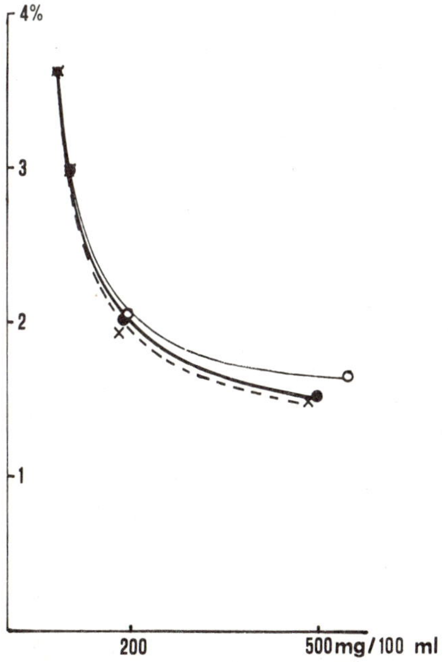

Fig. 1. Day-to-day coefficient of variation as a function of substrate concentration
X - - - X: Monitrol I, Qualtrol, Monitrol II, and 500 mg glucose in 100 ml of aqueous solution without correction for nonlinearity; ●—●: same samples, but corrected for nonlinearity by using a KT of 86 as previously described (*1*); O—O: same samples, but corrected for nonlinearity by using a KT of 326. Each point represents a mean of 20 measurements

References

1. Lutz, R. A., and Flückiger, J., Kinetic determination of glucose with the GEMSAEC (ENI) centrifugal analyzer by the glucose dehydrogenase reaction and comparison with two commonly used procedures. *Clin. Chem.* **21**, 1372 (1975).

2. Müller-Matthesius, R., Enzymkinetische Glucosebestimmung nach der Glucose-Dehydrogenase-Methode. *Z. Klin. Chem. Klin. Biochem.* **13**, 187 (1975).

R. A. Lutz

Laboratory Dr. Otto Lutz AG
Graben 35
CH-8402 Winterthur
Switzerland

Evaluation of the Chemical Activation Procedure (Rao's Method) for the Measurement of the MB Isoenzyme of Creatine Kinase

To the Editor:

I have compared the Calbiochem "CPK/MB" method, which is based on the method of Rao (*1*) et al., with a modification of the column-chromatographic procedure of Mercer (*2*). In the latter procedure the MM isoenzyme of CK is eluted with three 5.0-ml volumes of the buffer for MM. The MB isoenzyme is then eluted with two 2.5-ml volumes of the buffer for MB. The MB fractions were kinetically assayed with a LKB 8600 Reaction Rate Analyzer, with use of creatine phosphate to initiate the reaction. The Calbiochem CPK/MB procedure was performed according to the manufacturer's instructions, with use of a Beckman Model 24 spectrophotometer and recorder. All assays were done at 37 °C. The blood samples were specimens for which CK-MB activity measurements were requested. The normal range for CK-MB by the column method is 0–5 U/liter (*3*) and for the Calbiochem method 0–17 U/liter (*4*). The normal range for total CK by the Calbiochem method is 9–138 U/liter (*4*).

The correlation between results by the column method (x) and the Rao method (y) was poor ($n = 46, r = 0.4258, y = 1.88x + 56$). Two samples that had been treated with dithiothreitol gradually became turbid when they were added to the reagents, resulting in erroneously high values for activity. This was demonstrated on the recorder by a gradual decrease in activity with time (decrease in rate of turbidity formation). With one sample this phenomenon was time dependent. For example, when assayed immediately after treatment with dithiothreitol, no turbidity was observed and the MB activity was 30 U/liter. However, after a 2-h incubation at room temperature in the presence of dithiothreitol, turbidity was observed and the MB activity was 120 U/liter. No turbidity was observed in samples not treated with dithiothreitol.

An additional five samples gave negative results by the Rao method, ranging from −5 U/liter to −20 U/liter.

Because of the strong diagnostic implication of abnormally high MB isoenzyme activity, I strongly urge that more studies be done comparing the method of Rao et al. with established procedures for determining the activity of the MB isoenzyme before this method is accepted for routine use.

References

1. Rao, P. S., Lukes, J. J., Ayres, S. M., and Mueller, H., New manual and automated method for determining activity of creatine kinase isoenzyme MB, by use of dithiothreitol: Clinical applications. *Clin. Chem.* **21**, 1612 (1975).

2. Mercer, D. W., Simultaneous separation of serum creatine kinase and lactate dehydrogenase isoenzymes by ion-exchange column chromatography. *Clin. Chem.* **21**, 1102 (1975).

3. Unpublished data (this laboratory).

4. Calbiochem CPK/MB package insert, October 1, 1975.

R. M. Balkcom

UCLA Hospital Clinical Laboratories
Clinical Chemistry Section
The Center for the Health Sciences
Los Angeles, Calif. 90024

Ed. note: In a paper to be presented at the forthcoming AACC National Meeting, Mercer concludes that the Selective Actuating technique cannot distinguish cardiac and noncardiac conditions, and therefore "cannot provide a specific measurement of the cardiac CK-MB isoenzyme."

To the Editor:

Recently Rao et al. (*1*) reported a differential activation method for determining the activity of creatine kinase isoenzyme MB, with glutathione and dithiothreitol as activators. Their contention was that glutathione did not activate isoenzyme MB when it was present in a mixture with MM, whereas dithiothreitol fully activated MB and MM under all conditions; and thus the activity of MB could be determined as the difference in activities of specimens activated first with glutathione and then with dithiothreitol. Using an automated enzyme analyzer, this approach appeared to offer substantial savings in time over other methods for determining MB activity, and we therefore attempted to evaluate its merits with the idea of replacing the more time-consuming ion-exchange method of Mercer (*2*) that we were currently using. Unfortunately, we found the differential activation approach to be totally lacking in specificity with respect to isoenzymes MM and MB, and the results we obtained indicate that it is highly doubtful that MB activity is being measured at all.

Creatine kinase assays are routinely performed in our laboratory on a Perkin-Elmer KA-150 enzyme analyzer at 30 °C by a modified Oliver procedure (*3*) similar to the one used by Rao et al. Reagent kits with (A) and without (B) dithiothreitol added were obtained from the Perkin-Elmer Corporation and reconstituted with the appropriate volume of a 9 mmol/liter solution of reduced glutathione instead of water. Several specimens were then analyzed for MB activity according to the approach of Rao et al., by ion-exchange chromatography according to the method of Mercer (*2*), and by electrophoresis according to the method of Elevitch (*4*). Table 1 compares the results from these studies. Patients 1–5 had normal electrocardiograms and no history of heart trouble, while patients 6–8 had abnormal electrocardiograms and were thought to have had myocardial infarctions within the previous 24 hours. As can be seen from Table 1, ion-exchange chromatography and electrophoresis clearly distinguish these two groups, whereas the differential activation method does not. Although we confirmed the finding that the MB isoenzyme is fully activated by glutathione when not mixed with MM, we also found that isoenzymes BB and MM were only partly activated in the pure state by 9 mmol/liter glutathione. It would seem from these findings that MM and not MB is being differentially activated when the two isoenzymes are present together in a mixture, and that what is being attributed to MB activity is actually the difference in the MM activities. Why isoenzymes MM and BB are only partially activated by glutathione may have to do with rates of reactivation rather than the redox potentials of the activators as ascribed to by Rao et al. In a recent study of the reactivation of creatine kinase by thiol compounds, Miyada et al. (*5*) found, using various concentrations of glutathione, that linearity could be obtained without attaining maximum enzymatic activity, and they speculated that the lower creatine kinase activities observed at the lower glutathione concentrations were due either to exhaustion of the thiol activator or the attainment of an active–inactive enzyme equilibrium. Rao et al. also mentioned this phenomenon in picking 8.7–9.7 mmol of glutathione per liter as the optimum range for activating MB. The fact that their "MB" activity decreased as the glutathione concentration was increased up to 20 mmol/liter can thus be explained as more complete activation of the MM isoenzyme. Whatever the reason for these differences, however, our results indicate that differences in creatine kinase activity when glutathione and dithiothreitol as activators should not be ascribed to "MB" activity.

Table 1. Comparison of Creatine Kinase Isoenzyme MB Activities, U/liter[a]

Specimen	Glutathione only (B)	Glutathione plus DTT (A)	Apparent MB level[b]	% MB by ion-exchange[c]	MB by electro-phoresis[d]
Pure MM[e]	444	509	65 (13%)	0	(−)
Pure MM[e]	277	313	36 (12%)	0	(−)
Pure MM[e]	40	48	8 (17%)	0	(−)
Pure MB[f]	40	43	—	100	(+)
Pure MB[f]	28	26	—	100	(+)
Pure MB[f]	11	12	—	100	(+)
Pure BB[g]	393	550	—	0	(−)
Pure BB[g]	310	400	—	0	(−)
Pure BB[g]	140	175	—	0	(−)
Patient 1	238	280	42 (15%)	0	(−)
Patient 2	318	450	132 (29%)	0	(−)
Patient 3	590	680	90 (13%)	0	(−)
Patient 4	200	227	27 (12%)	0	(−)
Patient 5	460	525	65 (12%)	0	(−)
Patient 6	420	450	30 (7%)	20	(+)
Patient 7	650	756	106 (14%)	10	(+)
Patient 8	481	530	49 (9%)	18	(+)

[a] Coefficient of variation less than 5%
[b] Defined by Rao et al. as A − B (not defined for pure MB or BB)
[c] By the method of Mercer (*2*)
[d] By the method of Elevitch (*4*)
[e] Isolated from skeletal muscle
[f] Isolated from myocardium and fractionated by ion-exchange chromatography
[g] Isolated from brain tissue

References

1. Rao, P. S., Lukes, J. J., Ayres, S. M. and Mueller, H. S., New manual and automated method for determining activity of creatine kinase isoenzyme MB, by use of dithiothreitol: Clinical applications. *Clin. Chem.* **21**, 1612 (1975).
2. Mercer, D. W., Separation of tissue and serum creatine kinase isoenzymes by ion-exchange column chromatography. *Clin. Chem.* **20**, 36 (1974).
3. Oliver, I. T., Spectrophotometric method for the determination of creatine phosphokinase and myokinase. *Biochem. J.* **61**, 119 (1955).
4. Elevitch, F. R., Isoenzymes. In *Fluorometric Techniques in Clinical Chemistry*, Little, Brown & Co., Boston, 1973, p 244.
5. Miyada, D. S., Dinovo, E. C., and Nakamura, R. M., Creatine kinase reactivation by thiol compounds. *Clin. Chim. Acta* **58**, 97 (1975).

Michael Sheehan
Kenneth Leipper

Dept. of Pathology
School of Medicine
University of California
Davis, Calif. 95616

To the Editor:

A rapid, simple method for determination of serum creatine kinase (CK) isoenzymes was recently described by Rao et al. (*1*). The method, which depends on the selective activation of CK-MB by dithiothreitol, is the basis of the "CPK/MB Stat-Pack" reagent kit currently manufactured by Calbiochem. We used Calbiochem's kit (cat. No. 869210) to assay 46 serum samples from coronary-care patients for CK-MM (range, 16–1535 U/liter) and CK-MB (range, 0–280 U/liter). The CK isoenzyme activity on these specimens had previously been determined in our clinical laboratory by discontinuous gradient elution from micro-columns of DEAE-Sephadex A-50, as described by Yasmineh and Hanson (*2*). In both methods, CK activity was measured by

Table 1. Comparison of CK Isoenzyme Determination on Four Patients' Sera

Specimen No.:	64097		44735		80028		79020	
	MM	MB	MM	MB	MM	MB	MM	MB
	Activity, U/liter							
Calbiochem	1535	280	253	31	522	1	676	0
Discontinuous column chromatography	1307	16	180	2	302	38	472	12
Continuous-gradient elution	1187	12	157	2	386	41	518	12
Electrophoresis: positive or negative for MB band	—	pos	—	neg	—	pos	—	pos

the kinetic method of Rosalki (*3*) with a centrifugal analyzer.

The CK-MM activities by the two methods correlated fairly well, as desibed by a simple regression equation of $y = 0.820x - 20.40$ (y = isoenzyme separation by discontinuous column chromatography, x = Calbiochem kit) and a correlation coefficient (r) of 0.989. CK-MB isoenzyme activities did not compare well ($y = 0.057x + 5.67$, $r = 0.403$). The data on four samples on which the correlation was very poor was confirmed by conventional electrophoresis on cellulose acetate and isoenzyme separation by continuous gradient elution from DEAE-Sephadex A-50 (*2*), and is shown in Table 1. The results clearly indicate that there is good correlation between the latter two methods and our clinical laboratory method, while the correlation with the Calbiochem method is very poor.

References

1. Rao, P. S., Lukes, J. J., Ayres, S. M., and Mueller, H. S., New manual and automated method for determining activity of creatine kinase isoenzyme MB, by use of dithiothreitol: Clinical applications. *Clin. Chem.* **21**, 1612 (1975).

2. Yasmineh, W. G., and Hanson, N. Q., Electrophoresis on cellulose acetate and chromatography on DEAE-Sephadex A-50 compared in the estimation of creatine kinase isoenzymes. *Clin. Chem.* **21**, 381 (1975).

3. Rosalki, S. B., An improved procedure for serum creatine phosphokinase determination. *J. Lab. Clin. Med.* **69**, 696 (1967).

B. K. Hultman
W. G. Yasmineh

Dept. of Lab. Med. and Pathol.
Univ. of Minn. Hospital
Minneapolis, Minn. 55455

To the Editor:

We have assayed one or more specimens from 23 patients in the Coronary Care Units at Abbott Hospital, Minneapolis, Minnesota, and St. Francis Hospital, Shakopee, Minnesota, for CK-MB activity by [the Rao et al.] technique. Enzyme activity was determined on an Abbott ABA-100 chemistry analyzer, according to the recommended procedure. Some of the specimens were also assayed by a modified Worthington DEAE Sephadex A-50 column method for CK isoenzymes. This modified method has been shown to agree closely with the column method of Yasmineh and Hanson (*2*). By this method, values of CK-MB activity greater than 3% of total activity are considered diagnostic of myocardial infarction. We find excellent clinical correlation with this test. Column eluates were also assayed on the ABA-100.

Twelve of our patients had myocardial infarcts documented by electrocardiogram findings, lactate dehydrogenase isoenzyme patterns, and clinical impression. All but one of these patients had an increase of "CPK/MB" above 15 U/liter. The exceptional case was represented by only one specimen, so that the peak value might have been missed. However, the result is interpreted as falsely negative for CK-MB, since the patient had a CK-MB value of 14.3% by the column method. The data are shown in Table 1, which lists the highest values of "CK/MB" where multiple specimens were obtained. Where available, Worthington column results and the qualitative results by agarose electrophoresis on the same specimens are also shown.

Eleven patients did not have myocardial infarction as assessed by EKG, LDH isoenzymes, or clinical impression. Of these, seven had elevation of "CPK/MB" above 15 U/liter by the DTT method. Of the others, one had very low total CK activity and three were in the 10–15 U/liter borderline range of "CPK/MB". All seven patients with values above 15 U/liter would have received a diagnosis of myocardial infarction had reliance been placed on the DTT test. All other tests for CK-MB in these patients were negative. The data are shown in Table 2.

Table 1. Results in Myocardial Infarction

Total CK DTT	"CPK/MB" DTT	% MB, column	MB electrophoresis
237	39	9.4	
434	29	3.6	
63	9	7.0	
881	33		Positive
425	28	6.4	Positive
335	26		Positive
303	27		Positive
369	67		
657	24		
348	61	7.2	
397	41	10.3	
333	27	8.5	

If the DTT method were measuring the MB fraction that is found by column methods, one would expect close numerical correlation between the two types of methods. The comparative values are shown in Table 3, in terms of percent of total activity. Linear regression analysis of these data, with the DTT values in the abscissa and the column method in the ordinate, indicate a slope of −0.155 and a y-intercept of 6.914. The coefficient of correlation is −0.224. This treatment of the data indicates a very poor correlation in percent of MB activity by the two methods.

Our data also indicate a poor correlation between the DTT method and the clinical status of the patient, since in 23 cases we found one false-negative and seven false-positive results. We had nearly twice as many false positives as true negative or borderline cases among the patients without myocardial infarction.

Because the method is so simple to perform, it is anticipated that many laboratories will consider its use. I suggest that they evaluate the method carefully, with particular attention to the clinical findings in the patient and to the problem of false-positive results before adopting it as a routine test.

I am indebted to Brenda J. Spitzer, M.T.(ASCP) for technical assistance in this work.

Table 2. Results in Patients without Myocardial Infarction

Total CK DTT	"CPK/MB" DTT	% MB, column	MB electro-phoresis	Diagnosis
925	56		Negative	Pulmonary embolism
112	13		Negative	Healed MI, no recent change
22	1		Negative	Angina
249	14			Post-exercise
8880	500		Negative	Contusions, pneumonia
3060	400	1.3		Acetabular fracture
480	46	1.0		CVA
400	49	2.0		Hypoglycemic coma
90	21	2.0		Congestive failure, arrhythmia
51	11	1.4		Esophagitis
294	44	2.5		Overdose

Table 3. CK-MB (%) by DTT and Column Methods

DTT	16.0	6.7	14.3	11.8	17.5	10.2	13.0
Column	9.4	3.6	7.0	6.4	7.2	10.3	1.3
DTT	12.0	9.5	23.4	15	21	8	
Column	1.0	2.0	2.0	2.5	1.4	8.5	

References

1. Rao, P. S., Lukes, J. J., Ayres, S. M., and Mueller, H., New manual and automated method for determining activity of creatine kinase isoenzyme MB by use of dithiothreitol: Clinical applications. *Clin. Chem.* **21**, 1612 (1975).

2. Yasmineh, W. G., and Hanson, N. Q., Electrophoresis on cellulose acetate and chromatography on DEAE Sephadex A-50 compared in the estimation of creatine kinase isoenzymes. *Clin. Chem.* **21**, 381 (1975).

F. Muschenheim

Pathology Dept.
Abbott Hospital
Minneapolis, Minn. 55403

Ed. note: These letters were preceded by a letter from Dr. Leo G. Morin (VA Hospital, Atlanta), dated August 5, 1975, in which much the same criticisms were leveled at the usefulness of the Calbiochem kit based on this paper. A correspondence ensued among the affected parties in an effort to resolve these questions before publishing Dr. Morin's letter, but as yet (April 10) no mutually agreeable and completely satisfactory solution has been reached, to our knowledge, and studies are still in progress. We anticipate that a letter commenting on this will appear in our next issue.

The authors of the paper in question respond:

To the Editor:

In reply to the preceding four letters, most of the discrepancies observed using the dithiothreitol method for CK-MB determination can be explained on the basis of the following requirements. Since the publication of our paper [*Clin. Chem.* **21**, 1612 (1975)], we found that special care should be taken regarding condition of the serum, activators used, storage conditions, etc., and we recommend the following criteria for best use of the method.

1. Based on broad experience with the ABA-100 we agree [that it is best] not to use the dithiothreitol method with any automated enzyme analyzers at the present time (Hultman, Sheehan, and Muschenheim). Many parameters—including higher sensitivity of instrumentation, variability of values of same serum analyzed on the manual spectrophotometer and ABA-100, probably caused by improper and unreliable mixing, and different lag times—result in big variations of normal expected values (−15 to +35 U/liter) and irreproducible CK activities (Hultman, Table 1, CK-MM). Presently we are looking into appropriate changes in assay medium and instrumentation that are needed to make this method available for routine use with the ABA-100.

2. The condition of the serum and sample handling are important when using the dithiothreitol method. None of the preceding letters mentioned condition of the serum used for CK-assay. (*a*) For best results, samples must be assayed immediately or within 48 h after separation of serum from the clot. (*b*) If CK-MB is inactivated below 50% of its initial activity because of excessive storage time or extreme temperature (−20 °C), it cannot be reactivated by addition of dithiothreitol, whereas other methods show positive CK-MB (Hultman, specimens 80028 and 79020). Serum should be stored at 4 °C and never be frozen. (*c*) We do not recommend incubation of serum with dithiothreitol. If incubation is necessary, it should be at 4 °C and not at 25 °C (Balkcom). In our experience, CK-MM and -MB are stable within 5% when incubated with or without dithiothreitol for 0 and 3 h at 4 °C in most sera ($n = 32$). However, sera that are deeply colored, even when fresh, lipemic, turbid, heat inactivated, and hemolyzed, can react with dithiothreitol (2.2%, $n = 1800$), giving falsely elevated positive CK-MB values. With the aforementioned sera and where storage conditions are unknown, one additional measurement of serum containing dithiothreitol (blank correction) should be done routinely using an assay medium that contains no creatine phosphate (Calbiochem Kit Nos. 869215 and 869247). This may possibly explain the false-positive CK-MB values reported by Muschenheim (Table 2, Total CK 300; Table 3, DTT values). It also corrects for any false MB elevation from turbidity in the assay medium during a kinetic run.

3. Expected values: We find the range of expected values for the CK-MB, with the dithiothreitol method, is −15 to +20 U/liter; this explains the negative CK-MB values found occasionally (1.1%, $n = 1800$) and observed by Balkcom. This is due to different lag times for the coupled enzyme reaction (with dithiothreitol very little lag time; without dithiothreitol in serum, lag time varies between 6–12 min depending on serum CK concentration), and may also be due to oxidation of glutathione in the reagent kit upon storage. Because of precision differences in each laboratory, and because the expected range will vary with instrumentation, each laboratory is advised to establish its own expected value range. Below total CK ≤300 U/liter (CK-MB ≤25 U/liter), where the method is not reliable, the data should be confirmed by electrophoresis to avoid false CK-MB values (Muschenheim, Table 1, false negative; Table 2, false positive). As a matter of routine, we confirm and check all dithiothreitol measurements for CK-MB (both serial and random samples) in our laboratory by electrophoretic visualization, and recommended this procedure.

4. In our experience, CK-MM and -MB from physiological human serum behave differently to dilution, heat, and reactivation compared to prepared mixtures of isolated MM and MB added to either inactivated human serum or 10 mmol/liter Tris buffer. We recommend that serum should not be diluted at all (Hultman), but instead appropriate amounts (10 to 100 μl) should be used to

obtain the true CK values and the temperature should be kept at 30 °C-(Balkcom). The CK-MB activities obtained with the dithiothreitol method are expected to be higher compared to both electrophoresis (appreciable losses owing to removal and reaction of CK from the strip prior to complete elution, resulting in kinetic assay outside the optimal linear range of the actual enzyme measurement) and column chromatography (with Worthington columns, incomplete separation of CK-MB, and part of MB, 12–15%, measured as BB; Muschenheim, Table 3). However, the dithiothreitol method compares well with electrophoretic quantitation where the strips are first eluted into an assay medium that does not contain creatine phosphate, but later added for kinetic assay.

5. We emphasize that Sheehan and Leipper do not follow our method at all (they have dithiothreitol in their reagent kit instead of adding it to the serum), and hence the results and conclusions are not pertinent. We specifically recommended that dithiothreitol should be added to serum and not to the reagent kit. Furthermore, the amount of glutathione added is specific for the Calbiochem kit. If other kits are used (Sheehan and Leipper) the optimal concentration of glutathione in the assay medium should be individually established and tested with human CK-MM (the activation by dithiothreitol added to serum should be within 5%, if any; Table 1, their data). Further, dithiothreitol used should be pure and not oxidized ($\epsilon_{240\ nm}$ = 62 liter mol^{-1} cm^{-1} at pH 6.8). With regard to their contention that dithiothreitol only reactivated CK-MM, we have repeatedly shown that inactivated human CK-MB (stored for 24 h at 4 °C) can be quantitatively reactivated by dithiothreitol (n = 40) as long as inactivation is ≥50% of initial activity. Glutathione does not reactivate the inactivated CK-MB but only CK-MM.

We understand that Calbiochem has recently devised a new, refined CK-MB reagent kit incorporating the various changes and taking into account the above criteria.

Parinam S. Rao
Hiltrud S. Mueller

Division of Cardiology
Department of Internal Medicine
St. Louis University Medical School
St. Louis, Mo. 63104

Interference in Drug Screening Assays

To the Editor:

In the course of examination of biological fluids for unknown drug ingestion in overdose cases, several urine samples were found to contain significant concentrations (up to 30 mg/l) of lignocaine [lidocaine]. The extraction procedure was as follows: Urine was made basic with solid sodium carbonate and extracted with ether. The organic phase was back-extracted with 1.8 mol/liter sulfuric acid and the acid made basic with sodium carbonate and extracted with ether. The organic phase was taken to dryness, 100 μl of ethanol added, and the solution gas chromatographed, with a temperature program of 150 °C isothermal for 2 min, increasing the temperature at 8 °C per min to 290 °C and then holding. The column used was a 1.2 m × 4 mm i.d. 3% OV 17 on Gas Chrom Q.

When the positive lignocaine results were reported, investigation showed that these patients had been in a comatose state upon admission into hospital and that the urine samples had been taken by catheter. In the normal method of catheterization it was found that 10 ml of Xylocaine jelly (2% lignocaine hydrochloride) was used as both a local anesthetic and as a lubricant. It appears that this can contaminate the first urine samples taken, thus accounting for the high values obtained.

Events such as this emphasize the close contact necessary between analysts and clinicians, as false results may possibly result in erroneous treatment of the patient. Further data on values obtained, duration of excretion, and its significance will be reported at a later date.

L. P. Hackett
L. J. Dusci

State Health Laboratory Services
Perth Medical Centre
Shenton Park, Western Australia

More on Adjusting Serum Ca for Protein

To the Editor:

The letter by Pain and Phillips (*1*) criticizing our paper (*2*) was based on their claim that the regression coefficients for serum calcium on albumin vary so widely among people that the use of an "average" regression coefficient to adjust serum calcium is incorrect. This conclusion was derived from their study published recently (*3*).

Although it is not our wish to prolong this correspondence, we regard adjustment of serum calcium for protein not as an academic exercise, but as a matter of considerable clinical importance. For this reason we feel that your readers would be interested in the correspondence to the Editor of the *British Medical Journal* (*4–7*) that has resulted from the publication of the above paper (*3*). To date, all the authors of these letters have disagreed with the criticisms advanced by Pain and Phillips.

References

1. Pain, R. W., and Phillips, P. J., Adjustment of serum calcium for protein. *Clin. Chem.* **22,** 282 (1976).
2. Husdan, H., Rapoport, A., Locke, S., and Oreopoulos, D., Effect of venous occlusion of the arm on the concentration of calcium in serum, and methods for its compensation. *Clin. Chem.* **20,** 529 (1974).
3. Pain, R. W., Rowland, K. M., Phillips, P. J., and Duncan, B. McL., Current "corrected" calcium concept challenged. *Br. Med. J.* **iv,** 617 (1975).
4. Payne, R. B., Little, A. J., Williams, R. B., and Milner, J. R., "Corrected" calcium concept. *Br. Med. J.* **i,** 153 (1976).
5. Webster, D., "Corrected" calcium concept. *Br. Med. J.* **i,** 154 (1976).
6. Ramsay, L. E., and Shelton, J. R., "Corrected" calcium concept. *Br. Med. J.* **i,** 219 (1976).
7. Hodkinson, H. M., "Corrected" calcium concept. *Br. Med. J.* **i,** 219 (1976).

Harry Husdan
Abraham Rapoport
Sandra Locke
Dimitrios Oreopoulos

Departments of Medicine and Clinical Biochemistry
University of Toronto and Metabolic-Renal Unit and
Laboratory of the Toronto Western Hospital
Toronto, Ontario, Canada M5T 2S8

To the Editor:

Letters have recently appeared in your columns discussing the adjustment of total serum calcium to take account of changes in protein concentration (*1, 2*). Husdan et al. (*3*) had advocated that any adjustment should be based on the mean regression coefficient of serum calcium on total protein. However, Pain and Phillips (*1*) preferred a regression coefficient based on albumin, and also recommended that *individual* regression coefficients of calcium on albumin should be determined for each patient by using sequential specimens obtained during venous occlusion (*1, 4*).

We have investigated the relationship between calcium and total protein, and between calcium and albumin, in specimens from 200 patients with a very wide range of abnormalities of protein concentration but who were likely to have had a low prevalence of disorders of calcium homeostasis (*5*). We found that adjustments based on total protein gave a wide range of calcium values that were particularly low in patients with hypergammaglobulinemia. However, an adjustment based on our average regression coefficient of calcium on albumin, 1.0 mg of calcium per gram of albumin (25 μmol/g), gave an adjusted range of calcium values in the 200 patients identical with our normal range. We therefore agree with Pain and Phillips' recommendation that albumin rather than total protein should be used to adjust calcium concentration.

We cannot agree with Pain and Phillips' second proposal that an individual's *own* rather than an *average* regression coefficient should be used (*1, 4*). It is based on the finding of individual regression coefficients ranging from 0.28 to 2.22 mg of calcium per gram of albumin (7–53 μmol/g) in posture and tourniquet experiments (*4, 6, 7*). We have given elsewhere our reasons for believing that this range of values is highly improbable, and that Pain and his colleagues have paid insufficient attention to the effect of analytical precision on individual regression coefficients (*8*). The smaller the change induced in albumin concentration, and therefore in calcium concentration, the larger will be the standard error of the regression coefficient. This has been demonstrated in a computer simulation by Hodgkinson (*9*). However, a striking feature of the individual regression coefficient data is that the overall median value is 1.0 mg of calcium per gram of albumin (25 μmol/g), a value identical with the overall regression coefficient we derived from our study on patients (*5*). This is illustrated in Figure 1.

A criticism of the use of an average regression coefficient is that patients with high or low values for ionized calcium would have higher or lower regression coefficients (*10, 11*). However, adjustment gives values that are higher than they should be when ionized calcium is high and lower when it is low (*12*). It thus fulfills its intended function, that of a screening procedure to detect patients who need further investigation of calcium homeostasis.

We therefore recommend that albumin rather than total protein should be used to adjust calcium concentration, and that the *average* regression coefficient of 1.0 mg calcium per gram of albumin should be retained.

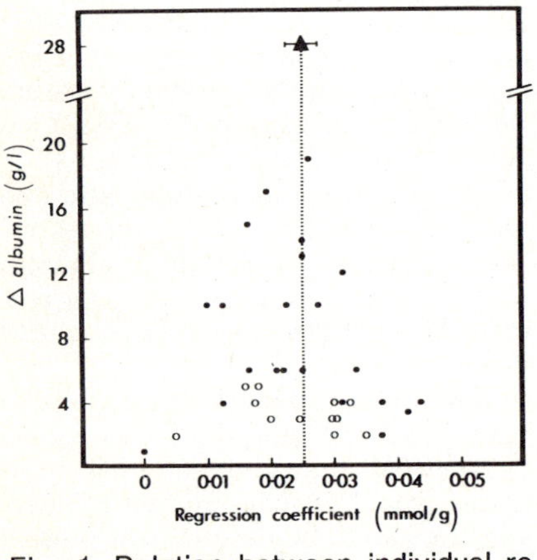

Fig. 1. Relation between individual regression coefficients and changes in serum albumin induced by posture (*open circles*) (*11*) and tourniquet (filled circles) (*12*)

The *dotted line* is the median value determined by Pain et al. (*4*) and the *triangle* at the top is the average regression coefficient ±2 SE determined by Payne et al. (*5*) for 200 patients with albumin values ranging from 20 to 48 g/liter. (Reproduced by kind permission of the Editor of the *British Medical Journal*)

References

1. Pain, R. W., and Phillips, P. J., Adjustment of serum calcium for protein. *Clin. Chem.* **22,** 282 (1976). Letter to the Editor.
2. Husdan, H., Rapoport, A., Locke, S., and Oreopoulos, D., Adjustment of serum calcium for protein. *Clin. Chem.* **22,** 282 (1976). Reply to *1*.
3. Husdan, H., Rapoport, A., Locke, S. and Oreopoulos, D., Effect of venous occlusion of the arm on the concentration of calcium in serum, and methods for its compensation. *Clin. Chem.* **20,** 529 (1974).
4. Pain, R. W., Rowland, K. M., Phillips, P. J., and Duncan, B. McL., Current "corrected" calcium concept challenged. *Br. Med. J.* **iv,** 617 (1975).
5. Payne, R. B., Little, A. J., Williams, R. B., and Milner, J. R., Interpretation of serum calcium in patients with abnormal serum proteins. *Br. Med. J.* **iv,** 643 (1973).
6. Pedersen, K. O., On the cause and degree of intra-individual serum calcium variability. *Scand. J. Clin. Lab. Invest.* **30,** 191 (1972).
7. Berry, E. M., Gupta, M. M., Turner, S. J., and Burns, R. R., Variation in plasma calcium with induced changes in plasma specific gravity, total protein and albumin. *Br. Med. J.* **iv,** 640 (1973).
8. Payne, R. B., Little, A. J., Williams, R. B., and Milner, J. R., "Corrected" calcium concept. *Br. Med. J.* **i,** 153 (1976).
9. Hodgkinson, H. M., "Corrected" calcium concept. *Br. Med. J.* **i,** 219 (1976).
10. Parfitt, A. M., Correction of plasma calcium measurements. *Br. Med. J.* **i,** 520 (1974).
11. Marshall, R. W., and Nordin, B. E. C., Adjustment of plasma calcium measurements. *Br. Med. J.* **ii,** 719 (1974).
12. Payne, R. B., Little, A. J., Williams, R. B., and Milner, J. R., Adjustment of plasma calcium measurements. *Br. Med. J.* **iii,** 345 (1974).

R. B. Payne
A. J. Little

Dept. of Chemical Pathology
St. Jame's University Hospital
Leeds LS9 7TF, U. K.

Bilirubin Standard Solutions

To the Editor:

Bilirubin standards prepared in bovine serum albumin (BSA) can be accurately analyzed by the Lathe and Ruthven (*1*) modification of the Malloy–Evelyn (*2*) bilirubin assay. This modification differs from the original in that the diazo reagent is prepared with sulfanilic acid in a concentration of 10 g/liter instead of 1 g/liter, and that the azobilirubin is measured at 560 nm instead of 540 nm. The modifications thus do not change the original method's manipulative simplicity.

Historically, the validity of standards prepared in an albumin matrix was questioned by Doumas et al. (*3*). These authors showed that serum bilirubin concentrations are overestimated by the Malloy–Evelyn method, which uses standards in bovine (BSA) or human serum albumin (HSA), because the molar absorptivity of the azobilirubin in either matrix is about 10% lower than the molar absorptivity in a whole serum base. This error is considered so serious by Doumas et al. that they recommend the Jendrassik–Grof method be substituted for the Malloy–Evelyn method; the former is not susceptible to this error. They would thus change methods to retain the advantages of an albumin standard matrix, which they cite as: (*a*) BSA and HSA contain no detectable bilirubin, (*b*) the resulting bilirubin standard solutions are transparent and not subject to turbidity artifacts after storage, and (*c*) the same protein matrix solutions can be used to dilute stock to working standard concentrations while retaining a constant protein content.

In studying this problem, we prepared stock bilirubin solutions at 202 and 244 mg/liter, using National Bureau of Standards (NBS) bilirubin (SRM No. 916, Office of Standard Reference Materials, Room B311 Chemistry Building, National Bureau of Standards, Washington, D.C. 20234) and either pooled human serum or 5% BSA ("Pentex" Fraction V Bovine Albumin; Research Products Division, Miles Laboratories, Kankakee, Ill. 60901).

Following NBS recommendations, we dissolved the bilirubin in 2.0 ml of 0.1 mol/liter Na_2CO_3 and in 1.5 ml of 0.1 mol/liter NaOH, and adjusted the pH with 0.1 mol/liter HCl to a phenolphthalein endpoint, pH 8.2–10.0. (The exact volume of HCl needed was determined in a separate titration experi-

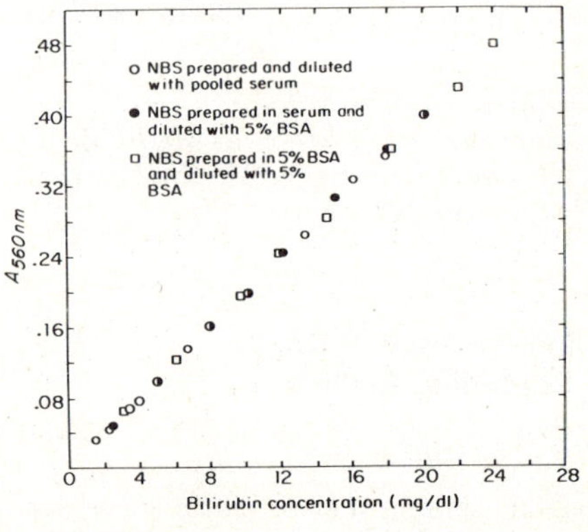

Fig. 1. Comparison of bilirubin standards in three matrices

Table 1. Parameters Obtained from a Linear Regression Analysis of Plots of Absorbance vs. Theoretical Bilirubin Concentration

Solvent for bilirubin	Slope	*Y*-Intercept	Standard error of estimate[a]	Correl. coeff.
Serum	1.99×10^{-2}	2.79×10^{-5}	2.75×10^{-3}	0.9998
BSA (50 g/l)	1.94×10^{-2}	4.90×10^{-3}	2.65×10^{-3}	0.9999
Serum (but diluted with BSA)	2.00×10^{-2}	7.50×10^{-4}	1.78×10^{-3}	0.9999

[a] Refers to the slope of the regression line.

ment.) After the pH of albumin–bilirubin solutions were adjusted, they were diluted to final volume.

From dilutions of these two stock bilirubin solutions, three sets of working standards were prepared: (*a*) the pooled human serum-based concentrate diluted with more human serum, (*b*) the pooled human serum-based concentrate diluted with 5% BSA, and (*c*) the 5% BSA-based concentrate diluted with 5% BSA. The standard curves generated by the Lathe and Ruthven (*1*) assay of these solutions are identical, all points of each concentration assayed agreeing within 3% (Figure 1). The curves are linear and pass through the origin of an absorbance versus bilirubin concentration plot. Table 1 gives the results of a linear regression analysis of these data. The molar absorptivity for azobilirubin, calculated from these data is 1130 ± 60 (range).

We conclude from these data that BSA is a suitable matrix for bilirubin stock and working standards used in the Lathe and Ruthven (*1*) method. Concentrated bilirubin solutions made in human serum may be validly diluted with BSA. This observation is relevant for analysts who wish to calibrate their assay by diluting the commercially prepared lyophilized human serum sold for this purpose.

However, during these experiments, we confirmed the further observation of Doumas et al. (*3*) that such commercial preparations are not acceptable substitutes for primary standards. One such serum, "Versatol Pediatric" (Lot No. 0350034; General Diagnostics, Division of Warner-Lambert Co., Morris Plains, N.J. 07950), was represented by the manufacturer as having a bilirubin concentration of 207 mg/liter, but under our assay conditions it was found to contain only 188 mg/liter. However, once the rated value was corrected to the observed value for this lot number, no subsequent anomalies were encountered. This experience demonstrates that commercial sera used to generate standard curves should be calibrated relative to standards prepared in solutions of BSA, or other suitable primary standards.

References

1. Lathe, G. H., and Ruthven, C. R. J., Factors affecting the rate of coupling of bilirubin and conjugated bilirubin in the Van Den Berg reaction. *J. Clin. Pathol.* **11**, 155 (1958).

2. Malloy, H. T., and Evelyn, K. A., The determination of bilirubin with the photoelectric colorimeter. *J. Biol. Chem.* **119**, 481 (1937).

3. Doumas, B. T., Perry, B. W., Sasse, E. A., and Straumfjord, J. V., Jr., Standardization in bilirubin assays: Evaluation of selected methods and stability of bilirubin solutions. *Clin. Chem.* **19**, 984 (1973).

Arthur M. Zebelman
Margaret A. Kenny
Catherine G. Sunday

Dept. of Laboratory Medicine
University of Washington
School of Medicine
Seattle, Wash. 98195

Effect of Mannitol (Osmitrol) Intoxication on Serum "Triglyceride" Values

To the Editor:

It is well recognized that numerous compounds, drugs and nonspecific chromogens in the blood may affect the determination of serum lipids (*1*). We have recently studied a 70-year-old female patient who was admitted to The Clinic with "Osmitrol" (Travenol Laboratories, Inc., Morton Grove, Ill. 60053) intoxication. Osmitrol (composed of 50–200 g of mannitol per liter) is an osmotic diuretic agent that frequently is administered to renal patients. The patient initially was azotemic and hypokalemic, with symptoms of urinary tract infection. The patient was treated with massive doses of Osmitrol infusion, which led to the lethargic and comatose condition. Further diagnosis indicated that the patient had diabetes mellitus, chronic renal failure, hypertension, severe electrolyte imbalance, and pulmonary congestion. The patient was maintained on renal dialysis for two sessions. The serum total cholesterol and "triglyceride" (glycerol) before dialysis was 0.89 and 9.80 g/liter, respectively.

The serum before renal dialysis was clear, with no evidence of chylomicra or pre-β-lipoprotein particles. This serum description did not agree with the increased "triglyceride" value of 9.80 g/liter. Furthermore, the lipoprotein pattern (Figure 1) did not demonstrate any elevation of the chylomicron or pre-β-lipoprotein band. Therefore, the value appeared to be in error. Serum aldehydes and ketones were in normal concentration. Because mannitol has been used in the past as a primary standard for triglyceride determination (*2*), we evaluated the adsorptive capacity of the zeolite mixture to remove this substance (Figure 2). Only 150 to 200 ml of mannitol per liter can be removed by the 2.0 g of zeolite mixture. Any mannitol concentration exceeding these limits will be measured as glycerol by our method (*3*) of triglyceride analysis, which is based on the Hantzsch reaction for formaldehyde. Mannitol is a hexahydroxy alcohol derived from mannose, which will form formaldehyde to produce the fluorescent compound, 3,5-diacetyl-1,4-dihydrolutidine, for triglyceride determination (*2*). After dialysis treatment the apparent serum triglyceride value decreased to 2.52 g/liter, a value in harmony with the lipoprotein profile of the patient. Total cholesterol was 740 mg/liter.

In conclusion, we have shown that while zeolite mixture can remove some

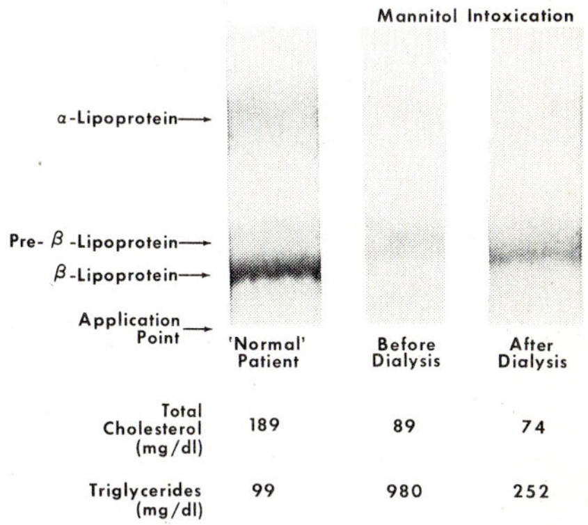

Fig. 1. Patient's lipoprotein pattern and lipid values

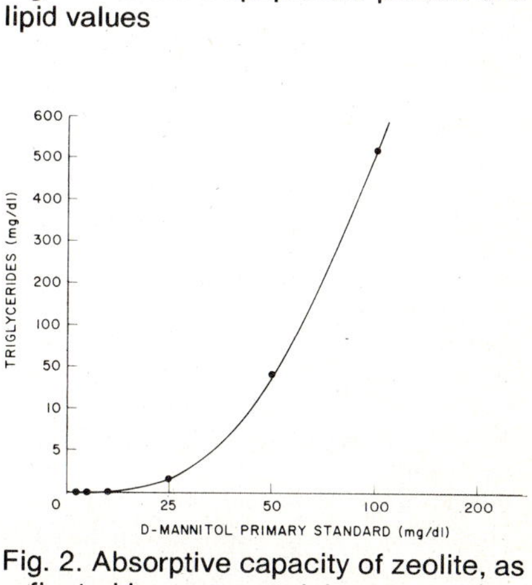

Fig. 2. Absorptive capacity of zeolite, as reflected in apparent triglyceride values

mannitol, excessive mannitol infusion to patients will result in falsely increased "triglyceride" results that will not be compatible with the lipoprotein profile. Under such conditions, true triglycerides can be estimated by running an unsaponified blank sample that will eliminate the free glycerol and mannitol interference of the test.

References

1. Young, D. S., Pestaner, L. C., and Gibberman, V., Effects of drugs on clinical laboratory tests. *Clin. Chem.* **21**, 1D (1975). Special issue.
2. Witter, R. F., and Whitner, V. S., Determination of serum triglycerides. In *Blood Lipids and Lipoproteins: Quantitation, Composition, and Metabolism*, G. J. Nelson, Ed., Wiley-Interscience, New York, N.Y., 1972, pp 75–111.
3. Technicon Autoanalyzer Clinical Method No. 24, Simultaneous Cholesterol and Triglyceride Analyses, Technicon Instruments Corp., Tarrytown, N.Y., 1972.

Herbert K. Naito
Vytenis J. Gatautis

Department of Atherosclerosis and Thrombosis Research, Division of Research; and Department of Biochemistry Division of Laboratory Medicine

Kathryn L. Popowniak

Department of Nephrology and Hypertension
The Cleveland Clinic Foundation
Cleveland, Ohio 44106

Effect of Two New Serum-Separating Devices on Results for Cholesterol and Triglyceride

To the Editor:

Since 1965, the use of many synthetic materials has been introduced to facilitate the separation of serum from the blood clot by (*a*) improving the yield of serum, (*b*) obtaining better separation of the serum from the blood cells, and (*c*) increasing the speed of the serum collection.

It is essential that when using such separator aids, there are no interferences with the analytes that are to be measured in the serum. Essentially, this means that the separatory material should be inert, have no effect on the concentration of the serum of plasma constituents, and not "trap" certain high-molecular-weight protein complexes seen in some disease states (i.e., cryoglobulins, lipoprotein–immune globulin complexes and certain 24S proteins).

Kaplan and Williamson (*1*) showed that when using the semi-automated cholesterol method of Block et al. (*2*) and the triglyceride method of Kessler and Lederer (*3*), there was a slight effect of "Serum Disc" (Whale Scientific, Denver, Colo.) on serum total cholesterol and triglyceride. They indicated a 2% difference in triglycerides and 1.5% difference in cholesterol when compared to the control sera. It was not stated whether the changes were increases or decreases in the samples prepared with "Serum Disc."

Mathies (*4*) evaluated the suitability of a new separatory device, "Sure-Sep" (General Diagnostics, Morris Plains, N.J.), and found that there was no effect of this silicone-polymer–silica barrier complex on serum lipids. This method is based on a container (filled with a semi-solid polymer) that is placed in the top of the blood-drawing tube before centrifugation. The polymer descends through the serum during centrifugation and becomes layered on the blood clot, which then separates the cells from the serum. Mathies reported that procedures for cholesterol (*2*), triglycerides (*5*), phospholipid (*6*, *7*), and total lipid (*6*) were not significantly affected as compared to the conventional method of double centrifugation of the serum samples.

Bernstein reported that using his enzymic assay for serum total cholesterol (*8*) the Sure-Sep technique for separation of serum caused no statistical significant differences when compared to the conventional method of serum separation.

Recently a new serum separation device has been introduced. It is a serum Vacutainer tube, "SST" (Becton-Dickinson, Rutherford, N.J.) which contains a semi-solid silicon-polymers–silica complex. During centrifugation, the silicon complex (relative density, 1.045) takes a position between the clot and the serum because its relative density is intermediate. Furthermore, the silicon complex floats along the side of the walls of the tube, following a course of least resistance to the blood cells, and layers itself at an angle, minimizing the trauma of the centrifugal force on the packed cells.

We compared the effects of these devices, Sure-Sep and SST, on serum total cholesterol and triglyceride determinations. The AutoAnalyzer II procedure for simultaneous determination of cholesterol and triglycerides was used for the study. A modification of the AutoAnalyzer II method (*9*) was run according to the procedure outlined by the Lipid Standardization Laboratory at the Center for Disease Control, Atlanta, Ga., for standardization and certification for total cholesterol and triglyceride determination.

Ninety-five patients were selected without conscious bias for the study; three tubes of blood were obtained from each patient. Serum was obtained in the following way in a random sequence: (*a*) conventional way, by double centrifugation; (*b*) by using Sure-Sep and single centrifugation; and (*c*) by using SST and single centrifugation. The results of the three methods of serum separation on results for lipid concentration are shown in Table 1.

By Students' *t*-test, the samples prepared with the SST showed no significant difference in concentration when compared to the conventional method, but showed a significant ($P < 0.001$) lowering when Sure-Sep was used. Values for triglycerides were 4.3% lower and for total cholesterol 4.2% lower than the values obtained from the serum obtained by the conventional method. The serum samples that were selected covered a triglyceride concentration range of 0.91 to 22.7 g/liter and cholesterol concentration range of 1.56 to 4.40 g/liter. When the difference in values between the Sure-Sep technique and conventional technique was plotted vs. concentration, the correlation coefficients for triglycerides and total cholesterol were 0.19 and 0.33, respectively. This indicates that the degree of decrease in lipid values caused by Sure-Sep was not related to the concentration of the serum lipids. The observed decrease in serum lipid values seen in our study with Sure-Sep is in contrast to the report of Bernstein (*8*) and Mathies (*4*), while our data indicating that the SST method does not interfere with triglyceride and cholesterol determinations agrees with the recent article of Laessig et al. (*10*). Further studies are necessary to fully assess the usefulness of any separator devices including the SST—i.e., the influence of such synthetic barrier complexes on cryoglobulins, macroglobulins, lipid-immunoglobulin complexes, and other high-molecular-weight protein or carbohydrate complexes. It has been our experience that when using Sure-Sep, the silicon-polymer complex will layer itself on the cryoglobulins, thereby "trapping" the cryoglobulins with the clot when the serum is decanted into another tube.

Table 1. Effect of Different Cell-Separation Methods on Serum Lipid Concentration[a]

Method of separation	Triglycerides (g/liter)	Cholesterol (g/liter)
Conventional	1.733 ± 0.130	2.456 ± 0.052
SST	1.744 ± 0.129[b]	2.486 ± 0.053[b]
Sure-Sep	1.658 ± 0.125[c]	2.353 ± 0.049[c]

[a] n = 95 samples
[b] Nonsignificant
[c] $P < 0.001$

Thus, while these unusual protein complexes are rare, they may not be detected when such serum-separator devices are used.

References

1. Kaplan, A., and Williamson, L., Effect on chemical values of using polystyrene beads for serum separation. *Clin. Chem.* **20,** 403 (1974). Letter to the Editor.
2. Block, W. D., Jarrett, K. J., Jr., and Levine, J. B., An improved automated determination of serum total cholesterol with single color reagent. *Clin. Chem.* **12,** 681 (1966).
3. Kessler, G., and Lederer, H., Fluorometric measurement of triglycerides. In *Automation in Analytical Chemistry, Technicon Symposia 1965,* L. T. Skeggs et al., Eds. Mediad Inc., New York, N. Y., 1966, p 341.
4. Mathies, J. C., Evaluation of a new device for rapidly separating serum or plasma from blood. *Clin. Chem.* **20,** 1573 (1974).
5. Soloni, F. G., Simplified manual micromethod for determination of serum triglycerides. *Clin. Chem.* **17,** 529 (1971).
6. Folch, J., Lees, M., and Sloane Stanley, G. H., A simple method for the isolation and purification of total lipids from animal tissues. *J. Biol. Chem.* **191,** 833 (1957).
7. King, E. J., The colorimetric determination of phosphorus. *Biochem. J.* **26,** 292 (1932).
8. Bernstein, R. E., Further use of the Sure-Sep technique for serum-plasma separation. *Clin. Chem.* **22,** 120 (1976). Letter to the Editor.
9. Technicon AutoAnalyzers II. Clinical Method No. 24, Simultaneous Cholesterol/Triglycerides. Technicon Instruments Corp., Tarrytown, N. Y., 1972.
10. Laessig, R. H., Westgard, J. O., Carey, R. N., et al., Assessment of a serum separator device for obtaining serum specimens suitable for clinical analyses. *Clin. Chem.* **22,** 235 (1976).

Herbert K. Naito
Vytenis J. Gatautis

Department of Atherosclerosis and Thrombosis Research
Division of Research, and
Department of Biochemistry
Division of Laboratory Medicine
The Cleveland Clinic Foundation
Cleveland, Ohio 44106

Data Handling and Reporting

To the Editor:

We read with interest the paper by Forrester et al. (*1*). However, inspection of the figures displaying the linearity and the patient comparison data raises several questions relating to data collection and interpretation. The authors are referred to Barnett and Youden (*2*) for the mechanics of methods comparison and Westgard and Hunt (*3*) for the use and interpretation of statistical tests in methods comparison. Westgard and

Hunt (*3*) conclude that least squares is the most useful statistical tool for estimating errors, but warn of limitations caused by nonlinearity, errant points, and a small range of patient values. Also, there should be a reasonably even distribution of the patient values at low, normal, and high ranges (*2*).

The authors present the upper limits of linearity in Table 1. However, inspection of Figure 2 indicates questionable linearity for glucose, calcium, and ALP, and definite nonlinearity for BUN and AST. For example, the authors state the upper limit of linearity for AST to be 900 U/liter. However, there appears to be deviation from linearity above 400 U/liter. If the extreme points had been successively excluded until the four high points had been eliminated then the slope would more closely approach 1 and the intercept 0. Since the nonlinear points are included, AST and BUN curves have proportional errors greater than 10%.

In the patient comparison data presented in Figure 1 there are serious method-comparison problems. There is not a reasonably even distribution of patient values into low, normal, and high ranges. For example, with the glucose data there is a paucity of samples at the low level and only a single point greater than 200 mg/dl even though the stated linearity is to 500 mg/dl. A point at the extreme can in effect act as a lever influencing the slope and intercept of the line. AST and bilirubin illustrate the same problem.

The calcium data illustrate a probable misuse of least-squares analysis. The range is very limited—approximately 6.0–10.4 mg/dl; i.e., there are no elevated calcium values. With such a limited range the 4.4% negative proportional error represented by the slope and the 0.44 mg/dl y intercept may be statistical artifacts. Westgard and Hunt (*3*) demonstrated that slope and intercept show large changes when the data points are restricted to the normal range. In this instance a comparison of the means by t-test may be more useful.

References

1. Forrester, R. L., Collinge, W., Hashimoto, P., and Worrall, J., Evaluation of a discrete-sample computer-directed clinical analyzer. *Clin. Chem.* **22,** 211 (1976).
2. Barnett, R. N., and Youden, W. J., A revised scheme for the comparison of quantitative methods. *Am. J. Clin. Pathol.* **54,** 454 (1970).
3. Westgard, J. O., and Hunt, M. R., Use and interpretation of common statistical tests in method-comparison studies. *Clin. Chem.* **19,** 49 (1973).

L. Brown
R. Feld

Dept. of Pathology
Univ. of Iowa Hospitals and Clinics
Iowa City, Iowa 52242

The authors' response follows:

To the Editor:

We sincerely appreciate this constructive criticism. We erred in not excluding the points beyond the range of linearity from the calculations and graphs presented in Figure 2 of the paper. However, we disagree with the comments regarding the range of linearity of glucose, calcium, ALP, BUN, and AST. Our conclusions were based upon recovery studies, the upper areas of which are presented in Table 1, and acceptability of recovery judged by the same criteria cited by Barnett and Youden (see below)—i.e., the differences between the recovered and the actual values must be within the precision of the method (2 SD) at the appropriate analytical value. In all cases, the differences between the recovered and the actual were within the precision of the method at that level.

We also include the least-squares calculations for calcium, ALP, BUN, and AST linearity after exclusion of those points above which we claim linearity and inclusion of some additional points for ALP and AST. Glucose was acceptable as published. As expected, the slope does more closely approach 1,

Table 1. Recovery Studies

	mg/liter				U/liter		
	Actual	Found	Recovery, %		Actual	Found	Recovery, %
Glucose	3,000	3,040	101.3	ALP	499	521	104.4
	4,000	3,940	98.5		566	576	101.8
	5,000	4,810	96.5		615	618	100.5
					943	947	100.4
Calcium	100	99	99.0				
	125	123	98.4	AST	420	435	103.6
					554	579	104.5
BUN	700	705	100.7		705	680	96.5
	1,000	960	96.0		953	884	92.8
	1,200	1,140	95.0				

except for calcium, and the intercept 0 (Table 2).

We also acknowledge the statistical weakness in the patient comparisons as presented and we are happy to have the opportunity to further substantiate our data. The data presented reflected our patient population only for the duration of a special time period when we were gathering data for the paper. We had previously gathered extensive data, not presented in the paper, which exhibit a much better distribution and wider range of values. We were comfortable with the small patient sampling because of our prior knowledge of the consistent agreement between the manual and the automated procedures in all ranges; we neglected to share our previous data and experience. We have recalculated the data in question, after inclusion of additional values in the low and high ranges, and in each case there is an improvement in the data (Table 3), strengthening our conclusions.

The comments on the calcium data prompted us to expand the comparison data to include some comparisons gathered in our early work with the instrument. The range of values is 59–129 mg/liter with a mean of 91.9 mg/liter; slope, 0.9728; y-intercept, 2.73; r, 0.9753; and n, 86. We also ran a t-test and found t to be 1.19. At the $P = 0.05$ level, t would have to be greater than 2.0 to indicate a significant difference.

We believe the data in the published paper and the additional data presented in this reply support our conclusions; we would, again, like to thank L. Brown and R. Feld for the opportunity to clarify any data that might have been misleading.

Reference

Barnett, R. N., and Youden, W. J., A revised scheme for the comparison of quantitative methods. *Am. J. Clin. Pathol.* **54,** 454 (1970).

Roger L. Forrester
Willa Collinge
Pattie Hashimoto
Jackie Worrall

Clinical Chemistry Laboratory
Mercy San Juan Hospital
Carmichael, Calif. 95608

Increased Purine-Nucleoside Phosphorylase Activity in Erythrocytes of Gouty Patients

To the Editor:

We have studied quantitative and qualitative modifications of purine-nucleoside phosphorylase (purine-nucleoside:orthophosphate ribosyltransferase, EC 2.4.2.1; PNP), in erythrocytes of 24 gouty patients being treated with uricosuric agents and in 30 controls. In

Table 2. Least-Squares Calculations for Linearity

	y-intercept	Slope	r	n
Calcium, mg/liter	4.10	0.9560	0.9991	5
ALP, U/liter	1.04	1.0064	0.9996	12
BUN, mg/liter	11.90	0.9499	0.9995	7
AST, U/liter	4.91	0.9540	0.9975	11

Table 3. Least-Squares Calculations for Patient Comparisons

	Range	Mean	y-intercept	Slope	r	n
Glucose, mg/liter	480–5340	1193	29.307	0.9896	0.9971	61
AST, U/liter	5–579	111.3	1.8334	0.9385	0.9992	58
Bilirubin, mg/liter	3–198	40	0.330	1.0028	0.9989	64

Table 1. Purine-Nucleoside Phosphorylase Activity in Erythrocytes from Normal and Gouty Subjects

		ΔA/min (mean ± SD) at 293 nm		
	No. samples	per g hemoglobin	per 10^9 cells	per ml packed cells
Normal subjects	30	149 ± 13.4	4.6 ± 0.46	47 ± 4.5
Gouty subjects	24	158 ± 12.3	4.9 ± 0.43	54 ± 4.8
P		<0.02	<0.02	<0.01

addition, PNP was determined in a juvenile gouty subject suffering from the Lesch-Nyhan syndrome.

The activity in erythrocytes was determined spectrophotometrically (*1*), and expressed as absorbance change (ΔA) per minute at 293 nm.

The following hematological variables were investigated for each blood sample: erythrocyte count, packed erythrocyte volume, hemoglobin, serum iron, and serum urate concentration (*2*).

Erythrocyte hypoxanthine phosphoribosyltransferase (EC 2.4.2.8; HPT) was also measured (*3*).

Horizontal electrophoresis of lysate on methyl cellulose (Cellogel) was done with use of a phosphate buffer system at pH 7.5 under a constant voltage of 12 V/cm for 1 h, PNP was made visible after electrophoresis, by using a specific mixture (inosine, phenazine methosulfate, nitro blue tetrazolium oxidase), as a single dark blue-purple zone, of mobility greater than A_1 hemoglobin.

The results are summarized in Table 1.

The increase in enzyme activity we observed in gouty patients is significant in whichever unit it is expressed: per gram of hemoglobin, per 10^9 cells, or per milliliter of packed erythrocytes. Evidently the increase is a real one and the conclusion was not biased by an eventual diminution of hemoglobin content or size of erythrocytes.

However, the increase observed was moderate, but significantly different, in comparison with the result obtained by Nishizawa et al. (*4*).

No correlation was found between PNP activity and serum urate concentration, PNP activity, or serum iron concentration.

No modification of the electrophoresis pattern was observed in common gout or HPT-deficient gouty subjects as compared with controls.

In the gouty patient with the Lesch-Nyhan syndrome, the results showed an even greater increase in activity (ΔA/min was 224 per gram of hemoglobin, 6.3 per 10^9 erythrocytes, or 71 per milliliter of packed erythrocytes). This patient had a slight anemia and a decreased serum iron value.

Ramachandran and Iyer (*5*) found a significantly increased PNP activity in erythrocytes of patients with anemia and low serum iron.

These modifications could explain the increase of activity observed in the HPT-deficient subject, but not the one observed in common gouty patients, whose erythrocyte count and serum iron concentration were normal.

Purine metabolism is accelerated in common gouty subjects. The increase of PNP activity we observed could be the result of enhanced activity of an enzymatic system in which PNP is implicated.

This work was supported by the Institut National de la Santé et de la Recherche Médicale.

We thank Dr. Claudine Auscher for her advice.

References

1. Marks, P. A., Red cell glucose-6-phosphate and 6-phosphogluconic dehydrogenase and nucleoside phosphorylase. *Science* **127,** 1338 (1958).

2. Praetorius, E., and Poulsen, H. E., Enzymatic determination of uric acid. *Scand. J. Clin. Lab. Invest.* **5,** 273 (1953).

3. Cartier, P., and Hamet, M., Les activités purine phosphorylase transférasiques dans les globules rouges humains: Technique de dosage. *Clin. Chim. Acta* **20,** 105 (1968).

4. Nishizawa, T., Nishida, Y., Akaoka, I., and Yoshimura, T., Erythrocyte adenosine deaminase and purine nucleoside phosphorylase activity in gout. *Clin. Chim. Acta* **58,** 277 (1975).

5. Ramachandran, M., and Iyer, G. Y. N., Purine nucleoside phosphorylase activity of human erythrocytes in iron deficiency anaemia. *Clin. Chim. Acta* **40,** 281 (1972).

Lucile Gerbaut
Elisabeth Rey
Georges Olive

Laboratoire de Biochimie
Hôpital Saint-Vincent de Paul
74, Avenue Denfert-Rochereau
75674 Paris Cedex 14, France

book reviews

Serum Protein Abnormalities. Diagnostic and Clinical Aspects. S. E. Ritzmann and J. C. Daniels, Ed. Little, Brown and Co., Boston, Mass. 02106, 1975, xxi + 550 pp.

This practical, useful, and timely reference book is a continuation of the *Series in Laboratory Medicine* edited by Leo P. Cawley, M.D. Intended primarily for the clinical pathologist, it will be helpful for clinicians at all stages of training, and can be heartily recommended for the clinical chemist and other laboratory personnel interested in the application of their efforts.

The first part of the book, on Methodology and Interpretation, is heavily weighted toward immunological techniques. Aside from immunochemistry, only protein electrophoresis and ultracentrifugation receive attention. This is understandable, since the authors are recognized experts in immunochemistry. Dr. Ritzmann is the Director for Consultation Laboratories of Behring Diagnostics. The detailed directions given for performing and interpreting methods of growing importance such as radial immunodiffusion and electroimmunodiffusion are welcome. The section on interpretation of electrophoretic patterns is excellent, and includes a useful diagnostic plan for followup analyses. The chemist will look in vain, however, for instructions for an assay for serum albumin, or for non-immunological assays for transferrin, haptoglobin, or ceruloplasmin other than literature references. But these are already well documented, and their omission is atoned for by down-to-earth hints on pitfalls such as "pseudohyperproteinemia" (caused by partial evaporation of the specimen) or "pseudomonoclonal gammopathies" (sharp electrophoretic bands caused by hemolysis, by absorption at the point of application, by the presence of lysozyme, etc.).

The major part of the volume deals with abnormalities of serum protein concentrations. It contains chapters on Albumin, Carrier Proteins, Protease Inhibitors, Complement, Immune-Complex Diseases, Acute-Phase Proteins, Immunoglobulins, Thermoproteins, and Embyronic and Fetal Proteins. The coverage is broad and thorough, with good descriptions of normal mechanisms, frequent use of clinical examples and cleverly-done original diagrams. Again, the sections dealing with immunology are noteworthy. Helpful charts of serial changes in acute-phase proteins following surgical procedures or infections are listed in the short chapter on Acute-Phase Proteins by C. L. Fischer and C. W. Gill. One even learns that piloting an Apollo lunar module caused serum antitrypsin and haptoglobin concentrations to rise.

As in any compendium in which information is assembled from various sources, there are weaknesses that might have been resolved by more careful editing. The molecular weights and normal ranges for individual proteins as tabulated throughout the text often conflict with the information in the composite table in the appendix. Ceruloplasmin, for instance, can be found to have a molecular weight of 150 000, 160 000, or 151 000, and a normal range of 10–40 or 15–60 mg/dl. But these are not serious deficiencies, and the real strength of this book is in its clinical applications and immunochemical details.

Theodore Peters, Jr.

The Mary Imogene Bassett Hospital
Cooperstown, N.Y. 13326

An Introduction to Bio-Inorganic Chemistry. D. R. Williams, Ed. Charles C Thomas, Springfield, Ill. 62703, 1976, x + 402 pp. $24.50.

This is a multi-author, interdisciplinary textbook of bio-inorganic chemistry dealing primarily with the role of metals in higher animals and man. It is written at an introductory level and neither an advanced knowledge of chemistry nor of mathematics is required for its understanding and appreciation. This book should appeal to all scientists who have an interest in the rapidly expanding field of trace element metabolism and requirement. It is a good general reference for those interested directly in medicine and approximately 20% of the 400 pages are addressed specifically to biomedical applications, which include Wilson's disease, therapeutic uses of metals, metal-induced toxicity, and chelation therapy. The remainder of the book is devoted to the general aspects and instrumental approaches to bio-inorganic chemistry. This book has some duplication, since most of the chapters are written by different scientists, but the multi-author nature of this book makes it more interesting and allows each chapter to be semi-independent, enabling one to comprehend individual chapters without reading the entire book. Parts of the book are of necessity very factual but others are speculative and thought provoking.

Richard A. Anderson

Vitamin and Mineral Nutrition Laboratory
Agricultural Research Center, USDA
Beltsville, Md. 20705

Enzyme Structure and Function (Enzymology Series, 3). S. Blackburn, Ed. Marcel Dekker, Inc., New York, N.Y. 10016, 1976, viii + 528 pp. $39.50.

This book offers the scientific public a close look at the advances in our understanding of the structure and function of enzymes during the past 10 years. The author is obviously familiar with the complex tools needed to elucidate enzyme structure and yet is a writer who can present this information to a wide audience in a direct and fairly simple manner. Each of twelve hydrolytic enzymes is considered individually and the similarities and differences in their active site structure and chemistry are examined. Each enzyme is systematically dissected with use of information provided by x-ray analysis as well as chemical and kinetic techniques, so that one gains a remarkably clear picture of the active site of most of these enzymes. Once descriptions of active-site structures have been developed, the author goes on to show feasible mechanisms for substrate hydrolyses based on sound principles of organic chemistry.

Chymotrypsin is the first enzyme considered, and it serves as a model for the other enzymes that follow: trypsin and several other well-characterized proteases, including the metalloenzymes carboxypeptidases A and B. Separate chapters are devoted to each of three nonproteases, ribonuclease, staphylococcal nuclease, and lysozyme.

There is little in this book that is currently applicable to clinical enzymology so that the practicing clinical chemist will find this text to be mainly of academic interest. However, for those of us who may be only vaguely aware of the advances in active-site chemistry that have come about in the last 10 years, this technically complex but quite readable text could be an invaluable aid to one's continuing education.

This book is strictly a "current state of knowledge text" and is probably not appropriate for one's personal library if for no other reason than its high cost. The quality of printing is poor but despite these shortcomings, the book should be a valuable addition to libraries serving those working in clinical enzymology.

Robert B. McComb

Hartford Hospital
Hartford, Conn.

Books Received

Phagocytic Engulfment and Cell Adhesiveness as Cellular Surface Phenomena, 2. C. J. Van Oss, C. F. Gillman, and A. W. Neumann, Eds, Marcel Dekker, Inc., New York, N. Y. 10016. vii + 160 pp. $19.50. Pub. Nov. 1975.

Eukaryotes at the Subcellular Level. Methods in Molecular Biology, 8. J. A. Last, Ed. Marcel Dekker, Inc., New York, N. Y. 10016. x + 460 pp. $32.50. Pub. Jan. 1976.

Technical Hematology. 2nd ed. A. Simmons. J. B. Lippincott Co., Philadelphia, Pa. 19105. xiii + 476 pp. $21.50. Pub. Jan. 1976.

Cyclic Nucleotides in Disease. B. Weiss, Ed. University Park Press, Baltimore, Md. 21202. xi + 396 pp. $24.50. Pub. Dec. 1975.

the clinical chemist

Compiled by J. S. King, Executive Editor

Neonate Released

The Neonate—Clinical Chemistry, Physiology, and Pathology, volume 2 in the AACC series *Current Topics in Clinical Chemistry* is expected to be released June 15 by the publisher, John Wiley and Sons. This 340-p book is priced at $19.50. AACC members who order it, either at the national meeting in Houston or through the AACC Business Office (1725 K Street, N.W., Washington, D. C. 20006), will receive a 25% discount. The book is an *updated* version of the proceedings of a conference held in Washington, D. C., Dec. 5–7, 1974 [*cf.* program in *Clin. Chem.* **20,** 1484 (1974)] and sponsored by the Capital Section. Drs. Donald Young and Jocelyn Hicks are the volume editors.

The first (1974) volume in this series was *Amniotic Fluid—Physiology, Biochemistry, and Clinical Chemistry,* so this is the second volume to deal with neonatology.

"And damn'd be him that first cries, 'Hold, enough!' "

The introductory editorial to this issue shows you the bright side of the information-explosion coin. The other side is less nitid, as one reviewer demonstrated in a way I should like to recount to you, even though you hardly will be surprised.

I sent him a paper for review, on the gas-chromatographic determination of drug A in serum. Our friend was so conscientious that he had a little chat with a computer (Medline and Chemcon) and ended up with a printout, which he sent to me, of several hundred papers published in the last five years or so on the determination of drug A (which was introduced in the late fifties). Among them were 27 that, judging from the titles, dealt specifically with GC determination of drug A, all published in the years 1970 to 1975, including four in *Clinical Chemistry.* The present manuscript differed insignificantly from published information, said our reviewer, giving the specifics but dryly adding that he thought this full paper, if published, might "expand the literature unnecessarily." One could only agree.

There is no particular reason to think that this case history is an unusual one. The reason for bringing it up here is that it provides a nice occasion to ask again some often-asked but tremendously important questions:

(*a*) Why would anyone, having done a similar search, undertake a research project on such a well-investigated subject?

(*b*) If the author had *not* done a proper literature search before setting out on the venture, why not?

(*c*) How many reviewers, selected for their expertise in GC of drugs in serum, could reasonably be expected to be aware of even a third, say, of these 27 papers in 15 different journals, and thus be fully prepared to assess the true novelty of this one? Small wonder that reviewing is subject to much criticism! But what substitute would you suggest?

(*d*) How many clinical chemists, wishing to analyze for drug A by this particular technique, have the time, energy, and facilities necessary to help them decide which of the 27 papers is the "best" one for their particular situation?

(*e*) Having finally selected one of the procedures (by reading tea leaves or gazing at chicken entrails) from among the 27 papers, what are the odds our chemist faces that it is so poorly described that he cannot make it work—or can do so only after long and exasperating efforts? One study concludes they are no better than 50-50. If there is anything some workers consider duller and more tedious than a literature search, it is the business of writing a clear, succinct account of their work for publication.

(*f*) Four sets of authors' names appear twice in the list of 27 papers—but not twice in the same journal. How many authors are truly reluctant to republish the same, or essentially the same, information (which is not to say that there are not sometimes, although rarely, compelling reasons for doing so)?

One of the several morals that may be drawn from this little story is a very practical editorial one: *critical* reviews of an important subject are becoming harder to prepare, but they are obviously welcome when they are well done, because of the untold man-hours they save.

The other morals I leave to you to draw.

—J.S.K.

Multiphasic Screening

In "A Controlled Trial of Multiphasic Screening" [*New Engl. J. Med.* **294,** 925 (1976)] the authors conclude that "the only significant difference found between screened and non-screened subjects was an increase in nights hospitalized for screened subjects. Previously unknown abnormalities prompted retesting for confirmation in only 28 per cent of the cases and even less often led to treatment (15 per cent)."

Meetings

Review of Clinical Chemistry for Practicing Pathologists and Clinical Chemists is a 5 h/day, weekdays, course being offered at Snowmass, Colo., on June 28–July 7 and July 12–21 and at Hanover, N. H., on August 2–11. Registration fee: $230. Write or phone Seymour Bakerman, Medical College of Virginia, Richmond, Va. 23298 (804/770-4121).

S. E. Chapter of Society of Nuclear Medicine will meet at Galt House, Louisville, Ky., on Oct. 13–16. Information from: T. J. Roper, Greenville General Hospital, 701 Grove Rd., Greenville, S. C. 29602

New Horizons in Clinical Chemistry is a course to be held at the Given Institute of Pathobiology, Aspen, Colo., August 30–Sept. 3, 1976. Tuition for resident physicians is $100, for others $200. Faculty includes M. D. Burke (Minneapolis), R. B. Conn (Baltimore), R. S. Galen (Hackensack), S. R. Gambino (New York), P. C. J. Ward (Minneapolis), and M. Werner (Washington, D. C.). For more information, write Dr. R. S. Galen, Dept. Pathology, Columbia-Presbyterian Medical Center, BHA-406, 630 W. 168th St., New York, N. Y. 10032. Registration deadline: July 15.

III Latin American Congress in Clinical Chemistry. Belatedly, we record that this meeting took place in Caracas, Venezuela, on May 2–7, 1976. Speakers from the U. S. A. at a quality-assurance seminar included V. Anido, K. Fallon, J. Hopkins, H. V. Nino, D. Plaret, H. Rahkemper, W. Sunderman, K. Vollmer, and D. S. Young.

8th Ohio Valley Chromatography Symposium, June 16–18, 1976, at Hueston Woods State Lodge, College Corner, Ohio 45003. Write to the Symposium, attention: Jean Weaver, Station B, Box 8, Dayton, Ohio 45407.

SI Units—More Support

No sooner had our comment appeared on the move of a pathology journal to the use of SI units (*Clin. Chem.* **22,** 565), than the April issue of *Analytical Chemistry* reached our desk. On p 633 of it was an editorial stating that all ACS publications will "move towards the usage of SI." This massive effort should speed the cause.

Cotlove Award

The first recipient of the Capital Section's Cotlove Award, for the best contributed paper, is Ulysses Smalls, a supervisory chemist in the clinical chemistry laboratory at Veterans Hospital, Baltimore. His paper dealt with an HPLC method for warfarin and its metabolites in serum.

Useful Publications

Patient Preparation and Specimen Collection and Handling, Including Storage Stability, a 58-p ($7.50) study by I. Schoen, C. Fischer, S. Winter and R. Barnett, of the Medical Usefulness Subcommittee of the CAP Standards Committee, was received in April by this office, together with a brochure listing "CAP Programs, Publications, and Services." Write H. E. Cartwright, Executive Director, College of American Pathologists, 7400 N. Skokie Blvd., Skokie, Ill. 60076.

Metric Glassware Brochure covering metric glassware meeting NBS specifications is available from SGA Scientific Inc., 734 Broad St., Bloomfield, N. J. 07003.

The Food and Drug Letter is a new independent newsletter launched to provide in-depth analysis and understanding of FDA policies. Subscription: $240 per year. Write: Washington Business Information, Inc., 1080 National Press Bldg., Washington, D. C. 20045.

Atomic Absorption Methods Manual, written around the IL X51 series but containing general information as well, is available for $50 (supplements free) from Instrumentation Laboratory Inc., Jonspin Road, Wilmington, Mass. 11887.

Comments from the Literature

I simply cannot imagine a state of affairs in which we still go on learning new things of such importance and profound meaning without uncovering at the same time the most detailed mechanisms of disease. This has not happened yet, except on a small and limited scale, but it seems to be a plain fact of life that it will happen, and when it does the science of medicine will become as powerful and effective as any other scientific enterprise known to the world. . . .

We are not on the verge of transforming the human condition. But for the limited mission of medicine, which is, as it has always been down the millenia, the prevention and relief of disease, the healing of sick people, the prospects for the future have never been as hopeful as they are today.

—Dr. Lewis Thomas
in *Hosp. Practice*
Jan. 1976, p 31.

. . . the ultimate "cross-fertilization" in medicine will occur when doctors and patients begin talking to one another, sharing a common language, reading one another's journals, respecting one another's observations, conclusions, and sense of what is true.

—Drs. Michael G. Michaelson, and
Carolyn E. Zelmanoff
in *New Engl. J. Med.* **294,** 563 (1976).

The DORA File—A Progress Report

Over 150 tests have now been entered into the directory of rare analyses maintained at the National Institutes of Health [see *Clin. Chem.* **21,** 1560 (1975)]. These include hematological and microbiological tests as well as clinical chemical and immunological tests. Indeed, the number of chemistry submissions is below that which we anticipated. The file has proved very useful in answering telephone queries and we hope to produce a published version by the time of the AACC National Meeting in August. We welcome contributions so that the usefulness of the file may be expanded. Forms for submission of items and further information may be obtained from: Jocelyn M. Hicks, Ph.D., Director, Clinical Laboratories, Children's Hospital National Medical Center, 2125 13th Street, N.W., Washington, D. C. 20009; D. S. Young, M.D., Ph.D., Chief, Clinical Chemistry Service, Clinical Pathology Department, Building 10, Room 4N-309, Bethesda, Md. 20014.

A representative entry follows:

Name of test: Transketolase
Fluids analyzed: Heparinized blood
Name and address of laboratory performing test: Regional Laboratory, Desk 50, The Cleveland Clinic, 9500 Euclid Ave., Cleveland, Ohio 44106
Individual to contact: Dr. Shamberger
Telephone of contact: (216) 229-2200, Ext. 2520
Volume of specimen: 10 ml heparinized blood
Special preparation of patient: None
Collection of specimen: Heparinized blood
Shipping instructions: Perform a hematocrit and then freeze blood and send frozen.
Fee for test: $20.00
Collaborative research: None
Prior notice required: None
Reference for procedure: *Am. J. Clin. Pathol.* **55,** No. 1, April 1971, pp 465–470.
"Normal" or reference values: 42.1–86.1 ml/7/min
Anticipated delay in reporting results: 3 days
Special restrictions: None

—D. S. Young